FOURTH EDITION

PEDIATRIC GASTROINTESTINAL DISEASE

Pathophysiology • Diagnosis • Management

VOLUME 2

W. Allan Walker, MD
Director, Mucosal Immunology Laboratory
Combined Program in Pediatric
Gastroenterology and Nutrition
Massachusetts General Hospital for Children
Conrad Taff Professor of Nutrition and Pediatrics
Harvard Medical School
Professor of Nutrition
Harvard School of Public Health
Boston, Massachusetts

Olivier Goulet, MD, PhD
Chief, In-patient Gastroenterology Unit
Necker-Enfants Malades Hospital
Professor of Pediatrics
Faculty of Medicine Necker
University of Paris V
Paris, France

Ronald E. Kleinman, MD
Chief, Division of Pediatric Gastroenterology
and Nutrition
Massachusetts General Hospital for Children
Professor of Pediatrics
Department of Pediatrics
Harvard Medical School
Boston, Massachusetts

Philip M. Sherman, MD, FRCPC
Research Institute, Hospital for Sick Children
Professor of Paediatrics and Microbiology
University of Toronto
Canada Research Chair in Gastrointestinal Disease
Toronto, Ontario, Canada

Benjamin L. Shneider, MD
Chief, Division of Pediatric Hepatology
Department of Pediatrics
Mount Sinai Medical Center
Professor
Department of Pediatrics
Mount Sinai School of Medicine
New York, New York

Ian R. Sanderson, MD, FRCP, FRCPCH
Professor of Paedatric Gastroenterology
Head, Research Centre in Gastroenterology
Institute of Cell and Molecular Science
St. Bartholomew's and the Royal London
School of Medicine and Dentistry
Queen Mary, University of London
London, England

BC Decker Inc
P.O. Box 620, LCD 1
Hamilton, Ontario L8N 3K7
Tel: 905-522-7017; 800-568-7281
Fax: 905-522-7839; 888-311-4987
E-mail: info@bcdecker.com
www.bcdecker.com

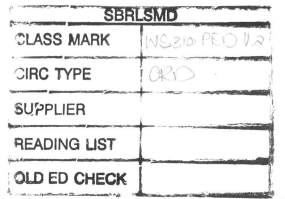

© 2004 by W. Allan Walker.

04 05 06 07 / WPC / 9 8 7 6 5 4 3 2 1

ISBN 1-55009-240-5
Printed in the United States

Sales and Distribution

United States
BC Decker Inc
P.O. Box 785
Lewiston, NY 14092-0785
Tel: 905-522-7017; 800-568-7281
Fax: 905-522-7839; 888-311-4987
E-mail: info@bcdecker.com
www.bcdecker.com

Canada
BC Decker Inc
20 Hughson Street South
P.O. Box 620, LCD 1
Hamilton, Ontario L8N 3K7
Tel: 905-522-7017; 800-568-7281
Fax: 905-522-7839; 888-311-4987
E-mail: info@bcdecker.com
www.bcdecker.com

Foreign Rights
John Scott & Company
International Publishers' Agency
P.O. Box 878
Kimberton, PA 19442
Tel: 610-827-1640
Fax: 610-827-1671
E-mail: jsco@voicenet.com

Japan
Igaku-Shoin Ltd.
Foreign Publications Department
3-24-17 Hongo
Bunkyo-ku, Tokyo, Japan 113-8719
Tel: 3 3817 5680
Fax: 3 3815 6776
E-mail: fd@igaku-shoin.co.jp

UK, Europe, Scandinavia, Middle East
Elsevier Science
Customer Service Department
Foots Cray High Street
Sidcup, Kent
DA14 5HP, UK
Tel: 44 (0) 208 308 5760
Fax: 44 (0) 181 308 5702
E-mail: cservice@harcourt.com

Singapore, Malaysia, Thailand, Philippines, Indonesia, Vietnam, Pacific Rim, Korea
Elsevier Science Asia
583 Orchard Road
#09/01, Forum
Singapore 238884
Tel: 65-737-3593
Fax: 65-753-2145

Australia, New Zealand
Elsevier Science Australia
Customer Service Department
STM Division
Locked Bag 16
St. Peters, New South Wales, 2044
Australia

Tel: 61 02 9517-8999
Fax: 61 02 9517-2249
E-mail: stmp@harcourt.com.au
www.harcourt.com.au

Mexico and Central America
ETM SA de CV
Calle de Tula 59
Colonia Condesa
06140 Mexico DF, Mexico
Tel: 52-5-5553-6657
Fax: 52-5-5211-8468
E-mail: editoresdetextosmex@prodigy.net.mx

Argentina
CLM (Cuspide Libros Medicos)
Av. Córdoba 2067 - (1120)
Buenos Aires, Argentina
Tel: (5411) 4961-0042/(5411) 4964-0848
Fax: (5411) 4963-7988
E-mail: clm@cuspide.com

Brazil
Tecmedd
Av. Maurílio Biagi, 2850
City Ribeirão Preto – SP – CEP: 14021-000
Tel: 0800 992236
Fax: (16) 3993-9000
E-mail: tecmedd@tecmedd.com.br

CONTRIBUTORS

Ana Abad-Sinden, MS, RD, CNSD
Director, Dietetic Internship Program
Pediatric Nutrition Support Specialist
Department of Nutrition Services
University of Virginia Health System
Charlottesville, VA
Nutritional Therapy: Nutrition Support: Enteral Nutrition

David W. K. Acheson, MD, FRCP
Chief Medical Officer
Food and Drug Administration, Center for Food Safety
   and Applied Nutrition
College Park, Maryland
Infections: Food- and Waterborne Infections

Nadeem Ahmad Afzal, MBBS, MRCPCH, MRCP(UK)
Specialist Registrar
Center for Pediatric Gastroenterology
Royal Free Hampstead National Health Service Trust
London, England
Drug Therapy: Alternative Medical Treatment

Stephen John Allen, MD, MRCP, DTM&H
Honorary Consultant Paediatrician
Department of Paediatrics
Singleton Hospital
Senior Lecturer in Paediatrics
The Clinical School
University of Wales, Swansea
Swansea, Wales
Malnutrition

Karin Andersson, MD
Clinical and Research Fellow
Gastrointestinal Unit
Medical Services
Massachusetts General Hospital
Fellow
Harvard Medical School
Boston, Massachusetts
Infections: Food- and Waterborne Infections

Robert D. Baker, MD, PhD
Co-Director, Digestive Diseases and Nutrition Center
Department of Pediatrics
Children's Hospital of Buffalo
Professor of Pediatrics
Department of Pediatrics
State University of New York at Buffalo
Buffalo, New York
Nutritional Therapy: Nutrition Support: Parenteral Nutrition

Susan S. Baker, MD, PhD
Co-Director, Digestive Diseases and Nutrition Center
Department of Pediatrics
Children's Hospital of Buffalo
Professor of Pediatrics
Department of Pediatrics
State University of New York at Buffalo
Buffalo, New York
Nutritional Therapy: Nutrition Support: Parenteral Nutrition

William F. Balistreri, MD
Director, Division of Pediatric Gastroenterology,
   Hepatology and Nutrition
Department of Pediatrics
Cincinnati Children's Hospital Medical Center
Dorothy M.M. Kersten Professor of Pediatrics
Department of Pediatrics
University of Cincinnati College of Medicine
Cincinnati, Ohio
Approach to Neonatal Cholestasis

Sanjay Bansal, MD, MRCP
Senior Registrar
Department of Paediatric Hepatology
King's College Hospital
London, England
Acute Liver Failure

Ronald G. Barr, MDCM, FRCPC
Director
BC Research Institute for Children's and Women's Health
Centre for Community Child Health Research
Professor of Pediatrics
Faculty of Medicine
University of British Columbia
Vancouver, British Columbia, Canada
Colic and Gas

Dorsey M. Bass, MD
Attending Physician
Division of Gastroenterology
Department of Pediatrics
Lucile Packard Children's Hospital at Stanford
Associate Professor of Pediatrics
Department of Pediatrics
Stanford University
Palo Alto, California
Infections: Viral Infections

Susan V. Beath, MB, BS, BSc, MRCP(UK), DTM, FRCPCH
Consultant Paediatric Hepatologist
The Liver Unit
The Birmingham Children's Hospital
Honorary Senior Lecturer
The Institute of Child Health
The University of Birmingham
Birmingham, England
Intestinal Failure: Small Bowel Transplant

Dominique C. Belli, MD
Associate Professor
Department of Pediatrics
University of Geneva
Geneva, Switzerland
Gastrointestinal Endoscopy: Upper Gastrointestinal Endoscopy

Suzanne Bender, MD
Staff Psychiatrist, Consultant GI Pediatric Clinic
Department of Psychiatry
Massachusetts General Hospital
Clinical Instructor
Department of Psychiatry
Harvard University Medical School
Boston, Massachusetts
Management of Surgical Patients: Psychological Aspects

Keith J. Benkov, MD
Chief of Pediatric Gastroenterology
Department of Pediatrics
Mount Sinai Medical Center
Associate Professor
Department of Pediatrics
Mount Sinai School of Medicine
New York, New York
Imaging: Cross-Sectional Imaging: Ultrasonography, Computed Tomography, Magnetic Resonance Imaging

Jorge A. Bezerra, MD
Staff Physician
Division of Pediatric Gastroenterology, Hepatology and Nutrition
Cincinnati Children's Hospital Medical Center
Associate Professor of Pediatrics
Department of Pediatrics
University of Cincinnati College of Medicine
Cincinnati, Ohio
Disorders of the Biliary Tract: Biliary Atresia

Julie E. Bines, MD, FRACP
Head of Clinical Nutrition, Consultant Gastroenterologist
Department of Gastroenterology and Clinical Nutrition
Royal Children's Hospital
Associate Professor
Department of Pediatrics
University of Melbourne
Victoria, Australia
Parenteral Nutrition–Associated Liver Disease

Billy Bourke, MD, FRCPI
Consultant Gastroenterologist
Department of Pediatrics
Our Lady's Hospital for Sick Children
Senior Lecturer
Department of Pediatrics
University College Dublin
Dublin, Ireland
Gastritis: Helicobacter pylori *and Peptic Ulcer Disease*

Athos Bousvaros, MD
Associate Director of the Inflammatory Bowel Disease Center
Combined Program in Pediatric Gastroenterology and Nutrition
Children's Hospital Boston
Assistant Professor of Pediatrics
Department of Pediatrics
Harvard Medical School
Boston, Massachusetts
Drug Therapy: Immunosuppressive Therapies

Kevin Bove, MD
Pathologist
Department of Pathology
Cincinnati Children's Hospital Medical Center
Professor
Department of Pathology
University of Cincinnati College of Medicine
Cincinnati, Ohio
Genetic and Metabolic Disorders: Lysosomal Acid Lipase Deficiencies: Wolman Disease and Cholesteryl Ester Storage Disease

John T. Boyle, MD
Division Chief
Division of Pediatric Gastroenterology & Nutrition
Children's Hospital of Alabama
Professor of Pediatrics
University of Alabama-Birmingham School of Medicine
Birmingham, Alabama
Abdominal Pain

Darla J. Bradshaw, BS, RD, CNSD
Clinical Dietitian
Department of Clinical Nutrition
The Children's Hospital of Philadelphia
Philadelphia, Pennsylvania
Nutritional Therapy: Special Dietary Therapy

Annemarie Broderick, MB, BCh, MRCPI, MMedSc
Department of Pediatrics
University College Dublin
Children's Research Centre, Our Lady's Hospital for Sick Children
Crumlin, Dublin, Ireland
Gallbladder Disease

Nicole Brousse, MD, PhD
Professor of Pathology
Department of Pathology
Hôpital Necker-Enfants Malades
Université René Descartes
Paris, France
Enteropathy: Autoimmune Enteropathy

Ross N. Butler, PhD
Chief Medical Scientist
Department of Gastroenterology
Women's and Children's Hospital
Doctor
Department of Paediatrics
University of Adelaide
North Adelaide, South Australia
Breath Analysis

Assad M. Butt, MB, BS, DCH(Lon), MRCP, CPCH
Consultant in Pediatric Gastroenterology and Nutrition
Department of Pediatrics
The Royal Alexandra Hospital for Sick Children
Consultant in Pediatric Gastroenterology and Nutrition
Department of Pediatrics
Brighton and Sussex University Hospitals
Brighton, England
Pancreas: Tumors

Kathleen M. Campbell, MD
Fellow
Division of Pediatric Gastroenterology, Hepatology,
    and Nutrition
Cincinnati Children's Hospital Medical Center
Fellow
Department of Pediatrics
University of Cincinnati College of Medicine
Cincinnati, Ohio
Disorders of the Biliary Tract: Biliary Atresia

Michael Caplan, MD
Chair, Department of Pediatrics
Evanston Northwestern Healthcare
Associate Professor of Pediatrics
Department of Pediatrics
Northwestern University, Feinberg School of Medicine
Evanston, Chicago, Illinois
Necrotizing Enterocolitis

Helen Carty, FRCR, FRCPI, FRCP, FRCPCH, FFRRCSI(Hon)
Professor of Paediatric Radiology
Department of Radiology
Royal Liverpool Children's Hospital NHS Trust-Alder Hey
Professor of Paediatric Radiology
Department of Medical Imaging
University of Liverpool
Liverpool, England
Imaging: Plain Radiographs and Contrast Studies

David Casson, BA, MBBS, MRCPI
Doctor
Department of Medicine
Royal Liverpool Children's Hospital National Health
    Service Trust-Alder Hey
Honorary Lecturer
Department of Medicine
University of Liverpool
Liverpool, England
Imaging: Radionuclide Diagnosis

Peter G. Chait, MBBCh(Rand)(D), SA, FRCPR(Eng)
Interventional Radiologist
Department of Diagnostic Imaging
Hospital for Sick Children
Professor
University of Toronto
Toronto, Ontario
Imaging: Interventional Gastrointestinal Radiology

Mei-Hwei Chang, MD
Chair, Department of Pediatrics
National Taiwan University Hospital
Professor
Department of Pediatrics
College of Medicine, National Taiwan University
Taipei, Taiwan
Postnatal Infections: Viral Hepatitis B

Denesh K. Chitkara, MD
Assistant in Medicine
Combined Program in Pediatric Gastroenterology
    and Nutrition
Children's Hospital Boston
Instructor
Department of Pediatrics
Harvard Medical School
Boston, Massachusetts
Genetic and Metabolic Disorders: Wilson Disease

Erika C. Claud, MD
Associate Neonatalogist
Division of Neonatology
University of Chicago Children's Hospital
Asssitant Professor of Pediatrics
University of Chicago School of Medicine
Chicago, Illinois
Necrotizing Enterocolitis

Geoffrey Cleghorn, MBBS, FRACP, FACG
Senior Specialist
Department of Gastroenterology
Royal Children's Hospital
Associate Professor and Head
Department of Pediatrics and Child Health
University of Queensland
Brisbane, Queensland, Australia
*Drug Therapy: Pharmacologic Therapy of Exocrine
    Pancreatic Insufficiency*

Mitchell B. Cohen, MD
Attending Physician
Division of Pediatric Gastroenterology, Hepatology
    and Nutrition
Cincinnati Children's Hospital Medical Center
Professor
Department of Pediatrics
University of Cincinnati College of Medicine
Cincinnati, Ohio
Secretory Tumors

Frances Laura Connor, MBBS, FRACP
Research Fellow
Division of Pediatric Gastroenterology
Children's Hospital of Pittsburgh
Research Fellow
Department of Pediatrics
University of Pittsburgh School of Medicine
Pittsburgh, Pennsylvania
Motility and *Drug Therapy: Motility*

Andrew B. Cooper, PhD
Research Assistant Professor
Department of Natural Resources
College of Life Sciences and Agriculture
University of New Hampshire
Durham, New Hampshire
*Study Design: Methodology (Statistical Analysis, Test
    Interpretation, Basic Principles of Screening with
    Application for Clinical Study)*

Catherine Cord-Udy, MBBS, FRACS(Paed Surg)
Consultant, Paediatric Surgeon
Department of Paediatric Surgery
The Royal London Hospital
London, England
Management of Surgical Patients: The Pediatric Ostomy

Richard T. Lee Couper, MD
Senior Paediatric Gastroenterologist
Department of Gastroenterology
Women's & Children's Hospital
Senior Paediatric Gastroenterologist
Department of Paediatrics
University of Adelaide
Adelaide, South Australia
Pancreatic Function Tests

Joseph M. Croffie, MD, MPH
Director, Pediatric GI Motility Laboratory
Division of Pediatric Gastroenterology, Hepatology and
    Nutrition
James Whitcomb Riley Hospital for Children
Associate Professor of Clinical Pediatrics
Department of Pediatrics
Indiana University School of Medicine
Indianapolis, Indiana
Hypomotility Disorders: Idiopathic Constipation

Carla D. Cuthbert, PhD
Fellow, Clinical-Biochemical Genetics
Department of Laboratory Medicine and Pathology
Mayo Medical School
Rochester, Minnesota
*Genetic and Metabolic Disorders: Inherited Abnormalities In
    Mitochondrial Fatty Acid Oxidation*

Steven J. Czinn, MD
Chief, Division of Pediatric Gastroenterology
Department of Pediatrics
Rainbow Babies and Children's Hospital
University Hospital Health System
Professor
Departments of Pediatrics and Pathology
Case Western Reserve University School of Medicine
Cleveland, Ohio
Inflammation

Danita I. Czyzewski, PhD
Pediatric Psychologist
Department of Psychiatry/Psychology Service
Texas Children's Hospital
Assistant Professor
Department of Psychiatry and Behavioral Science and
    Pediatrics
Baylor College of Medicine
Houston, Texas
Nutritional Therapy: Feeding Difficulties

Geoffrey P. Davidson, MBBS, MD, FRACP
Director
Centre for Paediatric and Adolescent Gastroenterology
Women's and Children's Hospital
Professor
Department of Paediatrics
University of Adelaide
North Adelaide, South Australia
Breath Analysis

Guilio De Marco, MD
Clinical Assistant
Department of Pediatrics
Division of Infectious Diseases
Research Assistant
Department of Pediatrics
University Federico II of Naples
Naples, Italy
Persistent Diarrhea

Gustavo Andrade de Paulo, MD, MSc
Hospital Albert Einstein
Endoscopy Unit
Universidad Federal de São Paolo-Escola Paulista
    de Medicina
Department of Gastroenterology
São Paolo, Brazil
*Gastrointestinal Endoscopy: Endoscopic Retrograde
    Cholangiopancreatography*

Lee A. Denson, MD
Attending Physician
Department of Pediatric Gastroenterology
Division of Pediatric Gastroenterology, Hepatology and
    Nutrition
Cincinnati Children's Hospital Medical Center
Assistant Professor
Department of Pediatrics
University of Cincinnati College of Medicine
Cincinnati, Ohio
Postnatal Infections of the Liver: Other Viral Infections

Anil Dhawan, MD, FRCPCH
Deputy Director
Paediatric Liver Services
King's College Hospital
Honorary Senior Lecturer
Department of Paediatrics
Guy's, King's and St. Thomas' School of Medicine
London, England
Acute Liver Failure

Carlo Di Lorenzo, MD
Director, Motility Center
Division of Pediatric Gastroenterology
Children's Hospital of Pittsburgh
Professor
Department of Pediatrics
University of Pittsburgh School of Medicine
Pittsburgh, Pennsylvania
Motility and *Drug Therapy: Motility*

Conor Doherty, MB, BS, MRCP, DTM&H
Clinical Scientist
Keneba Field Station
Medical Research Council (UK) Laboratories
The Gambia, Africa
Growth Failure

Ranjan Dohil, MBBCh, MRCP(UK)
Staff Physician
Division of Pediatric Gastroenterology
Children's Hospital and Health Center
Associate Clinical Professor
Department of Pediatrics
University of California, San Diego
San Diego, California
Gastritis: Other Causes

Malcolm Donaldson, MD, FRCP, FRCPCH, DCH
Doctor
Royal Hospital for Sick Children
Department of Child Health
Glasgow University
Glasgow, Scotland
Growth Failure

Brendan Drumm, MD, FRCPC, FRCPI
Head, Paediatrics
Department of Gastroenterology
Our Lady's Hospital for Sick Children
Professor
Department of Pediatrics
University College Dublin
Dublin, Ireland
Gastritis: Helicobacter pylori *and Peptic Ulcer Disease*

Hong Du, PhD
Assistant Professor
Division of Genetics
Cincinnati Children's Hospital Research Foundation
Department of Pediatrics
University of Cincinnati College of Medicine
Cincinnati, Ohio
*Genetic and Metabolic Disorders: Lysosomal Acid Lipase
    Deficiencies: Wolman Disease and Cholesteryl Ester
    Storage Disease*

Christopher Duggan, MD, MPH
Director, Clinical Nutrition Service
Combined Program in Pediatric Gastroenterology and
    Nutrition
Children's Hospital Boston
Assistant Professor of Pediatrics
Harvard Medical School
Assistant Professor of Nutrition
Harvard School of Public Health
Boston, Massachusetts
Nutritional Therapy: Nutritional Assessment and Requirements

Peter R. Durie, MD, FRCPC
Gastroenterologist
Division of Gastroenterology and Nutrition
Hospital for Sick Children
Professor
Department of Pediatrics
University of Toronto
Toronto, Ontario, Canada
*Exocrine Pancreatic Dysfunction: Shwachman-Diamond
    Syndrome*

Mounif El-Youssef, MD
Consultant
Division of Pediatric Gastroenterology and Nutrition
Mayo Clinic
Associate Professor
Department of Pediatrics
Mayo Medical School
Rochester, Minnesota
Systemic Conditions Affecting the Liver

Regina E. Ensenauer, MD
Fellow, Clinical-Biochemical Genetics
Department of Laboratory Medicine and Pathology
Mayo Medical School
Rochester, Minnesota
Genetic and Metabolic Disorders: Inherited Abnormalities in Mitochondrial Fatty Acid Oxidation

Mary K. Estes, PhD
Professor
Department of Virology and Microbiology
Baylor College of Medicine
Houston, Texas
Infections: Viral Infections

Michael J. G. Farthing, DSc(Med), MD, FRCP, FMedSci
Professor of Medicine
St. Georges Hospital Medical School
University of London
London, England
Infections: Parasitic and Fungal Infections

Alessio Fasano, MD
Director, Division of Pediatric GI & Nutrition
Director, Mucosal Biology Research Center
University Hospital
Professor
Department of Pediatrics
University of Maryland at Baltimore
Baltimore, Maryland
Infections: Bacterial Infections

Christophe Faure, MD
Physician
Division of Pediatric Gastroenterology
St. Justine Hospital
Associate Professor
Department of Pediatrics
University of Montreal
Montreal, Quebec, Canada
Hypomotility Disorders: Chronic Intestinal Pseudo-obstruction Syndrome and Drug Therapy: Acid-Peptic Disease

Ariel E. Feldstein, MD
Fellow, Division of Gastroenterology
Department of Pediatrics
Mayo Medical School
Rochester, Minnesota
Genetic and Metabolic Disorders: Wilson Disease

Milton J. Finegold, MD
Head, Department of Pathology
Texas Children's Hospital
Professor
Department of Pathology and Pediatrics
Baylor College of Medicine
Houston, Texas
Liver Tumors

Claudio Fiocchi, MD
Director, IBD Center
University Hospitals of Cleveland
Professor
Departments of Medicine, Pathology and Pediatrics
Case Western Reserve University School of Medicine
Cleveland, Ohio
Inflammation

Thomas M. Fishbein, MD
Director, Small Bowel Transplantation
Transplant Institute
Georgetown University
Washington, District of Columbia
Intestinal Failure: Outcomes

Joseph F. Fitzgerald, MD, MACG
Director, Division of Pediatric Gastroenterology, Hepatology and Nutrition
James Whitcomb Riley Hospital for Children
Professor
Department of Pediatrics
Indiana University School of Medicine
Indianapolis, Indiana
Hypomotility Disorders: Idiopathic Constipation

Judah Folkman, MD
Surgeon-In-Chief, Emeritus
Department of Surgery
Children's Hospital Boston
Andrus Professor of Pediatric Surgery
Department of Surgery
Professor of Cell Biology
Harvard Medical School
Boston, Massachusetts
Appendicitis

Victor L. Fox, MD
Director, Endoscopy Unit
Combined Program in Pediatric Gastroenterology and Nutrition
Children's Hospital Boston
Assistant Professor
Department of Pediatrics
Harvard Medical School
Boston, Massachusetts
Gastrointestinal Endoscopy: Patient Preparation and General Considerations

Thomas M. Foy, MD
Staff Physician
Division of Gastroenterology
Cardinal Glennon Children's Hospital
Associate Professor
Department of Pediatrics
St. Louis University
St. Louis, Missouri
Nutritional Therapy: Feeding Difficulties

Deborah K. Freese, MD
Consultant
Division of Pediatric Gastroenterology and Nutrition
Mayo Clinic
Associate Professor
Department of Pediatrics
Mayo Medical School
Rochester, Minnesota
Systemic Conditions Affecting the Liver

Narmer F. Galeano, MD
Attending Physician
Division of Pediatric Gastroenterology
Children's Hospital of New Jersey
Newark Beth Israel Medical Center
Newark, New Jersey
Mitochondrial Function and Dysfunction

Cheryl E. Gariepy, MD
Attending Physician
Divison of Gastroenterology and Nutrition
Department of Pediatrics
C.S. Mott Children's Hospital
Assistant Professor
Department of Pediatrics and Communicable Diseases
University of Michigan School of Medicine
Ann Arbor, Michigan
Hypomotility Disorders: Hirschsprung Disease

Kevin J. Gaskin, MD, FRACP
Professor
Departments of Gastroenterology and Nutrition
The Children's Hospital at Westmead
Professor
Department of Pediatrics
University of Sydney
Sydney, New South Wales, Australia
Exocrine Pancreatic Dysfunction: Cystic Fibrosis

Shuvo Ghosh, MD
Fellow, Department of Developmental-Behavioral
    Pediatrics
Montreal Children's Hospital, McGill University
    Health Center
Fellow, Department of Child Development
McGill University School of Medicine
Montreal, Quebec, Canada
Colic and Gas

Mark A. Gilger, MD
Director, Gastrointestinal Procedures Suite
Department of Gastroenterology
Texas Children's Hospital
Associate Professor
Department of Pediatrics
Baylor College of Medicine
Houston, Texas
Gastrointestinal Bleeding: Upper Gastrointestinal Bleeding

Praveen S. Goday, MB, BS
Consultant Pediatric Gastroenterologist
Department of Pediatrics
First Med Hospitals
Chennai, India
Secretory Tumors

Donald Goldmann, MD
Hospital Epidemiologist, Medical Director of Infection
    Control & Quality Improvement
Department of Medicine
Children's Hospital Boston
Professor
Department of Pediatrics
Harvard University Medical School
Boston, Massachusetts
*Study Design: Outcomes Research on Diagnostic and
    Therapeutic Procedures*

Regino P. González-Peralta, MD
Attending Physician and Medical Director, Pediatric Liver
    Transplant Program
Department of Pediatrics
Shands Children's Hospital
Associate Professor
Department of Pediatrics
University of Florida College of Medicine
Gainesville, Florida
Postnatal Infections of the Liver: Hepatitis C Virus

Frédéric Gottrand, MD, PhD
Professor of Medicine
Division of Gastroenterology, Hepatology and Nutrition
Department of Pediatrics
Jeanne de Flandre Hospital
Lille University
Lille, France
Drug Therapy: Acid-Peptic Disease

Olivier Goulet, MD, PhD
Chief, In-patient Gastroenterology Unit
Necker-Enfants Malades Hospital
Professor of Pediatrics
Faculty of Medicine Necker
University of Paris V
Paris, France
*Gastrointestinal Manifestations of Immunodeficiency:
    Primary Immunodeficiency Diseases* and *Congenital
    Disease of Dysfunction and Absorption: Congenital
    Enteropathy Involving Intestinal Mucosa Development*
    and *Enteropathy: Autoimmune Enteropathy*

Glenn R. Gourley, MD
Chief, Pediatric Gastroenterology Division
Department of Pediatrics
Doernbecher Children's Hospital
Adjunct Professor
Oregon Health & Science University School of Medicine
Portland, Oregon
Genetic and Metabolic Disorders: Bilirubin Metabolism

Gregory A. Grabowski, MD
Professor
Department of Pediatrics
Cincinnati Children's Hospital Research Foundation
University of Cincinnati College of Medicine
Cincinnati, Ohio
*Genetic and Metabolic Disorders: Lysosomal Acid Lipase
    Deficiencies: Wolman Disease and Cholesteryl Ester
    Storage Disease*

Fiona Graeme-Cook, MB, FRCP
Assistant in Pathology
Department of Pathology
Massachusetts General Hospital
Assistant Professor
Department of Pathology
Harvard Medical School
Boston, Massachusetts
Esophageal and Gastric Neoplasms

Richard J. Grand, MD
Director GCRC and IBD Center
Combined Program in Pediatric Gastroenterology and
    Nutrition
Children's Hospital Boston
Professor of Pediatrics
Department of Pediatrics
Harvard Medical School
Boston, Massachusetts
Genetic and Metabolic Disorders: Wilson Disease

Anne M. Griffiths, MD, FRCPC
Director, IBD Program
Gastrointestinal and Nutrition Division
Department of Pediatrics
Hospital for Sick Children
Professor
Department of Pediatrics
University of Toronto
Toronto, Ontario, Canada
Inflammatory Bowel Disease: Crohn Disease

Stefano Guandalini, MD
Section Chief
Division of Gastroenterology, Hepatology and Nutrition
University of Chicago Children's Hospital
Professor
Department of Pediatrics
University of Chicago
Chicago, Illinois
Acute Diarrhea

Alfredo Guarino, MD
Associate Professor of Pediatrics
Division of Infectious Diseases
Department of Pediatrics
University Federico II of Naples
Naples, Italy
Persistent Diarrhea

Joel E. Haas, MD
Chairman, Department of Pathology
The Children's Hospital
Professor
Department of Pathology
University of Colorado
Denver, Colorado
Liver Tumors

Eric Hassall, MBChB, FRCPC, FACG
Staff Physician
Division of Gastroenterology and Nutrition
BC Children's Hospital
Professor
Department of Pediatrics
University of British Columbia
Vancouver, British Columbia, Canada
Gastritis: Other Causes

Yves Heloury, MD
Professor
Department of Pediatric Surgery
Hôpital Mère-Enfant
Nantes, France
Peritonitis

**Robert B. Heuschkel, MB, BS, DRCOG,
    MRCPCH**
Pediatric Gastroenterologist
Center for Pediatric Gastroenterology
Royal Free Hampstead National Health Service Trust
Honorary Senior Lecturer
Department of Pediatrics
Royal Free and University College Medical School
London, England
Drug Therapy: Alternative Medical Treatment

Patricia L. Hibberd, MD, PhD
Director
Institute for Clinical Research and Health Policy Studies
Tufts New England Medical Center
Professor
Department of Geographic Medicine/Infectious Diseases
Tufts University School of Medicine
Boston, Massachusetts
*Study Design: Methodology (Statistical Analysis, Test
    Interpretation, Basic Principles of Screening with
    Application for Clinical Study)*

Leslie M. Higuchi, MD, MPH
Assistant in Medicine
Combined Program in Pediatric Gastroenterology and
    Nutrition
Children's Hospital Boston
Instructor
Department of Pediatrics
Harvard Medical School
Boston, Massachusetts
Inflammatory Bowel Disease: Ulcerative Colitis

Alison G. Hoppin, MD
Assistant Pediatrician
Combined Program in Pediatric Gastroenterology and
    Nutrition
Massachusetts General Hospital for Children
Instructor
Department of Pediatrics
Harvard Medical School
Boston, Massachusetts
Obesity and *Intestinal Tumors: Other Neoplasms*

Simon Horslen, MB, ChB, FRCPCH
Associate Professor
Department of Pediatrics
University of Nebraska Medical Center
Omaha, Nebraska
Genetic and Metabolic Disorders: Carbohydrate Metabolism

Sarah Hotchkin, RN
Specialist Sister, Paediatric Surgery and Stoma Care
The Royal London Hospital
London, England
Management of Surgical Patients: The Pediatric Ostomy

Jean-Pierre Hugot, MD, PhD
Professor
Department of Pediatric Gastroenterology and Nutrition
Hôpital Robert Debré
Professor
Faculté de Médecine Bichat
Université Paris VII
Paris, France
Inflammatory Bowel Disease: Crohn Disease

Essam Imseis, MD
Fellow, Divison of Gastroenterology and Nutrition
C. S. Mott Children's Hospital
Department of Pediatrics and Communicable Diseases
University of Michigan School of Medicine
Ann Arbor, Michigan
Hypomotility Disorders: Hirschsprung Disease

Elizabeth Iofel, MD
Attending Physician in Gastroenterology and Nutrition
Department of Pediatrics
Schneiders Children's Hospital North Shore/Long Island
    Jewish Health System
Assistant Professor
Department of Pediatrics
Albert Einstein College of Medicine
New Hyde Park/Bronx, New York
*Postnatal Infections of the Liver: AIDS and Other Immune
    Disorders*

Erika Isolauri, MD, PhD
Professor of Pediatrics
Department of Pediatrics
University of Turku
Turku, Finland
Drug Therapy: Modulation of Intestinal Flora: Probiotics

Shinya Ito, MD
Head, Division of Clinical Pharmacology and Toxicology
Hospital for Sick Children
Associate Professor
Department of Pediatrics
University of Toronto
Toronto, Ontario, Canada
Gastrointestinal Injury: Drug-Induced Bowel Injury

Tom Jaksic, MD, PhD
Attending Surgeon
Children's Hospital, Boston
Associate Professor
Department of Surgery
Harvard Medical School
Boston, Massachusetts
Benign Perianal Lesions

Dominique M. Jan, MD
Visiting Attending Surgeon
Department of Surgery, Center for Liver Disease and
    Transplantation
New York Presbyterian Hospital
Visiting Professor
Department of Surgery
Columbia University
New York, New York
Pancreas: Congenital Anomalies

Sidney Johnson, MD
Chief Surgical Resident
Department of Surgery
Children's Hospital Boston
Harvard Medical School
Boston, Massachusetts
Benign Perianal Lesions

Christopher D. Jolley, MD
Attending Physician
Division of Pediatric Gastroenterology
Department of Pediatrics
Shands Children's Hospital
Assistant Professor
Department of Pediatrics
University of Florida College of Medicine
Gainesville, Florida
Postnatal Infections of the Liver: Hepatitis C Virus

Nicola L. Jones, MD, FRCPC, PhD
Staff Gastroenterologist
Department of Paediatrics
Hospital for Sick Children
Assistant Professor
Departments of Paediatrics and Physiology
University of Toronto
Toronto, Ontario, Canada
Microbial Interactions with Gut Epithelium

Saul Karpen, MD, PhD
Director, Texas Children's Liver Center
Division of Gastroenterology, Hepatology and Nutrition
Texas Children's Hospital
Associate Professor
Departments of Pediatrics and Molecular and Cellular
    Biology
Baylor College of Medicine
Houston, Texas
*Liver Function and Dysfunction: Bile Formation and
    Cholestasis*

Stuart S. Kaufman, MD
Staff Physician
Department of Gastroenterology
Children's National Medical Center
Medical Director, Small Bowel Transplant Program
Transplant Institute
Georgetown University
Washington, District of Columbia
Intestinal Failure: Outcomes

Richard I. Kelley, MD, PhD
Director
Department of Metabolism
Kennedy Krieger Institute
Professor
Department of Pediatrics
Johns Hopkins University School of Medicine
Baltimore, Maryland
*Genetic and Metabolic Disorders: Zellweger Syndrome
    and Other Disorders of Peroxisomal Metabolism*

Deirdre Kelly, MD, FRCP, FRCPI, FRCPCH
Consultant Paediatric Hepatologist
Birmingham Children's Hospital
Professor of Paediatric Hepatology
University of Birmingham School of Medicine
Birmingham, England
Liver Transplant

Paul Kelly, MD, FRCP
Reader
Department of Gastroenterology
Barts & The London School of Medicine
London, England
*Gastrointestinal Manifestations of Immunodeficiency: HIV
    and Other Secondary Immunodeficiencies*

**Simon Edward Kenny, BSc(Hons), MB
    ChB(Hons), MD, FRCS(Paed Surg)**
Consultant Paediatric Surgeon
Department of Pediatric Surgery
Alder-Hey Children's Hospital
Honorary Senior Lecturer in Paediatric Surgery
Department of Child Health
University of Liverpool School of Medicine
Liverpool, England
Intestine: Congenital Anomalies

Seema Khan, MD
Attending Physician
Division of Gastroenterology and Nutrition
Children's Hospital of Pittsburgh
Assistant Professor
Department of Pediatrics
University of Pittsburgh School of Medicine
Pittsburgh, Pennsylvania
Gastroesophageal Reflux

Barbara S. Kirschner, MD
Director, The Pediatric Inflammatory Bowel Disease
    Center
Division of Pediatric Gastroenterology, Hepatology and
    Nutrition
The University of Chicago Children's Hospital
Professor
Departments of Pediatrics and Medicine
The University of Chicago School of Medicine
Chicago, Illinois
*Inflammatory Bowel Disease: Undetermined Colitis and
    Other Inflammatory Diseases*

Ronald E. Kleinman, MD
Chief, Division of Pediatric Gastroenterology and Nutrition
Massachusetts General Hospital for Children
Professor of Pediatrics
Department of Pediatrics
Harvard Medical School
Boston, Massachusetts
*Pediatric Gastroenterology: A Subspecialty in Pediatrics
    "Comes of Age"*

A. S. Knisely, MD
Consultant Histopathologist
Institute of Liver Studies
King's College Hospital
London, England
Liver Biopsy Interpretation

Sibylle Koletzko, MD
Department Head
Pediatric Gastroenterology and Hepatology
Dr. von Hauner Children's Hospital
Senior Lecturer in Pediatrics
Ludwig Maximilians University Munich
München, Germany
Hypomotility Disorders: Dysmotilities

Nancy F. Krebs, MD, MS
Director
Department of Nutrition
The Children's Hospital
Associate Professor
Department of Pediatrics
University of Colorado, Health Sciences Center
Denver, Colorado
Nutritional Therapy: Protective Nutrients

Amethyst C. Kurbegov, MD, MPH
Clinical Fellow
Division of Gastroenterology and Nutrition
Texas Children's Hospital
Clinical Fellow
Department of Pediatrics
Baylor College of Medicine
Houston, Texas
Liver Function and Dysfunction: Bile Formation and Cholestasis

Jacob C. Langer, MD, FRCSC
Chief, Pediatric General Surgery
Department of Surgery
Hospital for Sick Children
Professor of Surgery
Department of Surgery
University of Toronto
Toronto, Ontario, Canada
Inflammatory Bowel Disease: Surgical Aspects

Christophe Laplace, MD
Doctor
Department of Pediatric Surgery
Hôpital Mère-Enfant
Nantes, France
Peritonitis

Gregory Y. Lauwers, MD
Director
Gastrointestinal Pathology Service
Massachusetts General Hospital
Associate Professor
Department of Pathology
Harvard Medical School
Boston, Massachusetts
Esophageal and Gastric Neoplasms

Marc-David Leclair, MD
Doctor
Department of Pediatric Surgery
Hôpital Mère-Enfant
Nantes, France
Peritonitis

Alan M. Leichtner, MD
Clinical Director of Gastroenterology
Combined Program in Pediatric Gastroenterology and Nutrition
Children's Hospital Boston
Associate Professor
Department of Pediatrics
Harvard Medical School
Boston, Massachusetts
Inflammatory Bowel Disease: Ulcerative Colitis

Jeremiah J. Levine, MD
Director, Gastroenterology and Nutrition Division
Schneider Children's Hospital, North Shore/Long Island Jewish Health System
Professor
Department of Pediatrics
Albert Einstein College of Medicine
New Hyde Park/Bronx, New York
Postnatal Infections of the Liver: AIDS and Other Immune Disorders

Steven N. Lichtman, MD, FRCPC
Chief, Division of Pediatric Gastroenterology
University Hospital
Professor
Department of Pediatrics
University of North Carolina at Chapel Hill School of Medicine
Chapel Hill, North Carolina
Infections: Bacterial Overgrowth

Jenifer R. Lightdale, MD, MPH
Assistant in Medicine
Combined Program in Pediatric Gastroenterology and Nutrition
Children's Hospital Boston
Instructor
Department of Pediatrics
Harvard Medical School
Boston, Massachusetts
Study Design: Outcomes Research on Diagnostic and Therapeutic Procedures

Claude Liguory, MD
Director, Endoscopic Unit
Department of Gastroenterology
Alma Clinic
Paris, France
Gastrointestinal Endoscopy: Endoscopic Retrograde Cholangiopancreatography

David A. Lloyd, MChir, FRCS, FCS(SA)
Honorary Consultant Pediatric Surgeon
Department of Pediatric Surgery
Alder-Hey Children's Hospital
Professor of Pediatric Surgery
Department of Child Health
University of Liverpool School of Medicine
Liverpool, England
Intestine: Congenital Anomalies and *The Surgical Abdomen*

Olli Lohi, MD, PhD
Division of Pediatric Gastroenterology
Department of Pediatrics
Tampere University Hospital
University of Tampere Medical School
Tampere, Finland
Enteropathy: Celiac Disease

Mark E. Lowe, MD, PhD
Chief, Division of Gastroenterology
Children's Hospital of Pittsburgh
Professor
Department of Pediatrics
University of Pittsburgh School of Medicine
Pittsburgh, Pennsylvania
Pancreatic Function and Dysfunction and *Pancreatitis:
Acute and Chronic*

Dennis P. Lund, MD
Surgeon-In-Chief
University of Wisconsin Children's Hospital
Associate Professor
Department of Surgery
University of Wisconsin School of Medicine—Madison
Madison, Wisconsin
Appendicitis

Dilip Mahalanabis, MBBS, FRCP
President, Society for Applied Studies
Calcutta, India
President, Society for Essential Health
Action and Training
New Delhi, India
*Nutritional Therapy: Fluid and Dietary Therapy
of Diarrhea*

Markku Mäki, MD, PhD
Chief, Pediatric Gastroenterology
Department of Pediatrics
Tampere University Hospital
Professor of Pediatrics
University of Tampere Medical School
Tampere, Finland
Enteropathy: Celiac Disease

Martín G. Martín, MD, MPP
Gastroenterologist
Division of Gastroenterology
Associate Professor
Department of Pediatrics
David Geffen School of Medicine at University of
California, Los Angeles
Los Angeles, California
*Congenital Disease of Dysfunction and Absorption:
Congenital Intestinal Transport Defects*

Maria R. Mascarenhas, MBBS
Director, Nutrition Support Service
Department of Pediatrics
The Children's Hospital of Philadelphia
Associate Professor
Department of Pediatrics
University of Pennsylvania School of Medicine
Philadelphia, Pennsylvania
Nutritional Therapy: Special Dietary Therapy

Dietrich Matern, MD
Co-Director, Biochemical Genetics Laboratory
Department of Laboratory Medicine and Pathology
Mayo Clinic
Assistant Professor
Department of Laboratory Medicine and Pathology
Mayo Clinic College of Medicine
Rochester, Minnesota
*Genetic and Metabolic Disorders: Inherited Abnormalities In
Mitochondrial Fatty Acid Oxidation*

Suzanne V. McDiarmid, MB, CHB
Director, Hepatology Program
Division of Pediatric Gastroenterology
Professor
David Geffen School of Medicine at University of
California, Los Angeles
Los Angeles, California
Treatment of End-Stage Liver Disease

Valerie A. McLin, MD
Fellow
Division of Gastroenterology, Hepatology and Nutrition
Cincinnati Children's Hospital Medical Center
Department of Pediatrics
University of Cincinnati School of Medicine
Cincinnati, Ohio
Approach to Neonatal Cholestasis

Mini Mehra, MD
Staff Physician
Division of Gastroenterology and Nutrition
Assistant Professor
Department of Pediatrics
David Geffen School of Medicine at University of
California, Los Angeles
Los Angeles, California
*Gastrointestinal Endoscopy: Gastrointestinal
Endosonography*

Laurent Michaud, MD
Medical Doctor
Division of Gastroenterology, Hepatology and Nutrition
Department of Pediatrics
Hôpital Jeanne de Flandre
Lille, France
Gastrointestinal Bleeding: Lower Gastrointestinal Bleeding

Giorgina Mieli-Vergani, MD, PhD, FRCPCH
Alex Mowat Professor of Pediatric Hepatology
Department of Liver Studies and Transplantation
Guy's, King's, and St. Thomas' School of Medicine
London, England
Autoimmune Disease

Peter J. Milla, MSc, MB, BS, FRCP, FRCPCH
Honorary Consultant Pediatric Gastroenterologist
Great Ormond St. Hospital for Children
Professor in Pediatric Gastroenterology
Institute of Child Health
University of London School of Medicine
London, England
Motor Disorders including Pyloric Stenosis

Michael R. Millar, MB, ChB, PhD, FRCPath
Infection Control Doctor/Consultant Microbiologist
Department of Microbiology and Virology
Barts and The London National Health Service Trust
Honorary Senior Lecturer
Department of Microbiology
Queen Mary, University of London School of Medicine
London, England
*Drug Therapy: Modulation of Intestinal Flora:
    Antimicrobials*

Viswanathan Mohan, MD, MRCP, PhD, DSC
Director, M. V. Diabetes Specialties Centre
President, Madras Diabetes Research Foundation
Chennai, India
Pancreatitis: Juvenile Tropical Pancreatitis

Jean-François Mougenot, MD
Pediatric Gastroenterologist, Director of Pediatric
    Digestive Endoscopy Unit
Hôpital Robert Debré and Hôpital Necker-Enfants
    Malades
Paris, France
*Intestinal Tumors: Intestinal Polyps and Polyposis,
    Gastrointestinal Endoscopy: Upper Gastrointestinal
    Endoscopy, and Gastrointestinal Endoscopy: Endoscopic
    Retrograde Cholangiopancreatography*

Simon H. Murch, BSc, PhD, FRCP, FRCPCH
Consultant
Department of Paediatric Gastroenterology
Royal Free National Health Service Trust
Senior Lecturer
Centre for Paediatric Gastroenterology
Royal Free and University College School of Medicine
London, England
Enteropathy: Food-Allergic Enteropathy

Karen F. Murray, MD
Director, Hepatobiliary Program
Division of Gastroenterology
Department of Pediatrics
Children's Hospital and Regional Medical Center
Associate Professor of Pediatrics
Department of Pediatrics
University of Washington
Seattle, Washington
Genetic and Metabolic Disorders: Amino Acid Metabolism

Hassan Y. Naim, PhD
Professor and Chairman of Biochemistry
Department of Physiological Chemistry
School of Veterinary Medicine, Hannover
Hannover, Germany
*Congenital Disease of Dysfunction and Absorption:
    Genetically Determined Disaccharidase Deficiency*

Carla L. Nash, MD, FRCPC
Assistant Professor of Medicine
Division of Gastroenterology
University of Calgary School of Medicine
Calgary, Alberta, Canada
Intestinal Tumors: Other Neoplasms

Karen Norton, MD
Associate Professor
Departments of Radiology and Pediatrics
Mount Sinai School of Medicine
New York, New York
*Imaging: Cross-Sectional Imaging: Ultrasonography,
    Computed Tomography, Magnetic Resonance Imaging*

Samuel Nurko, MD, MPH
Director of Gastroenterology Motility Program
Combined Program in Pediatric Gastroenterology and
    Nutrition
Children's Hospital Boston
Assistant Professor
Department of Pediatrics
Harvard Medical School
Boston, Massachusetts
*Mouth and Esophagus: Other Motor Disorders,
    Gastrointestinal Manometry: Methodology and
    Indications, and Management of Surgical Patients:
    Complications after Gastrointestinal Surgery:
    A Medical Perspective*

Nancy C. O'Connell, MS, CCRC, CCRA
Research Assistant
Division of Clinical Mass Spectrometry
Children's Hospital Medical Center
St. Paul, Minnesota
*Genetic and Metabolic Disorders: Bile Acid Synthesis and
    Metabolism*

Judith A. O'Connor, MD, MS
Staff Physician
Division of Gastroenterology/Hepatology and Nutrition
The Children's Hospital of Colorado
Associate Professor
Department of Pediatrics
University of Colorado
Denver, Colorado
Nutritional Therapy: Protective Nutrients

P. Pearl O'Rourke, MD
Associate Professor Pediatrics
Department of Pediatrics
Harvard Medical School
Boston, Massachusetts
Study Design: Ethics and Regulatory Issues

Mark R. Oliver, MD, FRACP
Consultant Gastroenterologist
Department of Gastroenterology
Royal Children's Hospital
Senior Fellow
Department of Paediatrics
University of Melbourne
Melbourne, Victoria, Australia
Pancreatic Function Tests

Jean-Pierre Olives, MD
Chief, Medical Group of Specialties
Department of Pediatrics
Hôpital Des Enfants
Professor of Pediatrics
Department of Pediatrics
Université de Toulouse
Toulouse, France
Injuries of the Esophagus

Sylviane Olschwang, MD, PhD
Oncogenetics Counsellor
Researcher
INSERM U434
Paris, France
Intestinal Tumors: Intestinal Polyps and Polyposis

Susan R. Orenstein, MD
Pediatric Gastroenterology
Children's Hospital of Pittsburgh
Professor of Pediatrics
University of Pittsburgh School of Medicine
Pittsburgh, Pennsylvania
Gastroesophageal Reflux

Margarete Parrish, MSW, PhD
Assistant Professor
School of Social Work
University of Maryland, Baltimore
Baltimore, Maryland
Munchausen Syndrome by Proxy: Factitious Disorder by Proxy

Dinesh S. Pashankar, MD, MRCP
Pediatric Gastrenterologist
Department of Pediatrics
Children's Hospital of Iowa
Assistant Professor
Department of Pediatrics
University of Iowa School of Medicine
Iowa City, Iowa
Postnatal Infections of the Liver: Bacterial, Parasitic, and Other Infections

Wendy Paterson, BSc, MSc
Research Assistant
Royal Hospital for Sick Children
Honorary Research Associate
Department of Child Health
University of Glasgow
Glasgow, Scotland
Growth Failure

David H. Perlmutter, MD
Physician-in-Chief and Scientific Director
Children's Hospital of Pittsburgh
Vira I. Heinz Professor and Chair
Department of Pediatrics
University of Pittsburgh School of Medicine
Pittsburgh, Pennsylvania
Genetic and Metabolic Disorders: α_1-Antitrypsin Deficiency

Jay A. Perman, MD
Chief of Pediatrics
University of Maryland Medical System
Professor and Chair
Department of Pediatrics
University of Maryland School of Medicine
Baltimore, Maryland
Munchausen Syndrome by Proxy: Factitious Disorder by Proxy

Michel Peuchmaur, MD, PhD
Chief
Pathology Department
Hôpital Robert Debré
Professor of Pathology
Xavier Bichat University
Paris, France
Intestinal Tumors: Intestinal Polyps and Polyposis

David A. Piccoli, MD
Chief, Division of Gastroenterology and Nutrition
The Children's Hospital of Philadelphia
Professor
Department of Pediatrics
University of Pennsylvania School of Medicine
Philadelphia, Pennsylvania
Disorders of the Biliary Tract: Disorders of the Intrahepatic Ducts

Alan David Phillips, BA, PhD, FRCPCH
Consultant Clinical Scientist
Department of Pediatric Gastroenterology
Royal Free National Health Service Trust
Honorary Reader
Department of Pediatrics & Child Health
Royal Free and University College Medical School, University College London
London, England
Congenital Disease of Dysfunction and Absorption: Congenital Enteropathy Involving Intestinal Mucosa Development and Intestinal Biopsy

Hugues Piloquet, MD
Doctor
Service de Pédiatrie
Hôpital Mère-Enfant
Nantes, France
Peritonitis

C. S. Pitchumoni, MD, FRCPC, FACP, MACG, MPH
Chief of Gastroenterology, Hepatology, and Nutrition
Saint Peter's University Hospital
Professor of Medicine
Department of Medicine
Robert Wood Johnson School of Medicine
New Brunswick, New Jersey
Pancreatitis: Juvenile Tropical Pancreatitis

Randi Pleskow, MD
Associate in Medicine
Combined Program in Pediatric Gastroenterology
    and Nutrition
Children's Hospital Boston
Instructor
Department of Pediatrics
Harvard School of Medicine
Boston, Massachusetts
Genetic and Metabolic Disorders: Wilson Disease

Guillaume Podevin, MD
Doctor
Department of Pediatric Surgery
Hôpital Mère-Enfant
Nantes, France
Peritonitis

Stephen R. Porter, MD, PhD, FDS, RCS, FDS, RCSE
Associate Dean and Professor and Head of Department of
    Oral Medicine
Department of Oral Medicine
Eastman Dental Institute for Oral Health Care Sciences
London, England
Disorders of the Oral Cavity

Roy Proujansky, MD
Chief Executive, Nemours Children's Clinic—Wilmington
Associate Dean, Robert L. Brent Professor, and Chair
Department of Pediatrics
Jefferson Medical College
Philadelphia, Pennsylvania
Protein-Losing Enteropathy

Grant A. Ramm, PhD
Head, Hepatic Fibrosis Group
The Queensland Institute of Medical Research
Royal Brisbane Hospital
Brisbane, Queensland, Australia
Liver Function and Dysfunction: Fibrogenesis and Cirrhosis

Gerald V. Raymond, MD
Neurologist
Department of Neurogenetics
Kennedy Krieger Institute
Associate Professor
Department of Neurology
John Hopkins School of Medicine
Baltimore, Maryland
*Genetic and Metabolic Disorders: Zellweger Syndrome and
    Other Disorders of Peroxisomal Metabolism*

John Reilly, BSc, PhD
Division of Developmental Medicine
Queen Mother's Hospital
Reader
University of Glasgow
Glasgow, Scotland
Growth Failure

Sue J. Rhee, MD
Fellow
Combined Program in Pediatric Gastroenterology
    and Nutrition
Massachusetts General Hospital for Children
Fellow
Department of Pediatrics
Harvard Medical School
Boston, Massachusetts
Drug Therapy: Immunosuppressive Therapies

Piero Rinaldo, MD, PhD
Co-Director, Biochemical Genetics Laboratory
Department of Laboratory Medicine and Pathology
Mayo Clinic
Professor
Department of Laboratory Medicine and Pathology
Mayo Clinic College of Medicine
Rochester, Minnesota
*Genetic and Metabolic Disorders: Inherited Abnormalities
    in Mitochondrial Fatty Acid Oxidation*

Eve A. Roberts, MD, FRCPC
Staff Physician
Department of Pediatrics
Hospital for Sick Children
Professor
Department of Pediatrics, Medicine, and Pharmacology
University of Toronto School of Medicine
Toronto, Ontario, Canada
Drug-Induced Hepatotoxicity

Drucilla J. Roberts, MD
Associate Pathologist
Department of Pathology
Massachusetts General Hospital
Associate Professor
Department of Pathology
Harvard Medical School
Boston, Massachusetts
Stomach and Duodenum: Congenital Anomalies

Johanna M. Rommens, PhD
Senior Scientist
Program in Genetics and Genomic Biology
Associate Professor
Department of Molecular and Medical Genetics
University of Toronto School of Medicine
Toronto, Ontario, Canada
*Exocrine Pancreatic Dysfunction: Shwachman-Diamond
    Syndrome*

Rachel Rosen, MD
Fellow, Combined Program in Pediatric Gastroenterology
    and Nutrition
Children's Hospital Boston
Fellow, Department of Pediatrics
Harvard Medical School
Boston, Massachusetts
Mouth and Esophagus: Other Motor Disorders

Philip Rosenthal, MD
Medical Director, Pediatric Liver Transplant Program
Director, Pediatric Hepatology
Department of Pediatrics
University of California, San Francisco Children's
    Hospital
Professor
Department of Pediatrics and Surgery
University of California School of Medicine, San Francisco
San Francisco, California
Disorders of the Biliary Tract: Other Disorders

Marion Rowland, MB, MPH
Research Assistant
Division of Gastroenterology
Department of Pediatrics
University College Dublin
Dublin, Ireland
Gastritis: Helicobacter pylori *and Peptic Ulcer Disease*

Frank M. Ruemmele, MD, PhD
Department of Pediatrics
Hôpital Necker-Enfants Malades
Faculty of Medicine
René Descartes University
Paris, France
Enteropathy: Autoimmune Enteropathy

Pierre Russo, MD
Director, Division of Anatomic Pathology
The Children's Hospital of Philadelphia
Associate Professor
Department of Pathology and Laboratory Medicine
University of Pennsylvania School of Medicine
Philadelphia, Pennsylvania
*Disorders of the Biliary Tract: Disorders of the Intrahepatic
    Ducts*

Seppo Salminen, PhD
Professor
Functional Foods Forum, Health Biosciences Program
University of Turku
Turku, Finland
Drug Therapy: Modulation of Intestinal Flora: Probiotics

Ghislaine Sayer, MRCP, DMRD, FRCR
Specialist Registrar
Department of Radiology
University Hospital Aintree
Doctor
Department of Medical Imaging
University of Liverpool School of Medicine
Liverpool, England
Imaging: Plain Radiographs and Contrast Studies

Michela Schaeppi, MD
Registrar
Division of Gastroenterology
Department of Pediatrics
Hôpital Des Enfants Malades
Department of Public Instruction
University of Geneva
Geneva, Switzerland
*Gastrointestinal Endoscopy: Upper Gastrointestinal
    Endoscopy*

Steven Schlozman, MD
Staff Psychiatrist, Consultant, Pediatric Liver Transplant
    Program
Massachusetts General Hospital
Clinical Instructor in Psychiatry, Lecturer in Education
Department of Psychiatry
Harvard Medical School, Harvard Graduate School
    of Education
Boston, Massachusetts
Management of Surgical Patients: Psychological Aspects

Jacques Schmitz, MD
Chief, Ambulatory Pediatric Gastroenterology Unit
Hôpital Necker-Enfants Malades
Professor of Pediatrics
Faculty of Medicine
René Descartes University
Paris, France
Maldigestion and Malabsorption

Richard A. Schreiber, MD, FRCPC
Hepatologist
BC Children's Hospital
Clinical Associate Professor
Department of Pediatrics
University of British Columbia
Vancouver, British Columbia, Canada
*Postnatal Infections of the Liver: Bacterial, Parasitic, and
    Other Infections*

C. Ronald Scott, MD
Director
Biochemical Genetics Clinic, University of Washington
  Medical Center
Professor
Departments of Pediatrics and Medicine
University of Washington School of Medicine
Seattle, Washington
Genetic and Metabolic Disorders: Amino Acid Metabolism

Ernest G. Seidman, MD, FRCPC, FACG
Chief, Division of Gastroenterology and Nutrition
Ste Justine Hospital
Professor, Department of Pediatrics
University of Montreal
Montreal, Quebec, Canada
*Gastrointestinal Manifestations of Immunodeficiency:
  Primary Immunodeficiency Diseases*

Kenneth D. R. Setchell, PhD
Director, Clinical Mass Spectrometry
Children's Hospital Medical Center
Professor of Pediatrics
University of Cincinnati School of Medicine
Cincinnati, Ohio
*Genetic and Metabolic Disorders: Bile Acid Synthesis and
  Metabolism*

Eyal Shemesh, MD
Attending Physician
The Recanati-Miller Transplant Institute
Mount Sinai Medical Center
Assistant Professor
Department of Psychiatry and Pediatrics
Mount Sinai School of Medicine
New York, New York
Drug Therapy: Adherence to Medical Regimens

Ross W. Shepherd, MD, FRACP, FRCP
Director Liver Program
Division of Gastroenterology
St. Louis Children's Hospital
Professor
Department of Pediatrics
Washington University School of Medicine
St. Louis, Missouri
Liver Function and Dysfunction: Fibrogenesis and Cirrhosis

Philip M. Sherman, MD, FRCPC
Research Institute, Hospital for Sick Children
Professor of Paediatrics and Microbiology
University of Toronto
Canada Research Chair in Gastrointestinal Disease
Toronto, Ontario, Canada
Microbial Interactions with Gut Epithelium

Delane Shingadi, FRCPCH, MPH
Doctor
Department of Child Health
Barts and The London School of Medicine and Dentistry
Queen Mary, University of London
London, England
*Gastrointestinal Manifestations of Immunodeficiency:
  HIV and Other Secondary Immunodeficiencies*

Benjamin L. Shneider, MD
Chief, Division of Pediatric Hepatology
Department of Pediatrics
Mount Sinai Medical Center
Professor
Department of Pediatrics
Mount Sinai School of Medicine
New York, New York
Genetic and Metabolic Disorders: Biliary Transport

Virpi V. Smith, PhD
Clinical Scientist
Department of Histopathology
Great Ormond Street Hospital for Children
Honorary Lecturer
Gastroenterology Unit
Institute of Child Health, University College London
London, England
Intestinal Biopsy

John D. Snyder, MD
Gastroenterologist
Division of Pediatric Gastroenterology
Moffat Children's Hospital
Professor of Pediatrics
University of California School of Medicine
San Francisco, California
Nutritional Therapy: Fluid and Dietary Therapy of Diarrhea

Judith M. Sondheimer, MD
Chief of Gastroenterology, Hepatology and Nutrition
  Division
Children's Hospital
Professor of Pediatrics
University of Colorado Health Sciences Center
Denver, Colorado
Vomiting

Humberto Soriano, MD
Section Chief, Gastroenterology, Hepatology and
  Nutrition
Medical Director, Liver Transplant Program
St. Christopher's Hospital for Children
Associate Professor
Drexel University College of Medicine
Philadelphia, Pennsylvania
*Liver Function and Dysfunction: Normal Hepatocyte
  Function and Mechanisms of Dysfunction*

Robert H. Squires Jr, MD
Clinical Director
Division of Gastroenterology
Children's Hospital of Pittsburgh
Professor of Pediatrics
University of Pittsburgh School of Medicine
Pittsburgh, Pennsylvania
Abdominal Masses

Virginia A. Stallings, MD
Nutrition Center Director
Department of Pediatrics
The Children's Hospital of Philadelphia
Professor
Department of Pediatrics
University of Pennsylvania School of Medicine
Philadelphia, Pennsylvania
Nutritional Therapy: Special Dietary Therapy

Jennifer P. Stevens, MS
Medical Student
Harvard Medical School
Boston, Massachusetts
Study Design: Ethics and Regulatory Issues

James Sutphen, MD, PhD
Chief, Division of Pediatric Gastroenterology
University of Virginia Health Sciences Center
Professor
Department of Pediatrics
University of Virginia School of Medicine
Charlottesville, Virginia
Nutritional Therapy: Nutrition Support: Enteral Nutrition

Brian T. Sweeney, MB, BCh, Bao, MD
Fellow, Department of Pediatric Surgery
The Children's Hospital of Wisconsin
Milwaukee, Wisconsin
Gallbladder Disease

Jan A. J. M. Taminiau, MD, PhD
Doctor
Division of Pediatric Gastroenterology
Academisch Medisch Centrum Emma Kinderziekenhuis
Doctor
Department of Pediatrics
Amsterdam Municipal University
Amsterdam, Netherlands
Gastrointestinal Injury: Radiation Enteritis

Jonathan E. Teitelbaum, MD
Chief, Division of Pediatric Gastroenterology
Monmouth Medical Center
Long Branch, New Jersey
Assistant Professor
Department of Pediatrics
Drexel University College of Medicine
Philadelphia, Pennsylvania
Mouth and Esophagus: Congenital Anomalies and Systemic Endocrinopathies

Nikhil Thapar, BSc(Hons), BM(Hons), MRCP(UK), MRCPCH
Honorary Specialist Registrar in Pediatric Gastroenterology
Department of Adult and Paediatric Gastroenterology
St. Bartholomew's and the Royal London Hospitals
Research Fellow
Department of Enteric Neurodevelopment
National Institute for Medical Research
London, England
Stomach and Duodenum: Congenital Anomalies

Erica Thomas, RGN, RSCN, DPNS, BSc(Hons)
Senior Sister Paediatric Surgery
The Royal London Hospital
Department of Paediatric Nursing
City University London
London, England
Management of Surgical Patients: The Pediatric Ostomy

Mike Thomson, MB, ChB, DCH, FCRP, FRCPCH, MD
Consultant in Paediatric Gastroenterology and Nutrition
Royal Free Hospital National Health Service Trust
Honorary Senior Lecturer in Paediatric Gastroenterology
Royal Free and University College Medical School
London, United Kingdom
Esophagitis and *Gastrointestinal Endoscopy: Ileo-colonoscopy and Enteroscopy*

Franco Torrente, MD
Clinical Assistant
Department of Paediatric Gastroenterology
G. Gaslini Institute
Genoa, Italy
Genetic and Metabolic Disorders: Disorders of Carbohydrate Metabolism and *Enteropathy: Food-Allergic Enteropathy*

Silvia Tortorelli, MD, PhD
Fellow, Clinical-Biochemical Genetics
Department of Laboratory Medicine and Pathology
Mayo Clinic College of Medicine
Rochester, Minnesota
Genetic and Metabolic Disorders: Inherited Abnormalities in Mitochondrial Fatty Acid Oxidation

Juan A. Tovar, MD, PhD
Head, Department of Pediatric Surgery
Hospital Universitario La Paz
Professor of Pediatrics
Department of Pediatrics
Universidad Autónoma de Madrid
Madrid, Spain
Hernias

David N. Tuchman, MD
Director, Division of Pediatric Gastroenterology and
    Nutrition
Department of Pediatrics
Children's Hospital at Sinai
Assistant Professor
Department of Pediatrics
Johns Hopkins University
Baltimore, Maryland
Disorders of Deglutition

Dominique Turck, MD
Director, Division of Gastroenterology, Hepatology and
    Nutrition
Hôpital Jeanne de Flandre
Professor
Division of Gastroenterology, Hepatology and Nutrition
Lille University Faculty of Medicine
Lille, France
Gastrointestinal Bleeding: Lower Gastrointestinal Bleeding

Elizabeth C. Utterson, MD
Fellow, Division of Gastroenterology
The Children's Hospital
Department of Pediatrics
University of Colorado School of Medicine
Denver, Colorado
Nutritional Therapy: Protective Nutrients

Yvan Vandenplas, MD, PhD
Staff Gastroenterologist
Department of Pediatrics
Academisch Zeikenhuis-Vrye Universiteit Brussel
Professor
Department of Pediatrics
Vrye Univeriteit Brussel
Brussels, Belgium
pH Measurement

Jon A. Vanderhoof, MD
Vice President of Global Medical Affairs
Department of Global Medical Affairs
Mead Johnson Nutritionals
Evansville, Nebraska
Professor of Pediatrics
Department of Pediatrics
University of Nebraska
Omaha, Nebraska
*Intestinal Failure: Short-Bowel Syndrome and Intestinal
    Adaptation*

Jorge H. Vargas, MD
Gastroenterologist
Divison of Gastroenterology
Professor
Department of Pediatrics
David Geffen School of Medicine at University of
    California, Los Angeles
Los Angeles, California
*Gastrointestinal Endoscopy: Gastrointestinal
    Endosonography*

Diego Vergani, MD, PhD, FRCP
Professor of Liver Immunopathology
Department of Liver Studies and Transplantation
Guy's, King's, and St. Thomas' School of Medicine
London, England
Autoimmune Disease

Paul W. Wales, BSc, MD, MSc, FRCSC
Neonatal and Paediatric Surgeon; Coordinator, The Group
    for Improvement of Intestinal Function & Treatment
Department of Surgery
The Hospital for Sick Children
Assistant Professor
Department of Surgery
University of Toronto School of Medicine
Toronto, Ontario, Canada
Intestinal Failure: Aspects of Surgery

W. Allan Walker, MD
Director, Mucosal Immunology Laboratory
Combined Program in Pediatric Gastroenterology
    and Nutrition
Massachusetts General Hospital for Children
Conrad Taff Professor of Nutrition and Pediatrics
Harvard Medical School
Professor of Nutrition
Harvard School of Public Health
Boston, Massachusetts
*Pediatric Gastroenterology: A Subspecialty in Pediatrics
    "Comes of Age"*

Paul A. Watkins, MD, PhD
Associate Professor of Neurology
Johns Hopkins University School of Medicine
Baltimore, Maryland
*Genetic and Metabolic Disorders: Zellweger Syndrome and
    Other Disorders of Peroxisomal Metabolism*

Lawrence T. Weaver, MA, MD, FRCP, FRCPCH
Royal Hospital for Sick Children
Department of Gastroenterology
Professor
Department of Child Health
University of Glasgow
Glasgow, Scotland
Growth Failure

David C. Whitcomb, MD, PhD
Director, Medical Genomics; Chief, Division of
    Gastroenterology, Hepatology and Nutrition
Professor of Medicine, Cell Biology, Physiology, and
    Human Genetics
University of Pittsburgh School of Medicine
Pittsburgh, Pennsylvania
Pancreatic Function and Dysfunction and *Pancreatitis:
    Acute and Chronic*

Mark Wilks, BSc, Dip Bacteriol, PhD
Clinical Scientist
Department of Microbiology and Virology
Barts and The London National Health Service Trust
London, England
Drug Therapy: Modulation of Intestinal Flora:
  Antimicrobials

Helen J. Williams, MB ChB, MRCP, FRCR
Consultant Pediatric Radiologist
Radiology Department
Birmingham Children's Hospital
Birmingham, England
Imaging: Radionuclide Diagnosis

Michael Wilschanski, MD
Director, Department of Pediatric Gastroenterology
Hadassah Hospitals
Senior Lecturer
Department of Pediatrics
Hebrew University
Jerusalem, Israel
Exocrine Pancreatic Dysfunction: Other Hereditary and
  Acquired Disorders

Ernest M. Wright, PhD, DSc
Professor
Department of Physiology
David Geffen School of Medicine at University of
  California, Los Angeles
Los Angeles, California
Congenital Disease of Dysfunction and Absorption:
  Congenital Intestinal Transport Defects

Klaus-Peter Zimmer, MD
Professor
Division of Gastroenterology
Westfalische Wilhelms Universitat
Munster, Germany
Congenital Disease of Dysfunction and Absorption:
  Genetically Determined Disaccharidase Deficiency

DEDICATION

To Michael (Pic) Walker and Heather McDonald Walker in celebration of their union and as role models for life.

WAW

I wish to acknowledge my cherished French colleagues, professors Jean Rey, Claude Ricour, and Jacques Schmitz, who encouraged me to enter the exciting field of research and clinical practice in pediatric gastroenterology and nutrition, and Professor Allan Walker, who invited me to be one of the two European associate editors of this fourth edition. To my wife Véronique and our children, Pierre-Arthur, Charles, Alix, and Marine, who have supported me in my work for so many years.

OJG

To Allan Walker, who has inspired all of us in this discipline of pediatric gastroenterology and nutrition with his energy, wisdom, and imagination to dedicate our efforts to improving the lives of children with gastrointestinal, liver, pancreatic, and nutritional disorders; who has been and continues to be my mentor and close friend and a source of sage advice for over 25 years; and who remains the standard bearer for those who wish to advance the science and practice of medicine for pediatric patients. With deep gratitude.

REK

To Megan, David, and Rachael for their support.

PMS

To Julia and Vita with love.

IRS

To my wife Abigail and my daughters Caitlin and Elizabeth for their constant love and support, without which this and many of my other professional activities would not have been possible, and to my many mentors and colleagues in pediatric hepatology, including, most notably, Drs. Frederick Suchy, Peter Whitington, and Alex Mowat.

BLS

PREFACE TO THE FIRST EDITION

Over the last two decades, the field of pediatric gastroenterology has developed from an obscure subspecialty to an essential component of every major academic pediatric program throughout the world. Among the many pediatric texts available, none deals extensively with the pathophysiologic basis of gastrointestinal disease in children of all ages. Contributors to this text have been asked to undertake their writing with a plan to fill this void, extending pathophysiologic considerations to their coverage of diagnosis and management as well. In tandem with development of the subspecialty the literature of gastrointestinal and hepatic entities as they pertain to the pediatric patient has grown. Accordingly, we have prepared an approach to the subject that should provide a reference text for pediatricians, gastroenterologists, and pediatric gastroenterologists alike.

This new multivolume textbook is dedicated to establishing a comprehensive approach to pediatric gastroenterology. Each author was carefully selected to provide an authoritative, comprehensive, and complete account of his assigned topic. We have devised an approach to dealing with the families of children with gastrointestinal diseases, and a pathophysiologic section examines cardinal manifestations of gastrointestinal disease as well as the development of the gastrointestinal tract. These sections help to augment an in-depth approach to disease manifestations and management. A careful and unique approach to diagnosis of gastrointestinal diseases in children follows. Finally, the principles of therapy are explored. We hope and expect that this collective approach will be beneficial to all physicians dealing with gastrointestinal problems in children.

W. Allan Walker, M.D.
Peter R. Durie, B.Sc., M.D., FRCPC
J. Richard Hamilton, M.D., FRCPC
John A. Walker-Smith, M.D., (Syd.), F.R.C.P. (Lon., Edin.), F.R.A.C.P.
John B. Watkins, M.D.
1991

PREFACE TO THE FOURTH EDITION

The fourth edition of this textbook, published in time for the Second World Congress of Pediatric Gastroenterology, Hepatology, and Nutrition, to be held in Paris, France, in July 2004, has been planned to update pediatricians caring for children with gastrointestinal and liver diseases worldwide and to provide the most recent, cutting-edge developments in our field. In a recent article in *Pediatric Research* reviewing the development of our subspecialty, it was stated that evidence for the field "having arrived" as a discipline in pediatric medicine was the publication of a textbook exclusively devoted to pediatric gastroenterology.[1] This edition of the textbook has made major strides in covering the most important aspects of physiology and pathophysiology, clinical presentation of disease, clinical manifestations and management, diagnostic approach, and principles of therapy. As genetics and molecular biology, as well as areas of interest in certain aspects of disease, have expanded, we have added additional chapters to comprehensively cover these new developments. Conversely, as diseases have become less prevalent, we have decreased their emphasis in the textbook. Hence, we believe that the current edition is up to date with the needs of the field.

With this edition, the editorship of the textbook is being passed to a new generation of experts in the field. We thank Drs. Durie, Hamilton, Walker-Smith, and Watkins for their contributions over the last three editions. Dr. Walker has continued with the fourth edition to pave the way for the new editors: Drs. Kleinman and Shneider from the United States, Dr. Sherman from Canada, and Drs. Goulet and Sanderson from Europe. It is hoped that this textbook will continue in perpetuity under their able leadership.

To keep up with the ever-increasing growth of information in this rapidly advancing field, we have chosen to produce a fourth edition in 2004. The size and content of each section have been modified. This revision is dedicated to the maintenance of a comprehensive approach to the practice of pediatric gastroenterology. Each author, whether newly chosen or retained from the third edition, has been selected because of a particular expertise in a specific field. Each author has provided an authoritative and comprehensive account of his or her topic. For example, in the fourth edition, we have separated pathophysiology from clinical syndromes by establishing Section 2, "Clinical Presentation of Disease," and Section 3, "Clinical Manifestations and Management." We have also added new chapters on study design (outcomes, methodology, and ethics) to the diagnosis section entitled "Diagnosis of Gastrointestinal Diseases" to reflect increasing interest in clinical investigation and the evidence-based approach to disease management. We have also added a section on prebiotics and probiotics to reflect this alternative medical approach to the treatment of pediatric gastrointestinal diseases and have also extended the section devoted to clinical nutrition. We believe that these modifications have resulted in a more "user-friendly" textbook.

To give the readership a perspective on the evolution of this textbook, we have included the preface from the first edition published almost 13 years ago. It has been an exciting adventure for the editors to contribute in a small way to the overall development of the practice of gastroenterology by pediatricians. We hope that you enjoy this latest edition.

The editors wish to again thank Ms. Suzette McCarron for her organizational talents and her ability to liaise among authors, editors, and the publisher. Without her extensive efforts, this textbook would never have been possible. The editors are also grateful to Mr. Brian Decker, Patricia Bindner, and the able staff of BC Decker Inc for their help and support in further developing this edition and in the publication of this textbook.

W. Allan Walker
Olivier J. Goulet
Ronald E. Kleinman
Ian R. Sanderson
Philip M. Sherman
Benjamin L. Shneider
July 2004

REFERENCE

1. Walker-Smith JA, Walker WA. The development of pediatric gastroenterology: a historical overview. Pediatr Res 2003;53:706–15.

CONTENTS

VOLUME 2

The Liver

CHAPTER 49

APPROACH TO NEONATAL CHOLESTASIS

Valerie A. McLin, MD

William F. Balistreri, MD

Cholestasis, defined physiologically as a reduction in canalicular bile flow, is primarily manifested as conjugated hyperbilirubinemia. The major clinical consequences, however, are presumably related to retention of other substances, such as bile acids, which are dependent on bile flow for excretion. The attendant histopathologic features often reflect the nature and degree of the physiologic disturbance and imply the pathophysiologic basis.

There are multiple causes of cholestasis in early life, related either to the response of the neonatal liver to exogenous agents or to specific congenital pathologic conditions. Immature hepatic excretory function creates a milieu wherein infants are susceptible to further impairment of biliary excretion owing to infectious or metabolic insults. Although recognized disorders associated with neonatal cholestasis are numerous, the majority of cases fall into a few discrete and overlapping categories, one of the more frequent ones being the generic "neonatal hepatitis."

Efforts are being made to alert generalists and specialists worldwide to recognize the neonate with cholestasis at the earliest opportunity. Nevertheless, evaluation of the infant with cholestasis remains a difficult task owing to the diversity of cholestatic syndromes, to their obscure pathogenesis, and to the often nonspecific clinical and pathologic presentation. Prompt identification and diagnostic assessment of the infant with cholestasis are imperative to recognize disorders amenable either to specific medical therapy (eg, galactosemia, sepsis) or to early surgical intervention (eg, biliary atresia) and to institute effective nutritional and medical support to allow optimal growth and development. Although the advent of pediatric liver transplant has saved many, early intervention may avoid the need for organ replacement in some of these patients. For example, in tyrosinemia, a non-transplant option is now readily available and efficacious.

DEVELOPMENTAL PHYSIOLOGY OF HEPATOBILIARY FUNCTION

Although comprehension of liver and biliary development is still at the embryonal stage, it is known that the extrahepatic biliary tree develops from an outgrowth of the ventral foregut, whereas the intrahepatic tree differentiates from the multipotent hepatoblast in a centrifugal fashion.[1] Furthermore, the physiology of bile flow in the adult is well described, and its understanding may assist in the approach of the cholestatic infant and the interpretation of laboratory tests. However, it is paramount to remember that the liver of the term infant is "immature" both in its metabolic and excretory functions. With the increased survival of very premature infants, pediatricians, neonatologists, and gastroenterologists are more likely to be confronted by cholestasis and abnormal liver tests. Thus, a basic understanding of physiology, together with prompt recognition and management, should help improve the outcome of these patients. Our goal is to discuss the expeditious and cost-effective approach to the infant with conjugated hyperbilirubinemia, allowing recognition of those who need specialized care.

Bile flow has traditionally been divided into two components: (1) bile acid–dependent flow, which involves active canalicular transport of bile acids, accompanied by osmotic water flow and diffusion of other solutes, and (2) bile acid–independent flow, which is thought to be mediated by active transport of other anions and cations.[2] The primary motive force in the generation of bile flow in early life is the hepatocytic secretion of bile acids; there is little contribution of the bile acid–independent component during the neonatal period.[3] The hepatobiliary excretory system is both functionally and anatomically underdeveloped at birth, leaving the neonate with a unique propensity toward cholestasis.[4–6]

Substantial evidence supports the existence of a period of "physiologic cholestasis" associated with immature or altered metabolism and transport of bile acids at birth (Table 49-1). Serum bile acid concentrations, which reflect the net efficiency of intestinal absorption and hepatobiliary function, are maintained at low levels in the fetus by carrier-mediated transplacental transport to the mother.[7–9] Postnatally, in the normal infant, both fasting and postprandial serum bile acid concentrations are significantly higher than those found in older children. These levels are similar to those attained in adults with cholestatic disease[10,11] and persist through the first several months of life. Factors contributing to decreased bile flow and inefficient enterohepatic cycling of bile acids in the neonate include (1) inefficient intestinal and hepatic bile acid uptake owing to the pace of ontogenic expression of bile acid transport proteins, (2) qualitative and quantitative deficiencies of bile acid synthesis, (3) immature hepatic bile acid metabolism, and (4) inefficient hepatocellular secretion.[12]

The suckling rat model has been used extensively in studies of the developing hepatobiliary system.[13,14] Lower rates of hepatic uptake of bile acids have been demonstrated in experimental systems such as isolated hepatocytes[15] and purified basolateral (sinusoidal) membrane vesicles of developing rats,[16,17] reflecting immaturity of sodium-coupled bile acid transport. This appears to be secondary to reduced expression of specific transport proteins.[18] In the adult rat, avid extraction of bile acids by periportal hepatocytes results in a decreasing periportal to central lobular gradient for bile acid uptake.[19,20] Using similar radioautographic techniques, no acinar gradient could be demonstrated in the 14-day-old rat liver,[21] further supporting the concept of inefficient uptake of bile acids. There is enhanced efflux of taurocholate from suckling rat hepatocytes, which may represent back-diffusion across the sinusoidal membrane; this also contributes to the inefficient hepatic bile acid transport.[22] In the ileum, a similar developmental pattern for the transport of bile acids can be demonstrated, with decreased active bile acid uptake during the suckling period.[23,24] There is significant passive absorption of bile acids in the jejunum of suckling rats, which may combine with decreased hepatic uptake to lead to decreased intraluminal concentrations of some bile acids.[25] A recent study in rats looked at the correlation between intestinal resection

length and expression of the apical sodium bile acid transporter. The authors reasoned that there may be an intestinal length "threshold" that determines whether the apical sodium bile acid transporter is up- or down-regulated in response to ileal resection. In parallel, hepatic synthesis of bile acids increases to compensate for decreased absorption up to a certain level, later decreasing when the bile acid pool is severely reduced. These findings are important for two reasons: they illustrate the plasticity of infant bile acid physiology and they offer a hypothesis for the pathogenesis of cholestasis in patients with short bowel.[26]

Quantitative and qualitative differences in bile acid synthetic pathways are also apparent during early life. Bile acid synthesis begins on day 11 of the 21-day gestation in the rat[27] and near week 12 in the human fetus.[28] A decreased cholate-to-chenodeoxycholate ratio has been observed in the human fetus compared with that of the adult, indicating immaturity of hepatic α-hydroxylation.[29–31] It is believed that a "threshold" concentration of cholic acid, the primary bile acid, is needed to initiate and maintain bile flow. Cholic acid may be trophic to the developing hepatic excretory system. In the absence of sufficient quantities of cholic acid, there is decreased bile flow.

The immaturity of bile acid synthetic function is also reflected in the presence of "atypical" bile acids found in the fetus and normal neonate.[30,31] Certain of these atypical bile acids, such as the monohydroxylated compound 3-β-hydroxy-5-Δ-cholenoic acid, which has been detected in amniotic fluid[32] and meconium,[33,34] are thought to directly impair bile acid excretion. Significant amounts of nonsulfated tetrahydroxylated bile acids have been identified in the urine of healthy neonates[35] and in the urine of older children and adults with cholestatic liver disease.[33] This polyhydroxylation may increase bile acid solubility, providing a potential alternative pathway for excretion of "toxic" bile acids at a time when transformation and biliary secretion are not fully developed.

Although the mechanisms of intracellular biotransformation of bile acids are not well defined, there is evidence that both the conjugation and sulfation of these organic anions are underdeveloped in early life.[36,37] Conjugation of bile acids with the amino acids taurine and glycine provides a potential mechanism for detoxification and allows efficient intestinal fat digestion and absorption. In isolated hepatocytes obtained from fetal and suckling rats, the rate of conjugation of a radiolabeled bile acid was shown to increase with postnatal age.[37]

The development of effective bile acid secretion from the hepatocyte appears to lag behind the onset of bile acid synthesis, as would be expected if cholic acid truly plays a trophic role. This is suggested by studies of the distribution of the bile acid (taurocholate) pool in fetal and newborn rats.[38] In the fetus, more than 85% of the bile acid pool is localized in the liver, with only 10% found in the intestinal lumen. By postnatal day 5, this distribution is reversed, with more than 85% of the bile acid pool localized in the intestine. Canalicular excretion of bile acids appears to be the rate-limiting step. Reduced canalicular excretion of bile acids in the fetus appears to be related to an immaturity of the canalicular membrane transport sys-

TABLE 49-1   MANIFESTATIONS OF
UNDERDEVELOPED BILE ACID
TRANSPORT AND METABOLISM
IN EARLY LIFE

Increased serum bile acid levels (physiologic cholestasis)
Decreased hepatic uptake of bile acids from portal blood
Absent lobular gradient
Qualitative and quantitative differences in bile acid synthesis
Decreased conjugation, sulfation, and glucuronidation of bile acids
Enhanced bile acid efflux from hepatocyte
Decreased bile acid secretion rate
Decreased bile acid pool size
Low intraluminal concentrations of bile acids
Decreased ileal active transport of bile acids

tems for bile acids. The potential-dependent transport protein is not detected in rat liver until postnatal day 7, and transport does not occur until day 14.[39] The adenosine triphosphate–dependent portion of the transport system, however, appears to be functional in the neonatal period and may play a role in bile acid secretion.[40] It has been recognized recently that the regulation of bile acid synthesis occurs by a feedback mechanism involving the nuclear receptor farnesoid X.[41] One can speculate that as these feedback loops mature, they may participate in the imbalance between the hepatocellular bile acid pool and canalicular excretory function. Furthermore, the same ontogenic principles apply to other metabolic pathways and transporters localized on hepatocytes and biliary epithelial cells. Thus, metabolism and excretion of xenobiotics (eg, bacterial toxins, maternal drugs) into bile are likely to be both modified by and potentially exacerbate cholestasis by imposing further demand on the immature liver, especially in the sick newborn. Thus, when investigating an infant with cholestasis, especially a preterm infant, one must look beyond the liver because cholestasis is a nonspecific response to a wide variety of insults in the infant.[42]

During fetal development, canaliculi differentiate from simple intracellular invaginations of two adjacent cell membranes into well-defined structural lumina filled with microvilli.[43] Specific changes in the pericanalicular cytoskeleton, which has been implicated in promotion of bile formation, are also noted during development. Compared with adult cells, cultured fetal hepatocytes have a decreased frequency and force of canalicular contractions, which appear to be related to a lack of pericanalicular cytoplasmic actin.[44] Structural immaturity of both the canaliculi and the pericanalicular cytoskeleton may be significant factors in impaired bile acid secretion during development. Furthermore, studies in both preterm humans and newborn piglets suggest that gallbladder contractility and response to cholecystokinin are also slow to mature, adding an extrahepatic factor to the long list of intrahepatic mechanisms responsible for the increased susceptibility to cholestasis in the infant, in particular the patient dependent on total parenteral nutrition.[45,46]

Despite abundant data suggesting structural and functional immaturity of hepatic excretory function, the clinical and physiologic implications of "physiologic cholestasis" are unclear. However, a reasonable hypothesis could be advanced: in the presence of lower rates of bile flow, compounds destined for biliary excretion would accumulate in the hepatocyte.[11] Certain of these compounds, such as atypical bile acids, are damaging to the membrane or organelle, making hepatic injury likely. Exogenous factors, such as infusion of parenteral nutrition solutions, prolonged fasting, sepsis, or hypoxia, will perturb this already precarious situation and result in the anatomic and clinical manifestations of cholestasis.

DIFFERENTIAL DIAGNOSIS OF CHOLESTASIS

The causes of neonatal cholestasis are diverse (Table 49-2). These include structural anomalies of the biliary tract, both intrahepatic and extrahepatic, which result in obstruction of bile flow, and infectious, metabolic, hemodynamic, or toxic insults, which cause functional impairment of the hepatic excretory process and bile secretion.

Although the differential diagnosis of cholestasis in the neonate is varied, the clinical presentation is similar, reflecting the underlying decrease in bile flow. Specifically, infants with cholestasis present with variable degrees of jaundice, dark urine, light stools, and hepatomegaly. Synthetic dysfunction and hepatocellular necrosis may be present. In certain patients with rapid progression of hepatocellular disease, fibrosis occurs, with signs of decompensation, such as ascites, appearing early in life. Failure to thrive is not always manifest early in the course; normal development may be falsely reassuring and should not detract the clinician from initiating a workup. Similarly, although premature infants are at increased risk for cholestasis, gestational age and side effects of neonatal intensive care should remain a "default" diagnosis once surgical and medical emergencies have been ruled out. The diagnosis of "transient neonatal cholestasis," the most frequent form, may be a more limited subset of the generic "idiopathic" neonatal hepatitis.

Jacquemin and colleagues used the term "transient neonatal cholestasis" to describe a group of 92 patients with early-onset neonatal cholestasis, identifiable perinatal complications incriminated in cholestasis, and a spontaneously favorable outcome.[47] In 85% of the patients, there was a history consistent with acute or chronic perinatal distress. Mean gestational age was 37 weeks, and birth weight was 2,705 g, with one-third of the patients being small for gestational age. Histology was consistent with the previous description of "neonatal hepatitis." The authors did not identify a correlation between histologic findings and perinatal events. Jaundice resolved in all patients, together with normalization of liver biochemical markers and, importantly, growth. The mean duration of jaundice was 3.5 months, and hepatomegaly resolved at a mean age of 13 months. Most had a biphasic progression of their cholestatic markers, with γ-glutamyl transpeptidase reaching its peak as conjugated bilirubin levels normalized. The importance of this study lies in its description of a subset of patients with early-onset neonatal cholestasis and hepatomegaly, perinatal distress, and a characteristic pattern of biochemical markers, in whom it is appropriate to defer liver biopsy and offer supportive care only. It is all the more important that the population of premature babies is increasing, with numerous perinatal hypoxic and toxic insults. Special attention should be paid to those infants who do not have a clearly identifiable cause of prematurity and develop cholestasis or intrauterine growth retarded infants with cholestasis; together, these problems may be indicative of primary liver disease or of an underlying metabolic defect.

DIAGNOSTIC APPROACH

Because of the severity of many of the conditions leading to neonatal cholestasis, early recognition of cholestasis in an infant and prompt diagnosis of the underlying disorder are imperative to identify disorders that will respond to a specific treatment and to institute general supportive care that

TABLE 49-2   CLASSIFICATION OF DISORDERS ASSOCIATED WITH CHOLESTASIS IN THE NEWBORN

EXTRAHEPATIC DISORDERS
Biliary atresia
Bile duct stricture/neonatal sclerosing cholangitis
Choledochal cyst
Anomalies of the pancreaticoduodenal junction
Spontaneous perforation of the bile duct
Inspissated bile
Mass
   Intraductular: stone, rhabdomyosarcoma
   Extraductular: hepatoblastoma, neuroblastoma

INTRAHEPATIC DISORDERS
Idiopathic
   "Idiopathic" neonatal hepatitis
   Intrahepatic cholestasis, *persistent*
     Severe intrahepatic cholestasis with progressive hepatocellular disease
      (see Chapter 55.6, "Biliary Transport")
     Alagille syndrome (syndromic paucity of the intrahepatic bile ducts,
      arteriohepatic dysplasia)
     Nonsyndromic paucity of the intrahepatic bile ducts
   Intrahepatic cholestasis, *recurrent*
     Benign recurrent intrahepatic cholestasis
     Hereditary cholestasis with lymphedema (Aagenaes syndrome)
Anatomic
   Congenital hepatic fibrosis or infantile polycystic disease
     (liver and kidney)
   Caroli disease
Metabolic or endocrine disorders
   Disorders of amino acid metabolism
     Tyrosinemia
   Disorders of lipid metabolism
     Cholesterol ester storage disease (Wolman)
     Niemann-Pick disease
     Gaucher disease
   Disorders of carbohydrate metabolism
     Galactosemia
     Fructosemia
     Glycogen storage disease type IV
   Disorders of bile acid metabolism, primary
     3β-Hydroxysteroid Δ^5-C_{27} steroid dehydrogenase/isomerase
     Δ^5–3-Oxosteroid 5β-reductase (multiple mutations)
   Disorders of bile acid metabolism, secondary
     Zellweger syndrome (cerebrohepatorenal syndrome)
     Peroxisomal enzymopathies
   Disorders of bile acid transport
     Rotor syndrome
     Dubin-Johnson syndrome

Mitochondrial hepatopathies
Other metabolic defects
   α_1-Antitrypsin deficiency
   Cystic fibrosis
   Hypopituitarism
   Hypothyroidism
   Neonatal iron storage disease
   Infantile copper overload (Menkes syndrome)
   Hemophagocytic lymphohistiocytosis
   Arginase deficiency
Toxic
   Total parenteral nutrition–associated cholestasis
   Fetal alcohol syndrome
   Other drugs (maternal or used in neonatal intensive care)
Cholestasis associated with infection
   Sepsis with possible endotoxemia (urinary tract infection,
     gastroenteritis)
   Syphilis
   Toxoplasmosis
   Listeriosis
   Congenital viral infections
     Cytomegalovirus
     Herpesvirus (herpes simplex and human herpesvirus 6)
     Cocksackievirus
     Echoviruses
     Rubella virus
     Hepatitis B virus
     Other hepatitis viruses: C? nonAnonB?
     Human immunodeficiency virus (HIV)
     Parvovirus B19
Chromosomal
   Trisomy 18
   Trisomy 21 (Down syndrome)
   Donohue syndrome (leprechaunism)
Vascular disorders
   Budd-Chiari syndrome
   Perinatal asphyxia
   Multiple hemangiomata
   Cardiac insufficiency
Miscellaneous
   Congenital disorders of glycosylation
   Shock, hypoperfusion
   Intestinal obstruction
   Neonatal lupus
   ARC syndrome (arthrogryposis, renal tubular dysfunction,
     and cholestasis)

---

may ameliorate the clinical course. The majority of infants with prolonged cholestasis will be found to fall into the diagnostic category of either biliary atresia or "neonatal hepatitis" (Table 49-3); the latter is a "default diagnosis." As research progresses in pediatric liver disease, the number of cases falling into the "default" category are decreasing. However, at the present time, because of the preponderance of these disorders and the clinical importance of differentiating between them, this chapter focuses on neonatal hepatitis as we know it today; biliary atresia is covered elsewhere in this text. Other specific disorders associated with neonatal cholestasis are discussed in subsequent chapters.

IDIOPATHIC NEONATAL HEPATITIS VERSUS BILIARY ATRESIA

Extensive evaluation of the infant with cholestasis leads to a diagnosis of either idiopathic neonatal hepatitis or biliary atresia in approximately 40% of infants (see Table 49-3). These terms are descriptive and imply a clinical phenotype rather than an etiology. The precise etiology and mechanism of injury in the majority of cases of neonatal hepatitis and biliary atresia remain obscure. The term "idiopathic obstructive or obliterative cholangiopathy" has been used to include disorders that manifest a range of pathology from predominantly hepatocellular injury to predominantly extrahepatic biliary tract injury.

Several overlapping hypotheses attempt to conceptually unify the pathogenesis of these disorders:

1. The ductal plate malformation theory, proposed initially by Jorgensen,[48] suggests that altered embryogenesis may be partially responsible for clinically apparent disorders of cholestasis in the neonate. During normal embryogenesis, the earliest form of the bile duct is a cylindric ductal plate, which is remodeled through an

TABLE 49-3 ESTIMATED FREQUENCY OF VARIOUS CLINICAL FORMS OF NEONATAL CHOLESTASIS

CLINICAL FORM	CUMULATIVE PERCENTAGE
"Idiopathic" neonatal hepatitis	15
Extrahepatic biliary atresia	25–30
α_1-Antitrypsin deficiency	7–10
Intrahepatic cholestasis syndromes (eg, Alagille, PFIC type I)	20
Bacterial sepsis	2
Hepatitis	
Cytomegalovirus	3–5
Rubella, herpes	1
Endocrine (hypothyroidism, panhypopituitarism)	1
Galactosemia	1
Inborn errors of bile acid biosynthesis	2–5

PFIC = progressive familial intrahepatic cholestasis.

interaction between the ingrowing mesenchyme and disappearing ductal plate. Defective remodeling or incomplete dissolution, with failure of recanalization, has been postulated to lead to malformation of the ductal plate and subsequent anatomic abnormalities such as biliary atresia or cystic diseases of the hepatobiliary system. Desmet has suggested that ductal plate malformation is a basic morphologic lesion that occurs at different levels of the biliary tree and may be seen in a variety of disorders in addition to biliary atresia, including congenital hepatic fibrosis.[1]

On a molecular level, it was recently proposed by Clotman and colleagues that intra- and extrahepatic biliary tract development is regulated in part by a cascade involving hepatocyte nuclear factor (HNF) 6 and HNF1 and that ductal plate malformations are visible in knockout models of these transcription factors.[49] Similarly, McCright and colleagues created a mouse model of Alagille syndrome, which suggests that Notch-Jagged interactions are necessary for normal intrahepatic biliary development.[50]

2. Landing set forth the concept of infantile obstructive cholangiopathy, suggesting that these cholestatic disorders represent the pathophysiologic continuum of a single, underlying, obliterative process.[51] According to this hypothesis, an initial insult leads to inflammation at various levels of the hepatobiliary tract. The clinical sequelae represent a static or a progressive inflammatory process at the specific site of injury. If the site of injury is predominantly the bile duct epithelium, the resulting cholangitis could lead to progressive sclerosis and obliteration of the bile duct, clinically manifest as biliary atresia. If, on the other hand, the inflammation is primarily hepatocellular, the clinical picture may be one of neonatal hepatitis. The interrelation between these two processes is further supported by evidence of intrahepatic ductal injury in patients with biliary atresia.[52,53]

Although no specific virus has been consistently identified in patients with "obstructive cholangiopathies," there has been much interest in several specific potential pathogens in these disorders. The majority of studies dealing with viral etiologies in these conditions are related to biliary atresia and thus are discussed in that section. Inborn errors of bile acid synthesis associated with the clinical picture of neonatal hepatitis have also been identified.[6,54,55] As our understanding of immune dysregulation and autoimmunity evolves, it appears that in some cases, the primary insult directed against the hepatocyte or cholangiocyte may be (auto)immune,[56] not unlike diseases found in older subjects (autoimmune hepatitis, primary biliary cirrhosis, primary sclerosing cholangitis). Immunohistochemical analysis of the "giant cell" reveals that these cells likely result from hepatocellular fusion. However, these observations have not shed light on the underlying insult or trigger for this idiosyncratic cellular response.[57] These studies and others support the contention that the neonatal liver is uniquely susceptible to injury, which, in turn, is manifest in a unique fashion. The initial stereotypic histologic reaction and perpetual injury in infantile obstructive cholangiopathy may result from a wide variety of insults at any level of the hepatobiliary system or beyond in another organ system.

Distinguishing between the intrahepatic, hepatocellular process of neonatal hepatitis and the extrahepatic or mixed injury in biliary atresia is achieved through cholangiography and biopsy and is discussed below.

IDIOPATHIC NEONATAL HEPATITIS

Idiopathic neonatal hepatitis represents the third most common diagnosis in infants with neonatal cholestasis, accounting for 15% overall.[11,58,59] This relative percentage has steadily decreased since the initial description by Stokes and colleagues.[60] This shift is attributable to identification of specific disorders (such as α_1-antitrypsin deficiency and bile acid transport and synthesis defects, which present with a clinical picture of neonatal hepatitis) that were previously included in this category. This diagnosis should be restricted to cases of prolonged neonatal cholestasis in which the classic histologic changes described by Craig and Landing[61] are present on liver biopsy and known infectious or metabolic causes of neonatal hepatocellular disease have been excluded (see Table 49-2). Based on epidemiologic data, two categories of neonatal hepatitis have been proposed: sporadic and familial.[11] The increased incidence within certain families suggests that, at least in these cases, hereditary or metabolic factors are operant. In fact, recent studies have suggested that specific forms of intrahepatic cholestasis, previously included in the "idiopathic neonatal hepatitis" category, can be further subdivided based on the observed pathology and presumed pathophysiology (Table 49-4).[11] It is from this latter group that future discoveries related to the genetic and molecular basis of bile acid synthesis and transport are likely to be made. As research continues to make progress in these areas, the number of identifiable diseases will increase, and the category of idiopathic neonatal hepatitis will proportionately decrease.

TABLE 49-4   PROPOSED SUBTYPES OF INTRAHEPATIC
              CHOLESTASIS

Bile duct paucity
  Syndromic (Alagille)
  Nonsyndromic
Progressive (familial) intrahepatic cholestasis
  Disorders of canalicular transport
    Bile acid transport
    Phopholipid transport
  Disorders of bile acid biosynthesis
  Undefined

CLINICAL PRESENTATION

"Idiopathic" neonatal hepatitis appears to be associated with
low birth weight, but a cause and effect relationship is
unclear. The clinical course is highly variable: more than
50% develop jaundice, to a varying degree, within the first
week of life. In our experience, the majority appear well;
however, as much as one-third have evidence of chronic disease, such as failure to thrive. Acholic stools are uncommon
with this disorder but may be present if the cholestasis is
severe. The liver (and occasionally the spleen) is firm and
enlarged. Biochemical evaluation reveals bilirubin and
aminotransferase levels, which are mildly to moderately elevated (2 to 10 times the upper limit of normal). Alkaline
phosphatase and γ-glutamyl transpeptidase levels are variably increased (see below). Serum bile acid levels are
markedly elevated. A bleeding diathesis, resulting from vitamin K deficiency and/or decreased synthesis of clotting factors, may be present in those with a more fulminant course.
Other signs or associated abnormalities such as microcephaly, chorioretinitis, or vascular or skeletal anomalies are
unusual and should suggest alternative diagnoses. However,
if these signs are absent, the child appears well, and there is
a clear history of perinatal distress, "transient" neonatal
cholestasis is likely, and the child should be biopsied at the
earliest worrisome sign (failure to thrive, acholic stools).

PATHOLOGY

Although several histologic features such as giant cell
transformation and extramedullary hematopoiesis are
nonspecific and represent a stereotypic response of the
neonatal liver to injury, the biopsy can be helpful in
excluding other causes of neonatal hepatitis. In biopsy tissue obtained early (ie, within the first 2 months of life),
there is disarray of the lobular architecture with hepatocellular swelling (ballooning), focal hepatic necrosis, and
multinucleated giant cells (more than four nuclei per
cell), representing fusion of adjacent hepatocytes (Figure
49-1). Portal triads may be expanded with inflammatory
infiltrate of lymphocytes, neutrophils, and occasional
eosinophils. There is extramedullary hematopoiesis, as
well as varying degrees of portal fibrosis. Although hepa-
tocellular/canalicular bile stasis in the lobule may be
prominent, bile duct proliferation and bile duct plugging
in portal triads are usually absent. Interlobular bile
ducts/ductules are few in number in certain cases, suggesting paucity. The severity of hepatocellular injury usually correlates with the degree of cholestasis.[60,62]

MANAGEMENT

Neonatal hepatitis represents a heterogeneous disorder with
no specifically delineated causative or perpetuating factors
by definition. Management, therefore, is usually directed at
nutritional support, vitamin supplementation, and general
medical management of the clinical complications of
cholestasis, such as pruritus. General medical management
of chronic cholestasis is discussed in detail below.

PROGNOSIS

The overall prognosis in idiopathic neonatal hepatitis is
difficult to estimate owing to the variability of the clinical
course and the generally ill-defined pathogenesis. The factors that allow perpetuation of the cholestatic process and
hepatocyte injury are not fully understood. No specific
biochemical or histologic correlates with clinical outcome
have been identified. A composite of several large series
reviewing outcome of patients with idiopathic neonatal
hepatitis is presented in Table 49-5.[63–67] From these data, it
is clear that sporadic cases (classic giant cell hepatitis)
have a more favorable outcome than familial cases. The
poor prognosis in a number of familial cases presumably
relates to the presence of underlying inborn errors, specifically defects in bile acid metabolism or transport, as have
been described in familial cases of clinically defined neonatal hepatitis (eg, progressive familial intrahepatic cholestasis).[6,54,55] As the underlying causes and pathogenesis of
neonatal hepatitis are further defined, more precise prog-
noses can be established. It is therefore paramount to follow these patients well beyond the normalization of their
biochemical markers because neonatal cholestasis may be
the harbinger of a metabolic or immune defect manifesting
itself later in life. Repeating a liver biopsy for histology,
electron microscopy, and metabolic studies (respiratory
chain enzymes) is crucial for any child who does not follow a "normal" course, for example, by having a prolonged
cholestasis (> 3.5 months), by developing other symptoms
such as fasting hypoglycemia, or by presenting with a
recurrence of cholestasis.

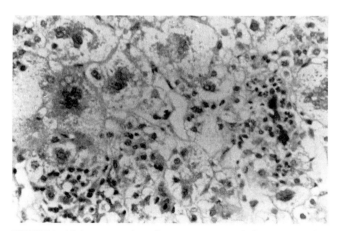

FIGURE 49-1 Liver histology in neonatal hepatitis. This
biopsy specimen demonstrates disruption of hepatic lobular
architecture with multinucleated giant cells. There are also
inflammatory cells within the portal area (hematoxylin and
eosin; ×400 original magnification).

TABLE 49-5   STAGED EVALUATION OF NEONATAL
              CHOLESTASIS

Differentiate cholestasis from physiologic breast milk jaundice and
  determine severity of disease
  Clinical evaluation (history, physical examination, stool color)
  Fractionated serum bilirubin (+ serum bile acids)
  Tests of hepatocellular and biliary disease (ALT, AST, alkaline
    phosphatase, GGT)
  Tests of hepatic function (serum albumin, prothrombin time, blood
    glucose, ammonia)
Exclude treatable and other specific disorders
  Bacterial cultures (blood, urine)
  VDRL test and viral serology as indicated (think HSV)
  α_1-Antitrypsin phenotype
  T_4 and TSH (rule out hypothyroidism)
  Metabolic screen: urine-reducing substances (drugs may cause false
    positives), urine bile acids, serum amino acids, ferritin,
    urine organic acids
  Sweat chloride/mutation analysis
Differentiate extrahepatic biliary obstruction from intrahepatic disorders
  Ultrasonography
  Hepatobiliary scintigraphy (not always essential)
  Liver biopsy

ALT = alanine transaminase; AST = aspartate transaminase; GGT = γ-glutamyl
transpeptidase; HSV = herpes simplex virus; T_4 = thyroxine; TSH = thyroid stimulating hormone; VDRL = Venereal Disease Research Laboratory.

EVALUATION OF THE INFANT WITH CHOLESTASIS

Conjugated hyperbilirubinemia in the newborn period always requires further evaluation, which must be prompt and decisive. Fractionation of the bilirubin, which allows identification of patients with cholestatic (as opposed to physiologic or breast milk) jaundice, should be obtained in any infant with prolonged (ie, more than 14 days) hyperbilirubinemia. Cholestasis traditionally is defined as the presence of a conjugated (or direct-acting) fraction of more than 2 mg/dL (35 μmol/L) or more than 20% of the total bilirubin[11]; however, we prefer to seriously regard any elevation of conjugated bilirubin. Cost-effectiveness should be considered, and a staged approach should be taken in the evaluation of neonatal cholestasis (see Table 49-5). First, treatable disorders such as sepsis, galactosemia, endocrinopathies, and inborn errors of bile acid synthesis must be identified to initiate appropriate therapy that may prevent further damage to the liver and/or reverse the existing injury. Next, biliary obstruction must be differentiated promptly from intrahepatic cholestatic disorders because early surgical intervention is associated with a better prognosis. Finally, the clinical complications of cholestasis, including coagulopathy owing to hypoprothrombinemia or vitamin K deficiency and the nutritional consequences of fat malabsorption, must be addressed because therapy may improve the ultimate outcome and the general quality of life.

HISTORY AND PHYSICAL EXAMINATION

During the evaluation of the infant with cholestasis, the family history, prenatal and postnatal clinical course, and physical examination on presentation may provide impor-

tant clues. Irritability, poor feeding, and vomiting may indicate a generalized infection or a metabolic disorder such as galactosemia or tyrosinemia or suggest encephalopathy, which is particularly difficult to identify in this age group. Vertebral arch anomalies, posterior embryotoxon, and the murmur of peripheral pulmonic stenosis suggest the diagnosis of Alagille syndrome.[68] Hepatomegaly is the norm. Splenomegaly should lead to the consideration of a systemic disease, infectious or other. Dysmorphic signs suggest chromosomal abnormalities.

It is important to consider that many cholestatic infants appear well at the onset of their disease: normal weight gain and development do not preclude a condition as severe as biliary atresia. In fact, the hallmark of these children is that, initially, many appear to be prospering in spite of their cholestasis.

In differentiating biliary obstruction from intrahepatic cholestasis, the presence of persistently acholic stools is suggestive but not diagnostic of biliary atresia because they may also be associated with severe intrahepatic cholestatic disease. Conversely, the presence of pigmented stools suggests patency of the biliary system and generally excludes the diagnosis of biliary atresia. Alagille identified four clinical features that, although nonspecific, supported the correct diagnosis of intrahepatic or extrahepatic cholestasis in 82% of the cases.[69] These clinical variables included stool color within 10 days of admission, birth weight, age at onset of acholic stools, and the features of hepatic involvement, specifically the presence of hepatomegaly and consistency of the liver on palpation. In this study, addition of liver histology to the evaluation increased the diagnostic accuracy by only 3%. In other studies, despite the use of this scoring system, 10% could not be differentiated,[70–72] also suggesting that further evaluation is sometimes necessary.

Recently, the North American Society for Pediatric Gastroenterology, Hepatology and Nutrition (NASPGHAN) published the Neonatal Cholestasis Clinical Practice Guidelines; these are available on-line(<www.naspgn/sub/positionpapers.asp>). These guidelines represent the current practice in most tertiary centers in North America and are thought to be the most efficient and cost-effective way to approach the complex problem of neonatal cholestasis.

LABORATORY EVALUATION

There is no pathognomonic or prognostic biochemical feature of neonatal cholestasis. There is no single test consistently reliable in differentiating neonatal hepatitis from biliary atresia. It is not possible to predict either clinically or based on the result of a neonatal screen which infant will develop cholestasis. Nevertheless, several tests may help identify specific causes of cholestasis and assess and monitor the degree of hepatobiliary dysfunction.[11,70] The laboratory data (see Table 49-5) must be analyzed in the context of the clinical setting. For example, urine-reducing substances may be falsely negative if the infant is not receiving a galactose-containing formula or is vomiting. In these situations, the diagnosis of galactosemia may be made by measuring the red blood cell galactose-1-phosphate uridyl transferase activity, provided that the infant has received no recent blood transfusions. Elevated serum methionine and tyrosine levels, detected during a metabolic screen, may reflect severe liver disease but not necessarily be diagnostic of an underlying metabolic defect. The diagnosis of tyrosinemia should be confirmed by identification of specific metabolites (succinylacetone, succinylacetoacetate). A phenotype is preferred in the evaluation for α_1-antitrypsin deficiency because neonates may have low levels of α_1-antitrypsin despite normal phenotypes, and heterozygotes may have elevated levels in the presence of inflammation. The traditionally requested TORCH (toxoplasmosis, other agents, rubella, cytomegalovirus, herpes simplex) titers have a low diagnostic yield and should be replaced by a request for specific viral titers or cultures only if there are suspicious features. For example, cytomegalovirus serologies should only be obtained based on maternal history and the clinical setting. It is sometimes difficult to obtain an adequate amount of sweat for a sweat chloride test in a neonate, but this test or more specific testing should be performed if the diagnosis of cystic fibrosis remains in question.

γ-Glutamyl transpeptidase, an enzyme located in the epithelial lining of the biliary tree and canaliculi, is elevated in most cholestatic disorders,[73] including biliary atresia, Alagille syndrome, α_1-antitrypsin deficiency, and idiopathic neonatal hepatitis. Normal levels, however, are seen in progressive familial intrahepatic cholestasis and disorders of bile acid synthesis,[74–76] where there is an abnormality of bile acid export into the canaliculus—hence, no bile acid–mediated injury of the canalicular membrane.[77]

As recommended in the NASPGHAN consensus guidelines, part of the stepwise workup always involves assessment of synthetic function by obtaining coagulation studies and metabolic function by measuring glucose and ammonia in serum. Although not used routinely in all centers, quantification of serum bile acids can help orient the diagnosis in neonatal cholestasis syndromes. Elevated levels are found in most forms of cholestasis; low serum bile acid concentration in the face of persistently elevated conjugated bilirubin levels should suggest an inborn error of bile acid synthesis. Other third-line investigations are warranted according to the clinical context: transferrin immunoelectrophoresis should be considered when the constellation of signs is consistent with a congenital defect in glycosylation. Serum α-fetoprotein should be measured especially when considering tyrosinemia because of the associated risk of malignancy. This test can be diagnostic and serve as a baseline for subsequent follow-up. In the presence of splenomegaly, Niemann-Pick disease should always be considered and appropriately addressed by performing a bone marrow aspirate. Similarly, neurologic findings should raise the question of mitochondriopathies and fatty acid oxidation defects. Finally, dysmorphic features, as always in pediatrics, should warrant evalutation. Unfortunately, at the present time, there is no reliable antenatal screening method for most of the conditions leading to neonatal cholestasis.

RADIOLOGIC EVALUATION

ULTRASONOGRAPHY

Real-time ultrasonography is an important adjunct in the diagnosis of neonatal cholestasis.[78] The study is most helpful in ascertaining the presence of a choledochal cyst, or, rarely, a tumor, which can have a clinical presentation similar to that of biliary atresia. The absence of a gallbladder on a fasting study is suggestive but not diagnostic of biliary atresia. Similarly, the presence of a gallbladder does not exclude this diagnosis. Dilated ducts are usually not present in biliary atresia, reflecting the fibro-obliterative or sclerotic nature of the coincident intrahepatic duct lesion.

In recent years, emphasis has been on trying to find a reliable, noninvasive method of diagnosing biliary atresia. The triangular cord sign, when performed by an experienced sonographer, is a potentially helpful diagnostic tool. In one small study, the characteristic cone-shaped finding cranial to the portal vein bifurcation demonstrated a positive predictive value of 100% when visualized together with an abnormal gallbladder and 88% when the gallbladder was normal.[79] The main disadvantage is that this ultrasonographic finding is operator dependent.

Recently, pediatric surgeons have also looked at the value of antenatal ultrasonography in the diagnosis and management of hepatobiliary lesions. Indeed, routine ultrasonography at 20 weeks gestation has led obstetricians and radiologists on occasion to find cystic lesions at the hepatic hilum.[80] Little is known about the natural history of these findings. As more experience is gained in imaging the hepatobiliary system antenatally, this tool may become part of the diagnostic algorithm of neonatal cholestasis.

Finally, a plain chest radiograph should be performed in investigating neonatal cholestasis to look for situs abnormalities, as well as butterfly vertebrae, or rickets, which may help orient the diagnosis.

RADIONUCLIDE IMAGING

Hepatobiliary scintigraphy, using technetium-labeled iminodiacetic acid analogs, may be used to differentiate biliary atresia from nonobstructive causes of cholestasis. The hepatic uptake and secretion into bile of these derivatives of iminodiacetic acid occur by a carrier-mediated organic anion pathway and depend on the structure of the specific analog, the integrity of hepatocellular function, and biliary tract patency.[81,82] In patients with biliary atresia, particularly early in the disorder, parenchymal function is not compromised; therefore, uptake of the radioisotope is unimpaired, although subsequent excretion into the intestine is absent (Figure 49-2A). Conversely, uptake is usually delayed in infants with neonatal hepatitis owing to hepatocellular dysfunction, but eventually excretion into the bile and intestine occurs (Figure 49-2B). Pretreatment with oral phenobarbital (5 mg/kg/d for 5 days) enhances biliary excretion of the isotope and can increase sensitivity to 94%.[81,82] There are limitations to this study, however; therefore, the diagnosis should not be made solely on the results of this test. Nonexcretion may be related to severe

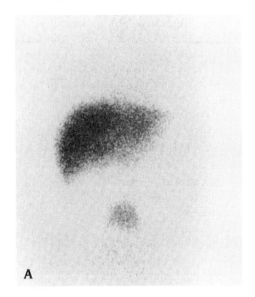
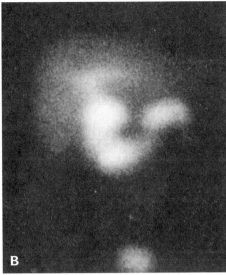

FIGURE 49-2 *A*, Radioisotope scan in biliary atresia. On a delayed scan, there is good uptake of the isotope by the liver, but there is no evidence of intestinal excretion. *B*, Radioisotope scan in neonatal hepatitis. Uptake of the isotope by the liver is delayed and decreased; however, excretion into the intestine is noted.

intrahepatic cholestasis rather than extrahepatic obstruction. In a retrospective study, 12 of 21 infants with intrahepatic causes of cholestasis had no excretion in their first study, despite the use of phenobarbital.[83] In our experience, one patient with isotopic demonstration of a "patent" biliary system was subsequently diagnosed with biliary atresia. In addition, the 5 days required for phenobarbital administration to optimize diagnostic yield may ultimately affect outcome by delaying surgical intervention. Whereas the passage of the tracer into the gastrointestinal tract is 100% sensitive in excluding biliary atresia, a nonexcreting result is only 60% specific for biliary atresia. This poor specificity, together with the time required to prepare for the study, is progressively excluding hepatobiliary scanning from the diagnostic algorithm.[77]

Although there has been much hope that magnetic resonance imaging would provide a means of exploring the biliary tract, there is no evidence at present to suggest that this method is of benefit in the diagnostic armamentarium when studying small infants.[84] Other radiographic studies, such as percutaneous transhepatic cholangiography or endoscopic retrograde cholangiopancreatography, are not only difficult to perform, but experience has been limited in these infants.[85–87]

LIVER BIOPSY

In our experience, the liver biopsy remains the most reliable and definitive procedure in the evaluation of the neonate with persistent conjugated hyperbilirubinemia. Tissue may be obtained, in most cases, using a percutaneous technique with local anesthesia.[11,70,88,89] Careful interpretation by an experienced pathologist yields the correct diagnosis in 90 to 95% of cases. Prompt diagnosis may expedite surgery for biliary atresia and preclude unnecessary surgical exploration. The typical findings in neonatal hepatitis are discussed above. Like the biochemical evaluation, the biopsy needs to be interpreted in the clinical context because the histology of neonatal hepatitis is nonspecific: giant cell transformation and hepatocyte ballooning with lobular disarray represent a nonspecific

response of the newborn liver to an insult. Many of the characteristic histologic findings stem from observational studies in term infants in their first few months of life. Less is known about the histology of the early course of some neonatal cholestasis syndromes or of preterm infants with cholestasis. These conditions are evolving processes, and more information may be gained by performing a repeat biopsy to look for more characteristic findings and to appreciate the evolution.

CONCLUSIONS REGARDING EVALUATION

In evaluating a neonate with cholestasis, both surgical and medical emergencies have to be excluded and attended to in a timely fashion. If galactosemia is suspected, appropriate dietary measures should be taken immediately. If sepsis is the likely cause of the cholestasis, this must be managed urgently. If biliary atresia is suggested, an exploratory laparotomy, often with an intraoperative cholangiogram, is performed to verify the nature and site of the obstruction prior to hepatoportoenterostomy. Finally, if no specific etiology is determined but extrahepatic obstruction is unlikely, the infant is followed and re-evaluated frequently. Empiric therapy may also be instituted to optimize growth and development and ameliorate the consequences of chronic cholestasis (discussed below).

The need to correctly differentiate biliary atresia from intrahepatic disorders is illustrated by a report from Markowitz and colleagues in which four patients who underwent hepatoportoenterostomies on the basis of hepatobiliary scans and intraoperative cholangiograms were subsequently found to have Alagille syndrome on histologic and clinical criteria.[90] None had adequate drainage postoperatively, two progressed to cirrhosis, and one died from hepatic failure, indicating that the intervening surgery had adversely altered the course of a usually benign disorder. If careful consideration is given to the history, physical examination, and these selected diagnostic tests (see Table 49-5), institution of appropriate surgery may be expedited, unnecessary surgery avoided, and, in many cases, the precise etiology determined.

MEDICAL MANAGEMENT OF CHRONIC CHOLESTASIS

In infants with intrahepatic cholestasis or those with biliary atresia in whom surgical attempts at establishing adequate biliary drainage are unsuccessful, the presence of the clinical consequences of persistent cholestasis directs medical therapy. These complications are related, either directly or indirectly, to diminished bile flow and reflect (1) retention of substances dependent on bile secretion, such as bile acids, bilirubin, and cholesterol; (2) decreased bile acid delivery to the intestine with resultant fat and fat-soluble vitamin malabsorption; and (3) progressive hepatocellular damage leading to portal hypertension and eventual liver failure (Figure 49-3). Currently, no specific therapy either reverses existing cholestasis or prevents ongoing damage; therefore, therapy is empiric and aimed at improving nutritional status, maximizing growth potential, and minimizing discomfort.[91] The success of this therapeutic intervention is limited by the residual capacity of the liver and by the rate of progression of the underlying disorder. The success is enhanced by introducing these measures in a timely fashion, namely as soon as abnormal weight gain is anticipated.

PRURITUS

Significant clinical morbidity may result from pruritus, and its management is a difficult and sometimes frustrating clinical problem. In some patients, the impairment in quality of life is so severe that liver transplant is indicated. The cause of cholestatic pruritus is not clear.[92,93] It has been reported that skin and serum levels of bile acids did not differentiate between patients with or without pruritus,[93] arguing against bile acids as direct pruritogens. Endogenous opioids have been implicated as mediators of pruritus, specifically cholestasis-induced pruritus.[94] Similarly, the serotonin neurotransmitter system has also been identified as one potential factor.[95] With these recent findings, new approaches to the management of cholestasis-induced pruritus are emerging.

Therapy directed at decreasing the concentrations of bile acids may be efficacious in some patients because of the nonspecific action of these agents. The anion exchange resion cholestyramine has been used historically to interrupt enterohepatic circulation. Because its use entails a complicated regimen, it is seldom used in pediatrics.

Phenobarbital, in therapeutic doses of 5 to 10 mg/kg/d, stimulates bile acid–independent flow and decreases the bile acid pool size.[96] The drug has not been consistently efficacious in relieving pruritus in intrahepatic cholestasis. The sedative side effects of phenobarbital may be a limiting factor in its usefulness. As a rule, its use in cholestasis is becoming more infrequent. The use of rifampin (10 mg/kg/d), which inhibits hepatic uptake of bile acids, has also been tried with variable success in relieving pruritus.[97,98] Like phenobarbital, it is a microsomal enzyme inducer, with the advantage of not having a sedative effect. Related side effects are minimal, but worsening biochemical liver markers can be suggestive of rifampin-induced hepatitis.[99]

Ursodeoxycholic acid (UDCA), which alters bile acid composition, has been shown to be beneficial in the relief of pruritus in studies of adults with primary biliary cirrhosis.[100] Preliminary studies, using 15 to 30 mg/kg/d, suggest that it may be of benefit in ameliorating pruritus in childhood cholestasis as well.[101,102] In our center, UDCA is routinely prescribed to all children with cholestasis for its potential cytoprotective effect on hepatocytes, as well as its

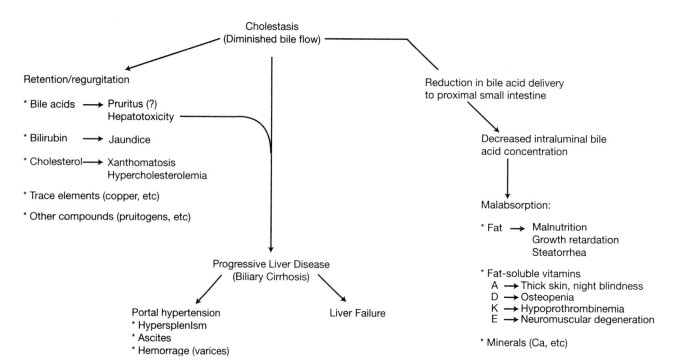

FIGURE 49-3 Clinical sequelae of chronic cholestasis. Numerous consequences of cholestasis become clinically manifest and result from retention of substances excreted in bile, reduction of intestinal bile acids, and progressive damage to the liver. See text for relationship between bile acids and pruritus.

role in relieving pruritus. The current trend is toward the higher dose of 30 mg/kg/d, although there is no documented evidence that the effect is dose dependent.

As mentioned above, interest in the role of the opiate receptor system in pruritus of cholestasis was prompted by the results of studies in which opioid antagonists relieved pruritus.[98,102] The presumed mechanism of action is that they prevent the binding of endogenous opioid agonists, which have been shown to be elevated in cholestasis. The three known opioid antagonists (naloxone, nalmefene, and naltrexone) have been studied and have demonstrated an alleviating effect, although none have completely abolished pruritus. There are problems associated with the use of opioid antagonists: they precipitate a withdrawal-like effect, and a "breakthrough" phenomenon has been described, which consists in an exacerbation of the pruritic symptoms after an initial improvement. Thus, determining the appropriate dose and management can be difficult, and consultation with anesthesia may be appropriate.[99] As mentioned earlier, there have been some studies implicating serotonin in the pathophysiology of pruritus. As such, the use of ondansetron in the relief of pruritus has been studied with some promising results, but more studies are required to confirm these findings.[99]

For those children with intrahepatic cholestasis and intractable pruritus unresponsive to therapy, partial external biliary diversion has been performed.[103] Patients with progressive intrahepatic cholestasis had a good response, with relief from itching and concomitant improvement in their biochemical tests of liver function and histology. In a retrospective review performed at our center, patients and parents reported a marked improvement in quality of life, as defined by school attendance and interactions with peers.[104] Finally, there have been anecdotal reports on the efficacy of a variety of other therapies, including phototherapy and plasmapheresis.

MALABSORPTION AND MALNUTRITION

Lipids. One of the major and more immediate complications of chronic cholestasis is fat malabsorption related to decreased intraluminal bile acids, which leads to malnutrition and fat-soluble vitamin deficiency. Decreased excretion of bile acids leads to a low intraluminal micellar concentration; therefore, long-chain triglyceride lipolysis and absorption are ineffective. Medium-chain triglycerides (MCTs) are more water soluble than their long-chain counterparts and are therefore readily absorbed by the gastric and intestinal mucosa in the face of low intraluminal concentrations of bile acids, making them a more adapted source of fat calories; MCTs can best be administered as MCT-containing formulas. MCT oil alone is insufficient because it does not contain essential fatty acids. In those children who are unable to take in sufficient calories orally, nocturnal enteral feeding has been shown to improve nutritional indices in many patients with chronic liver disease.[105]

Liposoluble Vitamins. Intestinal absorption of fat-soluble vitamins (A, D, E, and K) that require solubiliza-

tion by bile acids into mixed micelles is also compromised, and supplementation of at least two to four times the recommended daily allowance is often necessary (Table 49-6). Serum vitamin levels and laboratory tests such as serum calcium and phosphate levels and prothrombin time are useful indices of adequate supplementation. Chronic vitamin E (α-tocopherol) deficiency has been associated with a progressive neuromuscular syndrome characterized by areflexia, cerebellar ataxia, posterior column dysfunction, and peripheral neuropathy.[106,107] The most reliable index of vitamin E status is the ratio of serum vitamin E (mg/dL) to total serum lipids (g/dL) because elevated lipids, as seen in chronic cholestasis, allow vitamin E to partition into the nonpolar phase (plasma lipoprotein fraction), artificially raising the serum vitamin E concentration. In infants and children less than 12 years of age, a ratio of less than 0.6 mg/g indicates vitamin E deficiency.[108] In those children who do not respond to supplementation of vitamin E by traditional methods, oral administration of a water-soluble form of vitamin E, d-α-tocopherol polyethylene glycol 1000 succinate (TPGS), has been found to correct biochemical vitamin E deficiency in doses of 15 to 25 IU/kg/d.[109] In truly refractory cases, an admixture of all fat-soluble vitamins with TPGS may be more beneficial than administration of the supplement alone.[110] Although there are no data to support its use in neonatal cholestasis, vitamin E is part of the antioxidant armamentarium prescribed in many forms of acute and chronic liver disease.[111] Careful consideration should be given to fat-soluble vitamin replacement in the nutritional management of these patients because intracranial bleeding from vitamin K deficiency is still a frequent cause of death in infants and toddlers with cholestasis.

Carbohydrates. In animal models of biliary atresia, as much as a 20 to 30% decrease in brush border enzyme activity has been observed. Thus, although there is no published evidence to this effect in human subjects, one should consider changing the carbohydrate composition of the formula if the infant is demonstrating signs consistent with lactose intolerance. This is particularly important because the infant with cholestasis requires as much as 130% of the caloric intake of age-matched controls (as much as 150 kcal/kg/d), 60% of which should be in carbohydrate form.

TABLE 49-6   RECOMMENDED ORAL VITAMIN SUPPLEMENTATION

VITAMIN	PREPARATION, DOSE
Fat soluble	
Vitamin A	Aquasol A: 3,000–25,000 IU/d
Vitamin D	Cholecalciferol: 500–5,000 IU/d or 25-Hydroxycholecalciferol: 3–5 µg/kg/d
Vitamin K	Phytonadione (K1): 2.5–5 mg every other day
Vitamin E	Aquasol E: 50–400 IU/d or TPGS 15–25 IU/kg/d
Water soluble	Twice the recommended daily allowance

TPGS = d-α-tocopherol polyethylene glycol 1000 succinate.

Protein. Infants with cholestasis require a normal proportion (20–30%) of their diet in protein form. However, unless malnutrition is so severe, there is no evidence to suggest that protein hydrolysates are necessary. One study in a rat model suggested that adding branched-chain amino acids to the formula may impact growth and nitrogen retention favorably.[112] There is no such evidence in human subjects.

Other Vitamins and Nutrients.

1. Calcium. In spite of aggressive liposoluble enteral or parenteral vitamin replacement, most children with cholestasis suffer from severe osteopenia, often leading to pathologic fractures.[113,114] Thus, both additional calcium and magnesium[115] supplementation is advisable, ensuring that the child or infant receives at least 1,000 to 1,300 mg/d of calcium and 8 to 16 mg/kg/d of elemental magnesium. The time at which the supplement is taken is critical because it has been suggested that UDCA may affect calcium absorption negatively. Finally, monitoring a patient's calcium-phosphorus status using urinary indices and parathyroid hormone may be indicated because serum levels may not always be accurate because of acid-base abnormalities or hypoalbuminemia.

2. Zinc. Because of increased intestinal losses and fat malabsorption, zinc deficiency is more prevalent in cholestasis than is commonly thought. Because zinc is a common cofactor in numerous enzymatic reactions, including in the liver, zinc deficiency may further exacerbate the underlying liver disease.

3. Iron. Iron deficiency is common in these children. Early on, this may be due to insufficient dietary intake. As the course of the disease progresses, however, this is more often the sign of occult, or overt, gastrointestinal bleeding.

PORTAL HYPERTENSION

In most patients with biliary atresia, and in certain patients with intrahepatic cholestasis, progressive fibrosis and cirrhosis ultimately lead to the development of portal hypertension, the most clinically significant sequelae being ascites and variceal hemorrhage. The medical management of ascites should be dictated by patient comfort and by the relative risk of peritoneal bacterial infection. The judicious use of sodium restriction and diuretics may be helpful in controlling the accumulation of ascites. Initial steps include restricting dietary sodium intake to 1 to 2 mEq/kg/d and introducing a diuretic such as spironolactone, which inhibits the effects of aldosterone. We usually start with 3 to 5 mg/kg/d divided into 3 to 4 doses and increase the dose as needed up to 10 to 12 mg/kg/d to maintain an increased urinary sodium-to-potassium ratio. Refractory ascites with respiratory compromise may be managed by therapeutic paracentesis with concomitant administration of an intravenous colloid such as albumin.[11] Albumin has been shown in adult studies to play a role in the preservation of renal function in large-volume paracentesis and to have a protective effect against the risk of spontaneous bacterial peritonitis.[116] Used together with furosemide, it participates in the elimination of free water and sodium while avoiding the prompt recurrence of ascites.[116]

Esophageal and gastric varices are a potentially life-threatening complication of portal hypertension. Acute variceal hemorrhage is managed in an intensive care unit with intravenous fluids and blood products, gastric lavage, and intravenous vasopressin infusion (0.3 U/1.73 m²/min) as indicated. Balloon tamponade, used for severe or prolonged hemorrhage, may be associated with significant complications such as esophageal rupture, airway obstruction, and pulmonary aspiration. Endoscopic sclerotherapy is being used more extensively in infants and children for the acute and ongoing management of esophageal varices and may be superior to surgical alternatives,[117] particularly if eventual liver transplant is anticipated. Although not available for the infant population, banding is also used routinely in older children. However, to date, there is no literature to suggest that prophylactic banding or sclerotherapy is preferable to managing varices on an ad hoc basis following a bleed. This topic is covered in greater depth in Chapter 59, "Treatment of End-Stage Liver Disease." Gastric varices are not amenable to this therapy. There has also been interest in long-term administration of β-blocking agents such as propranolol to reduce portal pressure and prevent recurrent variceal bleeding in adults,[102,103] but the results have been variable, and there is limited experience in children. Furthermore, β-blockade may impede appropriate cardiovascular compensation in the event of an acute bleed and is therefore not used routinely in infants. In refractory hemorrhage, pediatric patients may be stabilized using intravenous octreotide, starting at 1 μg/kg/(min) and increasing as needed. Patients should be closely monitored for hyperglycemic side effects. The use of octreotide can be a convenient tool while the patient awaits emergent liver transplant.

Orthotopic liver transplant has become a viable option for infants and children who progress to end-stage liver disease.[118,119] The ability to determine the optimum time in the clinical course to pursue transplant requires careful monitoring and sequential evaluation of hepatic function. Although no one specific functional measure has been shown to reliably assess hepatocellular reserve, prognostic scores have been developed for predicting outcome without transplant. These scores may be compared with operative survival statistics for a particular patient group and thus aid in decision-making. In infants and children with end-stage liver disease, the deciding factor in timing organ transplant is usually organ availability. Therefore, it is important to carry out evaluation early in the course to develop supportive strategies and to stratify based on clinical criteria.

The major limiting factor for successful transplant in infants has been the supply of appropriately sized organs. This situation has been somewhat alleviated by introduction of the techniques of segmental or volume reduction liver transplant, living donor transplant, and "split" organ donation.[120] More effective means for supporting and monitoring infants with chronic liver disease are needed. Ultimately, a better understanding of the pathophysiology of specific underlying disease processes may lead to more efficacious treatment of the sequelae of persistent infantile cholestasis and to therapeutic interventions that will prevent or reverse the development of chronic liver disease.

ACKNOWLEDGMENTS

Special thanks go to Renée Wieman, RD, for her input regarding the nutritional management of cholestasis.

REFERENCES

1. Desmet VJ. Congenital diseases of intrahepatic bile ducts: variations on the theme "ductal plate malformation." Hepatology 1992;16:1069–83.
2. Trauner M, Meier PJ, Boyer JL, Molecular pathogenesis of cholestasis. N Engl J Med 1998;339:1217–27.
3. Shaffer EA, Zahavi I, Gall DG. Postnatal development of hepatic bile formation in the rabbit. Dig Dis Sci 1985;30:558–62.
4. Balistreri WF. Neonatal cholestasis: medical progress. J Pediatr 1985;106:171.
5. Suchy FJ. Hepatocellular transport of bile acids. Semin Liver Dis 1993;13:235–47.
6. Balistreri WF. Inborn errors of bile acid biosynthesis and transport: novel forms of metabolic liver disease. Gastroenterol Clin North Am 1999;28:145–72.
7. Itoh S, Onishi S, Isobe K, et al. Foetal maternal relationship of bile acid pattern estimated by high pressure liquid chromatography. Biochem J 1982;204:141–5.
8. Dumaswala R, Ananthanarayanan M, Suchy FJ. Characterization of a specific transport mechanism for bile acids on the brush border membrane of human placenta. Hepatology 1988;8:1260.
9. Marin JJ, Serrano MA, el-Mir MY, et al. Bile acid transport by basal membrane vesicles of human term placental trophoblast. Gastroenterology 1990;99:1431–5.
10. Suchy FJ, Balistreri WF, Heubi JE, et al. Physiologic cholestasis: elevation of primary bile acid concentrations in normal infants. Gastroenterology 1981;80:1037–41.
11. Balistreri WF. Liver disease in infancy and childhood. In: Schiff ER, Sorrell MF, Maddrey WC, editors. Schiffs diseases of the liver. 8th ed. Philadelphia: Lippincott-Raven; 1999. p. 1357–512.
12. Balistreri WF, Heubi JE, Suchy FJ. Immaturity of the enterohepatic circulation in early life: factors predisposing to "physiologic" malabsorption and cholestasis. J Pediatr Gastroenterol Nutr 1983;2:346–54.
13. Klaassen CD. Hepatic excretory function in the newborn rat. J Pharmacol Exp Ther 1975;184:721–8.
14. Belknap WM, Balistreri WF, Suchy FJ, Miller PC. Physiologic cholestasis. II. Serum bile acid levels reflect the development of the enterohepatic circulation in rats. Hepatology 1981;1:613–6.
15. Suchy FJ, Balistreri WF. Uptake of taurocholate by hepatocytes isolated from developing rats. Pediatr Res 1982;16:282–5.
16. Suchy FJ, Bucuvalas JC, Goodrich AL, et al. Taurocholate transport and Na + K + -ATPase activity in fetal and neonatal rat liver plasma membrane vesicles. Am J Physiol 1986;251:G655–73.
17. Suchy FJ, Courchene SM, Blitzer BL. Taurocholate transport by basolateral membrane vesicles isolated from developing rat liver. Am J Physiol 1985;248:G648–54.
18. von Dippe P, Levy D. Expression of the bile acid transport pro-

19. Jones AL, Hradek GT, Renston RH, et al. Autoradiographic evidence for hepatic lobular concentration gradient of bile acid derivative. Am J Physiol 1980;238:G233–7.
20. Groothius GM, Hardonk MJ, Keulemans KP, et al. Autoradiographic and kinetic demonstration of acinar heterogeneity of taurocholate transport. Am J Physiol 1982;243:G455–62.
21. Suchy FJ, Balistreri WF, Breslin JS, et al. Absence of an acinar gradient for bile acid uptake in developing rat liver. Pediatr Res 1987;21:417–21.
22. Belknap WM, Zimmer-Nechemias L, Suchy FJ, Balistreri WF. Bile acid efflux from suckling hepatocytes. Pediatr Res 1988;23:364–7.
23. de Belle RC, Vaupshas V, Vitullo BB, et al. Intestinal absorption of bile salts: immature development in the neonate. J Pediatr 1979;94:472–6.
24. Moyer MS, Heubi JE, Goodrich AL, et al. Ontogeny of bile acid transport in brush border membrane vesicles from rat ileum. Gastroenterology 1986;90:1188–96.
25. Stahl GE, Mascarenhas MR, Fayer JC, et al. Passive jejunal bile salt absorption alters the enterohepatic circulation in immature rats. Gastroenterology 1993;104:163–73.
26. Al-Ansari N, Xu G, Kollman-Bauerly K, et al. Analysis of the effect of intestinal resection on rat ileal bile acid transporter expression and on bile acid and cholesterol homeostasis. Pediatr Res 2002;52:286–91.
27. Danielsson H, Rutter WJ. The metabolism of bile acids in the developing rat liver. Biochemistry 1968;7:346–51.
28. Subbiah TR, Hassan AS. Development of bile acid biogenesis and its significance in cholesterol homeostasis. Adv Lipid Res 1982;19:137–61.
29. Colombo C, Zuliani G, Ronchi M, et al. Biliary bile acid composition of the human fetus in early gestation. Pediatr Res 1987;21:197–200.
30. Setchell KD, Dumaswala R, Colombo C, Ronchi H. Hepatic bile acid metabolism during early development revealed from the analysis of human fetal gall-bladder bile. J Biol Chem 1988;263:16637–44.
31. Wahlen E, Egestad B, Strandvik B, Sjoovall J. Ketonic bile acids in urine of infants during the neonatal period. J Lipid Res 1989;30:1847–57.
32. Deleze G, Paumgartner G, Karlaganis G, et al. Bile acid pattern in human amniotic fluid. Eur J Clin Invest 1978;8:41–5.
33. Back P, Walter K. Developmental pattern of bile acid metabolism as revealed by bile acid analysis of meconium. Gastroenterology 1980;78:671–6.
34. St. Pyrek J, Sterzycki R, Lester R, Adcock E. Constituents of human meconium. II. Identification of steroidal acids with 21 and 22 carbon atoms. Lipids 1982;17:241-9.
35. Strandvik B, Wikstrom SA. Tetrahydroxylated bile acids in healthy human newborns. Eur J Clin Invest 1982;12:301–5.
36. Balistreri WF, Zimmer L, Suchy FJ, Bove KE. Bile salt sulfotransferase: alteration during maturation and noninducibility during substrate ingestion. J Lipid Res 1984;25:228–35.
37. Suchy FJ, Courchene SM, Balistreri WF. Ontogeny of hepatic bile acid conjugation in the rat. Pediatr Res 1985;19:97–101.
38. Little JM, Richey JE, Van Thiel DH, Lester R. Taurocholate pool size and distribution in the fetal rat. J Clin Invest 1979;63:1042–8.
39. Novak DA, Sippel CJ, Ananthanarayanan M, Suchy FJ. Postnatal expression of the canalicular bile acid transport system of rat liver. Am J Physiol 1991;260:G743–51.
40. Ananthanarayanan M, Michaud G, Suchy FJ. Developmental

expression of ATP-dependent bile acid transport in rat liver canalicular membrane vesicles. Hepatology 1992;16:125A.

41. Denson LA, Sturm E, Echevarria W, et al. The orphan nuclear receptor, shp, mediates bile acid-induced inhibition of the rat bile acid transporter, ntcp. Gastroenterology 2001;121: 140–7.

42. Emerick KM, Whitington PF. Molecular basis of neonatal cholestasis. Pediatr Clin North Am 2002;49:221–35.

43. DeWolf-Peeters C, De Vos R, Desmet V, et al. Electron microscopy and morphometry of canalicular differentiation in fetal and newborn rat liver. Exp Mol Pathol 1974;21:339–50.

44. Miyairi M, Wantanabe S, Phillips MJ. Cell motility of fetal hepatocytes in short term culture. Pediatr Res 1985;19:1225–9.

45. Kaplan GS, Bhutani VK, Shaffer TH, et al. Gallbladder mechanisms in newborn piglets. Pediatr Res 1984;18:1181–4.

46. Lehtonen LSE, Svedstrom E, Kero P, Korvenranta H. Gallbladder contractility in preterm infants. Arch Dis Child 1993;68: 43–5.

47. Jacquemin E, Lykavieris P, Chaoui N, et al. Transient neonatal cholestasis: origin and outcome. J Pedriatr 1998;133:563–7.

48. Jorgensen MJ. The ductal plate malformation. Acta Pathol Microbiol Scand 1977;257:7–88.

49. Clotman F, Lannoy VJ, Reber M, et al. The onecut transcription factor HNF6 is required for normal development of the biliary tract. Development 2002;129:1819–28.

50. McCright B, Lozier J, Gridley T. A mouse model of Alagille syndrome: Notch2 as a genetic modifier of Jag1 haploinsufficiency. Development 2002;129:1075–82.

51. Landing BH. Consideration of the pathogenesis of neonatal hepatitis, biliary atresia and choledochal cyst: the concept of infantile obstructive cholangiopathy. Prog Pediatr Surg 1974;6:113–39.

52. Ito T, Horisawa M, Ando H. Intrahepatic bile ducts in biliary atresia: a possible factor determining the prognosis. J Pediatr Surg 1983;18:124.

53. Raweily EA, Gibson AAM, Burt AD. Abnormalities of intrahepatic bile ducts in extrahepatic biliary atresia. Histopathology 1990;17:521–7.

54. Clayton PT, Leonard JV, Lawson AM et al. Familial giant cell hepatitis associated with synthesis of 3β, 7α-dihydroxy- and 3β, 7α, 12α-tri-hydroxy-5-cholenoic acids. J Clin Invest 1987;79:1031–8.

55. Setchell KDR, Suchy FJ, Welsh MB, et al. D⁴-3 Oxosteroid 5β-reductase deficiency described in identical twins with neonatal hepatitis: a new inborn error in bile acid synthesis. J Clin Invest 1988;2:2148–57.

56. Bezerra JA, Tiao G, Ryckman FC, et al. Genetic induction of proinflammatory immunity in children with biliary atresia. Lancet 2002;360:1653–9.

57. Koukoulis G, Miegli-Vergani G, Portmann B. Infantile liver giant cells: immunohistological study of their proliferative state and possible mechanisms of formation. Pediatr Dev Pathol 1999;2:353–9.

58. Danks DM, Campbell PE, Jack I, et al. Studies of the aetiology of neonatal hepatitis and biliary atresia. Arch Dis Child 1977;52:360–7.

59. Henriksen NT, Drablos PA, Aegenaes O. Cholestatic jaundice in infancy: the importance of familial and genetic factors in aetiology and prognosis. Arch Dis Child 1981;56:62–7.

60. Stokes J Jr, Wolman IJ, Blanchar MC, Farquhar JD. Viral hepatitis in the newborn; clinical features, epidemiology and pathology. Am J Dis Child 1951;82:213–6.

61. Craig JM, Landing BH. Form of hepatitis in the neonatal period simulating biliary atresia. Arch Pathol 1952;54:321–33.

62. Montgomery CK, Ruebner BH. Neonatal hepatocellular giant cell transformation: a review. Perspect Pediatr Pathol 1976;3: 85–101.

63. Deutsch J, Smith AL, Danks DM, Campbell PE. Long-term prognosis for babies with neonatal liver disease. Arch Dis Child 1985;60:447–51.

64. Danks DM, Campbell PE, Smith AL, Rogers J. Prognosis of babies with neonatal hepatitis. Arch Dis Child 1977;52: 368–72.

65. Odievre M, Hadchouel M, Landrieu P, et al. Long-term prognosis for infants with intrahepatic cholestasis and patent extrahepatic biliary tract. Arch Dis Child 1981;56:373–6.

66. Lawson EE, Boggs JD. Long-term follow-up of neonatal hepatitis: safety and value of surgical exploration. Pediatrics 1974; 53:650–5.

67. Chang MH, Hsu HC, Lee CY, et al. Neonatal hepatitis: a follow-up study. J Pediatr Gastroenterol Nutr 1987;6:203–7.

68. Alagille D, Odievre M, Gautier M, Dommergues JP. Hepatic ductular hypoplasia associated with characteristic facies, vertebral malformations, retarded physical, mental and sexual development and cardiac murmur. J Pediatr 1975; 86:63–71.

69. Alagille D. Cholestasis in the first three months of life. Prog Liver Dis 1979;6:471–85.

70. Balistreri WF, Bove KE, Ryckman FC. Biliary atresia and other disorders of the extrahepatic bile ducts. In: Suchy FJ, editor. Liver disease in children. 2nd ed. Philadelphia: Lippincott Williams and Wilkins; 2000. p. 253–74.

71. Chiba T, Kasai M. Differentiation of biliary atresia from neonatal hepatitis by routine clinical examination. Tohoku J Exp Med 1988;154:149–56.

72. Hays DM, Woolley MM, Snyder WH Jr, et al. Diagnosis of biliary atresia: relative accuracy of percutaneous liver biopsy, open liver biopsy, and operative cholangiography. J Pediatr 1967;71:598.

73. Maggiore G, Bernard O, Hadchouel M, et al. Diagnostic value of serum gamma-glutamyl transpeptidase activity in liver disease in children. J Pediatr Gastroenterol Nutr 1991;12:21–6.

74. Bezerra JA, Balistreri WF. Intrahepatic cholestasis: order out of chaos [editorial]. Gastroenterology 1999;117:1496–8.

75. Shneider B. Genetic cholestasis syndromes. J Pediatr Gastroenterol Nutr 1999;28:124–31.

76. Spinner NB, Collins FS, Chandrasekharappa SC. Mutations in the human Jagged 1 gene are responsible for Alagille syndrome. Nat Genet 1997;16:235–42.

77. McKiernan PJ. Neonatal cholestasis. Semin Neonatol 2002;7: 153–65.

78. Franken EA, Smith WL, Siddiqui A. Noninvasive evaluations of liver disease in pediatrics. Radiol Clin North Am 1980;18: 239–52.

79. Park WH, Choi SO, Lee HJ. The ultrasonographic 'triangular cord' coupled with gallbladder images in the diagnostic prediction of biliary atresia from infantile intrahepatic cholestasis. J Pediatr Surg 1999;34:1706–10.

80. Redkar R, Davenport M, Howard ER. Antenatal diagnosis of congenital anomalies of the biliary tract. J Pediatr Surg 1998;33:700–4.

81. Miller JH, Sinatra FR, Thomas DW. Biliary excretion disorders in infants: evaluation using 99m Tc-PIPIDA. Am J Radiol 1980;135:47–52.

82. Johnson K, Alton HM, Chapman S. Evaluation of mebrofenin hepatoscintigraphy in neonatal-onset jaundice. Pediatr Radiol 1998;28:937–41.

83. Spivak W, Sarkar S, Winter D, et al. Diagnostic utility of hepa-

tobiliary scintigraphy with 99mTc-DISIDA in neonatal cholestasis. J Pediatr 1987;110:855–61.

84. Avni FE, Segers V, De Maertelaer V, et al. The evaluation by magnetic resonance imaging of hepatic periportal fibrosis in infants with neonatal cholestasis: preliminary report. J Pediatr Surg 2002;37:1128–33.

85. Guibaud L, Lachaud A, Touraine R, et al. MR cholangiography in neonates and infants: feasibility and preliminary applications. AJR Am J Roentgenol 1998;170:27–31.

86. Jaw TS, Kuo YT, Liu GC, et al. MR cholangiography in the evaluation of neonatal cholestasis. Radiology 1999;212:249–56.

87. Wilkinson ML, Mieli-Vergani G, Ball C, et al. Endoscopic retrograde cholangiopancreatography in infantile cholestasis. Arch Dis Child 1991;66:121–3.

88. Hong R, Schubert WK. Menghini needle biopsy of the liver. Am J Dis Child 1960;100:42–6.

89. Zerbini MC, Gallucci SD, Maezono R, et al. Liver biopsy in neonatal cholestasis: a review on statistical grounds. Mod Pathol 1997;10:793–9.

90. Markowitz J, Daum F, Kahn EI, et al. Arteriohepatic dysplasia. I. Pitfalls in diagnosis and management. Hepatology 1983;3:74–6.

91. Sokol RJ. Medical management of the infant or child with chronic liver disease. Semin Liver Dis 1987;7:155–67.

92. Ghent CN, Bloomer JR, Hsia YE. Efficacy and safety of long-term phenobarbital therapy of familial cholestasis. J Pediatr 1978;93:127–32.

93. Ghent CN, Bloomer JR, Klatskin G. Elevation in skin tissue levels of bile acids in human cholestasis: relation to serum levels and to pruritus. Gastroenterology 1977;73:1125–30.

94. Bergasa NV, Talbot TL, Alling DW, et al. A controlled trial of naloxone infusions for the pruritus of chronic cholestasis. Gastroenterology 1992;102:544–9.

95. Richardson BP. Serotonin and nociception. Ann N Y Acad Sci 1990;600:511–20.

96. Bloomer JR, Boyer JL. Phenobarbital effects in cholestatic liver disease. Ann Intern Med 1985;82:310–7.

97. Cynamon HA, Andres JM, Iafrate RP. Rifampin relieves pruritus in children with cholestatic liver disease. Gastroenterology 1990;98:1013–6.

98. Ghent CN, Carruthers SG. Treatment of pruritus in primary biliary cirrhosis with rifampin. Gastroenterology 1988;94:488–93.

99. Mela M, Mancuso A, Burroughs AK. Review article: pruritus in cholestatis and other liver diseases. Aliment Pharmacol Ther 2003;17:857–70.

100. Matsuzaki Y, Tanaka N, Osuga T, et al. Improvement of biliary enzyme levels and itching as a result of long-term administration of ursodeoxycholic acid in primary biliary cirrhosis. Am J Gastroenterol 1990;85:15–23.

101. Balistreri WF. Bile acid therapy in pediatric hepatobiliary disease: the role of ursodeoxycholic acid. J Pediatr Gastroenterol Nutr 1997;24:573–89.

102. Jones EA, Bergasa NV. The pruritus of cholestasis and the opioid system. JAMA 1992;269:3359–62.

103. Whitington PF, Whitington GL. Partial external diversion of bile for the treatment of intractable pruritus associated with intrahepatic cholestasis. Gastroenterology 1988;95:130–6.

104. Ng V, Ryckman FC, Porta G, et al. Long-term outcome after partial external biliary diversion for intractable pruritus in patients with intrahepatic cholestasis. J Pediatr Gastroenterol Nutr 2000;30:152–6.

105. Moreno LA, Gottrand F, Hoden S. Improvement of nutritional status in cholestatic children with supplemental nocturnal enteral nutrition. J Pediatr Gastroenterol Nutr 1991;12:213–6.

106. Rosenblum JL, Keating JP, Prensky AL, et al. A progressive neurologic syndrome in children with chronic liver disease. N Engl J Med 1981;304:503–8.

107. Sokol RJ, Heubi JE, Iannaccone S, et al. Mechanism causing vitamin E deficiency during chronic childhood cholestasis. Gastroenterology 1983;85:1172–82.

108. Sokol RJ, Heubi JE, Iannaccone ST, et al. Vitamin E deficiency with normal serum vitamin E concentrations in children with chronic cholestasis. N Engl J Med 1984;310:1209–12.

109. Sokol RJ, Butler-Simon N, Conner C, et al. Multicenter trial of d-alpha-tocopheryl polyethlene glycol 1000 succinate for treatment of vitamin E deficiency in children with chronic cholestasis, Gastroenterology 1993;104 1727–35.

110. Argao EA, Heubi JE. Fat-soluble vitamin deficiency in infants and children. Curr Opin Pediatr 1993;5:562–6.

111. Bucuvalas JC, Heubi JE, Specker BL, et al. Calcium absorption in bone disease associated with chronic cholestasis during childhood. Hepatology 1990;12:1200–5.

112. Floreani A, Baragiotta A, Martines D, et al. Plasma antioxidant levels in chronic cholestasic liver diseases. Aliment Pharmacol Ther 2000;4:353–8.

113. Sokal EM, Baudoux MC, Collette E, et al. Branched chain amino acids improve body composition and nitrogen balance in a rat model of extrahepatic biliary atresia. Pediatr Res 1996;40:66–71.

114. Argao EA, Specker BL, Heubi JE. Bone mineral content in infants and children with chronic cholestatic liver disease. Pediatrics 1993;91:1151–4.

115. Heubi JE, Higgins JV, Argao EA, et al. The role of magnesium in the pathogenesis of bone disease in childhood cholestatic liver disease: a preliminary report. J Pediatr Gastroenterol Nutr 1997;25:301–6.

116. Gines P, Guevara M, De Las Heras D, Arroyo V. Review article: albumin for circulatory support in patients with cirrhosis. Aliment Pharmacol Ther 2002;16 Suppl 5:24–31.

117. Howard ER, Stringer MD, Mowat AP. Assessment of injection sclerotherapy in the management of 152 children with oesophageal varices. Br J Surg 1988;75:404–8.

118. Whitington PF, Balistreri WF. Liver transplantation in pediatrics: indications, contraindications, and pre-transplant management. J Pediatr 1991;118:169–77.

119. Ryckman FC, Flake AW, Fisher RA, et al. Segmental orthotopic hepatic transplantation as a means to improve patient survival and diminish waiting-list mortality. J Pediatr Surg 1991;26:422–8.

120. Ryckman FC, Alonso MH. Liver transplantation (cadaveric). In: Balistreri WF, Ohi R, Todani T, Tsuchida Y, editors. Hepatobiliary, pancreatic and splenic disease in children: medical and surgical management. London: Elsevier Science BV; 1997. p. 391–432.

CHAPTER 50

DISORDERS OF THE BILIARY TRACT

1. Disorders of the Intrahepatic Ducts

David A. Piccoli, MD

Pierre Russo, MD

EMBRYOLOGY OF THE INTRAHEPATIC DUCTS

The development of the intrahepatic biliary tree begins between the fifth and ninth week postfertilization. The biliary epithelium is believed to arise from precursor bipotential hepatoblasts that can differentiate into either hepatocytes or biliary epithelial cells.[1] Genes and gene products regulating this process have been recently identified. HNF1β is required for the development of interlobular bile ducts and arteries in mice, and mutant mice lacking HNF1β in the liver have a paucity of intrahepatic bile ducts and absence of hepatic arteries.[2] HNF6 is believed to regulate the expression of HNF1β and is required for the development of the gallbladder and extrahepatic ducts.[3]

Differences in cytokeratin (CR) expression between hepatoblasts and biliary epithelial cells have been used to illustrate the development of intrahepatic bile ducts. Precursor hepatoblasts express CK 7, 8, 18, and 19; mature hepatocytes express CK 8 and 18 but not 19, whereas biliary epithelium expresses CK 8, 18, 19, and 20.[4] Around weeks 6 to 7, a prominent rim of CK19-positive cells forms along the outer boundary of the developing portal tracts, forming the so-called ductal plate.[5,6] During the next few weeks, the rim becomes a continuous double-layered saccular sleeve around each portal tract. Remodeling of the ductal plate, starting around week 12, results in the formation of discrete tubular spaces incorporated more centrally into the portal mesenchyme, with loss of excess epithelial elements (Figure 50.1-1). This process is believed to proceed from the hepatic hilum, extending centrifugally toward the periphery of the liver. It appears to continue into the first month of life ex utero. A delicate balance between cell proliferation and apoptosis appears to be a key element of this process.[7] The most cranial portions of the hepatic ducts, themselves derived from the cephalic portion of the hepatic diverticulum, would appear to be in direct continu-

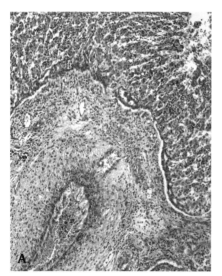 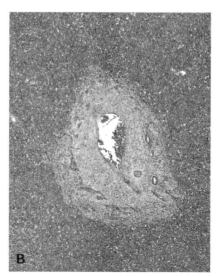 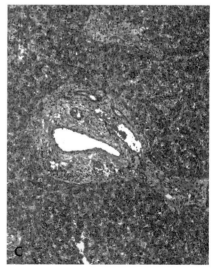

FIGURE 50.1-1   Development of the bile duct as illustrated in fetuses of different ages. A, Ten-week-old fetus. The portal vein is in the center of the portal tract. The ductal plate consists of a double-layered saccular sleeve that surrounds the portal tract. B, Sixteen weeks. Short segments of the ductal plate become tubules, which are incorporated toward the center of the portal tract. The ductal plate has become discontinuous. C, Twenty-five weeks. The ductal plate has largely involuted (hematoxylin and eosin; ×100 original magnification).

ity with converging ductules at the hepatic hilum, which, in turn, are continuous with the ductal plate.[7]

Persistence of the ductal plate in the postnatal liver, appearing as an excessive number of irregular, biliary structures at the site of the original ductal plate and accompanied by an increase in portal tract fibrous tissue, creates a lesion known as the ductal plate malformation (DPM),[8] biliary dysgenesis,[9] or congenital hepatic fibrosis[10] (Figure 50.1-2). The prominent duct elements should not be confused with the proliferating duct elements commonly seen as a response to a variety of hepatic insults, including mechanical obstruction. Jorgenson[8] recognized the similarity between these portal tracts and those seen in fetal life and coined the term "ductal plate malformation" to signify that the lesion represents an arrest in the development of normal portal tract and bile duct structures or, as characterized by Desmet,[11] a disruption of the normal "remodeling" of the embryonic bile duct and portal tract structures into their mature forms. The relevance of this lesion to cystic bile ducts lies in the fact that the abnormal ducts have a propensity to become dilated. This lesion is found in combination with renal abnormalities (usually cysts) in a number of heritable conditions in which there is actual or potential cystic dilatation of the biliary ducts. In addition to these heritable disorders, Desmet has suggested that persistence of the ductal plate can also be associated with extrahepatic biliary atresia,[11] which is not heritable and is not associated with renal disease.

The intrahepatic tree in humans can be divided into large bile ducts (300–800 μm), which include hepatic, segmental, and area ducts, which have associated mucous peribiliary glands, and small bile ducts (< 300 μm), which are not associated with peribiliary glands and include conducting and terminal (or interlobular) bile ducts.[12] Interlobular bile ducts link with intralobular canaliculi via bile ductules or canals of Hering, although the exact anatomy remains unclear. The biliary epithelia of small and large bile ducts express different enzymes and membrane proteins, suggesting that they repre-

sent distinct subpopulations.[13] Possible differences in disease susceptibility and responses to injury between epithelia of small and large bile ducts may explain why certain diseases preferentially target smaller bile ducts (primary biliary cirrhosis, graft-versus-host disease), whereas others (sclerosing cholangitis) are primarily directed at larger ducts.[14,15]

INTRAHEPATIC BILE DUCT CYSTIC CONDITIONS

Cystic diseases of the intrahepatic bile ducts present a wide range of disorders. They include both sporadically occurring and heritable conditions and extend from lesions typically discovered incidentally to frank malignancies. A classification scheme is presented in Table 50.1-1. Heritable cystic disease of bile ducts is also referred to as fibrocystic, or fibropolycystic, disease, reflecting the portal fibrosis and DPM that is the histologic hallmark of most of these disorders. The distinction between communicating and noncommunicating cysts is clinically significant because when duct cysts communicate with the biliary tree, they have a greater likelihood of causing clinical disease. Communicating duct cysts can be associated with cholangitis, stone formation, and (relatively uncommonly) neoplasia. Noncommunicating duct cysts are usually asymptomatic but, if sufficiently large, may present as an abdominal mass or biliary obstruction.

SOLITARY CYSTS

Solitary bile duct cysts are generally unilocular cysts lined by a single layer of cuboidal or columnar epithelium (Figure 50.1-3). They tend to present in the fourth to sixth decade with symptoms of fullness or a mass. They are rare in the pediatric age group, 31 having been diagnosed in 63 years at the Boston Children's Hospital.[16] They have been reported in newborns, including a case presenting as a con-

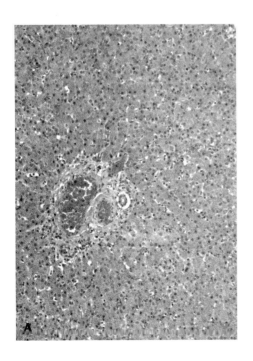

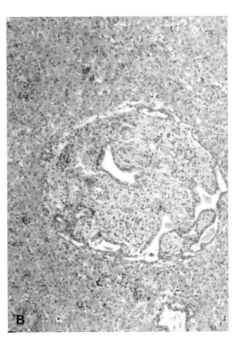

FIGURE 50.1-2 Congenital hepatic fibrosis (CHF). The left panel shows a normal portal tract from a newborn term infant. The right panel, taken at the same magnification, illustrates the hepatic histologic features from a 9-day-old infant with CHF and autosomal recessive polycystic kidney disease. The portal tract is expanded and fibrotic, and there is a proliferation of irregularly dilated biliary structures at the portal tract–lobular interface, a pattern known as "ductal plate malformation" (hematoxylin and eosin; ×100 original magnification).

TABLE 50.1-1   CLASSIFICATION OF HEPATIC CYSTS OF DUCTAL ORIGIN

SOLITARY NONPARASITIC CYSTS
Solitary bile duct cyst
Ciliated hepatic foregut cyst
Peribiliary cyst
Hepatobiliary cystadenoma

HERITABLE HEPATIC CYSTS—FIBROCYSTIC DISEASE
Communicating cysts
  Congenital hepatic fibrosis (CHF)
  CHF in association with
    Autosomal recessive polycystic kidney disease
    Nephronophthisis
    Malformation syndromes (see Table 50.1-2)
    Phosphomannose isomerase deficiency
    Caroli syndrome
Noncommunicating cysts
  Autosomal dominant polycystic kidney disease
  Isolated polycystic liver disease (chromosome 19p13.2-13.1)

genital diaphragmatic hernia.[17] The main differential diagnosis is with autosomal dominant polycystic disease. Imaging studies in the latter would show multiple cysts in the liver and kidney. The cystic structures of Caroli disease are usually part of a more diffuse involvement of the biliary tree (vide infra). In contrast, mesenchymal hamartomas, which are more common in the pediatric age group, have a more complex structure, with multiple cysts and a solid component. Ciliated hepatic foregut cysts, so named because of their alleged origin from the embryonic foregut, are characterized by a lining of ciliated pseudostratified columnar epithelium resting on a basement membrane and surrounded by smooth muscle bundles.[18] They seem to occur more commonly in males in the fourth to fifth decade. Peribiliary cysts are derived from dilatation of the peribiliary glands located in the hilum and large portal areas. They have been reported primarily as findings in autopsy or hepatectomy specimens and have been associated with a variety of liver disorders.[19] They have not been reported in childhood. Hepatobiliary cystadenomas are benign multilocular cystic neoplasms that tend to occur in middle-age women but have been reported in patients from 2 to 87 years of age.[20] They usually occur in the liver but may also arise within the extrahepatic biliary tree and gallbladder. They are lined by a flattened, occasionally papillary, mucin-producing columnar epithelium. In females, the cysts are surrounded by dense mesenchymal tissue resembling ovarian stroma. Its malignant counterpart, the biliary cystadenocarcinoma, has not been reported in children.

HERITABLE INTRAHEPATIC CYSTIC DISEASE

The major heritable conditions characterized by intrahepatic bile duct cysts are congenital hepatic fibrosis (CHF), autosomal recessive polycystic kidney disease (ARPKD), and autosomal dominant polycystic kidney disease (ADPKD). There are also a number of heritable malformation syndromes characterized by potential bile duct cysts and renal disease. The DPM is seen in essentially all of these disorders (least commonly in ADPKD). Whenever

the DPM is the basis for the cysts, the cysts communicate proximally and distally with the biliary tree. Renal cysts of tubular origin or other renal developmental lesions are typically present in most of these conditions. It is of note that the renal lesions tend to be dissimilar in the different clinical conditions.

CONGENITAL HEPATIC FIBROSIS

The term "congenital hepatic fibrosis" was coined by Kerr and colleagues[10] and is essentially defined by a characteristic hepatopathology, resulting in portal hypertension and an increased risk of ascending cholangitis. CHF is associated with a wide spectrum of disorders, the most frequent of which is ARPKD, but can also be an isolated condition.

The relationship of ARPKD to CHF is still somewhat controversial. Some investigators maintain that ARPKD and CHF represent a single disorder, whereas others suggest that they are distinct entities with overlapping hepatic histologic features.[5] The hepatic histomorphology in both lesions is essentially similar and is characterized by the DPM. The renal lesions, which also consist of tubular cysts in both, classically differ markedly in both pathology and clinical severity. In newborn patients with ARPKD, the renal lesions are diffuse and prominent clinically, whereas in patients who exhibit the clinical picture of CHF, the renal lesions are often not as evident in early life and are minor. Recently, a gene (*PKHD1*) that maps to the 6p21 locus and encodes a large, receptor-like protein, fibrocystin, has been identified as the site of mutations resulting in ARPKD.[21,22] The identification of this gene will prove to be valuable in the delineation of these two identities.

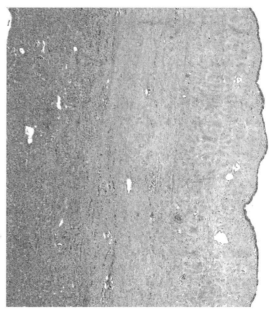

FIGURE 50.1-3 Hepatic cyst. Solitary hepatic cyst from a 9-year-old female. The cyst lining consists of a low cuboidal epithelium resting on a thick fibrous wall. Liver parenchyma can be noted toward the left of the picture (hematoxylin and eosin; ×40 original magnification).

CLINICAL FINDINGS

A considerable range of clinical presentations is observed in patients with CHF. Most patients present with portal hypertension in the first decades of life. Some patients present with cholangitis, whereas other patients are discovered only incidentally at autopsy (latent CHF).[23] The precise pathogenesis of the portal hypertension is unknown but is thought to be associated with the hepatic fibrosis and/or portal vein abnormalities. Hematemesis or melena is the presenting sign in 30 to 70% of patients from pediatric and mixed population studies.[24,25] In children, the age for presentation of hematemesis may be as early as the first year of life,[26] but it usually ranges from 5 to 13 years. Firm or hard hepatomegaly is present in nearly all patients, often with a prominent left lobe, and this is usually one of the presenting findings. Splenomegaly occurs in the majority, accompanied by hypersplenism with thrombocytopenia. Splenic pressure is elevated, and naturally occurring splenorenal or gastrorenal shunts are occasionally documented. Portal vein abnormalities, characteristically duplication of the intrahepatic branches, are common.[24,27] This is in contrast to histologic descriptions of hypoplastic portal vein branches by others.[5] Occasionally, portal vein thrombosis or cavernous transformation of the portal vein is documented. Renal lesions, when present, appear to be minimal and of little clinical significance. An appearance similar to medullary sponge kidney has been described.[28] Cases of renal insufficiency described in association with CHF may, in fact, represent "late-onset" ARPKD.[29]

PATHOLOGY

The cut surface of the liver is speckled with irregular, whitish areas of fibrosis. The characteristic lesion is the DPM, and parenchymal disease is usually absent. The degree of fibrosis is variable, from enlarged portal tracts to broad bands of connective tissue linking portal tracts. It is usually diffuse but occasionally confined to one lobe or even one segment of a lobe.[30,31] Because the lesion may not be equally prominent throughout the liver, needle biopsies may be unreliable in establishing the diagnosis. Although Jorgensen found an increase in the average diameter of bile ducts in patients with CHF compared with those in controls,[8] the exact incidence of gross cysts is not established, nor is it clear whether the incidence of cysts increases with age.[24] Dilatation of bile ducts becomes clinically significant when associated with either cholangitis or malignancy. Cholangitis may be occult, acute, or chronic in nature and contributes significantly to both the morbidity and mortality of CHF. Calculi may form in the dilated ducts, initiating or complicating preexisting cholangitis. Cholangiocarcinoma is an uncommon but serious complication of CHF,[32] and premalignant changes may be observed in the epithelium of cystically dilated ducts. Cholangiocarcinoma may also be found in association with choledochal cysts or dilated intrahepatic ducts in the absence of DPM.

Visceral abnormalities in addition to those in the liver and kidney, described in single or small groups of patients, include congenital heart disease,[33] pulmonary hypertension and arteriovenous fistulae,[34,35] berry aneurysms,[36,37]

and osteochondrodysplasia.[38] It is unclear whether these anomalies are intrinsic to the basic disease or coincidental. A syndrome of intestinal lymphangiectasia and protein-losing enteropathy in association with CHF, as described by Pedersen and Tygstrup[39] and by Pelletier and colleagues,[40] has now been demonstrated to be phosphomannose isomerase deficiency[41] (vide infra).

THERAPY FOR CHF

Portosystemic shunting has been the treatment of choice because there is a low incidence of postoperative encephalopathy or hyperammonemia.[24] Prospective trials of other alternative approaches, such as sclerotherapy, banding, or pharmacologic management of varices, are not yet available. Nevertheless, the presence of spontaneous portosystemic shunts in some children suggests that sclerotherapy or banding may be beneficial if either can be shown to hasten the development of hemodynamically significant shunts without surgery. If surgery is selected as the treatment for portal hypertension, the type of shunt should be carefully chosen to prevent the limitation of options for either hepatic or renal transplant in later life.

Prolonged cholangitis is a major complication and has been responsible for hepatic failure and death. Therefore, unexplained fever or serologic evidence of inflammation in the absence of fever warrants a diagnostic liver biopsy and aspirate for culture.[42] Manipulation of the extrahepatic biliary tree carries an increased risk of infection in patients with abnormal ducts or bile stasis.[43] In cases of refractory cholangitis, surgical management and external or internal drainage may be necessary to resolve the hepatobiliary infection. In patients with stasis and refractory cholangitis, a choleretic agent may significantly augment therapy. Ursodeoxycholic acid therapy and prophylactic antibiotic administration have not been adequately studied in CHF-related cholangitis but may have a role in selected patients.

PROGNOSIS FOR CHF

In general, the prognosis for those older children who present with CHF is good. The limitations are those imposed by complications of the disease, namely portal hypertension, cholangitis, and, occasionally, renal or hepatic failure. Chronic renal failure is most common in patients with a presentation in infancy. As noted, portal hypertension is usually successfully managed and rarely complicated by hepatic encephalopathy. Ascending cholangitis with sepsis and hepatic failure is a major cause of death in most series.[24,25,44] In those patients with chronic cholangitis and/or progressive hepatic dysfunction, liver transplant may prove to be the optimal therapy. Occasionally, patients have received combined renal and hepatic transplants for multiorgan failure.

CHF-NEPHRONOPHTHISIS

In this heritable group of disorders, there is a combination of hepatic lesions with some similarity to CHF with severe tubulointerstitial renal disease.[45-47] Its relation to the previously discussed disorders is not clear because the renal lesions differ considerably from those seen in the previously discussed disorders, and even the hepatic lesion sometimes does not show a completely typical DPM. These conditions are nonetheless discussed in this chapter given the combination of heredity and the simultaneous presence of renal and liver disease with DPM-like features. The renal lesions are quite different from those of CHF and ARPKD and are characterized by interstitial inflammation and fibrosis with tubular atrophy, cyst formation, and secondary glomerulosclerosis (nephronophthisis). There is usually progressive renal failure with uremia by 20 years of age. The hepatic lesion has features consistent with DPM, although the bile ducts may not feature the characteristic profiles of those in typical DPM, and portal inflammation has been noted in some instances. Morphometric studies by Landing and colleagues on the biliary profiles and portal tracts in some of these diseases suggested heterogeneity in expression and development.[48] These disorders bear some similarities to renal-retinal syndrome (Senior-Loken syndrome), which is characterized by nephronophthisis and retinitis pigmentosa or retinal aplasia. Recent studies have demonstrated significant genetic heterogeneity in Senior-Loken syndrome. The syndrome has been associated with homozygous mutations in the NPHP1[49] and NPHP4[50] genes. NPHP1 and NPHP4 code for nephrocystin and nephroretinin, highly conserved proteins important in cell-cell and cell-matrix recognition.[51] Some patients have also been mapped to a locus on 3q22, overlapping the NPHP3 locus.[52] Most of these patients do not seem to have liver involvement. It is currently unknown whether the patients with CHF nephronophthisis described in the past, before gene defects in cases of familial nephronophthisis were identified, have similar gene abnormalities.

PHOSPHOMANNOSE ISOMERASE DEFICIENCY

Phosphomannose isomerase deficiency, a disorder of glycosylation, has been associated with DPM and a protein-losing enteropathy.[41,53,54] Kidney disease has not been described in affected patients. Disease appears to result from hypoglycosylation of a number of serum and glycoproteins and suggests a metabolic anomaly leading to the development of the DPM. Phosphomannose isomerase deficiency is particularly interesting in light of the work of Terada and colleagues, who have highlighted cell-matrix interaction and the role of glycoproteins during development of the human intrahepatic biliary system.[55]

CHF AND MALFORMATION SYNDROMES

CHF accompanies a considerable number of malformation syndromes, usually in combination with cystic, dysplastic kidneys (Table 50.1-2). The pathogenetic implications of this coexistence of renal and hepatic cysts in these malformation syndromes and their relationship to ADPKD and ARPKD are not clear, particularly because the renal disease varies considerably in character among the various conditions. Although the literature is replete with descriptions

of syndromes with developmental liver lesions, in many reports, the liver findings are poorly defined, often superficially described as "liver fibrosis," "increased bile ducts," or "liver cysts," and lack adequate histologic analysis. Therefore, the syndromes briefly discussed here are those in which there is reasonable evidence that DPM frequently accompanies the other malformations.

Meckel-Gruber syndrome is a recessively inherited lethal condition characterized by a central nervous system malformation, usually an occipital meningoencephalocele, bilaterally large multicystic kidneys, CHF, and polydactyly.[56] There is considerable heterogeneity in clinical findings, and at least three different gene loci have been identified: MKS1 on 17q, MKS2 on 11q, and MKS3 on 8q.[57] Sergi and colleagues reviewed the liver sections of 30 fetuses with Meckel syndrome and found that DPM was a constant anomaly.[58] Two kinds of hepatic lesions were observed: 23 cases showed mainly a cystic dilatation of primitive biliary structures with little portal fibrosis, whereas 7 cases showed mainly rings of interrupted curved lumina around a central fibrovascular axis and pronounced portal fibrosis.

Jeune syndrome (asphyxiating thoracic dystrophy) is a rare autosomal recessive skeletal dysplasia that often leads to respiratory insufficiency because of a severely constricted thoracic cage. Renal disease, pancreatic insufficiency, and abnormalities of the retina, nails, and dental defects are also described.[59] Cystic lesions occur in the kidney and pancreas, whereas the liver changes are mostly characterized by DPM with progressive fibrosis.[60] Clinically significant liver dysfunction may not be apparent in the majority of patients who die in early life, although, among patients who survive beyond infancy, the liver fibrosis seems to be progressive.[61,62] Yerian and colleagues have described abnormalities of intrahepatic portal veins and vascular shunts in the resected liver of an older child who underwent transplant.[60]

Ivemark syndrome (renal-pancreatic-hepatic dysplasia) is one of the two syndromes described by Ivemark. One is usually sporadic and is characterized by asplenia

TABLE 50.1-2   MALFORMATION SYNDROMES WITH DUCTAL PLATE MALFORMATION

DPM AS A FREQUENT OCCURRENCE
Meckel-Gruber syndrome
Jeune syndrome
Ivemark syndrome
Bardet-Biedl syndrome

DPM—OCCASIONAL OR INSUFFICIENTLY DESCRIBED
Tuberous sclerosis
Smith-Lemli-Opitz syndrome
COACH syndrome
Ellis-van Creveld syndrome
Elejalde syndrome
Trisomy 9
Trisomy 13

Adapted from Ruchelli E. Normal and abnormal liver development. In: Russo P, Ruchelli E, Piccoli D, editors. Pathology of pediatric gastrointestinal and liver disease. New York: Springer-Verlag; 2004.
COACH = cerebellar aplasia, oligophrenia, ataxia, coloboma, hepatic fibrosis; DPM = ductal plate malformation.

with visceroatrial heterotaxy but no liver disease.[63] The other syndrome is characterized by dysplastic changes involving the kidneys and liver and pancreatic ducts and, frequently, polysplenia.[64] The liver lesions appear to be consistent with DPM. An autosomal recessive mode of inheritance has been proposed.[64] However, because similar renal, hepatic, and pancreatic abnormalities occur in other syndromes, including trisomy 9, Meckel, Jeune, Saldino-Noonan, and Elejalde types of chondrodysplasia, and glutaricaciduria type II, cases of renal-hepatic-pancreatic dysplasia do not necessarily constitute a homogeneous group.[65,66]

AUTOSOMAL RECESSIVE POLYCYSTIC KIDNEY DISEASE

ARPKD encompasses a spectrum of clinical and pathologic manifestations; however, the two invariant features are DPM and fusiform dilatation of the renal collecting ducts. The renal lesion, when identified in infancy, is characterized by radially arranged tubular cysts occupying most of the large externally smooth renal mass with widely spaced glomeruli (Figure 50.1-4). The longer patients survive, the less characteristic the renal lesions become because the cysts become more rounded, and in some cases with survival beyond the neonatal period, it may be difficult on

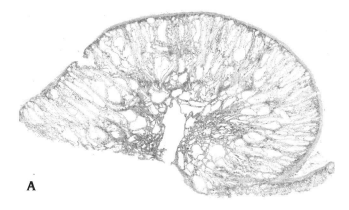

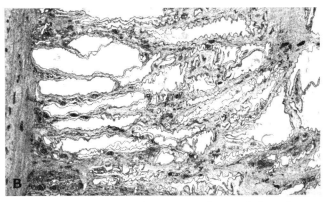

FIGURE 50.1-4   Autosomal recessive polycystic kidney disease. A, Low-power microphotograph of the kidney with diffuse fusiform dilatation of tubular segments in a radial arrangement. There is little residual normal parenchyma. B, Higher-power view. A few glomerular structures are seen between the dilated tubules and in the subcapsular area to the left of the picture (hematoxylin and eosin; whole mount section).

examination of biopsies to correctly classify the lesion.[67] Using linkage analysis in families with an affected child, prenatal diagnosis became possible.[68]

The renal disease may vary from a lethal perinatal disease to an incidental finding in older children. It has been estimated that 30 to 50% of infants affected with ARPKD will die in the perinatal period,[69] although recent studies suggest a better long-term prognosis.[70] In the infantile form, the kidneys are enlarged and severely dysfunctional. They may be palpable on examination, and an abdominal radiograph will demonstrate bilaterally enlarged kidneys. Excretory urography may only poorly visualize the collecting system. The nephrogram (characteristic of the neonatal presentation) demonstrates a radiolucent mottled parenchyma owing to the cystic changes of the nephrons. Many infants with ARPKD will develop uremia and chronic renal failure. Respiratory distress occurs from compression exerted by the enlarged kidneys, fluid retention, congestive heart failure, concomitant pulmonary hypoplasia, or pneumonia. Progressive renal failure and hypertension may occur over the first few weeks or months of life. Mortality is high in these patients. Patients who survive infancy may develop slowly progressive renal insufficiency and portal hypertension.[29]

The pathogenesis of the renal lesion is at least partially understood. It is tempting to speculate that closely related etiopathogeneses are responsible for both hepatic duct and renal tubular dilatation. Were this so, important insights regarding bile duct development and function might be gained. A variety of animal models have been developed to investigate the mechanisms of cystogenesis in the kidneys. These models have resulted in the speculation that abnormalities in epithelial cell growth, extracellular matrix composition, and fluid secretion are important in cyst formation.[71] Normal renal tubular absorptive epithelia can become cystic if (1) hyperplasia, localized to a distinct nephron segment, requires accommodation of an increased cell mass; (2) secretion, rather than absorption, leads to net accumulation of intratubular fluid; or (3) extracellular matrix abnormalities alter the epithelial microenvironment with resultant abnormal epithelial hyperplasia and secretory activity.[71] Evidence from several studies has suggested the role of the epidermal growth factor-α (EGFR) and transforming growth factor-α receptor axis in promoting epithelial hyperplasia and subsequent renal cyst formation in murine and human ADPKD and ARPKD.[72] Furthermore, similar abnormalities of EGFR expression have been suggested to mediate biliary epithelial hyperplasia and ductal ectasia in a mouse model.[73,74] An inhibitor of tyrosine EGFR tyrosine kinase activity has been shown to markedly reduce collecting tubule cystic lesions, improve renal function, decrease biliary epithelial abnormalities, and improve life span in a mouse model of ARPKD.[75] A murine model of ARPKD, characterized by a mutation in the mouse *cpk* gene, suggests that an inactivating mutation in the *cpk* allele interferes with normal tubular epithelial differentiation in the liver and kidney.[76] This rat model was a critical development in the identification of the *PKHD1* gene.

LIVER DISEASE IN ARPKD

The hepatic lesion is relatively uniform, and grossly visible cysts are uncommon. There is portal tract fibrous enlargement with numerous biliary profiles, as in CHF. Normal interlobular ducts in the center of the tracts are often missing.[5] As in CHF, the bile ducts are in continuity with the rest of the biliary system (communicating cystic disease). The precise incidence of portal hypertension in ARPKD is unclear and may be less than in CHF, although this may reflect the fact that children with ARPKD often die earlier in life. With increasing age of the patients, grossly visible cysts may become more frequent, and an increase in portal fibrosis may be noted.[77] CHF and its attendant complications appear to be a significant cause of mortality and morbidity in older children who have undergone renal transplant.[78] In addition to the renal and hepatic findings, pancreatic fibrosis with duct dilatation or proliferation has been reported occasionally in ARPKD.[79] Interestingly, the *PKHD1* gene has been found to be expressed in the pancreas, as well as in the liver and kidney.[21]

PKHD1 AND FIBROCYSTIN/POLYDUCTIN IN ARPKD

Genetic linkage studies of families with ARPKD allowed the mapping of the disease locus to the 6p21-cen region of chromosome 6.[80] This allowed prenatal diagnosis to be available for siblings of probands.[68] Subsequent studies demonstrated that the clinically diverse presentations of ARPKD, including the severe renal perinatal form, mapped to the same region of chromosome 6,[81] suggesting that mutations in a single gene are responsible for the varied clinical presentations and classifications of fibropolycystic disease. Of the different rodent models of ARPKD, only one rat model with similar manifestations to ARPKD, the Pck rat, mapped to a region syntenic to chromosome 6 in the human, and this model was used to localize and identify the human disease gene.[21] Independently, and using different strategies, Ward and colleagues[21] and Onuchic and colleagues[22] identified the gene *PKHD1*, which encodes a large receptor-like protein. The gene is extremely large, encompassing 67 coding exons spanning more than 469 kb of genomic deoxyribonucleic acid (DNA), and the human transcript is approximately 16 kb. The gene was expressed in the fetal kidney and in the adult kidney and pancreas, with lesser levels seen in the liver.[21,22] The massive protein encoded by *PKHD1*, termed by the authors fibrocystin[21] and polyductin,[22] was predicted to contain 4,074 amino acids with a molecular weight of at least 447 kD.[21,22] This protein has limited homology with other known protein domains but no homology with the polycystins of ADPKD.[22] In 11 of 14 studied kindreds, Ward and colleagues found 6 truncating and 12 missense mutations, with the majority of patients being compound heterozygotes.[21] In a patient group of 25 individuals, Onuchic and colleagues identified potentially pathologic variants in 21 (42%) of the 50 chromosomes, and there was some evidence supporting a genotype-phenotype correlation, with truncating mutations possibly being correlated with more severe manifestations.[22] Bergmann and colleagues[82] and

Rosetti and colleagues[83] reported further results of extensive screening for *PKHD1* mutations in ARPKD. In 90 patients, the mutation detection rate was 61%, and 45% of mutations were predicted to truncate the protein. The likelihood of mutation detection was higher for severely affected patients (85%) than for those with moderate ARPKD (41.9%) or for CHF with Caroli disease (32.1%).[83] In both studies, the type of mutation was somewhat correlated with the phenotype, with patients carrying two or one truncating mutation generally having more severe and earlier-onset disease. Except in cases of consanguinity, most patients with two identified mutations were compound heterozygotes.[82,83] The large size of the gene and the widespread location of mutations have, however, limited the applicability of mutation screening for many patients.

AUTOSOMAL DOMINANT POLYCYSTIC KIDNEY DISEASE

ADPKD is the most common hereditary kidney disorder, with a frequency estimated to be from 1 in 400 to 1 in 1,000 individuals worldwide.[84] In contrast, ARPKD is less common, with an incidence in the range of 1 in 6,000 to 1 in 40,000. Although the disease is clinically manifest primarily in adults, it can be anatomically identified even in fetal life. It is important to recognize for its genetic implications, even though the functional significance of the finding is not apparent until beyond childhood. The hepatic lesions are primarily duct cysts, which are readily demonstrated ultrasonographically. Cysts increase in size from childhood until 40 to 50 years of age (Figure 50.1-5). They are recognized and are perhaps present at an earlier age in women than in men. Commonly, the cysts in this condition are dilated ductal elements, which are not shown to communicate with the distal biliary tree and do not contain bile. However, there may also be portal tract lesions consistent with the (communicating) DPM in a smaller percentage of patients.[85] The

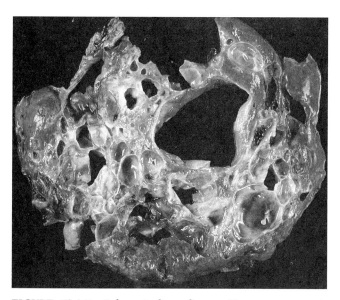

FIGURE 50.1-5 Polycystic liver disease. Hepatectomy specimen at transplant from a 37-year-old male. Photograph courtesy of Dr. Emma Furth, Hospital of the University of Pennsylvania.

significance of the association of communicating (DPM) and noncommunicating lesions for understanding the pathogenesis of the polycystic disease is unclear. Some authors consider the cysts in ADPKD the result of progressive dilatation of von Meyenburg complexes,[86] and Desmet has suggested that the cysts might become separated and noncommunicating as a result of kinks and strictures caused by the strangulating hyaline fibrosis that surrounds them.[5] The hepatic lesions in ADPKD have been thought to be insignificant clinically. However, as more patients with ADPKD survive for longer periods, it has become clear that a significant number of deaths result from hepatic complications.[87] Hepatic complications include infection of the cysts, cholangiocarcinoma, portal hypertension, and pressure effects owing to the cysts.

The renal lesion consists of cysts that appear to arise from multiple areas along the nephron and increase in size with age, eventuating in the kidneys and becoming large cystic reniform masses with inadequate numbers of functioning nephrons.[88]

Cysts may also be found in other organs, including the spleen, pancreas, thyroid, ovary, endometrium, seminal vesicles, and epididymis. Arterial aneurysms are present in up to 30% of cases.[89]

PKD1, PKD2, AND THE POLYCYSTINS

ADPKD results from mutations in one of at least three distinct genetic loci. Mutations in *PKD1*, mapped to chromosome 16p13.3, are responsible for the 85 to 90% of ADPKD in whites,[90,91] and prenatal diagnosis is thus possible. A second ADPKD gene, *PKD2*, has been localized to chromosome 4q13-4q23, and the mutant gene has been identified.[92] The products of *PKD1* and *PKD2* are polycystin 1 and polycystin 2, which have been hypothesized to be part of a common biologic pathway because mutations in these genes produce identical clinical manifestations. However, the onset of renal disease in polycystic kidney disease (PKD) type 2 occurs later in life than in PKD1. The genetic mechanism of disease in ADPKD seems to be a loss of heterozygosity caused by somatic mutations in the wild-type allele in renal epithelial cells. This "two-hit" hypothesis explains the focal nature of ADPKD in that cysts arise from only about 1% of the total nephrons in the kidney.[93] There is also evidence for a third locus for ADPKD, termed PKD3.[94]

ISOLATED HEPATIC POLYCYSTIC DISEASE

A number of reports derived from studies of medicolegal autopsies and occasional families suggested that a polycystic liver disease (PLD) might exist that occurs in the absence of renal disease and is dominantly inherited. Nevertheless, it has been uncertain whether such patients represent a discrete entity or patients with ADPKD, in whom renal cysts were overlooked or were inconspicuous. A study of over 30,000 medicolegal autopsies from Finland identified 22 cases with polycystic disease either of the liver or the kidneys. In only one case were cysts present in both organs, leading the authors to conclude that polycystic disease of the liver and polycystic disease of the kidney

were separate entities.[95] Strong genetic evidence that adult PLD is an entity distinct from either PKD1 or PKD2 was presented by Pirson and colleagues, who traced the disorder through three generations of a family and excluded the presence of kidney cysts and linkage of the disease to the genetic markers of PKD1 and PKD2.[96] The genetically distinct nature of isolated PLD is further supported by the finding of Reynolds and colleagues that the causative gene in two large families with PLD mapped to 19p13.2-p13.[97] A Finnish study achieved similar results and also suggested the possibility of a second locus.[98] Drenth and colleagues narrowed the linkage assignment of the PLD locus on 19p and detected a heterozygous mutation at the *PRKCSH* gene.[99] Li and colleagues identified the product of the *PRKCSH* gene as a highly conserved ubiquitous protein that is likely important in signal transduction.[100] Cysts in patients with PLD are believed to arise from dilatation of biliary microhamatomas (von Meyenburg complexes) and from peribiliary glands, as in ADPKD, suggesting that the hepatic cysts in both conditions have a similar pathogenesis.[101] The development of hepatic cysts in PLD appears to be age dependent and rare in childhood, coming to medical attention usually because of symptoms owing to mass effect or from complications such as hemorrhage, infection, or rupture. A relatively higher prevalence of mitral valve abnormalities was also found in patients with PLD.[101]

CAROLI SYNDROME AND CAROLI DISEASE

Caroli disease is a congenital dilatation of the larger intrahepatic bile ducts. Caroli described two variants.[102] One is characterized by pure ductal ectasia without other hepatic pathology, for which the term "Caroli disease" has been proposed. The other variant is a combined type in which Caroli disease is associated with the lesions of CHF, for which the term "Caroli syndrome" has been proposed.[11] Communicating duct cysts occur in both variants. The first variant is very rare and is not known to be heritable. The nature of the second variant, Caroli syndrome, is currently controversial. It is not clear whether Caroli syndrome represents a separate entity from CHF, a variant of it, or a mere radiologic appearance in a variety of biliary disorders. Caroli syndrome has been associated with ADPKD.[103] It has been postulated that Caroli disease represents developmental arrest at the level of the larger intrahepatic bile ducts, whereas Caroli syndrome involves the entire intrahepatic biliary tree such that smaller interlobular ducts are affected (Figure 50.1-6).[6] The mode of inheritance of Caroli syndrome has been reported to be autosomal recessive, although a recent report of a Japanese family suggests an autosomal dominant form of inheritance.[104]

The relationship between Caroli disease and choledochal cyst is also controversial. According to Todani and colleagues, the type V choledochal cyst (intrahepatic cysts) is similar to the appearance of Caroli disease, and they consider the two synonymous.[105] However, those cases described as choledochal cysts in association with

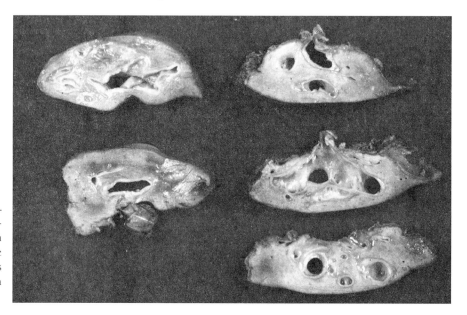

FIGURE 50.1-6 Caroli disease. Extensive intrahepatic bile duct dilatation involving primarily the left lobe of the liver, as illustrated by multiple sections from a partial hepatectomy specimen from a 9-year-old female.

CHF probably have a different pattern of inheritance and, thus, a different etiology and are considered to be a different entity by some authors.[84] Caroli disease typically becomes symptomatic in adults. Patients with Caroli syndrome may present earlier in life owing to the associated liver and renal abnormalities. The duct ectasias in both conditions predispose the patient to bile stasis and repeated attacks of cholangitis and complications such as intrahepatic lithiasis, biliary abscess, sepsis, amyloidosis, and cholangiocarcinoma (Figure 50.1-7).

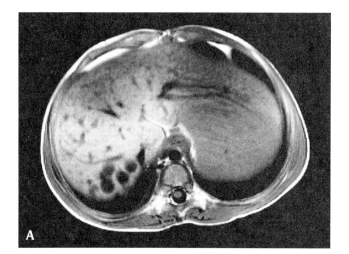

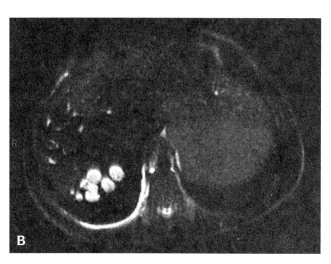

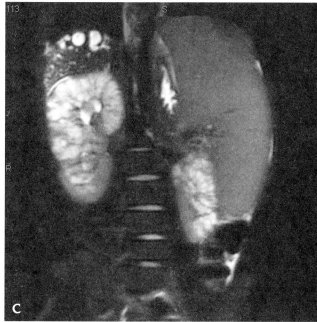

FIGURE 50.1-7 Hepatic magnetic resonance image (*A*) and magnetic resonance cholangiogram (*B*, *C*) demonstrating intrahepatic ductal dilatation in an child with autosomal recessive polycystic kidney disease and congenital hepatic fibrosis and unsuspected Caroli dilatation. Note also massive splenomegaly and nephromegaly with cysts. *A*, Transverse view; *B*, transverse view, enhanced; *C*, coronal view.

BILE DUCT PAUCITY

A decrease in the number of ducts (paucity) is one of the most significant abnormalities of the intralobular bile ducts in children.[106] Bile duct paucity can only be defined histologically. In patients at or beyond 37 weeks of gestational age, paucity is present when histologic examination demonstrates that the ratio of ducts to portal tracts is less than 0.9 (Figure 50.1-8). In determining this ratio, it should be kept in mind that (1) bile ductules should not be included in the counting, (2) counts must involve sufficient portal tracts to be representative of the liver as a whole, and (3) this ratio is not applicable in premature infants.[107] The standard for the number of portal tracts required is 20, although some authors suggest that as few as 5 portal tracts may be sufficient.[53,107] Because 20 portal tracts are obtainable only on an operative wedge biopsy, it is commonly necessary to make, or at least strongly suggest, the diagnosis of paucity with a smaller sample number.

Because there is little precise knowledge of the factors that influence the development, viability, and maintenance of the intrahepatic bile ducts, it is not possible to formulate a genuinely coherent classification of the duct paucity conditions. For example, in some situations, there is an active destruction of previously existing ducts. In others, paucity is associated with a primary disease. For this reason, the disorders outlined in Table 50.1-3 are more a list of conditions than a true classification. Furthermore, for a number of the primary disorders in the table, the incidence of paucity is so low as to perhaps be coincidental.

SYNDROMIC BILE DUCT PAUCITY (ALAGILLE SYNDROME)

Syndromic bile duct paucity, now referred to as Alagille syndrome (AGS), is defined by dominantly inherited bile duct paucity in conjunction with specific extrahepatic findings. It is a diagnosis that has both genetic and prog-

TABLE 50.1-3   DISORDERS ASSOCIATED WITH BILE DUCT PAUCITY IN CHILDREN

SYNDROMIC BILE DUCT PAUCITY—ALAGILLE SYNDROME
NONSYNDROMIC BILE DUCT PAUCITY
Metabolic and genetic disorders
  α_1-Antitrypsin deficiency
  Cystic fibrosis (rare)
  Peroxisomal disorders (rare)
  Progressive familial intrahepatic cholestasis (rare)
  Trisomy 21 (rare)
  Prune-belly syndrome (rare)
Infection
  Congenital cytomegalovirus infection (rare)
  Congenital syphilis (rare)
  Congenital rubella (rare)
Inflammatory and immune disorders
  Graft-versus-host disease
  Chronic hepatic allograft rejection
  Sclerosing cholangitis
  Sarcoidosis (rare)
Other
  Drug- or antibiotic-associated vanishing bile duct syndrome
  Familial idiopathic adulthood ductopenia
  Biliary atresia (late)
Panhypopituitarism (rare)
  Idiopathic

nostic implications.[108–120] Also known as Watson-Alagille syndrome, arteriohepatic dysplasia, syndromic intrahepatic biliary hypoplasia, intrahepatic biliary atresia, intrahepatic biliary dysgenesis, and syndromic paucity of the interlobular bile ducts, it is recognized as an important and relatively common cause of neonatal jaundice and cholestasis in older children. AGS is caused by mutations in the human gene *Jagged1* (*JAG1*), which is mapped to chromosome 20p12.[121,122] This gene encodes a ligand for the Notch signaling pathway, which is involved in cell fate determination.

DEFINITION

AGS is characterized by a marked reduction in the number of interlobular bile ducts and cholestasis, occurring in association with cardiovascular, skeletal, ocular, facial, renal, pancreatic, and neurodevelopmental abnormalities. These occur with variable frequency, and early in infancy, the duct paucity may be absent.

The condition was recognized independently by Watson and Miller[110] and by Alagille and colleagues.[108,109] It is a familial disease with a wide variability in its clinical spectrum, even within individual pedigrees. The list of abnormalities associated with the syndrome has steadily increased since the initial descriptions, but the principal manifestations have remained essentially unchanged (Table 50.1-4).

GENETICS OF AGS

The prevalence of AGS has been reported to be 1 per 100,000 births.[123] This certainly underestimates the true frequency because many symptomatic patients with cardiac disease and mildly affected individuals are not included. There is an equal gender incidence. The family

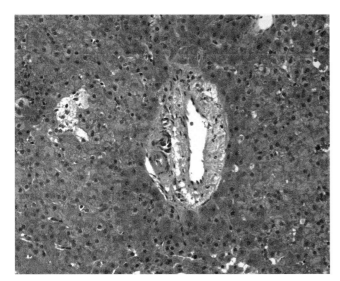

FIGURE 50.1-8   Alagille syndrome. Liver biopsy from a 1-year-old male. Bile ducts are absent from the portal tracts (hematoxylin and eosin; ×200 original magnification).

TABLE 50.1-4   FEATURES OF ALAGILLE SYNDROME

FEATURE	%
Paucity	89
Cholestasis	95
Murmur	94
Vertebral	68
Facies	94
Ocular	81
Renal	44
Growth retardation	68
Developmental delay	7.5
Intracranial bleeding	13

Adapted from references 111, 112, 116–119.

history is positive for related clinical features in at least 15 to 23% of pedigrees,[109,112,117] although this underestimates the number of family members with subclinical forms of the disease or with mutations in *JAG1*. Pedigree analysis in families with multiple affected members demonstrated an autosomal dominant pattern of inheritance, with low penetrance and a great variability of expression.[109,112,117,124–127] For probands with an identified mutation in *JAG1*, mutational analysis of the family members has recently demonstrated that 56 to 70% are new mutations, not present in either parent.[128,129]

A small number of patients have been reported to have cytogenetically visible deletions of chromosome 20. These visible deletions, however, are rare, occurring in 2 to 7% of patients.[128–130] A translocation that segregates concordantly with three affected family members confirmed the location of the Alagille gene region at 20p12.[131] Rare cytologically invisible microdeletions have been identified.[132] The multiple reports of 20p deletions led to the incorrect hypothesis that AGS is a contiguous gene deletion syndrome. In 1997, two groups, Li and colleagues and Oda and colleagues, reported that AGS is due to a single gene defect in *JAG1*.[121,122] *JAG1* encodes a cell-surface protein that functions as a ligand for the Notch transmembrane receptor. The Notch pathway has been well studied in *Drosophila melanogaster* and *Caenorhabditis elegans*.[133] The system is highly evolutionarily conserved. The Notch pathway is present in many cell types during development, where it serves to regulate cell fate decisions. The name was derived from the notched wing appearance seen in *D. melanogaster* mutants. The multiple manifestations of AGS in humans suggest that Jagged and Notch interactions are critical for normal embryogenesis of the heart, kidney, eye, face, skeleton, and other organs affected in AGS.[134,135] Multiple Notch receptors and ligands have been identified in humans. Defects in *Notch3* have been identified as the cause of cerebral autosomal dominant arteriopathy with subcortical infarcts and leukoencephalopathy (CADASIL) syndrome.[136] Mutations in another Notch pathway ligand, delta-like 3 (*DLL3*), have been linked to the skeletal disorder spondylocostal dysostosis.[137] The other Notch receptors and ligands have not, as yet, been linked to specific clinical syndromes in humans.

JAG1 encodes a protein with a large extracellular domain, a transmembrane domain, and a smaller intra-cellular portion. Several regions of the protein are similar in all species studied. Mutations in the gene, however, have not been confined to those regions. A large number of mutations in *JAG1* have now been reported[121,122,128,129,138,139] and are found in approximately 70% of individuals by current techniques.[140] Of these, approximately 4% are gene deletion, 49% are protein truncating frameshift or nonsense mutations, 9% are splice-site mutations, and 9% are missense mutations. In 30%, no mutation was identified.[141] The relatively low percentage of missense mutations is interesting. Although there does not appear to be any phenotypic difference between patients with total gene deletion and those with isolated defects, it is possible that missense mutations might cause milder variants of AGS or perhaps even single-organ abnormalities. Abnormalities in *JAG1* could theoretically cause disease by either of two mechanisms. It appears that having only one normal copy of *JAG1* (haploinsufficiency) is not sufficient for normal embryogenesis in humans. The alternative theory, a dominant negative effect caused by abnormal protein, is not supported by the presence of disease in humans with a total gene deletion. The role of *JAG1* in human embryogenesis is not understood, but studies are under way to assess its role in hepatic and cardiac development.[134,135,142]

Gene testing for AGS is currently available on a research basis. Evaluation by fluorescent in situ hybridization (FISH) for deletions at 20p12 is more widely available but is likely to identify only about 5% of mutations causing AGS. A negative result may be misleading. Molecular testing is available in several centers but is difficult owing to the large size of the gene and the lack of significant mutational hot spots. The majority of mutations identified to date are unique and scattered widely across the gene. In addition, current evaluations cannot identify a mutation in approximately 30% of clearly affected probands.[129] When a defect can be identified in a proband, however, it is then easy and useful to identify relatives who are minimally affected yet carry a significant risk to their offspring. Also, it can help to reassure parents of patients with de novo mutations. Prenatal testing is available but only if the mutation is identified in the proband. Testing has also aided in the diagnosis of AGS for patients with minor or atypical manifestations. Given the relatively large number of patients in whom no mutation has yet been identified, it remains possible that other Notch/ligand gene defects or other unrelated genes may account for some patients diagnosed clinically as having AGS. The similarities between AGS with the 22q contiguous gene deletion syndromes are instructive in that the features of heart disease, posterior embryotoxon, and butterfly vertebrae are common to both disorders.[143] A FISH analysis for 22q deletions should be completed in all patients with potentially overlapping syndromes, particularly if liver disease and duct paucity are not prominent features.

HISTOPATHOLOGY OF THE LIVER IN AGS

There are numerous publications describing the histopathologic features of the liver in AGS.[106,111,112,117,118,144–149] Although Alagille based his original diagnosis of the syndrome on a bile duct to portal tract ratio less than 0.5,[111] the presence and extent of bile duct paucity vary, largely as a result of the different ages of the patients at the time of biopsy.[112,117,118,149] There is ample evidence that the number of bile ducts may at first be normal in infants with AGS and that paucity develops with time.[112,144,148,149] Studies of serial liver biopsies have demonstrated that in up to 50% of initial biopsies of patients with AGS less than 6 months or 1 year of age, the bile duct to portal tract ratio is normal, with paucity observed in 90% of those older than 1 year of age.[117,118] The overall frequency of bile duct paucity in AGS also varies with the criteria used in establishing the diagnosis, being a requirement for diagnosis in older studies, whereas in more recent ones, which rely on nonhepatic manifestations and the presence of *JAG1* mutations, paucity is identified in 80 to 85% of patients.[140]

Proliferation of bile ducts has been reported in early biopsies of patients with AGS,[146,150] mimicking extrahepatic biliary obstruction, a diagnostic difficulty compounded by abnormal cholangiograms that fail to visualize the hypoplastic extrahepatic biliary tree.[117,148] Diagnostic confusion with extrahepatic biliary atresia has resulted in Kasai portoenterostomies being performed, with variable results in mortality and progression of disease. Evidence of bile duct damage may be inferred by the findings of a piling up of the epithelium, nuclear pyknosis and pleomorphism, epithelial vacuolization, lymphocytic infiltration of the biliary epithelium, and peribiliary fibrosis. Other morphologic changes observed in early infancy include hepatocellular giant cell transformation with extramedullary hematopoiesis (neonatal giant cell hepatitis) and intralobular cholestasis. Portal spaces are usually not expanded but may contain a mild mononuclear inflammatory infiltrate. A reduction in the number of portal spaces, as observed by Hadchouel and colleagues,[147] may reflect an abnormal vasculature.

Hepatectomy specimens obtained at transplant are typically nodular but variably cholestatic. Late histologic changes include portal expansion and fibrosis, with bridging in approximately 50% of patients and cirrhosis in up to one-quarter.[117] The fibrosis has been observed by Hashida and Yunis to be more severe at the hilum.[149] Paucity of bile ducts is by then usually well established, and there is prominent lobular cholestasis. Bile ductular proliferation at that late stage is uncommon and may indicate a concomitant process, such as cholangitis.[151] Edema of the portal spaces, with dilatation of the lymphatics and veins, has been noted.[149] Other changes noted include hepatocellular degeneration and "pseudoxanthomatous" transformation, pseudorosette formations, increased hepatocellular copper, and sinusoidal fibrosis.[144] Electron microscopic observation of bile pigment accumulation in the Golgi apparatus, in concert with normal-appearing canaliculi, was reported as distinctive ultrastructural features in AGS,[152] although its significance has been disputed by others.[153]

Narrowing and hypoplasia of the extrahepatic biliary tree have been observed by cholangiography in both autopsy and hepatectomy specimens[111,144,146,149,151] and decreased filling of intrahepatic branches by endoscopic retrograde cholangiopancreatography.[154]

Hepatocellular carcinomas have been reported with AGS in children as young as 4 years of age,[155–160] as well as later in life.[161,162] Familial occurrence of hepatocellular carcinomas has also been observed,[162] with three of four siblings affected in one family.[163] Nodular hyperplasia, in some cases involving an entire lobe, has been reported in a few cases.[164,165] The significance of reported associations with thyroid cancer[166] and colonic polyposis[167] awaits further studies.

RENAL HISTOMORPHOLOGY IN AGS

A variety of developmental and acquired renal abnormalities have been reported in AGS,[111,117,118,120,168–176] some leading to renal insufficiency, either early in infancy or later. These include medullary and cortical cysts,[171,174,175] renal hypoplasia,[169] ureteropelvic obstruction and bifid ureters, and renal artery stenoses.[176] The most frequently reported and most characteristic finding is deposition of lipids in the glomerular mesangium and basement membranes, resulting in a membranoproliferative pattern.[170–172] Lipid in the glomeruli can be demonstrated by histochemical stains on frozen sections or by electron microscopy.[171] According to Habib and colleagues, the glomerular lipidosis does not appear to be related either to the age of the patients or the degree of hypercholesterolemia but rather to the severity of cholestasis.[170]

CLINICAL MANIFESTATIONS OF AGS

AGS usually presents in the first 3 months of life in symptomatic patients. It is one of the more common etiologies of cholestasis and jaundice in the neonatal period and must be distinguished from biliary atresia and nonsyndromic bile duct paucity. In older children, AGS may present as a chronic hepatic disease. It is common for an adult to be diagnosed only after recognition of AGS in a severely affected child. The diagnosis is made when characteristic or compatible liver histology is accompanied by the major extrahepatic findings of the syndrome: chronic cholestasis, characteristic facies, cardiac murmur, vertebral anomalies, and posterior embryotoxon.

The extreme variability of the clinical manifestations and the incomplete penetrance of the syndrome obscure the diagnosis. Some patients demonstrate progressive pruritus, cirrhosis, or liver failure, resulting in liver transplant. Others have few or no symptoms and remain undiagnosed as adults.

Although most patients present with hepatic manifestations, the associated cardiac disease generally accounts for the majority of the early mortality.[111,112,117]

Hepatic Manifestations. The majority of symptomatic patients present in infancy and will have manifestations of hepatic disease ranging from mild cholestasis and pruritus to progressive liver failure. The severity of the disease in the parent is of no prognostic value as to severity in relatives or in subsequent children.[125] The degree of hepatic disease does not correlate with the severity of the other systemic manifestations, such as cardiac disease.

Hepatomegaly, with a firm or normal consistency, is recognized in nearly all patients.[61] Splenomegaly is rare in infancy but appears in one-third to two-thirds by the second decade.[111,112]

The most common laboratory abnormalities are elevations of serum bile aids, conjugated bilirubin, alkaline phosphatase, and γ-glutamyl transpeptidase, which suggest a defect in biliary excretion in excess of the abnormalities in hepatic metabolism or synthesis. There are elevations of the serum aminotransferases, up to 10-fold, which may persist throughout childhood. However, in general, metabolic regulation of transamination, urea synthesis, glucose homeostasis, and protein synthesis is well maintained.

Jaundice is present in the majority of symptomatic patients and presents as a conjugated hyperbilirubinemia in the neonatal period. In half of these infants, it is persistent, resolving only in later childhood. Jaundice commonly is noted during intercurrent illnesses, but the magnitude of the hyperbilirubinemia is minor compared with the degree of cholestasis. Cholestasis is manifest by pruritus and elevations in serum bile acid concentrations. This pruritus is among the most severe in any chronic liver disease. It is rarely present before 3 to 5 months of age[111,112] but is seen in nearly all symptomatic children by the third year of life, even in those who are anicteric.[111,112]

The presence of severe cholestasis results in the formation of xanthomas, characteristically on the extensor surfaces of the fingers, the palmar creases, nape of the neck, popliteal fossa, and buttocks and around inguinal trauma sites. The lesions persist throughout childhood but may gradually disappear after 10 years of age.[177] The timing for the formation of xanthomas relates to the severity of the cholestasis and correlates with a serum cholesterol greater than 500 mg/dL. Hypercholesterolemia and hypertriglyceridemia may be profound, reaching levels exceeding 1,000 mg/mL and 2,000 mg/mL, respectively, with the expected abnormalities in lipoproteinemia. The incidence of atheromata is unknown, but they have been reported as early as 4 years of age in a child found at autopsy to have extensive aortic and endocardial fat deposition.[112]

Hepatic synthetic function is usually well preserved. Serum albumin and ammonia are typically normal, as is the prothrombin time (with adequate vitamin K supplementation). Nevertheless, progression to cirrhosis and hepatic failure, initially reported to be uncommon, is recognized in approximately 20% of patients with AGS.

Malnutrition and Growth Failure. Diminished bile salt excretion and low intraluminal bile salt concentrations result in ineffective solubilization and absorption of dietary lipid, essential fatty acids, and fat-soluble vitamins. The deficiency of fat-soluble vitamins has profound systemic effects. Coagulopathy (vitamin K deficiency), rickets (vitamin D deficiency), retinopathy (vitamin E and A deficiency), and a peripheral neuropathy and myopathy (vitamin E deficiency) may occur.[178]

Growth failure is a common feature (50–90%) during childhood with delayed pubertal development. This is thought to be the result of caloric deprivation from fat malabsorption, the intrinsic vertebral and skeletal abnormalities, and perhaps a secondary abnormality in endocrine function

as demonstrated by elevated growth hormone levels with diminished somatomedin production.[179] Ponderal and linear growth is commonly delayed in the first 3 years of life, and this growth failure is due, at least in part, to significant acute and chronic wasting.[180] Patients with growth failure appear to be insensitive to exogenous growth hormone.[179]

Cardiovascular Manifestations. A wide range of cardiovascular abnormalities have been reported in patients with syndromic paucity.[111,117,181,182] An audible murmur is present at some time in 97% of patients.[117] The most common lesions are pulmonary artery stenoses at various sites in the proximal and distal tree, commonly at bifurcations. The entire pulmonary vascular tree may be hypoplastic, either alone or in association with other cardiovascular lesions. Among these, tetralogy of Fallot (TOF) is the most common (7–12%). Other lesions include truncus arteriosus, secundum atrial septal defect, patent ductus arteriosus, ventriculoseptal defects, and pulmonary atresia. Systemic vascular anomalies, including coarctation of the aorta, renal artery stenosis, and small carotid arteries, occur sporadically.[182] Although the majority of cardiac and vascular lesions are of no hemodynamic consequence, significant lesions do occur and in some series have been the predominant cause of early death.[111,112,117] In a large series of patients, Emerick and others demonstrated that only cardiac disease predicted increased mortality in AGS patients.[117] Many patients with intracardiac structural defects have concomitant pulmonic or peripheral pulmonic stenosis, and there is increased mortality following cardiac surgery for these lesions. Survival of AGS patients with TOF was 66% and with TOF with pulmonary atresia was only 25%.[117] In a recent, large study, McElhinney and colleagues reported the cardiac manifestions of 200 patients with a *JAG1* mutation or clinical AGS (or both), predominantly evaluated by cardiologists and/or by echocardiography.[182] A total of 187 subjects (94%) had evidence of cardiovascular involvement.[182] Of the 150 patients with anomalies characterized by imaging, right-sided anomalies were present in 123 and left-sided anomalies in 22, with both in 12.[182] The most common abnormality was stenosis or hyposplasia of the branch pulmonary arteries in 76%. TOF was seen in 23 (12% of all patients) and was accompanied by pulmonary atresia in one-third, a frequency higher than that seen in non-AGS TOF. The majority of patients with TOF-pulmonary atresia died early on. There was no clear difference in the cardiac disease seen in patients in whom a *JAG1* mutation was or was not identified.[182] Although, in general, genotype-phenotype correlations are rare with *JAG1* mutations, Eldadah and colleagues reported a large kindred with autosomal dominant TOF with reduced penetrance correlated with a missense mutation in *JAG1*.[183] Nine of 11 mutation carriers manifested cardiac disease, including TOF, pulmonic atresia, pulmonic stenosis, and absent pulmonary valve, yet none of the affected individuals met the diagnostic criteria for AGS.

Cardiac disease may also account in part for the increased post–liver transplant mortality seen in some series. Accordingly, it is advisable to seek formal diagnosis for any murmur in a patient with hepatic disease. Doppler echocardiography is usually sufficient in structural cardiac disease, but cardiac catheterization or digital subtraction arteriography may be necessary for diagnosis in some cases.[184]

Recently, patients with congenital cardiac disease but without apparent AGS have been evaluated by molecular techniques for mutations in *JAG1*. Patients with nonsyndromic TOF patients at one cardiac center were found to have unsuspected defects in *JAG1*.[185] Other lesions, such as multigenerational peripheral pulmonic stenosis without apparent AGS, have also been demonstrated to have defects in *JAG1* by mutational analysis.[185] Loomes and others have shown that the expression of *JAG1* in the developing mammalian heart correlates with the cardiovascular disease seen in AGS.[142] The similarity of the severe cardiac disease, particularly TOF, to other genetic syndromes such as 22q deletion is not yet understood.

Characteristic Facies. Characteristic facies are described in the original reports of syndromic bile duct paucity. These consist of a prominent forehead, moderate hypertelorism with deep-set eyes, a small pointed chin, and a saddle or straight nose that, in profile, may be in the same plane as the forehead (Figure 50.1-9).[111] The facies may be present at birth but, in general, become more obvious with increasing age. The usefulness of the facies as a major criterion for diagnosis of AGS has been challenged because of interobserver differences. It has been suggested that these facies are a common result of early and chronic cholestasis,[186] but the constellation of findings and the finding of typical facies in asymptomatic parents may be striking. In a recent study, clinical dysmorphologists were able to distinguish via photographs infants and children with AGS from others with liver disease with a high degree of sensitivity and specificity.[187] Identification of facies in adults was less accurate. Kamath and colleagues have emphasized that the facies change over time and that the characteristic facies of an adult do not, in fact, directly resemble the facies in childhood but do resemble other adults with the gene defect.[187] With time, the chin becomes

more prominent and the forehead becomes less dominant, resulting in a face with a predominant lower portion in contrast to the upper prominence of early childhood (Figure 50.1-10). Identification of these adults, who commonly have minimal signs and symptoms of AGS, would help hepatologists in the evaluation of adults with idiopathic cardiac, hepatic, or renal disease. Further evidence that *JAG1* mutations are directly involved in the development of characteristic facies include the demonstration of *JAG1* expression in the facial structures of developing mouse and human embryos[134,135] and the presence of characteristic facies in subjects with no history or evidence of clincal liver disease or cholestasis.

Vertebral and Musculoskeletal Abnormalities. Vertebral abnormalities are described in the initial reports of this syndrome.[109] The most characteristic finding is the sagittal cleft or butterfly vertebrae (Figure 50.1-11). This relatively uncommon anomaly may occur in normal individuals. The affected vertebral bodies are split sagittally into paired hemivertebrae owing to a failure of the fusion of the anterior arches of the vertebrae. Generally, these are asymptomatic and of no structural significance. The mildly affected vertebrae will have a central lucency. A fully affected vertebrae will have a pair of separate triangular hemivertebrae whose apices face each other like the wings of a butterfly. Although these abnormalities are present from birth, they are often unrecognized at the time of evaluation for neonatal hepatitis, only to be identified on spine films taken later. Other associated skeletal abnormalities include an abnormal narrowing of the adjusted interpeduncular space in the lumbar spine in half of the patients,[109,188] a pointed anterior process of C1, spina bifida occulta,[189] fusion of the adjacent vertebrae, hemivertebrae, and the presence of a bony connection between ribs.[110] The fingers may seem short, with short distal phalanges, broad thumbs, and fifth finger clinodactyly. A characteristic supernumerary digital flexion crease has been reported in 35% of AGS subjects compared with 1% of the general population.[190] Markedly decreased bone density and pathologic fractures are com-

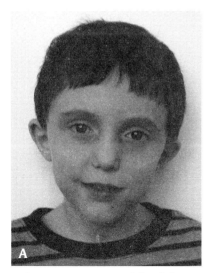
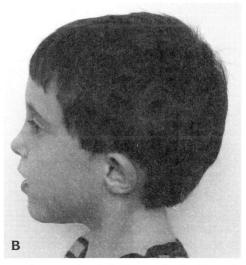
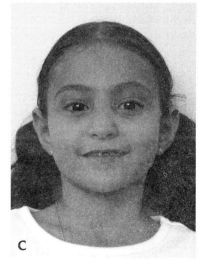

FIGURE 50.1-9   Typical facial characteristics of two unrelated children with Alagille syndrome.

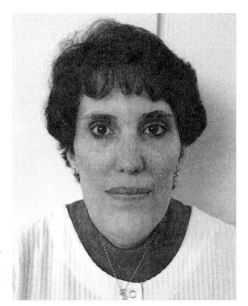
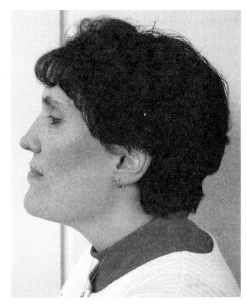

FIGURE 50.1-10 Typical facial characteristics of an adult with Alagille syndrome.

monly seen in patients with AGS and significant cholestasis. This may be due to a combination of fat and calcium malabsorption, vitamin D and K deficiency, magnesium[191] or zinc deficiency, copper excess, or chronic malnutrition.

Ocular Abnormalities. A large and varied number of abnormalities have been described in AGS, including abnormalities of the cornea, iris, retina, and optic disk. A

few of the findings are secondary to chronic vitamin deficiencies. Of the primary ocular abnormalities, posterior embryotoxon is the most important diagnostically. Posterior embryotoxon is a prominent, centrally positioned Schwalbe ring (or line), at the point where the corneal endothelium and the uveal trabecular meshwork join (Figure 50.1-12). Posterior embryotoxon occurs in up to 89% of patients with AGS,[111] but it also occurs in 8 to 15% of

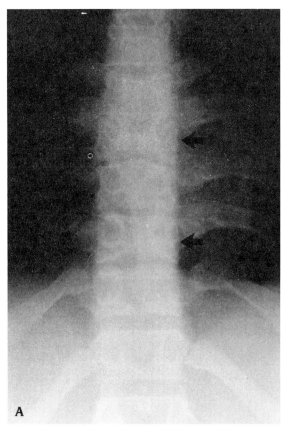
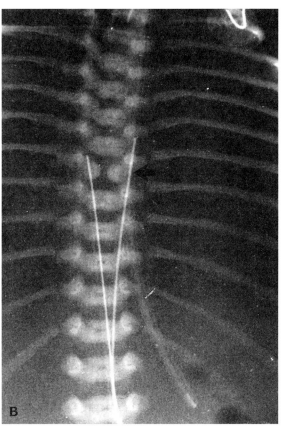

FIGURE 50.1-11 *A,* Multiple butterfly vertebrae (*arrows*) in an adolescent with Alagille syndrome. *B,* Fully affected vertebrae (*arrow*) with separate triangular vertebrae in a neonate with severe congenital heart disease and Alagille syndrome.

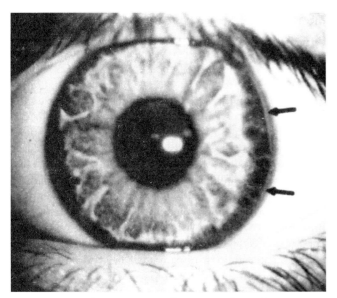

FIGURE 50.1-12   Posterior embryotoxon (*arrow*), prominent Schwalbe line.

normal eyes when evaluated by an ophthalmologist. Posterior embryotoxon can be part of an anterior chamber malformation syndrome. These malformations fall into three groups of peripheral and central abnormalities. Many of these abnormalities have now been reported in AGS. The Axenfeld anomaly is a prominent Schwalbe ring with attached iris strands. In general, about 50% of normal patients with this anomaly develop glaucoma, and glaucoma has been reported likewise in AGS.[192] The Rieger anomaly (primary mesodermal dysgenesis) is a prominent Schwalbe ring with attached iris strands and hypoplastic anterior iris stroma. This autosomal dominant inherited malformation has also been demonstrated in a patient with AGS.[193] Nischal found ultrasonographic evidence of optic disk drusen in at least one eye in 95% and bilateral disk drusen in 80% of patients with AGS but in none of the non-AGS liver patients they studied. This is markedly higher than the incidence in the normal population (0.3–2%), suggesting that this ophthalmologic sign may be an extremely useful diagnostic tool.[194] A peculiar mosaic pattern of iris stromal hypoplasia is present in many patients.[195] In addition, microcornea, keratoconus, congenital macular dystrophy, shallow anterior chambers, exotropia, ectopic pupil, band keratopathy, choroidal folds, and anomalous optic disks have been reported.[196,197] Other ocular findings, including retinal pigmentary changes, are identified in many patients with cholestasis but are not specific for the syndrome and are attributed to fat-soluble vitamin deficiencies.

Central and Peripheral Nervous System Abnormalities.
Significant mental retardation (IQ less than 80) is a prominent feature in the initial reports of syndromic paucity.[109,115] More recent estimates are lower, perhaps owing to earlier recognition of the syndrome, the identification of less severely affected individuals, or more aggressive nutritional management. Although only 2% of children had mild mental retardation in one series, 16% had delays in gross motor

skills.[117] Current studies emphasize the impact of chronic liver disease on brain development regardless of etiology[198,199] and focus on the role of vitamin E therapy and aggressive nutritional management with intervention programs to optimize outcome. No controlled trials are yet available to fully evaluate these claims. Abnormal visual, auditory, and somatosensory evoked potentials have been noted in AGS patients. These were not explained solely on the basis of fat-soluble vitamin deficiency. Visual evoked potentials returned to normal following resolution of the cholestasis with transplant. Dystonia and tremor associated with elevated whole-blood manganese levels and symmetric hyperintense basal ganglia magnetic resonance signals were seen in one patient with AGS.[200] This resolved following transplant. The possibility exists that neurologic findings in AGS are due to a combination of genetic and vascular abnormalities, chronic nutritional depletion, specific fat-soluble vitamin deficiencies, and toxins accumulated owing to deficient hepatic excretion and chronic cholestasis. A recent report details a family with dominantly inherited deafness, associated with congenital cardiac disease (including TOF) and posterior embryotoxon, without other features of AGS.[201] Affected individuals in this family had a missense mutation of *JAG1*, which segregated with the disease.

Intracranial bleeding has more recently been recognized to be a feature of AGS.[116,117] It occurs in up to 14% of patients and is a significant cause of morbidity and mortality. There is no pattern to the site of bleeding, which varies from epidural to subarachnoid to intraparenchymal. It may be associated with coagulopathy, although most patients had minimal or no abnormalities in clotting. Minor head trauma, to a degree unlikely to cause bleeding, was a factor in a minority of cases. Most were apparently spontaneous bleeds. A prospective study of magnetic resonance angiography was unable to identify any abnormalities, including one small aneurysm that resulted in a fatal subarachnoid hemorrhage (D. A. Piccoli, unpublished data, 1998). The data suggest that a central nervous system vasculopathy may be an intrinsic part of the multisystem abnormalities seen in AGS. Vascular abnormalities have been reported in other organs, including the kidneys and the lungs of patients with AGS. Furthermore, another Notch-related disorder in humans, CADASIL, is a dominantly inherited stroke disorder owing to defects in human *Notch3*. The occurrence and severity of strokes in AGS are not seen in other forms of pediatric liver diseases and thus should be considered as a primary complication of AGS. Careful correction of coagulopathy and observation after head trauma may decrease morbidity and mortality in some cases, but prediction or prevention of intracranial hemorrhage is not currently possible. Moyamoya syndrome, another form of vasculopathy, has been reported in children with AGS.[202] In addition, Lykavieris and colleagues reported a striking frequency of significant bleeding seen in 38 of 174 AGS patients not in liver failure who experienced a total of 49 significant events.[203] Although severe cholestasis was present in most, the majority of patients had normal coagulation and platelet studies. It is unclear if this bleeding tendency is a pleiotrophic consequence of cholestasis or a primary genetic defect in vascular integrity or hemostasis. In this study, however, eight patients died secondary to the bleeding, half following a surgical episode.

DIAGNOSIS: CLINICAL CRITERIA

The specific diagnosis of AGS can be established only by the clinical phenotype. Alagille and colleagues proposed diagnostic criteria for this disorder based on the presence of five major abnormalities. In addition to proper hepatic histopathology, the major criteria are chronic cholestasis, characteristic facies, cardiac murmur, vertebral abnormalities, and posterior embryotoxon.[111] The frequency of these abnormalities compiled from several large series is shown in Table 50.1-5.[111,112,117-119]

Because nearly all patients with significant bile duct paucity will manifest some degree of chronic cholestasis, Alagille and colleagues recommend the use of the other four criteria (facies, murmur, vertebral anomalies, and posterior embryotoxon) to define the syndrome.[111] In 36% of patients, all four features were present. Another 52% had three of the four features, and 12% had only two. Based on these data, Alagille and colleagues recommended that the diagnosis be made with cholestasis and two of the other four abnormalities. The need for more accurate criteria is emphasized by the 8 to 15% frequency of embryotoxon in the general population, the subjective nature of facies assessment, the potential difficulties in assigning a pathologic basis to a mild systolic flow murmur, and the incidence of cardiac disease in biliary atresia (10%), congenital rubella, and deletions of 22q. Furthermore, these data are derived only from significantly affected individuals, who, in

the majority of cases, are the affected proband in a family. It is clear from recent genetic studies that family members carrying a mutation in *JAG1* may have few, if any, overt signs of AGS. When tested, most relatives of AGS patients with even isolated manifestations have the mutation.[141] Thus, patients with isolated cardiac disease or apparently nonsyndromic paucity may have mutations in *JAG1*. Although the diagnosis of AGS in a proband should not be established on the basis of fewer than three clinical criteria, it can be suggested. Molecular testing should help to further define these mildly affected patients and their relatives.

In the majority of patients, the hepatic manifestations of the disease dominate the clinical picture. Patients may present with neonatal hepatitis, jaundice, pruritus, cholestasis, or cardiac disease or may be identified as asymptomatic siblings (or parents). The syndrome must be distinguished from other etiologies of neonatal hepatitis and from extrahepatic obstructions such as biliary atresia. The usual evaluation will include an initial laboratory evaluation to identify other etiologies, followed by a sonogram, nuclear scintiscan, liver biopsy, and possibly operative cholangiogram.

An infant with AGS will usually have an elevated conjugated bilirubin and moderately elevated levels of the aminotransferases. The γ-glutamyl transpeptidase, alkaline phosphatase, serum bile acids, and cholesterol may be dramatically elevated, but none of these findings aid in the discrimination of syndromic bile duct paucity from biliary atresia or other causes of extrahepatic obstruction.

Although there is no evidence of mechanical extrahepatic obstruction in AGS, differentiation from biliary atresia can be difficult.[110,111,117,204] Ultrasound examination may

TABLE 50.1-5   CLINICAL MANIFESTATIONS OF ALAGILLE SYNDROME

SYSTEM	FINDINGS
Hepatic	Duct paucity, cholestasis, neonatal hepatitis, fibrosis, cirrhosis, portal hypertension, liver failure, hepatocellular carcinoma, nodular hamartoma
Cardiac	Murmur, pulmonic valvular stenosis, tetralogy of Fallot, pulmonary atresia, truncus arteriosus, ventricular septal defect complex, ventricular septal defect, atrial septal defect, anomalous venous return
Vascular	Peripheral pulmonic stenosis, pulmonary outflow stenosis, coarctation, patent ductus arteriosus, renal artery stenosis, middle aorta syndrome, moyamoya
Skeletal	Butterfly vertebrae, shortened interpedicular distance, shortened phalanges, short stature, spina bifida occulta, fusion of adjacent vertebrae, absent twelfth rib, shortened distal ulna and radius, clubbing, pathologic fractures, osteopenia, rickets
Ocular	Posterior embryotoxon, Axenfeld anomaly, Rieger anomaly, shallow anterior chamber, cataracts, strabismus, exotropia, ectopic pupil, optic disk drusen, iris stromal hypoplasia, band keratopathy, glaucoma, microcornea, keratoconus, congenital macular dystrophy, anomalous optic disks, fundic hyperpigmentation, pigmentary retinopathy, night blindness
Facial/cranial	Characteristic pediatric "particular facies," adult "particular facies," sinus abnormalities, chronic sinusitis, thinned cortical bones, deafness, large ears, high-pitched voice, macrocephaly
Renal	Neonatal renal insufficiency, adult renal failure, solitary, ectopic, or horseshoe kidney, bifid pelvis, duplicated ureter, small kidney, cystic and multicystic kidney, dysplastic kidney, infantile renal tubular acidosis, juvenile nephronophthisis, lipidosis, tubulointerstitial nephropathy, interstitial fibrosis
Central nervous system	Intracranial epidural, subdural, subarachnoid, and intraparenchymal bleeding; stroke; vascular malformation; mental retardation; developmental delay; school dysfunction; abnormal visual, auditory, and somatosensory evoked potentials
Cutaneous	Jaundice, xanthomata, pruritus, thickened, lichenified hands and feet
Growth disorders	Failure to thrive, fat-soluble vitamin deficiency, protein-calorie malnutrition, short stature
Pancreatic	Exocrine insufficiency, diabetes mellitus, pancreatic fibrosis
Other	Tracheal and bronchial stenosis, jejunal atresia, ileal atresia, malrotation, microcolon, otitis media, extrahepatic malignancies

Adapted from references 111, 117, 119, 120, and 149.

not identify the extrahepatic tree owing to diminished gall-bladder size, and it is rarely diagnostic. Studies that may demonstrate patency of the extrahepatic biliary tree include technetium 99m disopropyl iminodiacetic acid (DISIDA) and similar scintiscans, radiologic cholangiography via either endoscopic retrograde cholangiopancreatography, percutaneous transhepatic cholangiography, gallbladder cholangiography, or operative cholangiography. A technetium-labeled scintiscan may show excretion into the duodenum in 39% of patients with AGS but in the remainder will not demonstrate communication (as is also seen in biliary atresia).[117]

In addition to the usefulness of DISIDA scintigraphy in the diagnosis of AGS in the neonatal period, there may be a characteristic pattern of excretion of tracer. Distinct retention of tracer in the periphery with central clearing in a young adult has been reported.[205] Studies have suggested that tracer excretion is uncommon in early infancy but may be demonstrable in the same patient later in childhood. In adults, tracer excretion is more common, and the pattern typically involves central clearing. This parallels the clinical progression of severe cholestasis seen in many patients with AGS and suggests that major ducts become the site of functional excretion in AGS.

The liver biopsy is the most useful preoperative study for the discrimination of syndromic bile duct paucity from extrahepatic biliary atresia. However, difficulties in histologic diagnosis may arise early in infancy because bile ductule proliferation may obscure duct paucity or because some ducts may, in fact, be present early in life. In very young infants in whom the percutaneous liver biopsy is not diagnostic, it may be helpful to delay exploration for 1 to 2 weeks and repeat the biopsy (while recognizing that the success of therapy for extrahepatic biliary atresia is correlated with surgery before 60 days of life).[206] If laparotomy is undertaken, an operative wedge biopsy should be obtained. An intraoperative cholangiogram performed by an experienced surgeon must be attempted and carefully interpreted prior to the construction of a portoenterostomy. The extrahepatic bile ducts are anatomically normal and patent in AGS but may be so narrow that operative cholangiography will fail to identify a patent system. Because operative cholangiography alone may result in an incorrect diagnosis of biliary atresia in up to 20% of cases,[117,204] a careful preoperative search should have been performed for the syndromic features. Hepatoportoenterostomy is inappropriate in AGS and may increase morbidity.[111,204] The correct diagnosis is also important for the genetic implications.

In older children, striking abnormalities are seen in fasting bile acid levels, serum lipids, γ-glutamyltransferase, and alkaline phosphatase. Bile acids in severe disease may be elevated 100-fold. The conjugated bilirubin is commonly moderately elevated. The magnitude of the hyperbilirubinemia is usually less than that of the bile acid elevation, and jaundice may disappear during childhood despite persistently elevated bile acids. Most patients have elevated triglyceride and cholesterol, which, in severe cases, may be from 1,000 to 2,000 mg/dL. Moderate elevations of the aminotransferases are common, although to lesser values than the γ-glutamyltransferase. In the majority of patients, the hepatic synthetic and metabolic functions are normal. Prothrombin time following parenteral vitamin K is usually normal. There may be deficiencies in substances requiring bile acids for absorption, such as vitamins A, D, E, and K, and essential fats.

TREATMENT

Infants with intrahepatic cholestasis may have significant fat malabsorption. Because half of the calories in infant formulas may be from fat, this defect contributes significantly to overall caloric deprivation. Medium-chain triglycerides are hydrolyzed and absorbed in the absence of bile salt micelle formation and thus are a significant caloric additive. Optimal diets include increased amounts of medium-chain triglycerides added to the diet and optimization of the carbohydrate and protein intake. Essential fatty acids may also be malabsorbed, resulting in clinically evident deficiency. This has resulted in acral lesions resembling porphyria, which have responded to parenteral supplementation of essential fatty acids.

Fat-soluble vitamin deficiency is present to a variable degree in most patients with bile duct paucity. Oral or parenteral supplementation is necessary for prevention of vitamin deficiencies. Further exacerbation of these deficiencies may be caused by therapy for cholestasis, such as phenobarbital or cholestyramine. Oral or intramuscular vitamin K will correct the coagulopathy in most patients, and its failure to do so may herald significant synthetic dysfunction. Aggressive therapy should be maintained in patients with clinical bleeding or evidence of significant hypersplenism. Rickets is seen in patients unless supplemented with oral or intramuscular vitamin D. Vitamin D absorption may be enhanced by administration of d-γ-tocopherol polyethylene glycol-1000 succinate (TPGS).[207] Early evidence of elevated serum alkaline phosphatase may be obscured, and serum levels of vitamin D should be checked at frequent intervals.

Deficiency of vitamins E and A may result in significant neurologic abnormalities, including cerebellar ataxia, peripheral neuropathy, abnormalities of extraocular movement, and retinopathy.[120,149,178,208] Vitamin E has been the most difficult to adequately supplement, although TPGS-soluble preparations are widely available. The TPGS is significantly more effective than other oral preparations and has been demonstrated to be effective in reversing neurologic damage in some patients.[209] The serum vitamin E level must be corrected for the serum lipid level in children with marked cholestasis. Vitamin A levels also should be monitored and oral or intramuscular replacement given as indicated. However, measurement of liver concentrations of vitamin A provides a more accurate indication of vitamin A status because serum levels of retinol and plasma retinol binding protein are still normal when hepatic stores of vitamin A are depleted.

Pruritus is the most significant symptom for many patients with chronic cholestasis. Antihistamines may give some relief, and care should be taken to keep the skin hydrated with emollients. Fingernails must be trimmed. Cholestyramine may improve pruritus in children who can be convinced to take sufficient amounts, but some children will develop a severe acidosis on this therapy.[210] Colesevelam is less well studied but may have some advantages over cholestyramine. Phenobarbital appears to have little effect on either jaundice or on pruritus, although it has proven effective in enhancing bile salt–independent bile formation. Ultraviolet therapy may give temporary relief of pruritus in some cases.[211] Rifampin, which inhibits uptake of bile acids into the hepatocyte, appears to provide significant relief of pruritus in approximately half of patients.[212,213] Ursodeoxycholic acid, a potent choleretic, may have a dramatic effect in reducing symptomatic cholestasis, although, in some patients, it appears to exacerbate pruritus. In other cholestatic diseases, such as sclerosing cholangitis and primary biliary cirrhosis, ursodeoxycholic acid has been demonstrated to improve biochemical parameters and symptoms and may possibly retard disease progression. Naltrexone, an opioid antagonist, has also been useful in some cases.[214] Emerick and Whitington treated nine patients with extreme cholestasis and pruritus with partial external biliary diversion and demonstrated a dramatic decrease in pruritus scores, mean serum bile salt levels, and serum cholesterol.[215] Surgical ileal exclusion has not been well studied in AGS but may provide a more cosmetically appealing alternative to external diversion.

PROGNOSIS

The outcome of syndromic bile duct paucity is highly variable and is most directly related to the severity of the hepatic and the cardiac lesions, with mortality predominantly attributable to these two organs. Complex congenital cardiac disease is a major cause of early mortality, although hepatic complications account for most of the later morbidity and mortality. These data are reflected in a follow-up study that reported a mortality rate of 26% (21 in 80) in 10 years, with only four deaths attributable to hepatic disease (portal hypertension in two and hepatic failure in two).[111] In another series, the predicted probability of survival to 20 years of age for all patients was 75%.[117] The probability of survival to age 20 was 80% for patients who did not require liver transplant and 60% in those who underwent transplant. Hepatic transplant may be required for chronic liver failure, portal hypertension, or severe intractable pruritus. Survival following transplant has varied significantly in different studies, from 45 to 100%.[60,61,116,117,156–158,216–218] Transplant does appear to have a higher risk for patients with AGS, owing in part to the severity of cardiopulmonary disease. Caution should be taken when considering relatives as potential donors for living-related transplant because unsuspected disease in the parent has thwarted donation.[219]

NONSYNDROMIC BILE DUCT PAUCITY

Nonsyndromic bile duct paucity is the term used to designate all instances of paucity except those occurring in AGS. It includes all nonsyndromic cases either with or without an associated primary disease. Thus defined, it covers such a great range of disorders that it is inappropriate to talk of a prognosis for nonsyndromic paucity generally. In some of these disorders, bile duct paucity is a characteristic feature (chronic allograft rejection) or a well-recognized association (α_1-antitrypsin deficiency) or outcome (biliary atresia). In others, bile duct paucity is an unusual and only infrequently reported finding. Most cases of nonsyndromic paucity are acquired, owing to either infections, immune-mediated injury (primary sclerosing cholangitis, primary biliary cirrhosis), or drugs and toxins, or in the setting of graft-versus-host disease (GVHD) or chronic allograft rejection. In those cases associated with a primary disorder, the principal determinant of outcome is usually the primary disease itself. In reviewing reports of supposed nonsyndromic paucity, it should also be kept in mind that there has been an inappropriate tendency to identify progressive intrahepatic cholestasis with paucity in the absence of histologic proof of paucity.

Only a few series of nonsyndromic cases have been published (earlier series of paucity probably include both syndromic and nonsyndromic cases because the syndrome has only relatively recently been recognized). Kahn and colleagues[220] and Alagille[221] have reported series based on histologic criteria. In the series of Kahn and colleagues, of 17 patients with nonsyndromic paucity, 9 were associated with well-defined primary diseases, including Down syndrome, hypopituitarism, cystic fibrosis, α_1-antitrypsin deficiency, cytomegalovirus (CMV) infection, and Ivemark syndrome. (In addition to these, other disorders, including congenital rubella, chromosomal abnormalities, GVHD, rejection of allograft livers, primary sclerosing cholangitis, and possibly Zellweger syndrome, have also been associated with paucity.[222]) In the remaining 8 cases in the series of Kahn and colleagues, the paucity was apparently primary or idiopathic (ie, not associated with any defined disease). The nonsyndromic cases had the clinical and general histopathologic picture of neonatal hepatitis. One of the most striking features in their series was that all of the nonsyndromic patients had paucity before the age of 90 days, whereas syndromic cases did not have paucity before 90 days of age. Their nonsyndromic cases also differed from their syndromic cases in that there was more portal fibrosis and less portal inflammation in the nonsyndromic cases. The clinical course of the patients with nonsyndromic paucity without underlying disease was not outlined in detail, but progressive liver disease was uncommon. Several aspects of this series deserve comment. Most authors have seen histologic paucity in occasional AGS patients before the age of 90 days, so this cannot be taken as an absolute criterion. It should also be noted that this study was conducted using needle biopsy specimens, and there is some lack of agreement as to how many portal tracts must be evaluated to obtain a statistically accurate estimate of bile duct numbers. As previously mentioned, in evaluating liver biopsies for paucity, it must be recognized, as pointed out by Kahn and colleagues, that in premature infants, a ratio of bile duct to portal tracts less than 0.9 may be normal.[107]

Alagille described 24 patients with nonsyndromic paucity who were classified into two groups: group I presented in the first few weeks of life with cholestasis, whereas group II presented later.[221] The groups differ histologically, with group I having portal inflammation, giant cell change, and minimal fibrosis and group II having more portal fibrosis and inflammation in relation to paucity. The outcome of these two groups is highly variable as half developed biliary cirrhosis and 38% died from hepatic failure. About one-third are anicteric, with only biochemical evidence of hepatic disease. Rubella was identified in one patient. It is of note that only 60% of these patients were screened for α_1-antitrypsin deficiency, but 29% of those tested were protease inhibitor type Z. Overall, therefore, it is not clear how many of the cases in this series were truly sporadic or idiopathic and how many were associated with primary diseases.

NONSYNDROMIC PAUCITY WITH PRIMARY DISEASE

Detailed discussions of the various primary diseases are presented elsewhere in this text, so the discussion here will be limited to the pathogenesis of paucity in those few primary conditions in which this pathogenesis is either partially understood or can be plausibly hypothesized.

In terms of paucity associated with well-defined primary diseases, it should be noted that (1) in virtually all of these, paucity is reported in only a small percentage of patients with these diseases, and (2) many of the diseases (eg, trihydroxycoprostanic acid excess, Ivemark syndrome) are themselves quite rare. From these facts, it is evident that a causal association between duct paucity and a number of these disorders is not well established.

BILE DUCT PAUCITY IN GVHD

Bile duct injury, sometimes eventuating in duct paucity, is one of the most distinctive hepatic lesions in GVHD. This injury is presumably the basis for the disappearance of ducts and potential paucity that occurs in some patients. It is unusual to find hepatic GVHD lesions in the absence of cutaneous manifestations of GVHD. The duct manifests injury by epithelial atypia, vacuolization, variable staining of nuclei and cytoplasm, and regeneration. Frank necrosis of epithelium can be seen on occasion. Accompanying the epithelial injury, there is often a lymphocytic infiltrate, sometimes with macrophages intermixed. On occasion, there is close proximity of lymphocytes and ducts and even invasion of the ducts by lymphocytes. In any single biopsy, however, it is not uncommon for the injury to be out of proportion to the inflammatory infiltrate, and the presence of endotheliilitis may be useful in indicating that the epithelial lesions reflect GVHD.[223] Centrilobular cholestasis is frequently present and is particularly intense when duct paucity has developed. The duct injury and paucity may be focal. Detailed reconstruction studies have suggested that the injury begins in relatively small ducts (± 30 μm in diameter).[224] When duct paucity is present in a patient with bone marrow transplant or when there is

prominent active duct destruction in such a patient, the diagnosis is quite straightforward, particularly in the absence of CMV infection. Reports of duct ultrastructure, which are uncommon, have described a number of rather nonspecific changes involving duct epithelium and basement membrane, as well as close contacts between epithelial cells and lymphocytes.[225,226] Immunohistochemical studies reveal increased numbers of HNK1+ (killer) cells, Leu 3+ cells, and expression of human leukocyte antigen (HLA)-DR (major histocompatibility complex class II) positivity by the epithelial cells.[224,227,228] The latter is not found in normal liver but is found in a variety of conditions affecting the bile ducts, many of which have been speculated to have an immune-related pathogenesis. The precise role and importance of these duct alterations in GVHD and the genesis of the duct lesions remain to be determined, but the effects may be mediated through the action of cytotoxic lymphocytes, as appears to be the situation in mucocutaneous GVHD.[229]

It is interesting to note that despite the rather common occurrence of bile duct injury in GVHD, including a number of cases with paucity of ducts, it is uncommon to find reports of cirrhosis, biliary or otherwise, in GVHD.[230,231] At least superficially, this seems analogous to the similarly infrequent development of progressive liver disease in syndromic bile duct paucity.

BILE DUCT PAUCITY IN LIVER ALLOGRAFT REJECTION

Bile duct injury is a significant element of the rejection of hepatic allografts,[223,232–235] and evidence of extensive damage (ie, involving greater than 50% of ducts) in a biopsy from a transplanted liver is regarded as strong evidence of acute rejection.[232] This damage is manifest by a variety of histologic features, including vacuolization of epithelial lining cells, variations in nuclei in these cells, and infiltration of the ducts by inflammatory cells. The latter are most commonly lymphocytes, but polys or eosinophils are not uncommon and may occasionally predominate. Active duct injury is accompanied by a lymphocytic or mixed portal infiltrate beyond the ducts. In a full-blown or classic case of cellular (acute) rejection, so-called endotheliilitis (together with duct injury and portal inflammatory infiltrate) forms the third element of a triad diagnostic for rejection.[232] If sufficiently severe, the injury may result in duct loss to the point of paucity, one of the histologic hallmarks of chronic rejection (Figure 50.1-13). The clinical presentation of chronic rejection may be either early or late, with the early-onset form typically occurring within 6 weeks of transplant. These patients often require urgent retransplant owing to the relentless progression of the liver disease. More commonly, patients with chronic rejection present between 6 weeks and 6 months following transplant with progressive jaundice and pruritus, following one or several episodes of acute rejection, or more insidiously, without apparent prior episodes of rejection. Histologically, chronic rejection is characterized by obliterative arteriopathy and bile duct injury, leading to bile duct loss. Degenerative changes in bile duct epithelium may be seen before significant bile duct loss.[236] Focal or transient paucity is not clinically or

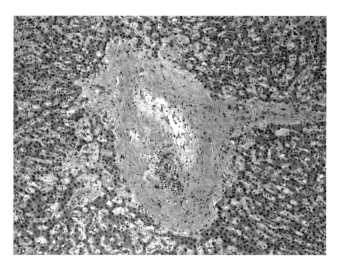

FIGURE 50.1-13   Bile duct paucity resulting from chronic rejection. Chronic rejection of a liver allograft 2 years following transplant. There is loss of bile ducts, with lymphocytic inflammation of the portal tracts and endotheliitis (hematoxylin and eosin; ×100 original magnification).

prognostically significant, but widespread persistent paucity is an ominous prognostic finding.[233] In hepatic allograft rejection, it is characteristic for portal tracts that have lost their ducts to show minimal or no inflammatory infiltrate. This probably speaks to the role of the infiltrating cells in the pathogenesis of the duct injury and loss.

BILE DUCT PAUCITY IN VIRAL INFECTIONS

Cholestatic liver disease with hepatocellular giant cell transformation and extramedullary hematopoiesis are frequent in congenital infection with CMV, among which are several well-documented cases of bile duct paucity, postulated to have resulted from an obliterative cholangitis.[237,238] Documentation of CMV-associated paucity in the preterm infant is more problematic because of the reasons stated earlier in the chapter.[239] Obliterative changes with focal loss of bile ducts have also been observed in congenital rubella[240] and in congenital syphilis.[241]

DRUG-ASSOCIATED BILE DUCT PAUCITY

Many different drugs have been reported to cause chronic cholestatic liver disease, defined as the persistence of jaundice for more than 6 months after withdrawal of the causative drug in a patient without previous hepatobiliary disease.[242] More recently, duct injury and loss have been documented, most frequently following the use of antibiotics such as penicillin derivatives, quinolones, tetracyclines, and sulfa drugs, among others.[243–247]

Early biopsies typically reveal an active nonsuppurative inflammatory destruction of bile ducts with evidence of epithelial damage such as vacuolization and nuclear pyknosis. The portal inflammatory infiltrate is usually lymphoid, occasionally with eosinophils, histiocytes, or small granulomas.[247–249] There typically is a lobular hepatic component with canalicular cholestasis. Persistent ductopenia with progression to fibrosis may evolve over the ensuing months even after the cessation of the medication. Pro-

gressive loss of intrahepatic bile ducts is noted in untreated cases, as early as 5 to 6 months, and occurs in most patients despite treatment, even when adequate biliary drainage is established.[250–253] Injury by bile stasis, peribiliary ischemia, and continuation of the original insult may all be contributing factors. Heterogeneity and unevenness in the distribution of bile duct loss and occasional nodules of better preserved parenchyma may reflect local differences in biliary obstruction or fibrosis.[250,254]

BILE DUCT PAUCITY IN EXTRAHEPATIC ATRESIA

The development of intrahepatic bile duct paucity in relatively long-surviving patients with biliary atresia was recognized prior to development of portoenterostomy and is also seen in patients following portoenterostomy, even when adequate biliary drainage is established.[250,251,253] Injury by bile stasis, peribiliary ischemia, and continuation of the original insult may all be contributing factors. Heterogeneity and unevenness in the distribution of bile duct loss and occasional nodules of better preserved parenchyma may reflect local differences in biliary obstruction or fibrosis.[250,254]

BILE DUCT PAUCITY IN PRIMARY SCLEROSING CHOLANGITIS

Primary sclerosing cholangitis is a chronic disorder of unknown etiology that is increasingly recognized in children. It is characterized by a generalized beading and stenosis of the biliary tree in the absence of choledocholithiasis, accompanied by histologic abnormalities of the bile ducts (Figure 50.1-14). It may occur in patients who are otherwise well but is often associated with inflammatory bowel disease. Secondary sclerosing cholangitis describes similar bile duct changes when a clearly predisposing factor such as choledocholithiasis or biliary surgery has been identified. There is progressive obliteration of the intra- and extrahepatic bile ducts, which may result in bile duct paucity, biliary cirrhosis, and liver failure.

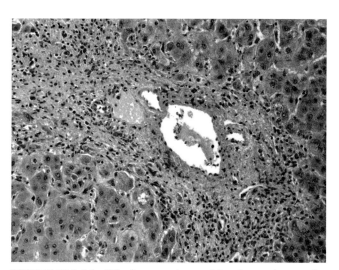

FIGURE 50.1-14   Bile duct paucity resulting from primary sclerosing cholangitis. Bile ducts are absent from the portal tracts. There is cholestasis in the adjacent hepatic lobule (hematoxylin and eosin; ×200 original magnification).

REFERENCES

1. Spagnoli FM, Amicone L, Tripodi M, Weiss MC. Identification of a bipotential precursor cell in hepatic cell lines derived from transgenic mice expressing cyto-Met in the liver. J Cell Biol 1998;143:1101–12.
2. Coffinier C, Gresh L, Fiette L, et al. Bile system morphogenesis defects and liver dysfunction upon targeted deletion of HNF1beta. Development 2002;129:1829–38.
3. Clotman F, Lannoy VJ, Reber M, et al. The onecut transcription factor HNF6 is required for normal development of the biliary tract. Development 2002;129:1819–28.
4. Desmet VJ. The cholangiopathies. In: Suchy FJ, Sokol R, Balistreri WF, editors. Liver disease in children. Philadelphia: Lippincott Williams and Wilkins; 2001. p. 39–63.
5. Desmet VJ. Ludwig symposium on biliary disorders—part I. Pathogenesis of ductal plate abnormalities. Mayo Clin Proc 1998;73:80–9.
6. Van Eyken P, Sciot R, Desmet V. Intrahepatic bile duct development in the rat: a cytokeratin-immunohistochemical study. Lab Invest 1988;59:52–9.
7. Nakanuma Y, Hoso M, Sanzen T, Sasaki M. Microstructure and development of the normal and pathologic biliary tract in humans, including blood supply. Microsc Res Tech 1997;38:552–70.
8. Jorgensen M. The ductal plate malformation. Acta Pathol Microbiol Scand Suppl 1977;257:1–87.
9. Bernstein J. Hepatic involvement in hereditary renal syndromes. Birth Defects 1987;21:115–30.
10. Kerr DNS, Harrison CV, Sherlock S, et al. Congenital hepatic fibrosis. QJM 1961;30:91–117.
11. Desmet VJ. Congenital diseases of intrahepatic bile ducts: variations on the theme "ductal plate malformation." Hepatology 1992;16:1069–83.
12. Crawford JM. Development of the intrahepatic biliary tree. Semin Liver Dis 2002;22:213–26.
13. Kanno N, LeSage G, Glaser S, et al. Functional heterogeneity of the intrahepatic biliary epithelium. Hepatology 2000;31:555–61.
14. Marzioni M, Glaser SS, Francis H, et al. Functional heterogeneity of cholangiocytes. Semin Liver Dis 2002;22:227–40.
15. Alpini G, McGill JM, Larusso NF. The pathobiology of biliary epithelia. Hepatology 2002;35:1256–68.
16. Donovan MJ, Kozakewich H, Perez-Atayde A. Solitary nonparasitic cysts of the liver: the Boston Children's Hospital experience. Pediatr Pathol Lab Med 1995;15:419–28.
17. Chu DY, Olson AL, Mishalany HG. Congenital liver cyst presenting as congenital diaphragmatic hernia. J Pediatr Surg 1986;21:897–9.
18. Vick DJ, Goodman ZD, Deavers MT, et al. Ciliated hepatic foregut cyst: a study of six cases and review of the literature. Am J Surg Pathol 1999;23:671–7.
19. Baron RL, Campbell WL, Dodd GD. Peribiliary cysts associated with severe liver disease: imaging-pathologic correlation. AJR Am J Roentgenol 1994;162:631–6.
20. Devaney K, Goodman ZD, Ishak KG. Hepatobiiary cystadenoma and cystadenocarcinoma. A light microscopic and immunohistochemical study of 70 patients. Am J Surg Pathol 1994;18:1078–91.
21. Ward CJ, Hogan MC, Rossetti S, et al. The gene mutated in autosomal recessive polycystic kidney disease encodes a large, receptor-like protein. Nat Genet 2002;30:259–69.
22. Onuchic LF, Furu L, Nagasawa Y, et al. PKHD1, the polycystic kidney and hepatic disease 1 gene, encodes a novel large protein containing multiple immunoglobulin-like plexin-transcription-factor domains and parallel beta-helix 1 repeats. Am J Hum Genet 2002;70:1305–17.
23. Fauvert R, Benhamou JP. Congenital hepatic fibrosis. In: Schaffner F, Scherlock S, Leery C, editors. The liver and its diseases. New York: Intercontinental Medical Book; 1974. p. 283.
24. Alvarez F, Bernard O, Brunelle F, et al. Congenital hepatic fibrosis in children. J Pediatr 1981;99:370–5.
25. Kerr DN, Okonkwo S, Choa RG. Congenital hepatic fibrosis: the long term prognosis. Gut 1978;19:514–20.
26. Fiorillo A, Migliorati R, Vajro P, et al. Congenital hepatic fibrosis with gastrointestinal bleeding in early infancy. Clin Pediatr 1982;21:183–5.
27. Odievre M, Chaumont P, Montagne JP, Alagille D. Anomalies of the intrahepatic portal venous system in congenital hepatic fibrosis. Radiology 1977;122:427–30.
28. Iitaka K, Sakai T. Clinical quiz. Renal tubular ectasia with congenital hepatic fibrosis. Pediatr Nephrol 1994;6:403–4.
29. Fonck C, Chauveau D, Gagnadoux MF, et al. Autosomal recessive polycystic kidney disease in adulthood. Nephrol Dial Transplant 2001;16:1648–52.
30. Hausner RJ, Alexander RW. Localized congenital hepatic fibrosis presenting as an abdominal mass. Hum Pathol 1978;9:473–6.
31. Leong AS. Segmental biliary ectasia and congenital hepatic fibrosis in a patient with chromosomal abnormality. Pathology 1980;12:275–81.
32. Daroca PJ Jr, Tuthill R, Reed RJ. Cholangiocarcinoma arising in congenital hepatic fibrosis. A case report. Arch Pathol 1975;99:592–5.
33. Naveh Y, Roguin N, Ludatscher R, et al. Congenital hepatic fibrosis with congenital heart disease. A family study with ultrastructural features of the liver. Gut 1980;21:799–807.
34. Dewhurst NG, Colledge NR, Miller HC. Severe pulmonary hypertension and multiple left coronary arterial fistulas in association with congenital hepatic fibrosis. Br Heart J 1987;58:525–7.
35. Maggiore G, Borgna-Pignatti C, Marni E, et al. Pulmonary arteriovenous fistulas: an unusual complication of congenital hepatic fibrosis. J Pediatr Gastroenterol Nutr 1983;2:183–6.
36. Kahn E, Markowitz J, Duffy L, et al. Berry aneurysms, cirrhosis, pulmonary emphysema, and bilateral symmetrical cerebral calcifications: a new syndrome. Am J Med Genet Suppl 1987;3:343–56.
37. Neumann HP, Krumme B, van Velthoven V, et al. Multiple intracranial aneurysms in a patient with autosomal recessive polycystic kidney disease. Nephrol Dial Transplant 1999;14:936–9.
38. Nishimura G, Nakayama M, Fuke Y, Suehara N. A lethal osteochondrodysplasia with mesomelic brachymelia, round pelvis, and congenital hepatic fibrosis: two siblings born to consanguineous parents. Pediatr Radiol 1998;28:43–7.
39. Pedersen PS, Tygstrup I. Congenital hepatic fibrosis combined with protein-losing enteropathy and recurrent thrombosis. Acta Paediatr Scand 1980;69:571–4.
40. Pelletier VA, Galeano N, Brochu P, et al. Secretory diarrhea with protein-losing enteropathy, enterocolitis cystica superficialis, intestinal lymphangiectasia, and congenital hepatic fibrosis: a new syndrome. J Pediatr 1986;108:61–5.
41. Vuillaumier-Barrot S, Le Bizec C, de Lonlay P, et al. Protein

losing enteropathy-hepatic fibrosis syndrome in Saguenay-Lac St-Jean, Quebec is a congenital disorder of glycosylation type Ib. J Med Genet 2002;39:849–51.

42. Alvarez F, Hadchouel M, Bernard O. Latent chronic cholangitis in congenital hepatic fibrosis. Eur J Pediatr 1982; 139:203–5.

43. Dusol M Jr, Levi JU, Glasser K, Schiff ER. Congenital hepatic fibrosis with dilation of intrahepatic bile ducts: a therapeutic approach. Gastroenterology 1976;71:839–43.

44. Murray Lyon IA, Shilkin KB, Laws JW, et al. Cholangitis complicating congenital hepatic fibrosis. Gut 1972;13:319.

45. Popovic-Rolovic M, Kostic M, Sundjic M, et al. Progressive tubulointerstitial nephritis and chronic cholestatic liver disease. Pediatr Nephrol 1993;7:396–400.

46. Hildebrandt F, Waldherr R, Kutt R, Brandis M. The nephronophthisis complex: clinical and genetic aspects. Clin Invest 1992;70:802–8.

47. Witzleben CL, Sharp AR. "Nephronophthisis-congenital hepatic fibrosis": an additional hepatorenal disorder. Hum Pathol 1982;13:728–33.

48. Landing BH, Wells TR, Lipsey AI, Oyemade OA. Morphometric studies of cystic and tubulointerstitial kidney diseases with hepatic fibrosis in children. Pediatr Pathol 1990;10:959–72.

49. Caridi G, Murer L, Bellantuono R, et al. Renal-retinal syndromes: association of retinal anomalies and recessive nephronophthisis in patients with homozygous deletion of the NPH1 locus. Am J Kidney Dis 1998;32:1059–62.

50. Schuermann MJ, Otto E, Becker A, et al. Mapping of gene loci for nephronophthisis type 4 and Senior-Loken syndrome, to chromosome 1p36. Am J Hum Genet 2002; 70:1240–6.

51. Otto E, Hoefele J, Ruf R, et al. A gene mutated in nephronophthisis and retinitis pigmentosa encodes a novel protein, nephroretinin, conserved in evolution. Am J Hum Genet 2002;71:1161–7.

52. Omran H, Sasmaz G, Haffner K, et al. Identification of a gene locus for Senior-Loken syndrome in the region of the nephronophthisis type 3 gene. J Am Soc Nephrol 2002;13:75–9.

53. De Koning TJ, Dorland L, van Berge Henegouwen GP. Phosphomannose isomerase deficiency as a cause of congenital hepatic fibrosis and protein losing enteropathy. J Hepatol 1999;31:557–60

54. De Koning TJ, Nikkels PG, Dorland L, et al. Congenital hepatic fibrosis in 3 siblings with phosphomannose isomerase deficiency. Virchows Arch 2000;437:101–5.

55. Terada T, Kitamura Y, Nakanuma Y. Normal and abnormal development of the human intrahepatic biliary system: a review. Tohoku J Exp Med 1997;181:19–32.

56. Salonen R, Paavola P. Meckel syndrome. J Med Genet 1998;35:497–501.

57. Morgan NV, Gissen P, Sharif SM, et al. A novel locus for Meckel-Gruber syndrome, MKS3, maps to chromosome 8q24. Hum Genet 2002;111:456–61.

58. Sergi C, Adam S, Kahl P, Otto HF. Study of the malformation of ductal plate of the liver in Meckel syndrome and review of other syndromes presenting with this anomaly. Pediatr Dev Pathol 2000;3:568–83.

59. Morgan NV, Bacchelli C, Gissen P, et al. A locus for asphyxiating thoracic dystrophy, ATD, maps to chromosome 15q13. J Med Genet 2003;40:431–5.

60. Yerian LM, Brady L, Hart J. Hepatic manifestations of Jeune syndrome (asphyxiating thoracic dystrophy). Semin Liver Dis 2003;23:195–200.

61. Whitley CB, Schwarzenberg SJ, Burke BA, et al. Direct hyperbilirubinemia and hepatic fibrosis: a new presentation of Jeune syndrome (asphyxiating thoracic dystrophy). Am J Med Genet Suppl 1987;3:211–20.

62. Labrune P, Fabre M, Trioche P, et al. Jeune syndrome and liver disease: report of three cases treated with ursodeoxycholic acid. Am J Med Genet 1999;87:324–8.

63. Noack F, Sayk F, Ressel A, et al. Ivemark syndrome with agenesis of the corpus callosum: a case report with a review of the literature. Prenat Diagn 2002;22:1011–5.

64. Torra R, Alos L, Ramos J, Estivill X. Renal-hepatic-pancreatic dysplasia: an autosomal recessive malformation. J Med Genet 1996;33:409–12.

65. Bernstein J, Chandra M, Creswell J, et al. Renal-hepatic-pancreatic dysplasia: a syndrome reconsidered. Am J Med Genet 1987;26:391–403.

66. Larson RS, Rudloff MA, Liapis H, et al. The Ivemark syndrome: prenatal diagnosis of an uncommon cystic renal lesion with heterogeneous associations. Pediatr Nephrol 1995;9:594–8.

67. Lieberman E, Salinas-Madrigal L, Gwinn JL, et al. Infantile polycystic disease of the kidneys and liver: clinical, pathological and radiologic correlations and comparisons with congenital hepatic fibrosis. Medicine 1971;50:277.

68. Zerres K, Mucher G, Becker J, et al. Prenatal diagnosis of autosomal recessive polycystic kidney disease (ARPKD): molecular genetics, clinical experience, and fetal morphology. Am J Med Genet 1998;76:137–44.

69. Guay-Woodford LM, Galliani CA, Musulman-Mroczek E, et al. Diffuse renal cystic disease in children: morphologic and genetic correlations. Pediatr Nephrol 1998;12:173–82.

70. Guay-Woodford LM, Desmond RA. Autosomal recessive polycystic kidney disease: the clinical experience in North America. Pediatrics 2003;111(5 Pt 1):1072–80.

71. Murcia NS, Sweeney WE Jr, Avner ED. New insights into the molecular pathophysiology of polycystic kidney disease. Kidney Int 1999;55:1187–97.

72. Richards WG, Sweeney WE, Yoder BK, et al. Epidermal growth factor receptor activity mediates renal cyst formation in polycystic kidney disease. J Clin Invest 1998;101:935–9.

73. Nauta J, Sweeney WE, Rutledge JC, Avner ED. Biliary epithelial cells from mice with congenital polycystic kidney disease are hyperresponsive to epidermal growth factor. Pediatr Res 1995;37:755–63.

74. Nauta J, Ozawa Y, Sweeney WE Jr, et al. Renal and biliary abnormalities in a new murine model of autosomal recessive polycystic kidney disease. Pediatr Nephrol 1993;7: 163–72.

75. Sweeney WE, Chen Y, Nakanishi K, et al. Treatment of polycystic kidney disease with a novel tyrosine kinase inhibitor. Kidney Int 2000;57:33–40.

76. Guay-Woodford LM, Green WJ, Lindsey JR, Beier DR. Germline and somatic loss of function of the mouse cpk gene causes biliary ductal pathology that is genetically modulated. Hum Mol Genet 2000;9:769–78.

77. Premkumar A, Berdon WE, Levy J, et al. The emergence of hepatic fibrosis and portal hypertension in infants and children with autosomal recessive polycystic kidney disease. Initial and follow-up sonographic and radiographic findings. Pediatr Radiol 1988;18:123–9.

78. Khan K, Schwarzenberg SJ, Sharp HL, et al. Morbidity from congenital hepatic fibrosis after renal transplantation for autosomal recessive polycystic kidney disease. Am J Transplant 2002;2:360–5.

79. Lieberman E, Salinas-Madrigal L, Gwinn JL, et al. Infantile polycystic disease of the kidneys and liver: clinical, pathological and radiological correlations and comparison with congenital hepatic fibrosis. Medicine (Baltimore) 1971;50:277–318.

80. Zerres K, Mucher G, Bachner L, et al. Mapping of the gene for autosomal recessive polycystic kidney disease (ARPKD) to chromosome 6p21-cen. Nat Genet 1994;7:429–32.

81. Guay-Woodford LM, Muecher G, Hopkins SD, et al. The severe perinatal form of autosomal recessive polycystic kidney disease maps to chromosome 6p21.1-p12: implications for genetic counseling. Am J Hum Genet 1995;56:1101–7.

82. Bergmann C, Senderek J, Sedlacek B, et al. Spectrum of mutations in the gene for autosomal recessive polycystic kidney disease (ARPKD/PKHD1). J Am Soc Nephrol 2003;14:76–89.

83. Rossetti S, Torra R, Coto E, et al. A complete mutation screen of PKHD1 in autosomal-recessive polycystic kidney disease (ARPKD) pedigrees. Kidney Int 2003;64:391–403.

84. D'Agata ID, Jonas MM, Perez-Atayde AR, Guay-Woodford LM. Combined cystic disease of the liver and kidney. Semin Liver Dis 1994;14:215–28.

85. Grunfeld JP, Albouze G, Junger P, et al. Liver changes and complications in adult polycystic disease. Adv Nephrol 1985;14:1.

86. Karhunen PJ. Adult polycystic liver disease and biliary microhamartomas (von Meyenburg's complexes). Acta Pathol Microbiol Immunol Scand [A] 1986;94:397–400.

87. Grunfeld JP, Chauveau D, Joly D, et al. Polycystic kidney disease: <<30 ans apres>>. J Nephrol 1999;12 Suppl 2:S42–6.

88. Kissane JM. Congenital malformations. In: Heptinstall RH, editor. Pathology of the kidney. 2nd ed. Boston: Little Brown and Co; 1974. p. 64.

89. Jennette JC, Olson JL, Schwartz MM, et al, editors. Heptinstall's pathology of the kidney. 5th ed. Philadelphia (PA): Lippincott Williams & Wilkins; 1998. p. 1183.

90. International Polycystic Kidney Disease Consortium. Polycystic kidney disease: the complete structure of the PKD1 gene and its protein. Cell 1995;8:289–98.

91. Hughes J, Ward CJ, Peral B, et al. The polycystic kidney disease 1 (PKD1) gene encodes a novel protein with multiple recognition domains. Nat Genet 1995;10:151–60.

92. Mochizuki T, Wu G, Hayashi T, et al. PKD2, a gene for polycystic kidney disease that encodes an integral membrane protein. Science 1996;272:1339–42.

93. Coffman TM. Another cystic mystery solved. Nat Genet 2002;30:247–8.

94. Daoust MC, Reynolds DM, Bichet DG, Somlo S. Evidence for a third genetic locus for autosomal dominant polycystic kidney disease. Genomics 1995;25:733–6.

95. Karhunen PJ, Tenhu M. Adult polycystic liver and kidney diseases are separate entities. Clin Genet 1986;30:29–37.

96. Pirson Y, Lannoy N, Peters D, et al. Isolated polycystic liver disease as a distinct genetic disease, unlinked to polycystic kidney disease 1 and polycystic kidney disease 2. Hepatology 1996;23:249–52.

97. Reynolds DM, Falk CT, Li A, et al. Identification of a locus for autosomal dominant polycystic liver disease, on chromosome 19p13.2-13.1. Am J Hum Genet 2000;67:1598–604.

98. Tahvanainen P, Tahvanainen E, Reijonen H, et al. Polycystic liver disease is genetically heterogeneous: clinical and linkage studies in eight Finnish families. J Hepatol 2003;38:39–43.

99. Drenth JP, te Morsche RH, Smink R, et al. Germline mutations in PRKCSH are associated with autosomal dominant polycystic liver disease. Nat Genet 2003;33:345–7.

100. Li A, Davila S, Furu L, et al. Mutations in PRKCSH cause isolated autosomal dominant polycystic liver disease. Am J Hum Genet 2003;72:691–703.

101. Qian Q, Li A, King BF, et al. Clinical profile of autosomal dominant polycystic liver disease. Hepatology 2003;37:164–71.

102. Caroli J. Diseases of the intrahepatic biliary tree. Clin Gastroenterol 1973;2:147–61.

103. Jordon D, Harpaz N, Thung SN. Caroli's disease and adult polycystic kidney disease: a rarely recognized association. Liver 1989;9:30–5.

104. Tsuchida Y, Sato T, Sanjo K, et al. Evaluation of long-term results of Caroli's disease: 21 years' observation of a family with autosomal "dominant" inheritance, and review of the literature. Hepatogastroenterology 1995;42:175–81.

105. Todani T, Watanabe Y, Narusue M, et al. Congenital bile duct cysts: classification, operative procedures, and review of thirty-seven cases including cancer arising from choledochal cyst. Am J Surg 1977;134:263–9.

106. Witzleben CL. Bile duct paucity ("intrahepatic atresia"). Perspect Pediatr Pathol 1982;7:185–201.

107. Kahn E, Markowitz J, Aiges H, Daum F. Human ontogeny of the bile duct to portal space ratio. Hepatology 1989; 10:21–3.

108. Alagille D, Habib EC, Thomassin N. L'atresie des voies biliares intra-hepatiques avec voies biliaires extra-hepatiques permeables chez l'enfant. J Paris Pediatr 1969; 301–24.

109. Alagille D, Odievre M, Gautier M, Dommergues JP. Hepatic ductular hypoplasia associated with characteristic facies, vertebral malformations, retarded physical, mental, and sexual development, and cardiac murmur. J Pediatr 1975; 86:63–71.

110. Watson GH, Miller V. Arteriohepatic dysplasia: familial pulmonary arterial stenosis with neonatal liver disease. Arch Dis Child 1973;48:459–66.

111. Alagille D, Estrada A, Hadchouel M, et al. Syndromic paucity of interlobular bile ducts (Alagille syndrome or arteriohepatic dysplasia): review of 80 cases. J Pediatr 1987;110:195–200.

112. Deprettere A, Portmann B, Mowat AP. Syndromic paucity of the intrahepatic bile ducts: diagnostic difficulty; severe morbidity throughout early childhood. J Pediatr Gastroenterol Nutr 1987;6:865–71.

113. Deutsch J, Smith AL, Danks DM, Campbell PE. Long term prognosis for babies with neonatal liver disease. Arch Dis Child 1985;60:447–51.

114. Mueller RF. The Alagille syndrome (arteriohepatic dysplasia). J Med Genet 1987;24:621–6.

115. Odievre M, Hadchouel M, Landrieu P, et al. Long term prognosis for infants with intrahepatic cholestasis and patent extrahepatic biliary tract. Arch Dis Child 1981;56:373–6.

116. Hoffenberg EJ, Narkewicz MR, Sondheimer JM, et al. Outcome of syndromic paucity of interlobular bile ducts (Alagille syndrome) with onset of cholestasis in infancy. J Pediatr 1995;127:220–4.

117. Emerick KM, Rand EB, Goldmuntz E, et al. Features of Alagille syndrome in 92 patients: frequency and relation to prognosis. Hepatology 1999;29:822–9.

118. Quiros-Tejeira RE, Ament ME, Heyman MB, et al. Variable morbidity in Alagille syndrome: a review of 43 cases. J Pediatr Gastroenterol Nutr 1999;29:431–7.

119. Crosnier C, Lykavieris P, Meunier-Rotival M, Hadchouel M.

Alagille syndrome. The widening spectrum of ateriohepatic dysplasia. Clin Liver Dis 2000;4:765–78.

120. Lykavieris P, Hadchouel M, Chardot C, Bernard O. Outcome of liver disease in children with Alagille syndrome: a study of 163 patients. Gut 2001;49:431–5.

121. Li L, Krantz ID, Deng Y, Genin A, et al. Alagille syndrome is caused by mutations in human Jagged1, which encodes a ligand for Notch1. Nat Genet 1997;16:243–51.

122. Oda T, Elkahloun AG, Meltzer PS, et al. Mutations in the human Jagged1 gene are responsible for Alagille syndrome. Nat Genet 1997;16:235–42.

123. Danks DM, Campbell PE, Jack I, et al. Studies of the aetiology of neonatal hepatitis and biliary atresia. Arch Dis Child 1977;52:360–7.

124. LaBrecque DR, Mitros FA, Nathan RJ, et al. Four generations of arteriohepatic dysplasia. Hepatology 1983;2:467–74.

125. Shulman SA, Hyams JS, Gunta R, et al. Arteriohepatic dysplasia (Alagille syndrome): extreme variability among affected family members. Am J Med Genet 1984;19:325–32.

126. Mueller RF, Pagon RA, Pepin MG, et al. Arteriohepatic dysplasia: phenotypic features and family studies. Clin Genet 1984;25:323–31.

127. Dhorne-Pollet S, Deleuze JF, Hadchouel M, Bonaiti-Pellie C. Segregation analysis of Alagille syndrome. J Med Genet 1994;31:453–7.

128. Krantz ID, Colliton RP, Genin A, et al. Spectrum and frequency of Jagged1 (JAG1) mutations in Alagille syndrome patients and their families. Am J Hum Genet 1998;62:1361–9.

129. Crosnier C, Driancourt C, Raynaud N, et al. Mutations in JAGGED1 gene are predominantly sporadic in Alagille syndrome. Gastroenterology 1999;116:1141–8.

130. Desmaze C, Deleuze JF, Dutrillaux AM, et al. Screening of microdeletions of chromosome 20 in patients with Alagille syndrome. J Med Genet 1992;29:233–5.

131. Spinner NB, Rand EB, Fortina P, et al. Cytologically balanced t(2;20) in a two-generation family with Alagille syndrome: cytogenetic and molecular studies. Am J Hum Genet 1994;55:238–43.

132. Rand EB, Spinner NB, Piccoli DA, et al. Molecular analysis of 24 Alagille syndrome families identifies a single submicroscopic deletion and further localizes the Alagille syndrome region within 20p12. Am J Hum Genet 1995;57:1068–73.

133. Artavanis-Tsakonas S, Rand MD, Lake RJ. Notch signaling: cell fate control and signal integration in development. Science 1999;284:770–6.

134. Crosnier C, Attie-Bitach T, Encha-Razavi F, et al. JAGGED1 gene expression during human embryogenesis elucidates the wide phenotypic spectrum of Alagille syndrome. Hepatology 2000;32:574–81.

135. Jones EA, Clement-Jones M, Wilson DI. JAGGED1 expression in human embryos: correlation with the Alagille syndrome phenotype. J Med Genet 2000;37:663–8.

136. Joutel A, Vahedi K, Corpechote C, et al. Strong clustering and stereotyped nature of Notch3 mutations in CADASIL patients. Lancet 1997;350:1511–5.

137. Bulman MP, Kusumi K, Frayling TM, et al. Mutations in the human Delta homologue, DLL3, cause axial skeletal defects in spondylocostal dysostosis. Nat Genet 2000;24:438–41.

138. Yuan ZR, Kohsaka T, Ikegaya T, et al. Mutational analysis of the Jagged 1 gene in Alagille syndrome families. Hum Mol Genet 1998;7:1363–9.

139. Pilia G, Uda M, Macis D, et al. Jagged-1 mutation analysis in Italian Alagille syndrome patients. Hum Mutat 1999;14:394–400.

140. Piccoli DA, Spinner NB. Alagille syndrome and the Jagged1 gene. Semin Liver Dis 2001;21:525–34.

141. Krantz ID, Piccoli DA, Spinner NB. Clinical and molecular genetics of Alagille syndrome. Curr Opin Genet 1999;11:558–64.

142. Loomes KM, Underkoffler LA, Morabito J, et al. The expression of Jagged1 in the developing mammalian heart correlates with cardiovascular disease in Alagille syndrome. Hum Mol Genet 1999;8:2443–9.

143. McDonald-McGinn DM, La Rossa D, Goldmuntz E, et al. The 22q11.2 deletion: screening, diagnostic workup, and outcome of results; report on 181 patients. Genet Test 1997;1:99–108.

144. Dahms BB, Petrelli M, Wyllie R, et al. Arteriohepatic dysplasia in infancy and childhood: a longitudinal study of six patients. Hepatology 1982;2:350–8.

145. Russo P, Loomes KM. Diseases of the intrahepatic biliary tree—paucity of intrahepatic bile ducts. In: Russo P, Ruchelli ED, Piccoli DA, editors. Pathology of pediatric gastrointestinal and liver disease. New York: Springer Verlag; 2004. [In press]

146. Ghishan FK, LaBrecque DR, Mitros FA, Younoszai MK. The evolving nature of "infantile obstructive cholangiopathy." J Pediatr 1980;97:27–32.

147. Hadchouel M, Hugon RN, Gautier M. Reduced ratio of portal tracts to paucity of intrahepatic bile ducts. Arch Pathol Lab Med 1978;102:402.

148. Kahn EI, Daum F, Markowitz J, et al. Arteriohepatic dysplasia. II. Hepatobiliary morphology. Hepatology 1983;3:77–84.

149. Hashida Y, Yunis EJ. Syndromatic paucity of interlobular bile ducts: hepatic histopathology of the early and end-stage liver. Pediatr Pathol 1988;8:1–15.

150. Deutsch, GH, Sokol RJ, Stathos TH, Knisely AS. Proliferation to paucity: evolution of bile duct abnormalities in a case of Alagille syndrome. Pediatr Dev Pathol 2001;4:559–63.

151. Kahn E. Paucity of interlobular bile ducts. Arteriohepatic dysplasia and nonsyndromic duct paucity. Perspect Pediatr Pathol 1991;14:168–215.

152. Valencia-Mayoral P, Weber J, Cute E, et al. Possible defect in the bile secretory apparatus in arteriohepatic dysplasia (Alagille's syndrome): a review with observations on the ultrastructure of liver. Hepatology 1984;4:691–8.

153. Witzleben CL, Finegold M, Piccoli DA, Treem WR. Bile canalicular morphometry in arteriohepatic dysplasia. Hepatology 1987;7:1262–6.

154. Morelli A, Pelli MA, Vedovelli A, et al. Endoscopic retrograde cholangiopancreatography study in Alagille's syndrome: first report. Am J Gastroenterol 1983;78:241–4.

155. Adams PC. Hepatocellular carcinoma associated with arteriohepatic dysplasia. Dig Dis Sci 1986;31:438–42.

156. Kaufman SS, Wood RP, Shaw BWJ, et al. Hepatocellular carcinoma in a child with the Alagille syndrome. Am J Dis Child 1987;141:698–700.

157. Ong E, Williams SM, Anderson JC, Kaplan PA. MR imaging of a hepatoma associated with Alagille syndrome. J Comput Assist Tomogr 1986;10:1047–9.

158. Keeffe EB, Pinson CW, Ragsdale J, Zonana J. Hepatocellular carcinoma in arteriohepatic dysplasia. Am J Gastroenterol 1993;88:1446–9.

159. Rabinovitz M, Imperial JC, Schade RR, Van Thiel DH. Hepatocellular carcinoma in Alagille's syndrome: a family study. J Pediatr Gastroenterol Nutr 1989;8:26–30.

160. Bekassy AN, Garwicz S, Wiebe T, et al. Hepatocellular carcinoma associated with arteriohepatic dysplasia in a 4-year-old girl. Med Pediatr Oncol 1992;20:78–83.

161. Chiaretti A, Zampino G, Botto L, Polidori G. Alagille syndrome and hepatocarcinoma: a case report. Acta Paediatr 1992;81:937.

162. Perez Becerra E, Fuster M, Fraga M, et al. [Alagille's syndrome: a family case and its association with hepatocellular carcinoma]. Rev Clin Esp 1991;188:459–62.

163. Rabinovitz M, Imperial JC, Schade RR, Van Thiel DH. Hepatocellular carcinoma in Alagille's syndrome: a family study. J Pediatr Gastroenterol Nutr 1989;8:26–30.

164. Nishikawa A, Mori H, Takahashi M, et al. Alagille's syndrome. A case with a hamartomatous nodule of the liver. Acta Pathol Jpn 1987;37:1319–26.

165. Tuset E, Ribera JM, Domenech E, et al. [Pseudotumorous hyperplasia of the caudate lobe of the liver in a patient with Alagille syndrome]. Med Clin (Barc) 1995;104:420–2.

166. Kato Z, Asano J, Kato T, et al. Thyroid cancer in a case with the Alagille syndrome. Clin Genet 1994;45:21–4.

167. Dufour JF, Pratt DS. Alagille syndrome with colonic polyposis. Am J Gastroenterol 2001;96:2775–7.

168. Dommergues JP, Gubler MC, Habib R, et al. [Renal involvement in the Alagille syndrome]. Arch Pediatr 1994;1:411–3.

169. Wolfish NM, Shanon A. Nephropathy in arteriohepatic dysplasia (Alagille's syndrome). Child Nephrol Urol 1988; 9:169–72.

170. Habib R, Dommergues JP, Gubler MC, et al. Glomerular mesangiolipidosis in Alagille syndrome (arteriohepatic dysplasia). Pediatr Nephrol 1987;1:455–64.

171. Russo PA, Ellis D, Hashida Y. Renal histopathology in Alagille's syndrome. Pediatr Pathol 1987;7:557–68.

172. Chung Park M, Petrelli M, Tavill AS, et al. Renal lipidosis associated with arteriohepatic dysplasia (Alagille's syndrome). Clin Nephrol 1982;18:314–20.

173. Schonck M, Hoorntje S, van Hooff J. Renal transplantation in Alagille syndrome. Nephrol Dial Transplant 1998;13: 197–9.

174. Martin SR, Garel L, Alvarez F. Alagille's syndrome associated with cystic renal disease. Arch Dis Child 1996;74:232–5.

175. Devriendt K, Dooms L, Proesmans W, et al. Paucity of intrahepatic bile ducts, solitary kidney and atrophic pancreas with diabetes mellitus: atypical Alagille syndrome? Eur J Pediatr 1996;155:87–90.

176. Berard E, Sarles J, Triolo V, et al. Renovascular hypertension and vascular anomalies in Alagille syndrome. Pediatr Nephrol 1998;12:121–4.

177. Weston CF, Burton JL. Xanthomas in the Watson Alagille syndrome. J Am Acad Dermatol 1987;16:1117–21.

178. Alvarez F, Landrieu P, Laget P, et al. Nervous and ocular disorders in children with cholestasis and vitamin A and E deficiencies. Hepatology 1983;3:410–4.

179. Bucuvalas JC, Horn JA, Carlsson L, et al. Growth hormone insensitivity associated with elevated circulating growth hormone-binding protein in children with Alagille syndrome and short stature. J Clin Endocrinol Metab 1993;76:1477–82.

180. Sokol RJ, Stall C. Anthropometric evaluation of children with chronic liver disease. Am J Clin Nutr 1990;52:203–8.

181. Silberbach M, Lashley D, Reller MD, et al. Arteriohepatic dysplasia and cardiovascular malformations. Am Heart J 1994;127:695–9.

182. McElhinny DB, Krantz ID, Bason L, et al. Analysis of cardiovascular phenotype and genotype-phenotype correla-

tion in individuals with a JAG1 mutation and/or Alagille syndrome. Circulation 2002;106:2567–74.

183. Eldadah ZA, Hamosh A, Biery NJ, et al. Familial tetralogy of Fallot caused by mutation in the Jagged1 gene. Hum Mol Genet 2001;10:163–9.

184. Brindza D, Moodie DS, Wyllie R, Sterba R. Intravenous digital subtraction angiography to assess pulmonary artery anatomy in patients with the Alagille syndrome. Cleve Clin Q 1984;51:493–7.

185. Krantz ID, Smith R, Colliton RP, et al. Jagged1 mutations in patients ascertained with isolated congenital heart defects. Am J Med Genet 1999;84:56–60.

186. Sokol RJ, Heubi JE, Balistreri WF. Intrahepatic "cholestasis facies": is it specific for Alagille syndrome? J Pediatr 1983;103:205–8.

187. Kamath BM, Loomes KM, Oakey RJ, et al. Facial features in Alagille syndrome: specific or cholestasis facies? Am J Med Genet 2002;112:163–70.

188. Rosenfield NS, Kelley MJ, Jensen PS, et al. Arteriohepatic dysplasia: radiologic features of a new syndrome. AJR Am J Roentgenol 1980;135:1217–23.

189. Berman MD, Ishak KG, Schaefer CJ, et al. Syndromatic hepatic ductular hypoplasia (arteriohepatic dysplasia): a clinical and hepatic histologic study of three patients. Dig Dis Sci 1981;26:485–97.

190. Kamath BM, Loomes KM, Oakey RJ, Krantz ID. Supernumerary digital flexion creases: an additional clinical manifestation of Alagille syndrome. Am J Med Genet 2002; 112:171–5.

191. Heubi JE, Higgins JV, Argao EA, et al. The role of magnesium in the pathogenesis of bone disease in childhood cholestatic liver disease: a preliminary report. J Pediatr Gastroenterol Nutr 1997;25:301–6.

192. Potamitis T, Fielder AR. Angle closure glaucoma in Alagille syndrome. A case report. Ophthalm Paediatr Genet 1993; 14:101–4.

193. Johnson BL. Ocular pathologic features of arteriohepatic dysplasia (Alagille's syndrome). Am J Ophthalmol 1990; 110:504–12.

194. Nischal KK. Ocular ultrasound in Alagille syndrome: a new sign. Ophthalmology 1997;104:79–85.

195. Brodsky MC, Cunniff C. Ocular anomalies in the Alagille syndrome (arteriohepatic dysplasia). Ophthalmology 1993;100:1767–74.

196. Romanchuk KG, Judisch GF, LaBrecque DR. Ocular findings in arteriohepatic dysplasia (Alagille's syndrome). Can J Ophthalmol 1981;16:94–9.

197. Wells KK, Pulido JS, Judisch GF, et al. Ophthalmic features of Alagille syndrome (arteriohepatic dysplasia). J Pediatr Ophthalmol Strabismus 1993;30:130–5.

198. Sokol RJ, Gruggenheim MA, Iannaccone ST, et al. Improved neurologic function after long-term correction of vitamin E deficiency in children with chronic cholestasis. N Engl J Med 1985;313:1580–6.

199. Stewart SM, Uauy R, Kennard BD, et al. Mental development and growth in children with chronic liver disease of early and late onset. Pediatrics 1988;82:167–72.

200. Devenyi AG, Barron TF, Mamourian AC. Dystonia, hyperintense basal ganglia, and high whole blood manganese levels in Alagille's syndrome. Gastroenterology 1994;106: 1068–71.

201. Le Caignec C, Lefevre M, Schott JJ, et al. Familial deafness, congenital heart defects, and posterior embryotoxon caused by cysteine substitution in the first epidermal-

growth-factor-like domain of Jagged 1. Am J Hum Genet 2002;71:180–6.

202. Woolfenden AR, Albers GW, Steinberg GK, et al. Moyamoya syndrome in children with Alagille syndrome: additional evidence of a vasculopathy. Pediatrics 1999;103:505–8.

203. Lykavieris P, Crosnier C, Trichet C, et al. Bleeding tendency in children with Alagille syndrome. Pediatrics 2003;111: 167–70.

204. Markowitz J, Daum F, Kahn EI, et al. Arteriohepatic dysplasia, I. Pitfalls in diagnosis and management. Hepatology 1983;3:74–6.

205. Aburano T, Yokoyama K, Takayama T, et al. Distinct hepatic retention of Tc-99m IDA in arteriohepatic dysplasia (Alagille syndrome). Clin Nucl Med 1989;14:874–6.

206. Hitch DC, Shikes RH, Lilly JR. Determinants of survival after Kasai's operation in biliary atresia using actuarial analysis. J Pediatr Surg 1979;14:310–4.

207. Argao EA, Heubi JE, Hollis BW, Tsang RC. d-Alpha-tocopherol polyethylene glycol-1000 succinate enhances the absorption of vitamin D in chronic cholestatic liver disease of infancy and childhood. Pediatr Res 1992;31:146–50.

208. Sokol RJ, Bove KE, Heubi JE, Iannaccone ST. Vitamin E deficiency during chronic childhood cholestasis—presence of sural nerve lesion prior to 1½ years of age. J Pediatr 1983;103:197–204.

209. Sokol RJ, Bulter-Simon N, Conner C, et al. Multicenter trial of d-alpha-tocopherol polyethylene glycol 1000 succinate for treatment of vitamin E deficiency in children with chronic cholestasis. Gastroenterology 1993;104:1727–35.

210. Sharp HL, Carey JB, White JG, Krivit W. Cholestyramine therapy in patients with a paucity of intrahepatic bile ducts. J Pediatr 1967;71:723–36.

211. Person JR. Ultraviolet A (UV-A) and cholestatic pruritus. Arch Dermatol 1982;117:684.

212. Cynamon HA, Andres JM, Iafrate RP. Rifampin relieves pruritus in children with cholestatic liver disease. Gastroenterology 1990;98:1013–6.

213. Gregorio GV, Ball CS, Mowat AP, Mieli Vergani G. Effect of rifampicin in the treatment of pruritus in hepatic cholestasis. Arch Dis Child 1993;69:141–3.

214. Jones EA, Bergasa NV. The pruritus of cholestasis. Hepatology 1999;29:1003–6.

215. Emerick KM, Whitington PF. Partial external biliary diversion for intractable pruritus and xanthomas in Alagille syndrome. Hepatology 2002;35:1501–6.

216. Tzakis AG, Reyers J, Tepetes K, et al. Liver transplantation for Alagille's syndrome. Arch Surg 1993;128:337–9.

217. Andrews W, Sommersauer J, Roden J, et al. 10 years of pediatric liver transplantation. J Pediatr Surg 1996;31:619–24.

218. Cardona J, Houssin D, Gauthier F, et al. Liver transplantation in children with Alagille syndrome—a study of twelve cases. Transplantation 1995;60:339–42.

219. Gurkan A, Emre S, Fishbein TM, et al. Unsuspected bile duct paucity in donors for living-related liver transplantation: two cases reports. Transplantation 1999;67:416–8.

220. Kahn E, Daum F, Markowitz J, et al. Nonsyndromatic paucity of interlobular bile ducts: light and electron microscopic evaluation of sequential liver biopsies in early childhood. Hepatology 1986;6:890–901.

221. Alagille D. Cholestasis in children. In: Alagille D, Odievre M, editors. Liver and biliary tract disease in children. New York: John Wiley and Sons; 1979. p. 185.

222. Witzleben CL. Bile duct paucity ("intrahepatic atresia"). Perspect Pediatr Pathol 1982;7:185–201.

223. Snover DC, Freese DK, Sharp HL, et al. Liver allograft rejection. An analysis of the use of biopsy in determining outcome of rejection. Am J Surg Pathol 1987;11:1–10.

224. Tanaka M, Umihara J, Chiba S, Ishikawa E. Intrahepatic bile duct injury following bone marrow transplantation. Analysis of pathological features based on three-dimensional and histochemical observation. Acta Pathol Jpn 1986;36:1793–806.

225. Bernuau D, Feldmann G, Degott C, Gisselbrecht C. Ultrastructural lesions of bile ducts in primary biliary cirrhosis. A comparison with the lesions observed in graft-versus-host disease. Hum Pathol 1981;12:782–93.

226. Bernuau D, Gisselbrecht C, Devergie A, et al. Histological and ultrastructural appearance of the liver during graft-versus-host disease complicating bone marrow transplantation. Transplantation 1980;29:236–44.

227. Dilly SA, Sloane JP. An immunohistological study of human hepatic graft-versus-host disease. Clin Exp Immunol 1985;62:545–53.

228. Miglio F, Pignatelli M, Mazzeo V, et al. Expression of major histocompatibility complex class II antigens on bile duct epithelium in patients with hepatic graft-versus-host disease after bone marrow transplantation. J Hepatol 1987; 5:182–9.

229. Sale GE. Direct ultrastructural evidence of target-directed polarization by cytotoxic lymphocytes in lesions of human graft-versus-host disease. Arch Pathol Lab Med 1987;111:333–6.

230. Yau JC, Zander AK, Srigley JR, et al. Chronic graft-versus-host disease complicated by micronodular cirrhosis and esophageal varices. Transplantation 1986;41:129–30.

231. Knapp AB, Crawford JM, Rappeport JM, Gollan JL. Cirrhosis as a consequence of graft-versus-host disease. Gastroenterology 1987;92:513–9.

232. Snover DC, Weisdorff SA, Ramsay NK, et al. Hepatic graft-versus-host disease: a study of the predictive value of liver biopsy in diagnosis. Hepatology 1984;4:123–30.

233. Snover DC, Sibley RK, Freese DK, et al. Orthotopic liver transplantation: a pathological study of 63 serial liver biopsies from 17 patients with special reference to the diagnostic features and natural history of rejection. Hepatology 1984;4:1212–22.

234. Demetris AJ, Lasky S, Vanthoel DH, et al. Pathology of hepatic transplantation. A review of 62 adult allograft recipients immunosuppressed with cyclosporine/steroid regimen. Am J Pathol 1985;118:151–61.

235. Vierling JM, Fennel RH Jr. Histopathology of early and late human hepatic allograft rejection: evidence of progressive destruction of interlobular bile ducts. Hepatology 1985;5:1076–82.

236. Demetris AJ, Seaberg EC, Batts KP, et al. Chronic liver allograft rejection: a National Institute of Diabetes and Digestive and Kidney Diseases interinstitutional study analyzing the reliability of current criteria and proposal of an expanded definition. National Institute of Diabetes and Digestive and Kidney Diseases Liver Transplantation Database. Am J Surg Pathol 1998;22:28–39.

237. Dimmick JE. Intrahepatic bile duct paucity and cytomegalovirus infection. Pediatr Pathol 1993;13:847–52.

238. Kage M, Kosai K, Kojiro M, et al. Infantile cholestasis due to cytomegalovirus infection of the liver. A possible cause of paucity of interlobular bile ducts. Arch Pathol Lab Med 1993;117:942–4.

239. Finegold MJ, Carpenter RJ. Obliterative cholangitis due to

cytomegalovirus: a possible precursor of paucity of intra-hepatic bile ducts. Hum Pathol 1982;13:662–5.

240. Strauss L, Bernstein J. Neonatal hepatitis in congenital rubella. A histopathological study. Arch Pathol 1968;86:317–27.

241. Sugiura HM, Hayashi R, Koshida R, et al. Nonsyndromatic paucity of intrahepatic bile ducts in congenital syphilis. A case report. Acta Pathol Jpn 1988;38:1061–8.

242. Hunt CM, Washington K. Tetracycline-induced bile duct paucity and prolonged cholestasis. Gastroenterology 1994;107:1844–7.

243. Davies MH, Harrison RF, Elias E, Hubscher SG. Antibiotic-associated acute vanishing bile duct syndrome: a pattern associated with severe, prolonged, intrahepatic cholesta-sis. J Hepatol 1994;20:112–6.

244. Chawla A, Kahn E, Yunis EJ, Daum F. Rapidly progressive cholestasis: an unusual reaction to amoxicillin/clavulanic acid therapy in a child. J Pediatr 2000;136:121–3.

245. Richardet JP, Mallat A, Zafrani ES, et al. Prolonged cholestasis with ductopenia after administration of amoxicillin/clavulanic acid. Dig Dis Sci 1999;44:1997–2000.

246. Bataille L, Rahier J, Geubel A. Delayed and prolonged cholesta-tic hepatitis with ductopenia after long-term ciprofloxacin therapy for Crohn's disease. J Hepatol 2002;37:696–9.

247. Altraif I, Lilly L, Wanless I, Heathcote J. Cholestatic liver disease with ductopenia (vanishing bile duct syndrome) after administration of clindamycin and trimethoprim-sulfamethoxazole. Am J Gastroenterol 1994;89:1230–4.

248. Desmet VJ, van Eyken P, Roskams T. Histopathology of van-ishing bile duct diseases. Adv Clin Pathol 1998;2:87–99.

249. Degott C, Feldmann G, Larrey D, et al. Drug-induced pro-longed cholestasis in adults: a histological semiquantita-tive study demonstrating progressive ductopenia. Hepa-tology 1992;15:244–51.

250. Nietgen GW, Vacanti JP, Perez-Atayde A. Intrahepatic bile duct loss in biliary atresia despite portoenterostomy: a consequence of ongoing obstruction? Gastroenterology 1992;102:2126–33.

251. Bates MD, Bucuvalas JC, Alonso MH, Ryckman FC. Biliary atresia: pathogenesis and treatment. Semin Liver Dis 1998;18:281–93.

252. Sokol RJ, Mack C. Etiopathogenesis of biliary atresia. Semin Liver Dis 2001;21:517–24.

253. Balistreri WF, Grand R, Hoofnagle J, et al. Biliary atresia: current concepts and research directions. Summary of a symposium. Hepatology 1996;23:1682–92.

254. Ijiri R, Tanaka Y, Kato K, et al. Clinicopathological study of a hilar nodule in the livers of long-term survivors with biliary atresia. Pathol Int 2001;51:16–9.

2. Biliary Atresia

Kathleen M. Campbell, MD

Jorge A. Bezerra, MD

Biliary atresia is a progressive fibroinflammatory cholangiopathy of infancy that results in complete obliteration of the entire or portions of the extrahepatic biliary tree within weeks of birth. This obstruction results in impaired bile flow, reactive proliferation of intrahepatic bile ducts, chronic cholestasis, and ongoing hepatocellular injury. In general, infants appear well but display the classic features of jaundice, acholic stools, and hepatomegaly, features shared with other causes of neonatal cholestasis. Therefore, the initial task is to differentiate biliary atresia from other forms of neonatal cholestasis; timely diagnosis is vital because early surgical relief of biliary obstruction may improve long-term outcome. In the absence of surgical intervention, ongoing injury leads to biliary cirrhosis, portal hypertension, and end-stage liver disease. At this stage, liver transplant is the only therapeutic option for long-term survival.

Biliary atresia is the most common cause of prolonged conjugated hyperbilirubinemia in neonates and is the most frequent indication for liver transplant in the pediatric population, accounting for 40 to 50% of all pediatric liver transplants.[1] The health care costs associated with biliary atresia are significant, reaching $65 million/year in the United States alone.[1] Despite the obvious adverse impact to children's health, advances in understanding of the etiology and pathogenesis of biliary atresia have not kept pace with progress in other cholestatic disorders of childhood.[2] The lack of progress reflects the multifactorial nature of the disease, which has challenged physicians since it was recognized early in the nineteenth century (Table 50.2-1).[3] The development of surgical approaches to re-establish biliary drainage and the acceptance of liver transplant as a treatment for end-stage liver disease owing to biliary atresia have markedly improved clinical outcome. Yet multiple challenges remain, such as early recognition of pathologic jaundice by health care providers, accurate diagnosis of biliary atresia, identification of predictors of outcome and optimal timing of transplant, and design of novel and effective medical therapies. The recent development of research agendas to sponsor multicenter studies in Europe and the United States promises to bring biliary atresia to the forefront of patient- and laboratory-based research priorities. Although the biologic basis of biliary atresia is not yet known, important data exist on epidemiology, clinical course, pathology, treatment, and outcome. A review of these data is the focus of this chapter.

EPIDEMIOLOGY

Biliary atresia respects no geographic boundaries; it occurs worldwide and affects 1 in 8,000 to 1 in 15,000 live births. Within regions, there appears to be a higher incidence of the disease in nonwhite populations (African American, French Polynesian, Chinese). Some studies have suggested time-space clustering of cases and seasonal variation, with the majority of cases occurring in the fall and winter months (December to March).[4,5] Two large population-based studies from France and Sweden, however, failed to identify a significant seasonal variation or time-space clustering.[4–7] After controlling for geographic and racial factors, associations have been observed with advanced maternal age and increased parity, and with a tendency for early fetal losses in mothers of infants with biliary atresia.[4,7] In this context, the disease is rarely seen in stillborns or premature infants, although some patients have a low birth weight for gestational age.[4,8] A slight female predominance (1.25:1) may be present among affected infants, particularly in the "embryonic" form of the disease.[9,10] Although the overwhelming majority of cases of biliary atresia are sporadic, there are reports of apparent recurrences within families.[11–13] This may reflect a shared genetic predisposition, but studies of twins have demonstrated that most sets are discordant for the disease.[14,15]

TABLE 50.2-1 HISTORICAL LANDMARKS FOR BILIARY ATRESIA

YEAR	LANDMARK
1817	Burns's description of an infant with features suggestive of biliary atresia
1892	Review of 50 cases by Thomson
1916	Review of anatomic findings and discussion of surgical approach by Holmes
1928	Ladd reports surgical success in selected infants with biliary atresia
1959	Kasai describes hepatoportoenterostomy in infants with biliary atresia
1982	NIH Consensus Conference: liver transplant as an acceptable treatment modality for end-stage liver disease owing to biliary atresia
1999	European Biliary Atresia Registry: European initiative for collaborative research in biliary atresia
2002	NIH-Biliary Atresia Research Consortium: multicenter consortium to foster clinical, epidemiologic, and therapeutic research in biliary atresia

Adapted from Bates MD et al.[3]
NIH = National Institutes of Health.

Taken together, these epidemiologic data suggest that environmental factors and genetic predisposition may be important determinants of disease. They also highlight the widespread occurrence of biliary atresia and underscore the need for physicians to be knowledgeable of the clinical features of the disease so that a diagnosis can be reached in a timely fashion.

CLINICAL PRESENTATION

COMMON FEATURES

Despite variability in age at onset of symptoms, extent of hepatobiliary involvement, and presence of nonhepatic abnormalities, infants with biliary atresia share the cardinal features of jaundice (owing to conjugated hyperbilirubinemia), acholic stools, and hepatomegaly. This triad presents in infants who otherwise appear well. Although weight gain is initially adequate, it becomes suboptimal with progression of disease. In addition to these common features, variability in clinical presentation results from complications of liver disease or nonhepatic abnormalities. For example, (1) splenomegaly is common at the time of diagnosis and reflects the degree of hepatic fibrosis and portal hypertension, (2) lethargy is uncommon and when present should trigger evaluation of clotting function and of the central nervous system integrity because coagulopathy owing to vitamin K deficiency may result in intracranial hemorrhage, and (3) poor feeding and recurrent emesis may signal the coexistence of intestinal malrotation or hemodynamic instability secondary to a severe cardiac defect (Table 50.2-2).

Other signs and symptoms may develop with progression of liver disease. Ascites is rarely present at the time of diagnosis but may develop in infants with advanced fibrosis, bacterial peritonitis, or obstruction of portal blood flow (owing to portal vein thrombosis). Sometimes the presence of ascites is suggested by the appearance of inguinal or umbilical hernia, which is treated more appropriately by management of ascites rather than herniorrhaphy. When infants have impaired biliary drainage despite portoenterostomy, progression of liver disease is manifest by variable signs of malnutrition, with decreased subcutaneous mass and muscle weakness. In this setting, infants may also have dilated vascular collaterals ascending from the anterior abdominal wall toward the chest in a distended abdomen (caput medusae) because of intra- and/or extrahepatic portal venous hypertension. Careful evaluation and monitoring of these common clinical features are important for appropriate diagnosis and provide critical clues about the state of evolution of the liver disease. The rate of disease progression may also depend on specific clinical forms that have been identified by the systematic cataloguing of clinical features at the time of diagnosis.

CLINICAL FORMS

There are two well-recognized clinical forms of biliary atresia: embryonic and perinatal.[10,16,17] These forms share the cardinal features of jaundice, acholic stools, and hepatomegaly but differ in the presence of associated anomalies, the timing of onset of jaundice, and perhaps clinical outcome. The embryonic form of biliary atresia (also referred to as "congenital" or "fetal") accounts for 10 to 20% of cases and is defined by the presence of congenital nonhepatic anomalies and earlier onset of disease. Infants present with pathologic jaundice at birth or shortly thereafter, frequently overlapping with physiologic jaundice, such that there is no jaundice-free interval. In addition, affected infants are more likely to have birth weights below the 50th percentile for age, even in the presence of maternal diabetes.[10] Notably, these infants may have complete absence of extrahepatic bile ducts, even a fibrous cord, suggesting a true defect in embryogenesis of the biliary system in a subset of patients.

Although the genetic basis for this form is unknown, hepatic and nonhepatic malformations may result from defects in molecules regulating embryonic development of the hepatobiliary system and the asymmetric organization of single organs, a process named laterality. Analysis of a large cohort identified nonhepatic malformations in 20% of the patients with biliary atresia.[18] Among these patients, defects in laterality were present in 29%, whereas isolated gastrointestinal or cardiovascular anomalies occurred in 59% and intestinal malrotation (with or without preduodenal portal vein; Figure 50.2-1A) was present in 12%. Splenic abnormalities (asplenia, double spleen, and polysplenia) may be present in up to 7.5% of patients with biliary atresia (Figure 50.2-1B), occurring in isolation or in combination with one or more additional defects in a variant known as biliary atresia splenic malformation (BASM) syndrome.[10] This syndrome includes polysplenia/asplenia, preduodenal portal vein, intestinal malrotation, abdominal situs inversus, midline liver, hepatic artery abnormalities, absent inferior vena cava, abnormal lung lobation, annular pancreas, and congenital heart disease. Although infants with the embryonic form of biliary atresia, with or without the BASM syndrome, had no obvious clinical or biochemical differences at the time of diagnosis, 15% were born to mothers with diabetes.[10] There is some evidence that patients with the embryonic form of biliary atresia have

---

TABLE 50.2-2   MAIN (TYPICAL AND ATYPICAL) CLINICAL FEATURES OF BILIARY ATRESIA

TYPICAL FEATURES FOR INFANTS AT THE TIME OF DIAGNOSIS
Jaundice (secondary to direct or conjugated hyperbilirubinemia)
Acholic stools
Hepatomegaly—with variable degrees of splenomegaly

CLINICAL SIGNS SUGGESTIVE OF NONHEPATIC COMPLICATIONS
Easy bruising, central nervous system hemorrhage—coagulopathy owing to vitamin K deficiency
Poor feeding, vomiting—cardiac insufficiency owing to structural defects
Recurrent (bilious) emesis—intestinal malrotation and midgut volvulus

FEATURES OF ADVANCED DISEASE
Moderate to severe splenomegaly owing to progressive hepatic fibrosis
Growth failure—poor caloric intake, decreased absorption, or increased metabolic needs
Ascites—secondary to portal hypertension
Caput medusae—secondary to portal hypertension
Umbilical and/or inguinal hernia—complication of ascites
Coagulopathy not responsive to vitamin K—hepatocellular failure

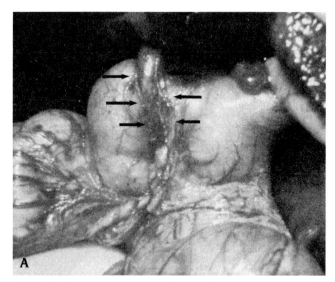 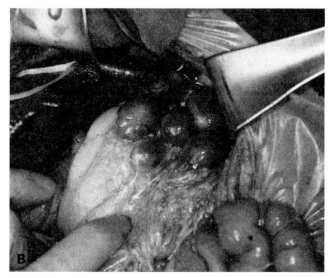

FIGURE 50.2-1   *A*, Operative findings of a preduodenal portal vein (*arrows*) in an infant with the embryonic form of biliary atresia at the time of portoenterostomy. *B*, Polysplenia in an infant with the embryonic form of biliary atresia at the time of portoenterostomy. Courtesy of Dr. Frederick Ryckman, Cincinnati Children's Hospital Medical Center, Cincinnati, OH.

worse outcome following portoenterostomy, with a decrease in actuarial survival (defined as death or transplant) within the first 2 years after surgery.[10] In addition to the challenges that extrahepatic malformations add to the care of infants with biliary atresia, more rapid progression of the hepatobiliary disease in this clinical form may account for a worse outcome.[19]

The perinatal form of biliary atresia (also referred to as "acquired" or "postnatal") accounts for the majority of the cases (80–90%) and occurs in the absence of other congenital anomalies. Most of the infants are born at term with an appropriate weight for gestational age. They have a variable jaundice-free interval after birth but develop jaundice, acholic stools, and dark-colored urine within the first few weeks of life. In contrast to the clinical setting observed in infants with the embryonic form, the combination of jaundice in an otherwise healthy infant and a history of a jaundice-free period is more consistent with a biliary injury that results from a perinatal or early postnatal insult. Efforts to determine the biologic relationship of potential pathogenic mechanisms are particularly important to understand the molecular basis of the clinical forms and to develop new diagnostic/therapeutic modalities for infants with biliary atresia.

PATHOGENIC MECHANISMS OF DISEASE

Any proposed pathogenic mechanism of disease must take into account important clinical features that are exclusive to biliary atresia: (1) onset of disease restricted to the neonatal period, (2) target of injury limited to the biliary system, and (3) lack of recurrence of hepatobiliary lesions typical of biliary atresia following liver transplant. Although inflammation of intra- and extrahepatic biliary tree is universal in biliary atresia, conflicting evidence exists with regard to triggering events, pre- and postnatal timing of onset, and the factors that promote ongoing hepatobiliary inflamma-

tion. However, careful observations based largely on epidemiologic and clinical features reported predisposing genetic factors, and the pace of disease progression provided valuable insight into the pathogenesis of disease. Based on these observations, five mechanisms have been proposed: (1) a defect in morphogenesis of the biliary tract, (2) a defect in fetal/prenatal circulation, (3) environmental toxin exposure, (4) viral infection, and (5) immunologic/inflammatory dysregulation (Table 50.2-3).[20]

EVIDENCE FOR DEFECTIVE MORPHOGENESIS

Biliary atresia may belong to a spectrum of diseases involving inappropriate persistence or lack of remodeling of the embryonic ductal plate. This concept of ductal plate malformation as a contributing or causative factor for biliary atresia is supported by the persistence of the embryonic shape of interlobular bile ducts in some infants at the time of diagnosis.[17] Also, comparative analyses of the normal embryonic development of the ductal plate and the extrahepatic biliary tree between 11 and 13 weeks of gestation with biliary structures from 205 infants with biliary atresia revealed morphologic similarities in periductular mesenchyme and fibrosis.[21] During this phase of embryogenesis, the ductal plate undergoes remodeling to form large tubular structures surrounded by thick mesenchyme, with shared morphologic similarities to abnormal ductules within the porta hepatis of livers from infants with biliary atresia. Together, these data suggest that abnormal mesenchymal support and improper remodeling of hilar ducts may be important pathogenic factors in early stages of disease development. In agreement with a prenatal onset in some cases, a recent report described segmental cystic dilatation of the biliary system in three fetuses during routine prenatal ultrasonography; postnatally, only duct remnants were detected proximally and distally to the cysts in a fashion similar to the histologic features of biliary atresia.[22]

There is a growing body of evidence pointing to possible roles of specific genes in the control of hepatobiliary

TABLE 50.2-3   POTENTIAL MECHANISMS INVOLVED IN THE PATHOGENESIS OF BILIARY ATRESIA

MECHANISM	SUPPORTING DATA
Defect in morphogenesis	Development of jaundice soon after birth; coexistence of other embryologic abnormalities; polymorphisms in the *Jag1* gene; abnormal remodeling of the "ductal plate"; *inv* mouse: model of biliary obstruction and situs inversus
Defect in prenatal circulation	Intrauterine devascularization results in abnormal extrahepatic bile ducts
Toxin exposure	Time-space clustering of cases
Viral infection	CMV, HPV, reovirus, rotavirus, HHV6 detected in infants with biliary atresia; models of virus-induced injury to biliary tract in suckling mice
Immunologic dysregulation	Increased expression of intercellular adhesion molecules; infiltration of biliary structures by CD4+ and CD8+ lymphocytes; increased frequency of the HLA-B12 allele; expression of proinflammatory cytokines

Adapted from Balistreri WF et al.[20]
CMV = cytomegalovirus; HHV6 = human herpesvirus 6; HLA = human leukocyte antigen; HPV = human papillomavirus.

morphogenesis. From clinical observations, the earlier onset of disease and the presence of nonhepatic malformations in the embryonic form of biliary atresia suggest a prenatal onset and a pathogenesis that differs, at least in part, from that of infants with the perinatal form. The main associated malformations, poly- or asplenia, cardiovascular defects, abdominal situs inversus, intestinal malrotation, and anomalies of the portal vein and hepatic artery, point to potential defects in embryogenesis and asymmetric left-right determination of visceral organs.[18] In support of this concept, abnormalities in organ symmetry and biliary drainage have been identified in the *inv* mouse. In this transgenic mouse line, a recessive insertional mutation of the inversin gene results in complete abdominal situs inversus, severe jaundice, poor weight gain, and death within the first week of life in 100% of homozygous mice.[23] Polysplenia is also occasionally present. In a detailed morphologic analysis of the hepatobiliary system in the *inv* mouse, a defect in patency of the extrahepatic ductular system was identified by trypan blue cholangiography and absent excretion of technetium 99m–labeled tracer.[24] In addition, intrahepatic ductular proliferation was described similar to that seen in biliary atresia. However, the complete absence of inflammation or necrosis within the hepatic parenchyma and the absence of inflammation and fibrosis of the extrahepatic biliary tree are in stark contrast to the histologic features of infants with biliary atresia.[24,25] Furthermore, mutational analyses in children with laterality defects and biliary atresia failed to identify mutations in the inversin gene.[26]

More recently, genetic inactivation of the transcription factors hepatocyte nuclear factor (HNF)-6 and HNF-1β in mice resulted in neonatal cholestasis and growth retardation.[27,28] Morphologic analysis of the HNF-6–deficient mice showed an abnormal development of intrahepatic bile ducts, with a transient formation of cystic structures followed by a new phase of ductular development, with loss of cysts and persistence of a discontinuous ductal plate through the first week of life.[28] In addition, these mice

lacked the gallbladder, the extrahepatic bile ducts were replaced by an enlarged structure that connected the liver to the duodenum, and jaundice was present in the first few days of life. Jaundice also developed in HNF-1β–deficient mice but at a later stage of postnatal development. Interestingly, the biliary system of HNF-1β–deficient mice appeared patent, but the gallbladder had a disorganized epithelium, there were variable cystic changes in the extrahepatic bile ducts, and there was a paucity of small intrahepatic ducts.[27] Based on the time-specific onset of biliary abnormalities during fetal development in both mouse lines and on additional gene expression studies in HNF-6–deficient mice, it appears that the development of the biliary system is controlled by a HNF-6 βHNF-1β cascade.[28]

In a different set of experiments, double heterozygosity for the *Jag1* and *Notch2* genes resulted in paucity of intrahepatic ducts in mice, which exhibited some of the cardinal phenotypic features observed in patients with Alagille syndrome.[29–31] Jag1-Notch signaling pathways define a fundamental mechanism controlling cell fate during embryogenesis by modifying the ability of a broad spectrum of precursor cells to progress to a more differentiated state. Although the developmental abnormalities reported for heterozygous *Jag1/Notch2* mice are not similar to those of infants with biliary atresia, the *Jag1* gene may be a modifier of liver disease, as demonstrated by the identification of a high frequency of single-nucleotide polymorphisms of the *Jag1* gene in infants with biliary atresia with poor outcome.[32] Taken together, these data suggest that genetic factors governing morphogenesis of the biliary system may play an important role in development and/or progression of liver disease in biliary atresia.

EVIDENCE FOR DEFECTIVE FETAL/PRENATAL CIRCULATION

Early interruption to flow in the hepatic artery, which supplies the intra- and extrahepatic biliary system, has been proposed to be an initiating factor in the fibroinflammatory injury of biliary atresia. This is an attractive concept based on the presence of hepatic artery and portal vein abnormalities associated with biliary atresia and the arterial hyperplasia and hypertrophy described in liver specimens of affected infants.[33] Additional data from humans or the development of experimental models to study the impact of blood flow on biliary development are necessary to further validate a potential role of impaired circulation in the pathogenesis of biliary atresia.

EVIDENCE FOR ENVIRONMENTAL TOXIN EXPOSURE

To date, the only supportive patient-based data for a role of a toxic insult as a causative factor of biliary atresia are the time-space clustering of cases. In animals, unusual outbreaks of hepatobiliary injury in lambs and calves in New South Wales, Australia, occurred in 1964 and 1988, with pathologic specimens displaying features akin to the pathology seen in humans with biliary atresia. Despite the localized geographic distribution of the outbreaks, an extensive investigation for causative phytotoxins or mycotoxins was unrevealing.[34]

EVIDENCE FOR VIRAL INFECTION

Another environmental factor that may play an important initiating role in biliary atresia is viral infection. The possible role of viral infection as an initiating event in the pathogenesis of biliary atresia was initially suggested by Landing, who viewed biliary atresia as existing along a continuum with choledochal cyst and neonatal intrahepatic cholestasis, which could be linked by a shared infectious insult.[35] Consistent with this concept, different viruses have been detected in the liver of infants with biliary atresia sporadically. For example, hepatitis B virus antigens were detected in the liver of infants with biliary atresia in Japan, but these findings were not reproduced in the United States.[36,37] Likewise, there is little evidence to support the role of hepatitis A or C virus in spite of histologic findings suggesting the presence of non-A, non-B viruses in the liver.[37–39] Subsequent reports using a variety of techniques and substrates for viral detection have implicated cytomegalovirus, retrovirus, human papillomavirus, human herpesvirus 6, reovirus, and rotavirus in specific groups of patients not only with biliary atresia but also with neonatal intrahepatic cholestasis and choledochal cyst.[40–50] The etiologic role for a single agent, however, has not been supported owing to the inability to reproduce the association in other patient populations.[50–54] Nevertheless, among these viruses, reovirus type 3 and rotavirus type C continue to emerge as potential triggering agents for biliary atresia.

Prevalence of antibodies against reovirus type 3 and the detection of the virus in hepatobiliary specimens of patients with biliary atresia have varied according to patient population and laboratory techniques. This is demonstrated by a high prevalence of immunoglobulins G and M to reovirus in infants with biliary atresia,[47–49,55] but at least two studies could not find such an association.[52,56] More recently, the use of virus-specific amplification by reverse transcription–polymerase chain reaction identified reovirus in hepatobiliary samples of 55% of patients with biliary atresia and 78% with choledochal cyst, whereas the virus was present in tissues of only 8 to 21% of appropriately matched controls.[44] The putative association between reovirus and biliary atresia was initially suspected based on studies in young mice, which showed that reovirus infection in the weanling period resulted in the "oily fur syndrome," which is marked by growth failure, jaundice, and oily fur. Histologically, reovirus induced hepatitis and intra- and extrahepatic biliary epithelial necrosis with surrounding edema and inflammation.[57–59] With repeated intraperitoneal injections, weanling mice develop fibrosis of the extrahepatic biliary tree but do not progress to irreversible luminal obstruction.[57]

Administration of rhesus rotavirus type A to newborn mice orally or intraperitoneally produces a notable phenotype resembling biliary atresia, with progressive jaundice, acholic stools, bilirubinuria, and growth failure, eventually culminating in death in many infected animals.[60–62] The histologic appearance of the liver and biliary tree is remarkably similar to that seen in biliary atresia, with inflammation and edema of the intra- and extrahepatic bile ducts 7 days after infection, progressing to sloughing of the biliary epithelium, concentric fibrosis of the extrahepatic bile ducts, and segmental or continuous obstruction of the extrahepatic ductal lumen by cellular debris and inflammatory cells. The precise mechanisms of virus-induced injury have not yet been established, but studies on the potential tropism of the virus to cholangiocytes, the role of inflammatory cells in biliary injury, and the identification of host factors that restrict disease susceptibility of biliary injury by rhesus rotavirus type A to only the immediate postnatal period may provide unique insight into the pathogenic mechanisms of biliary atresia in humans.[60–63]

EVIDENCE FOR INFLAMMATORY/IMMUNOLOGIC DYSREGULATION

Several patient-based studies suggest that the inflammation observed in the biliary system is not simply a biologic response to an as yet unidentified insult but rather that it may play a primary role in the targeted destruction of extrahepatic and intrahepatic bile ducts. For example, cholangiocyte pyknosis and necrosis have been associated with infiltration of mononuclear cells into the walls of interlobular bile ducts, as well as lymphocytic infiltration into portal tracts, the duct walls at the porta hepatis, and common hepatic duct remnants of infants with biliary atresia.[64–66] Phenotypic characterization of these inflammatory cells has identified CD8+ T cells infiltrating proliferated bile ducts, although the cells did not express perforin or granzyme B, markers of activated cytotoxic T lymphocytes.[67] In general, however, the lymphocytes infiltrating portal tracts in biliary atresia are CD4+ rather than CD8+ T cells. These cells express markers of T helper (Th) lymphocyte activation and proliferation, such as the interleukin (IL)-2 receptor CD25 and the transferrin receptor CD71.[68–70]

Th lymphocytes are broadly divided into two subtypes: Th1 cells, which regulate cell-mediated immunity, and Th2 cells, which regulate humoral immunity. To initiate a Th-mediated immune response, CD4+ T cells must encounter exogenous antigens complexed with a major histocompatibility complex (MHC) class II molecule on the surface of an antigen-presenting cell. In the context of biliary atresia, cholangiocytes, which normally express MHC class I but not class II antigens, are induced to aberrantly express human leukocyte antigen (HLA)-DR (a major MHC class II molecule) and act as antigen-presenting cells.[68,71,72] Furthermore, intercellular adhesion molecule 1 is expressed on the bile duct cells of patients with biliary atresia, whereas one of its ligands, leukocyte functional antigen 1, is expressed on infiltrating mononuclear cells.[70,73] Interaction between these two molecules is one of the mechanisms necessary for inflammatory cell recruitment and perpetuation of the immune response.

A potential role for Kupffer cells (resident hepatic macrophages) in promoting inflammation and fibrosis has been inferred from their increased number and size in the livers of infants with biliary atresia, as well as from their expression of the MHC class II antigen HLA-DR.[70,74,75] A potential pathway that would explain the interaction of Kupffer cells and lymphocytes in the pathogenesis of biliary atresia involves infiltration of portal tracts by CD14+ Kupffer cells, which are induced to express IL-18, a proinflammatory cytokine that promotes interferon-γ production and Th1-differentiation of lymphocytes.[74,75] Further evidence to support a Th1 proinflammatory immunity in the pathogenesis of biliary atresia has been provided by large-scale gene expression analyses of liver tissue from infants with biliary atresia and neonatal intrahepatic cholestasis. This approach identified a genetic footprint in which genes involved in lymphocyte differentiation (including the regulators of Th1 response osteopontin and interferon-γ) are activated in the early stages of biliary atresia, with simultaneous but transient suppression of markers of humoral immunity.[76] Although circumstantial, these findings point to a potential functional synergism of inflammatory effectors in the development of biliary injury in infants with biliary atresia.

PROPOSED MODEL OF DISEASE PATHOGENESIS

The five proposed mechanisms of disease reviewed above can be grouped into environmental factors (toxins and infections) and processes directly dependent on the host (defective morphogenesis, abnormal fetal/prenatal circulation, and immunologic dysregulation). Collectively, they can be unified in a "working model" in which a toxic or infectious insult to the hepatobiliary system triggers a normal reactive inflammatory response. This response effectively clears the insulting agent and, in the normal infant, stops the injury, repairs the tissue, and restores physiologic homeostasis. In the genetically susceptible infant, however, the injury is perpetuated by a preexisting developmental abnormality or by the predisposition to a proinflammatory differentiation of T lymphocytes, which targets the extrahepatic biliary tract (Figure 50.2-2). Injury to the biliary cells may secondarily result in accumulation of bile acids and activation of apoptosis, which may further exacerbate the tissue injury. As a consequence, the ductular epithelium is destroyed, fibrous material obliterates the lumen, and biliary drainage ceases. The fact that these processes occur in the first few weeks after birth suggests that developmental forces play a key role in disease onset and/or progression.

It remains possible that in a very small number of patients, the biliary injury does not completely destroy the biliary epithelium and allows for the development of different phenotypes: choledochal cyst and chronic hepatitis. This setting is consistent with the model of "infantile obstructive cholangiopathy" proposed by Landing in 1974.[35] Landing's theory was based on several premises. First, biliary atresia is not predominantly a congenital malformation but is probably an acquired obliterative process. Second, biliary atresia displays histopathologic features often found in livers of infants with intrahepatic cholestasis (idiopathic neonatal hepatitis), such as giant cell transformation of hepatocytes and variable degrees of lobular hepatitis. Third, the basic process leading to biliary atresia is inflammatory/immunologic in nature, which is common not only to intrahepatic cholestasis but also to choledochal cyst. Fourth, the inflammation present in choledochal cyst may act in a different manner than in biliary atresia, weakening the duct wall and allowing for aneurysmal dilatation of the affected portion of the duct rather than obliteration

of the ductal lumen. Although highly speculative, this theory remains attractive, at least in part, and might be corroborated by recent data from the rotavirus-induced model of biliary injury in neonatal mice. Anatomic analysis of the extrahepatic biliary system in these mice clearly demonstrates a spectrum of hepatobiliary abnormalities, including intrahepatic changes of reactive necrosis and proliferation of small bile ducts, obstruction of the extrahepatic biliary system, and cystic dilatation resembling choledochal cyst.[77]

We have been able to independently reproduce the findings of rotavirus-induced injury in our laboratory. In one set of experiments, intraperitoneal administration of rotavirus type A on the first day of life resulted in biliary injury affecting predominantly the extrahepatic bile ducts, with segmental stenosis, focal dilatation, or complete atresia in 24 of 27 of the mice (Campbell and Bezerra, unpublished data, July 2003). One of the other three mice had a large cystic dilatation of the common bile duct resembling a choledochal cyst and the other two had resolution of acholic stools but continued with jaundice and bilirubinuria. Notably, histopathologic examination of the liver of these two mice with partial improvement of symptoms showed lymphocytic infiltrate in the portal tracts and extensive fibrosis. These data support the concept that one single agent (in this case, rotavirus) induces

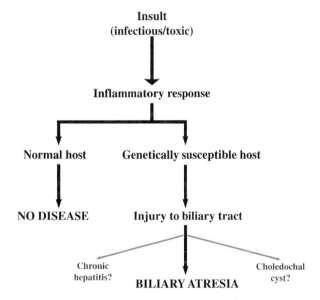

FIGURE 50.2-2 Proposed pathogenic model for biliary atresia. In this model, an infectious or toxic insult to the hepatobiliary system triggers a normal inflammatory response, which results in the clearance of the insulting agent, tissue repair, and restoration of biliary drainage in normal infants. Although the insulting agent may also be cleared in the genetically susceptible infant, a developmental abnormality of the bile ducts and/or a predisposition to a proinflammatory response lead to an ongoing injury that results in the obstruction of the extrahepatic bile ducts by fibrosis (biliary atresia). This model also depicts the potential development of chronic hepatitis or choledochal cyst, rather than biliary atresia, in a very small number of susceptible infants, in whom the injury/inflammation leads to an ongoing injury of intrahepatic bile ducts (chronic hepatitis) or the aneurysmal dilatation of a weak extrahepatic bile duct (choledochal cyst).

a primary phenotype (fibroinflammatory obstruction of the biliary tree) and two secondary phenotypes (choledochal cyst and chronic hepatitis) (see Figure 50.2-2). The use of this animal model and of other in vivo and in vitro models may provide unique insight into the interplay of different factors triggering the biliary injury, modulating the proinflammatory response, and perpetuating disease progression.

DIAGNOSTIC APPROACH

Proper and prompt identification of biliary atresia in the neonate with cholestasis is a high priority because the success of portoenterostomy to restore biliary flow rapidly declines with age.[78–80] Yet the lack of disease-specific clinical signs and laboratory tests makes it difficult to reliably distinguish between biliary atresia, other causes of extrahepatic obstruction, and intrahepatic cholestasis (Table 50.2-4). Therefore, the clinician is challenged to develop a diagnostic algorithm that incorporates ancillary tests with high predictive value for biliary atresia; the approach should be tailored to make full use of center-specific expertise. Our approach to any neonate with cholestasis obeys three diagnostic priorities. First, we establish whether jaundice is due to impaired excretion of conjugated or direct bilirubin. In practice, it is difficult to precisely define the onset of jaundice in the neonate because physiologic and breast milk jaundice may overlap with early phases of pathologic jaundice, defined as serum conjugated or direct bilirubin > 20% of total bilirubin and > 2 mg/dL. Thus, if the neonate is jaundiced beyond 2 weeks, fractionation of serum bilirubin is warranted. Identification of unconjugated hyperbilirubinemia most often points to benign processes, whereas high levels of serum conjugated bilirubin reveal the first clue to an underlying hepatobiliary pathology.

Second, we search for any evidence of systemic or metabolic diseases that may present with neonatal cholestasis and that require immediate treatment. For example, septicemia, galactosemia, and panhypopituitarism are disorders that may present with jaundice and require targeted therapeutics (antibiotics, avoidance of lactose-containing formulas, and thyroid hormone replacement, respectively) to improve survival and optimize long-term outcome. Third, we focus on those diagnostic tools that enable us to differentiate biliary atresia from other causes of neonatal jaundice in a timely fashion. In this context, it must be kept in mind that the most accurate diagnosis derives from careful histopathology combined with intraoperative examination of the extrahepatic ductular system.

HISTORY AND PHYSICAL EXAMINATION

Infants with biliary atresia typically present with jaundice between 3 and 8 weeks of age. They often appear well and develop acholic stools, but in the early stages of disease, the stools may have some bile pigment. Family history of cholestasis is almost always negative in biliary atresia, whereas the history may be positive in 15 to 20% of the cases of intrahepatic cholestasis.[4,81,82] Variable levels of lethargy, emesis, and abdominal distention and a history of bleeding or seizures often reflect coagulopathy secondary to vitamin K deficiency or potentially devastating nonhepatic conditions, such as intestinal volvulus owing to malrotation. On physical examination, hepatosplenomegaly is frequently present; nodular liver surface, prominent splenomegaly, digital clubbing, and arterial desaturation may be seen with advanced disease. Notably, the findings of a liver that is mostly palpable at midline (below the xyphoid process), pathologic murmurs, and dextrocardia in the setting of neonatal cholestasis are highly indicative of biliary atresia, specifically the embryonic form.

BIOCHEMICAL ANALYSIS

Routine indicators of liver function and injury are helpful but not diagnostic. Although some infants may have prolonged prothrombin time, normalization of coagulopathy following administration of vitamin K and serum levels of albumin above 3 g/dL indicate normal synthetic function. The usual markers of hepatocellular injury, serum alanine and aspartate aminotransferases, are mildly to moderately elevated, whereas the serum levels of alkaline phosphatase and γ-glutamyl transpeptidase (γ-GTP) progressively

---

TABLE 50.2-4   INTRA- AND EXTRAHEPATIC DISEASES THAT MAY PRESENT
IN THE NEONATAL PERIOD AND LEAD TO CHRONIC CHOLESTASIS

INTRAHEPATIC CHOLESTASIS*	EXTRAHEPATIC CHOLESTASIS
α_1-Antitrypsin deficiency	Biliary atresia
Alagille syndrome	Choledochal cyst
Transport defects	Type I: cystic dilatation of the common bile duct
Chronic cholestasis owing to *FIC* mutations	Type II: diverticulum of common duct and/or gallbladder
Chronic cholestasis owing to *BSEP* mutations	Type III: choledochocele
MDR3 deficiency	Type IV: multiple cysts
Cystic fibrosis	Type V: fusiform intrahepatic dilatations (variant of Caroli disease?)
Defects in bile acid synthesis	Spontaneous perforation of the common bile duct
Hypopituitarism/hypothyroidism	Neonatal sclerosing cholangitis
	Biliary sludge and cholelithiasis
	Acalculous gallbladder disease[†]

BSEP = bile salt export pump gene; *FIC* = familial intrahepatic cholestasis type 1 gene; MDR3 = multidrug resistance protein type 3.
*Detailed differential diagnosis for intrahepatic cholestasis is discussed elsewhere in this book.
[†]Uncommon in the neonatal period.

increase, indicating more profound biliary injury. γ-GTP levels may have some discriminatory value, with low γ-GTP rarely seen in infants with biliary atresia.[83–85] If infants are evaluated before 4 months of age, conjugated or direct hyperbilirubinemia is present but rarely above 7 mg/dL, despite the existence of an obliterative fibrosis and severe impairment to biliary drainage.

RADIOLOGIC STUDIES AND PROCEDURES

A sonographic examination of the upper abdomen is particularly useful in the search for potential causes of anatomic obstruction or cystic abnormalities of the biliary system, such as choledochal cyst, and to survey for congenital malformations, such as midline liver, polysplenia, and vascular malformations. Absence of the gallbladder suggests biliary atresia, but its presence does not rule it out. Examining the hilar structures, the ultrasonographic appearance of a "triangular cord" is suggestive of biliary atresia, with a negative predictive value of over 95% for intrahepatic cholestasis ("neonatal hepatitis").[86,87] This finding corresponds to the fibrous cone of tissue at the bifurcation of the portal vein and is often not present in infants with intrahepatic cholestasis.[86] An evolving technology with a great potential to identify the ductular structures is magnetic resonance cholangiography, but its value is largely unproven to date.[88,89] Despite remarkable improvements in sonographic and magnetic resonance cholangiographic techniques, the main limitation resides in the inability to directly visualize discontinuity of extrahepatic bile ducts with available imaging tools. This can potentially be established using hepatobiliary scintigraphy, a nuclear medicine scan that measures hepatic uptake and excretion of analogs of iminodiacetic acid into the intestine. In infants with intrahepatic cholestasis, uptake is delayed secondary to impaired hepatic function but excretion is not impaired, whereas prompt uptake is not followed by excretion into the duodenum in neonates with biliary atresia. To increase the discriminatory value of the test, phenobarbital may be given at a dose of 5 mg/kg/d for 5 days prior to the study to enhance hepatic uptake and excretion through the biliary system.[90] Despite the potential value of hepatic scintigraphy in establishing patency of the biliary system, the time required for the test may significantly delay the diagnosis.

Aspiration of duodenal fluid is another indirect measure of extrahepatic bile duct patency. If bile-stained fluid is present in a 24-hour collection of duodenal contents, biliary atresia is unlikely.[91,92] A more direct examination can be obtained by endoscopic retrograde cholangiography, which is very useful in adults to determine the patency of extrahepatic ducts but requires an experienced endoscopist for careful examination of the neonate.[93–96]

The combination of specific clinical features and ancillary tests/procedures discussed above may offer a high likelihood of an accurate diagnosis. This was documented in a retrospective review of 288 infants presenting with jaundice before 3 months of age that reported lower birth weight, later onset of jaundice, later onset of acholic stools, and the appearance of pigmented stools within 10 days

after admission occurring more frequently in infants with intrahepatic cholestasis rather than in those with biliary atresia.[97] Because of the limited predictive value of scoring systems, however, caution must be exercised and more definitive diagnostic modalities must be pursued because in approximately 10% of infants, intrahepatic disease cannot be reliably distinguished from biliary atresia.[98]

HISTOPATHOLOGY

Microscopic examination of a liver biopsy sample is a critical component of the diagnostic approach to the neonate with cholestasis. The initial biopsy is obtained percutaneously and typically shows preservation of basic lobular organization in infants with biliary atresia, with prominent abnormalities in the portal tracts and, to a lesser extent, in the lobule. Portal tracts are expanded by variable levels of edema, proliferation of bile ducts, and fibrosis (Figure 50.2-3). When present, bile plugs within proliferated ducts are highly suggestive of biliary atresia but occur in only about half of the biopsies. Inflammation in the portal space and giant cell transformation of hepatocytes may be seen but are not the dominant features and are more commonly seen in other causes of intrahepatic cholestasis.[99] Canalicular cholestasis, lobular disarray, and extramedullary hematopoiesis do not have discriminatory value between biliary atresia and other causes of neonatal cholestasis. In very young infants, the initial liver biopsy may be inconclusive, in which case, a repeat liver biopsy in 1 to 3 weeks may be necessary before the diagnosis is fully established. Whether these cases represent the sampling error inherent in percutaneous biopsies or the true progression of disease remains to be determined.

EXPLORATORY LAPAROTOMY WITH CHOLANGIOGRAPHY

When histopathologic features are suggestive of biliary atresia or the diagnostic workup is inconclusive, exploratory laparotomy must be performed in a timely manner. During laparotomy, direct inspection of the gallbladder and ductular system is the best approach to (1) determine if the ductular system is obstructed, (2) define the site of obstruction, and (3) create a conduit to re-establish biliary drainage. In most cases of biliary atresia, the gallbladder is small and fibrotic, along with diffuse fibrosis of the extrahepatic system extending to or above the level of the porta hepatis. If the gallbladder has a lumen, it may be filled with mucoid clear secretions.

For the cholangiogram, a needle or catheter is inserted into the gallbladder so that diluted contrast material can be injected to document the extent of obstruction and the anatomic variants of extrahepatic disease. These anatomic variants have been proposed by the Japanese Society of Pediatric Surgeons[100] and consist of three main types: type 1, atresia involving primarily the common bile duct; type 2, atresia extending up to the common hepatic duct; and type 3, atresia involving the whole extrahepatic ductular system (Figure 50.2-4). Sometimes a cholangiogram may not be possible owing to extensive fibrosis of the gallbladder or because of an absence of the biliary tree, a condition that has been termed "biliary agenesis." If the contrast delineates the cystic and

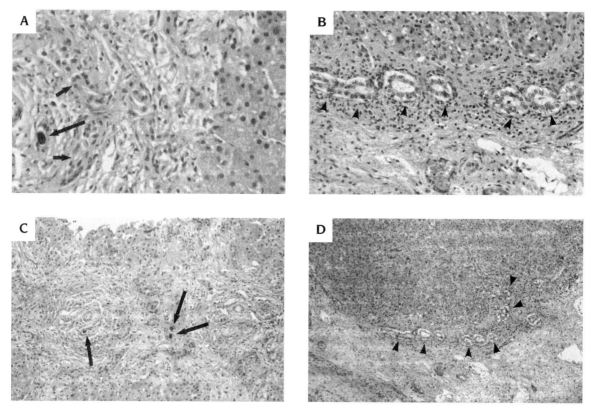

FIGURE 50.2-3   Hematoxylin and eosin staining of liver sections from infants with biliary atresia. *A* and *C* show edema, fibrosis, bile duct proliferation (*short arrows*, *A*) and a bile plug (*long arrow*, *A*) in the liver of an infant with the perinatal form of biliary atresia. In addition to edema and fibrosis, *B* and *D* also show ductal plate malformation (*arrowheads*) in an infant with the embryonic form of biliary atresia. *A* and *B* = ×200 original magnification; *C* and *D* = ×100 original magnification. Courtesy of Dr. Kevin Bove, Cincinnati Children's Hospital Medical Center, Cincinnati, OH.

common bile ducts but fails to show the patency of the hepatic and intrahepatic ducts, gentle and transient clamping of the common duct may be necessary to direct the contract upward, which may enable better filling and visualization of the proximal ductular system by the contrast. Poor filling of intrahepatic bile ducts should be interpreted with caution to avoid the creation of portoenterostomy in patients without biliary atresia. In at least one series, four patients underwent portoenterostomy after inadequate filling of intrahepatic bile ducts at intraoperative cholangiography and were later found to have the phenotypic features of Alagille syndrome.[101] In these patients, portoenterostomy may lead to biliary cirrhosis and a worse prognosis.

Histologically, the extrahepatic biliary remnants show the most typical finding of complete fibrous obliteration of the bile duct at one or more levels (Figure 50.2-5). In some patients, small single-lumen ducts that are present in biliary remnants close to the hilum may show active cholangitis. In other patients, the main duct may be reduced to smaller channels surrounded by moderate chronic inflammatory infiltrate. Although the histologic examination of the biliary structures is essential for a definitive diagnosis, the decision to proceed with portoenterostomy is not delayed until the histologic examination is completed; instead, it is made at the time of laparotomy and is based on data obtained prior to surgery, visual inspection of the biliary tree, and the results of the cholangiogram.

TREATMENT

No medical therapy has been developed to date that effectively halts or reverses cholestasis and hepatic injury in children with biliary atresia. The only therapeutic choice to increase biliary flow and improve jaundice is the portoenterostomy. Prior to the development of this surgical procedure, the mortality from biliary atresia was virtually 100%. Early attempts to relieve obstruction were limited to infants with the "correctable" forms, in which only the common bile duct was obstructed, with patent ducts proximally (type 1 of Figure 50.2-4). In the 1950s, Kasai and Suzuki noted that minute, patent bile duct remnants were present in the fibrous tissue at the porta hepatis. They reasoned that dissection into the liver parenchyma would allow drainage of bile through these ducts, whereas failure to re-establish biliary flow would lead to progressive intrahepatic ductal obliteration. This led to the development of the Kasai portoenterostomy, in which the fibrotic extrahepatic bile ducts are completely excised and an intestinal conduit is anastomosed to the transected surface of the porta hepatis in a Roux-en-Y fashion.[102]

Portoenterostomy

Although there have been numerous modifications to the original procedure of portoenterostomy described by Kasai, the concept remains the same: to bypass the fibrotic extra-

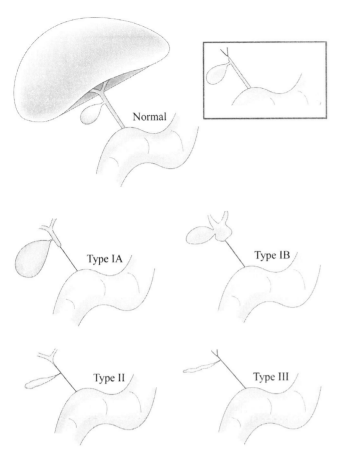

FIGURE 50.2-4 Anatomic variants of the extrahepatic biliary system in infants with biliary atresia. In type 1, the main site of obliteration is the common bile duct, which extends to the hepatic duct in type 2. Type 3, the most common variant, has complete obliteration of the entire biliary system. In the *inset*, a patent common bile duct and gallbladder may be used in lieu of an intestinal conduit to improve biliary drainage by anastomosis of the gallbladder to the hilum ("gallbladder Kasai").

hepatic biliary tree and re-establish bile drainage through intrahepatic ducts that remain patent. On entry into the abdominal cavity, the liver is firm to the touch and appears brown-green, with varying degrees of subcapsular telangiectasia. The liver and intestine are mobilized to expose the ductular and vascular structures, and the gallbladder and extrahepatic ducts are examined. Hilar structures may be edematous in the early phases of disease but are likely fibrotic and more difficult to identify in older infants.

If careful inspection of ductular structures and cholangiography are diagnostic of biliary atresia, the (fibrotic) common bile duct is transected just above the duodenal margin. Next, the gallbladder is mobilized from its hepatic bed, and the bile duct is dissected away from the anterior portal vein wall. Careful dissection toward the hilum is guided by the principle that fibrotic ducts follow the normal biliary position within the portal triad. Therefore, the dissection of the fibrous triangular mass proceeds toward the level of the liver capsule, where the fibrous remnants are transected at the level of the portal vein bifurcation on the right and the umbilical point of the portal vein on the left. Dissection deeper into the

hepatic parenchyma has not been shown to significantly increase biliary drainage. At this time, Roux-en-Y anastomosis is achieved with a 35 to 40 cm isoperistaltic retrocolic jejunal limb, which extends from the hilum to the most proximal portion of the jejunum. The Roux-hilar anastomosis is constructed just outside the margin of the hilum where the tissue has been dissected, using absorbable monofilament suture material to avoid the formation of a nidus for future infection. Distally, the intestinal conduit is anastomosed to the proximal jejunum so that biliary drainage optimizes nutrient digestion and absorption. For a small number of infants with anatomic variants of atresia in which there is a patent gallbladder and distal ducts, a "gallbladder Kasai" may be performed (see Figure 50.2-4). In this procedure, the gallbladder is mobilized from its fossa (maintaining intact the cystic artery), the fundus of the gallbladder is transected, and the opening is sutured to the biliary hilum (rather than the use of an intestinal segment). Although logical, this approach may not allow for efficient long-term biliary drainage owing to a potential dysfunction or subsequent obliteration of the common duct.

MEDICAL TREATMENT
FOLLOWING PORTOENTEROSTOMY

The goals of postoperative management of infants with biliary atresia are threefold: (1) prevention of cholangitis, (2) stimulation of choleresis, and (3) nutritional support. Infants typically receive parenteral broad-spectrum antibiotics for 3 to 5 days postoperatively, followed by oral prophylaxis with trimethoprim-sulfamethoxazole (TMP-SMX; 5 mg TMP/kg/d) or another antibiotic initiated after the patient resumes oral feedings and continued for a variable period of time (3–12 months).[100] Studies do not conclusively demonstrate the efficacy of this approach, but at least one open-label study reported lower recurrence rates of cholangitis when infants received prophylaxis with either TMP-SMX or neomycin.[103]

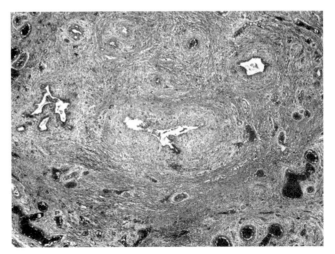

FIGURE 50.2-5 Photomicrograph of a remnant of the extrahepatic bile duct showing marked fibrosis, minute ductules, and vascular channels in a surgical specimen from an infant with biliary atresia. Courtesy of Dr. Kevin Bove, Cincinnati Children's Hospital Medical Center, Cincinnati, OH

Choleretic and Immunomodulatory Agents. Ursodeoxycholic acid (UDCA; 10–20 mg/kg/d) has been used by many centers to improve choleresis; however, very few studies have documented the efficacy of this approach. In two of these studies, use of UDCA was associated with improved weight gain and decreased levels of serum bilirubin and bile acids in more than half of the patients.[104,105] A similar trend toward improved weight gain, a decrease in the levels of serum aminotransferases and bilirubin, and a reduction in the degree of pruritus has also been reported in infants receiving UDCA, but there were no obvious differences in long-term survival or the need for transplant between treated and nontreated patients.[106]

Corticosteroids are another class of drugs used postoperatively in many centers. At pharmacologic doses, corticosteroids stimulate bile salt–independent bile flow by inducing expression of hepatic Na-K adenosine triphosphatase, a sinusoidal transporter that helps maintain the osmotic and electrical forces necessary for bile formation.[107] In addition, corticosteroids have well-described anti-inflammatory and immunomodulatory properties, including inhibition of leukocyte infiltration and down-regulation of inflammatory mediators, which may lead to decreased hilar edema and scar formation. Dosing regimens and duration of treatment with corticosteroids vary remarkably among published reports. In two early reports, administration of methylprednisolone or prednisolone either the week after portoenterostomy or later in the postoperative course when the infant developed jaundice (3 months to 4 years after surgery) induced a decrease in the levels of serum bilirubin in at least 50% of the patients.[108,109] More recently, two studies in which corticosteroid therapy was initiated soon after portoenterostomy reported improved clinical outcome, as defined by clearance of jaundice and increased survival with native liver, in over 70% of patients.[110,111] Unfortunately, these studies are limited by the use of varying dosing regimens, different indications and timing of treatment, lack of appropriate randomization, and small cohorts of patients. Despite these limitations, the results are promising and provide the basis for future multicenter randomized controlled clinical trials to objectively determine the role of corticosteroids in the treatment of infants following portoenterostomy.

Nutritional Support. Plans for adequate nutritional management should begin at the time of diagnosis and should follow the same general principles for patients with chronic cholestasis: caloric intake to meet energy needs and promote growth and supplementation with fat-soluble vitamins. Serial weight- and height-for-age and weight-for-height measurements are helpful but should be interpreted carefully if the infant develops significant hepatosplenomegaly or ascites. In this setting, high percentiles may derive from organomegaly or fluid retention rather than adequate nutrition. Anthropometrics with triceps and subscapular skin fold thickness may offer more reliable indices. Infants should receive approximately 125% of the Recommended Dietary Allowance based on weight for height at the 50th percentile, with additional calories often needed if biliary drainage is marginal (Table 50.2-5). Breastfeeding should be continued if it fosters adequate weight gain; if weight gain is inadequate or the infant is formula-fed, the use of formulas enriched with medium-chain triglycerides, which are relatively water soluble and directly absorbed into the portal circulation, will increase the pool of available energy and minimize steatorrhea. Intestinal absorption of fat-soluble vitamins A, D, E, and K is strongly dependent on adequate intraluminal concentration of bile acids. Therefore, if cholestasis is present, infants require supplementation and close monitoring to prevent the consequences of vitamin deficiencies. Unfortunately, malnutrition and progressive coagulopathy frequently develop if cholestasis is severe, and liver disease progresses despite adequate nutritional support.

COMPLICATIONS AND SEQUELAE

Most infants with biliary atresia have successful bile drainage after portoenterostomy, but adequate bile flow may be transient. If bile drainage is not achieved, progressive cholestasis and rapid progression to end-stage liver disease are the rule, at which time, orthotopic liver transplant offers the only chance for long-term survival. In the remaining majority of the patients, the clinical course is variable and is often marked by episodes of cholangitis and progressive accumulation of components of the extracellular matrix, which leads to sinusoidal obstruction and portal hypertension.

ASCENDING CHOLANGITIS
Cholangitis is the rule rather than the exception in infants with successful biliary drainage after portoenterostomy, with an incidence ranging from 40 to 60%.[100,112] Although the pathogenesis is not well defined, clinical observations point to an interplay between the patency of biliary chan-

TABLE 50.2-5   NUTRITIONAL MANAGEMENT OF INFANTS WITH BILIARY ATRESIA

NUTRIENT	TREATMENT OPTIONS	CONSEQUENCES OF DEFICIT
Energy	125% of RDA based on 50th percentile weight for height; protein: 2–3 g/kg/d; lipid: MCT enriched (~ 50% of fat calories)	Malnutrition*
Vitamin A	5,000–25,000 IU/d of water-miscible preparation of vitamin A	Punctate keratopathy[155]
Vitamin D	3–10× RDA for age; 3–5 μg/kg/d as 25-hydroxyvitamin D if rickets is present	Rickets, osteomalacia
Vitamin E	15–25 IU/kg/d TPGS	Neurologic dysfunction
Vitamin K	2.5 mg/twice a week to 5.0 mg/d	Coagulopathy

MCT = medium-chain triglyceride; RDA = Recommended Dietary Allowance; TPGS = d-α-tocopheryl polyethylene glycol-1000 succinate.
*Malnutrition may develop in patients with chronic cholestasis and progressive liver disease despite high caloric intake.

nels and enteric pathogens in the development of cholangitis. Pathogens have been proposed to ascend through the intestinal biliary conduit at the porta hepatis, translocate from other intestinal segments, or result from overgrowth favored by bile stasis that may exist in the intestinal conduit regardless of the type of surgical approach.[113-116] One strategy of unproven efficacy, but in widespread use, is the prophylactic administration of TMP-SMX for variable lengths of time during the first year of life to prevent cholangitis. Surgical modifications of the Roux-en-Y, such as partially diverted stoma for decompression of biliary conduit or valve formation in the conduit, have also been employed but have not consistently decreased the incidence of cholangitis.[100] It remains undefined whether the potential immunologic dysfunction that may play a role in disease pathogenesis also makes infants more susceptible to infectious cholangitis.

Typically, infants with cholangitis present with the triad of fever, acholic stools, and increased levels of serum bilirubin. These symptoms can also occur in isolation; therefore, the clinician must keep a high degree of suspicion so that prompt diagnosis is made and antibiotic therapy is initiated. In this context, ascending cholangitis should be suspected following portoenterostomy in any infant with irritability and poor feeding or who suddenly develops fever without an obvious source of infection; acholic stools and jaundice may lag behind by 24 hours. Sudden onset of acholic stools and jaundice in an infant with initial drainage following portoenterostomy should also be considered highly suspicious for cholangitis, even in the absence of fever or additional symptoms. Biochemically, conjugated bilirubin rises and levels of serum aminotransferases, γ-GTP, and alkaline phosphatase may increase above baseline values; leukocytosis with or without immature cells (left shift) may also be present.

Once the presumptive diagnosis of cholangitis is made, blood cultures are obtained, and patients are treated with broad-spectrum intravenous antibiotics. If an organism is identified, dosage and choice of antibiotics should be adjusted based on antimicrobial sensitivity. Intravenous antibiotics are continued for 2 to 3 days after fever resolves. In the event that stools remain acholic and conjugated hyperbilirubinemia persists, a short course of high-dose corticosteroids may be helpful.[108] Surgical revision of the portoenterostomy should be considered when evidence of cholestasis persists despite medical treatment. The surgical approach is made through the anterior wall of the portoenterostomy, followed by débridement of the scarred areas at the porta hepatis. This approach is successful in more than half of patients when they have a history of initial bile flow after primary portoenterostomy, a favorable hepatic histology, and biliary ductal remnants at initial operation or when there is a suspicion of mechanical obstruction in the intestinal conduit.[79,117,118] If revision does not result in improved biliary flow, repeated attempts are discouraged. Repeated revisions and recurrent episodes of bacterial peritonitis may produce perihepatic and intraperitoneal adhesions, which significantly complicate the surgical approach during liver transplant.

PORTAL HYPERTENSION

In addition to the fibro-obliterative changes in the extrahepatic ducts, variable degrees of intrahepatic fibrosis and portal hypertension are also present at the time of diagnosis of biliary atresia.[119] This fibrosis progresses even in the infants with improved biliary flow[120]; portal pressure gradually increases, and significant portal hypertension develops in 34 to 76% of infants with biliary atresia.[119,121] The clinical consequences of portal hypertension are variable, often resulting in the development of esophageal varices. Interestingly, portal hypertension may resolve spontaneously in older patients. Therefore, the initial approach to portal hypertension in infants with biliary atresia is directed at preventing and treating complications, such as gastrointestinal hemorrhage. A study of a single center's experience in Japan reported esophageal varices in 25% and hypersplenism in 14% of 106 children with biliary atresia without jaundice.[100] Notably, esophageal bleeding occurs in approximately 19% of all long-term survivors[122] and at a higher rate (20–60%) when studies include only those children with esophageal varices.[123]

Primary therapy for children with biliary atresia and hemorrhage from esophageal varices is endoscopic injection sclerotherapy or variceal band ligation.[124-127] Before endoscopy, the patient should be monitored closely, be evaluated for coagulopathy, and receive an infusion of packed red blood cells to restore normal blood pressure. Packed red blood cells should be transfused slowly to avoid sudden expansion of intravascular volume and a new onset of variceal hemorrhage. Continuous infusion of somastatin analogs to decrease the severity of the bleeding may be particularly valuable to stabilize the patient in preparation for endoscopy. In the setting of active bleeding or in small infants, sclerotherapy is the treatment of choice.

β-Blockers represent another therapeutic option for primary prophylaxis or after an episode of variceal hemorrhage (secondary prophylaxis). Although their use is well accepted in adults, there are few data regarding the efficacy of β-blockers in children. In the one published study to date, 6 of 17 children subjected to primary prophylaxis with propanolol had variceal hemorrhage, whereas 1 of 4 patients receiving secondary prophylaxis bled.[128] In the absence of a control group, it is unclear whether this represents a decrease in the incidence of variceal hemorrhage. Likewise, questions regarding optimum dosage and dosing schedule in children also need to be addressed prospectively. For those patients with recurrent or severe hemorrhage, the utility of the traditional portal shunt (with or without esophageal transection) and transjugular intrahepatic portosystemic shunt should be considered. Decisions regarding these therapies should be made on an individual basis and take into account the available expertise in the medical center. The best therapeutic choice for these patients is timely liver transplant if a suitable organ is available. This is particularly relevant based on recent data suggesting that the outcome of children following the first episode of variceal hemorrhage is related to the coexisting degree of hyperbilirubinemia, with a 12-fold increase in the risk of death or need for transplant if the serum total bilirubin is > 10 mg/dL versus a 0.6-fold risk when the serum bilirubin was ≤ 4 mg/dL, when compared with children with biliary atresia and no history of variceal hemorrhage.[129]

OTHER COMPLICATIONS

Hypersplenism is another complication in long-term survivors and is especially problematic in those infants with significant thrombocytopenia and a history of bleeding from esophageal varices. If hypersplenism significantly worsens coagulopathy, splenic embolization has been shown to result in improved blood cell count and hemorrhagic tendency in 60 to 70% of patients, but high fever and abdominal pain are universal complications.[100] Another potential complication in long-term survivors is the development of the hepatopulmonary syndrome, which results from intrapulmonary vascular dilatation with shunting. These patients typically have exercise intolerance, digital clubbing, and cutaneous spider telangiectasia. Currently, no medical therapy alleviates hepatopulmonary syndrome; a definitive cure can be achieved by liver transplant, although children with the syndrome may be more susceptible to complications.[130,131] Lastly, children with biliary atresia may rarely develop cystic dilatation of intrahepatic bile ducts or hepatocellular carcinoma.[132–134]

LONG-TERM OUTCOME

Most patients with biliary atresia have improved biliary drainage following portoenterostomy. Long-term outcome, however, may be better predicted by the serum level of bilirubin 3 months after surgery. In those infants with serum bilirubin levels below 1 mg/dL 3 months after portoenterostomy, 53% had normal growth, no esophageal varix, or hyperplenism at 12 or more years after portoenterostomy.[135] Although the precise mechanisms regulating progression of liver disease are not well defined, ongoing cholestasis, intrahepatic cholangiopathy, persistent inflammatory processes, and progressive fibrosis appear to be important factors.[118,136–139] Specific markers for disease progression and predictors of long-term outcome may emerge from studies of the pathogenesis of biliary atresia. For example, serial levels of serum hyaluronic acid and procollagen propeptides may be unique markers of hepatic fibrogenesis and disease progression.[140]

Actuarial survival with native liver has been estimated at 32 to 61% at 5 years and 27 to 54% at 10 years of life.[100,141,142] Among the several factors that may influence long-term outcome, age and the size of the ductules in biliary remnants at the time of portoenterostomy have been systematically examined. Collectively, studies point to better outcome when portoenterostomy is performed in infants ≤ 60 days of age and when the size of ductules within the biliary remnant measures ≥ 150 μm (Table 50.2-6). The patient's age at operation alone, however, may not be a reliable predictor of outcome, as suggested by a study of infants who underwent portoenterostomy before 30 days of age. In this group, 78% of the patients required liver transplant at a mean age of 6.8 ± 2.3 months.[19] This

outcome may reflect a more severe form of disease that leads to early jaundice and early diagnosis of biliary atresia. Other factors that contribute to long-term outcome include episodes of cholangitis after surgery, the decade when surgery was performed, and the experience of the surgical team.[141,143] For example, at Tohoku University Hospital (Japan), actuarial survival of 307 patients treated with the Kasai portoenterostomy improved from ~ 20% before 1971 to ~ 70% between 1971 and 1998.[100] An effect of the "center experience" in achieving high success rates has been emphasized by an improved survival rate to 78% in centers in which a large number of portoenterostomies are performed by the surgical team.[6,144] As long-term survival increases, the quality of life in children with biliary atresia has become a focus of studies designed to improve outcome. In this context, 44 to 47 of 108 patients reported development of pruritus, reduced physical fitness, and the inability to attend school regularly.[143] These results clearly identify areas requiring additional support and therapeutic targets for long-term survivors.

LIVER TRANSPLANT

Liver transplant is a well-accepted treatment option for children with biliary atresia and end-stage liver disease. Access to transplant by a greater number of children has been driven by remarkable improvements in surgical techniques, which have led to the development of reduced-size and living-related donor transplant and to improved immunosuppression.[145–147] As a consequence, biliary atresia has become the most frequent indication for liver transplant in children.[118,148–151] For example, biliary atresia has been the primary indication for liver transplant at the Cincinnati Children's Hospital Medical Center (July 1985 to May 2003), accounting for 44% of 255 transplanted children. Although effective, the timely use of the technique in children with end-stage liver disease is significantly limited by an ever-increasing number of pediatric patients on transplant waiting lists and the scarcity of suitable organs. This is particularly important because the outcome in our center appears to be related to the severity of the patient's illness at the time of transplant.[148,152]

With limited organ availability, the clinician is challenged to identify those patients who may best benefit from liver transplant. In this context, the primary goal should be

TABLE 50.2-6   FACTORS INFLUENCING LONG-TERM OUTCOME OF INFANTS WITH BILIARY ATRESIA

FACTOR	% WITH BILE FLOW	REFERENCE
Age at the time of portoenterostomy		78, 100, 112
< 60 d	67–82	
60–90 d	45–62	
> 90 d	10–44	
Morphology of duct remnants		156
≥ 150 μm lumen size	92	
50–150 μm lumen size	81	
No identified epithelium-lined ducts	18	

to optimize the clinical status and quality of life of all children with their native liver and stay vigilant for the primary indications for transplant evaluation: (1) persistent cholestasis associated with severe malnutrition, growth failure, and hepatocellular dysfunction and (2) decompensated cirrhosis, as evidenced by intractable ascites and hemorrhage. For all children, the overall goals of transplant include restoration of hepatic function, improved nutritional status, adequate growth and development, and improved quality of life with full social reintegration.[149,153]

One additional indication for transplant that generates a significant debate is the use of transplant as the primary treatment modality for infants with biliary atresia who are diagnosed beyond 90 to 120 days of age and have established cirrhosis. Although portoenterostomy in this group has been associated with low incidence of improved biliary flow and poor long-term outcome, data analysis from a large cohort of patients showed a 5-year survival with native liver of ~ 31% when surgery was performed beyond 45 days of age in comparison with ~ 41% when portoenterostomy was performed before 45 days.[144] Therefore, portoenterostomy should remain the first line of therapy in infants with biliary atresia.[154] With appropriate management after portoenterostomy, improved surgical techniques, effective post-transplant immunosuppression, and aggressive management of infectious complications, the overall survival and quality of life of children with biliary atresia will continue to increase.

SUMMARY

Biliary atresia is the most common cause of pathologic jaundice in young infants and results from obliteration of the extrahepatic bile ducts by an inflammatory and fibro-obliterative process. Although the pathogenesis is not fully elucidated, patient- and animal-based studies point to a possible pathogenic model in which a genetically susceptible subject abnormally destroys the extrahepatic biliary system in response to environmental factors. Clinically, the disease is manifest by the triad of jaundice, acholic stools, and hepatosplenomegaly. In approximately one-fifth of the cases, infants also have nonhepatic malformations, such as laterality defects. Because many of the initial features are shared by other causes of neonatal cholestasis, the clinician is challenged to develop a diagnostic algorithm that facilitates the diagnosis so that portoenterostomy is performed in a timely fashion. Postoperatively, infants often require a high-calorie diet, supplementation with fat-soluble vitamins, and medications to induce choleresis and prevent cholangitis. Despite medical and surgical treatments, the disease commonly progresses, with hepatic fibrosis, portal hypertension, and end-stage liver disease occurring in at least half of the patients by 2 years of age. At this stage, liver transplant is an effective treatment modality, but the surgical success presents the infants with new morbidities and carries a high monetary cost to society. Therefore, we are challenged to systematically search for pathogenic mechanisms so that prevention can be attempted and new therapeutic strategies can be developed to stop disease progression and improve long-term outcome.

REFERENCES

1. Schreiber RA, Kleinman RE. Biliary atresia. J Pediatr Gastroenterol Nutr 2002;35 Suppl 1:S11–6.
2. Balistreri WF. Pediatric hepatology. A half-century of progress. Clin Liver Dis 2000;4:191–210.
3. Bates MD, Bucuvalas JC, Alonso MH, Ryckman FC. Biliary atresia: pathogenesis and treatment. Semin Liver Dis 1998;18:281–93.
4. Danks DM, Campbell PE, Jack I, et al. Studies of the aetiology of neonatal hepatitis and biliary atresia. Arch Dis Child 1977;52:360–7.
5. Strickland AD, Shannon K. Studies in the etiology of extrahepatic biliary atresia: time-space clustering. J Pediatr 1982;100:749–53.
6. Chardot C, Carton M, Spire-Bendelac N, et al. Epidemiology of biliary atresia in France: a national study 1986-96. J Hepatol 1999;31:1006–13.
7. Fischler B, Haglund B, Hjern A. A population-based study on the incidence and possible pre- and perinatal etiologic risk factors of biliary atresia. J Pediatr 2002;141:217–22.
8. Yoon PW, Bresee JS, Olney RS, et al. Epidemiology of biliary atresia: a population-based study. Pediatrics 1997;99:376–82.
9. Balistreri WF. Neonatal cholestasis. J Pediatr 1985;106:171–84.
10. Davenport M, Savage M, Mowat AP, Howard ER. Biliary atresia splenic malformation syndrome: an etiologic and prognostic subgroup. Surgery 1993;113:662–8.
11. Cunningham ML, Sybert VP. Idiopathic extrahepatic biliary atresia: recurrence in sibs in two families. Am J Med Genet 1988;31:421–6.
12. Lachaux A, Descos B, Plauchu H, et al. Familial extrahepatic biliary atresia. J Pediatr Gastroenterol Nutr 1988;7:280–3.
13. Smith BM, Laberge JM, Schreiber R, et al. Familial biliary atresia in three siblings including twins. J Pediatr Surg 1991;26:1331–3.
14. Hyams JS, Glaser JH, Leichtner AM, Morecki R. Discordance for biliary atresia in two sets of monozygotic twins. J Pediatr 1985;107:420–2.
15. Strickland AD, Shannon K, Coln CD. Biliary atresia in two sets of twins. J Pediatr 1985;107:418–20.
16. Schweizer P. Treatment of extrahepatic bile duct atresia: results and long-term prognosis after hepatic portoenterostomy. Pediatr Surg Int 1986;1:30–6.
17. Desmet VJ. Congenital diseases of intrahepatic bile ducts: variations on the theme "ductal plate malformation." Hepatology 1992;16:1069–83.
18. Carmi R, Magee CA, Neill CA, Karrer FM. Extrahepatic biliary atresia and associated anomalies: etiologic heterogeneity suggested by distinctive patterns of associations. Am J Med Genet 1993;45:683–93.
19. Volpert D, White F, Finegold MJ, et al. Outcome of early hepatic portoenterostomy for biliary atresia. J Pediatr Gastroenterol Nutr 2001;32:265–9.
20. Balistreri WF, Grand R, Hoofnagle JH, et al. Biliary atresia: current concepts and research directions. Summary of a symposium. Hepatology 1996;23:1682–92.
21. Tan CE, Driver M, Howard ER, Moscoso GJ. Extrahepatic biliary atresia: a first-trimester event? Clues from light microscopy and immunohistochemistry. J Pediatr Surg 1994;29:808–14.
22. Hasegawa T, Sasaki T, Kimura T, et al. Prenatal ultrasonographic appearance of type IIId (uncorrectable type with cystic dilatation) biliary atresia. Pediatr Surg Int 2002;18:425–8.
23. Yokoyama T, Copeland NG, Jenkins NA, et al. Reversal of left-right asymmetry: a situs inversus mutation. Science 1993;260:679–82.
24. Mazziotti MV, Willis LK, Heuckeroth RO, et al. Anomalous development of the hepatobiliary system in the Inv mouse. Hepatology 1999;30:372–8.

25. Perlmutter DH, Shepherd RW. Extrahepatic biliary atresia: a disease or a phenotype? Hepatology 2002;35:1297–304.

26. Schon P, Tsuchiya K, Lenoir D, et al. Identification, genomic organization, chromosomal mapping and mutation analysis of the human INV gene, the ortholog of a murine gene implicated in left-right axis development and biliary atresia. Hum Genet 2002;110:157–65.

27. Coffinier C, Gresh L, Fiette L, et al. Bile system morphogenesis defects and liver dysfunction upon targeted deletion of HNF1-beta. Development 2002;129:1829–38.

28. Clotman F, Lannoy VJ, Reber M, et al. The onecut transcription factor HNF6 is required for normal development of the biliary tract. Development 2002;129:1819–28.

29. McCright B, Lozier J, Gridley T. A mouse model of Alagille syndrome: Notch2 as a genetic modifier of Jag1 haploinsufficiency. Development 2002;129:1075–82.

30. Oda T, Elkahloun AG, Pike BL, et al. Mutations in the human Jagged1 gene are responsible for Alagille syndrome. Nat Genet 1997;16:235–42.

31. Li L, Krantz ID, Deng Y, et al. Alagille syndrome is caused by mutations in human Jagged1, which encodes a ligand for Notch1. Nat Genet 1997;16:243–51.

32. Kohsaka T, Yuan ZR, Guo SX, et al. The significance of human jagged 1 mutations detected in severe cases of extrahepatic biliary atresia. Hepatology 2002;36(4 Pt 1):904–12.

33. Ho CW, Shioda K, Shirasaki K, et al. The pathogenesis of biliary atresia: a morphological study of the hepatobiliary system and the hepatic artery. J Pediatr Gastroenterol Nutr 1993;16:53–60.

34. Harper P, Plant JW, Unger DB. Congenital biliary atresia and jaundice in lambs and calves [published erratum appears in Aust Vet J 1990;67:167]. Aust Vet J 1990;67:18–22.

35. Landing BH. Considerations of the pathogenesis of neonatal hepatitis, biliary atresia and choledochal cyst—the concept of infantile obstructive cholangiopathy. Prog Pediatr Surg 1974;6:113–39.

36. Tanaka M, Ishikawa T, Sakaguchi M. The pathogenesis of biliary atresia in Japan: immunohistochemical study of HBV-associated antigen. Acta Pathol Jpn 1993;43:360–6.

37. Balistreri WF, Tabor E, Gerety RJ. Negative serology for hepatitis A and B viruses in 18 cases of neonatal cholestasis. Pediatrics 1980;66:269–71.

38. Scotto JM, Alvarez F. Biliary artresia and non-A, non-B hepatitis? Gastroenterology 1982;82:393–4.

39. HH AK, Nowicki MJ, Kuramoto KI, et al. Evaluation of the role of hepatitis C virus in biliary atresia. Pediatr Infect Dis J 1994;13:657–9.

40. Gomez MA, Drut R, Lojo MM, Drut RM. Detection of human papillomavirus in juvenile laryngeal papillomatosis using polymerase chain reaction. Medicina 1995;55:213–7.

41. Riepenhoff-Talty M, Gouvea V, Evans MJ, et al. Detection of group C rotavirus in infants with extrahepatic biliary atresia. J Infect Dis 1996;174:8–15.

42. Tarr PI, Haas JE, Christie DL. Biliary atresia, cytomegalovirus, and age at referral. Pediatrics 1996;97(6 Pt 1):828–31.

43. Fischler B, Ehrnst A, Forsgren M, et al. The viral association of neonatal cholestasis in Sweden: a possible link between cytomegalovirus infection and extrahepatic biliary atresia. J Pediatr Gastroenterol Nutr 1998;27:57–64.

44. Tyler KL, Sokol RJ, Oberhaus SM, et al. Detection of reovirus RNA in hepatobiliary tissues from patients with extrahepatic biliary atresia and choledochal cysts. Hepatology 1998;27:1475–82.

45. Drut R, Drut RM, Gomez MA, et al. Presence of human papillomavirus in extrahepatic biliary atresia. J Pediatr Gastroenterol Nutr 1998;27:530–5.

46. Mason AL, Xu L, Guo L, et al. Detection of retroviral antibodies in primary biliary cirrhosis and other idiopathic biliary disorders [published erratum appears in Lancet 1998;352:152]. Lancet 1998;351:1620–4.

47. Glaser JH, Balistreri WF, Morecki R. Role of reovirus type 3 in persistent infantile cholestasis. J Pediatr 1984;105:912–5.

48. Morecki R, Glaser JH, Cho S, et al. Biliary atresia and reovirus type 3 infection. N Engl J Med 1984;310:1610.

49. Morecki R, Glaser JH, Johnson AB, Kress Y. Detection of reovirus type 3 in the porta hepatis of an infant with extrahepatic biliary atresia: ultrastructural and immunocytochemical study. Hepatology 1984;4:1137–42.

50. Domiati-Saad R, Dawson DB, Margraf LR, et al. Cytomegalovirus and human herpesvirus 6, but not human papillomavirus, are present in neonatal giant cell hepatitis and extrahepatic biliary atresia. Pediatr Dev Pathol 2000;3:367–73.

51. Jevon GP, Dimmick JE. Biliary atresia and cytomegalovirus infection: a DNA study. Pediatr Dev Pathol 1999;2:11–4.

52. Brown WR, Sokol RJ, Levin MJ, et al. Lack of correlation between infection with reovirus 3 and extrahepatic biliary atresia or neonatal hepatitis. J Pediatr 1988;113:670–6.

53. Steele MI, Marshall CM, Lloyd RE, Randolph VE. Reovirus 3 not detected by reverse transcriptase-mediated polymerase chain reaction analysis of preserved tissue from infants with cholestatic liver disease. Hepatology 1995;21:697–702.

54. Bobo L, Ojeh C, Chiu D, et al. Lack of evidence for rotavirus by polymerase chain reaction/enzyme immunoassay of hepatobiliary samples from children with biliary atresia. Pediatr Res 1997;41:229–34.

55. Richardson SC, Bishop RF, Smith AL. Reovirus serotype 3 infection in infants with extrahepatic biliary atresia or neonatal hepatitis. J Gastroenterol Hepatol 1994;9:264–8.

56. Dussaix E, Hadchouel M, Tardieu M, Alagille D. Biliary atresia and reovirus type 3 infection. N Engl J Med 1984;310:658.

57. Bangaru B, Morecki R, Glaser JH, et al. Comparative studies of biliary atresia in the human newborn and reovirus-induced cholangitis in weanling mice. Lab Invest 1980;43:456–62.

58. Wilson GA, Morrison LA, Fields BN. Association of the reovirus S1 gene with serotype 3-induced biliary atresia in mice. J Virol 1994;68:6458–65.

59. Szavay PO, Leonhardt J, Czech-Schmidt G, Petersen C. The role of reovirus type 3 infection in an established murine model for biliary atresia. Eur J Pediatr Surg 2002;12:248–50.

60. Riepenhoff-Talty M, Schaekel K, Clark HF, et al. Group A rotaviruses produce extrahepatic biliary obstruction in orally inoculated newborn mice. Pediatr Res 1993;33(4 Pt 1):394–9.

61. Petersen C, Biermanns D, Kuske M, et al. New aspects in a murine model for extrahepatic biliary atresia. J Pediatr Surg 1997;32:1190–5.

62. Petersen C, Kuske M, Bruns E, et al. Progress in developing animal models for biliary atresia. Eur J Pediatr Surg 1998;8:137–41.

63. Czech-Schmidt G, Verhagen W, Szavay P, et al. Immunological gap in the infectious animal model for biliary atresia. J Surg Res 2001;101:62–7.

64. Bill AH, Haas JE, Foster GL. Biliary atresia: histopathologic observations and reflections upon its natural history. J Pediatr Surg 1977;12:977–82.

65. Ohya T, Fujimoto T, Shimomura H, Miyano T. Degeneration of intrahepatic bile duct with lymphocyte infiltration into biliary epithelial cells in biliary atresia. J Pediatr Surg 1995;30:515–8.

66. Gosseye S, Otte JB, De Meyer R, Maldague P. A histological study of extrahepatic biliary atresia. Acta Paediatr Belg 1977;30:85–90.

67. Ahmed AF, Ohtani H, Nio M, et al. CD8+ T cells infiltrating into bile ducts in biliary atresia do not appear to function as cytotoxic T cells: a clinicopathological analysis. J Pathol 2001;193:383–9.

68. Broome U, Nemeth A, Hultcrantz R, Scheynius A. Different expression of HLA-DR and ICAM-1 in livers from patients with biliary atresia and Byler's disease. J Hepatol 1997;26:857–62.

69. Dillon PW, Belchis D, Minnick K, Tracy T. Differential expression of the major histocompatibility antigens and ICAM-1 on bile duct epithelial cells in biliary atresia. Tohoku J Exp Med 1997;181:33–40.

70. Davenport M, Gonde C, Redkar R, et al. Immunohistochemistry of the liver and biliary tree in extrahepatic biliary atresia. J Pediatr Surg 2001;36:1017–25.

71. Kobayashi H, Puri P, O'Brian DS, et al. Hepatic overexpression of MHC class II antigens and macrophage-associated antigens (CD68) in patients with biliary atresia of poor prognosis. J Pediatr Surg 1997;32:590–3.

72. Nakada M, Nakada K, Kawaguchi F, et al. Immunologic reaction and genetic factors in biliary atresia. Tohoku J Exp Med 1997;181:41–7.

73. Dillon P, Belchis D, Tracy T, et al. Increased expression of intercellular adhesion molecules in biliary atresia. Am J Pathol 1994;145:263–7.

74. Tracy TF Jr, Dillon P, Fox ES, et al. The inflammatory response in pediatric biliary disease: macrophage phenotype and distribution. J Pediatr Surg 1996;31:121–5; discussion 125–6.

75. Urushihara N, Iwagaki H, Yagi T, et al. Elevation of serum interleukin-18 levels and activation of Kupffer cells in biliary atresia. J Pediatr Surg 2000;35:446–9.

76. Bezerra JA, Tiao G, Ryckman FC, et al. Genetic induction of proinflammatory immunity in children with biliary atresia. Lancet 2002;360:1653–9.

77. Petersen C, Biermanns D, Kuske M, et al. New aspects in a murine model for extrahepatic biliary atresia. J Pediatr Surg 1997;32:1190–5.

78. Kasai M. Treatment of biliary atresia with special reference to hepatic porto-enterostomy and its modifications. Prog Pediatr Surg 1974;6:5–52.

79. Ohi R, Hanamatsu M, Mochizuki I, et al. Reoperation in patients with biliary atresia. J Pediatr Surg 1985;20:256–9.

80. Karrer FM, Price MR, Bensard DD, et al. Long-term results with the Kasai operation for biliary atresia. Arch Surg 1996;131:493–6.

81. Danks D, Bodian M. A genetic study of neonatal obstructive jaundice. Arch Dis Child 1963;38:378–87.

82. Mowat AP, Psacharopoulos HT, Williams R. Extrahepatic biliary atresia versus neonatal hepatitis. Review of 137 prospectively investigated infants. Arch Dis Child 1976;51:763–70.

83. Fung KP, Lau SP. Gamma-glutamyl transpeptidase activity and its serial measurement in differentiation between extrahepatic biliary atresia and neonatal hepatitis. J Pediatr Gastroenterol Nutr 1985;4:208–13.

84. Sinatra FR. The role of gamma-glutamyl transpeptidase in the preoperative diagnosis of biliary atresia. J Pediatr Gastroenterol Nutr 1985;4:167–8.

85. Tazawa Y, Yamada M, Nakagawa M, et al. Significance of serum lipoprotein-X and gammaglutamyltranspeptidase in the diagnosis of biliary atresia. A preliminary study in 27 cholestatic young infants. Eur J Pediatr 1986;145:54–7.

86. Choi SO, Park WH, Lee HJ, Woo SK. 'Triangular cord': a sonographic finding applicable in the diagnosis of biliary atresia. J Pediatr Surg 1996;31:363–6.

87. Choi SO, Park WH, Lee HJ. Ultrasonographic "triangular cord": the most definitive finding for noninvasive diagnosis of extrahepatic biliary atresia. Eur J Pediatr Surg 1998;8:12–6.

88. Guibaud L, Lachaud A, Touraine R, et al. MR cholangiography in neonates and infants: feasibility and preliminary applications. AJR Am J Roentgenol 1998;170:27–31.

89. Jaw TS, Kuo YT, Liu GC, et al. MR cholangiography in the evaluation of neonatal cholestasis. Radiology 1999;212:249–56.

90. Ohi R, Klingensmith WC III, Lilly JR. Diagnosis of hepatobiliary disease in infants and children with Tc-99m-diethyl-IDA imaging. Clin Nucl Med 1981;6:297–302.

91. Greene HL, Helinek GL, Moran R, O'Neill J. A diagnostic approach to prolonged obstructive jaundice by 24-hour collection of duodenal fluid. J Pediatr 1979;95:412–4.

92. Faweya AG, Akinyinka OO, Sodeinde O. Duodenal intubation and aspiration test: utility in the differential diagnosis of infantile cholestasis. J Pediatr Gastroenterol Nutr 1991;13:290–2.

93. Lebwohl O, Waye JD. Endoscopic retrograde cholangiopancreatography in the diagnosis of extrahepatic biliary atresia. Am J Dis Child 1979;133:647–9.

94. Heyman MB, Shapiro HA, Thaler MM. Endoscopic retrograde cholangiography in the diagnosis of biliary malformations in infants. Gastrointest Endosc 1988;34:449–53.

95. Wilkinson ML, Mieli-Vergani G, Ball C, et al. Endoscopic retrograde cholangiopancreatography in infantile cholestasis. Arch Dis Child 1991;66:121–3.

96. Shirai Z, Toriya H, Maeshiro K, Ikeda S. The usefulness of endoscopic retrograde cholangiopancreatography in infants and small children. Am J Gastroenterol 1993;88:536–41.

97. Alagille D. Cholestasis in the first three months of life. Prog Liver Dis 1979;6:471–85.

98. Hays DM, Woolley MM, Snyder WH Jr, et al. Diagnosis of biliary atresia: relative accuracy of percutaneous liver biopsy, open liver biopsy, and operative cholangiography. J Pediatr 1967;71:598–607.

99. Brough AJ, Bernstein J. Conjugated hyperbilirubinemia in early infancy. A reassessment of liver biopsy. Hum Pathol 1974;5:507–16.

100. Ohi R. Biliary atresia: a surgical perspective. Clin Liver Dis 2000;4:779–804.

101. Markowitz J, Daum F, Kahn EI, et al. Arteriohepatic dysplasia. I. Pitfalls in diagnosis and management. Hepatology 1983;3:74–6.

102. Kasai M, Suzuki S. A new operation for "non-correctable" biliary atresia, hepatic portoenterostomy [in Japanese]. Shujutsu 1959;13:733–9.

103. Bu L, Chen H, Chang C, et al. Prophylactic oral antibiotics in prevention of recurrent cholangitis after the Kasai portoenterostomy. J Pediatr Surg 2003;48:590–3.

104. Nittono H, Tokita A, Hayashi M, et al. Ursodeoxycholic acid therapy in the treatment of biliary atresia. Biomed Pharmacother 1989;43:37–41.

105. Ullrich D, Rating D, Schroter W, et al. Treatment with ursodeoxycholic acid renders children with biliary atresia suitable for liver transplantation. Lancet 1987;ii:1324.

106. Balistreri W, Setchell K, Ryckman F, and the UDCA study group. Bile acid therapy in paediatric liver disease. London: Kluwer Academic Publishers; 1993.

107. Miner PB Jr, Sutherland E, Simon FR. Regulation of hepatic sodium plus potassium-activated adenosine triphosphatase activity by glucocorticoids in the rat. Gastroenterology 1980;79:212–21.

108. Karrer F, Lilly JR. Corticosteroid therapy in biliary atresia. J Pediatr Surg 1985;20:693–5.

109. Muraji T, Higashimoto Y. The improved outlook for biliary atresia with corticosteroid therapy. J Pediatr Surg 1997;32:1103–7.

110. Dillon P, Owings E, Cilley R, et al. Immunosuppression as adjuvant therapy for biliary atresia. J Pediatr Surg 2001;36:80–5.

111. Meyers R, Book L, O'Gorman M, et al. High-dose steroids, ursodeoxycholic acid, and chronic intravenous antibiotics improve bile flow after Kasai procedure in infants with biliary atresia. J Pediatr Surg 2003;38:406–11.

112. Howard ER. Extrahepatic biliary atresia: a review of current management. Br J Surg 1983;70:193–7.

113. Danks DM, Campbell PE, Clarke AM, et al. Extrahepatic biliary atresia: the frequency of potentially operable cases. Am J Dis Child 1974;128:684–6.

114. Hirsig J, Kara O, Rickham PP. Experimental investigations into the etiology of cholangitis following operation for biliary atresia. J Pediatr Surg 1978;13:55–7.

115. Welsh FK, Ramsden CW, MacLennan K, et al. Increased intestinal permeability and altered mucosal immunity in cholestatic jaundice. Ann Surg 1998;227:205–12.

116. Hitch DC, Lilly JR. Identification, quantification, and significance of bacterial growth within the biliary tract after Kasai's operation. J Pediatr Surg 1978;13:563–9.

117. Ohi R, Ibrahim M. Biliary atresia. Semin Pediatr Surg 1992; 1:115–24.

118. Ryckman F, Fisher R, Pedersen S, et al. Improved survival in biliary atresia patients in the present era of liver transplantation. J Pediatr Surg 1993;28:382–6.

119. Ohi R, Mochizuki I, Komatsu K, Kasai M. Portal hypertension after successful hepatic portoenterostomy in biliary atresia. J Pediatr Surg 1986;21:271–4.

120. Altman RP, Chandra R, Lilly JR. Ongoing cirrhosis after successful porticoenterostomy in infants with biliary atresia. J Pediatr Surg 1975;10:685–91.

121. Stringer MD, Howard ER, Mowat AP. Endoscopic sclerotherapy in the management of esophageal varices in 61 children with biliary atresia. J Pediatr Surg 1989;24:438–42.

122. Howard ER, Davenport M. The treatment of biliary atresia in Europe 1969-1995. Tohoku J Exp Med 1997;181:75–83.

123. Lilly JR, Stellin G. Variceal hemorrhage in biliary atresia. J Pediatr Surg 1984;19:476–9.

124. Hall RJ, Lilly JR, Stiegmann GV. Endoscopic esophageal varix ligation: technique and preliminary results in children. J Pediatr Surg 1988;23:1222–3.

125. Howard ER, Stamatakis JD, Mowat AP. Management of esophageal varices in children by injection sclerotherapy. J Pediatr Surg 1984;19:2–5.

126. Howard ER, Stringer MD, Mowat AP. Assessment of injection sclerotherapy in the management of 152 children with oesophageal varices. Br J Surg 1988;75:404–8.

127. Paquet KJ, Lazar A. Current therapeutic strategy in bleeding esophageal varices in babies and children and long-term results of endoscopic paravariceal sclerotherapy over twenty years. Eur J Pediatr Surg 1994;4:165–72.

128. Shashidhar H, Langhans N, Grand RJ. Propranolol in prevention of portal hypertensive hemorrhage in children: a pilot study. J Pediatr Gastroenterol Nutr 1999;29:12–7.

129. Miga D, Sokol RJ, Mackenzie T, et al. Survival after first esophageal variceal hemorrhage in patients with biliary atresia. J Pediatr 2001;139:291–6.

130. Yonemura T, Yoshibayashi M, Uemoto S, et al. Intrapulmonary shunting in biliary atresia before and after living-related liver transplantation. Br J Surg 1999;86:1139–43.

131. Egawa H, Kasahara M, Inomata Y, et al. Long-term outcome of living related liver transplantation for patients with intrapulmonary shunting and strategy for complications. Transplantation 1999;67:712–7.

132. Kohno M, Kitatani H, Wada H, et al. Hepatocellular carcinoma complicating biliary cirrhosis caused by biliary atresia: report of a case. J Pediatr Surg 1995;30:1713–6.

133. Saito S, Nishina T, Tsuchida Y. Intrahepatic cysts in biliary atresia after successful hepatoportoenterostomy. Arch Dis Child 1984;59:274–5.

134. Tsuchida Y, Honna T, Kawarasaki H. Cystic dilatation of the intrahepatic biliary system in biliary atresia after hepatic portoenterostomy. J Pediatr Surg 1994;29:630–4.

135. Ohhama Y, Shinkai M, Fujita S, et al. Early prediction of long-term survival and the timing of liver transplantation after the Kasai operation. J Pediatr Surg 2000;35:1031–4.

136. Ito T, Horisawa M, Ando H. Intrahepatic bile ducts in biliary atresia—a possible factor determining the prognosis. J Pediatr Surg 1983;18:124–30.

137. Raweily EA, Gibson AA, Burt AD. Abnormalities of intrahepatic bile ducts in extrahepatic biliary atresia. Histopathology 1990;17:521–7.

138. Grosfeld JL, Fitzgerald JF, Predaina R, et al. The efficacy of hepatoportoenterostomy in biliary atresia. Surgery 1989;106: 692–700; discussion 700–1.

139. Lally KP, Kanegaye J, Matsumura M, et al. Perioperative factors affecting the outcome following repair of biliary atresia. Pediatrics 1989;83:723–6.

140. Trivedi P, Dhawan A, Risteli J, et al. Prognostic value of serum hyaluronic acid and type I and III procollagen propeptides in extrahepatic biliary atresia. Pediatr Res 1995;38:568–73.

141. Altman RP, Lilly JR, Greenfield J, et al. A multivariable risk factor analysis of the portoenterostomy (Kasai) procedure for biliary atresia. Ann Surg 1997;226:348–55.

142. Chiba T, Mochizuki I, Ohi R. Postoperative gastrointestinal hemorrhage in biliary atresia. Tohoku J Exp Med 1990;162:255–9.

143. Schweizer P, Lunzmann K. Extrahepatic bile duct atresia: how efficient is the hepatoportoenterostomy? Eur J Pediatr Surg 1998;8:150–4.

144. Chardot C, Carton M, Spire-Bendelac N, et al. Prognosis of biliary atresia in the era of liver transplantation: French national study from 1986 to 1996. Hepatology 1999;30:606–11.

145. Bismuth H, Houssin D. Reduced-sized orthotopic liver graft in hepatic transplantation in children. Surgery 1984;95:367–70.

146. Otte JB, de Ville de Goyet J, Sokal E, et al. Size reduction of the donor liver is a safe way to alleviate the shortage of size-matched organs in pediatric liver transplantation. Ann Surg 1990;211:146–57.

147. Tanaka K, Uemoto S, Tokunaga Y, et al. Surgical techniques and innovations in living related liver transplantation. Ann Surg 1993;217:82–91.

148. Ryckman FC, Fisher RA, Pedersen SH, Balistreri WF. Liver transplantation in children. Semin Pediatr Surg 1992;1:162–72.

149. Whitington PF, Balistreri WF. Liver transplantation in pediatrics: indications, contraindications, and pretransplant management. J Pediatr 1991;118:169–77.

150. Millis JM, Brems JJ, Hiatt JR, et al. Orthotopic liver transplantation for biliary atresia. Evolution of management. Arch Surg 1988;123:1237–9.

151. Goss JA, Shackleton CR, Swenson K, et al. Orthotopic liver transplantation for congenital biliary atresia. An 11-year, single-center experience. Ann Surg 1996;224:276–84; discussion 284–7.

152. Ryckman FC, Alonso MH, Bucuvalas JC, Balistreri WF. Long-term survival after liver transplantation. J Pediatr Surg 1999; 34:845–9; discussion 849–50.

153. Zitelli BJ, Miller JW, Gartner JC Jr, et al. Changes in life-style after liver transplantation. Pediatrics 1988;82:173–80.

154. Ryckman FC, Alonso MH, Bucuvalas JC, Balistreri WF. Biliary atresia—surgical management and treatment options as they relate to outcome. Liver Transplant Surg 1998;4(5 Suppl 1):S24–33.

155. Amedee-Manesme O, Furr HC, Alvarez F, et al. Biochemical indicators of vitamin A depletion in children with cholestasis. Hepatology 1985;5:1143–8.

156. Chandra RS, Altman RP. Ductal remnants in extrahepatic biliary atresia: a histopathologic study with clinical correlation. J Pediatr 1978;93:196–200.

3. Other Disorders

Philip Rosenthal, MD

CHOLEDOCHAL CYST

Although uncommon, choledochal cysts are classified as congenital anomalies of the biliary tract with varying degrees of cystic dilatation occurring at varying segments of the biliary tree (extrahepatic or intrahepatic). In general, the term "choledochal cyst" refers to all cystic dilatations of the biliary tree; others, however, restrict the term to only cystic abnormalities of the common bile duct.

EPIDEMIOLOGY

Choledochal cysts occur four times more frequently in girls than in boys regardless of racial differences. It is more frequently diagnosed in Asians, with an estimated incidence of 1 in 1,000 live births in Japan.[1] In the United States, the incidence is estimated at 1 in 13,000 live births.[2] About half of the cases are diagnosed in children before the age of 10 years, and another 25% of cases are diagnosed by 20 years of age. Thus, choledochal cysts are predominantly a disorder of children and young adults.[3,4]

CLASSIFICATION

Choledochal cysts have been categorized into several different types.[3] Anatomic classification is of practical importance in the planning of surgical intervention and treatment (Figure 50.3-1).

Type I, which is the most common type encountered, consists of a cystic dilatation of the common bile duct. Observed may be (1) a large saccular cystic dilatation, (2) small segmental cystic dilatation, or (3) diffuse or cylindrical fusiform dilatation. Type I cysts account for 75 to 85% of biliary cysts.

Type II cysts are diverticuli in the extrahepatic ducts. They may be seen in the common bile duct and/or the gallbladder. They represent only 2 to 3% of reported cases.

Type III cysts are choledochoceles. They are also rare, occurring in only about 3.5% of reported cases. A further anatomic classification of type III cysts has been proposed by Sarris and Tsang.[5] In type A, the ampulla opens into the choledochocele, which communicates with the duodenum via another small opening. Type A choledochoceles can be subclassified into A_1, in which the pancreatic and common bile duct share a common opening into the cyst; A_2, in which the openings are distinct; and A_3, in which the choledochocele is small and entirely intramural. In type B, the ampulla opens directly into the duodenum, with the choledochocele communicating only with the distal common duct.

Type IV cysts are multiple cysts. In type IV A, the multiple cysts are in the intra- and extrahepatic bile ducts and account for about 20% of reported cases. Type IV B cysts are rare and include multiple cysts found only in the extrahepatic system.

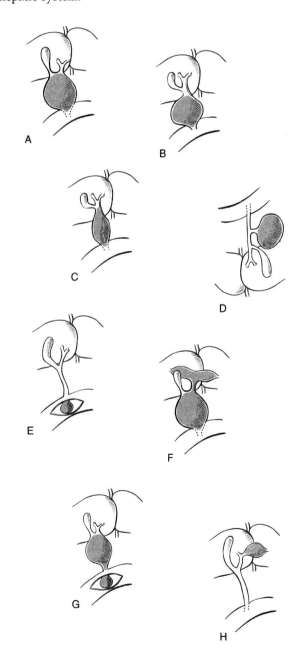

FIGURE 50.3-1 Diagrams demonstrating typing of ductal cysts. Reproduced from Todani T et al[3] with permission from Excerpta Medica.

Type V cysts are either single or multiple intrahepatic bile duct cysts. These are also rare. Type V cysts are identical to the original description of Caroli disease.

CLINICAL PRESENTATION

Choledochal cysts present clinically with two distinct constellations determined primarily by patient age.[6,7] In infants, jaundice, the result of a conjugated hyperbilirubinemia with or without acholic stools, is observed. The presentation may be indistinguishable from biliary atresia, which is sometimes associated with a choledochal cyst. Abdominal pain may or may not be present. Hepatomegaly may be commonly found, and about half of the children have a palpable abdominal mass if carefully examined. The mass is typically in the right hypochondrium, soft, elastic, round, and mobile and may move with respiration. The classic triad of pain, jaundice, and a palpable abdominal mass occurs in anywhere from 13 to 63% of reported series. Biliary cirrhosis and portal hypertension may also be seen.

In older children and adults, many asymptomatic patients have been reported. Chronic or intermittent abdominal pain is the most common presenting symptom. Also, a history of intermittent jaundice or recurrent cholangitis is obtained. Palpation of an abdominal mass and the presence of cirrhosis or portal hypertension are infrequent in these older individuals compared with infants. However, recurrent pancreatitis is reported only in older children and adults. Frequently, abnormalities of the pancreatic duct system are found. Carcinoma associated with choledochal cysts has been reported only in patients over 10 years of age.

Spontaneous perforation of a choledochal cyst in infancy can occur. In one series, 7% (13/187) of infants with choledochal cysts were encountered with spontaneous perforation of the cyst.[8] Eight patients had biliary peritonitis, and five had sealed perforation. The postulated cause of perforation was biliary epithelial irritation from refluxed pancreatic juice, the result of malformed biliary and pancreatic ducts.

PATHOGENESIS

The etiology of choledochal cysts is unknown. Theories suggest either a congenital cause or an acquired cause.[9–11] The congenital theory postulates an unequal epithelial cell proliferation during embryogenesis while the embryonic bile ducts are still solid. In support of the congenital theory is the fact that biliary cysts have been reported in utero as early as 15 weeks gestation.[11] Further, after decompression surgery, many cysts fail to shrink, supporting inherently abnormal ductal wall development. The acquired injury theory proposes that choledochal cysts develop owing to an anomalous arrangement of the distal pancreaticobiliary tree. The anomalous merger of the common bile duct and the pancreatic duct proximal to the sphincter of Oddi permits reflux of pancreatic enzymes into the common bile duct, resulting in inflammation, edema, fibrosis, obstruction to bile flow, localized weakness, and dilatation. It is apparent that several factors may be important in the pathogenesis of biliary cysts. No single explanation supports each type of biliary cyst observed.

DIAGNOSIS

Choledochal cysts in the majority of patients are recognized during infancy.[6,7] The diagnosis is suggested if noninvasive imaging studies are sought for vague right upper quadrant symptoms. Ultrasonography is a valued and preferred method to screen for a choledochal cyst (Figure 50.3-2A). Differentiation of a cystic structure that is not the gallbladder is an important consideration (Figure 50.3-2B). Although upper gastrointestinal tract radiographs may outline a mass that displaces the first or second portion of the duodenum, they are unnecessary. If there is doubt following ultrasound examination, the use of nuclear hepatobiliary scans, computed tomography, or magnetic resonance imaging (magnetic resonance cholangiography) may provide important discriminatory information.[12–14]

Percutaneous transhepatic cholangiography (PTC) and endoscopic retrograde cholangiopancreatography (ERCP) can provide excellent detailed information.[15] PTC may be especially helpful in defining complex intrahepatic cysts, whereas ERCP may provide the best visualization of the distal biliary tree. Obviously, PTC and ERCP are more invasive. Ultimate diagnosis can be confirmed by an intraoperative cholangiogram at surgery.

PATHOLOGY

The wall of a choledochal cyst is often thickened because of productive fibrosis and inflammation. Histologic examination reveals dense connective tissue, fibrocollagen, and, occasionally, smooth muscle and elastic elements.[16] Often there is no epithelial lining, but islets of preserved cylindrical or columnar epithelium may be found. Externally, duodenal mucosa covers choledochoceles, and, internally, there may be duodenal mucosa, bile duct mucosa, or unclassified glandular epithelium.

Hepatic changes owing to choledochal cyst frequently occur. Biliary cirrhosis, portal fibrosis, or evidence of bile duct obstruction with bile duct proliferation, cholestasis, parenchymal damage, and inflammatory cell infiltration may be seen.[17] Obviously, these changes may simulate biliary atresia.

TREATMENT

Therapy for choledochal cysts is complete surgical excision.[18,19] It is important that the entire cyst mucosa be removed. Historically, cyst aspiration, external drainage, internal decompression, and drainage into the duodenum or direct anastomosis of the cyst to a jejunal Roux-en-Y loop were used. Each of these techniques retained the cyst abnormal mucosal wall. Poor drainage resulted in stricture formation, biliary lithiasis, and an increased risk of malignant potential in the retained mucosal wall. It is imperative that the extent of any intrahepatic cystic disease be defined at the time of choledochal cyst excision. An intraoperative cholangiogram is well suited for this task. Segmental multifocal cystic disease isolated to a single hepatic lobe can be treated with lobectomy. If the intrahepatic disease is dif-

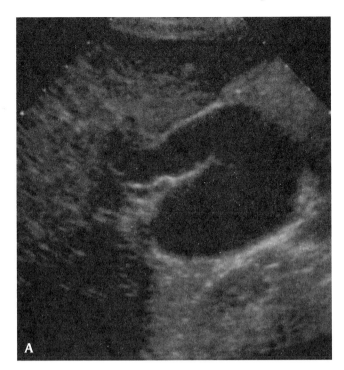

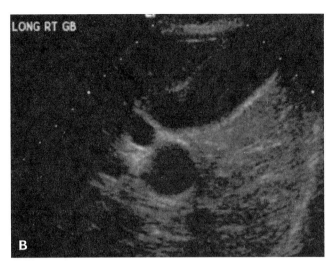

FIGURE 50.3-2 *A*, Choledochal cyst. Ultrasonographic findings of a choledochal cyst in an infant. *B*, Gallbladder and choledochal cyst. Ultrasonographic findings of the gallbladder (upper cystic structure) and choledochal cyst (lower cystic structure) in an infant. Courtesy of Dr. Ruth Goldstein, University of California, San Francisco.

fuse, involving all hepatic lobes, then liver transplant may be required. Following surgery, complications include cholangitis, stricture formation, and pancreatitis. These can be significantly decreased by total cyst excision and careful surgical dissection. Recently, a report of the complete laparoscopic management of choledochal cysts was published.[20] The authors concluded that although feasible, this technique is technically difficult and should currently be restricted to specialized centers dealing with advanced laparoscopic surgery.

MALIGNANCY

The most alarming complication of choledochal cyst is malignancy. Carcinoma has been reported in remaining cystic tissue in up to 26% of patients.[21–24] Although the overall incidence of biliary carcinoma in association with biliary cysts is about 2.5%, the overall incidence of biliary carcinoma in the general population is only about 0.012 to 0.5%. The typical malignancy is adenocarcinoma of the bile duct or gallbladder. Squamous cell carcinoma and cholangiocarcinoma have also been observed. The risk of developing malignancy increases with age. Malignant change can also occur in areas of the biliary tree remote from the cyst. The prognosis if such malignancies develop is grim. Thus, complete cyst removal, even in asymptomatic patients, including those with prior cyst surgery, is warranted.

SPONTANEOUS PERFORATION OF THE COMMON BILE DUCT

Spontaneous perforation of the bile ducts is a rare but well-documented condition in neonates.[25–27] Typically, these infants present with cholestatic jaundice following a postnatal symptom-free interval. There is associated mild jaundice, ascites, acholic stools, poor weight gain, vomiting, and evolving abdominal distention. The combination of a

mildly elevated conjugated hyperbilirubinemia with minimally elevated serum transaminases and acholic stools in a neonate should suggest the possibility of the diagnosis. Ultrasonography may reveal ascites or a loculated fluid collection. Nuclear hepatobiliary scintigraphy may demonstrate activity of the isotope outside the biliary tree in the abdomen.[28] Abdominal paracentesis may aid in the diagnosis, revealing clear, bile-stained ascites. Treatment requires surgical intervention to either attempt to repair the perforation or to re-establish bile flow from the liver to the intestine while decompressing the biliary tract. Operative cholangiography may demonstrate the site of the perforation. Often there is stenosis of the distal end of the common bile duct, segmental atresia, or inspissated bile. There is a predilection for the perforation to occur at the confluence of the cystic duct and the common bile duct, suggesting a particular susceptibility to weakness or injury at this site.[29]

NEONATAL SCLEROSING CHOLANGITIS

Sclerosing cholangitis refers to a disorder with irregular narrowing of either the intrahepatic or extrahepatic bile ducts, the result of inflammation and subsequent fibrosis. Obliteration of the bile ducts eventually results in biliary cirrhosis. Cholangiography demonstrates the typical "beading" pattern with alternating areas of strictures and dilatations in the intrahepatic and extrahepatic bile ducts. A neonatal form of sclerosing cholangitis has been reported in infants.[30–35] Jaundice, cholestasis, and acholic stools were observed within the first weeks of life. Cholecystography disclosed abnormal intrahepatic and extrahepatic bile ducts with rarefaction of segmental branches, stenosis, and focal dilation. The early clinical symptoms following birth suggest the possibility of a congenital onset. A history of consanguinity in many of the affected infants suggests an inherited or genetic basis for this disorder. A case of neonatal sclerosing cholangitis associated with a positive anti–smooth muscle antibody titer (1:320) and elevated immunoglobulin has been reported.[34] Although the cause of neonatal sclerosing cholangitis is unknown, genetic or immunologic factors may be important in its etiology. In all cases of neonatal sclerosing cholangitis reported, jaundice resolved within the first year of life. However, the disease progressed to cirrhosis. Liver transplant has been used to treat some cases of neonatal sclerosing cholangitis.[33] To date, there has been no report of recurrence of disease following transplant. The role of medical therapy, such as ursodeoxycholic acid (UDCA) administration, to alter the progression of neonatal sclerosing cholangitis is unknown.

SCLEROSING CHOLANGITIS

Although more frequently diagnosed in adults, sclerosing cholangitis may also be seen in childhood. Sclerosing cholangitis is defined as a chronic hepatobiliary disorder with inflammation of the intrahepatic and extrahepatic bile ducts. The subsequent periductular fibrosis results in narrowing and dilatation of the bile ducts. Progression of the disorder results in cirrhosis and portal hypertension. Diagnosis can be made by cholangiography and/or histology of the liver parenchyma.

The nomenclature for sclerosing cholangitis is a bit confusing. Primary sclerosing cholangitis (PSC) is the most frequent liver disorder associated with inflammatory bowel disease (IBD). However, PSC may occur in the absence of IBD. Cholangitis related to chronic ascending bacterial infection, stones, bile duct surgery, congenital anomalies of the bile ducts, ischemic injury, neoplasms, or infectious cholangiopathy owing to acquired immune deficiency syndrome (AIDS) is referred to as primary cholangitis. This designation assumes that prior to the onset of PSC, the bile duct anatomy was normal. Secondary sclerosing cholangitis is associated with bile duct injury, the result of choledocholithiasis, postoperative stricture formation, or specific duct involvement from systemic disease. Rather than categorizing sclerosing cholangitis as primary or secondary, Debray and colleagues divide sclerosing cholangitis into three groups: neonatal, postneonatal associated with a disease, and postneonatal not associated with a disease.[36]

The distinction between sclerosing cholangitis and the obstructive cholangiopathies of infancy (ie, biliary atresia, syndromic and nonsyndromic paucity of intrahepatic ducts) is vague. There are histologic and radiographic similarities, suggesting common etiologies. In biliary atresia, there is an inflammatory, progressive, and obliterative destruction of the extrahepatic and intrahepatic bile ducts. Infants with the neonatal form of sclerosing cholangitis may have pathologic and radiographic features that are very similar to biliary atresia early in the course of the disease that do not become characteristic of sclerosing cholangitis until the disease evolves.[31,32] Further, a report of siblings, one with biliary atresia and the other with PSC, has been published.[37]

SCLEROSING CHOLANGITIS AND ASSOCIATED CONDITIONS

Reports of PSC associated with both ulcerative colitis and Crohn disease in children are becoming more frequent, potentially as a result of improved cholangiographic techniques being used.[38–50] In adults, PSC is often associated with other disorders with an autoimmune basis, including diabetes mellitus, pancreatitis, and thyroid diseases. These disorders may precede or follow the diagnosis of PSC. In children, besides an association with IBD, PSC may be associated with a wide variety of disorders.[51–58]

CLINICAL PRESENTATION

Although PSC can occur in infancy, the majority of cases in childhood occur in young adults. As in older adults, there may be a gradual onset of fatigue, malaise, anorexia, and weight loss. Pruritus and intermittent jaundice may then occur. Cholangitis recognized by right upper quadrant pain, fever, and conjugated hyperbilirubinemia is often encountered. In children, growth failure and delayed puberty may also be presenting symptoms. Many children with PSC are clinically asymptomatic, and the disease is detected only as a result of screening serum biochemical abnormalities, which prompts further investigation. There are no pathognomonic laboratory findings in PSC. Commonly in adults, there is an elevated serum alkaline phosphatase. Although this may be variable in children, elevated alkaline phosphatase levels may be difficult to interpret because of growth. An elevated serum γ-glutamyltransferase level appears to be a sensitive indicator for PSC in children. Other variably abnormal biochemical tests include high immunoglobulin G concentrations, positive antinuclear antibodies, anti–smooth muscle antibodies, and antineutrophil cytoplasmic antibodies, suggesting an autoimmune connection. Although the physical examination may be completely normal, often hepatomegaly, splenomegaly, or jaundice is noted.[36,50]

DIAGNOSIS

Cholangiography is considered essential in the diagnosis of PSC (Figure 50.3-3). This may be accomplished by ERCP, PTC, intraoperative cholangiography, or, more recently, magnetic resonance cholangiopancreatography.[38] Characteristic findings are irregular narrowing and stricturing of the hepatic and common bile ducts owing to inflammation and fibrosis. There may be concomitant involvement of the intrahepatic ducts. The strictures may be localized, diffuse, or multifocal. Strictures may be short, with intervening normal duct segments producing the characteristic beaded appearance. The intrahepatic bile ducts may show decreased peripheral arborization, which is referred to as the pruned tree appearance.

PATHOLOGY

The characteristic histologic findings in PSC may not be present in many cases in children, limiting the usefulness of this modality for diagnosis.[36,50] Classically, there are focal concentric edema and fibrosis around interlobular bile ducts. This is referred to as an onion skin appearance. Typically, there is portal to portal variability in the biopsy, and a review

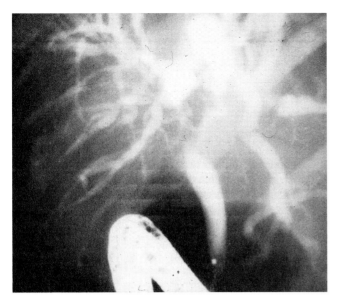

FIGURE 50.3-3   Primary sclerosing cholangitis. Cholangiogram demonstrating irregular narrowing and stricturing of the hepatic and common bile ducts owing to inflammation and fibrosis. Courtesy of Dr. Roy Gordon, University of California, San Francisco.

of serial sections may be required. Serial biopsies demonstrating progressive ductal changes may also be necessary to establish the diagnosis. A fibro-obliterative cholangitis may progress over time to solid cords of connective tissue and loss of interlobular bile ducts, giving the appearance of a paucity of bile ducts per portal zone (Figure 50.3-4). This may continue to progress to frank biliary cirrhosis.

PATHOGENESIS

The etiology of PSC is unknown. The association of PSC with IBD may suggest potential etiologic mechanisms, but PSC may occur in the absence of IBD.

To incorporate the various proposed theories into a unifying hypothesis, perhaps an immune-mediated destruction of the biliary tree initiated by an infectious agent in a susceptible host with or without intestinal involvement best describes the process. To this end, there is exciting new evidence implicating a retrovirus in the pathogenesis of primary biliary cirrhosis, another obliterative ductal disease.[59] Further, pilot studies using antiviral therapy with lamivudine and zidovudine in adult patients demonstrated significant biochemical and histologic improvement with reversal of ductopenia and normalization of liver function tests.[60] Whether antiviral therapy has a role in PSC remains speculative.

Alterations in the immune system are also proposed to be important in the initiation or perpetuation of PSC (see Chapter 52, "Autoimmune Disease").

TREATMENT

Unfortunately, there have been no large randomized controlled trials of any potential therapeutic agents for the treatment of PSC in children. UDCA therapy has been used in children with PSC.[40] There were no side effects reported in its use in nine children. There were significant reduc-

tions in serum alkaline phosphatase, alanine aminotransferase, aspartate aminotransferase, and γ-glutamyltransferase levels with up to 20 months of treatment. The long-term effect of UDCA therapy for children with PSC awaits further trials.

Immunosuppressive therapy has long been used for PSC therapy in children.[61,62] Certainly, there is a rationale for this in children with PSC with IBD. Those children with autoimmune features of disease might also be expected to respond to this therapy. Oral vancomycin was reported to normalize serum transaminase levels in three children with PSC.[45] Although provocative and supporting a role for intraluminal bacteria, further confirmation is awaited before oral vancomycin therapy can be recommended for routine use in children with PSC.

Surgical options have been used predominantly to relieve biliary obstruction, reduce the occurrence of cholangitis, and combat the consequences of cirrhosis and portal hypertension. Procedures performed either surgically, by interventional radiology, or endoscopically range from drainage procedures, stent placement, balloon dilatation of strictures, resection, and transplant.[33,63–67] Certainly, surgical intervention should be avoided if at all possible and reserved for refractory patients after attempts at dilatation and stent placement have been exhausted. Transplant is appropriate for children with PSC who have progressed to cirrhosis and who have developed portal hypertension in the absence of refractory complications. Unfortunately, recurrence of PSC in the transplanted liver has been reported.[68,69] Recently, a report of a 15-year-old boy who underwent liver transplant for PSC was published.[70] What was novel about this case and another five adult cases in this report was the sequential occurrence of autoimmune hepatitis that evolved to PSC over several years.

PROGNOSIS

The true rate of progression of PSC in children is unknown. Presumably, the rate of progression is slow because PSC is

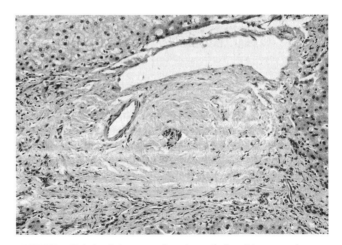

FIGURE 50.3-4   Primary sclerosing cholangitis: portal zone shows prominent periductal fibrosis (onion skin–like fibrosis) around the interlobular bile duct. Ductal remnant remains in this example but can disappear completely. Hematoxylin and eosin stain; ×40 original magnification. Courtesy of Dr. Linda Ferrell, University of California, San Francisco.

not one of the leading indications for pediatric liver transplant. The prognosis may be better for children than for adults, based on the study by Floreani and colleagues.[41] In the larger pediatric series, about a third of children died, the result of cirrhosis and portal hypertension, and another third either were listed for transplant or went on to transplant.[36,50]

REFERENCES

1. Yamaguchi M. Congenital choledochal cyst: analysis of 1,433 patients in the Japanese literature. Am J Surg 1980;140:653–7.

2. Kim SH. Choledochal cyst: survey by the surgical section of the American Academy of Pediatrics. J Pediatr Surg 1981;16: 402–7.

3. Todani T, Watanabe Y, Narusue M, et al. Congenital bile duct cysts: classification, operative procedures, and review of thirty-seven cases including cancer arising from choledochal cyst. Am J Surg 1977;134:263–9.

4. Babbitt DP, Starshak RJ, Clement AR. Choledochal cyst: a concept of etiology. AJR Am J Roentgenol 1973;119:57–62.

5. Sarris GE, Tsang D. Choledochocele: case report, literature review, and a proposed classification. Surgery 1989;105:408–14.

6. Sherman P, Kolster E, Davies C, et al. Choledochal cysts: heterogeneity of clinical presentation. J Pediatr Gastroenterol Nutr 1986;5:867–72.

7. Kasai M, Asakura Y, Taira Y. Surgical treatment of choledochal cyst. Ann Surg 1970;172:844–51.

8. Ando K, Miyano T, Kohno S, et al. Spontaneous perforation of choledochal cyst: a study of 13 cases. Eur J Pediatr Surg 1998;8:23–5.

9. Okada A, Nakamura T, Higaki J, et al. Congenital dilatation of the bile duct in 100 instances and its relationship with anomalous junction. Surg Gynecol Obstet 1990;17:291–8.

10. Wood WJJ, Trump DS. Pancreaticobiliary common channel associated with common duct stricture. J Pediatr Surg 1986; 21:738–40.

11. Schroeder D, Smith L, Prain HC. Antenatal diagnosis of choledochal cyst at 15 weeks' gestation: etiologic implications and management. J Pediatr Surg 1989;24:936–8.

12. Camponovo E, Buck JL, Drane WE. Scintigraphic features of choledochal cyst. J Nucl Med 1989;30:622–8.

13. Gupta RK, Kakar AK, Jena A, et al. Magnetic resonance in obstructive jaundice. Australas Radiol 1989;33:245–51.

14. Kim SH, Lim JH, Yoon HK, et al. Choledochal cyst: comparison of MR and conventional cholangiography. Clin Radiol 2000;55:378–83.

15. Shemesh E, Czerniak A, Klein E, et al. The role of endoscopic retrograde cholangiopancreatography in the diagnosis and treatment of adult choledochal cyst. Surg Gynecol Obstet 1988;167:423–6.

16. Alonso-Lej F, Rever WBJ, Pessagno DJ. Congenital choledochal cyst, with a report of 2 and analysis of 94 cases. Int Abstr Surg 1959;108:1–30.

17. Nambirajan L, Taneja P, Singh MK, Mitra DK, Bhatnagar V. The liver in choledochal cyst. Trop Gastroenterol 2000;21:135–9.

18. McWhorter GL. Congenital cystic dilatation of the bile and pancreatic ducts. Arch Surg 1939;38:397–411.

19. Lilly JR. Total excision of choledochal cyst. Surg Gynecol Obstet 1978;146:254–6.

20. Chowbey PK, Katrak MP, Sharma A, et al. Complete laparoscopic management of choledochal cyst: report of two cases. J Laparoendosc Adv Surg Tech A 2002;12:217–21.

21. Todani T, Watanabe Y, Toki A, et al. Carcinoma related to choledochal cysts with internal drainage operations. Surg Gynecol Obstet 1987;164:61–4.

22. Yoshida H, Itai Y, Minami M, et al. Biliary malignancies occurring in choledochal cysts. Radiology 1989;173:389–92.

23. Bismuth H, Krissat J. Choledochal cystic malignancies. Ann Oncol 1999;10:94–8.

24. Watanabe Y, Toki A, Todani T. Bile duct cancer developed after cyst excision for choledochal cyst. J Hepatobiliary Pancreat Surg 1999;6:207–12.

25. Chardot C, Iskandarani F, De Dreuzy O, et al. Spontaneous perforation of the biliary tract in infancy: a series of 11 cases. Eur J Pediatr Surg 1996;6:341–6.

26. Davenport M, Heaton ND, Howard ER. Spontaneous perforation of the bile duct in infants. Br J Surg 1991;78:1068–70.

27. Niedbala A, Lankford A, Boswell WC, Rittmeyer C. Spontaneous perforation of the bile duct. Am Surg 2000;66:1061–3.

28. Kumar R, Sriram M, Bhatnagar V, et al. Spontaneous perforation of the common bile duct in infancy: role of Tc-99m mebrofenin hepatobiliary imaging. Clin Nucl Med 1999;24:847–8.

29. Hasegawa T, Udatsu Y, Kamiyama M, et al. Does pancreaticobiliary maljunction play a role in spontaneous perforation of the bile duct in children? Pediatr Surg Int 2000;16:550–3.

30. Mieli-Vergani G, Vergani D. Sclerosing cholangitis in the paediatric patient. Best Pract Res Clin Gastroenterol 2001;15: 681–90.

31. Amedee-Manesme O, Bernard O, Brunelle F, et al. Sclerosing cholangitis with neonatal onset. J Pediatr 1987;111:225–9.

32. Baker AJ, Portmann B, Westaby D, et al. Neonatal sclerosing cholangitis in two siblings: a category of progressive intrahepatic cholestasis. J Pediatr Gastroenterol Nutr 1993;17:317–22.

33. Ewart-Toland A, Enns GM, Cox VA, et al. Severe congenital anomalies requiring transplantation in children with Kabuki syndrome. Am J Med Genet 1998;80:362–7.

34. Bar Meir M, Hadas-Halperin I, Fisher D, et al. Neonatal sclerosing cholangitis associated with autoimmune phenomena. J Pediatr Gastroenterol Nutr 2000;30:332–4.

35. Gauthier F, Hadchouel M. Congenital disorders of the biliary ducts. Rev Prat 2000;50: 2142–5.

36. Debray D, Pariente D, Urvoas E, et al. Sclerosing cholangitis in children. J Pediatr 1994;124: 49–56.

37. Isoyama K, Yamada K, Ishikawa K, Sanada Y. Coincidental cases of primary sclerosing cholangitis and biliary atresia in siblings? Acta Paediatr 1995;84:1444–6.

38. Ferrara C, Valeri G, Salvolini L, Giovagnoni A. Magnetic resonance cholangiopancreatography in primary sclerosing cholangitis in children. Pediatr Radiol 2002;32:413–7.

39. Faubion WA Jr, Loftus EV, Sandborn WJ, et al. Pediatric "PSC-IBD": a descriptive report of associated inflammatory bowel disease among pediatric patients with PSC. J Pediatr Gastroenterol Nutr 2001;33:296–300.

40. Gilger MA, Gann ME, Opekun AR, Gleason WA Jr. Efficacy of ursodeoxycholic acid in the treatment of primary sclerosing cholangitis in children. J Pediatr Gastroenterol Nutr 2000; 31: 136–41.

41. Floreani A, Zancan L, Melis A, et al. Primary sclerosing cholangitis (PSC): clinical, laboratory and survival analysis in children and adults. Liver 1999;19:228–33.

42. Roberts EA. Primary sclerosing cholangitis in children. J Gastroenterol Hepatol 1999;14:588–93.

43. Lin WT, Lin SJ, Ni YH, et al. Primary sclerosing cholangitis in a child. J Formos Med Assoc 1999;98:209–13.

44. Siegel EG, Folsch UR. Primary sclerosing cholangitis mimicking choledochal cyst type 1 in a young patient. Endoscopy 1999;31:200–3.

45. Cox KL, Cox KM. Oral vancomycin: treatment of primary scle-

rosing cholangitis in children with inflammatory bowel disease. J Pediatr Gastroenterol Nutr 1998;27:580–3.

46. Kozaiwa K, Tajiri H, Sawada A, et al. Three paediatric cases of primary sclerosing cholangitis treated with ursodeoxycholic acid and sulphasalazine. J Gastroenterol Hepatol 1998;13:825–9.

47. Vajro P, Cucchiara S, Vegnente A, et al. Primary sclerosing cholangitis preceding Crohn's disease in a child with Down's syndrome. Dig Dis Sci 1998;43:166–9.

48. Kagalwalla AF, Altraif I, Shamsan L, et al. Primary sclerosing cholangitis in Arab children: report of four cases and literature review. J Pediatr Gastroenterol Nutr 1997;24:146–52.

49. Lacaille F, Canioni D, Bernard O, et al. Celiac disease, inflammatory colitis, and primary sclerosing cholangitis in a girl with Turner's syndrome. J Pediatr Gastroenterol Nutr 1995; 21:463–7.

50. Wilschanski M, Chait P, Wade JA, et al. Primary sclerosing cholangitis in 32 children: clinical, laboratory, and radiographic features, with survival analysis. Hepatology 1995;22:1415–22.

51. Bucuvalas JC, Bove KE, Kaufman RA, et al. Cholangitis associated with *Cryptococcus neoformans*. Gastroenterology 1985;88:1055–9.

52. Davis JJ, Heyman MB, Ferrell L, et al. Sclerosing cholangitis associated with chronic cryptosporidiosis in a child with a congenital immunodeficiency disorder. Am J Gastroenterol 1987;82:1196–202.

53. DiPalma JA, Strobel CT, Farrow JG. Primary sclerosing cholangitis associated with hyperimmunoglobulin M immunodeficiency (dysgammaglobulinemia). Gastroenterology 1986;91: 464–8.

54. Braier J, Ciocca M, Latella A, et al. Cholestasis, sclerosing cholangitis, and liver transplantation in Langerhans cell histiocytosis. Med Pediatr Oncol 2002;38:178–82.

55. Goddard EA, Mouton SC, Westwood AT, et al. Cryptosporidiosis of the gastrointestinal tract associated with sclerosing cholangitis in the absence of documented immunodeficiency: *Cryptosporidium parvum* and sclerosing cholangitis in an immunocompetent child. J Pediatr Gastroenterol Nutr 2000;31:317–20.

56. Neveu I, Labrune P, Huguet P, et al. Sclerosing cholangitis revealing histiocytosis X. Arch Fr Pediatr 1990;47:197–9.

57. Puel O, Guillard JM. Sclerosing cholangitis in the course of histiocytosis X. Arch Fr Pediatr 1990;47:155–6.

58. Waldram R, Kopelman H, Tsantoulas D, Williams R. Chronic pancreatitis, sclerosing cholangitis, and sicca complex in two siblings. Lancet 1975;i:550–2.

59. Mason A, Xu L, Guo L, et al. Detection of retroviral antibodies in primary biliary cirrhosis and other idiopathic biliary disorders. Lancet 1998;351:1620–4.

60. Mason A, Nair S. Primary biliary cirrhosis: new thoughts on pathophysiology and treatment. Curr Gastroenterol Rep 2002;4:45–51.

61. El-Shabrawi M, Wilkinson ML, Portmann B, et al. Primary sclerosing cholangitis in childhood. Gastroenterology 1987;92: 1226–35.

62. Kane W, Miller K, Sharp HL. Inflammatory bowel disease presenting as liver disease during childhood. J Pediatr 1980;97:775–8.

63. Stoker J, Lameris JS, Robben SGF, et al. Primary sclerosing cholangitis in a child treated by nonsurgical balloon dilatation and stenting. J Pediatr Gastroenterol Nutr 1993;17: 303–6.

64. Lee JG, Schutz SM, England RE, et al. Endoscopic therapy of sclerosing cholangitis. Hepatology 1995;21:661–7.

65. Wagner S, Gebel M, Meier P, et al. Endoscopic management of biliary tract strictures in primary sclerosing cholangitis. Endoscopy 1996;28:546–51.

66. Martin FM, Rossi RL, Nugent FW, et al. Surgical aspects of sclerosing cholangitis: results in 178 patients. Ann Surg 1990; 212:551–8.

67. Ismail T, Angrisani L, Powell JF, et al. Primary sclerosing cholangitis: surgical options, prognostic variables and outcome. Br J Surg 1991;78:564–7.

68. Graziadei IW, Wiesner RH, Batts KP, et al. Recurrence of primary sclerosing cholangitis following liver transplantation. Hepatology 1999;29:1050–6.

69. Vera A, Moledina S, Gunson B, et al. Risk factors for recurrence of primary sclerosing cholangitis of liver allograft. Lancet 2002;360:1943–4.

70. Abdo AA, Bain VG, Kichian K, Lee SS. Evolution of autoimmune hepatitis to primary sclerosing cholangitis: a sequential syndrome. Hepatology 2002;36:1393–9.

CHAPTER 51

POSTNATAL INFECTIONS

1A. *Viral Hepatitis B*

Mei-Hwei Chang, MD

Hepatitis viruses can infect individuals of any age. Although most of the complications manifest mainly in adulthood, primary infection may occur in infancy or childhood. Among the hepatotrophic viral infections (A through E), hepatitis A and E run an acute self-limited or fulminant course, whereas hepatitis B, C, and D may follow either an acute or a chronic course. Chronic hepatitis D is very rare in children all over the world, except in a few endemic areas, whereas chronic infection of hepatitis B virus (HBV) is more prevalent and can occur in children of any age, even in the perinatal period. Chronic infection of HBV during childhood may cause chronic hepatitis, cirrhosis, and liver cancer during childhood or later in adulthood. HBV-related carcinogenesis requires time; hepatocellular carcinoma may occur much earlier in those infected in childhood than in those infected in adulthood.

HBV infection is a worldwide health problem. Approximately 2 billion people in the world have been infected by HBV, and 350 million of them are chronic hepatitis B antigen carriers. In hyperendemic areas, where most of the complications of chronic HBV infection develop in adulthood, primary HBV infection occurs mainly during infancy or early childhood.[1] Understanding the long-term natural course of chronic HBV infection in children is very important to evaluate the efficacy and determine the strategy of antiviral therapy for chronic HBV infection in children.

Hepatitis B immunization has effectively reduced the infection and carrier rate of HBV. Immunization is the most important method to achieve the eradication of hepatitis B–related diseases.

HEPATITIS B VIRUS

Hepatitis B virus is a 3.2 kb, circular, partially double-stranded deoxyribonucleic acid (DNA) virus. During active replication in the early phase of infection, viral particles appear in large quantity in the serum in two forms: one is the complete virion of 42 nm diameter, which consists of an envelope, a capsid with capsid protein, a circular DNA molecule, and a DNA polymerase,[2,3] and the other is a 22 nm empty viral envelope, which contains only the hepatitis B surface antigen (HBsAg). In addition, a soluble antigen, hepatitis B e antigen (HBeAg), which is closely related to the nonsecretory capsid antigen (hepatitis B core antigen [HBcAg]), also appears in the serum during the highly replicative phase of HBV infection (Table 51.1A-1).

HBV contains four open reading frames, which encode major structural and nonstructural proteins for HBV. These are the polymerase gene region for polymerase, surface gene region for three surface proteins, precore and core gene regions for HBcAg and HBeAg, and X gene region for

TABLE 51.1A-1   CLINICAL SIGNIFICANCE OF HEPATITIS B VIRUS ANTIGENS, ANTIBODIES, AND DNA

ANTIGEN	CLINICAL SIGNIFICANCE	ANTIBODY	CLINICAL SIGNIFICANCE
HBsAg	Acute or chronic infection	Anti-HBs	Protection by vaccination recovery from infection
HBeAg	Active viral replication	Anti-HBe	Inactive viral replication
HBcAg	Not detectable in the serum	Anti-HBc	Present (IgM, IgG) or detectable in the liver Past infection (IgG)
HBV DNA	Presence of HBV		

Anti-HBc = hepatitis B core antibody; Anti-HBe = hepatitis B e antigen; Anti-HBs = hepatitis B surface antibody; DNA = deoxyribonucleic acid; HBcAg = hepatitis B core antigen; HBeAg = hepatitis B e antigen; HBsAg = hepatitis B surface antigen; HBV = hepatitis B virus; Ig = immunoglobulin.

hepatitis B X protein.[4] HBV has a restricted host range. It infects only humans and chimpanzees.

EPIDEMIOLOGY OF HBV INFECTION IN CHILDREN

HBV infection is prevalent in Asia, Africa, Southern Europe, and Latin America, where the HBsAg-seropositive rate ranges from 2 to 20% in most regions. In hyperendemic areas, HBV infections occur mainly during infancy and early childhood. In Taiwan, the HBsAg carrier rate is approximately 10 to 20%. Before the implementation of a universal HBV immunization program, the HBsAg-seropositive rate in this population was 5% in infants and increased to 10% at 2 years of age, remaining at the same rate thereafter. However, the infection rate, measured by hepatitis B core antibody (anti-HB$_c$) seropositivity, reached 50% by the age of 15 years. This suggests that most chronic HBsAg carriers are infected before 2 years of age in this population.[1]

Perinatal transmission from HBsAg carrier mothers to their infants is a very important route of transmission, leading to chronicity, in Asia. This mode of transmission accounts for 40 to 50% of HBsAg carriers in Taiwan and many other hyperendemic areas. Approximately 90% of the infants of HBeAg-seropositive carrier mothers become HBsAg carriers,[5] irrespective of a high or low HBsAg carrier rate in the population. The age of infection is an important factor in determining the outcome of infection.[6,7]

In areas of low endemicity, horizontal infection is the main route of transmission. Although Africa is an area of high endemicity, horizontal infection in early childhood is the main route of HBV transmission. The two most important routes of horizontal transmission in children are highly infectious family members, such as siblings, and improperly sterilized syringes.[8] Other sources of horizontally transmitted infections include institutionalized children and multiple or large-volume blood transfusions. In the United States and Europe, HBV is highly prevalent among adopted children from endemic areas of the world.

PATHOGENESIS AND NATURAL COURSE OF HBV INFECTION IN CHILDREN

HBV has an incubation period of 2 to 6 months. Following a primary HBV infection, the host may run an acute, fulminant, or chronic course. The interaction between the host and virus determines the outcome of infection.

ACUTE AND FULMINANT HEPATITIS B
Acute hepatitis runs a self-limited course. Recovery is marked by hepatitis B surface antibody (anti-HB$_s$) seroconversion. Fulminant hepatitis is signaled by pathologic mental status changes within 2 to 8 weeks after the initial symptoms in an otherwise healthy child. Trey and Davison defined fulminant hepatic failure as the onset of altered metal status within 8 weeks of initial symptoms in an otherwise healthy individual.[9] Later Bernuau and colleagues defined fulminant hepatitis as hepatic encephalopathy developing within 2 weeks after the onset of jaundice and subfulminant hepatitis as hepatic encephalopathy developing between 2 and 12 weeks after the onset of jaundice.[10]

Symptoms of acute or fulminant hepatitis B may develop as early as 2 months of age in infants of HBsAg carrier mothers. In areas hyperendemic for HBV infection, HBV accounts for around 65% of the etiologic agents for fulminant hepatitis in children. Approximately 65% of pediatric patients with fulminant hepatitis B present in infancy. Maternal transmission is the most important route of transmission in infants with acute or fulminant hepatitis,[11] mainly in infants of hepatitis B e antibody (anti-HB$_e$)-seropositive mothers.[12]

Fulminant hepatitis carries a very high mortality rate of 55 to 70% without transplant and 30 to 50% with transplant.[11,13] Those who survive usually recover without sequelae. In both acute and fulminant hepatitis B, HBV is cleared rapidly from the host.

Precore mutations have been associated with fulminant hepatitis B in adults, but this has not been confirmed by more recent studies.[14,15] Thirty-three percent of the children with fulminant hepatitis B have the hepatitis B precore stop codon mutant, a prevalence rate similar to that (30%) in children with acute hepatitis B.[16] This suggests that precore stop codon mutations alone do not explain the severe clinical course in fulminant hepatitis B.

CHRONIC HBV INFECTION
Children with chronic HBV infection are mostly asymptomatic. They are generally active and grow well, with very rare exceptions. Even with acute exacerbation of liver inflammation, jaundice or growth failure is rare. Although liver damage is usually mild during childhood, serious sequelae, including cirrhosis and hepatocellular carcinoma, may develop insidiously at any age.

The coexistence of high rates of viral replication, normal liver function profiles, and minimal hepatic hisopathology for many years in children with chronic HBV infection suggests that HBV may not be directly cytopathic. An immune-mediated process is the main mechanism for cell damage. During acute exacerbations of chronic HBV infections, CD8-positive cytotoxic T lymphocytes are the predominant cells in the liver in the areas of piecemeal necrosis. As hepatocellular necrosis occurs, there is a gradual decrease of HBV replication and HBeAg serocoversion occurs, along with a decrease in hepatic inflammation (Figure 51.1A-1).

Spontaneous Hepatitis B e Seroconversion. HBeAg is an important marker reflecting active viral replication and infectivity. Its clearance is therefore used as a marker for the success of antiviral therapy. Children with chronic HBV infection are HBeAg seropositive at the initial stage of infection. During this stage, the child is tolerant to HBV, the virus is highly replicative, and serum HBV DNA levels are usually high. The child is thus an important source of horizontal infection in the family and community. Aminotransferase levels fluctuate but are usually normal or mildly elevated, with mean levels higher than those in noncarrier healthy children.[17] Peak alanine aminotrans-

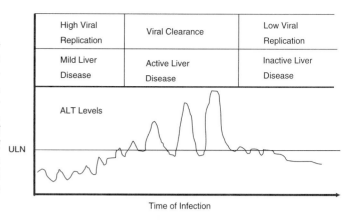

FIGURE 51.1A-1 Natural course of chronic hepatitis B virus infection acquired in childhood. During the early phase of infection, the amount of virus in the liver and blood is usually large, whereas the liver damage is mostly mild. The host immune system gradually recognizes the virus and starts to clear the virus. It results in active inflammation of the liver and elevation of serum aminotransferases. Repeated episodes of elevation of aminotransferases may be followed by hepatitis B e antigen (HBeAg) seroconversion. After HBeAg seroconversion, viral replication declines and the liver inflammation gradually becomes inactive. ULN = upper limit of normal.

ferase (ALT) levels > 100 IU/L are uncommon in this phase. Hepatitis B e antigenemia can persist for years after primary infection.

Spontaneous clearance of serum HBeAg occurs gradually as the child ages. Viral replication is reduced during this process. This process of HBeAg clearance is usually preceded by an elevation of aminotransferases. The peak level of aminotransferase elevation can be mild, transient, and fluctuating. An ALT level > 1,000 IU/mL is unusual. This process of HBeAg seroconversion takes place subclinically in most individuals for a period of 2 to 7 years.[18] After the detection of elevated levels of aminotransferases, around 40% of children will clear HBeAg within 1 year. Children with elevated aminotransferase levels of > 100 IU/mL and HBV DNA levels of < 1,000 pg/mL often seroconvert during the subsequent 1 to 3 years.[17] After HBeAg clearance, aminotransferase levels gradually return to normal limits, and anti-HBe develops spontaneously. In our series, HBV DNA was detectable in only 1% of the anti-HBe–positive sera. However, using polymerase chain reaction (PCR), HBV DNA persists long term in the serum of children with chronic hepatitis B after HBeAg seroconversion. Bortolotti and colleagues. studied 39 children after hepatitis B e seroconversion.[19] They found that 87% of children had detectable HBV DNA by PCR within 5 years of follow-up and in 58% of cases 10 years after seroconversion. ALT levels were persistently normal in 92%, whereas 8% had slightly elevated ALT.

Acute exacerbation of inflammation with reactivation of HBV replication and a rise in aminotransferases is not common in children after hepatitis B e seroconversion.[18,20] Permanent liver damage has occurred, and integration of the genome of HBV has occurred insidiously and gradually, despite clearance of HBeAg. Development of cirrhosis or hepatocellular carcinoma is occasionally observed but is rare during childhood. Most of those who develop these complications of chronic HBV infection are anti-HBe seropositive.[21]

Factors Affecting Hepatitis B e Seroconversion. Age is an important determinant of the rate of HBeAg seroconversion.[22] Before 3 years of age, the spontaneous HBeAg clearance rate is very low (< 2% per year). The hepatitis B e seroconversion rate gradually increases to around 5% per year after 3 years of age. This might be due to immune tolerance to HBcAg and HBeAg in infected children. Immune

tolerance owing to transplacental e antigen has been demonstrated by the absence of a T-cell response to HBcAg in infants and children of HBeAg-positive HBsAg carrier mothers, whereas the T lymphocytes from infants with acute hepatitis of hepatitis B e–negative HBsAg carrier mothers respond very well to HBcAg.[23] The age of hepatitis B e seroconversion varies, ranging from infancy to more than 40 years of age. The most common period is from 15 to 30 years of age. Before 15 years of age, the majority (85% in Taiwan) of HBsAg carrier children are HBeAg seropositive.

Another factor affecting the hepatitis B e seroconversion rate in children is maternal HBsAg.[22] Those with HBsAg carrier mothers have a lower rate of HBeAg clearance than those whose mothers were not HBsAg carriers. Maternal carrier state reflects perinatal transmission or early infection, which will lead to a longer duration of immune tolerance to HBV (Figure 51.1A-2).

HBsAg/Antibody Seroconversion. In our long-term follow-up of HBsAg carrier children, the annual HBsAg clearance rate was very low (only 0.56%),[24] occurring only after clearance of HBeAg. After loss of HBsAg, its antibody (anti-HBs) remains low or undetectable in the majority (0 to < 100 mIU/mL). The underlying mechanisms of a poor anti-HBs response in HBsAg carriers who lost HBsAg are multifactorial, including specific failure of antigen presentation or T-cell activation or the lack of a T helper cell–like response to HBsAg.[25] Hepatitis B immunization is not beneficial in these individuals.

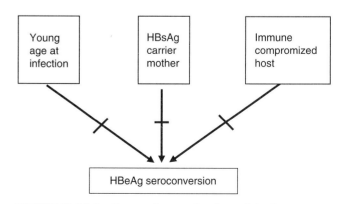

FIGURE 51.1A-2 Factors that may hinder or delay hepatitis B e antigen (HBeAg) seroconversion and viral clearance.

Histopathologic Findings in Children with Chronic HBV Infection. Liver histology in HBeAg-positive HBsAg carrier children generally reveals very mild inflammation and fibrosis.[26] During the process of HBV and HBeAg clearance, the abnormal changes include lobular changes with portal inflammation and fibrosis, with or without piecemeal necrosis. The inflammation is usually milder than that observed in adults. Bridging hepatic necrosis may occur but is uncommon. Within 6 months of hepatitis B e seroconversion, the inflammation is less active and, beyond 6 months, becomes inactive, with mild to minimal inflammation and fibrosis in most children.

The authors have studied the liver histology in 41 asymptomatic HBsAg children at 1 to 9 years of age who were perinatally infected by their HBeAg-positive HBsAg carrier mothers. The histologic findings included chronic active hepatitis (n = 1), chronic persistent hepatitis (n = 8), chronic nonspecific hepatitis (n = 30), and normal histology (n = 2). The histologic abnormalities in the liver begin early in life and may progress to severe liver impairment in later life.

Virologic Factors That May Affect the Clinical Course. During the course of infection, HBV may undergo mutations, which accumulate particularly in some DNA hot spots. Mutations of HBV may affect the outcome of infection or, more commonly, are the result of host immune pressure. HBV precore G to A stop codon mutations at nucleotide 1896 are a common site of mutations detected in patients with fulminant hepatitis, acute hepatitis, chronic hepatitis with acute exacerbation, cirrhosis, or hepatocellular carcinoma in adults.[27,28] We have studied the temporal changes of this mutation in children with chronic HBV infection and found that it emerged before hepatitis B e seroconversion. The proportion of positive precore stop codon mutations increased gradually after HBeAg seroconversion to around 50% of the children.[29]

HBcAg is the target in HBV-infected hepatocytes for cytotoxic T lymphocyte–mediated cell lysis. Mutation of the HBV core gene may change the conformation of core protein and allow the hepatocytes to escape the immune surveillance of the host. Among 31 Taiwanese children with chronic HBV infection, HBV core gene codons 21 (29%), 147 (29%), and 65 (15%) were the frequent sites of mutation.[30]

Genotypes of HBV were reported to correlate with the clinical outcome in patients with chronic hepatitis B. Genotype C was more prevalent in patients with cirrhosis and hepatocellular carcinoma, whereas patients with genotype B experienced earlier hepatitis B e seroconversion and slower progression of liver fibrosis and development of hepatomas.[31,32]

Hepatocellular Carcinoma. Hepatocellular carcinoma is 1 of the 10 most common cancers in the world. In areas prevalent for HBV infection, hepatocellular carcinoma is not rare in children. The rate of seroprevalence of hepatitis B surface antigenemia approaches 100% in children with hepatocellular carcinoma in Taiwan. Maternal transmission or infection in early childhood is an important risk factor.[21,23] Integration of HBV DNA has been detected in the tumor and nonmalignant liver tissue of children with chronic HBV infection and hepatocellular carcinoma.[33]

Core gene mutations were identified much more commonly at some codons (codons 74, 87, and 159) in children with hepatoma than in children with chronic HBV infection but without cancer. Those core gene mutations may induce persistent host immune attacks and lead to severe liver damage, as observed in children with hepatocellular carcinoma.[30]

HEPATITIS B IMMUNOPROPHYLAXIS

Prevention of HBV infection can be achieved by passive and active immunization. Passive immunization using hepatitis B immunoglobulin (HBIg) provides temporary immunity. After hepatitis B vaccine became available in 1982, active immunization with three or four doses of HBV vaccine without HBIg has proved to be immunogenic in more than 90% of neonates of noncarrier mothers or HBeAg-negative carrier mothers. In infants of HBeAg-seropositive mothers, it decreased the carrier rate to 24%. Injection of HBIg within 24 hours after birth followed by three doses of HBV vaccine further reduces the carrier rate down to 3% in pilot studies[34] and to 14% in a study of the general population.[35] According to a random sampling study of children in Taiwan 3 years after implementing a universal HBV vaccination program, the protective efficacy was found to be 86% from HBIg plus HBV vaccine and 78% from three doses of HBV vaccine alone.[35]

The first universal hepatitis B vaccination program in the world was launched in Taiwan in July 1984.[36] Pregnant women are screened for both serum HBsAg and HBeAg or titers of HBsAg by a reverse passive hemagglutination test. Infants of mothers with negative serum HBeAg with a reciprocal HBsAg titer lower than 1:2,560 or with negative serum HBsAg receive plasma-derived hepatitis B vaccine at 0, 1, 2, and 12 months for those born before July 1992 or a recombinant hepatitis B vaccine at 0, 1, and 6 months for those born after July 1992. Infants of mothers with positive serum HBeAg or with reciprocal titers of HBsAg by reverse passive hemagglutination ≥ 2,560 receive HBIg within 24 hours after birth in addition to doses of hepatitis B vaccine. The coverage rate of hepatitis B vaccine for neonates is around 94%.

Different immunization strategies are used in different countries, depending on their basic epidemiologic features of HBV infection and available resources. In many hyperendemic countries, HBV vaccination consists of three doses of hepatitis B vaccine and no HBIg for all infants, including infants of an HBsAg carrier mother This has an efficacy of around 75 to 80%. Using this HBV immunization program, the cost of maternal screening and HBIg can be minimized. Other countries, such as the United States, give one dose of HBIg to infants of HBsAg-positive mothers, regardless of their HBeAg status, and three doses of HBV vaccine to all infants.

IMPACT OF UNIVERSAL HEPATITIS B IMMUNIZATION ON HEPATITIS B ERADICATION

The seroprevalence rates of HBsAg and anti-HB$_c$ in Taiwanese children before and 15 years after the initiation of a universal vaccination program were remarkably reduced.[37] The HBsAg carrier rate in Taipei in children < 15 years old decreased significantly from around 10% before to < 1% after the vaccination program (see Table 51.1A-2). The infection rate, measured by the seropositive prevalence of anti-HBc, was decreased in all of the children (anti-HB$_c$ seropositivity declined from 38 to 16% in children below 13 years of age), even in those above 15 years of age who were not vaccinated during infancy. This vaccination program has indeed reduced both the perinatal and the horizontal transmission of HBV.[38] The decrease in horizontal transmission was a result of a decline in the prevalence of sources of infection and the vaccination of the older children.

Although immunoprophylaxis for HBV infection is very successful, around 2.4% of infants of HBeAg-positive mothers still had HBsAg in the serum at birth or shortly after birth.[39] They became HBsAg carriers in spite of complete immunoprophylaxis. Intrauterine HBV infection, although infrequent, is possible. Risk factors for failure of immunoprophylaxis include a high level of maternal HBV DNA, a low level of maternal anti-HB$_c$, and uterine contraction and placental leakage during the process of delivery.[40,41]

VACCINE PREVENTION OF HEPATOCELLULAR CARCINOMA

After the implementation of the universal vaccination program for HBV in Taiwan, we have successfully demonstrated a decline in the incidence of hepatocellular carcinoma in children. The average annual incidence of hepatocellular carcinoma in children of 6 to 14 years declined from 0.70 per 100,000 children between 1981 and 1986, to 0.57 between 1986 and 1990, and to 0.36 between 1990 and 1994.[42] In contrast, the incidence of hepatoblastoma in children and the incidence of hepatocellular carcinoma in adults during the same study period were not reduced. Analyzing the incidence of hepatocellu-

lar carcinoma according to the birth cohort, the reduction effect is even more impressive. The incidence of hepatocellular carcinoma in children 6 to 9 years of age declined from 0.52 in 100,000 children for those born between 1974 and 1984 to 0.13 in 100,000 children for those born between 1984 and 1986.

Boys may benefit more from HBV vaccination than girls in the prevention of hepatocellular carcinoma.[43] The boy-to-girl incidence of hepatocellular carcinoma decreased steadily from 4.5 in 1981 to 1984 (before the launch of a universal HBV vaccination program) to 1.9 in 1990 to 1996 (6–12 years after the launch of a universal HBV vaccination program) (Table 51.1A-3).

LONG-TERM VACCINE IMMUNOGENICITY

A large-scale prospective community-based study enrolling 1,200 children with complete HBV immunization in infancy was conducted until the children were 14 years of age. Eleven children had new HBV infections with anti-HB$_c$ seropositivity. None of them became positive for HBsAg or HBV DNA by PCR. The proportion of children with protective anti-HB$_s$ gradually decreased from 71% at age 7 years to 37% at age 12 years in 951 children who did not receive booster doses of HBV vaccine during follow-up. Among the 458 children with anti-HB$_s$ levels lower than the protective level at age 7 years, only 1 of the 200 children in the group that received booster doses and 2 of the 258 children in the group that did not developed a new infection with anti-HB$_c$ positivity during follow-up to age 14 years.[44]

REMAINING BARRIERS TO ERADICATION OF HBV

Further investigation into the mechanisms of HBV vaccine failures or nonresponders is critical. Interventions to prevent intrauterine infection, the development of HBV vaccines against surface antigen gene mutants, and better vaccines for immunocompromised individuals will further reduce the incidence of new infections.

Those opposed to the HBV vaccines may be reduced in number by a better understanding of vaccine-related side effects. For instance, although there is little supporting evidence, an association between central nervous system demyelinating diseases and hepatitis B vaccine has been suggested.[45] Clarification of this and other poorly documented side effects of the vaccines may help to reduce anxiety about the risks of the vaccine and enhance an appreciation of HBV vaccine benefits. Finally, it is extremely important to find ways to reduce the cost of HBV vaccines and to increase funding for HBV vaccination of children living in hyperendemic areas under poor economic conditions

TREATMENT

The goal of antiviral therapy for HBV infection is to eradicate HBV and to prevent its related liver damage. However, current antiviral regimens are not completely effective in this regard. Inhibition of viral replication with prevention of liver damage and related consequences is also important and is more achievable with available antiviral agents (Table 51.1A-4).

TABLE 51.1A-2   HBSAG-SEROPOSITIVE RATES BEFORE AND AFTER IMPLEMENTATION OF A UNIVERSAL HEPATITIS B VACCINATION PROGRAM IN TAIWAN

	HBSAG-SEROPOSITIVE RATE (%)			
AGE (YR)	1984	1989	1994	1999
< 1	5.1	3.0	0.0	0.0
1–2	10.7	1.5	0.5	1.2
3–4	10.1	2.2	0.3	0.0
5–6	10.6	3.9	0.8	0.0
7–8	9.7	4.7	0.9	2.0
9–10	11.0	9.8	1.5	1.3
11–12	9.1	10.5	6.8	0.0

Universal hepatitis B vaccination was implemented in Taiwan in July 1984.
Adapted from Ni YH et al.[37]

TABLE 51.1A-3   EFFECT OF UNIVERSAL HEPATITIS B VACCINATION ON THE PREVENTION OF HEPATOCELLULAR CARCINOMA IN CHILDREN IN TAIWAN

YEAR OF DIAGNOSIS	BOYS	GIRLS	TOTAL INCIDENCE OF HCC*	MALE/FEMALE
1981–84[†]	1.08	0.24	0.67	4.5
1984–90	0.87	0.32	0.61	2.7
1990–96	0.49	0.26	0.38	1.9

HCC = hepatocellular carcinoma.
*Per 100,000 population of children aged 6 to 14 years.
[†]Before the hepatitis B virus vaccination program (universal vaccination was implemented in July 1984).

STRATEGIES FOR THE TREATMENT OF CHRONIC VIRAL HEPATITIS

Interferon Therapy. Interferons are antiviral and immunomodulatory proteins.[46] They interact with cells by binding to specific receptors on the cell surface. Interferon-α is produced by leukocyte or lymphoblastoid cells when they are stimulated by virus-infected or tumor cells, bacteria, or viral envelopes. In virus-infected cells, interferons can produce antiviral proteins, inhibit synthesis of viral ribonucleic acid, and enhance the expression of human leukocyte antigen class I antigens, thus allowing recognition of the infected hepatocytes by cytotoxic T lymphocytes. Interferon therapy is employed worldwide and is the most frequently used therapeutic antiviral agent for hepatitis B and C. The disadvantages of this drug are the parenteral route of administration and mostly tolerable but frequent adverse reactions (Table 51.1A-5).

Overall, approximately 30 to 40% of adults with chronic hepatitis B achieve a sustained response to interferon-α at a usual dosage of 5 MU/d or 10 MU three times a week for 3 to 4 months. Evidence for the efficacy of interferon therapy in children with chronic HBV is limited by the small number of children enrolled in most reported studies. As shown in Table 51.1A-6, interferon therapy is not effective for hepatitis B e seroconversion in carrier children with normal liver enzymes. In those with elevated aminotransferases, the results of interferon treatment are similar to those in adults, with a rate of hepatitis B e seroconversion and normalization of aminotransferase levels 20 to 40%

higher in the treatment group than in the control group.[47–54] A systematic review of the world literature has shown a significant benefit of interferon therapy for chronic HBV infection in children.[55]

Factors that are predictive for a positive response to interferon include high pretreatment levels of aminotransferase, low pretreatment HBV DNA levels, late acquisition of HBV infection, and hepatocellular inflammation.

The recommended dose of interferon for children is 0.1 MU/kg or 3 to 6 MU/m² three times a week for 4 to 6 months. Some studies in a small number of children, using higher doses, 6 to 10 MU/m², have shown a higher rate of sustained responses but also a higher rate of adverse effects. If severe reactions to interferon occur, the dose should be modified (50% reduction) or discontinued. Extending the duration of therapy for a total of 12 months may be beneficial for those who have a partial response to initial interferon therapy.

Pegylated interferon is a long-acting interferon successfully used in treating chronic hepatitis C[56] and has also been used in treating hepatitis B in adults.[57] The safety and efficacy have not been reported in children.

Nucleoside Analogs. Lamivudine is a 2′,3′-dideoxynucleoside that is phosphorylated by intracellular enzymes to form lamivudine triphosphate. Lamivudine triphosphate can inhibit DNA synthesis by terminating the nascent proviral DNA chain and interfere with the reverse transcriptase activity of HBV. After oral administration, lamivudine is well absorbed and has a mean absolute bioavailability of > 80% in adults and 68% in infants and children.[58] In clinical trials in adults, lamivudine rapidly reduced HBV DNA to undetectable levels in a daily dose of 100 mg or more.[59,60]

TABLE 51.1A-4   THERAPIES FOR CHRONIC VIRAL HEPATITIS B

INTERFERON
ANTIVIRAL AGENTS
Nucleoside analog
   Lamivudine
   Adefovir dipivoxil
   Entecavir
   Emtricitabine
Gene therapy
   Antisense oligonucleotide
   Ribozyme
   Interfering proteins or peptides
IMMUNOMODULATORY THERAPY
Thymosin
DNA vaccine
COMBINATION THERAPY

TABLE 51.1A-5   ADVERSE EFFECTS OF INTERFERON, LAMIVUDINE, AND ADEFOVIR DIPIVOXIL

AGENT	ADVERSE EFFECTS
Interferon	Flu-like symptoms, depression, anorexia, weight loss, hair loss, bone marrow suppression, autoantibody induction
Lamivudine	Ear, nose, and throat problems; gastrointestinal symptoms; malaise and fatigue; lower respiratory tract symptoms; pancreatitis; neutropenia; elevation of liver enzyme
Adefovir	Nephrotoxicity

TABLE 51.1A-6   INTERFERON THERAPY FOR HEPATITIS B VIRUS INFECTION IN CHILDREN

| PLACE AND STUDY | ALT AT THERAPY | RATE OF HBEAG SEROCLEARANCE | |
		CONTROL GROUP	IFN THERAPY GROUP
SPAIN			
Ruiz-Moreno et al,[51] 1995	> 45 IU/L	—	34% (17/50)
ITALY			
Barbera et al,[49] 1994	No limit	14% (5/37)	26% (10/39)
Vajro et al,[53] 1996	> 1.5 × of ULN	11% (1/9)	48% (10/21)
Gregorio et al,[52] 1996	No limit	13% (4/31)	38% (24/64)
UNITED STATES			
Narkewicz et al,[50] 1995	> 2 × of ULN	—	78% (7/9)
HONG KONG			
Lai et al,[47] 1987	Normal	8% (1/12)	8% (1/12)
Lai et al,[48] 1991	No limit	0% (0/30)	8% (5/60)
TAIWAN			
Chang et al,[42] 1997	> 80 IU/L	46% (6/13)	73% (8/11)
EUROPE + AMERICA (MULTICENTERED)			
Sokal et al,[54] 1998	> 1.3 × ULN	11% (8/74)	26% (18/70)
META-ANALYSIS			
Torre and Tambini,[55] 1996	No limit	11% (12/113)	23% (29/126)*

ALT = alanine aminotransferase; IFN = interferon; ULN = upper limit of normal.
*p = .026.

Lamivudine 0.7 to 8 mg/d was well tolerated in 53 European and Canadian children aged 2 to 17 years.[61] Around one-fifth of patients who received 1 month of lamivudine therapy experienced drug-related adverse events. The most common adverse events were ear, nose, and throat problems; gastrointestinal symptoms; general symptoms (malaise and fatigue); and lower respiratory symptoms (see Table 51.1A-5). No serious side effects or need for withdrawal occurred during therapy or follow-up.

Lamivudine was able to eliminate or reduce HBV DNA in pediatric patients after 1 month of therapy in a multicentered study in European and Canadian children.[61] A dramatic fall of HBV DNA of 99.9% and a reduction in HBV DNA of approximately 1,000-fold was noted. However, HBV DNA returned to the pretreatment levels in all patients after cessation of lamivudine. The HBeAg loss rate remained low after 3 months of follow-up. The efficacy of 52 weeks of lamivudine therapy was evaluated in 286 children in a multicentered placebo-controlled study. The complete virologic response (with HBeAg clearance and negative HBV DNA) at the end of treatment was achieved in 23% of the treatment group (191 children) and 13% of the placebo group (95 children). The anti-HB$_e$ seroconversion rate was 22% versus 13% in the treatment group versus the control group. ALT normalization was noted in 55% of the treatment group and 12% of the placebo group. The HBsAg loss rate was minimal (2% in the treatment group and 0% in the placebo group).[62] Higher ALT levels and liver histologic inflammation scores and lower HBV DNA levels before treatment predict a better treatment response.

Lamivudine, at 100 mg/d, is the recommended dose for adults.[60] The recommended dose for children is 3 mg/kg/d up to a maximal dose of 100 mg/day.[61] There is no added benefit to dividing the total daily dose. The optimal duration of treatment requires further investigation. At this time, treatment for 1 year is recommended.

Children aged 2 to 17 years of age who are HBsAg seropositive for more than 6 months with elevated aminotransferase levels and HBV DNA in their serum for more than 3 months may be candidates for lamivudine therapy. This includes HBV carriers who are waiting for a liver transplant, children with repeated acute exacerbations of HBV infections, children with HBV infection < 2 years of age, and children with fibrosing cholestatic HBV hepatitis. Drug compliance should be monitored carefully, particularly in adolescents. Regular physical examinations are mandatory, along with monitoring of serum biochemical markers of inflammation and viral infection, including aminotransferases, coagulation profiles, complete blood cell count, amylase, lipase, urea nitrogen, and creatinine. Liver histology, quantified by the Knodell score, before and 1 year after starting therapy provides valuable information regarding viral clearance, necroinflammatory activity, and fibrosis. Lamivudine should be discontinued if any related adverse reactions develop. HBV DNA, HBeAg, and anti-HB$_e$ should be monitored after discontinuing use of lamivudine because HBV replication frequently resumes.

Mutants of the HBV polymerase gene at the reverse transcriptase region may develop after use of lamivudine for more than 9 months.[63,64] The mutations most frequently found are methionine to valine or methionine to isoleucine mutations at the YMDD (tyrosine-methionine-aspartate-aspartate) motif. The second common site of mutagenesis is leucine to methionine at the polymerase gene nucleotide 528 for gentoype A or nucleotide 526 for genotypes B, C, and F (or reverse transcriptase nucleotide 180).[65] The clinical relevance of these mutations in children infected with HBV is poorly understood at this time. Among the 166 children treated with lamivudine in a muticentered study, 31 developed YMDD mutations at the end of 52 weeks of therapy. Those with YMDD mutants had a higher (1.5 times) median level of ALT and HBV DNA (19 times) than those without this mutant.[62]

Lamivudine-associated HBV YMDD mutant strains have been reported to be less replicable than the wild-type virus. In fact, the long-term use of lamivudine after the emergence of the YMDD motif mutation may lead to acute exacerbation and subsequent HBV clearance.[66] However, there is a risk of liver failure during these acute exacerbations of infection. Careful monitoring of the quantity of HBV DNA and signs of clinical or biochemical deterioration of liver function is mandatory in children infected with mutant strains.

Adefovir dipivoxil, a nucleoside analog recently approved by the US Food and Drug Administration, is effective in inhibiting the replication of the YMDD motif mutants[67-69] and can be used in patients with acute exacerbation of inflammation during lamivudine therapy. It is an acyclic analog of deoxyadenosine monophosphate that can competitively inhibit deoxyadenosine triphosphate and the first-strand synthesis. It can inhibit > 95% of viral DNA and 30% of pregenomic ribonucleic acid, pre-S (gene of hepatitis B virus middle and large surface protein gene), core proteins, and covalently closed circular hepatitis B virus DNA. Adefovir is nephrotoxic. Other nucleoside analogs, including entecavir and emtricitabine, have good antiviral potential, but their therapeutic benefit in children remains unclear.

GENE THERAPY AND IMMUNOTHERAPY

Gene therapy for HBV infection is still under investigation.[70] Antisense oligonucleotides can inhibit hepatitis viral gene expression and may provide a new therapeutic choice for patients with chronic HBV infections.[71] Thymosin α is an immune modifier that has been shown to trigger maturational events in lymphocytes, augment T-cell function, and promote reconstitution of immune defects. It has been reported to be effective in treating chronic HBV infections with clearance of HBeAg and normalization of aminotransferase levels in some[72] but not all studies. DNA vaccines are still in the experimental stage. Injection into mice of a plasmid expressing HBV DNA encoding HBV proteins, under the cytomegalovirus promoter, may induce both cellular and humoral immune responses against this viral antigen.[73,74]

COMBINATION THERAPIES

Combination therapies are increasingly used for the management of persistent viral infections. The synergistic effect of ribavirin and interferon in treating chronic hepatitis C is one example of successful combination antiviral therapy.

The benefit of different combinations of doses and schedules for interferon plus lamivudine therapy has been controversial in adults.[75] Comparisons between interferon alone versus lamivudine plus interferon have been conducted in children (n = 15 to 47 in each group of treatment) with no statistically significant differences in the outcomes measured. These studies used interferon-α 5 to 10 MU/m² three times per week for 6 to 12 months plus lamivudine 4 mg/kg daily (maximun 100 mg daily) for 12 months. A complete virologic response rate of 37 to 47% at 6 months was seen after the end of treatment. It was similar to the 30 to 40% complete virologic response in children treated with interferon alone for 6 to 12 months.[76,77] The use of lamivudine alone for 2 months, then interferon-α 10 MU/m² plus lamivudine for 6 months, and then lamivudine alone again for additional 4 months versus interferon plus lamivudine simultaneously for 6 months and then lamivudine alone for another 6 months also showed no differences between the two treatment groups (47% versus 46% complete elimination of HBV).[78] Large-scale studies using other combination schedules or regimens are needed to clarify the efficacy of combination therapy.

FUTURE PROSPECTS

The World Health Organization (WHO) recommended in 1997 that universal hepatitis B immunization should be introduced in all countries. WHO also established the objective to reduce the incidence of new HBV carriers among children by 80% by year 2001 and eventually to eliminate the more than a million deaths that occur annually from HBV-associated cirrhosis and hepatocellular carcinoma.[79,80] Up to now, a total of approximately 140 countries have followed this recommendation. With the integration of the hepatitis B vaccination program into the Expanded Immunization Program in most countries in the world, chronic HBV infection will be further reduced in the twenty-first century. The major issues that remain for hepatitis B prevention include vaccine failure and noncompliance with vaccination programs. Further understanding of the immune defects and pathogenesis of chronic HBV infection will enhance the development of better therapeutic and preventive agents and vaccines focused on the T-cell epitopes of HBV that can be recognized by convalescent patients.

REFERENCES

1. Hsu HY, Chang MH, Chen DS, et al. Baseline seroepidemiology of hepatitis B viurs infection in children in Taipei, 1984: a study just before mass hepatitis B vaccination program in Taiwan. J Med Virol 1986;18:301–7.
2. Tiollais P, Pourcel C, Dejean A. The hepatitis B virus. Nature 1985; 317:489–95.
3. Seeger C, Ganem D, Varmus HE. Biochemical and genetic evidence for the hepatitis B virus replication strategy. Science 1986;232:477–84.
4. Lau JYN, Wright TL. Molecular virology and pathogenesis of hepatitis B. Lancet 1993;342:1335–44.
5. Stevens CE, Beasley RP, Tsui J, Lee WC. Vertical transmission of hepatitis B antigen in Taiwan. N Engl J Med 1975;292:771–4.
6. Beasley RP, Hwang LY, Lin CC, et al. Incidence of hepatitis B virus infection preschool children in Taiwan. J Infect Dis 1982;146:198–204.
7. Beasley RP, Hwang LY, Lin CC, et al. Incidence of hepatitis among students at a university in Taiwan. Am J Epidemiol 1983;117:213–22.
8. Hsu SC, Chang MH, Ni YH, et al. Horizontal transmission of hepatitis B virus in children. J Pediatr Gastroenterol Nutr 1993;292:771–4.
9. Trey C, Davison CS. The management of fulminant hepatic failure. In: Popper H, Schaffner F, editors. Progress in liver diseases. New York: Grune & Stratton; 1970. p. 282–98.

10. Bernuau J, Rueff B, Benhamou JP. Fulminant and subfulminant liver failure: definitions and causes. Semin Liver Dis 1986;6: 97–106.

11. Shiraki K, Yoshihara N, Sakurai M, et al. Acute hepatitis B in infants born to carrier mothers with the antibody t hepatitis B e antigen. J Pediatr 1980;97:768–70.

12. Chang MH, Lee CY, Chen DS, et al. Fulminant hepatitis in children in Taiwan: the important role of hepatitis B virus. J Pediatr 1987;111:34–9.

13. Durand P, Debray D, Mandel R, et al. Acute liver failure in infancy: a 14-year experience of a pediatric liver transplantation center. J Pediatr 2001;139:871–6.

14. Carman W, Fagan EA, Hadziyannis S, et al. Association of a pre-core genomic variant of hepatitis B virus with fulminant hepatitis. Hepatology 1991;14:219–22.

15. Feray C, Gigou M, Samuel D, et al. Low prevalence of precore mutations in hepatitis B virus DNA in fulminant hepatitis type B in France. J Hepatol 1993;18:119–22.

16. Hsu HY, Chang MH, Lee CY, et al. Precore mutant of hepatitis B virus in childhood fulminant hepatitis B: an infrequent association. J Infect Dis 1995;171:776–81.

17. Lee PI, Chang MH, Lee CY, et al. Changes of serum hepatitis B virus DNA and aminotransferase levels during the course of chronic hepatitis B virus infection in children. Hepatology 1990;12:657–60.

18. Chang MH, Hsu HY, Hsu HC, et al. The significance of spontaneous hepatitis B antigen seroconversion in childhood: with special emphasis on the clearance of hepatitis B e antigen before three years of age. Hepatology 1995;22:1387–92.

19. Bortolotti F, Wirth S, Crivellaro C, et al. Long-term persistence of hepatitis B virus DNA in the serum of children with chronic hepatitis B after hepatitis B e antigen to antibody seroconversion. J Pediatr Gastroenterol Nutr 1996;22:270–4.

20. Bortolotti F, Cadrobbi M, Crivellaro C, et al. Long-term outcome of chronic type B hepatitis in patients who acquire hepatitis B virus infection in childhood. Gastroenterology 1990;99:805–10.

21. Chang MH, Chen DS, Hsu HC, et al. Maternal transmission of hepatitis B virus in childhood hepatocellular carcinoma. Cancer 1989;64:2377–80.

22. Chang MH, Sung JL, Lee CY, et al. Factors affecting clearance of hepatitis B e antigen in hepatitis B surface antigen carrier children. J Pediatr 1989;115:385–90.

23. Hsu HY, Chang MH, Hsieh KH, et al. Cellular immune response to hepatitis B core antigen in maternal-infant transmisson of hepatitis B virus. Hepatology 1992;15:770–6.

24. Hsu HY, Chang MH, Lee CY, et al. Spontaneous loss of HBsAg in children with chronic hepatitis B virus infection. Hepatology 1992;15:380–6.

25. Hsu HY, Chang MH, Hsieh RP, et al. Humoral and cellular immune response to hepatitis B vaccination in hepatitis B surface antigen-carrier children who cleared serum-hepatitis B surface antigen. Hepatology 1996;24:1355–60.

26. Chang MH, Hwang LY, Hsu HC, et al. Prospective study of asymptomatic HBsAg carrier children infected in the perinatal period: clinical and liver histologic studies. Hepatology 1988;8:374–7.

27. Carman WF, Jacyna MR, Hadziyannis S, et al. Mutation prevalence reventing formation of hepatitis B e antigen in patients with chronic hepatitis B infection. Lancet 1989;ii:588–90.

28. Chan HLY, Hussain M, Lok AS. Different hepatitis B virus genotypes are associated with different mutations in the core promoter and precore regions during hepatitis B e antigen seroconversion. Hepatology 1999;29:976–84.

29. Chang MH, Hsu HY, Ni YH, et al. Precore stop codon mutant in chronic hepatitis B virus infection in children: its relation to hepatitis B e seroconversion and maternal hepatitis B surface antigen. J Hepatol 1998;28:915–22.

30. Ni YH, Chang MH, Hsu HY, Tsuei DJ. Different hepatitis B virus core gene mutations in children with chronic infection and hepatocellular carcinoma. Gut 2003;52:122–5.

31. Kao JH, Chen PJ, Lai MY, Chen DS. Hepatitis B genotypes correlate with clinical outcomes in patients with chronic hepatitis B. Gastroenterology 2000;118:554–9.

32. Sumi H, Yokosuka O, Seki N, et al. Influence of hepatitis B virus genotypes on the progression of chronic type B hepatitis liver disease. Hepatology 2003;37:19–26.

33. Chang MH, Chen PJ, Chen JY, et al. Hepatitis B virus integration in hepatitis B virus-related hepatocellular carcinoma in childhood. Hepatology 1991;13:316–4.

34. Beasley RP, Hwang LY, Lin CC, et al. Hepatitis B immune globulin (HBIG) efficacy in the interruption of perinatal transmission of hepatitis B virus carrier state. Lancet 1981;i:388–93.

35. Hsu NHM, Chen DS, Chuang CH, et al. Efficacy of a mass hepatitis B vaccination program in Taiwan: studies on 3464 infants of hepatitis B surface antigen-carrier mothers. JAMA 1988;260:2231–5.

36. Chen DS, Hsu NHM, Sung JL, et al. A mass vaccination program in Taiwan against hepatitis B virus infection in infants of hepatitis B surface antigen-carrier mothers. JAMA 1987;257: 2597–603.

37. Ni YH, Chang MH, Huang LM, et al. Hepatitis B virus infection in children and adolescents in a hyperendemic area: 15 years after mass hepatitis B vaccination. Ann Intern Med 2001; 135:796–800.

38. Chen HL, Chang MH, Ni YH, et al. Seroepidemiology of hepatitis B virus infection in children-ten years of mass vaccination in Taiwan. JAMA 1996;276:906–8.

39. Tang JR, Hsu HU, Lin HH, et al. Hepatitis B surface antigenemia at birth: a long-term follow-up study. J Pediatr 1998;133: 374–7.

40. Lin HH, Chang MH, Chen DS, et al. Early predictor of the efficacy of immunoprophylaxis against perinatal hepatitis B transmission: analysis of prophylaxis failure. Vaccine 1991;9:457–60.

41. Chang MH, Hsu HY, Huang LM, et al. The role of transplacental hepatitis B core antibody in the mother-to-infant transmission of hepatitis B virus. J Hepatol 1996;24:674–9.

42. Chang MH, Chen CJ, Lai MS, et al. Universal hepatitis B vaccination in Taiwan and the incidence of hepatocellular carcinoma in children. N Engl J Med 1997;336:1855–9.

43. Chang MH, Shau WY, Chen CJ, et al. The effect of universal hepatitis B vaccination on hepatocellular carcinoma rates in boys and girls. JAMA 2000;284:3040–2.

44. Lin YC, Chang MH, Ni YH, et al. Long-term immunogenicity and efficacy of universal hepatitis B virus vaccination in Taiwan. J Infect Dis 2003;187:134–8.

45. Halsey NA, Duclos P, van Damme P, Margolis H, on behalf of the Viral Hepatitis Prevention Board. Hepatitis B vaccine and central nervous system demyelinating diseases. Pediatr Infect Dis J 1999;18:23–4.

46. Dianzani F, Antonelli G, Capobianchi MR. The biological basis for the clinical use of interferon. J Hepatol 1990;11 Suppl 1:S5–10.

47. Lai CL, Lok ASF, Lin HJ, et al. Placebo-controlled trial of recombinant α2-interferon in Chinese HBsAg-carrier children. Lancet 1987;17:877–80.

48. Lai CL, Lin HJ, Lau JY-N, et al. Effect of recombinant alpha2 interferon with or without prednisone in Chinese HBsAg carrier children. QJM 1991;286:155–63.

49. Barbera C, Bortolotti F, Crivellaro C, et al. Recombinant interferon-2a hastens the rate of HBeAg clearance in children with chronic hepatitis B. Hepatology 1994;20:287–90.

50. Narkewicz MR, Smith D, Silverman A, et al. Clearance of chronic hepatitis B virus infection in young children after alpha interferon treatment. J Pediatr 1995;127:815–8.

51. Ruiz-Moreno M, Camps T, Jimenez J, et al. Factors predictive of response to interferon therapy in children with chronic hepatitis B. J Hepatol 1995;22:540–4.

52. Gregorio GV, Jara P, Hierro L, et al. Lymphoblastoid interferon alfa with or without steroid pretreatment in children with chronic hepatitis B: a multicenter controlled trial. Hepatology 1996;23:700–7.

53. Vajro P, Tedesco M, Fontanella A, et al. Prolonged and high dose recombinant interferon alpha-2b alone or after prednisone priming accelerates termination of active viral replication in children with chronic hepatitis B infection. Pediatr Infect Dis J 1996;15:223–31.

54. Sokal EM, Conjeevaram HS, Roberts EA, et al. Interferon alfa therapy for chronic hepatitis B in children: a multinational randomized controlled trial. Gastroenterology 1998;114:988–95.

55. Torre D, Tambini R. Interferon-α therapy for chronic hepatitis B in children: a meta-analysis. Clin Infect Dis 1996;23:131–7.

56. Zeuzem S, Feinman SV, Rasenack J, et al. Peginterferon alfa-2a in patients with chronic hepatitis C. N Engl J Med 2000;343:1666–72.

57. Cooksley WG, Piratvisuth T, Lee SD, et al. Peginterferon alpha-2a (40 kDa): an advance in the treatment of hepatitis B e antigen-positive chronic hepatitis B. J Viral Hepatitis 2003;10:298–305.

58. Perry CM, Faulds D. Lamivudine: a review of its antiviral activity, pharmacokinetic properties, and therapeutic efficacy in the management of HIV infection. Drugs 1997;53:657–80.

59. Dienstag JL, Perillo RP, Schiff ER, et al. A preliminary trial of lamivudine for chronic hepatitis B infection. N Engl J Med 1995;333:1657–61.

60. Lai CL, Chen RN, Leung NWY, et al. A one-year trial of lamivudine for chronic hepatitis B. N Engl J Med 1998;339:61–8.

61. Sokal E, Roberts EA, Mieli-Vergani G, et al. Dose finding and safety of lamivudine (LAM) in children and adolescents with chronic hepatitis B. Hepatology 1998;28:489A.

62. Jonas M, Kelly DA, Mizerski J, et al. Clinical trial of lamivudine in children with chronic hepatitis B. N Engl J Med 2002;346:1706–13.

63. Zoulin F, Trepo C. Drug therapy for chronic hepatitis B: antiviral efficacy and influence of hepatitis B virus polymerase mutations on the outcome of therapy. J Hepatol 1998;29:151–68.

64. Melegari M, Scaglioni PP, Wands JR. Hepatitis B virus mutants associated with 3TC and famciclovir administration are replication defective. Hepatology 1998;27:628–33.

65. Stuyver LJ, Locarnini SA, Lok A, et al. Nomenclature for antiviral-resistant human hepatitis B virus mutations in the polymerase region. Hepatology 2001;33:751–7.

66. Liaw YF, Chien RN, Yeh CT, et al. Acute exacerbation and hepatitis B virus clearance after emergence of YMDD motif mutation during lamivudine therapy. Hepatology 1999;30:567–72.

67. Ono-Nita SK, Kato N, Shiratori Y, et al. Susceptibility of lamivudine resistant hepatitis B virus to other reverse transcriptase inhibitors. J Clin Invest 1999;103:1635–40.

68. Perrillo R, Schiff E, Yoshida E, et al. Adefovir dipivoxil for the treatment of lamivudine-resistant hepatitis B mutants. Hepatology 2000;32:129–34.

69. Malik AH, Lee W. Chronic hepatitis B virus infection: treatment strategies for the next millennium. Ann Intern Med 2000;132:723–31.

70. Von Weizsacker F, Wieland S, Kock J, et al. Gene therapy for chronic viral hepatitis: ribozymes, antisense oligonucleotides, and dominant negative mutants. Hepatology 1997;26:251–5.

71. Putlitz JZ, Wieland S, Blum HE, Wands JR. Antisense RNA complimentary to hepatitis B virus specifically inhibits viral replication. Gastroenterology 1998;115:702–13.

72. Chien RN, Liaw YF, Chen TC, et al. Efficacy of thymosin α1 in patients with chronic hepatitis B: a randomized, controlled trial. Hepatology 1998;27:1383–7.

73. Rollier C, Sunyach C, Barraud L, et al. Protective and therapeutic effect of DNA-based immunization against hepadnavirus large envelope protein. Gastroenterology 1999;116:658–65.

74. Chow YH, Huang WL, Chi WK, et al. Improvement of hepatitis B virus DNA vaccines by plasmas coexpressing hepatitis B surface antigen and interleukin-2. J Virol 1997;71:169–78.

75. Schalm SW, Heathcote J, Cianciara J, et al. Lamivudine and α-interferon combnation therapy of patients with chronic hepatitis B infection: a randomized trial. Gut 2000;46:562–8.

76. Dikici B, Bosnak M, Bosnak V, et al. Comparison of treatments of chronic hepatitis B in children with lamivudine and α-interferon combination and with α-interferon alone. Pediatr Int 2002;44:517–21.

77. Selimoglu MA, Aydogdu S, Unal F, et al. Alpha-interferon and lamivudine combination therapy for chronic hepatitis B in children. Pediatr Int 2002;44:404–8.

78. Dikici B, Bosnak M, Bosnak V, et al. Combination therapy for children with chronic hepatitis B virus infection. J Gastroenterol Hepatol 2002;17:1087–91.

79. Kane MA. Global status of hepatitis B immunization. Lancet 1996;348:696.

80. Kane M. Hepatitis B control through immunization. In: Rizzetto M, Purcell RH, Gerin JL, Verme G, editors. Viral hepatitis and liver diseases. Turin: Edizioni Minerva Medica; 1997. p. 57–66.

1B. *Hepatitis C Virus*

Regino P. González-Peralta, MD

Christopher D. Jolley, MD

Although non-A, non-B hepatitis was recognized some 30 years ago,[1,2] its major causative agent was identified only in 1989 and was named hepatitis C virus (HCV).[3,4] Since the discovery of HCV, significant advances have been made in our understanding of the molecular virology and pathobiology of this important viral pathogen. In adults, the epidemiology and natural history of HCV infection are well defined, and approved efficient treatment strategies are available. In contrast, we know much less about the evolution and treatment of HCV infection in children. This part of the chapter summarizes our current understanding of the epidemiology, natural history, and treatment of HCV infection in this young population.

THE VIRUS

HCV is an enveloped, single-stranded, positive-sense ribonucleic acid (RNA) virus that is the major causative agent of non-A, non-B hepatitis. Besides humans, chimpanzees are the only other animals permissive to HCV infection. Based on nucleotide sequence analysis and genetic organization of the viral genome, HCV is classified as an independent genus (*Hepacivirus*) within the Flavivirus family.[5] The HCV genome is approximately 10,000 kb long with one open reading frame that encodes for a polyprotein containing approximately 3,000 amino acids (Figure 51.1B-1).[6,7] The recent detection of a previously unrecognized viral peptide putatively within the core region suggests the presence of a second open reading frame.[8] This new finding, which challenges the prevalent contemporary assertion that the HCV genome consists of only one reading frame, awaits further confirmation. The large viral polyprotein undergoes proteolysis by viral and host-encoded proteases, which results in the formation of the various HCV proteins. The proteolytic processing occurs as the nascent viral polyprotein is newly synthesized (cotranslation) and after it is completely formed (posttranslation). The HCV genome is organized so that its 5' end encodes for the structural proteins. including the core (or capsid) and envelope proteins (E1 and E2), whereas the nonstructural (NS) or functional viral proteins (NS2-NS5) are encoded by the larger subsequent 3' segment. There are two well-conserved noncoding areas (untranslated regions [UTRs]) flanking the HCV open reading frame that are critically important for the initiation of efficient viral protein synthesis (5'-UTR) and RNA replication (3'-UTR).

The core protein is a highly basic, hydrophobic, and relatively conserved protein that is intimately associated with the viral RNA and forms its "inner shell" or nucleocapsid. In addition to being the integral structural component of HCV, the core protein interacts with several cellular proteins, including apolipoprotein A-2, 60S ribosomal Sub U, hetero-

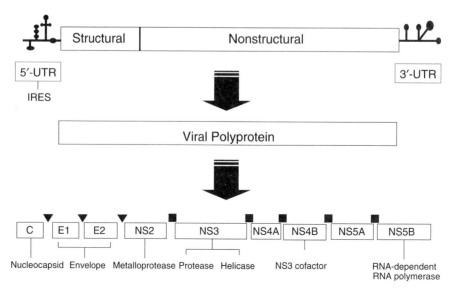

FIGURE 51.1B-1   Processing of hepatitis C virus polypeptide by host (▼) and viral (■) encoded proteases into the various viral proteins. IRES = internal ribosomal entry site; UTR = untranslated region.

geneous nuclear ribonuclear protein, tumor necrosis factor-α receptor, and lymphotoxin-β receptor. Although the precise pathogenetic mechanisms are largely unknown, these virus–host interactions suggest that the HCV core protein may play an important role in directly mediating liver cell damage. Indeed, the HCV core protein has been implicated in the development of hepatic steatosis and liver cancer in a transgenic mouse model.[9] The HCV E1 and E2 proteins are glycoproteins embedded within the viral lipid envelope and are integral constituents of the HCV "outer shell." In contrast to the core protein, the envelope proteins are very heterogeneous and display extensive nucleotide and antigenic variability. This antigenic diversity, greatest within a small area of the 5' end of the E2 gene (the hypervariable region), is believed to be an important mechanism by which HCV evades host immunologic surveillance, facilitating the establishment of chronic infection. The NS2 segment encodes for a metalloproteinase whose function is limited to specifically cleave the NS2-NS3 site. The 5' and 3' ends of the HCV NS3 encode for proteins with serine protease and helicase activities, respectively. The HCV serine protease is the major viral peptidase because it is required for the precise processing of a large segment of the viral polyprotein, including all cleavage sites within the NS3-NS5 segment. The NS3 serine protease interacts with an NS4-derived peptide (NS4 cofactor), which, although not essentially required, augments the proteolytic activity of the viral protease. The HCV helicase encoded by the 3' end of the NS3 segment is an enzyme that unwinds RNA-RNA duplexes formed during viral replication. Proteolytic hydrolysis of the NS4-encoded protein by viral serine protease yields two peptides, denoted NS4A and NS4B, respectively. In addition to enhancing the activity of the HCV NS3 serine protease activity, as mentioned above, the NS4A product appears to facilitate phosphorylation of the NS5A product. In a similar fashion, NS3-dependent protease cleavage of the NS5 gene results in the elaboration of two viral proteins, NS5A and NS5B. Increased nucleotide heterogeneity within the NS5A product is associated with lower serum HCV RNA levels and more favorable responses to interferon-based therapy,[10,11] suggesting that this protein may be involved in the transcriptional regulation of viral RNA. However, others have not found a link between NS5A mutations and a therapeutic response to antiviral agents[12,13]; the precise function of this gene product remains to be elucidated. The NS5B is an RNA-dependent RNA polymerase, the enzyme responsible for viral replication. The 5'-UTR is an internal ribosomal entry site (IRES) component through which HCV RNA binds to host cellular ribosomes, a necessary step for the initiation of viral protein synthesis. Finally, the 3'-UTR contains a highly conserved region of nucleotide known as the "X region," whose predicted stem-loop structure plays an important role in initiating viral RNA and in enhancing IRES-driven protein synthesis.

VIRAL HETEROGENEITY

The NS5B-encoded HCV RNA-dependent RNA polymerase lacks proofreading ability. As a result, like many other RNA viruses, HCV is genetically heterogeneous. Based on phylogenetic analysis of HCV sequences, six major HCV genotypes

are currently recognized, and there are multiple subtypes within each viral genotype.[5] Although HCV genotypes 1 and 2 are the most prevalent worldwide, there are unique geographic variations in the global distribution of viral genotypes. Accordingly, HCV genotype 3 is most common in Australia and the Indian subcontinent, and genotypes 4, 5, and 6 are almost exclusively seen in individuals from sub-Saharan Africa, South Africa, and Southeast Asia, respectively. In the United States, HCV genotypes 1, 2, and 3 account for approximately 70%, 15%, and 10% of adult infections, respectively.[14] More recently, some have proposed to divide HCV into six phylogenetically distinct groups called clades. In this new classification scheme, clades 1, 2, 4, and 5 correspond to genotypes 1, 2, 4, and 5; clade 3 comprises genotypes 3 and 10; and clade 6 includes genotypes 6, 7, 8, 9, and 11.[5] The relationship between viral genotypic diversity and clinical disease outcome is a controversial issue because some, but not all, studies correlate HCV genotype 1 infection with more aggressive liver disease and a higher risk for the development of hepatocellular carcinoma.[15] However, HCV genotype 1 is consistently associated with higher serum HCV RNA levels and a significantly poorer response to currently available antiviral regimens than HCV genotype 2 or 3. In fact, based on the results of recent clinical trials in adults, some authorities advocate a shorter duration of therapy for individuals with HCV genotype 2 or 3 than for those infected with HCV genotype 1.[16] Accordingly, determining the HCV genotype has become an essential component of the medical evaluation of infected adults, particularly those who are contemplating initiating antiviral therapy. Much less is known about the geographic distribution of HCV genotypes in children or its impact on the clinical evolution of liver disease in this population. Nevertheless, the viral genotypic distribution in children generally parallels that reported regionally in adults.[17–23] Furthermore, as in adults, HCV genotype 1 correlates with higher serum viral levels and a less favorable response to antiviral treatment.

The degree of genetic heterogeneity is such that even within persons infected with a unique viral genotype, HCV exists as a highly heterogeneous population of different but closely related genomes, which are called quasispecies.[24] HCV quasispecies play an important role in the pathobiology of HCV infection in adults as increased heterogeneity correlates with less favorable response rates to interferon given alone or in combination with ribavirin.[25–27] Assessment of HCV quasispecies by molecular evolutionary analysis has been instrumental in selected situations, such as in verifying the transmission of virus by accidental needle-stick exposures[28,29] or by infected mothers to their offspring (vertical transmission).[30,31] However, little is known about the clinical significance of HCV quasispecies in childhood infection; therefore, its assessment is not currently a component of the routine medical management of patients with HCV infection.

PATHOGENESIS OF LIVER DISEASE

In general, viral infections lead to cellular damage in vivo by either direct cytopathicity or immune-mediated injury, targeted against either viral or autoantigens. HCV may be directly cytopathic in situations that allow unusually high levels of viral replication and antigen expression, such as in immunosuppressed patients.[32,33] However, a significant amount of accumulating experimental evidence suggests that immune-mediated mechanisms play a more critical role in the controlling and mediating liver cell damage in chronic HCV infection in adults.[34,35] In contrast, our understanding of the pathogenesis of childhood HCV infection is very limited.[36] A Spanish study compared clinical, virologic, and immunohistochemical parameters between 12 children and 24 adults with chronic hepatitis C.[23] Although the HCV genotype distribution and estimated duration of infection were similar between these groups, children had statistically lower serum HCV RNA levels and more benign histologic disease than adults. More importantly, expression of all immunohistochemical markers studied, including CD2+, CD4+ (helper), and activated CD8+ (cytotoxic) lymphocytes; β_2-microglobulin; intercellular adhesion molecule 1; vascular cell adhesion molecule 1; platelet–endothelial cell adhesion molecule 1; and endoglin, were significantly lower in children than in adults. Although limited by the small number of children and adults analyzed, these data suggest that immunologic mechanisms are important in mediating liver cell damage in chronically infected children and that young patients may be more immunologically tolerant to HCV than similarly infected adults.

EPIDEMIOLOGY

The worldwide prevalence of HCV infection is approximately 3%, which represents an estimated 170 million infected persons.[37] Wasley and Alter described several patterns of geographic and temporal variation in the global prevalence of HCV.[37] In the pattern seen in the United States and Australia, individuals younger than 20 years have the lowest prevalence rates, whereas those between the ages of 30 and 49 years have the highest, suggesting that HCV infection is primarily acquired in early adulthood.

Variations in global prevalence rates are observed in children as well and may reflect differences in socioeconomic status. Studies of general pediatric populations have yielded seroprevalence rates as low as 0% (Egypt, Japan, United States) and as high as 14.5% (Cameroon).[38–40] In the United States, the estimated seroprevalence is 0.2% for those children less than 12 years of age and 0.4% among those 12 to 19 years of age.[41] Based on current population statistics, this prevalence rate indicates that there are about 150,000 to 200,000 children who are infected with HCV in the United States.

The prevalence of HCV in the general population of the United States is 1.8% based on serologic analysis from approximately 21,000 subjects in the Third National Health and Nutrition Examination Survey (NHANES III) data, collected between 1988 and 1994.[42] This prevalence rate corresponds to approximately 3.9 million persons nationwide being positive for anti-HCV. It should be noted that children younger than 6 years of age were not represented in this large cohort. The prevalence of viremia as measured by detectable serum HCV RNA among anti-HCV–positive subjects was 73.9%; therefore, an estimated 2.7 million people nationwide are chronically infected with HCV. The factors most strongly associated with HCV infection in persons 17 to 59 years old were illicit drug abuse and practicing high-risk sexual behavior. Age at first sexual encounter was also an important epidemiologic factor because persons who had a first sexual intercourse before the age of 18 years had significantly higher rates of HCV infection than those whose initial sex activity occurred at a later age. Subjects reporting greater use of marijuana had a higher prevalence of HCV infection than those who did not. Because there is no apparent reason to explain the association between increased transmission of HCV and marijuana use, it is presumed that larger amounts of marijuana use serve as a surrogate for other high-risk behaviors such as injection drug abuse or high-risk sexual practices.

Although the seroprevalence among incarcerated adults is as high as 82%,[43] this population was not included in the NHANES III analysis. The prevalence of anti-HCV positivity in incarcerated juveniles in the United States (2%) is significantly higher than that observed in the general adolescent population.[44] High-risk behaviors, which correlated with HCV infection in this confined population, included being sexually active and a history of body piercing. Interestingly, only 6% of the juveniles studied acknowledged injection drug abuse, a well-defined parenteral risk associated with the acquisition of HCV. However, this information was collected by voluntary self-reporting in this study and therefore likely underestimates the prevalence of this illicit practice. Of note, the HCV seroprevalence rate of 2% among incarcerated juveniles in this report is lower than that observed in other studies of homeless or confined young persons, which included a higher proportion of injection drug abusers.[45–47]

Saiman and colleagues retrospectively studied a cohort of 504 internationally adopted children from China, Russia, Southeast Asia, Eastern Europe, and Latin America.[48] Only four children, or 0.8% of the 496 tested, were anti-HCV positive, and none were positive for HCV RNA, compared with 2.8% who tested positive for hepatitis B surface antigen. A study of 169 Romanian orphans found that 36% were positive for hepatitis B surface antigen, whereas only 1 child was anti-HCV positive.[49] Therefore, the seroprevalence of HCV in international adoptees appears to be quite low.

Children who received transfusions of potentially contaminated blood products prior to the institution of routine screening have seroprevalence rates that vary depending on their degree of exposure. Seroprevalence rates of 50 to 95% have been reported in those receiving multiple transfusions or transfusions from pooled plasma, such as factor concentrates.[50–52] Children with fewer but repeated exposures, including those undergoing hemodialysis and cancer survivors, have intermediate seroprevalence rates of 18 to 52%.[53–55]

Since the initiation of routine blood screening in 1992, perinatal transmission has become the predominant source of new HCV infections (see "Natural History"); the seroprevalence of HCV in pregnant women is 1 to 2%.[56,57]

Household nonsexual contacts of infected individuals have a seroprevalence rate of 7%, although this appears to increase with longer duration of exposure to the index patient.[58]

CLINICAL ASPECTS

The mean incubation period of post-transfusion acute HCV infection is 7 to 8 weeks, with a range of 2 to 26 weeks.[59] The majority of acute HCV infections appear within 5 to 12 weeks following transfusion. Acute HCV is usually anicteric or subclinical, and only one-third of patients will develop jaundice or symptoms.[60] Fulminant hepatic failure owing to HCV is exceedingly rare. In adults, 85% of patients exposed to HCV will develop chronic infection, of whom approximately 10 to 20% develop cirrhosis and 1% develops liver cancer. Although the precise mechanisms are unknown, it is now clear that concurrent alcohol ingestion and immunodeficiency accelerate the rate of HCV-related liver disease and thus have a negative impact on its outcome.

In children, the course of HCV infection is generally benign. Most children with acute hepatitis C are asymptomatic and go unnoticed. When symptoms are present, they are often nonspecific (malaise, anorexia) or mild. Jaundice may be evident in only 25% of patients.[41] Children with chronic HCV infection may also remain asymptomatic. Progression to decompensated liver disease (variceal bleeding, ascites) in children can occur, but this is the exception. As in adults, children with immunodeficiency may progress to serious liver disease more rapidly.[61,62]

Biochemical markers such as serum alanine aminotransferase (ALT) typically fluctuate in HCV patients. Normal or only minimally increased ALT levels are usually reported with chronic HCV infection, and serum ALT levels can remain elevated despite anti-HCV seronegativity.[63,64] The histopathologic features of chronic hepatitis C in children are similar to those found in adults.[65–67] Histologic characteristics include portal lymphoid aggregates, bile duct injury, and prominent steatosis. Necroinflammatory activity is commonly mild. Varying degrees of fibrosis and, less commonly, cirrhosis have also been described.

NATURAL HISTORY

The clinical evolution of HCV infection in adults is well defined, but much less is known about the natural history of the disease in children. As in adults, the course of infection in children with parenteral or perinatally acquired HCV may be influenced by host factors such as immunologic status, underlying disease, or the deleterious effects of transfusion-related iron overload on the liver, which further hinders the ability to precisely determine the evolution of this viral infection.

Despite these potential shortcomings, several studies have delineated the clinical impact and evolution of childhood parenteral and perinatal HCV infection (Table 51.1B-1).[68–74] In an early analysis, Chang and colleagues prospectively studied 88 children at risk for HCV infection because of either periodic blood transfusion for hemolytic anemia (33 children), transfusion for cardiac surgery (38 children), or maternal chronic HCV infection (17 infants).[63] Of these, 10 children contracted HCV infection, including 5 with hemolytic anemia, 2 after cardiac surgery, and 3 with HCV-infected mothers. Five children, including the three perinatally infected infants, had detectable HCV RNA and anti-HCV antibodies in serum without symptoms of acute hepatitis. Two of the five patients who developed acute hepatitis exhibited jaundice and malaise. Sixty percent of the 10 children developed chronic infection, and half of these maintained normal ALT during the 3-year follow-up period. As suggested by the authors, these data demonstrate that host factors such as iron overload may play a significant role in the evolution of childhood hepatitis C. This report also shows that HCV seroconversion is a clinically silent process in many exposed children.

In one of the largest natural history reports published to date, Jara and colleagues retrospectively investigated 224 children who were HCV RNA positive.[75] None of the children studied had underlying disease such as malignancy or hemophilia, and the diagnosis of chronic hepatitis was defined by persistently abnormal ALT for more that 6 months or by histologic assessment of liver tissue. Of the 224 children, 45% had an HCV-infected mother and 39% had received transfusion of blood products. At study entry,

TABLE 51.1B-1 SELECTED STUDIES OF THE NATURAL HISTORY OF HCV INFECTION IN CHILDREN

STUDY	NUMBER STUDIED*	TRANSMISSION ROUTE	MEAN FOLLOW-UP PERIOD (RANGE; YR)	CLINICALLY SILENT (%)	PROGRESSIVE HISTOLOGIC DISEASE†	HCV RNA POSITIVE AT END OF FOLLOW-UP (%)
Palomba et al[68]	7	Perinatal	5.4 (2.2–7.5)	100	0/5‡	100
Bortolotti et al[69]	30	Perinatal	1.8 (1–4)	100	0/7	80
Tovo et al[70]	104	Perinatal	4.1 (0.5–12.8)	98	3/20	94
Ni et al[71]	8	Parenteral	NR	100	NR	88
Matsuoka et al[72]	29	Parenteral	7.1 (4–13)	100	1/19	45
Vogt et al[73]	67	Parenteral	17 (12–27)	NR	3/17	55
Sasaki et al[74]	11	Perinatal	3.2 (1.4–5.0)	100	NR	64
	14	Parenteral	4.0 (2.6–6.1)	100	NR	100

HCV = hepatitis C virus; NR = not reported; RNA = ribonucleic acid.
*Number of HCV infected patients included.
†Number with severe hepatitis, fibrosis, or cirrhosis of those who underwent histologic assessment.
‡Complicated by congestive heart disease or hepatitis B virus infection in all cases.

all of the perinatally infected children were asymptomatic, and none of the children exhibited jaundice. Hepatomegaly was a presenting feature in only 15%. The course of infection was studied in 200 of the original 224 children for a period of 1 to 17.5 years (mean 6.2 years). During this time, serum ALT levels normalized and HCV RNA became undetectable in 12 (6%) patients, including 17% of those with perinatal infection. Most children with chronic hepatitis had mild histologic disease, and only one patient, a transfusion recipient, developed cirrhosis and subsequent liver failure in this study. However, older adolescents had greater degrees of hepatic fibrosis than younger children, suggesting that gradual progression of histologic liver disease occurs in young patients.

In general, then, most children exposed to HCV become chronically infected based on persistently detectable serum anti-HCV antibodies and HCV RNA. Acute and chronic hepatitis C in children is usually subclinical, characterized by fluctuating serum ALT and mild histologic abnormalities. However, significant liver disease, including cirrhosis, can occur.

PARENTERAL TRANSMISSION

Liver disease in children with concurrent systemic illness may be related to factors other than HCV infection, and these patients are discussed separately.[76]

Hemophilia. HCV infection is noted in 50 to 98% of children with hemophilia treated with factor concentrates prepared from suboptimally decontaminated pooled plasma.[77-81] The high prevalence rate is particularly important because HCV infection strongly correlates with liver dysfunction in this population.[77,79] In a study from Japan, anti-HCV antibodies were found in 32 of 45 children (80%) with hemophilia who were followed for 1 to 4 years. Twenty-seven of these 32 HCV-seropositive patients were assayed for HCV RNA by polymerase chain reaction. Liver disease was observed in 18 of 22 patients (82%) with detectable HCV RNA but in none of 5 children without this viral marker.[78] In another investigation, HCV infection was demonstrated in nearly 40% of patients with hemophilia with abnormal liver tests, whereas serologic viral markers were found in only 17% of those with normal liver biochemistry.[80] Percutaneous liver biopsies are not usually done in children with hemophilia owing to the potential risk for bleeding. As a result, little is known about the histologic progression of HCV in this group. However, a recent report demonstrated that this procedure can be safely accomplished with appropriate factor replacement therapy.[81] More importantly, mild histologic abnormalities were noted in most of the children with hemophilia analyzed in this report. These data suggest that HCV is associated with liver disease and that clinical and histologic abnormalities are mild in most infected children with hemophilia. In contrast, HCV infection is associated with the development of liver cancer in adults with hemophilia,[82,83] suggesting that earlier viral eradication during childhood may result in reduced HCV-related morbidity later in life.

Thalassemia. Serologic markers of HCV infection are noted in up to 80% of multitransfused children with thalassemia.[84-89] In one prospective 8-year study, 75 of 135 newly diagnosed patients acquired HCV infection, which became chronic in nearly 80% of them, based on persistently elevated transaminase levels. In another prospective study, HCV-infected children were found to have significantly higher levels of transaminases than those without detectable markers of viral infection.[88] The severity of liver disease was not related to HCV genotypes or to HCV RNA levels. Furthermore, hepatic fibrosis was more commonly noted in patients with HCV infection than in uninfected children. To better delineate the rate of liver fibrosis progression, 211 children who had received bone marrow replacement for the treatment of thalassemia underwent serial histologic assessment of the liver by percutaneous biopsy.[90] Of these, 46 (22%) had evidence of fibrosis progression during a median follow-up of 64 months. Using multivariate analysis, hepatic iron overload and HCV infection were noted to be independent risk factors for the progression of liver fibrosis, and their concomitant presence resulted in a striking increase in this risk.

Cancer Survivors. HCV infection has been demonstrated in up to 50% of pediatric cancer survivors and is an important cause of liver disease in this population.[91-94] As a result of an impaired humoral immune response, anti-HCV antibodies are often not detected, despite the presence of HCV RNA in these patients.[91] Thus, the diagnosis of HCV in this population should rely on the detection of HCV RNA by nucleic amplification tests such as polymerase chain reaction or transcription-mediated assays. The clinical impact of HCV infection has been difficult to determine in this group of patients, in whom the pathogenesis of liver disease is likely related to multiple factors. Although elevations of aminotransferase levels are commonly noted during the course of cancer treatment, the biochemical profile and clinical outcomes are similar for children with and without HCV infection.[94,95] These initial retrospective observations, which are limited by the small number of patients included in these reports and relatively brief observation periods, have been verified in large prospective studies. In an Italian study of 114 leukemia survivors, 56 had detectable HCV RNA in serum at the end of chemotherapy, of which 40 had persistent viremia after a mean follow-up of 17 years.[94] At the completion of chemotherapy, a significantly higher proportion of HCV RNA–positive children had elevated serum aminotransferase levels than those without detectable virus. Most patients who underwent liver biopsy at this point had mild histologic abnormalities and the severity of liver disease was similar between HCV RNA–positive and –negative children. During follow-up, all HCV-infected children remained clinically stable, and none developed evidence of decompensated liver disease. Liver tests remained normal in approximately 71% of patients with detectable HCV RNA in serum, whereas 25% and 4% had fluctuating and persistently abnormal levels of serum aminotransferase, respectively. In a preliminary report from a similar ongoing trial, 77 of 1,175 cancer survivors tested had detectable HCV antibodies.[96] Persistent viral infection, defined by the presence of circulating HCV RNA, was verified in 65 of those with serologic evidence of HCV, most of whom were clinically asymptomatic and had normal liver tests. Although histologic abnormalities were common among the 35 patients who underwent liver biopsy in this report, the degree of disease was mild in most patients at a mean of 6 years after diagnosis of cancer. Of note, three patients had histologic evidence of cirrhosis, and two patients died of complications of HCV-related hepatocellular carcinoma. The two reported cases of hepatocellular carcinoma were leukemia survivors who were transfused prior to routine blood screening.[97] Both patients presented 25 years after their last blood transfusion and were approximately 28 to 30 years old on diagnosis of liver cancer. One of the patients with hepatocellular carcinoma also had chronic HBV infection, another well-known risk factor for this disease. We have also cared for one cancer-surviving adolescent with HCV-related cirrhosis who died of complications of liver cancer, which was discovered while she was being evaluated for liver transplant (R. González-Peralta, personal observation, 1994).

Hemodialysis and Renal Disease. Similar to prevalence rates in adults, anti-HCV antibodies have been detected in 20 to 45% of pediatric patients undergoing hemodialysis but in only 0 to 4% of those on peritoneal dialysis.[98–102] The lower prevalence rate in patients on peritoneal dialysis is likely the result of less exposure to blood products in this group. Most HCV antibody–reactive children develop chronic infection based on persistent detection of viral RNA in serum. More importantly, the majority of children on hemodialysis have persistently normal aminotransferase levels. However, systematic assessment of hepatic histology, a more reliable indicator of liver disease than aminotransferase levels in chronic HCV infection, has not been reported in these children.

PERINATAL TRANSMISSION

Since the implementation of routine and effective screening strategies, perinatal or vertical transmission has become the primary cause of new HCV infections in children.[103] Perinatal transmission of HCV, suspected even before the virus was discovered,[104,105] has been subsequently confirmed in numerous studies by the detection of HCV RNA in infants born to infected mothers.[106–115] The average rate of vertical transmission is approximately 5 to 6%, which is low compared with those observed for hepatitis B virus and human immunodeficiency virus (HIV). The precise timing and process by which the virus is transmitted from mother to infant are unknown, but high-titer maternal viremia consistently correlates with higher transmission rates and thus appears to facilitate the process. Although the rates of vertical transmission are generally higher in infants born to mothers coinfected with HIV (0–36%; mean 16%),[116–120] other researchers have not documented this correlation.[106,114] Similarly, there are conflicting reports on the influence of mode of delivery on the risk of perinatal trans-

mission of HCV, with increased rates after vaginal delivery noted in some[107,108,115] but not all[112,114] studies. In one report, exposure to contaminated maternal blood and placement of fetal scalp probes during delivery were associated with increased risk for perinatal HCV infection.[121] Interestingly, a recent report noted that human leukocyte antigen DR13–positive infants born to mothers with HCV were less likely to become infected than those who did not express this marker, implying that immunologic mechanisms may play an important role in the transmission of HCV from mother to infant.[122] Of note, there appears to be no increased risk of HCV transmission by breast milk because the rate of viral infection transmission is similar between breast- and formula-fed infants.[110–112,114,115]

LIVER TRANSPLANT

HCV-related chronic liver disease is a leading indication for liver transplant in adults.[123] However, little is known about the risks, significance, and evolution of HCV infection in children undergoing liver transplant. In a cross-sectional study, the overall prevalence of HCV was found to be 6.5% among 65 children who underwent liver transplant by detection of HCV RNA.[124] All HCV-positive children had undergone liver replacement before the initiation of routine screening for HCV in blood donors. In this cohort, serum transaminase levels were significantly higher in young patients with HCV infection than they were in uninfected children. Recurrent HCV infection is nearly universal after liver transplant, but infection arising de novo is now rare because of improved donor screening.[125] The course of HCV-related liver disease appears to be particularly aggressive in children with de novo infection following liver transplant.[126] In this series, viral infection was verified in 14 of 117 patients who underwent liver replacement before the availability of reliable screening tests for HCV. Nearly all of the children with HCV infection had evidence of histologic progression, varying from nonspecific inflammation to cirrhosis. The overall mortality rate in this group of patients was high (23%), despite intense therapeutic interventions including antiviral treatment and, in a few cases, retransplant.

DIAGNOSIS

The diagnosis of HCV infection is based on detection of antibodies directed against recombinant HCV antigens by enzyme immunoassay (EIA) or recombinant immunoblot assay (RIBA) or by detection of HCV RNA using nucleic acid tests (NATs).

SEROLOGIC TESTS

Initial, first-generation EIAs were licensed by the US Food and Drug Administration (FDA) in 1990 and detected immunoreactivity against a single viral polypeptide (Figure 51.1B-2).[127] Although the assay provided the first reliable means to easily detect HCV infection, it was limited by occasional false-negative[128] and frequent false-positive results, particularly in patients with elevated globulin levels such as those with autoimmune hepatitis.[129,130] Subsequent

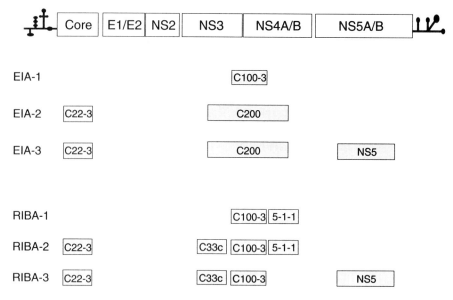

FIGURE 51.1B-2   Hepatitis C virus antigens used in different enzyme immunoassay (EIA) tests. RIBA = recombinant immunoblot assay.

incorporation of additional HCV antigens in second-generation EIAs significantly enhanced the accuracy of the assays (Table 51.1B-2).[131,132] As a result, these more reliable tests were approved by the FDA in 1992 and quickly replaced earlier test versions for the routine detection of anti-HCV antibodies in clinical and laboratory practice. In 1997, the FDA approved a third-generation EIA containing an additional NS5 antigen and reconfigured HCV core and NS3 antigens.[133] However, these modifications did not significantly improve sensitivity and specificity over earlier versions of EIA, and both second- and third-generation assays are currently used. In general, EIAs are easy to perform, yield reproducible results, and are relatively inexpensive, which makes them excellent tools in the initial diagnostic evaluation of and screening for HCV infection. Therefore, the detection of anti-HCV antibodies by these methods in persons with evidence of liver disease and a parenteral risk factor for the virus is probably sufficient to establish the diagnosis of active viral infection. However, the Centers for Disease Control and Prevention advises that anti-HCV EIA–reactive samples be verified by supplemental testing to more precisely identify those harboring HCV.[134]

Like the Western blot test for the detection of HIV antibodies, RIBA detects HCV immunoglobulin (Ig)G antibodies against synthetic HCV recombinant antigens and synthetic peptides immobilized on a solid matrix (nitrocellulose strip) (see Figure 51.1B-2). As in the case of EIAs, more reliable second- and third-generation RIBAs have replaced earlier forms of the test.[135] RIBAs are less sensitive but more specific than EIAs in detecting anti-HCV antibodies. Therefore, RIBAs are not recommended for initial HCV screening and are particularly suited to confirm viral infection.[134]

In addition to IgG anti-HCV antibodies, IgM anti-HCV antibodies are also detected during viral infection. Although the presence of IgM antibodies by EIA correlates well with active viral infection,[136] these are detected in a relatively small proportion of HCV-infected persons. As a result, tests that rely on the detection of IgM anti-HCV antibodies offer little advantage to currently available assays and are not currently used for the diagnosis or clinical management of HCV.

NUCLEIC ACID TESTS

NATs are assays that directly detect circulating virus. There are two NATs currently used for the detection of HCV that rely on different amplification schemes, namely target and signal amplification. In the target amplification process, extracted HCV RNA is transcribed to deoxyribonucleic acid (DNA), which is then directly amplified (polymerase chain reaction) or is converted to RNA during amplifica-

TABLE 51.1B-2   SENSITIVITY AND PREDICTED VALUE OF SEROLOGIC TESTS FOR HCV INFECTION

| ASSAY | SENSITIVITY (%) | POSITIVE PREDICTIVE VALUE (%) | | TIME TO POSITIVE AFTER INFECTION (WK) |
		LOW-PREVALENCE GROUPS	HIGH-PREVALENCE GROUPS	
EIA-1	70–80	30–50	70–85	16
EIA-2	92–95	50–60	88–95	10
EIA-3	97	25	98	7–8

Adapted with permission from Davis GL. Hepatitis C. In: Schiff ER, Sorrell MF, Maddrey WC, editors. Schiff's diseases of the liver. Vol. 1, 9th ed. Philadelphia: Lippincott, Williams and Wilkins; 2003. p. 819.
EIA = enzyme immunoassay; HCV = hepatitis C virus.

tion (transcription-mediated assay). Both quantitative and qualitative (generally more sensitive) versions of target amplification tests are available. By contrast, for signal amplification (branched DNA assay, Bayer Diagnostics, Tarrytown, NJ), extracted HCV RNA is captured by specific oligonucleotides fixed on a solid matrix (Microwell). After incubation with amplifying enzyme–labeled probes and specific substrate, viral levels are determined by comparing the chemiluminescence of test samples to those of controls with known HCV RNA concentrations.

Technical advancements in recent years, in particular the development of automated equipment capable of rapidly and accurately analyzing a large number of samples in a standardized format, have led to widespread use of NATs for the routine laboratory evaluation of HCV in clinical practice. Equally important, the results obtained by different commercial NATs are now normalized against a well-characterized HCV RNA standard developed by the World Health Organization.[137,138] Because these assays were initially developed using different HCV standards, conversion factors are necessary to compare the concentration of HCV RNA copies obtained by the various methods (Table 51.1B-3). One of the major advantages of NATs is their ability to provide direct assessment for the presence of circulating virus, which is only indirectly inferred with serologic assays. Therefore, positive HCV NAT results more precisely reflect active viremia than do antibody-based tests. In addition, exceedingly low levels of circulating virus are detected with currently available NATs, with a detection limit in the range of 30 to 50 IU/mL (see Table 51.1B-3).[139] As a result, NATs markedly reduce the time during which HCV infection can be detected.[140] The ability to recognize HCV infection at the earliest possible phase is particularly important in the clinical practice of transfusion medicine, where the use of NATs has led to reductions in the incidence of post-transfusion hepatitis.[141] Like RIBAs, NATs are also used to confirm HCV infection in anti-HCV EIA–reactive individuals in low-prevalence groups. To minimize the possibility of HCV RNA degradation and thereby avert false-negative results, only serum separated within 4 to 8 hours of venesection and those samples that have not undergone repeated cycles of freeze-thaw should be used for NAT.[134,142]

Nuclear amplification tests are particularly useful in certain clinical scenarios. First, because NATs identify the presence of HCV very early in the course of infection, they can be used to diagnose HCV even before the anti-HCV antibodies have appeared.[139] Therefore, NATs are recommended in HCV EIA–negative patients in whom clinical suspicion for HCV exists. Second, NATs are necessary to detect HCV in infants born to infected mothers, in whom HCV antibodies may be of maternal origin and in immunocompromised patients whose ability to produce HCV antibodies may be impaired. Finally, by identifying persons with active viremia, NATs are critically important to select appropriate candidates for, and monitor the response to, antiviral treatment.

MANAGEMENT

SCREENING FOR HCV INFECTION

HCV testing should be considered for children with risk factors for HCV infection, including recipients of blood product transfusions and organ transplants before the implementation of effective routine donor screening strategies (1992) or of clotting factor concentrates before the widespread use of reliable sterilizing techniques (1987), infants born to HCV-infected mothers, and those with a history of injection drug use. Routine screening of internationally adopted children for HCV is generally not recommended unless the biologic mother has a known high-risk factor, such as injection drug use.[143]

GENERAL CARE GUIDELINES

Periodic examination of children with chronic HCV infection is recommended, although there is a lack of consensus about which tests to monitor and how often to check them.[143] In our center, infants, children, and adolescents who are newly diagnosed with HCV undergo thorough medical evaluation to determine the risk factor(s) for infection and detect the presence of liver disease or associated sequelae. This is accomplished by a detailed history and physical examination and comprehensive laboratory evaluation, including complete blood count, liver tests, and coagulation studies. In our practice, any abnormal result promptly triggers further serologic evaluation aimed at excluding other potential concomitant causes of liver

TABLE 51.1B-3   CHARACTERISTICS OF QUANTITATION TESTS FOR HCV

ASSAY	MANUFACTURER	FORMAT	DYNAMIC RANGE (IU/ML)	CONVERSION FACTOR*
Amplicor HCV Monitor V2.0	Roche Molecular Systems (Pleasanton, CA, USA)	Manual RT-PCR	600–500,000	0.9
COBAS Amplicor HCV Monitor V2.0	Roche Molecular Systems	Semiautomated RT-PCR	600–500,000	2.7
LCx HCV RNA	Abbott Diagnostics (Abbott Park, IL, USA)	Semiautomated RT-PCR	25–2,630,000	3.8
SuperQuant	National Genetics Institute (Los Angeles, CA, USA)	Semiautomated RT-PCR	30–1,470,000	3.4
Versant HCV RNA 2.0	Bayer Corporation (Tarrytown, NY, USA)	Manual branched DNA	—	None
Versant HCV RNA 3.0	Bayer Corporation	Semiautomated branched DNA	615–7,700,000	5.2

Adapted from Pawlotsky JM.[139]

DNA = deoxyribonucleic acid; HCV = hepatitis C virus; RNA = ribonucleic acid; RT-PCR = reverse transcriptase polymerase chain reaction.

*HCV RNA IU/mL multiplied by conversion factor = HCV copies/mL.

disease, including other viral hepatitides, autoimmune hepatitis, α_1-antitrypsin deficiency, Wilson disease, and hemochromatosis, as clinically appropriate. Although an arguable practice, histologic assessment of the liver by percutaneous tissue sampling may be valuable in excluding comorbid diseases and determining the severity of liver damage, particularly in those in whom antiviral treatment is being entertained.

Because patients and their families are frequently ill-informed about HCV at the time of diagnosis, an equally critical component of the management of children with HCV is to provide basic concepts about the virus, including ways to prevent its spread and the implications of infection as they specifically relate to potential clinical outcomes and antiviral treatment. Adolescents, in particular, need to clearly understand the negative impact of alcohol on the course of HCV infection (accelerates progression)[144] and should be counseled to abstain from its consumption. The importance of avoiding high-risk behavior such as sharing of intravenous needles needs to be openly discussed and appropriate psychosocial assistance offered to those actively engaged in such practices. The American Academy of Pediatrics also discourages sharing of personal items such as toothbrushes or razors, which may be contaminated. Exclusion of HCV-infected children from child care centers is not justified.[143] Finally, successful completion of hepatitis B virus vaccination should be objectively ascertained and hepatitis A virus immunization should be offered as necessary.

ANTIVIRAL THERAPY

In an ideal world, the selection of individuals for antiviral therapy would strictly depend on a well-defined propensity to develop severe, chronic liver disease. In such an ideal approach, patients whose liver disease would be more likely to progress would be treated, whereas those expected to have a benign course would be spared treatment and would thereby avert potential treatment-related adverse effects. Unfortunately, the natural history of hepatitis C is incompletely understood, especially in children in whom precise rates of spontaneous viral remission are not reliably known.[103] Accordingly, determining if and when to treat a child or adolescent for chronic hepatitis C is, at the moment, a challenging and controversial task. Nevertheless, compelling reasons exist to consider treating this unique young population with chronic hepatitis C. First, a significant proportion of children exposed to HCV, particularly infants born to infected mothers, develop chronic infection (see Table 51.1B-1). Second, although chronic hepatitis C is usually a mild disease in children with few, if any, symptoms, significant liver damage, including severe hepatitis, cirrhosis, and liver cancer, can occur, as already noted. Finally, factors associated with a favorable response to antiviral therapy in adults, such as short duration of infection, young age, mild histologic inflammation, and absence of cirrhosis, are commonly noted in children with HCV infection. On a theoretical basis, then, a greater global reduction in HCV-related morbidity and mortality may be attainable by treating children (in whom HCV may be easier to eradicate) than adults.

Interferons are a group of naturally occurring agents with antiviral, antineoplastic, and immunomodulatory properties. Multiple large prospective randomized trials confirm that recombinant interferon therapy results in normalization of aminotransferase levels and reductions in serum HCV RNA below detectable levels in approximately 40 to 50% of adults by the end of treatment. Unfortunately, most of these patients relapse, as manifested by elevations of serum aminotransferases and reappearance of serum HCV RNA within 6 months after discontinuation of therapy. Therefore, sustained virologic responses are achieved in only 8 to 35% of adults given interferons alone.[145] Attempts to improve treatment efficacy by using higher interferon doses and prolonging duration of therapy lead to only marginal improvements in virologic responses at the expense of higher rates of side effects. However, significantly higher sustained virologic responses are attained (30–40%) by combining interferons with ribavirin, a guanosine analog. Longer-acting pegylated interferons have been subsequently developed based on the premise that more sustained drug levels would result in greater antiviral activity. Indeed, several randomized clinical trials in adults verify considerably better virologic responses (50–60%) with the use of pegylated interferons, particularly when given in conjunction with ribavirin.[146,147]

Multiple studies have evaluated the efficacy and safety of interferon alone for the treatment of childhood hepatitis C, as comprehensively reviewed.[148] The use of multiple treatment regimens in mostly small and uncontrolled clinical trials in children makes direct comparisons with adult data difficult. However, in general, sustained virologic response rates in children treated with interferon alone (30–60%) appear to be two- to threefold higher than in similarly treated adults.[148] Importantly, biochemical and virologic responses have been accompanied by significant histologic improvement in all treated patients included in these trials, and interferon has been well tolerated in children.

Based on the observed synergy between interferons and ribavirin in adults with chronic hepatitis C, the efficacy and safety of this combination treatment in children have been assessed in several clinical trials. In an initial dose-finding study, sustained virologic response rates were noted in 33%, 35%, and 45% of children treated with interferon and ribavirin 8, 12, or 15 mg/kg/d, respectively.[149] There were no significant differences in the rate of adverse events between the treatment groups. Because a greater sustained virologic response is achieved with the highest dose while maintaining a safety profile similar to that of the lower ribavirin regimens, ribavirin 15 mg/kg/d has become the standard dose for treating children with chronic hepatitis C. Two subsequent pilot studies of childhood cancer survivors with transfusion-acquired HCV given standard interferon and ribavirin doses further verified these initial results because 50% and 64% of treated children had a sustained response, respectively.[150,151] These preliminary results were further confirmed in two subsequent larger studies, which together included a total of 110 chronically infected European and North American children and adolescents.[152,153] In a study from Germany, 25 of 40 children (62%) had a sustained response,[152] whereas this was accomplished in 34 of 70 (49%) of young persons in the other trial.[153] As in adults, several important factors are associated with a favorable therapeutic response to interferon therapy given alone or in combination with ribavirin, including infection with an HCV genotype other than type 1, low pretreatment serum HCV RNA levels, younger age, and absence of cirrhosis.[148-153]

Adverse events such as fever, headache, and influenza-like symptoms, ascribed to interferons, are common during the first two to three treatments and generally improve or resolve afterward.[148-153] These frequent side effects may be minimized by administering interferon in the evenings and prescribing routine acetaminophen or nonsteroidal anti-inflammatory agents during the initial weeks of therapy. Hematologic abnormalities are common with antiviral therapy. Ribavirin-induced anemia occurs in nearly all treated patients within 4 to 8 weeks of initiating treatment and then stabilizes, in association with a reactive reticulocytosis. Concomitantly with a reduction in hemoglobin, mild elevations in serum bilirubin and uric acid levels rarely occur. In a similar fashion, neutropenia is consistently seen with antiviral therapy, but this is not associated with clinically significant infections. Mild thrombocytopenia occurs infrequently. Persistent complications include anorexia, weight loss, and depression. It is important to point out that ribavirin is clearly associated with the development of fetal malformations in many animal species tested. Therefore, it is critical that women of childbearing years avoid pregnancy by effective contraception techniques during ribavirin therapy and for up to 6 months after its discontinuation. Finally, there are reported cases of spastic diplegia and seizures occurring in young infants given interferon for treatment of cutaneous vascular anomalies.[154] Although these infants generally received higher doses of interferon than those proposed for chronic hepatitis C, this medication should probably not be used in the very young patient for the treatment of HCV infection.

Because pegylated interferon–based regimens are better than those that rely on conventional interferon in adults, clinical trials are currently under way to assess the efficacy and safety of pegylated interferon in combination with ribavirin in children with chronic hepatitis C. With the development of novel antiviral agents such as HCV protease, helicase, and polymerase inhibitors and efficient immunomodulatory strategies, the future for the eradication of HCV is promising.

REFERENCES

1. Feinstone SM, Kapikian AZ, Purcell RH, et al. Transfusion associated hepatitis not due to viral hepatitis type A or B. N Engl J Med 1975;292:767–70.
2. Dienstag JL, Feinstone SM, Purcell RH, et al. Non-A, non-B post-transfusion hepatitis. Lancet 1977;i:560–62.
3. Choo QL, Weiner AJ, Overby LR, et al. Hepatitis C virus: the major causative agent of viral non-A, non-B hepatitis. Br Med Bull 1990;46:423–41.
4. Choo QL, Kuo G, Weiner AJ, et al. Isolation of a cDNA clone derived from a blood-borne non-A, non-B viral hepatitis genome. Science 1989;244:359–61.
5. Robertson B, Myers G, Howard C, et al. Classification, nomenclature, and database development for hepatitis C virus (HCV) and related viruses: proposals for standardization. Arch Virol 1998;143:2493–503.
6. Thomson M, Liang TJ. Molecular biology of hepatitis C virus. In: Liang TJ, Hoofnagle JH, editors. Hepatitis C. San Diego (CA): Academic Press; 2000. p. 1–23.
7. Smith RM, Wu GY. Molecular virology of hepatitis B and C. In: Koff RS, Wu GY, editors. Chronic viral hepatitis: diagnosis and therapeutics. Totowa (NJ): Humana Press; 2002. p. 1–24.
8. Walewski JL, Keller TR, Stump DD, Branch AD. Evidence for a new hepatitis C virus antigen encoded in an overlapping reading frame. RNA 2001;7:710–21.
9. Moriya K, Fujie H, Shintani Y, et al. The core protein of hepatitis C virus induces hepatocellular carcinoma in transgenic mice. Nat Med 1998;4:1065–7.
10. Kurosaki M, Enomoto N, Murakami T, et al. Analysis of genotypes and amino acid residues 2209 to 2248 of the NS5A region of hepatitis C virus in relation to the response to interferon-beta therapy. Hepatology 1997;25:750–3.
11. Enomoto N, Sakuma I, Asahina Y, et al. Mutations in the nonstructural protein 5A gene and response to interferon in patients with chronic hepatitis C virus 1b infection. N Engl J Med 1996;334:77–81.
12. Squadrito G, Leone F, Sartori M, et al. Mutations in the nonstructural protein 5A region of hepatitis C virus and response of chronic hepatitis C to interferon alfa. Gastroenterology 1997;113:567–72.
13. Murphy MD, Rosen HR, Marousek GI, Chou S Analysis of sequence configurations of the ISDR, PKR-binding domain, and V3 region as predictors of response to induction interferon-alpha and ribavirin therapy in chronic hepatitis C infection. Dig Dis Sci 2002;47:1195–205.
14. Lau JYN, Davis GL, Prescott LE, et al. Distribution of hepatitis C virus genotypes determined by line probe assay in patients with chronic hepatitis C seen at tertiary referral centers in the United States. Ann Intern Med 1996;124:868–76.
15. González-Peralta RP, Lau JYN. Do viral genotypes and HLA matching influence the outcome of recurrent HCV infection after liver transplantation? Liver Transplant Surg 1998;4:104–8.
16. Abdelmalek M, Davis GL. Treatment of chronic hepatitis C infection. In: Koff RS, Wu GY, editors. Chronic viral hepatitis: diagnosis and therapeutics. Totowa (NJ): Humana Press; 2002. p. 145–67.
17. Jara P, Resti M, Hierro L, et al. Chronic hepatitis C virus infection in childhood: clinical patterns and evolution in 224 white children. Clin Infect Dis 2003;36:275–80.
18. Wirth S, Lang T, Gehring S, Gerner P. Recombinant alfa-interferon plus ribavirin therapy in children and adolescents with chronic hepatitis C. Hepatology 2002;36:1280–4.
19. González-Peralta RP, Haber B, Jonas M, et al. Interferon alfa-2b in combination with ribavirin for the treatment of chronic hepatitis C in children. Hepatology 2002;36:311A.
20. Jacobson KR, Murray K, Zellos A, Schwarz KB. An analysis of published trials of interferon monotherapy in children with chronic hepatitis C. J Pediatr Gastroenterol Nutr 2002;34:52–8.
21. Jonas MM, Ott MJ, Nelson SP, et al. Interferon-alpha treatment

of chronic hepatitis C virus infection in children. Pediatr Infect Dis J 1998;17:241–6.

22. Matsuoka S, Tatara K, Hayabuchi Y, et al. Serologic, virologic, and histologic characteristics of chronic phase hepatitis C virus disease in children infected by transfusion. Pediatrics 1994;94:919–22.

23. Garcia-Monzon C, Jara P, Fernandez-Bermejo M, et al. Chronic hepatitis C in children: a clinical and immunohistochemical comparative study with adults patients. Hepatology 1998;28: 1696–701.

24. Martell M, Esteban JI, Quer J, et al. Hepatitis C virus circulates as a population of different but closely related genomes: quasi-species nature of HCV genome distribution. Virology 1992; 66:3225–9.

25. Moribe T, Hayashi N, Kanasawa Y, et al. Hepatitis C viral complexity detected by single strand conformational polymorphism and response to interferon therapy. Gastroenterology 1995;108:789–95.

26. González-Peralta RP, Qian K, She JY, et al. Clinical implications of viral quasispecies in chronic hepatitis C. J Med Virol 1996;49:242–7.

27. González-Peralta RP, Liu WZ, Davis GL, et al. Modulation of hepatitis C virus quasispecies heterogeneity by interferon-α and ribavirin. J Viral Hepatitis 1997;4:99–106.

28. Mizuno Y, Suzuki K, Mori M, et al. Study of needlestick accidents and hepatitis C virus infection in healthcare workers by molecular evolutionary analysis. J Hosp Infect 1997;35: 149–54.

29. Weiner AJ, Thaler MM, Crawford K, et al. A unique, predominant hepatitis C virus variant found in an infant born to a mother with multiple variants. J Virol 1993;67:4365–8.

30. Suzuki K, Mizokami M, Lau JY, et al. Confirmation of hepatitis C virus transmission through needlestick accidents by molecular evolutionary analysis. J Infect Dis 1994;170:1575–8.

31. Gish RG, Cox KL, Mizokami M, et al. Vertical transmission of hepatitis C. J Pediatr Gastroenterol Nutr 1996;22:118–9.

32. Dickson RC, Caldwell SH, Ishitani MB, et al. Clinical and histologic patterns of early graft failure due to recurrent hepatitis C in four patients after liver transplantation. Transplantation 1996;61:701–5.

33. Schluger LK, Sheiner PA, Thung SN, et al. Severe recurrent cholestatic hepatitis C following orthotopic liver transplantation. Hepatology 1996;23:971–6.

34. Nelson DR. The immunopathogenesis of hepatitis C virus infection. Clin Liver Dis 2001;5:931–53.

35. Cerny A, Chisari FV. Pathogenesis of chronic hepatitis C: immunological features of hepatic injury and viral persistence. Hepatology 1999;30:595–601.

36. Li DY, Schwarz KB. Immunopathogenesis of chronic hepatitis C virus infection. J Pediatr Gastroenterol Nutr 2002;35:260–7.

37. Wasley A, Alter MJ. Epidemiology of hepatitis C: geographic differences and temporal trends. Semin Liver Dis 2000;20:1–16.

38. Khalifa AS, Mitchell BS, Watts DM, et al. Prevalence of hepatitis C viral antibody in transfused and nontransfused Egyptian children. Am J Trop Med Hyg 1993;49:316–21.

39. Tanaka E, Kiyosawa K, Sodeyama T, et al. Prevalence of antibody to hepatitis C virus in Japanese schoolchildren: comparison with adult blood donors. Am J Trop Med Hyg 1992;46:460–4.

40. Ngatchu T, Stroffolini T, Rapicetta M, et al. Seroprevalence of anti-HCV in an urban child population: a pilot survey in a developing area, Cameroon. J Trop Med Hyg 1992;95:57–61.

41. Chesney PJ, Fisher MC, Gerber MA, et al. Hepatitis C virus infection. Pediatrics 1998;101:481–5.

42. Alter MJ, Kruszon-Moran D, Nainan OV, et al. The prevalence of hepatitis C virus infection in the United States, 1988 through 1994. N Engl J Med 1999;341:556–62.

43. Samuel MC, Doherty PM, Bulterys M, Jenison SA. Association between heroin use, needle sharing and tattoos received in prison with hepatitis B and C positivity among street-recruited injecting drug users in New Mexico, USA. Epidemiol Infect 2001;127:475–84.

44. Murray KF, Richardson LP, Morishima C, et al. Prevalence of hepatitis C virus infection and risk factors in an incarcerated juvenile population: a pilot study. Pediatrics 2003;111:153–7.

45. Ogilvie EL, Veit F, Crofts N, Thompson SC. Hepatitis infection among adolescents resident in a Melbourne juvenile justice centre: risk factors and challenges. J Adolesc Health 1999; 25:46–51.

46. Hahn JA, Page-Shafer K, Lum PJ, et al. Hepatitis C virus infection and needle exchange use among young injection drug users in San Francisco. Hepatology 2001;34:180–7.

47. Noell J, Rohde P, Ochs L, et al. Incidence and prevalence of *Chlamydia*, herpes, and viral hepatitis in a homeless adolescent population. Sex Transm Dis 2001;28:4–10.

48. Saiman L, Aronson J, Zhou J, et al. Prevalence of infectious diseases among internationally adopted children. Pediatrics 2001;108:608–12.

49. Rudin C, Berger R, Tobler R, et al. HIV-1, hepatitis (A, B, and C), and measles in Romanian children [letter]. Lancet 1990; 336:1592–3.

50. Resti M, Azzari C, Rossi ME, et al. Hepatitis C virus antibodies in a long-term follow-up of beta-thalassemic children with acute and chronic non-A non-B hepatitis. Eur J Pediatr 1992; 151:573–6.

51. Lai ME, DeVirgilis S, Argiolu F, et al. Evaluation of antibodies to hepatitis C virus in a long-term prospective study of post-transfusion hepatitis among thalassemic children: comparison between first- and second-generation assay. J Pediatr Gastroenterol Nutr 1993;16:458–64.

52. Blanchette VS, Vorstman E, Shore A, et al. Hepatitis C infection in children with hemophilia A and B. Blood 1991;78:285–9.

53. Greco M, Cristiano K, Leozappa G, et al. Hepatitis C infection in children and adolescents on haemodialysis and after renal transplant. Pediatr Nephrol 1993;7:424–7.

54. Jonas MM, Zilleruelo GE, Larue SI, et al. Hepatitis C infection in a pediatric dialysis population. Pediatrics 1992;89:707–9.

55. Rossetti F, Cesaro S, Pizzocchero P, et al. Chronic hepatitis B surface antigen-negative hepatitis after treatment of malignancy. J Pediatr 1992;121:39–43.

56. Roudot-Thoraval F, Pawlotsky J-M, Thiers V, et al. Lack of mother-to-infant transmission of hepatitis C virus in human immunodeficiency virus-seronegative women: a prospective study with hepatitis C virus RNA testing. Hepatology 1993;17:772–7.

57. Bohman VR, Stettler RW, Little BB, et al. Seroprevalence and risk factors for hepatitis C virus antibody in pregnant women. Obstet Gynecol 1992;80:609–13.

58. Chang T-T, Liou T-C, Young K-C, et al. Intrafamilial transmission of hepatitis C virus: the important role of inapparent transmission. J Med Virol 1994;42:91–6.

59. Dienstag JL. Non-A, non-B hepatitis. I. Recognition, epidemiology, and clinical features. Gastroenterology 1983;85:439–62.

60. Hoofnagle JH. Hepatitis C: the clinical spectrum of disease. Hepatology 1997;26:15S–20S.

61. Alter MJ. Epidemiology of hepatitis C in the west. Semin Liver Dis 1995;15:41–63.

62. Jonas MM, Baron MJ, Breese JS, et al. Clinical and virologic features of hepatitis C virus infection associated with intravenous immunoglobulin. Pediatrics 1996;98:211–5.

63. Chang M-H, Ni Y-H, Hwang L-H, et al. Long term clinical and virologic outcome of primary hepatitis C virus infection in children: a prospective study. Pediatr Infect Dis J 1994;13:769–73.

64. Locasciulli A, Gornati G, Tagger A, et al. Hepatitis C virus infection and chronic liver disease in children with leukemia in long-term remission. Blood 1991;78:1619–22.

65. Guido M, Rugge M, Jara P, et al. Chronic hepatitis C in children: the pathological and clinical spectrum. Gastroenterology 1998;115:1525–9.

66. Badizadegan K, Jonas MM, Ott MJ, et al. Histopathology of the liver in children with chronic hepatitis C viral infection. Hepatology 1998;28:1416–23.

67. Kage M, Fujisawa T, Shiraki K, et al. Pathology of chronic hepatitis C in children. Hepatology 1997;26:771–5.

68. Palomba E, Manzini P, Fiammengo P, et al. Natural history of perinatal hepatitis C virus infection. Clin Infect Dis 1996; 23:47–50.

69. Bortolotti F, Resti M, Giacchino R, et al. Hepatitis C virus infection and related liver disease in children of mothers with antibodies to the virus. J Pediatr 1997;130:990–3.

70. Tovo P-A, Pembrey LJ, Newell M-L. Persistence rate and progression of vertically acquired hepatitis C infection. J Infect Dis 2000;181:419–24.

71. Ni YH, Chang MH, Lue HC, et al. Posttransfusion hepatitis C infection in children. Pediatrics 1994;124:709–13.

72. Matsuoka S, Tatara K, Hayabuchi Y, et al. Serologic, virologic, and histologic characteristics of chronic phase hepatitis C virus disease in children infected by transfusion. Pediatrics 1994;94:919–22.

73. Vogt M, Lang T, Frosner G, et al. Prevalence and clinical outcome of hepatitis C infection in children who underwent cardiac surgery before the implementation of blood-donor screening. N Engl J Med 1999;341:866–70.

74. Sasaki N, Matsui A, Momoi M, et al. Loss of circulating hepatitis C virus in children who developed a persistent carrier state after mother-to-baby transmission. Pediatr Res 1997;42:263–7.

75. Jara P, Resti M, Hierro L, et al. Chronic hepatitis C virus infection in childhood: clinical patterns and evoluation in 224 white children. Clin Infect Dis 2003;36:275–80.

76. González-Peralta RP. Hepatitis C virus infection in pediatric patients. Clin Liver Dis 1997;3:691–705.

77. Blanchette VS, Vortsman E, Shore A, et al. Hepatitis C infection in children with hemophilia A and B. Blood 1991;78:285–9.

78. Kanesaki T, Kinoshita S, Tsujino G, et al. Hepatitis C virus infection in children with hemophilia: characterization of antibody response to four different antigens and relationship of antibody response, viremia, and hepatic dysfunction. J Pediatr 1993;123:381–7.

79. Leslie DE, Rann S, Nicholson S, et al. Prevalence of hepatitis C antibodies in patients with clotting disorders in Victoria. Med J Aust 1992;156:789–92.

80. Wagner N, Rotthauwe HW. Hepatitis C contributes to liver disease in children and adolescents with hemophilia. Klin Pediatr 1994;206:40–4.

81. Zellos A, Thomas DL, Mocilnikar C, et al. High viral load and mild liver injury in children with hemophilia compared with other children with chronic hepatitis C virus infection J Pediatr Gastroenterol Nutr 1999;29:418–23.

82. Tradati F, Colombo M, Mannucci PM, et al. A prospective multicenter study of hepatocellular carcinoma in Italian hemophiliacs with chronic hepatitis C. The Study Group of the Association of Italian Hemophilia Centers. Blood 1998;91:1173–7.

83. Darby SC, Ewart DW, Giangrande PL, et al. Mortality from liver cancer and liver disease in haemophilic men and boys in UK given blood products contaminated with hepatitis C. Lancet 1997;350:1425–31.

84. Al-Fawaz I, Rasheed S, Al-Mugeiren M, et al. Hepatitis E virus infection in patients from Saudi Arabia with sickle cell anaemia and beta-thalassaemia major: possible transmission by blood transfusion. J Viral Hepat 1996;3:203–5.

85. Al-Mahroos FT, Ebrahim A. Prevalence of hepatitis B, hepatitis C, and human immunodeficiency virus markers among patients with hereditary haemolytic anaemias. Ann Trop Paediatr 1995;15:121–8.

86. Lai ME, DeVirgilis S, Argiolu F, et al. Evaluation of antibodies to hepatitis C virus in a long-term prospective study of posttransfusion hepatitis among thalassemic children: comparison between first- and second-generation assay. J Pediatr Gastroentrerol Nutr 1993;16:458–64.

87. El-Nanawy AA, el-Azzouni OF, Soliman AT, et al. Prevalence of hepatitis C antibody seropositivity in healthy Egyptian children and four high risk groups. J Trop Pediatr 1995;41:341–3.

88. Ni YH, Chang MH, Lin KH, et al. Hepatitis C viral infection in children: clinical and molecular studies. Pediatr Res 1996; 39:323–8.

89. Resti M, Azzari C, Rossi ME, et al. Hepatitis C virus antibodies long-term follow-up of beta-thalassemic children. Eur J Pediatr 1992;151:573–6.

90. Angelucci E, Muretto P, Nicolucci A, et al. Effects of iron overload and hepatitis C virus positivity in determining progression of liver fibrosis in thalassemia following bone marrow transplantation. Blood 2002;100:17–21.

91. Arico M, Maggiore G, Silini E, et al. Hepatitis C virus infection in children treated for acute lymphoblastic leukemia. Blood 1994;84:2919–22.

92. Dibenedetto SP, Ragusa R, Sciacca A, et al. Incidence and morbidity of infection by hepatitis C virus in children with acute lymphoblastic leukaemia. Eur J Pediatr 1994;153:271–5.

93. Fink FM, Hocker-Schulz S, Mor W, et al. Association of hepatitis C virus infection with chronic liver disease in paediatric cancer patients. Eur J Pediatr 1993;152:490–2.

94. Locasciulli A, Testa M, Pontisso P, et al. Prevalence and natural history of hepatitis C infection in patients cured of childhood leukemia. Blood 1997;90:4628–33.

95. Rosetti F, Cesaro S, Pizzocchero P, et al. Chronic hepatitis B surface antigen-negative hepatitis after treatment of malignancy. J Pediatr 1992;121:39–43.

96. Strickland DK, Riely CA, Patrick CC, et al. Hepatitis C infection among survivors of childhood cancer. Blood 2000;95:3065–70.

97. Strickland DK, Jenkins JJ, Hudson MM. Hepatitis C infection and hepatocellular carcinoma after treatment of childhood cancer. J Pediatr Hematol Oncol 2001;23:527–9.

98. Al-Mugeiren M, al-Faleh FZ, Ramia S, et al. Seropositivity to hepatitis C virus in Saudi children with chronic renal failure. Ann Trop Paediatr 1992;12:217–9.

99. Bdour S. Hepatitis C virus infection in Jordanian haemodialysis units: serological diagnosis and genotyping. J Med Microbiol 2002;51:700–4.

100. Molle ZL, Baqi N, Gretch D, et al. Hepatitis C infection in children and adolescents with end-stage renal disease. Pediatr Nephrol 2002;17:444–9.

101. Greco M, Cristiano K, Leozappa G, et al. Hepatitis C infection in children and adolescents on haemodialysis and after renal transplant. Pediatr Nephrol 1993;7:424–7.

102. Jonas MM, Zilleruelo GE, LaRue SI, et al. Hepatitis C infection in a pediatric dialysis population. Pediatrics 1992;89:707–9.

103. Jonas MM. Children with hepatitis C. Hepatology 2002;36 Suppl 1:S173–8.

104. Wejstal R, Norkrans G. Chronic non-A, non-B hepatitis in pregnancy: outcome and possible transmission to the offspring. Scand J Infect Dis 1989;21:485–90.

105. Tong MJ, Thursby M, Rakela J, et al. Studies on the maternal-infant transmission of the viruses which cause acute hepatitis. Gastroenterology 1981;80:999–1004.

106. Resti M, Azzari C, Galli L, et al. Maternal drug use is a preeminent risk factor for mother-to-child hepatitis C virus transmission: results from a multicenter study of 1372 mother-infant pairs. J Infect Dis 2002;185:567–72.

107. Ceci O, Margiotta M, Marello F, et al. Vertical transmission of hepatitis C virus in a cohort of 2,447 HIV-seronegative pregnant women: a 24-month prospective study. J Pediatr Gastroenterol Nutr 2001;33:570–5.

108. Okamoto M, Nagata I, Murakami J, et al. Prospective reevaluation of risk factors in mother-to-child transmission of hepatitis C virus: high virus load, vaginal delivery, and negative anti-NS4 antibody. J Infect Dis 2000;182:1511–4.

109. Lin H-H, Kao J-H, Hsu H-Y, et al. Possible role of high-titer maternal viremia in perinatal transmission of hepatitis C virus. J Infect Dis 1994;169:638–41.

110. Moriya T, Sasaki F, Mizui M, et al. Transmission of hepatitis C virus from mothers to infants: its frequency and risk factors revisited. Biomed Pharmacother 1995;49:59–64.

111. Lin HH, Kao JH, Hsu HY, et al. Absence of infection in breast-fed infants born to hepatitis C virus-infected mothers. J Pediatr 1995;126:589–91.

112. Tajiri H, Miyoshi Y, Funada S, et al. Prospective study of mother-to-infant transmission of hepatitis C virus. Pediatr Infect Dis J 2001;20:10–4.

113. Ohto H, Terazawa S, Sasaki N, et al. Transmission of hepatitis C virus from mothers to infants. The Vertical Transmission of Hepatitis C Virus Collaborative Study Group. N Engl J Med 1994;330:744–50.

114. Conte D, Fraquelli M, Prat D, et al. Prevalence and clinical course of chronic hepatitis C virus infection and rate of HCV vertical transmission in a cohort of 15,250 pregnant women. Hepatology 2000;31:751–5.

115. Gibb DM, Goodall RL, Dunn DT, et al. Mother-to-child transmission of hepatitis C virus: evidence for preventable peripartum transmission. Lancet 2000;356:904–7.

116. Thaler MM, Park CK, Landers DV, et al. Vertical transmission of hepatitis C virus. Lancet 1991;338:17–8.

117. Zanetti AR, Tanzi E, Pacccagnini S, et al. Mother-to-infant transmission of hepatitis C virus. Lombardi Study Group on Vertical HCV Transmission. Lancet 1995;345:289–91.

118. Novati R, Thiers V, Monforte AD, et al. Mother-to-child transmission of hepatitis C virus detected by nested polymerase chain reaction. J Infect Dis 1992;165:720–3.

119. Lam JPH, McOmish F, Burns SM, et al. Infrequent vertical transmission of hepatitis C virus. J Infect Dis 1993;167:572–6.

120. Harland L, Enockson E, Nemeth A. Vertical transmission of hepatitis C virus. Scand J Infect Dis 1996;28:353–6.

121. Steininger C, Kundi M, Jatzo G, et al. Increased risk of mother-to-infant transmission of hepatitis C virus by intrapartum infantile exposure to maternal blood. J Infect Dis 2003;187:345–51.

122. Bosi I, Ancora G, Mantovani W, et al. HLA DR13 and HCV vertical infection. Pediatr Res 2002;51:746–9.

123. Charlton M. Hepatitis C infection in liver transplantation. Am J Transplant 2001;1:197–203.

124. Nowicki MJ, Ahmad N, Heubi JE, et al. The prevalence of hepatitis C virus in infants and children after liver transplantation. Dig Dis Sci 1994;39:2250–4.

125. Everhart JE, Wei Y, Eng H, et al. Recurrent and new hepatitis C virus infection after liver transplantation. Hepatology 1999;29:1220–6.

126. McDiarmid SV, Conrad A, Ament ME, et al. De novo hepatitis C in children after liver transplantation. Transplantation 1998;66:311–8.

127. Kuo G, Choo QL, Alter HJ, et al. An assay for circulating antibodies to a major etiologic virus of human non-A, non-B hepatitis. Science 1989;244:362–64.

128. Gretch DR, Lee W, Corey L. Use of aminotransferase, hepatitis C antibody and hepatitis C polymerase chain reaction RNA assays to establish the diagnosis of hepatitis C virus infection in a diagnostic virology laboratory. J Clin Microbiol 1992;30:2145–9.

129. McFarlane IG, Smith HM, Johnson PJ, et al. Hepatitis C virus antibodies in chronic active hepatitis: pathogenetic factor or false positive? Lancet 1990;335:754–7.

130. Alvarez F, Martres P, Maggiore G, et al. False-positive result of hepatitis C enzyme-linked immunosorbent assay in children with autoimmune hepatitis. J Pediatr 1991;119:75–7.

131. Kleinman S, Alter H, Busch M, et al. Increased detection of hepatitis C virus-infected blood donors by multiple-antigen HCV enzyme immunoassay. Transfusion 1992;32:805–13.

132. Alter H. New kit on the block: evaluation of second-generation assays for detection of antibody to the hepatitis C virus. Hepatology 1992;15:350–3.

133. Vrielink H, Reesink HW, van den Burg PJ, et al. Performance of three generations of anti-hepatitis C virus enzyme-linked immunosorbent assays in donors and patients. Transfusion 1997;37:845–9.

134. Alter MJ, Kuhnert WL, Finelli L, Centers for Disease Control and Prevention. Guidelines for laboratory testing and result reporting of antibody to hepatitis C virus. MMWR Morb Mortal Wkly Rep 2003;52:1–13.

135. Uyttendale S, Claeys H, Mertens W, et al. Evaluation of third-generation screening and confirmatory assays for HCV antibodies. Vox Sang 1994;66:122–9.

136. Powlotsky JM. Hepatitis C: viral markers and quasispecies. In: Liang TJ, Hoofnagle JH, editors. Hepatitis C. San Diego (CA): Academic Press; 2000. p. 25–52.

137. Saldanha J, Lelie N, Heath A. Establishment of the first international standard for nucleic acid amplification technology (NAT) assays for HCV RNA. WHO Collaborative Study Group. Vox Sang 1999;76:149–58.

138. Saldanha J, Heath A, Lelie N, et al. Calibration of HCV working reagents for NAT assays against the HCV international standard. The Collaborative Study Group. Vox Sang 2000;78:217–24.

139. Pawlotsky JM. Use and interpretation of virological tests for hepatitis C. Hepatology 2002;36 Suppl 1:S65–73.

140. Kolk DP, Dockter J, Linnen J, et al. Significant closure of the human immunodeficiency virus type 1 and hepatitis C virus preseroconversion detection windows with a transcription-mediated-amplification-driven assay. J Clin Microbiol 2002;40:1761–6.

141. Dodd RY, Notari EP IV, Stramer SL. Current prevalence and incidence of infectious disease markers and estimated window-period risk in the American Red Cross blood donor population. Transfusion 2002;42:994–8.

142. Davis GL, Lau JYN, Urdea MS, et al. Quantitative detection of hepatitis C virus RNA by solid phase branched DNA amplification method: definition and optimal conditions for specimen collection and clinical application in interferon-treated patients. Hepatology 1994;19:1337–41.

143. Chesney PJ, Fisher MC, Gerber MA, et al. Hepatitis C virus infection. Pediatrics 1998;101:481–5.

144. Peters MG, Terrault NA. Alcohol use and hepatitis C. Hepatology 2002;36 Suppl 1:S220–5.

145. Davis GL. Treatment of acute and chronic hepatitis C. Clin Liver Dis 1997;1:615–30.

146. Davis GL, Esteban-Mur R, Rustgi V, et al. Interferon alfa-2b alone or in combination with ribavirin for the treatment of relapse of chronic hepatitis C. N Engl J Med 1998;339:1493–9.

147. McHutchison JG, Gordon SC, Schiff ER, et al. Interferon alfa-2b alone or in combination with ribavirin as initial treatment for chronic hepatitis C. N Engl J Med 1998;339:1485–92.

148. Jacobson KR, Murray K, Zellos A, Schwarz KB. An analysis of published trials of interferon monotherapy in children with chronic hepatitis C. J Pediatr Gastroenterol Nutr 2002; 34:52–8.

149. Kelly DA, Bunn SK, Apelian D, et al. Safety, efficacy and phar-macokinetics of interferon alfa-2b plus ribavirin in children with chronic hepatitis C. Hepatology 2001;34:680A.

150. Lackner H, Moser A, Deutsch J, et al. Interferon-alpha and ribavirin in treating children and young adults with chronic hepatitis C after malignancy. Pediatrics 2000;106:E53–6.

151. Christensson B, Wiebe T, Akesson A, Widell A. Interferon-alpha and ribavirin treatment of hepatitis C in children with malignancy in remission. Clin Infect Dis 2000;30:585–6.

152. Wirth S, Lang T, Gehring S, Gerner P. Recombinant alfa-interferon plus ribavirin therapy in children and adolescents with chronic hepatitis C. Hepatology 2002;36:1280–4.

153. González-Peralta RP, Haber B, Jonas M, et al. Interferon alfa-2b in combination with ribavirin for the treatment of chronic hepatitis C in children. Hepatology 2002;36:311A.

154. Barlow CF, Priebe CJ, Mulliken JB, et al. Spastic diplegia as a complication of interferon alfa-2a treatment of hemangiomas of infancy. J Pediatr 1998;132:527–30.

1C. Other Viral Infections

Lee A. Denson, MD

Numerous viruses have been implicated in causing hepatitis. With the exception of hepatitis B and C, which are covered in the preceding parts of this chapter, these are typically acute, self-limited infections. This part reviews the route of transmission, presentation, and diagnosis for the most important agents in immunocompetent individuals (Table 51.1C-1).

Of the known hepatotropic viruses, hepatitis A virus (HAV) causes the majority of cases of community-acquired viral hepatitis in children throughout the world, whereas hepatitis E virus (HEV) plays a significant role in regions where it is endemic.[1] Because a significant number of cases of both post-transfusion and community-acquired hepatitis are not identified as being caused by hepatitis A–E, investigators have sought to identify additional potentially hepatotropic viral agents. In recent years, candidates have included hepatitis G virus (HGV), TT virus (TTV), and SEN virus (SENV). Whether these agents actually do replicate in the liver and cause hepatitis is now in question; however, the current evidence for and against this is briefly summarized. Finally, a number of viral agents can cause what is typically a milder, nonicteric hepatitis as part of an overall viral syndrome in immunocompetent hosts. The presentation and diagnosis of hepatitis owing to cytomegalovirus (CMV) and Epstein-Barr virus (EBV) are reviewed in this regard. Viral hepatitis as part of a congenital or perinatal infection and in the immunocompromised host is reviewed in Chapter 49, "Approach to Neonatal Cholestasis," and Chapter 51.3, "AIDS and Other Immune Disorders," respectively.

HEPATITIS A

HAV is a nonenveloped ribonucleic acid (RNA) virus in the Picornaviridae family.[2] Within this family, which also includes the rhinoviruses, poliovirus, coxsackievirus, echoviruses, and enteroviruses, HAV is classified in the genus *Hepatovirus*.[3] Oral ingestion of infected material leads to absorption from the stomach or intestine, replication in the liver, secretion into bile, and then either excretion in stool or reabsorption.[2] HAV may also replicate in the intestinal epithelial cells.[4] Viral particles may be detected in the bile and blood, and high titers are present in stool for 2 to 3 weeks before symptomatic liver injury as detected by elevated transaminases has occurred.[5] Fecal excretion then persists for an additional 2 weeks. The hepatitis is due to both a direct cytopathic effect of the virus and the resultant immune-mediated injury, although recent studies have favored the importance of the immune-mediated mechanisms.[6,7]

Hepatitis A is the most common cause of acute hepatitis in the United States; however, in recent years, the incidence in the United States has been declining (Figure 51.1C-1). In 2001, 10,616 cases were reported to the Centers for Disease Control and Prevention. From this, it was estimated that there were 45,000 acute clinical cases and 93,000 new infections in the United States that year.[8] This is as compared with 30,021 reported and 128,000 estimated cases in 1997. The reduction in incidence has been particularly striking in children aged 5 to 14 years. Transmission is primarily via the fecal-oral route, with the most common identifiable source being via personal contact. This includes primarily household contacts and day-care centers. In fact, approximately 10% of cases in the United States each year occur in day-care centers in children who are not toilet trained. Because of the risk of transmission to adults, it is recommended that an index case with hepatitis A be excluded from day-care centers and preschools for 1 week.[9] Foodborne epidemics have been associated with contaminated shellfish and have been transmitted in the United States via produce.[10,11] Waterborne transmission is less important in the United States. Although much less common than fecal-oral transmission, parenteral transmission has also been reported.[12]

Immunoglobulin (Ig)M antibodies directed against HAV are usually present in serum when patients present

TABLE 51.1C-1   AGENTS ASSOCIATED WITH NON-B/C VIRAL HEPATITIS

VIRUS	FAMILY	TYPE	ROUTE OF SPREAD	DISEASE
Hepatitis A	Picornavirus	RNA	Oral/fecal	Acute
Hepatitis E	Hepatitis E–like viruses	RNA	Oral/fecal	Acute
Hepatitis G	Flavivirus	RNA	Parenteral	Unlikely
TT	Circovirus	DNA	Parenteral and nonparenteral	Unlikely
SEN	Circovirus	DNA	Parenteral and nonparenteral	Acute/chronic
Cytomegalovirus	Herpesvirus	DNA	Parenteral and nonparenteral	Acute
Epstein-Barr	Herpesvirus	DNA	Nonparenteral	Acute

DNA = deoxyribonucleic acid; RNA = ribonucleic acid.

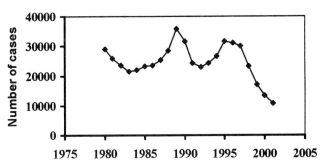

FIGURE 51.1C-1 The annual incidence of reported cases of acute hepatitis A virus (HAV) infection in the United States for the period between 1980 and 2002 is shown. Adapted from the Centers for Disease Control and Prevention.[8]

with clinical symptoms and can first be detected 5 to 10 days after exposure.[13] These are therefore diagnostic of acute infection. An IgG response then occurs that is long-lived and provides resistance against reinfection. The liver injury is likely due primarily to the associated cellular immune response to HAV rather than a direct cytopathic effect of the virus.[6,7] The diagnostic accuracy of the commercially available IgM-specific anti-HAV assay is quite good, with a sensitivity approaching 100%, a specificity of 99%, and a positive predictive value of 88%.[14] Rarely, the test may be negative at the time of presentation but should become positive within 1 to 2 weeks.[15] IgM titers will be detectable for several weeks and then become undetectable. The typical time course of the clinical presentation and viral serology is shown in Figure 51.1C-2.

The clinical presentation of hepatitis A may be classified as sporadic, endemic, or epidemic.[2] Sporadic cases typically occur in older patients and manifest the expected viral prodrome and icteric phase. The endemic form includes a large number of asymptomatic and anicteric cases occurring in younger children.[2] For

example, fewer than 10% of children less than 6 years of age will become jaundiced with HAV infection compared with 40% of children between the ages of 6 and 14 years and 70% of children older than 14 years. In endemic areas, 73 to 100% of children have been shown to have been infected in early childhood.[16,17] Epidemics owing to HAV have been reported to have a seasonal pattern, beginning in the fall and peaking in the winter, although the reason for this is not known.[2] The clinical presentation is like that in sporadic cases, with a prodrome featuring anorexia, nausea, vomiting, and malaise leading to the icteric phase. The incubation period averages 30 days, with the prodromal period averaging 7 days. Dark urine is then typically noted before scleral icterus. The duration of jaundice is quite variable but has been reported to range from 7 to 21 days on average.[2] The most prominent finding on physical examination is tender hepatomegaly. The peak bilirubin is typically around 10 mg/dL, and peak alanine transaminase (ALT) is around 3,000 mIU/L (ranging from 20 to 100 times the upper limit of normal). The serum transaminases usually normalize within 2 to 3 weeks, although minor elevations may persist for months, whereas the bilirubin usually normalizes within 4 weeks.

Hepatitis A infections may also follow a relapsing, prolonged, or cholestatic course (see Table 51.1C-1). In these individuals, the IgM anti-HAV may persist for 6 to 12 months. Relapses resembling the initial presentation have been documented in 2 to 10% of reported adult series.[18] A prolonged course, with laboratory abnormalities lasting more than 10 weeks, has also been reported in around 9% of cases.[18] Biochemical abnormalities have resolved in these cases by 20 weeks and almost all clinical symptoms by 24 weeks.[2] A cholestatic variant with prominent pruritis, diarrhea, and weight loss has also been described, with eventual complete resolution, although this may take more than 12 weeks.[19] Both the cholestatic and relapsing variants have been associated with an increased frequency of disorders mediated by immune-complex deposition, including cutaneous vasculitis, arthritis, and cryoglobulinemia (see Table 51.1C-1).[20] Finally, there is some evidence that acute HAV infection may trigger an autoim-

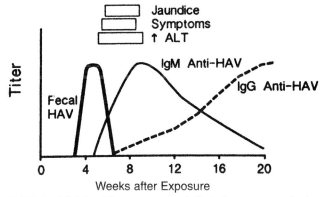

FIGURE 51.1C-2 The sequence and clinical events seen during hepatitis A are shown in this schematic illustration. Fecal hepatitis A virus (HAV) appears during the late phase of the incubation period, peaks near the onset of symptoms, and then declines rapidly; detection of fecal HAV is not used in clinical diagnosis. Diagnosis of acute hepatitis A is usually based on detection of immunoglobulin (Ig)M anti-HAV. Courtesy of the Clinical Teaching Project, American Gastroenterological Association. ALT = alanine transaminase.

TABLE 51.1C-2   ATYPICAL MANIFESTATIONS OF HAV INFECTION

CHOLESTATIC HEPATITIS
Jaundice persists for more than 12 wk
Accompanied by severe pruritis

RELAPSING HEPATITIS
Multiple courses of acute hepatitis
Persistence of IgM anti-HAV in serum
Recurrence of fecal excretion of HAV

IMMUNE COMPLEX DISORDERS
Cutaneous vasculitis
Arthritis
Cryoglobulinemia

AUTOIMMUNE HEPATITIS
Trigger of autoimmune hepatitis in susceptible individuals

HAV = hepatitis A virus; IgM = immunoglobulin M.

mune hepatitis in susceptible individuals.[21] The fatality rate for hepatitis A infection is quite low, reaching a maximum of 1.8% in adults older than age 50 years and less than 0.3% in children under 14 years of age.[8] Older age and underlying liver disease (eg, chronic hepatitis B or C infection) have been associated with more severe disease.

Passive immunoprophylaxis with immune serum globulin is useful for preventing transmission to close contacts of an index case (when given within 2 weeks of exposure) or when traveling to an endemic area. The effectiveness of this strategy has been estimated to be around 90%, although the overall waning of anti-HAV seropositivity in the general population may render this less effective.[22] The US Food and Drug Administration (FDA) has licensed a formalin-inactivated hepatitis A vaccine (Havrix) for administration to children 2 years of age and older. The most recent US recommendations for immunization target children in states with rates of HAV infection twice the national average, or approximately 20 cases per 100,000. Other high-risk populations for which immunization is recommended include travelers to endemic areas (when given within 2–4 weeks of travel), men who have sex with men, users of illegal drugs, persons who are at occupational risk for infection, persons with clotting factor disorders, and persons with chronic liver disease.[23] Individuals with chronic liver diseases should be particularly identified for immunization because coinfection with HAV has been shown to cause more severe liver injury in this setting.[24] However, a recent survey indicated that, in the adult population, HAV immunization in this patient group has not yet been consistently performed.[25] Reported adverse reactions with the vaccine have been minimal, and the seroconversion rate after two doses is 99.8% in healthy individuals.[2] Recent reports have indicated that immunization of the entire population in nonendemic countries would be cost-effective, which may become the policy in the United States in the future.[26,27] Recently, a combination vaccine directed against HAV and hepatitis B virus (HBV) has been approved by the FDA that will be useful in this regard.[28,29]

HEPATITIS E

HEV is a nonenveloped single-stranded RNA virus. It is currently classified within a separate *Hepatitis E–like viruses* genus.[30] Although the general fecal-oral mode of transmission and clinical presentation are quite similar to those in HAV, there are significant differences in its geographic distribution, with endemic areas in subtropical and tropical parts of the world.[31] In contrast to HAV, many outbreaks have been attributable to contaminated water sources, and the highest attack rate is in young adults aged 15 to 40 years.[31] The rate of person to person transmission is relatively lower for HEV relative to HAV, and the prevalence of anti-HEV IgG in endemic areas is much lower, usually not more than 25% for HEV versus 90% for HAV. The case-fatality rate during epidemics is between 0.2% and 4%, with a much higher rate (10–20%) in pregnant women.[31] Endemic areas include parts of India, areas of central and Southeast Asia, northwest China, and parts of Africa (Figure 51.1C-3).

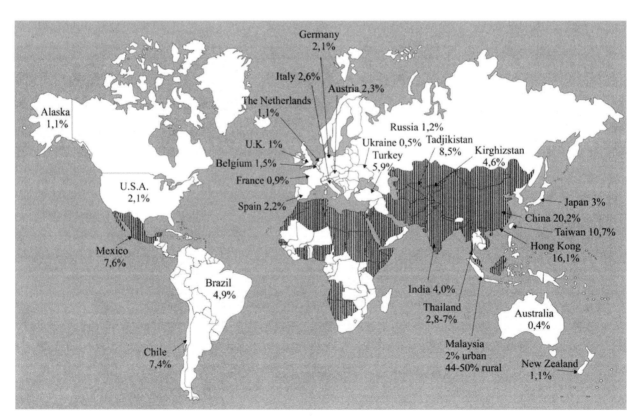

FIGURE 51.1C-3   The prevalence of positive hepatitis E virus serology in various countries is shown. Endemic regions are indicated by the dark vertical bars. Reprinted from Worm HC et al,[30] with permission from Elsevier.

As for HAV, the major mode of transmission for HEV is via the fecal-oral route. Secondary cases in household contacts occur in only 1 to 2% compared with 15% for HAV.[32] Interestingly, cases have not been associated with a foodborne mechanism of transmission. The probability of parenteral transmission is quite low.[33] The prevalence of anti-HEV does not typically exceed 25%, even in endemic areas.[30,31] The reported prevalence in children is much lower (not more than 9%) and increases in adulthood.[34] This is in contrast to other enteric viruses such as HAV, for which the prevalence of anti-HAV may exceed 90% in young children in endemic areas.[35] A low prevalence of anti-HEV ranging from 0.5 to 2% has been consistently detected in the United States and Europe. However, there have been no outbreaks of HEV, and the rare sporadic cases have been primarily limited to travelers to endemic areas. Recent reports have indicated that HEV may also circulate in domestic animals such as swine and in rodents native to industrialized countries; this may represent an increased risk for exposed individuals.[36,37] A recent cross-sectional study identified seropositivity for HEV in 10.9% of North Carolina swine workers compared with 2.4% of nonexposed individuals.[36] This compared with a prevalence of anti-HEV in 34.5% of swine. However, no associated history of past clinical hepatitis or unexplained jaundice was reported in seropositive individuals.

In areas with a low incidence of sporadic HEV, such as the United States and Europe, patients with a recent travel history and acute hepatitis should be evaluated for HEV infection. Otherwise, more common causes should be ruled out first. HEV enters by the oral route and then replicates in the liver.[30] The incubation period ranges from 2 to 9 weeks. The clinical presentation is quite similar to HAV and includes jaundice, malaise, nausea, anorexia, and a variable degree of hepatomegaly. Pruritus may be a prominent feature of the cholestatic form. A flu-like prodrome precedes the acute hepatitic phase. The incubation time is in the range of 15 to 60 days, and the virus is excreted in the stool for an average of 2 weeks after the onset of the illness.[30,32] Abnormalities in transaminases and alkaline phosphatase typically normalize within 1 to 6 weeks.[30] HEV infection may be diagnosed through detection of anti-HEV IgM in serum at the onset of symptoms; this remains positive for 2 to 3 months. Anti-HEV IgG persists long term in about 50% of infected individuals. Although prolonged cases lasting up to 6 months have been reported, there is no evidence that HEV causes chronic hepatitis.[30] As for HAV, HEV superinfection has been reported to worsen liver injury in chronic HBV infection.[38] Although this is typically self-limited, cases of severe liver decompensation have been reported.[39] Thus, patients with chronic liver diseases traveling to or living in endemic areas will be candidates for HEV immunization when a vaccine becomes available.

Strategies to reduce the number of HEV outbreaks and sporadic cases include improved sanitation in endemic areas and the development of an HEV vaccine. This is particularly necessary in endemic areas because of the relatively low prevalence of natural immunity to HEV and the high fatality rate in pregnant women. Because of its high prevalence, HEV is the leading cause of fulminant hepatitis in endemic areas such as India.[40,41] Several efforts are currently under way to develop an effective HEV vaccine, and a candidate vaccine has been evaluated in clinical trials.[42–44]

GB VIRUS C/HEPATITIS G VIRUS

Despite significant advances in the molecular characterization of the primary hepatotropic viruses, A–E, there is still a significant proportion of cases of both post-transfusion and community-acquired hepatitis that are of unknown origin.[45] This includes approximately 10% of cases of transfusion-associated hepatitis and, in some series, up to 20% of cases of community-acquired hepatitis. This and the next two sections briefly summarize the evidence for and against the potential contribution of three recently characterized viruses to these cases: HGV, TTV, and SENV. GB virus C (GBV-C), or HGV, is a recently discovered enveloped RNA virus that belongs to the Flavivirus family.[46] GBV-C and HGV were independently isolated and reported by two different groups; they are 96% homologous, indicating that they are two genotypes of the same virus.[47] Most reported cases have involved parenteral transmission through contaminated blood or blood products; however, cases attributable to intravenous drug use, vertical transmission from mother to child, and sexual transmission have also been reported.[48–50] The risk of vertical transmission is on the order of 50 to 60%, which is much higher than for HCV.[51]

HGV is found throughout the world, with a high prevalence in both healthy populations and in different patient groups.[52–56] This has called into question its actual role in acute or chronic hepatitis.[57–59] Active infection has been detected using a polymerase chain reaction (PCR) assay for HGV RNA in serum, whereas past exposure has been detected using an antibody against the envelope 2 (E2) protein.[50,60] Prevalence rates in healthy populations of 1 to 4% have been reported in Europe and North America and 10 to 33% in South America and Africa.[46] Supporting the parenteral mode of transmission, prevalence rates of 24 to 49% have been reported in intravenous drug use and 18% in polytransfused patients. Rates ranging from 2 to 39% have been reported for acute non-A–E hepatitis and 16 to 43% for fulminant hepatic failure.[46] The majority of adults have a transient infection with clearance of the virus and the appearance of E2 antibodies. However, persistent infections lasting for years in the absence of liver disease have been documented. This has been particularly true in cases of vertical or perinatal transmission.

Although the tissue tropism of HGV is not clearly established, it may replicate in human mononuclear cells rather than in hepatocytes.[61] In this regard, it is interesting to note that coinfection with HGV has been shown to slow the progression of HIV infection, with coinfected patients having higher CD4 counts.[61] Other recent studies have indicated that HGV may also infect and replicate in hepatocytes, albeit without causing any detectable liver injury.[62] Although HGV infection has been implicated in cases of acute, chronic, and fulminant non-A–E hepatitis, whether it is clearly the cause of these cases has become much less likely with additional negative reports. In most subjects, liver histology has been normal despite evidence of HGV infection in hepatocytes.[62] There is no increase in HGV infection in children with liver disease compared with children without liver disease.[63] Moreover, HGV superinfection has not been shown to worsen liver disease in HCV infection.[64] Overall, most infections are asymptomatic, and whether HGV is truly a cause of non–A-E hepatitis is unlikely.

TT VIRUS

TTV is a nonenveloped single-stranded deoxyribonucleic acid (DNA) virus that was originally identified in an adult with nontypable post-transfusion hepatitis.[65] Although TTV has subsequently been found in patients with non-A–E hepatitis, its overall prevalence has not been different between healthy individuals and patients with liver disease.[66,67] Like HGV, TTV has been detected using PCR from serum samples. A recent study determined the prevalence of TTV in healthy children and children with non-A–E hepatitis and/or a history of transfusion.[68] Depending on the PCR primers used, from 27 to 89% of healthy children had evidence of TTV infection. Children with a history of transfusion had a higher prevalence, ranging from 46 to 100%.[68] However, children with non-A–E hepatitis, whether acute, chronic, or fulminant, did not have a significantly higher prevalence of TTV infection than healthy controls.[68] There was no increase in serum transaminases in children coinfected with TTV and HBV or HCV relative to HBV or HCV alone. Moreover, the treatment response in HCV infection was not affected by coinfection with TTV.[69] Importantly, the data in healthy children also supported a significant nonparenteral route of transmission, beginning in the first year of life and peaking by 4 to 6 years of age. Thus, the data as a whole support both parenteral and nonparenteral routes of transmission for TTV but do not support a significant role for TTV in non-A–E hepatitis in children.[70,71] In fact, more recently, it has been proposed that TTV may represent part of the normal human "viral flora."

SEN VIRUS

The most recent agent to be implicated in non-A–E hepatitis is SENV. SENV is a single-stranded DNA virus from the newly characterized Circovirus family that bears some homology to TTV.[72] Five strains have been characterized, with total SENV detected in 13% of healthy blood donors and up to 70% of transfused patients.[72] The SENV-D and SENV-H strains have been felt to be more promising in terms of potentially causing liver disease, with a prevalence of less than 1% in healthy blood donors and up to 50% in cases of transfusion-associated non-A–E hepatitis.[72] The prevalence of SENV infection was shown to increase with the volume of transfused blood, supporting the parenteral mode of transmission.[72]

In a recent prospective study, 11 of 12 patients who developed nontypable post-transfusion hepatitis were infected with SENV-D and/or SENV-H.[72] However, 55 of 225 patients who did not develop post-transfusion hepatitis were also acutely infected with SENV-D and/or SENV-H. None of the patients were jaundiced; the mean peak ALT level was 396 U/L. In some cases, there was concordance between the level of viremia and ALT. The severity of HCV cases detected in this study was not affected by coincident SENV infection. Most patients cleared SEN-V infection, although 15% were chronic carriers for several years. In two of these patients, chronic viremia was associated with a persistently elevated level of ALT. Overall, this study demonstrated the relatively common occurrence of post-transfusion SENV infection in 30% of patients. Whereas a minority (11/86) of SENV-infected patients did develop acute non-A–E hepatitis temporally related to the appearance of viremia, the majority (75/86) did not. Several recent retrospective studies similarly documented a high prevalence of SENV infection in both healthy individuals and those with acute or chronic liver diseases and also supported a nonparenteral route of transmission.[73–75] Therefore, it is unlikely that SENV infection causes non-A–E hepatitis in most cases. As for TTV, coinfection with SENV has not been shown to affect the severity or response to treatment of HCV; SENV, however, has been shown to be sensitive to interferon therapy.[76] However, further data regarding hepatotrophism and replication will be required to determine whether SENV infection does cause hepatitis in a minority of cases.

CYTOMEGALOVIRUS

It has been estimated that up to 10% of cases of acute viral hepatitis in immunocompetent individuals may be due to non-A–E agents. These may include EBV, herpesviruses, CMV, adenovirus, and parvovirus. The clinical presentation, diagnosis, and management of acute hepatitis associated with CMV and EBV are summarized in the next two sections. A detailed discussion of hepatitis owing to the other viral agents is beyond the scope of this section.

CMV is one of seven members of the herpesvirus family, each of which may infect the liver. Although CMV and other herpes family member infections are a more significant problem in immunocompromised hosts, they may also cause a variety of clinical diseases in immunocompetent patients. This includes what is typically an acute anicteric hepatitis as part of a systemic infection.

By the age of 15 years, approximately 20% of children will have been infected; this reaches a maximum of 50 to 60% by 25 to 30 years of age.[77] The consequences of CMV infection in immunocompromised patients and infants are covered in another chapter. CMV may infect and replicate in both hepatocytes and cholangiocytes.[78] However, whether the resulting liver injury is due to a direct cytopathic effect of the virus or the host immune response is not clear. In fact, this may vary depending on the clinical situation.[78] Whether hepatocytes may harbor CMV in a latent infection is also not well understood and is currently being studied. Finally, it has recently been reported that patients with other forms of chronic viral hepatitis and cirrhosis may be more susceptible to developing acute CMV infections that cause additional liver injury.[78]

Although acute primary CMV infection in immunocompetent hosts is usually asymptomatic, it may result in a syndrome similar to EBV mononucleosis.[78] This includes fever, malaise, cervical lymphadenopathy, and splenomegaly. Liver involvement is indicated by a modest elevation in serum transaminases (usually less than threefold) and minimal hepatomegaly.[79] Overt jaundice is rare.[79] The diagnosis of CMV infection may be made by detecting anti-CMV IgM antibodies or CMV antigen in serum or CMV cultured from urine. Typical viral cytomegalic cells or CMV early antigens are rarely detected on liver biopsy, perhaps indicating a vigorous immune response in the normal host leading to destruction of infected hepatocytes. By comparison, cytomegalic cells and both CMV early and late antigens are frequently detected on liver biopsy of transplant patients infected with CMV.[78] Therefore, the liver injury in the normal host may be due primarily to the host immune response, whereas viral cytopathic injury may be more important in the immunocompromised host.[78]

Compared with infection with HAV, patients with hepatitis owing to CMV tend to have fever longer and more prominent cervical lymphadenopathy and splenomegaly.[78] The incubation period ranges from 3 to 12 weeks.[80] Jaundice is much less common, and the maximum elevation in serum transaminases is typically less than 200 U.[80] Transaminases typically peak 2 to 3 weeks after disease onset and normalize by the fifth week.[80] Very rarely, however, acute CMV infection has been reported to cause massive hepatocellular necrosis in a normal host, with attendant fever, jaundice, highly elevated transaminases, and coagulopathy. In severe cases, therapy with ganciclovir or foscarnet may be effective.[81,82]

Ordinarily, CMV infection leads to a lifelong latent phase in the normal host. CMV can then become reactivated in immunocompromised individuals.[78] Patients with chronic liver disease, particularly when it has advanced to cirrhosis, develop a condition of impaired cellular immunity. This may make them more susceptible to CMV reactivation or reinfection. Coincident CMV infection is then associated with an additional impairment in liver function.[78] The specific effect of CMV infection on the progression of chronic liver diseases, including HBV and HCV, is currently the subject of active investigation.[78] A recombinant CMV vaccine has recently completed phase I trials in seronegative toddlers and may prove useful in terms of preventing transmission to woman of childbearing age and other individuals for whom the consequences of primary CMV infection may be severe.[83]

EPSTEIN-BARR VIRUS

As for CMV, EBV may also affect the liver as part of a generalized mononucleosis syndrome in the normal host. This section is limited to a brief review of the hepatitis associated with infectious mononucleosis; the role of EBV in post-transplant lymphoproliferative disease, lymphoma, and acquired immune deficiency syndrome (AIDS) is discussed elsewhere.

Like CMV, EBV is ubiquitous and will have infected over 80% of individuals by the time they are adults.[84] It is a double-stranded DNA virus. Infection of the oropharynx results in ongoing shedding of virus during an active infection. EBV DNA is subsequently incorporated into B cells, resulting in lifelong latent infection. The primary infection in young children is usually asymptomatic.[84] Infection in adolescents leads to the classic infectious mononucleosis syndrome, with fever, cervical lymphadenopathy, sore throat, fatigue, and splenomegaly. Primary infection is confirmed by detection of antiviral capsid antigen IgM in the serum.[84] Liver involvement is similar to CMV, with a mild anicteric hepatitis in most cases. However, from 5 to 10% may develop jaundice.[79,85] Rarely, in about 1 in 3,000 cases of infectious mononucleosis, this may take a more fulminant course, with severe hepatitis, bone marrow failure, and acute respiratory distress syndrome.[84,86] Death may result in these cases from massive hepatocellular necrosis and liver failure. Liver injury owing to EBV is likely secondary to infected cytotoxic T lymphocytes rather than a direct cytopathic effect of the virus on hepatocytes.[87]

FULMINANT HEPATITIS

A more detailed discussion related to evaluation of the child with fulminant hepatic failure is presented in Chapter 58, "Acute Liver Failure." Although each of the viruses previously reviewed may rarely cause fulminant hepatitis in children, a number of cases do not have an identifiable cause. This has led a number of investigators to search for additional causes of severe viral hepatitis.[88] The reported contribution of HAV in developed countries has ranged from < 5% (United States) to 26 to 31% (France and England).[88] Although the reported prevalence of HBV infection in adult fulminant hepatic failure has ranged from 25 to 75%, making it the most common identified viral cause, it remains an uncommon cause in children in nonendemic areas, including the United States.[88] In endemic areas, it plays a significant role, equivalent to the prevalence reported for adults. Also in endemic areas, infection with HEV alone or in combination with HAV has commonly been implicated in pediatric cases of fulminant hepatic failure. This has not been reported in children in the United States or western Europe.[88] As previously reviewed, it is unlikely that HGV or TTV causes fulminant hepatic failure; the potential role of specific strains of SENV remains under investigation. Viruses in the herpes family, including CMV, EBV, herpes simplex virus, and varicella-zoster virus, have each been implicated in causing fulminant hepatic failure, although almost always in an immunocompromised host.

Therefore, a significant proportion of cases of severe hepatitis and, in particular, fulminant hepatic failure in children are presumed to be due to an as yet unidentified virus(es). Survival without liver transplant is lower for this entity than for fulminant hepatitic failure owing to HAV or HBV.[88] The association with aplastic anemia has strengthened the hypothesis that this is a viral infection. In this regard, parvovirus B19 infection has been implicated in some cases, although its overall contribution is unclear.[89,90] A recent study from Japan identified human herpesvirus 6 in 7 of 11 patients (5 children and 2 adults) with fulminant hepatic failure.[91] With continued improvements in molecular techniques, additional potential viral causes of non-A–E hepatitis will likely be identified in the near future. However, rigorous methods will be required to determine whether these agents are causative or innocent bystanders.

REFERENCES

1. Poovorawan Y, Chatchatee P, Chongsrisawat V. Epidemiology and prophylaxis of viral hepatitis: a global perspective. J Gastroenterol Hepatol 2002;17 Suppl:S155–66.

2. Cuthbert JA. Hepatitis A: old and new. Clin Microbiol Rev 2001;14:38–58.

3. Lemon SM, Jansen RW, Brown EA. Genetic, antigenic and biological differences between strains of hepatitis A virus. Vaccine 1992;10 Suppl 1:S40–4.

4. Asher LV, Binn LN, Mensing TL, et al. Pathogenesis of hepatitis A in orally inoculated owl monkeys (Aotus trivirgatus). J Med Virol 1995;47:260–8.

5. Coulepis AG, Locarnini SA, Lehmann NI, Gust ID. Detection of hepatitis a virus in the feces of patients with naturally acquired infections. J Infect Dis 1980;141:151–6.

6. Siegl G, Weitz M. Pathogenesis of hepatitis A: persistent viral infection as basis of an acute disease? Microb Pathog 1993;14:1–8.

7. Vallbracht A, Maier K, Stierhof YD, et al. Liver-derived cytotoxic T cells in hepatitis A virus infection. J Infect Dis 1989;160:209–17.

8. Centers for Disease Control and Prevention. Viral hepatitis A. Available at:www.cdc.gov/nciod/diseases/hepatitis (accessed Sept 8, 2003).

9. Richardson M, Elliman D, Maguire H, et al. Evidence base of incubation periods, periods of infectiousness and exclusion policies for the control of communicable diseases in schools and preschools. Pediatr Infect Dis J 2001;20:380–91.

10. Rosenblum LS, Mirkin IR, Allen DT, et al. A multifocal outbreak of hepatitis A traced to commercially distributed lettuce. Am J Public Health 1990;80:1075–9.

11. Halliday ML, Kang LY, Zhou TK, et al. An epidemic of hepatitis A attributable to the ingestion of raw clams in Shanghai, China. J Infect Dis 1991;164:852–9.

12. Noble RC, Kane MA, Reeves SA, Roeckel I. Posttransfusion hepatitis a in a neonatal intensive care unit. JAMA 1984;252:2711–5.

13. Stapleton JT. Host immune response to hepatitis a virus. J Infect Dis 1995;171 Suppl 1:S9–14.

14. Storch GA, Bodicky C, Parker M, et al. Use of conventional and IgM-specific radioimmunoassays for anti-hepatitis A antibody in an outbreak of hepatitis A. Am J Med 1982;73:663–8.

15. Hirata R, Hoshino Y, Sakai H, et al. Patients with hepatitis A with negative IgM-HA antibody at early stages. Am J Gastroenterol 1995;90:1168–9.

16. Perez OM, Morales W, Paniagua M, Strannegard O. Prevalence of antibodies to hepatitis A, B, C, and E viruses in a healthy population in Leon, Nicaragua. Am J Trop Med Hyg 1996;55:17–21.

17. Darwish MA, Faris R, Clemens JD, et al. High seroprevalence of hepatitis A, B, C, and E viruses in residents in an Egyptian village in the Nile Delta: a pilot study. Am J Trop Med Hyg 1996;54:554–8.

18. Glikson M, Galun E, Oren R, et al. Relapsing hepatitis A. Review of 14 cases and literature survey. Medicine (Baltimore) 1992;71:14–23.

19. Gordon SC, Reddy KR, Schiff L, Schiff ER. Prolonged intrahepatic cholestasis secondary to acute hepatitis A. Ann Intern Med 1984;101:635–7.

20. Inman RD, Hodge M, Johnston ME, et al. Arthritis, vasculitis, and cryoglobulinemia associated with relapsing hepatitis a virus infection. Ann Intern Med 1986;105:700–3.

21. Vento S, Garofano T, Di Perri G, et al. Identification of hepatitis A virus as a trigger for autoimmune chronic hepatitis type 1 in susceptible individuals. Lancet 1991;337:1183–7.

22. Behrens RH, Doherty JF. Severe hepatitis A despite passive immunisation. Lancet 1993;341:972.

23. Koff RS. Hepatitis A, hepatitis B, and combination hepatitis vaccines for immunoprophylaxis: an update. Dig Dis Sci 2002;47:1183–94.

24. Kyrlagkitsis I, Cramp ME, Smith H, et al. Acute hepatitis A virus infection: a review of prognostic factors from 25 years experience in a tertiary referral center. Hepatogastroenterology 2002;49:524–8.

25. Arguedas MR, Mcguire BM, Fallon MB. Implementation of vaccination in patients with cirrhosis. Dig Dis Sci 2002;47:384–7.

26. Rosenthal P. Cost-effectiveness of hepatitis A vaccination in children, adolescents, and adults. Hepatology 2003;37:44–51.

27. Jacobs RJ, Meyerhoff AS. Comparative cost effectiveness of varicella, hepatitis A, and pneumococcal conjugate vaccines. Prev Med 2001;33:639–45.

28. Levie K, Beran J, Collard F, Nguyen C. Long term (24 months) follow-up of a hepatitis A and B vaccine, comparing a two and three dose schedule in adolescents aged 12-15 years. Vaccine 2002;20:2579–84.

29. Koff RS. Risks associated with hepatitis A and hepatitis B in patients with hepatitis C. J Clin Gastroenterol 2001;33:20–6.

30. Worm HC, Van Der Poel WH, Brandstatter G. Hepatitis E: an overview. Microb Infect 2002;4:657–66.

31. Krawczynski K, Kamili S, Aggarwal R. Global epidemiology and medical aspects of hepatitis E. Forum (Genova) 2001;11:166–79.

32. Khuroo MS. Study of an epidemic of non-A, non-B hepatitis. Possibility of another human hepatitis virus distinct from posttransfusion non-A, non-B type. Am J Med 1980;68:818–24.

33. Robson SC, Adams S, Brink N, et al. Hospital outbreak of hepatitis E. Lancet 1992;339:1424–5.

34. Colak D, Ogunc D, Gunseren F, et al. Seroprevalence of antibodies to hepatitis A and E viruses in pediatric age groups in turkey. Acta Microbiol Immunol Hung 2002;49:93–7.

35. Batra Y, Bhatkal B, Ojha B, et al. Vaccination against hepatitis A virus may not be required for schoolchildren in northern India: results of a seroepidemiological survey. Bull World Health Organ 2002;80:728–31.

36. Withers MR, Correa MT, Morrow M, et al. Antibody levels to hepatitis E virus in North Carolina swine workers, non-swine workers, swine, and murids. Am J Trop Med Hyg 2002;66:384–8.

37. Smith HM, Reporter R, Rood MP, et al. Prevalence study of antibody to ratborne pathogens and other agents among patients using a free clinic in downtown Los Angeles. J Infect Dis 2002;186:1673–6.

38. Shang Q, Yu J, Xiao D, et al. The effects of hepatitis E virus superinfection on patients with chronic hepatitis B: a clinicopathological study. Zhonghua Nei Ke Za Zhi 2002;41:656–9.

39. Hamid SS, Atiq M, Shehzad F, et al. Hepatitis E virus superinfection in patients with chronic liver disease. Hepatology 2002;36:474–8.

40. Acharya S, Batra Y, Hazari S, et al. Etiopathogenesis of acute hepatic failure: eastern versus western countries. J Gastroenterol Hepatol 2002;17 Suppl 3: S268–73.

41. Sheikh A, Sugitani M, Kinukawa N, et al. Hepatitis E virus infection in fulminant hepatitis patients and an apparently healthy population in Bangladesh. Am J Trop Med Hyg 2002;66:721–4.

42. Kamili S, Spelbring J, Krawczynski K. DNA vaccination against hepatitis E virus infection in cynomolgus macaques. J Gastroenterol Hepatol 2002;17 Suppl 3:S365–9.

43. Che XY, Qian QJ, Liu SX, et al. Construction of specifically targeted chimeric hepatitis E virus DNA vaccine and its efficacy assessment. Di Yi Jun Yi Da Xue Xue Bao 2002;22:97–101.

44. Hyams KC. New perspectives on hepatitis E. Curr Gastroenterol Rep 2002;4:302–7.

45. Chu CM, Lin DY, Yeh CT, et al. Epidemiological characteristics, risk factors, and clinical manifestations of acute non-A-E hepatitis. J Med Virol 2001;65:296–300.

46. Halasz R, Weiland O, Sallberg M. GB virus C/hepatitis G virus. Scand J Infect Dis 2001;33:572–80.

47. Muerhoff AS, Simons JN, Leary TP, et al. Sequence heterogeneity within the 5′-terminal region of the hepatitis GB virus C genome and evidence for genotypes. J Hepatol 1996;25:379–84.

48. Linnen J, Wages J Jr, Zhang-Keck ZY, et al. Molecular cloning and disease association of hepatitis G virus: a transfusion-transmissible agent. Science 1996;271:505–8.

49. Fischler B, Lara C, Chen M, et al. Genetic evidence for mother-to-infant transmission of hepatitis G virus. J Infect Dis 1997;176:281–5.

50. Lara C, Halasz R, Sonnerborg A, Sallberg M. Detection of hepatitis G virus RNA in persons with and without known risk factors for blood-borne viral infections in Sweden and Honduras. J Clin Microbiol 1998;36:255–7.

51. Hino K, Moriya T, Ohno N, et al. Mother-to-infant transmission occurs more frequently with GB virus C than hepatitis C virus. Arch Virol 1998;143:65–72.

52. Bjorkman P, Widell A, Veress B, et al. GB virus C/hepatitis G virus infection in patients investigated for chronic liver disease and in the general population in southern Sweden. Scand J Infect Dis 2001;33:611–7.

53. Dai CY, Yu ML, Chang WY, et al. The prevalence of TT virus and GB virus C/hepatitis G virus infection in individuals with raised liver enzymes but without HBV or HCV infection in Taiwan. Epidemiol Infect 2002;129:307–13.

54. Cacopardo B, Nunnari G, Berger A, et al. Acute non A-E hepatitis in eastern Sicily: the natural history and the role of hepatitis G virus. Eur Rev Med Pharmacol Sci 2000;4:117–21.

55. Di SR, Ferraro D, Bonura C, et al. Are hepatitis G virus and TT virus involved in cryptogenic chronic liver disease? Dig Liver Dis 2002;34:53–8.

56. Kondili LA, Chionne P, Dettori S, et al. GB virus C/hepatitis G virus exposure in Italian pediatric and young adult thalassemic patients. Infection 2001;29:219–21.

57. Kleinman S. Hepatitis G virus biology, epidemiology, and clinical manifestations: implications for blood safety. Transfus Med Rev 2001;15:201–12.

58. Kapoor S, Gupta RK, Das BC, Kar P. Clinical implications of hepatitis G virus (HGV) infection in patients of acute viral hepatitis and fulminant hepatic failure. Indian J Med Res 2000;112:121–7.

59. Sathar M, Soni P, York D. GB virus C/hepatitis G virus (GBV-C/HGV): still looking for a disease. Int J Exp Pathol 2000;81:305–22.

60. Pilot-Matias TJ, Carrick RJ, Coleman PF, et al. Expression of the GB virus C E2 glycoprotein using the Semliki Forest virus vector system and its utility as a serologic marker. Virology 1996;225:282–92.

61. George SL, Wunschmann S, McCoy J, et al. Interactions between GB virus type C and HIV. Curr Infect Dis Rep 2002;4:550–8.

62. Halasz R, Sallberg M, Lundholm S, et al. The GB virus C/hepatitis G virus replicates in hepatocytes without causing liver disease in healthy blood donors. J Infect Dis 2000;182:1756–60.

63. Halasz R, Fischler B, Nemeth A, et al. A high prevalence of serum GB virus C/hepatitis G virus RNA in children with and without liver disease. Clin Infect Dis 1999;28:537–40.

64. Strauss E, Da Costa Gayotto LC, Fay F, et al. Liver histology in co-infection of hepatitis C virus (HCV) and hepatitis G virus (HGV). Rev Inst Med Trop Sao Paulo 2002;44:67–70.

65. Nishizawa T, Okamoto H, Konishi K, et al. A novel DNA virus (TTV) associated with elevated transaminase levels in post-transfusion hepatitis of unknown etiology. Biochem Biophys Res Commun 1997;241:92–7.

66. Simmonds P, Davidson F, Lycett C, et al. Detection of a novel DNA virus (TTV) in blood donors and blood products. Lancet 1998;352:191–5.

67. Naoumov NV, Petrova EP, Thomas MG, Williams R. Presence of a newly described human DNA virus (TTV) in patients with liver disease. Lancet 1998;352:195–7.

68. Hsu HY, Ni YH, Chen HL, et al. TT virus infection in healthy children, children after blood transfusion, and children with non-A to E hepatitis or other liver diseases in Taiwan. J Med Virol 2003;69:66–71.

69. Kawanaka M, Niiyama G, Mahmood S, et al. Effect of TT virus co-infection on interferon response in chronic hepatitis C patients. Liver 2002;22:351–5.

70. Kadayifci A, Guney C, Uygun A, et al. Similar frequency of TT virus infection in patients with liver enzyme elevations and healthy subjects. Int J Clin Pract 2001;55:434–6.

71. Luo K, Zhang L. Enteric transmission of transfusion-transmitted virus. Chin Med J (Engl) 2001;114:1201–4.

72. Umemura T, Yeo AE, Sottini A, et al. SEN virus infection and its relationship to transfusion-associated hepatitis. Hepatology 2001;33:1303–11.

73. Mikuni M, Moriyama M, Tanaka N, et al. SEN virus infection does not affect the progression of non-A to -E liver disease. J Med Virol 2002;67:624–9.

74. Wong SG, Primi D, Kojima H, et al. Insights into SEN virus prevalence, transmission, and treatment in community-based persons and patients with liver disease referred to a liver disease unit. Clin Infect Dis 2002;35:789–95.

75. Yoshida H, Kato N, Shiratori Y, et al. Weak association between SEN virus viremia and liver disease. J Clin Microbiol 2002;40:3140–5.

76. Umemura T, Alter HJ, Tanaka E, et al. SEN virus: response to interferon alfa and influence on the severity and treatment response of coexistent hepatitis C. Hepatology 2002;35:953–9.

77. Stern H. Cytomegalovirus and EB virus infections of the liver. Br Med Bull 1972;28:180–5.

78. Varani S, Landini MP. Cytomegalovirus as a hepatotropic virus. Clin Lab 2002;48:39–44.

79. Cohen JI, Corey GR. Cytomegalovirus infection in the normal host. Medicine (Baltimore) 1985;64:100–14.

80. Zuschke CA, Herrera JL, Pettyjohn FS. Cytomegalovirus hepatitis mimicking an acute exacerbation of chronic hepatitis B. South Med J 1996;89:1213–6.

81. Eddleston M, Peacock S, Juniper M, Warrell DA. Severe cytomegalovirus infection in immunocompetent patients. Clin Infect Dis 1997;24:52–6.

82. Nigro G, Krzysztofiak A, Bartmann U, et al. Ganciclovir therapy for cytomegalovirus-associated liver disease in immunocompetent or immunocompromised children. Arch Virol 1997;142:573–80.

83. Mitchell DK, Holmes SJ, Burke RL, et al. Immunogenicity of a recombinant human cytomegalovirus GB vaccine in seronegative toddlers. Pediatr Infect Dis J 2002;21:133–8.

84. Markin RS. Manifestations of Epstein-Barr virus-associated disorders in liver. Liver 1994;14:1–13.

85. Jacobson IM, Gang DL, Schapiro RH. Epstein-Barr viral hepatitis: an unusual case and review of the literature. Am J Gastroenterol 1984;79:628–32.

86. Okano M, Gross TG. Epstein-Barr virus-associated hemophagocytic syndrome and fatal infectious mononucleosis. Am J Hematol 1996;53:111–5.

87. Kimura H, Nagasaka T, Hoshino Y, et al. Severe hepatitis caused by Epstein-Barr virus without infection of hepatocytes. Hum Pathol 2001;32:757–62.

88. Whitington PF, Alonso EM. Fulminant hepatitis in children: evidence for an unidentified hepatitis virus. J Pediatr Gastroenterol Nutr 2001;33:529–36.

89. Karetnyi YV, Beck PR, Markin RS, et al. Human parvovirus B19 infection in acute fulminant liver failure. Arch Virol 1999;144:1713–24.

90. Naides SJ, Karetnyi YV, Cooling LL, et al. Human parvovirus B19 infection and hepatitis. Lancet 1996;347:1563–4.

91. Ishikawa K, Hasegawa K, Naritomi T, et al. Prevalence of herpesviridae and hepatitis virus sequences in the livers of patients with fulminant hepatitis of unknown etiology in Japan. J Gastroenterol 2002;37:523–30.

2. Bacterial, Parasitic, and Other Infections

Dinesh S. Pashankar, MD, MRCP

Richard A. Schreiber, MD, FRCPC

The epidemiology of postnatal nonviral infections of the liver varies throughout the world. Whereas in the United States, most nonviral infections of the liver are bacterial, parasites are especially important etiologic agents in developing countries. Although the incidence of hepatic abscesses postappendicitis has decreased substantially owing to the advent of broad-spectrum antibiotics and improvements in surgical care, liver infections in immunocompromised hosts are on the rise. The clinical presentation of hepatic infections may be subtle, and a high index of suspicion is necessary, especially in those patients at high risk. Modern diagnostic techniques and novel therapeutic interventions have afforded significant improvements in mortality rates.[1,2] This chapter discusses the assessment and management of pyogenic liver abscess and some of the other more common nonviral infectious causes of postnatal liver infection.

PYOGENIC ABSCESS

INCIDENCE AND PATHOGENESIS

Pyogenic liver abscess is an uncommon infection in children. The incidence was reported as 0.35% in all pediatric cases coming to autopsy in St. Louis prior to 1967 and as 0.03% of all admissions to Milwaukee Children's Hospital between 1957 and 1977.[3,4] Whereas pyogenic liver abscess in South Africa and India can account for 0.015% and 0.078% of hospital admissions, respectively,[1,5] a hospital rate of 0.025% was noted in a pediatric population from Florida.[6] It is suspected that the incidence of hepatic abscess in children is on the rise, likely owing to improved diagnostic imaging techniques and the changing complexity and survival of pediatric patients at high risk for developing liver abscess, such as those with leukemia or immunodeficiency. Pyogenic liver abscess does occur in neonates, accounting for 0.026% of admissions to a neonatal intensive care unit in one study.[7]

Pyogenic bacteria can reach the liver via the portal vein or hepatic artery from structures adjacent or contiguous to the liver or by direct hepatic trauma. Infections originating within the abdominal cavity (eg, appendicitis, omphalitis, or perforated viscus) can seed to the liver, resulting in abscess formation. Although biliary tract disorders are less common in pediatric patients compared with adults, children who have undergone hepatic portoenterostomy are predisposed to developing ascending cholangitis and liver abscess.[3] In developing countries, malnutrition and helminthic (ascariasis) infestations are the major risk factors associated with liver abscess in children.[1,8] In developed countries, pyogenic liver abscesses occur most frequently in immunocompromised hosts. A review of 92 children with chronic granulomatous disease (CGD) found that 45% of cases were complicated by hepatic or perihepatic abscesses.[9] Children with leukemia on chemotherapy are predisposed to developing bacterial or fungal liver abscesses.[3,10] Patients with congenital neutropenia,[4] hyperimmunoglobulinemia E syndrome,[11] or other congenital or acquired immune deficiency syndromes[12] are also at risk for developing liver abscess. In a review of adult liver transplant recipients, allograft abscess was reported in 1% of cases, with hepatic arterial thrombosis being a significant risk factor.[13] Hepatic "mini-microabscess syndrome" has recently been described in pediatric liver transplant recipients.[14] Liver abscesses have been reported in children with Crohn disease[15] and sickle cell anemia.[16] Ingestion of sharp objects,[17] penetrating injuries to the liver,[18] and the presence of a ventriculoperitoneal shunt[19] can be complicated by the development of liver abscesses. Pyogenic liver abscess also occurs in healthy immunocompetent children, yet no specific etiology is identified in many of these "cryptogenic" cases.[20] The development of liver abscess in neonates is usually associated with umbilical venous catheterization, prematurity, and necrotizing enterocolitis requiring surgical intervention.[7]

MICROBIOLOGY

A number of pathogenic bacteria can cause pyogenic liver abscess; in some cases, more than one pathogen is recovered (Table 51.2-1). In a review of 96 children with pyogenic liver abscess, Staphylococcus aureus was the most common pathogen, seen in 44% of the cases, followed by gram-negative enteric organisms such as Escherichia coli, Pseudomonas, and Klebsiella in 25% of cases and anaerobic organisms in 10% of cases.[21] An increasing role for anaerobes as a source of infection has been appreciated in both adults and children, probably owing to improvement in anaerobic culture techniques.[22] Recently, a severe form of liver abscess owing to Klebsiella pneumoniae along with endophthalmitis has been reported in diabetic adults from Taiwan.[23] In neonates with liver abscess, gram-negative enteric organisms are the most common pathogens isolated.[7] Patients with CGD have a high frequency of S. aureus, but gram-negative enteric organisms that produce catalase have also been noted.

Knowledge of the source or route of infection can be helpful in predicting a particular pathogen. S. aureus is the

TABLE 51.2-1   INFECTIONS OF THE LIVER

BACTERIA
Staphylococcus aureus
Streptococci
Escherichia coli
Pseudomonas aeruginosa
Klebsiella
Proteus
Enterococcus fecalis
Serratia
Salmonella
Brucella
Gonococci
Bartonella

RICKETTSIA
R. rickettsii
Coxiella

PARASITES
Amebiasis
Malaria
Ascariasis
Echinococcosis
Clonorchiasis
Fascioliasis
Schistosomiasis

FUNGI
Candida
Histoplasma
Aspergillus
Cryptococci
Coccidiodes

ANAEROBES
Peptostreptococci
Bacteroides
Clostridium

SPIROCHETES
Leptospira
Borrelia

most likely organism in children with liver abscess following bacteremia or in those who are immunocompromised. Gram-negative enteric organisms and anaerobes are likely culprits when infection spreads to the portal venous system from the gastrointestinal tract. Fungal liver abscesses may occur in neutropenic children with leukemia who have been on broad-spectrum antibiotics.[10] Patients with acquired immune deficiency syndrome (AIDS) are at increased risk for mycobacterial abscesses owing to *Mycobacterium tuberculosis* and *Mycobacterium avium-intracellulare.*[12]

CLINICAL FEATURES

In children, the clinical manifestations of pyogenic liver abscesses are nonspecific. A high index of suspicion is necessary to establish the diagnosis, particularly in those patients with predisposing risk factors. The presentation may be acute, with rapid onset of severe symptoms, or chronic, with a more insidious onset over weeks to months. The most common presenting complaints are fever and abdominal pain. Many patients have other associated symptoms, including nausea, vomiting, anorexia, malaise, and weakness. Some children present only with

fever of unknown origin. Hepatomegaly is present in 50 to 73% of children with hepatic abscess,[6,20] and right upper quadrant tenderness is noted in 40% of cases.[20] Other findings such as abdominal distention or evidence of pleuropulmonary involvement are uncommon on physical examination. The diagnosis of liver abscess in neonates is especially difficult because the presentation is often similar to neonatal sepsis.[24] Children from developing countries tend to have a more acute presentation, with fever, abdominal pain, tender hepatomegaly, and septic shock.[1,25]

DIAGNOSIS

Routine laboratory tests, like the clinical presentation, are nonspecific and are of little value for establishing the diagnosis of liver abscess. Anemia and leukocytosis are typically seen; however, children with underlying malignancy on chemotherapy may be leukopenic.[3] Hepatic transaminases are usually normal or only mildly elevated. Elevation in serum alkaline phosphatase and bilirubin is present in cases secondary to biliary obstruction. Although the yield of aerobic and anaerobic blood cultures is variable and may be quite low, the documentation of bacteremia with the identification of a specific organism is most helpful for directing treatment. Patients with multiple abscesses are more likely to have positive blood cultures than those with a solitary abscess. In a review of neonates with liver abscesses, half of the patients were bacteremic with the same organism that was eventually cultured from the liver abscess.[7]

Radiologic imaging is the most important tool for establishing the diagnosis of liver abscess. Plain chest radiographs may be abnormal, with the presence of an elevated right hemidiaphragm, right pleural effusion, or air in the abscess cavity. Historically, radioactive-isotope liver-spleen scanning or angiography was used to establish the diagnosis. However, the recent advent of noninvasive imaging techniques, including ultrasonography and computed tomography (CT), has allowed for easy, quick, and accurate diagnosis. Ultrasonography is the imaging study of choice in suspected liver abscess because of its high sensitivity and the relative ease with which it can be performed, even in very young infants. On ultrasonography, abscesses appear as hypoechoic lesions with irregular borders (Figure 51.2-1). In children, a solitary (rather than multiple) abscess located in the right (rather than left) lobe of the liver is the most common finding.[25] The differential diagnosis of a solitary hypoechoic liver lesion includes congenital hepatic cyst, liver tumor, or hydatid cyst. On ultrasonography, pyogenic abscesses are more likely to have a "honeycomb" pattern with irregular margins compared with amebic abscesses.[26] CT (Figure 51.2-2) should be requested in the face of a normal sonogram if the clinical suspicion remains high. Magnetic resonance imaging of a hepatic abscess offers no significant advantage over CT or ultrasonography for detecting or characterizing liver abscess.[27]

TREATMENT

Antibiotic therapy with drainage of the pus collection is the mainstay of therapy for liver abscess. Supportive management in the form of intravenous hydration and analge-

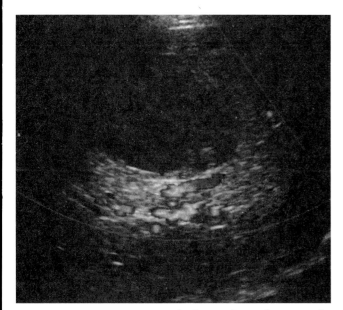

FIGURE 51.2-1 A sonogram of a large solitary abscess in the right lobe of the liver. The abscess appears as a hypoechoic lesion with irregular borders. Courtesy of Dr. D. H. Jamieson, British Columbia's Children's Hospital, Vancouver, BC.

sia may be required. Initial antibiotic therapy should be empiric, broad spectrum, and based on knowledge of the organisms most commonly involved, as discussed earlier. A penicillinase-resistant penicillin should be used, along with an aminoglycoside or third-generation cephalosporin for gram-negative flora, whereas clindamycin, cefoxitin, and metronidazole are appropriate for anaerobes. Empiric parenteral antibiotic therapy should not be delayed, pending the abscess drainage procedure. Once pathogens are identified in blood or abscess cultures, antibiotic therapy can be tailored to susceptibility.

Drainage of the liver abscess can be performed by needle aspiration, percutaneous catheter, or an open surgical approach. In a recent controlled trial, percutaneous continuous catheter drainage was more effective than therapeutic large-needle aspiration.[28] Other reports have documented the safety and efficacy of percutaneous drainage, although left lobe abscesses are more difficult to treat by this route.[6,29] The duration of continuous percutaneous drainage is usually 2 to 3 weeks, whereas parenteral antibiotic therapy should be maintained for at least 2 to 4 weeks, followed by oral antibiotics for a total of 4 to 6 weeks. Longer treatment may be required in immunocompromised children. In a recent report of pyogenic liver abscess in adults, sequential intravenous therapy for 3 weeks followed by oral antibiotics for 3 weeks was safe and equally effective compared with 6-week intravenous antibiotic therapy.[30] Serial ultrasonographic imaging of the abscess cavity and clinical response are helpful in deciding the duration of antibiotic therapy. In a recent series of adults with pyogenic liver abscesses, percutaneous drainage of liver abscesses was associated with a success rate of 90%.[2] Open surgical drainage should be reserved for those cases in which percutaneous drainage is not feasible or fails or cases in which other intra-abdominal pathology is sus-

pected. Drainage procedures may be associated with complications. In a large series of children who were treated with open surgical drainage for pyogenic and amebic liver abscesses, complications such as adhesive intestinal obstruction, incisional hernia, and colonic fistula resulting from erosion of the drain were reported.[25]

Multiple hepatic microabscesses or those abscesses not amenable to continuous drainage have been successfully treated with prolonged antibiotic therapy alone. However, in a large series of South African children with pyogenic or amebic liver abscesses, conservative treatment with antibiotics was successful in only 37% of cases[25]; the remaining cases eventually required surgical drainage owing to worsening of the clinical picture. If a conservative approach is taken, close clinical monitoring with surgical backup is mandatory. The management of children with CGD is difficult. Whereas small abscesses (< 5 cm) may be treated with antibiotics alone, surgical management of larger hepatic abscesses in patients with CGD is crucial for survival.[31] Despite aggressive management, children with CGD may be resistant to the standard therapeutic options of antibiotics and drainage. In this instance, interferon-γ has been employed successfully.[32] Following the successful treatment of a child with liver abscess, appropriate immunologic investigations should be planned because liver abscess may be the presenting manifestation of an immunodeficiency disorder.

OUTCOME

The complications of pyogenic liver abscess include pleural and pericardial effusions, rupture leading to peritonitis, septicemia, and shock.[25] The mortality associated with pyogenic liver abscess before 1977 was high: up to 27% in children with CGD and 42% in children without CGD.[4] The diagnosis was often missed and was established only at autopsy in many cases. A review of 109 cases of liver abscess in children (excluding neonates) from 1977 to 1988 reported a drop in mortality to 15%.[6] Recently, a mortality figure of 11% was quoted from a series from India of 18 children with pyogenic liver abscesses.[1] Recent

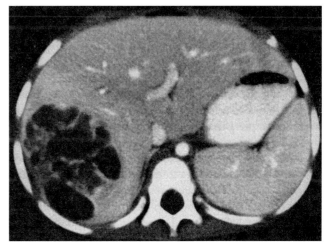

FIGURE 51.2-2 Abdominal computed tomographic scan showing a large multiloculated abscess in the right lobe of the liver.

studies in adults have also reported improvement in mortality rates.[2] In adults, the most important determinant of mortality is the presence of major underlying disease such as malignancy or severe organ dysfunction.[2] Early diagnosis and prompt therapeutic intervention are also important determinants for survival.[2] Thus, the overall outcome for pyogenic liver abscess has been improving in recent years. The principal reasons for this are improvements in imaging techniques (allowing for prompt diagnosis), the introduction of efficacious antibiotic therapy, and novel interventional radiologic techniques.

OTHER BACTERIAL INFECTIONS

TYPHOID FEVER

Typhoid fever (enteric fever) is an acute systemic illness usually caused by *Salmonella typhi*. It is a major health problem in tropical and developing countries but is uncommon in developed countries. The presenting symptoms, reported in a series of 94 children with typhoid fever from Florida, included fever, diarrhea, vomiting, abdominal pain, and anorexia.[33] Hepatomegaly and splenomegaly were noted in 52% and 23% of children, respectively. A mild elevation of serum hepatic transaminases was noted in the majority of patients in that series, but clinical jaundice was uncommon.[33] In developing countries, clinical and biochemical evidence of hepatic dysfunction is much more obvious, particularly in multidrug-resistant typhoid fever.[34] In one series of adult patients, abnormal liver enzymes were noted in 100% of cases after the first week of typhoid fever, and it was proposed that the liver is always affected to some degree in these patients.[35] Rarely, typhoid fever can mimic an acute viral hepatitis, with fever and moderately abnormal liver enzymes being the sole clinical features.[36] Histologic features on liver biopsy are nonspecific and include focal necrosis with mononuclear infiltrate, inflammation of the portal area, and hyperplasia of Kupffer cells.[35] Other organ complications of typhoid fever in children include encephalopathy, seizures, myocarditis, and circulatory failure. The serodiagnosis of *S. typhi* infection using the Widal agglutination assay is unreliable and not recommended. The diagnosis can be established by positive blood culture or through novel molecular biologic techniques using deoxyribonucleic acid (DNA) probes and polymerase chain reaction (PCR). The abnormal liver function tests seen in typhoid fever completely resolve with appropriate antibiotic treatment.[35] Multidrug-resistant typhoid fever is an increasing problem in tropical countries, and ciprofloxacin and ceftriaxone have been used in such cases.[37] The chronic carrier state for typhoid fever is thought to be due to persistent infection in the liver or gallbladder.

BRUCELLOSIS

Brucellosis is primarily a zoonotic infection, caused by *Brucella melitensis*, *Brucella abortus*, or *Brucella suis*.[38] The mode of transmission to humans is direct contact with infected animals, such as cattle and sheep, or consumption of infected unpasteurized milk or milk products. Brucellosis in childhood can present with nonspecific symptoms. In a series of 102 children with brucellosis, the common

symptoms were fever, malaise, arthralgia, weight loss, and anorexia.[39] Hepatomegaly was noted in 28% of children in that series, and splenomegaly was present in 35% of cases. Complications of brucellosis include osteomyelitis, pneumonitis, meningitis, and endocarditis. Hepatosplenic abscess has been reported in a 3-year-old child, but this appears to be a rare complication.[40] Common laboratory features include leukocytosis and an elevated erythrocyte sedimentation rate. Elevated hepatic transaminases and alkaline phosphatase were noted in 58% of children.[38] Histopathologic findings in the liver are variable and include inflammation of the portal tract, hepatocellular necrosis, and noncaseating epithelioid granuloma.[41]

The diagnosis of brucellosis should be suspected with a history of exposure, and diagnosis is confirmed by isolation of the organisms in blood or bone marrow cultures. A presumptive diagnosis can be made by high or rising titers of *Brucella* antibodies. Brucellosis responds well to antibiotic therapy, and the prognosis is excellent. In a large multicenter study of children with brucellosis, tetracycline for 3 weeks with initial gentamicin therapy was recommended as the most appropriate therapy for children older than 8 years.[42] For younger children, trimethoprim-sulfamethoxazole can be used in place of tetracycline.

PERIHEPATITIS (FITZ-HUGH–CURTIS SYNDROME)

Perihepatitis, or Fitz-Hugh–Curtis syndrome, occurs as a complication of pelvic inflammatory disease in young adolescent females. Although the classic cause is *Neisseria gonorrhoeae*, this syndrome has also been described with *Chlamydia trachomatis* infection.[43] The pathophysiology of this syndrome is uncertain, and direct extension of the infection from the genital tract to the hepatic capsule is a possible mechanism.[44] The clinical presentation is one of acute, sharp, right upper quadrant abdominal pain, with or without fever, mimicking the signs of acute cholecystitis.[45,46] Clinical findings may include hepatomegaly, tenderness in the right upper quadrant, and a "friction rub" over the liver. Serum hepatic enzymes and bilirubin are normal.[45]

The history and physical findings of the associated pelvic inflammatory disease are suggestive of the diagnosis, and isolation of the causative organisms from the cervix or urethra confirms the diagnosis. Laparoscopic findings include classic "violin string" adhesions from the liver to the right costal wall.[47] The hepatic parenchyma does not appear to be involved, and liver biopsy findings are normal. Treatment with appropriate antibiotics for the causative organisms is associated with an excellent response.

CAT-SCRATCH DISEASE

Cat-scratch disease is an infective illness caused by the gram-negative bacillus *Bartonella* (previously *Rochalimaea*) *hensalae*. Following inoculation of the bacillus, a papule occurs locally, which vesiculates and then encrusts. Within a few days, regional lymphadenopathy (which may suppurate or remain enlarged for a few months) is noted. Although cat-scratch disease occurs in persons of all ages, the highest incidence is among children under 10 years of age.[48] In more than 75% of children, the illness is mild, with generalized myalgias, malaise, anorexia, fever, and abdominal pain.[49] Unusual clinical manifestations include preauricular lymphadenopathy and conjunctivitis (Parinaud oculoglandular syndrome), pneumonia, erythema nodosum, encephalitis, and granulomatous hepatitis. Cat-scratch disease can also present as a prolonged fever of unknown origin, with or without any obvious adenopathy.[50,51]

Serum hepatic transaminases, alkaline phosphatase, and bilirubin are usually normal, and the erythrocyte sedimentation rate is often elevated. Abdominal imaging (ultrasonography and CT), usually performed as part of the evaluation for fever of unknown origin, may reveal multiple small hypoechogenic lesions in the liver and spleen, with mild enlargement of both organs.[50,52] In a recent retrospective study of 13 children with hypoechogenic liver lesions, 70% were found to have *Bartonella* infection.[51] Liver histology showed epithelioid granuloma with central necrosis and chronic inflammation. Warthin-Starry–stained bacilli may be found in the biopsy specimen. The indirect fluorescence antibody test for *B. henselae* provides a rapid and reliable diagnostic test.[51] The disease is self-limiting in nature, and complete resolution, without any therapy, of radiographically detected hepatic lesions has been reported.[50] However, antibiotics such as ciprofloxacin, azithromycin, and doxycycline have been used in severe cases with good response.[48,53] In a recent report from Texas, 2-week rifampicin therapy resulted in rapid improvement in symptoms and was recommended as an initial antimicrobial treatment of hepatosplenic cat-scratch disease in children.[54]

SPIROCHETAL INFECTIONS

Leptospirosis. Leptospirosis is caused by one of several serotypes of *Leptospira interrogans*. Humans acquire infection by exposure to urine or other body fluids of infected animals such as dogs, cattle, hogs, and rats. Leptospirosis is usually a biphasic illness with an initial septicemic or leptospiremic phase lasting 4 to 7 days, characterized by fever, chills, headache, anorexia, abdominal pain, rash, and lymphadenopathy.[55] A second or immune phase, thought to be caused by the host response to the infection, is heralded by a lower-grade fever and complications including hepatitis, jaundice, renal dysfunction, thrombocytopenia, and meningitis. In one series from Brazil, significant jaundice was noted in 70% of infected children, and abnormal liver transaminases were seen in 56%.[56] In another series, 55% of children with leptospirosis had hepatomegaly and acalculus cholecystitis.[57]

Weil syndrome is a rare severe form of leptospirosis associated with hepatic dysfunction, renal failure, hemorrhagic manifestations, and pulmonary involvement, and it portends a high mortality rate.[55] Abnormal laboratory findings in Weil syndrome include direct hyperbilirubinemia, elevated serum transaminases, and prolonged prothrombin time.[55] Histologic changes in the liver include multinucleated cells, proliferation of Kupffer cells, erythrophagocytosis, and cholestasis.[55] Severe hepatic necrosis is unusual, and complete recovery of liver function is seen in those who survive. The diagnosis of leptospirosis requires a high

index of suspicion and is confirmed by isolating the organism from blood, cerebrospinal fluid, or urine. A fourfold increase in antibody titers between acute and convalescent sera also establishes the diagnosis.[56] Optimal treatment of leptospirosis is with penicillin or ampicillin, along with supportive management. Antibiotics have been shown to be of significant benefit even in late-presenting or severe cases of leptospirosis.[58] The mortality in children has been reported as 2% in one series, with death owing to respiratory failure secondary to pulmonary hemorrhage.[56]

Lyme Disease. Lyme disease is a multisystem infection caused by *Borrelia burgdorferi*. It is transmitted to humans through the bite of a deer tick. Lyme disease is the most common vectorborne disease among children in the United States.[59] The clinical presentation includes nonspecific symptoms of fever, malaise, and headache associated with a characteristic annular erythematous skin rash (erythema chronicum migrans), which is present in approximately 68% of infected children.[60] The complications of Lyme disease in children include arthritis, facial palsy, aseptic meningitis, and carditis.

Rarely, Lyme disease can present in childhood as acute hepatitis with fever, jaundice, and elevated liver transaminases.[61] In a large prospective series of adults with Lyme disease, 40% of patients had at least one liver test abnormality, whereas 27% had more than one abnormality.[62] These improved significantly or resolved completely after antibiotic therapy. The diagnosis of Lyme disease should be suspected with a history of a tick bite in an endemic area and with finding the classic skin rash on examination. Serologic testing for *B. burgdorferi* is diagnostic. Treatment is with tetracycline except for children under 9 years of age, in whom cefuroxime, amoxicillin, or erythromycin should be used.[63] The prognosis for children adequately treated for Lyme disease is excellent, with no long-term morbidity.[59]

RICKETTSIAL INFECTIONS

Rocky Mountain Spotted Fever. Rocky Mountain spotted fever is a clinical syndrome characterized by fever, headache, and a classic maculopapular rash that begins peripherally and spreads to involve the entire body. The disease is caused by *Rickettsia rickettsii*, and ticks serve as vectors for transmission. The clinical presentation is usually with fever, myalgia, rash, headache, abdominal pain, and vomiting.[64] Hepatic involvement may occur in the form of hepatomegaly and jaundice. Variable elevations of serum hepatic transaminases and alkaline phosphatase have been reported.[64] Pathologic changes in one postmortem pediatric study revealed marked inflammation of the portal triad with portal vasculitis and sinusoidal erythrophagocytosis.[65] Rickettsiae have been found in portal blood vessels and in cells of the sinusoidal lining.

A diagnosis of Rocky Mountain spotted fever requires a high index of clinical suspicion. Disease confirmation is established by demonstrating a fourfold rise in antibody titer in the second or third week of illness, using a complement fixation serologic test. About 70 to 80% of patients will have a positive Weil-Felix reaction, but the test is not specific. Treatment with tetracycline or chloramphenicol is most effective. The treatment should not be delayed pending laboratory diagnosis because untreated infection can lead to severe ilness and fatal outcome.[66]

Q Fever. Q fever is a febrile illness caused by *Coxiella burnetii*. The usual mode of transmission is inhalation, and the animal hosts include cattle, sheep, and goats. The disease presents in acute and chronic forms. Hepatic involvement is common in the acute form, heralded by fever, headache, malaise, vomiting, abdominal pain, and respiratory symptoms. Hepatosplenomegaly may be present on physical examination. In one series, 11 of 13 children with Q fever had elevation of hepatic transaminases.[67] Although quite rare, fulminant hepatic failure and death have been reported in childhood.[68] Liver histology in Q fever shows fatty change with diffuse granulomatous lesions.[69] A classic histopathologic finding is fibrin ring granuloma with a central clear space (Figure 51.2-3). The diagnosis of Q fever is confirmed by serologic testing. The treatment of choice is tetracycline, although most patients recover uneventfully without any specific treatment.

PARASITIC INFECTIONS

AMEBIASIS

Amebiasis is caused by the protozoan *Entamoeba histolytica*. It occurs in all parts of the world and is endemic in southern and western Africa, the Far East, South and Central America, and the Indian subcontinent. In the United States, the prevalence of amebiasis is estimated to be about 4%.[70] The epidemiologic risk factors predisposing to amebiasis are lower socioeconomic status, crowding, poor sanitation, immigration from an area of endemicity, and young age, including infancy.[70] *E. histolytica* is an enteric pathogen that exists in either trophozoite or cyst form. Transmission is by the fecal-oral route, and the infection is acquired by the ingestion of cysts. Cysts dissolve during passage through the small bowel and mature into trophozoites. Trophozoites colonize the colon and may encyst or invade the colonic epithelium, resulting in colitis. Trophozoites reach the liver via the portal venous system and penetrate into the hepatic parenchyma, leading to hepatic abscess. An amebic abscess cavity contains acellular proteinaceous debris surrounded by necrotic hepatic tissue.[71] Fever and right upper quadrant pain are the most common symptoms of hepatic amebic abscess. A history of dysentery may be present; it was reported in up to 16% of childhood cases in one series.[72] On examination, tender hepatomegaly and abdominal distention are usually seen. Clinical jaundice is uncommon. Patients may also present with respiratory symptoms secondary to rupture of the abscess into the pleura or tracheobronchial tree. Rupture of the abscess into the peritoneum may lead to an acute abdomen, and intrapericardial rupture may present as shock.[73]

Routine laboratory tests are of limited value in the diagnosis of hepatic amebic abscess. In one large series, anemia and leukocytosis were seen in more than 90% of children,

whereas abnormality of serum transaminases and alkaline phosphatase was observed in only 16% of cases.[72] Examination of stool for cysts or trophozoites is positive in only a minority of cases. Ultrasonography or CT can provide anatomic verification and intrahepatic localization of the abscess cavity. Amebic abscess is usually solitary and is seen in the right hepatic lobe in 75% of cases.[72] Reliable differentiation between amebic and pyogenic abscess is difficult on ultrasonographic appearance alone, but an amebic abscess is likely to have a better defined margin with a peripheral "halo."[26] If a diagnosis of amebic liver abscess cannot be made on the basis of serology and clinical features, needle aspiration of the abscess can exclude the possibility of pyogenic abscess. Aspiration of an amebic abscess yields a reddish brown fluid that has the appearance of anchovy paste.[21] Amebae are usually not recovered from the abscess fluid, and the pus is sterile.

The development of serologic tests for the diagnosis of amebiasis has virtually eliminated the need for needle aspiration. These tests include indirect immunofluorescence, indirect hemagglutination, and enzyme-linked immunosorbent assay.[71] In a recent study, elevated indirect hemagglutination titers (> 1:250) were seen in all children with amebic liver abscess.[72] However, serologic testing may not be as reliable in young infants. In one review, only 62% of infants with amebic abscess had a positive serologic test at presentation.[74] Because each individual test is not always positive, the use of at least two different serologic tests is recommended for diagnostic purposes.

In contrast to pyogenic liver abscess, amebic liver abscess can be successfully treated with antibiotics alone, without aspiration or drainage. Metronidazole (30–50 mg/kg/d in three divided doses for 10 days) is the therapy of choice. A course of intestinal amebicide such as diloxanide furoate (10 mg/kg/d for 10 days) or iodoquinol (30–40 mg/kg/d [maximum 2 g/d] in three doses for 20 days) should be given following metronidazole therapy to eradicate the intraluminal infection.[70] Needle aspiration is recommended when a clinical response is not evident within 48 hours after

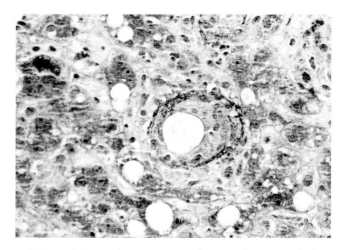

FIGURE 51.2-3 Fibrin ring granuloma with a central clear space in a patient with Q fever (hematoxylin and eosin; ×400 original magnification). Courtesy of Dr. F. A. Mitros, University of Iowa Hospital, Iowa City, IA.

starting medical therapy.[72] Other indications for needle aspiration include an abscess cavity larger than 7 cm and abscesses located in the left lobe (because of the higher risk for pericardial involvement).[72] Surgical intervention is necessary for ruptured amebic abscesses.[73] In one large series, antibiotic therapy along with timely aspiration of the abscess obviated the need for surgical intervention, even in malnourished children who presented late for treatment.[72] The prognosis for uncomplicated amebic abscess is usually good.[71] In infancy, however, the clinical course can be fulminant, with a high mortality rate.[74]

MALARIA

Malaria is caused by *Plasmodium vivax*, *Plasmodium falciparum*, *Plasmodium ovale*, and *Plasmodium malariae*. Malaria is an important cause of morbidity and mortality in tropical and subtropical countries, with an estimated incidence of 300 to 500 million cases per year. Malaria is acquired from the bite of infected female anopheline mosquitoes. Sporozoites injected into the bloodstream reach hepatocytes, where further division and maturation take place. Merozoites released from the hepatocytes invade erythrocytes. The symptoms of malaria include fever, abdominal pain, vomiting, and diarrhea.[75] Fever and chills may be periodic (every 48 to 72 hours) or may occur daily. *P. falciparum* infection can result in severe life-threatening disease with complications such as seizures, coma, renal failure, severe anemia, shock, and (rarely) hepatic failure.[76] On examination, tender hepatosplenomegaly is a common finding. Jaundice, usually owing to hemolysis, and mild elevation of liver enzymes may be seen.[75]

Histologic findings in the liver include hyperplasia of Kupffer cells and diffuse periportal infiltration with mononuclear cells.[76] The diagnosis of malaria is established by the detection of parasites in thin and thick peripheral blood smears prepared with Giemsa stains. The drug of choice for all uncomplicated malaria except chloroquine-resistant *P. falciparum* is chloroquine phosphate (10 mg of base per kilogram to a maximum of 600 mg of base [a 1 g tablet] and then half the dose [maximum 500 mg] given once daily beginning 6 hours later, for 2 days). For severe and complicated malaria, quinine is the parenteral drug of choice supplemented with aggressive supportive management.[77] For chloroquine-resistant strains, quinine or mefloquine may be used.

ASCARIASIS

Ascariasis, caused by *Ascaris lumbricoides* (roundworm), is the most prevalent helminthic infection in the world. Although cases have been reported worldwide, ascariasis mostly occurs in developing tropical and subtropical countries. Ascariasis is most common in childhood and is endemic to areas with poor sanitation. The transmission is via the fecal-oral route. Ingested eggs eventually mature into the adult worm in the small intestine. The clinical manifestations of ascariasis depend on whether the worms reside in the intestinal lumen or whether they invade the pancreatic and biliary ductal system. The usual symptoms are vague abdominal pain and distention.[78] Some heavily

infected children may present with an acute abdomen secondary to intestinal obstruction from the mass of worms.[79] Worms invading the ampullary orifice can induce biliary colic or acute pancreatitis.[80] Worm obstruction of the bile duct system can cause acalculous cholecystitis, pyogenic cholangitis, or acute pancreatitis in children.[78] In a report from a children's hospital in Burma, ascariasis was the culprit in acute surgical cases such as biliary obstruction, volvulus, and intestinal obstruction and perforation, accounting for 26.3% of emergency abdominal laparotomies in children.[79] Hepatic abscess has been reported in children and adults owing to worms obstructing the intrahepatic bile ducts.[5,80] In children from developing countries, ascariasis has been considered a predisposing factor for pyogenic liver abscess.[1,5]

The diagnosis of ascariasis is made by the finding of ova in the stools or by a history of passing worms. Elevation of liver enzymes and serum bilirubin may be seen in cases of biliary ascariasis. Ultrasonography of the abdomen is very useful in diagnosing complications, including cholecystitis, biliary tract dilatation, and hepatic abscess.[78] Rarely, an echogenic wormlike structure may be seen within the bile duct on ultrasonography.[81] Worms may also be seen on endoscopic retrograde cholangiopancreatography, and *Ascaris* ova can be found in the bile sample.[80] The treatment of ascariasis is with mebendazole (100 mg twice daily for 3 days) or piperazine salts (50–75 mg/kg/d for 2 days). Surgery may be required for selective obstructive cases, although biliary obstruction and colic symptoms have been treated by the removal of worms with endoscopic retrograde cholangiopancreatography.[80]

ECHINOCOCCOSIS

Echinococcus granulosus infection is found throughout the world and is endemic in sheep- and cattle-raising areas, including the Mediterranean, Australia, New Zealand, and parts of Asia, Europe, and South and North America. Echinococci are small tapeworms that inhabit the intestine of the definitive host, usually dogs, and humans acquire the infection by the ingestion of ova. The parasites may lodge in the liver or lungs of affected patients, leading to the formation of hydatid cysts. The cyst has a thick lamellar layer that supports a thin germinal layer of cells responsible for the budding and production of protoscoleces (Figure 51.2-4). The cyst is surrounded by a fibrous capsule produced by the host. Hydatid cysts may occur in other sites, such as the kidney, spleen, brain, eyes, and pancreas. Although the infection is acquired in childhood, symptoms may not occur for many years owing to the slow growth of hydatid cysts (1 cm in diameter per year).[82]

The clinical presentation of a hydatid cyst of the liver depends on the size of the cyst and on the complications arising owing to the cyst. Common symptoms in children with hepatic hydatid cysts include abdominal pain, abdominal mass, fever, and anorexia.[83] Some children are totally asymptomatic, with the abdominal mass detected incidentally on physical examination. Large hepatic cysts may compress on the venous system or the biliary tract, leading to portal hypertension or obstructive jaundice,[79]

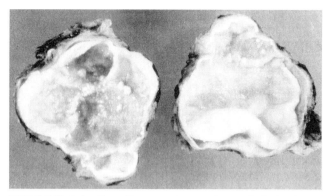

FIGURE 51.2-4   Gross liver resection specimen of a hydatid cyst.

respectively.[84] Cysts may rupture into the biliary tract or the peritoneal or pleural cavities. Anaphylaxis may occur owing to the release of the highly antigenic cystic fluid.[82] Laboratory tests are not specific for the diagnosis of echinococcosis. Eosinophilia, elevated liver enzymes, and hyperbilirubinemia may be present. Plain abdominal radiographs of the abdomen or chest may show a calcified mass. Ultrasonography is useful for diagnosing and localizing the cyst, but imaging does not readily differentiate echinococcal disease from other solitary cysts of the liver unless daughter cysts are present or intracystic septations or calcification of the cyst wall are recognized (see Figure 51.2–4). Definitive diagnosis can be made either by positive serology to *E. granulosus* or by demonstrating the presence of scoleces in the cystic fluid.

Historically, the optimal treatment for hepatic hydatid cyst was surgical, with care taken to avoid spillage of cystic fluid. However, novel reports favor conservative management for uncomplicated cysts. Careful percutaneous drainage combined with albendazole therapy was found to be an effective and safe alternative to surgery in adults.[84] In one long-term follow-up study from Israel, the use of albendazole therapy alone was associated with a cure in 41% of patients with hepatic hydatid cysts and with improvement in another 41% of adult patients.[85] In a recent report from Turkey, 3-month albendazole therapy resulted in successful resolution of hepatic cysts in 27% of children, and medical therapy was recommended as an initial therapy prior to surgery.[86] Medical therapy has also been suggested for children with hydatid cysts under 5 cm in size or for cases in which multiple cysts or multiorgan involvement occurs.[83]

LIVER FLUKE INFECTION

Clonorchiasis. Clonorchiasis, caused by *Clonorchis sinensis*, a liver fluke, is endemic throughout the Far East. Infection is acquired by the consumption of raw infected fish, which act as one of the intermediate hosts, along with snails.[87] The parasite migrates from the duodenum into the biliary ductal system and matures in the intrahepatic bile ducts. The injury to bile ducts manifests as adenomatous proliferation and goblet cell metaplasia.[88] Secondary infection occurs frequently, and recurrent pyogenic cholangitis can lead to stricture, periductal fibrosis, and hepatic

abscess.[88] Patients with mild disease may be asymptomatic, whereas more severe cases present with recurrent cholangitis, biliary duct obstruction, or portal hypertension.[89] Cholangiocarcinoma has been reported with long-standing disease in adults.[90] Laboratory findings include variable elevation of liver enzymes and bilirubin. Ultrasonography is useful for assessing abnormalities in the biliary ductal system. The diagnosis is made by stool or duodenal aspirate examination for *Clonorchis* eggs. Praziquantel is the drug of choice for treatment.[89]

Fascioliasis. Fascioliasis is caused by *Fasciola hepatica*, the sheep liver fluke, and is found worldwide. Human infection is acquired by ingestion of infected watercress or water. The parasites penetrate the duodenal wall, traverse the peritoneal cavity, and penetrate the hepatic capsule to reach the bile ducts. The disease has two phases: an acute invasive phase, during which the parasite is migrating through the liver, and a chronic phase, during which it resides in the biliary tract.[91] Acute clinical manifestations in childhood include prolonged fever, abdominal pain, and tender hepatomegaly.[92] Significant eosinophilia, raised sedimentation rate, and elevated serum alkaline phosphatase are typically seen. Serum hepatic transaminases are usually normal or only mildly elevated.[91] CT may show abscess-like nodular lesions or multiple hypodense areas in the liver.[93] Liver biopsy findings include eosinophilic abscess (parasitic granuloma) and coagulative necrosis. Chronic fascioliasis can cause biliary colic, jaundice, cholangitis, and pancreatitis owing to obstruction of the bile ducts.[91] The diagnosis is by serologic testing or by finding *F. hepatica* ova in the stool. In a recent report from Egypt, triclabendazole (10 mg/kg single dose) was highly effective and was recommended as the treatment of choice in children.[94]

Schistosomiasis. Schistosomiasis is an important cause of morbidity and mortality in tropical countries. Hepatic schistosomiasis is caused by *Schistosoma mansoni* and *Schistosoma japonicum*. Endemic areas for *S. mansoni* include Africa, the Middle East, and South America, whereas *S. japonicum* infection is endemic in Central and Southeast Asia. Human infection occurs when schistosomes, released from a snail host, penetrate intact human skin. The parasites then migrate to the liver, enter into the portal venous system, and finally reside in the mesenteric veins.[95] Granulomatous hepatic lesions occur as a result of the host's immunologic response to the ova in the portal venous system (Figure 51.2-5). Fibrosis around branches of the portal veins subsequently leads to portal hypertension. Hepatic parenchymal function is usually preserved.

Infection occurs mainly in childhood or adolescence. Acute schistosomiasis (also known as Katayama fever), presumably a consequence of the host's immunologic response to mature worms and eggs, occurs about 4 to 6 weeks after exposure. Clinical features vary and include fever, cough, edema, lymphadenopathy, and eosinophilia.[95] Untreated acute schistosomiasis progresses to chronic disease, resulting in portal hypertension. Children may present with upper gastrointestinal bleeding owing to esophageal varices.

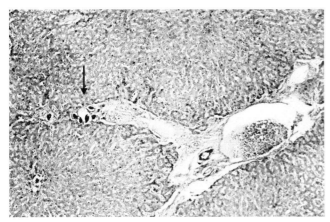

FIGURE 51.2-5 Schistosomiasis with multiple ova (*arrow*) embedded in a fibrotic portal triad (hematoxylin and eosin; ×200 original magnification). Courtesy of Dr. F. A. Mitros, University of Iowa Hospital, Iowa City, IA.

Hepatosplenomegaly can reach massive proportions, and ascites is present in some cases.[95] Other potential complications associated with hepatosplenic schistosomiasis are pulmonary hypertension, myocarditis, and transverse myelitis. Prolonged *Salmonella* infection may be a concurrent feature.

Laboratory features of anemia, leukopenia, and thrombocytopenia may be seen owing to hypersplenism. Eosinophilia and hyperglobulinemia may also occur, but liver function tests are usually normal.[96] Ultrasonography has been used to detect and grade the degree of periportal fibrosis and portal hypertension.[97] Serologic studies using *S. mansoni* egg antigen are helpful for diagnosis. The diagnosis is confirmed by detecting *Schistosoma* eggs in stool or in a rectal biopsy tissue sample. The treatment of choice is a single dose of praziquantel (20–40 mg/kg three times a day for 1 day), resulting in eradication of the parasite in 90% of cases[95] and reversal of periportal fibrosis in some children.[97] The management of portal hypertension and esophageal variceal bleeding may be difficult; however, in most instances, sclerotherapy has been effective. The use of propranolol for the management of portal hypertension in children has not been well studied.[98]

FUNGAL INFECTIONS

CANDIDIASIS
Candida infections are the most frequently encountered systemic fungal infections, with infection of the liver and spleen occurring as a consequence of seeding during fungemia. Candidiasis usually occurs in immunocompromised patients, particularly those on chemotherapy for malignancy. Acute leukemia was the most common malignancy seen in children with hepatosplenic candidiasis.[10] Other risk factors for hepatosplenic candidiasis include neutropenia, recent chemotherapy, and the use of broad-spectrum antibiotics.[10] Clinical symptoms are nonspecific and usually include fever and abdominal pain. On examination, jaundice, hepatomegaly, splenomegaly, and abdominal tenderness may be found. The white blood cell count may be normal, although a history of prolonged neutropenia is usually pre-

sent. The diagnosis should be suspected in patients with persisting fever and abdominal pain even after resolution of the neutropenia.[99] *Candida* may be isolated from blood, urine, throat, or stool. Serum hepatic transaminases, alkaline phosphatase, and bilirubin are often elevated. Abdominal ultrasonography may show several hypoechoic areas throughout an enlarged liver (Figure 51.2-6). Abdominal CT features include liver enlargement with multiple well-circumscribed low-density areas of 0.5 to 2 cm in diameter, often with accompanying splenic involvement. The appearance of *Candida* abscesses is usually distinct from that of bacterial abscesses, the latter being larger and fewer in number on imaging studies.[100] A percutaneous liver biopsy can confirm the diagnosis in 70% of cases, whereas a laparoscopic or an open liver biopsy provides an even better diagnostic yield.[99] Grossly, the liver surface is studded with yellow to white nodules ranging in size from 1 mm to 2 cm.[99] Histologically, *Candida* abscesses show fungal elements in the necrotic center, surrounded by inflammatory cells and a ring of fibrosis.[101] Granulomatous lesions with occasional giant cells in the liver have also been observed.[10]

The treatment of choice is the use of antifungal agents such as amphotericin B, 5-flurocytosine, or fluconazole. In a recent international consensus conference, fluconazole was favored as first-line therapy for stable patients, whereas amphotericin B was considered the drug of choice for life-threatening infections.[102] The optimal duration of therapy is controversial, and treatment for several months may be required.[103] In the vast majority of cases, drainage of the pus is impractical because of the small size and diffuse nature of the hepatic abscesses. Many of these patients have multisystem disease, and the outcome is poor, with mortality rates in children reported as high as 20%.[10]

OTHER FUNGAL INFECTIONS
Other fungal organisms such as *Histoplasma capsulatum*, *Aspergillus* species, *Cryptococcus neoformans*, and *Coccidioides immitis* may also infect liver. Similar to candidiasis, these infections usually occur in immunocompromised patients. Children with cancer on chemotherapy are par-

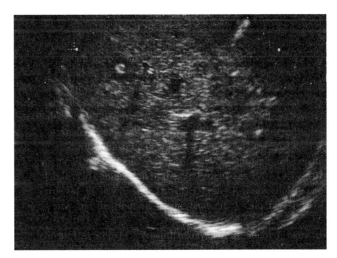

FIGURE 51.2-6 Sonogram of the liver showing multiple foci of *Candida* abscesses in a child with leukemia.

ticularly at risk.[104] Most systemic fungal infections involve organs such as the lungs, skin, central nervous system, and bones, and liver involvement is part of disseminated disease. Hepatic involvement may manifest as hepatomegaly, elevated serum hepatic transaminases, hyperbilirubinemia, and liver abscess formation.[100,105] Histologic findings in the liver include granuloma, inflammatory cells, and fungal organisms.[106] The diagnosis is made by serology or by isolation of the organisms from tissue or body fluids. Optimal treatment is with antifungal agents such as amphotericin B.

REFERENCES

1. Kumar A, Srinivasan S, Sharma AK. Pyogenic liver abscess in children—South Indian experiences. J Pediatr Surg 1998; 33:417–21.

2. Seeto RK, Rockey DC. Pyogenic liver abscess. Changes in etiology, management, and outcome. Medicine 1996;75:99–113.

3. Dehner LP, Kissane JM. Pyogenic hepatic abscesses in infancy and childhood. J Pediatr 1969;74:763–73.

4. Chusid MJ. Pyogenic hepatic abscess in infancy and childhood. Pediatrics 1978;62:554–9.

5. Hendricks MK, Moore SW, Miller AJW. Epidemiological aspects of liver abscesses in children in the Western Cape Province of South Africa. J Trop Pediatr 1997;43:103–5.

6. Pineiro-Carrero VM, Andres JM. Morbidity and mortality in children with pyogenic liver abscess. Am J Dis Child 1989; 143:1424–7.

7. Doerr CA, Demmler GJ, Garcia-Prats JA, Brandt ML. Solitary pyogenic liver abscess in neonates: report of three cases and review of the literature. Pediatr Infect Dis J 1994;13:64–9.

8. Moreira-Silva SF, Pereira FEL. Intestinal nematodes, *Toxocara* infection, and pyogenic liver abscess in children: a possible association. J Trop Pediatr 2000;46:167–72.

9. Johnston RB Jr, Baehner RL. Chronic granulomatous disease: correlation between pathogenesis and clinical findings. Pediatrics 1971;48:730–9.

10. Carstensen H, Wedding E, Storm K, et al. Hepatosplenic candidiasis in children with cancer. Three cases in leukemic children and a literature review. Pediatr Hematol Oncol 1990;7:3–12.

11. Fanconi S, Seger RA, Willi U, et al. Oral chloramphenicol therapy for multiple liver abscesses in hyperimmunoglobulinemia E syndrome. Eur J Pediatr 1984;142:292–5.

12. Pottipati AR, Dave PB, Gumaste V, Vieux U. Tuberculous abscess of the liver in acquired immunodeficiency syndrome. J Clin Gastroenterol 1991;13:549–53.

13. Rabkin JM, Orloff SL, Corless CL, et al. Hepatic allograft abscess with hepatic arterial thrombosis. Am J Surg 1998;175:354–9.

14. MacDonald GA, Greenson JK, DelBuono EA, et al. Mini-microabscess syndrome in liver transplant recipients. Hepatology 1997;26:192–7.

15. Tung JY, Johnson JL, Liacouras CA. Portal-mesenteric pylephlebitis with hepatic abscesses in a patient with Crohn's disease treated successfully with anticoagulation and antibiotics. J Pediatr Gastroenterol Nutr 1996;23:474–8.

16. Lama M. Hepatic abscess in sickle cell anemia: a rare manifestation. Arch Dis Child 1993;69:242–3.

17. Lowry P, Rollins NK. Pyogenic liver abscess complicating ingestion of sharp objects. Pediatr Infect Dis J 1993;12:348–50.

18. Taguchi T, Ikeda K, Yakabe S, Kimura S. Percutaneous drainage for post-traumatic hepatic abscess in children under ultrasound imaging. Pediatr Radiol 1988;18:85–7.

19. Meyers RL, Scaife ER. Benign liver and biliary tract masses in infants and toddlers. Semin Pediatr Surg 2000;9:146–55.

20. Bilfinger TV, Hayden K, Oldham KT, Lobe TE. Pyogenic liver abscesses in nonimmunocompromised children. South Med J 1986;79:37–40.

21. Kays DW. Pediatric liver cysts and abscesses. Semin Pediatr Surg 1992;1:107–14.

22. Brook I, Fraizer EH. Role of anaerobic bacteria in liver abscesses in children. Pediatr Infect Dis J 1993;12:743–6.

23. Fung CP, Chang FY, Lee SC, et al. A global emerging disease of *Klebsiella pneumoniae* liver abscess: is serotype K1 an important factor for complicated endophthalmitis? Gut 2002;50:420–4.

24. DeFranco PE, Shook LA, Goebel J, Lee B. Solitary hepatic abscess with associated glomerulonephritis in a neonate. J Perinatol 2000;20:384–6.

25. Moore SW, Millar AJW, Cywes S. Conservative initial treatment for liver abscesses in children. Br J Surg 1994;81:872–4.

26. Oleszczuk-Raszke K, Cremin BJ, Fisher RM, et al. Ultrasonic features of pyogenic and amoebic hepatic abscesses. Pediatr Radiol 1989;19:230–3.

27. Mendez RJ, Schiebler ML, Outwater EK, Kressel HY. Hepatic abscesses: MR imaging findings. Radiology 1994;190:431–6.

28. Rajak CL, Gupta S, Jian S, et al. Percutaneous treatment of liver abscess: needle aspiration versus catheter drainage. Am J Radiol 1998;170:1035–9.

29. Vachon L, Diament MJ, Stanley P. Percutaneous drainage of hepatic abscesses in children. J Pediatr Surg 1986;21:366–8.

30. Ng FH, Wong WM, Wong BCY, et al. Sequential intravenous/oral antibiotic vs. continuous intravenous antibiotic in the treatment of pyogenic liver abscess. Aliment Pharmacol Ther 2002;16:1083–90.

31. Lubin M, Bartlett DL, Danforth DN, et al. Hepatic abscess in patients with chronic granulomatous disease. Ann Surg 2002;235:383–91.

32. Hague RA, Eastham EJ, Lee REJ, Cant AJ. Resolution of hepatic abscess after interferon gamma in chronic granulomatous disease. Arch Dis Child 1993;69:443–5.

33. Colon AR, Gross DR, Tamer MA. Typhoid fever in children. Pediatrics 1975;56:606–9.

34. Jagadish K, Patwari AK, Sarin SK, et al. Hepatic manifestations in typhoid fever. Indian Pediatr 1994;31:807–11.

35. Morgenstern R, Hayes PC. The liver in typhoid fever: always affected, not just a complication. Am J Gastroenterol 1991; 86:1235–9.

36. El-Newihi HM, Alamy ME, Reynolds TB. *Salmonella* hepatitis: analysis of 27 cases and comparison with acute viral hepatitis. Hepatology 1996;24:516–9.

37. Gupta A, Swarnkar NK, Choudhary SP. Changing antibiotic sensitivity in enteric fever. J Trop Pediatr 2001;47:369–71.

38. Dios Colmenero J, Queipo-Ortuno MI, Reguera M, et al. Chronic hepatosplenic abscesses in brucellosis. Clinicotherapeutic features and molecular diagnostic approach. Diag Microbiol Infect Dis 2002;42:158–67.

39. Al-Eissa YA, Kambal AM, Al-Nasser MN, et al. Childhood brucellosis: a study of 102 cases. Pediatr Infect Dis J 1990;9:74–9.

40. Vallejo JG, Stevens AM, Dutton RV, Kaplan SL. Hepatosplenic abscesses due to *Brucella melitensis*: report of a case involving a child and review of the literature. Clin Infect Dis 1996;22:485–9.

41. Young EJ. An overview of human brucellosis. Clin Infect Dis 1995;21:283–90.

42. Lubani MM, Dudin KI, Sharda DC, et al. A multicenter therapeutic study of 1100 children with brucellosis. Pediatr Infect Dis J 1989;8:75–8.

43. Wolner-Hanssen P, Westrom L, Mardh PA. Perihepatitis and chlamydial salpingitis. Lancet 1980;i:901–3.

44. McLain LG, Decker M, Nye D, et al. Gonococcal perihepatitis in a female adolescent. Fitz-Hugh–Curtis syndrome. JAMA 1978;239:339–40.

45. Katzman DK, Friedman IM, McDonald CA, Litt IF. Chlamydia trachomatis Fitz-Hugh-Curtis syndrome without salpingitis in female adolescents. Am J Dis Child 1988;142:996–8.

46. Tsubuku M, Hayashi S, Terahara A, et al. Fitz Hugh Curtis syndrome: linear contrast enhancement of the surface of the liver on CT. J Comp Assist Tomogr 2002 26:456–8

47. Cano A, Fernandez C, Scapa M, et al. Gonococcal perihepatitis: diagnostic and therapeutic value of laparoscopy. Am J Gastroenterol 1984;79:280–2.

48. Centers for Disease Control and Prevention. Cat-scratch disease in children-Texas, September 2000-August 2001. JAMA 2002;287:2647–9.

49. Carithers HA. Cat scratch disease. An overview based on a study of 1,200 patients. Am J Dis Child 1985;139:1124–33.

50. Malatack JJ, Jaffe R. Granulomatous hepatitis in three children due to cat-scratch disease without peripheral adenopathy. An unrecognized cause of fever of unknown origin. Am J Dis Child 1993;147:949–53.

51. Ventura A, Massei F, Not T, et al. Systemic Bartonella henselae infection with hepatosplenic involvement. J Pediatr Gastroenterol Nutr 1999;29:52–6.

52. Estrella M, Cosgrove SE. Cases from the Osler medical service at John Hopkins University. Am J Med 2002;113:344–6.

53. Holley HP Jr. Successful treatment of cat-scratch disease with ciprofloxacin. JAMA 1991;265:1563–5.

54. Arisoy ES, Correa AG, Wagner ML, Kaplan SL. Hepatosplenic cat-scratch disease in children: selected clinical features and treatment. Clin Infect Dis 1999;28:778–84.

55. Feigin RD, Anderson DC. Leptospirosis. In: Feigin RD, Cherry RD, editors. Textbook of pediatric infectious diseases. 4th ed. Philadelphia: WB Saunders; 1998. p. 1529–42.

56. Marotto PCF, Marotto MS, Santos DL, et al. Outcome of leptospirosis in children. Am J Trop Med Hyg 1997;56:307–10.

57. Wong ML, Kaplan S, Dunkle LM, et al. Leptospirosis: a childhood disease. J Pediatr 1977;90:532–7.

58. Watt G, Padre LP, Tuazon ML, et al. Placebo-controlled trial of intravenous penicillin for severe and late leptospirosis. Lancet 1988;i:433–5.

59. Shapiro ED. Lyme disease in children. Am J Med 1995;98 (4 Suppl 1):69S–73S.

60. Williams CL, Strobino B, Lee A, et al. Lyme disease in childhood: clinical and epidemiologic features of ninety cases. Pediatr Infect Dis J 1990;9:10–4.

61. Edwards KS, Kanengiser S, Li KI, Glassman M. Lyme disease presenting as hepatitis and jaundice in a child. Pediatr Infect Dis J 1990;9:592–3.

62. Horowitz HW, Dworkin B, Forseter G, et al. Liver function in early Lyme disease. Hepatology 1996;23:1412–7.

63. Eppes SC, Childs JA. Comparative study of cefuroxime axetil versus amoxicillin in children with early Lyme disease. Pediatrics 2002;109:1173–7.

64. Zaidi SA, Singer C. Gastrointestinal and hepatic manifestations of tickborne diseases in the United States. Clin Infect Dis 2002;34:1206–12.

65. Jackson MD, Kirkman C, Bradford WD, Walker DH. Rocky Mountain spotted fever: hepatic lesions in childhood cases. Pediatr Pathol 1986;5:379–88.

66. Centers for Disease Control and Prevention. Consequences of delayed diagnosis of Rocky Mountain spotted fever in chil-dren—West Virginia, Michigan, Tennessee, and Oklahoma, May-July 200. JAMA 2000;284:2049–50.

67. Ruiz-Contreras J, Montero RG, Amador TR, et al. Q fever in children. Am J Dis Child 1993;147:300–2.

68. Berkovitch M, Aladiem M, Beer S, Cohar K. A fatal case of Q fever hepatitis in a child. Helv Paediatr Acta 1985;40:87–91.

69. Hoffman CE, Heaton JW Jr. Q fever hepatitis. Clinical manifestations and pathological findings. Gastroenterology 1982;83:474–9.

70. Ravdin JI. Amebiasis. Clin Infect Dis 1995;20:1453–66.

71. Hughes MA, Petri WA. Amebic liver abscess. Infect Dis Clin North Am 2000;14:565–82.

72. Moazam F, Nazir F. Amebic liver abscess: spare the knife but save the child. J Pediatr Surg 1998;33:119–22.

73. Porras-Ramirez G, Hernandez-Herrera H, Porras-Hernandez JD. Amebic hepatic abscess in children. J Pediatr Surg 1995;30:662–4.

74. Johnson JL, Baird JS, Hulbert TV, Opas LM. Amebic liver abscess in infancy: case report and review. Clin Infect Dis 1994;19:765–7.

75. Waller D, Krishna S, Crawley J, et al. Clinical features and outcome of severe malaria in Gambian children. Clin Infect Dis 1995;21:577–87.

76. Fitch CD. Malaria. In: Feigin RD, Cherry JD, editors. Textbook of pediatric infectious diseases. 4th ed. Philadelphia: WB Saunders; 1998. p. 2437–51.

77. Murphy S, English M, Omar A, et al. The management of severe malaria in children: a review. East Afr Med J 1995;72:536–9.

78. Bahu MGS, Baldisseroto M, Custodio CM, et al. Hepatobiliary and pancreatic complications of ascariasis in children: a study of seven cases. J Pediatr Gastroenterol Nutr 2001;33:271–5.

79. Thein-Hlaing, Myat-Lay-Kyin, Hlaing-Mya, Maung-Maung. Role of ascariasis in surgical abdominal emergencies in the Rangoon Children's Hospital, Burma. Ann Trop Pediatr 1990;10:53–60.

80. Khuroo MS, Zargar SA, Mahajan R. Hepatobiliary and pancreatic ascariasis in India. Lancet 1990;335:1503–6.

81. Deeg KH. Sonographic diagnosis of biliary ascariasis. Eur J Pediatr 1990;150:95–6.

82. American Academy of Pediatrics, Committee on Infectious Diseases. Other tapeworm infections (including hydatid disease). In: Report of the Committee on Infectious Diseases. Elk Grove Village (IL): American Academy of Pediatrics; 2000. p. 562–3.

83. Senyuz OF, Celayir AC, Killic N, et al. Hydatid disease of the liver in childhood. Pediatr Surg Int 1999;15:217–20.

84. Khuroo MS, Wani NA, Javid G, et al. Percutaneous drainage compared with surgery for hepatic hydatid cysts. N Engl J Med 1997;337:881–7.

85. Nahmias J, Goldsmith R, Soibelman M, El-On J. Three to 7 year follow-up after albendazole treatment of 68 patients with cystic echinococcosis (hydatid disease). Ann Trop Med Parasitol 1994;88:295–304.

86. Demirbilek S, Sander S, Atayurt HF, Aydm G. Hydatid disease of the liver in childhood: the success of medical therapy and surgical alternatives. Pediatr Surg Int 2001;17:373–7.

87. Schantz PM. The dangers of eating raw fish. N Engl J Med 1989;320:1143–5.

88. Sun T. Pathology and immunology of Clonorchis sinensis infection of the liver. Ann Clin Lab Sci 1984;14:208–15.

89. Lin AC, Chapman SW, Turner HR, Wofford JD Jr. Clonorchiasis: an update. South Med J 1987;80:919–22.

90. Ona FV, Dytoc JNT. Clonorchis-associated cholangiocarcinoma: a report of two cases with unusual manifestations. Gastroenterology 1991;101:831–9.

91. Roig GVG. Hepatic fascioliasis in the Americas: a new challenge for therapeutic endoscopy. Gastrointest Endosc 2002;56: 315–7.

92. El-Shabrawi M, El-Karasky H, Okasha S, El-Hennawy A. Human fascioliasis: clinical features and diagnostic difficulties in Egyptian children. J Trop Pediatr 1997;43:162–6.

93. Case records of the Massachusetts General Hospital. Weekly clinicopathological exercises: case 12-2002: a 50-year-old man with eosinophilia and fluctuating hepatic lesions. N Engl J Med 2002;346:1232–9.

94. El-Karaksy H, Hassanein B, Okasha S, et al. Human fascioliasis in Egyptian children: successful treatment with triclabendazole. J Trop Pediatr 1999;45:135–8.

95. Doehring E. Schistosomiasis in childhood. Eur J Pediatr 1988; 147:2–9.

96. Strickland GT. Gastrointestinal manifestations of schistosomiasis. Gut 1994;35:1334–7.

97. Doehring-Schwerdtfeger E, Abdel-Rahim IM, Kardorff R, et al. Ultrasonographical investigation of periportal fibrosis in children with *Schistosoma mansoni* infection: reversibility of morbidity twenty-three months after treatment with praziquantel. Am J Trop Med Hyg 1992;46:409–15.

98. Schreiber RA. Propranolol and portal hypertension: should kids be on the block? J Pediatr Gastroenterol Nutr 1999; 29:10–1.

99. Thaler M, Pastakia B, Shawker TH, et al. Hepatic candidiasis in cancer patients: the evolving picture of the syndrome. Ann Intern Med 1988;108:88–100.

100. Marcus SG, Walsh TJ, Pizzo PA, Danforth DN. Hepatic abscess in cancer patients. Characterization and management. Arch Surg 1993;128:1358–64.

101. Johnson TL, Barnett JL, Appelman HD, Nostrant T. *Candida* hepatitis. histopathologic diagnosis. Am J Surg Pathol 1988; 12:716–20.

102. Edwards JE Jr, Bodey GP, Bowden RA, et al. International conference for the development of a consensus on the management and prevention of severe candidial infections. Clin Infect Dis 1997;25:43–59.

103. Sallah S, Semelka RC, Wehibie R, et al. Hepatosplenic candidiasis in patients with acute leukaemia. Br J Haematol 1999; 106:697–701.

104. Pizzo PA, Rubin M, Freifeld A, Walsh TJ. The child with cancer and infection. II. Nonbacterial infections. J Pediatr 1991; 119:845–57.

105. Goenka M, Mehta S, Yachha SK, et al. Hepatic involvement culminating in cirrhosis in a child with disseminated cryptococcosis. J Clin Gastroenterol 1995;20:57–60.

106. Lamps LW, Molina CP, West AB, et al. The pathologic spectrum of gastrointestinal and hepatic histoplasmosis. Am J Clin Pathol 2000;113:64–72.

3. AIDS *and* Other Immune Disorders

Elizabeth Iofel, MD

Jeremiah J. Levine, MD

Immunodeficiency predisposes the host to the development of recurrent and unusual infections. Liver involvement in these infectious processes is commonly observed. This chapter describes liver infections in three major groups of immunodeficient states: human immunodeficiency virus (HIV) infection, congenital primary immunodeficiencies, and secondary immunodeficiency states associated with bone marrow and solid organ transplant.

As of the end of 2001, the Joint United Nations Programme on HIV-AIDS estimated that more than 40 million adults and children were living with HIV–acquired immune deficiency syndrome (AIDS). In children, there are two important routes of transmission: maternal transfer of virus during pregnancy or in the perinatal period and transmission through blood products. Approximately 90% of pediatric AIDS infections are acquired by the perinatal route.[1] Clinical symptoms in this situation can develop as early as 1 month of age, but the median interval from birth to symptom onset is 8 months. Gastrointestinal problems are typical in patients with HIV, and the liver is commonly involved. Hepatomegaly and abnormal liver function tests are frequently observed in HIV patients.[2–4] Acute hepatitis can be the first manifestation of HIV infection in early infancy.[5] However, significant abnormalities in liver synthetic function, complicated by cirrhosis, hypoalbuminemia, ascites, and portal hypertension, are rare.[2,6]

With newer treatment regimens for HIV, opportunistic infections are decreasing in frequency. On the other hand, mortality from end-stage liver disease among adult patients with HIV is on the rise.[7] Chronic coinfections with hepatitis B and C are the most frequent causes of chronic liver disease in adults with HIV.[3] Because no comparable data are available in the pediatric population, this discussion, for the most part, provides information based on extrapolations from the adult literature. Liver disease in the HIV-infected patient may be caused by a variety of pathogens. The most important ones are listed in Table 51.3-1. Liver damage in HIV-infected patients may also be caused by antiretroviral drugs and medications used for the treatment and prevention of opportunistic infections (Table 51.3-2), as well as tumors. Tumors are exceedingly rare in pediatric patients.

In the earlier stages of HIV infection, liver disease is usually related to drug hepatotoxicity or coinfection with hepatotropic viruses. With disease progression, the systemic opportunistic infections become more problematic. The clinical findings of liver disease in HIV patients are similar, regardless of underlying cause. Fever, malaise,

hepatomegaly, right-sided or epigastric abdominal pain, and nausea have all been described. Jaundice is unusual, even in patients with biliary tract disease.

HIV virus has been observed within Kupffer cells and in hepatic endothelial cells,[8] and HIV messenger ribonucleic acid (RNA) has been detected within hepatocytes.[9] Hepatic macrophages and endothelial cells express the CD4 surface molecule and have been shown to support viral replication in vitro.[10] It remains unclear, however, whether HIV can damage the liver directly. There is no correlation between the amount of HIV antigens in the liver and the severity of histologic abnormality, and normal histology can also be seen.[11] There are limited data about hepatic histology in children with HIV disease.[12–14] Steatosis, Kupffer cell hyperplasia, portal inflammation, and focal necrosis are common but nonspecific findings.[15] Certain pathologic features appear somewhat unique to the pediatric age group. The presence of giant cells is common, even in children older than 6 months. The giant cells may be associated with cytomegalovirus (CMV) infection or Kaposi sarcoma but can also be a reaction of the liver to HIV infection.[13,14] Dense lymphoid infiltration of portal spaces with features of chronic active hepatitis has been described in several

TABLE 51.3-1 COMMON PATHOGENS CAUSING LIVER DISEASE IN PATIENTS WITH HIV

HIV VIRUS

COINFECTIONS NONSPECIFIC TO HIV
Hepatitis A
Hepatitis B
Hepatitis C
Adenovirus
Herpes viruses group (EBV, HSV, VZV)

OPPORTUNISTIC INFECTIONS
Viruses
   Herpes group (CMV, HHV-6, HHV-8)
Protozoa
   Pneumocystis carinii
   Cryptosporidium
   Microsporida
Fungi
   Cryptococcus
   Histoplasma
   Candida
Bacteria
   Mycobacterium-avium
   Mycobacterium intracellulare
   Mycobacterium tuberculosis

CMV = cytomegalovirus; EBV = Epstein-Barr virus; HHV = human herpesvirus; HIV = human immunodeficiency virus; HSV = herpes simplex virus; VZV = varicella zoster virus.

cases.[12–14] Cholestatic hepatitis, unique to children less than 1 year of age, has been reported in association with nonspecific or giant cell hepatitis.[5,15–17] A severe course

TABLE 51.3-2   PATTERNS OF BIOCHEMICAL ABNORMALITIES OF DRUGS COMMONLY USED IN PATIENTS WITH HIV

HEPATOCELLULAR
Acetaminophen
Aminosalicylic acid
Ciprofloxacin
Clarithromycin
Clindamycin
Dilantin
Ethionamide
Fluconazole
Foscarnet
Ganciclovir
Itraconazole
Ketoconazole
Mebendazole
Oxacillin
Pentamidine
Pyrazinamide
Ranitidine
Rifabutin
Sulfonamides
Sulfones
Tetracycline
Trimethoprim-sulfamethoxazole
Vitamin A
Zalcitabine
Zidovudine

CHOLESTATIC
Amitriptyline
Carbenicillin
Cimetidine
Clarithromycin
Diazepam
Doxepin
Erythromycin
Naprosyn
Prochlorperazine
Ranitidine
Thiabendazole
Zidovudine

STEATOSIS
Glucocorticoids
Tetracycline
Valproic acid
Zidovudine

MIXED
Amitriptyline
Carbamazepine
Clarithromycin
Diazepam
Doxepin
Naprosyn
Phenobarbitol
Piroxicam
Prochlorperazine
Sulfonamides
Sulfones
Trimethoprim-sulfamethoxazole

Adapted from Weiner FR, Simon D. Liver disease in patients with acquired immunodeficiency syndrome. In: Brandt LJ, editor. Clinical practice of gastroenterology. Vol. 2. Philadelphia: Churchill Livingstone; 1999. p. 975.
HIV = human immunodeficiency virus.

with quick progression is typical for these patients.[15] Peliosis hepatitis has not yet been reported in children.[15]

Pitlick and colleagues[18,19] and Guarda and colleagues[20] were the first to report biliary tract involvement in patients with AIDS. The reported infectious agents in these cases include CMV, *Cryptosporidium*,[21] *Microsporida*,[22] and *Isospora*.[23] The spectrum of HIV-related biliary tract disorders includes acalculous cholecystitis, papillary stenosis, and sclerosing cholangitis. Four distinct cholangiographic patterns have been described by Cello.[24] Papillary stenosis occurs in 15 to 20% of patients, sclerosing cholangitis in 20%, and a combination of both in 50% of patients. The pattern of long, 1 to 2 cm extrahepatic bile duct strictures occurs in 15% of cases.

The pathogenesis of the biliary disease in HIV patients is not well understood. It is possible that HIV itself infects and damages the biliary tract. However, to date, HIV has not been isolated from the biliary epithelium.[25] It has been suggested that patients with certain human leukocyte antigen types may develop an immunologic reaction in response to pathogens directed against the biliary epithelium. It is also possible that enteric infection in AIDS patients may lead to portal bacteremia and bile duct injury.[26] Damage to the sphincter of Oddi caused by different pathogens has also been proposed as a possible mechanism.[27,28] The clinical picture of HIV-related cholangitis is similar regardless of the pathogenic organism involved.[24,29] Anicteric cholangitis is a predominant finding. Elevation of serum amylase has also been described, although its significance is unclear.

EVALUATION OF HIV-INFECTED PATIENTS WITH SUSPECTED HEPATOBILIARY DISEASE

Given the wide variety of possible etiologic agents and nonspecific clinical findings of liver disease in patients with HIV infection, an organized approach to the investigation of elevated transaminases, hepatomegaly, and unexplained fever is important. Figure 51.3-1 provides an algorithm for the approach to these patients. The history should focus on prior infections (CMV, hepatitis B or C), recent travel (exposure to tuberculosis, hepatitis A, or parasites), and a history of contact with individuals with highly contagious illnesses (varicella, roseola). Use of potentially toxic medications also has to be evaluated. A complete physical examination can often detect an extrahepatic site of opportunistic infections. Attention should also be paid to the nutritional status of the patient because acute weight loss or precipitous weight gain may cause hepatosteatosis and present as elevated liver function tests.

Although routine liver function tests are of limited value in identifying a specific infection, the magnitude of injury and pattern of injury may be suggested.[4] Two main patterns can be differentiated: hepatocellular dysfunction and cholestasis. With a pattern suggesting predominantly hepatocellular disease, viral hepatitis or drug toxicity should be considered. A cholestatic pattern with right upper quadrant pain, with or without jaundice, should raise suspicion of AIDS cholangiopathy. A markedly elevated serum alkaline phosphatase level in the absence of bile duct obstruction is suggestive of mycobacterial or fungal infection.[2] Elevation of serum bilirubin and alkaline phosphatase levels without ductal dilatation suggests drug- or virus-induced cholestasis.

The CD4 cell count should be part of the laboratory evaluation because it reflects the degree of immunosuppression. Certain infections, such as *Pneumocystis carinii*

and *Mycobacterium avium-intracellulare* complex (MAC), usually occur in severely immunocompromised patients. In contrast, tuberculosis and hepatotropic viruses (hepatitis A, B, or C) can be symptomatic at earlier stages of immunocompromise. Blood cultures, serology, and fungal and viral cultures may help elucidate specific pathogens causing liver dysfunction.

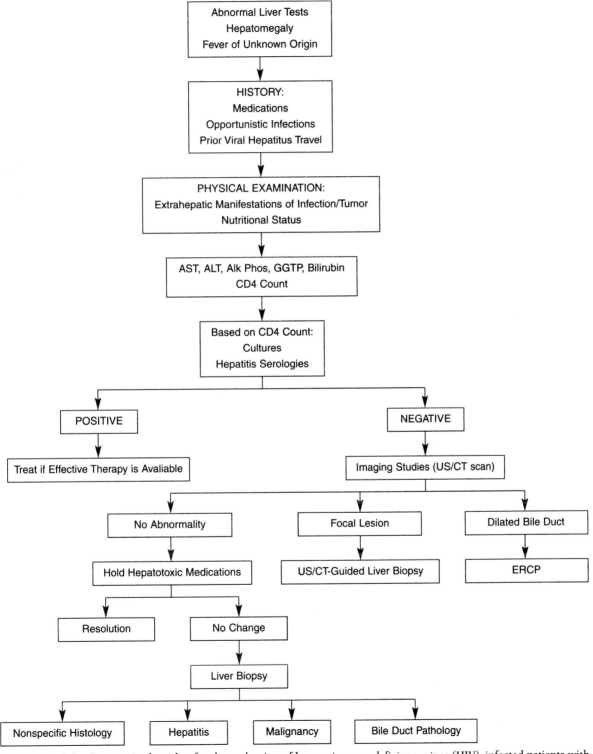

FIGURE 51.3-1   Diagnostic algorithm for the evaluation of human immunodeficiency virus (HIV)–infected patients with hepatobiliary disease. Alk phos = alkaline phosphatase; ALT = alanine transaminase; AST = aspartate transaminase; CD4 count = CD4 count lymphocyte cell count; CT = computed tomography; ERCP = endoscopic retrograde cholangiopancreatography; GGTP = γ-glutamyl transpeptidase; US = ultrasonography.

Ultrasonography is useful in the initial evaluation of suspected biliary tract disease. Although it may miss up to 25% of cases of HIV-related biliary tract disease diagnosed by endoscopic retrograde cholangiopancreatography,[30] it is easily available and inexpensive. Computed tomography (CT) offers a better delineation of focal lesions and intra-abdominal lymph nodes. Both ultrasonography and CT may be useful in performing a liver biopsy. The role of liver biopsy in the evaluation of HIV patients with parenchymal liver disease is controversial. A specific diagnosis may be made by liver biopsy in up to 50% of adult AIDS patients.[31,32] No comparable data are available in the pediatric patient population.

The risk of bleeding after liver biopsy is much increased in AIDS patients, even with normal coagulation. The rate of significant hemorrhage following liver biopsy is described to be as high as 5 to 10%.[15,33,34] Finally, it has not been demonstrated that findings on liver biopsy result in improved quality of life or survival of these patients.[4,35] Despite these issues, a liver biopsy is useful in certain situations. A recent pediatric study has suggested two groups for whom liver biopsy may be very useful when other non-invasive tests are negative: those patients with suspected mycobacterial infections and patients with jaundice.[15] Symptomatic hepatomegaly and persistent fever with a negative noninvasive workup have also been mentioned in the adult literature as indications for biopsy.[4] When a liver biopsy is performed, cultures and special stains should be obtained in addition to routine histology.

In contrast to hepatocellular disease, biliary tract complications of AIDS require an aggressive approach. Patients are frequently symptomatic, and effective palliation is available by endoscopic and surgical means. Endoscopic retrograde cholangiopancreatography remains the gold standard in diagnosing AIDS cholangiopathy.

HIV COINFECTIONS

HEPATITIS B

Hepatitis B virus (HBV) and HIV have similar routes of transmission and so frequently coexist. It is unclear whether HIV alters the natural history of chronic HBV infection.[36] Following acute HBV infection, the virus is cleared in 95% of immunocompetent patients. In contrast, 50% of HIV coinfected patients develop chronic infection.[37] Individual case reports suggest that reactivation of HBV infection is associated with progression of the HIV disease.[38–42] Loss of naturally acquired anti–hepatitis B surface antibodies (HBsAB), even in patients who remain hepatitis B surface antigen (HBsAg) negative, has also been described.[43] Increased prevalence of hepatitis B e antigen (HBeAg) expression and elevated levels of deoxyribonucleic acid (DNA) polymerase in HIV-positive patients has been reported.[37,41,44,45] Therefore, more patients with HIV-HBV coinfection are in a chronic HBV carrier state, with highly infectious serum and body fluids, compared with the HIV-negative population.[45]

Patients with early or well-controlled HIV infection tend to have milder HBV infection, whereas those severely immunosuppressed tend to have severe HBV disease.[46] Spontaneous resolution of chronic HBV infection with an improved immune response in treated HIV patients has also been described.[47] Thus, aggressive treatment of HIV appears to be an important factor in the control of HBV infection. Although HIV-positive patients with HBV may express higher HBV DNA levels and increased HbeAg titers,[36] they often have lower serum transaminases and less histologic damage.[48] Despite these findings, HBV infection in these patients has a greater risk of progression to cirrhosis and development of hepatocellular carcinoma.[49]

The results of interferon treatment in the HIV population are controversial.[50–54] In general, for hepatitis B, response rates to interferon therapy have been less impressive than those seen in the HIV-negative group. Lamivudine significantly lowers HBV DNA and serum transaminases and may result in seroconversion from HBsAg to HB$_s$ antibody.[54,55] Unfortunately, reactivation of hepatitis B may occur following withdrawal of therapy; therefore, long-term treatment appears to be necessary.[38] Mutation of the viral polymerase gene occurs at a rate of approximately 20% per year, similar to that of an immunocompetent host.[56] This mutation leads to antiviral resistance in up to one-third of the patients.[57] The dosage of lamivudine used for HBV treatment in HIV-positive patients is similar to that used for HIV treatment alone (150 mg twice daily) to avoid development of HIV resistance to lamivudine. Minimal published information is available about the role of other nucleoside analogs in the treatment of HBV infection.[47,58–60]

Vaccination against HBV has been recommended for all patients infected with HIV. Unfortunately, HIV infection reduces the efficacy of vaccination in these patients. Several studies demonstrated suboptimal response in both the magnitude and duration of antibody response.[61–64] Loss of anti-HB$_s$ in HIV-infected patients is seen in 43% of persons by 4 years compared with an 8% loss in immunocompetent controls.[65]

HEPATITIS C

Hepatitis C virus (HCV) infects an estimated 170 million people worldwide and is five times more widespread than infection with HIV.[66] In the United States alone, approximately 300,000 to 400,000 individuals are HIV-HCV coinfected.[67] For children infected with hepatitis C through vertical transmission, the prevalence of HCV infection is estimated at 8 to 17%.[68,69] With the introduction of highly active antiretroviral therapy (HAART) and improvement in survival, HCV infection has become a major contributor to morbidity and mortality in patients with HIV. End-stage liver disease has become a frequent complication,[67,70,71] and cases of hepatocellular carcinoma (HCC) in HIV-HCV–coinfected adults have been described.[72] HCV also has been implicated as a cause of increased hepatotoxicity of HAART in coinfected patients.[73–75]

In children, HCV is acquired primarily through perinatal transmission. The rate of vertical transmission of HCV alone is 5 to 11%.[76] Maternal coinfection with HIV increases the rate of perinatal HCV transmission even without simultaneous HIV transmission.[77,78] Likewise, maternal HCV infection has been associated with a higher likelihood of vertical HIV transmission. Perinatal transmission of HIV is approximately two times more frequent in mothers who are infected with both hepatitis C and HIV.[79]

There are no data on the natural history of HCV in HIV-infected children. In adults, HCV infection appears to be more aggressive in HIV-positive patients compared with immunocompetent adults. Hepatic damage from HCV infection is primarily due to direct viral damage. However, an immunologic response is important in the elimination of HCV. Therefore, the rate of HCV replication and levels of HCV viremia are much higher in immunosuppressed individuals.[80] Several studies demonstrated a more rapid progression and more severe course of HCV infection in the HIV population.[81,82]

The US Public Health Service and National Institutes of Health consensus panel has recommended anti-HCV enzyme-linked immunosorbent assay III as a screening test for HCV regardless of the HIV status of the patient.[70] A recent study showed a sensitivity of this test of over 99% in both HIV-infected and HIV-negative patients.[83] The recombinant immunoblot assay produced indeterminate results in 10 to 23% of coinfected subjects.[84] False-negative HCV serology may be associated with CD4 counts less than 200 cells/mm[3]. If suspicion of the liver disease is high in those patients, an HCV-RNA test should be performed. The liver biopsy is considered the gold standard for clinical assessment of individuals with chronic HCV infection. Both inflammation and fibrosis tend to be greater in HIV-infected patients, primarily in those with low CD4 counts.[84]

Until recently, treatment of HCV-HIV coinfected patients was with antiretroviral drugs alone. It now has been well documented that HAART does not have any beneficial suppressive effect on HCV.[85] With the improved survival of HIV-positive patients, an aggressive approach to the treatment of HCV infection in this population has been advocated. Monotherapy with interferon-α results in a poor sustained response (0–20%).[79,86] Recent studies with the combination of interferon and ribavirin have demonstrated an end of treatment response rate of 50%, with up to 28% of the patients remaining HCV-RNA negative 3 months after treatment.[86–88] Introduction of pegylated interferon has led to a sustained viral response in 30 to 45%.[89,90] No treatment data are available in the pediatric population.

HEPATITIS A, E, AND G

The prevalence, morbidity, and mortality of hepatitis A infection are not altered by HIV infection.[91] Vaccination of the HIV-infected patients against hepatitis A is recommended. Vaccination appears to be safe but may be less effective. Prevaccination screening is cost-effective in adults.[91] Hepatitis E virus, a waterborne, fecally-orally transmitted virus, usually causes acute self-limited disease. One study showed an increased incidence of hepatitis E in HIV-infected patients but without clinical significance.[92] Hepatitis G virus (HGV) is present in approximately 20 to 40% of HIV-infected patients.[80] The presence of HGV does not alter

the levels of the serum transaminases, CD4 cell count, or plasma HIV-1 levels.[80] Some studies suggest that coinfection of HGV and HIV is a favorable prognostic factor, correlating with a slower progression of HIV disease.[93]

ADENOVIRUS

Adenovirus infections in healthy children usually present as a self-limited upper respiratory tract infection, gastroenteritis, maculopapular rash, and conjunctivitis. In HIV-infected individuals, fulminant multiorgan involvement with bilateral pneumonia, gastroenteritis or colitis, and urinary tract infection is typical.[94–96] Hepatic involvement with rapid progression to liver failure is not uncommon.[95] Ulcerations of the gallbladder wall have also been linked to adenoviral infection.[97] The difference in serotypes affecting healthy and immunocompromised patients may be responsible for the differences in clinical presentation.[98] In adenoviral hepatitis, there is lobular necrosis of the hepatocytes with Cowdry type A basophilic nuclear inclusion bodies. Portal tracts are usually speared. Adenoviral virions can be detected in the hepatocytes by electron microscopy; adenoviral disease is usually more severe. Diagnosis is usually made by viral isolation or histologic examination.

Currently, no effective treatment against adenovirus is available. Use of immunoglobulin (Ig) therapy[99] and intravenous ribavirin[100,101] has been advocated.

HERPES GROUP VIRUS INFECTION

Herpes Simplex Virus (1 and 2). Herpes simplex virus (HSV) dissemination to the liver has been described in patients with HIV.[102] Significant dissemination more commonly occurs with primary infection, although it has also been observed with reactivation. Fulminant liver disease may be the only presenting symptom because mucocutaneous lesions may be absent in up to 50% of the patients.[103] Patients present with significantly elevated transaminases, jaundice, and rapidly progressive liver failure.[80] Liver biopsy demonstrates characteristic intranuclear inclusions (Cowdry type A bodies) in hepatocytes. The intranuclear inclusion bodies produce a typical ground-glass appearance. Although a mild neutrophilic infiltrate is sometimes described, a notable feature of HSV disease is the absence of a significant inflammatory cell response in either the portal areas or parenchyma. Fatty degeneration is frequently observed. Electron microscopy is confirmatory and demonstrates typical intranuclear herpes virions. Viral cultures are usually positive (in more than two-thirds of cases) and should always be obtained.[104] Prompt initiation of acyclovir treatment, as well as discontinuation of all potentially hepatotoxic medications, is recommended.

Human Herpesvirus 3 (Varicella-Zoster Virus). Dissemination of varicella-zoster virus (VZV) infection may occur with primary infection or with reactivation. Certain clinical features distinguish severe VZV and HSV infections. In contrast to HSV, VZV disease is typically accompanied by classic skin and mucous membrane lesions. These lesions are usually obvious on presentation but may be delayed by

3 to 4 days. The main target organ of VZV is the lung. Although the liver is commonly involved in disseminated VZV disease, fulminant hepatitis without significant pulmonary disease is rare.[103] Abdominal pain, nausea, and vomiting are common. Elevated transaminases, with or without bilirubin elevation, and leukocytosis are common with VZV disease, in contrast to the leukopenia associated with HSV dissemination. Coagulopathy, renal failure, and multiorgan system failure are typical of severe VZV.

Immediate administration of varicella-zoster Ig to individuals with no history of chickenpox or without vaccination is recommended within 96 hours of exposure.[103] Prophylactic acyclovir should be prescribed. Intravenous acyclovir is reserved for patients with clinical signs of VZV, and the recommended doses are higher than those for HSV disease.[103]

Among HIV-positive patients, only asymptomatic, nonimmunosuppressed patients should be vaccinated against VZV. Vaccination is contraindicated in all other HIV-positive children.

Human Herpesvirus 4 (Epstein-Barr Virus). Epstein-Barr virus (EBV) infection may present as an acute mononucleosis syndrome, but it has also been implicated in the pathogenesis of non-Hodgkin lymphoma, leiomyomas, and leiomyosarcomas of the liver in children with AIDS.[104,105] If acute mononucleosis syndrome occurs, low-grade fever, abdominal discomfort, nausea, mild hepatomegaly, and lymphadenopathy are common. Hepatitis is frequently present but usually resolves completely. Minimal swelling and vacuolization of hepatocytes associated with lymphocytic and monocytic infiltration of the portal areas are noted in the liver biopsy. Extensive liver necrosis has also been described in HIV patients.

Non-Hodgkin lymphoma is a common feature of AIDS and has been associated with EBV infection. The EBV viral genome has been found within tumor cells by DNA hybridization.[105] It may occur at any stage of AIDS but usually occurs late in the disease. The prevalence of non-Hodgkin lymphoma in HIV is increasing, leading some to suggest that it is the most common AIDS-related neoplasm.[4] Isolated liver involvement without extrahepatic disease has been reported in up to 14% of AIDS patients.[2] Elevation of serum alkaline phosphatase is a very sensitive marker of hepatic involvement; elevation of transaminases and bilirubin is usually observed in the advanced disease. The typical symptoms seen in immunocompetent patients, such as weight loss, night sweats, and fever, are often absent.[105] An abdominal CT scan may help with the diagnosis of non-Hodgkin lymphoma.[4]

Leiomyomas and leiomyosarcomas are extremely rare tumors in children. The incidence of these lesions is increased in pediatric HIV patients. Quantitative polymerase chain reaction (PCR) analysis demonstrated very high levels of EBV in tumor tissue from these patients. No EBV was detected in normal tissues of the same patients or in the tumor tissue of subjects not affected by HIV.[104] The lesions in HIV patients tend to involve the gastrointestinal tract, liver, and lungs.

Human Herpesvirus 6B. Human herpesvirus 6B (HHV-6B) has been implicated in causing roseola (exanthem subitum) in immunocompetent patients. In immunocompromised patients, severe disseminated HHV-6B infection occurs with primary infection and may cause fulminant hepatitis.[106,107] Transaminase elevation, cholestasis, thrombocytopenia, and leukopenia have been reported. There is focal hepatocyte necrosis with mild lymphocytic infiltration of the portal tracts and sinusoids. HHV-6 is detectable in the lymphocytes. The clinical manifestations of HHV-6/-7 reactivation have not been described. Indications for therapy are not clearly defined, but in vitro susceptibility to ganciclovir has been described.[108]

Human Herpesvirus 8. Human herpesvirus 8 viral infection is associated with Kaposi sarcoma, a neoplasm involving skin, mucous membranes, and internal organs. Liver involvement usually occurs as part of a disseminated process, although primary liver disease has also been described.[3,109] Patients are rarely symptomatic from liver disease, although an elevated serum alkaline phosphatase level may be present. Owing to significant sampling error, the diagnosis may be missed if an unguided liver biopsy is performed. Histologically, the lesions appear as dark red to purple nodules in the portal regions, filled with spindle-shaped endothelial cells.

OPPORTUNISTIC INFECTIONS

CYTOMEGALOVIRUS

CMV is one of the most common hepatic infections in HIV-positive adults. CMV is seen in 33 to 44% of all patients and in close to 100% of those who are severely immunosuppressed (CD4 count < 100 cells/mm³).[80] The incidence of CMV infection associated with symptomatic disease has not been well documented in the pediatric HIV population, with a range of 30 to 60% cited in the literature.[110] The presentation of CMV hepatitis is usually mild, with fever, malaise, hepatomegaly, and transaminitis. CMV typically infects hepatocytes and Kupffer cells, as well as endothelial cells. Inflammation in the portal and periportal areas is usually observed. Intranuclear and intracytoplasmic inclusion bodies are often surrounded by a clear halo ("owl-eye" appearance), and giant cells may be seen in the biopsies.[3,4,13] Less frequently, CMV may affect the biliary epithelium, leading to acalculous cholecystitis, papillary stenosis, and sclerosing cholangitis.[3,4,111]

The diagnosis of CMV may be difficult. The significance of a positive urine culture is unclear because viruria may represent asymptomatic shedding and may persist for months to years.[110] CMV viremia is a much better predictor of active disease.[112] In one study, CMV disease was evident in 57% of children with blood cultures positive for CMV compared with 17% of children with positive urine cultures.[110] There are no controlled trials addressing the use of foscarnet or ganciclovir in the setting of CMV hepatitis. The experience treating nonhepatic infections may suggest their use in hepatitis patients.

PROTOZOA

Pneumocystis carinii. *Pneumocystis carinii* pneumonia (PCP) is the most common protozoal pathogen among patients with AIDS. The incidence of PCP infection has decreased dramatically, first with the institution of routine PCP prophylaxis and later with the introduction of the HAART regimen. Pulmonary symptoms are the hallmark of *P. carinii* infection. Disseminated infection is not common. Only a few cases of isolated hepatic involvement have been described.[113] It has been suggested that widespread use of aerosolized pentamidine for PCP prophylaxis has contributed to the appearance of *P. carinii* infections of other organs.[114,115] Clinical findings are limited to mild abdominal pain with variable elevation of transaminases. Isolated cases of an obstructive process with increased γ-glutamyl transpeptidase have been reported.[116] Abdominal CT may reveal diffuse punctate calcifications of the liver.[80] Pathology from liver biopsy specimens demonstrates foamy eosinophilic exudate, with the organism demonstrable on silver stain. Acellular nodules in a random or periportal distribution in the lobule, with or without infiltration of the hepatic sinusoids, have also been described.[116,117]

Cryptosporidium. *Cryptosporidium* is the most commonly identified cause of AIDS-related cholangitis. It has been identified in the bile ducts or stools from 20 to 62% of patients with AIDS-related cholangitis.[24] It has been estimated that 10 to 16% of patients with intestinal cryptosporidiosis may develop biliary tract symptoms.[118] Infiltration of portal spaces with eosinophils, plasma cells, and lymphocytes is observed in liver biopsies. Ulceration of the duct epithelium with basophilic Giemsa stain–positive organisms, attached to the luminal surface of the epithelial cells, may be noted.[119]

Microsporida. *Microsporida* is a less common cause of AIDS cholangitis, occurring in less than 10% in most series.[120] The incidence of this infection may be underestimated because techniques for the detection of *Microsporida* are not well developed.[25] The two microsporidia most commonly associated with the disease are *Enterocytozoon bieneusi* and *Enterocytozoon intestinalis*. Clinical symptoms are not different from the cholangitis caused by other organisms and include right upper quadrant pain, nausea, vomiting, and fever. Many patients have associated diarrhea and weight loss. Jaundice is present in only 10% of patients.[121] The diagnosis is based on the detection of *Microsporida* in the stool or bile aspirates. Tissue obtained from the duodenum, ampulla, bile duct, or liver may also be used. Pathogens identified in stools or bile may provide circumstantial evidence that the organism is the etiology of cholangitis. A biopsy specimen from the bile duct revealing the pathogen and inflammation suggests that this pathogen is actually causing cholangitis. Pathogens may be identified in up to 75% of cases.[121]

FUNGI

Fungal infections involve the liver only in disseminated disease. These infections share a nonspecific clinical presentation, including fever, hepatomegaly, elevated alkaline phosphatase, and bilirubin.[3] Hepatic involvement may accompany cryptococcal meningitis in the setting of hematogenous dissemination. Opportunistic infections with *Histoplasma*, *Coccidioides*, *Candida*, and *Sporothrix* occur less commonly.[80] Imaging studies may demonstrate diffuse irregularity of the liver parenchyma or, rarely, a formed fungal abscess. Liver biopsy demonstrates nonspecific poorly formed granulomata with minimal inflammatory response.[122] The response to prolonged antifungal therapy is variable, with death resulting from disseminated infection rather than from hepatic involvement itself.

MYCOBACTERIA

MAC includes two closely related species: *M. avium* and *M. intracellulare*. These organisms are small, gram-positive, acid-fast bacilli. Bacterial proliferation typically occurs in the macrophages and is controlled by cell-mediated immunity. With a decrease of the CD4 count, proliferation of the bacteria becomes poorly controlled, and patients are at risk for disseminated MAC infection. CD4 counts of less than 50 cells/mm^3 have been described in patients with disseminated MAC.[123] It is the most common opportunistic pathogen found in AIDS patients. In one series, MAC was found in 38% of cases when liver biopsy was performed.[3] The clinical presentation of disseminated infection is nonspecific and may be attributable to the advanced HIV. Fever, weight loss, hepatomegaly, and anemia have been described. A unique feature of MAC disease in HIV patients is marked elevation of alkaline phosphatase. The enzyme may reach 20 to 40 times the normal level, with little elevation of transaminases, bilirubin, or other parameters of hepatic function.[3] Fractionation shows it to be hepatic in origin. The histologic picture does not show marked abnormalities. This disparity between measured levels and histology suggests interference with enzyme metabolism rather than hepatic destruction.[124]

Diagnosis of MAC infection is based on cultivation of *M. avium* from the liver tissue.

Histology of the liver reveals diffuse, poorly formed noncaseating granulomata, composed mainly of foamy histiocytes. In MAC infection of patients with AIDS, granulomas usually do not contain multinuclear giant cells. Granuloma may be absent in up to 25% of patients. Acid-fast bacilli are found within and around granulomas.

In contrast, *Mycobacterium tuberculosis* is found in patients who are less immunosuppressed (CD4 > 200 cells/mm^3).[3] Extrapulmonary infection with *M. tuberculosis* is seen in over 50% of adult AIDS patients with lung disease.[80] In one study, 7.5% of patients with extrapulmonary disease had hepatic infection.[125] The clinical presentation in these patients is similar to *M. avium* infection; in addition, cough, night sweats, and sputum production may be noted. Tuberculous abscess and biliary obstruction owing to bile duct tuberculoma have rarely been described in adult HIV patients. Liver biopsy reveals well-formed caseating granuloma with a lesser load of acid-fast bacilli compared with MAC infection. Other mycobacteria implicated in liver disease are *Mycobacterium xenopi*, *Mycobacterium genavese*, and *Mycobacterium kansasii*

Before the availability of HAART, the median survival time in patients with disseminated MAC infection ranged from 5 to 11 months.[123,126] Clinical manifestations of MAC in children receiving HAART have not been described. Treatment regimens have been evaluated in the adult population,[127] with gastrointestinal tuberculosis usually responding to 9 to 12 months of combination antibiotic therapy. Current recommendations for the initial treatment include clarithromycin and azithromycin in combination with ethambutol and rifabutin.[128]

PRIMARY IMMUNODEFICIENCY

Patients with primary immunodeficiency syndromes may have liver disease. Liver infections in these patients can occur due to an increased predisposition to a variety of infectious processes. Causative organisms may vary, based on the type of immunologic defect (Table 51.3-3).

CHRONIC GRANULOMATOUS DISEASE

Chronic granulomatous disease (CGD) is characterized by the inability of phagocytic cells to reduce molecular oxygen and create the active oxygen metabolites that are necessary for efficient intracellular microbicidal activity. CGD is inherited in an autosomal recessive or X-linked manner. CGD represents a group of four related disorders. The types of infections most frequently encountered include pneumonia, osteomyelitis, skin and soft tissue abscesses, and liver abscess. The increased susceptibility to infection among patients who have CGD is limited to bacteria and fungi that are catalase positive and do not themselves have any production of reduced oxygen metabolites, such as hydrogen peroxide. Catalase-positive organisms are not killed efficiently by the phagocytic cells in patients who have CGD. In contrast, microorganisms that are catalase negative and can produce hydrogen peroxide supply the necessary reactive oxygen metabolites when they are ingested, thereby contributing to their own demise. *Staphylococcus aureus* and *Pseudomonas aeruginosa* are the two most common isolates from a liver abscess in patients with CGD.[129] Needle aspiration of the abscess is needed for the etiologic diagnosis. The use of drainage procedures is limited by poor healing.

Antibiotic therapy should always include penicillinase-resistant penicillin such as nafcillin or oxacillin. These medications may be combined with gentamicin for synergism. Reports of utility of interferon-γ[130] and granulocyte transfusion[131] combined with surgical drainage[132] are present in the literature. Antibiotic prophylaxis with trimethoprim-sulfamethoxazole[133] and use of interferon-γ[130] appear to decrease the incidence of serious infections, including liver abscess, in patients with CGD.

SHWACHMAN SYNDROME

Shwachman syndrome primarily affects the exocrine pancreas, bone marrow, and skeleton. The most prominent features seen in this disorder include neutropenia, pancreatic insufficiency, and short stature. Hepatic involvement has frequently been reported with this syndrome and usually manifests as hepatomegaly and elevated transaminases.

Biopsy specimens demonstrate steatosis and mild fibrosis. Progression of the liver disease is uncommon.[134,135]

X-LINKED AGAMMAGLOBULINEMIA

X-linked agammaglobulinemia presents with recurrent infections in male infants after 9 months of age owing to a failure to synthesize all classes of Igs. Recurrent otitis, sinusitis, pneumonias, and diarrhea are typical. An association with sclerosing cholangitis has occasionally been described. It is not clear whether sclerosing cholangitis is associated with increased autoimmunity in these patients[136] or is caused by opportunistic infections such as cryptosporidiosis.[137]

An unusual syndrome of severe enteroviral infection, most commonly caused by echovirus type 11, has been described in these patients.[138] Patients usually present with meningoencephalitis that has a progressive, usually fatal course. Typical manifestations include fever, dermatomyositis, and significant hepatitis. These symptoms may precede the development of neurologic symptoms. The neurologic disease usually determines survival in these patients.

COMMON VARIABLE IMMUNODEFICIENCY

Common variable immunodeficiency is an uncommon disorder with more than 95% of the patients presenting with recurrent sinopulmonary infections. The liver is usually affected by a granulomatous process. This process is thought to be caused by a cytokine disturbance, especially increased production of tumor necrosis factor-α.[139] Approximately 20% of patients have elevated alkaline phosphatase levels that are thought to represent presinusoidal granuloma formation. Most of the patients with liver involvement will develop portal hypertension, esophageal varices, and cirrhosis.

SEVERE COMBINED IMMUNODEFICIENCY

Severe combined immunodeficiency (SCID) is a group of genetic disorders characterized by a block in T-lymphocyte differentiation and may be associated with abnormalities in other lymphocyte lines. At least eight separate diseases comprise this category. Findings indicating combined immunodeficiency include lymphocytopenia; absence of lymph nodes, tonsil tissue, and a thymic shadow on radiographs; low levels of serum Igs; and absent in vitro B- and T-lymphocyte responses to antigens and mitogens. Owing to profound immunosuppression, frequent and severe infections caused by pathogens and opportunistic organisms are commonly observed and may include the liver. In addition, sclerosing cholangitis, possibly caused by biliary tract infection with *Cryptosporidium*, has been reported. Two disorders in this group deserve separate mention with regard to liver disease.

Adenosine deaminase (ADA) deficiency is a systemic metabolic disorder. The enzymatic defect is expressed in all cells, and deoxyadenosine triphosphate, a by-product produced in this disorder, is built up in all cells. Deoxyadenosine triphosphate is extremely toxic to lymphocytes, so 85 to 90% of patients who are ADA deficient present with a picture consistent with severe combined immunodeficiency. These patients are lymphopenic at birth and are pre-

TABLE 51.3-3 COMMON PATHOGENS IN CONGENITAL IMMUNOLOGIC DEFECTS

			PATHOGENS			
ABNORMALITY	EXAMPLE	LIVER DISEASE	BACTERIA	FUNGI	VIRUSES	PROTOZOA
Phagocyte defects						
Quantitative	Neutropenia	Rare	Staphylococci, streptococci,	Candida, Aspergillus		
Qualitative	CGD	Common				
	Shwachman syndrome	Common	Nocardia,			
	Leukocyte adhesion defect	Rare	Escherichia coli, Klebsiella			
Immunoglobulin deficiencies	X-linked agammaglobulinemia	Rare	Klebsiella,		Enteroviruses, echoviruses, CMV, HSV	Giardia
	Common variable immunodeficiency	Common	Haemophilus influenzae,			
	Hyper IgE (Job) syndrome	Rare	Streptococcus pneumoniae			
Complement deficiencies		Rare	S. pneumoniae, H. influenzae, Neisseria			
Cellular and combined immunodeficiencies	SCID	Common	Mycobacteria,	Candida, Histoplasma, Cryptococcus	CMV, VZV, HSV, EBV	Pneumocystis carinii, Toxoplasma gondii, Cryptosporidium, Microsporida, Isospora spp
	DiGeorge syndrome	Rare	Salmonella spp,			
	Wiskott-Aldrich syndrome	Rare	Listeria spp,			
	X-linked lymphoprolipherative syndrome	Common	Legionella spp			

CGD = chronic granulomatous disease; CMV = cytomegalovirus; EBV = Epstein-Barr virus; HSV = herpes simplex virus; IgE = immunoglobulin E; SCID = severe combined immunodeficiency; VZV = varicella-zoster virus.

disposed to recurrent illnesses caused by both pathogens and opportunistic organisms. Symptoms often begin within a few weeks of birth. Pneumonia, intractable diarrhea, and extensive candidiasis are common. Profound failure to thrive is also frequently present. A growth abnormality of costochondral junctions causing cupping and flaring of rib ends on radiograph has been associated specifically with ADA deficiency. Elevated serum levels of hepatic transaminases are not uncommon in ADA-deficient patients, but the cause usually is not determined. Severe bridging fibrosis has been described in liver specimens during autopsy.[140] Bollinger and colleagues described a patient with ADA deficiency and persistent neonatal hepatitis, apparently unrelated to infection or graft-versus-host disease (GVHD), that responded to ADA replacement therapy.[141] It is thus possible that the toxic effects of ADA substrates may be responsible for the liver disease in these patients.

Omenn syndrome is another variant of SCID. T-lymphocyte infiltration of the skin and gut is the hallmark of this condition. Patients present with erythroderma, alopecia, protein-losing enteropathy, and failure to thrive. Life-threatening infections are common. Marked hepatosplenomegaly and lymphadenopathy may be present within the first weeks of life. Laboratory evaluation usually demonstrates elevated white blood cell and eosinophil counts, increased IgE, hypogammaglobulinemia, and histiocytosis. Severe liver disease, likely owing to infiltration with T cells and histiocytes, is associated with this condition.[142]

X-Linked Lymphoproliferative Syndrome

In 1975, Purtilo and colleagues described a kindred with 18 boys, of whom 6 died of a lymphoproliferative disorder.[143] This syndrome has since been linked to infection with EBV. The affected boys had a T-cell regulatory defect that made them extremely vulnerable to EBV infection, which often is fatal.[144] The immune defect allows an explosive proliferation of B cells after exposure to EBV. Liver involvement is a prominent feature, with progression to multiorgan system failure, and death is typical. Of the patients who survive the initial infection with EBV, 24% will acquire a malignant lymphoproliferative disorder at a median age of 4.9 years. All neoplasms have a B-cell phenotype. The majority of the non-Hodgkin lymphomas occur in the intestinal region, especially the ileocecal area. The overall risk of having a lymphoma has been estimated to be 200 times higher than that for the general population.[144]

INFECTIONS IN TRANSPLANT RECIPIENTS

Infectious complications following solid organ transplant may be divided into three time periods.[145] The early post-transplant period (first 4 weeks) is characterized by nosocomial bacterial and fungal infections. The only significant viral infection observed during the early period after transplant is caused by recurrent HSV.

The risk of infection is directly related to the surgical procedure itself, invasive monitoring with intravascular catheters, or preexisting infection in the donor or recipient. Typically, the specific sites of transplant and allograft are the most likely sites of infection. For example, liver transplant recipients are at risk for biliary sepsis and liver abscesses.

From 1 to 6 months post-transplant, infections are often related to the use of immunosuppressive agents. CMV is the dominant pathogen causing disease during this period. Other major pathogens are *Cryptococcus*, *Candida*, tuberculosis, HBV and HCV, and EBV. Infectious complications that occur later than 6 months after transplant are usually due to one of two factors: the effect of chronic viral infection acquired earlier or chronic graft dysfunction, which requires repeated courses of immunosuppression and puts patients at risk for infection with opportunistic organisms.

The course of the patients who undergo bone marrow transplant may also be divided into three phases.[146] The early phase corresponds to the first 2 to 4 weeks post-transplant. The predominant risk factor in this period is profound neutropenia and damage to mucosal surfaces. Invasive fungal and bacterial infections predominate during this period.

Between the period of engraftment and weeks 15 to 20 post-transplant, infections with opportunistic pathogens (CMV, *P. carinii*) predominate. The major predisposing factors for these infections are the immunosuppressive effects of acute GVHD and its treatment. Serious infections occurring 4 to 6 months after transplant are seen predominantly in patients with chronic GVHD.[146] Liver infections are rare in this period, with the most common being EBV infection.

The majority of patients undergoing solid organ or bone marrow transplant show evidence of CMV infection (a rise in titers or viral isolation from the urine or blood). However, not all patients develop clinical disease. The major determinant of the progression to disease is whether the infection with CMV is primary or secondary. If the organ from a CMV-positive donor is transplanted into a CMV-negative recipient, this will result in primary infection. Primary infection is more likely to be associated with the disease than is CMV reactivation.[147] The severity of the immunosuppression is another determining factor. In general, bone marrow transplant patients have more severe manifestations of CMV disease compared with solid organ transplant patients. Clinical manifestations of CMV infection in transplant recipients are usually a mononucleosis-type syndrome with fever, leukopenia, and elevated transaminases. Interstitial pneumonitis may be life threatening. Liver disease is rarely severe.[146] CMV infection in liver transplant patients may be associated with a higher risk of acute rejection[148] and possibly with an increased incidence of hepatic artery thrombosis owing to endothelial cell infection.[149] HSV and VZV infections are also common during this time, with a clinical course that is similar to that in HIV-infected patients.

EBV is responsible for a number of disorders, but the major concern in solid organ transplant recipients is post-transplant lymphoproliferative disorder (PTLD). Acute infection with EBV leads to polyclonal activation of B cells with expansion of lymphoid tissues. Because the cellular immune responses provided by natural killer and cytotoxic T cells are critical to clearing the virus, the T cell–targeted immunosuppression used in organ transplant puts allograft recipients at risk for PTLD.[150] It has now been well established that as the level of immunosuppression increases, so does the incidence of PTLD.[151,152]

Primary EBV infection, young age, and receiving an EBV-positive donor organ are interrelated predisposing factors to PTLD and are particularly important in pediatric transplant recipients.[153] Many young children, usually EBV negative, receive grafts from older donors who are much more likely to have had previous EBV infection.

Sites of involvement include the small bowel, the intra-abdominal lymph nodes, the tonsillar bed, and the liver. Patients may present immediately post-transplant or months to years after successful transplant. Fever, weight loss, lymphadenopathy, hepatosplenomegaly, and abdominal pain are typical presenting findings. Hepatitis may resemble rejection episodes in liver transplant patients.[150]

How best to prevent EBV infection in the EBV-naive recipient is debatable.[154] Some protocols use intravenous ganciclovir for variable lengths of time; others rely primarily on CMV hyperimmunoglobulin. Along with a preventive strategy, there should be a method of detecting when EBV infection or reactivation first occurs so that immunosuppression levels can be decreased promptly. This determination is best accomplished by serially monitoring the peripheral blood for EBV by quantitative PCR techniques.[155–157]

Hepatitis B infection tends to be more aggressive in immunosuppressed patients. An accelerated course of the disease was described after kidney transplant.[158]

Reactivation of previously quiescent disease has been described in children undergoing chemotherapy[159] and in patients after bone marrow transplant.[160] Hepatitis B may result in mortality rates as high as 12% in bone marrow transplant patients.[161] Increased mortality from liver disease in recipients of kidney transplants has been found in some studies, but if it occurs, it is seen 10 years or more following renal transplant.[162] Fibrosing cholestatic hepatitis is a rare, early, severe complication of renal transplant in HBV-infected recipients of kidney transplants.[163] It is characterized by cholestasis, with only a mild to moderate increase in aminotransferase levels, and by a rapid deterioration in liver function that can lead to short-term liver failure. The liver histology demonstrates periportal and perisinusoidal cholestasis, scarce mixed infiltrates, hepatocellular ballooning, and histologic cholestasis.

In addition, the acquisition of HBV soon after renal transplant carries a risk of early death from liver failure.[162] Reactivation of HBV after renal transplant in patients with preexisting HBV surface antibodies has been reported.[164] Use of immunosuppressive medications has been demonstrated to increase viral replication in vitro.[165] Viral mutations may also be responsible for the more aggressive course of the disease.[166] Hepatitis B–induced chronic liver disease is one of the main indications for liver transplant in adults. Thus, viral reinfection of the allograft is a major challenge in this population but is a less common issue in pediatrics.

The use of hepatitis B immunoglobulin during and after transplant has been proven to decrease the incidence of the recurrence rate in up to 80% of the patients.[167] The limitations of this treatment are indefinite length of the therapy, need for parenteral administration, and drug cost.[168] Other medications used to prevent HBV include agents used in the treatment of HBV in the nontransplant setting. Interferon-α is poorly tolerated and has limited efficacy in this population. Lamivudine and adefovir have been successfully used to prevent HBV recurrence.[58,169] The combination of lamivudine with hepatitis B immunoglobulin has completely eliminated recurrent HBV disease in some series.[170] Previously vaccinated patients who are HBsAg negative should be tested annually for anti-HBV antibodies and should receive booster vaccinations[171] when the titer decreases to < 10 mIU/mL. Allografts from donors who are positive for HBsAg should not be used. Controversy exists with respect to whether allografts from donors who are HBV core antibody positive should be used.

Hepatitis C infection may be caused either by exposure to contaminated blood products or tissues or via recurrence of preexisting HCV infection following liver transplant. In the pediatric population, the former is the more common route. HCV can also be transmitted with other allografts in addition to the liver. In one study, 42% of patients receiving kidneys from donors seropositive for HCV developed clinical hepatitis.[172] Organs from donors with HCV antibody who are HCV RNA positive are most likely to transmit HCV infection, but organs from donors who are HCV antibody positive and HCV RNA negative cannot be regarded as completely safe.[173]

Virtually all liver transplant recipients who are viremic with HCV at the time of transplant will become reinfected.[174–176] Factors associated with a more rapid progression of the disease after transplant may include the degree of immunosuppression,[177] coinfection with CMV,[178] and HCV genotype 1b.[179] In bone marrow transplant patients, HCV infection is a major cause of post-transplant cirrhosis. Clear association with veno-occlusive disease has also been observed.[180] The evolution of the liver disease is typically slow, with the disease following a similar course in liver, heart,[181] kidney,[182] and bone marrow transplant patients. Short-term survival is not affected in kidney transplant patients, but long-term (10 and 20 years) outcome was significantly worse in HCV antibody–positive patients.[183,184] Fibrosing cholestatic hepatitis is the only early but serious complication of HCV infection observed in transplant patients.[180] The clinical and pathologic features are similar to the one described in hepatitis B. Diagnosis is made by detection of HCV RNA by reverse transcriptase PCR and other assays because serology is a poor marker of HCV infection in transplant recipients.[185,186] Liver biopsy is important to confirm the diagnosis histologically and to delineate the severity of the disease.

Treatment is similar to that in the normal host. Interferon alone or in combination with ribavirin is typically used. The concern with the use of interferon is its association with graft rejection in renal transplant; however, these issues do not appear to be valid in liver transplant recipients. The response rates to treatment are lower than those seen in immunocompetent patients.[187] Preemptive therapy prior to liver transplant tends to reduce the viral load and is associated with milder disease and slower progression.

Invasive candidiasis is a major cause of mortality and morbidity in patients with hematologic malignancies. Hepatosplenic involvement is typical, as was initially described by Bodey and colleagues.[188] Risk factors for invasive disease include the presence of acute leukemia, prolonged neutropenia, intravascular catheters, disruption of mucosal barriers, and the administration of broad-spectrum antibiotics.[189] Invasive candidal infection is extremely rare in nonleukemic patients.

Hepatosplenic candidiasis initially presents as neutropenia and fever without focal signs or symptoms that fails to respond to broad-spectrum antibiotics. Liver function tests, as well as ultrasonography and CT scan of the abdomen, are generally normal at this point. Often the patient's leukemia goes into remission, and the neutrophil count recovers. However, high fever, anorexia, and weight loss persist. Right-sided abdominal pain or pleuritic chest pain may be present. Substantial elevation of alkaline phosphatase is noted and may persist for months. Elevation of other liver function tests is usually present but is less impressive.[189]

CT scan identifies lesions in about 90% of the patient, and ultrasonography visualizes pathology in 70 to 75% of patients.[190] CT scan demonstrates small, round, low-attenuation lesions scattered throughout the liver and spleen. The appearance on CT scan is not pathognomonic and may mimic metastatic disease or bacterial abscesses. Histologically, three patterns have been observed: necrosis with minimal inflammatory reaction, microabscesses with severe inflammation, and granulomas.[191] Granulomatous inflammation is usually seen in the liver. Central areas of necrosis or fibrosis, surrounded by granulation tissue, are seen; macrophages, fibroblasts, and giant cells are typically observed.[189]

The diagnosis of invasive candidiasis requires a high index of suspicion. No single noninvasive study is sufficient to establish a diagnosis, and liver biopsy is frequently performed. Because many infections may cause granulomatous inflammation, and given the small size of the lesions, percutaneous liver biopsy may fail to establish the diagnosis. Open liver biopsy is considered by many to be the most reliable way of diagnosing hepatosplenic candidiasis.[192] The optimal management of this condition is not yet established. The response rate to the liposomal formulation of amphotericin B is much better than the response rate to the regular formulation: 85 to 90% versus 50%.[193–195] Fluconazole has a response rate of about 80% and may be effective even in patients who failed to respond to amphotericin B treatment.[193,194,196] It is believed that fluconazole should be the drug of choice for hepatosplenic candidiasis because it is at least as effective as amphotericin B, is less toxic, may be given orally, and is less expensive than liposomal amphotericin B.[197] Usually, it takes 2 to 3 weeks to see a measurable response.

REFERENCES

1. Centers for Disease Control and Prevention. US HIV and AIDS cases reported through June 1999. HIV/AIDS Surveillance Report 1999;11(No.1):1–24.
2. Schneiderman DJ, Arenson DM, Cello JP. Hepatic disease in patients with acquired immunodeficiency syndrome (AIDS). Hepatology 1987;7:925–30.
3. Bonacini M. Hepatobiliary complications in patients with human immunodeficiency virus infection. Am J Med 1992;92:404–11.
4. American Gastroenterological Association technical review. Malnutrition and cachexia, chronic diarrhea, and hepatobiliary disease in patients with human immunodeficiency virus infection. Gastroenterology 1996;111:1724–52.
5. Persaud D, Bangaru B, Greco A, et al. Cholestatic hepatitis in children infected with the human immunodeficiency virus. Pediatr Infect Dis J 1993;12:492–8.
6. Kahn SA, Saltzman BR, Klein RS, et al. Hepatic syndromes in the acquired immunodeficiency syndrome: a clinical and pathological study. Am J Gastroenterol 1986;81: 1145–8
7. Puoti M, Spinetti A, Ghezzi A, et al. Mortality for liver disease in patients with HIV infection: a cohort study. J AIDS 2000;24:211–7.
8. Housset C, Boucher O, Girard P. Immunohistochemical evidence for human immunodeficiency virus-1 infection of liver Kupffer cells. Hum Pathol 1990;21:404–8.
9. Lafon ME, Kirn A. Human immunodeficiency virus infection of the liver. Semin Liver Dis 1992;12:197–204.
10. Schmitt M, Lafon M, Gendrault J. Primary cultures of endothelial cells from the human liver sinusoid are permissible for human immunodeficiency virus type 1. Proc Natl Acad Sci U S A 1992;89:1582–6.
11. Lebovics E, Dwrkin BM, Heier SK, et al. The hepatobiliary manifestations of human immunodeficiency virus infection. Am J Gastroenterol 1988;83:1–7.
12. Duffy LF, Daum F, Kahn E, et al. Hepatitis in children with acquired immunodeficiency syndrome: histopathologic and immunocytologic features. Gastroenterology 1986;90:173–81.
13. Jonas MM, Roldan EO, Lyons HJ, et al. Histopathologic features of the liver in pediatric acquired immunodeficiency syndrome. J Pediatr Gastroenterol Nutr 1989;9:73–81.
14. Kahn E, Greco MA, Daum F, et al. Hepatic pathology in pediatric acquired immunodeficiency syndrome. Hum Pathol 1991;22:1111–9.
15. Lacaille F, Fournet J-C, Blanche S. Clinical utility of liver biopsy in children with acquired immunodeficiency syndrome. Pediatr Infect Dis J 1999;18:143–7.
16. Witzleben CL, Marshall GS, Wenner W, et al. HIV as a cause of giant cell hepatitis. Hum Pathol 1988;19:603–5.
17. Gaur S, Rosenthal S, Dadhania J, et al. Cholestatic giant cell hepatitis associated with ultrastructural evidence of intrahepatic retroviral infection in a human immunodeficiency virus-positive infant. J Pediatr Gastroenterol Nutr 1993;16:199–202.
18. Pitlik S, Fainstein V, Garza D, et al. Human cryptosporidiosis: spectrum of disease: report of 6 cases and review of the literature. Arch Intern Med 1983;143:2269–75.
19. Pitlick S, Fainstein V, Rios A, et al. Cryptosporidial cholecystitis. N Engl J Med 1983;308:967.
20. Guarda LA, Stein SA, Cleary KA, Ordonez NG. Human cryptosporidiosis in the acquired immunodeficiency syndrome. Arch Pathol Lab Med 1983;107:562–6.
21. Margulis SJ, Honig CL, Souve R, et al. Biliary tract obstruction in the acquired immunodeficiency syndrome. Ann Intern Med 1986;105:207–10.
22. Pol S, Romana C, Richard S, et al. Enterocytozoan bienusi infection in acquired immunodeficiency syndrome related sclerosing cholangitis. Gastroenterology 1992;102:1178–81.

23. Benator DA, French AL, Beaudet LM, et al. *Isospora belli* infection associated with acalculous cholecystitis in a patient with AIDS. Ann Intern Med 1994;121:663–4.

24. Cello JP. Acquired immunodeficiency syndrome cholangiopathy: spectrum of disease. Am J Med 1989;86:539–46.

25. Nash JA, Cohen SA. Gallbladder and biliary tract disease in AIDS. Gastroenterol Clin North Am 1997;26:323–35.

26. Cello JP. Human immunodeficiency virus associated biliary tract disease. Semin Liver Dis 1992;12:213–8.

27. Auer P, Lubke HJ, Frieling T, et al. Sphincter of Oddi dysfunction in AIDS related autonomic failure. Gastroenterology 1995;108:A404.

28. Levenson SD, Koch J, Shlueck G, et al. Sphincter of Oddi dysfunction in patients with suspected AIDS cholangiopathy [abstract]. Gastrointest Endosc 1994;40:116.

29. Benhamou Y, Caumes E, Gerosa Y, et al. AIDS-related cholangiopathy: critical analysis of a perspective series of 26 patients. Dig Dis Sci 1993;38:1113–8.

30. Grumback K, Coleman RG, Gal AA. Hepatic and biliary tract abnormalities in patients with AIDS. Sonographic-pathologic correlation. J Ultrasound Med 1989;8:247–54.

31. Capell MS, Schwartz MS, Biempica L. Clinical utility of liver biopsy in patients with serum antibodies to the human immunodeficiency virus. Am J Med 1990;88:123–30.

32. Beale TJ, Wetton CW, Crofton ME. A sonographic-pathological correlation of liver biopsy in patients with acquired immune deficiency syndrome (AIDS). Clin Radiol 1995;50:761–4.

33. Churchill DR, Mann D, Coker RJ, et al. Fatal hemorrhage following liver biopsy in patients with HIV infection. Genitourin Med 1996;72:62–4.

34. Gordon SC, McFadden RF, Reddy KR, et al. Major hemorrhage after percutaneous liver biopsy in patients with AIDS. Gastroenterology 1991;30:1787.

35. Poles MA, Dieterich DT, Schwarz ED, et al. Liver biopsy findings in 501 patients with the human immunodeficiency virus (HIV). J Acquir Immune Defic Retrovirol 1996;11:170–7.

36. Housset C, Pol S, Carnot F, et al. Interactions between human immunodeficiency virus-1, hepatitis delta virus and hepatitis B virus infections in 260 chronic carriers of hepatitis B virus. Hepatology 1992;15:578–83.

37. Lazizi Y, Grangeot-Keros L, Delfraissy J. Reappearance of hepatitis B virus in immune patients infected with human immunodeficiency virus type 1. J Infect Dis 1988;158:666–7.

38. Altfeld M, Rockstroh JK, Addo M, et al. Reactivation of hepatitis B in a long-term anti-HBs-positive patient with AIDS following lamivudine withdrawal. J Hepatol 1998;29:306–9.

39. Lau D, Bianchine P, Mican J, et al. Liver disease in patients with hepatitis B and human immunodeficiency virus co-infection. Gastroenterology 1997;112:A1313.

40. Rusnak JM, Hong G. Reactivation vs. reinfection of hepatitis B in HIV seropositive individuals with previous natural immunity to hepatitis B. In: Programs and Abstracts of the 11th International Conference on AIDS 1996. Vancouver, July 1996.

41. Waite J, Gilson R, Weller I. Hepatitis B reactivation or reinfection associated with HIV-1 infection. AIDS 1988;2:443–8.

42. Laukam-Josten U, Muller O, Bienzle U. Decline of naturally acquired antibodies to hepatitis B surface antigen in HIV-1 infected homosexual men. AIDS 1988;2:400–1.

43. Biggar R, Goedert J, Hoofnagle J. Accelerated loss of antibody to hepatitis B surface antigen among immunodeficient homosexual men infected with HIV. N Engl J Med 1987;316:630–1.

44. Scharschmidt B, Held M, Hollander H. Hepatitis B in patients with HIV infection: relationship to AIDS and patient survival. Ann Intern Med 1992;117:837–8.

45. Bodsworth N, Donovan B, Nightingale B. The effect of concurrent human immunodeficiency virus infection on chronic hepatitis B: a study of 150 homosexual men. J Infect Dis 1989;160:577–82.

46. Befeler AS, Di Bisceglie AM. Hepatitis B. Infect Dis Clin North Am 2000;14:617–32.

47. Velasco M, Moran A, Jesus Tellez M. Resolution of chronic hepatitis B after ritonavir treatment in an HIV-infected patient. N Engl J Med 1999;340:1765–6.

48. Goldin RD, Fish DE, Hay A, et al. Histological and immunohistochemical study of hepatitis B virus in human immunodeficiency virus infection. J Clin Pathol 1990;43:203–5.

49. Colin JF, Cazals-Hatem D, Loriot MA, et al. Influence of human immunodeficiency virus infection on chronic hepatitis B in homosexual men. Hepatology 1999;29:1306–10.

50. Di Martino V, Lunel F, Cadranel JF, et al. Long-term effects of interferon-alpha in five HIV-positive patients with chronic hepatitis B. J Viral Hepat 1996;3:253–60.

51. McDonald JA, Caruso L, Karayiannis P, et al. Diminished responsiveness of male homosexual chronic hepatitis B virus carriers with HTLV-III antibodies to recombinant alpha-interferon. Hepatology 1987;7:719–23.

52. Wong DK, Yim C, Naylor CD, et al. Interferon alfa treatment of chronic hepatitis B: randomized trial in a predominantly homosexual male population. Gastroenterology 1995;108:165–71.

53. Zylberberg H, Jiang J, Pialoux G, et al. Alpha-interferon for chronic active hepatitis B in human immunodeficiency virus-infected patients. Gastroenterol Clin Biol 1996;20:968–71.

54. Dore GJ, Cooper DA, Barrett C, et al. Dual efficacy of lamivudine treatment in human immunodeficiency virus/hepatitis B virus-coinfected persons in a randomized, controlled study (CAESAR). The CAESAR Coordinating Committee. J Infect Dis 1999;180:607–13.

55. Dienstag JL, Schiff ER, Wright TL, et al. Lamivudine as initial treatment for chronic hepatitis B in the United States. N Engl J Med 1999;341:1256–63.

56. Benhamou Y, Bochet M, Thibault V, et al. Long-term incidence of hepatitis B virus resistance to lamivudine in human immunodeficiency virus-infected patients. Hepatology 1999;30:1302–6.

57. Dusheiko G. Lamivudine treatment of chronic hepatitis B. Rev Med Virol 1998;8:153–9.

58. Ono-Nita SK, Kato N, Shiratori Y, et al. Susceptibility of lamivudine-resistant hepatitis B virus to other reverse transcriptase inhibitors. J Clin Invest 1999;103:1635–40.

59. Eison RC, Dieterich DT. Adefovir and abacavir combination therapy for chronic HBV: a case report of successful treatment [abstract]. Presented at Digestive Diseases Week; 1999, May 16–19; Orlando, FL.

60. Marcellin P, Boyer N, Colin JF, et al. Recombinant alpha interferon for chronic hepatitis B in anti-HIV positive patients receiving zidovudine. Gut 1993;34(2 Suppl):S106.

61. Mannuci M, Zanetti A, Gringeri A. Long-term immunogenicity of a plasma-derived hepatitis B vaccine in HIV-seropositive and HIV-negative hemophiliacs. Arch Intern Med 1989;149:1333–7.

62. Carne C, Weller I, Waite J. Impaired responsiveness of homosexual men with HIV antibodies to plasma-derived hepatitis B vaccine. BJM 1987;294:866–8.

63. Collier A, Corey L, Murphy V. Antibody to human immunodeficiency virus and suboptimal response to hepatitis B vaccination. Ann Intern Med 1988;109:101–5.

64. Wong D, Cheung A, O'Rourke K, et al. Effect of alpha-interferon treatment in patients with hepatitis Be antigen-positive chronic hepatitis B: a meta-analysis. Ann Intern Med 1993;119:312–23.

65. Perillo R, Regeenstein F, Roodman S. Chronic hepatitis B in asymptomatic homosexual men with antibody to the human immunodeficiency virus. Ann Intern Med 1986;105:382–3.

66. Bruno R, Sacchi P, Puoti M, et al. HCV chronic hepatitis in patients with HIV: clinical management issues. Am J Gastroenterol 2002;97:1598–606.

67. Sherman KE, Rouster SD, Chung R, et al. Hepatitis C. Prevalence in HIV infected patients: a cross sectional analysis of the US adult clinical trials Group. Presented at: 10th International Symposium on Viral Hepatitis and Liver Disease; 2000 Apr 9–14; Atlanta, GA.

68. Thomas DL, Villano SA, Riester KA, et al. Perinatal transmission of hepatitis C virus from human immunodeficiency virus type 1-infected mothers. Women and Infants Transmission Study. J Infect Dis 1998;177:1480–8.

69. Nigro G, D'Orio F, Catania S, et al. Mother to infant transmission of co-infection by human immunodeficiency virus and hepatitis C virus: prevalence and clinical manifestations. Arch Virol 1997;142:453–7.

70. National Institutes of Health. Consensus development conference panel statement: management of hepatitis C. Hepatology 1997;26 Suppl 1:2–10.

71. Consensus statement: EASL International Consensus Conference on Hepatitis C. J Hepatol 1999;30:956–61.

72. Garcia-Samaniego J, Rodriguez M, Berenguer J, et al. Hepatocellular carcinoma in HIV-infected patients with chronic hepatitis C. Am J Gastroenterol 2001;96:179–83.

73. Benhamou Y, Di Martino V, Bochet M, et al. Factors affecting liver fibrosis in human immunodeficiency virus- and hepatitis C virus-coinfected patients: impact of protease inhibitor therapy. Hepatology 2001;34:283–7.

74. Sulkowski MS, Thomas DL, Chaisson RE, et al. Hepatotoxicity associated with antiretroviral therapy in adults infected with human immunodeficiency virus and the role of hepatitis C or B virus infection. JAMA 2000;283:74–80.

75. Bruno R, Sacchi P, Filice G. Hepatitis C virus RNA dynamics during antiretroviral therapy. Blood 2001;97:3318–9.

76. Jonas MM. Treatment of chronic hepatitis C in pediatric patients. Clin Liver Dis 1999;3:855–67.

77. Giovannini M, Tagger A, Ribero ML, et al. Maternal-infant transmission of hepatitis C virus and HIV infections: a possible interaction. Lancet 1990;335:1166.

78. Paccagnini S, Principi N, Massironi E, et al. Perinatal transmission and manifestation of hepatitis C virus infection in a high risk population. Pediatr Infect Dis J 1995;14:195–9.

79. Dodig M, Tavill A. Hepatitis C and human immunodeficiency virus coinfections. J Clin Gastroenterol 2001;33:367–74.

80. Poles MA, Dieterich DT. Infections of the liver in HIV-infected patients. Infect Dis Clin North Am 2000;14:741–59.

81. Benhamou Y, Bochet M, Di Martino V, et al. Liver fibrosis progression in human immunodeficiency virus and hepatitis C virus coinfected patients. Hepatology 1999;30:1054–8.

82. Bierhoff E, Fischer HP, Willsch E, et al. Liver histopathology in patients with concurrent chronic hepatitis C and HIV infection. Virchows Arch 1997;430:271–7.

83. Thio CL, Nolt KR, Astemborski J, et al. Screening for hepatitis C virus in human immunodeficiency virus-infected individuals. J Clin Microbiol 2000;38:575–7.

84. Cribier B, Rey D, Schmitt C, et al. High hepatitis C viremia and impaired antibody response in patients coinfected with HIV. AIDS 1995;9:1131–6.

85. Zylberger H, Chaix Ml, Rabian C, et al. Tritherapy for human immunodeficiency virus infection does not modify replication of hepatitis C virus in coinfected subjects. Clin Infect Dis 1998;26:1104–6.

86. Bonacini M, Puoti M. Hepatitis C in patients with human immunodeficiency virus infection: diagnosis, natural history, meta-analysis of sexual and vertical transmission, and therapeutic issues. Arch Intern Med 2000;160:3365–73.

87. Sauleda S, Juarez A, Esteban JI, et al. Interferon and ribavirin combination therapy in chronic hepatitis C in human immunodeficiency virus infested patients with congenital coagulopathy disorders. Hepatology 2001;3:1035–40.

88. Landau A, Batisse D, Piketty C, et al. Long term efficacy of combination therapy with interferon alpha 2b and ribavirin for severe chronic hepatitis C in HIV-infected patients. AIDS 2001;15:2149–55.

89. Reddy KR, Wright TL, Pockros PJ, et al. Efficacy and safety of pegylated (40-kd) interferon alpha-2a compared with interferon alpha-2a in noncirrhotic patients with chronic hepatitis C. Hepatology 2001;33:433–8.

90. Heathcote EJ, Shiffman ML, Cooksley WG, et al. Peginterferon alpha-2a patients with chronic hepatitis C and cirrhosis. N Engl J Med 2000;43:1673–80.

91. 1999 US Public Health Service/Infectious Disease Society of America. Guidelines for the prevention of opportunistic infections in persons infected with HIV: part II. Prevention of the first episode of the disease. Am Fam Physician 2000;61:441–2, 445–9, 453–4.

92. Balayan MS, Fedorova OE, Mikhailov MI, et al. Antibody to hepatitis E virus in HIV-infected individuals and AIDS patients. J Viral Hepatol 1997;4:279–83.

93. Lefrere JJ, Roudot-Thoraval F, Morand-Joubert L, et al. Carriage of GB virus C/hepatitis G virus RNA is associated with a slower immunologic, virologic, and clinical progression of human immunodeficiency virus disease in co-infected persons. J Infect Dis 1999;179:783–9.

94. Janner D, Petru AM, Belchis D, et al. Fatal adenovirus infections in a child with acquired immunodeficiency syndrome. Pediatr Infect Dis J 1990;9:434–6.

95. Krilov LR, Kaplan MH, Frogel M, et al. Disseminated adenoviral infection with hepatic necrosis in patients with HIV infection and other immunodeficiency states. Rev Infect Dis 1990;12:303–7.

96. Janoff EN, Orenstein JM, Manischewitz JF, et al. Adenovirus colitis in the acquired immunodeficiency syndrome. Gastroenterology 1991;100:976–9.

97. Hedderwick SA, Greenson JK, McGaughy VR, Clark NM. Adenovirus cholecystitis in a patient with AIDS. Clin Infect Dis 1998;26:997–9.

98. Hierholzer LC. Adenoviruses in the immunocompromised host. Clin Microbiol Rev 1992;5:262–74.

99. Dagan R, Schwartz RH, Insel RA, et al. Severe diffuse adenovirus 7a pneumonia in a child with combined immunodeficiency: possible therapeutic effects of human serum globulin containing specific neutralizing antibody. Pediatr Infect Dis J 1984;3:246–9.

100. Cassano WF. Intravenous ribavirin therapy for adenovirus cystitis after allogenic bone marrow transplantation. Bone Marrow Transplant 1991;7:247–8.

101. Munoz FM, Piedra PA, Demmler GJ. Disseminated adenovirus disease in immunocompromised and immunocompetent children. Clin Infect Dis 1998;27:1194–200.

102. Zimmerli W, Bianchi L, Gudat F, et al. Disseminated herpes simplex type 2 and systemic *Candida* infection in a patient with

previous asymptomatic human immunodeficiency virus infection. J Infect Dis 1988;157:597–8.

103. Fingeroth J. Herpesvirus infection of the liver. Infect Dis Clin North Am 2000;14:689–719.

104. McClain KL, Leach CT, Jenson HB, et al. Association of Epstein-Barr virus with leiomyosarcomas in children with AIDS. N Engl J Med 1995;332:12–8.

105. Herndier BG, Friedman SL. Neoplasms of the gastrointestinal tract and hepatobiliary system in acquired immunodeficiency syndrome. Semin Liver Dis 1992;12:128–41.

106. Sobue R, Miyazaki H, Okamoto M, et al. Fulminant hepatitis in primary human herpesvirus-6 infection [letter]. N Engl J Med 1991;324:1290.

107. Asano Y, Yoshikawa T, Suga S, et al. Fatal fulminant hepatitis in an infant with human herpesvirus-6 infection [letter]. Lancet 1990;335:862–3.

108. Yoshida M, Yamada M, Tsukazaki T, et al. Comparison of antiviral compounds against human herpesvirus 6 and 7. Antiviral Res 1998;40:73–84.

109. Hasan FA, Jeffers LJ, Welsh SW, et al. Hepatic involvement as the primary manifestation of Kaposi's sarcoma in the acquired immunodeficiency syndrome. Am J Gastroenterol 1989;84:1449–51.

110. Kitchen BJ, Engler HD, Gill VJ, et al. Cytomegalovirus infection in children with human immunodeficiency virus syndrome. Pediatr Infect Dis J 1997;16:358–63.

111. Burgart LJ. Cholangitis in viral disease. Mayo Clin Proc 1998; 73:479–82.

112. Salmon D, Lacassin F, Harzic M, et al. Predictive value of cytomegalovirus viraemia for the occurrence of CMV organ involvement in AIDS. J Med Virol 1990;32:160–3.

113. Capell MS. Hepatobiliary manifestations of the acquired immunodeficiency syndrome. Am J Gastroenterol 1991;86:1–15.

114. Hagovian WA, Huseby JS. Pneumocystis hepatitis despite successful aerosolized pentamedine pulmonary prophylaxis. Chest 1989;96:949–51.

115. Raviglione MC, Mariuz P, Sugar J, Mullen MP. Extrapulmonary Pneumocystis infection. Ann Intern Med 1989;111:339–40.

116. Merkel IS, Good CB, Nalesnik M, et al. Chronic Pneumocystis carinii infection of the liver. J Clin Gastroenterol 1992;15:55–8.

117. Lebovics ES, Thung S, Schaffner F, et al. The liver in acquired immunodeficiency syndrome: a clinical and histologic study. Hepatology 1985;5:293–8.

118. Forbes A, Blanshard C, Gazzard B. Natural history of AIDS-related sclerosing cholangitis: a study of 20 cases. Gut 1993;34:116–21.

119. Kahn E, Ishak KG. Hepatic system. In: Morgan C, Mullick FG, editors. Systemic pathology of HIV infection and AIDS in children. Washington (DC): Armed Forces Institute of Pathology, American Registry of Pathology; 1997. p. 193.

120. Bouche H, Housset C, Dumont JL, et al. AIDS related cholangitis: diagnostic features in course of 15 patients. J Hepatol 1993;17:34–9.

121. Sheikh RA, Prindville TP, Yenamandra S, et al. Microsporidial AIDS cholangiopathy due to Encephalitozoon intestinalis: case report and review. Am J Gastroenterol 2000;95:2364–71.

122. Bonacini M, Nussbaum J, Ahluwalia C. Gastrointestinal, hepatic, and pancreatic involvement with Cryptococcus neoformans in AIDS. J Clin Gastroenterol 1990;12:295–7.

123. Horsburgh CR Jr, Cladwell MB, Simonds RJ. Epidemiology of disseminated nontuberculous mycobacterial disease in children with acquired immunodeficiency syndrome. Pediatr Infect Dis J 1993;12:219–22.

124. Horsburgh CR Jr. The pathophysiology of disseminated Mycobacterium avium complex disease in AIDS. J Infect Dis 1999;179 Suppl 3:S461–5.

125. Chaisson RE, Schecter GF, Theuer CP, et al. Tuberculosis in patients with the acquired immunodeficiency syndrome. Clinical features, response of therapy and survival. Am Rev Respir Dis 1987;136:570–4.

126. Rutstein RM, Cobb P, McGowan KL, et al. Mycobacterium avium intracellulare complex infection in HIV-infected children. AIDS 1993;7:507–12.

127. Shafran SD, Singer J, Zarowny DP, et al. A comparison of two regimens for the treatment of Mycobacterium avium complex bacteremia in AIDS: rifabutin, ethambutol, and clarithromycin versus rifampin, ethambutol, clofazimine, and ciprofloxacin. N Engl J Med 1996;335:377–83.

128. Working Group on Antiretroviral Therapy and Medical Management of HIV-Infected Children. Antiretroviral therapy and medical management of pediatric HIV infection. Pediatrics 1998;102 Suppl:1.

129. Barton L, Moussa SL, Villar R, Hulett RL. Gastrointestinal complications of chronic granulomatous disease. Case report and literature review. Clin Pediatr 1998;37:231–6.

130. Conte D, Fraquelli M, Capsoni F, et al. Effectiveness of IFN-γ for liver abscesses in chronic granulomatous disease. J Interferon Cytokine Res 1999;19:705–10.

131. Buescher ES, Gallin JI. Leukocyte transfusions in chronic granulomatous disease. N Engl J Med 1982;307:800–3.

132. von Planta M, Ozsahin H, Schroten H, et al. Greater omentum flaps and granulocyte transfusions as combined therapy of liver abscesses in chronic granulomatous disease. Eur J Pediatr Surg 1997;7:234–6.

133. Forrest CB, Forehand JR, Axtell RA, et al. Clinical features and current management of chronic granulomatous disease. Hematol Oncol Clin North Am 1988;2:253–65.

134. Aggett PJ, Cavanagh NPC, Matthew DJ, et al. Shwachman's syndrome, a review of 21 cases. Arch Dis Child 1980;55:331–47.

135. Mack DR, Forstner GG, Wilschanski M, et al. Shwachman syndrome: exocrine pancreatic dysfunction and variable phenotypic expression. Gastroenterology 1996;111:1593–602.

136. Sisto A, Feldman P, Garel L, et al. Primary sclerosing cholangitis in children: study of five cases and review of the literature. Pediatrics 1987;80:918–23.

137. Davis JJ, Heyman MB, Ferrell L, et al. Sclerosing cholangitis associated with chronic cryptosporidiosis in a child with a congenital immunodeficiency disorder. Am J Gastroenterol 1987;82:1196–202.

138. McKinney R, Katz S, Wilfert C. Chronic enteroviral meningoencephalitis in agammaglobulinemia patients. Rev Infect Dis 1987;9:334.

139. Webster AB. Common variable immunodeficiency. Immunol Allergy Clin North Am 2001;21:1–22.

140. Ratech H, Greco MA, Gallo G, et al. Pathologic findings in adenosine deaminase-deficient severe combined immunodeficiency. Kidney, adrenal, and chondro-osseous tissue alterations. Am J Pathol 1985;120:157–69.

141. Bollinger ME, Arredono-Vega FX, Sentisteban I. Brief report: hepatic dysfunction as a complication of adenosine deaminase deficiency. N Engl J Med 1996;334:1367–71.

142. Aleman K, Noordzij J, De Groot R, et al. Reviewing Omenn syndrome. Eur J Pediatr 2001;160:718–25.

143. Purtilo DT, Yang JPS, Cassel CK, et al. X-linked recessive progressive combined variable immunodeficiency (Duncan's disease). Lancet 1975;i:935–41.

144. Seibel NL, Cossman J, Magrath IT. Lymphoproliferative disorders. In: Pizzo PA, Poplack DG, editors. Principles and prac-

tice of pediatric oncology. 2nd ed. Philadelphia: JB Lippincott; 1993. p. 595–616.

145. Fishman JA, Rubin RH. Infection in organ-transplant recipients. N Engl J Med 1998;338:1741.

146. Sneller M, Lane C. Infections in the immunocompromised host. In: Rich RR, editor. Clinical immunology: principles and practice. Vol. 1. London: Mosby; 2001. p. 32.11–3.

147. Singh N, Dummer JS, Kusne S, et al. Infections with cytomegalovirus and other herpesviruses in 121 liver transplant recipients: transmission by donated organ and the effect of OKT3 antibodies. J Infect Dis 1988;158:124–31.

148. Rosen HR, Corless CL, Rabkin J, et al. Association of cytomegalovirus genotype with graft rejection after liver transplantation. Transplantation 1998;66:1627–31.

149. Madalosso C, De Souza NF, Ilstrup DM, et al. Cytomegalovirus and its association with hepatic artery thrombosis after liver transplantation. Transplantation 1998;66:294–7.

150. McDiarmid SV. Liver transplantation. The pediatric challenge. Clin Liver Dis 2000;4:879–927.

151. Cox KL, Lawrence-Miyasaki LS, Garcia-Kennedy R, et al. An increased incidence of Epstein-Barr virus infection and lymphoproliferative disorder in young children on FK506 after liver transplantation. Transplantation 1995;4:524–9.

152. Renard TH, Andrews WS, Foster ME. Relationship between OKT3 administration, EBV seroconversion, and the lymphoproliferative syndrome in pediatric liver transplant recipients. Transplant Proc 1991;23:1473–6.

153. Ho M, Jaffe R, Miller G, et al. The frequency of Epstein-Barr virus infection and associated lymphoproliferative syndrome after transplantation and its manifestations in children. Transplantation 1988;45:719–27.

154. Green M, Michaels MG, Webber SA, et al. The management of Epstein-Barr virus associated post-transplant lymphoproliferative disorders in pediatric solid-organ transplant recipients. Pediatr Transplant 1999;3:271–81.

155. Cacciarelli TV, Reyes J, Mazariegos GV, et al. Natural history of Epstein-Barr viral load in peripheral blood of pediatric liver transplant recipients during treatment for posttransplant lymphoproliferative disorder. Transplant Proc 1999;31:488–9.

156. Rowe DT, Qu L, Reyes J, et al. Use of quantitative competitive PCR to measure Epstein-Barr virus genome load in the peripheral blood of pediatric transplant patients with lymphoproliferative disorders. J Clin Microbiol 1997;135:1612–5.

157. Kogan DL, Burroughs M, Emre S, et al. Prospective longitudinal analysis of quantitative Epstein-Barr virus polymerase chain reaction in pediatric liver transplant recipients. Transplantation 1999;67:1068–70.

158. Fornairon S, Pol S, Legendre C, et al. The long-term virologic and pathologic impact of renal transplantation on chronic hepatitis B infection. Transplantation 1996;62:297–9.

159. Alexopoulos CG, Valslamatzis M, Hatzidimitrou G. Prevalence of hepatitis B virus marker positivity and evolution of hepatitis B virus profile, during chemotherapy, in patients with solid tumors. Br J Cancer 1999;67:69–74.

160. Reed EC, Myerson D, Corey L, et al. Allogenic marrow transplantation in patients positive for hepatitis B surface antigen. Blood 1991;77:195–200.

161. Lau GK, Liang R, Chiu EK, et al. Hepatic events after bone marrow transplantation in patients with hepatitis B infection: a case control study. Bone Marrow Transplant 1997;19:797–9.

162. Davis C, Gretch DR, Carithers RL. Hepatitis B and transplantation. Infect Dis Clin North Am 1995;9:925–41.

163. Kairaitis LK, Gottlieb T, George CR. Fatal hepatitis B virus infection with fibrosing cholestatic hepatitis following renal transplantation. Nephrol Dial Transplant 1998;13:1571–3.

164. Blanpain C, Knoop C, Delforge ML, et al. Reactivation of hepatitis B after transplantation in patients with pre-existing anti-hepatitis B surface antigen antibodies: report on three cases and review of the literature. Transplantation 1998;66:883–6.

165. McMillan JS, Shaw T, Angus PW, Locarnini SA. Effect of immunosuppressive and antiviral agents on hepatitis B virus replication in vitro. Hepatology 1995;22:36–43.

166. Angus P, Locarnini SA, McCaughan GW, et al. Hepatitis B virus pre-core mutant infection in association with severe recurrent disease after liver transplantation. Hepatology 1995;21:14–8.

167. Terrault NA, Zhou S, Combs C, et al. Prophylaxis in liver transplant recipients using a fixed dosing schedule of hepatitis B immunoglobulin. Hepatology 1996;24:1327–33.

168. Rosen HR, Martin P. Viral hepatitis in the liver transplant recipient. Infect Dis Clin North Am 2000;14:761–84.

169. Wedemeyer H, Boker KH, Pethig K, et al. Famciclovir treatment of chronic hepatitis B in heart transplant recipients: a prospective trial. Transplantation 1999;68:1503–11.

170. Markowitz JS, Martin P, Conrad AJ, et al. Prophylaxis against hepatitis B recurrence following liver transplantation using combination lamivudine and hepatitis B immune globulin. Hepatology 1998;28:585–9.

171. Kasiske BL, Vazguez MA, Harmon WE, et al. Recommendations for the outpatient surveillance of renal transplant recipients. American Society for Transplantation. J Am Soc Nephrol 2000;11 Suppl 15: S1–S86.

172. Kirk AD, Heisey DM, D'Alessandro AM, et al. Clinical hepatitis after transplantation of hepatitis C virus-positive kidneys: HLA-DR3 as a risk factor for the development of posttransplant hepatitis. Transplantation 1996;62:1758–62.

173. Terrault NA, Wright TL, Pereira BJG. Hepatitis C infection in the transplant recipient. Infect Dis Clin North Am 1995;4:943–64.

174. Wright T, Donegan E, Hsu HH, et al. Recurrent and acquired hepatitis C viral infection in liver transplant recipients. Gastroenterology 1992;103:317–22.

175. Everhart JE, Wei Y, Eng H, et al. Recurrent and new hepatitis C virus infection after liver transplantation. Hepatology 1999;29:1220–6.

176. Boker KH, Dalley G, Bahr MJ, et al. Long-term outcome of hepatitis C virus infection after liver transplantation. Hepatology 1997;25:203–10.

177. Papatheodoridis GV, Barton SG, Andrew D, et al. Longitudinal variation in hepatitis C (HCV) viraemia and early course of HCV infection after liver transplantation for HCV cirrhosis: the role of different immunosuppressive regimens. Gut 1999;45:427–34.

178. Rosen HR, Chou S, Corless DR, et al. Cytomegalovirus viraemia. Risk factor for allograft cirrhosis after liver transplantation for hepatitis C. Transplantation 1997;64:721–6.

179. Feray C, Gigou M, Samuel D, et al. Influence of genotypes of hepatitis C virus on the severity of recurrent liver disease after liver transplantation. Gastroenterology 1995;108:1088–96.

180. Locasciulli A, Testa M, Pontisso P, et al. Hepatitis C virus genotypes and liver disease in patients undergoing allogeneic bone marrow transplantation. Bone Marrow Transplant 1997;19:237–40.

181. Ong JP, Barnes DS, Younossi ZM, et al. Outcome of de novo hepatitis C virus infection in heart transplant recipients. Hepatology 1999;30:1293–8.

182. Mathurin P, Mouquet C, Poynard T, et al. Impact of hepatitis B and C virus on kidney transplantation outcome. Hepatology 1999;29:257–63.

183. Gentil MA, Rocha JL, Rodriguez-Algarra G, et al. Impaired kidney transplant survival in patients with antibodies to hepatitis C virus. Nephrol Dial Transplant 1999;14:2455–60.

184. Hanafusa T, Ichikawa Y, Kishikawa H, et al. Retrospective study on the impact of hepatitis C virus infection on kidney transplant patients over 20 years. Transplantation 1998;66: 471–6.

185. Maple PAC, McKee T, Desselberger U, Wreghitt TG. Hepatitis C virus infections in transplant patients: serological and virological investigations. J Med Virol 1994;44:43–8.

186. Chan TM, Wu PC, Lok AS, et al. Clinicopathological features of hepatitis C virus antibody negative fatal chronic hepatitis C after renal transplantation. Nephron 1995;71:213–7.

187. Wright T, Combs C, Kim M, et al. Interferon-alpha therapy for hepatitis C infection after liver transplantation. Hepatology 1994;20:773–9.

188. Bodey GP, DeJongh D, Isassi A, et al. Hypersplenism due to disseminated candidiasis in a patient with acute leukemia. Cancer 1969;26:417.

189. Kontoyiannis DP, Luna MA, Samuels BI, Bodey GP. Hepatosplenic candidiasis. A manifestation of chronic disseminated candidiasis. Infect Dis Clin North Am 2000;14:721–39.

190. Samuels BI, Pagani JJ, Libshitz HI. Radiologic features of *Candida* infections. In: Bodey GP, editor. Candidiasis: pathogenesis, diagnosis and treatment. New York: Raven Press; 1993. p. 137.

191. Luna MA, Tortoledo ME. Histologic identification and pathologic patterns of disease caused by *Candida*. In: Bodey GP, editor. Candidiasis: pathogenesis, diagnosis and treatment. New York: Raven Press; 1993. p. 21.

192. Anttila VJ, Ruutu P, Bondestam S, et al. Hepatosplenic yeast infection in patients with acute leukemia: a diagnostic problem [review]. Clin Infect Dis 1994;18:979–81.

193. Anaissie E, Bodey GP, Kantarjian H, et al. Fluconazole therapy for chronic disseminated candidiasis in patients with leukemia and prior amphotericin B therapy. Am J Med 1991; 91:142–50.

194. Kauffman CA, Bradley SF, Ross SC, et al. Hepatosplenic candidiasis: successful treatment with fluconazole. Am J Med 1991;91:137–41.

195. Lopez-Berestein G, Bodey GP, Frankel LS, et al. Treatment of hepatosplenic candidiasis with liposomal-amphotericin B. J Clin Oncol 1987;5:310–7.

196. de Pauw BE, Raemaekers JM, Donnelly JP, et al. An open study on the safety and efficacy of fluconazole in the treatment of disseminated *Candida* infections in patients treated for hematological malignancy. Ann Hematol 1995;70:83–7.

197. Edwards JE Jr, Bodey GP, Bowden RA, et al. International conference for the development of a consensus on the management and prevention of severe candidal infections [review]. Clin Infect Dis 1997;25:43–59.

CHAPTER 52

AUTOIMMUNE DISEASE

Diego Vergani, MD, PhD, FRCP

Giorgina Mieli-Vergani, MD, PhD, FRCPCH

Autoimmune liver disorders are inflammatory liver diseases characterized histologically by a dense mononuclear cell infiltrate in the portal tract and serologically by the presence of nonorgan and liver-specific autoantibodies and increased levels of immunoglobulin G (IgG), all in the absence of a known etiology. These disorders usually respond to immunosuppressive treatment, which should be instituted as soon as a diagnosis is made. The onset of these conditions is often ill-defined, and they frequently mimic acute hepatitis; the previously accepted requirement of 6 months duration of symptoms before a diagnosis of autoimmune disease can be made has been abandoned.[1,2]

There are three liver disorders in which liver damage is likely to arise from an autoimmune attack: autoimmune hepatitis (AIH), autoimmune sclerosing cholangitis (ASC), and de novo autoimmune hepatitis after liver transplant.

According to data collected at our tertiary center, there appears to be an increase in the yearly incidence of AIH and ASC in childhood. Thus, in the 1990s, these conditions represented 2.3% of children older than 4 months referred to our unit during 1 year, whereas in the past 3 years, their incidence has increased to 12%.

AUTOIMMUNE HEPATITIS

CLINICAL FEATURES

Two types of AIH are recognized according to the presence of smooth muscle antibody (SMA) and/or antinuclear antibody (ANA) or liver/kidney microsomal type 1 antibody (LKM-1). A major target of SMA is the actin of smooth muscle,[3] whereas the molecular target of LKM-1 is cytochrome P-4502D6 (CYP2D6).[4] Pediatric series, including our own, report a similarly severe disease in ANA/SMA-positive and LKM-1–positive patients.[5,6] We reviewed the clinical, biochemical, and histologic features and outcomes of ANA/SMA-positive or LKM-1–positive AIH in 52 children referred between 1973 and 1993 (Table 52-1).[6] Thirty-two patients were ANA and/or SMA positive, and 20 were LKM-1 positive. All other known causes of liver disease were excluded. Only one child with the LKM-1 antibody presented with acute liver failure and had received plasma transfusions abroad before referral, as well as had evidence of exposure to hepatitis C virus (HCV) infection, being positive for anti-HCV antibody by second-generation assay. There was a predominance of girls (75%) in both groups.

Although LKM-1–positive patients presented at a younger age (median 7.4 versus 10.5 years), the duration of symptoms before diagnosis and the frequency of hepatosplenomegaly were similar in the two groups. There was also no significant difference in the frequency of associated autoimmune disorders and a family history of autoimmune disease between the two groups. Associated autoimmune disorders included nephrotic syndrome, thyroiditis, Behçet's disease, ulcerative colitis, insulin-dependent diabetes, and urticaria pigmentosa in ANA/SMA patients and thyroiditis, vitiligo, hypoparathyroidism, and Addison disease in LKM-1 patients.

We observed three clinical patterns of disease: (1) In 50% of ANA/SMA-positive and 65% of LKM-1–positive patients, the presentation was indistinguishable from that of acute viral hepatitis (nonspecific symptoms of malaise, nausea/vomiting, anorexia, and abdominal pain, followed by jaundice, dark urine, and pale stools); six children (five LKM-1 positive) developed acute hepatic failure with grade II to IV hepatic encephalopathy from 2 weeks to 2 months (median 1 month) after onset of symptoms. In the remaining children, the duration of disease before diagnosis ranged from 10 days to 5 months (median 1.8 months). (2) Twenty-five percent of LKM-1–positive and 38% of ANA/SMA-positive patients had an insidious onset, with an illness characterized by progressive fatigue, relapsing jaundice, headache, anorexia, and weight loss, lasting from 6 months to 2 years (median 9 months) before diagnosis. (3) In six patients (two LKM-1 positive), there was no history of jaundice, and the diagnosis followed presentation with complications of portal hypertension, such as hematemesis from esophageal varices, bleeding diathesis, chronic diarrhea, weight loss, and vomiting.

The mode of presentation of AIH in childhood is therefore variable, and the disease should be suspected and excluded in all children presenting with symptoms and signs of prolonged or severe liver disease.

Laboratory features at presentation are summarized in Table 52-2. Overall, LKM-1–positive patients had higher median levels of bilirubin and aspartate aminotransferase than those who were ANA/SMA positive, but if the six patients presenting with acute hepatic failure are excluded, the differences for these two parameters are not significant. A severely impaired hepatic synthetic function, as assessed by the presence of both prolonged prothrombin time and

TABLE 52-1 CLINICAL FEATURES AT PRESENTATION IN 52 PATIENTS WITH AUTOIMMUNE HEPATITIS DIVIDED ACCORDING TO ASSOCIATED AUTOANTIBODIES

FEATURE	ANA/SMA POSITIVE AIH (n = 32)	LKM-1 POSITIVE AIH (n = 20)	p VALUE
Age at diagnosis (yr), median (range)	10.5 (2.3–14.9)	7.4 (0.8–14.2)	.011
Female n (%)	24 (75)	15 (75)	1.00
Duration of illness before diagnosis (mo; median [range])	4 (0.2–24.6)	1.7 (0.03–15.4)	.06
Fulminant liver failure n (%)	1 (3)	5 (25)	.05
Associated autoimmune disorders before or after diagnosis of AIH, n (%)[*]	7 (22)	4 (20)	.85
Nephrotic syndrome	1	0	
Autoimmune thyroiditis	1	2	
Behçet disease	1	0	
Ulcerative colitis	3	0	
Insulin-dependent diabetes	2	0	
Urticaria pigmentosa	1	0	
Vitiligo	0	1	
Hypoparathyroidism and Addison disease (APS-1)	0	1	
Autoimmune disorders in first-degree relatives, n (%)[*]	13 (43)	8 (40)	.81
Thyroid disease	3	4	
Insulin-dependent diabetes	3	4	
Autoimmune hepatitis	3	0	
Crohn disease	2	0	
Behçet disease	1	0	
Rheumatoid arthritis	1	1	
Psoriasis	0	1	
Systemic lupus erythematosus	0	1	

AIH = autoimmune hepatitis; ANA/SMA = nuclear and/or smooth muscle antibody; APS-1 = autoimmune polyendocrine syndrome type 1; GGT = γ-glutamyl transpeptidase; LKM-1 = liver kidney microsomal type 1 antibody.
*Some subjects have more than one disorder.

hypoalbuminemia, tended to be more common in ANA/SMA-positive patients (53%) than in LKM-1–positive patients (30%). The majority (80%) of the patients had increased levels of IgG, but 10 (5 LKM-1 positive) had a normal serum IgG level for age, including 3 patients who presented with acute hepatic failure, indicating that normal IgG values do not exclude the diagnosis of AIH. As previously reported, we found that partial IgA deficiency is significantly more common in LKM-1–positive patients than in ANA/SMA-positive patients (45% versus 9%).[7]

When compared with those of controls, the frequencies of the human leukocyte antigen (HLA)-DR3 were significantly higher in patients with ANA/SMA-positive AIH but not in those with LKM-1–positive AIH. Recent data suggest that possession of DR7 predisposes the patient to type 2 AIH.[8] Although these results should be confirmed in a

TABLE 52-2 LABORATORY FEATURES AT PRESENTATION IN 52 PATIENTS WITH AUTOIMMUNE HEPATITIS DIVIDED ACCORDING TO ASSOCIATED AUTOANTIBODIES

	ANA/SMA POSITIVE AIH (n = 32)	LKM-1 POSITIVE AIH (n = 20)	p VALUE
Total bilirubin, μmol/L (nv: 20)	62 (6–462)	188 (13–773)	.007
Aspartate aminotransferase, IU/L (nv: 50)	632 (81–2,500)	1,146 (93–2440)	.047
GGT, IU/L (nv: 50)	126 (11–871), n = 26	91 (36–299), n = 17	.055
Alkaline phosphatase, IU/L (nv: 350)	376 (131–1,578)	377 (102–1,677)	.87
Total protein, g/L (nv: 60–80)	75 (58–117)	72 (45–92)	.20
Albumin, g/L (nv: 35–50)	32 (20–43)	38 (25–54)	.02
International normalized ratio (nv: 0.9–1.2)	1.6 (1–2.5)	1.6 (1–8.6)	.39
Immunoglobulin G, g/L (nv: 5–18)	28 (13.4–73.3)	21 (10.2–40)	.06
Immunoglobulin A, g/L (nv: 0.8–4.8)	2.3 (0.9–4.2)	1.4 (0.07–3.6)	.059
Immunoglobulin M, g/L (nv: 0.5–2)	1.7 (0.4–9.3)	2.0 (1.05–8.0)	.53
C3, g/L (nv: 0.6–1.2)	0.7 (0.03–1.6), n = 19	0.7 (0.2–1.2), n = 12	.79
C4, g/L (nv: 0.2–0.6)	0.1 (0.03–0.34), n = 19	0.1 (0.03–0.24), n = 12	.52
ANA titer	120 (10–5,120), n = 20	NA	
SMA titer	160 (10–2,560), n = 26	NA	
LKM-1 titer	NA	640 (40–10,400), n = 19	
Anti-LSP titer	1,000 (0–3,300), n = 21	1,250 (0–2,400), n = 7	.61
Anti-ASGPR titer	0 (0–1,500), n = 21	200 (0–750), n = 7	.27

AIH = autoimmune hepatitis; ANA/SMA = nuclear and/or smooth muscle antibody; ASGPR = asialoglycoprotein receptor; LKM-1: liver kidney microsomal type 1 antibody; LSP = liver-specific lipoprotein; NA = not applicable; nv = normal value.

larger number of patients and in different centers, they suggest that the immunopathogenic mechanisms involved in the development of the two forms of AIH may be different. Patients with AIH, whether LKM-1 or ANA/SMA positive, have isolated partial deficiency of the HLA class III complement component C4, which is genetically determined, being associated with the possession of the silent gene C4AQ0 at the C4A locus.[9,10] C4AQ0, either in linkage with DR3 or on its own, has been reported in association with other autoimmune disorders.[11]

The severity of portal tract inflammation, lobular activity, and periportal necrosis, features characteristic of interface hepatitis, at diagnosis was similar in both groups. Cirrhosis on initial biopsy was more frequent in ANA/SMA-positive patients (69%) than in LKM-1–positive patients (38%). Of note is that 57% of patients already cirrhotic at diagnosis presented with a clinical picture reminiscent of that of prolonged acute virus-like hepatitis. Multiacinar or panacinar collapse, which suggests an acute liver injury, was present in eight patients (five LKM-1 positive), six of whom had acute liver failure. In these patients, it was not possible to ascertain the degree of fibrosis or the presence or absence of cirrhosis. The question as to whether the acute presentation in these patients represented a sudden deterioration of an underlying unrecognized chronic process or a genuinely acute liver damage remains open. Progression to cirrhosis was noted in four of seven ANA/SMA-positive patients and in two of five LKM-1–positive patients on follow-up biopsies done between 17 and 56 months from the initial biopsy. Overall, 74% of ANA/SMA-positive and 44% of LKM-1–positive patients showed evidence of cirrhosis on initial or follow-up histologic assessment, indicating that, apart from the higher tendency to present as acute liver failure, the severity of LKM-1–positive disease is not worse than that of ANA/SMA-positive disease. Recently, we have demonstrated that a more severe disease and a higher tendency to relapse are associated with the possession of antibodies to soluble liver antigen, which are present in about half of the patients with AIH type 1 or 2 at diagnosis.[12]

PATHOPHYSIOLOGY

The typical histologic picture of AIH, which is characterized by a dense mononuclear cell infiltrate eroding the limiting plate and invading the parenchyma (interface hepatitis), first suggested that autoaggressive cellular immunity might be involved in its causation.[13,14] Immunocytochemical studies have identified the phenotype of the infiltrating cells. T lymphocytes mounting the alpha/beta T-cell receptor predominate. Among the T cells, a majority are positive for the CD4 helper/inducer phenotype, and a sizable minority are positive for the CD8 cytotoxic phenotype. Lymphocytes of non–T-cell lineage are fewer and include (in decreasing order of frequency) natural killer cells (CD16/CD56 positive), macrophages, and B lymphocytes.[15] The recently described natural killer T cells, which express simultaneously markers of both natural killer (CD56) and T cells (CD3), are involved in liver damage in an animal model of autoimmune hepatitis.[16]

A powerful stimulus must be promoting the formation of the massive inflammatory cell infiltrate present at diagnosis. Whatever the initial trigger, it is most probable that such a high number of activated inflammatory cells cause liver damage. There are different possible pathways that an immune attack can follow to inflict damage on the hepatocyte (Figure 52-1). Liver damage is believed to be orchestrated by CD4-positive T lymphocytes recognizing a self-antigenic peptide. To trigger an autoimmune response, the peptide must be embraced by an HLA class II molecule and presented to uncommitted T helper (Th)0 cells by professional antigen-presenting cells (APCs), with the costimulation of ligand–ligand (CD28 on Th0, CD80 on APC) interaction between the two cells. The Th0 cells become activated, differentiate into functional phenotypes according to the cytokines prevailing in the microenvironment and the nature of the antigen, and initiate a cascade of immune reactions determined by the cytokines they produce. Arising in the presence of the macrophage-produced interleukin-12, Th1 cells secrete mainly interleukin-2 and interferon-γ, which activate macrophages, enhance expression of HLA class I (increasing the vulnerability of liver cells to cytotoxic attack), and induce expression of HLA class II molecules on hepatocytes, which then become able to present the autoantigenic peptide to Th cells, thus perpetuating the immune recognition cycle. Th2 cells, which differentiate from Th0 if the microenvironment is rich in interleukin-4, produce mainly interleukin-4, -5, and -10, which induce autoantibody production by B lymphocytes. Physiologically, Th1 and Th2 cells antagonize each other. The process of autoantigen recognition is strictly controlled by regulatory mechanisms. If these regulatory mechanisms fail, the autoimmune attack is perpetuated. Over the past two decades, different aspects of the above pathogenic scenario have been investigated.

An impairment of immunomodulatory mechanisms, which would enable the autoimmune response to develop, has been described in several reports. Children and young adults with AIH have low levels of T lymphocytes expressing the CD8 marker.[17] The notion of defective immunoregulation is supported by the finding that suppressor cell function is also impaired in AIH.[18] Nouri-Aria and colleagues[19,20] have shown that (1) the impairment of immunoregulation segregates with the possession of the HLA haplotype B8/DR3,[19] the haplotype that predisposes to AIH,[21] and (2) this immunoregulatory defect is correctable by therapeutic doses of corticosteroids.[20] In addition, it has been shown that patients with AIH have a specific defect in a subpopulation of T cells controlling the immune response to liver-specific membrane antigens.[22]

Lobo-Yeo and colleagues have shown that hepatocytes from patients with AIH, in contrast to normal hepatocytes, express HLA class II molecules.[23] These hepatocytes, although lacking the antigen-processing machinery typical of APCs, may present peptides through a bystander mechanism.[24] Given the impaired regulatory function and the inappropriate expression of HLA class II antigens on the hepatocytes, the question arises as to whether an autoantigenic peptide is presented to the helper/inducer

Autoimmune hepatitis

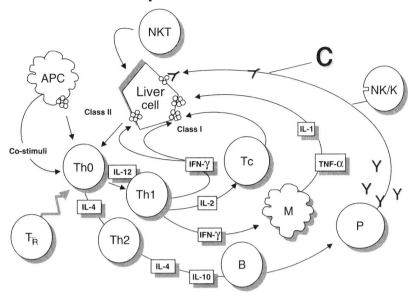

FIGURE 52-1 Autoimmune attack on the liver. A specific autoantigenic peptide is presented to an uncommitted T helper (Th0) lymphocyte within the human leukocyte antigen (HLA) class II molecule of an antigen-presenting cell (APC). Th0 cells become activated and, according to the presence in the microenvironment of interleukin (IL)-12 or IL-4 and nature of antigen, differentiate into Th1 or Th2 and initiate a series of immune reactions determined by the cytokines they produce: Th2 secrete mainly IL-4 and IL-10 and direct autoantibody production by B lymphocytes; Th1 secrete IL-2 and interferon-γ (IFN-γ), which stimulate T cytotoxic (Tc) lymphocytes, enhance expression of class I and induce expression of class II HLA molecules on hepatocytes and activate macrophages; activated macrophages release IL-1 and tumour necrosis factor-α (TNF-α). If T "regulatory" (T_R) lymphocytes do not oppose, a variety of effector mechanisms are triggered: liver cell destruction could derive from the action of Tc lymphocytes; cytokines released by Th1 and recruited macrophages; complement (C) activation or engagement of killer (NK/K) lymphocytes by the autoantibody (Y) bound to the hepatocyte surface. Natural killer T cells (NKT), cells with markers of both natural killer and T cells, are involved in liver damage in an animal model of autoimmune hepatitis. Adapted from Vergani D, Chodhuri K, Bogdanos DP, Mieli-Vergani G. Pathogenesis of autoimmune hepatitis. Clin Liver Dis 2002;6:439–49.

cells, leading to their activation. Although there is no direct evidence as yet that an autoantigenic peptide is presented and recognized, activation of helper cells has been documented in AIH.[15,25] These activated cells possess the CD4 phenotype, and their numbers are highest when the disease is most active.

What triggers the immune system to react to an autoantigen is unknown. A lesson may be learned by the study of humoral autoimmune responses during viral infections. Thus, recent studies aimed at determining the specificity of the LKM-1 antibody, present in both the juvenile form of AIH and in some patients with chronic HCV infection, have shown a high amino acid sequence homology between the HCV polyprotein and CYP2D6, the molecular target of LKM-1, thus implicating a mechanism of molecular mimicry as a trigger for the production of LKM-1 in HCV infection.[4,26,27] It is therefore conceivable that an as yet unknown virus infection may be at the origin of the autoimmune attack in AIH.

Titers of antibodies to liver-specific lipoprotein, a macromolecular complex present on the hepatocyte membrane, and to its well-characterized component asialoglycoprotein receptor, correlate with the biochemical and histologic severity of AIH.[28,29] Antibodies to alcohol dehydrogenase, a

second well-defined component of liver-specific lipoprotein, have been described in patients with AIH.[30] Immunofluorescence studies on monodispersed suspensions of liver cells obtained from patients with AIH showed that these cells are coated with antibodies in vivo.[31] A pathogenic role for these autoantibodies has been indicated by cytotoxicity assays showing that autoantibody-coated hepatocytes from patients with AIH are killed when incubated with autologous or allogeneic[32] lymphocytes. The effector cell was identified as an Fc receptor–positive mononuclear cell.[32] More recently, T-cell clones obtained from liver biopsies of children with AIH and expressing the gamma/delta T-cell receptor have been shown to be cytotoxic to a variety of targets but to preferentially kill liver-derived cells as opposed to cell lines derived from other organs.[33–35]

Data from our laboratory show an elevation of the circulating levels of cytokines produced by both Th1 and Th2 cells at diagnosis of AIH, whereas Th1 cytokine levels significantly decrease and Th2 cytokines remain elevated during remission (D. Vergani and colleagues, unpublished data, 2001). This observation, implicating Th1 cytokines in the causation of liver damage, finds support in immunohistochemical studies showing a significantly higher number of cells that produce interferon-γ and interleukin-2 in the liver tissue of patients with active disease, whereas the number of cells producing interleukin-4 and interleukin-10 is similar in active and inactive biopsies (D. Vergani and colleagues, unpublished data, 2001).

The establishment of cell lines and clones has enabled Wen and colleagues[33,34] and Löhr and colleagues[36,37] to show that the majority of T-cell clones obtained from the peripheral blood and a proportion of those from the liver of patients with AIH are CD4 positive and use the conventional alpha/beta T-cell receptor. Some of these CD4-positive clones were further characterized and were found to react with partially purified antigens, such as crude preparations of liver cell membrane or liver-specific lipoprotein,[34] and with purified asialoglycoprotein receptor[34,37] or recombinant CYP2D6[36] and to be restricted by HLA class II molecules in their response. Because CD4 is the phenotype of Th cells, both Wen and colleagues[34] and Löhr and colleagues[37] investigated whether these clones were able to help autologous B lymphocytes in the production of immunoglobulin in vitro and found that their coculture with B lymphocytes resulted in a dramatic increase in autoantibody production. All of the above experimental evidence suggests that cellular immune responses are involved in the liver damage of AIH even though the evidence that the trigger is an autoantigen is still incomplete.

TREATMENT

Unless it presents with acute liver failure (which usually requires urgent transplant), AIH responds satisfactorily to immunosuppression. Treatment should be started with prednisolone 2 mg/g/d (maximum 60 mg/d), which is gradually decreased over a period of 4 to 8 weeks if there is progressive normalization of the transaminases, and then the patient is maintained on the minimal dose able to sustain normal transaminase levels, usually 5 mg/d. During the first 6 to 8 weeks of treatment, liver function tests are checked weekly to allow a constant and frequent fine-tuning of the treatment, avoiding severe steroid side effects. If progressive normalization of the liver function tests is not obtained over this period of time or if too high a dose of prednisolone is required to maintain normal transaminases, azathioprine is added at a starting dose of 0.5 mg/g/d, which, in the absence of signs of toxicity, is increased up to a maximum of 2 mg/g/d until biochemical control is achieved. Azathioprine is not recommended as first-line treatment because of its hepatotoxicity, particularly in severely jaundiced patients. A preliminary report in a cohort of 30 children with AIH suggests that the measurements of the azathioprine metabolites 6-thioguanine and 6-methylmercaptopurine are useful in identifying drug toxicity and nonadherence and in achieving a level of 6-thioguanine considered therapeutic for inflammatory bowel disease.[38]

In our experience, although an 80% decrease of initial transaminase levels is obtained within 6 weeks from starting treatment in most patients, complete normalization of liver function may take several months. In our own series, normalization of transaminase levels occurred at medians of 0.5 years (range 0.2–7 years) in ANA/SMA-positive children and 0.8 years (range 0.02–3.2 years) in LKM-1–

positive children.[6] Relapse while on treatment is common, affecting about 40% of the patients and requiring a temporary increase of the steroid dose. The risk of relapse is higher if steroids are administered on an alternate-day schedule, often instituted in the unsubstantiated belief that it has a less negative effect on the child's growth. Small daily doses should be used because they are more effective in maintaining disease control and minimize the need for high-dose steroid pulses during relapses (with attendant more severe side effects). If a liver biopsy shows minimal or no inflammatory changes after 1 year of normal liver function tests, cessation of treatment should be considered but not during or immediately before puberty, when relapses are more common. In 13 children (4 LKM-1 positive), the only ones fulfilling these criteria in our series, discontinuation of treatment was attempted. This was successful in six children, all ANA/SMA positive, after a median duration of 3.2 (range 1–11) years of treatment. All six have remained in remission for a period of 9 to 13 years. The remaining children (three ANA/SMA positive and four LKM-1 positive) relapsed between 1 and 15 months (median 2 months) after immunosuppression was discontinued. They all responded to the reintroduction of treatment. These data indicate that most children with AIH, particularly those who are LKM-1 positive, are likely to require lifelong immunosuppressive treatment. An important role in monitoring the response to treatment is the measurement of autoantibody titers and IgG levels, the fluctuation of which is correlated with disease activity.[39] Despite the efficacy of current treatment, severe hepatic decompensation may develop even after many years of apparently good biochemical control. Thus, four of our patients who responded satisfactorily to immunosuppression ultimately required transplant 8 to 14 years after diagnosis. Overall, in our series, 46 of the 47 patients treated with immunosuppression were alive between 0.3 and 19 years (median 5 years) after diagnosis, including 5 patients after liver transplant.

Sustained remission of AIH has been reported in adult patients maintained on azathioprine alone.[40] Following this observation, we have attempted to stop prednisolone, maintaining azathioprine, in five children, two who were ANA/SMA positive and three who were LKM-1 positive. Although the attempt was successful in the ANA/SMA-positive cases, all LKM-1–positive children relapsed and required reinstitution of steroid treatment.

Remission was achieved in 25 of 32 children with AIH treated with cyclosporin A alone for 6 months followed by combined low-dose prednisone and azathioprine for 1 month, after which cyclosporin A was stopped and the other two drugs were continued.[41] The side effects of cyclosporin A were mild, and high-dose steroid side effects were avoided. A disadvantage of this schedule was that all patients were eventually treated with the prednisone-azathioprine combination, whereas by using the conventional treatment schedule, about a third of the children can maintain remission with very-low-dose steroids alone. In addition, longer follow-up of the patients is necessary to establish possible long-term toxicity of cyclosporin A.

Mycophenolate mofetil has been successfully used in adult patients with type 1 AIH who have been either intolerant of or not responsive to azathioprine.[42] Mycophenolate mofetil is an inhibitor of purine nucleotide synthesis and has a mechanism of action similar to that of azathioprine. It is not hepatotoxic or nephrotoxic, and its main side effects are diarrhea, vomiting, and bone marrow suppression. In our experience, the drug was able to resolve laboratory abnormalities in 5 of 12 children who did not tolerate or respond to azathioprine. In four others, it reduced serum aminotransferase levels to a degree that allowed a decrease in the dose of prednisolone. Only three patients did not respond to mycophenolate mofetil, and the side effects were minor, apart from severe nausea and dizziness in one of these three children.

Children who present with acute hepatic failure pose a particularly difficult therapeutic problem. Although it has been reported that they may benefit from conventional immunosuppressive therapy,[43,44] only one of the six children with acute liver failure in our own series responded to immunosuppression and survived without transplant. Of the four LKM-1–positive patients, one died before a donor organ could be found and two died soon after transplant. Encouraging results have been reported using cyclosporin A in LKM-1–positive patients presenting with fulminant hepatitis.[44,45] These results should be evaluated on a larger number of patients because our own experience has not confirmed the value of this therapeutic approach.

AUTOIMMUNE SCLEROSING CHOLANGITIS

CLINICAL FEATURES

Sclerosing cholangitis is an uncommon disorder, characterized by chronic inflammation and fibrosis of the intrahepatic and/or extrahepatic bile ducts. In childhood, sclerosing cholangitis may occur as an individual disease or may develop in association with a wide variety of disorders, including Langerhans cell histiocytosis, immunodeficiency, psoriasis, cystic fibrosis, and chronic inflammatory bowel disease. An overlapping syndrome between AIH and sclerosing cholangitis has been reported both in adults[46–48] and children.[49–52] In a retrospective study, we have shown that 40% of patients with sclerosing cholangitis have clinical, biochemical, immunologic, and histologic features that are indistinguishable from those of AIH.[49] In both AIH and sclerosing cholangitis, the serum IgG level is similarly increased, and non–organ-specific ANA and/or SMA are frequently present. Both diseases also commonly have portal tract inflammation and interface hepatitis. Most of the reported cases of overlap were originally diagnosed as AIH.[46–48,51] Typically, the overlap with sclerosing cholangitis was not recognized until years later, when biliary features on follow-up liver biopsy examination justified the performance of cholangiography. The sequence of diagnoses was then interpreted as an evolution from AIH to sclerosing cholangitis, when, in fact, the concurrence of these diseases had not been excluded by cholangiographic studies performed at presentation.

In a prospective study over a period of 16 years, we found that 27 of 55 children who presented with clinical and/or laboratory features characteristic of AIH had evidence of sclerosing cholangitis when assessed by cholangiography at presentation.[53] Bile duct abnormalities on cholangiography were both intra- and extrahepatic in two-thirds of patients and intrahepatic in one-third. Because of the cholangiographic changes, a diagnosis of ASC was made in these patients (Figure 52-2).

Of the 27 patients with ASC, 26 were seropositive for ANA and/or SMA and 1 for LKM-1.[53] Fifty-five percent were girls, and the mode of presentation was similar to that of 28 patients with typical AIH. Symptoms were those of acute hepatitis or chronic liver dysfunction. In some instances, symptoms were absent, and the diagnosis was revealed after the incidental discovery of abnormal liver tests. Inflammatory bowel disease was present in 44% of children with cholangiopathy compared with 18% of those with typical AIH, and more than 75% of children with ASC had greatly increased serum IgG levels. Perinuclear antineutrophil cytoplasmic antibodies were present in 74% of patients with ASC compared with 36% of patients with typical AIH.

There was only a partial concordance between the histologic and radiologic findings, and six patients with an abnormal cholangiogram had histologic features more compatible with AIH than sclerosing cholangitis.[53] Interestingly, all patients fulfilled the criteria for the diagnosis of "definite" or "probable" AIH established by the International Autoimmune Hepatitis Group.[1] Indeed, the diagnosis of sclerosing cholangitis was possible only because of the cholangiographic studies. The similarities and differences between type 1 AIH, type 2 AIH, and ASC are summarized in Table 52-3.

TREATMENT

Children with ASC respond to the same immunosuppressive treatment described above for typical AIH.[53] The liver test abnormalities resolved in almost 90% of our patients within a median of 2 months after starting treatment. This good response is in contrast to the outcome in adults with primary sclerosing cholangitis (PSC) who have no beneficial effects from corticosteroid treatment.[54,55] The PSC of adults, however, is usually diagnosed at an advanced stage and may be the result of various etiologies. Disappointing results with immunosuppressive agents have been reported in a small number of children with sclerosing cholangitis associated with autoimmune features, but these children may have had more advanced disease than those recruited into our prospective study.[51]

Ursodeoxycholic acid (UDCA) was added to our treatment schedule in 1992 following preliminary reports of its value in the treatment of adult PSC.[56,57] The small number of patients and the relatively short follow-up period do not allow us to determine whether treatment with UDCA from onset is successful in arresting the progression of ASC. In adults with well-established PSC, UDCA treatment has been disappointing, possibly because of the advanced stage of the disease at the time of diagnosis.[58]

Measurement of autoantibody titers and IgG levels is useful in monitoring disease activity and response to treatment, not only in AIH but also in ASC.[39]

Follow-up liver biopsies in our series have shown no progression to cirrhosis, although one patient did develop vanishing bile duct syndrome. Follow-up endoscopic retrograde cholangiograms have shown static bile duct disease in half of our patients with ASC and progression of the bile duct abnormalities in the other half. Interestingly, one of the children with AIH who was followed prospectively developed sclerosing cholangitis 8 years after presentation despite treatment with corticosteroids and no biliary changes on several follow-up liver biopsies. This observation suggests that AIH and ASC are part of the same pathogenic process and that prednisolone and azathioprine may be more effective in controlling the liver parenchyma inflammatory changes than the bile duct disease.

The medium-term prognosis of ASC is good.[53] All patients in our series were alive after a median follow-up of 7 years. Four patients with ASC, however, required liver transplant after 2 to 11 years of observation (median interval of follow-up 7 years). In contrast, liver transplant has not been required by any of the 28 children with typical AIH who have been followed for this same time.

PATHOPHYSIOLOGY

It is unclear if the juvenile autoimmune form of sclerosing cholangitis and AIH are two distinct entities or different aspects of the same condition. Akin to AIH, liver-specific autoantibodies, including antibodies to liver-specific lipoprotein, asialoglycoprotein receptor, alcohol dehydrogenase, and soluble liver antigen, are found in ASC.[12,30,59] HLA-DR3, -DR13, and -DR15 occur as commonly in patients with ASC as in healthy control subjects, but HLA-DR4 occurs less commonly. This HLA profile has also been associated with susceptibility to sclerosing cholangitis in adults.[60]

DE NOVO "AUTOIMMUNE" HEPATITIS AFTER LIVER TRANSPLANT

CLINICAL FEATURES

Late graft dysfunction not attributable to recognized causes such as rejection, infection, or vascular and/or biliary complications may occur after liver transplant. We have observed and reported a particular type of graft dysfunction associated with autoimmune features in 7 (4%) of 180 children transplanted at our center between 1991 and 1996.[61] They developed an unexplained but characteristic form of graft dysfunction at a median postsurgery period of 24 months (range 6–45 months). Of the seven children, five were boys, and the median age at presentation was 10.3 years (range 2–19.4 years). None of the children had been transplanted for autoimmune liver disease. Indications for transplant were extrahepatic biliary atresia in four children, Alagille syndrome in one child, drug-induced acute liver failure in one child, and α$_1$-antitrypsin deficiency in one child. At the time of graft dysfunction, four were on triple immunosuppression with cyclosporin A,

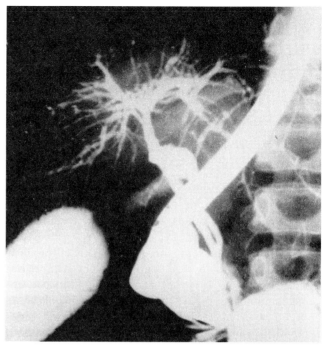

FIGURE 52-2 Endoscopic cholangiography demonstrating widespread intrahepatic changes predominantly affecting the second- and third-order bile ducts.

azathioprine, and prednisolone, whereas three were on tacrolimus. Common causes of graft dysfunction, such as infectious and surgical complications, were excluded. Liver biopsy showed the histologic changes of chronic hepatitis, including portal and periportal hepatitis with lymphocytes and plasma cells, bridging collapse, and perivenular cell necrosis, without changes typical of acute or chronic rejection. All patients had increased levels of IgG and positive autoantibodies, ANAs, SMAs, or atypical liver/kidney microsomal antibodies (LKMs, which, on immunofluorescence, stain the proximal renal tubules similarly to LKM-1, in the absence of liver staining).

Following this report,[61] autoimmune phenomena and liver disease mimicking AIH after liver transplant have been described in adults and children.[62–66] The graft dysfunction has been responsive to therapy with corticosteroids and azathioprine but not to increased doses of cyclosporin A or tacrolimus.[62–66]

TREATMENT

In our study, all patients but one responded to the conventional treatment regimen for AIH based on prednisolone (2 mg/kg/d) and azathioprine (1.5 mg/kg/d).[61] Antirejection therapy with cyclosporin A or tacrolimus was not changed. Serum aminotransferase abnormalities resolved within a median treatment period of 32 days (range 7–316 days). The one child who did not respond had a history of poor compliance with therapy. One responder relapsed owing to poor compliance, but remission was again obtained after retreatment. All six responders remained in remission on a reduced dose of prednisolone (5–10 mg/d) and azathioprine (1.5 mg/kg/d) during a median follow-up interval of 283 days (range 108–730 d). Similar satisfactory results

TABLE 52-3 COMPARISON BETWEEN AUTOIMMUNE HEPATITIS AND AUTOIMMUNE SCLEROSING CHOLANGITIS

CLINICAL FEATURES AT PRESENTATION	TYPE 1 AIH	TYPE 2 AIH	ASC
Median age (yr)	11	7	12
Females (%)	75	75	55
Mode of presentation (%)			
Acute hepatitis	47	40	37
Acute liver failure	3	25	0
Insidious onset	38	25	37
Complication of chronic liver disease	12	10	26
Associated immune diseases (%)	22	20	48
Inflammatory bowel disease (%)	20	12	44
Family history autoimmune disease (%)	43	40	37
Abnormal cholangiogram (%)	0	0	100
ANA/SMA (%)	100	25	96
LKM-1	0	100	4
pANCA	45	11	74
Increased IgG level (%)	84	75	89
Partial IgA deficiency (%)	9	45	5
Low C4 level (%)	89	83	70
Increased frequency of HLA-DR3	Yes	No	No
Increased frequency of HLA-DR7	No	Yes	—
Interface hepatitis (%)	66	72	35
Biliary features (%)	28	6	31
Cirrhosis (%)	69	38	15
Remission after immunosuppressive treatment (%)	97	87	89

Adapted from Mieli-Vergani G, Vergani D. Autoimmune hepatitis in children. Clin Liver Dis 2002;6:335–45.

AIH = autoimmune hepatitis; ANA = antinuclear antibodies; ANCA = antineutrophil cytoplasmic antibody; ASC = autoimmune sclerosing cholangitis; C4 = C4 component of complement; HLA = human leukocyte antigen; IgA = immunoglobulin A; IgG = immunoglobulin G; LKM-1 = anti–liver/kidney microsomal type 1 antibody; SMA = anti–smooth muscle antibody.

have been reported by other authors using prednisolone and azathioprine,[62–66] whereas the condition has worsened in the absence of such treatment.[66] These findings underscore the importance of prompt recognition of the condition and institution of appropriate treatment.

PATHOPHYSIOLOGY

Whether the liver damage observed in these patients is a form of rejection or the consequence of an "autoimmune" injury, possibly triggered by drugs or viral infection, remains to be established. Further characterization of the target specificity of intrahepatic lymphocytes may provide information regarding its pathogenesis. The administration of cyclosporin A or tacrolimus to rodents after bone marrow transplant can result in a "paradoxical" autoimmune syndrome in which the immunosuppressive drugs interfere with maturation of T lymphocytes and favor the emergence of autoaggressive T-cell clones.[67–69] This experience in animals may explain, in part, the development of this disorder in immunosuppressed children after liver transplant.

The manifestations of the autoimmune condition in rodents vary in different strains and depend on genetic factors possibly encoded by the major histocompatibility complex.[67] Analysis of the HLA phenotypes of the recipients and donors in our study did not show an association between the development of autoimmune features, the possession of either HLA-DR3 or -DR4, or the degree of donor-recipient HLA mismatch.[61] Five of the seven patients, however, had received livers from donors with HLA markers known to be associated with susceptibility to

AIH, including two with DR4, one with DR3, and two with DR3 and DR4.[21]

RECURRENCE OF AUTOIMMUNE LIVER DISEASE AFTER LIVER TRANSPLANT

Recurrence of AIH after transplant has been repeatedly reported in some 30% of patients.[70–75] The recurrence rate may be as high as 68% 5 years after transplant.[76] The diagnosis is based on the reappearance of clinical symptoms and signs, histologic features of periportal hepatitis, raised transaminases, circulating autoantibodies, and elevated IgG, associated with a response to prednisolone and azathioprine. Possession of the HLA-DR3 allele appears to confer predisposition to disease recurrence, as it does to the original AIH,[71] but this has not been universally confirmed.[75] Recurrence has been noted both in adult and pediatric series, and although the rate of this complication increases with the post-transplant interval, it may appear as early as 35 days postsurgery.[77] The reported recurrence rates are likely to be influenced by differences in study design, immunosuppressive regimens, and lengths of follow-up. Most transplant recipients with recurrent AIH respond to an increase in the dose of corticosteroids and azathioprine, but AIH recurrence can lead to graft failure and to the need for retransplant. Caution should be taken in weaning immunosuppression in patients who undergo transplant for AIH because discontinuation of corticosteroid therapy may increase the risk for recurrent disease.

Recurrence of sclerosing cholangitis after transplant has also been reported in 6 to 20% of patients transplanted for this condition, but it is particularly difficult to prove.[78-81] The diagnosis of sclerosing cholangitis is based on the radiographic documentation of biliary tree lesions, which can also arise as a consequence of the transplant surgery or post-transplant complications. Most patients transplanted for sclerosing cholangitis have a Roux-en-Y loop rather than a duct-to-duct anastomosis, with an increased risk of biliary obstruction and radiographic appearances of sclerosing cholangitis in the graft, making it difficult to distinguish secondary from recurrent disease. Moreover, radiologic and histologic features indistinguishable from sclerosing cholangitis may result from ischemic biliary complications.[82] Whether patients with the autoimmune form of sclerosing cholangitis are more likely to experience recurrence than those without is unclear at the present time. Similarly to AIH, immunosuppression may modify or delay the disease expression within the graft. Patient and graft survival, however, do not appear to be affected by recurrence of sclerosing cholangitis in the intermediate term.

REFERENCES

1. Johnson PJ, McFarlane IG. Meeting report: International Autoimmune Hepatitis Group. Hepatology 1993;18:998–1005.
2. International Autoimmune Hepatitis Group report: review of criteria for diagnosis of autoimmune hepatitis. J Hepatol 1999;31:929–38.
3. Johnson GD, Holobrow EJ, Glynn LE. Antibody to smooth muscle in patients with liver disease. Lancet 1965;ii:878–9.
4. Manns MP, Griffin KJ, Sullivan KF, Johnson EF. LKM-1 autoantibodies recognize a short linear sequence in P450IID6, a cytochrome P-450 monooxygenase. J Clin Invest 1991;88:1370–8.
5. Maggiore G, Veber F, Bernard O, et al. Autoimmune hepatitis associated with anti-actin antibodies in children and adolescents. J Pediatr Gastroenterol Nutr 1993;17:376–81.
6. Gregorio GV, Portmann B, Reid F, et al. Autoimmune hepatitis in childhood: a 20-year experience. Hepatology 1997;25:541–7.
7. Homberg JC, Abuaf N, Bernard O, et al. Chronic active hepatitis associated with antiliver/kidney microsome antibody type 1: a second type of "autoimmune" hepatitis. Hepatology 1987;7:1333–9.
8. Underhill J, Ma Y, Bogdanos DP, et al. Different immunogenetic background in autoimmune hepatitis type 1, type 2 and autoimmune sclerosing cholangitis. J Hepatol 2002;36 Suppl 1:156A.
9. Vergani D, Wells L, Larcher VF, et al. Genetically determined low C4: a predisposing factor to autoimmune chronic active hepatitis. Lancet 1985;ii:294–8.
10. Doherty DG, Underhill JA, Donaldson PT, et al. Polymorphism in the human complement C4 genes and genetic susceptibility to autoimmune hepatitis. Autoimmunity 1994;18:243–9.
11. Lachmann PJ. Complement. In: Lachmann PJ, Peters DK, editors. Clinical aspects of immunology. Oxford (UK): Blackwell; 1982. p. 18–49.
12. Ma Y, Okamoto M, Thomas MG, et al. Antibodies to conformational epitopes of soluble liver antigen define a severe form of autoimmune liver disease. Hepatology 2002;35:658–64.
13. De Groote JD. A classification of chronic hepatitis. Lancet 1968;ii:626.
14. Scheuer P. Chronic aggressive hepatitis. In: Liver biopsy interpretation. 2nd ed. Philadelphia: Balliere Tindall; 1973.
15. Senaldi G, Portmann B, Mowat AP, et al. Immunohistochemical features of the portal tract mononuclear cell infiltrate in chronic aggressive hepatitis. Arch Dis Child 1992;67:1447–53.
16. Takeda K, Hayakawa Y, Van Kaer L, et al. Critical contribution of liver natural killer T cells to a murine model of hepatitis. Proc Natl Acad Sci U S A 2000;97:5498–503.
17. Nouri-Aria KT, Lobo Yeo A, Vergani D, et al. T suppressor cell function and number in children with liver disease. Clin Exp Immunol 1985;61:283–9.
18. Nouri-Aria KT, Lobo Yeo A, Vergani D, et al. Immunoregulation of immunoglobulin production in normal infants and children. Clin Exp Immunol 1985;59:679–86.
19. Nouri-Aria KT, Donaldson PT, Hegarty JE, et al. HLA A1-B8-DR3 and suppressor cell function in first-degree relatives of patients with autoimmune chronic active hepatitis. J Hepatol 1985;1:235–41.
20. Nouri-Aria KT, Hegarty JE, Alexander GJ, et al. Effect of corticosteroids on suppressor-cell activity in "autoimmune" and viral chronic active hepatitis. N Engl J Med 1982;307:1301–4.
21. Donaldson PT, Doherty DG, Hayllar KM, et al. Susceptibility to autoimmune chronic active hepatitis: human leukocyte antigens DR4 and A1-B8-DR3 are independent risk factors. Hepatology 1991;13:701–6.
22. Vento S, Hegarty JE, Bottazzo G, et al. Antigen specific suppressor cell function in autoimmune chronic active hepatitis. Lancet 1984;i:1200–4.
23. Lobo-Yeo A, Senaldi G, Portmann B, et al. Class I and class II major histocompatibility complex antigen expression on hepatocytes: a study in children with liver disease. Hepatology 1990;12:224–32.
24. Chen M, Shirai M, Liu Z, et al. Efficient class II major histocompatibility complex presentation of endogenously synthesized hepatitis C virus core protein by Epstein-Barr virus-transformed B-lymphoblastoid cell lines to CD4(+) T cells. J Virol 1998;72:8301–8.
25. Lobo-Yeo A, Alviggi L, Mieli-Vergani G, et al. Preferential activation of helper/inducer T lymphocytes in autoimmune chronic active hepatitis. Clin Exp Immunol 1987;67:95–104.
26. Vento S, Cainelli F, Renzini C, Concia E. Autoimmune hepatitis type 2 induced by HCV and persisting after viral clearance. Lancet 1997;350:1298–9.
27. Kerkar N, Choudhuri K, Ma Y, et al. CYP2D6193-212: a new immunodominant epitope and target of virus/self cross-reactivity in LKM1 positive liver disease. J Immunol 2003;170:1481–9.
28. Jensen DM, McFarlane IG, Portmann BS, et al. Detection of antibodies directed against a liver-specific lipoprotein in patients with acute and chronic active hepatitis. N Engl J Med 1978;299:1–7.
29. McFarlane BM, McSorley CG, Vergani D, et al. Serum autoantibodies reacting with the hepatic asialoglycoprotein receptor protein (hepatic lectin) in acute and chronic liver disorders. J Hepatol 1986;3:196–205.
30. Ma Y, Gaken J, McFarlane BM, et al. Alcohol dehydrogenase: a target of humoral autoimmune response in liver disease. Gastroenterology 1997;112:483–92.
31. Vergani D, Mieli-Vergani G, Mondelli M, et al. Immunoglobulin on the surface of isolated hepatocytes is associated with antibody-dependent cell-mediated cytotoxicity and liver damage. Liver 1987;7:307–15.
32. Mieli-Vergani G, Vergani D, Jenkins PJ, et al. Lymphocyte cytotoxicity to autologous hepatocytes in HBsAg-negative chronic active hepatitis. Clin Exp Immunol 1979;38:16–21.

33. Wen L, Peakman M, Mowat AP, et al. Gamma/delta+ T cell clones from liver biopsies of children with autoimmune chronic active hepatitis (aCAH) and primary sclerosing cholangitis (aPSC) are cytotoxic to human liver target cells. J Hepatol 1991;13 Suppl 2:S80.

34. Wen L, Peakman M, Lobo-Yeo A, et al. T-cell-directed hepatocyte damage in autoimmune chronic active hepatitis. Lancet 1990;336:1527–30.

35. Wen L, Ma Y, Bogdanos DP, et al. Pediatric autoimmune liver diseases: the molecular basis of humoral and cellular immunity. Curr Mol Med 2001;1:379–89.

36. Löhr H, Manns M, Kyriatsoulis A, et al. Clonal analysis of liver-infiltrating T cells in patients with LKM-1 antibody-positive autoimmune chronic active hepatitis. Clin Exp Immunol 1991;84:297–302.

37. Löhr H, Treichel U, Poralla T, et al. Liver-infiltrating T helper cells in autoimmune chronic active hepatitis stimulate the production of autoantibodies against the human asialoglycoprotein receptor in vitro. Clin Exp Immunol 1992;88:45–9.

38. Rumbo C, Emerick KM, Emre S, Shneider BL. Azathioprine metabolite measurements in the treatment of autoimmune hepatitis in pediatric patients: a preliminary report. J Pediatr Gastroenterol Nutr 2002;35:391–8.

39. Gregorio GV, McFarlane B, Bracken P, et al. Organ and non-organ specific autoantibody titres and IgG levels as markers of disease activity: a longitudinal study in childhood autoimmune liver disease. Autoimmunity 2002;35:515–9

40. Johnson PJ, McFarlane IG, Williams R. Azathioprine for long-term maintenance of remission in autoimmune hepatitis. N Engl J Med 1995;333:958–63.

41. Alvarez F, Ciocca M, Canero-Velasco C, et al. Short-term cyclosporine induces a remission of autoimmune hepatitis in children. J Hepatol 1999;30:222–7.

42. Richardson PD, James PD, Ryder SD. Mycophenolate mofetil for maintenance of remission in autoimmune hepatitis in patients resistant to or intolerant of azathioprine. J Hepatol 2000;33:371–5.

43. Maggiore G, Hadchouel M, Alagille D. Life-saving immunosuppressive treatment in severe autoimmune chronic active hepatitis. J Pediatr Gastroenterol Nutr 1985;4:655–8.

44. Debray D, Maggiore G, Girardet JP, et al. Efficacy of cyclosporin A in children with type 2 autoimmune hepatitis. J Pediatr 1999;135:111–4.

45. Debray D, Bernard O. Autoimmune hepatitis (AIH) in children. Cyclosporin treatment of autoimmune hepatitis. J Pediatr Gastroenterol Nutr 1995;20:470.

46. Gohlke F, Lohse AW, Dienes HP, et al. Evidence for an overlap syndrome of autoimmune hepatitis and primary sclerosing cholangitis. J Hepatol 1996;24:699–705.

47. McNair AN, Moloney M, Portmann BC, et al. Autoimmune hepatitis overlapping with primary sclerosing cholangitis in five cases. Am J Gastroenterol 1998;93:777–84.

48. Rabinovitz M, Demetris AJ, Bou-Abboud CF, et al. Simultaneous occurrence of primary sclerosing cholangitis and autoimmune chronic active hepatitis in a patient with ulcerative colitis. Dig Dis Sci 1992;37:1606–11.

49. el-Shabrawi M, Wilkinson ML, Portmann B, et al. Primary sclerosing cholangitis in childhood. Gastroenterology 1987;92:1226–35.

50. Debray D, Urvoas E, Hadchouel M, Bernard O. Sclerosing cholangitis in children. J Pediatr 1994;124:49–56.

51. Wilschanski M, Chait P, Wade JA, et al. Primary sclerosing cholangitis in 32 children: clinical, laboratory, and radiographic features, with survival analysis. Hepatology 1995;22.1413–22.

52. Sisto A, Feldman P, Garel L, et al. Primary sclerosing cholangitis in children: study of five cases and review of the literature. Pediatrics 1987;80:918–23.

53. Gregorio GV, Portmann B, Karani J, et al. Autoimmune hepatitis/sclerosing cholangitis overlap syndrome in childhood: a 16-year prospective study. Hepatology 2001;33:544–53.

54. Czaja AJ. Frequency and nature of the variant syndromes of autoimmune liver disease. Hepatology 1998;28:360–5.

55. Lee YM, Kaplan MM. Primary sclerosing cholangitis. N Engl J Med 1995;332:924–33.

56. Beuers U, Spengler U, Kruis W, et al. Ursodeoxycholic acid for treatment of primary sclerosing cholangitis: a placebo-controlled trial. Hepatology 1992;16:707–14.

57. Lebovics E, Salama M, Elhosseiny A. Resolution of radiographic abnormalities with ursodeoxycholic acid therapy of primary sclerosing cholangitis. Gastroenterology 1992;102:2143–7.

58. Lindor KD. Ursodiol for primary sclerosing cholangitis. Mayo Primary Sclerosing Cholangitis-Ursodeoxycholic Acid Study Group. N Engl J Med 1997;336:691–5.

59. Mieli-Vergani G, Lobo-Yeo A, McFarlane BM, et al. Different immune mechanisms leading to autoimmunity in primary sclerosing cholangitis and autoimmune chronic active hepatitis of childhood. Hepatology 1989;9:198–203.

60. Donaldson PT, Manns MP. Immunogenetics of liver disease. In: Bircher J, Benhamou J-P, McIntyre N, et al, editors. Oxford textbook of clinical hepatology. Oxford (UK): Oxford University Press; 1999. p. 173–88.

61. Kerkar N, Hadzic N, Davies ET, et al. De-novo autoimmune hepatitis after liver transplantation. Lancet 1998;351:409–13.

62. Andries S, Casamaiou L, Sempoux C, et al. Posttransplant immune hepatitis in pediatric liver transplant recipients: incidence and maintenance therapy with azathioprine. Transplantation 2001;72:267–72.

63. Duclos-Vallee JC, Johanet C, Bach JF, et al. Autoantibodies associated with acute rejection after liver transplantation for type-2 autoimmune hepatitis. J Hepatol 2000;33:163–6.

64. Heneghan MA, Portmann BC, Norris SM, et al. Graft dysfunction mimicking autoimmune hepatitis following liver transplantation in adults. Hepatology 2001;34:464–70.

65. Hernandez HM, Kovarik P, Whitington PF, et al. Autoimmune hepatitis as a late complication of liver transplantation. J Pediatr Gastroenterol Nutr 2001;32:131–6.

66. Salcedo M, Vaquero J, Banares R, et al. Response to steroids in de novo autoimmune hepatitis after liver transplantation. Hepatology 2002;35:349–56.

67. Bucy RP, Xu XY, Li J, et al. Cyclosporin A-induced autoimmune disease in mice. J Immunol 1993;151:1039–50.

68. Cooper MH, Hartmann GG, Starzl TE, et al. The induction of pseudo-graft-versus-host disease following syngeneic bone marrow transplantation using FK 506. Transplant Proc 1991;23:3234–5.

69. Hess AD, Fischer AC, Horwitz LR, et al. Cyclosporine-induced autoimmunity: critical role of autoregulation in the prevention of major histocompatibility class II-dependent autoregression. Transplant Proc 1993;25:2811–3.

70. Neuberger J, Portmann B, Calne R, Williams R. Recurrence of autoimmune chronic active hepatitis following orthotopic liver grafting. Transplantation 1984;37:363–5.

71. Wright HL, Bou-Abboud CF, Hassanein T, et al. Disease recurrence and rejection following liver transplantation for autoimmune chronic active liver disease. Transplantation 1992;53:136–9.

72. Birnbaum AH, Benkov KJ, Pittman NS, et al. Recurrence of autoimmune hepatitis in children after liver transplantation. J Pediatr Gastroenterol Nutr 1997;25:20–5.

73. Sempoux C, Horsmans Y, Lerut J, et al. Acute lobular hepatitis as the first manifestation of recurrent autoimmune hepatitis after orthotopic liver transplantation. Liver 1997;17:311–5.

74. Narumi S, Hakamada K, Sasaki M, et al. Liver transplantation for autoimmune hepatitis: rejection and recurrence. Transplant Proc 1999;31:1955–6.

75. Milkiewicz P, Hubscher SG, Skiba G, et al. Recurrence of autoimmune hepatitis after liver transplantation. Transplantation 1999;68:253–6.

76. Prados E, Cuervas-Mons V, de la Mata M, et al. Outcome of autoimmune hepatitis after liver transplantation. Transplantation 1998;66:1645–50.

77. Ayata G, Gordon FD, Lewis WD, et al. Liver transplantation for autoimmune hepatitis: a long-term pathologic study. Hepatology 2000;32:185–92.

78. Letourneau JG, Day DL, Hunter DW, et al. Biliary complications after liver transplantation in patients with preexisting sclerosing cholangitis. Radiology 1988;167:349–51.

79. McEntee G, Wiesner RH, Rosen C, et al. A comparative study of patients undergoing liver transplantation for primary sclerosing cholangitis and primary biliary cirrhosis. Transplant Proc 1991;23:1563–4.

80. Harrison RF, Davies MH, Neuberger JM, Hubscher SG. Fibrous and obliterative cholangitis in liver allografts: evidence of recurrent primary sclerosing cholangitis? Hepatology 1994;20:356–61.

81. Marsh JW Jr, Iwatsuki S, Makowka L, et al. Orthotopic liver transplantation for primary sclerosing cholangitis. Ann Surg 1988;207:21–5.

82. Sebagh M, Farges O, Kalil A, et al. Sclerosing cholangitis following human orthotopic liver transplantation. Am J Surg Pathol 1995;19:81–90.

CHAPTER 53

DRUG-INDUCED HEPATOTOXICITY

Eve A. Roberts, MD, FRCPC

The liver plays a central role in drug action. It chemically transforms many drugs to their active form and acts on most drugs to expedite their excretion from the body. These functions put the liver at risk for toxicity from these chemicals and their metabolites. Because of its anatomic and physiologic complexity, drug-induced liver disease represents a broad spectrum of biochemical, histologic, and clinical abnormalities. This can make it difficult to diagnose drug-induced liver disease or determine its pathogenesis. The problem of drug-induced liver disease in children is further complicated by a widely held notion that drug hepatotoxicity does not happen very often in children. Children may indeed be protected in some way from drug hepatotoxicity. Whether or not this is true, because the child's liver is in the process of metabolic maturation, the manifestations of drug-induced liver disease may differ in children from those in adults. Because drug hepatotoxicity often imitates other more common diseases, arriving at a diagnosis of drug hepatotoxicity in a child can be especially difficult.

The purpose of this chapter is to address special features of drug hepatotoxicity in children. Mechanistic information gained from studying such processes in children is important for understanding the pathogenesis of drug hepatotoxicity. However, much more is known about the diversity of hepatic drug reactions in adults than that in children. For encyclopedic reviews of which hepatotoxicities a given drug has caused in patients of any age, the reader should consult broader references[1–3] or computerized adverse drug reaction indices (such as <www.fda.gov/medwatch> and <www.pharmacovigilance.org>).

ROLE OF THE LIVER IN DRUG METABOLISM

Hepatic drug metabolism, or biotransformation, contributes to drug hepatotoxicity and to some hepatic neoplasia. Biotransformation in the liver is divided into two broad aspects: activation (phase I) and detoxification (phase II) (Figure 53-1). For hepatotoxicity, the balance between these two processes is critical. Factors that influence this balance include age or stage of development, fasting or undernutrition, coadministered drugs, and immunomodulators resulting from viral infection. Induc-

ing chemicals may affect phase I and phase II processes differently. The pharmacokinetics of the toxic drug also affects hepatic biotransformation. Whether the drug is taken as a single dose or many doses chronically may change its hepatic metabolism. Finally, polymorphisms of cytochromes P-450 and various phase II enzymes also influence this balance.

The cytochromes P-450 are hemoproteins that are found in numerous body tissues but are particularly important in the liver. They carry out most phase I reactions. These reactions are diverse and include various types of hydroxylation, dealkylation, and dehalogenation. The common feature in all reactions is that one atom of molecular oxygen is inserted into the substrate, whereas the other combines with protons to form water. Hence these enzyme activities are monooxygenases. Cytochromes P-450 themselves are diverse and have overlapping substrate specificity. An important characteristic of many cytochromes P-450 is inducibility. Another is functional polymorphism.

The cytochromes P-450 were initially classified on the basis of the predominant inducing chemical: basically either phenobarbital or the polycyclic aromatic hydrocarbon 3-methylcholanthrene.[4] Thirty-six subfamilies of cytochromes P-450 have been distinguished on the basis of similarities in primary amino acid sequence. The cytochrome P-450 1A (CYP1A) subfamily includes those cytochromes induced by polycyclic aromatic hydrocarbons. Two major forms within the CYP1A subfamily have been identified in the rat, mouse, and rabbit and in humans. Apart from various carcinogens, other chemicals, such as caffeine and theophylline, are metabolized by these cytochromes to a varying extent. Induction of the cytochromes in the CYP1A subfamily is regulated through a cytoplasmic receptor protein, the Ah receptor, which has been characterized in humans. The cytochrome P-450 2B (CYP2B) subfamily includes cytochromes induced by phenobarbital. Cytochrome P-450 2E1 (CYP2E1) represents ethanol-inducible cytochrome P-450. The cytochrome P-450 3A (CYP3A) subfamily includes cytochromes induced by pregnenolone and by glucocorticoids. CYP3A4 is the most abundant cytochrome P-450 in human liver. Induction of cytochromes P-450 by phenobarbital involves

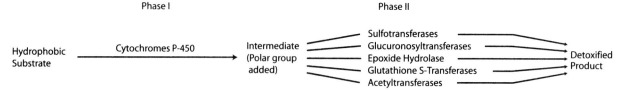

FIGURE 53-1 Phase I and phase II metabolism. Although the main objective is to convert a hydrophobic substance to a detoxified, water-soluble product so that it can be excreted from the body, phase I metabolism is also capable of converting some drugs to their active form or transforming other chemicals to toxic intermediates.

the constitutive active receptor (CAR) for CYP2B cytochromes and the pregnane X receptor (PXR) for CYP3A cytochromes through response elements, but not all details of these regulatory mechanisms are yet known.[5] Drugs that cause proliferation of peroxisomes appear to induce yet another cytochrome P-450 subfamily, P-450 4A (CYP4A). As the hepatic metabolism of common drugs is studied more extensively, these subfamilies, as well as CYP2C cytochromes and CYP2D6, are found to be involved. This has important implications for hepatotoxicity.

Polymorphisms for certain cytochromes P-450 have also been identified in human populations and in laboratory animals. In general, these polymorphisms relate to differences in the rate of enzyme action. An important polymorphism is that for debrisoquine 4-hydroxylation, for which individuals may be "extensive metabolizers" or "poor metabolizers." Other drugs whose metabolism shows the same pattern include sparteine, metoprolol, and dextromethorphan. The poor metabolizer phenotype is associated with absence of cytochrome CYP2D6 protein; several different mutations in the structural gene for CYP2D6 have been described, which account for this phenotype.[6] Poor metabolizers appear to be at greater risk for adverse drug reaction from drugs that are metabolized by this route, although clear relationships to any specific hepatotoxicity have been difficult to prove.[7]

For many drugs, the effect of phase I biotransformation reactions is to create a more polar chemical with a substituent poised for conjugation via a phase II reaction. Phase II detoxifying reactions are performed by a variety of different types of enzymes, including glutathione S-transferases, glucuronosyl transferases, epoxide hydrolase, sulfotransferases, and N-acetyltransferases. In general, these reactions complete the transformation of a hydrophobic chemical to a hydrophilic one that can be excreted easily in urine or bile. Certain phase II enzymes, such as some glucuronosyl transferases, are subject to induction. Some are polymorphic, notably N-acetyltransferase (either rapid or slow acetylators). In some metabolic diseases, the activity of phase II enzymes may be abnormal; for example, in 5-oxoprolinuria, conjugation to glutathione is reduced because of deficiency of glutathione owing to decreased levels of glutathione synthetase.[8] In hereditary tyrosinemia, glutathione S-transferase activity is depressed because intermediates in the abnormal tyrosine pathway consume glutathione.

Hepatic drug metabolism shows developmental changes. Caffeine, which is metabolized in part by cytochromes P-450 in the 1A subfamily, exemplifies these changes. The elimina-

tion half-life is very long in the newborn period[9] and drops to approximately 3 to 4 hours around 6 months of age.[10] For the balance of childhood, that is, until puberty, caffeine metabolism remains somewhat more rapid than in adults.[11] Clearance of many drugs is more rapid in children than in adults. Prominent examples include theophylline, phenobarbital, and phenytoin. Among phase II processes, a well-known example of late maturation of a detoxifying enzyme is the glucuronosyl transferase for bilirubin conjugation, which is frequently deficient for a short time after birth. Hepatic bile acid metabolism also shows maturational changes in the first months of life. These variations may influence the occurrence and character of hepatotoxicity in children.

The product of a phase I reaction may be an unstable or reactive metabolite. Phase II reactions may inactivate such chemicals before they do much harm. However, it is possible, as in the case of benzo[a]pyrene, for the product of phase I to recycle through the same cytochrome a second time and then be metabolized to a proximate carcinogen. Apart from the adequacy of the detoxification systems, whether reactive metabolites actually damage the cell will also depend on how much reactive metabolite actually binds to cellular components, whether these components are critical to cellular function, and whether they can be repaired. If the reactive metabolite binds to intracellular proteins or membranes that are vital to cellular integrity, the hepatocyte may die. If it binds to a genetic apparatus, mutagenesis, carcinogenesis, or teratogenesis may ensue (Figure 53-2).

Toxic metabolites are electrochemically unstable, and thus highly reactive, species derived from drugs, xenobiotics, or endogenous chemicals. Electrophilic intermediates (or electrophiles) are formed when electrons are lost from the original chemical; they carry a net positive charge. Examples include hydroxylamines, quinoneimines, and arene oxides. Tissue nucleophiles, such as glutathione, preferentially combine with these species. Not all nucleophiles are necessarily protective. For example, reactions that involve activation of oxygen produce negatively charged species, which are nucleophiles. They tend to bind to intracellular lipids, leading to lipid peroxidation. Examples include halocarbon and nitroso radicals. Besides lipid peroxidation, membranes can be altered by alkylation (addition of an aliphatic radical such as methyl or ethyl groups), arylation (addition of an aromatic group such as a phenyl group), or acylation (adding a radical derived from a carboxy acid). Glutathione, which is found in most mammalian cells in high concentrations, can react with electrophiles via conjugation reactions catalyzed by glutathione S-trans-

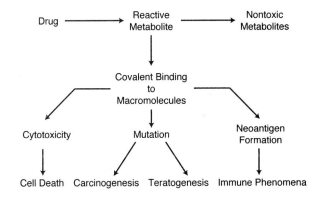

FIGURE 53-2 The potential fates of a toxic intermediate.

ferases. It can also interact with hydrogen peroxide and activated oxygen species via a different enzyme, glutathione peroxidase. In general, when toxic metabolites are the important cause of cell damage, high tissue concentrations of the parent drug are not found. Metabolite(s) covalently bound to cellular constituents may be detected.

The cellular specialization of hepatocytes accounts in part for the diversity of patterns of hepatotoxicity. Binding to certain subcellular elements may interfere with specific metabolic functions such as protein or lipid synthesis or energy production. The parent compound or its reactive metabolites may interfere with biliary excretion or damage proteins within the biliary excretion apparatus, thus leading to cholestasis.[12] In particular, the bile salt excretory pump (BSEP; abnormal in progressive familial intrahepatic cholestasis type 2) appears to be an important target in forms of drug hepatotoxicity with prominent cholestatic features. Additionally, polymorphisms in the genes for these bile canalicular transporters may influence their susceptibility to damage by toxic intermediates. Binding to nuclear deoxyribonucleic acid (DNA) may lead to carcinogenesis. Binding to mitochondrial DNA or otherwise interfering with production of normal mitochondrial DNA may have important consequences for hepatocellular metabolism because, unlike nuclear DNA, mitochondrial DNA has limited resources for DNA repair. Drug-induced injury may occur to other cells in the liver besides hepatocytes. Cytotoxic damage to biliary epithelial cells, hepatic stellate cells, or endothelial cells accounts for some of the clinical diversity of drug-induced liver disease. For example, damage to sinusoidal endothelial cells by reactive metabolites leads to veno-occlusive disease.

CLASSIFICATION OF DRUG HEPATOTOXICITY

The clinical spectrum of drug hepatotoxicity in adults is wide. The clinical patterns of drug hepatotoxicity presented in Table 53-1 form the basis for considering hepatotoxicity in children. It encompasses a combination of clinical presentations, histologic findings, and other factors. Nonspecific elevation of serum aminotransferases is omitted. This form of hepatotoxicity is probably the most common of all, but its causes are extremely heterogeneous and the least understood.

Most drug-induced liver disease is cytotoxic. Clinically, serum aminotransferases are elevated, and hepatic insufficiency may develop. Hepatocellular damage is classically defined in adults as having an alanine aminotransferase (ALT) level greater than two times the upper limit of normal or the ALT-to-alkaline phosphatase (ALP) ratio is ≥ 5.[13] The exact mechanism of cell death is not known and is probably different for different drugs and toxins. Hepatocyte damage may be zonal, reflecting metabolic specialization in various parts of the hepatic lobule. Specifically, hepatocytes in zone 3 of the Rappaport acinus have the highest concentration of drug-metabolizing enzymes and thus the greatest potential for producing toxic intermediates. Zonal hepatocellular necrosis suggests that metabolic activation of toxic metabolites has an important role in the pathogenesis of the toxicity, but spotty necrosis scattered throughout the lobule does not necessarily exclude a mechanism involving toxic metabolites. The same drugs that can cause this spotty hepatocyte damage can, on occasion, cause damage affecting most hepatocytes, leading to massive hepatocellular necrosis. Whenever hepatocellular damage is sufficiently severe, some degree of cholestasis will develop.

Some drug-induced liver disease, however, is predominantly cholestatic. For adults, this is classically defined as serum ALP greater than two times the upper limit of normal or the ALT-to-ALP ratio is ≤ 2.[13] Clinically, this type of reaction is characterized by jaundice, pruritus, prominent elevation of ALP, and mild elevations of serum aminotransferases. Traditionally, these cholestatic injuries have been classified on the basis of histologic inflammation. In hepatocanalicular jaundice, with agents such as chlorpromazine or erythromycin, liver cell injury and inflammation

TABLE 53-1 SPECTRUM OF DRUG-INDUCED LIVER DISEASE

TYPE	EXAMPLES
Acute hepatitis	Methyldopa, isoniazid, halothane, phenytoin
Hepatitis-cholestasis	Erythromycin, chlorpromazine, azathioprine, nitrofurantoin, cimetidine
Zonal liver cell necrosis	Acetaminophen
Bland cholestasis	Estrogens, cyclosporines
Steatonecrosis (like alcoholic hepatitis)	Perhexiline, amiodarone
Phospholipidosis	Amiodarone
Microvesicular steatosis	Valproic acid, tetracycline
Granulomatosis	Sulfonamides, phenylbutazone, carbamazepine
Biliary cirrhosis	Practolol, chlorpropamide
Sclerosing cholangitis	Floxuridine via hepatic artery
Hepatic vascular changes	
Peliosis	Estrogens, androgens
Hepatic vein thrombosis	Estrogens (oral contraceptives)
Veno-occlusive disease	Thioguanine, busulfan, pyrrolizidine (*Senecio*) alkaloids
Noncirrhotic portal hypertension	Vinyl chloride, arsenic
Liver cell adenoma	Estrogens (oral contraceptives), anabolic steroids
Malignant tumors	Estrogens, anabolic steroids, vinyl chloride
Porphyria	2,3,7,8-Tetrachlorodibenzo-*p*-dioxin, chloroquine

are relatively prominent. This mixed picture is characterized biochemically in adults because the ALT-to-ALP ratio is 2–5, and the ALT and ALP are each at least twice the upper limit of normal. In bland cholestasis, with agents such as contraceptive steroids, inflammation is minimal.

It is sometimes useful to think about drug hepatotoxicity in terms of the duration of the hepatotoxic process. Acute hepatotoxic injuries develop over a relatively short time and cause a lesion without any features of chronicity. Subacute hepatotoxicity refers to lesions that have developed over weeks to months as indicated by areas of fibrosis and possibly regeneration. Chronic hepatotoxic lesions include those with fibrosis or cirrhosis, vascular changes, and neoplasia. Some drugs can cause clinical liver disease indistinguishable from autoimmune hepatitis (the so-called "chronic active hepatitis" picture): these include oxyphenisatin, methyldopa, isoniazid, nitrofurantoin, and minocycline.

Our knowledge of the mechanisms of hepatotoxicity is evolving. For many years, hepatotoxicity has been categorized on the basis of predictability. Intrinsic hepatotoxins are differentiated from idiosyncratic heptatotoxins. The intrinsic hepatotoxin causes predictable hepatic damage in almost any individual. The toxicity is dose related: higher doses cause worse damage. Animal models can be developed that exhibit the same type of hepatotoxicity. However, most instances of hepatotoxicity, mainly those associated with medications, are unpredictable, infrequent, and apparently sporadic. If such a reaction is accompanied by systemic features such as fever, rash, eosinophilia, atypical lymphocytosis, and possibly other major organ involvement, then, classically, it has been regarded as an idiosyncratic hypersensitivity reaction, where hypersensitivity, with its connotation of allergy, is left undefined.

An alternate explanation is that idiosyncratic hepatotoxicity has a biochemical basis and is due to metabolic idiosyncrasy. It occurs in individuals who have specific abnormalities in drug metabolism. If this abnormal metabolism is expressed in liver cells, then these rare individuals will develop hepatotoxicity if exposed to the appropriate drug. In most instances, a metabolite, not the drug itself, is responsible for hepatotoxicity (see Figure 53-2). Frequently, the problem seems to be a defect in detoxification of the reactive metabolite because the detoxification system is itself focally defective and cannot meet the normal demands of metabolite production. Sometimes these individuals show systemic features interpreted as hypersensitivity: it is likely that interaction of the reactive metabolite with cellular components, such as the cell membrane, elicits an immune response. In such cases, hypersensitivity is itself the consequence of metabolic idiosyncrasy, not a separate mechanism of drug hepatotoxicity. There may be strictly allergic drug hepatotoxicity, but investigations of the mechanism of drug-induced hepatotoxicity suggest that metabolic idiosyncrasy is much more common than formerly supposed. It seems likely to account for hepatotoxicity with drugs that show two main patterns of toxicity: mild reversible toxicity in a comparatively large segment of patients and severe hepatotoxicity in a few individuals. Toxic metabolites are probably involved in both patterns of toxicity. Severe reactions occur in rare persons with abnormal generation of toxic metabolites or detoxification, irrespective of the appearance of drug allergy. Transient reaction may reflect spontaneous adjustments in hepatic biotransformation for the particular drug.

The major implication of the metabolic idiosyncrasy thesis is that most drug hepatotoxicity is predictable if one understands the pathways of hepatic biotransformation and detoxification for each drug. Given the plethora of drugs and hepatic biotransformation pathways, it is no wonder that most clinically important drug hepatotoxicity appears sporadic and fortuitous. However, enough experimental data are available now to warrant rethinking the standard classification of drug hepatotoxicity that regards all drug-associated hepatotoxicity as either intrinsic, owing to the drug being a poison, or else idiosyncratic-allergic. The definable metabolic defects in hepatic drug metabolism are particularly common in the types of drug hepatotoxicity that occur in children.

Recent research has focused on the role of the immune system in drug hepatotoxicity.[14] It seems likely that for many, if not most, individuals, drug hepatotoxicity depends on immune reactivity as well as personal peculiarities of drug biotransformation. With some drugs, the connection between immune-mediated mechanisms and hepatic damage may be very direct: autoantibodies are elaborated against specific components of the hepatic biotransformation machinery. The target cytochrome P-450 varies with different drugs: CYP2C9 for tienilic acid, CYP1A2 for dihydralazine, and CYP2E1 for halothane. In addition, the herb germander is associated with antibodies directed against the phase II enzyme epoxide hydrolase.[15] Reactive metabolites may alter other components of hepatocytes to form neoantigens. Hepatocyte damage mediated through immune mechanisms involves apoptosis or necrosis. Bile acid–associated hepatocyte injury involves Fas (CD95) activation leading to apoptosis. When toxic metabolites or reactive oxygen species or cytokines stimulate Kupffer cells, specific mechanisms of cell damage are set into motion involving tumor necrosis factor-α or nitric oxide produced by Kupffer cells. Nitric oxide elaborated by Kupffer cells and hepatocytes appears to play a role in acetaminophen hepatotoxicity. Other cytokines, including interleukin-8[16] and other CXC chemokines regulating leukocyte action, may modulate these effects. Moreover, Kupffer cells also elaborate a number of factors that are cytoprotective to hepatocytes.[17] The vigor of the immune response in general, an individual polygenic trait, may also determine the importance of immune mechanisms in drug hepatotoxicity. Thus, the individual's "immunogenetic" makeup and "pharmacogenetic" makeup are important.

In summary, as our knowledge of the complex and numerous individual mechanisms of drug hepatotoxicity continues to evolve, it remains useful to categorize drugs as follows: intrinsic hepatotoxins, contingent hepatotoxins, and drugs eliciting an immunoallergic response. The intrinsic toxin is a true poison and causes predictable damage in all persons in a dose-dependent fashion. The contingent hepatotoxin causes drug hepatotoxicity in individuals who are susceptible under circumstances that favor imbalance of production of a toxic intermediate and its detoxification. These circumstances may be inborn (such as genetic defects in a phase II detoxification enzyme or genetic polymorphism in a cytochrome P-450) or acquired (such as induction of CYP2E1 by chronic ethanol abuse or depletion of hepatic glutathione by fasting and malnutrition). Genetic variations in expression of cytokines that effect hepatic cytoprotection (such as interleukin-10 promoter region polymorphisms, which regulate its expression) also contribute to the mechanism of contingency. Drugs eliciting an immune response can produce a variety of clinical phenomena: the drug hypersensitivity syndrome (fever, rash, atypical lymphocytosis, eosinophilia, lymphadenopathy, multisystem involvement including hepatitis, renal dysfunction, myocarditis, thyroiditis), hepatic granulomatosis, autoantibodies, and "chronic active hepatitis" fully resembling idiopathic autoimmune hepatitis. Individual immunogenetic makeup probably determines the pattern and extent of this response. These categories are not mutually exclusive. Acetaminophen is an intrinsic toxin at very high doses and a contingent toxin at therapeutic doses. Phenytoin is a contingent hepatotoxin and the archetypal drug for eliciting an immunoallergic response.

INCIDENCE OF DRUG-INDUCED LIVER DISEASE IN CHILDREN

Drug-induced liver disease is generally regarded as rare in children. In a survey of 10,297 pediatric hospital admissions to teaching and community hospitals in Boston, Mitchell and colleagues found that only 2% of hospital admissions were due to any sort of adverse drug reaction.[18] In a subset of 725 patients with cancer, however, 22% of admissions were related to adverse drug reactions. Adverse drug reactions in the whole population were somewhat more common in the 0- to 5-year-old age group than in older children. The most commonly implicated drugs included phenobarbital, aspirin, phenytoin, ampicillin or amoxicillin, and sulfa. Only phenytoin-associated hepatitis was specifically mentioned in this large survey as drug hepatotoxicity. An outpatient study of 1,590 children in Britain also failed to detect drug hepatotoxicity as a problem in children.[19] A recent review of the Yellow Card Scheme for reporting adverse drug reactions in the United Kingdom revealed that between 1964 and December 2000, there were 331 deaths in children possibly owing to drug toxicity, and 50 of these involved hepatic failure.[20] The median age was 5 years old, and the types of drugs most often associated with fatal adverse events were anticonvulsants and antineoplastic drugs. Despite the limitations of this tracking system, these data help to objectify this problem in the pediatric age bracket.

Why childhood drug hepatotoxicity seems uncommon is not certain. Underdiagnosis and underreporting remain a possibility. Another simple reason is that most children take relatively few medications. They do not use ethanol chronically or smoke cigarettes; most are not obese. Thus, they are free of many predisposing factors to drug hepato-

toxicity. Interestingly, where drug therapy plays a key role—epilepsy and childhood neoplasia—drug hepatotoxicity is somewhat frequent. Advanced age is a risk factor for severe hepatotoxic reactions. The aging liver metabolizes some drugs more slowly. In view of the increased risk attached to some drug hepatotoxicities in women, one can speculate that changes in drug metabolism possibly associated with puberty may influence the differing incidence of drug hepatotoxicity in childhood and adulthood.

SPECIFIC DRUG HEPATOTOXICITIES IN CHILDREN

Drug hepatotoxicity does occur in children. Hepatotoxicity attributable to most of the following drugs has been diagnosed in children at the Hospital for Sick Children in Toronto in the past 15 to 20 years. Other drugs are included because they are commonly used in pediatric practice and are known to be hepatotoxic in children.

ACETAMINOPHEN

Acetaminophen is commonly used in children as an effective antipyretic and analgesic because its metabolism is rapid enough in most children that it does not accumulate and is not influenced by dehydration. A single large dose is extremely hepatotoxic. The mechanism for this toxicity involves the formation of a toxic metabolite.[21–24] The important role of drug metabolism in this hepatotoxicity is reflected in the predominance of hepatocellular injury in zone 3 (Figure 53-3). Acetaminophen is usually metabolized via sulfation and glucuronidation (Figure 53-4). If a sufficiently large amount is taken, these pathways are saturated, and an otherwise relatively minor pathway through

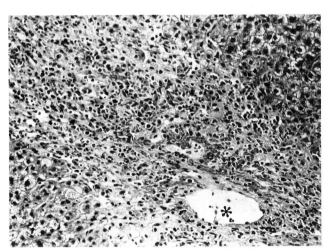

FIGURE 53-3 Liver biopsy in acetaminophen hepatotoxicity. There is a wide zone of necrosis occupying zone 3 of the liver, to which there is only a modest inflammatory cell response. The transition between the necrotic cells and the surrounding hepatocytes, which are swollen, vacuolated, and contain fat, is abrupt. In zone I (not shown), the liver parenchyma is normal. This zonal distribution of necrosis surrounded by swollen fatty hepatocytes is characteristic of acetaminophen hepatotoxicity. Terminal hepatic venule (*asterisk*) (hematoxylin and eosin, ×250 original magnification). Courtesy of Dr. M. J. Phillips.

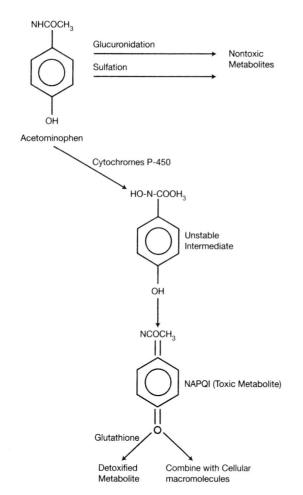

FIGURE 53-4 Metabolism of acetaminophen.

cytochromes P-450 (CYP3A4, CYP2E1, and CYP1A2) becomes quantitatively important. The product of this pathway is a highly reactive species N-acetyl-p-benzo-quinoneimine (NAPQI),[25] a potent electrophile. It is conjugated by glutathione as long as sufficient glutathione is available; otherwise, NAPQI reacts with cellular proteins, causing cell damage and cell death. N-Acetylcysteine acts by providing substrate for making more glutathione[26] and thus can minimize hepatotoxicity if given early enough. It does not reverse the toxic effects of the toxic intermediate once they have occurred. Other factors may influence the metabolism of acetaminophen. Cimetidine, which inhibits cytochromes P-450, interferes with acetaminophen toxicity in laboratory animals if given early, but the comparable dose for humans is probably toxic in itself. Concomitant drug treatment may induce cytochromes P-450 involved in the production of NAPQI. Fasting decreases the amount of glutathione in cells and thus increases acetaminophen toxicity. Additionally, recent reports indicate that nitric oxide may play a role in the mechanism of acetaminophen hepatotoxicity[27,28] and that interleukin-10 acts as an immunologic cytoprotective mediator by interfering with nitric oxide production and possibly with the action of other proinflammatory cytokines.[29]

The clinical course of single high-dose acetaminophen hepatotoxicity is distinctive. Immediately after taking a large single dose of the drug, there is nausea and vomiting. These symptoms clear, and then there is an interval before hepatic toxicity becomes clinically apparent. At that point, jaundice, abnormal serum aminotransferases, and coagulopathy develop. Serum aminotransferases may be extremely high in this condition, and the degree of abnormality is not necessarily predictive of outcome. Finally, hepatic failure may supervene with progressive coma. In adults, clinical findings predicting poor outcome (ie, extremely severe hepatic failure) are the concurrent findings of serum creatinine > 300 μmol/L *and* prothrombin time > 100 seconds (international normalized ratio > 7) *and* grade 3 or 4 hepatic encephalopathy in patients with a normal pH or the single finding of arterial pH < 7.3 in a patient who is not hypovolemic.[30]

Whether to use N-acetylcysteine can be decided on the basis of plotting on a semilogarithmic graph the patient's plasma acetaminophen concentration against time[31]; if it falls in the zone for probable hepatic toxicity, N-acetylcysteine should be given. N-Acetylcysteine is most effective if given within 10 hours of acetaminophen ingestion and may be of less benefit if given more than 24 hours after ingestion of the acetaminophen. However, even if there is doubt as to its usefulness, it should be given anyway. Indeed, there is a strong case for treating all patients with N-acetylcysteine because some patients who appear to be at low risk by the nomogram develop severe hepatotoxicity.[32] In adults, late administration of N-acetylcysteine has been associated with greater survival after acute acetaminophen intoxication; no adverse side effects of the N-acetylcysteine were observed.[33,34] A 72-hour regimen of oral N-acetylcysteine appears to be as effective as the 20-hour intravenous regimen; the oral regimen may be more effective if treatment is delayed.[35] This regimen consists of a loading dose of 140 mg of oral N-acetylcysteine per kilogram of body weight, followed 4 hours later by 70 mg per kilogram given every 4 hours for an additional 17 doses, and it can be given by a nasogastric tube. A recent retrospective study of children 1 to 17 years old who presented with acetaminophen poisoning showed that the best predictor for low risk of acetaminophen hepatotoxicity in this setting was normal prothrombin time *and* aspartate aminotransferase *and* ALT at 48 hours after ingestion, and these authors concluded that treatment with N-acetylcysteine should be used for at least 48 hours in children—longer if the clinical situation warranted it.[36] Activated charcoal may be effective but only if administered early (less than 1 hour after the ingestion); interaction with N-acetylcysteine reduces the effectiveness of charcoal.[37] Inducing vomiting may not provide any benefit. Hemodialysis, if it is to be effective at all, must be used early when acetaminophen plasma concentrations are high.

Extensive reviews of acetaminophen poisoning in children suggest that younger children tend to be resistant to this hepatotoxicity.[38,39] The incidence of hepatotoxicity was 5.5% in a study of 417 children 5 years old or less compared with 29% in adolescents and adults at comparable toxic blood levels.[38] Various studies of acetaminophen pharmacokinetics, metabolism, and toxicity in children suggest a biochemical basis for this observation. The elimination half-life is essentially the same in children and adults, although, with interindividual variation, it ranges as much as 1 to 3.5 hours.[40] The elimination half-life is somewhat longer (2.2–5.0 hours) in neonates. The profile of metabolites differs greatly in early childhood from adolescence and adulthood: sulfation predominates over glucuronidation.[41] The switch to the adult pattern seems to occur around 12 years of age. However, even in newborns, urinary metabolites reflecting cytochrome P-450–generated intermediates can be found; thus, the capacity for producing toxic metabolites seems to be present from an early age.[42,43] In vitro studies with fetal human hepatocytes have shown that the cytochrome P-450–generated intermediates can be formed and conjugated to glutathione as early as at 18 weeks of gestation, but the rate of formation is approximately 10% of that in adult human hepatocytes; sulfation, but not glucuronidation, of acetaminophen also can be detected in human fetal liver cells.[44] Studies in young rats showed less susceptibility to hepatotoxicity in the 11-day-old rat compared with the adult rat.[45] In other studies, hepatocytes from young rats were shown to have a higher capacity for synthesizing glutathione than those from older rats and to be able to also increase synthesis when glutathione is depleted.[46] Perhaps human infants also have a greater capacity for synthesis of glutathione than adults and thus can detoxify acetaminophen toxic metabolites more effectively.

Despite their relative resistance to acetaminophen hepatotoxicity, young children definitely can develop severe hepatotoxicity from acetaminophen. The threshold dose for severe toxicity in children has not been determined but is probably in the range of a single dose of 120 to 150 mg/kg.[47] In contrast to single high-dose ingestion, therapeutic misadventure is an important pattern of hepatotoxicity in young children. This term denotes hepatotoxicity that develops after taking repeated doses of relatively small amounts of acetaminophen (three to four times the recommended dose) for a short time, usually a few days.[48–52] Typically, the improper use of acetaminophen occurs because the dosage schedule was not understood, a different preparation of acetaminophen was substituted for the age-appropriate version (eg, tablet substituted for elixir), or the wrong measuring device was used. Incorrect use of sustained-release preparations or inadvertent overdosing because it was not appreciated that many over-the-counter cold remedies contain acetaminophen may also lead to hepatotoxicity. The threshold dose for hepatotoxicity under these circumstances has been estimated at 90 mg/kg/d.[53] The liver disease presents as acute liver failure, which is often attributed to another etiology, usually viral hepatitis. The typical clinical course of the single large-dose ingestion is either not present or not noticed. Serum concentrations of acetaminophen are frequently not in a toxic range. Diagnosis requires an extremely meticulous drug history to find out exactly what preparation of acetaminophen was used and how often. The nomogram for treatment with N-acetylcysteine does not apply; however, finding a detectable concentration of acetaminophen

at 24 hours or more after the last dose suggests this etiology. An estimated elimination half-life > 4 hours also suggests acetaminophen hepatotoxicity. Detection of serum acetaminophen-cysteine conjugates by high-performance liquid chromatography is a sensitive diagnostic test.[54] These children should be treated with N-acetylcysteine as soon as possible. The intercurrent illness for which the acetaminophen was used may have caused enough anorexia to deplete normal glutathione stores. Hepatotoxicity with extreme prolongation of the elimination half-life of acetaminophen has been reported in infants born after maternal self-poisoning with acetaminophen.[43,44]

Rectal administration of acetaminophen may also cause hepatotoxicity. Absorption from the suppository is often highly variable. In general, it takes longer to attain peak blood levels, but bioavailability can vary within the length of a single suppository and between different types of suppository depending on carrier composition. Overall, this appears to be a highly unsatisfactory way to give the drug because it is difficult to predict efficacy, determine dosing interval, and calculate cumulative dose. Hepatic failure associated with rectal acetaminophen has been reported, probably owing to high-dose acetaminophen, although the child also received diclofenac and underwent appendectomy.[55]

Initial studies on the mechanism of acetaminophen toxicity showed that toxicity was worse when animals were pretreated with the polycyclic aromatic hydrocarbon 3-methylcholanthrene, a potent inducer of CYP1A1. It has become evident that chronic alcoholics are more sensitive to acetaminophen than nonalcoholics in that they can develop subacute acetaminophen hepatotoxicity after taking ordinary therapeutic doses over time because of induction of CYP2E1.[56] Some adolescents may be at risk for this type of acetaminophen hepatotoxicity. Whether exposure to environmental toxins such as polychlorinated biphenyls or aromatic hydrocarbons, cigarette smoking, or chronic use of proton pump inhibitors that induce CYP1A2 increases susceptibility to acetaminophen hepatotoxicity remains unproved. Whether obesity (often associated with CYP2E1 induction) enhances the risk of acetaminophen hepatotoxicity has not been established. Available data relevant to children do show that concomitant treatment with medications that induce cytochromes P-450 lowers the threshold for acetaminophen hepatotoxicity. These drugs include phenobarbital, carbamazepine, phenytoin, rifampin, and isoniazid (INH). Mercury poisoning through exposure to elemental mercury apparently enhanced acetaminophen hepatotoxicity in one child.[57]

PHENYTOIN

Although the commonly used anticonvulsant diphenylhydantoin has been associated with a broad range of adverse effects, phenytoin-induced hepatitis is important because severe hepatic necrosis and liver failure often develop. The perception that it is rare in children is misleading. Phenytoin-associated hepatitis was the only hepatitis mentioned specifically among adverse drug reactions in a large prospective study of adverse drug reactions in children.[18] There are at least 30 cases in the literature[58,59] and an additional 18 cases of hepatic dysfunction in patients (9 of whom were children) whose adverse reaction to phenytoin was dominated by other organ system involvement.[60]

Phenytoin hepatotoxicity typically presents as part of a systemic disease with fever, rash (including morbilliform rash, Stevens-Johnson syndrome, and toxic epidermal necrolysis), lymphadenopathy, leukocytosis, eosinophilia, and atypical lymphocytosis. Serum aminotransferases are elevated, and the patient may be moderately jaundiced. In severe cases, clinical features of hepatic failure (coagulopathy, ascites, altered level of consciousness) are also present. Histopathologic examination of the liver shows spotty necrosis of hepatocytes, along with features reminiscent of mononucleosis in some cases or of viral hepatitis in others; cholestasis may complicate more severe hepatocellular injury; granulomas are sometimes found.[61] Although treatment of severe phenytoin hepatitis with high-dose intravenous corticosteroids has not been tested in a controlled trial and anecdotal reports do not uniformly show clear benefit, intravenous methylprednisolone 2 mg/kg/d has been effective in some patients. In patients with severe Stevens-Johnson syndrome, use of intravenous gammaglobulin has also been advocated.[62]

The typical clinical presentation of phenytoin hepatotoxicity is termed a "drug hypersensitivity reaction." There is reason to believe that this clinical syndrome develops as a result of abnormal handling of a toxic metabolite of phenytoin. Phenytoin is metabolized via an arene oxide intermediate that is ordinarily metabolized and thus detoxified by epoxide hydrolase.[63] When lymphocytes, which are readily isolated cells complete with most phase II biotransformation pathways, are incubated in vitro with phenytoin and a murine microsomal system that can generate the intermediate metabolites of phenytoin, lymphocytes from persons who have developed the drug hypersensitivity syndrome to phenytoin are killed in excess of control lymphocytes.[63] If lymphocytes from normal individuals are pretreated with chemicals that inhibit cellular epoxide hydrolase, these lymphocytes behave like those from affected individuals.[64] Studies of parents indicate an intermediate sensitivity to the toxic metabolite(s), consistent with an inherited defect in drug detoxification. Instead of causing cell death, binding of the toxic metabolite may create haptens for initiating an immune response. This may account for the appearance of hypersensitivity clinically and for positive immune challenges noted by others.[65] More recent studies have failed to confirm the thesis that deficient epoxide hydrolase activity is responsible for phenytoin hepatotoxicity.[66] Others have shown elaboration of reactive intermediates, including quinone derivatives.[67,68]

Three of four children reported with fatal diphenylhydantoin hepatotoxicity were taking phenobarbital at the same time. Because in vitro studies indicate that some patients who cannot detoxify toxic intermediates of phenytoin are similarly sensitive to phenobarbital, this combined treatment may have made the liver damage worse. Another patient was switched from phenytoin to phenobarbital and then relapsed; he improved when high-dose corticosteroids were given along with phenobarbital.[58]

CARBAMAZEPINE

Carbamazepine is a dibenzazepine derivative, similar structurally to imipramine in that it has fundamentally a tricyclic chemical structure. Hepatotoxicity is relatively uncommon. In adults, the predominant hepatotoxicity has been granulomatous hepatitis presenting with fever and right upper quadrant pain, suggestive of cholangitis.[69,70] In children, the clinical picture has been more of a hepatitis, sometimes dominating a drug hypersensitivity syndrome like that of phenytoin. One child died of progressive liver failure when carbamazepine was not stopped in time.[71] Four children with fatal acute liver failure were taking carbamazepine, phenytoin, and primidone.[72] More recently, severe hepatitis was reported in three children taking only carbamazepine: one recovered with corticosteroid treatment, but the others died or required liver transplant.[73] Another child developed acute severe hepatitis 5 months after beginning treatment with carbamazepine; she survived with prednisone treatment.[74] Two other children presented with a mononucleosis-like illness with rash, lymphadenopathy, hepatosplenomegaly, hepatosplenomegaly, and, eventually, neutropenia.[75,76] This is similar to a child treated at the Hospital for Sick Children in Toronto (Figure 53-5), who presented with fever, rash, incipient liver failure, lymphopenia, and eosinophilia. In vitro rechallenge of her lymphocytes with metabolites of carbamazepine provided evidence of defective detoxification mechanisms. An infant boy also presented here with only hepatotoxicity and three other children with drug hypersensitivity to carbamazepine, with hepatitis not the dominant feature, have been described.[60] Carbamazepine may also be metabolized via arene oxides, although not all data support this thesis.[77]

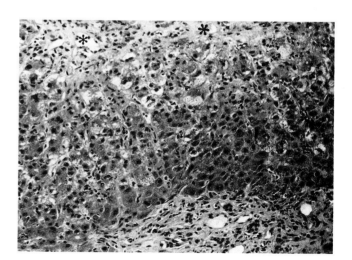

FIGURE 53-5 Liver biopsy in carbamazepine hepatotoxicity. The portal area shows widening with fibrosis, ductular proliferation, and mild chronic inflammatory changes. The lobular parenchyma shows variability in the size of the hepatocytes, with many swollen ballooned hepatocytes in zones 2 and 3 and occasional inflammatory cells. In zone 3, there is central bridging necrosis (asterisks). The pathologic diagnosis is drug-induced acute hepatitis with bridging necrosis; these findings are fully representative of the hepatic lesion with carbamazepine (hematoxylin and eosin, ×250 original magnification). Courtesy of Dr. M. J. Phillips.

Recent work indicates that carbamazepine is metabolized to a reactive iminoquinone species that can react with glutathione.[78] Persons with the metabolic idiosyncrasy that renders them susceptible to carbamazepine hepatotoxicity may also be susceptible to phenytoin and phenobarbital hepatotoxicity.

PHENOBARBITAL

Hepatitis is a rare complication of phenobarbital use. When it occurs, it, too, is usually part of a multisystemic drug hypersensitivity reaction, but it may dominate the clinical picture. Seven of 13 patients reported in the world literature were children.[79] Two additional children, a girl aged 3 years and a boy aged 18 months, have been treated at the Hospital for Sick Children in Toronto; both had severe hepatic dysfunction with coagulopathy or ascites but ultimately survived. Two further cases in children have been treated at the Hospital for Sick Children in Toronto, but hepatitis was not the dominant clinical feature.[60] In most cases of major hepatotoxicity, jaundice began 1 to 8 weeks after starting phenobarbital, along with generalized rash and fever. Usually, the liver disease was moderately severe but self-limited; however, a few patients developed severe hepatitis with coagulopathy and ascites, and one died fulminantly. One child developed chronic liver disease. Severe phenobarbital hepatitis may be treated with intravenous methylprednisolone.[79]

The mechanism of this hepatotoxicity remains unclear. Results from in vitro rechallenge indicate an inherited defect in detoxification of active metabolite. Phenobarbital may also be metabolized via arene oxide intermediates, which are typically detoxified via epoxide hydrolase. In in vitro rechallenge, if lymphocyte epoxide hydrolase is inhibited, the extent of cytotoxicity of metabolites generated from phenobarbital, as from phenytoin, increases.[64]

Persons who develop hepatotoxicity from phenobarbital also cannot detoxify other barbiturates and may get worse if so treated. Sedation for a diagnostic procedure in a child is an important opportunity for such a drug exposure. It is also important to bear in mind that persons who cannot detoxify the toxic metabolite(s) of phenobarbital often cannot detoxify those of carbamazepine or phenytoin either.[60] Thus, substituting either may worsen the hepatitis.

LAMOTRIGINE

Lamotrigine may cause hepatotoxicity with a typical anticonvulsant hypersensitivity syndrome clinically.[80–82] Hepatic involvement varies from elevated serum aminotransferases to severe acute hepatitis. Lamotrigine can generate an arene oxide intermediate, which is a candidate for mediating this hepatotoxicity.[83] Whether cross-reactivity between lamotrigine and the phenytoin-carbamazepine-phenobarbital anticonvulsant group exists has not been conclusively proven.

VALPROIC ACID

Valproic acid (VPA) is chemically very different from the other anticonvulsants above: it is an eight-carbon, branched fatty acid. Hepatotoxicity is mild or severe. In a certain proportion of patients, estimated at 11% overall,[84] serum aminotransferase levels become abnormal, typically within a short time of starting treatment. This biochemical abnormality returns to normal when the dose of VPA is decreased. Much more rarely, patients develop progressive liver failure that, in some cases, looks similar clinically to Reye syndrome. This severe hepatotoxicity does not always regress when the drug is withdrawn. Its occurrence cannot be predicted by regular monitoring of serum aminotransferases and other liver function tests.[85] The time from initiating treatment with VPA and onset of liver disease is usually less than 4 months, but hepatotoxicity may develop later in treatment. A distinctive feature of severe VPA hepatotoxicity is that it is more common in children than in adults.[86] Special identifiable risk factors include age less than 2 years, multiple anticonvulsant treatment along with VPA, and coexistent medical problems such as mental retardation, developmental delay, or congenital abnormalities.[87] In children with these predisposing factors, the risk of fatal hepatotoxicity is 1 in 600.[88] Hyperammonemia, not associated with liver failure, is another metabolic adverse effect of VPA.[89,90]

Severe hepatotoxicity was described with rising use of VPA,[91,92] and the total experience has been reviewed in detail.[84,93,94] The severe hepatotoxicity typically presents with a hepatitis-like prodrome, mainly malaise, anorexia, nausea, and vomiting. Seizure control is often found to deteriorate over the same time period. An intercurrent illness with fever may precede the onset of liver failure. Coagulopathy is often present early; jaundice and other signs of progressive hepatic insufficiency, such as ascites and hypoglycemia, develop later. Death owing to liver failure, complicated by renal failure or infection, is the frequently reported outcome; liver transplant may be performed. Liver histology reviewed in one large series shows evidence of hepatocellular necrosis, which may be zonal, with extensive loss of hepatocytes and severe damage to those remaining.[93] Acidophilic bodies, ballooned hepatocytes, and cholangiolar proliferation may be present. Microvesicular steatosis is the most common finding overall and is often present in addition to the features of cell necrosis. Hepatocellular mitochondria may be prominent on light microscopy so that the hepatocytes have a granular, very eosinophilic appearance (Figure 53-6). In cases presenting clinically like Reye syndrome, fever, coagulopathy, progressive loss of consciousness, severe acidosis, and variably abnormal serum aminotransferases are present, but the patient is not jaundiced.[92] Hepatocellular necrosis, as well as microvesicular fat, is found on histologic examination of the liver, unlike the histologic findings of Reye syndrome. Electron microscopically, the mitochondrial changes associated with VPA toxicity differ from those of Reye syndrome.

The mechanism of this severe hepatotoxicity is thought to involve generation of toxic metabolite(s) plus some type of metabolic idiosyncrasy. Metabolic idiosyncrasy is probable not only because severe hepatotoxicity is rare but because toxic ingestions do not necessarily lead to liver necrosis.[95] VPA is related structurally to two known hepatotoxins: hypoglycin, which causes Jamaican vomiting sickness, characterized by microvesicular steatosis, and 4-pentenoic acid,

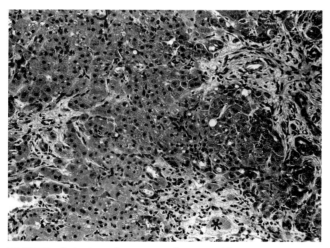

FIGURE 53-6   Liver biopsy in valproic acid hepatotoxicity. The liver lobule shows great reduction in the number of hepatocytes. There is portal tract widening with increased numbers of bile ducts. Hepatocytes are swollen, and most contain multiple microvesicular fat droplets. In zone 3, there is an area of necrosis (*asterisk*) with tubular transformation of hepatocytes surrounding the necrotic zone (hematoxylin and eosin, ×250 original magnification). Courtesy of Dr. M. J. Phillips.

which causes microvesicular steatosis in rat liver and inhibits β-oxidation. The partly unsaturated metabolite 4-ene-valproic acid (4-ene-VPA), produced by Ω-oxidation, which is a minor pathway of VPA metabolism, is chemically very similar to these toxins. Formation of 4-ene-VPA has been demonstrated in a primate model[96] and in patients with liver failure developing on VPA treatment.[97] Administration of 4-ene-VPA to rats caused accumulation of microvesicular fat in hepatocytes along with changes in hepatocyte organelles, including mitochondrial abnormalities and elaboration of myeloid bodies,[98] as well as inhibition of β-oxidation.[99] Both VPA and 4-ene-VPA inhibit β-oxidative metabolism of decanoic acid, a fatty acid of medium length; in contrast, 4-pentenoic acid is only a weak inhibitor in this system.[100] Thus, VPA and its metabolite(s) are capable of causing adverse changes in liver cell metabolism, which may lead to the observed features of this hepatotoxicity. The similarities and differences in these metabolic toxicities compared with those of hypoglycin and 4-pentenoic acid merely reflect the complexity of this metabolic system. The β-oxidation metabolite of 4-ene-VPA, (*E*)-2,4-diene-VPA, may also mediate VPA hepatotoxicity as a toxic intermediate. Urinary levels of thiol conjugates of 4-ene-VPA and (*E*)-2,4-diene-VPA were found to be elevated in children less than 7.5 years old receiving VPA monotherapy and were also elevated in older children if they were receiving treatment with an antiepileptic drug capable of inducing cytochromes P-450 along with the VPA.[101] Concentrations of the thiol conjugates of (*E*)-2,4-diene-VPA were higher than those of 4-ene-VPA.

VPA is capable of inhibiting β-oxidation in humans. Investigations of VPA metabolism in patients with severe hepatotoxicity indicate that β-oxidation is inhibited in these patients,[102] although the step in β-oxidation at which the apparent block occurred varied individually.[103]

Increased amounts of 4-ene-VPA were detected in some cases.[97,104,105] Biochemical abnormalities indicating inhibition of β-oxidation have also been found in children on VPA treatment at low risk for hepatotoxicity.[106] These observations suggest a complex pattern of inhibited β-oxidation and increased utilization of alternative pathways, including those associated with cytochromes P-450 and δ-dehydrogenation to produce, among other metabolites, 4-ene-VPA.

In VPA hepatotoxicity, the target organelle appears to be the mitochondrion. An individual who develops severe VPA hepatotoxicity may not be able to detoxify these metabolites or subsequent toxic intermediates before significant mitochondrial damage occurs. The defective detoxification pathway is not yet known. Studies of VPA toxicity in vitro in human liver slices indicate important interindividual variation in susceptibility to toxicity.[107] The metabolic idiosyncrasy might be a functional defect in the mitochondrion itself. An intercurrent environmental problem, such as a viral illness, might additionally inhibit β-oxidation. Experimental data in the ornithine transcarbamylase–deficient mouse support the hypothesis of an intrinsic metabolic defect in the mitochondrion. The ornithine transcarbamylase–deficient mouse develops hepatocellular necrosis and microvesicular steatosis at doses of VPA that do not affect the normal control adversely.[108] Individuals who develop severe VPA hepatotoxicity may have mitochondria biochemically predisposed to this injury. Ornithine transcarbamylase deficiency may be one such definable abnormality and has been suspected in one instance.[109,110] Other mitochondrial abnormalities may have predisposed some patients to VPA hepatotoxicity.[111]

Serum carnitine has been found to be abnormally low in persons with Reye syndrome. Decreased serum carnitine has also been found in VPA hepatotoxicity.[102,112] Serum carnitine is also low in patients treated chronically, without evidence clinically of hepatotoxicity.[112–114] Conjugation to carnitine is a unique metabolic pathway for VPA.[115] Whether this pathway is important for the development of hepatotoxicity is not known. Equally, the value of carnitine repletion as treatment for severe hepatotoxicity remains unproven, and most evidence to date suggests that it is ineffective.[106,116] However, a recent retrospective study indicated efficacy if carnitine was started very early in the course of severe hepatotoxicity.[117]

SULFONAMIDES

Hepatotoxicity may occur with any sulfonamide antibiotic. In children, this problem arises most commonly in connection with treatment for otitis media and upper respiratory infections or for inflammatory bowel disease. Sulfanilamide, trimethoprim-sulfamethoxazole, and pyrimethamine-sulfadoxine have all been associated with major hepatic injury.[118,119] Sulfasalazine has been associated with severe liver disease in adolescents and young adults.[120–123] Although the liver abnormality may be manifested only by elevated serum aminotransferases or may be a granulomatous hepatitis, the hepatic dysfunction may be severe enough to cause acute hepatic failure, which is fatal in some cases. In general, hepatotoxicity is part of a clinical drug hypersensitivity reaction. Fever, significant rash, periorbital edema, atypical lymphocytosis, lymphadenopathy, and renal dysfunction with proteinuria have all been described.

Sulfonamide hepatotoxicity is due to elaboration of an electrophilic toxic metabolite in the liver. The intermediate appears to be the hydroxylamine derived from the particular sulfonamide or, more likely, the nitroso species derived from the hydroxylamine.[124–126] Patients who develop severe adverse reactions, including significant hepatotoxicity, have been shown to be slow acetylators (in the rapid/slow polymorphism for N-acetyltransferase) and are also unable to detoxify this reactive metabolite. On in vitro rechallenge of their lymphocytes with sulfonamide and a metabolite-generating system, the patient's lymphocytes show significantly more cytotoxicity than controls.[119] Glutathione S-transferases may be important for detoxifying the toxic intermediate.[127,128] How this reactive intermediate causes hepatocellular damage is not yet known. The multisystemic hypersensitivity features of this adverse drug reaction appear to be subsequent to metabolic events in that the reactive metabolite probably acts as a hapten to initiate the immune response. Thus, sulfa hepatotoxicity fundamentally represents metabolic idiosyncrasy, not simply allergy.

ERYTHROMYCIN

Erythromycin estolate and other salts are used frequently in children. Although the estolate was originally associated with a cholestatic hepatic lesion, it is now clear that the ethylsuccinate and other salts are also potentially hepatotoxic.[129–132] Indeed, all forms of erythromycin are potentially hepatotoxic. The clinical presentation includes anorexia, nausea, predominantly right upper quadrant abdominal pain, and jaundice. Pruritus owing to cholestasis has been reported in some adults. Hepatomegaly, sometimes accompanied by splenomegaly, appears to be frequent in children. Erythromycin ethylsuccinate hepatotoxicity in a child was a relatively mild, self-limited disease.[130]

Histologic findings include prominent cholestasis, which is particularly severe in zone 3, focal necrosis of hepatocytes also tending to predominate in zone 3, and eosinophils in the portal infiltrates and in the sinusoids.[129] These histologic findings are different from those of extrahepatic biliary tract obstruction, although the clinical presentation may suggest biliary tract obstruction.

The mechanism of this hepatotoxicity remains obscure. Erythromycin itself, not a specific erythromycin salt, may be the cause of the hepatotoxicity. However, in the perfused rat liver model, erythromycin estolate led to decreased bile secretion, altered canalicular permeability, and decreased activities of Na/K–adenosine triphosphatase and Mg++–adenosine triphosphatase, unlike erythromycin base.[133] Earlier studies in Chang liver cells suggested that erythromycin derivatives cause intrinsic hepatocellular damage. In various types of primary rat hepatocyte culture systems, erythromycin estolate leads to cytotoxicity.[134,135] Erythromycin and other macrolide antibiotics are metabolized in the liver by the CYP3A subfamily. Hepatocellular damage may be due to a toxic metabolite, but this is by no

means proven. Cholestasis may also reflect damage to the cellular biliary apparatus. The association of eosinophilia with erythromycin hepatotoxicity in some patients probably represents a forme fruste of a drug hypersensitivity syndrome.

PROPYLTHIOURACIL

Hepatitis is a rare complication of propylthiouracil treatment for hyperthyroidism. It tends to occur in girls, but this may reflect the greater frequency of thyroid disease in girls.[136–140] The clinical picture typically was a nonspecific hepatitic presentation with anorexia, nausea, vomiting, and jaundice. Serum aminotransferases were moderately elevated. Symptoms began typically within 2 to 3 months of starting treatment, but in one child, liver disease began at least 9 months after starting treatment and in another after 15 months. A more cholestatic picture has been reported in some adults. Liver histology shows mild to severe hepatocellular necrosis, which was characterized as submassive in three cases.

A single case of propylthiouracil hepatotoxicity associated with chronic active hepatitis has been reported in a child.[141] Hepatomegaly with elevated serum aminotransferases developed after more than 1 year of treatment. Both anti–smooth muscle antibodies and anti–liver/kidney microsomal (anti-LKM1) antibodies were negative. Liver biopsy showed portal inflammation with moderate piecemeal necrosis.

ASPIRIN

Hepatotoxicity has been associated with high-dose aspirin treatment. Approximately 60% of the 300 reported cases have been in patients with juvenile rheumatoid arthritis (JRA) (not necessarily all children), and a further 10% have occurred in children with acute rheumatic fever.[142] Hepatotoxicity may be more frequent in girls. The hepatotoxicity appears to be dose dependent, and patients without rheumatoid disease can develop hepatotoxicity. The preponderance of cases in patients with rheumatologic diseases, however, raises the possibility that these patients have a predisposition to this toxicity. One theory is that chronic inflammation favors generation of oxygen radicals.[143]

In most cases, salicylate hepatotoxicity presents with anorexia, nausea, vomiting, and abdominal pain, along with elevated serum aminotransferases.[144–148] Hepatomegaly is usually present, and the liver may be tender. Progressive signs of liver damage, such as jaundice and coagulopathy, are rare, occurring in approximately 4% of all reported cases.[142] However, even in uncomplicated cases, serum aminotransferase levels may be quite high, greater than 1,000 IU.[146] In some cases, encephalopathy (not related to Reye syndrome) was present.[149,150] Clinical and laboratory abnormalities resolve when aspirin is stopped. Rechallenge with aspirin may lead to recurrent hepatotoxicity. Liver histology frequently shows a rather nonspecific picture with acute, focal hepatocellular necrosis.[144]

A different clinical syndrome with hepatotoxicity has been reported in seven children with JRA, of whom all but one received aspirin.[151] Clinical features included high fever, drowsiness, vomiting, hepatosplenomegaly, and bleeding owing to disseminated intravascular coagulation and suboptimal clotting factor synthesis. Liver histology showed steatosis (predominantly large droplet) and prominence of reticuloendothelial cells in the liver. Rechallenge with aspirin did not reproduce this syndrome, and it may have been related to other drug treatment or to intercurrent infection. Two children died of coma, but there was neither cerebral edema nor severe hyperammonemia noted, and other features were not typical of Reye syndrome. However, Reye syndrome can occur in children with rheumatologic diseases who receive aspirin chronically,[152] and its clinical presentation may be atypical.

METHOTREXATE

Methotrexate hepatotoxicity in children appears to be similar to that in adults. Chronic low-dose treatment used for treatment of psoriasis or connective tissue disease can cause hepatic fibrosis with steatosis.[153,154] Histologically, it may resemble alcoholic hepatitis with fibrosis. Cirrhosis can develop, and liver transplant has been performed in some adults treated for psoriasis.[155] In adults, obesity, diabetes, chronic alcohol abuse, older age, and large cumulative dose appear to be factors associated with increased risk of methotrexate hepatotoxicity. Serum aminotransferase levels may not indicate reliably the extent of ongoing liver damage, and liver biopsy prior to treatment and at regular intervals during prolonged treatment has been advised. Recent guidelines for monitoring methotrexate hepatotoxicity in adults with rheumatoid arthritis advocate a more formal approach to monitoring aspartate aminotransferase, ALT, ALP, albumin, and bilirubin (γ-glutamyltransferase to corroborate hepatic origin of ALP should be added to this list) every 4 to 8 weeks; liver biopsy is performed only when sustained abnormalities are found.[156] Liver biopsy prior to starting treatment is reserved for patients with known liver disease or specific risk (chronic hepatitis B or C infection). Meta-analysis indicates that there is a tangible risk in adults for significant hepatotoxicity owing to long-term, low-dose methotrexate.[157]

It is difficult to transpose these data from adults with various diseases directly to children. The risk factors identified in adults have limited applicability to children except for obesity. Regular monitoring of liver function tests in children receiving chronic methotrexate treatment is advisable. Children with JRA on methotrexate should have serum aminotransferases checked frequently (monthly or bimonthly). Those with elevated aspartate aminotransferase or ALT on ≥ 40% of tests in 1 year should be considered for liver biopsy. Generally, the surveillance regimen should be individualized for each child, depending on many variables, such as existence of previous liver disease (including chronic viral infection), concomitant drug therapy, cumulative methotrexate dose, chronic hypoalbuminemia, obesity, and diabetes mellitus. Liver biopsy is indicated to determine the extent of liver damage. Performing a liver biopsy after a large cumulative dose of methotrexate has been taken may be appropriate in some cases, especially if continued treatment is anticipated. A pretreatment liver biopsy is also sometimes appropriate since several studies indicate that hepatic abnormalities may be present prior to treatment, which would otherwise be wrongly attributed to methotrexate hepatotoxicity.

Several recent studies have examined the occurrence of hepatotoxicity in children with JRA treated with methotrexate over the long term. The risk of methotrexate hepatotoxicity in JRA appears to be comparatively low. No child in a cross-sectional study of 14 children with JRA who had received a methotrexate cumulative dose > 3,000 mg or > 4,000 mg/1.73 m² body surface area had significant fibrosis; one had moderate to severe fatty or inflammatory changes or hepatocellular necrosis on liver biopsy.[158] In a study of 37 liver biopsies from 25 patients with JRA, most were normal or near normal; 4 had moderate to severe fatty or inflammatory changes, and 2 had mild portal fibrosis. Weak yet statistically significant correlations were found between abnormal histology and percent frequency of serum aminotransferase elevations and body mass index.[159] In similar previous studies, normal or near-normal liver histology was found.[160,161] Two patients with JRA treated with methotrexate have been reported as developing some degree of liver fibrosis.[162]

High-dose methotrexate treatment used in some oncology regimens may cause acute hepatitis.[163,164] After more protracted treatment, hepatic damage may be relatively slight, apart from ultrastructural changes including steatosis, fibrosis, and damage to some hepatocellular organelles.[165] Others have also found steatosis, portal inflammation, or portal fibrosis on light microscopic examination of liver biopsies from children with acute lymphoblastic leukemia, treated with various drugs, including methotrexate.[166] Serum aminotransferase abnormalities did not predict histologic findings, which were, in general, mild after 2 years of treatment.[166,167]

The mechanism of this hepatotoxicity is not known. The dosage schedule may be important. Chronic intermittent administration of methotrexate may lead to recurrent hepatocellular damage superimposed on partial repair and regeneration, not unlike experimental models of carbon tetrachloride–induced hepatic fibrosis.

ANTINEOPLASTIC DRUGS

Besides methotrexate, many drugs used to treat neoplasia in childhood can cause hepatotoxicity.[168,169] A common and perplexing problem is elevation in serum aminotransferases without other evidence of severe liver toxicity. Antineoplastic drugs that commonly produce this reaction include nitrosoureas, 6-mercaptopurine, cytosine arabinoside, cisplatinum, and dacarbazine. Doxorubicin, cyclophosphamide, dactinomycin (actinomycin D), and vinca alkaloids are infrequently associated with hepatotoxicity, although drug interactions may increase their hepatotoxicity. Indeed, the difficulty in assessing the hepatotoxic potential of all of these drugs is that they are rarely used separately, and patients receiving them are usually at risk for multiple types of liver injury.

In children and adults, L-asparaginase has been associated with more severe damage characterized by severe steatosis, hepatocellular necrosis, and fibrosis. This is usually reversible after the L-asparaginase is stopped.[170] The most likely mechanism for this hepatotoxicity is a profound interference with hepatocellular protein metabolism. Dactinomycin (actinomycin D) is exceptionally associated with severe liver damage. Several patients treated with dactinomycin at the Hospital for Sick Children in Toronto developed acute severe hepatitis, with extremely elevated serum aminotransferases and coagulopathy, all of which resolved spontaneously off the drug. The mechanism is not known. Mithramycin has been associated with acute hepatic necrosis. Thrombocytopenia and acute liver failure have been reported in an 18-year-old patient receiving carboplatin.[171]

Thioguanine and other antineoplastic agents, including cyclophosphamide, cytosine arabinoside, busulfan, dacarbazine, and carmustine, have been associated with veno-occlusive disease (VOD) at conventional or high doses.[172] It most frequently develops after allogeneic bone marrow transplant. It presents acutely with an enlarged tender liver, ascites or unexplained weight gain, and jaundice; serum aminotransferases may be elevated; it may progress to cirrhosis. Although irradiation can, in itself, lead to this type of hepatic vascular damage,[173] the combination of irradiation and chemotherapy in conditioning regimens may lead to earlier development of VOD than after single-agent (irradiation or chemical) injury.[174] Clinical predictors of likelihood for development of VOD in children have not yet been identified, but patients with chronic hepatitis, for example, owing to chronic hepatitis C or possibly nonalcoholic steatohepatitis, preceding bone marrow transplant are at increased risk.

The pathogenesis of VOD involves direct toxicity to the sinusoidal endothelial cells in the liver. When it is due to dacarbazine, the damage to endothelial cells occurs through production of toxic metabolite(s) in the endothelial cells; glutathione appears to protect against toxicity.[175] With cyclophosphamide, the toxic intermediate may be produced in hepatocytes.[176] Treatment with N-acetylcysteine may reverse the process.[177] Unchecked, the damage progresses from congestion and hemorrhage into the space of Disse in zone 3 of the Rappaport acinus to damage to terminal hepatic venules, which has been described as sinusoidal obstruction syndrome, and, subsequently, to fibrosis.[178] The term sinusoidal obstruction syndrome emphasizes that damage to sinusoidal endothelial cells is the initiating event in this kind of hepatotoxicity and that terminal hepatic venules may be patent as the lesions evolve; however, in many patients, only the resulting lesion with obliterative damage to terminal hepatic venules (namely, VOD) is identified.

CYCLOSPORINE

Cyclosporine is a calcineurin inhibitor with potent immunosuppressive effects. It is extremely lipophilic and has a novel cyclic structure composed of 11 amino acids. It is metabolized in humans by CYP3A4. Although, at high dosage, jaundice with abnormal serum aminotransferases may develop, the more common hepatic abnormality is mainly cholestasis, direct hyperbilirubinemia without

other evidence of hepatocellular damage.[179] Cholestasis without biochemical or histologic evidence of hepatotoxicity after cyclosporine administration has been demonstrated in a rat model.[180] Cyclosporine inhibits the bile salt excretory pump (BSEP) directly,[181] down-regulates expression of the multidrug resistance–associated protein (Mrp2), which is located on the apical membrane, and interferes with enzymes responsible for synthesizing glutathione.[182] It may also affect membrane fluidity and thus impair canalicular transporter function indirectly.[183] Increased incidence of gallstones has been reported in children receiving cyclosporine after organ transplant.[184]

PEMOLINE

Pemoline, a second-line drug for treatment of attention-deficit disorders, has been associated with significant hepatotoxicity: asymptomatic elevation of serum aminotransferases, hepatitis with jaundice, and acute liver failure.[185–190] The largest series documented hepatitis of variable severity, including one patient who died with fulminant hepatic failure[191]; male patients predominated. Two other deaths associated with hepatic dysfunction while on pemoline have been reported. Both patients were boys: one may have had previous chronic liver disease, and the other may have taken an overdose of pemoline.[192] Other cases of severe hepatotoxicity leading to liver transplant have been reported. Pemoline has been withdrawn in some countries. If it is used, serum aminotransferases and other liver function tests must be monitored frequently throughout the entire term of treatment. When pemoline is associated with elevated serum aminotransferases, it must be discontinued. The mechanism of this hepatotoxicity is not known but is probably related to the hepatic metabolism of the drug, not to immune response. Pemoline should not be combined with other hepatotoxic drugs and should not be used in patients with a history of liver disease.

RISPERIDONE

Risperidone is a new drug for various psychiatric problems, including autistic disorders. A few cases of possible hepatotoxicity in children have been reported in adults,[193,194] although they are difficult to interpret because of prior liver disease or concomitant drug treatment. A report of risperidone hepatotoxicity in two children may actually have been concurrence of nonalcoholic steatohepatitis and possible drug toxicity,[195] and a subsequent case series review did not corroborate these findings.[196] Nevertheless, serum aminotransferase elevations after starting risperidone have been observed in children. Risperidone typically leads to weight gain. Body mass index should be assessed before and during treatment. Children taking risperidone should have serum aminotransferases and bilirubin monitored regularly until the risk of hepatotoxicity is determined.

ISONIAZID

In adults, INH is capable of causing a wide spectrum of toxic liver disease.[197,198] Clinically, the common finding is an asymptomatic patient with elevated serum aminotransferases. The development of a hepatitis-like illness with fatigue, anorexia, nausea, and vomiting is ominous. On histologic examination, INH hepatotoxicity frequently looks like acute viral hepatitis. Submassive hepatic necrosis can occur, and, occasionally, the hepatocellular damage is zonal.

There have been scattered reports of INH hepatotoxicity, including fatal hepatic necrosis, occurring both in children being treated for tuberculosis and in those receiving prophylaxis.[199–205] The overall incidence of symptomatic INH hepatitis in children is 0.1 to 7.1%.[206] Large studies of INH hepatotoxicity as evidenced by abnormal serum aminotransferases in children receiving INH alone as prophylaxis showed a 7% incidence in a series of 369 children[207] and a 17.1% incidence in 239 patients aged 9 to 14 years.[208] The discrepancy in these two studies is partly methodologic. However, these findings are nearly the same as in adults, where the incidence of transiently elevated serum aminotransferases is estimated at 10 to 20%.[198] Several studies of children being treated with INH and rifampicin for tuberculosis also show a high incidence of hepatic dysfunction. Thirty-six of 44 patients receiving INH and rifampicin had some elevation of serum aminotransferases and 15 patients (42%) had elevated AST and were jaundiced.[209] These children received comparatively high doses of INH and rifampicin, and many had severe infection. In another study, 37% had hepatotoxicity, including four of seven under 17 months old.[210] These children received conventional, lower doses of INH and rifampicin and brief sequential courses of streptomycin and ethambutal. Inducers of cytochromes P-450 may contribute to INH hepatotoxicity. Severe INH hepatotoxicity occurred in a 10-year-old boy concurrently treated with carbamazepine.[211] As in adults, hepatotoxicity typically developed in children in the first 8 to 10 weeks of treatment. In most children, it resolved with either no change in dose or else a modest dose reduction. Children with more severe tuberculosis, such as tuberculous meningitis, seemed to be at greater risk for hepatotoxicity.

INH hepatotoxicity appears to be due to a toxic metabolite, although the mechanism remains obscure. Acetylisoniazid or its derivatives have been thought to be the toxic intermediate. Susceptibility to hepatotoxicity has been linked to the polymorphism for N-acetylation—rapid acetylators being at greater risk.[198] Clinical studies in children have not shown a universal trend implicating rapid acetylators as more susceptible.[210,212] Metabolism by cytochromes P-450 may also be implicated because pretreatment with phenobarbital appears to increase toxicity in laboratory animal models. Rifampicin may enhance INH toxicity by inducing certain cytochromes P-450.[204]

It is probably inaccurate to regard INH hepatotoxicity as uncommon in children. Some of the hepatotoxicity appears to be dose related, and recent downward revisions of dosage recommendations may eliminate some instances of hepatotoxicity. Children who have more severe tuberculosis or who receive simultaneous treatment with rifampicin, phenytoin, or phenobarbital may be at increased risk. The genetic predisposing factors remain

unclear. Monitoring with frequent measurement of serum aminotransferases and direct inquiry for symptoms of hepatitis is important in the first 10 to 12 weeks of treatment. INH should be discontinued if anorexia, nausea, or vomiting develops.

HALOTHANE

Halothane hepatotoxicity shows two major clinical patterns. One is hepatitis indicated by abnormal serum aminotransferases in the first or second week after the anesthetic exposure. The other pattern is severe hepatitis with extensive hepatocyte necrosis and liver failure.[213] It is remarkably infrequent in children. Large retrospective studies in children estimate that the incidence is approximately 1 in 80,000 to 1 in 200,000,[214,215] in contrast to an incidence of 1 in 7,000 to 1 in 30,000 in adults.[216] The infrequency of this hepatotoxicity is not due to lack of exposure to the drug because halothane is a mainstay of pediatric anesthetic practice. However, despite its rarity, it is evident that halothane hepatitis can occur in children. Eight cases have been documented in detail in children aged 11 months to 15 years, all of whom had multiple exposures to halothane; one died of fulminant liver failure, but all others recovered.[217,218] In addition, three cases of halothane hepatitis were found retrospectively,[214,215] as well as three further children who succumbed to fulminant hepatic failure after halothane.[219–221] Perhaps an additional eight cases may be found among other reports of hepatitis or hepatic failure in children after halothane anesthesia where inadequate data or the presence of complicated, and thus confounding, systemic disease make evaluation difficult. Clearly, this problem cannot be discounted in children. There has been some speculation that children with α_1-antitrypsin deficiency may tolerate halothane poorly.

Halothane is metabolized by various cytochromes P-450, and toxic metabolites are generated.[222–224] Depending on the prevailing tissue oxygen tension, oxidative or reductive metabolic pathways predominate (Figure 53-7). The reductive pathway generates a toxic intermediate identified as a chlorotrifluoroethyl radical, which leads to lipid peroxidation,[222] and the oxidative pathway generates a trifluoroacetyl intermediate, which can acetylate cellular membranes. The contribution of these metabolic systems to halothane hepatotoxicity in humans is complex. The oxidative pathway is probably predominant in humans. CYP2A6 and CYP3A4 are associated with the reductive metabolism,[225] and CYP2A6 and CYP2E1 (mainly the latter) are associated with the oxidative pathway.[226]

Recent studies of the mechanism of halothane hepatotoxicity are beginning to show the connection between cytotoxic damage from reactive intermediates and immunologic phenomena often associated with this hepatotoxicity. Patients surviving halothane hepatotoxicity have been found to have an antibody to altered hepatocyte membrane constituents.[227] In rabbits, only oxidative metabolism of halothane has been associated with production of this altered hepatocyte membrane antigen, and the effect is greater after pretreatment with the polycyclic aromatic hydrocarbon β-naphthaflavone.[228] Other investigators have shown that tri-

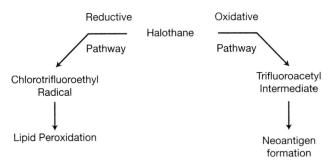

FIGURE 53–7 Metabolic fates of halothane. Whether the reductive or oxidative pathway predominates depends on the prevailing tissue oxygen tension.

fluoroacetyl adducts can be identified with fluorescent-tagged antibodies, mainly in zone 3 hepatocytes in the rat after phenobarbital pretreatment and also on the hepatocyte plasma membrane.[229] Antibodies to these neoantigens have been identified in sera from patients with halothane hepatitis.[230] Further studies have shown that neoantigens, analogous to these neoantigens derived from halothane-treated animals, are expressed in human liver in individuals exposed to halothane.[231] One of these neoantigens has been purified and identified as a microsomal carboxylesterase.[232] Kupffer cells may participate in the process by which the trifluoroacetyl adducts initiate an immune response.[233] Other studies in rats suggest that factors such as gender and previous exposure to specific inducers of cytochromes P-450 may influence the expression of halothane-associated neoantigens.[234] Thus, the oxidative pathway appears to be associated with hepatocellular membrane damage and immune phenomena typical of the clinical hepatotoxic syndrome.

In summary, severe halothane hepatotoxicity involves several factors whose interdependence can be partly defined. Formation of toxic metabolites depends on tissue oxygenation and possibly on which cytochromes P-450 are involved. Idiosyncratic susceptibility with inadequate detoxification of an electrophilic intermediate may play a role.[216] The extent of immune phenomena may further depend on the immunogenicity of adducts formed and the innate immune responsiveness of the host.[229] Halothane hepatotoxicity provides the best example currently available for demonstrating a link between drug metabolism and an immune reaction in hepatotoxicity.

PENICILLINS

Semisynthetic derivatives of penicillin may cause liver damage. Amoxicillin-clavulinic acid has also been associated with cholestasis[235] or a mixed hepatic-cholestatic reaction.[236,237] The cholestatic effect of flucloxacillin may be mediated by an intermediate produced by hepatocellular cytochromes P-450 that may be toxic to bile duct epithelial cells.[238] With prolonged cholestasis owing to semisynthetic penicillins, the development of small portal ("interlobular") bile duct paucity, known as ductopenia, has been observed in adults.[239] Although small bile duct paucity has been associated with amoxicillin alone,[240] the combination drug containing clavulinic acid appears to be

more toxic.[241] Hepatotoxicity has been reported in children with intravenous oxacillin.[242] Ductopenia has been reported with amoxicillin-clavulinic acid in one child, who eventually required liver transplant.[243]

MINOCYCLINE

The tetracycline derivative minocycline is often used to treat acne in adolescents. It appears to have a greater potential for causing liver damage than is generally appreciated. Several cases of hepatotoxicity in teenagers have been reported: symptoms of hepatitis, jaundice, elevated serum aminotransferases, and positive antinuclear antibodies were common.[244-248] One typical presentation was polyarthritis with biochemical hepatitis; jaundice was present when hepatitis was severe. Some cases had features of autoimmune hepatitis. In many patients, liver damage resolved when the drug was discontinued. Two cases of acute liver failure in adolescents have been reported[249,250]: one died before transplant and the other underwent liver transplant. Careful monitoring of liver function is indicated when minocycline is used chronically.

HERBALS

Complementary medicines are frequently used, usually without a physician's knowledge or review. Problems relating to the purity and strength of the specific preparation and to potential drug interactions complicate the issue of inherent risk for hepatotoxicity.[251] Children may be given herbal medications as tonics, and adolescents may choose to take them on their own. Herbal drugs known to be hepatotoxic include bush teas containing pyrrolizidine alkaloids, comfrey,[252] germander,[253,254] chaparral leaf,[255] kava-kava,[256,257] jin bu huan,[258-260] and ma huang (Ephedra). Comfrey also contains pyrrolizidine alkaloids, which can cause sinusoidal obstruction syndrome.[261] Germander undergoes biotransformation by CYP3A4, leading to diterpenoid toxic metabolites.[262,263] Some of these herbal medications are taken to promote weight loss, and the role of obesity in predisposing patients to hepatotoxicity deserves consideration.

"ECSTASY" (3,4-METHYLENEDIOXYMETHAMPHETAMINE)

This drug is frequently used by adolescents as a recreational drug. It can have severe multisystemic adverse effects, including cardiac arrhythmias, hyperthermia, and rhabdomyolysis. The severity of hepatotoxicity can be extremely variable, including mild to moderate elevations of serum aminotransferases with acute or chronic hepatitis, fibrosis, and, occasionally, a picture resembling autoimmune hepatitis.[264] Acute liver failure occurs, sometimes at the first use, and is either fatal or requires liver transplant.[265,266] This has become an important problem for young adults and, to a lesser extent, adolescents. The mechanism of hepatotoxicity remains unclear. Hepatic biotransformation pathways are complex and involve CYP2D6 as the high-affinity component for the major pathway and also CYP1A2, CYP3A4, and CYP2B6.[267] Whether slow metabolizers in the CYP2D6 polymorphism are at greater risk for Ecstasy-associated hepatotoxicity is disputed.[268,269] Production of Ecstasy is clandestine; thus, drug potency and purity are always uncertain, factors that may also contribute to hepatotoxicity.

PRINCIPLES OF TREATMENT

Most drug-induced liver disease resolves spontaneously when the hepatotoxic drug is withdrawn. Severe chronic changes should not be expected to regress. However, the histologic finding of bridging necrosis on liver biopsy does not tend to presage aggressive chronic liver damage in drug-induced liver disease. Certain hepatotoxins require timely treatment with specific antidotes, such as N-acetylcysteine for acetaminophen hepatotoxicity. Intravenous steroid treatment has been beneficial when severe acute hepatitis dominates a multisystemic hypersensitivity reaction, as with phenytoin, carbamazepine, or phenobarbital. In general, the use of steroids in drug-induced liver disease remains controversial. The treatment of fulminant hepatic failure owing to drug hepatotoxicity is otherwise essentially the same as in viral hepatitis. Liver transplant may be lifesaving in these circumstances.

When the major intervention is to stop a drug treatment, arriving at the diagnosis of drug-induced liver disease becomes all important. A high index of clinical suspicion is critical to making the diagnosis. A meticulous history of the illness with detailed attention to all drugs taken, including over-the-counter preparations, and to the potential for exposure to environmental or industrial toxins is of utmost importance. In children, it is important to ensure that the appropriate dosage was actually given. Liver biopsy, with electron microscopic examination if possible, is often very informative and sometimes definitive. Algorithms for determining the likelihood of an adverse drug reaction,[270] especially those specifically developed for drug hepatotoxicity,[271–273] may be helpful diagnostically. A recent study[274] showed that the Council for International Organizations of Medical Sciences scoring system[271] is superior to that of Maria and Victorino[273]; however, neither is specifically geared for children. In vitro rechallenge of the patient's lymphocytes with generated toxic metabolites usually provides important corroborative evidence,[275] but this remains a research investigation. Rechallenge assays using immunologic end points are often difficult to interpret.

SUMMARY

Drug-induced hepatotoxicity is more common in children than is generally thought. As in adults, the spectrum of disease is wide. Although cytotoxic processes, presenting as hepatitis, predominate, virtually every major type of hepatic pathology can occur. Hepatic drug metabolism has an important role in most of the drugs that most frequently cause hepatotoxicity in children: an imbalance between generation of toxic metabolite and detoxification processes can be identified. Focal defects in detoxification, often responsible for this imbalance, may be inherited. Developmental changes in drug disposition and metabolism further complicate the clinical spectrum of drug hepatotoxicity in children. Developmental and genetically determined aspects of immune function may also play a role. The possibility of drug hepatotoxicity should be considered in every instance of childhood liver disease.

REFERENCES

1. Zimmerman HJ. Hepatotoxicity: the adverse effects of drugs and other chemicals on the liver. 1st ed. New York: Appleton-Century-Crofts; 1978.
2. Farrell GC. Drug induced liver disease. New York: Churchill Livingstone; 1994.
3. Kaplowitz N, DeLeve L. Drug hepatotoxicity. New York: Marcel Dekker; 2002.
4. Okey AB, Roberts EA, Harper PA, Denison MS. Induction of drug-metabolizing enzymes: mechanisms and consequences. Clin Biochem 1986;19:132–41.
5. Sueyoshi T, Negishi M. Phenobarbital response elements of cytochrome P450 genes and nuclear receptors. Annu Rev Pharmacol Toxicol 2001;41:123–43.
6. Gonzalez FJ, Meyer UA. Molecular genetics of the debrisoquin-sparteine polymorphism. Clin Pharmacol Ther 1991;50:233–8.
7. Lennard MS. Genetic polymorphism of sparteine/debrisoquine oxidation: a reappraisal. Pharmacol Toxicol 1990;67:273–83.
8. Spielberg SP, Gordon GB. Glutathione synthetase-deficient lymphocytes and acetaminophen toxicity. Clin Pharmacol Ther 1981;29:51–5.
9. Aranda JV, Cook CE, Gorman A, et al. Pharmacokinetic profile of caffeine in the premature newborn with apnea. J Pediatr 1979;94:663–8.
10. Aranda JV, Collinge JM, Zinman R, Watters G. Maturation of caffeine elimination in infancy. Arch Dis Child 1979;54:946–9.
11. Lambert GH, Schoeller DA, Kotake AN, et al. The effect of age, gender, and sexual maturation on the caffeine breath test. Dev Pharmacol Ther 1986;9:375–88.
12. Bohan A, Boyer JL. Mechanisms of hepatic transport of drugs: implications for cholestatic drug reactions. Semin Liver Dis 2002;22:123–36.
13. Benichou C. Criteria of drug induced liver disorders: report of an international consensus meeting. J Hepatol 1990;11:272–6.
14. Jaeschke H, Gores GJ, Cederbaum AI, et al. Mechanisms of hepatotoxicity. Toxicol Sci 2002;65:166–76.
15. De Berardinis V, Moulis C, Maurice M, et al. Human microsomal epoxide hydrolase is the target of germander-induced autoantibodies on the surface of human hepatocytes. Mol Pharmacol 2000;58:542–51.
16. James LP, Farrar HC, Darville TL, et al. Elevation of serum interleukin 8 levels in acetaminophen overdose in children and adolescents. Clin Pharmacol Ther 2001;70:280–6.
17. Ju C, Reilly TP, Bourdi M, et al. Protective role of Kupffer cells in acetaminophen-induced hepatic injury in mice. Chem Res Toxicol 2002;15:1504–13.
18. Mitchell AA, Lacouture PG, Sheehan JE, et al. Adverse drug reactions in children leading to hospital admission. Pediatrics 1988;82:24–9.
19. Woods CG, Rylance ME, Cullen RE, Rylance GW. Adverse reactions to drugs in children. BMJ 1987;294:689–90.
20. Clarkson A, Choonara I. Surveillance for fatal suspected adverse drug reactions in the UK. Arch Dis Child 2002;87:462–7.
21. Mitchell JR, Jollow DJ, Potter WZ, et al. Acetaminophen-induced hepatic necrosis. I. Role of drug metabolism. J Pharmacol Exp Ther 1973;187:185–94.
22. Jollow DJ, Mitchell JR, Potter WZ, et al. Acetaminophen-induced hepatic necrosis. II. Role of covalent binding in vivo. J Pharmacol Exp Ther 1973;187:195–202.

23. Potter WZ, Davis DC, Mitchell JR, et al. Acetaminophen-induced hepatic necrosis. III. Cytochrome P-450-mediated covalent binding in vitro. J Pharmacol Exp Ther 1973;187:203–10.

24. Mitchell JR, Jollow DJ, Potter WZ, et al. Acetaminophen-induced hepatic necrosis. IV. Protective role of glutathione. J Pharmacol Exp Ther 1973;187:211–7.

25. Dahlin DC, Miwa GT, Lu AYH, Nelson SD. N-Acetyl-p-benzoquinone imine: a cytochrome P450-mediated oxidation product of acetaminophen. Proc Natl Acad Sci U S A 1984; 81:1327–31.

26. Corcoran CB, Todd EL, Racz WJ, et al. Effects of N-acetylcysteine on the disposition and metabolism of acetaminophen in mice. J Pharmacol Exp Ther 1985;232:857–63.

27. Knight TR, Kurtz A, Bajt ML, et al. Vascular and hepatocellular peroxynitrite formation during acetaminophen toxicity: role of mitochondrial oxidant stress. Toxicol Sci 2001;62:212–20.

28. Knight TR, Ho YS, Farhood A, Jaeschke H. Peroxynitrite is a critical mediator of acetaminophen hepatotoxicity in murine livers: protection by glutathione. J Pharmacol Exp Ther 2002;303:468–75.

29. Bourdi M, Masubuchi Y, Reilly TP, et al. Protection against acetaminophen-induced liver injury and lethality by interleukin 10: role of inducible nitric oxide synthase. Hepatology 2002;35:289–98.

30. Makin AJ, Wendon J, Williams R. A 7-year experience of severe acetaminophen-induced hepatotoxicity (1987-1993). Gastroenterology 1995;109:1907–16.

31. Rumack BH, Matthew H. Acetaminophen poisoning and toxicity. Pediatrics 1975;55:871–6.

32. Schmidt LE, Dalhoff K, Poulsen HE. Acute versus chronic alcohol consumption in acetaminophen-induced hepatotoxicity. Hepatology 2002;35:876–82.

33. Harrison PM, Keays R, Bray GP, et al. Improved outcome of paracetamol-induced fulminant hepatic failure by late administration of acetylcysteine. Lancet 1990;335:1572–73.

34. Keays R, Harrison PM, Wendon JA, et al. Intravenous acetylcysteine in paracetamol induced fulminant hepatic failure: a prospective controlled trial. BMJ 1991;303:1026–9.

35. Smilkstein MJ, Knapp GL, Kulig KW, Rumack BH. Efficacy of oral N-acetylcysteine in the treatment of acetaminophen overdose. N Engl J Med 1988;319:1557–62.

36. James LP, Wells E, Beard RH, Farrar HC. Predictors of outcome after acetaminophen poisoning in children and adolescents. J Pediatr 2002;140:522–6.

37. Tenenbein PK, Sitar DS, Tenenbein M. Interaction between N-acetylcysteine and activated charcoal: implications for the treatment of acetaminophen poisoning. Pharmacotherapy 2001;21:1331–6.

38. Rumack BH. Acetaminophen overdose in young children. Treatment and effects of alcohol and other additional ingestants in 417 cases. Am J Dis Child 1984;138:428–33.

39. Meredith TJ, Newman B, Goulding R. Paracetamol poisoning in children. BMJ 1978;2:478–9.

40. Peterson RG, Rumack BH. Pharmacokinetics of acetaminophen in children. Pediatrics 1978;62:877–9.

41. Miller RP, Roberts RJ, Fischer LF. Acetaminophen elimination kinetics in neonates, children and adults. Clin Pharmacol Ther 1976;19:284–94.

42. Lederman S, Fysh WJ, Tredger M, Gamsu HR. Neonatal paracetamol poisoning: treatment by exchange transfusion. Arch Dis Child 1983;58:631–3.

43. Roberts I, Robinson MJ, Mughal MZ, et al. Paracetamol metabolites in the neonate following maternal overdose. Br J Clin Pharmacol 1984;18:201–6.

44. Rollins DE, Von Bahr C, Glaumann H, et al. Acetaminophen: potentially toxic metabolites formed by human fetal and adult liver microsomes and isolated fetal liver cells. Science 1979;205:1414–6.

45. Green MD, Shires TK, Fischer LJ. Hepatotoxicity of acetaminophen in neonatal and young rats. I. Age-related changes in susceptibility. Toxicol Appl Pharmacol 1984;74:116–24.

46. Lauterburg BH, Vaishnav Y, Stillwell WG, Mitchell JR. The effect of age and glutathione depletion on hepatic glutathione turnover in vivo determined by acetaminophen probe analysis. J Pharmacol Exp Ther 1980;213:54–8.

47. Ward RM, Bates BA, Benitz WE, et al. American Academy of Pediatrics Committee on Drugs statement: acetaminophen toxicity in children. Pediatrics 2001;108:1020–24.

48. Alonso EM, Sokol RJ, Hart J, et al. Fulminant hepatitis associated with centrilobular hepatic necrosis in young children. J Pediatr 1995;127:888–94.

49. Rivera-Penera T, Gugig R, Davis J, et al. Outcome of acetaminophen overdose in pediatric patients and factors contributing to hepatotoxicity. J Pediatr 1997;130:300–4.

50. Heubi JE, Barbacci MB, Zimmerman HJ. Therapeutic misadventures with acetaminophen: hepatoxicity after multiple doses in children. J Pediatr 1998;132:22–7.

51. Anderson BD, Shepherd JG, Klein-Schwartz W. Outcome of acetaminophen overdose. J Pediatr 1998;132:1080.

52. Pershad J, Nichols M, King W. "The silent killer": chronic acetaminophen toxicity in a toddler. Pediatr Emerg Care 1999; 15:43–6.

53. Kearns GL, Leeder JS, Wasserman GS. Acetaminophen overdose with therapeutic intent. J Pediatr 1998;132:5–8.

54. Muldrew KL, James LP, Coop L, et al. Determination of acetaminophen-protein adducts in mouse liver and serum and human serum after hepatotoxic doses of acetaminophen using high-performance liquid chromatography with electrochemical detection. Drug Metab Dispos 2002;30:446–51.

55. Bruun LS, Elkjaer S, Bitsch-Larsen D, Andersen O. Hepatic failure in a child after acetaminophen and sevoflurane exposure. Anesth Analg 2001;92:1446–8.

56. Seeff LB, Cuccherini BA, Zimmerman HJ, et al. Acetaminophen hepatotoxicity in alcoholics. A therapeutic misadventure. Ann Intern Med 1986;104:399–404.

57. Zwiener RJ, Kurt TL, Day LC, et al. Potentiation of acetaminophen hepatotoxicity in a child with mercury poisoning. J Pediatr Gastroenterol Nutr 1994;19:242–5.

58. Powers NG, Carson SH. Idiosyncratic reactions to phenytoin. Clin Pediatr 1987;26:120–4.

59. Bessmertny O, Hatton RC, Gonzalez-Peralta RP. Antiepileptic hypersensitivity syndrome in children. Ann Pharmacother 2001;35:533–8.

60. Shear NH, Spielberg SP. Anticonvulsant hypersensitivity syndrome. In vitro assessment of risk. J Clin Invest 1988;82: 1826–32.

61. Mullick FG, Ishak KG. Hepatic injury associated with diphenylhydantoin therapy. Am J Clin Pathol 1980;74:442–52.

62. Scheuerman O, Nofech-Moses Y, Rachmel A, Ashkenazi S. Successful treatment of antiepileptic drug hypersensitivity syndrome with intravenous immune globulin. Pediatrics 2001; 107:e14–5.

63. Spielberg SP, Gordon GB, Blake DA, et al. Predisposition to phenytoin hepatotoxicity assessed in vitro. N Engl J Med 1981;305:722–7.

64. Spielberg SP, Gordon GB, Blake DA, et al. Anticonvulsant toxicity in vitro: possible role of arene oxides. J Pharmacol Exp Ther 1981;217:386–9.

65. Kahn HD, Faguet GB, Agee JF, Middleton HM. Drug-induced liver injury. In vitro demonstration of hypersensitivity to both phenytoin and phenobarbital. Arch Intern Med 1984;144:1677–9.

66. Gaedigk A, Spielberg S, Grant D. Characterization of the microsomal epoxide hydrolase gene in patients with anticonvulsant adverse drug reactions. Pharmacogenetics 1994;4:142–53.

67. Panman T, Chen G, Wells P. Free radical intermediates of phenytoin and related teratogens. Prostaglandin H synthase-catalyzed bioactivation, electron paramagnetic resonance spectrometry and photochemical product analysis. J Biol Chem 1998;273:25079–88.

68. Munns A, De Voss J, Hooper W, et al. Bioactivation of phenytoin by human cytochrome P450: characterization of the mechanism and targets of covalent adduct formation. Chem Res Toxicol 1997;10:1049–58.

69. Mitchell MC, Boitnott JK, Arregui A, Maddrey WC. Granulomatous hepatitis associated with carbamazepine therapy. Am J Med 1981;71:733–5.

70. Williams SJ, Ruppin DC, Grierson JM, Farrell GC. Carbamazepine hepatitis: the clinicopathological spectrum. J Gastroenterol Hepatol 1986;1:159–68.

71. Zucker P, Daum F, Cohen MI. Fatal carbamazepine hepatitis. J Pediatr 1977;91:667–8.

72. Smith DW, Cullity GJ, Silberstein EP. Fatal hepatic necrosis associated with multiple anticonvulsant therapy. Aust N Z J Med 1988;18:575–81.

73. Hadzic N, Portmann B, Davies ET, et al. Acute liver failure induced by carbamazepine. Arch Dis Child 1990;65:315–7.

74. Morales-Diaz M, Pinilla-Roa E, Ruiz I. Suspected carbamazepine-induced hepatotoxicity. Pharmacotherapy 1999;19:252–5.

75. Lewis IJ, Rosenbloom L. Glandular fever-like syndrome, pulmonary eosinophilia and asthma associated with carbamazepine. Postgrad Med J 1982;58:100–1.

76. Brain C, MacArdle B, Levin S. Idiosyncratic reactions to carbamazepine mimicking viral infection in children. BMJ 1984;289:354.

77. Green V, Pirrnohamed M, Kitteningham N, et al. Genetic analysis of microsomal epoxide hydrolase in patients with carbamazepine hypersensitivity. Biochem Pharmacol 1995;50:1353–9.

78. Ju C, Uetrecht J. Detection of 2-hydroxyiminostilbene in the urine of patients taking carbamazepine and its oxidation to a reactive iminequinone intermediate. J Pharmacol Exp Ther 1999;288:51–6.

79. Roberts EA, Spielberg SP, Goldbach M, Phillips MJ. Phenobarbital hepatotoxicity in an 8-month-old infant. J Hepatol 1990;10:235–9.

80. Schlienger R, Knowles S, Shear N. Lamotrogine-associated anticonvulsant hypersensitivty syndrome. Neurology 1998;51:1172–5.

81. Brown TS, Appel JE, Kasteler JS, Callen JP. Hypersensitivity reaction in a child due to lamotrigine. Pediatr Dermatol 1999;16:46–9.

82. Fayad M, Choueiri R, Mikati M. Potential hepatotoxicity of lamotrigine. Pediatr Neurol 2000;22:49–52.

83. Maggs JL, Naisbitt DJ, Tettey JN, et al. Metabolism of lamotrigine to a reactive arene oxide intermediate. Chem Res Toxicol 2000;13:1075–81.

84. Powell-Jackson PR, Tredger JM, Williams R. Hepatotoxicity to sodium valproate: a review. Gut 1984;25:673–81.

85. Green SH. Sodium valproate and routine liver function tests. Arch Dis Child 1984;59:813–4.

86. Zafrani ES, Berthelot P. Sodium valproate in the induction of unusual hepatotoxicity. Hepatology 1982;2:648–9.

87. Koenig SA, Siemes H, Blaker F, et al. Severe hepatotoxicity during valproate therapy: an update and report of eight new fatalities. Epilepsia 1994;35:1005–15.

88. Bryant AE III, Dreifuss FE. Valproic acid hepatic fatalities. III. U.S. experience since 1986. Neurology 1996;46:465–9.

89. Coulter DR, Allen RJ. Hyperammonemia with valproic acid therapy. J Pediatr 1981;99:317–9.

90. Kondo T, Ishida M, Kaneko S, et al. Is 2-propyl-4-pentenoic acid, a hepatotoxic metabolite of valproate, responsible for valproate-induced hyperammonemia? Epilepsia 1992;33:550–4.

91. Suchy FJ, Balistreri WF, Buchino J, et al. Acute hepatic failure associated with the use of sodium valproate. Report of two fatal cases. N Engl J Med 1979;300:962–6.

92. Gerber N, Dickinson RG, Harland RC, et al. Reye-like syndrome associated with valproic acid therapy. J Pediatr 1979;95:142–4.

93. Zimmerman HJ, Ishak KG. Valproate-induced hepatic injury: analysis of 23 fatal cases. Hepatology 1982;2:591–7.

94. Scheffner D, Konig ST, Rauterberg-Ruland I, et al. Fatal liver failure in 16 children with valproate therapy. Epilepsia 1988;29:530–42.

95. Schnabel R, Rambeck B, Janssen F. Fatal intoxication with sodium valproate. Lancet 1984;i:221–2.

96. Rettenmeier AW, Gordon WP, Prickett KS, et al. Metabolic fate of valproic acid in the rhesus monkey. Formation of a toxic metabolite, 2-n-propyl-4-pentenoic acid. Drug Metab Dispos 1986;14:443–53.

97. Kochen W, Schneider A, Ritz A. Abnormal metabolism of valproic acid in fatal hepatic failure. Eur J Pediatr 1983;14:30–5.

98. Kesterson JW, Granneman GR, Machinist JM. The hepatotoxicity of valproate in rats. I. Toxicologic, biochemical and histopathologic studies. Hepatology 1984;4:1143–52.

99. Granneman GR, Wang SI, Kesterson JW, Machinist JM. The hepatotoxicity of valproic acid and its metabolites in rats. II. Intermediary and valproic acid metabolism. Hepatology 1984;4:1153–8.

100. Bjorge SM, Baillie TA. Inhibition of medium-chain fatty acid beta-oxidation in vitro by valproic acid and its unsaturated metabolite, 2-n-propyl-4-pentenoic acid. Biochem Biophys Res Commun 1985;132:245–52.

101. Gopaul S, Farrell K, Abbott F. Effects of age and polytherapy, risk factors of valproic acid (VPA) hepatotoxicity, on the excretion of thiol conjugates of (E)-2,4-diene VPA in people with epilepsy taking VPA. Epilepsia 2003;44:322–8.

102. Böhles H, Richter K, Wagner-Thiessen E, Shaefer H. Decreased serum carnitine in valproate induced Reye syndrome. Eur J Pediatr 1982;139:185–6.

103. Eadie MJ, McKinnon GE, Dunstan PR, et al. Valproate metabolism during hepatotoxicity associated with the drug. QJM 1990;77:1229–40.

104. Keulen FP, Kochen W. Hepatotoxität unter Valproinsaure Behandlung. Klin Pädiatr 1985;197:431–6.

105. Dickinson RG, Bassett ML, Searle J, et al. Valproate hepatotoxicity: a review and report of two instances in adults. Clin Exp Neurol 1985;21:79–91.

106. Kossak BD, Schmidt-Sommerfeld E, Schoeller DA, et al. Impaired fatty acid oxidation in children on valproic acid and the effect of L-carnitine. Neurology 1993;43:2362–8.

107. Fisher R, Nau H, Gandolfi AJ, et al. Valproic acid hepatotoxicity in human liver slices. Drug Chem Toxicol 1991;14:375–94.

108. Qureshi IA, Letarte J, Tuchweber B, et al. Heptotoxicology of sodium valproate in ornithine transcarbamylase-deficient mice. Toxicol Lett 1985;25:297–306.

109. Hjelm M, De Silva LVK, Seakins IWT, et al. Evidence of inherited urea cycle defect in a case of fatal valproate toxicity. BMJ 1986;292:23–4.

110. Kay JDS, Hilton-Jones D, Hyman N. Valproate toxicity and ornithine carbamoyltransferase deficiency. Lancet 1986;ii: 1283–4.

111. Chabrol B, Mancini J, Chretien D, et al. Valproate-induced hepatic failure in a case of cytochrome c oxidase deficiency. Eur J Pediatr 1994;153:133–5.

112. Murphy JV, Maquardt KM, Shug AL. Valproic acid associated abnormalities of carnitine metabolism. Lancet 1985;i:820–1.

113. Matsuda I, Ohtani Y, Ninoniya N. Renal handling of carnitine in children with carnitine deficiency and hyperammonemia associated with valproate therapy. J Pediatr 1986;109:131–4.

114. Beghi E, Bizzi A, Codegoni AM, et al. Valproate, carnitine metabolism, and biochemical indicators of liver function. Epilepsia 1990;31:346–52.

115. Millington DS, Bohan TP, Roe CR, et al. Valproylcarnitine: a novel drug metabolite identified by fast atom bombardment and thermospray liquid chromatography-mass spectroscopy. Clin Chim Acta 1985;145:69–76.

116. Laub MC, Paetzke-Brunner I, Jaeger G. Serum carnitine during valproic acid therapy. Epilepsia 1986;27:559–62.

117. Bohan TP, Helton E, McDonald I, et al. Effect of L-carnitine treatment for valproate-induced hepatotoxicity. Neurology 2001;56:1405–9.

118. Poland GA, Love KR. Marked atypical lymphocytosis, hepatitis and skin rash in sulfasalazine drug allergy. Am J Med 1986;81:707–8.

119. Shear NH, Spielberg SP, Grant DM, et al. Differences in metabolism of sulfonamides predisposing to idiosyncratic toxicity. Ann Intern Med 1986;105:179–84.

120. Sotolongo RP, Neefe LI, Rudzki C, Ishak KG. Hypersensitivity reaction to sulfasalazine with severe hepatotoxicity. Gastroenterology 1978;75:95–9.

121. Losek JH, Werlin SL. Sulfasalazine hepatotoxicity. Am J Dis Child 1981;135:1070–2.

122. Ribe J, Benkov KJ, Thung SN, et al. Fatal massive hepatic necrosis: a probable hypersensitivity reaction to sulfasalazine. Am J Gastroenterol 1986;81:205–8.

123. Gremse DA, Bancroft J, Moyer SA. Sulfasalazine hypersensitivity with hepatotoxicity, thrombocytopenia, and erythroid hypoplasia. J Pediatr Gastroenterol Nutr 1989;9:261–3.

124. Rieder MJ, Uetrecht J, Shear NH, et al. Diagnosis of sulfonamide hypersensitivity reactions by in-vitro "rechallenge" with hydroxylamine metabolites. Ann Intern Med 1989;110:286–9.

125. Cribb AE, Spielberg SP. Hepatic microsomal metabolism of sulfamethoxazole to the hydroxylamine. Drug Metab Dispos 1990;18:784–7.

126. Cribb AE, Spielberg SP. Sulfamethoxazole is metabolized to the hydroxylamine in humans. Clin Pharmacol Ther 1992;51: 522–6.

127. Shear NH, Spielberg SP. In vitro evaluation of a toxic metabolite of sulfadiazine. Can J Physiol Pharmacol 1985;63:1370–2.

128. Rieder MJ, Uetrecht J, Shear NH, Spielberg SP. Synthesis and in vitro toxicity of hydroxylamine metabolites of sulfonamides. J Pharmacol Exp Ther 1988;244:724–8.

129. Zafrani ES, Ishak KG, Rudzki C. Cholestatic and hepatocellular injury associated with erythromycin esters. Report of nine cases. Dig Dis Sci 1979;24:385–96.

130. Phillips KG. Hepatotoxicity of erythromycin ethylsuccinate in a child. Can Med Assoc J 1983;129:411–2.

131. Diehl AM, Latham P, Boitnott JK, et al. Cholestatic hepatitis from erythromycin ethylsuccinate. Am J Med 1984;76:931–4.

132. Principi N, Esposito S. Comparative tolerability of erythromycin and newer macrolide antibacterials in paediatric patients. Drug Saf 1999;20:25–41.

133. Gaeta GB, Utili R, Adinolfi LE, et al. Characterization of the effects of erythromycin estolate and erythromycin base on the excretory function of the isolated rat liver. Toxicol Appl Pharmacol 1985;80:185–92.

134. Villa P, Begue JM, Guillouzo A. Erythromycin toxicity in primary cultures of rat hepatocytes. Xenobiotica 1985;15:767–73.

135. Sorensen EMB, Acosta A. Erythromycin toxicity in primary cultures of rat hepatocytes. Toxicol Lett 1985;27:73–82.

136. Garty BZ, Kauli R, Ben-Ari J, et al. Hepatitis associated with propylthiouracil treatment. Drug Intell Clin Pharm 1985;19:740–2.

137. Jonas MM, Edison MS. Propylthiouracil hepatotoxicity: two pediatric cases and review of the literature. J Pediatr Gastroenterol Nutr 1988;7:776–9.

138. Kirkland JL. Propylthiouracil-induced hepatic failure and encephalopathy in a child. Ann Pharmacother 1990;24:470–1.

139. Levy M. Propylthiouracil hepatotoxicity. A review and case presentation. Clin Pediatr 1993;32:25–9.

140. Williams KV, Nayak S, Becker D, et al. Fifty years of experience with propylthiouracil-associated hepatotoxicity: what have we learned? J Clin Endocrinol Metab 1997;82:1721–33.

141. Maggiore G, Larizza D, Lorini R, et al. PTU hepatotoxicity mimicking autoimmune chronic active hepatitis in a girl. J Pediatr Gastroenterol Nutr 1989;8:547–8.

142. Benson GD. Hepatotoxicity following the therapeutic use of antipyretic analgesics. Am J Med 1983;75:85–93.

143. Parke DV. Activation mechanisms to chemical toxicity. Arch Toxicol 1987;60:5–15.

144. Seaman WE, Ishak KG, Plotz PH. Aspirin-induced hepatotoxicity in patients with systemic lupus erythematosus. Ann Intern Med 1974;80:1–8.

145. Zucker P, Daum F, Cohen MI. Aspirin hepatitis. Am J Dis Child 1975;129:1433–4.

146. Doughty R, Giesecke L, Athreya B. Salicylate therapy in juvenile rheumatoid arthritis. Am J Dis Child 1980;134:461–3.

147. Barron KS, Person DA, Brewer EJ. The toxicity of non-steroidal anti-inflammatory drugs in juvenile rheumatoid arthritis. J Rheumatol 1982;9:149–55.

148. Hamdan JA, Manasra K, Ahmed M. Salicylate-induced hepatitis in rheumatic fever. Am J Dis Child 1985;139:453–5.

149. Ulshen MH, Grand RJ, Crain JD, Gelfand EW. Hepatotoxicity with encephalopathy associated with aspirin therapy in rheumatoid arthritis. J Pediatr 1978;93:1034–7.

150. Petty BG, Zahka KG, Bernstein MT. Aspirin hepatitis associated with encephalopathy. J Pediatr 1978;93:881–2.

151. Hadchouel M, Prieur AM, Griscelli C. Acute hemorrhagic, hepatic, and neurologic manifestations in juvenile rheumatoid arthritis: possible relationship to drugs or infection. J Pediatr 1985;106:561–6.

152. Hanson JR, McCray PB, Bole JF Jr, et al. Reye syndrome associated with aspirin therapy for systemic lupus erythematosus. Pediatrics 1985;76:202–5.

153. Van de Kerkhof PCM, Hoegnagels WHL, Van Haelst UJGM, Mali JWH. Methotrexate maintenance therapy and liver damage in psoriasis. Clin Exp Dermatol 1985;10:194–200.

154. Kremer JM, Lee RG, Tolman KG. Liver histology in rheumatoid arthritis patients receiving long-term methotrexate therapy. A prospective study with baseline and sequential biopsy samples. Arthritis Rheum 1989;32:121–7.

155. Gilbert SC, Klintmalm G, Mentor A, Silverman A. Methotrexate-induced cirrhosis requiring liver transplantation in three patients with psoriasis: a word of caution in light of the expanding use of this 'steroid sparing' agent. Arch Intern Med 1990;150:889–91.

156. Kremer JM, Alarcón GS, Lightfoot RWJ, et al. Methotrexate for rheumatoid arthritis. Suggested guidelines for monitoring liver toxicity. Arthritis Rheum 1994;37:316–28.

157. Whiting-O'Keefe QE, Fye KH, Sack KD. Methotrexate and histologic hepatic abnormalities: a meta-analysis. Am J Med 1991;90:711–6.

158. Hashkes PJ, Balistreri WF, Bove KE, et al. The long-term effect of methotrexate therapy on the liver in patients with juvenile rheumatoid arthritis. Arthritis Rheum 1997;40:2226–34.

159. Hashkes PJ, Balistreri WF, Bove KE, et al. The relationship of hepatotoxic risk factors and liver histology in methotrexate therapy for juvenile rheumatoid arthritis. J Pediatr 1999;134: 47–52.

160. Graham LD, Myones BL, Rivas-Chacon RF, Pachman LM. Morbidity associated with long-term methotrexate therapy in juvenile rheumatoid arthritis. J Pediatr 1992;120:468–73.

161. Kugathasam S, Newman AJ, Dahms BB, Boyle JT. Liver biopsy findings in patients with juvenile rheumatoid arthritis receiving long-term, weekly methotrexate therapy. J Pediatr 1996;128:149–51.

162. Keim D, Ragsdale C, Heidelberger K, Sullivan D. Hepatic fibrosis with the use of methotrexate for juvenile rheumatoid arthritis. J Rheumatol 1990;17:846–8.

163. Jolivet J, Cowan KH, Curt GA, et al. The pharmacology and clinical use of methotrexate. N Engl J Med 1983;309:1094–104.

164. Banerjee AK, Lakhani S, Vincent M, Selby P. Dose-dependent acute hepatitis associated with administration of high dose methotrexate. Hum Toxicol 1988;7:561–2.

165. Harb JM, Werlin SL, Camitta BM, et al. Hepatic ultrastructure in leukemic children treated with methotrexate and 6-mercaptopurine. Am J Pediatr Hematol Oncol 1983;5: 323–31.

166. Topley J, Benson J, Squier MV, Chessells JM. Hepatotoxicity in the treatment of acute lymphoblastic leukemia. Med Pediatr Oncol 1979;7:393–9.

167. McIntosh S, Davidson DL, O'Brien RT, Pearson HA. Methotrexate hepatotoxicity in children with leukemia. J Pediatr 1977; 90:1019–21.

168. Perry MC. Hepatotoxicity of chemotherapeutic agents. Semin Oncol 1982;9:65–74.

169. Sznol M, Ohnuma T, Holland JF. Hepatic toxicity of drugs used for hematologic neoplasia. Semin Liver Dis 1987;7:237–56.

170. Pratt CB, Johnson WW. Duration and severity of fatty metamorphosis of the liver following L-asparaginase therapy. Cancer 1971;28:361–4.

171. Hruban RH, Sternberg SS, Meyers P, et al. Fatal thrombocytopenia and liver failure associated with carboplatin therapy. Cancer Invest 1991;9:263–8.

172. Rollins BJ. Hepatic veno-occlusive disease. Am J Med 1986; 81:297–306.

173. Fajardo LF, Colby TV. Pathogenesis of veno-occlusive disease after radiation. Arch Pathol Lab Med 1980;104:584–8.

174. McDonald GB, Sharma P, Matthews DE, et al. The clinical course of 53 patients with veno-occlusive disease of the liver after marrow transplantation. Transplantation 1985;39:603–8.

175. DeLeve LD. Dacarbazine toxicity in murine liver cells: a model of hepatic endothelial injury and glutathione defense. J Pharmacol Exp Ther 1994;268:1261–70.

176. DeLeve LD. Cellular target of cyclophosphamide toxicity in the murine liver: role of glutathione and site of metabolic activation. Hepatology 1996;24:830–7.

177. Ringden O, Remberger M, Lehmann S, et al. N-Acetylcysteine for hepatic veno-occlusive disease after allogeneic stem cell transplantation. Bone Marrow Transplant 2000;25:993–6.

178. Shulman HM, Fisher LB, Schoch HG, et al. Veno-occlusive disease of the liver after marrow transplantation: histological correlates of clinical signs and symptoms. Hepatology 1994; 19:1171–81.

179. Kassianides C, Nussenblatt R, Palestine AG, et al. Liver injury from cyclosporine A. Dig Dis Sci 1990;35:693–7.

180. Stone BG, Udani M, Sanghvi A, et al. Cyclosporin A-induced cholestasis. The mechanism in a rat model. Gastroenterology 1987;93:344–51.

181. Stieger B, Fattinger K, Madon J, et al. Drug- and estrogen-induced cholestasis through inhibition of the hepatocellular bile salt export pump (BSEP) of rat liver. Gastroenterology 2000;118:422–30.

182. Bramow S, Ott P, Thomsen Nielsen F, et al. Cholestasis and regulation of genes related to drug metabolism and biliary transport in rat liver following treatment with cyclosporine A and sirolimus (Rapamycin). Pharmacol Toxicol 2001;89:133–9.

183. Yasumiba S, Tazuma S, Ochi H, et al. Cyclosporin A reduces canalicular membrane fluidity and regulates transporter function in rats. Biochem J 2001;354:591–6.

184. Weinstein S, Lipsitz EC, Addonizio L, Stolar CJ. Cholelithiasis in pediatric cardiac transplant patients on cyclosporine. J Pediatr Surg 1995;30:61–4.

185. Pratt DS, Dubois RS. Hepatotoxicity due to pemoline (Cylert). A report of two cases. J Pediatr Gastroenterol Nutr 1990; 10:239–41.

186. Elitsur Y. Pemoline (Cylert)-induced hepatotoxicity. J Pediatr Gastroenterol Nutr 1990;11:143–4.

187. Adcock KG, MacElroy DE, Wolford ET, Farrington EA. Pemoline therapy resulting in liver transplantation. Ann Pharmacother 1998;32:422–5.

188. Marotta PJ, Roberts EA. Pemoline hepatotoxicity in children. J Pediatr 1998;132:894–7.

189. Rosh JR, Dellert SF, Narkewicz M, et al. Four cases of severe hepatotoxicity associated with pemoline: possible autoimmune pathogenesis. Pediatrics 1998;101:921–3.

190. Safer DJ, Zito JM, Gardner JE. Pemoline hepatotoxicity and postmarketing surveillance. J Am Acad Child Adolesc Psychiatry 2001;40:622–9.

191. Nehra A, Mullick F, Ishak KG, Zimmerman HJ. Pemoline-associated hepatic injury. Gastroenterology 1990;99:1517–9.

192. Jaffe SL. Pemoline and liver function. J Am Acad Child Adolesc Psychiatry 1989;28:457–8.

193. Krebs S, Dormann H, Muth-Selbach U, et al. Risperidone-induced cholestatic hepatitis. Eur J Gastroenterol Hepatol 2001;13:67–9.

194. Fuller MA, Simon MR, Freedman L. Risperidone-associated hepatotoxicity. J Clin Psychopharmacol 1996;16:84–5.

195. Kumra S, Herion D, Jacobsen LK, et al. Case study: risperidone-induced hepatotoxicity in pediatric patients. J Am Acad Child Adolesc Psychiatry 1997;36:701–5.

196. Szigethy E, Wiznitzer M, Branicky LA, et al. Risperidone-induced hepatotoxicity in children and adolescents? A chart review study. J Child Adolesc Psychopharmacol 1999;9:93–8.

197. Maddrey WC, Boitnott JK. Isoniazid hepatitis. Ann Intern Med 1973;79:1–12.

198. Mitchell J, Zimmerman H, Ishak K, et al. Isoniazid liver injury: clinical spectrum, pathology and probable pathogenesis. Ann Intern Med 1976;84:181–96.

199. Rudoy R, Stuemky J, Poley R. Isoniazid administration and liver injury. Am J Dis Child 1973;125:733–6.

200. Casteels-Van Daele M, Igodt-Ameye L, Corbell L, Eeckels R. Hepatotoxicity of rifampicin and isoniazid in children. J Pediatr 1975;86:739–41.

201. Vanderhoof JA, Ament ME. Fatal hepatic necrosis due to isoniazid chemoprophylaxis in a 15-year-old girl. J Pediatr 1976; 88:867–8.

202. Litt IF, Cohen MI, McNamara H. Isoniazid hepatitis in adolescents. J Pediatr 1976;89:133–5.

203. Walker A, Park-Hah J. Possible isoniazid-induced hepatotoxicity in a two-year-old child. J Pediatr 1977;91:344–5.

204. Pessayre D, Bentata M, Degott C, et al. Isoniazid-rifampin fulminant hepatitis. A possible consequence of the enhancement of isoniazid hepatotoxicity by enzyme induction. Gastroenterology 1977;72:284–9.

205. Gal AA, Klatt EC. Fatal isoniazid hepatitis in a child. Pediatr Infect Dis 1986;5:490–1.

206. Palusci VJ, O'Hare D, Lawrence RM. Hepatotoxicity and transaminase measurement during isoniazid chemoprophylaxis in children. Pediatr Infect Dis J 1995;14:144–8.

207. Beaudry P, Brickman H, Wise M, MacDougall D. Liver enzyme disturbances during isoniazid chemoprophylaxis in children. Am Rev Respir Dis 1974;110:581–4.

208. Spyridis P, Sinantios C, Papadea I, et al. Isoniazid liver injury during chemoprophylaxis in children. Arch Dis Child 1979; 54:65–7.

209. Tsagaropoulou-Stinga H, Mataki-Emmanouilidou T, Karadi-Kavalioti S, Manios S. Hepatotoxic reactions in children with severe tuberculosis treated with isoniazid-rifampin. Pediatr Infect Dis 1985;4:270–3.

210. Martinez-Roig A, Cami J, Llorens-Teroi J, et al. Acetylation phenotype and hepatotoxicity in the treatment of tuberculosis of children. Pediatrics 1986;77:912–5.

211. Berkowitz FE, Henderson SL, Fajman N, et al. Acute liver failure caused by isoniazid in a child receiving carbamazepine. Int J Tuberc Lung Dis 1998;2:603–6.

212. Seth V, Beotra A. Hepatic function in relation to acetylator phenotype in children treated with antitubercular drugs. Ind J Med Res 1989;89:306–9.

213. Moult PJ, Sherlock S. Halothane-related hepatitis. A clinical study of twenty-six cases. QJM 1975;44:99–114.

214. Wark HJ. Postoperative jaundice in children. Anaesthesia 1983;38:237–42.

215. Warner LO, Beach TP, Gariss JP, Warner EJ. Halothane and children: the first quarter century. Anesth Analg 1984;63:838–40.

216. Farrell G, Prendergast D, Murray M. Halothane hepatitis: detection of a constitutional susceptibility factor. N Engl J Med 1985;313:1310–4.

217. Kenna JG, Newberger J, Mieli-Vergani G, et al. Halothane hepatitis in children. BMJ 1987;294:1209–11.

218. Hassall E, Israel DM, Gunasekaran T, Steward D. Halothane hepatitis in children. J Pediatr Gastroenterol Nutr 1990; 11:553–7.

219. Psacharopoulos HJ, Mowat AP, Davies M, et al. Fulminant hepatic failure in childhood: an analysis of 31 cases. Arch Dis Child 1980;55:252–8.

220. Inman WHV, Mushin WW. Jaundice after repeated exposure to halothane: a further analysis of reports to the Committee of Safety of Medicines. BMJ 1978;2:1455–6.

221. Campbell RL, Small EW, Lesesne HR, et al. Fatal hepatic necrosis after halothane anesthesia in a boy with juvenile rheumatoid arthritis: a case report. Anesth Analg 1977;56:589–93.

222. DeGroot H, Noll T. Halothane hepatotoxicity: relation between metabolic activation, pyrexia, covalent binding, lipid peroxidation and liver cell damage. Hepatology 1983;3:601–6.

223. Neuberger J, Williams R. Halothane hepatitis. Dig Dis 1988;6: 52–64.

224. Farrell GC. Mechanism of halothane-induced liver injury: is it immune or metabolic idiosyncrasy? J Gastroenterol Hepatol 1988;3:465–82.

225. Spracklin DK, Thummel KE, Kharasch ED. Human reductive halothane metabolism in vitro is catalyzed by cytochrome P450 2A6 and 3A4. Drug Metab Dispos 1996;24:976–83.

226. Spracklin DK, Hankins DC, Fisher JM, et al. Cytochrome P450 2E1 is the principal catalyst of human oxidative halothane metabolism in vitro. J Pharmacol Exp Ther 1997;281:400–11.

227. Vergani D, Mieli-Vergani G, Alberti A, et al. Antibodies to the surface of halothane-altered rabbit hepatocytes in patients with severe halothane-associated hepatitis. N Engl J Med 1980;303:66–71.

228. Neuberger J, Mieli-Vergani G, Tredger JM, et al. Oxidative metabolism of halothane in the production of altered hepatocyte membrane antigens in acute halothane-induced hepatic necrosis. Gut 1981;22:669–72.

229. Satoh H, Fukada Y, Anderson DK, et al. Immunological studies on the mechanism of halothane-induced hepatotoxicity: immunohistochemical evidence of trifluoroacetylated hepatocytes. J Pharmacol Exp Ther 1985;233:857–62.

230. Kenna JG, Satoh H, Christ DD, Pohl LR. Metabolic basis for a drug hypersensitivity: antibodies in sera from patients with halothane hepatitis recognize liver neoantigens that contain the trifluoroacetyl group derived from halothane. J Pharmacol Exp Ther 1988;245:1103–9.

231. Kenna JG, Neuberger J, Williams R. Evidence for expression in human liver of halothane-induced neoantigens recognized by antibodies in sera from patients with halothane hepatitis. Hepatology 1988;8:1635–41.

232. Satoh H, Martin BM, Schulick AH, et al. Human antiendoplasmic reticulum antibodies in sera of patients with halothane-induced hepatitis are directed against a trifluoroacetylated carboxylesterase. Proc Natl Acad Sci U S A 1989;86:322–6.

233. Christen U, Buergin M, Gut J. Halothane metabolism: Kupffer cells carry and partially process trifluoroacetylated protein adducts. Biochem Biophys Res Commun 1991;175:256–62.

234. Kenna JG, Martin JL, Satoh H, Pohl LR. Factors affecting the expression of trifluoroacetylated liver microsomal protein neoantigens in rats treated with halothane. Drug Metab Dispos 1990;18:788–93.

235. Reddy CM. Propylthiouracil and hepatitis: a case report. J Natl Med Assoc 1979;72:1185–6.

236. Verhamme M, Ramboer C, Van De Bruaene P, Inderadjaja N. Cholestatic hepatitis due to an amoxicillin/clavulanic acid preparation. J Hepatol 1989;9:260–4.

237. Larrey D, Vial T, Babany G, et al. Hepatitis associated with amoxicillin-clavulanic acid combination report of 15 cases. Gut 1992;33:368–71.

238. Lakehal F, Dansette PM, Becquemont L, et al. Indirect cytotoxicity of flucloxacillin toward human biliary epithelium via metabolite formation in hepatocytes. Chem Res Toxicol 2001;14:694–701.

239. Degott C, Feldmann G, Larrey D, et al. Drug-induced prolonged cholestasis in adults: a histological semiquantitative study demonstrating progressive ductopenia. Hepatology 1992; 15:244–51.

240. Davies MH, Harrison RF, Elias E, Hübscher SG. Antibiotic-associated acute vanishing bile duct syndrome: a pattern associated with severe, prolonged, intrahepatic cholestasis. J Hepatol 1994;20:112–6.

241. Alexander P, Roskams T, Van Steenbergen W, et al. Intrahepatic cholestasis induced by amoxicillin/clavulinic acid (Augmentin): a report on two cases. Acta Clin Belg 1991;46: 327–32.

242. Maraqa NF, Gomez MM, Rathore MH, Alvarez AM. Higher occurrence of hepatotoxicity and rash in patients treated with oxacillin compared with those treated with nafcillin and other commonly used antimicrobials. Clin Infect Dis 2002;34:50–4.

243. Chawla A, Kahn E, Yunis EJ, Daum F. Rapidly progressive cholstasis: an unusual reaction to amoxicillin/clavulinic acid in a child. J Pediatr 2000;136:121–3.

244. Malcolm A, Heap TR, Eckstein RP, Lunzer MR. Minocycline-induced liver injury. Am J Gastroenterol 1996;91:1641–3.

245. Bhat G, Jordan JJ, Sokalski S, et al. Minocycline-induced hepatitis with autoimmune features and neutropenia. J Clin Gastroenterol 1998;27:74–5.

246. Gough A, Chapman S, Wagstaff K, et al. Minocycline induced autoimmune hepatitis and systemic lupus erythematosus-like syndrome. BMJ 1996;312:169–72.

247. Lawrenson RA, Seaman HE, Sundstrom A, et al. Liver damage associated with minocycline use in acne: a systematic review of the published literature and pharmacovigilance data. Drug Saf 2000;23:333–49.

248. Goldstein NS, Bayati N, Silverman AL, Gordon SC. Minocycline as a cause of drug-induced autoimmune hepatitis. Report of four cases and comparison with autoimmune hepatitis. Am J Clin Pathol 2000;114:591–8.

249. Davies MG, Kersey PJW. Acute hepatitis and exfoliative dermatitis associated with minocycline. BMJ 1989;298:1523–4.

250. Boudreaux JP, Hayes DH, Mizrahi S, et al. Fulminant hepatic failure, hepatorenal syndrome, and necrotizing pancreatitis after minocycline hepatotoxicity. Transplant Proc 1993;25:1873.

251. Stickel F, Egerer G, Seitz HK. Hepatotoxicity of botanicals. Public Health Nutr 2000;3:113–24.

252. Yeong ML, Swinburn B, Kennedy M, Nicholson G. Hepatic veno-occlusive disease associated with comfrey ingestion. J Gastroenterol Hepatol 1990;5:211–4.

253. Laliberte L, Villeneuve JP. Hepatitis after the use of germander, a herbal remedy. Can Med Assoc J 1996;154:1689–92.

254. Larrey D, Vial T, Pauwels A, et al. Hepatitis after germander (Teucrium chamaedrys) administration: another instance of herbal medicine hepatotoxicity. Ann Intern Med 1992;117:129–32.

255. Katz M, Saibil F. Herbal hepatitis: subacute hepatic necrosis secondary to chaparral leaf. J Clin Gastroenterol 1990;12:203–6.

256. Campo JV, McNabb J, Perel JM, et al. Kava-induced fulminant hepatic failure. J Am Acad Child Adolesc Psychiatry 2002;41:631–2.

257. Wooltorton E. Herbal kava: reports of liver toxicity. Can Med Assoc J 2002;166:777.

258. Divinsky M. Case report: jin bu huan—not so benign herbal medicine. Can Fam Physician 2002;48:1640–2.

259. Woolf GM, Petrovic LM, Rojter SE, et al. Acute hepatitis associated with the Chinese herbal product jin bu huan. Ann Intern Med 1994;121:729–35.

260. Horowitz RS, Feldhaus K, Dart RC, et al. The clinical spectrum of jin bu huan toxicity. Arch Intern Med 1996;156:899–903.

261. Rode D. Comfrey toxicity revisited. Trends Pharmacol Sci 2002;23:497–9.

262. Lekehal M, Pessayre D, Lereau JM, et al. Hepatotoxicity of the herbal medicine germander: metabolic activation of its furano diterpenoids by cytochrome P450 3A depletes cytoskeleton-associated protein thiols and forms plasma membrane blebs in rat hepatocytes. Hepatology 1996;24:212–8.

263. Fau D, Lekehal M, Farrell G, et al. Diterpenoids from germander, an herbal medicine, induce apoptosis in isolated rat hepatocytes. Gastroenterology 1997;113:1334–6.

264. Jones AL, Simpson KJ. Review article: mechanisms and management of hepatotoxicity in ecstasy (MDMA) and amphetamine intoxications. Aliment Pharmacol Ther 1999;13:129–33.

265. Andreu V, Mas A, Bruguera M, et al. Ecstasy: a common cause of severe acute hepatotoxicity. J Hepatol 1998;29:394–7.

266. Ellis AJ, Wendon JA, Portmann B, Williams R. Acute liver damage and Ecstasy ingestion. Gut 1996;38:454–8.

267. Kreth K-P, Kovar K-A, Schwab M, Zanger UM. Identification of the human cytochromes P450 involved in the oxidative metabolism of "Ecstasy"-related designer drugs. Biochem Pharmacol 2000;59:1563–71.

268. Gilhooly TC, Daly AK. CYP2D6 deficiency, a factor in Ecstasy related deaths? Br J Clin Pharmacol 2002;54:69–70.

269. Ramamoorthy Y, Yu A-M, Suh N, et al. Reduced +/–3,4-methylenedioxymethampetamine ("Ecstasy") metabolism with cytochrome P450 2D6 inhibitors and pharmacogenetic variants in vitro. Biochem Pharmacol 2002;63:2111–9.

270. Naranjo CA, Busto U, Sellers EM, et al. A method for estimating the probability of adverse drug reactions. Clin Pharmacol Ther 1981;30:239–45.

271. Danan G, Benichou C. Causality assessment of adverse reactions to drugs—I. A novel method based on the conclusions of international consensus meetings: application to drug-induced liver injuries. J Clin Epidemiol 1993;46:1323–30.

272. Benichou C, Danan G, Flahault A. Causality assessment of adverse reactions to drugs—II. An original model for validation of drug causality assessment methods: case reports with positive rechallenge. J Clin Epidemiol 1993;46:1331–6.

273. Maria VAJ, Victorino RMM. Development and validation of a clinical scale for the diagnosis of drug-induced liver injuries. Hepatology 1997;26:664–9.

274. Lucena MI, Camargo R, Andrade RJ, et al. Comparison of two clinical scales for causality assessment in hepatotoxicity. Hepatology 2001;33:123–30.

275. Spielberg SP. In vitro assessment of pharmacogenetic susceptibility to toxic drug metabolites in humans. Fed Proc 1984;43:2308–13.

CHAPTER 54

LIVER TUMORS

Milton J. Finegold, MD

Joel E. Haas, MD

Understanding and treating liver tumors in children continues to be a formidable task. The very rarity of such tumors contributes to the difficulty because few individuals or centers compile sufficient experience to provide definitive direction. Additionally, the remarkable diversity of conditions that fall under the term "tumor" makes it difficult to design a unifying formula to approach the subject or individual patient. Another problem is the extraordinary functional capacity of the liver to compensate for the intruding mass, so clues to the presence of a tumor are often few and so late as to make simple removal impossible. Finally, the liver's anatomy encourages internal dissemination of neoplasms and taxes the skills of the most experienced surgeon. Nevertheless, recent advances in knowledge of the molecular biology of gene expression and cellular differentiation, experimental carcinogenesis, monoclonal antibodies for diagnosis and perhaps even treatment, imaging techniques and anesthesia, and transplant immunology make this a time for optimism. But of all of the scientific advances, the single most important advance has already been achieved and is being implemented: vaccination against hepatitis B virus (HBV). In regions where hepatitis B is endemic, such as Taiwan, hepatocellular carcinoma (HCC) has accounted for 13% of all cancers in patients less than 15 years of age. By interrupting the cycle of mother to newborn transmission, vaccination has already begun to eliminate the most important single cause of hepatic malignancy.[1] Prevention of hepatitis C virus (HCV) transmission in blood products will further reduce the incidence of cirrhosis and HCC in adults. Thus far, no children with HCV and liver cancer have been reported. However, two 20-year childhood leukemia survivors developing HCC exhibited antibodies to hepatitis C at the time of diagnosis.[2]

Estimates of the incidence of primary hepatic tumors suggest that they account for about 0.04 to 0.16% of 1,000 US hospital admissions and 0.5 to 2.0% of all pediatric cancers. About three-quarters of the collected tumors in large series worldwide (Table 54-1) are malignant, and 85% of those are of hepatocellular origin.[3] Hepatoblastomas comprise about 43% of all primary hepatic tumors. They occur in about one child per million under the age of 15 years (about 100 cases per year) in the United States.[4]

There is a strong possibility that all series and reports are biased toward malignancy, unusual cases, and unusual circumstances. The relative contribution of referral centers to surgical surveys and national statistics is uncertain, and the use of death certificates without autopsy verification is unreliable. The incidence of hepatoblastoma appears to be increasing,[4] possibly because of the survival of extremely premature infants (< 1,000 g).[5] It was found that 58% of all hepatoblastomas in the Japanese Children's Cancer Registry occurred in children who weighed less than 1,500 g at birth.[6] The relative risk for hepatoblastoma in premature versus term infants was 15.6 for those weighing less than 1,000 g, 2.5 for birth weights of 1,000 to 1,499 g, and 1.2 for birth weights in the 2,000 to 2,499 g range. The Children's Cancer Group (CCG) of the United States found that 13.9% of 72 patients who had gestational histories recorded in their series were premature.[7] Ten of the 18 patients weighed less than 1,000 g at birth—a 16- to 23-fold excess versus term infants. Four percent of the hepatoblastoma patients in the German Registry (3 of 77) were premature infants who required parenteral nutrition,[8] suggesting a potential source of mutagens. Three premature infants treated with long-term parenteral nutrition have developed hepatocarcinoma,[9] but the German Registry reports the first hepatoblastoma–parenteral nutrition association.

ETIOLOGY

Worldwide, HBV has been responsible for more malignancy than any other environmental agent. Among adults, there is a definite relationship to chronic hepatitis and macronodular cirrhosis, and at least 20 years of infection

TABLE 54-1 PRIMARY LIVER TUMORS IN CHILDREN (18 SERIES WORLDWIDE)

TUMOR	NUMBER (%)
Hepatoblastoma	539 (43)
Hepatocarcinoma	287 (23)
Adenoma	23 (2)
Hemangioma, hemangioendothelioma	171 (13)
Mesenchymal hamartoma	76 (6)
Sarcoma	80 (6)
Focal nodular hyperplasia	22 (2)
Other	58 (5)
Total	1,256 (100)

Adapted from Weinberg AG and Finegold MJ.[3]

seem to be required for neoplastic transformation. The occurrence of HCC in children as young as 3 years of age following perinatal exposure to carrier mothers is surely an important clue to the carcinogenic process. Only 2 of 173 black South Africans with HCC under age 30 lacked serologic evidence of HBV infection. One hundred percent of Taiwanese children with HCC are HBV carriers.[10] The younger the child, the less often there is evidence of active hepatitis and cirrhosis. HBV functions like a retrovirus, with reverse transcriptase activity providing the means toward deoxyribonucleic acid (DNA) replication. As with other carcinogenic retroviruses, the DNA may become integrated into the host genome, and there may be associated deletions of portions of the cellular genome, but the integration site is variable, and mutations in the virus may be important.[11] Increasing reports of cell-cycle gene disruptions[12,13] may lead us to anticipate additional specific mutations as molecular methods are applied to HBV-associated HCC. The reason why children exposed to HBV as infants develop HCC so quickly may be that the integration of viral DNA is facilitated by the rapid rate of cell division in the developing liver. Perhaps the effects of early viral DNA integration on hepatocyte differentiation would explain why three of the five HCCs in children with HBV infection described by Ohaki and colleagues[14] contained primitive hepatoblastic foci. We have examined seven tumors containing both HCC and hepatoblastoma in children having a mean age of 8.5 years. All were HBV positive.

At least three-quarters of the mothers of children with HBV infection and HCC in Africa, China, and Japan display hepatitis B surface (HB$_s$) antigenemia. Curiously, only a minority of the fathers have antigenemia.[10] Even more perplexing is the observation that 27 of 28 fathers of children with HCC in Senegal lacked antibody to the HB$_s$ antigen compared with 48% of age-controlled males in the same population.[15] Eighteen percent of those fathers had HB$_s$ antigenemia, in contrast to 71% of the mothers. The role of gender in the development of liver tumors is indeed noteworthy. Among adults, the male-to-female HCC ratio is said to be 8:1 to 10:1. Most of the difference is attributed to chronic HBV hepatitis with cirrhosis, industrial or occupational exposure, and alcoholism. Only 1 of 15 HB$_s$ antigen–positive mothers of Taiwanese children with HCC had HCC herself, and no malignancy developed in any of their 9 HB$_s$ antigen–positive sisters. However, 5 of 13 HBV-carrying brothers had HCC.[10] Even with underlying genetic diseases and metabolic errors having an autosomal recessive (sex neutral) basis, such as familial adenomatous polyposis,[16] familial cholestatic cirrhosis,[17] and type I glycogen storage disease, the incidence of hepatocellular malignancy in boys is at least double that of girls. Coire and colleagues described liver adenomas in 24 males and 12 females with von Gierke disease.[18] All four patients who later developed carcinomas were males (Figure 54-1).

It is stimulating to consider these clinical observations in light of studies on steroid hormone receptors in normal and neoplastic liver tissue. Iqbal and colleagues found androgen receptors in fetal liver and HCC but not in normal adult liver, whereas estrogen receptors were detected

in both tumor and adjacent liver.[19] Nagasue and colleagues were able to detect androgen receptors in normal male liver, and 18 of 23 carcinomas had a significantly higher concentration.[20] The cirrhotic liver of one woman also had androgen receptors. But one of two HCCs in that same liver lacked androgen receptors. Both Nagasue and colleagues[20] and Ohnishi and colleagues[21] found a loss of estrogen receptor activity in HCC versus the surrounding liver tissue. When aplastic or Fanconi anemia patients of either sex are treated with C17–alkylated anabolic steroids, tumors develop with significant frequency, and tumors have also been observed when testosterone was given to correct sexual immaturity in boys.[3] Boys accounted for 25 of the 34 androgen-associated liver tumors in patients less than 20 years of age reviewed by Chandra and colleagues.[22] Although half were discovered at autopsy, just two were judged to be carcinomas. Some of the benign tumors regressed on withdrawal of steroids.

Estrogens in oral contraceptives are definitely associated with hepatic adenoma development. After 8 years of oral contraceptive use, the incidence of hepatic carcinoma in women is 4 to 20 times that of age-matched controls when alcoholism, hepatitis, and cirrhosis are excluded.[23] Focal nodular hyperplasia is a non-neoplastic process that has to be distinguished from adenomas and carcinomas.[24] For a short time, it appeared that this lesion was more common in women. It now seems that the lesion is more often symptomatic in women because oral contraceptives make it more vascular and more likely to bleed. Case reports associate angiosarcoma and cholangiocarcinoma with oral contraceptives. Additionally a 19-year-old girl was found to have a hepatoblastoma after 15 months of "pill" use.[25] Prenatal exposure to synthetic estrogens or gonadotropins has been reported in two infants with hepatoblastoma[3] and one with angiosarcoma.[26] The Children's Cancer Study Group (CCSG) looked for risk factors in

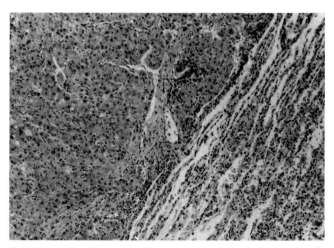

FIGURE 54-1 Hepatocarcinoma metastatic to the lung. A well-differentiated malignancy from a 17-year-old boy who had glucose-6-phosphatase deficiency, managed successfully by frequent and nocturnal feedings. Adenomas were recognized in this liver 3 years earlier. If the illustrated tumor were in the liver, it would be impossible to predict its behavior from histology alone (hematoxylin and eosin; ×63 original magnification).

75 cases of hepatoblastoma versus age-matched controls and found a significantly higher frequency of maternal exposure to metals and petroleum products. Paternal exposure to metals was also excessive.[27]

The importance of oncogene expression in the genesis of hepatic malignancy has been augmented by recent studies of tumor suppressor genes, cell-cycle genes, and growth factors. Baffett and colleagues found expression of N-ras messenger ribonucleic acid (RNA) in 11 of 11 hepatocarcinomas.[28] In 7 of 11 tumors, c-Ki-ras and c-Ha-ras were detected, whereas c-myc and fos were expressed in 2 of 11 tumors. The finding that *c-met* is overexpressed in a significant (8 of 18) proportion of HCCs is intriguing because the protein is a receptor for hepatocyte growth factor, a potent stimulant of hepatocyte mitosis.[29] Overexpression of c-met conferred a worse prognosis (33% 5-year survival versus 80% in low expressors).[30] Likewise, the role of transforming growth factor-α (TGF-α) in hepatocellular malignancy appears to be important. It is produced by fetal hepatoblastoma cells with low proliferative activity[31] and by 65% of hepatocarcinomas.[32] It is a strong stimulus of hepatocyte replication,[33] and, interestingly, only male mice overexpressing TGF-α develop hepatocarcinomas.[34] Telomerase activity in nontumoral regenerative nodules of patients with cirrhosis and hepatocarcinoma was equal to that in the neoplasm and predictive of early recurrence or second primaries.[35] In hepatoblastomas, the most significant genetic abnormalities involve the chromosome 11p15 region, in which the Beckwith-Wiedemann locus is found (see below). Genes for insulin and insulin-like growth factor 2 (IGF-2), both stimulants of fetal cell growth, are located in the same region. Loss of imprinting and loss of heterozygosity for IGF-2 and IGF-2 receptor have both been observed in hepatoblastoma.[36,37] Overexpression of IGF-2 has also been demonstrated in hepatoblastomas by microarray expression technology.[38] That report also revealed surprising breast cancer (BRCA2) expression in hepatoblastomas and binding of antibody to BRCA2 protein by six of six hepatoblastomas but not normal fetal liver.[38]

The exact role of *p53* in the pathogenesis of hepatic neoplasia remains uncertain. No liver tumors were found when the *p53* gene was inactivated by homologous recombination in mice (in whom several other cell types developed neoplasms).[39] When small early HCCs in humans were examined, *p53* expression was normal, whereas 8 of 22 cancers at an advanced stage had mutations.[40] Interestingly, six of those eight cases that were informative also had deletions of the retinoblastoma gene product. The activation of HIC-1, hypermethylated in cancer, a candidate tumor suppressor, by *p53* may be meaningful because messenger RNA for HIC-1 is markedly reduced in precancerous nodules of cirrhosis and even more so in poorly differentiated carcinomas.[41] In Japan, serum antibodies to *p53* were associated with decreased survival.[42]

Many metabolic defects and congenital malformations are associated with and possibly contribute to hepatocellular malignancy.[3] They are listed in Table 54-2. The highest frequency of HCC in a metabolic disease of childhood was found with tyrosinemia type 1, owing to inactivity of

fumarylacetoacetate hydrolase.[43] The 18 to 37% incidence of HCC reported in survivors of the infantile period has been reduced by the recent discovery that an inhibitor of an upstream enzyme (4-hydroxyphenylpyruvate dioxygenase) reversed the clinical and chemical abnormalities in four of five children with fumarylacetoacetate hydrolase deficiency.[44] By 2000, over 200 children with tyrosinemia were treated with the inhibitor 2-(2-nitro-4-trifluoromethyl benzoyl)-1,3 cyclohexane dione prior to the age of 2 years. Just two have developed hepatocarcinoma, one of whom (whose treatment began at 5 months of age) was 15 months old when the malignancy was discovered.[45]

Kingston and colleagues found that hepatoblastoma occurred in five families with intestinal polyposis.[46] With an incidence of familial adenomatous polyposis of 1 per 8,300 and an incidence of hepatoblastoma of one per million children under the age of 15 years, this cannot be coincidental. One of 20 hepatoblastomas occurs in a polyposis kindred. Hughes and Michels have pointed out that despite the 500 to 1,000 excess of hepatoblastoma in families with familial adenomatous polyposis, less than 1% of the families are at risk.[47] Garber and colleagues expanded the number of affected families to 25; there were 18 boys and 7 girls.[48] Eleven of the 25 patients have survived, including all but one of the girls but only five of the boys. Six of the seven survivors examined developed colonic polyps as early as 7 years of age. Bodmer and colleagues localized the adenomatous polyposis coli gene (APC) for familial polyposis to chromosome 5q21,[49] and it is now possible to screen young children in families with polyposis (Gardner syndrome) for the presence of the gene by a variety of molecular tools. Mutations of APC were found in 8 of 13 sporadic hepatoblastomas,[50] but no cytogenetic

---

TABLE 54-2   PRECURSORS OF HEPATIC NEOPLASIA

PERINATAL EXPOSURE
Oral contraceptives
Phenytoin
Ethyl alcohol

NEONATAL FACTORS
Extreme prematurity

METABOLIC DISEASE
Tyrosinemia
von Gierke disease, glycogenosis type I
Glycogenosis III and IV (case reports)

MALFORMATIONS
Hemihypertrophy, Beckwith-Wiedemann syndrome
Von Recklinghausen neurofibromatosis
Soto syndrome
Multiple hemangiomatosis
Ataxia-telangiectasia
Fanconi syndrome
Budd-Chiari syndrome

BILIARY TRACT DISEASE
Extrahepatic atresia
Familial cholestatic cirrhosis
Alagille syndrome
Parenteral alimentation

DRUGS
Oral contraceptives
Anabolic steroids

abnormalities at chromosome 5q21 have been described (Table 54-3). The mechanism of carcinogenesis by germline *APC* mutations appears to be mediated via a cell adhesion protein that accumulates in cells with the mutation.[51] Activating mutations in β-catenin have been observed in 48% of sporadic hepatoblastomas[52] and 20 to 26% of hepatocarcinomas.[53,54]

Several other cytogenetic abnormalities have been seen in children with hepatic neoplasms (see Table 54-3). Trisomy 2 was complete or partial in 26 of 40 hepatoblastomas, and trisomy 20 was found in 29 of 40 cases.[55,56] A unique t(10;22) was reported in one small cell hepatoblastoma.[57] The relatively small number of reported cytogenetic aberrations in hepatoblastoma may relate to the lack of suitable dividing cell samples. When conventional cytogenetic analyses are limited by the lack of suitable metaphase cells, fluorescent in situ hybridization techniques applied to frozen or paraffin-embedded tissues may reveal abnormalities in chromosome number and structure.[58] Among HCCs, the frequent allelic deletions at 17p (38 to 54%) correlate with deficient p53 function.[59] Among the many other deletions observed in HCC, those at chromosomes 16q and 4q have not been observed in other cancers, so they may be the most meaningful. Molecular genetic analysis of hepatocellular neoplasms has begun to provide important insights into dysregulation of growth. Those occurring with significant frequency are shown in Table 54-4.

Also noteworthy are reports of HCC in relation to chronic biliary tract disease, including extrahepatic biliary atresia, Byler disease, and bile salt export protein deficiency.[60,61] A 6-month-old boy received parenteral alimentation all his life and was found at autopsy to have a microscopic focus of carcinoma.[62] Two more cases have been described.[8] Arteriohepatic dysplasia (Alagille syndrome) was previously not regarded as a preneoplastic condition because 85 to 90% of affected individuals survive without serious hepatic complications of their childhood-onset cholestasis and bile duct paucity. But several patients with the syndrome have been described with HCC, even in the absence of biliary cirrhosis; the youngest was a 3½-year-old girl,[63] and there were three affected siblings in one family.[64]

CLINICAL MANIFESTATIONS

Regardless of cell type, the great majority of hepatic tumors are first detected as a mass or abdominal swelling. Upper abdominal pain is the next most frequent presenting complaint, followed by anorexia and weight loss, vomiting, and diarrhea. Infants with vascular hamartomas (hemangiomas) may display signs of congestive heart failure, as have rare patients with mesenchymal hamartomas. Pruritus and frank jaundice are observed when tumors obstruct bile flow. In children, obstruction suggests rhabdomyosarcoma at any level of the biliary tract. Minor blunt trauma or apparently spontaneous hemorrhage of a liver tumor can be the earliest sign of its presence, especially among adolescent girls and young women taking estrogens for oral contraception, when tumors are especially vascular.

Several metabolic effects or paraneoplastic syndromes occur with a variety of hepatic tumors. Hypercalcemia with marked osteopenia can be very severe in children with hepatoblastoma, carcinoma, or sarcoma. As in other malignancy-related hypercalcemias, the mechanism is not fully understood, but ectopic parathormone production is not the reason.[65] Hyperlipidemia has been associated with epithelial malignancies; when caused by hepatoblastoma in infants, it has been associated with early fatality.[66] Both hyperlipidemia and hypoglycemia are thought to be secondary to injury to the remaining liver or dysfunction of the neoplastic epithelial cells rather than a sign of underlying enzymatic error, such as glucose-6-phosphatase deficiency. The rare carcinomas in von Gierke disease do not appear until the midteens or early adulthood.[18] A few case reports of HCC in children and adults with debrancher and

---

TABLE 54-3   CYTOGENETIC ABNORMALITIES IN LIVER NEOPLASMS

NEOPLASM	ABNORMALITY	INCIDENCE (%)
Hepatoblastoma	Trisomy 20	72 (40 cases)*
	Trisomy 2	65 (40 cases)*
	Trisomy 8	32.5 (40 cases)
	Chromosome 1 translocation	8 cases
	Trisomy 18	3 cases
Hepatocarcinoma	1q excess by CGH	58–72
	4q losses by CGH or LOH	43–77
	8q excess by CGH or LOH	48-77
	16q LOH	52–70
	17p loss or LOH	49–51
Mesenchymal hamartoma	Translocations of 19q13.4	3 cases
	Aneuploidy	2 of 8 cases
Undifferentiated (embryonal)	Monosomy 20	2 cases
	Sarcoma aneuploidy dicentric telomeric association (4;22)(p16;q13)	1 case
Inflammatory myofibroblastoma (pseudotumor)	Hyperdiploidy	4 of 9 cases
	2p23 rearrangements (*ALK* abnormalities)	Unknown for liver

CGH = comparative genomic hybridization; LOH = loss of heterozygosity.
*Two cases each in which trisomy 20 or 2 was the only karyotypic abnormality.[55,56]

TABLE 54-4   MOLECULAR GENETICS OF HEPATOCELLULAR NEOPLASMS

GENE OR LOCUS	ABNORMALITY	TUMOR TYPE	TUMORS AFFECTED (%)
HIC1 (17p13.3)	Hypermethylation, LOH, ↓ expression	HCC	90
CDK4 (12q13–15)	↑ Expression	HB	88
Telomerase (3q26.3)	↑ Expression	HCC	74
Cyclin D₁ (11q13)	↑ Expression	HB	70
p53 (17p13)	Codon 249 mutation	HCC	67 in aflatoxin regions, < 15 elsewhere
FAS (CD95L)	↓ Expression	HCC	64
IGF2 (11p15.5)	LOH or LOI	HB	64
E-cadherin (16q22.1)	Hypermethylation ↓ Expression	HCC	58
TGF-β (2p13)	↑ Expression	HCC	54
β-catenin (3p22–p21.3)	↑ Expression	HB	48
RB (13q14)	LOH	HCC	47

HB = hepatoblastoma; HCC = hepatocellular carcinoma; IGF = insulin-like growth factor; LOH = loss of heterozygosity; LOI = loss of imprinting; TGF = transforming growth factor.

branching enzyme deficiencies (glycogen storage disease III and IV) have appeared recently. Thrombocytosis and polycythemia have been observed in some HCC patients, and some 60% of children with hepatoblastoma have thrombocytosis at presentation. Precocious puberty in males has been observed with hepatoblastomas and carcinomas. In most cases, ectopic gonadotropin production is responsible, but a few instances of tumor testosterone synthesis have been reported.[67]

IMAGING TECHNIQUES

Real-time ultrasonography is the hepatologist's "stethoscope." In Japan, where the incidence of hepatic malignancy is high and screening resources are readily available, Okuda compared the various imaging modalities in adults.[68] They found none to be sufficiently sensitive to detect HCCs smaller than 2 cm or to discriminate between regenerating nodules or adenomas and HCCs. Repeat ultrasonography has shown the doubling time for carcinomas to be variable, with growth from 1 to 2 cm taking an average of 3 months. The most proliferative tumors grew from 1 to 3 cm in 4.6 months. Ultrasonography, combined with serum α-fetoprotein measurements, can detect early lesions susceptible to resection in the presence of cirrhosis. Intraoperative ultrasonography has proven a useful aid to partial hepatectomy in children.[69]

Arterial injections of enhancing compounds during computed tomography (CT) or magnetic resonance imaging (MRI) provide more expensive and complex means of detecting small intrahepatic lesions with questionably greater sensitivity than ultrasonography. The application of MRI is especially useful for distinguishing small and common hemangiomas from solid tumors.[70] MRI also shows spread of tumor into large abdominal veins very clearly. By including iodized oil (Lipiodol) in the arterial infusate and taking delayed CT images, cancers as small as 3 mm have been observed because the oily material is retained only by the tumor. CT is useful for scanning the chest and abdomen for other sites of involvement when a liver mass is present. Enhanced CT and MRI have superseded angiography in delineating the extent of disease prior to partial hepatectomy (Figure 54-2).[70] Scintigraphy with radio-

labeled sulfur colloids has been used to distinguish lesions containing Kupffer cells (focal nodular hyperplasia) from those without Kupffer cells (adenomas and carcinomas).[71] However, some hepatoblastomas have produced scintigraphic images indistinguishable from those of benign masses. Imaging with radiolabeled monoclonal antibody to α-fetoprotein proved helpful in managing a child whose hepatoblastoma could not be fully resected.[72]

LABORATORY TESTS

Serum α-fetoprotein measurement is the most useful marker of malignant liver tumors. Eighty to 90% of hepatoblastoma patients and 60 to 90% of HCC patients have elevated levels at diagnosis. Small cell undifferentiated hepatoblastomas and rhabdoid tumors in infancy do not produce α-fetoprotein.[73,74] Except for a very few infant mesenchymal hamartomas and germ cell and yolk sac tumors, there are no false indications of hepatocellular malignancy when serum α-fetoprotein levels exceed

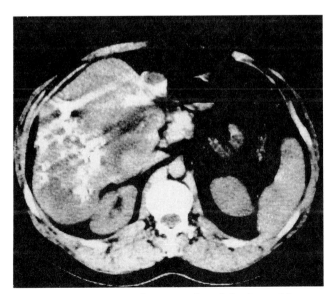

FIGURE 54-2 Computed tomography of the hepatoblastoma shown in Figure 58-4. The larger inner zones of calcification are visualized as stellate radiopaque zones, whereas the epithelial portions of the mass are difficult to distinguish from host liver.

500 ng/mL after 3 months of age. Serum α-fetoprotein is elevated, although not to such high levels, in the absence of demonstrable carcinomas in both hereditary tyrosinemia and ataxia-telangiectasia.[3] Both conditions are associated with a high frequency of hepatic malignancy, and the secretion of the fetal protein is indicative of defective regulation of gene expression in the hepatocyte. Regrettably, α-fetoprotein levels may not be elevated in time for effective therapy. For example, elevations may not occur until ordinary HCCs exceed 4 to 5 cm in diameter, which can take several years.[68] Intrahepatic portal vein dissemination has been observed in both hepatoblastomas and primary carcinomas less than 3 cm in diameter. Measuring serum α-fetoprotein to follow recurrences of resected liver tumors can be helpful. However, a return to normal levels has been observed in some patients even though their tumors continued to grow.

Pseudouridine, a catabolic product of transfer RNA, was detectable in the urine of 9 of 13 patients with HCC whose serum α-fetoprotein concentration was normal.[75] Plasma transcobalamin I (vitamin B_{12}–binding protein) and neurotensin have been elevated in patients with fibrolamellar carcinoma (FLC), which is potentially very useful because only 10% of those tumors have increased α-fetoprotein.[71,76,77] An abnormal form of prothrombin, desgamma-carboxyprothrombin, was present in the serum of 74% of 70 adult HCC patients and in blood and tumor cells of three children with hepatoblastoma.[78] Coagulation tests were unaffected. There was no correlation with serum α-fetoprotein levels, and the test was insensitive for carcinomas less than 3 cm in diameter.

Because of the low incidence of childhood hepatocellular malignancy in the United States, screening of children in the United States or elsewhere would be unrewarding. But application of some of these sensitive tools to the small groups of patients with precursor or associated conditions, such as extreme prematurity, tyrosinemia, hepatic glycogenoses, and chronic cholestatic conditions, could be lifesaving.

PATHOLOGY

HEPATOBLASTOMA

This is an embryonal tumor in the classic sense of incomplete differentiation. Ninety percent of the cases are manifest by the fourth birthday, and several have been present at birth. The usual composition reflects the complex origin of the organ, with endodermal derivatives from the original midgut outgrowth and mesodermally derived offspring of the septum transversum. Thus, parenchymal elements include hepatocytes of varying maturity, resembling the early embryonal or later fetal liver, in association with hematopoietic cells (Figure 54-3). Primitive ducts are characteristic of the embryonal pattern, but well-differentiated ductal elements are unusual except in relation to diffusely infiltrating mesenchymal or blastemal cells. In that situation, they represent residual and sometimes proliferating cholangioles of the host liver because they are not found in metastases. However, when ductal epithelium and tumor cells in the middle of a mass are in continuity on ultra-

structural examination, it is difficult to regard them as normal remnants.[79] It is not unusual to find portions of the epithelial hepatoblastoma to be indistinguishable from HCC, even in the youngest patients.[3] Undifferentiated mesodermal and/or mature stromal derivatives are present in 20 to 30% of cases. The differentiated stroma usually includes osteoid-like material but less often skeletal muscle or cartilage (see Figure 54-3). The osteoid is clearly related to epithelial rather than mesenchymal cells. Not infrequently, keratinizing squamous nests are found among the embryonal cells. Rarely, ducts resembling primitive intestine, neural rosettes, and melanocytes suggest the possibility of a true teratoma.[80]

Depending on the proportions and degree of maturation of the various elements, the gross appearance ranges from yellow-brown (well-differentiated epithelium) to pink-gray (undifferentiated mesenchyme). Focal necrosis and hemorrhage are found in rapidly growing tumors, and firm, even gritty, areas are present when osteoid is abundant. Generally large multinodular expansile masses, hepatoblastomas appear to be well demarcated from the normal host liver but are not encapsulated (Figure 54-4). They may invade hepatic veins and disseminate to the lungs by the time of discovery or penetrate the capsule to reach contiguous tissues and the peritoneum. Hilar lymph nodes are early targets. Staging of hepatoblastomas is done at diagnosis. Stage I indicates complete resection; II, microscopic residual tumor (IIA, inside the liver; IIB, outside the liver); III, gross residual tumor (IIIA, spillage during surgery or gross nodal involvement; IIIB, incomplete resection with or without spillage or node involvement); and IV, metastatic disease (IVA, primary completely resected; IVB, primary not completely resected). Our review of 316 hepatoblastomas from US Pediatric Oncology Group (POG) contributors from 1986 to 2002 had 79 (25%) stage I, 24 (7.5%) stage II, 153 (48%) stage III, and 60 (19%) stage IV cases. The hepatoblastoma histology classifications by Ishak and

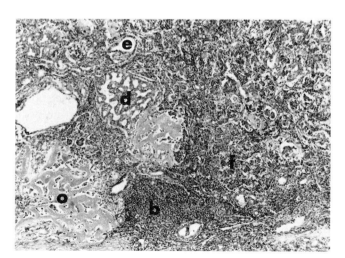

FIGURE 54-3 Hepatoblastoma. The diversity of cell types and varying degrees of maturation are demonstrated in this classic embryonal neoplasm. b = undifferentiated blastemal cells; d = ductular epithelium; e = embryonal epithelium; f = fetal epithelium; o = osteoid (hematoxylin and eosin; × 63 original magnification).

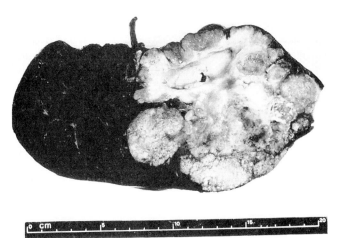

FIGURE 54-4 Hepatoblastoma. A multilobular expansile yellowish tan mass of mixed epithelial and mesenchymal tissues has foci of cystic degeneration and bone. It appears clearly demarcated from the host liver, which is normal, but there is no encapsulation.

TABLE 54-5	CLASSIFICATION OF HEPATOBLASTOMA

MAJOR CATEGORIES
Epithelial
  Fetal, well differentiated (mitotically inactive, diploid)
  Crowded fetal (mitotically active)
  Embryonal
  Macrotrabecular
  Small cell undifferentiated
Mixed
Undifferentiated mesenchymal-blastemal

MINOR COMPONENTS
Ductal (cholangioblastic)
Osteoid
Keratinizing squamous epithelium
Intestinal glandular epithelium
Neuroid-melanocytic (teratoid)
Rhabdomyoblastic
Chondroid

EXCEPTION
Rhabdoid

Glunz[81] and Kasai and Watanabe[82] provide the foundation for current microscopic assessment of hepatoblastoma. Incorporating minor modifications from Gonzalez-Crussi and colleagues[83] and Manivel and colleagues,[80] we evaluated tumors in the POG-CCG intergroup study according to the scheme shown in Table 54-5. In the current US intergroup study, the stage I (well-differentiated fetal hepatoblastoma with less than 2 mitoses per 10 high-power fields) has been singled out for surgical treatment without adjuvant therapy. Only 9 of the 316 cases (2.8%) in the POG series qualified, but the decision to spare children with such completely resected tumors the morbidity of adjuvant therapy seems soundly based. Early observations of 100% survival rate in a small group of such tumors treated with surgery alone[3] were augmented by similar cures when surgery was combined with minimal doses of doxorubicin[84,85] or standard chemotherapy.[86]

Quantification of DNA by image analysis and flow cytometry demonstrated good correlation with prognosis (71% 3-year survival for diploid tumors versus 31% for aneuploid lesions).[87] Six of seven pure fetal tumors were diploid (ie, "favorable"), whereas each of two embryonal epithelial tumors was aneuploid. Ruck and colleagues described another important correlation: p53 expression by immunostaining was lacking in fetal areas of eight tumors and mesenchymal areas of four tumors.[88] However, p53 was expressed in both small cell tumors and in embryonal regions of two of eight tumors examined.

Unresolved questions about the relation of histology to outcome relate to the following:

1. The prognostic import of the degree of differentiation of the fetal epithelial component, which often displays gradual but sometimes abrupt transition from a uniformly well-differentiated pattern with few mitoses to a more crowded but still cord- or plate-like architecture in which nuclei are more pleomorphic and mitoses are more numerous (Figure 54-5). Do such tumors require standard chemotherapy if totally resected?

2. The significance of the proportion of prognostically important histology. Rowland recently provided insightful quantitative analysis pertinent to the limitations of prior published associations between histology and outcome.[89] The relation of completely excised well-differentiated pure fetal histology with low mitotic activity to outcome is unquestionable. However, the lack of uniformity in definition of other histotypes combined with limited sampling of unresectable tumors prior to chemotherapy presents challenges to the desired histology outcome paradigm.

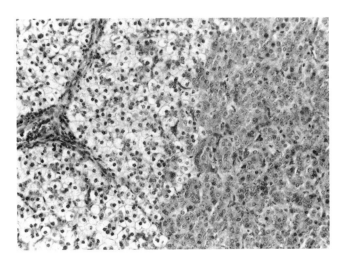

FIGURE 54-5 Hepatoblastoma. The well-differentiated fetal pattern is on the left. Regular cords or plates, one to three cells thick, contain hepatocytes having glycogen-rich clear cytoplasm and regular uniform nuclei and rare mitoses (none in this picture). Immediately adjacent, on the right, the regular cordlike pattern is maintained, but the cells are more numerous and crowded without being macrotrabecular (five to six cells in thickness) or primitive, as in embryonal tumors. The growth rate is increased, as reflected by the presence of two mitoses. A well-differentiated fetal pattern has been associated with an excellent rate of resection and cure. The "crowded" pattern is of uncertain prognostic significance (hematoxylin and eosin; ×160 original magnification).

3. The influence of the differentiated stromal derivatives on prognosis. Muraji and colleagues[66] and Haas and colleagues[84] found that mixed tumors, particularly in stage II–III cases, responded better to chemotherapy than did pure epithelial lesions. However, the impossibility of determining the totality or proportion of all histologic constituents from biopsies of unresectable tumors must be acknowledged.

4. The impact of small undifferentiated cells on prognosis. As the name indicates, these cells fail to demonstrate histologic or ultrastructural features of any known hepatocellular or ductal element, but they contain both cytokeratin filaments typical of epithelial cells and vimentin, a mesenchymal component.[74] Their mitotic activity is variable. Of the 5% of hepatoblastomas that are pure small cell, all but two cases occurred in infants less than 6 months of age, and all such patients have died of disease despite chemotherapy that is highly effective for other histologic subtypes.[85] The role of small cell undifferentiated histology in completely resected hepatoblastoma is becoming more clear.[90] Ten patients with such tumors suffered a relapse in periods ranging from 2 to 21 months. Five whose tumor recurred died. The proportion of small cell histology in four of the fatal cases exceeded 75% of the tissue available for examination, whereas the other fetal case and all of the five survivors had less than 5% small cells. It may be important to note that just three of eight such patients treated with contemporary adjuvant therapy suffered relapse, but none died.[90]

5. The histogenesis of the "rhabdoid" cell type. These monomorphic malignancies of diffusely infiltrating, noncohesive cells with large quantities of intermediate filaments have arisen in several tissues. They tend to occur in young infants, to disseminate widely, and to resist chemotherapy.[73] Immunohistochemical and ultrastructural studies indicate the cells to have both epithelial and mesenchymal characteristics.[91] In the liver, this cell may represent a neoplastic derivative of a stage in the maturation of the undifferentiated mesoderm to the hepatocyte. Except for the presence of epithelial membrane antigen, the immunohistochemical reactions resemble the small undifferentiated or "blastemal" cells of the hepatoblastoma exactly.[92] We have observed transition to "rhabdoid" morphology in otherwise typical hepatoblastomas (Figure 54-6).[3]

6. The significance of postchemotherapy microscopic residual disease. In addition to the greater abundance of osteoid, it is common to find complete necrosis of tumor within hepatic and portal vein branches that are obliterated by scar.[93,94] Nevertheless, nodules of viable tumor are usually found despite marked clinical regression. Most often these have bland fetal histology, but all patterns may be observed, as they are in metastases. The expression of the cell-cycle regulatory protein kinase inhibitory protein (Kip 1 or P27) was markedly reduced in nuclei of residual fetal hepatoblasts after chemotherapy compared with the same cell type before

treatment: from a mean of 75% positive tumor cells to 12%.[95] This difference was not associated with increased DNA synthesis, as determined by Mib1 immunostaining. It is not clear which factors govern the susceptibility or resistance of hepatoblasts to current therapeutic regimens, but von Schweinitz and colleagues have emphasized the importance of postchemotherapy complete resection before development of drug resistance.[96]

HEPATOCARCINOMA

The frequency of cirrhosis in pediatric patients with HCC is much less than in adults (20–25% versus 60–70%), but its presence compounds the therapeutic problem. The appearance of the tumor is similar in children and adults. HCC has a higher frequency of multiple nodules than does hepatoblastoma and exhibits intrahepatic portal vein and lymphatic dissemination more often at the time of diagnosis. A wide range of histologic appearance seems to have little or no influence on resectability or responsiveness to therapy, with one possible exception: the FLC may express different behavior in adults than it does in children.

FLC is rarely associated with cirrhosis, rarely produces α-fetoprotein, and tends to affect young persons. In contrast to the more typical HCCs, just one FLC has been associated with Fanconi anemia.[97] Thirty-nine percent of FLC patients are less than 20 years old, and 90% are less than 25 years of age. Forty-five of 80 tumors occurred in girls, and Malt has called attention to the high incidence of reproductive dysfunction among the group.[71]

The POG-CCG intergroup study has demonstrated that children with FLC do not have a favorable prognosis and do not respond any differently to current therapeutic regi-

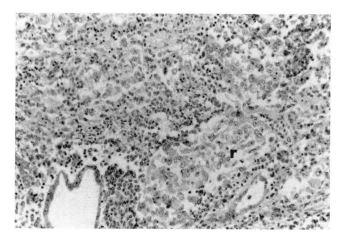

FIGURE 54-6   Hepatoblastoma with focal "rhabdoid" transformation. On the left, fetal-type epithelial components of the neoplasm admixed with hematopoietic cells abut what is probably a residual (non-neoplastic) bile duct. A transition to noncohesive cells of uncertain differentiation is seen in the center right (r). Those cells have larger, vesicular nuclei with prominent nucleoli and perinuclear cytoplasm that is rich in intermediate filaments, producing eosinophilic inclusions in some cells. When tumors are homogeneous for such cells, they are called "rhabdoid." In the liver, they tend to occur in infants younger than 1 year of age, and they behave badly (hematoxylin and eosin; ×160 original magnification).

mens when compared with typical HCC.[98] Although children with initially resectable typical HCC or FLC have a good prognosis (75% 5-year event free survival) irrespective of histologic subtype, outcome is uniformly poor for children with advanced-stage disease.

FLC tends to be a single large bulky light tan to yellow-orange mass with distinct borders. Histologically, large polygonal cells cluster in small groups separated by bands of well-organized collagen (Figure 54-7). Carcinoembryonic antigen and fibrinogen are abundant in the tumor, and the serum concentration of carcinoembryonic antigen has been observed to fall after resection.[99] The tumor cells also tend to be rich in copper and to express the biliary cytokeratin 7 that is not found in ordinary HCC.[100] Intense immunohistochemical staining of TGF-β demonstrable in 9 of 11 FLCs was present in just 3 of 14 typical hepatocarcinomas.[101] The morphologic differences between FLC and ordinary HCC are further reflected in the secretion of neurotensin and by histochemical and ultrastructural evidence of neurosecretory granules.[102] None of these tumors has been associated with clinically evident hormonal effects, and they do not morphologically resemble any of the several cases of primary hepatic carcinoid tumors examined.[3] The exact histogenesis of this epithelial neoplasm is unresolved.

ADENOMA AND FOCAL NODULAR HYPERPLASIA

Each condition contributes 2% of the collected series of childhood liver tumors (see Table 54-1). Both adenomas and focal nodular hyperplasia have been observed in patients with glycogen storage disease[18] and in women using oral contraceptives, but only adenoma seems to be causally related to "the pill."[23,24] Both are usually solitary and expansile, but adenoma is more often multiple and is generally encapsulated. Both consist primarily of well-differentiated hepatocytes arranged in cords or plates but

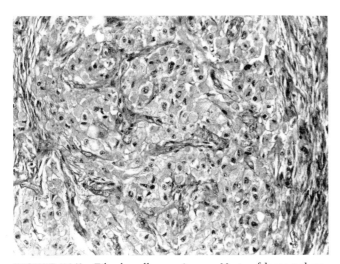

FIGURE 54-7 Fibrolamellar carcinoma. Nests of large polygonal cells with abundant eosinophilic cytoplasm and slightly pleomorphic nuclei are separated by distinct bundles of collagen. Ordinary hepatocarcinomas have little fibrous tissue unless there is a ductal (cholangiolar) component. This was from a 19-year-old girl with normal serum α-fetoprotein. Resection was curative (trichrome, ×160 original magnification).

without the normal lobular pattern. However, the cells of adenomas may be slightly larger than normal hepatocytes, and their nuclei can be slightly pleomorphic. Adenomas lack bile ducts or portal tracts, and focal nodular hyperplasia has septa radiating from a central region of scarring in which ducts can be numerous. In a needle biopsy, these distinguishing features may be unavailable.

VASCULAR TUMORS

Hemangioendotheliomas of infancy are the most common benign tumors of the liver and are generally regarded as hamartomas rather than neoplasms. Nevertheless, they may be symptomatic as mass lesions or may produce high-output congestive heart failure owing to arteriovenous shunting. They may rupture and cause intraperitoneal hemorrhage. Occasionally, thrombocytopenia and intravascular coagulation have been observed.[103] Classification depends on the degree of endothelial cell proliferation and the size of the channels. When actively dividing vasoformative cells are plentiful and not quite organized into channels, the lesions are called type II hemangioendotheliomas.[104] The type II lesions have reportedly disseminated occasionally.[104] Type I lesions consist of definite vessels, with few mitoses and no nuclear atypia. Calcification is frequent. Most cases of both types regress spontaneously or respond well to corticosteroid therapy. However, perfectly bland type I lesions have been followed, on at least four occasions, by hepatic angiosarcomas. At that point, atypical rapidly dividing neoplastic cells were widely dispersed through the sinusoids as well as filling vascular lumens and replacing parenchymal tissues.[3] Two additional angiosarcomas in children appeared histologically to have arisen in preexisting hemangioendotheliomas.[26] Sometimes the spleen and other organs have been involved. One infant had documented exposure to arsenicals. The other had been exposed to metals, glue, and oral contraceptives during the first trimester.[26] Two young adults with neurofibromatosis have had hepatic angiosarcomas.[105] A lymphangioendothelioma confined to the liver almost completely replaced the hepatic parenchyma of a newborn.[106] Hepatic angiomyolipomas have been reported in 24% of children with tuberous sclerosis.[107]

MESENCHYMAL TUMORS

The mesenchymal hamartoma of infancy can be present at birth, grow to an enormous size, and cause heart failure because of arteriovenous shunting. Over 90% of cases are manifest in infancy, but individual cases have been observed in adults, the oldest patient being 28 years old.[108] The mass may bulge from the liver and even become pedunculated, but it has no capsule (Figures 54-8 and 54-9). Typically, there are multiple large cystic spaces with a flat endothelial or biliary epithelial lining and serous fluid content (Figure 54-10). The stroma is myxomatous and bland. At the interface with the remaining parenchyma, bile ducts proliferate actively. Seven reports document simultaneous occurrence or subsequent development of undifferentiated or embryonal hepatic sarcoma in mesenchymal hamartoma.[109–115] The frequently observed translocation

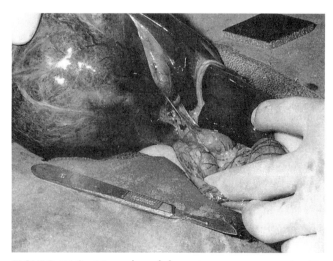

FIGURE 54-8   Mesenchymal hamartoma at surgery. An 11-month-old boy presented with a distended abdomen. Ultrasonography revealed a multilocular cystic mass. It protruded from the right lobe inferiorly and was completely resectable.

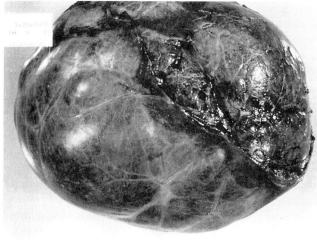

FIGURE 54-9   Mesenchymal hamartoma after resection. The huge bulging mass weighed 1,250 g and consisted mainly of tense cysts. The patient had about 35% of the liver left and recovered uneventfully.

involving chromosome 19q 13.4 in mesenchymal hamartomas has not been described in sarcomas, however. The treatment of unresectable cystic lesions by drainage and marsupialization is undesirable in light of this association.

Malignant mesenchymomas were so named because of the multiple derivatives of stromal cells they contain, including myxoid, chondroid, muscular, bony, and fibrous tissues. Since the report by Stocker and Ishak,[116] most authors have referred to the lesion as an undifferentiated or embryonal sarcoma, even though many of the tumors have indeed had regions of fibrous histiocytoma, liposarcoma, and even benign pericytoma.[117] Half of the cases have presented in children between the ages of 6 and 10 years. Embryonal undifferentiated sarcoma tends to be huge and unresectable at presentation. The liver is found to be replaced by a variegated, hemorrhagic, cystic mass of gray-white soft tissue (Figure 54-11). Microscopically, the undifferentiated aspect is characterized by huge bizarre cells having prominent glycoprotein inclusions associated with small nondescript cells and abundant myxoid stroma (Figure 54-12). One case has occurred in a family with Li-Fraumeni syndrome, in which germline mutations of *p53* have been found.[118] Comparative genomic hybridization of sarcomas has revealed multiple amplifications and deletions, none of which involve the locus affected in mesenchymal hamartoma.[119] The prognosis of these lesions was generally very poor, but reports from Germany,[120] Italy,[121] and the United States[122] indicate that these sarcomas may respond to intensive chemotherapy, with cisplatinum, doxorubicin, and ifosfamide in most regimens.

Rhabdomyosarcomas of the biliary tract tend to form polypoid masses of soft, gelatinous, pink-gray tissue that

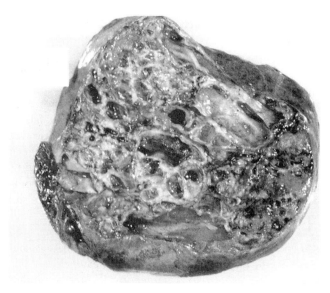

FIGURE 54-10   Mesenchymal hamartoma after sectioning. Multiple cysts filled with serous fluid are separated by myxomatous stroma.

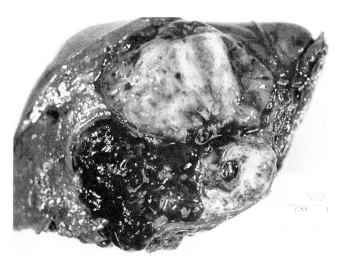

FIGURE 54-11   Undifferentiated sarcoma replaces most of the right lobe in a 6-year-old boy. A multinodular fleshy mass with large areas of hemorrhage and cystic degeneration, it gives the impression of encapsulation but, in fact, insinuates into the surrounding host liver.

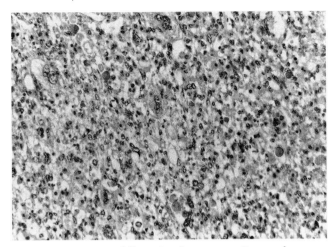

FIGURE 54-12 Undifferentiated sarcoma. Scattered among numerous small and nondescript cells are several giant cells with multilobate vesicular nuclei having prominent nucleoli. Large globular inclusions of glycoprotein are regularly present in the cytoplasm of such cells and sometimes spill out into the adjacent loose ground substance. Portions of such tumors have differentiated into fibroblasts and fibrohistiocytic, lipoblastic, and chondroid cells (hematoxylin and eosin; ×160 original magnification).

tend to obstruct bile flow. The cells are generally primitive embryonal forms with rare, ill-defined muscle filaments. All bile ducts, from ampulla and gallbladder, can be affected. Patients have ranged in age from infancy to the teens. Two of the eight cases reported by Geoffray and colleagues were resectable, but both recurred.[123] In the series of Mihara and colleagues, six of nine patients responded well to vigorous chemotherapy and radiotherapy.[124]

Rhabdoid tumors of the liver were mentioned in the discussion of hepatoblastoma. One such tumor was found in a 14-day-old boy with a primitive neuroectodermal tumor of the cerebrum that contained similar cells,[125] just as has been observed for renal rhabdoid tumors.

A 9-year-old girl with acquired immune deficiency syndrome (AIDS) is the twentieth and youngest child with leiomyosarcoma arising in the liver.[126] No human immunodeficiency virus (HIV) DNA was detected in her tumor. Unlike most such tumors in immunodeficient children,[127] this one was negative for Epstein-Barr virus. Granular cell myoblastomas, which actually arise from Schwann cells, are benign tumors that can arise in the bile ducts. Eighty-seven percent of the cases in the United States have been in the black population. Two have been described in teenagers.[128]

BILE DUCT EPITHELIAL TUMORS
Biliary cystadenomas with mesenchymal stroma are benign tumors in young women but have malignant potential in middle-aged women. Cholangiocarcinomas have occurred in three adults with congenital hepatic fibrosis, the mild form of infantile polycystic disease.[129] We have observed cholangiocarcinoma in a 1-year-old boy with bile salt excretory protein deficiency. Carcinomas have been observed in the remnants of choledochal cysts, so surgeons have learned to excise the affected region.[130] Two cases of cholangiocarcinoma have been reported in young women

with chronic ulcerative colitis and sclerosing cholangitis. One patient was 17 years old.[131]

TERATOMAS
Primary teratomas are rare and usually affect females; half contain undifferentiated elements. When yolk sac tissue (endodermal sinus tumor) is present or the tumor is wholly yolk sac in type, α-fetoprotein levels can be strikingly increased. It was extremely high (77,000 μg/L) in a 17-month-old child with adjoining benign cystic teratoma and mixed hepatoblastoma and whose preoperative imaging studies identified only the benign tumor.[132] Ninety percent of teratomas are in infants. Treatment is surgical.

INFLAMMATORY MYOFIBROBLASTIC TUMOR, LYMPHOMA, AND LEUKEMIA
Inflammatory myofibroblastic tumor was originally called inflammatory pseudotumor or plasma cell granuloma. Anthony and Telesinghe described 17 patients with liver involvement, 6 of whom were less than 12 years old.[133] They presented with fever, abdominal pain, and/or vomiting. Jaundice was evident in four patients. Weight loss and diarrhea were also noted. There were solitary masses in eight patients and multiple nodules in four. The clinical impression and initial pathologic diagnosis may be confused with malignancy, but the histologic features of dense plasma cell infiltrates associated with active fibroplasia are indications of a chronic inflammatory process. The etiology is unknown, but some tumors have regressed with steroid therapy. On the other hand, the finding of hyperdiploidy in four of nine inflammatory pseudotumors, three of which recurred or metastasized,[134] suggested a neoplastic process. Rearrangements of the ALK gene at chromosome 2p23 have been observed in several inflammatory myofibroblastic tumors but not specifically in those involving the liver.[135] Portoenterostomy has been required for biliary obstruction in some cases. Transplant was needed for an 8-year-old girl whose hilar region was so extensively involved as to preclude resection.[136] Primary lymphomas of the liver of children are very rare and have monomorphous infiltrates without fibrosis.[137] Involvement of the liver in various forms of leukemia is common but only rarely of clinical significance. An exception is the megakaryoblastic leukemia of infancy, which can present with hepatomegaly and abnormal liver function tests prior to peripheral blood manifestations.[86] Liver biopsy shows diffuse infiltration of sinusoids by blast cells whose nature may not immediately be apparent. Platelet glycoprotein 2b immunostaining will be diagnostic. Diffuse scarring is prominent and a useful clue to the diagnosis.

NON-NEOPLASTIC HEPATIC MASSES
Non-neoplastic tumors include parasitic cysts, biliary and simple cysts, and nodular regenerative hyperplasia. All but the latter tend to present as masses and rarely because of jaundice. Most are diagnosed readily by a combination of imaging techniques, particularly ultrasonography. Nodular regeneration may present with signs of portal hypertension and is sometimes associated with collagen-vascular dis-

ease. The diagnosis is difficult even on biopsy, but neoplasia can be excluded. Two cases of maldeveloped fetuses with nodular regeneration have been described.[138]

SECONDARY NEOPLASIA OF THE LIVER

Neuroblastoma is the most common solid tumor metastasis in children. The primitive cells infiltrating sinusoids may be mistaken for hepatoblastoma in routine microscopic studies of small biopsies. Other malignancies spreading to the liver include Wilms tumor, rhabdomyosarcoma, Ewing sarcoma, intra-abdominal small cell desmoplastic tumor, and ovarian germ cell tumors. Among the 123 cases submitted for review to CCG and POG pathologists in the hepatoblastoma/hepatocarcinoma 1986 to 1989 intergroup study, 13 incorrectly diagnosed cases (10.6%) included examples of each of the above.[86]

TREATMENT

The primary goal in treating liver neoplasms is complete surgical removal. The tendency of tumors to reach very large size before discovery and an anatomy that allows interlobar spread are handicaps. For benign tumors, such as vascular hamartoma, focal nodular hyperplasia, and adenoma, extensive surgery may be unnecessary. Many benign lesions have responded to medical management or arterial embolization, and many are stable indefinitely.[103] Therefore, vigorous efforts are made to reach a diagnosis preoperatively and intraoperatively. When that is not possible or when malignancy is suspected, surgical resection is attempted. Newer imaging modalities have been helpful in delineating the extent of involvement preoperatively[70] and intraoperatively.[69] When initial surgery for a malignancy is deemed to be too risky, preoperative chemotherapy has proven effective in shrinking many hepatoblastomas and some sarcomas to the point of resectability. Beginning in 1981, Gauthier and colleagues have routinely used doxorubicin in combination with vincristine, cyclophosphamide, 5-fluorouracil, or cisplatinum, achieving resectability in over 80% of cases.[139] The POG was able to achieve resectability 29 of 37 (79%) hepatoblastomas with cisplatinum, vincristine, and 5-fluorouracil.[140] Seventy-seven percent of those resected had no evidence of disease at 13 to 54 months, a result identical to that observed among 26 patients who had primary resections. These good results have led some centers to treat all new cases with chemotherapy, sometimes without even a biopsy if the imaging studies and serum α-fetoprotein point to neoplasia.[141,142] This approach is deemed undesirable for three reasons.[143] The first is based on the concept of "favorable" histology discussed (above and) below. Primary resection of a stage I tumor permits a thorough histologic study. If such a tumor has favorable histology, toxic chemotherapy can be minimized or even eliminated. Second, in both the latest CCG[144] and POG[140] trials, the major surgical complications after chemotherapy (hemorrhage or bile duct injury) were significantly greater than those occurring after primary resections (CCG, 25% versus 8%; POG, 23% versus 0%). Finally, small cell undifferentiated histology in otherwise

typical, completely resected hepatoblastomas was associated with recurrence and fatality in at least 6 of 10 patients.[86,91] This unfavorable histology requiring alternative adjuvant therapy can easily be missed in a small biopsy.

The same chemotherapeutic regimens used preoperatively for unresectable tumors are then employed postoperatively. Nine patients with hepatoblastoma so treated by Gauthier and colleagues were cured,[139] and there have been case reports of pulmonary metastases being eliminated by such intense regimens. Recently, irinotecan has been added for unresponsive hepatoblastomas by the US Children's Oncology Group. The incidence of severe hematologic toxicity in the CCSG–Southwest Oncology Group study of 57 patients with hepatic malignancies given combination chemotherapy was 50%, and 3 children died of the complication.[145]

When completely resected lesions (stage I), which comprise 15 to 50% of different series, have been reviewed according to histologic subtype, the "pure" or "predominantly" fetal tumors were found in several series to have a good prognosis even without adjuvant therapy.[82,87] An analysis of 168 hepatoblastomas collected by the US Intergroup Study found 28 of 90 fetal cases to be resectable, and 87% of them survived 48 months.[85] In those series, the fetal cases were not further classified into "well-differentiated with low mitotic rate," a requirement that Weinberg and Finegold emphasize is necessary for a "favorable" designation.[3] Only 15% of 333 hepatoblastomas in the Intergroup,[85] Armed Forces Institute of Pathology,[146] and POG studies through 1989[140] were primarily resectable, but 92% (47 of 51) were disease free beyond 2 years. Embryonal tumors behaved less well in the early Intergroup series, with 20 of 50 cases being resectable and 63% of those surviving 48 months. All received combination chemotherapy. Tumors with a macrotrabecular growth pattern were uniformly unresectable, but 9 of 18 survived 48 months, which also is much more favorable than in all other reports to date. Just one of the small cell undifferentiated tumors was resectable, but all 10 children with small cell undifferentiated histology died within 24 months.[86] The POG and CCSG have since treated nine stage I well-differentiated fetal hepatoblastomas with doxorubicin for 4 months, with no recurrences in 5 years.[87] Patients with more advanced disease and unfavorable histologic patterns were treated with cisplatinum, vincristine, and 5-fluorouracil or cisplatinum and doxorubicin by continuous infusion; both groups had excellent results for stage I and II tumors and 64% event-free survival even for stage III. The former regimen had lesser toxicity.[87]

HCCs are resectable only 10 to 20% of the time. Nine of 46 HCCs in the latest intergroup study were resectable. Eighty-eight percent of those patients survived 5 years without disease on the same regimens as above. Neither regimen was beneficial for the higher stages of disease.[147] A better result was reported from Johns Hopkins University School of Medicine, where external beam radiation (2,100 cGy), chemotherapy, and radioiodinated antiferritin antibody were combined.[148] Forty-eight percent of the patients survived 5 years without evidence of tumor. Starzl and colleagues have performed liver transplants in selected cases with modest success.[149] Many of the failures were in the precyclosporine era, so early death owing to graft rejection or other complications limited evaluation. Starzl and colleagues reported transplant success in three of six patients with unresectable FLCs.[149] On the other hand, they also concluded that aggressive resection was preferable because only one of eight patients with a subtotal hepatectomy suffered a recurrence. A more recent review of the University of Pittsburgh School of Medicine experience with orthotopic liver transplant for liver cancers includes six children with hepatoblastomas, of whom five are alive with no evidence of disease at 1.9 ± 0.5 years, and nine with HCCs, with four being disease free for 1.2 years.[150] One additional patient with HCC who had upper abdominal exenteration is alive 14 months later. Six transplanted patients died of malignancy, five with recurrences and one of lymphoma. More recent transplant data indicate improved transplant expectations for HCC provided that tumors were not multicentric, larger than 5 cm, and did not exhibit vascular invasion, metastasis, or positive margins at initial surgery.[151] There is active discussion among surgeons caring for children with hepatic neoplasms about the potential benefits of primary transplant versus attempted resections in anatomically problematic cases.

CONCLUSION

The likelihood of new metabolic interventions to prevent hepatic malignancies, such as that for tyrosinemia, is currently highly speculative. However, rapidly increasing knowledge about molecular interactions of growth control and gene expression, as in the APC–β-catenin pathway, offers great promise for targeting loci that might be sensitive to manipulation, perhaps by specific inhibitory RNA, for example. Until these measures became clinically applicable, however, the potential benefits of careful periodic screening with the existing tools of ultrasonography and serum α-fetoprotein in susceptible populations such as survivors of extreme prematurity, chronic cholestasis, and the glycogenoses seem worthy of general application.

REFERENCES

1. Chang MH, Chen CJ, Lai MS, et al. Universal hepatitis B vaccination in Taiwan and the incidence of hepatocellular carcinoma in children. Taiwan Childhood Hepatoma Study Group. N Engl J Med 1997;336:1855–9.
2. Strickland DK, Jenkins JJ, Hudson MM. Hepatitis C infection and hepatocellular carcinoma after treatment of childhood cancer. J Pediatr Hematol Oncol 2001;23:527–9.
3. Weinberg AG, Finegold MJ. Primary hepatic tumors in childhood. In: Finegold MJ, editor. Pathology of neoplasia in children and adolescents. Philadelphia: WB Saunders; 1986. p. 333.
4. Ross JA, Gurney JG. Hepatoblastoma incidence in the United States from 1973 to 1992. Med Pediatr Oncol 1998;30:141–2.
5. Ikeda H, Matsuyama S, Tanimura M. Association between hepatoblastoma and very low birth weight: a trend or a chance? J Pediatr 1997;130:557–60.
6. Ikeda H, Hachitanda Y, Tanimura M, et al. Development of

7. Feusner J, Buckley J, Robison L, et al. Prematurity and hepatoblastoma: more than just an association? J Pediatr 1998;133:585–6.
8. von Schweinitz D, Byrd DJ, Hecker H, et al. Efficiency and toxicity of ifosfamide, cisplatin and doxorubicin in the treatment of childhood hepatoblastoma. Study Committee of the Cooperative Paediatric Liver Tumour Study HB89 of the German Society for Paediatric Oncology and Haematology. Eur J Cancer 1997;33:1243–9.
9. Ribons LA, Slovis TL. Hepatoblastoma and birth weight. J Pediatr 1998;132:750.
10. Chen WJ, Lee JC, Hung WT. Primary malignant tumor of liver in infants and children in Taiwan. J Pediatr Surg 1988;23:457–61.
11. Baptista M, Kramvis A, Kew MC. High prevalence of 1762(T) 1764(A) mutations in the basic core promoter of hepatitis B virus isolated from black Africans with hepatocellular carcinoma compared with asymptomatic carriers. Hepatology 1999;29:946–53.
12. Wang J, Chenivesse X, Henglein B, Brechot C. Hepatitis B virus integration in a cyclin A gene in a hepatocellular carcinoma. Nature 1990;343:555–7.
13. Nishida N, Fukuda Y, Ishizaki K, Nakao K. Alteration of cell cycle-related genes in hepatocarcinogenesis. Histol Histopathol 1997;12:1019–25.
14. Ohaki Y, Misugi K, Sasaki Y, Tsunoda A. Hepatitis B surface antigen positive hepatocellular carcinoma in children. Report of a case and review of the literature. Cancer 1983;51:822–8.
15. Larouze B, Saimot G, Lustbader ED, et al. Host responses to hepatitis-B infection in patients with primary hepatic carcinoma and their families. A case/control study in Senegal, West Africa. Lancet 1976;ii:534–8.
16. Giardiello FM, Petersen GM, Brensinger JD, et al. Hepatoblastoma and APC gene mutation in familial adenomatous polyposis. Gut 1996;39:867–9.
17. Dahms BB. Hepatoma in familial cholestatic cirrhosis of childhood: its occurrence in twin brothers. Arch Pathol Lab Med 1979;103:30–3.
18. Coire CI, Qizilbash AH, Castelli MF. Hepatic adenomata in type Ia glycogen storage disease. Arch Pathol Lab Med 1987;111:166–9.
19. Iqbal MJ, Wilkinson ML, Johnson PJ, Williams R. Sex steroid receptor proteins in foetal, adult and malignant human liver tissue. Br J Cancer 1983;48:791–6.
20. Nagasue N, Yukaya H, Chang YC, et al. Active uptake of testosterone by androgen receptors of hepatocellular carcinoma in humans. Cancer 1986;57:2162–7.
21. Ohnishi S, Murakami T, Moriyama T, et al. Androgen and estrogen receptors in hepatocellular carcinoma and in the surrounding noncancerous liver tissue. Hepatology 1986;6:440–3.
22. Chandra RS, Kapur SP, Kelleher J Jr, et al. Benign hepatocellular tumors in the young. A clinicopathologic spectrum. Arch Pathol Lab Med 1984;108:168–71.
23. Neuberger J, Forman D, Doll R, Williams R. Oral contraceptives and hepatocellular carcinoma. BMJ 1986;292:1355–7.
24. Stocker JT, Ishak KG. Focal nodular hyperplasia of the liver: a study of 21 pediatric cases. Cancer 1981;48:336–45.
25. Meyer P, LiVolsi V, Cornog JL. Hepatoblastoma associated with an oral contraceptive [letter]. Lancet 1974;ii:1387.
26. Selby DM, Stocker JT, Ishak KG. Angiosarcoma of the liver in childhood: a clinicopathologic and follow-up study of 10 cases. Pediatr Pathol 1992;12:485–98.
27. Buckley JD, Sather H, Ruccione K, et al. A case control study of

risk factors for hepatoblastoma. A report from the Children's Cancer Study Group. Cancer 1989;64:1169–76.

28. Baffet G, Deugnier Y, Lehry D. A study of oncogene activation in human hepatocellular carcinoma. Hepatology 1986;6:1212.

29. Boix L, Rosa JL, Ventura F, et al. c-met mRNA overexpression in human hepatocellular carcinoma. Hepatology 1994;19:88–91.

30. Ueki T, Fujimoto J, Suzuki T, et al. Expression of hepatocyte growth factor and its receptor c-met proto-oncogene in hepatocellular carcinoma. Hepatology 1997;25:862–6.

31. Kiss A, Szepesi A, Lotz G, et al. Expression of transforming growth factor-alpha in hepatoblastoma. Cancer 1998;83:690–7.

32. Sirica AE. The role of cell types in hepatocarcinogenesis. Boca Raton (FL): CRC Press; 1992. p. 291–2.

33. Sandgren EP, Luetteke NC, Qiu TH, et al. Transforming growth factor alpha dramatically enhances oncogene-induced carcinogenesis in transgenic mouse pancreas and liver. Mol Cell Biol 1993;13:320–30.

34. Takagi H, Sharp R, Hammermeister C, et al. Molecular and genetic analysis of liver oncogenesis in transforming growth factor alpha transgenic mice. Cancer Res 1992;52:5171–7.

35. Ohta K, Kanamaru T, Morita Y, et al. Telomerase activity in hepatocellular carcinoma as a predictor of postoperative recurrence. J Gastroenterol 1997;32:791–6.

36. Kim KS, Lee YI. Biallelic expression of the H19 and IGF2 genes in hepatocellular carcinoma. Cancer Lett 1997;119:143–8.

37. Piao Z, Choi Y, Park C, et al. Deletion of the M6P/IGF2r gene in primary hepatocellular carcinoma. Cancer Lett 1997;120:39–43.

38. Schofield D, Jackson G, Wetzel J, Triche T. Patterns of gene expression in hepatoblastoma and hepatocellular carcinoma. Lab Invest 1999;59:5P.

39. Donehower LA, Harvey M, Slagle BL, et al. Mice deficient for p53 are developmentally normal but susceptible to spontaneous tumours. Nature 1992;356:215–21.

40. Murakami Y, Hayashi K, Hirohashi S, Sekiya T. Aberrations of the tumor suppressor p53 and retinoblastoma genes in human hepatocellular carcinomas. Cancer Res 1991;51:5520–5.

41. Kanai Y, Hui AM, Sun L, et al. DNA hypermethylation at the D17S5 locus and reduced HIC-1 mRNA expression are associated with hepatocarcinogenesis. Hepatology 1999;29:703–9.

42. Shiota G, Kishimoto Y, Suyama A, et al. Prognostic significance of serum anti-p53 antibody in patients with hepatocellular carcinoma. J Hepatol 1997;27:661–8.

43. Labelle Y, Phaneuf D, Leclerc B, Tanguay RM. Characterization of the human fumarylacetoacetate hydrolase gene and identification of a missense mutation abolishing enzymatic activity. Hum Mol Genet 1993;2:941–6.

44. Lindstedt S, Holme E, Lock EA, et al. Treatment of hereditary tyrosinaemia type I by inhibition of 4-hydroxyphenylpyruvate dioxygenase. Lancet 1992;340:813–7.

45. Holme E, Lindstedt S. Nontransplant treatment of tyrosinemia. Clin Liver Dis 2000;4:805–14.

46. Kingston JE, Herbert A, Draper GJ, Mann JR. Association between hepatoblastoma and polyposis coli. Arch Dis Child 1983;58:959–62.

47. Hughes LJ, Michels VV. Risk of hepatoblastoma in familial adenomatous polyposis. Am J Med Genet 1992;43:1023–5.

48. Garber JE, Li FP, Kingston JE, et al. Hepatoblastoma and familial adenomatous polyposis. J Natl Cancer Inst 1988;80:1626–8.

49. Bodmer WF, Bailey CJ, Bodmer J, et al. Localization of the gene for familial adenomatous polyposis on chromosome 5. Nature 1987;328:614–6.

50. Oda H, Imai Y, Nakatsuru Y, et al. Somatic mutations of the APC gene in sporadic hepatoblastomas. Cancer Res 1996;56:3320–3.

51. Munemitsu S, Albert I, Souza B, et al. Regulation of intracellular beta-catenin levels by the adenomatous polyposis coli (APC) tumor-suppressor protein. Proc Natl Acad Sci U S A 1995;92:3046–50.

52. Koch A, Denkhaus D, Albrecht S, et al. Childhood hepatoblastomas frequently carry a mutated degradation targeting box of the beta-catenin gene. Cancer Res 1999;59:269–73.

53. de La CA, Romagnolo B, Billuart P, et al. Somatic mutations of the beta-catenin gene are frequent in mouse and human hepatocellular carcinomas. Proc Natl Acad Sci U S A 1998;95:8847–51.

54. Miyoshi Y, Iwao K, Nagasawa Y, et al. Activation of the beta-catenin gene in primary hepatocellular carcinomas by somatic alterations involving exon 3. Cancer Res 1998;58:2524–7.

55. Mascarello JT, Jones MC, Kadota RP, Krous HF. Hepatoblastoma characterized by trisomy 20 and double minutes. Cancer Genet Cytogenet 1990;47:243–7.

56. Tonk VS, Wilson KS, Timmons CF, Schneider NR. Trisomy 2, trisomy 20, and del(17p) as sole chromosomal abnormalities in three cases of hepatoblastoma. Genes Chromosomes Cancer 1994;11:199–202.

57. Hansen K, Bagtas J, Mark HF, et al. Undifferentiated small cell hepatoblastoma with a unique chromosomal translocation: a case report. Pediatr Pathol 1992;12:457–62.

58. Surace C, Leszl A, Perilongo G, et al. Fluorescent in situ hybridization (FISH) reveals frequent and recurrent numerical and structural abnormalities in hepatoblastoma with no informative karyotype. Med Pediatr Oncol 2002;39:536–9.

59. Slagle BL, Zhou YZ, Butel JS. Hepatitis B virus integration event in human chromosome 17p near the p53 gene identifies the region of the chromosome commonly deleted in virus-positive hepatocellular carcinomas. Cancer Res 1991;51:49–54.

60. Tatekawa Y, Asonuma K, Uemoto S, et al. Liver transplantation for biliary atresia associated with malignant hepatic tumors. J Pediatr Surg 2001;36:436–9.

61. Fabre M, Gauthier F, Martin V, et al. Hepatocarcinoma and preneoplastic lesions in chronic advanced liver disease in children. International Society of Pediatric Oncology XXVI Meeting; Paris; 1998 Sept 20–24;233.

62. Patterson K, Kapur SP, Chandra RS. Hepatocellular carcinoma in a noncirrhotic infant after prolonged parenteral nutrition. J Pediatr 1985;106:797–800.

63. Kaufman SS, Wood RP, Shaw BW Jr, et al. Hepatocarcinoma in a child with the Alagille syndrome. Am J Dis Child 1987;141:698–700.

64. Rabinovitz M, Imperial JC, Schade RR, Van Thiel DH. Hepatocellular carcinoma in Alagille's syndrome: a family study. J Pediatr Gastroenterol Nutr 1989;8:26–30.

65. Mundy GR. Hypercalcemia of malignancy revisited. J Clin Invest 1988;82:1–6.

66. Muraji T, Woolley MM, Sinatra F, et al. The prognostic implication of hypercholesterolemia in infants and children with hepatoblastoma. J Pediatr Surg 1985;20:228–30.

67. Galifer RB, Sultan C, Margueritte G, Barneon G. Testosterone-producing hepatoblastoma in a 3-year-old boy with precocious puberty. J Pediatr Surg 1985;20:713–4.

68. Okuda K. Early recognition of hepatocellular carcinoma. Hepatology 1986;6:729–38.

69. Thomas BL, Krummel TM, Parker GA, et al. Use of intraoperative ultrasound during hepatic resection in pediatric patients. J Pediatr Surg 1989;24:690–2.

70. Mortele KJ, Mergo PJ, Urrutia M, Ros PR. Dynamic gadolinium-enhanced MR findings in infantile hepatic hemangioendothelioma. J Comput Assist Tomogr 1998;22:714–7.

71. Malt RA. Fibrolamellar hepatocellular carcinoma (CPC). N Engl J Med 1987;317:556.

72. Kairemo KJ, Lindahl H, Merenmies J, et al. Anti-alpha-fetoprotein imaging is useful for staging hepatoblastoma. Transplantation 2002;73:1151–4.

73. Scheimberg I, Cullinane C, Kelsey A, Malone M. Primary hepatic malignant tumor with rhabdoid features. A histological, immunocytochemical, and electron microscopic study of four cases and a review of the literature. Am J Surg Pathol 1996;20:1394–400.

74. Ruck P, Xiao JC, Kaiserling E. Small epithelial cells and the histogenesis of hepatoblastoma. Electron microscopic, immunoelectron microscopic, and immunohistochemical findings. Am J Pathol 1996;148:321–9.

75. Tamura S, Amuro Y, Nakano T, et al. Urinary excretion of pseudouridine in patients with hepatocellular carcinoma. Cancer 1986;57:1571–5.

76. Collier NA, Weinbren K, Bloom SR, et al. Neurotensin secretion by fibrolamellar carcinoma of the liver. Lancet 1984;i:538–40.

77. Wheeler K, Pritchard J, Luck W, Rossiter M. Transcobalamin I as a "marker" for fibrolamellar hepatoma. Med Pediatr Oncol 1986;14:227–9.

78. Weitz IC, Liebman HA. Des-gamma-carboxy (abnormal) prothrombin and hepatocellular carcinoma: a critical review. Hepatology 1993;18:990–7.

79. Zimmermann A. Hepatoblastoma with cholangioblastic features ('cholangioblastic hepatoblastoma') and other liver tumors with bimodal differentiation in young patients. Med Pediatr Oncol 2002;39:487–91.

80. Manivel C, Wick MR, Abenoza P, Dehner LP. Teratoid hepatoblastoma. The nosologic dilemma of solid embryonic neoplasms of childhood. Cancer 1986;57:2168–74.

81. Ishak KG, Glunz PR. Hepatoblastoma and hepatocarcinoma in infancy and childhood. Report of 47 cases. Cancer 1967;20:396–422.

82. Kasai M, Watanabe I. Histologic classification of liver-cell carcinoma in infancy and childhood and its clinical evaluation. A study of 70 cases collected in Japan. Cancer 1970;25:551–63.

83. Gonzalez-Crussi F, Upton MP, Maurer HS. Hepatoblastoma. Attempt at characterization of histologic subtypes. Am J Surg Pathol 1982;6:599–612.

84. Haas JE, Muczynski KA, Krailo M, et al. Histopathology and prognosis in childhood hepatoblastoma and hepatocarcinoma. Cancer 1989;64:1082–95.

85. Finegold MJ. Tumors of the liver. Semin Liver 1994;14:270.

86. Ortega JA, Douglass EC, Feusner JH, et al. Randomized comparison of cisplatin/vincristine/fluorouracil and cisplatin/continuous infusion doxorubicin for treatment of pediatric hepatoblastoma: a report from the Children's Cancer Group and the Pediatric Oncology Group. J Clin Oncol 2000;18:2665–75.

87. Schmidt D, Wischmeyer P, Leuschner I, et al. DNA analysis in hepatoblastoma by flow and image cytometry. Cancer 1993;72:2914–9.

88. Ruck P, Xiao JC, Kaiserling E. P53 protein expression in hepatoblastoma: an immunohistochemical investigation. Pediatr Pathol 1994;14:79–85.

89. Rowland JM. Hepatoblastoma: assessment of criteria for histologic classification. Med Pediatr Oncol 2002;39:478–83.

90. Haas JE, Feusner JH, Finegold MJ. Small cell undifferentiated histology in hepatoblastoma may be unfavorable. Cancer 2001;92:3130–4.

91. Parham DM, Peiper SC, Robicheaux G, et al. Malignant rhabdoid tumor of the liver. Evidence for epithelial differentiation. Arch Pathol Lab Med 1988;112:61–4.

92. Abenoza P, Manivel JC, Wick MR, et al. Hepatoblastoma: an immunohistochemical and ultrastructural study. Hum Pathol 1987;18:1025–35.

93. Saxena R, Leake JL, Shafford EA, et al. Chemotherapy effects on hepatoblastoma. A histological study. Am J Surg Pathol 1993;17:1266–71.

94. Heifetz SA, French M, Correa M, Grosfeld JL. Hepatoblastoma: the Indiana experience with preoperative chemotherapy for inoperable tumors; clinicopathological considerations. Pediatr Pathol Lab Med 1997;17:857–74.

95. Brotto M, Finegold MJ. Distinct patterns of p27/KIP 1 gene expression in hepatoblastoma and prognostic implications with correlation before and after chemotherapy. Hum Pathol 2002;33:198–205.

96. von Schweinitz D, Hecker H, Harms D, et al. Complete resection before development of drug resistance is essential for survival from advanced hepatoblastoma—a report from the German Cooperative Liver Tumor Study. J Pediatr Surg 1995;30:845–52.

97. LeBrun DP, Silver MM, Freedman MH, Phillips MJ. Fibrolamellar carcinoma of the liver in a patient with Fanconi anemia. Hum Pathol 1991;22:396–8.

98. Katzenstein HM, Krailo MD, Malogolowkin MH, et al. Fibrolamellar hepatocellular carcinoma in children and adolescents. Cancer 2003;97:2006–12.

99. Berman MA, Burnham JA, Sheahan DG. Fibrolamellar carcinoma of the liver: an immunohistochemical study of nineteen cases and a review of the literature. Hum Pathol 1988;19:784–94.

100. Van Eyken P, Sciot R, Brock P, et al. Abundant expression of cytokeratin 7 in fibrolamellar carcinoma of the liver. Histopathology 1990;17:101–7.

101. Orsatti G, Hytiroglou P, Thung SN, et al. Lamellar fibrosis in the fibrolamellar variant of hepatocellular carcinoma: a role for transforming growth factor beta. Liver 1997;17:152–6.

102. Payne CM, Nagle RB, Paplanus SH, Graham AR. Fibrolamellar carcinoma of liver: a primary malignant oncocytic carcinoid? Ultrastruct Pathol 1986;10:539–52.

103. Holcomb GW III, O'Neill JA Jr, Mahboubi S, Bishop HC. Experience with hepatic hemangioendothelioma in infancy and childhood. J Pediatr Surg 1988;23:661–6.

104. Dehner LP, Ishak KG. Vascular tumors of the liver in infants and children. A study of 30 cases and review of the literature. Arch Pathol 1971;92:101–11.

105. Lederman SM, Martin EC, Laffey KT, Lefkowitch JH. Hepatic neurofibromatosis, malignant schwannoma, and angiosarcoma in von Recklinghausen's disease. Gastroenterology 1987;92:234–9.

106. Peters ME, Gilbert-Barness EF, Rao B, Odell GB. Lymphangioendothelioma of the liver in a neonate. J Pediatr Gastroenterol Nutr 1989;9:115–8.

107. Jozwiak S, Michalowicz R, Pedich M, Rajszys P. Hepatic hamartoma in tuberous sclerosis. Lancet 1992;339:180.

108. Gramlich TL, Killough BW, Garvin AJ. Mesenchymal hamartoma of the liver: report of a case in a 28-year-old. Hum Pathol 1988;19:991–2.

109. de Chadarevian JP, Pawel BR, Faerber EN, Weintraub WH. Undifferentiated (embryonal) sarcoma arising in conjunction with mesenchymal hamartoma of the liver. Mod Pathol 1994;7:490–3.

110. Corbally MT, Spitz L. Malignant potential of mesenchymal hamartoma: an unrecognized risk. Pediatr Surg Int 1992;7:321.

111. Walker NI, Horn MJ, Strong RW, et al. Undifferentiated (embryonal) sarcoma of the liver. Pathologic findings and long-term survival after complete surgical resection. Cancer 1992;69:52–9.

112. Lauwers GY, Grant LD, Donnelly WH, et al. Hepatic undiffer

entiated (embryonal) sarcoma arising in a mesenchymal hamartoma. Am J Surg Pathol 1997;21:1248–54.

113. Begueret H, Trouette H, Vielh P, et al. Hepatic undifferentiated embryonal sarcoma: malignant evolution of mesenchymal hamartoma? Study of one case with immunohistochemical and flow cytometric emphasis. J Hepatol 2001;34:178–9.

114. Bove KE, Blough RI, Soukup S. Third report of t(19q)(13.4) in mesenchymal hamartoma of liver with comments on link to embryonal sarcoma. Pediatr Dev Pathol 1998;1:438–42.

115. O'Sullivan MJ, Swanson PE, Knoll J, et al. Undifferentiated embryonal sarcoma with unusual features arising within mesenchymal hamartoma of the liver: report of a case and review of the literature. Pediatr Dev Pathol 2001;4:482–9.

116. Stocker JT, Ishak KG. Undifferentiated (embryonal) sarcoma of the liver: report of 31 cases. Cancer 1978;42:336–48.

117. Aoyama C, Hachitanda Y, Sato JK, et al. Undifferentiated (embryonal) sarcoma of the liver. A tumor of uncertain histogenesis showing divergent differentiation. Am J Surg Pathol 1991;15:615–24.

118. Lack EE, Schloo BL, Azumi N, et al. Undifferentiated (embryonal) sarcoma of the liver. Clinical and pathologic study of 16 cases with emphasis on immunohistochemical features. Am J Surg Pathol 1991;15:1–16.

119. Sowery RD, Jensen C, Morrison KB, et al. Comparative genomic hybridization detects multiple chromosomal amplifications and deletions in undifferentiated embryonal sarcoma of the liver. Cancer Genet Cytogenet 2001;126:128–33.

120. Urban CE, Mache CJ, Schwinger W, et al. Undifferentiated (embryonal) sarcoma of the liver in childhood. Successful combined-modality therapy in four patients. Cancer 1993; 72:2511–6.

121. Bisogno G, Pilz T, Perilongo G, et al. Undifferentiated sarcoma of the liver in childhood: a curable disease. Cancer 2002; 94:252–7.

122. Harris MB, Shen S, Weiner MA, et al. Treatment of primary undifferentiated sarcoma of the liver with surgery and chemotherapy. Cancer 1984;54:2859–62.

123. Geoffray A, Couanet D, Montagne JP, et al. Ultrasonography and computed tomography for diagnosis and follow-up of biliary duct rhabdomyosarcomas in children. Pediatr Radiol 1987; 17:127–31.

124. Mihara S, Matsumoto H, Tokunaga F, et al. Botryoid rhabdomyosarcoma of the gallbladder in a child. Cancer 1982; 49:812–8.

125. Chang CH, Ramirez N, Sakr WA. Primitive neuroectodermal tumor of the brain associated with malignant rhabdoid tumor of the liver: a histologic, immunohistochemical, and electron microscopic study. Pediatr Pathol 1989;9:307–19.

126. Ross JS, Del Rosario A, Bui HX, et al. Primary hepatic leiomyosarcoma in a child with the acquired immunodeficiency syndrome. Hum Pathol 1992;23:69–72.

127. Timmons CF, Dawson DB, Richards CS, et al. Epstein-Barr virus-associated leiomyosarcomas in liver transplantation recipients. Origin from either donor or recipient tissue. Cancer 1995;76:1481–9.

128. Butler JD Jr, Brown KM. Granular cell tumor of the extrahepatic biliary tract. Am Surg 1998;64:1033–6.

129. Daroca PJ Jr, Tuthill R, Reed RJ. Cholangiocarcinoma arising in congenital hepatic fibrosis. A case report. Arch Pathol 1975; 99:592–5.

130. Bloustein PA. Association of carcinoma with congenital cystic conditions of the liver and bile ducts. Am J Gastroenterol 1977;67:40–6.

131. Ham JM, MacKenzie DC. Primary carcinoma of the extrahepatic bile ducts. Surg Gynecol Obstet 1964;118:977.

132. Conrad RJ, Gribbin D, Walker NI, Ong TH. Combined cystic teratoma and hepatoblastoma of the liver. Probable divergent differentiation of an uncommitted hepatic precursor cell. Cancer 1993;72:2910–3.

133. Anthony PP, Telesinghe PU. Inflammatory pseudotumour of the liver. J Clin Pathol 1986;39:761–8.

134. Biselli R, Ferlini C, Fattorossi A, et al. Inflammatory myofibroblastic tumor (inflammatory pseudotumor): DNA flow cytometric analysis of nine pediatric cases. Cancer 1996;77:778–84.

135. Coffin CM, Patel A, Perkins S, et al. ALK1 and p80 expression and chromosomal rearrangements involving 2p23 in inflammatory myofibroblastic tumor. Mod Pathol 2001;14:569–76.

136. Heneghan MA, Kaplan CG, Priebe CJ Jr, Partin JS. Inflammatory pseudotumor of the liver: a rare cause of obstructive jaundice and portal hypertension in a child. Pediatr Radiol 1984;14:433–5.

137. Miller ST, Wollner N, Meyers PA, et al. Primary hepatic or hepatosplenic non-Hodgkin's lymphoma in children. Cancer 1983;52:2285–8.

138. Galdeano S, Drut R. Nodular regenerative hyperplasia of fetal liver: a report of two cases. Pediatr Pathol 1991;11:479–85.

139. Gauthier F, Valayer J, Thai BL, et al. Hepatoblastoma and hepatocarcinoma in children: analysis of a series of 29 cases. J Pediatr Surg 1986;21:424–9.

140. Reynolds M, Douglass EC, Finegold M, et al. Chemotherapy can convert unresectable hepatoblastoma. J Pediatr Surg 1992;27:1080–3.

141. Fuchs J, Rydzynski J, von Schweinitz D, et al. Pretreatment prognostic factors and treatment results in children with hepatoblastoma: a report from the German Cooperative Pediatric Liver Tumor Study HB 94. Cancer 2002;95:172–82.

142. Ehrlich PF, Greenberg ML, Filler RM. Improved long-term survival with preoperative chemotherapy for hepatoblastoma. J Pediatr Surg 1997;32:999–1002.

143. Finegold MJ. Chemotherapy for suspected hepatoblastoma without efforts at surgical resection is a bad practice. Med Pediatr Oncol 2002;39:484–6.

144. Ortega JA, Krailo MD, Haas JE, et al. Effective treatment of unresectable or metastatic hepatoblastoma with cisplatin and continuous infusion doxorubicin chemotherapy: a report from the Children's Cancer Study Group. J Clin Oncol 1991;9:2167–76.

145. Evans AE, Land VJ, Newton WA, et al. Combination chemotherapy (vincristine, adriamycin, cyclophosphamide, and 5-fluorouracil) in the treatment of children with malignant hepatoma. Cancer 1982;50:821–6.

146. Conran RM, Hitchcock CL, Waclawiw MA, et al. Hepatoblastoma: the prognostic significance of histologic type. Pediatr Pathol 1992;12:167–83.

147. Katzenstein HM, Krailo MD, Malogolowkin MH, et al. Hepatocellular carcinoma in children and adolescents: results from the Pediatric Oncology Group and the Children's Cancer Group intergroup study. J Clin Oncol 2002;20:2789–97.

148. Sitzmann JV, Abrams R. Improved survival for hepatocellular cancer with combination surgery and multimodality treatment. Ann Surg 1993;217:149–54.

149. Starzl TE, Iwatsuki S, Shaw BW Jr, et al. Treatment of fibrolamellar hepatoma with partial or total hepatectomy and transplantation of the liver. Surg Gynecol Obstet 1986;162: 145–8.

150. Tagge EP, Tagge DU, Reyes J, et al. Resection, including transplantation, for hepatoblastoma and hepatocellular carcinoma: impact on survival. J Pediatr Surg 1992;27:292–6.

151. Iwatsuki S, Dvorchik I, Marsh JW, et al. Liver transplantation for hepatocellular carcinoma: a proposal of a prognostic scoring system. J Am Coll Surg 2000;191:389–94.

CHAPTER 55

GENETIC AND METABOLIC DISORDERS

1. *Carbohydrate Metabolism*

Simon Horslen, MB, ChB, FRCPCH

An infant is brought into the office or seen as an inpatient consultation. You ask yourself, "Is this conglomeration of clinical features the result of a defect of hepatic carbohydrate metabolism? If it is, how do I make the diagnosis? How do I manage the infant in the short term? What are the long-term consequences of this disease state? And how do I explain the disease to the family?" The intention of this chapter is to assist in answering these questions.

A brief review of normal hepatic glucose, fructose, and galactose metabolism will allow the individual metabolic defects that have been identified in humans to be placed within a physiologic context. Each enzyme defect is explored in terms of clinical presentation, genetics, pathogenesis and clinical consequences, treatment, and prognosis.

Apart from the classic pathways of carbohydrate metabolism (ie, glycolysis/gluconeogenesis), other pathways involve carbohydrate moieties. Examples include defects of glucuronidation, as in Crigler-Najjar syndrome, in which glucuronide conjugation with bilirubin is interrupted; defective glycosylation of intracellular proteins, as in I-cell disease, in which mannose 6-phosphate fails to be added to proteins intended for lysosomal compartmentalization; and defective glycosylation of glycoproteins, as occurs in the carbohydrate-deficient glycoprotein syndromes. Defects in these pathways may have hepatic implication but lie outside the scope of this chapter.

INITIAL MANAGEMENT OF SUSPECTED CASES OF INBORN ERRORS OF CARBOHYDRATE METABOLISM

The first suspicion that a defect in carbohydrate metabolism may be underlying a child's illness arises from the understanding of the presenting features of this group of conditions. Clinical features that may be associated with disorders of hepatic carbohydrate metabolism are shown in Table 55.1-1. Initial investigations may include those suggested in Table 55.1-2. In many circumstances, an infant may be acutely unwell and in need of care prior to the results of diagnostic tests being available. The following steps should be taken while awaiting the results of diagnostic investigations:

- Measure the blood glucose and correct hypoglycemia with intravenous (IV) glucose solutions aiming at 8 to 9 mg of glucose/kg/min, an infant's normal rate for hepatic glucose synthesis. Avoid protein and lipid input until more diagnostic information is available (there may be an inborn error of metabolism other than one affecting carbohydrate metabolism).
- Collect blood and urine cultures followed by empiric broad-spectrum antibiotics. *Escherichia coli* sepsis is a particular association with galactosemia. Rule out disseminated viral syndromes, particularly herpesviruses.
- Measure prothrombin time and partial thromboplastin time and consider correcting coagulopathy if present.
- Manage any other features of liver failure.
- Provide general supportive measures such as rehydration and management of acidosis.

The approach to investigation and management of infants with potential metabolic defects has been excellently reviewed in a number of publications.[1-3]

TABLE 55.1-1	POSSIBLE PRESENTING FEATURES OF DEFECTS OF CARBOHYDRATE METABOLISM
Neonate	Hypoglycemia, vomiting, diarrhea, lethargy, poor feeding, sepsis syndrome, lactic acidosis, jaundice, hemolysis, hypotonia, seizures, liver failure
Infant	Hypoglycemia or hypoglycemic seizure, failure to thrive, episodic vomiting, hepatomegaly, abnormal liver function tests, chronic liver disease, cataracts
Child	Hepatomegaly, failure to thrive, short stature, anomalous eating behavior/sugar avoidance, developmental delay

TABLE 55.1-2   SUGGESTED INITIAL INVESTIGATIONS

Blood/plasma/serum samples
 Electrolytes
 Liver function tests
 Coagulation studies (prothrombin time/partial thromboplastin time)
 Blood gases
 Blood glucose
 Insulin level
 Lactate and pyruvate
 Free fatty acid and 3-OH-butyrate
 Urate
 Triglycerides and cholesterol
 Phosphate and magnesium
 Red blood cell galactose 1-phosphate uridyl transferase activity
 Sugar chromatography
 Urine sample
 Ketones
 Reducing substances

Many of these investigations will be most informative if collected at the time of hypoglycemia. Therefore, when suspecting an inborn error of carbohydrate metabolism in a sick infant, it is important to attempt to collect the samples immediately at presentation because the opportunity for "safe" hypoglycemia may not present itself for some time. In other cases, a controlled fast should be arranged. In many cases, this list will be in addition to specific investigations of infantile liver disease and/or a full metabolic workup depending on specific clinical features.

NORMAL CARBOHYDRATE METABOLISM IN HUMANS

Glucose is the main energy source for most tissues in the human body; therefore, the liver's role in maintaining glucose homeostasis is one of fundamental importance. Glucose derived from dietary intake is intermittent, and it is the responsibility of the liver to maintain the circulating glucose pool within relatively confined limits during fasting and following a feed. To do this, the liver needs to be able to take up and store excess carbohydrate to be released as glucose at times of need. Glucose can be generated either through the pathways of gluconeogenesis or by the degradation of stored glycogen. Although there are gluconeogenic tissues other than liver, such as muscle and kidney, the only cell type capable of exporting free glucose in significant amounts is the hepatocyte. Regulation of glucose uptake and release is under hormonal control. At times of high dietary glucose intake, insulin increases and promotes the uptake of glucose and the laying down of glycogen by the liver cells. As the time from the last feed increases, insulin levels fall, glucagon levels increase, and

FIGURE 55.1-1 Major pathways of normal hepatic carbohydrate metabolism. Enzymes known to be affected in inborn errors of hepatic carbohydrate metabolism are shown. GLUT = glucose transporter; UDP = uridine diphosphate.

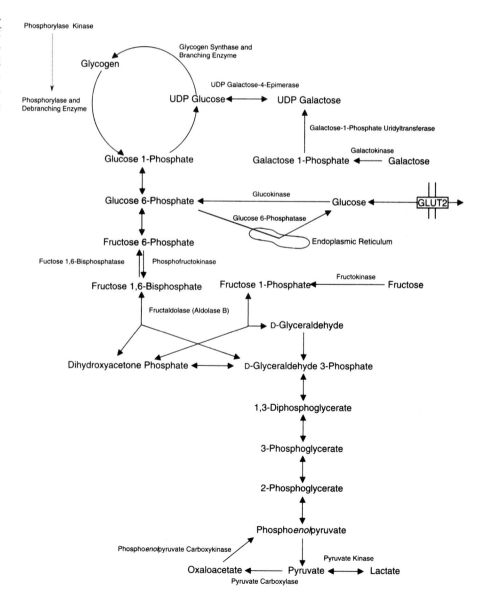

glucose synthesis and release by the liver cells increase. Hepatocytes will also synthesize and release glucose in response to epinephrine as part of the "fight or flight" response. The ability of hepatocytes to generate free glucose is due to the expression of glucose 6-phosphatase, the enzyme required for the dephosphorylation of glucose 6-phosphate. The pathways of normal carbohydrate metabolism are outlined in Figure 55.1-1.

The majority of dietary carbohydrates are absorbed in the form of glucose, galactose, and fructose. Glucose and galactose primarily enter the hepatocytes via the facultative glucose transport (GLUT) protein GLUT2. The GLUT proteins, a family of transmembrane monosaccharide transporters, are present in all human tissues. GLUT isoforms vary by tissue type, with hepatocytes expressing primarily GLUT2. The 12 transmembrane domains are thought to form a hydrophilic tunnel through the hydrophobic lipid cell membrane. Alteration in protein configuration, triggered by the concentration gradient, exposes the specific monosaccharide-binding site either inside or outside the membrane, allowing movement of glucose in both directions. GLUT proteins transport glucose only into most cells because, unlike hepatocytes, they lack net synthesis of glucose. Exceptions to the one-way transport of glucose include, in addition to the hepatocyte, enterocytes and kidney tubular cells. Fructose transport is less clearly understood. All three sugars ultimately enter the common pathway of glycolysis/gluconeogenesis following phosphorylation by specific kinases.

To enable a rapid and consistent generation of free glucose during periods of fasting, a form of storage is essential. This is primarily in the form of glycogen, a branched-chain glucose polymer. Many other tissues in the body have the enzymes required for synthesis and breakdown of glycogen, but most glycogen is found in liver and muscle. In muscle, glycogen is stored as an energy source to be used at times of high energy expenditure by muscle fibers themselves, whereas liver exports glucose to maintain circulating glucose pool and supply the other tissues of the body. Glycogen can be seen on electron microscopy in the form of β particles in muscle and liver and also as larger α particles in liver. The chemical differences to account for the morphologic difference between α and β particles have not been explained. The β particle consists of one molecule of glycogen with the proteins required for glycogen metabolism and some minor constituents, such as glucosamine and inorganic phosphate, the function of which is not clear.

The initiating event in glycogen synthesis is autoglycosylation of the protein glycogenin.[4] This protein not only acts as the substrate to which a glucose residue is covalently bound, it also actively catabolizes the reactions for the polymerization of the growing glucose chain up to a length of 6 to 10 glucose residues. At this stage, further chain lengthening is controlled by glycogen synthase, using uridine diphosphate (UDP) glucose and catalyzing the formation of 1,4-α linkages with the terminal glucose residue of the growing polymer. This produces straight-chain lengthening; the characteristic branching of these chains is catalyzed by another enzyme, amylo-(1,4),(1,6)-transglucosidase ("branching enzyme"). Branching enzyme disrupts 1,4-α

bonds, at least six glucose residues from the terminal residue, and reforms a branch point with 1,6-α linkages.

Under hormonal control, glycogen metabolism is able to switch rapidly from net synthesis to net breakdown. Insulin induces glycogen synthesis, but both glucagon and epinephrine can override this mechanism and induce glycogen breakdown to increase glucose production. The hormonal signals have opposing effects on the phosphorylation of key enzymes for both synthesis and breakdown of glycogen. Following a feed, under the influence of elevated insulin levels, glycogen synthase is activated by dephosphorylation, whereas glycogen phosphorylase (responsible for glycogen degradation) is inhibited. In the fasting state, with glucagon predominating, the enzymes are again phosphorylated, which reduces the activity of glycogen synthase, and glycogen phosphorylase is activated.

Glycogen degradation requires two enzymes. Phosphorylase cleaves the 1,4-α link of terminal glycosyl units, releasing glucose 1-phosphate. Phosphorylase is activated by the action of phosphorylase kinase. This cytosolic protein kinase is itself activated by phosphorylation, via cyclic adenosine monophosphate–dependent protein kinase, and by binding ionic calcium. Phosphorylase continues degrading glycogen, one residue at a time, until only four glycosyl residues remain beyond a branch point. At this stage, debranching enzyme is needed for further degradation of the glycogen molecule. Debranching enzyme uniquely possesses two independent catalytic sites on a single polypeptide strand. Initially, the three terminal residues beyond the branch point are moved to the end of another chain using transferase activity. The actual debranching activity (amylo-1,6-glucosidase) then hydrolyzes the 1,6-α branch point, releasing a single molecule of glucose (Figure 55.1-2).

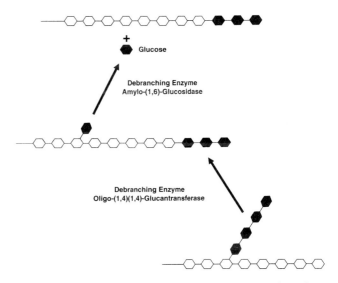

FIGURE 55.1-2 Action of debranching enzyme. Debranching enzyme has two catalytic sites on a single protein strand. When the action of glycogen phosphorylase has reduced a glycogen side chain to just four glycosol residues, the transferase activity of debranching enzyme transfers the three terminal residues to the end of an adjacent branch. The final residue is released as a single molecule of free glucose by glucosidase activity of the debranching enzyme.

Conversion of glucose 1-phosphate to glucose 6-phosphate enables the production of free glucose by the glucose 6-phosphatase system. Unlike other enzymes involved in glycolysis or gluconeogenesis, which are located in cytosol, glucose 6-phosphatase activity is found in the endoplasmic reticulum. This compartmentalization implies the need for a glucose 6-phosphate transporter, as well as the catalytic enzyme itself. These two enzymes, along with a putative phosphate transporter and a glucose transporter, are the proposed components of the "translocase-catalytic unit model" of the glucose 6-phosphatase system (Figure 55.1-3). To date, only the glucose 6-phosphatase and glucose 6-phosphate translocase units have been cloned and characterized. Glucose 6-phosphate can also be catabolized via the glycolysis pathway. This proceeds via triose phosphate to pyruvate and lactate or to acetyl coenzyme A (CoA) and entry into the tricarboxylic acid (TCA) cycle for oxidative phosphorylation and energy production.

In addition to glycogen breakdown, free glucose can also be synthesized via the gluconeogenic pathway. This is essentially the reverse of the glycolytic pathway, using all of the reversible enzyme steps from pyruvate back to glucose 6-phosphate. There are two steps in the glycolytic pathway that are irreversible, and alternate enzymes are used to bypass these steps. The first enzyme of the gluconeogenic pathway is pyruvate carboxylase, which catalyzes the conversion of pyruvate to oxaloacetate. This, in addition to phospho-*enol*pyruvate carboxykinase (PEPCK), is essential for bypassing the irreversible action of pyruvate kinase. Pyruvate carboxylase is an intramitochondrial biotin-containing protein and a key regulator of gluconeogenesis. The conversion from oxaloacetate to phospho*enol*pyruvate is catalyzed by PEPCK.

The second irreversible enzymatic reaction in glycolysis involves phosphofructokinase, the conversion of fructose

1-phosphate to fructose 1,6-bisphosphate. Reversal of this, that is, splitting fructose 1,6-bisphosphate to fructose 1-phosphate and ionic phosphate, involves a Mg-dependent enzyme, fructose 1,6-bisphosphatase. The determination of overall flux in the direction of gluconeogenesis or glycolysis involves another isomeric form of fructose diphosphate. Fructose 2,6-bisphosphate inhibits the activity of fructose 1,6-bisphosphatase and activates phosphofructokinase, increasing flux through the glycolytic pathway. Fructose 2,6-bisphosphate synthesized from glucose is present in increased concentrations in the fed state and thus blocks gluconeogenesis.

DEFECTS OF HEPATIC CARBOHYDRATE METABOLISM

INBORN ERRORS OF GLYCOGEN METABOLISM

Glycogen Storage Disease Type I: Glucose 6-Phophatase Deficiency (von Gierke Disease). The usual presentation of glycogen storage disease (GSD) I is an infant of a few months with a protuberant abdomen, short stature, and fasting hypoglycemia.[5,6] An overview of hepatic defects of glycogen metabolisms is given in Table 55.1-3. Frequent breast- or bottle-feeding of newborns often protects them during early infancy. A neonatal presentation is recognized with severe metabolic decompensation, hypoglycemia, and lactic acidosis.[7] Such a fulminant presentation may be fatal even with aggressive management.

At the time of presentation, an infant may be noted to have the characteristic "doll's" facies with big cheeks owing to excessive subcutaneous fat deposition. The protuberant abdomen is due to massive hepatomegaly, with-

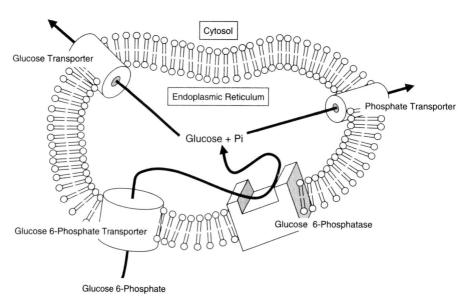

FIGURE 55.1-3 Translocase-catalytic model of the glucose 6-phosphatase system. Glucose 6-phosphatase is transported into the lumen to where the catalytic activity of the enzyme system resides. Free glucose and inorganic phosphate produced by the actions of glucose 6-phosphatase need to be removed from the endoplasmic reticulum because they inhibit the further action of glucose 6-phosphatase. The phosphate transporter remains to be fully characterized and the glucose transporter remains hypothetical at present. Pi = inorganic phosphate.

TABLE 55.1-3   GLYCOGEN STORAGE DISEASES

	EPONYM	ENZYME DEFECT	PRINCIPAL TISSUES AFFECTED
GSD I	von Gierke disease		
a		Glucose 6-phosphatase	Liver, kidney
b		Glucose 6-phosphate transporter	Liver, kidney, neutrophils
c		Phosphate transporter	
d		Glucose transporter	
GSD II	Pompe disease	Acid α-glucosidase	Heart, muscle
GSD III	Forbes or Cori disease	Debrancher enzyme	
a			Liver, muscle
b			Liver
GSD IV	Andersen disease	Brancher enzyme	Liver, heart
GSD V	McArdle disease	Muscle phosphorylase	Muscle
GSD VI	Hers disease	Hepatic phosphorylase	Liver
GSD VII	Tarui disease	Phosphofructokinase	Muscle
GSD IX (VIII McKusick)		Phosphorylase kinase	Liver
FBS	Fanconi-Bickel syndrome	GLUT 2	Liver, kidney
GSD 0		Glycogen synthase	Liver

GLUT = glucose transporter; GSD = glycogen storage disease.

out splenomegaly. Kidney enlargement is also present but is usually noted only on ultrasonography. The characteristic biochemical features of GSD I are fasting hypoglycemia with elevated plasma lactate, urate, and triglycerides. Cholesterol is also elevated, but not to the same extent as triglycerides. Mucosal bleeding or excessive bruising may be noted owing to platelet dysfunction as a consequence of hyperlipidemia.

Liver histology shows swollen hepatocytes with apparent cell wall thickening owing to peripheral displacement of organelles by the stored glycogen, which produces an appearance likened to plant cells. The excessive cytoplasmic glycogen stains with periodic acid–Schiff (PAS) and is readily digested by diastase. Microvesicular fat is almost invariably seen in the biopsy, but there is little in the way of inflammatory activity or fibrosis. These changes, although characteristic, are not pathognomonic, and differentiating the type of GSD on histologic criteria is not reliable.

A German pathologist, Edgar Otto Conrad von Gierke, first described GSD I in 1929.[8] Later it was demonstrated that the disease was due to the lack of activity of hepatic glucose 6-phosphatase activity.[9] There were, however, many patients who shared the phenotype but who still had glucose 6-phosphatase activity on frozen liver specimens. These patients were said to have GSD Ib. The hypothesis that this subtype was due to a defect in microsomal membrane transport was eventually proven with the identification of glucose 6-phosphate translocase (see Figure 55.1-3).[10-12] A third subtype, GSD Ic, has been shown to be genetically separate from types Ia and Ib and is thought to be a defect in a microsomal phosphate/pyrophosphate transporter.[13] Finally, it has been proposed that a microsomal glucose transporter is also part of the glucose 6-phosphatase system, and although a deficiency of this glucose transporter has been postulated (GSD Id), it has not been convincingly demonstrated.[14,15]

Both GSD Ia and GSD Ib are autosomal recessive conditions. The catalytic unit of glucose 6-phosphatase is located at chromosome 17q21 and encodes an endoplasmic reticulum membrane protein with nine transmembrane domains

and a catalytic site on the luminal side of the endoplasmic reticulum membrane.[16] Over 70 separate mutations have been identified, and there is generally no genotype–phenotype correlation.[6] Glucose 6-phosphatase maintains latent activity and is dependent on transport of substrate from the cytosol into the endoplasmic reticulum lumen.[17] If the endoplasmic reticulum membrane is disrupted, either by freezing or detergent action, the catalytic activity is released and becomes apparent on enzymologic testing. The gene encoding glucose 6-phosphate translocase is located at chromosome 11q23. The protein has 10 transmembrane domains and is expressed in many human cell types, unlike glucose 6-phosphatase, which is expressed only in gluconeogenic tissues such as liver and kidney tubular cells.[18] Specifically, the glucose 6-phosphate transporter has been demonstrated in human neutrophils, where it may have a second, unspecified function, the lack of which presumably is the cause for the immune dysfunction seen in GSD Ib.[19,20]

The metabolic consequences of GSD Ia and Ib are similar, with the exception of the neutrophil dysfunction seen in GSD Ib (Figure 55.1-4).[21] Glucose 6-phosphatase is the only enzyme system capable of producing significant amounts of free glucose; therefore, the liver in GSD I is unable to maintain circulating glucose levels when the supply from a feed has been exhausted. The block in the last step of gluconeogenesis leads to excessive hepatic and renal accumulation of glycogen, which is the main cause of hepatomegaly and nephromegaly in this condition.[6] Recurrent hypoglycemia leads to increased glucagon production, which stimulates glycogen breakdown with accumulation of glucose 6-phosphate. As glucose 6-phosphate enters the glycolytic pathways, excess lactate is produced, giving rise to acidosis.

Lactate competes with urate for tubular excretion in the kidney.[5] Increased urate levels are, therefore, in part attributable to decreased urate excretion but may also be due to increased urate production. Glucose 6-phosphate may be shunted into the pentose-phosphate cycle, which stimulates synthesis of PP-ribose-P, degradation of which leads to further urate production. Finally, depletion of intrahepatic phosphate, as a result of production of glucose 6-phosphate

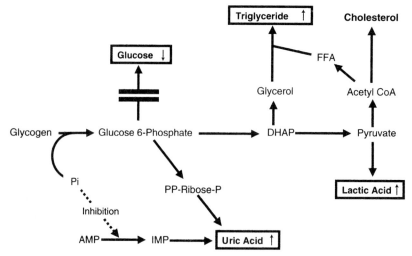

FIGURE 55.1-4 Schematic representation of the biochemical derangements responsible for the metabolic consequences of glycogen storage disease 1, namely hypoglycemia, lactic acidosis, hyperuricemia, and hypertriglyceridemia. AMP = adenosine monophosphate; CoA = coenzyme A; DHAP = dihydroxyacetone phosphate; FFA = free fatty acids; IMP = inosine monophosphate; Pi = inorganic phosphate.

from both dietary glucose and glycogen breakdown, relieves inhibition on adenosine monophosphate (AMP) deaminase, which converts AMP to inosine 5-monophosphate (IMP), which is metabolized to uric acid.[22,23]

Excess glucose 6-phosphate feeding into the glycolysis pathway increases production of glycerol and acetyl CoA and the energy precursors reduced oxidized nicotinamide adenine dinucleotide (NADH+) and reduced oxidized nicotinamide adenine dinucleotide phosphate (NADPH+), which provide substrates and cofactors for hepatic triglyceride production. Decreased peripheral use of fatty acids and increased lipolysis can result from low insulin levels. Bandsma and colleagues conclude that increased free fatty acid flux from adipose tissue to the liver probably makes the major contribution to hyperlipidemia and hepatic steatosis seen in GSD I.[24]

A diagnosis of GSD is usually suspected on the basis of clinical and biochemical features. Liver histology will suggest GSD but is not specific for the type. Glucagon stimulation is rarely carried out now, but in GSD I, there is little or no elevation in the plasma glucose following glucagon infusion, but lactic acid levels increase.[25] Enzyme assays on fresh (intact microsomes) and frozen (disrupted microsomes) liver biopsy specimens will diagnose and differentiate GSD Ia and Ib. Recent recommendations suggest that mutational analysis should precede liver enzymology (Table 55.1-4), with liver biopsy reserved for cases in which mutations in glucose 6-phosphatase or glucose 6-phosphate translocase genes cannot be identified but the diagnosis is still suspected.[6]

The clinical consequences of GSD I largely mirror the metabolic features discussed earlier. Recurrent hypoglycemia necessitates frequent feeding because the liver is unable to maintain glucose levels when the dietary supply of carbohydrates dissipates. Newborn infants often feed every 1 to 2 hours on demand, without significant periods of fasting, so that features of hypoglycemia may not appear. In addition, possibly because the brain can use lactate as an energy source, infants with GSD are often remarkably tol-

erant of hypoglycemia.[26] Hypoglycemia may first be manifest at several months of age because feeding frequency tends to decrease or at times of an intercurrent illness when dietary intake is impaired. There is an unexplained increase in fasting tolerance with age, and it may be that there is recruitment of other mechanisms for free glucose production. It is known, for example, that small amounts of free glucose can be produced by α-glucosidase, a lysosomal enzyme, deficiency of which produces GSD II, Pompe disease, and that a single molecule of free glucose is produced when debranching enzyme cleaves an 1,6-α branch point on a glycogen chain.

Untreated, massive hepatomegaly is the rule through childhood but tends to be relatively less significant in adults. There is often a modest increase in transaminases, but features of chronic liver disease are absent. Fibrosis is unusual, as is portal hypertension, but hepatic adenomas are very commonly found in untreated adults with GSD I. Adenomas in the liver are prone to bleeding and may undergo malignant transformation to hepatocellular carcinoma.[7,27]

There is slow linear growth in untreated children seen in infancy and childhood.[28] Adults tend to be short. There is frequently pubertal delay, and females have polycystic ovaries. With increasing body stores of uric acid, gout was frequently seen (before modern therapy) occurring initially at or around the time of puberty.[29] Xanthomata and lipemia retinalis may be seen at the time of presentation in infancy.[5] Massive hypertriglyceridemia is the cause proposed for the increased cases of pancreatitis seen in uncontrolled GSD I and also contributes to the platelet dysfunction responsible for the increased bleeding tendency.[30] The risk of atherosclerosis may be increased owing to the hyperlipidemia associated with GSD I.[31]

Renal dysfunction is first manifest with hyperperfusion and hyperfiltration causing an increase in creatinine clearance, but actual renal damage is heralded by microalbuminuria that may progress to frank proteinuria.[32] Chronic

TABLE 55.1-4   DIAGNOSTIC INVESTIGATIONS

DISEASE	TISSUE FOR ENZYME STUDIES	ROUTINE DNA TESTING AVAILABLE	HUMAN GENE LOCUS
GSD Ia	Liver	Yes	17q21
Ib	Liver	Yes	11q23
III	Liver and muscle	Exon 3 mutations only (ie, GSD IIIb)	1q21
IV Liver and other affected tissues	No	3p12	
VI	Liver	No	14q21–22
IX	Liver, erythrocytes, leukocytes, other affected tissues	No	Product of multiple genes
Glycogen synthase deficiency	Liver	No	12p12.2
Fanconi-Bickel syndrome	Liver, kidney	No	3q26.1–26.3
Fructosuria	Liver	No	2p23.3–23.2
Hereditary fructose intolerance	Liver	No	9q22.3
Fructose 1,6-bisphosphatase deficiency	Liver	No	9q22.2–22.3
D-Glyceric acid	Liver?	No	Unknown
Galactokinase deficiency	Erythrocytes	No	17q24
Galactose 6-phosphate uridyl transferase deficiency	Erythrocytes	Yes	9p13
UDP galactose 4-epimerase deficiency	Erythrocytes	No	1p36-35
Pyruvate carboxylase deficiency	Fibroblasts	No	11q13.4–13.5
Phosphoenolpyruvate carboxykinase deficiency	Liver?	No	20q13.31 (soluble) Unknown (mitochondrial)

GSD = glycogen storage disease; UDP = uridine diphosphate.
Tissues primarily tested for enzyme activity in defects of hepatic carbohydrate metabolism. Few of these conditions can presently be diagnosed routinely by deoxyribonucleic acid (DNA) analysis, although the loci for most genes are known.

renal failure may ensue with hypertension, hypercalciuria, and nephrocalcinosis. Renal calculi may occur. Acidosis and renal Fanconi syndrome can accompany the renal dysfunction. Osteopenia, rickets, and fractures are also commonly seen. Histologic changes on kidney biopsy are those of focal segmental glomerular sclerosis.

In addition to the above features, there is a tendency to recurrent bacterial infections with neutropenia in GSD Ib, which may be cyclical or persistent.[21] Mucosal inflammation is common, and overt inflammatory bowel disease may be present.

It has been demonstrated that avoidance of hypoglycemia and maintenance of normoglycemia improve overall metabolic control.[33] This can be achieved with frequent enteral feeds, total parenteral nutrition, or continuous nasogastric tube feedings. The standard approach at diagnosis is now continuous overnight nasogastric feeding with glucose polymer solution or a specialized infant formula aiming to supply glucose at rates equivalent to normal hepatic synthesis, which for infants is 8 to 9 mg/kg/min and for older children is in the range of 5 to 7 mg/kg/min. During the day, frequent feeds are given. The patient should avoid galactose and fructose because these are converted to glucose 6-phosphate without contributing free glucose. In older children, the diet should be rich in complex carbohydrates. Uncooked cornstarch given every 4 hours to young children at a dose of 1 to 2 g/kg can act as a slow-release form of glucose.[34] It is slowly hydrolyzed in the gut and improves the duration of normoglycemia.[35] The period between cornstarch feeds can be extended as the child gets older, and some adults can tolerate a full 8 hours sleep on a single intake of cornstarch. Care needs to be taken when patients with GSD I are unwell. IV fluids should always contain appropriate amounts of glucose. Lactated Ringer

solution should not be used. Metabolic control should be achieved and strictly maintained prior to surgery to limit bleeding problems. Successful pregnancies have been documented in women with GSD I, but strict dietary control is recommended prior to and during pregnancy.[36–38]

The use of diazoxide has been suggested to increase fasting tolerance, and Nuoffer and colleagues showed an impressive response in terms of normoglycemic control and linear growth in two patients treated with this drug.[39] Allopurinol is useful in the management of hyperuricemia, and evidence is accumulating that angiotensin-converting enzyme inhibitors may be helpful in treating the proteinuria, an early indicator of renal dysfunction.[29,40,41] With regard to the management of neutropenia and recurrent infections in patients with GSD Ib, granulocyte colony-stimulating factor has been demonstrated to increase the neutrophil counts and reduce the frequency and severity of bacterial infections.[42,43]

Orthotopic liver transplant has been carried out in patients with GSD I, usually for multiple adenomas and fear of malignant change.[44] Hypoglycemia and metabolic control are improved with successful liver transplant.[45] Hyperuricemia, lactic acidosis, and hypertriglyceridemia clear; however, it is unclear whether liver transplant influences the progression of renal disease. In those patients with end-stage renal disease, kidney transplant has been performed, but this does not improve the systemic manifestations of deranged hepatic metabolism.[46] There is one report of isolated hepatocyte transplant for this condition in an adult with poor compliance to dietary management.[47] The authors documented improved glycemic control but did not demonstrate that infused hepatocytes had, in fact, engrafted or that enzyme activity on liver biopsy had increased. Gene therapy is presently confined to laboratory studies on animal models of GSD Ia.[48,49]

Prior to modern treatment, patients frequently died soon after presentation. If they survived, they were likely to live through to adulthood with short stature and multiple complications, as discussed previously. Modern therapy, with the maintenance of normoglycemia and metabolic stability, has changed this dramatically. Although some infants succumb to acute metabolic collapse and lactic acidosis in the neonatal period, with urgent attention to glucose replacement and appropriate intensive management, these children should survive. With aggressive dietary management, overnight tube feedings, and cornstarch feeds, metabolic control can be maintained, avoiding hyperuricemia, lactic acidosis, hypertriglyceridemia, and recurrent hypoglycemia and allowing the children to achieve normal growth velocities.

Obesity can be a problem with the high carbohydrate intake, and hyperlipidemia may not be fully ameliorated.[31] Long-term sequelae such as adenomas appear to be less frequent, and adenomas already present may regress when appropriate treatment is started in teenagers and adults.[50] In spite of adequate therapy, there are suggestions that renal dysfunction may not be completely prevented; specifically, hyperfiltration does not appear to be affected even by excellent glycemic control.[5]

GSD III: Debranching Enzyme Deficiency (Cori Disease, Forbes Disease, Limit Dextrinosis).

GSD III, like GSD I, commonly presents in infancy with signs and symptoms of hypoglycemia and a protuberant abdomen owing to hepatomegaly. Growth retardation is common, as is hyperlipidemia. Hypoglycemia and hyperlipidemia are frequently less severe than in GSD I and occasionally are absent completely. In addition, children may present later in childhood with isolated hepatomegaly or abnormal liver enzymes, which, in some cases, may be very high.[51] Some patients present first in adulthood with a distal myopathy.[52,53] Liver biopsy in early childhood tends to show a typical glycogenosis but is more likely to show diffuse fibrosis and less steatosis than is seen typically in GSD I. Based on clinical phenotypes, GSD III has been divided into subtypes a and b. GSD IIIa has typical liver involvement with later muscle involvement. GSD IIIb accounts for about 15% of cases, with only the liver affected by this deficiency.[5]

Snappes and Van Creveld described the first cases of this condition in 1928, and because most patients with GSD III survive into adulthood, the authors were able to demonstrate a deficiency of the debranching enzyme in the original cases 35 years later.[54] This was after Illingworth and colleagues had identified that the deficiency of this enzyme was the cause of GSD III.[55] GSD III has been identified in all races, but there is a higher incidence in Faroe Islanders (incidence 1:3,600) and North African Jews (incidence 1:5,400).[56,57] Differential translation of a single gene, located on chromosome 1p21, is responsible for the liver and muscle isoforms of this enzyme.[58,59] This gene encodes a single polypeptide that possesses two separate catalytic sites that can function independently (see Figure 55.1-2), and occasional case reports have suggested

selective absence of either the glucosidase activity or the transferase activity. These cases have been termed GSD IIIc and GSD IIId, respectively.[60–62]

Glucagon stimulation gives differing results in GSD III depending on whether it is carried out in the fed or fasting state.[63] After a feed, glucagon stimulation leads to a rise in plasma glucose because hepatic phosphorylase is able to release glucose from the end-chains of glycogen. However, if the glucagon challenge takes place after an 8-hour fast, no rise in glucose is seen because the side chains have already been shortened as far as the branch points, and no further degradation can be effected in the absence of debranching enzyme. Fasting hypoglycemia results from incomplete glycogen degradation, lactic acidosis is not seen because there is no block in gluconeogenesis, and ketosis is more apparent during hypoglycemia than in GSD I.

Although hypoglycemia and hepatomegaly tend to recede with age, hepatic fibrosis and even micronodular cirrhosis can be seen in this condition.[64–66] Adenomas have been reported, but in GSD III, hepatocellular carcinoma appears to be associated only with cirrhosis.[67,68] Progressive myopathy and occasionally cardiomyopathy can occur in GSD IIIa patients, being an infrequent finding in childhood but often becoming a significant functional impairment by the third or fourth decade.[52] It is usually manifest by slowly progressive weakness and muscle atrophy. Ventricular hypertrophy is commonly seen, but frank cardiac dysfunction is the exception.[69] Polycystic ovaries have been noted in affected females; however, fertility appears to be unaffected.[70,71]

The diagnosis of GSD III is suspected on clinical and biochemical grounds, and the diagnosis is confirmed by liver enzymology, although the enzyme is expressed in other tissues such as fibroblasts. Differentiation of GSD IIIa from GSD IIIb requires a muscle biopsy. Deoxyribonucleic acid (DNA) techniques are now available for mutational analysis (see Table 55.1-4), and there appears to be a special association between exon 3 mutations and GSD IIIb.[62] More studies are needed before the type of GSD III can be ensured purely by mutational analysis.

Treatment of GSD III is similar to GSD I in that hypoglycemia needs to be effectively managed with frequent feeds, nighttime nasogastric tube feeding, and the introduction of cornstarch as the patients get older. It has been suggested that a high-protein diet can be helpful because amino acids can act as a gluconeogenic precursor and that a high-protein diet may be useful in the slowing of the progression of the myopathy even though long-term outcome studies are not available.[72] Similarly, there may be no need to restrict galactose and fructose intake because there is no impairment to their conversion to free glucose, as there is in GSD I.

Most patients with this condition survive into adulthood, usually with minimal hepatic symptoms and with an ability to tolerate a normal diet. The myopathy is slowly progressive but may become debilitating in later adulthood.

GSD IV: Branching Enzyme Deficiency (Andersen Disease, Amylopectinosis).

In 1956, Andersen described a

child with progressive hepatomegaly and a hepatic storage substance similar to amylopectin, the insoluble component of plant starch.[73] In 1966, the defect in the branching enzyme was reported.[5] Although this remains the characteristic form of GSD IV, this condition has an extremely variable phenotype.[74] In addition to Andersen disease, there have been cases described with nonprogressive hepatic disease, patients with associated cardiomyopathy, or multiple system involvement including neuromuscular involvement in the form of peripheral myopathy and neuropathy with or without cardiomyopathy. A severe neonatal form with hypotonia, muscle atrophy, cardiomyopathy, arthrogryposis, pulmonary hypoplasia, and hydrops fetalis has also been attributed to mutations within the gene responsible for GSD IV. Finally, an adult-onset disease called polyglucosan body disease, a severe progressive neurologic condition with peripheral neuropathy, seizures, and dementia, has been identified to be due to a defect of branching enzyme.

GSD IV is the least common of the hepatic GSDs, and the variants are still more rare. In the classic form of this disease, the affected infant is normal at birth; however, liver disease progresses rapidly through infancy with hepatosplenomegaly, cirrhosis, and portal hypertension. Without liver transplant, death usually occurs between the ages of 2 and 5 years. Fasting hypoglycemia and massive hepatomegaly are generally absent. Liver histology differs from other forms of hepatic GSD as well, with interstitial and portal fibrosis leading to micronodular cirrhosis. Hepatocytes are enlarged and stain PAS positive but are only partially digested by diastase. On electron microscopy, aggregates reminiscent of amylopectin are visible, along with more normal-appearing glycogen particles.

The mechanism by which the abnormal unbranched glycogen leads to hepatocyte damage is not clear. It is presumably related to abnormal and insoluble glycogen inducing a foreign body reaction within hepatocytes, leading to individual hepatocyte death with an inflammatory response and fibrosis thereafter. GSD IV is an autosomal recessive condition. The gene coding for the branching enzyme has been localized to chromosome 3p12.[75] Although the enzyme is usually assayed on liver, it is also expressed in leukocytes, red blood cells, and fibroblasts (see Table 55.1-4). In addition, branching enzyme can be assayed in amniocytes and chorionic villous cells, facilitating prenatal diagnosis.[76]

There is no specific treatment for this condition. General supportive measures are recommended to maintain growth. Liver transplant has been shown to be both feasible and effective.[44] However, there are a few cases in which, after transplant, progressive cardiomyopathy has occurred, leading to death.[77,78] The situation is difficult because there is no predictor as to which patients will proceed to a progressive cardiomyopathy. Starzl and colleagues have reported patients who had evidence of cardiac involvement that regressed after liver transplant.[79] It is possible that, with further molecular studies, genotype–phenotype correlations may help to understand and predict the outcome in these patients after liver transplants.

GSD VI: Phosphorylase Deficiency (Hers Disease). Diminished phosphorylase activity in patients with excessive hepatic glycogen storage was first ascribed the term GSD VI in 1960.[5] Many of these patients have since been shown to have a defect in activation of glycogen phosphorylase rather than a defect in the gene coding for glycogen phosphorylase itself, localized to chromosome 14q21-22.[80] The number of cases with proven mutations in the phosphorylase gene is small.[81,82] Usually, GSD VI is a benign condition and affects only liver because other tissues express glycogen phosphorylases that are the products of completely separate genes. If present at all, hypoglycemia is mild and present only in infancy and early childhood. Similarly, ketosis and hyperlipidemia are minimal. Lactate and urate levels are normal. Hepatomegaly and poor growth in early childhood are the most notable features, and both tend to improve with age. In most cases, treatment is not required. If hypoglycemia is present, it can be managed with frequent feeds and nighttime tube feeding. Prognosis is excellent, and normal growth velocities can be expected beyond the first few years of life.

GSD IX: Phosphorylase Kinase Deficiency (GSD VIII according to McKusick's Online Mendelian Inheritance in Man). Of the group of mild GSDs with decreased phosphorylase activity, family studies showed that a significant proportion of these were X-linked. Defective activation of hepatic phosphorylase was demonstrated, as well as deficiency of phosphorylase kinase activity within the blood cells of these patients.[83,84] A smaller number of patients, also with measurable deficiencies of phosphorylase kinase, have an autosomal recessive mode of inheritance.[85,86] The classification of this condition (strictly a group of conditions) is a little confused; most authorities refer to phosphorylase kinase deficiency as GSD IX, but McKusick's Online Mendelian Inheritance in Man[87] categorizes it as GSD VIII.

The common presentation for this condition is that of a young child, usually not an infant, with a protuberant abdomen and moderate growth retardation. Laboratory testing may show elevated transaminases, modestly elevated cholesterol and triglycerides, and fasting ketosis. Hypoglycemia is uncommon. Like GSD VI, growth retardation is confined to early childhood. Hepatomegaly is the most dramatic finding, but this resolves with age. Curiously, the liver biopsy may show mild inflammatory changes with some fibrosis in addition to glycogen-distended hepatocytes (Figure 55.1-5). Steatosis is not usually apparent.

In the majority of cases, GSD IX is a benign condition; there are, however, a few descriptions of more significant disease with symptomatic hyperglycemia requiring dietary management as described for other GSDs.[88,89] Other patients have had more aggressive liver disease, with progression to cirrhosis, and still others have had muscle involvement.[86,90–92] The variable phenotype is largely explained by the complex nature of the phosphorylase kinase protein, which consists of multiple copies of four separate gene products: the α, β, γ, and δ subunits.[5] The α and β subunits are regulatory subunits, regulated by phos-

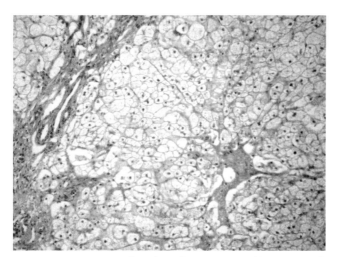

FIGURE 55.1-5   Liver histology from a 2-year-old patient with X-linked phosphorylase kinase deficiency. Note distended hepatocytes and mild periportal, pericentral, and intralobular fibrosis (hematoyxylin and eosin stain; ×20 original magnification).

phorylation and dephosphorylation. There are two genes, both on the X chromosome for the α subunit, one predominantly a muscle subunit (pHka1) and the other mainly expressed in liver phosphorylase kinase (pHka2, locus Xp22.2-22.1). The β subunit is coded at chromosome 16q12-13. The γ subunit is the catalytic subunit, and, again, there are two genes on separate chromosomes for this subunit: pHkg1 (muscle) on chromosome 7 and pHkg2 (testis and liver subunit) at chromosome 16p12.1-12.2. The δ subunit is the calcium binding protein calmodulin.

Over 75% of described cases of phosphorylase kinase deficiency have defects in the α liver subunit and produce the benign hepatic form of GSD IX. Patients with β subunit defects are more likely to have evidence of muscle involvement, and cirrhosis is characteristic of the defect in the liver/testis subunit gene *PHKG2*.[85,86] Diagnosis depends on enzyme assay, which can be carried out either in red cells or liver (see Table 55.1-4). Management is generally symptomatic, but the majority of patients require no intervention. The prognosis for the X-linked glycogenosis is excellent, with hepatomegaly receding certainly by teenage years, and final adult height within the normal range. Prognosis for the variant forms is presently unclear.

Fanconi-Bickel Syndrome (Hepatorenal Glycogenosis with Renal Fanconi Syndrome). In 1949, Fanconi and Bickel described a 3-year-old boy, born to consanguineous parents from a small alpine village, with renal Fanconi syndrome and hepatomegaly.[93] He had increased liver glycogen, fasting hypoglycemia, hyperlipidemia, and renal tubular defects. Santer and colleagues reviewed this patient, with over 50 years of follow-up.[94] The same group reported knowledge of 112 patients, the vast majority being white.[95] Presentation is usually in the first year, with failure to thrive, vomiting and diarrhea, rickets and polyuria, and a protuberant abdomen. Findings include glycosuria, generalized aminoaciduria, phosphaturia, and calciuria with renal tubular acidosis. There is increased

plasma alkaline phosphatase, mild to moderate fasting hypoglycemia, and hyperlipidemia; however, plasma lactate and uric acid levels are usually normal. Of particular note are postprandial hyperglycemia and hypergalactosemia. Later clinical features include a moon-shaped face, truncal obesity, retarded growth and puberty, bone problems associated with hypophosphatemic rickets, and dental caries. Cataracts from hypergalactosemia have only rarely been described, and the renal lesion is usually not progressive in nature.

The facultative glucose transporter GLUT2 was localized to chromosome 3q26.1–26.3 in 1988 and is expressed on hepatocytes, renal tubular cells, enterocytes, and pancreatic β islet cells.[95,96] It was not, however, until 1997 that a defect in GLUT2 was proposed as the possible metabolic basis for Fanconi-Bickel syndrome (FBS).[97] Mutations in the gene for GLUT2 have been demonstrated in FBS subjects, including the original patient described by Fanconi and Bickel.[98]

The features of FBS can be explained by the loss of GLUT2 function. GLUT proteins are membrane-bound monosaccharide transporters that transport sugars in an energy-independent manner. GLUT2 is responsible for transport of glucose (and galactose) into hepatocytes after feeding and export of free glucose out of hepatocytes during fasting. The hyperglycemia and hypergalactosemia seen postprandially are due to reduced uptake of these monosaccharides by the liver and may be enhanced by the poor insulin response to elevated blood glucose levels demonstrated in patients with FBS.[95] Glucose is transported inefficiently into pancreatic β cells because of the defect in GLUT2, thus failing to provoke an appropriate insulin response. Fasting hypoglycemia results from defective export of free glucose from hepatocytes when peripheral glucose supplies have been exhausted. Elevated intracellular levels of glucose stimulate increased glycogen production. Glycosuria is the result of failure to export glucose across the basolateral membranes of renal tubular cells. This again leads to an increased intracellular glucose and stimulates glycogen production. The excessive intracellular glycogen may be responsible for the other features of renal Fanconi syndrome. Finally, defective transport of glucose and galactose across enterocytes may be responsible for the diarrhea and malabsorption seen.

The treatment of patients with FBS is based on the management of renal Fanconi syndrome with maintenance of water and electrolyte balance; supplementation of vitamin D, calcium, phosphorus, and bicarbonate; and the management of the deranged glucose homeostasis. The ideal diet has not yet been decided on, but suggestions have included frequent small meals, the ketogenic diet, or uncooked cornstarch, as is used in GSD I.[95,99] On these diets, the hepatomegaly has been seen to diminish. It has also been noted that fructose metabolism does not appear to be affected by the defect in GLUT2; therefore, the use of fructose may be useful in the dietary management of patients with FBS.[100]

The prognosis for this condition appears to be generally good in terms of survival, but adults are universally short in stature. Many also have ongoing bony problems related to rickets and osteomalacia. Hepatomegaly tends to recede after puberty.[95]

GLYCOGEN SYNTHASE DEFICIENCY

Although referred to as GSD 0, there is no excessive storage of glycogen, and, in fact, there is a demonstrable reduction in hepatic glycogen in this condition. Like many enzymes for glycogen metabolism, separate gene products account for glycogen synthase activity in muscle and liver, GYS1 and GYS2, respectively.[87]

The deficiency state of GYS2 is very rare in humans.[101,102] Although Aynsley-Green and colleagues have reported apparent asymptomatic patients with this condition, on the whole, patients have presented in infancy with features of fasting hypoglycemia.[103] The characteristic biochemical features are fasting ketotic hypoglycemia with low alanine and lactate levels and postprandial hyperglycemia with increased circulating lactate levels. There is no hepatomegaly in this condition because there is no glycogen storage, and hyperlipidemia does not occur. Liver biopsy is required for enzymologic diagnosis (see Table 55.1-4). The gene locus is chromosome 12p12.2, and mutational analysis has been conducted on affected subjects.[104] With avoidance of symptomatic hypoglycemia, the prognosis is good.

INBORN ERRORS OF FRUCTOSE METABOLISM

FRUCTOSURIA

Essential fructosuria is due to deficiency of fructokinase, which converts free fructose to fructose 1-phosphate.[105] It was first revealed in a patient checked for glycosuria while being investigated for possible diabetes.[106] Fructose, although containing no aldehyde group, becomes a reducing sugar in basic solution and will give a positive test when urine is checked for reducing substances but gives a negative reaction on glucose oxidase stick testing. Fructokinase deficiency is an autosomal recessive condition, but it is likely that many cases go undetected because of its entirely benign nature.

HEREDITARY FRUCTOSE INTOLERANCE

In contrast to the previous condition, hereditary fructose intolerance (HFI) is a potentially life-threatening condition. The defect is due to absence of aldolase B (fructose 1,6-bisphosphate aldolase) from the liver, kidney, and small intestine. Other tissues in the body express aldolase A or C. This enzyme catalyzes the conversion of fructose 1,6-phosphate and fructose 1-phosphate to triose phosphates.[106]

Patients with this condition remain entirely healthy provided that they do not ingest significant amounts of fructose or sucrose. The infant is protected from harm by breastfeeding, and modern infant formulas no longer contain fructose or sucrose as a sweetener. Problems may occur on weaning to solid foods, particularly with the introduction of fruit and baby food sweetened with sucrose. Symptoms include poor feeding, vomiting, failure to thrive, and abdominal pain. If intake of fructose persists, acute hypoglycemia, bleeding, hepatomegaly, and trembling or jerking can occur. This may proceed to metabolic collapse with liver and kidney failure and, ultimately, death. With acute illness, laboratory findings are consistent with liver failure, lactic acidosis, hyperuricemia, and proximal renal tubular dysfunction. The histology of the liver at this stage shows isolated hepatocyte necrosis with intralobular and periportal fibrosis and diffuse fatty change.

If the diagnosis is not made, but the patient survives, the course may be intermittent and chronic.[106] As these children grow, they develop a dramatic aversion to sweet foods, and sometimes their odd eating habits are the reason for medical attention. Dentists have noted complete absence of caries in adult patients, and this has, on occasion, prompted the diagnosis.[107] Others have been diagnosed in adulthood after metabolic collapse, or even death, when intravenous fluids containing fructose or sorbitol have been given for routine surgeries.[108,109]

With intermittent exposure to fructose in HFI, many nonspecific symptoms may occur, such as poor feeding, intermittent vomiting, failure to thrive, irritability or apathy, and diarrhea. Chronic liver disease can also occur with hepatomegaly and cirrhosis. Symptoms are related to the fundamental toxicity of fructose. It has been demonstrated in animals and humans that large infusions of fructose are, in themselves, toxic and produce many of the features seen in patients with hereditary fructose intolerance, particularly increased circulating lactic acid and hyperuricemia.[110] The mechanism for this commences with the rapid and irreversible conversion of free fructose to fructose 1-phosphate by fructokinase.[111] Further metabolism of fructose 1-phosphate to D-glyceraldehyde and dihydroxyacetone phosphate is prevented. Production of large amounts of fructose 1-phosphate effectively sequestrates inorganic phosphate, causing a drastic reduction in cytoplasmic phosphate concentrations. This leads to a depletion of adenosine triphosphate (ATP) because of irreversible deamination of AMP to IMP. Further mitochondrial regeneration of ATP is prevented by the lack of inorganic phosphate. Elevation in Mg^{2+} seen in acute episodes is related to the fact that a large quantity of Mg is bound to ATP, and with the loss of ATP, Mg^{2+} is released.[106] The overall effect of this is a loss of cellular energy supply, and studies using ^{31}P magnetic resonance spectroscopy are providing direct proof of this mechanism.[112,113] Hypoglycemia during acute exposure to fructose is due both to deranged gluconeogenesis because of the increased fructose 1-phosphate levels and to failure of glycogenolysis because inorganic phosphate deficiency inhibits glycogen phosphorylase. Hypoglycemia can be reversed by galactose infusion, implying that there is no inhibition of the glucose 6-phosphatase pathway. Glucagon cannot correct hypoglycemia during these episodes because of the deranged gluconeogenic pathways.[114]

Aldolase B gene is located on the long arm of chromosome 9 (9q22.3).[115] The incidence of this condition in Switzerland, from where many cases have been described, is estimated at about 1 in 20,000.[116] However, the incidence in other populations is unknown and is complicated by the fact that many affected individuals may live a long life without the diagnosis being made.

The diagnosis of HFI is dependent on the physician having a high degree of awareness of this condition. A careful nutritional history will solidify the suspicions, and the urine can be checked for non–glucose-reducing substances; however, absence does not rule out the diagnosis. On initial suspicion, all dietary fructose, sucrose, and sorbitol should be excluded from the diet. Infants presenting with severe toxic episodes may need intensive support for an extended period. Once recovered, the child should be maintained on a fructose-free diet for several weeks to ensure recovery and improved growth. A fructose tolerance test can then be carried out.[117] A small dose, standardized at 200 mg/kg, is infused while monitoring laboratory parameters such as glucose, plasma phosphate, uric acid, lactate, and Mg^{2+}. A characteristic response is an increase in plasma urate and magnesium with a corresponding fall in phosphorus and glucose. Aldolase B can be assayed on liver biopsy, and DNA mutational analysis is now also available.[118,119]

Treatment involves removal of all known dietary sources of fructose, sucrose, and sorbitol, which are found naturally in fruits, vegetables, and honey, as well as in processed food. Fructose is so widespread that patients should be very open about their intolerance so as not to be inadvertently exposed. This is especially true in any contact with medical professionals. Medicines may be sweetened with sucrose. IV fluids or parenteral nutritional supplements using fructose or sorbitol have been advocated in the past but should be avoided in all patients. When recovery occurs, it is complete, with reversal of hepatic histologic changes and renal dysfunction. Growth and development become normal.

FRUCTOSE 1,6-BISPHOSPHATASE DEFICIENCY

Fewer than 100 cases of fructose 1,6-biphosphatase deficiency have been reported. Affected individuals may present with neonatal jaundice, but, more commonly, episodic bouts of hyperventilation around the time of weaning from frequent milk feeds are seen.[120] The hallmark is ketotic hypoglycemia, lactic acidosis on fasting, and elevated uric acid. Metabolic collapse may be rapidly lethal, and fasting or infections often trigger late episodes.

After stabilization and avoidance of dietary fructose, an IV fructose tolerance test is abnormal, but unlike HFI, there is no aversion to sweet foods and no proximal renal tubular signs. Liver biopsy shows steatosis but no fibrosis. Again, this enzyme can be assayed in liver biopsy. The condition is inherited as autosomal recessive, and the gene has been localized to the almost identical locus to aldolase B on the long arm of chromosome 9. Treatment consists of IV glucose for the acute episode and long-term avoidance of fasting. Fructose should be limited, but complete avoidance is probably unnecessary. When the diagnosis is made and treated appropriately, the course is said to be favorable.[106]

D-GLYCERICACIDURIA

This extremely rare condition is due to the absence of D-glycerate kinase, which is required in the pathway of metabolism of D-glyceraldehyde, which, in turn, is derived from the metabolism of fructose 1-phosphate or glycerol. The presence of D-glyceric acid in urine is associated with hyperglycinemia, metabolic acidosis, and neurologic features that include hypotonia, seizures, severe developmental delay, and spastic quadriplegia. However, other cases have been relatively asymptomatic.[121,122] Dietary restriction of fructose has been suggested as management for this condition.

INBORN ERRORS OF GALACTOSE METABOLISM

GALACTOKINASE DEFICIENCY

The first step in the hepatic metabolism of free galactose is the conversion to galactose 1-phosphate catalyzed by galactokinase, the deficiency of which was first described in a child with bilateral cataracts.[123] This has been a consistent feature in all cases described since, and it is notable that the other features of classic galactosemia do not occur. There is no acute metabolic episode associated with this condition. Ovarian failure and growth failure do not occur. Galactokinase deficiency is not thought to pose neurodevelopment problems, although pseudotumor cerebri has been described in a few cases.[124,125] Galactokinase deficiency is probably less common than classic galactosemia, based on neonatal screening data, but its true incidence is undetermined.

The diagnosis is suspected either on the basis of neonatal screening or because of infantile cataracts and is confirmed by demonstrating deficient galactokinase activity with normal galactose 1-phosphate uridyl transferase (GALT) activity in red blood cells (see Table 55.1-4). The cause of the cataracts appears to be galactitol, the product of reduction of galactose by aldose reductase.[126] High concentrations of this enzyme occur within the ocular lens and lead to accumulation of galactitol. Galactitol is poorly mobilized from the lens media and exerts an osmotic effect.[127] Cataracts can be prevented in experimental animal models of galactokinase deficiency by inhibiting aldose reductase.[128] The management of this condition involves dietary galactose exclusion and is highly effective provided that the vision has not been permanently damaged prior to diagnosis.

GALT DEFICIENCY

GALT deficiency is the most common defect of galactose metabolism, and the clinical picture was first described by Goppert in 1917.[129] The frequency of GALT deficiency varies in different populations, with the highest incidence in Irish travelers of 1 in 480 and an estimated prevalence overall of 1 in 62,000.[125,130] In the United States, most infants with galactosemia are now diagnosed on infant screening. Often the patients are asymptomatic at diagnosis. Some infants present acutely within days of birth with vomiting and diarrhea, irritability, or lethargy with hypotonia, and the rapid diagnosis allowed by the early neonatal screening may assist in the care of these sick infants. If galactose ingestion continues, this progresses to hemolysis with jaundice and acidosis. There may be acute metabolic collapse with liver and kidney failure leading to death. Many of the fulminant early infantile cases are related to the high incidence of bacterial septicemia, with the causative organism most commonly being *E. coli*.[131] *E. coli* sepsis is so characteristic that any neonate so affected should be investigated for underlying galactosemia. Other infants follow a more chronic course with poor feeding and growth and progressive liver disease leading to cirrhosis. In surviving children, mental retardation is almost universal, although this is rarely at a profound level. Cataracts have been observed within days of birth but are more commonly seen later in infancy in those on an unrestricted diet.

GALT catalyzes the reaction that converts galactose 1-phosphate to UDP galactose (Figure 55.1-6). The acute metabolic syndrome is probably due to sequestration of inorganic phosphate as galactose 1-phosphate, with resulting deficiency in cellular energy owing to loss and insufficient restitution of ATP supply, possibly analogous to the demonstrated acute effects of fructose intake in patients with HFI. Galactose 1-phosphate itself inhibits a number of enzymes, in vitro, involved in glucose metabolism. The acute disturbance leads to liver disease, hemolysis, lactic acidosis and renal tubular acidosis, proteinuria, and aminoaciduria.

With the introduction of neonatal screening, individuals were identified with milder disease.[132] The "Duarte" variants identified on neonatal screening have structurally altered GALT that is functionally deficient, at least in young infants. However, after a few months, GALT activity can often be measured in the 50% range. Development in patients with a Duarte variant is normal, and they can tolerate an unrestricted diet. It had also been noted that galactosemia was commonly less severe in black individuals. Despite complete peripheral GALT deficiency, such patients are able to tolerate a normal diet. This so-called "Negro" variant has zero activity of GALT in erythrocytes but up to 10% GALT activity when measured on liver biopsy.

The GALT gene is located at chromosome 9p13. A large number of mutations have been identified (some are specifically associated with variants); the most common mutation in Caucasians causing classic galactosemia is Q188R. The "Negro" variant is associated with the most common mutation in the GALT gene found in black populations, *S135L*.

The diagnosis is frequently made on the basis of a neonatal screen. Positive neonatal screens should always be followed up with assay of red blood cell GALT activity (see Table 55.1-4). Isoelectric focusing of GALT will identify the Duarte variant, which has a faster electrophoretic mobility than normal GALT. In the unscreened population, the clinical presentation with metabolic collapse and/or *E. coli* sepsis is a clue to check for nonglucose urinary reducing substances (remember that this will become negative following the cessation of galactose-containing feeds). With clinical suspicion, milk feeds should be discontinued and IV glucose given until enzyme activity can be proven to be present.

The treatment for galactosemia is dietary galactose restriction, which, for an infant, means removal of breast milk or regular formula feeds and substitution with a galactose-free formula. The elimination of galactose will lead to a fall in red cell galactose and urinary excretion of metabolites such as galactitol and galactinate within a few days. However, red cell galactose 1-phosphate levels remain high and fall only gradually, and red cell galactose 1-phosphate levels never return fully to normal. The introduction of a galactose-exclusion diet allows recovery from the initial acute illness and prevents further acute metabolic episodes. It will reverse liver and renal dysfunction and prevent the formation of cataracts. Unfortunately, the diet as it exists presently appears to do little for the long-term complications of mental retardation or ovarian dysfunction in females.[133] In addition, growth failure, speech delay, and delayed-onset neurologic lesions are also not obviously affected by diet.[134] Waggoner and colleagues have shown that the incidence of these complications in patients who start a galactose-free diet later after a clinical presentation is not significantly different from those children on galactose elimination prior to the onset of symptoms because of neonatal screening or because of a previously affected sibling.[135]

Therefore, if galactose restriction does not alter long-term outcome, what is the pathogenesis of these long-term complications? The answers remain to be elucidated, but the debate revolves around a number of questions. The first is, Does the insult or injury occur before or after birth? Amniotic fluid of fetuses with classic galactosemia has been demonstrated to have increased levels of galactitol,

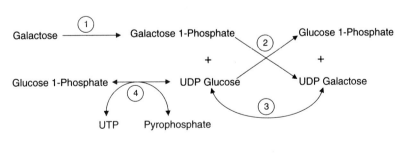

1. Galactokinase
2. Galactose 1-Phosphate Uridyl Transferase
3. UDP Galactose 4-Epimerase
4. UDP Glucose Pyrophosphorylase

FIGURE 55.1-6 Metabolism of galactose to uridyl diphosphogalactose. UDP glucose = uridyl diphosphoglucose; UTP = uridyl triphosphate.

and cord blood has increased galactose 1-phosphate, even if the mother is on a galactose-restricted diet, suggesting in utero metabolic derangement.[136] To support the idea of postnatal injury, it has been noted in a number of studies that mental retardation measured by DQ/IQ is not a fixed defect but falls progressively with age and may not be affected by the patient's compliance with galactose restriction.[137] Similarly, ovarian failure common in affected females is not always manifest with primary amenorrhea; secondary amenorrhea may even occur after a successful pregnancy. It would seem quite possible that there is a contribution to the long-term complications of galactosemia, both from antenatal and postnatal insults.

The second question is, If the diet is adequately restricted, where does the toxic galactose come from? Are there unrevealed dietary sources of galactose, or is this some form of "autointoxication" with de novo synthesis of galactose or galactose 1-phosphate in the body? In practical terms, a completely galactose-free diet is effectively impossible. Although the vast majority of galactose in the diet comes from milk and dairy products, there are other sources of dietary galactose. Free galactose exists in some fruit and vegetables, and galactose can be derived from animal glycoproteins, galactolipids, and galactosides.[138] It has been suggested that plant oligosaccharides, which contain galactose such as raffinose and stachyose, may contribute to galactose intake. However, humans do not possess the digestive oligosaccharides to free galactose from these sugars. On the other hand, a female volunteer with classic galactosemia had no change in galactose metabolites when taking a diet rich in fruit and vegetables known to contain free galactose compared with when she adhered strictly to a galactose exclusion of less than 8 mg galactose/d.[139] This implied to the authors de novo synthesis of galactose, giving support to the "autointoxication" hypothesis. Galactose 1-phosphate can be synthesized through cleavage of UDP galactose. These metabolites are produced by the reversible actions of UDP galactose 4-epimerase from UDP glucose (see Figure 55.1-6). The flux through this pathway in the absence of GALT activity is not known.

The third question is, Are the long-term complications attributable to the toxic effects of galactose 1-phosphate and other aberrant metabolites or to defective synthesis of glycoproteins and other essential galactose-containing molecules owing to a relative depletion of UDP galactose? This, again, depends on whether the flux through the pyrophosphorylase pathway can make up for the lack of UDP galactose, which, under normal circumstances, appears predominantly to come from metabolism of free galactose. These questions are, as yet, unanswered.

Current recommendations are to maintain galactose restriction as severely as possible, especially in early infancy, while the prognosis in terms of growth and development remains guarded.

UDP Galactose 4-Epimerase Deficiency

This condition was again identified as a result of newborn screening for galactosemia. The initial patients were noted to have normal growth and development. The enzyme deficiency in these patients is restricted to circulating red blood cells and leukocytes, with normal activity of the epimerase enzyme in liver and fibroblasts.[126] This condition is entirely benign.

In contrast, a severe form has been reported in only three families, each with highly consanguineous lineages.[140] The clinical features are those of severe classic galactosemia with early metabolic dysfunction and liver disease. Galactose restriction prevents the acute syndrome but does not influence the growth and mental retardation observed. Walter and colleagues have given small amounts of lactose to these patients in an attempt to maintain essential glycoprotein synthesis because, unlike in GALT deficiency, UDP galactose cannot be generated via the pyrophosphorylase pathway (see Figure 55.1-6).[140]

INBORN ERRORS OF PYRUVATE METABOLISM

Pyruvate Carboxylase Deficiency

Pyruvate carboxylase is key to the initiation and regulation of gluconeogenesis, as well as maintaining cellular concentrations of oxaloacetate. Deficiency of pyruvate carboxylase has been identified in only a small number of patients, but there appear to be three distinct phenotypes.[141] The first group presents in infancy, with lactic acidosis, organicaciduria, elevated plasma levels of pyruvate and alanine, and severe mental retardation. Of particular note is the frequency of this condition among Canadian Natives.[142] The second group is a severe neonatal form, with macrocephaly, intractable lactic acidemia with elevated lactate-to-pyruvate ratios, hyperammonemia, hypercitrullinemia, and hepatomegaly.[143] Death usually occurs by 3 months. Finally, there are two cases described of children with intermittent acidosis but normal development.[144,145] Pyruvate carboxylase activity in fibroblasts is low in all groups of patients, but only in the severe neonatal group are cases found in which no pyruvate carboxylase activity, protein, or messenger RNA can be detected.[146] The variation in phenotype is possibly related to the amount of residual pyruvate carboxylase activity.

Lactic acidosis and elevated alanine levels are related to excess pyruvate accumulation, but the more severe symptoms of hyperammonemia and deranged lactate-to-pyruvate ratios seen in the neonatal form result from an inability to maintain cellular concentrations of oxaloacetate, which is necessary to maintain the TCA cycle and to synthesize aspartate.[141] Aspartate is an essential nitrogen donor for the urea cycle; therefore, citrulline and ammonia accumulate. Aspartate depletion also disrupts transport of reducing equivalents (NADH+ and NADPH+) into the mitochondria, which is reflected in the deranged lactate-to-pyruvate ratio.

Dietary treatment with correction of acidosis and addition of aspartate to supplement the cellular amino acid depletions has been tried.[147] Thiamine, a cofactor for pyruvate dehydrogenase complex, and dichloroacetate, which stimulates pyruvate dehydrogenase activity, may allow more pyruvate to be metabolized through to acetyl CoA. Biotin, although a cofactor for pyruvate carboxylase, has not been shown to have benefit. There is one report of orthotopic liver transplant in a child with a severe form of pyruvate carboxylase deficiency, and although transplant was unable to reverse preexisting neurologic damage, much of the systemic metabolic disturbance was corrected.[148] There was some optimism that the neurologic progression of this disease may have been slowed.

PEPCK Deficiency

PEPCK, the second enzyme in the gluconeogenic pathway from pyruvate, is dependent on guanosine triphosphate for the conversion of oxaloacetate to phospho*enol*pyruvate. There are two forms of this enzyme: one soluble or cytosolic and the other mitochondrial, which are products of different genes. A number of cases of PEPCK deficiency have been described in children.[149–152] Certain cases have since been demonstrated to be due to generalized mitochondrial defects.[153] The features attributed to the cases that remain are infantile hypoglycemia, fatty infiltration of both liver and kidneys, and liver failure. The extent of the phenotype is not well defined owing to the difficulty of the enzyme assays and the extreme rarity of the cases.

REFERENCES

1. Clayton PT. Inborn errors presenting with liver dysfunction. Semin Neonatol 2002;7:49–63.
2. Saudubray JM, Nassogne MC, de Lonlay P, et al. Clinical approach to inherited metabolic disorders in neonates: an overview. Semin Neonatol 2002;7:3–15.
3. Ellaway CJ, Wilcken B, Christodoulou J. Clinical approach to inborn errors of metabolism presenting in the newborn period. J Paediatr Child Health 2002;38:511–7.
4. Roach PJ. Glycogen and its metabolism. Curr Mol Med 2002;2:101–20.
5. Chen YT. Glycogen storage diseases. In: Scriver C, Beaudet A, Sly W, et al, editors. The metabolic and molecular bases of inherited disease. Vol 1. 8th ed. New York: McGraw-Hill; 2000. p. 1521–51.
6. Chou JY, Matern D, Mansfield BC, et al. Type I glycogen storage diseases: disorders of the glucose-6-phosphatase complex. Curr Mol Med 2002;2:121–43.
7. Rake JP, Visser G, Labrune P, et al. Glycogen storage disease type I: diagnosis, management, clinical course and outcome. Results of the European Study on Glycogen Storage Disease Type I (ESGSD I). Eur J Pediatr 2002;161 Suppl 1:S20–34.
8. von Gierke E. Hepato-nephromegalia Glycogenica (Glycogenspeicherkrankheit der Leber und Nieren). Beitr Pathol Anat 1929;82:497–513.
9. Cori GT, Cori CF. Glucose-6-phosphatase of the liver in glycogen storage disease. J Biol Chem 1952;199:661–7.
10. Gerin I, Veiga-da-Cunha M, Achouri Y, et al. Sequence of a putative glucose 6-phosphate translocase, mutated in glycogen storage disease type Ib. FEBS Lett 1997;419:235–8.
11. Kure S, Suzuki Y, Matsubara Y, et al. Molecular analysis of glycogen storage disease type Ib: identification of a prevalent mutation among Japanese patients and assignment of a putative glucose-6-phosphate translocase gene to chromosome 11. Biochem Biophys Res Commun 1998;248:426–31.
12. Annabi B, Hiraiwa H, Mansfield BC, et al. The gene for glycogen storage disease type 1b maps to chromosome 11q23. Am J Hum Genet 1998;62:400–5.
13. Lin B, Hiraiwa H, Pan CJ, et al. Type-1c glycogen storage disease is not caused by mutations in the glucose-6-phosphate transporter gene. Hum Genet 1999;105:515–7.
14. Foster JD, Nordlie RC. The biochemistry and molecular biology of the glucose-6-phosphatase system. Exp Biol Med (Maywood) 2002;227:601–8.
15. Burchell A. A re-evaluation of GLUT 7. Biochem J 1998;331:973.
16. Pan CJ, Lei KJ, Annabi B, et al. Transmembrane topology of glucose-6-phosphatase. J Biol Chem 1998;273:6144–8.
17. Narisawa K, Otomo H, Igarashi Y, et al. Glycogen storage disease type 1b due to a defect of glucose-6-phosphate translocase. J Inherit Metab Dis 1982;5:227–8.
18. Pan CJ, Lin B, Chou JY. Transmembrane topology of human glucose 6-phosphate transporter. J Biol Chem 1999;274:13865–9.
19. Verhoeven AJ, Visser G, van Zwieten R, et al. A convenient diagnostic function test of peripheral blood neutrophils in glycogen storage disease type Ib. Pediatr Res 1999;45:881–5.
20. Lin B, Annabi B, Hiraiwa H, et al. Cloning and characterization of cDNAs encoding a candidate glycogen storage disease type 1b protein in rodents. J Biol Chem 1998;273:31656–60.
21. Visser G, Rake JP, Fernandes J, et al. Neutropenia, neutrophil dysfunction, and inflammatory bowel disease in glycogen storage disease type Ib: results of the European Study on Glycogen Storage Disease type I. J Pediatr 2000;137:187–91.
22. Roe TF, Kogut MD. The pathogenesis of hyperuricemia in glycogen storage disease, type I. Pediatr Res 1977;11:664–9.
23. Cohen JL, Vinik A, Faller J, et al. Hyperuricemia in glycogen storage disease type I. Contributions by hypoglycemia and hyperglucagonemia to increased urate production. J Clin Invest 1985;75:251–7.
24. Bandsma RH, Smit GP, Kuipers F. Disturbed lipid metabolism in glycogen storage disease type 1. Eur J Pediatr 2002;161 Suppl 1:S65–9.
25. Dunger DB, Leonard JV. Value of the glucagon test in screening for hepatic glycogen storage disease. Arch Dis Child 1982;57:384–9.
26. Fernandes J, Berger R, Smit GP. Lactate as a cerebral metabolic fuel for glucose-6-phosphatase deficient children. Pediatr Res 1984;18:335–9.
27. Bianchi L. Glycogen storage disease I and hepatocellular tumours. Eur J Pediatr 1993;152 Suppl 1:S63–70.
28. Mundy HR, Hindmarsh PC, Matthews DR, et al. The regulation of growth in glycogen storage disease type 1. Clin Endocrinol (Oxf) 2003;58:332–9.
29. Cameron JS, Moro F, Simmonds HA. Gout, uric acid and purine metabolism in paediatric nephrology. Pediatr Nephrol 1993;7:105–18.
30. Herman TE. Type IA glycogenosis with acute pancreatitis. J Radiol 1995;76:51–3.
31. Levy E, Letarte J, Lepage G, et al. Plasma and lipoprotein fatty acid composition in glycogen storage disease type I. Lipids 1987;22:381–5.
32. Chen YT. Type I glycogen storage disease: kidney involvement, pathogenesis and its treatment. Pediatr Nephrol 1991;5:71–6.
33. Wolfsdorf JI, Crigler JF Jr. Effect of continuous glucose therapy begun in infancy on the long-term clinical course of patients with type I glycogen storage disease. J Pediatr Gastroenterol Nutr 1999;29:136–43.
34. Chen YT, Bazzarre CH, Lee MM, et al. Type I glycogen storage disease: nine years of management with cornstarch. Eur J Pediatr 1993;152 Suppl 1:S56–9.

35. Bodamer OA, Feillet F, Lane RE, et al. Utilization of cornstarch in glycogen storage disease type Ia. Eur J Gastroenterol Hepatol 2002;14:1251–6.

36. Ryan IP, Havel RJ, Laros RK Jr. Three consecutive pregnancies in a patient with glycogen storage disease type IA (von Gierke's disease). Am J Obstet Gynecol 1994;170:1687–90; discussion 1690–1.

37. Farber M, Knuppel RA, Binkiewicz A, et al. Pregnancy and von Gierke's disease. Obstet Gynecol 1976;47:226–8.

38. Johnson MP, Compton A, Drugan A, et al. Metabolic control of von Gierke disease (glycogen storage disease type Ia) in pregnancy: maintenance of euglycemia with cornstarch. Obstet Gynecol 1990;75:507–10.

39. Nuoffer JM, Mullis PE, Wiesmann UN. Treatment with low-dose diazoxide in two growth-retarded prepubertal girls with glycogen storage disease type Ia resulted in catch-up growth. J Inherit Metab Dis 1997;20:790–8.

40. Ozen H, Ciliv G, Kocak N, et al. Short-term effect of captopril on microalbuminuria in children with glycogen storage disease type Ia. J Inherit Metab Dis 2000;23:459–63.

41. Pela I, Donati MA, Zammarchi E. Effect of ramipril in a patient with glycogen storage disease type I and nephrotic-range proteinuria. J Inherit Metab Dis 2001;24:681–2.

42. Latger-Cannard V, Marchand-Arvier M, Vidailhet M, et al. Neutrophil adherence receptor deficiency regressing with granulocyte-colony stimulating factor therapy in a case of glycogen storage disease type Ib. Eur J Pediatr 2002; 161:87–93.

43. Boneh A, Auldist AW, Francis DE, et al. Splenectomy in two siblings with G-CSF-dependent glycogen storage disease type Ib. J Inherit Metab Dis 2001;24:419–21.

44. Matern D, Starzl TE, Arnaout W, et al. Liver transplantation for glycogen storage disease types I, III, and IV. Eur J Pediatr 1999;158 Suppl 2:S43–8.

45. Koestinger A, Gillet M, Chiolero R, et al. Effect of liver transplantation on hepatic glucose metabolism in a patient with type I glycogen storage disease. Transplantation 2000;69:2205–7.

46. Labrune P. Glycogen storage disease type I: indications for liver and/or kidney transplantation. Eur J Pediatr 2002;161 Suppl 1:S53–5.

47. Muraca M, Gerunda G, Neri D, et al. Hepatocyte transplantation as a treatment for glycogen storage disease type 1a. Lancet 2002;359:317–8.

48. Beaty RM, Jackson M, Peterson D, et al. Delivery of glucose-6-phosphatase in a canine model for glycogen storage disease, type Ia, with adeno-associated virus (AAV) vectors. Gene Ther 2002;9:1015–22.

49. Zingone A, Seidel J, Aloj L, et al. Monitoring the correction of glycogen storage disease type 1a in a mouse model using [(18)F]FDG and a dedicated animal scanner. Life Sci 2002; 71:1293–301.

50. Lee PJ. Glycogen storage disease type I: pathophysiology of liver adenomas. Eur J Pediatr 2002;161:S46–9.

51. Coleman RA, Winter HS, Wolf B, et al. Glycogen debranching enzyme deficiency: long-term study of serum enzyme activities and clinical features. J Inherit Metab Dis 1992;15: 869–81.

52. Kiechl S, Kohlendorfer U, Thaler C, et al. Different clinical aspects of debrancher deficiency myopathy. J Neurol Neurosurg Psychiatry 1999;67:364–8.

53. Cornelio F, Bresolin N, Singer PA, et al. Clinical varieties of neuromuscular disease in debrancher deficiency. Arch Neurol 1984;41:1027–32.

54. Van Creveld S, Huijing F. Differential diagnosis of the type of glycogen storage disease in two adult patients with a long history of glycogenosis. Metabolism 1964;13:191.

55. Illingworth B, Cori G, Cori C. Amylo-1,6-glucosidase in muscle tissue in generalized glycogen storage disease. J Biol Chem 1956;218:123.

56. Santer R, Kinner M, Steuerwald U, et al. Molecular genetic basis and prevalence of glycogen storage disease type IIIA in the Faroe Islands. Eur J Hum Genet 2001;9:388–91.

57. Parvari R, Moses S, Shen J, et al. A single-base deletion in the 3′-coding region of glycogen-debranching enzyme is prevalent in glycogen storage disease type IIIA in a population of North African Jewish patients. Eur J Hum Genet 1997;5:266–70.

58. Shen J, Bao Y, Liu HM, et al. Mutations in exon 3 of the glycogen debranching enzyme gene are associated with glycogen storage disease type III that is differentially expressed in liver and muscle. J Clin Invest 1996;98:352–7.

59. Fukuda T, Sugie H, Ito M. Novel mutations in two Japanese cases of glycogen storage disease type IIIa and a review of the literature of the molecular basis of glycogen storage disease type III. J Inherit Metab Dis 2000;23:95–106.

60. Sugie H, Fukuda T, Ito M, et al. Novel exon 11 skipping mutation in a patient with glycogen storage disease type IIId. J Inherit Metab Dis 2001;24:535–45.

61. Ding JH, de Barsy T, Brown BI, et al. Immunoblot analyses of glycogen debranching enzyme in different subtypes of glycogen storage disease type III. J Pediatr 1990;116:95–100.

62. Shen JJ, Chen YT. Molecular characterization of glycogen storage disease type III. Curr Mol Med 2002;2:167–75.

63. Fernandes J, Huijing F, van de Kamer JH. A screening method for liver glycogen diseases. Arch Dis Child 1969;44:311–7.

64. Hashimoto M, Watanabe G, Yokoyama T, et al. Case report: rupture of a gastric varix in liver cirrhosis associated with glycogen storage disease type III. J Gastroenterol Hepatol 1998;13: 232–5.

65. Okuda S, Kanda F, Takahashi K, et al. Fatal liver cirrhosis and esophageal variceal hemorrhage in a patient with type IIIa glycogen storage disease. Intern Med 1998;37:1055–7.

66. Markowitz AJ, Chen YT, Muenzer J, et al. A man with type III glycogenosis associated with cirrhosis and portal hypertension. Gastroenterology 1993;105:1882–5.

67. Haagsma EB, Smit GP, Niezen-Koning KE, et al. Type IIIb glycogen storage disease associated with end-stage cirrhosis and hepatocellular carcinoma. The Liver Transplant Group. Hepatology 1997;25:537–40.

68. Siciliano M, De Candia E, Ballarin S, et al. Hepatocellular carcinoma complicating liver cirrhosis in type IIIa glycogen storage disease. J Clin Gastroenterol 2000;31:80–2.

69. Lee PJ, Deanfield JE, Burch M, et al. Comparison of the functional significance of left ventricular hypertrophy in hypertrophic cardiomyopathy and glycogenosis type III. Am J Cardiol 1997;79:834–8.

70. Lee PJ, Patel A, Hindmarsh PC, et al. The prevalence of polycystic ovaries in the hepatic glycogen storage diseases: its association with hyperinsulinism. Clin Endocrinol (Oxf) 1995;42:601–6.

71. Mendoza A, Fisher NC, Duckett J, et al. Successful pregnancy in a patient with type III glycogen storage disease managed with cornstarch supplements. Br J Obstet Gynaecol 1998; 105:677–80.

72. Slonim AE, Weisberg C, Benke P, et al. Reversal of debrancher deficiency myopathy by the use of high-protein nutrition. Ann Neurol 1982;11:420–2.

73. Andersen DH. Familial cirrhosis of the liver with storage of abnormal glycogen. Lab Invest 1956;5:11–20.

74. Moses SW, Parvari R. The variable presentations of glycogen storage disease type IV: a review of clinical, enzymatic and molecular studies. Curr Mol Med 2002;2:177–88.

75. Thon VJ, Khalil M, Cannon JF. Isolation of human glycogen branching enzyme cDNAs by screening complementation in yeast. J Biol Chem 1993;268:7509–13.

76. Brown BI, Brown DH. Branching enzyme activity of cultured amniocytes and chorionic villi: prenatal testing for type IV glycogen storage disease. Am J Hum Genet 1989;44:378–81.

77. Sokal EM, Van Hoof F, Alberti D, et al. Progressive cardiac failure following orthotopic liver transplantation for type IV glycogenosis. Eur J Pediatr 1992;151:200–3.

78. Rosenthal P, Podesta L, Grier R, et al. Failure of liver transplantation to diminish cardiac deposits of amylopectin and leukocyte inclusions in type IV glycogen storage disease. Liver Transplant Surg 1995;1:373–6.

79. Starzl TE, Demetris AJ, Trucco M, et al. Chimerism after liver transplantation for type IV glycogen storage disease and type 1 Gaucher's disease. N Engl J Med 1993;328:745–9.

80. Billingsley GD, Cox DW, Duncan AM, et al. Regional localization of loci on chromosome 14 using somatic cell hybrids. Cytogenet Cell Genet 1994;66:33–8.

81. Chang S, Rosenberg MJ, Morton H, et al. Identification of a mutation in liver glycogen phosphorylase in glycogen storage disease type VI. Hum Mol Genet 1998;7:865–70.

82. Burwinkel B, Bakker HD, Herschkovitz E, et al. Mutations in the liver glycogen phosphorylase gene (PYGL) underlying glycogenosis type VI. Am J Hum Genet 1998;62:785–91.

83. Hug G, Schubert WK, Chuck G. Phosphorylase kinase of the liver: deficiency in a girl with increased hepatic glycogen. Science 1966;153:1534–5.

84. Huijing F, Fernandes J. X-chromosomal inheritance of liver glycogenosis with phosphorylase kinase deficiency. Am J Hum Genet 1969;21:275–84.

85. Burwinkel B, Shiomi S, Al Zaben A, et al. Liver glycogenosis due to phosphorylase kinase deficiency: PHKG2 gene structure and mutations associated with cirrhosis. Hum Mol Genet 1998;7:149–54.

86. van den Berg IE, van Beurden EA, de Klerk JB, et al. Autosomal recessive phosphorylase kinase deficiency in liver, caused by mutations in the gene encoding the beta subunit (PHKB). Am J Hum Genet 1997;61:539–46.

87. McKusick VA. Online Mendelian Inheritance in Man. Vol. NCBI; 2003. Available at: http://www.ncbi.nlm.nih.gov/omim/ (accessed Oct 10, 2003).

88. Nakai A, Shigematsu Y, Takano T, et al. Uncooked cornstarch treatment for hepatic phosphorylase kinase deficiency. Eur J Pediatr 1994;153:581–3.

89. Ficicioglu C, Aydin A, Mikla S, et al. Neonatal-onset severe recurrent hypoglycaemia in an infant with hepatic phosphorylase kinase deficiency with normal enzyme activity in erythrocytes. J Inherit Metab Dis 1996;19:84–5.

90. Burwinkel B, Tanner MS, Kilimann MW. Phosphorylase kinase deficient liver glycogenosis: progression to cirrhosis in infancy associated with PHKG2 mutations (H144Y and L225R). J Med Genet 2000;37:376–7.

91. Buhrer C, van Landeghem F, Bruck W, et al. Fetal-onset severe skeletal muscle glycogenosis associated with phosphorylase-B kinase deficiency. Neuropediatrics 2000;31:104–6.

92. Bak H, Cordato D, Carey WF, et al. Adult-onset exercise intolerance due to phosphorylase B kinase deficiency. J Clin Neurosci 2001;8:286–7.

93. Fanconi G, Bickel H. Die chronische Aminoaciduria (Aminosaurediabetes oder nephrotisch-glukosurischer Zwergwuchs) bei der Glykogenose und der Cystinkrankheit. Helv Paediat Acta 1949;4:359–96.

94. Santer R, Schneppenheim R, Suter D, et al. Fanconi-Bickel syndrome—the original patient and his natural history, historical steps leading to the primary defect, and a review of the literature. Eur J Pediatr 1998;157:783–97.

95. Santer R, Steinmann B, Schaub J. Fanconi-Bickel syndrome—a congenital defect of facilitative glucose transport. Curr Mol Med 2002;2:213–27.

96. Fukumoto H, Seino S, Imura H, et al. Sequence, tissue distribution, and chromosomal localization of mRNA encoding a human glucose transporter-like protein. Proc Natl Acad Sci U S A 1988;85:5434–8.

97. Santer R, Schneppenheim R, Dombrowski A, et al. Mutations in GLUT2, the gene for the liver-type glucose transporter, in patients with Fanconi-Bickel syndrome. Nat Genet 1997; 17:324–6.

98. Santer R, Groth S, Kinner M, et al. The mutation spectrum of the facilitative glucose transporter gene SLC2A2 (GLUT2) in patients with Fanconi-Bickel syndrome. Hum Genet 2002; 110:21–9.

99. Lee PJ, Van't Hoff WG, Leonard JV. Catch-up growth in Fanconi-Bickel syndrome with uncooked cornstarch. J Inherit Metab Dis 1995;18:153–6.

100. Manz F, Bickel H, Brodehl J, et al. Fanconi-Bickel syndrome. Pediatr Nephrol 1987;1:509–18.

101. Bachrach BE, Weinstein DA, Orho-Melander M, et al. Glycogen synthase deficiency (glycogen storage disease type 0) presenting with hyperglycemia and glucosuria: report of three new mutations. J Pediatr 2002;140:781–3.

102. Rutledge SL, Atchison J, Bosshard NU, et al. Case report: liver glycogen synthase deficiency—a cause of ketotic hypoglycemia. Pediatrics 2001;108:495–7.

103. Aynsley-Green A, Williamson DH, Gitzelmann R. Asymptomatic hepatic glycogen-synthetase deficiency. Lancet 1978;i:147–8.

104. Orho M, Bosshard NU, Buist NR, et al. Mutations in the liver glycogen synthase gene in children with hypoglycemia due to glycogen storage disease type 0. J Clin Invest 1998; 102:507–15.

105. Bonthron DT, Brady N, Donaldson IA, et al. Molecular basis of essential fructosuria: molecular cloning and mutational analysis of human ketohexokinase (fructokinase). Hum Mol Genet 1994;3:1627–31.

106. Steinmann B, Gitzelmann R, Van den Berghe G. Disorders of fructose metabolism. In: Scriver C, Beaudet A, Sly W, et al, editors. The metabolic and molecular bases of inherited disease. Vol 1. 8th ed. New York: McGraw-Hill; 2000. p. 1489–520.

107. Newbrun E, Hoover C, Mettraux G, et al. Comparison of dietary habits and dental health of subjects with hereditary fructose intolerance and control subjects. J Am Dent Assoc 1980; 101:619–26.

108. Muller-Wiefel DE, Steinmann B, Holm-Hadulla M, et al. [Infusion-associated kidney and liver failure in undiagnosed hereditary fructose intolerance]. Dtsch Med Wochenschr 1983;108:985–9.

109. Schulte MJ, Lenz W. Fatal sorbitol infusion in patient with fructose-sorbitol intolerance. Lancet 1977;ii:188.

110. Woods HF, Alberti KG. Dangers of intravenous fructose. Lancet 1972;ii:1354–7.

111. van den Berghe G, Bronfman M, Vanneste R, et al. The mechanism of adenosine triphosphate depletion in the liver after a load of fructose. A kinetic study of liver adenylate deaminase. Biochem J 1977;162:601–9.

112. Buemann B, Gesmar H, Astrup A, et al. Effects of oral D-tagatose, a stereoisomer of D-fructose, on liver metabolism in

man as examined by ^{31}P-magnetic resonance spectroscopy. Metabolism 2000;49:1335–9.

113. Oberhaensli RD, Rajagopalan B, Taylor DJ, et al. Study of hereditary fructose intolerance by use of ^{31}P magnetic resonance spectroscopy. Lancet 1987;ii:931–4.

114. Levin B, Snodgrass GJ, Oberholzer VG, et al. Fructosaemia. Observations on seven cases. Am J Med 1968;45:826–38.

115. Henry I, Gallano P, Besmond C, et al. The structural gene for aldolase B (ALDB) maps to 9q13-32. Ann Hum Genet 1985;49:173–80.

116. Cox TM. Hereditary fructose intolerance. Baillieres Clin Gastroenterol 1990;4:61–78.

117. Steinmann B, Gitzelmann R. The diagnosis of hereditary fructose intolerance. Helv Paediatr Acta 1981;36:297–316.

118. Sanchez-Gutierrez JC, Benlloch T, Leal MA, et al. Molecular analysis of the aldolase B gene in patients with hereditary fructose intolerance from Spain. J Med Genet 2002;39:e56.

119. Dursun A, Kalkanoglu HS, Coskun T, et al. Mutation analysis in Turkish patients with hereditary fructose intolerance. J Inherit Metab Dis 2001;24:523–6.

120. el-Maghrabi MR, Lange AJ, Jiang W, et al. Human fructose-1,6-bisphosphatase gene (FBP1): exon-intron organization, localization to chromosome bands 9q22.2-q22.3, and mutation screening in subjects with fructose-1,6-bisphosphatase deficiency. Genomics 1995;27:520–5.

121. Topcu M, Saatci I, Haliloglu G, et al. D-Glyceric aciduria in a six-month-old boy presenting with West syndrome and autistic behaviour. Neuropediatrics 2002;33:47–50.

122. Bonham JR, Stephenson TJ, Carpenter KH, et al. D(+)-Glyceric aciduria: etiology and clinical consequences. Pediatr Res 1990;28:38–41.

123. Gitzelmann R. Deficiency of erythrocyte galactokinase in a patient with galactose diabetes. Lancet 1965;ii:670–1.

124. Litman N, Kanter AI, Finberg L. Galactokinase deficiency presenting as pseudotumor cerebri. J Pediatr 1975;86:410–2.

125. Dunger DB, Holton JB. Disorders of carbohydrate metabolism. In: Holton JB, editor. The inherited metabolic diseases. London: Churchill Livingstone; 1994. p. 21–65.

126. Segal S, Berry GT. Disorders of galactose metabolism. In: Scriver C, Beaudet A, Sly W, Valle D, editors. The metabolic and molecular bases of inherited disease. Vol 1. 7th ed. New York: McGraw-Hill; 1995. p. 967–1000.

127. Hightower KR, Misiak P. The relationship between osmotic stress and calcium elevation: in vitro and in vivo rat lens models. Exp Eye Res 1998;66:775–81.

128. Hu TS, Datiles M, Kinoshita JH. Reversal of galactose cataract with sorbinil in rats. Invest Ophthalmol Vis Sci 1983;24:640–4.

129. Goppert F. Galaktosurie nach Milchzuckergabe bei angeborenem, familiaerem chronischem Leberleiden. Klin Wschr 1917;54:473–7.

130. Murphy M, McHugh B, Tighe O, et al. Genetic basis of transferase-deficient galactosaemia in Ireland and the population history of the Irish Travellers. Eur J Hum Genet 1999;7:549–54.

131. Barr PH. Association of Escherichia coli sepsis and galactosemia in neonates. J Am Board Fam Pract 1992;5:89–91.

132. Tyfield L, Reichardt J, Fridovich-Keil J, et al. Classical galactosemia and mutations at the galactose-1-phosphate uridyl transferase (GALT) gene. Hum Mutat 1999;13:417–30.

133. Widhalm K, Miranda da Cruz BD, Koch M. Diet does not ensure normal development in galactosemia. J Am Coll Nutr 1997;16:204–8.

134. Gitzelmann R, Steinmann B. Galactosemia: how does long-term treatment change the outcome? Enzyme 1984;32:37–46.

135. Waggoner DD, Buist NR, Donnell GN. Long-term prognosis in galactosaemia: results of a survey of 350 cases. J Inherit Metab Dis 1990;13:802–18.

136. Holton JB. Effects of galactosemia in utero. Eur J Pediatr 1995;154:S77–81.

137. Schweitzer S, Shin Y, Jakobs C, et al. Long-term outcome in 134 patients with galactosaemia. Eur J Pediatr 1993;152:36–43.

138. Acosta PB, Gross KC. Hidden sources of galactose in the environment. Eur J Pediatr 1995;154:S87–92.

139. Berry GT, Palmieri M, Gross KC, et al. The effect of dietary fruits and vegetables on urinary galactitol excretion in galactose-1-phosphate uridyltransferase deficiency. J Inherit Metab Dis 1993;16:91–100.

140. Walter JH, Roberts RE, Besley GT, et al. Generalised uridine diphosphate galactose-4-epimerase deficiency. Arch Dis Child 1999;80:374–6.

141. Robinson BR. Lactic acidemia (disorders of pyruvate carboxylase, pyruvate dehydrogenase). In: Scriver C, Beaudet A, Sly W, Valle D, editors. The metabolic and molecular bases of inherited disease. Vol 1. 7th ed. New York: McGraw-Hill; 1995. p. 1479–99.

142. Carbone MA, MacKay N, Ling M, et al. Amerindian pyruvate carboxylase deficiency is associated with two distinct missense mutations. Am J Hum Genet 1998;62:1312–9.

143. Brun N, Robitaille Y, Grignon A, et al. Pyruvate carboxylase deficiency: prenatal onset of ischemia-like brain lesions in two sibs with the acute neonatal form. Am J Med Genet 1999;84:94–101.

144. Van Coster RN, Fernhoff PM, De Vivo DC. Pyruvate carboxylase deficiency: a benign variant with normal development. Pediatr Res 1991;30:1–4.

145. Hamilton J, Rae MD, Logan RW, et al. A case of benign pyruvate carboxylase deficiency with normal development. J Inherit Metab Dis 1997;20:401–3.

146. Robinson BH, Oei J, Saudubray JM, et al. The French and North American phenotypes of pyruvate carboxylase deficiency, correlation with biotin containing protein by 3H-biotin incorporation, 35S-streptavidin labeling, and Northern blotting with a cloned cDNA probe. Am J Hum Genet 1987;40:50–9.

147. Ahmad A, Kahler SG, Kishnani PS, et al. Treatment of pyruvate carboxylase deficiency with high doses of citrate and aspartate. Am J Med Genet 1999;87:331–8.

148. Nyhan W, Khanna A, Barshop B, et al. Pyruvate carboxylase deficiency—insights from liver transplantation. Mol Genet Metab 2002;77:143.

149. Hommes FA, Bendien K, Elema JD, et al. Two cases of phosphoenolpyruvate carboxykinase deficiency. Acta Paediatr Scand 1976;65:233–40.

150. Clayton PT, Hyland K, Brand M, et al. Mitochondrial phosphoenolpyruvate carboxykinase deficiency. Eur J Pediatr 1986;145:46–50.

151. Matsuo M, Maeda E, Nakamura H, et al. Hepatic phosphoenolpyruvate carboxykinase deficiency: a neonatal case with reduced activity of pyruvate carboxylase. J Inherit Metab Dis 1989;12:336–7.

152. Vidnes J, Sovik O. Gluconeogenesis in infancy and childhood. III. Deficiency of the extramitochondrial form of hepatic phosphoenolpyruvate carboxykinase in a case of persistent neonatal hypoglycaemia. Acta Paediatr Scand 1976;65:307–12.

153. Leonard JV, Hyland K, Furukawa N, et al. Mitochondrial phosphoenolpyruvate carboxykinase deficiency. Eur J Pediatr 1991;150:198–9.

2. Amino Acid Metabolism

Karen F. Murray, MD

C. Ronald Scott, MD

Vomiting, irritability, and failure to thrive are frequent symptoms for which consultation with a pediatric gastroenterologist is sought. Especially when the child is an infant, inborn errors of metabolism must be included in the list of potential diagnoses. Discussed in this chapter are those errors of metabolism that occur in the use or breakdown of amino acids—frequent disorders that can result in common symptoms encountered in pediatric gastroenterology practice. Additionally, because the liver is the main site for many of these metabolic processes, other nonspecific findings, such as hepatomegaly or hepatic dysfunction, may precipitate referral erroneously for evaluation of primary liver disease. Understanding the most common conditions, their forms of presentation, and the methods with which they can be quickly distinguished and diagnosed is the main goal of this chapter.

The metabolic conditions can be categorized into (1) disorders of the aromatic amino acids, of which hereditary tyrosinemia is the most common disorder encountered by gastroenterologists; (2) disorders of branched-chain amino acids (BCAAs), including maple syrup urine disease (MSUD), isovalericaciduria (IVA), propionicaciduria (PA), and methylmalonicaciduria (MMA); and (3) the urea cycle defects, including ornithine transcarbamylase (OTC) deficiency, carbamyl phosphate synthetase (CPS) deficiency, citrullinemia, argininosuccinicaciduria, N-acetylglutamate synthetase deficiency, and argininemia. It should be noted that other amino acid metabolic disturbances have been identified in rare subjects; consequently, unusual patterns of metabolite profiles could be encountered for which additional consultation for diagnosis should be considered.

For each condition, the molecular basis of the disease is reviewed, the common clinical presentations are discussed, the method of diagnosis and the distinguishing patterns of metabolites detected with each condition are reviewed, and the effective therapies are covered. Additionally, it is important to understand that nonspecific amino acid disturbances occur with liver disease in general, and the bases for these changes are discussed so that they may be properly interpreted when encountered.

DISORDERED AMINO ACID PROFILES SEEN WITH HEPATIC DISEASE

Hepatic dysfunction with or without hyperammonemia, severe hepatitis, and cholestatic liver disease may cause nonspecific abnormalities in serum and urine amino acid profiles. In the setting of hyperammonemia, concentra-

tions of glutamine, alanine, and sometimes aspartic acid are elevated. With cholestatic liver disease, severe hepatitis and hepatic dysfunction elevation of tyrosine and methionine are frequently seen as a consequence of a nonspecific reduction of tyrosine aminotransferase enzyme activity. Tyrosine aminotransferase is the rate-limiting step in tyrosine metabolism, and its activity can be reduced by as much as 50% with liver disease.

DISORDERS OF AROMATIC AMINO ACIDS

HEREDITARY TYROSINEMIA
Disorders of aromatic amino acids are the most common of the inborn errors of amino acid metabolism owing to the high frequency of phenylketonuria in the population and frequency of alkaptonuria and tyrosinemia, types II and III. However, for the gastroenterologist, it is the disorder of tyrosinemia type I that is of major concern.

Tyrosinemia type I is a devastating disease of childhood that causes liver failure, painful neurologic crises, hepatocarcinoma, and usually death prior to the age of 10 years. It is a rare disorder in the general population, with an incidence no greater than 1 in 100,000 newborns.[1] However, because of the inconsistent and confusing nature of its clinical presentation, it is estimated that less than 50% of cases are diagnosed before their demise. Children born with tyrosinemia type I typically develop severe liver disease at less than 6 months of age and, if unrecognized or untreated, die within a few weeks to months. A more chronic form of the disorder exists in which children develop first symptoms older than 6 months and have a better short-term prognosis. These patients typically present with a Fanconi-like renal syndrome, rickets, and growth failure. They may have repetitive bouts of neurologic crises that are similar in nature to those seen in older patients with acute intermittent porphyria (changes in mental status, abdominal pain, peripheral neuropathy, respiratory depression). In all cases, the symptoms are severe, leading either to death in infancy or to chronic early childhood morbidity, with the eventual development of hepatocarcinoma and death in the later years of childhood.

MOLECULAR DEFECT
Tyrosinemia type I occurs because of a deficiency of fumarylacetoacetate hydrolase (FAH),[2,3] the terminal enzyme in the tyrosine catabolic pathway (Figure 55.2-1). With the deficiency of FAH, the immediate precursor, fumarylacetoacetate (FAA), is prevented from being con-

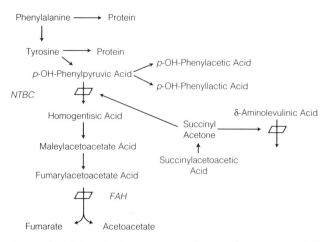

FIGURE 55.2-1 Tyrosine pathway indicating the enzymatic deficiency in tyrosinemia type I and the sites of succinylacetone inhibition. 2-(2-Nitro-4-trifluoromethylbenzoyl)-1,3-cyclohexanedione (NTBC) acts as an inhibitor of *p*-hydroxyphenylpyruvate oxidase. FAH = fumarylacetoacetate hydrolase.

verted to fumerate and acetoacetate, and FAA is instead diverted to succinylacetoacetate and succinylacetone. These two compounds, particularly succinylacetone, are believed to be the toxic metabolites in tyrosinemia. It is known that succinylacetone interferes with two enzymatic reactions, *p*-hydroxyphenylpyruvic acid dioxygenase (*p*-HPPD) and δ-aminolevulinic acid (δ-ALA). The elevation of plasma tyrosine observed in tyrosinemia is secondary to the inhibition to *p*-HHPD by succinylacetone.

Succinylacetone is also a potent inhibitor of δ-ALA hydratase.[4] It is the inhibition of this enzyme that precipitates the acute neurologic episodes. δ-ALA dehydratase activities have been shown to be reduced in liver and circulating red cells, and δ-ALA is excreted in high levels in children with tyrosinemia type I.[5] There are also suggestions that succinylacetone may interfere with immune functions, cell functions, heme synthesis, and renal tubular function.[6–8]

Two regions of the world have a higher than expected frequency of tyrosinemia type I. In Norway and Finland, the incidence at birth is estimated to be approximately 1 in 60,000 live births, and within the Saguenay-Lac Saint-Jean region of Quebec, Canada, there is an incidence of 1 in 1,846 live births that has occurred because of a founder effect.[9] A common mutation exists within the latter population (IVS12+5 G→A). Within the United States, only a few mutations account for the majority of cases, with these mutations introduced from the populations of northern and southern Europe and from Mexico.

CLINICAL FEATURES

The clinical presentation of patients with tyrosinemia can be divided into two main groups: those presenting at less than 6 months of age with severe liver involvement and those presenting after 6 months of age with either mild liver dysfunction or renal involvement, growth failure, and rickets (Table 55.2-1). Children less than 6 months of age typically have acute liver failure, with a markedly

prolonged prothrombin time and partial thromboplastin time that are not corrected by vitamin K supplementation. The analysis of other clotting factors indicates the preservation of factor V and factor VIII levels but a decrease in factors II, VII, IX, XI, and XII. Serum transaminase levels may be modestly elevated, and serum bilirubin may be normal or only slightly elevated. Thus, the loss of clotting factors from synthetic function is the major abnormality in the early phases of the disorder.[11] The other striking biochemical feature is a markedly elevated α-fetoprotein that averages approximately 160,000 ng/mL at the time of diagnosis. For those children presenting in the acute phase of their illness, appropriate intervention strategies are essential to prevent their demise. This early phase can progress to loss of liver function and the appearance of ascites, jaundice, and gastrointestinal bleeding. There may be a characteristic odor of "boiled cabbage" or "rotten mushrooms." The odor and elevation of α-fetoprotein often lead to the recognition and eventual documentation of elevations of plasma methionine and tyrosine and the identification of succinylacetone in urine or plasma.

In the more chronic form of the disorder, renal involvement is the major manifestation. The renal tubular dysfunction involves a generalized aminoaciduria, phosphate loss, and, for many, renal tubular acidosis. The continued renal loss of phosphate is believed to be the mechanism for the development of rickets because abnormal calcium levels have not been systematically documented. Growth failure can be ascribed to the chronic illness from poor nutritional intake, liver involvement, or chronic renal disease.

Repeated episodes of neurologic crises often go unrecognized. Mitchell and colleagues reported that 42% of the patients in the French Canadian population had experienced these episodes.[5] They often are associated with excruciating pain and posturing and can last 1 to 7 days. They are associated with weakness or paralysis that, in some cases, may require mechanical ventilation for survival. Van Spronsen and colleagues reported in the international survey that 10% of deaths occurred during a neurologic crisis, representing a major life-threatening mechanism independent of liver failure.[10]

DIAGNOSIS

The pathognomonic metabolite for the confirmation of the diagnosis is succinylacetone. Succinylacetone can be detected in the urine of all untreated patients with tyrosinemia type I. Organic acid analysis by gas chromatography–mass spectroscopy will identify an organic acid pattern with elevations of parahydroxyphenylacetic acid, parahydroxyphenyllactic acid, and significant elevations of succinylacetone. Succinylacetone may need to be requested specifically on laboratory request forms.

The measurement of FAH in cultured skin fibroblasts can be used as a confirmatory test or, potentially, the identification of an abnormal mutation within the FAH gene. These latter approaches are not readily available as a common clinical assay.

TABLE 55.2-1 COMPARATIVE FEATURES OF THE MOST COMMON DISORDERS OF AMINO ACID METABOLISM

DIAGNOSIS	PHENOTYPE	CLINICAL FEATURES	SERUM GLUCOSE	SERUM AMMONIA	METABOLIC ACIDOSIS	URINE KETONES	SERUM AMINO ACIDS	URINE AMINO ACIDS	URINE ORGANIC ACIDS	DIAGNOSIS
Tyrosinemia type I	Acute chronic	Acute liver failure or renal Fanconi syndrome with rickets	Normal	Normal	Absent or mild	None	Elevated methionine and tyrosine	Elevated methionine and tyrosine	Succinylacetone	Succinylacetone in urine or plasma
Maple syrup urine disease	Classic	Neonatal encephalopathy; "maple syrup" urine odor	Sometimes low	Normal	Prominent	Elevated	Markedly increased alloisoleucine, BCAAs	Elevated BCAAs	Elevated BCKAs	BCKD activity in cultured fibroblasts or lymphocytes < 2%
	Intermediate	Developmental delay, seizures	Normal	Normal	Prominent during symptoms	Elevated	Same as above	Same as above	Same as above	3–30%
	Intermittent	Episodic ataxia and lethargy	Normal	Normal	Prominent during symptoms	Elevated during symptoms	Elevated BCAA during symptoms	Elevated BCAA during symptoms	Elevated BCAA during symptoms	5–20%
Isovalericaciduria, propionicaciduria, methylmalonicaciduria	Same as above	Same as above; dehydration, hepatomegaly; "sweaty feet" odor in IVA	Variable	Elevated	Prominent	Elevated	Nonspecific elevations of glycine	Nonspecific elevations	Specific OA patterns	Cultured fibroblast enzyme activity
Ornithine transcarbamylase deficiency	Classic	Lethargy; poor feeding, coma, seizures, developmental delay	Normal	Elevated	Absent	None		Nonspecific elevation	Orotic acid elevation	Small intestine or liver biopsy enzyme activity
Carbamyl phosphate synthetase deficiency	Same as above	Same as above	Normal	Elevated	Absent	None	Absent citrulline	Nonspecific elevation	Nonspecific elevation	Same as above
Citrullinemia	Same as above	Same as above	Normal	Elevated	Absent	None	Elevated citrulline	Elevated citrulline	Nonspecific elevation	Cultured fibroblast or lymphocyte enzyme activity
Argininosuccinicaciduria	Neonatal	Same as above; fragile hair	Normal	Elevated	Absent	None	Elevation of glutamine and argininosuccinic acid	Elevated arginine-succinate	Nonspecific elevation	Cultured fibroblast or erythrocyte enzyme activity
	Late onset	Developmental delay; hepatomegaly; fragile hair	Normal	Episodically elevated		None	Same as above	Same as above	Nonspecific elevation	Same as above
Arginase		Developmental delay, spasticity	Normal	Moderately elevated	Absent	None	Elevated arginine	Elevated lysine, arginine, ornithine, cystine	Orotic acid elevation	Erythrocyte enzyme activity

BCAA = branched-chain amino acid; BCKA = branched-chain α-keto acids; BCKD = branched-chain α-keto dehydrogenase; IVA = isovalericaciduria; OA = organic acid.

TREATMENT

Prior to 1995, there was no effective medical treatment for tyrosinemia type I. Dietary interventions using an artificial formula, low in phenylalanine and tyrosine, were modestly helpful in reducing the formation of succinylacetone and were of some benefit in the more chronic forms of the disease. They were not very effective, however, in managing the acute stage of the disease of young children presenting with liver failure or in the long-term prevention of hepatocarcinoma for those children who survived their early presentation. Data supplied by van Spronsen and colleagues in 1994 showed that for those children diagnosed at less than 2 months of age, there was a 75% mortality rate by 2 years; for those diagnosed between 2 and 6 months of age, there was a 70% mortality by 6 years; and for those diagnosed older than 6 months of age, there was a 40% mortality by 10 years.[11] The only effective therapy was liver transplant to remove the genetic burden of FAH deficiency from the host.

In 1992, Lindstedt and colleagues reported preliminary data on the use of an inhibitor called NTBC [2-(2-nitro-4-trifluoromethylbenzoyl)-1,3-cyclohexanedione] (or nitisinone; available as Orfadin from Rare Disease Therapeutics, Nashville, TN) as an effective inhibitor of parahydroxyphenylpyruvic acid oxidase for the treatment of tyrosinemia.[11] This inhibitor blocks the enzyme proximal in the catabolic pathway of tyrosine and prevents substrate from reaching the FAH enzyme. Thus, succinylacetoacetate and succinylacetone are unable to be formed, and this prevents the deleterious consequences of their existence. In studies in Europe and the United States, over 250 children with documented tyrosinemia type I have now received this compound (E. Holme, personal communication, 2001). It has reduced the mortality of children with tyrosinemia type I and has dramatically affected the natural history of the disease. Within the United States, of 63 children placed acutely on the medication, there have been 5 deaths. Each death occurred within the first 2 weeks of drug administration, all in children in acute liver failure who were unable to recover from the acute stage of their disease. For the remainder of the children, there was a dramatic improvement (C. R. Scott, unpublished data, 2004). Liver function begins to recover within a week, prothrombin and thromboplastin times return to normal values within 1 month and 2 months, respectively, high levels of α-fetoprotein return to normal levels between 6 months and 1 year, and detectable succinylacetone in the urine disappears within 1 to 2 days of initiation of oral treatment. Normal growth has been demonstrated in children following treatment for a period of 5 to 7 years (C. R. Scott, unpublished data, 2004).

Dietary intervention remains an important aspect of treatment, even with the use of nitisinone. Because nitisinone blocks p-hydroxyphenylpyruvic acid oxidase, tyrosine values in blood can rise to levels that cause tyrosine crystals to be deposited in tissue. Tyrosine has a low degree of solubility and readily crystallizes in tissue at concentrations that exceed its solubility. The major complication from nitisinone therapy is tyrosine crystal deposition in the cornea, which leads to photophobia and an inflammatory response in the eye. To prevent this, it is recommended that tyrosine concentrations be monitored in children on a tyrosine-restricted diet and nitisinone to maintain the tyrosine concentration at less than 500 µM. At this level, no eye complications have been observed. To achieve a satisfactory plasma concentration of tyrosine requires special formulas deficient in phenylalanine and tyrosine, coupled with a low-protein diet, not dissimilar to that given to children with phenylketonuria. For young children under the age of 6 months, this is usually not a problem; however, for older children, it may require significant nutritional skills and counseling to achieve these goals.

Monitoring of the liver for the potential development of hepatocarcinoma is essential. It is recommended that magnetic resonance images or computed tomographic scans of the liver be obtained on an annual basis. Given that the liver texture is frequently nodular, monitoring for interval changes that could suggest emerging or enlarging hepatocarcinoma, in the setting of persistently elevated α-fetoprotein, is imperative. This, coupled with monitoring of α-fetoprotein as an indicator of tumor formation, is necessary. Radiographic monitoring should continue until the α-fetoprotein has persistently returned to normal.

Liver transplant still remains an option for eventual treatment but is not as emergent as in the past. Longer-term studies are necessary at this time to make a value judgment on whether liver transplant will be necessary in a significant percentage of affected children, depending on their age of diagnosis or the eventual formation of hepatic nodules with transformation. Of the 19 patients who underwent liver transplant, only 5 patients were operated on for the possibility of hepatocarcinoma, and 4 of these were confirmed to have carcinomatous changes.

DISORDERS OF BCAAS

MAPLE SYRUP URINE DISEASE (BRANCHED-CHAIN KETOACIDURIA)

The cases of four siblings with cerebral degeneration within the first weeks of life and death within months, all with urine smelling of maple syrup, were first reported in 1954.[12] Westall and colleagues subsequently studied another child with the same clinical features and found high levels of serum BCAAs, and coined the term "maple syrup urine disease."[13] High levels of the branched-chain α-keto acids (BCKAs) derived from the BCAA were then isolated in the urine of these patients, implicating the decarboxylation step as the blocked step in the metabolism of the α-keto acids—hence the alternate name "branched-chain ketoaciduria."[14]

Hepatic presentations may occur with MSUD and other organicacidurias with a Reye-like syndrome characterized by coma, cerebral edema, hepatomegaly, liver dysfunction, hypoglycemia, and hyperammonemia with liver histology showing macro- or microvesicular fatty infiltration.[15] Additionally, pancreatitis is sometimes observed with MSUD and other organicacidurias.[16]

MSUD is an autosomal recessive panethnic metabolic disorder caused by a deficiency in activity of the mitochondrial branched-chain α-keto acid dehydrogenase (BCKD) complex. The worldwide frequency is approximately 1 in 185,000 live births. In select genetically isolated populations such as the Old Order Mennonite populations of Pennsylvania, however, MSUD occurs as frequently as 1 in 176 live births.[17]

MOLECULAR DEFECT

MSUD results from a deficiency in the activity of the BCKD multienzyme complex (Figure 55.2-2). In normal catabolism of BCAAs, the amino acids are transported into the cell by a cytosolic membrane transporter. Inside the cell, they are reversibly transaminated by the cytosolic or mitochondrial isoforms of the BCAA aminotransferase to produce the BCKA. The BCKAs are then translocated by a specific transporter into the mitochondria, where they are oxidatively decarboxylated by the single BCKD complex. These reactions generate the corresponding branched-chain acyl CoAs, which are further metabolized to acetyl CoA and acetoacetic acid (leucine), acetyl CoA and succinyl CoA (isoleucine), and succinyl CoA (valine). These end products are used in fatty acid and cholesterol synthesis and adenosine triphosphate synthesis. In the human, the skeletal muscle is the main site of BCAA transamination and oxidation, but there is also BCKD activity in the liver, kidney, heart, brain, and adipose tissue.

Deficiency of the BCKD complex results in inadequate oxidative decarboxylation of the BCKAs, causing the accumulation of BCAAs (leucine, isoleucine, valine) and the associated BCKAs (α-ketoisocaproic acid, α-keto-α-methylvaleric acid, α-ketoisovaleric acid).

The mitochondrial BCKD is an enzyme complex macromolecule with three catalytic components: a thiamine pyrophosphate–dependent decarboxylase, a transacylase, and a dehydrogenase. Additionally, the complex has two regulatory enzymes, a kinase and a phosphatase, which control the complex's activity through reversible phosphorylation-dephosphorylation. Each component is coded for by a separate characterized gene, leading to wide genetic heterogenicity underlying the MSUD phenotype.

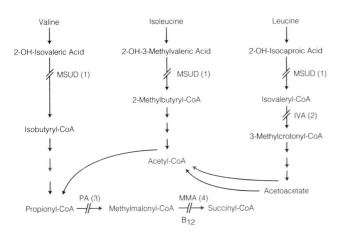

FIGURE 55.2-2 Branched-chain amino acid metabolism. IVA = isovalericaciduria; MMA = methylmalonicaciduria; MSUD = maple syrup urine disease; PA = propionicaciduria. 1 = branched-chain ketoacid decarboxylase; 2 = isovaleryl-CoA dehydrogenase; 3 = propionyl-CoA carboxylase; 4 = methylmalonyl-CoA mutase.

CLINICAL FEATURES

Multiple clinical phenotypes of MSUD are described based on the biochemical and clinical features (see Table 55.2-1). Distinction based on the patient's responsiveness to thiamine is also made in practice.

Classic. The "classic" form of MSUD is both the most common and most severe form of the disease. It is characterized by the onset of encephalopathy in the neonatal period with high levels of BCAAs, particularly of leucine, in the blood, cerebrospinal fluid, and urine. The presence of alloisoleucine is also characteristic. Symptoms usually develop toward the end of the first week of life, but breast-feeding may delay the onset into the second week. Lethargy and apathy toward feeding are followed by progressive neurologic signs of alternating hyper- and hypotonia, with dystonic extension of the upper extremities and weight loss. It is at this stage that ketosis and the maple syrup or burnt sugar odor to the urine become apparent. Hypoglycemia is not a prominent feature but can be observed. Ultimately, seizures and coma followed by death will occur unless treatment is instituted. Untreated, most patients die in the first months of life from repeated bouts of metabolic crisis and ongoing neurologic deterioration precipitated by infection or other stresses. Surviving individuals may suffer from mental retardation and spasticity. Early treatment has greatly improved the complications faced by these patients, but patients are still at high risk of neurologic sequelae. Even in apparent metabolic control, transient ataxia can occur, and visual hallucinations are frequently experienced in periods of ketonemia.[18] Metabolic crises induced by physical stress can cause encephalopathy and death.[18,19] These patients usually have less than 2% of the normal BCKD activity in cultured fibroblasts or lymphoblasts.

Intermediate. These rare patients are spared the catastrophic neonatal neurologic crises but do have persistently elevated BCAAs. Neurologic impairment with developmental delay and seizures are still a risk. In these subjects, the BCKD activity is roughly 3 to 30% of normal. Few patients have been diagnosed with this form of MSUD, most in the 5-month to 7-year age range during evaluations for their neurologic abnormalities.

Intermittent. Children with this variant usually present between 5 months and 2 years of age. Earlier in life, they have normal growth and development; however, with infectious stresses such as normal childhood illnesses, they develop metabolic decompensation, exhibited most commonly as ataxia and lethargy. More subtle findings of unsteady gait or behavioral changes may progress to seizures, stupor, and coma. Although the plasma BCAAs are normal during well, nonstressed times, the classic findings of maple syrup urine odor and elevated plasma BCAAs and BCKAs occur during symptomatic periods and can be detected in serum amino acid and urine organic acid profiles. The BCKD complex activity typically ranges between 5 and 20% of normal.[17]

Thiamine-Responsive MSUD. Some individuals who have a chronic elevation of BCAAs and gradual advancement of neurologic involvement without crises (intermediate variant) will have enhanced responsiveness with thiamine administration in addition to the usual protein restriction therapy. The patient population is heterogeneous, and none have been able to be treated with thiamine alone.

DIAGNOSIS

Detection of elevated BCKAs by gas chromatography–mass spectroscopy analysis of urine and elevated BCAAs in the blood by amino acid analysis is indicative of the disorder. The presence of alloisoleucine is pathognomonic for MSUD. Definitive diagnosis is established by a low measured activity of BCKD in cultured lymphocytes or fibroblasts.

NEWBORN SCREENING AND PRENATAL DIAGNOSIS

In some states, MSUD may be detected by newborn screening. The fragmentation pattern of the protonated molecular ions of leucine, isoleucine, and alloisoleucine is measurable by tandem mass spectroscopy. Classic and intermediate variants can be detected through newborn screening; however, the intermittent variant may be missed if their levels of BCAAs in the newborn period are normal.

Prenatal diagnosis is possible by measuring the BCKD activity from cultured cells obtained through amniocentesis (amniocytes) or chorionic villus sampling. The BCKD activity from these cultured cells is in the same range as found with cultured fibroblasts and can be performed from amniotic fluid cells obtained at midtrimester (weeks 14 to 18 of gestation).

TREATMENT

Both removal of the toxic metabolites and minimizing catabolism and promoting anabolism are important in the initial phase of management. In the acute symptomatic situation, treatment must be instituted emergently to prevent or limit the rapid neurologic deterioration that will otherwise occur. Hemodialysis and continuous venovenous hemofiltration are the most efficient methods for BCAA and BCKA clearance from very high levels.

Dietary therapy is the mainstay of acute and chronic management. Initially, the BCAAs are totally omitted from the diet for a few days to allow for correction of their elevated levels. When enteral intake is possible, this can be achieved with BCAD 1 or 2 (Mead Johnson and Company, Evansville, IN) or Ketonex 1 or 2 (Ross Pediatrics, Abbott Laboratories, Columbus, OH), formulas that are leucine, isoleucine, and valine free (Table 55.2-2). The plasma levels of isoleucine, followed by valine, and then leucine 7 to 10 days later, will normalize with proper management. Because leucine is the most neurologically toxic metabolite, its normalization is imperative. Leucine-level normalization can be accelerated by adding isoleucine and valine into the diet to maintain their plasma concentration above normal. When parenteral nutrition is necessary, a BCAA-free L-amino acid mixture in combination with glucose, lipid, electrolytes, and vitamins can provide balanced nutrition. Again, isoleucine and valine supplementation after the first few days of therapy can expedite the return to normal levels of leucine. With either parenteral or enteral nutrition, special attention to the changing protein requirements of the subject must occur to properly adjust their dietary therapy.

During stable metabolism, the daily requirements for the BCAA vary dramatically with age, the severity of the enzyme deficiency, and the child's growth rate. The leucine requirement is highest in the first 6 months of life and then falls to stable requirements around the second and third year of life, remaining relatively stable through the first decade. Although the normal daily leucine requirement is between 300 and 600 mg, the optimal intake of this BCAA in subjects with MSUD must be individualized because their requirements may be a fraction of those for normal children. Plasma levels should be kept as close to normal as possible but less than 300 μM, with special attention to avoiding the situation of high leucine in relation to valine and isoleucine. Frequent monitoring of these levels is advisable during the first year of life.

In some subjects, pharmacologic doses of thiamine (5 mg/kg/d) for 3 weeks may improve BCAA tolerance[20] and biochemical stability. Consequently, a trial of thiamine is usually warranted.

TABLE 55.2-2   ENTERAL FORMULAS FOR METABOLIC DISEASE

METABOLIC DISORDER	DESCRIPTION	FORMULAS	
		MEAD JOHNSON NUTRITIONALS*	ROSS PEDIATRICS*†
Tyrosinemia	Phenyalanine and tyrosine free	TYR 1† and Tyros 2, 3200AB§	Tyrex 1 and 2
Maple syrup urine disease	Leucine, isoleucine, and valine free	BCAD 2,‖ MSUD diet†	Ketonex 1 and 2
Propionicaciduria, Methylmalonicaciduria	Isoleucine, valine, methionine, and threonine free	OS 1 and 2#	Propimex 1 and 2
Isovalericaciduria	Leucine free		I-Valex 1 and 2
Urea cycle defects	Contains only essential and some conditionally essential amino acids	UCD 1,# WND 2§	Cyclinex 1 and 2

*"1" formulas are for infants under 1 year of age and "2" formulas are for children over 1 year of age.
†Ross products contain carbohydrate: hydrolyzed cornstarch; fat: coconut, soy, and palm oil; electrolytes, minerals, vitamins, and trace elements.
†Contains carbohydrate: sucrose; fat: corn oil; electrolytes, minerals, vitamins, and trace elements. Formula names and formulas are subject to change.
§Contains corn syrup solids, modified tapioca starch, corn oil; electrolytes, minerals, vitamins, and trace elements.
‖Contains corn syrup solids, sugar, modified corn starch, soy oil; electrolytes, minerals, vitamins, and trace elements.
#Contains sucrose, no fat; electrolytes, minerals, vitamins, and trace elements.

In severe cases of the neonatal (classic) form of MSUD, liver transplant has been used successfully to correct the metabolic perturbations and allow an unrestricted diet with neurologic stability.[21]

ISOVALERICACIDURIA, PROPIONICACIDURIA, AND METHYLMALONICACIDURIA

Like MSUD, these organicacidurias result from defects in the catabolism of the BCAAs. They, too, can present clinically with severe neonatal crisis, intermittent and late forms, and chronically progressive forms with developmental delay, hypotonia, failure to thrive, and seizures.

Molecular Defects. Isovalericaciduria. The first children described with IVA were siblings with an odor of "sweaty feet" or "cheese."[22,23] IVA is now known to be an autosomal recessive inherited disorder caused by a deficiency in the mitochondrial flavoprotein isovaleryl-CoA dehydrogenase apoprotein, which transfers electrons to the respiratory chain via the electron transfer flavoprotein (see Figure 55.2-2, enzyme 2). This deficiency results in the accumulation of isovaleryl-CoA derivatives, including isovaleric acid, 3-hydroxyvaleric acid, N-isovalerylglycine, and isovaleryl-carnitine; the latter two forms are nontoxic, readily excreted derivatives of the toxic isovaleric acid; hence, glycine and carnitine can be used therapeutically to aid in isovaleric acid excretion.

Propionicaciduria. PA is an autosomal recessive disorder with an incidence of less than 1 in 100,000 live births.[16] It is caused by a deficiency in the mitochondrial biotin-dependent enzyme propionyl-CoA carboxylase (see Figure 55.2-2, enzyme 3). This enzyme defect results in elevated levels of free propionate, propionylcarnitine, 3-hydroxypropionate, and methylcitrate in the urine and blood. More rarely combined defects that are partly responsive to biotin have been described.

Methylmalonicaciduria. MMA is an autosomal recessive disorder, with an incidence of 1 in 100,000 live births, caused by a deficiency in vitamin B$_{12}$–dependent methylmalonyl-CoA mutase apoenzyme (see Figure 55.2-2, enzyme 4). The resultant metabolic block results in elevated levels of methylmalonyl CoA, methylmalonic acid, and, secondarily, the same elevations as seen with PA in plasma and urine. In subjects in whom elevated methylmalonic acid is found, vitamin B$_{12}$ deficiency must be ruled out.

Clinical Features. The clinical presentations of patients with IVA, PA, or MMA follow the same patterns as those in subjects with MSUD. Patients presenting with IVA, PA, or MMA are frequently dehydrated and commonly have moderate hepatomegaly. They have a metabolic acidosis from hyperlactacidemia, elevated anion gap, and ketonuria. Hyperammonemia is uniformly present with IVA, PA, and MMA and, if severe enough, can cause a confounding picture that may lead the clinician to erroneously diagnose a urea cycle defect (Figure 55.2-3). Moderate hypocalcemia and variable glucose levels (hypo-, normal, or hyper-) are common, and cytopenias are frequent with IVA, PA, and MMA. IVA can be distinquished by its "sweaty feet" unpleasant odor.

Diagnosis and Prenatal Diagnosis. Diagnosis in IVA, PA, and MMA is based on the detection of the elevated organic acids in the plasma or urine in the pattern specific for the different disorders.

For those states or countries using tandem mass spectroscopy as a component of newborn screening, each of these organic acid disorders will be detected from submitted blood spots. An abnormal profile of acylcarnitine will detect increased concentrations of propionyl-, methylmalonyl-, or isovalerylcarnitine.

In the case of IVA, PA, and MMA, reliable and fast prenatal diagnosis is possible by the twelfth to fourteenth week of gestation by directly measuring the metabolites in the amniotic fluid. Direct enzyme analysis can also be performed from fresh or cultured chorionic villi or cultured amniocytes.

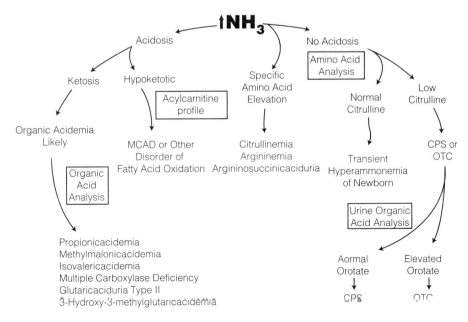

FIGURE 55.2-3 Diagnostic evaluation of the hyperammonemic infant. CPS = carbamyl phosphate synthetase; MCAD = medium-chain acyl-CoA dehydrogenase deficiency; OTC = ornithine transcarbamylase deficiency.

Treatment. The same principles as with the treatment of MSUD apply to the treatment of these disorders. Protein restriction, specifically BCAA restriction, is required. Specialty formulas with supplemental amino acids or protein as indicated are again effective (see Table 55.2-2) with attention to maintaining anabolism even in the face of metabolic crisis. In the case of IVA, leucine restriction is required. For patients with defects of PA, the administration of biotin (5 mg/d orally) may help in clinical and biochemical improvement.

In acute metabolic crisis, hemodialysis or continuous venous-venous hemoperfusion is effective, and for IVA, oral L-glycine (250–600 mg/kg/d) and intravenous L-carnitine (100–400 mg/kg/d) may assist with toxin removal.

DISORDERS OF THE UREA CYCLE

The urea cycle serves to convert the ammonia into nontoxic and readily excreted urea. Ammonia is produced continuously from degradation of the amino groups of amino acids and purines and from the amide groups of glutamine and asparagine. Although some is reused in the synthesis of nonessential amino acids and pyrimidines, the majority of ammonia is excreted as urea. The urea cycle is found in its entirety only in the liver and is composed of both cytosolic and mitochondrial enzymes. Patients with defects at each step in the cycle have been detected, resulting in disorders of the urea cycle. Although there are clinical distinctions between these conditions, they all result in significant hyperammonemia, neurologic compromise, and significant morbidity and mortality. Presentation with these disorders can occur at any time, but they typically become apparent with higher protein intake or metabolic stress from infection; hence, infancy, the toddler years, and puberty are the greatest risk periods. The distinction in infancy between the different disorders of hyperammonemia resulting in coma can be important for therapeutic intervention (see Figure 55.2-3).

The mainstay of therapy involves protein restriction, but pharmacologic interventions are also effective with many of these disorders. Despite therapy and dietary control, however, many of these conditions will result in repeated episodes of hyperammonemia and mental deficiency. Consequently, liver transplant has been offered and has been successful for many of the more aggressive conditions to ameliorate the metabolic deficiency.[24–29]

OTC DEFICIENCY

Molecular Defect. OTC deficiency is an X-linked disorder of the mitochondrial enzyme OTC (Figure 55.2-4, enzyme 2). Enzyme activity is found exclusively in the liver, although some activity is in the small intestine, and a minimal amount is found in the brain. The enzyme catalyzes the formation of citrulline from carbamyl phosphate and ornithine. Its absence results in the accumulation of not only ammonia but also orotic acid and other pyrimidine derivatives, including uracil and uridine, which are derived from the excessive carbamyl phosphate.[30] These accumulated compounds can be detected in blood and urine.

Clinical Features. Males. The classic and severe form of OTC deficiency results in an enzyme activity level of less than 2% of normal and the death of 75% of the affected male infants in the first months of life.[30] Within hours or days of birth, poor feeding, lethargy, and tachypnea with labored breathing become apparent. Seizures and coma subsequently develop, and cerebral edema and death follow without treatment. In those patients who survive, severe neurologic impairment with mental retardation is common.

A milder variant occurs in males who present at a later age, usually precipitated by a protein challenge either from a dietary change, infection, or concomitant illness. These individuals generally have a higher level of enzyme activity. Hepatomegaly may be observed in these older patients.

Heterozygous Females. In females, the most common presenting symptoms are those of vomiting, feeding difficulties, headache, or tiredness after a protein-containing meal. Onset is in infancy or during the first decade most commonly. In older subjects, again, hepatomegaly may be observed.

Diagnosis. The condition should be suspected in any male infant with hyperammonemia without acidosis (see Figure 55.2-3). The presence of oroticaciduria and the absence of citrulline in plasma are diagnostic. Enzyme analysis from duodenal or rectal mucosal biopsy or liver tissue will confirm the diagnosis and determine the degree of enzyme deficiency.

Heterozygosity for OTC deficiency in females may be detected by assaying the urine for orotic acid following a protein load of 1 g/kg. The urine is collected in three 4-hour aliquots after the protein ingestion.[30,31] Loading with alanine has alternatively been used; however, false-positive results are more common.[32] The allopurinol test is also a

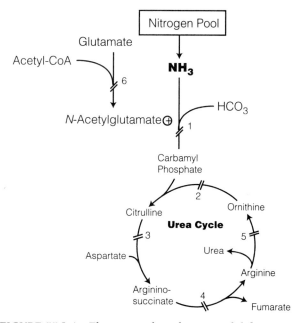

FIGURE 55.2-4   The urea cycle and associated defects. 1 = carbamyl phosphate synthetase; 2 = ornithine transcarbamylase; 3 = argininosuccinate synthetase; 4 = argininosuccinase; 5 = arginase; 6 = N-acetylglutamate synthetase.

common way to detect heterozygotes. Allopurinol inhibits the decarboxylation of orotidine monophosphate, a breakdown product of ototic acid. This accumulation of orotidine monophosphate can then be detected in the urine as orotic acid and orotidine.[33] In all cases, an experienced laboratory is required to perform and interpret these tests.

Treatment. The goal of treatment of patients with urea cycle defects is to eliminate the accumulated ammonia and precursors to its formation, decrease ureagenesis by a low-protein diet, and increase arginine levels (except in arginase deficiency) for the conversion of waste nitrogen into urea.

In the acute setting with hyperammonemia causing life-threatening symptoms, rapid and effective ammonia removal can be achieved with hemodialysis or continuous venous-venous hemoperfusion.[34,35] All protein intake should be stopped and an infusion of 10% glucose initiated.

The pharmacologic provision of alternative routes for waste nitrogen excretion is also effective after the acute removal of ammonia (NH_3) (Figure 55.2-5). Glycine and glutamine can be removed from the nitrogen pool by giving benzoate and phenylbutyrate, respectively. Benzoate conjugates to glycine, forming hippurate, and phenybutyrate conjugates to glutamine, forming phenylacetylglutamine. Each mole of glycine conjugated to benzoate removes one mole of NH_3, and each mole of glutamine conjugated to phenylacetate removes two moles of NH_3. Hippurate and phenylacetylglutamine are excreted in the urine without the need for conversion to urea.[30,35,36] Providing arginine as a substrate for ornithine in those without complete deficiency in OTC can help in urea synthesis and hence further enhance nitrogen excretion, but this is far more helpful in those with citrullinemia or argininosuccinicaciduria. Practically, these compounds are delivered by a loading infusion of 200 to 800 mg/kg arginine hydrochloride, 250 mg/kg sodium benzoate, and 250 mg/kg sodium phenylacetate in 20 mL/kg of 10% glucose over 1 to 2 hours intravenously. A continuous infusion of 250 mg/kg/d each of sodium benzoate and sodium phenylacetate and 200 to 800 mg/kg/d of arginine hydrochloride in 10% glucose with maintenance electrolytes

is then provided until the ammonia level is normal.[30] The 10% glucose further limits hyperammonemia by minimizing catabolism and hence ammonia production. The additional use of mannitol in the setting of cerebral edema may further aid in nitrogen excretion by promoting diuresis.

The long-term management of the chronically hyperammonemic child usually requires a combination of dietary and pharmacologic manipulations. Phenylbutyrate 250 mg/kg/d (less odoriferous than phenylacetate) can be given alone or in combination with sodium benzoate (250 mg/kg/d) and arginine (200 mg/kg/d). The diet is usually restricted to protein of 700 mg/kg/d, with the essential amino acids added at 700 mg/kg/d total through a combination of regular formula and the specialty formulas (see Table 55.2-2).

CPS Deficiency

Molecular Defect. CPS I (CPS) is a liver mitochondrial enzyme that catalyzes the formation of carbamyl phosphate from ammonia using acetylglutamate as an activator and is the first step in the urea cycle (see Figure 55.2-4, enzyme 1). There also exists cytosolic CPS, designated CPS II, which is involved in pyrimidine biosynthesis and is largely responsible for the formation of orotic acid in the face of carbamyl phosphate excess with OTC deficiency. CPS I deficiency is a rare condition resulting from an autosomal recessive mutation. This mutation gives rise to a wide clinical heterogenicity in the patients affected depending on the degree of enzyme deficiency. Owing to the early block in the urea cycle caused by this deficiency, subjects have high ammonia in the face of low orotic acid, citrulline, and arginine.

Clinical Features. Children affected with CPS deficiency typically present in the first days of life after feeds are initiated. Drowsiness, poor feeding, lethargy, vomiting, and hypo- or hypertonia become apparent, followed by seizures, hypothermia, and coma. Death usually occurs in the first 2 to 18 months without treatment. Untreated survivors are typically mentally retarded, with neurologic complications.

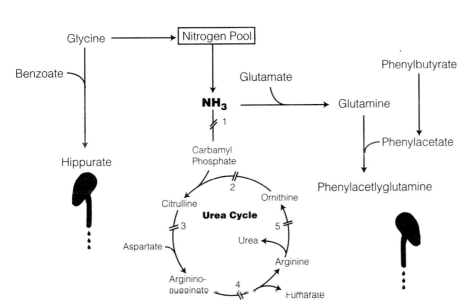

FIGURE 55.2-5 Alternative routes of waste N_2 excretion. 1 = carbamyl phosphate synthetase; 2 = ornithine transcarbamylase; 3 = argininosuccinate synthetase; 4 = argininosuccinase; 5 = arginase; 6 = N-acetylglutamate synthetase.

More rarely, a partial deficiency of CPS I results in older individuals having episodic lethargy and vomiting associated with high protein intake or states of catabolism, usually with progressive, severe neurologic consequences.

Diagnosis. CPS deficiency should be suspected in the young infant with hyperammonemia in the absence of a metabolic acidosis, low orotic acid, low citrulline, and low arginine. The diagnosis can be confirmed and enzyme activity measured from biopsy material from the liver, small intestine, or rectal mucosa.

Treatment. The treatment of CPS is the same as that for OTC deficiency.

CITRULLINEMIA

Citrullinemia was first reported in 1963[37] and is now known to be secondary to deficiency of argininosuccinate synthetase, a widely expressed enzyme.

Molecular Defect. Citrullinemia is an autosomal recessive disorder resulting from a mutation in the gene for the cytosolic enzyme argininosuccinate (argininosuccinic acid) synthetase, mapped to chromosome 9 at q34.[38] This enzyme catalyzes the formation of argininosuccinic acid from citrulline and aspartic acid (see Figure 55.2-4, enzyme 3). Argininosuccinate synthetase is widely distributed and has been measured in cultured fibroblasts and in liver.

Clinical Features. The clinical presentation of patients with citrullinemia is heterogeneous. The majority of subjects present in infancy either with the classic neonatal form or later in the first year with a more subacute form. Patients with the neonatal form resemble infants with OTC deficiency. After the first few days, infants develop poor feeding, lethargy, and irritability; seizures are common, followed by coma and death within weeks, if not treated. Hepatomegaly is sometimes observed. In infants with the classic neonatal form, the enzyme activity is usually zero. The subacute form may present later in the first year with developmental delay, failure to thrive, recurrent vomiting, ataxia, or seizures. Presentations in late childhood or early adulthood have been reported in some patients.[39]

Diagnosis and Prenatal Diagnosis. Diagnosis should be suspected in the hyperammonemic infant without metabolic acidosis and with elevation of plasma and urine citrulline. The diagnosis can be confirmed and level of enzyme activity determined from cultured fibroblasts or lymphocytes.

Prenatal diagnosis is possible by analyzing the amniotic fluid for citrulline or by assay of the enzyme from cultured amniocytes or, less reliably, chorionic villi.

Treatment. The general principles of treatment are the same as in the treatment of patients with OTC deficiency. In citrullinemia, however, the administration of arginine can dramatically lower the level of ammonia by providing this compound as the backbone for urea synthesis. Furthermore, as the elevated citrulline is not thought to be the toxic metabolite (ammonia causes the toxicity), and citrulline itself is excreted in the urine, the provision of arginine allows for increased synthesis of citrulline, use of ammonia, and its subsequent excretion. Citrulline adds only one N atom to ornithine and hence is not as efficient as urea in waste nitrogen excretion but is adequate in times of anabolism. Arginine can be provided along with sodium benzoate and phenylacetate in both the loading solution and continuous infusion solution at a dose of at least 660 mg/kg.[39] Sodium bicarbonate and chloride monitoring may be necessary because arginine is supplied as arginine hydrochloride for intravenous use.

ARGININOSUCCINICACIDURIA

Argininosuccinicaciduria is somewhat unique compared with the previous urea cycle defects discussed in that many patients with this disorder come to attention for chronic, more indolent complaints of alopecia or mild retardation, and most have hepatomegaly. The majority, however, do present in the neonatal period with symptoms typical of the urea cycle disorders.

Molecular Defect. This condition results from a defect in the enzyme argininosuccinate lyase (argininosuccinase), which catalyzes the conversion of argininosuccinic acid (ASA, formed from aspartate and citrulline) to fumarate and arginine (see Figure 55.2-4, enzyme 4). These patients have marked elevations in the levels of ASA in blood, urine, and cerebrospinal fluid and also may have elevations of orotic acid because this is created from the combination of aspartate and carbamyl phosphate.

Deficiency of argininosuccinate activity is inherited in an autosomal recessive manner, and the gene for this enzyme has been localized to chromosome 7.[40] The enzyme deficiency has been demonstrated in the liver, red blood cells, and cultured fibroblasts.[41]

Clinical Features. Neonatal. This is a relatively rare condition in which infants present in the first days of life with the classic symptoms of a urea cycle defect and similar to those with OTC deficiency. Differing features have been observed, however, including hepatomegaly and abnormally fragile hair by weeks of age.

Infantile. Patients present at months of life with failure to thrive, feeding difficulties, and, later, seizures and psychomotor retardation.

Late Onset. This is the most common form of presentation. In the second year of life, patients are noted to have developmental delay and frequently develop feeding difficulties, irritability, and seizures. Symptoms more attributable to hyperammonemia, such as episodic ataxia, lethargy, and seizures, are provoked by infection or increased protein in the diet. Many of these subjects have hepatomegaly, and roughly 50% have abnormally fragile hair. The hepatomegaly is usually associated with elevation of transaminases, but the synthetic capacity of the liver is generally preserved.[42,43]

The fragile hair is trichorrhexis nodosa, short dry hair that never needs to be cut because it breaks easily. Microscopically, the hair shafts have nodules.

Diagnosis and Prenatal Diagnosis. The diagnosis is made by demonstrating an excess of ASA in urine or plasma. The diagnosis can then be confirmed by assaying ASA lyase in red blood cells or cultured fibroblasts.[41]

Prenatal diagnosis is possible by assaying for enzyme activity in cultured amniocytes[44] or by the detection of ASA in amniotic fluid.

Treatment. Treatment is similar to that of citrullinemia. Providing arginine enables forward cycling of the urea cycle using ammonia in the formation of ASA. ASA is effectively excreted in the urine and is as effective in N removal as urea. Sodium benzoate and phenylacetate are not generally needed; however, sodium bicarbonate and chloride monitoring may be necessary because arginine is supplied as the hydrochloride for intravenous use.

N-Acetylglutamate Synthetase Deficiency

Few patients have been reported with deficiency of hepatic N-acetylglutamate synthetase. This mitochondrial enzyme catalyzes the combination of acetyl CoA and glutamate to form acetylglutamate, which, in turn, is required for activation of CPS I (see Figure 55.2-4, enzyme 6). The clinical phenotype and treatment are similar to those observed with CPS deficiency.

Argininemia

Argininemia is the least common of the urea cycle defects and was initially reported in 1965 and 1969.[45,46]

Molecular Defect. Argininemia is an autosomal recessive disorder caused by a deficiency of arginase, an enzyme coded for on chromosome 6 at band q23.[47] Arginase is responsible for the conversion of arginine to ornithine and urea (see Figure 55.2-4, enzyme 5). Individuals with arginase deficiency have a nearly complete absence of enzyme activity and have predictably elevated levels of arginine. They may also have elevated levels of orotic acid, however, because arginine serves an effector function toward N-acetylglutamate synthetase, which, in turn, stimulates CPS to form carbamyl phosphatase. Because ornithine is lacking in the face of arginase deficiency, the carbamyl phosphate flows in the pathway of pyrimidine synthesis and orotic acid is formed.

Clinical Features. Symptomatic onset is usually in infancy, with irritability, poor feeding, vomiting, lethargy, seizures, and coma. Unlike with the other urea cycle defects, however, survivors have spasticity or opisthotonos with developmental delay and may be thought initially to have cerebral palsy. Although ammonia levels elevate intermittently with infection or increased protein in the diet, the degree of ammonia elevation in this condition is not as dramatic as with the other urea cycle defects.

Diagnosis. Elevated plasma arginine levels are diagnostic, and the enzyme activity can be assayed in erythrocytes.

Treatment. The principle of treatment is to restrict arginine from the diet by providing a mixture of amino acids at an equivalent of 2 g/kg of protein, fat and carbohydrates to supply 125 kcal/kg/d, and vitamins and minerals. As the child ages, fruits, low-protein vegetables, and cereals can be introduced and then later the protein types liberalized but to never exceed 5 g/d of high biologic protein (300 mg arginine). Arginine intake must be episodically reduced in the face of infection or illness and blood levels of arginine and ammonia monitored regularly.[43]

REFERENCES

1. Mitchell GA, Grompe M, Lambert M, Tanguay RM. Hypertyrosinemia. In: Scriver CR, Beaudet AL, Sly WS, Valle D, editors. The metabolic and molecular bases of inherited disease. New York: McGraw Hill; 2001. p. 1777–806.
2. Lindblad B, Lindstedt S, Steen G. On the enzymic defects in hereditary tyrosinemia. Proc Natl Acad Sci U S A 1977;74:4641–5.
3. Fällström SP, Lindblad B, Lindstedt S, Steen G. Hereditary tyrosinemia-fumarylacetoacetate deficiency. Pediatr Res 1979;13:78.
4. Sassa S, Kappas A. Hereditary tyrosinemia and the heme biosynthetic pathway. Profound inhibition of delta-aminolevulinic acid dehydratase activity by succinylacetone. J Clin Invest 1983;71:625.
5. Mitchell G, Larochelle J, Lambert M, et al. Neurologic crises in hereditary tyrosinemia. N Engl J Med 1990;322:432–7.
6. Tschudy DP, Hess RA, Frykholm BC, Blaese RM. Immunosuppressive activity of succinylacetone. J Lab Clin Med 1982;99:526-32.
7. Roth KS, Carter BE, Higgins ES. Succinylacetone effects on renal tubular phosphate metabolism: a model for experimental renal Fanconi syndrome. Proc Soc Exp Biol Med 1991;196:428–31.
8. Roth KS, Carter BE, Moses LC, Spencer PD. On rat renal aminolevulinate transport and metabolism in experimental Fanconi syndrome. Biochem Med Metab Biol 1990;44:238–46.
9. Grompe M, St-Louis M, Demers SI, et al. A single mutation of the fumarylacetoacetate hydrolase gene in French Canadians with hereditary tyrosinemia type I. N Engl J Med 1994;331:353–7.
10. Van Spronsen FJ, Thomasse Y, Smit GP, et al. Hereditary tyrosinemia type I: a new clinical classification with difference in prognosis on dietary treatment. Hepatology 1994;20:1187–91.
11. Lindstedt S, Holme E, Lock EA, et al. Treatment of hereditary tyrosinaemia type I by inhibition of 4-hydroxyphenylpyruvate dioxygenase. Lancet 1992;340:813–7.
12. Menkes JH, Hurst PL, Craig JM. A new syndrome: progressive familial infantile cerebral dysfunction associated with an unusual urinary substance. Pediatrics 1954;14:462–7.
13. Westall RG, Dancis J, Miller S. Maple syrup urine disease. Am J Dis Child 1957;94:571–2.
14. Dancis J, Levitz M, Westall RG. Maple syrup urine disease: branched-chain keto-aciduria. Pediatrics 1960;25:72–9.
15. Ogier de Baulny H, Saudubray J-M. Branched-chain organic acidurias. In: Fernandes J, Saudubray J-M, Van den Berghe G, editors. Inborn metabolic diseases, diagnosis and treatment. 3rd ed. New York: Springer; 2000. p. 197–212.
16. Friedrich CA, Marble M, Maher J, Valle D. Successful control of branched-chain amino acids (BCAA) in maple syrup urine disease using elemental amino acids in total parenteral nutrition during acute pancreatitis. Am J Hum Genet 1992;51:A350.
17. Chuang DT, Shih VE. Maple syrup urine disease (branched-chain ketoaciduria). In: Scriver CR, Beaudet AL, Sly WS, Valle D, editors. The metabolic and molecular bases of inherited disease. 8th ed. New York: McGraw-Hill; 2001. p. 1971–2005.

18. Treacy E, Clow CL, Reade TR, et al. Maple syrup urine disease: interrelations between branched-chain amino-, oxo- and hydroxyacids; implications for treatment; associations with CNS dysmyelination. J Inherit Metab Dis 1992;15:121–35.

19. Riviello JJ Jr, Rezvani I, Digeorge AM, Foley CM. Cerebral edema causing death in children with maple syrup urine disease. J Pediatr 1991;119:42–5.

20. Elsas LJ, Danner DJ, Lubitz D, et al. Metabolic consequence in inherited defects in branched chain a-ketoacid dehydrogenase: mechanism of thiamine action. In: Walser M, Williamson JR, editors. Metabolism and clinical implications of branched chain amino and ketoacids. New York: Elsevier/North-Holland; 1981. p. 369–82.

21. Kaplan P, Mazur A, Smith R, et al. Liver transplantation for maple syrup urine disease (MSUD) and methylmalonic acidopathy (MMA). Am J Hum Genet 1997;61:A254.

22. Budd MA, Tanaka K, Holmes LB, et al. Isovaleric acidemia: clinical features of a new genetic defect of leucine metabolism. N Engl J Med 1967;277:321–7.

23. Tanaka K, Budd MA, Efron ME, Isselbacher KJ. Isovaleric acidemia: a new genetic defect of leucine metabolism. Proc Natl Acad Sci U S A 1966;56:236.

24. Whitington PF, Alonso EM, Boyle JT, et al. Liver transplantation for the treatment of urea cycle disorders. J Inherit Metab Dis 1998;21 Suppl 1:112–8.

25. Kayler LK, Merion RM, Lee S, et al. Long-term survival after liver transplantation in children with metabolic disorders. Pediatr Transplant 2002;6:295–300.

26. Florman S, Shneider B. Living-related liver transplantation in inherited metabolic liver disease: feasibility and cautions. J Pediatr Gastroenterol Nutr 2001;33:520–1.

27. Fletcher JM, Couper R, Moore D, et al. Liver transplantation for citrullinemia improves intellectual function. J Inherit Metab Dis 1999;22:581–6.

28. Ban K, Sugiyama N, Sugiyama K, et al. A pediatric patient with classical citrullinemia who underwent living-related partial liver transplantation. Transplantation 2001;71:1495–7.

29. Saudubray JM, Touati G, Delonlay P, et al. Liver transplantation in urea cycle disorders. Eur J Pediatr 1999;158 Suppl 2: S55–9.

30. Nyhan WL, Ozand PT. Ornithine transcarbamylase deficiency. In: Nyhan WL, Ozand PT, editors. Atlas of metabolic diseases. London: Chapman & Hall Medical; 1998. p. 168–77.

31. Haan EA, Danks DM, Grimes A, Hoogenraad NJ. Carrier detection in ornithine transcarbamylase deficiency. J Inherit Metab Dis 1982;5:37–40.

32. Winter S, Sweetman L, Batshaw ML. Carrier detection in ornithine carbamylase deficiency using L-alanine loading test [abstract]. Clin Res 1983;31:112A.

33. Hauser ER, Finkelstein JE, Valle D, Brusilow SW. Allopurinol-induced orotidinuria: a test for mutations at the ornithine carbamoyl transferase locus in women. N Engl J Med 1990; 322:1641–5.

34. Wiegand C, Thompson T, Bock GH, et al. The management of life-threatening hyperammonemia: a comparison of several therapeutic modalities. J Pediatr 1980;96:142–4.

35. Batshaw ML, Brusilow SW. Treatment of hyperammonemic coma caused by inborn errors of urea synthesis. J Pediatr 1980;97:893–900.

36. Brusilow SW, Tinker J, Batshaw ML. Amino acid acylation: a mechanism of nitrogen excretion in inborn errors of urea synthesis. Science 1980;207:659.

37. McMurray WC, Rathbun JC, Mohyuddin F, Koegler SJ. Citrullinemia. Pediatrics 1963;32:347–57.

38. Su TS, Nussbaum RL, Airpart S, et al. Human chromosomal assignments for 14 argininosuccinate synthetase pseudogenes: cloned DNAs as reagents for cytogenetic analysis. Am J Hum Genet 1984;36:954–64.

39. Nyhan WL, Ozand PT. Citrullinemia. In: Nyhan WL, Ozand PT, editors. Atlas of metabolic diseases. London: Chapman & Hall Medical; 1998. p. 182–7.

40. Lambert MA, Simard LR, Ray PN, McInnes RR. Molecular cloning of cDNA for rat hepatoma cell lines. Mol Cell Biol 1986;6:1722–8.

41. Fensom AH, Benson PF, Baker JA, Mutton DE. Prenatal diagnosis of argininosuccinic aciduria: effect of Mycoplasma contamination on the indirect assay for argininosuccinate lyase. Am J Hum Genet 1980;32:761–3.

42. Nyhan WL, Ozand PT. Argininosuccinic aciduria. In: Nyhan WL, Ozand PT, editors. Atlas of metabolic diseases. London: Chapman & Hall Medical; 1998. p. 188–93.

43. Benson PF, Fensom AH. Genetic biochemical disorders. 1st ed. Oxford: Oxford University Press; 1985.

44. Fleisher LD, Rassin DK, Desnick RH, et al. Argininosuccinic aciduria: prenatal studies in a family at risk. Am J Hum Genet 1979;31:439–45.

45. Serrano AP. Argininuria, convulsiones y oligofrenia; unnuevo error innato del metabolismo? Rev Clin Esp 1965;97:176.

46. Terheggen HG, Schwenk A, Lowenthal A, et al. Argininaemia with arginase deficiency. Lancet 1969;ii:748–9.

47. Sparkes RS, Dizikes GJ, Klisak I, et al. The gene for human liver arginase (ARG1) is assigned to chromosome band 6q23. Am J Hum Genet 1986;39:186–93.

3. Inherited Abnormalities in Mitochondrial Fatty Acid Oxidation

Carla D. Cuthbert, PhD

Silvia Tortorelli, MD, PhD

Regina E. Ensenauer, MD

Piero Rinaldo, MD, PhD

Dietrich Matern, MD

Mitochondrial fatty acid β-oxidation (FAO) plays a pivotal role in energy production and homeostasis once glycogen stores are depleted owing to fasting, during febrile illness, and owing to increased muscular activity. Mitochondrial fatty acid β-oxidation provides as much as 80% of energy for heart and liver functions at all times.[1] In the liver, the oxidation of fatty acids fuels the synthesis of ketone bodies, 3-hydroxybutyrate and acetoacetate. Ketones are used as an alternative energy source by extrahepatic organs, particularly the brain, and the oxidation of long-chain fatty acids also provides the energy required for nonshivering thermogenesis by brown adipose tissue.

The first genetic defect of FAO in humans was recognized in 1973 as a disorder of skeletal muscle presenting with exercise-induced rhabdomyolysis and myoglobinuria.[2] Many additional FAO disorders covering a wide spectrum of phenotypes have since been discovered. A growing number of clinical entities such as Reye syndrome, sudden infant death syndrome, cyclic vomiting syndrome, liver failure, and maternal complications of pregnancy have been associated with various FAO disorders.[1]

BIOCHEMISTRY OF MITOCHONDRIAL FATTY ACID METABOLISM

LIPID MOBILIZATION AND TRANSPORT

Glycogen serves as the primary energy source, but once glycogen stores become depleted, energy must be acquired by alternative means. Decreasing blood glucose concentrations cause a reduction of the insulin-to-glucagon ratio and subsequent lipid mobilization from adipose tissue. Free fatty acids are released into the plasma following the hydrolysis of triglycerides by endothelial-bound lipoprotein lipase and hepatic lipase. The most abundant species are long-chain fatty acids, in particular palmitic ($C_{16:0}$), stearic ($C_{18:0}$), oleic ($C_{18:1}$), and linoleic ($C_{18:2}$) acids.[3,4]

Long-chain fatty acids are weakly soluble in plasma and readily bind to albumin. Two models, involving both saturable (protein mediated) and nonsaturable (nonprotein mediated) components, specific for cellular long-chain fatty acid uptake exist.[5] In a non–protein-mediated model, fatty acids partition into membranes and become protonated, and the neutral molecule is translocated across the membrane into the cytosol.[6] Growing evidence also supports the presence of high-affinity tissue-specific fatty acid transporters on liver and muscle cell membranes (Figure 55.3-1).[7] A family of fatty acid transport proteins (FATPs) has been characterized in different species, and in vitro experiments demonstrated increased fatty acid import when expressed in cultured cells and reduced uptake when the *FATP1* gene was disrupted.[8,9] To date, however, mutations in the *FATP1* gene have not been associated with a disease.

Inside the cytosol, fatty acid binding proteins play a similar role as plasma albumin in the binding and transportation of intracellular fatty acids.[10] Eventually, the intracellular fatty acids are esterified by acyl coenzyme A (CoA) synthetases to fatty acyl CoAs. These can bind to ubiquitously expressed, high-affinity acyl-CoA binding proteins (ACBPs) or to the lower-affinity fatty acid binding proteins (~ 1,000-fold lower affinity than the ACBPs). Bound to ACBPs, acyl-CoA esters are delivered to carnitine palmitoyltransferase (CPT) 1.[11]

ROLE OF CARNITINE

Whereas short- and medium-chain fatty acyl-CoA esters are able to passively cross the mitochondrial membranes, long-chain fatty acyl-CoA esters are actively transported. This transport mechanism requires intracellular carnitine as a cofactor and involves three steps mediated by two CPTs (1 and 2) and a carnitine acylcarnitine translocase (CACT) (see Figure 55.3-1).[12]

Carnitine (β-hydroxytrimethylaminobutyrate) is an essential molecule in intermediary metabolism.[13] It is involved in the transfer of cytosolic fatty acids across the mitochondrial membrane for β-oxidation. Products of peroxisomal β-oxidation are also transported by carnitine to the mitochondria for further oxidation. Carnitine influences the acetyl CoA to free CoA ratio by acting as a reservoir for activated acetyl groups. Finally, carnitine influences the toxicity associated with abnormal accumulation of fatty acids and organic acids by forming carnitine esters, which can be removed from the intracellular environment.

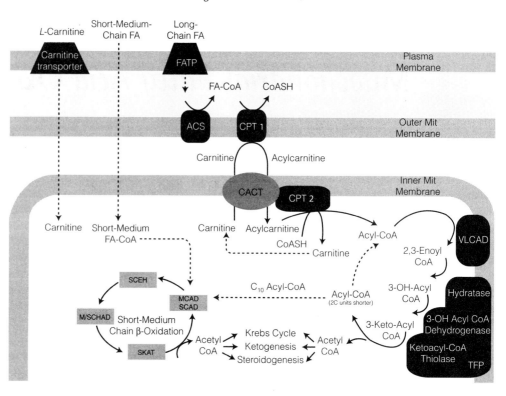

FIGURE 55.3-1 Overview of fatty acid import and metabolism. ACS = acyl-CoA synthetase; CACT = carnitine acylcarnitine translocase; CoA = coenzyme A; CoASH = unacylated coenzyme A; CPT1 = carnitine palmitoyltransferase 1; CPT2 = carnitine palmitoyltransferase 2; FA = fatty acid; FA-CoA = fatty acyl CoA; FATP = fatty acid transport protein; MCAD = medium-chain acyl-CoA dehydrogenase; Mit = mitochondrial; M/SCHAD = medium-/short-chain 3-hydroxyacyl-CoA dehydrogenase; SCAD = short-chain acyl-CoA dehydrogenase; SCEH = short-chain enoyl-CoA hydratase; SKAT = short-chain ketoacyl-CoA thiolase; TFP = trifunctional protein; VLCAD = very-long-chain acyl-CoA dehydrogenase.

Carnitine originates to about 75% from dietary intake of meat, fish, and dairy products. Under normal conditions, endogenous synthesis from lysine and methionine plays a minor role but can be stimulated by a diet low in carnitine. Carnitine is not further metabolized and is excreted in urine as free carnitine or as conjugated carnitine esters. Adequate intracellular levels of carnitine are therefore maintained by mechanisms that modulate dietary intake, endogenous synthesis, reabsorption, and cellular uptake.

PLASMA MEMBRANE UPTAKE OF CARNITINE

Only the kidney, liver, and brain have the full complement of enzymes necessary to synthesize carnitine. Other tissues depend on carnitine from the circulation. Carnitine uptake is an active process and occurs against a gradient to concentrate intracellular levels as free carnitine or carnitine esters. In humans, concentrations of carnitine in skeletal and cardiac muscle tissue exceed levels in plasma by 50-fold.

Muscle, heart, placenta, and fibroblasts have been shown to possess high-affinity carnitine transport systems with Michaelis constant (Km) values ranging between 6 and 60 μM. The best characterized member of this family is the organic cation transporter 2 (OCTN2) (encoded by the *SLC22A5* gene), a low-Km (2–6 μM), high-affinity, sodium-dependent active transporter present in muscle, heart, and renal tubule cells.[13] OCTN2 dysfunction, particularly in the kidney, results in excessive carnitine losses to the urine and consequently reduced plasma and tissue carnitine levels, affecting particularly those tissues relying heavily on ketogenesis as an energy source.

CARNITINE CYCLE

CPT1 is located in the outer mitochondrial membrane and converts long-chain acyl-CoA intermediates into the corresponding acylcarnitine. There are muscle and liver isoforms of this enzyme, the latter also being expressed in fibroblasts and amniocytes. CACT mediates the transfer of acylcarnitine species from the intermembrane space into the mitochondrial matrix in exchange for free carnitine, thereby maintaining the mitochondrial and cytosolic carnitine pools. CPT2 is located on the matrix aspect of the inner mitochondrial membrane and converts the translocated long-chain acylcarnitine back into its corresponding acyl-CoA ester, releasing free carnitine.

MITOCHONDRIAL β-OXIDATION

Substrates for β-oxidation are fatty acyl-CoA esters, which repeatedly undergo four chain-shortening steps, each cycle resulting in the removal of a 2-carbon acetyl group (Figure 55.3-2). The four steps of each cycle require the action of four enzymatic activities, each with overlapping chain-length specificities for very-long-, long-, medium-, and short-chain acyl-CoA fatty acid substrates. They include (1) acyl-CoA dehydrogenases (ACADs), (2) 2-enoyl-CoA hydratases, (3) 3-hydroxyacyl-CoA dehydrogenases, and (4) 3-ketoacyl-CoA thiolases. The enzymes with specificity for very-long-chain and long-chain fatty acid substrates are membrane associated, whereas the enzymes recognizing the medium- and short-chain fatty acids are soluble mitochondrial matrix enzymes. The genes for most enzymes involved in FAO have been cloned and pathogenic mutations identified.[14]

Acyl-CoA Dehydrogenases. ACADs are flavin adenine dinucleotide (FAD)-requiring oxidoreductases that catalyze the first dehydrogenation step in the β-oxidation of fatty acids, resulting in the formation of a double bond between the 2 and 3 position of the fatty acyl-CoA derivative. Very-long-chain acyl-CoA dehydrogenase (VLCAD) is

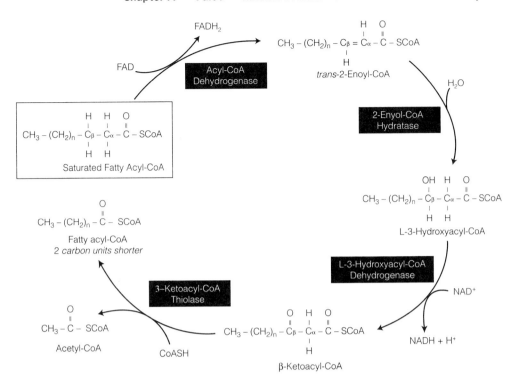

FIGURE 55.3-2 Reactions involved in β-oxidation of saturated fatty acids. CoA = coenzyme A; CoASH = unacylated coenzyme A; FAD = flavin adenine dinucleotide (oxidized form); FADH₂ = flavin adenine dinucleotide (reduced form); NAD = nicotinamide adenine dinucleotide (oxidized form); NADH = nicotinamide adenine dinucleotide (reduced form).

a 154 kD heterodimer associated with the matrix surface of the inner mitochondrial membrane.[15] Medium- and short-chain acyl-CoA dehydrogenases (MCAD and SCAD, respectively) are located within the mitochondrial matrix and are homotetramers with subunits ranging from 43 to 45 kD.[16,17] Chain-length specificities for the various ACADs are C_{14} to C_{20} fatty acyl CoA for VLCAD, C_{12} to C_{18} for long-chain acyl CoA dehydrogenase (LCAD), C_6 to C_{10} for MCAD, and C_4 to C_6 for SCAD.

Enoyl-CoA Hydratases. The second step of β-oxidation is catalyzed by 2-enoyl-CoA hydratase and results in the hydration of the double bond of the 2-trans-enoyl-CoA ester to form L-3-hydroxyacyl CoA. There are two different hydratases with different substrate specificities. The short-chain enoyl-CoA hydratase, also referred to as crotonase, acts on substrates with short chain lengths with reduced activity as chain length increases. The hydratase with specificity for longer-chain substrates is part of the trifunctional protein (TFP).

Trifunctional Protein. TFP is a hetero-octamer ($\alpha_4\beta_4$) that catalyzes three steps in the mitochondrial β-oxidation of long-chain fatty acids. Long-chain enoyl-CoA hydratase (LCEH) and long-chain 3-hydroxyacyl-CoA dehydrogenase (LCHAD) activities are located at the amino- and carboxy-terminal domains, respectively, of the four α subunits, whereas the four β subunits contain long-chain ketoacyl-CoA thiolase (LCKAT) activity.[18]

L-3-Hydroxyacyl-CoA Dehydrogenases. The conversion of L-3-hydroxyacyl CoA to the corresponding 3-ketoacyl-CoA derivative is mediated by L-3-hydroxyacyl-CoA dehydrogenase and occurs with the concomitant reduction of

oxidized nicotinamide adenine dinucleotide (NAD⁺) to reduced nicotinamide adenine dinucleotide. Long-chain 3-hydroxyacyl-CoA substrates are metabolized by LCHAD, which is part of the aforementioned TFP. The medium-/short-chain L-3-hydroxyacyl-CoA dehydrogenase (M/SCHAD) has highest activity toward 3-hydroxybutyryl CoA but will also recognize substrates with higher chain lengths with reducing activity as chain length increases.

3-Ketoacyl Thiolase. The last reaction in the β-oxidation spiral is performed in the presence of CoA and involves a thiolytic cleavage between C-2 and C-3 atoms of the 3-ketoacyl-CoA intermediate with the release of acetyl CoA and the generation of an acyl-CoA product shortened by two carbons. There are two mitochondrial thiolases. The ketothiolase that resides in the β subunit of the TFP cleaves long-chain substrates, whereas the remaining keto acyl-CoA derivatives of shorter chain lengths are substrates for medium-chain ketoacyl thiolase (MCKAT).[18]

OXIDATION OF UNSATURATED FATTY ACIDS

Unsaturated dietary fatty acids such as oleic ($C_{18:1}$), linoleic ($C_{18:2}$), and linolenic ($C_{18:3}$) acids undergo β-oxidation in a manner similar to saturated fatty acids, sequentially releasing acetyl CoA with each round until the formation of intermediates, which are not recognized by the enzymes of β-oxidation (Figure 55.3-3). Unsaturated fatty acids with double bonds located at odd-numbered and even-numbered positions, respectively, generate intermediates with the double bond between the C-3 and C-4 atoms (cis-3-enoyl CoA) and between the C-2 and C-3 atoms (cis-2-enoyl CoA). Further metabolism requires modification by ancillary enzymes. The cis-2-enoyl-CoA esters can be hydrated and either be epimerized to form L (ɪ) 3-hydroxy intermediates or converted to

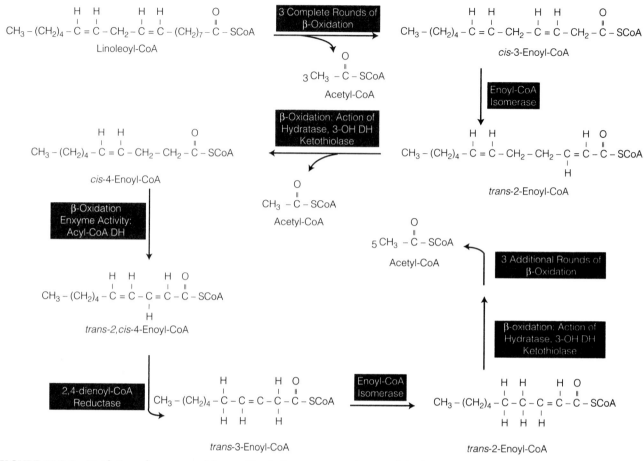

FIGURE 55.3-3 Oxidation of unsaturated fatty acids. CoA = coenzyme A; DH = dehydrogenase.

3-*trans*-enoyl-CoA esters by the action of 2,4-dienoyl-CoA reductase. Re-entry of 3-enoyl-CoA intermediates into the β-oxidation pathway is accomplished by a reaction mediated by 3,2-*trans*-enoyl-CoA isomerase, which results in a shift of the double bond from the C-3 position to the C-2 position. In this step, all 3-enoyl-CoA intermediates, occurring in either the *cis* or *trans* configuration, are converted into their corresponding 2-*trans*-enoyl-CoA intermediates, which can subsequently be metabolized by the enoyl-CoA hydratase of the β-oxidation pathway.

Only one patient has been described with 2,4-dienoyl-CoA reductase deficiency.[19] No defect of enoyl-CoA isomerase has been reported to date.

OXIDATION OF ODD-CHAIN FATTY ACIDS

Fatty acids with an odd number of carbons undergo β-oxidation as described above until the 3-carbon propionyl-CoA molecule is formed. Propionyl CoA is also generated by the metabolism of amino acids and is decarboxylated to methylmalonyl CoA by propionyl-CoA carboxylase. Methylmalonyl CoA is further metabolized by methylmalonyl-CoA mutase to form succinyl CoA, an intermediate of the Krebs cycle.

KETONE BODY METABOLISM

The three compounds referred to as ketone bodies are acetoacetate (AcAc), 3-hydroxybutyrate (3HB), and acetone.

They represent the physiologic products of the metabolism of fatty acids and ketogenic amino acids. The two predominant ketone bodies are AcAc and 3HB, and they share a metabolic relationship in the mitochondria similar to that of pyruvate and lactate in the cytoplasm. 3HB is a stable, nonvolatile metabolite that arises only through the reduction of AcAc. Acetone, formed by the decarboxylation of the chemically unstable AcAc, is responsible for the fruity smell recognized in ketoacidotic individuals.

Acetyl CoA generated by fatty acid β-oxidation is converted to acetoacetyl CoA by the action of β-ketothiolase (Figure 55.3-4). This reaction marks both the first step in ketogenesis and the last step in ketolysis. This enzyme can also catalyze the conversion of the isoleucine intermediate 2-methylacetoacetyl CoA to acetyl-CoA and propionyl CoA. Human β-ketothiolase is a homotetramer composed of 41 kD subunits, and two isoenzymes have been described. The human β-ketothiolase gene is known, and pathogenic mutations have been described in deficient patients.[20]

Acetoacetyl CoA thus formed is transformed into 3-hydroxy-3-methylglutaryl (HMG)-CoA by mitochondrial HMG-CoA synthase. Two HMG-CoA synthase isoenzymes are encoded by distinct genes. One is located inside the mitochondria and is involved in ketogenesis; the other is located in the cytoplasm and plays a role in cholesterol synthesis. Patients with mitochondrial HMG-CoA synthase deficiency have been described clinically and confirmed at the molecular level.[21]

In the last step of ketogenesis, HMG-CoA is irreversibly converted to AcAc by HMG-CoA lyase. The mitochondrial HMG-CoA lyase is a homodimer, the gene of which has been identified.[22] The HMG-CoA lyase enzyme is also targeted to the peroxisome, where its physiologic role is as yet undefined.[23]

The interconversion between AcAc and 3HB is mediated by 3HB dehydrogenase (3HBD). This protein is located on the inner mitochondrial membrane and has an absolute requirement for phosphatidylcholine as an allosteric activator. Highest activity has been described in the liver, with lower activity present in the heart, adrenal glands, and kidney.

Ketolysis involves the metabolism of AcAc and 3HB and occurs in the mitochondrial compartment of extrahepatic tissue (see Figure 55.3-4). The action of 3HBD converts 3HB to AcAc, which can subsequently be metabolized by succinyl-CoA oxoacid transferase (SCOT) to AcAc-CoA. β-Ketothiolase present in these cells converts AcAc-CoA into Ac-CoA, which subsequently enters the Krebs cycle. SCOT is a monomer that assembles into a homodimer. Although highly expressed in heart muscle, kidney, adrenal glands, and brain, SCOT is not present in liver.[24]

ELECTRON TRANSFER TO THE RESPIRATORY CHAIN COMPLEX

The electron transfer flavoprotein (ETF) and ETF-ubiquinone oxidoreductase (ETF-QO) function together to transfer electrons from at least nine flavoprotein dehydrogenases.[25] Electrons are transferred between the two flavin moieties in the dehydrogenases and ETF. The reduced ETF is subsequently reoxidized by ETF-QO activity, with the concomitant reduction of ubiquinone.[26]

ETF is a mitochondrial matrix heterodimer consisting of α and β subunits, which are encoded by different genes.[27,28] ETF-QO is a monomer associated with the inner mitochondrial membrane. It contains two redox groups, a FAD cofactor and an iron-sulfur prosthetic group, which are thought to act as entry and exit sites, respectively, for electron transfer.[29] The gene for ETF-QO and pathogenic mutations have also been identified.[30]

PATHOPHYSIOLOGY AND CLINICAL PRESENTATION

Typically prompted by increased energy requirements during fever, fasting, or prolonged exercise, an enzyme defect in the FAO pathway leads to energy depletion owing to inadequate production of acetyl CoA, ketone bodies, and, ultimately, adenosine triphosphate in tissues with high energy demands, such as liver, heart, skeletal muscle, and brain.[1,31] Transient to fulminant liver failure, hepatic encephalopathy, dilated or hypertrophic cardiomyopathy, skeletal myopathy, and sudden, unexpected death at any age are the major clinical manifestations. The biochemical hallmark of FAO defects is hypo- or nonketotic hypoglycemia resulting from two different mechanisms: glucose depletion and secondary impairment of gluconeogenesis owing to a lack of reducing equivalents. Nonmetabolized free fatty acids are incorporated into triglycerides and can account for the observed fat storage in liver and muscle.[32]

Intracellular toxicity is triggered by the accumulation of acyl-CoA intermediates upstream of the block and the secondary depletion of carnitine and CoA. The metabolites may have toxic effects either directly (ie, membrane disruption) and/or by the inhibition of other enzymes. For example, cardiac arrhythmias are thought to be caused by long-chain acylcarnitine accumulation in mitochondrial fatty acid transport and β-oxidation defects.[33]

COMPLICATIONS OF PREGNANCY

A peculiar association between FAO disorders and severe complications during pregnancy has been well documented in women carrying LCHAD-deficient fetuses.[34,35] Preeclampsia, HELLP (hemolysis, elevated liver enzymes,

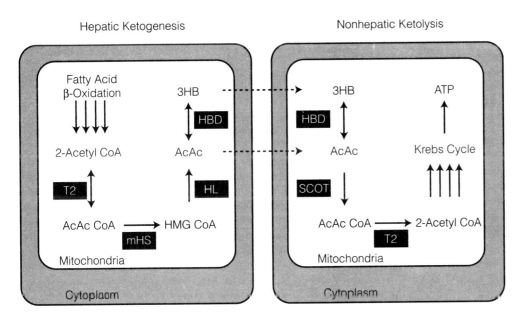

FIGURE 55.3-4 Ketone body metabolism: hepatic ketogenesis and ketolysis in nonhepatic tissue. AcAc = acetoacetate; ATP = adenosine triphosphate; CoA = coenzyme A; 3HB = 3-hydroxybutyrate; HBD = 3-hydroxybutyrate dehydrogenase; HL = HMG-CoA lyase; HMG = 3-hydroxy-3-methylglutarate; mHS = mitochondrial HMG-CoA synthase; SCOT = succinyl-CoA oxoacid transferase; T2 = β-ketothiolase.

and low platelets) syndrome, acute fatty liver of pregnancy (AFLP), and placental floor infarction are the observed maternal phenotypes (Table 55.3-1).[36] The mechanism of this association is not clearly understood. A combination of different factors might result in hepatic dysfunction during the third trimester of pregnancy.[1]

It is possible that the placenta, which shares the same genetic makeup as the fetus, is responsible for the production and accumulation of abnormal fatty acid metabolites.[37] These metabolites pass into the maternal circulation and overwhelm the β-oxidation pathway of the heterozygote mother, who has reduced capacity to oxidize long-chain fatty acids. In addition, during the latter trimester of pregnancy, β-oxidation in the mother is already challenged by the shifting of maternal metabolism toward ketogenesis. This metabolic imbalance is also harmful for the fetus, making it difficult to receive enough energy from the placenta.

Intrauterine growth retardation and premature delivery are relatively common observations. Although there is a predominant association with LCHAD deficiency, severe complications during pregnancy have been reported also in other FAO.[36]

OTHER CLINICAL MANIFESTATIONS

Less frequently observed and poorly understood clinical manifestations have also been described. Hyperinsulinism, described in a case of SCHAD deficiency, supports the hypothesis of the existence of a lipid signaling pathway, strictly related to the β-oxidation spiral, which intervenes in the control of insulin secretion.[38] Hypoparathyroidism has been an occasional finding in patients affected with LCHAD or TFP deficiency.[39]

GENERAL APPROACH TO THE DIAGNOSIS

The approach to the diagnosis of patients at risk for FAO disorders should involve a combination of routine, specialized, and in vitro analyses, with careful consideration of the clinical condition at the time of sample acquisition (Table 55.3-2). When the patient is clinically stable and in an anabolic state, the concentration of key metabolites may not be significant. Patient samples collected under these conditions may not be informative because the metabolic

intermediates may be absent or undetectable. The most useful specimens for evaluation are typically acquired during periods of metabolic decompensation, before the initiation of treatment. Because metabolic status has such critical consequences on the metabolite profiles, the interpretation of biochemical parameters relies heavily on the clinical and therapeutic context at sample procurement. Accordingly, it must be remembered that although metabolite analyses can be diagnostic, negative or inconclusive results in cases of high clinical suspicion should be followed up by in vitro investigations that are independent of patient status.

ROUTINE TESTING

During episodes of metabolic decompensation, plasma and urine specimens should be collected at the earliest possible opportunity. Hypoketotic hypoglycemia is a hallmark of most, but not all, FAO disorders. Routine chemistries include blood gases, electrolytes, glucose, ammonia, uric acid, liver function tests, creatine kinase, ratio of lactic to pyruvic acid, 3-hydroxybutyric and acetoacetic acids, and urinalysis. These more readily available analyses help to assess the extent of organ involvement and often allow for initiation of adequate treatment, while awaiting the results of more specialized metabolite analyses in plasma and urine. Careful consideration of the patient's personal (eg, preceding fever, fasting), pregnancy (eg, maternal liver disease during pregnancy, intrauterine growth retardation, prematurity), and family history (ie, sudden unexpected death in a sibling) may also provide important clues that should trigger inclusion of FAO disorders into the differential diagnosis.[40,41]

SPECIALIZED METABOLITE ANALYSES

Defects associated with mitochondrial FAO result in the accumulation of fatty acids and acyl-CoA intermediates proximal to the metabolic block. These intermediates can be converted into dicarboxylic and hydroxydicarboxylic acids through peroxisomal ω- and ω-1-oxidation. Mechanisms to detoxify these accumulating metabolites and to restore the depleted pool of CoA result in the formation of acylglycine conjugates and acylcarnitine species from their respective acyl-CoA esters. Abnormal accumulation of these acyl-

TABLE 55.3-1   DISORDERS OF FATTY ACID TRANSPORT AND MITOCHONDRIAL OXIDATION ASSOCIATED WITH MATERNAL COMPLICATIONS OF PREGNANCY

MATERNAL COMPLICATION	DISORDERS OF FATTY ACID TRANSPORT AND MITOCHONDRIAL OXIDATION						
	LCHAD	TFP	CPT1	CACT	MCAD	SCAD	UNKNOWN*
Acute fatty liver of pregnancy	+++	+	(+)	−	(+)	+	+
HELLP syndrome	+++	−	−	−	+	+	+
Preeclampsia	+++	−	(+)	(+)	−	−	−
Placenta floor infarction	(+)	−	−	−	−	−	−

CACT = carnitine acylcarnitine translocase; CPT = carnitine palmitoyltransferase; HELLP = hemolysis, elevated liver enzymes, low platelets; LCHAD = long-chain 3-hydroxyacyl-CoA dehydrogenase; MCAD = medium-chain acyl-CoA dehydrogenase; SCAD = short-chain acyl-CoA dehydrogenase; SCHAD = short-chain 3-hydroxyacyl-CoA dehydrogenase; TFP = trifunctional protein; + = association reported in more than one case; (+) = association reported in one case, possibly a coincidental event; +++ = association reported in multiple cases; − = association not reported.
*Mothers of children with unspecified disorders but with clinical manifestations and strong biochemical evidence in vivo and in vitro of an underlying fatty acid oxidation disorder (P. Rinaldo et al, unpublished observations, 2003).

TABLE 55.3-2   CLINICAL PRESENTATION AND BIOCHEMICAL DIAGNOSIS OF DISORDERS OF THE CARNITINE CYCLE, FATTY ACID TRANSPORT AND MITOCHONDRIAL OXIDATION, AND KETOGENESIS

TRANSPORTER/ENZYME	FASTING HYPOGLYCEMIA	LIVER	GI	MUSCLE	HEART	CNS	SUDDEN DEATH	OTHER	URINE OA	URINE AG	PLASMA AC	FC	AC/FC	FFA	PRENATAL DIAGNOSIS*	POSSIBLE	EFFICACY OF EARLY THERAPY	RISK FOR ACUTE CRISIS	PM DIAGNOSIS†
Carnitine uptake defect	+	+	+	+	++	+	+	Hypochromic anemia	–	–	–	↓↓	–	–	+	+	++	+	+
Carnitine palmitoyltransferase 1 (liver)	+	++	+	+	+/–	+	+	Respiratory failure, renal tubulopathy	–	–	+	N–↑	–	–	(+)	+	+	+	+
Carnitine acylcarnitine translocase	+	+	+	+	++	–	+	–	–	+	N–↓	↑	–	+	+	–	+	+	
Carnitine palmitoyltransferase 2 (type 1)	+	–	–	+	+	+	+	Renal abnormalities	–	–	+	N–↓	↑	–	(+)	+	–	+	+
Carnitine palmitoyltransferase 2 (type II)	+	–	–	+	+	–	+	+/–	–	+	N–↓	↑	–	(+)	+	+	+	+	
Carnitine palmitoyltransferase 2 (type III)	–	–	+	+	–	–	–	+/–	–	+	N–↓	↑	–	(+)	+	+	+	+	
Very-long-chain acyl-CoA dehydrogenase (early onset)	+	+	–	+	++	+	++	+ (acute)	+ (acute)	+	+	↑	+	+	+	+	+	+	+
Very-long-chain acyl-CoA dehydrogenase (late onset)	+	–	+	+	+	–	–		+ (acute)	–	+	N–↓	↑	+	+	+	+	+	
Isolated long-chain 3-hydroxyacyl-CoA dehydrogenase	+	++	–	+	++	+	++	Peripheral neuropathy, retinopathy	+ (acute)	+	+	N–↓	↑	+	+	+	+	+	+
Trifunctional protein (α and β subunits)	+	–	–	+	–	–	–	Peripheral neuropathy, retinopathy	+ (acute)	–	+	N–↓	↑	+	+	+	+	+	
Medium-chain acyl-CoA dehydrogenase	++	++	–	–	–	–	++	Asymptomatic to fulminant course	+ (acute)	+	+	N–↓	↑	+	+	+	+	+	+
Medium-/short-chain 3-hydroxyacyl-CoA dehydrogenase	+	+/–	–	+	+	–	+	Hyper-insulinism	+ (acute)	–	+	N–↓	↑	+	(+)	+	+	+	
Medium-chain ketoacyl-CoA thiolase	+	+	++	–	–	–	–		+ (acute)	+	+	N–↓	↑	–	–	+			
Short-chain acyl-CoA dehydrogenase	+	–	+	+	+	+	–	Asymptomatic to fulminant course (+)	+ (acute)	+	+	N–↓	↑	–	–	+	+	+	+
3-Hydroxy-3-methylglutaryl-CoA synthase	++	+	–	–	–	+	–		–	–	N	–	–	–	+	+	+		
3-Hydroxy-3-methylglutaryl-CoA lyase	++	+/–	–	–	+/–	++	+	Pancreatitis, + deafness, retinopathy	+ (acute)	–	N	–	–	+	+	+	+		
Succinyl-CoA oxoacid transferase	+	–	–	–	+/–	+	–	Intermittent ketoacidosis	(+)	N	–	+	+	–					
Acetoacetyl-CoA thiolase	+	–	+	–	+	+	+/–	Neutropenia, thrombocytopenia	+	N	+	+	+						
Electron transfer flavoprotein (ETF): α or β subunit	++	+	+	+	+	+	+	Congenital anomalies	+	+	+	N–↓	↑	+	+	+	+/–	+	+
ETF-quinone oxidoreductase	++	+	+	+	+	+	+	Renal cysts, Congenital anomalies	+	+	+	N–↓	↑	+	+	+	+/–	+	+
2,4-Dienoyl-CoA reductase	–	–	++	–	–	–	–		+	N–↓	↑	–	–	?	?				

AC = acylcarnitines; AC/FC = acylcarnitine-to-free carnitine ratio; AG = acylglycine; CNS = central nervous system; FC = free carnitine; FFA = free fatty acids; GI = gastrointestinal involvement; N–↓ = normal to reduced; N–↑ = normal to elevated; OA = organic acid; – = not described; + = common manifestation; ++ = frequent manifestation; + (acute) = present usually during episodes of acute decompensation; +/– = may or may not be present; (+) = not described but theoretically possible; ? = not known.
*Prenatal diagnosis reported by biochemical and/or molecular genetic analysis of amniotic fluid, cultured amniocytes, or chorionic villus samples.
†Postmortem diagnosis reported by biochemical and/or molecular genetic analysis of blood, bile, cultured fibroblasts, liver, or muscle.

glycine and acylcarnitine metabolites can therefore assist in the evaluation of the metabolic defect in these patients. Of note, the buildup of esterified carnitine fractions can subsequently result in secondary L-carnitine deficiency, a condition frequently observed in patients with FAO disorders.

Urinary Organic Acid Analysis. Organic acids are water-soluble compounds that have at least one carboxyl group. They are best detected in urine by gas chromatography–mass spectrometry (GC-MS).[42] Urine organic acid analysis plays an important role in the diagnosis of FAO disorders. Especially during metabolic stress, the finding of inadequate ketonuria in the presence of particular excretion patterns of medium-chain saturated and unsaturated dicarboxylic acids and acylglycines provides strong evidence for an underlying mitochondrial FAO disorder. Nonspecific and even normal organic acid profiles are typically encountered in defects of fatty acid transport, carnitine uptake, and HMG-CoA synthase.

Urinary Acylglycine Analysis. Stable isotope dilution GC-MS allows for quantitative determination of specific urinary acylglycines at concentrations below the detection limit of routine organic acid analysis. MCAD deficiency can be diagnosed reliably by the findings of elevated excretions of hexanoylglycine, phenylpropionylglycine, and suberylglycine in random specimens of asymptomatic patients.[43] Other FAO disorders with informative acylglycine profiles are SCAD deficiency, MCKAT deficiency, and glutaricaciduria type II (ETF and ETF-QO deficiencies).[44–46]

Acylcarnitine Analysis. Acylcarnitine analysis has become the most widely used tool for the investigation of FAO disorders. However, although it is capable of identifying and distinguishing most of the different FAO defects, limitations of this methodology are frequently overlooked. Because adequate tissue levels of free L-carnitine are necessary to form carnitine esters, patients with FAO disorder and severe secondary carnitine deficiency may not exhibit diagnostic or even abnormal acylcarnitine accumulations.[47] Patients with primary carnitine deficiency are also expected to have overall low concentrations of acylcarnitine species.[48] In addition, acylcarnitine analysis cannot differentiate between isomeric carnitine esters, making the performance of other biochemical investigations a necessity to provide appropriate interpretation.[49,50]

Free and Total Carnitine Analysis. Determination of total and free carnitine as well as the acylcarnitine fraction aids in the diagnosis of primary carnitine deficiency and CPT1 deficiency, which are not readily identified by the above-mentioned analyses. Furthermore, carnitine analysis is useful when deciding whether L-carnitine supplementation is warranted in disorders associated with secondary carnitine deficiency and for monitoring patients on carnitine supplementation.[51]

Fatty Acid Analysis. Quantitative determination of plasma fatty acid profiles, in particular C_8 to C_{18} species and

3-hydroxy fatty acids, also provides useful and complementary information when assessing patients suspected of having an FAO defect.[52] Abnormal profiles may be observed in patients with MCAD, LCHAD/TFP, SCHAD, and VLCAD deficiencies as well as glutaricacidemia type II.[53,54]

BIOCHEMICAL IN VITRO STUDIES

Cell-based biochemical in vitro assays are used to confirm a preliminary diagnosis suggested by clinical findings and biochemical data. With the ability to establish fibroblast cultures from small skin punch biopsies, assays were developed allowing metabolic in vitro challenges for the diagnosis of most FAO disorders in a single test.[55,56] Only those few FAO disorders not expressed in fibroblasts (ie, the muscle form of CPT1) are not amenable to this approach and require more specific enzyme investigations in other tissues or a molecular genetic approach. Assays for direct enzyme and transporter analyses are available in a few laboratories worldwide.[57]

MOLECULAR GENETIC STUDIES

Genes harboring disease-carrying mutations responsible for FAO disorders have been identified, and a genotype-phenotype correlation is emerging in a few disorders as well. Accordingly, mutation analysis can principally confirm a tentative diagnosis and facilitate counseling. However, such studies are available for only relatively common mutations that have been described in a few defects. In many cases, deoxyribonucleic acid (DNA) sequencing of the complete gene would be required to reach a conclusive diagnosis by identification of private mutations, which hinders the broad application of molecular genetic analysis to the diagnosis of FAO disorders.[14]

PRENATAL DIAGNOSIS

All known FAO disorders have an autosomal recessive mode of inheritance, carrying with it a recurrence risk of 25% in another pregnancy of the same couple. A rare exception was recently described in two unrelated cases with fatal TFP deficiency whose etiology was found to be associated with uniparental disomy for chromosome 2, which has a significantly lower recurrence risk.[58] Parental investigations are therefore a prerequisite for the provision of comprehensive genetic counseling. Because FAO disorders cover a wide spectrum of clinical presentations and treatability, and disease status in the fetus may even have consequences on the mother's well-being, several criteria must be considered before seeking prenatal diagnostic testing.[36]

Treatment of most FAO disorders is simple and results in a normal life when initiated early. However, an ethical issue may arise when families who suffered the tragic loss of an undiagnosed child are reluctant to accept that simple treatment is indeed available. The decision is easier for disorders in which the outcome must be considered dismal based on the absence of significant treatment options. A prerequisite for all prenatal diagnostic considerations is a related index case with a well-established diagnosis and the availability of a diagnostic test that can be performed on amniotic fluid, amniocytes, or chorionic villi samples using any or a combination of metabolite, protein, and molecular analyses.[59-62]

With the exception of cases in which the prognosis is clearly poor or the mother's health is a significant cause for concern, it is recommended that newborns suspected of having an FAO disorder should undergo a comprehensive evaluation and be managed aggressively immediately after birth until the FAO in question has been excluded.

NEWBORN SCREENING

Newborn screening is a public health program whose mandate is the early identification of diseases in newborns in whom timely intervention could significantly improve the prognosis for their long-term health. Guthrie's innovative application of the bacterial inhibition assay to the detection of levels of phenylalanine in dried blood spots on filter paper led to the establishment of the first newborn screening assay for phenylketonuria.[63] In the following decades, additional tests were added to screening panels using similar or entirely new technology for the detection of key metabolites or enzymatic activity.

The introduction of tandem mass spectrometry (MS/MS) to newborn screening as a sensitive and specific means for the simultaneous detection of key diagnostic metabolites has significantly increased the number of metabolic diseases that could be screened for in a single process using dried blood spot specimens.[64] Currently, over 30 diseases can be screened for, and in addition to several organic acidemias and aminoacidopathies, the ability to quantify acylcarnitine species has also enabled the detection of FAO disorders.[31] However, there is no uniformity in the panel of disorders that each state screens for, with the number of diseases ranging from 4 to over 30.[65]

The prognosis for most patients with FAO disorders who are identified presymptomatically and managed appropriately is generally favorable and suggests benefit from early diagnosis and treatment.

POSTMORTEM SCREENING

The period after birth is a critical time for infants with FAO disorders, and episodes of hypoglycemia can be triggered by inadequate food intake and limited glycogen stores.[66] The severity of these episodes is variable, with symptoms resolving in response to either intravenous glucose or feeding in some patients, whereas, on the other end of the spectrum, the decompensation events may be fatal, resulting in sudden and unexpected death.[67] An estimated 5% of sudden, unexpected deaths in children less than 1 year of age and an even higher percentage of deaths observed in the 1- to 5-year age group are caused by FAO disorders.[68-70] Postmortem studies involving histochemical and biochemical analyses of liver specimens,[70] organic and fatty acid analysis of urine and plasma specimens,[69] analysis of acylcarnitine profiles in dried blood and bile spots,[71,72] and the determination of FAO rates using cultured skin fibroblasts[73] have all been used to investigate sudden unexpected death in previously healthy patients.

An approach for the investigation of such a patient suspected of having an FAO disorder has been described.[74]

We propose a complete postmortem investigation and genetic counseling of parents who lost a child suddenly and/or unexpectedly. Blood and bile could be conveniently collected on the same filter paper card, one identical to those used for newborn screening, which can be shipped at room temperature. Liver and skin biopsies should also be collected and kept until the blood and bile samples have been analyzed. Both of these specimens should be collected to provide a better chance to detect and independently confirm the largest possible number of disorders. In cases with a higher level of suspicion, an effort should be made to collect a frozen specimen of liver and a skin biopsy. Although fatty infiltration of the liver and/or other organs (heart, kidneys) is a common finding in FAO disorders, caution should be exercised not to use steatosis as the sole criteria to indicate a possible underlying FAO disorder during the postmortem evaluation of a case of sudden death.[70] Additional risk factors include a family history of sudden death, Reye syndrome, or maternal pregnancy complication and evidence of lethargy, vomiting, and/or fasting in the 48 hours prior to death. To ensure that all possible avenues are covered, cases of alleged child abuse should also be fully investigated. The frozen liver and skin biopsy could be discarded at a later time without further testing when a credible cause of death has been established but could otherwise be crucial to reach a proper diagnosis and conclusive confirmation in vitro.

These studies are important in providing the basis for appropriate genetic counseling and even testing of family members because the identification of affected, healthy appearing siblings is not uncommon.[75]

DISORDERS OF PLASMA MEMBRANE FUNCTIONS

LONG-CHAIN FATTY ACID TRANSPORT/BINDING DEFECT

Two patients have been described who presented with episodes of acute liver failure and mild acute encephalopathy associated with nonketotic hypoglycemia and hyperammonemia.[76] Both of them received liver transplants, and their further development was normal. The biochemical phenotype of these patients was nonspecific, and steatosis was not observed in either patients' livers. In cultured skin fibroblasts, reduced intracellular concentration of C_{14} to C_{18} fatty acids and reduced cellular oxidation of palmitate and oleate were found. The latter finding was normalized by permeabilization of the plasma membrane with digitonin. No mutations were found by sequencing of several target genes involved in fatty acid transport. The exact defect in these patients remains to be determined.

CARNITINE UPTAKE DEFECT

Carnitine uptake defect is the only cause of primary carnitine deficiency and is due to a defective plasma membrane carnitine transporter. Renal reabsorption and intestinal uptake are impaired, with subsequent tissue depletion of carnitine. Intracellular carnitine deficiency impairs the entry of long-chain fatty acids into the mitochondrial matrix and therefore compromises FAO, particularly in tissues that are most reliant on this pathway. Patients present with progressive cardiomyopathy, episodes of hypoketotic hypoglycemia associated with encephalopathy, and hepatomegaly. Skeletal myopathy is also a common clinical manifestation. Some patients had episodes of abdominal pain and diarrhea owing to gastrointestinal dysmotility; others had hypochromic anemia.[77,78] Several cases of sudden and unexpected death at variable ages have also been reported.[67,79] Microvesicular steatosis and lipid infiltration may be seen in liver and muscle biopsies, respectively. Plasma carnitine concentrations are less than 10% of normal and typically associated with increased urinary carnitine excretion. The diagnosis is confirmed either by determination of carnitine uptake in fibroblasts or molecular genetic analysis of the gene (SLC22A5) encoding the sodium ion-dependent carnitine transporter OTCN2. A genotype-phenotype correlation is not apparent.[80] Presymptomatic identification through newborn screening using tandem mass spectrometry has been reported.[48] Heterozygotes for OTCN2 mutations show moderately reduced plasma carnitine levels and reduced rates of carnitine uptake,[79] increased urinary carnitine losses,[81] and predisposition to late-onset benign cardiac hypertrophy.[82]

DISORDERS OF THE CARNITINE CYCLE

CPT1 DEFICIENCY

CPT1 exists as two tissue-specific and genetically distinct isoforms, a hepatic (CPT1A) and a muscle type (CPT1B).[83,84] CPT1A is expressed in liver and other tissues except muscle, whereas CPT1B is primarily expressed in skeletal and cardiac muscle. Accordingly, CPT1A deficiency is characterized primarily by nonketotic hypoglycemia and liver dysfunction, which may result in a fatal Reye-like encephalopathy. Several cases were reported with cardiac (cardiomegaly, arrhythmia) and renal involvement (distal renal tubular acidosis).[85,86] AFLP was reported in two subsequent pregnancies, both resulting in CPT1A-deficient offspring.[87]

The biochemical diagnosis is not straightforward. Organic acid analysis of urine collected during clinically significant episodes is not informative. Blood acylcarnitine analysis may reveal an elevation of free and acetylcarnitine in the presence of relatively low concentrations of long-chain acylcarnitines allowing the calculation of a ratio specific for CPT1 deficiency.[88] In contrast to other FAO defects, CPT1A deficiency is associated with an elevated level of plasma carnitine, in particular free carnitine. This is probably caused by the unusually high renal threshold for free carnitine and secondary increase in carnitine transport.[89] Accordingly, high plasma concentrations of total and free carnitine in a patient with a suspicious clinical presentation should lead to the inclusion of CPT1 in the differential diagnosis. CPT1A can be confirmed by enzyme assay in fibroblasts and molecular genetic analysis of the CPT1A gene. However, most mutations are private, with the exception of the G710E mutation, which is common in

the Hutterite communities of North America.[90] Treatment is based on strict avoidance of fasting and subsequent hypoglycemia and a low-fat diet supplemented with medium-chain triglycerides (MCTs). Patients with CPT1B deficiency have not been reported to date.

CACT DEFICIENCY

Patients with CACT deficiency typically present in the neonatal period with hypoketotic hypoglycemia, liver failure accompanied by hyperammonemia, and/or hypertrophic cardiomyopathy.[91] Impaired motility of the whole gastrointestinal tract has been reported in one patient.[92] Frequent feedings of a low-fat diet, with most fat consisting of MCTs, which do not require CACT to cross the mitochondrial membranes, are the mainstay of treatment. Nevertheless, despite therapeutic efforts, most patients will die following the development of cardiac arrhythmias, possibly caused by an accumulation of arrhythmogenic long-chain acylcarnitines.[33] Autopsy reveals fatty infiltration in liver, kidney, and muscle and hypertrophic cardiomyopathy.[92,93] Outcome has been more favorable for patients, with in vitro evidence of some residual enzyme activity.[91,94,95] Because CACT deficiency is identifiable through expanded newborn screening using tandem mass spectrometry, it is expected that in the future, more patients will be identified and treated before the onset of symptoms. Whether the prognosis can be improved by presymptomatic initiation of treatment, however, remains to be seen. Acylcarnitine analysis in plasma or dried blood spots reveals markedly elevated long-chain acylcarnitines, with C_{16} and C_{18} species being particularly prominent. However, because CPT2 deficiency (see below) results in virtually the same acylcarnitine profile, further biochemical testing by enzyme assay or molecular genetic analysis of the CACT gene is necessary to arrive at the correct diagnosis. Molecular analysis usually requires gene sequencing owing to significant allelic heterogeneity.[91]

CPT2 DEFICIENCY

CPT2 deficiency can be differentiated into several clinical presentations. A relatively mild, adult-onset form of CPT2 deficiency was the first mitochondrial FAO defect to be described.[96] It is typically limited to the skeletal muscle, with episodes of myopathy and rhabdomyolysis usually triggered by prolonged exercise combined with either fasting or cold exposure. One patient had recurrent pancreatitis with intermittent myoglobinuria; another's myopathic crises appeared to be induced by valproate therapy.[97,98]

A recently proposed classification is based on organ involvement, residual enzyme activity, and genotype.[99] Accordingly, CPT2 type I is the most severe form that presents in the neonatal period and affects the liver, skeletal muscle, and heart and is associated with congenital brain and kidney abnormalities.[100,101] CPT2 type II involves the liver, skeletal muscle, and heart and presents in the first few years of life. Type III is limited to skeletal muscle, presents in early adulthood, and, relative to types I and II, is associated with the highest residual enzyme activity. Because of several patients having experienced malignant hyperthermia during surgery, it has been suggested to include CPT2 deficiency in the differential diagnosis of this anesthetic complication.[102]

Myoglobinuria and markedly elevated serum creatine phosphokinase levels are hallmarks of CPT2 deficiency. Acylcarnitine profiles are also abnormal but identical to those observed in CACT deficiency. More specific enzyme assays or molecular genetic tests are needed to verify a presumptive diagnosis. The most common mutation in CPT2 type III is S113L, whereas 413delAG appears to be common in the Ashkenazi Jewish population.[103] Symptomatic heterozygotes for particular mutations have also been described.[104]

DISORDERS OF LONG-CHAIN FATTY ACID METABOLISM

VLCAD Deficiency

The first patients with VLCAD deficiency were described as having LCAD deficiency, based on the ETF reduction assay using palmitoyl CoA as a substrate.[105] However, once molecular genetic studies of the LCAD gene were possible and the VLCAD protein was identified, patients previously labeled as LCAD deficient were shown to have no mutations in the LCAD gene, whereas they had no detectable VLCAD protein by immunoblot analysis.[106] A patient with true LCAD deficiency has not yet been described. However, an LCAD knockout mouse model features typical symptoms of an FAO disorder, suggesting that LCAD is indeed a critical enzyme and will likely be demonstrated in humans eventually.[107]

VLCAD catalyzes the first step of the fatty acid β-oxidation spiral. The severity of the phenotype seems to correlate with specific genotypes.[108] The most severe phenotype manifests early in life and is associated with nonsense mutations, resulting in complete loss of enzyme activity. Morbidity and mortality are significant owing to involvement of multiple organ systems, in particular the liver and heart, resulting in recurrent metabolic crises and cardiomyopathy.[109] Patients carrying missense mutations or with single amino acid deletions permitting some residual enzyme activity are at high risk of metabolic decompensation with nonketotic hypoglycemia and a Reye-like syndrome triggered by increased energy demands (eg, prolonged fasting, fever).[110] The phenotype switches from a more hepatic presentation to muscle weakness as patients become older; some are able to sustain metabolic stress during childhood and do not present until adulthood with exercise-induced myopathy and rhabdomyolysis.

Laboratory hallmarks during acute episodes include hypoketotic hypoglycemia and creatine phosphokinase elevations. Urine organic acid analysis is nonspecific, with hypoketotic dicarboxylicaciduria. Acylcarnitine analysis is most informative, revealing a characteristic profile with elevated levels of saturated and unsaturated C_{14} to C_{18} carnitine esters, the predominant species being tetradecenoylcarnitine ($C_{14:1}$).[57] The diagnosis can be confirmed by specific enzyme assay or FAO in vitro probing in fibroblast cultures[111] or by molecular genetic analysis of the VLCAD gene. Because

acylcarnitine analysis can be performed in newborn screening blood spots, early identification and treatment of affected patients are generally possible.[112,113]

TFP and LCHAD

The TFP is a hetero-octamer containing four α and four β subunits encoded by two different genes. The α subunit harbors the activities of the second and third steps of fatty acid β-oxidation, LCEH and LCHAD. The β subunit harbors LCKAT, which catalyzes the last step in β-oxidation of long-chain fatty acids. Although mutations in either gene may cause complete TFP deficiency, a few mutations in the α subunit cause isolated LCHAD deficiency. In keeping with the previously mentioned disorders, a genotype-phenotype correlation has also emerged for TFP deficiency, with residual enzyme activity being associated with a milder, later-onset phenotype. Patients with late-onset TFP deficiency present with a progressive peripheral neuropathy and episodic rhabdomyolysis.[114] Recently, two patients with lethal TFP deficiency owing to isodisomy for chromosome 2 were described. This finding is of great importance in particular for genetic counseling of families because the recurrence risk in future pregnancies would be significantly lower than the 25% risk typical for FAO disorders, which are generally autosomal recessive.[58]

Although the phenotype of both disorders includes all of the symptoms expected in a FAO disorder, patients with LCHAD and TFP deficiencies may also develop pigmentary retinitis and a peripheral neuropathy, the pathophysiology of which remains obscure. In addition, many patients are born prematurely and small for gestational age. The initial hypothesis that a secondary deficiency of docosahexaenoic acid may cause the retinal changes and may be treatable by dietary supplementation has not been proven conclusively.[115]

A recent study described the clinical and biochemical abnormalities in 50 patients with isolated LCHAD deficiency.[116] All patients presented by 26 months, and most became symptomatic within the first 6 months of life. Thirty-nine patients had episodes of acute metabolic decompensation, with symptoms of hepatic dysfunction (79%), coma (56%), seizures (38%), and apnea (23%). Fewer patients experienced cardiorespiratory arrest, arrhythmia, and sudden death. Hypoglycemia was a key laboratory finding in all 39 patients, and most of the patients showed decreases in total carnitine and significant elevations in plasma lactate, aspartate aminotransferase, creatine kinase, and ammonia levels. The 11 patients who did not experience an acute metabolic decompensation before diagnosis of LCHAD deficiency were also found to have a range of more chronic symptoms, which included hepatomegaly, cholestasis and hepatic dysfunction, cardiomyopathy, feeding difficulties, failure to thrive, hypotonia and lethargy, psychomotor retardation, peripheral neuropathy, and microcephaly. This spectrum of clinical signs before and at the time of diagnosis was similar for both groups of patients presenting with or without acute metabolic crisis. With more newborn screening laboratories introducing tandem mass spectrometry for acylcarnitine analysis into their programs, patients should come to attention earlier in life, and follow-up studies will have to determine whether presymptomatic initiation of treatment is beneficial.[50,117]

Patients with isolated LCHAD deficiency have a reduction in LCHAD activity with normal LCEH and LCKAT activities. The most common cause of isolated LCHAD deficiency is the 1528G→C mutation, which changes a glutamate to a glutamine residue (E474Q) in the active site of the α subunit of the LCHAD gene. The replacement of the acidic residue with a neutral amide amino acid is thought to affect the NAD$^+$-binding site of the enzyme and subsequently results in an isolated reduction of LCHAD activity without affecting the activities of LCEH and LCKAT.

Another feature that was thought to be specific to LCHAD deficiency was the observation that approximately 20% of patients were born following pregnancies complicated with maternal liver disease, in particular AFLP and HELLP syndrome. However, several other FAO disorders have meanwhile been implicated as possible triggers of maternal liver disease during pregnancy.[36] The simplified hypothesis is that pathologic fatty acid metabolites accumulating in the affected fetus eventually overwhelm the obligate heterozygous mother's FAO capacity, which already is reduced in the third trimester of pregnancy.[34]

DISORDERS OF MEDIUM-CHAIN FATTY ACID METABOLISM

MCAD DEFICIENCY

MCAD is responsible for the initial dehydrogenation of acyl CoAs with a chain length between 4- and 12-carbon atoms. MCAD deficiency is probably the best known FAO defect because it has gained prominent attention over the last decade as a disorder fulfilling all classic criteria for inclusion into newborn screening programs.[118,119] Early diagnosis is crucial because MCAD is a potentially lethal disease, documented by the fact that up to at least 20% of undiagnosed patients die during their first metabolic decompensation.[120] A common missense mutation (985A→G; K304E) has been identified in whites of Northern European descent that results in reduced production of an unstable protein. But patients homozygous for this mutation may present at any time during life—typically, when a metabolic stressor is experienced (fever, prolonged fasting) that triggers an acute manifestation. However, identification of patients by newborn screening has led to the discovery of cases with only mild biochemical abnormalities and specific genotypes involving mutations that preserve significant enzyme activity in vitro. Whether patients with such genotypes will remain asymptomatic even during times of increased energy demands remains to be determined either by long-term follow-up or by carefully conducted fasting challenges.

A defect of the MCAD enzyme leads to fasting-induced hypoglycemia and accumulation of medium-chain fatty acids. The latter are further metabolized not only to dicarboxylic and carnitine esters but also to glycine esters, which can be determined in urine by organic acid analysis or more accurately by stable isotope dilution methods and GC-MS.[43] Analysis of plasma acylcarnitines by MS/MS reveals accumulation of C_6 to C_{10} acylcarnitine species, with prominent octanoylcarnitine.[121] Detection of these metabolites is the basis for newborn screening for MCAD deficiency by MS/MS.[64,118] Affected individuals may develop secondary carnitine deficiency; thus, the characteristic metabolites may not be reliably detectable.[47] Urine acylglycine analysis should therefore be pursued in carnitine-deficient and asymptomatic patients, making obsolete previously advocated provocative tests in most cases.[43] The biochemical diagnosis of MCAD deficiency can be confirmed by measurement of the activity of the MCAD enzyme in fibroblasts and other tissues and by molecular genetic testing of the ACADM gene; both test methods can be used for prenatal diagnosis. MCAD deficiency has been observed in all populations but Asians.[122]

M/SCHAD DEFICIENCY

Previously, the clinical entity now known as M/SCHAD deficiency was described as a defect of SCHAD, an enzyme of the mitochondrial short-chain fatty acid β-oxidation pathway converting L-3-hydroxybutyryl CoA to acetoacetyl CoA.[123] However, our present understanding of the protein encoded by the SCHAD gene suggests a chain-length specificity toward C_8 to C_{10} acyl CoA.[124] At the clinical and biochemical levels, a deficiency of this enzyme has been described with three different phenotypes. The first one presented with cardiomyopathy and recurrent rhabdomyolysis, culminating in death as a teenager.[125] Enzyme activity was reduced in skeletal muscle but not in skin fibroblasts; other tissues were not studied enzymatically. A second phenotype was described with a presentation similar to that seen in ketotic hypoglycemia, and enzyme deficiency was described in isolated mitochondria from cultured skin fibroblasts.[126] Other tissues were not analyzed in these patients. A third group of patients had hepatic involvement and steatosis; the catalytic activity with the C_4 substrate was deficient in liver but normal in muscle and fibroblasts.[127] Mutation analysis of the SCHAD gene in these patients has been inconclusive, suggesting the existence of another protein with high activity toward acetoacetyl CoA.[128]

Recently, however, five patients in two unrelated families were reported who presented with hypoketotic hypoglycemia associated with hyperinsulinism, reduced M/SCHAD activity in fibroblast mitochondria, and mutations in the SCHAD gene.[38,129,130] Further molecular information and detailed studies of M/SCHAD protein interactions will hopefully improve our understanding of the function, substrate specificity, and tissue expression of this peculiar enzyme.

In addition to hypoglycemia, which may be either ketotic or hypoketotic, elevated transaminases, creatine phosphokinase, and hyperammonemia may be present during acute episodes of metabolic decompensation in affected patients. Specific laboratory findings include various chain-length dicarboxylic and 3-hydroxydicarboxylicaciduria. Plasma acylcarnitine analysis may be normal or show an elevated concentration of 3-hydroxybutyryl carnitine.[38]

MCKAT DEFICIENCY

Only one patient with this disorder has been described to date.[131] This Japanese male newborn presented at 2 days of life with emesis, dehydration, liver dysfunction, and terminal rhabdomyolysis and died several days later. Laboratory findings included hypoglycemia, hyperammonemia, metabolic acidosis, and elevated creatine phosphokinase levels. Urine organic acid analysis showed ketotic lacticaciduria and significant C_6 to C_{12} dicarboxylicaciduria, with prominent C_{10} and C_{12} species. Whereas palmitate oxidation on skin fibroblasts was normal, octanoate oxidation was reduced to 31% of controls. An isolated deficiency of MCKAT was demonstrated in fibroblasts. This result was supported by the findings of immunoprecipitation studies, which demonstrated a 60% reduction in protein signal. A better understanding of this disorder will require the elucidation of the molecular basis and identification of additional patients.

DISORDERS OF SHORT-CHAIN FATTY ACID METABOLISM

SCAD DEFICIENCY

Initially suggested in 1984,[132] SCAD deficiency has been reported in less than 30 patients.[1,14] The first SCAD-deficient patients reported were two newborns with unusually large urinary excretion of ethylmalonic acid (EMA). One of these patients died during the neonatal period, whereas the other suffered only one metabolic decompensation in the newborn period and remained asymptomatic thereafter.[133]

EMA is an alternative metabolite of butyryl CoA that accumulates when β-oxidation of fatty acids cannot proceed in shortening fatty acyl CoAs with four carbons owing to inactivity of SCAD. Butyryl CoA is then carboxylated by propionyl-CoA carboxylase to EMA, which is readily excreted in urine, where it can be measured by organic acid or acylglycine analysis. Butyryl CoA can also be esterified with carnitine to facilitate egress out of the mitochondria and eventually into the blood, where it is measurable as a C_4-acylcarnitine by MS/MS. An increased concentration of butyrylcarnitine in blood and excretion of EMA into urine are considered biochemical markers of SCAD deficiency, although these findings are not specific for this disorder.

A variety of symptoms have been described, the most common being developmental delay and muscle hypotonia.[134] The laboratory confirmation of SCAD deficiency is difficult and should include both biochemical and molecular genetic studies. Most conveniently, fibroblasts can be used to first assess FAO,[135,136] followed by SCAD gene sequencing. However, although several pathogenic, mostly missense mutations have been identified, molecular genetic testing for SCAD deficiency is complicated by two SCAD gene variants, $511C \rightarrow T$ (R147W) and $625G \rightarrow A$ (G185S), which occur in the homozygous or compound heterozygous state in 7% of the US population.[137] Among patients overexcreting EMA, these variants are even more frequent.[138,139] In addition, some patients with biochemical evidence of SCAD deficiency do not carry any other SCAD gene mutations.[134,140] In vitro studies revealed that these variants compromise SCAD activity owing to abnormal protein folding and thermolability, respectively.[139,141] All of these findings considered, these variants are believed to

confer disease susceptibility in combination with other, as yet unidentified genetic or environmental factors.

DISORDERS OF KETOGENESIS

HMG-CoA SYNTHASE DEFICIENCY

Only six patients with HMG-CoA synthase deficiency have been described to date.[21,142–145] All patients presented with recurrent hypoketotic hypoglycemic episodes leading to coma, usually triggered by prolonged fasting owing to gastroenteritis.

This diagnosis may be underestimated because of the relatively nonspecific biochemical phenotype during an acute episode with hypoketotic hypoglycemia, dicarboxylicaciduria, and normal blood acylcarnitine profile in the presence of elevated free fatty acids.[21]

Enzymatic analysis is difficult because HMG-CoA synthase is expressed in the liver, and its substrates and products are also used or synthesized by other proteins. The human *HMGCS2* gene, however, has been isolated, and the diagnostic potential of a molecular approach has been documented by the detection of disease-causing mutations.[21,146]

HMG-CoA LYASE DEFICIENCY

HMG-CoA lyase is the second mitochondrial enzyme that mediates ketogenesis from fatty acids (see Figure 55.3-4). It also catalyzes the final step of leucine catabolism. Approximately 60 patients described presented with acute, often lethal episodes of hypoketotic hypoglycemia and acidosis.[147] Fifty percent of the cases presented in the first weeks of life acutely, triggered by fasting or intercurrent illness. Exceptionally, the onset is after 2 years of age. The central nervous system appears to be particularly vulnerable during metabolic crises, but abnormal magnetic resonance imaging signal abnormalities in white matter were observed even in asymptomatic patients.[148] In addition to possible neurologic sequelae, pancreatitis, cardiomyopathy, and deafness associated with retinopathy have been described.[149–151]

The urine organic acid profile is characteristic, with abnormal excretion of 3-hydroxy-3-methylglutaric, 3-methylglutaconic, 3-methylglutaric, and 3-hydroxyisovaleric acids. Acylcarnitine analysis in plasma and newborn screening blood spots is remarkable for elevated 3-methylglutarylcarnitine.[152] The diagnosis should be confirmed by measurement of enzymatic activity in fibroblast cultures or molecular genetic testing. The defect appears to be relatively frequent in Saudi Arabia, where it accounts for about 16% of inherited metabolic diseases.[153]

SCOT DEFICIENCY

Succinyl-CoA:3-oxoacid-CoA transferase is the first step of ketone body use in extrahepatic tissues, particularly the heart, kidney, and brain (see Figure 55.3-4). The typical clinical presentation includes recurrent episodes of severe ketoacidosis, with persistent ketonuria and hyperketonemia even during the fed state. In almost all described patients, the onset was in the first year of life.[154] In two cases, cardiomegaly was noted,[155] and behavioral problems have also been reported.[156]

Urine organic acid analysis reveals persistent, although nonspecific, ketonuria. A tentative diagnosis should be confirmed by enzyme assay or molecular genetic analysis.[157]

The disease is potentially fatal. Treatment relies on limitation of protein intake, provision of adequate calories, and alkaline therapy to prevent aggravation of ketosis at the onset of any intercurrent infection.[158]

MITOCHONDRIAL β-KETOTHIOLASE DEFICIENCY

β-Ketothiolase is a ketogenic and ketolytic enzyme that also intervenes in isoleucine catabolism (see Figure 55.3-4). Although variable, most patients present with acute ketoacidosis accompanying infections and vomiting. Dilated cardiomyopathy, neutropenia, and thrombocytopenia are also possible.[147] Neurologic complications, such as mental retardation and basal ganglia involvement, have been described in a few patients.[159,160] However, asymptomatic affected individuals have been documented in families with an affected case.[161]

Urine organic acid analysis is diagnostic with the documentation of a large excretion of 2-methyl-3-hydroxybutyric acid and tiglylglycine, reflecting a block in isoleucine catabolism. The enzymatic assay presents some technical difficulties because of the presence of three other thiolases. Significant genetic heterogeneity hinders a rapid molecular genetic approach to the diagnosis.[162]

Key biochemical findings associated with the disorders of ketone body metabolism are presented in Table 55.3-3.

OTHER DISORDERS

GLUTARIC ACIDEMIA TYPE II

Primary defects of ETF or ETF-QO result in glutaric acidemia type II. This disorder is also known as multiple acyl-CoA dehydrogenase deficiency because the reoxidation of several mitochondrial dehydrogenases is impaired owing to the inability of their cofactor, FAD, to transfer electrons to ETF. The clinical phenotype is variable, with an early-onset, severe form with or without congenital anomalies and a milder, later-onset form of the disease.[162] The milder phenotype has also been described as ethylmalonic-adipicaciduria.

The severe, neonatal-onset form with congenital anomalies is often associated with prematurity. Patients generally present with overwhelming illness within the first 2 days of life and die shortly thereafter. Hypotonia, severe hypoglycemia, metabolic acidosis, large kidneys, and renal dysgenesis have also been described. Congenital

anomalies include dysmorphic facial features, rocker-bottom feet, muscular and abdominal wall defects, and genital anomalies.[163–165]

Patients with early neonatal onset without congenital abnormalities also initially present with hypotonia, metabolic acidosis, hypoglycemia, tachypnea, hepatomegaly, and the odor of sweaty feet. These patients may survive for a few months with treatment. Death is often due to severe cardiomyopathy. An even longer survival was noted in patients who initially presented with hypoglycemia in the newborn period followed by episodes of Reye-like illness.[164–168]

There is considerable variability in patients with the milder, late-onset phenotype.[165] The clinical presentation may include episodic vomiting, hypoglycemia, and acidosis. Hepatomegaly, carnitine deficiency, and lipid storage myopathy have also been described. Whereas some patients present clinically within the first few years of life,[169] others may remain symptom free until adulthood.[170]

Mutations in ETF-QO but not ETF are associated with renal cysts. Although several mutations have been described in the genes for the ETF α subunit and ETF-QO, there are no common mutations. Olsen and colleagues examined the genetic basis of nine patients with the three different clinical phenotypes of glutaric acidemia type II and showed a relationship between the genotype and the phenotype.[171] The three patients with neonatal-onset and congenital anomalies were homozygous for null mutations and demonstrated palmitate oxidation levels of less than 5% of control cell lines in metabolic flux studies. The milder clinical phenotypes are associated with mutations that result in residual enzymatic activity, which itself may be modulated by environmental factors, such as fever.

Glutaric acidemia type II has a characteristic biochemical phenotype, primarily associated with the secondarily altered metabolism of its related dehydrogenases.[172] Urinary organic acid profiles demonstrate an accumulation of EMA, glutaric acid, and 2-hydroxyglutaric acid. Isovalerylglycine and hexanoylglycine accumulation is notable, particularly by urinary acylglycine analysis, and elevated levels of butyrylcarnitine, isovalerylcarnitine, glutarylcarnitine, and several other medium- and long-chain acylcarnitine species are observed by acylcarnitine analysis in plasma and newborn screening blood spots.

2,4-DIENOYL-COA REDUCTASE DEFICIENCY

There has only been one published case of 2,4-dienoyl-CoA reductase deficiency.[19] The patient was a term female who presented at 2 days of age with hypotonia. Notable

TABLE 55.3-3   DISORDERS OF KETONE BODY METABOLISM AND CHARACTERISTIC BIOCHEMICAL ABNORMALITIES

DISORDER	KETOSIS	ACIDOSIS	BLOOD GLUCOSE	BLOOD AMMONIA	PLASMA LACTATE
KETOGENESIS					
HMG-CoA synthase deficiency	−	−	↓	N	N
HMG-CoA lyase deficiency	−	+	↓	N	↑
KETOLYSIS					
SCOT deficiency	+++	+	N/↓	N	N
β-Ketothiolase deficiency	+++	+	↑/N/↓	N	N

HMG-CoA = 3-hydroxy-3-methylglutaryl coenzyme A; N = normal; SCOT = succinyl-CoA oxoacid transferase; ↓ = reduced; ↑ = elevated.

physical features included microcephaly; a large face; small arms, feet, and fingers; and a small trunk. The biochemical phenotype consisted of hyperlysinemia, carnitine deficiency, and a normal urinary organic acid profile. Acylcarnitine analysis, however, revealed an abnormal accumulation of decadienoylcarnitine ($C_{10:2}$) in blood and urine. The infant was placed on a lysine-restricted diet with MCTs and carnitine supplementation. Although this diet resulted in some weight gain, at 4 months of age, the patient ultimately suffered a fatal episode of respiratory distress. Autopsy findings also demonstrated pulmonary vascular congestion and bilateral hypertrophy. It is surprising that no additional cases have been found after the initial report despite the routine application of acylcarnitine analysis in the laboratory evaluation of metabolic patients.

GENERAL APPROACH TO TREATMENT

The mainstay of treatment is the avoidance of fasting. Frequent feedings are recommended to avoid accumulation of toxic metabolites resulting from peripheral lipolysis and hypoglycemia that may occur in affected patients when hepatic glycogen stores become depleted during prolonged fasting and periods of higher energy demands.[173] Infants should be fed every 3 to 4 hours, and older patients may be given uncooked cornstarch as a source of complex carbohydrates, which are slowly released into the bloodstream, allowing longer feeding intervals and prolonged nighttime rest. The initial dose is 1.0 to 1.5 g/kg, which can be slowly increased to 1.75 to 2 g/kg by 2 years of age.[174] If this is not tolerated well, a bedtime snack rich in complex carbohydrates should be provided. In severe cases with a high risk of recurrent hypoglycemia, continuous overnight administration of carbohydrates by nasogastric or gastrostomy tube may be required.

RESTRICTION OF FAT INTAKE
A dietary regimen of fat restriction and high carbohydrate intake has been generally recommended for the long-term management of FAO disorders. The exact limitations, however, have not been studied systematically and vary, ranging from 10 to 35%, with a median fat restriction of 29%.[173] Depending on the severity of the disorder, a reasonable approach appears to be the reduction to 25 to 30% of total calories from fat. The substitution of MCTs as a lipid substrate has been suggested for patients with long-chain FAO defects because medium-chain fatty acids do not require the carnitine cycle to cross the mitochondrial membranes and enter the β-oxidation pathway downstream of the defective enzyme.[175] Ten to 20% of total calories should come from MCT oil in these disorders.[173,176] However, MCT oil must not be prescribed for patients with deficiencies of medium- and short-chain fatty acid metabolism and ketogenesis. Supplementation of essential fatty acids at 1 to 2% of total energy intake by the use of flaxseed, canola, walnut, or safflower oils has been suggested, particularly when MCT oil is a significant part of the diet and because deficiency of docosahexaenoic acid has been hypothesized as a possible cause for the development of pigmentary

retinopathy in patients with LCHAD deficiency.[115,173,177] Fat-soluble vitamins should also be supplemented to meet Recommended Dietary Allowance standards.[173]

CARNITINE SUPPLEMENTATION
Primary carnitine deficiency (carnitine uptake defect) is the only disorder for which the supplementation of L-carnitine is proven to be essential and lifesaving.[78] In this condition, oral doses of 100 mg/kg/d and higher are required to maintain plasma carnitine levels in the normal range. The use of carnitine in other disorders of FAO that are associated with secondary carnitine deficiency is controversial. Arguments in support of carnitine are based on its potentially beneficial role in the removal of accumulated toxic acyl-CoA intermediates and repletion of the intramitochondrial carnitine pool. However, neither protective nor deleterious effects of carnitine have been proven conclusively. Treem and colleagues reported a study of one patient with MCAD deficiency who was fasted before and on carnitine supplementation.[178] Treatment did not prolong the period of fasting tolerance or prevent the accumulation of abnormal metabolites. Furthermore, the benefit of L-carnitine supplementation has been questioned for long-chain FAO disorders in particular because the accumulation of long-chain fatty acylcarnitines may cause fatal cardiac arrhythmias.[33,179] On the other hand, L-carnitine has been proposed as an antiarrhythmic medication.[180] Den Boer and colleagues did not find evidence that carnitine supplementation had any effect on the number of metabolic decompensations in LCHAD-deficient patients.[114] In a few patients with LCHAD deficiency, a positive response to carnitine administration was reported with respect to serum carnitine values and clinical status.[181,182] Other patients with FAO disorders died while treated with carnitine,[183–185] whereas the clinical condition improved for others who did not receive carnitine.[186]

OTHER TREATMENT MODALITIES
Although no data regarding efficacy are available, riboflavin is sometimes prescribed (100 mg/d) for SCAD and ETF/ETF dehydrogenase deficiencies. The rationale is that riboflavin, a cofactor of dehydrogenases, may boost any residual enzyme activity. More recently, Roe and colleagues reported the use of an anaplerotic odd-chain triglyceride, triheptanoin, in three patients with VLCAD deficiency.[187] It is postulated that triheptanoin increases the concentration of oxaloacetate (derived from propionic acid) that can serve to favor oxidation of acetyl CoA by the Krebs cycle or enter gluconeogenesis. This anaplerotic effect was found to be effective in the normalization of the acylcarnitine profile and some clinical symptoms in patients with VLCAD deficiency.[187] It is unclear whether odd-chain fatty acids offer any therapeutic advantage over the widely available MCT-rich diet for patients with carnitine or acylcarnitine translocase deficiency. Cardiomyopathy and muscle weakness resolved in these patients, and rhabdomyolysis did not occur at least during the 26 months of treatment with this dietary modification. Side effects were also not observed, but a larger, longer-term study has not been reported, and

studies using many available mouse models for FAO disorders have not yet been conducted.

Future pharmacologic approaches to the treatment of FAO disorders may also include the use of fibrates, which have been shown in vitro to increase enzyme activity at least in patients with some residual enzyme activity. So far, this has only been shown to be of potential benefit in CPT2–deficient fibroblast cultures.[188] The beneficial effect of increased enzyme activity appears to be related to fibrate acting as a ligand of peroxisome proliferator–activated receptor α, which induces expression of β-oxidation enzyme genes.

MANAGEMENT DURING INTERCURRENT ILLNESS

The most pressing issue in a patient with an impending or present metabolic decompensation is the reversal of catabolism by provision of energy in the form of glucose. When oral intake of adequate amounts of carbohydrates cannot be achieved, intravenous glucose (8–10 mg/kg/min) should be administered. This should stimulate insulin secretion and hence suppress peripheral lipolysis. Some, particularly newborn, patients do not appear to clinically improve despite the development of even hyperglycemia. However, hyperglycemia may not be a reflection of a glucose overload but can be caused by an inadequate insulin response. In such cases, glucose should not be reduced, but insulin therapy should be carefully initiated to allow the patient's metabolism to use the administered glucose.

Once diagnosed, all patients should be provided with a frequently updated "emergency" letter to be given, if needed, to health care providers who may not be familiar with the patient's disorder. This letter should include a detailed explanation of the management of acute metabolic decompensation, emphasizing the importance of preventive measures (eg, intravenous glucose regardless of "normal" laboratory results, overnight in-hospital observation), and the telephone numbers of the patient's metabolic specialist.

REFERENCES

1. Rinaldo P, Matern D, Bennett MJ. Fatty acid oxidation disorders. Annu Rev Physiol 2002;64:477–502.
2. DiMauro S, DiMauro PM. Muscle carnitine palmityltransferase deficiency and myoglobinuria. Science 1973;182:929–31.
3. Schaffer JE. Fatty acid transport: the roads taken. Am J Physiol Endocrinol Metab 2002;282:E239–46.
4. Eaton S. Control of mitochondrial beta-oxidation flux. Prog Lipid Res 2002;41:197–239.
5. Abumrad NA, Perkins RC, Park JH, Park CR. Mechanism of long chain fatty acid permeation in the isolated adipocyte. J Biol Chem 1981;256:9183–91.
6. Stump DD, Fan X, Berk PD. Oleic acid uptake and binding by rat adipocytes define dual pathways for cellular fatty acid uptake. J Lipid Res 2001;42:509–20.
7. Brinkmann JF, Abumrad NA, Ibrahimi A, et al. New insights into long-chain fatty acid uptake by heart muscle: a crucial role for fatty acid translocase/CD36. Biochem J 2002;367(Pt 3):561–70.
8. Stahl A, Hirsch DJ, Gimeno RE, et al. Identification of the major intestinal fatty acid transport protein. Mol Cell 1999;4:299–308.
9. Faergeman NJ, DiRusso CC, Elberger A, et al. Disruption of the *Saccharomyces cerevisiae* homologue to the murine fatty acid transport protein impairs uptake and growth on long-chain fatty acids. J Biol Chem 1997;272:8531–8.
10. McArthur MJ, Atshaves BP, Frolov A, et al. Cellular uptake and intracellular trafficking of long chain fatty acids. J Lipid Res 1999;40:1371–83.
11. Abo-Hashema KA, Cake MH, Lukas MA, Knudsen J. Evaluation of the affinity and turnover number of both hepatic mitochondrial and microsomal carnitine acyltransferases: relevance to intracellular partitioning of acyl-CoAs. Biochemistry 1999;38:15840–7.
12. McGarry JD, Brown NF. The mitochondrial carnitine palmitoyltransferase system. From concept to molecular analysis. Eur J Biochem 1997;244:1–14.
13. Vaz FM, Wanders RJ. Carnitine biosynthesis in mammals. Biochem J 2002;361(Pt 3):417–29.
14. Gregersen N, Andresen BS, Bross P. Prevalent mutations in fatty acid oxidation disorders: diagnostic considerations. Eur J Pediatr 2000;159 Suppl 3:S213–8.
15. Aoyama T, Souri M, Ushikubo S, et al. Purification of human very-long-chain acyl-coenzyme A dehydrogenase and characterization of its deficiency in seven patients. J Clin Invest 1995;95:2465–73.
16. Matsubara Y, Kraus JP, Yang-Feng TL, et al. Molecular cloning of cDNAs encoding rat and human medium-chain acyl-CoA dehydrogenase and assignment of the gene to human chromosome 1. Proc Natl Acad Sci U S A 1986;83:6543–7.
17. Naito E, Ozasa H, Ikeda Y, Tanaka K. Molecular cloning and nucleotide sequence of complementary DNAs encoding human short chain acyl-coenzyme A dehydrogenase and the study of the molecular basis of human short chain acyl-coenzyme A dehydrogenase deficiency. J Clin Invest 1989;83:1605–13.
18. Uchida Y, Izai K, Orii T, Hashimoto T. Novel fatty acid beta-oxidation enzymes in rat liver mitochondria. II. Purification and properties of enoyl-coenzyme A (CoA) hydratase/3-hydroxyacyl-CoA dehydrogenase/3-ketoacyl-CoA thiolase trifunctional protein. J Biol Chem 1992;267:1034–41.
19. Roe CR, Millington DS, Norwood DL, et al. 2,4-Dienoyl-coenzyme A reductase deficiency: a possible new disorder of fatty acid oxidation. J Clin Invest 1990;85:1703–7.
20. Fukao T, Scriver CR, Kondo N. The clinical phenotype and outcome of mitochondrial acetoacetyl-CoA thiolase deficiency (beta-ketothiolase or T2 deficiency) in 26 enzymatically proved and mutation-defined patients. Mol Genet Metab 2001;72:109–14.
21. Zschocke J, Penzien JM, Bielen R, et al. The diagnosis of mitochondrial HMG-CoA synthase deficiency. J Pediatr 2002;140:778–80.
22. Mitchell GA, Robert MF, Hruz PW, et al. 3-Hydroxy-3-methylglutaryl coenzyme A lyase (HL). Cloning of human and chicken liver HL cDNAs and characterization of a mutation causing human HL deficiency. J Biol Chem 1993;268:4376–81.
23. Ashmarina LI, Pshezhetsky AV, Branda SS, et al. 3-Hydroxy-3-methylglutaryl coenzyme A lyase: targeting and processing in peroxisomes and mitochondria. J Lipid Res 1999;40:70–5.
24. Fukao T, Song XQ, Mitchell GA, et al. Enzymes of ketone body utilization in human tissues: protein and messenger RNA levels of succinyl-coenzyme A (CoA):3-ketoacid CoA transferase and mitochondrial and cytosolic acetoacetyl-CoA thiolases. Pediatr Res 1997;42:498–502.
25. Fraaije MW, Mattevi A. Flavoenzymes: diverse catalysts with recurrent features. Trends Biochem Sci 2000;25:126–32.

26. Beckmann JD, Frerman FE. Reaction of electron-transfer flavo-protein with electron-transfer flavoprotein-ubiquinone oxi-doreductase. Biochemistry 1985;24:3922–5.

27. Finocchiaro G, Ito M, Ikeda Y, Tanaka K. Molecular cloning and nucleotide sequence of cDNAs encoding the alpha-subunit of human electron transfer flavoprotein. J Biol Chem 1988; 263:15773–80.

28. Finocchiaro G, Colombo I, Garavaglia B, et al. cDNA cloning and mitochondrial import of the beta-subunit of the human electron-transfer flavoprotein. Eur J Biochem 1993;213: 1003–8.

29. Beard SE, Goodman SI, Bemelen K, Frerman FE. Characteriza-tion of a mutation that abolishes quinone reduction by elec-tron transfer flavoprotein-ubiquinone oxidoreductase. Hum Mol Genet 1995;4:157–61.

30. Goodman SI, Binard RJ, Woontner MR, Frerman FE. Glutaric acidemia type II: gene structure and mutations of the elec-tron transfer flavoprotein:ubiquinone oxidoreductase (ETF:QO) gene. Mol Genet Metab 2002;77:86–90.

31. Rinaldo P, Matern D. Disorders of fatty acid transport and mito-chondrial oxidation: challenges and dilemmas of metabolic evaluation. Genet Med 2000;2:338–44.

32. Tein I. Neonatal metabolic myopathies. Semin Perinatol 1999;23:125–51.

33. Bonnet D, Martin D, Pascale De L, et al. Arrhythmias and con-duction defects as presenting symptoms of fatty acid oxida-tion disorders in children. Circulation 1999;100:2248–53.

34. Ibdah JA, Yang Z, Bennett MJ. Liver disease in pregnancy and fetal fatty acid oxidation defects. Mol Genet Metab 2000; 71:182–9.

35. Ibdah JA, Bennett MJ, Rinaldo P, et al. A fetal fatty-acid oxida-tion disorder as a cause of liver disease in pregnant women. N Engl J Med 1999;340:1723–31.

36. Rinaldo P, Studinski AL, Matern D. Prenatal diagnosis of disor-ders of fatty acid transport and mitochondrial oxidation. Pre-natal Diagn 2001;21:52–4.

37. Rakheja D, Bennett MJ, Foster BM, et al. Evidence for fatty acid oxidation in human placenta, and the relationship of fatty acid oxidation enzyme activities with gestational age. Pla-centa 2002;23:447–50.

38. Clayton PT, Eaton S, Aynsley-Green A, et al. Hyperinsulinism in short-chain L-3-hydroxyacyl-CoA dehydrogenase deficiency reveals the importance of beta-oxidation in insulin secretion. J Clin Invest 2001;108:457–65.

39. Dionisi-Vici C, Garavaglia B, Burlina AB, et al. Hypoparathy-roidism in mitochondrial trifunctional protein deficiency. J Pediatr 1996;129:159–62.

40. Rinaldo P. Fatty acid transport and mitochondrial oxidation dis-orders. Semin Liver Dis 2001;21:489–500.

41. Sim KG, Hammond J, Wilcken B. Strategies for the diagnosis of mitochondrial fatty acid beta-oxidation disorders. Clin Chim Acta 2002;323:37–58.

42. Lehotay DC, Clarke JT. Organic acidurias and related abnor-malities. Crit Rev Clin Lab Sci 1995;32:377–429.

43. Rinaldo P, O'Shea JJ, Coates PM, et al. Medium-chain acyl-CoA dehydrogenase deficiency. Diagnosis by stable-isotope dilution measurement of urinary n-hexanoylglycine and 3-phenylpropionylglycine. N Engl J Med 1988;319:1308–13.

44. Costa CG, Guerand WS, Struys EA, et al. Quantitative analysis of urinary acylglycines for the diagnosis of beta-oxidation defects using GC-NCI-MS. J Pharm Biomed Analysis 2000;21:1215–24.

45. Kimura M, Yamaguchi S. Screening for fatty acid beta oxidation disorders. Acylglycine analysis by electron impact ionization

gas chromatography-mass spectrometry. J Chromatogr B Bio-med Sci Appl 1999;731:105–10.

46. Bonafe L, Troxler H, Kuster T, et al. Evaluation of urinary acyl-glycines by electrospray tandem mass spectrometry in mito-chondrial energy metabolism defects and organic acidurias. Mol Genet Metab 2000;69:302–11.

47. Clayton PT, Doig M, Ghafari S, et al. Screening for medium chain acyl-CoA dehydrogenase deficiency using electrospray ionisation tandem mass spectrometry. Arch Dis Child 1998;79:109–15.

48. Wilcken B, Wiley V, Sim KG, Carpenter K. Carnitine transporter defect diagnosed by newborn screening with electrospray tandem mass spectrometry. J Pediatr 2001;138:581–4.

49. Koeberl DD, Young SP, Gregersen NS, et al. Rare disorders of metabolism with elevated butyryl- and isobutyryl-carnitine detected by tandem mass spectroscopy newborn screening. Pediatr Res 2003;54:219–23.

50. Matern D, He M, Berry SA, et al. Prospective diagnosis of 2-methylbutyryl-CoA dehydrogenase deficiency in the Hmong population by newborn screening using tandem mass spec-trometry. Pediatrics 2003;112:74–8.

51. Scaglia F, Wang Y, Longo N. Functional characterization of the carnitine transporter defective in primary carnitine defi-ciency. Arch Biochem Biophys 1999;364:99–106.

52. Costa CG, Dorland L, Holwerda U, et al. Simultaneous analysis of plasma free fatty acids and their 3-hydroxy analogs in fatty acid beta-oxidation disorders. Clin Chem 1998;44:463–71.

53. Lagerstedt SA, Hinrichs DR, Batt SM, et al. Quantitative deter-mination of plasma C_8-C_{26} total fatty acids for the biochem-ical diagnosis of nutritional and metabolic disorders. Mol Genet Metab 2001;73:38–45.

54. Jones PM, Quinn R, Fennessey PV, et al. Improved stable iso-tope dilution-gas chromatography-mass spectrometry method for serum or plasma free 3-hydroxy-fatty acids and its utility for the study of disorders of mitochondrial fatty acid beta-oxidation. Clin Chem 2000;46:149–55.

55. Shen JJ, Matern D, Millington DS, et al. Acylcarnitines in fibro-blasts of patients with long-chain 3-hydroxyacyl-CoA dehy-drogenase deficiency and other fatty acid oxidation disor-ders. J Inherit Metab Dis 2000;23:27–44.

56. Olpin SE, Manning NJ, Pollitt RJ, et al. The use of [9,10-3H]myristate, [9,10-3H]palmitate and [9,10-3H]oleate for the detection and diagnosis of medium and long-chain fatty acid oxidation disorders in intact cultured fibroblasts. Adv Exp Med Biol 1999;466:321–5.

57. Wanders RJ, Vreken P, den Boer ME, et al. Disorders of mito-chondrial fatty acyl-CoA beta-oxidation. J Inherit Metab Dis 1999;22:442–87.

58. Spiekerkoetter U, Eeds A, Yue Z, et al. Uniparental disomy of chromosome 2 resulting in lethal trifunctional protein defi-ciency due to homozygous alpha-subunit mutations. Hum Mutat 2002;20:447–51.

59. Ibdah JA, Zhao Y, Viola J, et al. Molecular prenatal diagnosis in families with fetal mitochondrial trifunctional protein muta-tions. J Pediatr 2001;138:396–9.

60. Jakobs C, Sweetman L, Wadman SK, et al. Prenatal diagnosis of glutaric aciduria type II by direct chemical analysis of dicar-boxylic acids in amniotic fluid. Eur J Pediatr 1984;141:153–7.

61. Shigematsu Y, Hata I, Nakai A, et al. Prenatal diagnosis of organic acidemias based on amniotic fluid levels of acylcar-nitines. Pediatr Res 1996;39(4 Pt 1):680–4.

62. Bennett MJ, Allison F, Lowther GW, et al. Prenatal diagnosis of medium-chain acyl-coenzyme A dehydrogenase deficiency. Prenatal Diagn 1987;7:135–41.

63. Guthrie RS. A simple phenylalanine method for detecting phenylketonuria in large populations of newborn infants. Pediatrics 1963;32:338–43.

64. Matern D. Tandem mass spectrometry in newborn screening. Endocrinologist 2002;12:50–7.

65. National Newborn Screening and Genetics Resource Center. <http://genes-r-us.uthscsa.edu/resources/newborn/screenstatus.htm> (accessed Dec 9, 2003).

66. Seashore MR, Rinaldo P. Metabolic disease of the neonate and young infant. Semin Perinatol 1993;17:318–29.

67. Rinaldo P, Stanley CA, Hsu BY, et al. Sudden neonatal death in carnitine transporter deficiency. J Pediatr 1997;131:304–5.

68. Bennett MJ, Allison F, Pollitt RJ, Variend S. Fatty acid oxidation defects as causes of unexpected death in infancy. Prog Clin Biol Res 1990;321:349–64.

69. Bennett MJ, Powell S. Metabolic disease and sudden, unexpected death in infancy. Hum Pathol 1994;25:742–6.

70. Boles RG, Buck EA, Blitzer MG, et al. Retrospective biochemical screening of fatty acid oxidation disorders in postmortem livers of 418 cases of sudden death in the first year of life. J Pediatr 1998;132:924–33.

71. Rashed MS, Ozand PT, Bennett MJ, et al. Inborn errors of metabolism diagnosed in sudden death cases by acylcarnitine analysis of postmortem bile. Clin Chem 1995;41(8 Pt 1):1109–14.

72. Chace DH, DiPerna JC, Mitchell BL, et al. Electrospray tandem mass spectrometry for analysis of acylcarnitines in dried postmortem blood specimens collected at autopsy from infants with unexplained cause of death [erratum appears in Clin Chem 2001;47:1748]. Clin Chem 2001;47:1166–82.

73. Lundemose JB, Kolvraa S, Gregersen N, et al. Fatty acid oxidation disorders as primary cause of sudden and unexpected death in infants and young children: an investigation performed on cultured fibroblasts from 79 children who died aged between 0-4 years. Mol Pathol 1997;50:212–7.

74. Rinaldo P, Yoon HR, Yu C, et al. Sudden and unexpected neonatal death: a protocol for the postmortem diagnosis of fatty acid oxidation disorders. Semin Perinatol 1999;23:204–10.

75. Gregersen N, Winter V, Jensen PK, et al. Prenatal diagnosis of medium-chain acyl-CoA dehydrogenase (MCAD) deficiency in a family with a previous fatal case of sudden unexpected death in childhood. Prenatal Diagn 1995;15:82–6.

76. Odaib AA, Shneider BL, Bennett MJ, et al. A defect in the transport of long-chain fatty acids associated with acute liver failure. N Engl J Med 1998;339:1752–7.

77. Scaglia F. Carnitine deficiency. eMed J [Serial online] 2002;3(3). http://www.emedicine.com/ (accessed March 4, 2004).

78. Lamhonwah AM, Olpin SE, Pollitt RJ, et al. Novel OCTN2 mutations: no genotype-phenotype correlations: early carnitine therapy prevents cardiomyopathy. Am J Med Genet 2002;111:271–84.

79. Stanley CA, DeLeeuw S, Coates PM, et al. Chronic cardiomyopathy and weakness or acute coma in children with a defect in carnitine uptake. Ann Neurol 1991;30:709–16.

80. Wang Y, Korman SH, Ye J, et al. Phenotype and genotype variation in primary carnitine deficiency. Genet Med 2001;3:387–92.

81. Scaglia F, Wang Y, Singh RH, et al. Defective urinary carnitine transport in heterozygotes for primary carnitine deficiency. Genet Med 1998;1:34–9.

82. Koizumi A, Nozaki J, Ohura T, et al. Genetic epidemiology of the carnitine transporter OCTN2 gene in a Japanese population and phenotypic characterization in Japanese pedigrees with primary systemic carnitine deficiency. Hum Mol Genet 1999;8:2247–54.

83. Britton CH, Schultz RA, Zhang B, et al. Human liver mitochondrial carnitine palmitoyltransferase I: characterization of its cDNA and chromosomal localization and partial analysis of the gene. Proc Natl Acad Sci U S A 1995;92:1984–8.

84. Britton CH, Mackey DW, Esser V, et al. Fine chromosome mapping of the genes for human liver and muscle carnitine palmitoyltransferase I (CPT1A and CPT1B). Genomics 1997;40:209–11.

85. Falik-Borenstein ZC, Jordan SC, Saudubray JM, et al. Brief report: renal tubular acidosis in carnitine palmitoyltransferase type 1 deficiency. N Engl J Med 1992;327:24–7.

86. Olpin SE, Allen J, Bonham JR, et al. Features of carnitine palmitoyltransferase type I deficiency. J Inherit Metab Dis 2001;24:35–42.

87. Innes AM, Seargeant LE, Balachandra K, et al. Hepatic carnitine palmitoyltransferase I deficiency presenting as maternal illness in pregnancy. Pediatr Res 2000;47:43–5.

88. Fingerhut R, Roschinger W, Muntau AC, et al. Hepatic carnitine palmitoyltransferase I deficiency: acylcarnitine profiles in blood spots are highly specific. Clin Chem 2001;47:1763–8.

89. Stanley CA, Sunaryo F, Hale DE, et al. Elevated plasma carnitine in the hepatic form of carnitine palmitoyltransferase-1 deficiency. J Inherit Metab Dis 1992;15:785–9.

90. Prasad C, Johnson JP, Bonnefont JP, et al. Hepatic carnitine palmitoyl transferase 1 (CPT1 A) deficiency in North American Hutterites (Canadian and American): evidence for a founder effect and results of a pilot study on a DNA-based newborn screening program. Mol Genet Metab 2001;73:55–63.

91. Costa C, Costa JM, Slama A, et al. Mutational spectrum and DNA-based prenatal diagnosis in carnitine-acylcarnitine translocase deficiency. Mol Genet Metab 2003;78:68–73.

92. Roschinger W, Muntau AC, Duran M, et al. Carnitine-acylcarnitine translocase deficiency: metabolic consequences of an impaired mitochondrial carnitine cycle. Clin Chim Acta 2000;298:55–68.

93. Chalmers RA, Stanley CA, English N, Wigglesworth JS. Mitochondrial carnitine-acylcarnitine translocase deficiency presenting as sudden neonatal death. J Pediatr 1997;131:220–5.

94. al Aqeel AI, Rashed MS, Wanders RJ. Carnitine-acylcarnitine translocase deficiency is a treatable disease. J Inherit Metab Dis 1999;22:271–5.

95. Olpin SE, Bonham JR, Downing M, et al. Carnitine-acylcarnitine translocase deficiency—a mild phenotype. J Inherit Metab Dis 1997;20:714–5.

96. DiMauro S, DiMauro PM. Muscle carnitine palmityltransferase deficiency and myoglobinuria. Science 1973;182:929–31.

97. Tein I, Christodoulou J, Donner E, McInnes RR. Carnitine palmitoyltransferase II deficiency: a new cause of recurrent pancreatitis. J Pediatr 1994;124:938–40.

98. Kottlors M, Jaksch M, Ketelsen UP, et al. Valproic acid triggers acute rhabdomyolysis in a patient with carnitine palmitoyltransferase type II deficiency. Neuromuscul Disord 2001;11:757–9.

99. Thuillier L, Rostane H, Droin V, et al. Correlation between genotype, metabolic data, and clinical presentation in carnitine palmitoyltransferase 2 (CPT2) deficiency. Hum Mutat 2003;21:493–501.

100. North KN, Hoppel CL, De Girolami U, et al. Lethal neonatal deficiency of carnitine palmitoyltransferase II associated with dysgenesis of the brain and kidneys. J Pediatr 1995;127:414–20.

101. Pierce MR, Pridjian G, Morrison S, Pickoff AS. Fatal carnitine palmitoyltransferase II deficiency in a newborn: new phenotypic features. Clin Pediatr (Phila) 1999;38:13–20.

102. Vladutiu GD, Hogan K, Saponara I, et al. Carnitine palmitoyl

transferase deficiency in malignant hyperthermia. Muscle Nerve 1993;16:485–91.

103. Bonnefont JP, Demaugre F, Prip-Buus C, et al. Carnitine palmitoyltransferase deficiencies. Mol Genet Metab 1999;68:424–40.

104. Vladutiu GD, Bennett MJ, Smail D, et al. A variable myopathy associated with heterozygosity for the R503C mutation in the carnitine palmitoyltransferase II gene. Mol Genet Metab 2000;70:134–41.

105. Treem WR, Witzleben CA, Piccoli DA, et al. Medium-chain and long-chain acyl CoA dehydrogenase deficiency: clinical, pathologic and ultrastructural differentiation from Reye's syndrome. Hepatology 1986;6:1270–8.

106. Yamaguchi S, Indo Y, Coates PM, et al. Identification of very-long-chain acyl-CoA dehydrogenase deficiency in three patients previously diagnosed with long-chain acyl-CoA dehydrogenase deficiency. Pediatr Res 1993;34:111–3.

107. Kurtz DM, Rinaldo P, Rhead WJ, et al. Targeted disruption of mouse long-chain acyl-CoA dehydrogenase gene reveals crucial roles for fatty acid oxidation. Proc Natl Acad Sci U S A 1998;95:15592–7.

108. Andresen BS, Olpin S, Poorthuis BJ, et al. Clear correlation of genotype with disease phenotype in very-long-chain acyl-CoA dehydrogenase deficiency. Am J Hum Genet 1999;64:479–94.

109. Mathur A, Sims HF, Gopalakrishnan D, et al. Molecular heterogeneity in very-long-chain acyl-CoA dehydrogenase deficiency causing pediatric cardiomyopathy and sudden death. Circulation 1999;99:1337–43.

110. Takusa Y, Fukao T, Kimura M, et al. Identification and characterization of temperature-sensitive mild mutations in three Japanese patients with nonsevere forms of very-long-chain acyl-CoA dehydrogenase deficiency. Mol Genet Metab 2002;75:227–34.

111. Roe DS, Vianey-Saban C, Sharma S, et al. Oxidation of unsaturated fatty acids by human fibroblasts with very-long-chain acyl-CoA dehydrogenase deficiency: aspects of substrate specificity and correlation with clinical phenotype. Clin Chim Acta 2001;312:55–67.

112. Wood JC, Magera MJ, Rinaldo P, et al. Diagnosis of very long chain acyl-dehydrogenase deficiency from an infant's newborn screening card. Pediatrics 2001;108:E19.

113. Spiekerkoetter U, Sun B, Zytkovicz T, et al. MS/MS-based newborn and family screening detects asymptomatic patients with very-long-chain acyl-CoA dehydrogenase deficiency. J Pediatr 2003;143:335–42.

114. Spiekerkoetter U, Sun B, Khuchua Z, et al. Molecular and phenotypic heterogeneity in mitochondrial trifunctional protein deficiency due to beta-subunit mutations. Hum Mutat 2003;21:598–607.

115. Harding CO, Gillingham MB, van Calcar SC, et al. Docosahexaenoic acid and retinal function in children with long-chain 3-hydroxyacyl-CoA dehydrogenase deficiency. J Inherit Metab Dis 1999;22:276–80.

116. den Boer ME, Wanders RJ, Morris AA, et al. Long-chain 3-hydroxyacyl-CoA dehydrogenase deficiency: clinical presentation and follow-up of 50 patients. Pediatrics 2002;109:99–104.

117. Hintz SR, Matern D, Strauss A, et al. Early neonatal diagnosis of long-chain 3-hydroxyacyl coenzyme A dehydrogenase and mitochondrial trifunctional protein deficiencies. Mol Genet Metab 2002;75:120–7.

118. Chace DH, Hillman SL, Van Hove JL, Naylor EW. Rapid diagnosis of MCAD deficiency: quantitative analysis of octanoylcarnitine and other acylcarnitines in newborn blood spots by tandem mass spectrometry. Clin Chem 1997;43:2106–13.

119. Charrow J, Goodman SI, McCabe ERG, Rinaldo P. Tandem mass spectrometry in newborn screening. Genet Med 2000;2:267–9.

120. Iafolla AK, Thompson RJ Jr, Roe CR. Medium-chain acyl-coenzyme A dehydrogenase deficiency: clinical course in 120 affected children. J Pediatr 1994;124:409–15.

121. Van Hove JL, Zhang W, Kahler SG, et al. Medium-chain acyl-CoA dehydrogenase (MCAD) deficiency: diagnosis by acylcarnitine analysis in blood. Am J Hum Genet 1993;52:958–66.

122. Tanaka K, Gregersen N, Ribes A, et al. A survey of the newborn populations in Belgium, Germany, Poland, Czech Republic, Hungary, Bulgaria, Spain, Turkey, and Japan for the G985 variant allele with haplotype analysis at the medium chain Acyl-CoA dehydrogenase gene locus: clinical and evolutionary consideration. Pediatr Res 1997;41:201–9.

123. Hale DE, Bennett MJ. Fatty acid oxidation disorders: a new class of metabolic diseases. J Pediatr 1992;121:1–11.

124. Kobayashi A, Jiang LL, Hashimoto T. Two mitochondrial 3-hydroxyacyl-CoA dehydrogenases in bovine liver. J Biochem (Tokyo) 1996;119:775–82.

125. Tein I, De Vivo DC, Hale DE, et al. Short-chain L-3-hydroxyacyl-CoA dehydrogenase deficiency in muscle: a new cause for recurrent myoglobinuria and encephalopathy. Ann Neurol 1991;30:415–9.

126. Bennett MJ, Weinberger MJ, Kobori JA, et al. Mitochondrial short-chain L-3-hydroxyacyl-coenzyme A dehydrogenase deficiency: a new defect of fatty acid oxidation. Pediatr Res 1996;39:185–8.

127. Bennett MJ, Spotswood SD, Ross KF, et al. Fatal hepatic short-chain L-3-hydroxyacyl-coenzyme A dehydrogenase deficiency: clinical, biochemical, and pathological studies on three subjects with this recently identified disorder of mitochondrial beta-oxidation. Pediatr Dev Pathol 1999;2:337–45.

128. Vredendaal PJ, van den Berg IE, Malingre HE, et al. Human short-chain L-3-hydroxyacyl-CoA dehydrogenase: cloning and characterization of the coding sequence. Biochem Biophys Res Commun 1996;223:718–23.

129. Molven A, Rishaug U, Matre GE, et al. Hunting for a hypoglycemia gene: severe neonatal hypoglycemia in a consanguineous family. Am J Med Genet 2002;113:40–6.

130. Sovik O, Matre G, Rishaug U, et al. Familial hyperinsulinemic hypoglycemia with a mutation in the gene encoding short-chain 3-hydroxyacyl-CoA dehydrogenase. J Inherit Metab Dis 2002;25 Suppl 1:63.

131. Kamijo T, Indo Y, Souri M, et al. Medium chain 3-ketoacyl-coenzyme A thiolase deficiency: a new disorder of mitochondrial fatty acid beta-oxidation. Pediatr Res 1997;42:569–76.

132. Turnbull DM, Bartlett K, Stevens DL, et al. Short-chain acyl-CoA dehydrogenase deficiency associated with a lipid-storage myopathy and secondary carnitine deficiency. N Engl J Med 1984;311:1232–6.

133. Amendt BA, Greene C, Sweetman L, et al. Short-chain acyl-coenzyme A dehydrogenase deficiency. Clinical and biochemical studies in two patients. J Clin Invest 1987;79:1303–9.

134. Corydon MJ, Vockley J, Rinaldo P, et al. Role of common gene variations in the molecular pathogenesis of short-chain acyl-CoA dehydrogenase deficiency. Pediatr Res 2001;49:18–23.

135. Roe CR, Roe DS. Recent developments in the investigation of inherited metabolic disorders using cultured human cells. Mol Genet Metab 1999;68:243–57.

136. Young SP, Matern D, Gregersen N, et al. A comparison of in vitro acylcarnitine profiling methods for the diagnosis of classical and variant short chain acyl-CoA dehydrogenase deficiency. Clin Chim Acta 2003;337:103–13.

137. Nagan N, Kruckeberg KE, Tauscher AL, et al. The frequency of

short-chain acyl-CoA dehydrogenase gene variants in the US population and correlation with the C(4)-acylcarnitine concentration in newborn blood spots. Mol Genet Metab 2003;78:239–46.

138. Corydon MJ, Gregersen N, Lehnert W, et al. Ethylmalonic aciduria is associated with an amino acid variant of short chain acyl-coenzyme A dehydrogenase. Pediatr Res 1996;39:1059–66.

139. Gregersen N, Winter VS, Corydon MJ, et al. Identification of four new mutations in the short-chain acyl-CoA dehydrogenase (SCAD) gene in two patients: one of the variant alleles, 511C→T, is present at an unexpectedly high frequency in the general population, as was the case for 625G→A, together conferring susceptibility to ethylmalonic aciduria. Hum Mol Genet 1998;7:619–27.

140. Matern D, Hart P, Murtha AP, et al. Acute fatty liver of pregnancy associated with short-chain acyl-coenzyme A dehydrogenase deficiency. J Pediatr 2001;138:585–8.

141. Pedersen CB, Bross P, Winter VS, et al. Misfolding, degradation and aggregation of variant proteins—the molecular pathogenesis of short chain acyl-CoA dehydrogenase (SCAD) deficiency. J Biol Chem 2003;23:23.

142. Morris AA, Lascelles CV, Olpin SE, et al. Hepatic mitochondrial 3-hydroxy-3-methylglutaryl-coenzyme a synthase deficiency. Pediatr Res 1998;44:392–6.

143. Aledo R, Zschocke J, Pie J, et al. Genetic basis of mitochondrial HMG-CoA synthase deficiency. Hum Genet 2001;109:19–23.

144. Wolf NG, Rahman S, Clayton PG, Zschocke J. Mitochondrial HMG-CoA synthase deficiency: identification of two further patients carrying two novel mutations. Eur J Pediatr 2003;162:279–80.

145. Thompson GN, Hsu BY, Pitt JJ, et al. Fasting hypoketotic coma in a child with deficiency of mitochondrial 3-hydroxy-3-methylglutaryl-CoA synthase. N Engl J Med 1997;337:1203–7.

146. Boukaftane Y, Mitchell GA. Cloning and characterization of the human mitochondrial 3-hydroxy-3-methylglutaryl CoA synthase gene. Gene 1997;195:121–6.

147. Mitchell AG, Fukao T. Inborn errors of ketone body metabolism. In: Scriver CR, Beaudet AL, Valle D, et al, editors. Metabolic and molecular basis of inherited disease. Vol. II. New York: McGraw-Hill; 2002. p. 2327–56.

148. van der Knaap MS, Bakker HD, Valk J. MR imaging and proton spectroscopy in 3-hydroxy-3-methylglutaryl coenzyme A lyase deficiency. AJNR Am J Neuroradiol 1998;19:378–82.

149. Wilson WG, Cass MB, Sovik O, et al. A child with acute pancreatitis and recurrent hypoglycemia due to 3-hydroxy-3-methylglutaryl-CoA lyase deficiency. Eur J Pediatr 1984;142:289–91.

150. Gibson KM, Cassidy SB, Seaver LH, et al. Fatal cardiomyopathy associated with 3-hydroxy-3-methylglutaryl-CoA lyase deficiency. J Inherit Metab Dis 1994;17:291–4.

151. Jones KJ, Wilcken B, Kilham H. The long-term evolution of a case of 3-hydroxy-3-methylglutaryl-coenzyme A lyase deficiency associated with deafness and retinitis pigmentosa. J Inherit Metab Dis 1997;20:833–4.

152. Rashed MS, Ozand PT, Bucknall MP, Little D. Diagnosis of inborn errors of metabolism from blood spots by acylcarnitines and amino acids profiling using automated electrospray tandem mass spectrometry. Pediatr Res 1995;38:324–31.

153. Ozand PT, al Aqeel A, Gascon G, et al. 3-Hydroxy-3-methylglutaryl-coenzyme A (HMG-CoA) lyase deficiency in Saudi Arabia. J Inherit Metab Dis 1991;14:174–88.

154. Niezen-Koning KE, Wanders RJ, Ruiter JP, et al. Succinyl-CoA:acetoacetate transferase deficiency: identification of a new patient with a neonatal onset and review of the literature. Eur J Pediatr 1997;156:870–3.

155. Morris AAM. Disorders of ketogenesis and ketolysis. In: Fernandes J, Saudubray JM, van der Berghe G, editors. Inborn metabolic diseases. Berlin: Springer; 2000. p. 151–6.

156. Berry GT, Fukao T, Mitchell AG, et al. Neonatal hypoglycemia in severe succinyl-CoA: 3-oxoacid CoA-transferase deficiency. J Inherit Metab Dis 2001;24:587–95.

157. Fukao T, Mitchell GA, Song XQ, et al. Succinyl-CoA:3-ketoacid CoA transferase (SCOT): cloning of the human SCOT gene, tertiary structural modeling of the human SCOT monomer, and characterization of three pathogenic mutations. Genomics 2000;68:144–51.

158. Snyderman SE, Sansaricq C, Middleton B. Succinyl-CoA:3-ketoacid CoA-transferase deficiency. Pediatrics 1998;101 (4 Pt 1):709–11.

159. Ozand PT, Rashed M, Gascon GG, et al. 3-Ketothiolase deficiency: a review and four new patients with neurologic symptoms. Brain Dev 1994;16 Suppl:38–45.

160. Yalcinkaya C, Apaydin H, Ozekmekci S, Gibson KM. Delayed-onset dystonia associated with 3-oxothiolase deficiency. Mov Disord 2001;16:372–5.

161. Fukao T, Kodama A, Aoyanagi N, et al. Mild form of beta-ketothiolase deficiency (mitochondrial acetoacetyl-CoA thiolase deficiency) in two Japanese siblings: identification of detectable residual activity and cross-reactive material in EB-transformed lymphocytes. Clin Genet 1996;50:263–6.

162. Fukao T, Yamaguchi S, Orii T, Hashimoto T. Molecular basis of beta-ketothiolase deficiency: mutations and polymorphisms in the human mitochondrial acetoacetyl-coenzyme A thiolase gene. Hum Mutat 1995;5:113–20.

163. Mitchell G, Saudubray JM, Gubler MC, et al. Congenital anomalies in glutaric aciduria type 2. J Pediatr 1984;104:961–2.

164. Bohm N, Uy J, Kiessling M, Lehnert W. Multiple acyl-CoA dehydrogenation deficiency (glutaric aciduria type II), congenital polycystic kidneys, and symmetric warty dysplasia of the cerebral cortex in two newborn brothers. II. Morphology and pathogenesis. Eur J Pediatr 1982;139:60–5.

165. al-Essa MA, Rashed MS, Bakheet SM, et al. Glutaric aciduria type II: observations in seven patients with neonatal- and late-onset disease. J Perinatol 2000;20:120–8.

166. Przyrembel H, Wendel U, Becker K, et al. Glutaric aciduria type II: report on a previously undescribed metabolic disorder. Clin Chim Acta 1976;66:227–39.

167. Sweetman L, Nyhan WL, Tauner DA, et al. Glutaric aciduria type II. J Pediatr 1980;96:1020–6.

168. Rose M, Matern D, Millington DS, Lehnert W. [Atypical course of a multiple acyl-CoA-dehydrogenase deficiency]. Klin Padiatr 1999;211:413–6.

169. Verjee ZH, Sherwood WG. Multiple acyl-CoA dehydrogenase deficiency: a neonatal onset case responsive to treatment. J Inherit Metab Dis 1985;8 Suppl 2:137–8.

170. Dusheiko G, Kew MC, Joffe BI, et al. Recurrent hypoglycemia associated with glutaric aciduria type II in an adult. N Engl J Med 1979;301:1405–9.

171. Olsen RK, Andresen BS, Christensen E, et al. Clear relationship between ETF/ETFDH genotype and phenotype in patients with multiple acyl-CoA dehydrogenation deficiency. Hum Mutat 2003;22:12–23.

172. Goodman SI, Loehr JP, Frerman FE. Clinical and biochemical aspects of glutaric acidemia type II. Prog Clin Biol Res 1990; 321:465–76.

173. Solis JO, Singh RH. Management of fatty acid oxidation disorders: a survey of current treatment strategies. J Am Diet Assoc 2002;102:1800–3.

174. Vockley J, Singh RH, Whiteman DA. Diagnosis and manage-

ment of defects of mitochondrial beta-oxidation. Curr Opin Nutr Metab Care 2002;5:601–9.

175. Pollitt RJ. Disorders of mitochondrial long-chain fatty acid oxidation. J Inherit Metab Dis 1995;18:473–90.

176. Gillingham MB, Connor WE, Matern D, et al. Optimal dietary therapy of long-chain 3-hydroxyacyl-CoA dehydrogenase deficiency. Mol Genet Metab 2003;79:114–23.

177. Gillingham M, Van Calcar S, Ney D, et al. Dietary management of long-chain 3-hydroxyacyl-CoA dehydrogenase deficiency (LCHADD). A case report and survey. J Inherit Metab Dis 1999;22:123–31.

178. Treem WR, Stanley CA, Goodman SI. Medium-chain acyl-CoA dehydrogenase deficiency: metabolic effects and therapeutic efficacy of long-term L-carnitine supplementation. J Inherit Metab Dis 1989;12:112–9.

179. Corr PB, Creer MH, Yamada KA, et al. Prophylaxis of early ventricular fibrillation by inhibition of acylcarnitine accumulation. J Clin Invest 1989;83:927–36.

180. Rizzon P, Biasco G, Di Biase M, et al. High doses of L-carnitine in acute myocardial infarction: metabolic and antiarrhythmic effects. Eur Heart J 1989;10:502–8.

181. Duran M, Wanders RJ, de Jager JP, et al. 3-Hydroxydicarboxylic aciduria due to long-chain 3-hydroxyacyl-coenzyme A dehydrogenase deficiency associated with sudden neonatal death: protective effect of medium-chain triglyceride treatment. Eur J Pediatr 1991;150:190–5.

182. Przyrembel H, Jakobs C, Ijlst L, et al. Long-chain 3-hydroxyacyl-CoA dehydrogenase deficiency. J Inherit Metab Dis 1991; 14:674–80.

183. Green A, Preece MA, de Sousa C, Pollitt RJ. Possible deleterious effect of L-carnitine supplementation in a patient with mild multiple acyl-CoA dehydrogenation deficiency (ethylmalonic-adipic aciduria). J Inherit Metab Dis 1991;14:691–7.

184. Ribes A, Riudor E, Navarro C, et al. Fatal outcome in a patient with long-chain 3-hydroxyacyl-CoA dehydrogenase deficiency. J Inherit Metab Dis 1992;15:278–9.

185. Rocchiccioli F, Wanders RJ, Aubourg P, et al. Deficiency of long-chain 3-hydroxyacyl-CoA dehydrogenase: a cause of lethal myopathy and cardiomyopathy in early childhood. Pediatr Res 1990;28:657–62.

186. Moore R, Glasgow JF, Bingham MA, et al. Long-chain 3-hydroxyacyl-coenzyme A dehydrogenase deficiency—diagnosis, plasma carnitine fractions and management in a further patient. Eur J Pediatr 1993;152:433–6.

187. Roe CR, Sweetman L, Roe DS, et al. Treatment of cardiomyopathy and rhabdomyolysis in long-chain fat oxidation disorders using an anaplerotic odd-chain triglyceride. J Clin Invest 2002;110:259–69.

188. Djouadi F, Bonnefont JP, Thuillier L, et al. Correction of fatty acid oxidation in carnitine palmitoyl transferase 2-deficient cultured skin fibroblasts by bezafibrate. Pediatr Res 2003; 54:446–51.

4. Bile Acid Synthesis and Metabolism

Kenneth D. R. Setchell, PhD

Nancy C. O'Connell, MS, CCRC, CCRA

For several decades, bile acids have been implicated in the pathogenesis of liver disease; however, their exact role in initiating or perpetuating liver injury has proven difficult to discern. Nonspecific alterations in serum, urinary, and biliary bile acid composition are found in infants and children with neonatal cholestasis. However, until recently, it was difficult to determine whether such changes were primary or secondary to the cholestatic condition. Largely as a consequence of methodologic advances,[1] specific inborn errors in bile acid biosynthesis have been recently recognized[2–5] that appear to be causal in the pathogenesis of the idiopathic and familial forms of neonatal hepatitis.[6–13] Although the exact genetic basis for these defects is still to be established, the deficiency in activity of specific enzymes involved in bile acid synthesis results in diminished production of the primary bile acids that are essential for promoting bile flow[14] and the concomitant production of atypical bile acids with the potential for causing liver injury.[15] This chapter outlines the pathways for bile acid synthesis, highlights the features of bile acid metabolism in early life, and describes the clinical and biochemical characteristics of inborn errors in bile acid synthesis.

CHEMISTRY

The bile acids are a group of compounds that belong to the steroid class.[16] Structurally, they consist of a four-ringed, cyclopentanoperhydrophenanthrene nucleus (ABCD rings) with a side chain, most commonly of five carbon atoms length, terminating in a carboxylic acid (Figure 55.4-1); they are therefore classified as acidic steroids. A great variety of bile acids can be found in biologic fluids, and significant species differences exist with regard to the synthesis and metabolism of the bile acids.[17] The vast majority of naturally occurring bile acids have the C-5 hydrogen oriented in the 5β-configuration, thereby confirming a cis-A/B ring structure. Bile acids with a 5α-H are referred to as allo-bile acids,[18] and these are found as minor metabolites in biologic fluids. In humans, the principal bile acids synthesized by the liver[3,19] have hydroxyl groups substituted in the nucleus at the carbon positions C-3, C-7, and C-12. Additional reactions involving other hydroxylations, epimerization, and oxidoreduction also take place, leading to a complex array of structures (see Figure 55.4-1). Although many of the products of these reactions may be of negligi-

ble quantitative importance in health, they are found in substantial concentrations in cholestatic syndromes, arising out of the induction of cytochrome P-450 hydroxylations.[1] During early development, alternative pathways for bile acid synthesis and metabolism become quantitatively important, as is evident from the findings of relatively high proportions of bile acids hydroxylated at the C-1, C-2, C-4, and C-6 positions of the nucleus.[20,21]

The two principal bile acids synthesized by the liver and referred to as the "primary" bile acids are cholic acid (3α,7α,12α-trihydroxy-5β-cholanoic acid) and chenodeoxycholic acid (3α,7α-dihydroxy-5β-cholanoic acid; a description of the conventions used for the systematic nomenclature of bile acids is reviewed elsewhere.[22] These bile acids are extensively conjugated to the amino acids glycine and taurine.[23] To a lesser extent, conjugation occurs with glucuronic acid to form glucuronide ethers[24] and esters[25] and with sulfuric acid to form sulfate conjugates.[26] More recently, bile acid conjugates of glucosides,[27,28] N-acetylglucosaminides,[29] and drugs[30] have also been recognized (see Figure 55.4-1). The diversity in bile acid structure is further increased by the fact that unsaturation (double bonds) in the steroid nucleus and side chain and substitution of oxo-groups also occurs, whereas bile

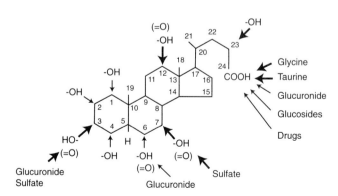

FIGURE 55.4-1 Chemical structure of the bile acid (5β-cholanoic acid) nucleus indicating the numbering system for each carbon atom and the various positions of the substituent groups for the majority of bile acids found in normal and pathophysiologic conditions. The size of the arrows indicates the relative importance of each of the substituent groups. Bile acids can additionally possess unsaturation in a number of positions in the nucleus and the side chain, but for simplicity, this is not indicated.

acids may be found with side chains longer or shorter than the usual 5-carbon side-chain length.[1]

The bile acids perform several important functions. They represent one of the major catabolic pathways for the elimination of cholesterol from the body.[3,19] From the standpoint of hepatobiliary disease, bile acids provide the primary driving force for the promotion and secretion of bile[14] and are essential to the development of the biliary excretory route for the elimination of endogenous and exogenous toxic substances, including bilirubin, xenobiotics, and drug metabolites. Within the intestinal lumen, the detergent action of bile acids facilitates the absorption of fats and fat-soluble vitamins, and the importance of this role becomes apparent in chronic cholestasis, where failure to thrive, fat malabsorption, and fat-soluble vitamin deficiency present significant clinical management problems. Indeed, the measurement of fat-soluble vitamin status is a very sensitive marker of disturbances in bile acid synthesis and secretion, as is evident from the manifestation of inborn errors in bile acid synthesis.[6,7,9–11,13]

Physiologically, the normal bile acid pool size is 2 to 4 g, but the effectiveness of this pool is increased by an efficient enterohepatic recycling (10–12 times/d) stimulated by postprandial gallbladder contraction.[31] Conservation of the bile acid pool occurs by an efficient reabsorption, principally from the small intestine, and an effective hepatic extraction from the portal venous circulation so that each day less than 5% of the pool is lost in the stool.[32] This bile acid loss is compensated for by hepatic synthesis of newly formed bile acids; therefore, in the steady state, determination of fecal bile acid excretion provides a reliable estimate of daily bile acid synthesis rates.[32]

PATHWAYS FOR BILE ACID SYNTHESIS

The biochemical pathways for bile acid synthesis in the adult have been relatively well defined and are reviewed in detail elsewhere.[3,19] Much of our understanding of these pathways results from in vitro and in vivo studies of precursor-product relationships in various animal species, most notably the rat and rabbit, and from studies of pathologic disorders affecting bile acid production. This discussion therefore serves to indicate only the salient features of the pathways. The conversion of cholesterol, a C_{27} sterol, to the two primary bile acids, cholic and chenodeoxycholic acids, requires significant alterations to the steroid nucleus (Figure 55.4-2) and side chain (Figure 55.4-3) of the molecule. These include (1) the introduction of additional hydroxyl groups at positions C-7 (for both chenodeoxycholic and cholic acids) and C-12 (for cholic acid); (2) epimerization of the 3β-hydroxyl group; (3) reduction of the Δ^5 bond; (4) reduction in length of the side chain from C_8 to C_5, with the formation of a terminal carboxylic acid; and (5) conjugation to the amino acids glycine and taurine.

Several pathways are responsible for bile acid synthesis from cholesterol.[33–35] Beginning from cholesterol, two reactions are possible: 7α-hydroxylation, initiating bile acid synthesis via the classic pathway, now referred to as the

neutral pathway, or 27-hydroxylation, referred to as the acidic pathway. Although, classically, the 7α-hydroxylation pathway has been considered the major pathway for primary bile acid synthesis and cholesterol 7α-hydroxylase the accepted rate-limiting enzyme, more recently, the quantitative importance of the acidic pathway has been realized.[9,33,35–37] Nevertheless, irrespective of the route by which primary bile acids are synthesized, common reactions occur, and the enzymes catalyzing these reactions have broad specificity.[3] For the sake of simplicity, this review highlights the individual reactions involved in the classic (neutral) pathway, but it should be pointed out that these reactions do not necessarily occur in this orderly fashion. Indeed, permutations of these sequences of reactions give rise to the complex array of bile acids typically found in physiologic and pathophysiologic states, highlighting the promiscuity of these enzymes.

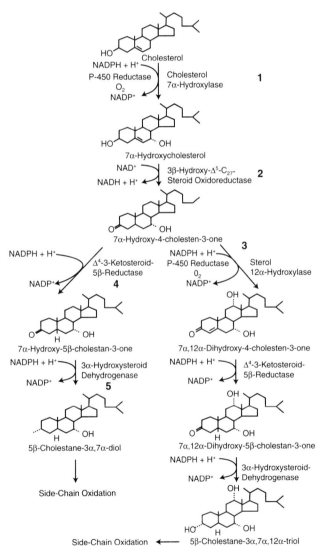

FIGURE 55.4-2 Metabolic pathway for the biosynthesis of the primary bile acids indicating the reactions involved in modifying the steroid nucleus in the conversion of cholesterol to 5β-cholestane-3α,7α,12α-triol. In the classic (neutral) pathway, these reactions were considered to precede side-chain oxidation. NADP = nicotinamide adenine dinucleotide phosphate; NADPH = reduced nicotinamide adenine dinucleotide phosphate.

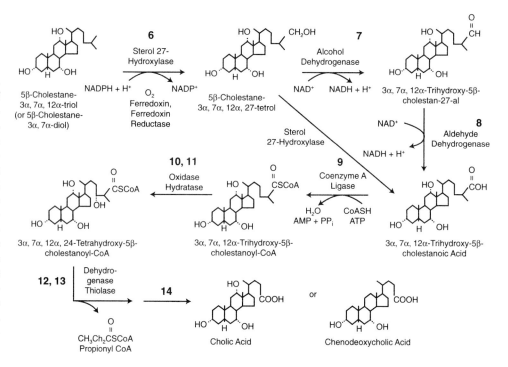

FIGURE 55.4-3 Sequence of reactions involved in the side-chain oxidation of 5β-cholestane-3α,7α,12α-triol to yield cholic or chenodeoxycholic acids, which are then conjugated with glycine and taurine. AMP = adenosine monophosphate; ATP = adenosine triphosphate; CoA = coenzyme A; NAD = nicotinamide adenine dinucleotide; NADH = reduced nicotinamide adenine dinucleotide; NADP = nicotinamide adenine dinucleotide phosphate; NADPH = reduced nicotinamide adenine dinucleotide phosphate.

In the classic pathway for bile acid synthesis from cholesterol, nine principal steps occur. All of the enzymes responsible for catalyzing these reactions are located in various subcellular fractions within the hepatocyte; consequently, there is considerable intracellular trafficking of the products of these reactions. Additionally, several of the enzymes are expressed in extrahepatic organs and tissues, including fibroblasts, macrophages, brain, lung, kidney, and vascular endothelia.[38-45] Why these enzymes are located in these tissues is unclear, but they are considered to play an important role in cholesterol homeostasis independent of their primary function, which is to catalyze reaction rates for primary bile acid synthesis.

STEP 1: CHOLESTEROL 7α-HYDROXYLASE

The first step in bile acid synthesis involves the introduction of a hydroxyl group at the C-7 position of the nucleus.[46] This reaction is catalyzed by a microsomal cholesterol, 7α-hydroxylase,[47] a cytochrome P-450 liver-specific enzyme with a molecular weight of 57 kD. A vast literature exists on the role of cholesterol 7α-hydroxylase in bile acid synthesis and the factors involved in its regulation that cannot be covered within the scope of this review, and the reader is directed to several excellent articles on this topic.[3,19,47,48] This step is potentially the most important because it is rate limiting for bile acid synthesis[49] and is subject to negative feedback regulation by the flux of bile acids returning to the liver. Differences exist, however, in the ability of different bile acids to regulate this enzyme.[50] For example, unlike primary bile acids, bile acids possessing a 7β-hydroxyl group (such as ursodeoxycholic acid [UDCA]) are unable to down-regulate bile acid synthesis,[51] and UDCA may even be mildly stimulatory.[52] Biliary drainage increases cholesterol 7α-hydroxylase activity approximately 10-fold in rats,[53,54] whereas taurochenodeoxycholic acid infusion restores activity to normal.[55]

Likewise, cholestyramine administration increases the activity of cholesterol 7α-hydroxylase. Because bile acid synthesis is self-regulated via the activity of cholesterol 7α-hydroxylase, this provides the basis for the feeding of oral primary bile acids for the treatment of metabolic defects involving enzymes in the pathway.[56-60]

Changes in the activity of cholesterol 7α-hydroxylase parallel changes in 3-hydroxy-3-methylglutaryl coenzyme A (HMG-CoA) reductase activity; consequently, these two key enzymes regulate the cholesterol pool size.[61] A diurnal rhythm in cholesterol 7α-hydroxylase activity occurs synchronously with the diurnal rhythm in the activity of the HMG-CoA reductase.[62-64] Bile acid synthesis increases nocturnally[65] and may be regulated by glucocorticoids.[66]

Cholesterol 7α-hydroxylase has been isolated and purified from rat liver,[67] the protein structure has been sequenced, and complementary deoxyribonucleic acids (cDNAs) have been prepared for the rat and human enzymes.[68-70] This enzyme has been shown to be exclusively of hepatic origin. With molecular tools, many studies of the gene, the messenger ribonucleic acid (mRNA), and the protein have been carried out.[71-74] These studies have also heightened awareness of the complexity in the regulation of bile acid synthesis and have led to the realization that the classic neutral pathway is not the sole contributing pathway for bile acid synthesis. When the gene for cholesterol 7α-hydroxylase is knocked out in a mouse,[37,75] most of the animals die within the first few weeks of life from liver failure and the consequences of fat-soluble vitamin malabsorption, highlighting the importance of bile acids for lipid absorption. However, if these animals are fed fat-soluble vitamins and cholic acid, they survive, the symptoms resolve,[76] and primary bile acid synthesis takes place via the developmental expression of an oxysterol 7α-hydroxylase specific to the acidic pathway.[37] Furthermore, in rats, if activity of cholesterol 7α-hydroxylase is completely repressed by continuous infusion of squalestatin, bile acid synthesis 24 hours later is still 43% of preinfusion levels, indicating that the acidic pathway accounts for almost half of the total bile acid synthesis in the rat.[36] Our recent discovery of a genetic defect in the oxysterol 7α-hydroxylase causing fatal liver disease[9] suggests that the acidic pathway is quantitatively the most important, at least in early infancy. This contention is based on the fact that even though the patient had a normal cholesterol 7α-hydroxylase gene, there was no detectable mRNA or enzyme activity. Also, cholesterol 7α-hydroxylase activity was not detected or was very low in liver samples from infants of less than 1 year of age, confirming earlier reports that have shown cholesterol 7α-hydroxylase enzyme activity to be low or undetectable in human fetal and infant liver.[77,78] What triggers the increased activity in cholesterol 7α-hydroxylase during development is uncertain. Overall, it appears that there are significant species differences with regard to the developmental expression of the neutral and acidic pathways.

It has been shown that bile acids and their oxysterol intermediates interact with a number of nuclear orphan receptors.[79–81] Furthermore, bile acids are present in the nucleus of hepatocytes.[82] At least four such orphan receptors have been identified: liver X receptor, farnesoid X receptor (FXR), pregnane X receptor, and constitutive androstane receptor; there may be others yet to be identified.[79,80,83,84] It appears that these may be important at two levels of regulation: in the liver by transcriptional regulation of cholesterol 7α-hydroxylase[85–87] and at the intestinal level by inducing transcription of the ileal bile acid binding protein that is involved in the ileal uptake and conservation of the bile acid pool.[88] The importance of these orphan receptors in regulating bile acid synthesis and expression of bile acid transporters is illustrated from significant changes observed in studies of gene knockout models of these orphan receptors.[83,89] It is now evident that bile acid synthesis and transport may, in the future, be manipulated by the use of specific ligands for these orphan receptors to treat cholestatic liver diseases and disorders of cholesterol metabolism. Chenodeoxycholic and cholic acids have a high affinity for FXR,[81,88,90,91] and this dihydroxy bile acid is also a potent regulator of cholesterol synthesis.[88] UDCA, on the other hand, has little affinity.

STEP 2: 3β-HYDROXY-C$_{27}$-STEROID OXIDOREDUCTASE (3β-HYDROXY-C$_{27}$-STEROID DEHYDROGENASE/ISOMERASE)

The conversion of 7α-hydroxycholesterol to 7α-hydroxy-4-cholesten-3-one is catalyzed by a microsomal 3β-hydroxy-C$_{27}$-steroid oxidase (previousy referred to as a 3β-hydroxy-C$_{27}$-steroid dehydrogenase/isomerase enzyme, and considerable effort has gone into understanding the mechanism of this relatively complex two-step reaction[92,93] that involves oxidation of the 3β-hydroxyl group and isomerization of the Δ^5 bond. It is possible that 7α-hydroxy-5-cholesten-3-one is formed as an intermediate, but attempts to isolate this compound have proved unsuccessful. In 1981, Wikvall isolated what appeared to be a single, highly specific enzyme of molecular weight 46 kD respon-

sible for catalyzing this reaction in rabbits.[94] The enzyme was later isolated and purified to homogeneity from pig liver and shown to have a molecular weight of 36 kD.[95] More recently, a single gene (HSD3B7) on chromosome 16p11.2-12 encoding the enzyme was identified and sequenced, and a number of mutations associated with progressive familial cholestatic liver disease were described.[96,97] The enzyme only catalyzes the conversion of 7α-hydroxylated sterols or bile acid intermediates with a 3β-hydroxy-Δ^5 structure to the corresponding 3-oxo-Δ^4 metabolites. It shows no activity toward corresponding 7β-hydroxy analogs. Comparable reactions occur in the biosynthetic pathways for steroid hormones, but the enzyme active on the sterol intermediates of bile acid synthesis differs from the isozymes described for C$_{19}$ and C$_{21}$ neutral steroids, for which cDNAs are described.[98–101] The 3β-hydroxy-C$_{27}$-steroid oxidoreductase enzyme is expressed in fibroblasts,[102] although its function is unknown. Nevertheless, this does enable its activity to be determined in patients in whom there is a evidence of a deficiency in this enzyme; however, sequencing of the DNA is a preferred approach to accurately confirming a biochemical defect in this reaction step.

STEP 3: 12α-HYDROXYLATION

The conversion of 7α-hydroxy-4-cholesten-3-one into 7α, 12α-dihydroxy-4-cholesten-3-one is catalyzed by cytochrome P-450–dependent microsomal 12α–hydroxylase, which has a relatively broad substrate specificity. This reaction is responsible for diverting sterol intermediates into the cholic acid pathway. The enzyme was purified from rabbit liver and shows specificity toward 5α-cholestane-3α,7α-diol and 7α-hydroxycholesterol in rabbits.[103] The primary structure of the rabbit, mouse, and human enzymes has been deduced by molecular cloning of the cDNAs, and the enzyme has been expressed in COS cells.[104,105] There is little similarity in its peptide sequence with other cytochrome P-450 enzymes involved in bile acid synthesis, and because it shows a 43% homology with prostacyclin synthase (CYP8A1), it has been designated as CYP8B1.[105] The human gene has been localized to chromosome 3p21.3-p22 and structurally has been found to be the first cytochrome P-450 enzyme to lack introns. The enzyme is well expressed in rabbit and human liver, two species in which deoxycholic acid is quantitatively important, and to a lesser extent in rats and mice. Studies in rats have shown that the introduction of a C-27 hydroxyl group prevents subsequent 12α-hydroxylation and that thyroid hormone inhibits its activity while stimulating microsomal C-27 hydroxylase activity.[106,107] It is also transcriptionally downregulated by hydrophobic bile acids.[108] Both enzymes may therefore be of importance in regulating the synthesis of cholic acid in rats.[107] This, however, seems not to be the case for humans, in whom the introduction of a C-27 hydroxyl group has no inhibitory effect on the microsomal 12α-hydroxylase activity and thyroid hormone has only a small influence on the cholic-to-chenodeoxycholic acid ratio. These differences highlight species variations[17] that require consideration when using animal models. Other factors influencing microsomal 12α-hydroxylase include bile acid feeding,[109,110] which has an inhibitory effect, and cholestyramine administration, which increases the ratio of cholic-to-chenodeoxycholic acid[111] owing to an interruption of the normal enterohepatic circulation of bile acids. Similarly, biliary drainage[49] and starvation[103,112] increase its activity, the latter by an increase in mRNA levels. There appears to be no correlation between 12α-hydroxylase activity and the ratio of biliary cholic acid to chenodeoxycholic acid in humans,[113] indicating that other factors, such as the extent of enterohepatic recycling, intestinal metabolism, and absorption, may be important in regulating the relative proportions of intermediates that are diverted to each pathway. Additionally, the existence of alternative pathways for bile acid synthesis, particularly chenodeoxycholic acid,[33–35] which may be under separate regulatory control, could explain this lack of relationship.

STEP 4: Δ⁴-3-OXOSTEROID 5β-REDUCTASE

A soluble reduced nicotinamide adenine dinucleotide phosphate (NADPH)-dependent Δ⁴-3-oxosteroid 5β-reductase enzyme is responsible for catalyzing the reaction that leads to the saturation of the Δ⁴-bond and the formation of the 5β-(H) configuration at the AB-ring junction[114,115] that is common to the majority of bile acids found in most animal species, including humans. The Δ⁴-3-oxosteroid 5β-reductase has been purified,[116] and sequence analysis of both the human[117] and rat[118,119] cDNA encoding this enzyme indicates its molecular weight to be 37 to 38 kD, being made up of 327 amino acids. The rat and human enzymes show similar homology but differ significantly in structure from the analogous 5α-reductase enzyme responsible for the formation of *allo*-bile acids. The activity of this enzyme parallels that of cholesterol 7α-hydroxylase, as indicated from the finding that the plasma concentration of 7α-hydroxy-4-cholesten-3-one correlates with hepatic cholesterol 7α-hydroxylase activity.[120] Although this enzyme does not appear to be of regulatory importance for bile acid synthesis under normal conditions, the finding of significantly elevated levels of Δ⁴-3-oxo-bile acids in severe cholestasis[121] would suggest that under pathologic conditions, it may become rate limiting for primary bile acid synthesis.

STEP 5: 3α-HYDROXYSTEROID DEHYDROGENASE

Conversion of 7α-hydroxy-5β-cholestan-3-one and 7α,12α-dihydroxy-5β-cholestan-3-one by reduction into the respective 3α-hydroxy analogues takes place in the cytosolic fraction under the influence of a NADPH-dependent 3α-hydroxysteroid dehydrogenase enzyme.[114,115] This enzyme, which has broad substrate specificity, has been purified to homogeneity, and a number of cDNAs have been sequenced.[122–125] In addition to its role in metabolism, 3α-hydroxysteroid dehydrogenase was shown to be identical to the 33 kD Y' bile acid binders involved in the intracellular transport of bile acids.[126] The enzyme is inhibited by indomethacin, and bile acid binding to this protein is a major determinant of the intracellular distribution.[127]

STEP 6: STEROL 27-HYDROXYLASE

The mechanism by which oxidation of the C_{27} sterol side chain occurs has been the subject of extensive study. Under normal conditions, it would appear that the first step involves the introduction of a hydroxyl group at the C-27 position (see Figure 55.4-3). This reaction can take place in both the microsomal and mitochondrial fractions[3,19]; for humans, the mitochondrial C-27 hydroxylase (formerly referred to as a C-26 hydroxylase) is quantitatively more important. The mitochondrial C-27 hydroxylation has been shown to be stereospecific, involving hydroxylation of the 25-pro-S methyl group to yield the 27-hydroxylated product with a 25(R) configuration. On the other hand, the microsomal C-27 hydroxylation seems to involve the formation of the 25(S) product. The mitochondrial C-27 sterol hydroxylase exhibits a broad substrate specificity toward many sterols, including cholesterol and vitamin D,[128–130] but is particularly active toward 5β-cholestan-3α,7α-diol, 5β-cholestan-3α,7α,12α-triol, and 7α-hydroxy-4-cholesten-3-one.[131,132] The reaction involves a cytochrome P-450 species,[133] and the enzyme can be induced by phenobarbital treatment and by starvation. In addition to 27-hydroxylation, this enzyme is capable of catalyzing multiple oxidation reactions that give rise to 3α,7α,12α-trihydroxy-5β-cholestanoic acid (THCA).[134]

Although the microsomal C-27 hydroxylase (which is also cytochrome P-450 dependent) is of minor quantitative importance in humans, compared with the mitochondrial enzyme, it has a higher substrate specificity in the rat.[131] The microsomal fraction of rat liver, however, catalyzes the hydroxylation of the C-23, C-24 (α and β), and C-25 carbons, with the latter being as efficient as C-27 hydroxylation.[135]

It would appear that the 27-hydroxylation of cholesterol that drives the acidic pathway is catalyzed by the very same sterol 27-hydroxylase enzyme that is active on cholestane-3α,7α,12α-triol in the neutral pathway. This is in contrast to 7α-hydroxylation, in which there are separate and distinct enzymes in both pathways.[9] The sterol 27-hydroxylase is expressed in many extrahepatic tissues,[35,39,40,43,44,128,136,137] but especially in the adrenals, intestine, and lung, where its activity is highest. Its function appears to be one of facilitating the removal of cellular cholesterol for subsequent oxidation to bile acids. In the lung, where it is highly expressed, the ratio of 27-hydroxycholesterol to cholesterol is high. It appears that this organ accounts for most of the production of 3β-hydroxy-5-cholestenoic acid[38]; interestingly, removal of one lung reduces the level of this cholestenoic acid by half.

cDNAs encoding the rat, rabbit, and human C-27 hydroxylase have been isolated,[128,136,138,139] and whereas the activity and message for the sterol 27-hydroxylase have been determined in many tissues, its role in regulating bile acid synthesis is unclear, and it is evident that there are significant species differences. In the rabbit, the activity of cholesterol 27-hydroxylase is unaffected by bile acids,[140,141] whereas in rat hepatocytes transfected with the sterol 27-hydroxylase gene, bile acids repress transcription.[142] Sterol 27-hydroxylase appears to be much more important for bile acid synthesis in the mouse than in the human. When the gene was disrupted in the mouse, the formation of bile acids was shown to be markedly reduced.[143] This is not the case in humans, in whom mutations in the cholesterol 27-hydroxylase gene account for the lipid storage disease of cerebrotendinous xanthomatosis (CTX). In CTX, bile acids are produced by a compensatory pathway involving the 25-hydroxylation pathway leading to cholic acid, but chenodeoxycholic acid synthesis is markedly impaired.[144–146]

STEP 7: FORMATION OF CHOLESTANOIC ACIDS

The oxidation of the C-27 hydroxylated sterol intermediates to the respective cholestanoic (C_{27}) acids takes place in two steps[147] with the formation of an aldehyde as the intermediate. After purification of the enzymes responsible for these reactions, it was concluded that they were identical to the hepatic alcohol dehydrogenase and aldehyde dehydrogenase enzymes.[148–152] The relative importance of these enzymes in the oxidation of the side chain compared with that of the C-27 hydroxylase catalyzed reaction is unknown,[152] but the resulting product formed is the enantiomer (25R)$3\alpha,7\alpha,12\alpha$-trihydroxy-5β-cholestanoic acid ((25R)THCA).

STEP 8: OXIDATION OF THE SIDE CHAIN

Initiation of side-chain oxidation occurs with the formation of the CoA ester of (25R)THCA, a reaction that takes place in the endoplasmic reticulum and is catalyzed by a THCA-CoA synthetase.[153,154] Racemization of (25R)THCA-CoA to (25S)THCA-CoA takes place, catalyzed by 2-methylacyl-CoA racemase,[155] and this is an obligatory step to enable subsequent peroxisomal β-oxidation to occur because only the (25S)-enantiomers are substrates for the peroxisomal branched-chain acyl-CoA oxidase that leads to primary bile acid formation. 2-Methylacyl-CoA racemase is also responsible for catalyzing the stereoisomerization of the branched-chain fatty acid (2R)pristanoyl-CoA to its corresponding (S)-isomer.[156] The gene encoding this enzyme has been sequenced, and mutations have been reported in three adult patients with sensory neuropathies[155] and in two infants with liver disease and fat-soluble vitamin malabsorption.[13] Once formed, (25S)THCA-CoA undergoes oxidation by a series of reactions analogous to those responsible for the mitochondrial β-oxidation of fatty acids, involving the formation of 24α-hydroxylated and CoA derivatives with subsequent release of propionic acid to yield the cholanoic (C_{24}) acid CoA ester.[157,158] These reactions occur in the peroxisome, although, at one time, they were thought to be of microsomal origin.[152,158] Once within the peroxisome, the rate-limiting enzyme in side-chain oxidation, THCA-CoA oxidase, yields a Δ^{24} intermediate. A cDNA encoding the THCA-CoA oxidase was recently cloned and characterized in the rat, rabbit, and human.[159–162] This enzyme is distinct from the very-long-chain fatty acid (VLCFA) CoA oxidase that performs an analogous reaction[163] but is common to the oxidation of 2-methyl branched-chain fatty acids.[156] The Δ^{24} product of this reaction is then hydrated to form 24-hydroxy-THCA-CoA, which, in turn, is dehydrogenated to yield 24-oxo-THCA-CoA.[10,156,158,163,164] These two reactions are catalyzed by a

multifunctional protein,[165–167] of which two forms are known, multifunctional enzyme (MFE)-I and MFE-II, the latter being the one responsible for the degradation of bile acids and branched-chain fatty acids.[168] It is possible that the sterol carrier protein SCP-2/SCPx, which binds and complexes acyl CoAs and acyl-CoA oxidases within the peroxisome, may play a role in side-chain oxidation of bile acids, at least in the mouse, because when the gene was knocked out, an accumulation of $3\alpha,7\alpha,12\alpha$-trihydroxy-27-nor-5β-cholestan-24-one occurred.[169] The final step in the sequence of reactions for side-chain oxidation involves thiolytic cleavage of propionic acid, and this yields cholanoyl CoA.[170,171] The mechanisms involved in these reactions are described in more detail in a separate chapter on peroxisomes in this book.

STEP 9: CONJUGATION OF BILE ACIDS

The CoA derivatives of cholic and chenodeoxycholic acids are finally conjugated with the amino acids glycine and taurine. It is not known whether this reaction takes place exclusively within the peroxisome[172,173] or, as was originally thought, the cytosol, or both of these compartments.[174,175] A microsomal bile acid–CoA synthetase has been isolated,[175] which may be involved in the hydrolysis of the CoA ester and subsequent transport of cholic and chenodeoxycholic acids between these compartments.

Bile acid amino acid conjugates are formed in two consecutive enzymic reactions. The unconjugated bile acid is first converted to an acyl-CoA thioester,[174,176–178] a reaction that is catalyzed by a rate-limiting hepatic microsomal[179] bile acid CoA ligase (EC 6.2.1.7). This enzyme has also been identified in a rat kidney.[180] It has been purified and characterized from rat liver and found to have a molecular weight of 65 kD, and, more recently, its cDNA has been cloned and expressed in insect Sf9 cells.[181] It shows activity toward chenodeoxycholic and cholic acids but is inhibited by more hydrophobic bile acids, especially lithocholic and deoxycholic acids. Although the gene for the human hepatic enzyme has yet to be identified and sequenced, a gene encoding a 58 kD protein, recognized as a bile acid CoA ligase, was interestingly identified from *Eubacterium* sp strain VPI 12708.[182]

In the second reaction, the bile acid CoA thioester, catalyzed by a cytosolic bile acid–CoA:amino acid N-acyltransferase (EC 2.3.1.65),[183] is coupled to the amino acids glycine and taurine. This enzyme has been purified from human liver,[184] and its substrate specificity has been well characterized.[184–186] A cDNA encoding the human bile acid CoA:amino acid N-acyltransferase has been isolated, characterized, and expressed in bacteria,[187] as has a cDNA for the corresponding mouse enzyme, the gene for the latter being localized to chromosome 4.[188] The human cDNA encoded a monomeric protein of 46,296 D, and although there was reported close homology with the mouse enzyme[188] and with *kan-1*, a putative rat liver N-acyltransferase,[189] a significant species difference in substrate specificity was demonstrated. The human bile acid–CoA:amino acid N-acyltransferase is capable of conjugating cholic acid with both glycine and taurine, whereas the mouse enzyme showed selectivity toward taurine only. This is consistent with the fact that the mouse is an obligate taurine conjugator of bile acids, as are the rat and the dog.[190] The human bile acid–CoA:amino acid N-acyltransferase was recently found to be capable of conjugating fatty acids with glycine,[191] and because it is expressed in many tissues that play no role in bile acid synthesis, it was suggested that its function in extrahepatic tissues may be one of regulating intracellular levels of VLCFA.

Bile acids with a side-chain length of four carbon atoms (nor-bile acids) and six carbon atoms (homo-bile acids) are poor substrates for the enzymes; however, cholestanoic acids (C_{27} bile acids) are conjugated efficiently with taurine, as evidenced from their conjugation patterns in patients with peroxisomal defects.[2,192] The final products of the above-described multiple reactions, glycocholic, taurocholic, and chenodeoxycholic acids, are referred to as primary bile acids and are secreted in bile. In the normal adult, the ratio of glycine to taurine conjugated bile acids is 3:1,[23] but this can be altered by an increased availability of taurine, as occurs during taurine feeding[193] or in early life,[21] when hepatic taurine stores are high[194] because of selective placental transfer.[195] Unusual amidated conjugates are formed in some species, as evidenced by the finding that 3% of the biliary deoxycholic acid of the domestic rabbit is a glycyltaurine conjugate.[196]

Other bile acid conjugates occur naturally, and these include sulfates,[26] glucuronide ethers and esters,[24,25,197–200] glucosides,[27,28,199] N-acetylglucosaminides,[29,201] and conjugates of some drugs.[30,202,203] These metabolic pathways serve to increase the polarity of the molecule, thereby facilitating its renal excretion, and to decrease the membrane-damaging potential of the more hydrophobic unconjugated species.[204,205] Under normal conditions, these pathways are of minor quantitative importance but are activated in early life in the diseased state, particularly cholestasis, in the presence of an increased bile acid load such as exogenous bile administration or by drug administration.

A sulfotransferase enzyme catalyzes the formation of bile acid sulfates, most commonly at the C-3 position, but C-7 and C-12 sulfates are also found.[206–208] This enzyme shows sex-dependent differences in rats[208] but not in humans. Its activity has been shown to be low in the fetus compared with the adult,[209] as is evident from the finding of relatively small proportions of bile acid sulfates in fetal bile.[21] Although sulfation of bile acids has traditionally been considered to occur in the liver, it is evident that renal sulfation is important,[210,211] and most probably accounts for the increased concentrations of urinary bile acid sulfates in cholestasis.[212]

Glucuronidation is catalyzed by a number of glucuronyl transferase isozymes[199] that give rise to glucuronide ethers (ring conjugation) and esters (side-chain carboxyl conjugates). The affinity of this conjugation system is relatively specific[213]; short-chain bile acids are preferentially glucuronidated,[214] whereas bile acids possessing a 6α-hydroxyl group form the 6-O-ethers.[200,215]

Several other conjugation pathways for bile acids have been recently recognized. Glucosides[27,28,216] and N-acetylglucosaminides[29,201] of nonamidated and glycine- and taurine-conjugated bile acids have been found in normal human urine,[28,217] and quantitative excretion (1 μmol/d) approximates that of bile acid glucuronides.[198,218] A microsomal glucosyltransferase from human liver has been isolated and characterized and found in extrahepatic tissues.[216] This enzyme exhibits substrate specificity toward 7β-hydroxylated bile acids,[29] which explains why N-acetylglucosaminide conjugates of UDCA are found in large proportions in the urine of patients undergoing UDCA therapy.[212,219]

The identification of bile acid conjugates of fluorouracil[30,203,216] demonstrates that drug interactions with hepatic conjugation enzymes can take place and may play a role in the development of drug-induced cholestasis.

ALTERNATIVE PATHWAYS FOR BILE ACID SYNTHESIS

The simplified view of the pathways for bile acid synthesis described above assumes that the sequence of reactions occurs in an orderly manner, with changes to the steroid nucleus preceding side-chain oxidation. This, of course, is not the case, as is apparent from in vitro studies of enzyme kinetics using radiolabeled intermediates, which demonstrate the existence of alternative pathways for primary bile acid synthesis (Figure 55.4-4).[220–222] This is reinforced by the finding that patients with T tubes converted radiolabeled 27-hydroxycholesterol to chenodeoxycholic acid to a greater extent than 7α-hydroxycholesterol.[223] This pathway was denoted the acidic pathway[33] and is under separate regulatory control to the classic cholesterol 7α-hydroxylase (neutral) pathway. The relative importance of alternative pathways for primary bile acid synthesis, which mainly relate to initiating hydroxylation reactions on the side chain followed by 7α-hydroxylation, has become more recently appreciated.[33,35] These reactions occur in the liver and in many different extrahepatic tissues, including the brain, alveolar macrophages, vascular endothelia, and fibroblasts.[41,45,224] Their extrahepatic function may be related in some way to the regulation of cholesterol homeostasis because of their ability to generate significant amounts of oxysterols that are potent repressors of cholesterol synthesis.[35,44,225,226]

Under normal conditions, the neutral pathway is still considered to be quantitatively the most important one for cholic acid synthesis in adults. Recent studies, however, now indicate that the acidic pathway contributes significantly to overall total bile acid synthesis, especially to chenodeoxycholic acid synthesis.[33,35] It has also become evident that the acidic pathway, although being developmentally induced in the rodent,[37] is possibly the most important one for bile acid synthesis in early human life.[9] This contention is based on the finding that an infant having a mutation in the oxysterol 7α-hydroxylase gene but a normal cholesterol 7α-hydroxylase gene failed to synthesize primary bile acids[9] and instead accumulated massive quantities of 24-hydroxy-, 25-hydroxy-, and 27-hydroxycholesterol. Although the sterol 27-hydroxylase directs intermediates into the acidic pathway, it is the subsequent 7α-hydroxylation that is the most important step in this pathway because

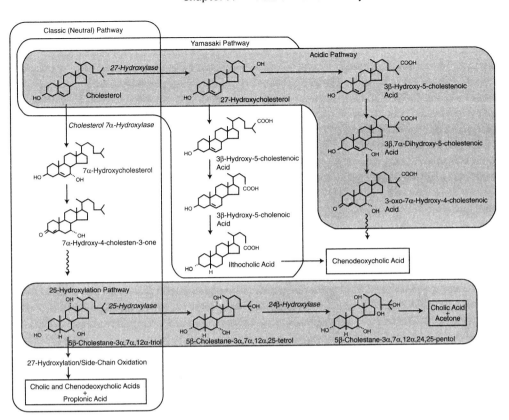

FIGURE 55.4-4 Alternative pathways for bile acid synthesis and their relationship to the classic "neutral" pathway.

it is essential to protect the liver from the toxicity of mono-hydroxy bile acids,[227–230] which would otherwise be formed if 7α-hydroxylation did not take place.[9]

For some time, it was evident that there were separate 7α-hydroxylases[33,231–233] and that bile acid synthesis via the acidic pathway was regulated differently and independently of the microsomal cholesterol 7α-hydroxylase.[35,50–52] The enzyme, referred to as oxysterol 7α-hydroxylase (*CYP7B1*), has a high activity in human liver,[233] but its regulation is not fully understood.[234,235] At least in the cholesterol 7α-hydroxylase (*CYP7A1*) knockout mouse, it is not affected by changes in the enterohepatic flux of cholesterol or bile acids induced by cholesterol or cholestyramine feeding.[236] It shows broad substrate specificity, being active on both 27- and 25-hydroxycholesterol[42,45,232,233] and 3β-hydroxy-5-cholenoic and 3β-hydroxy-5-cholestenoic acids.[231] The cDNA encoding the rat,[41] mouse,[235] and human[9,234] hepatic oxysterol 7α-hydroxylase (*CYP7B1*) has recently been reported. Translation of the human cDNA revealed the enzyme to have 506 amino acids, and there is a 56% and 66% homology with the rat and mouse enzymes, respectively.[9] The gene is localized to chromosome 8q21.3 and in close proximity to the gene encoding cholesterol 7β-hydroxylase (*CYP7A1*). Evidence for yet a further 7α-hydroxylase became apparent from studies of the *CYP7B1* knockout mouse,[237] which, unlike the human infant with a defect in this enzyme,[9] did not exhibit liver disease or accumulate to the same extent the oxysterols. This suggested that there was a third enzyme capable of 7α-hydroxylation, and, subsequently, *CYP39A1* was isolated[238] and shown to be active on 24-hydroxycholesterol. This enzyme is also present in humans, but its role is unclear.

The quantitative importance of the acidic pathway for bile acid synthesis has been hotly debated. When the cholesterol 7α-hydroxylase gene is knocked out in a mouse model, by 3 weeks of life, almost normal levels of bile acids are synthesized. This occurs following the developmental expression of the oxysterol 7α-hydroxylase.[37] In the rat, when cholesterol 7α-hydroxylase is chemically inhibited by continuous infusion of squalestatin, bile acid synthesis is still 43% of preinfusion levels after 24 hours.[36] These findings suggest that the acidic pathway accounts for about half of the total bile acid synthesis in the rodent. Under normal conditions, both the acidic and neutral pathways lead to the formation of cholic and chenodeoxycholic acids; however, it is suggested that 50% of the chenodeoxycholic acid synthesis is derived via this acidic pathway.[33]

As detailed above, side-chain oxidation proceeds with an initial C-27 hydroxylation and release of propionic acid; however, a pathway involving microsomal C-25 hydroxylation followed by 24-hydroxylation and release of acetone has been described. The cDNAs have been cloned of the cholesterol 25- and 24-hydroxylases,[239] and these enzymes have been found to play a key role in regulating lipid metabolism, particularly in the brain. The relative quantitative importance of this pathway to bile acid synthesis in healthy adults has been controversial.[144–146] Available evidence overwhelmingly supports 27-hydroxylation as the more important reaction initiating side-chain oxidation in normal humans.[240–242] This was confirmed in vivo by measuring the production of [14C]acetone following prior labeling of the cholesterol pool with [26-14C]cholesterol[145]; the 25-hydroxylation pathway accounted for less than 2% and 5% of the total bile acid synthesis in adult rats and humans, respectively.[145,146]

An alternative pathway for chenodeoxycholic acid synthesis[222] that is seemingly important in early life involves side-chain shortening prior to nuclear modifications, reactions that are initiated via a cholesterol C-27 hydroxylase.[34,210] In this pathway (often termed the Yamasaki pathway),[222] 27-hydroxycholesterol is oxidized directly to 3β-hydroxy-5-cholenoic acid, lithocholic acid, and, finally, chenodeoxycholic acid.[223,243–247] Although this pathway could be of minor importance in the adult, it may account for the increased levels of 3β-hydroxy-5-cholenoic and lithocholic acids in early life and in severe cholestatic conditions.

In many lower vertebrates, allo(5α-H)-bile acids are the major species of bile acids.[17,18] However, in humans, they are normally present in relatively small proportions and are generally believed to result from bacterial metabolism of 3-oxo-5β-bile acids during the course of their enterohepatic circulation. Studies of rodents have indicated that allo-bile acids may also be derived from 5α-cholestanol,[248,249] which can be efficiently 7α-hydroxylated in rat liver[250] and subsequently converted to 7α-hydroxy-5α-cholestan-3-one and then to 5α-cholestane-3α,7α-diol.[251] The 12α-hydroxylase enzyme shows a high specificity toward 5α-sterols,[252–254] and 5α-cholestane-3α,7α,12α-triol is readily formed from 5α-cholestane-3α,7α-diol and converted to allo-cholic acid in the bile fistula rat.[251]

A further mechanism for the formation of allo-bile acids involves their direct conversion from 7α-hydroxy-4-cholesten-3-one and 7α,12α-dihydroxy-4-cholesten-3-one by the action of an active Δ⁴-3-oxosteroid 5α-reductase. The enzyme shows a three- to fourfold higher activity in female rats compared with male rats,[255] but no gender differences have been demonstrated for humans. The quantitative importance of this reaction in humans is uncertain. Large amounts of allo-bile acids are found in patients with a deficiency in the bile acid Δ⁴-3-oxosteroid 5β-reductase.[7]

Intestinal microflora play an important role in bile acid metabolism[256] and therefore in the maintenance of the integrity of the enterohepatic circulation. Lithocholic (3α-hydroxy-5β-cholanoic) and deoxycholic (3α,12α-dihydroxy-5β-cholanoic) acids, the major bile acids excreted in feces,[32] are referred to as "secondary" bile acids. Both are formed from conjugated chenodeoxycholic and cholic acids by deconjugation and 7α-dehydroxylation, by enzymes found in a variety of organisms, such as Bacteroides, clostridia, bifidobacteria, and Escherichia coli. The mechanism by which 7α-dehydroxylation occurs has been extensively investigated by Hylemon, who purified a bile acid–CoA hydrolase from a strain of Eubacterium sp.[257] The dehydroxylation reaction involves a series of steps and appears to be initiated from the CoA thioester of the unconjugated bile acid but proceeds only following deconjugation.

Lithocholic acid is relatively insoluble and is consequently poorly absorbed from the intestinal lumen. It is found in relatively high proportions in meconium[258] and amniotic fluid[259,260] but is barely detectable in fetal bile.[21] In severe cholestatic conditions, deoxycholic acid levels in the serum become undetectable, and this bile acid is a useful marker of the extent of impairment of the enterohepatic circulation. Conversely, elevations in the serum unconjugated bile acid concentrations,[261] particularly secondary bile acids, reflect bacterial overgrowth of the small bowel.[262,263] Elevations in lithocholic acid sulfate, which occur in severe cholestasis,[264] demonstrate that lithocholic acid is also a primary product of hepatic synthesis and under such circumstances arises via the alternative pathways discussed previously.

BILE ACID SYNTHESIS DURING EARLY DEVELOPMENT

Knowledge of hepatic bile acid synthesis and metabolism during human development is limited and is derived largely from analysis of biologic fluids[21,265–271] and in vitro studies of the enzymes in fetal liver homogenates.[77,272–274] Ontogenic studies have been carried out in several animal species.[209,272,275–281] Detailed analytic studies of human fetal gallbladder bile[21,270] and in vitro studies of hepatic subcellular fractions[273,274] established significant qualitative and quantitative differences in bile acid synthesis and metabolism between the developing and adult liver. Because biliary excretion is the principal route for bile acid secretion, analysis of gallbladder bile permits a direct means of assessing hepatic synthesis and secretion.

The earliest studies of human fetal gallbladder bile used methodology less advanced than is currently available but nevertheless established primary bile acid synthesis to be relatively well developed during early gestation.[266,270] These early studies showed the concentration of chenodeoxycholic acid to be greater than cholic acid at midgestation, and primary bile acids were conjugated mainly with taurine. These findings were later corroborated using improved methodology, which confirmed that for humans, pathways for primary bile acid synthesis are developed as early as the twelfth week of gestation.[21] The activities of enzymes catalyzing 7α-hydroxylation, 12α-hydroxylation, side-chain oxidation, and conjugation of the primary bile acids and bile acid intermediates in homogenates of rat liver from rat embryos and suckling rats were found to increase 30-fold from day 15 after fertilization to day 5 of life.[275] Studies of preterm and older infants have found that the bile acid pool size is only one-sixth that of adults, and a rapid expansion of the pool occurs over the first year of life.[282–285] The chenodeoxycholic acid concentration in human fetal bile is relatively low in early gestation and exceeds the cholic acid concentration. This is in marked contrast to the biliary bile acid composition of the full-term infant and the adult, in whom cholic acid is the predominant bile acid.[265,267] Similar developmental differences in bile acid composition are found in amniotic fluid collected at different times of gestation.[260] There are several possible explanations for these differences: (1) cholic acid synthesis would be reduced in early life if there was an immaturity in hepatic 12α-hydroxylase activity; however, in vitro studies have established the activity of this enzyme to be relatively well developed[77,275]; (2) preferential clearance of cholic acid by metabolism to more polar C-1, C-2, C-4, or C-6 tetrahydroxylated bile acids would lead to a relative increase in the proportion of chenodeoxycholic acid; however, tetrahydroxy bile acids constitute less than 2% of the total biliary bile acids of the human fetus[21]; (3) chenodeoxycholic acid synthesis occurs via the C-27 hydroxylase pathway, which is under separate regulatory control and appears to be up-regulated when the activity of cholesterol 7α-hydroxylase is low, as would be expected in utero. This latter explanation is most likely and would explain the increased amounts of monohydroxy bile acids found in meconium.[258]

A conspicuous feature of bile acid synthesis and metabolism during development is the relatively large proportion of a complex array of bile acids not typically found in adult bile.[20,21] Interestingly, the profile of biologic fluids of the newborn and fetus[20,21,270,286] resembles that observed for adult patients with severe cholestasis.[287,288] Analysis of human fetal gallbladder bile[21,270] and in vitro incubations of hepatic subcellular fractions with radiolabeled bile acids[273,274] has served to confirm the quantitative importance of several hepatic hydroxylation pathways, including C-6 and C-1 hydroxylation. Hyocholic acid (3α,6α,7α-trihydroxy-5β-cholanoic acid) is a major biliary bile acid of the fetus, and concentrations often exceed cholic acid concentrations,[21] whereas a series of C-1 hydroxylated isomers can also be found.[21,270]

1β-Hydroxylation has been demonstrated in vitro by human fetal microsomes,[273] and several C-1 hydroxylated bile acid isomers have been found in the urine of healthy adults[287] and infants,[286,289] in meconium,[2,20,258,268] and in biologic fluids from patients with liver disease.[288,290] A novel and prominent C-4 hydroxylation pathway was recently discovered and suggested to be unique to early human development.[21,271] 3α,4β,7α-Trihydroxy-5β-cholanoic acid was identified and found to account for 5 to 15% of the total biliary bile acids in early gestation.[271]

Newborn infants in the first few days of life excrete significant amounts of 3-oxo-Δ^4 bile acids, and this is indicative of an immaturity in bile acid synthesis.[286,291] The levels of these unsaturated bile acids typically decline rapidly in the first few months of life, but when high levels persist, a "primary" deficiency in the Δ^4-3-oxosteroid 5β-reductase enzyme should be suspected.[7] High levels of 3-oxo-Δ^4 bile acids are also associated with a severe loss of hepatic synthetic function, and differentiating the primary from the secondary deficiency in the Δ^4-3-oxosteroid 5β-reductase enzyme can be difficult.[8,121]

Secondary bile acids can be found in fetal bile but only in very small proportions. This is consistent with the lack of bacterial flora in the fetal gut and the maternal-fetal placental transport of secondary bile acids that has been demonstrated in vivo[277,278] and in vitro.[292]

The principal bile acid conjugation reaction of the fetal liver is amidation with taurine. In fetal bile, 85% of the total biliary bile acids are taurine conjugates,[21] which contrasts to the pattern for adult bile, for which the glycine-to-taurine ratio is approximately 3:1.[20,23] This reflects the increased accumulation and availability of taurine in the fetal liver[194] resulting from selective placental transport.[195]

Bile acid sulfates, which are generally increased in cholestatic conditions in adults,[264,287,293–295] are virtually absent in early gestation.[21] This probably reflects an immaturity in the bile acid sulfotransferase enzyme or may be a

consequence of additional and preferential metabolism of bile acids by hydroxylation. Lithocholic acid sulfate and 3β-hydroxy-5-cholenoic acid sulfate are found in relatively large proportions in the meconium[258] and amniotic fluid[259,260,296] as a result of accumulation and sequestration during gestation.

Meconium also contains a series of short-chain monohydroxylated bile acids.[297–299] These compounds possess a steroid nucleus of 20-, 21-, and 22-carbon atoms and are predominantly found as glucuronide or sulfate conjugates.[214,299] In contrast to the monohydroxy-C_{24} bile acids, which are cholestatic, etianic acid (3α-hydroxy-5β-androstan-17β-carboxylic acid) produces a marked choleresis in the rat,[214] illustrating how relatively small changes to the structure of the steroid nucleus can cause marked differences in physiologic actions. The origin of short-chain bile acids is unknown, but their close similarity in structure to steroid hormones suggests that they may be metabolic end products of steroid hormones formed during pregnancy.

INBORN ERRORS IN BILE ACID SYNTHESIS

Disorders in bile acid synthesis and metabolism can be broadly classified as primary or secondary. Primary enzyme defects involve congenital deficiencies in enzymes responsible for catalyzing key reactions in the synthesis of cholic and chenodeoxycholic acids, and, to date, the following such defects have been described:

- Cholesterol 7α-hydroxylase (*CYP7A1*) deficiency leading to disturbances in lipid metabolism but not manifest as liver disease[300]
- 3β-Hydroxy-C_{27}-steroid dehydrogenase/isomerase (3β-hydroxy-C_{27}-steroid oxidoreductase) deficiency[6] involving the conversion of 7α-hydroxycholesterol into 7α-hydroxy-4-cholesten-3-one caused by mutations in the *HSD3B7* gene encoding this enzyme[97]
- Δ^4-3-Oxosteroid 5β-reductase deficiency[7] involving the cytosolic enzyme that catalyzes the reduction of the Δ^4-bond to give rise to a 5β-H and consequently the *cis*-configuration of the A/B rings of the bile acid nucleus
- Oxysterol 7α-hydroxylase deficiency[9] caused by a mutation in the gene encoding the enzyme catalyzing the 7α-hydroxylation of 27-hydroxycholesterol in the "acidic" pathway for bile acid synthesis
- CTX, a rare lipid storage disease[301] caused by mutations in the sterol 27-hydroxylase gene
- 2-Methylacyl-CoA racemase deficiency causing liver disease and fat-soluble vitamin malabsorption in early life[13] and late-onset sensory motor neuropathy in adults[155]
- Trihydroxycholestanoic acid CoA oxidase deficiency involving an initial step in the side-chain oxidation[10,12,302–305]
- An amidation defect involving a deficiency in the bile acid–CoA ligase, the rate-limiting enzyme for conjugation of cholic and chenodeoxycholic acids with glycine and taurine[11]

- Side-chain oxidation defect in the 25-hydroxylation pathway for bile acid resulting in an overproduction of bile alcohols[306]

Secondary metabolic defects that impact on primary bile acid synthesis include the following:

- The cerebrohepatorenal syndrome of Zellweger[307] and related disorders[308] involving enzymes responsible for β-oxidation of the side chain of cholestanoic acids, which result from abnormal peroxisomal assembly, structure, or function
- Mutations in the genes encoding organic anion transport proteins,[309,310] in particular progressive familial intrahepatic cholestasis (PFIC) type 1 or Byler disease, a familial and fatal progressive intrahepatic cholestatic syndrome
- RSH/Smith-Lemli-Opitz syndrome,[311] a disorder caused by a deficiency of Δ^7-desaturase that results in reduced cholesterol synthesis and therefore has a knock-on effect in the bile acid pathway by limiting the available supply of cholesterol

Hepatic synthesis of the primary bile acids cholic and chenodeoxycholic acids is critical to the development and maintenance of the enterohepatic circulation because of the pivotal role of bile acids in promoting the secretion of bile.[14] Progressive cholestatic liver disease is consequently a striking clinical manifestation of patients presenting with severely impaired primary bile acid synthesis, and this includes patients with both of the steroid nuclear defects and those patients with the more severe peroxisomopathies.[2,4,9,13,312] The recent identification of single-enzyme defects in side-chain oxidation and conjugation presenting as disorders of fat-soluble vitamin malabsorption or rickets[10,13] attests to the importance at the intestinal level of adequate concentrations of primary bile acids for lipid absorption.

The biochemical presentation of these bile acid synthetic defects includes a markedly reduced or complete lack of cholic and chenodeoxycholic acids in the serum, bile, and urine and greatly elevated concentrations of atypical bile acids and sterols that retain the characteristic structure of the substrates for the deficient enzyme. These signature metabolites are generally not detected by the routine or classic methods for bile acid measurement, and mass spectrometric techniques presently provide the most appropriate means of characterizing defects in bile acid synthesis. Screening procedures using liquid secondary ionization mass spectrometry (LSIMS) indicate that inborn errors in bile acid synthesis probably account for 2 to 5% of the cases of liver disease in infants, children, and adolescents, making this an important and specific category of metabolic liver disease.

PRIMARY ENZYME DEFECTS

CEREBROTENDINOUS XANTHOMATOSIS

CTX is a rare inherited lipid storage disease, first described by Van Bogaert and colleagues,[301] with an estimated preva-

lence of 1 in 70,000.[4] Characteristic features of the disease in adults include progressive neurologic dysfunction, dementia, ataxia, cataracts, and the presence of xanthomatous lesions in the brain and tendons; however, in infants, we have characterized this defect in a number of patients with neonatal cholestasis (K. D. R. Setchell, unpublished data, 2003). Biochemically, the disease can be distinguished from other conditions involving xanthomatous deposits by (1) significantly reduced primary bile acid synthesis; (2) elevations in biliary, urinary, and fecal excretion of bile alcohol glucuronides; (3) low plasma cholesterol concentration, with deposition of cholesterol and cholestanol in the tissues; and (4) marked elevations in cholestanol. Elegant studies by Salen and colleagues demonstrated the metabolic defect to be an impairment in oxidation of the cholesterol side chain,[313,314] and chenodeoxycholic acid synthesis is reduced to a greater extent than cholic acid synthesis.[315–317] Initially, it was thought to be due to a defect in sterol 24-hydroxylase,[313] but later studies indicated the primary defect to be a deficiency in the mitochondrial sterol 27-hydroxylase (Figure 55.4-5).[318] The following evidence supports this contention: (1) the mitochondrial fraction of the liver from a patient with CTX was shown to be completely devoid of sterol 27-hydroxylase activity[318]; (2) in liver homogenates, the amount of 5β-cholestane-3α,7α,12α-triol, the substrate for this enzyme, was 50-fold higher than normal[318]; (3) 27-hydroxycholesterol in the serum of patients with CTX is markedly reduced or undetectable[319]; (4) intravenous administration of radiolabeled precursors showed that only precursors with a C-27 hydroxy group were converted to cholic acid[318]; (5) the increased amounts of bile alcohol glucuronides synthesized in this defect are polyhydroxylated in the side chain and mainly at positions other than the C-27 carbon.

To explain the findings of greatly increased amounts of 5β-cholestane-3α,7α,12α,25-tetrol, Salen initially proposed a deficiency in microsomal 24(S)hydroxylation; this reaction normally yields 5β-cholestane-3α,7α,12α,24,25-pentol.[316] Studies using this radiolabeled cholestane-pentol showed that it was converted to cholic acid, indicating an alternative pathway to the classic C-27 hydroxylation pathway for cholic acid synthesis,[144,313] but the quantitative importance of this pathway in health has since been established to be relatively minor.[145,146] Furthermore, if the primary defect in CTX was a deficiency in 24(S)-hydroxylase, this would not explain the greatly reduced synthesis of chenodeoxycholic acid,[320] which, in humans, is synthesized in significant amounts via the C-27 hydroxylation pathway. A deficiency in sterol 27-hydroxylase, on the other hand, would lead to elevations in 5β-cholestane-3α,7α-diol and 7α-hydroxy-4-cholesten-3-one[321]; thus, these intermediates are available for 12α-hydroxylation and preferential conversion to cholic acid via the C-25 hydroxylation pathway.[322] Interestingly, microsomal 12α-hydroxylase activity has been shown to be threefold higher in patients with CTX.[317] Evidence reinforcing a sterol 27-hydroxylase deficiency as the primary enzyme defect in CTX was established following the cloning of the cDNA for

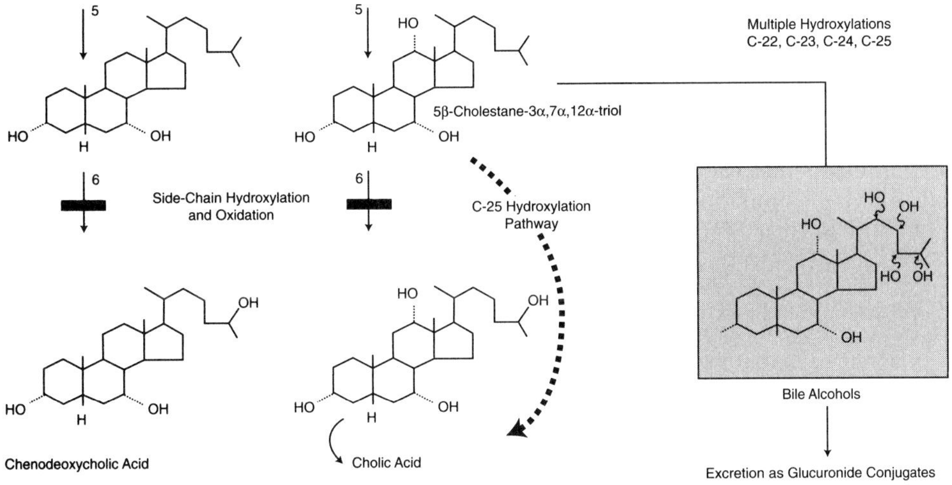

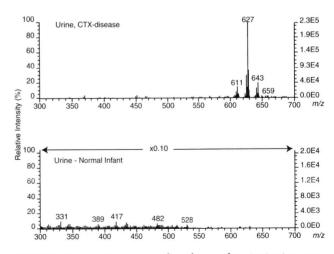

FIGURE 55.4-5 Biochemical defect in the sterol 27-hydroxylase deficiency of cerebrotendinous xanthomatosis.

this enzyme.[128,136,138,139] Using this probe, the mRNA was isolated from fibroblasts of two CTX patients, and the corresponding cDNA was synthesized by reverse transcription. Point mutations in the gene located on the long arm of chromosome 2 were identified and expressed in COS cells, and the resulting sterol 27-hydroxylase enzyme was found to be inactive.[139] These molecular studies clearly establish the primary defect in CTX to be due to a deficiency in the mitochondrial C-27 hydroxylase. In recent years, several types of mutations have been identified in CTX patients from different countries, and these include insertion, deletion, and point mutations.[323–344]

Impaired oxidation of the cholesterol side chain results in accelerated cholesterol synthesis and metabolism that leads to greatly increased production and excretion of bile alcohol glucuronides,[314,345–349] which can be readily detected in urine by fast atom bombardment ionization mass spectrometry (FAB-MS) (Figure 55.4-6).[2,350] These bile alcohols have the common 5β-cholestane-3α,7α,12α-triol nucleus, with additional hydroxyl groups in the side chain, mainly at the C-22, C-23, C-24, and C-25 positions (see Figure 55.4-5). The major bile alcohol excreted in bile and feces is the 5β-cholestane-3α,7α,12α,25-tetrol,[314,347,351,352] whereas the more polar 5β-cholestane-3α,7α,12α,23,25-pentol predominates in urine.[348,351,353] It has been suggested that the difference in these patterns could be due to more efficient renal excretion of the more polar pentol or a result of renal C-23 hydroxylation of 5β-cholestane-3α,7α,12α,25-tetrol.[351,352]

The elevation in 5α-cholestan-3β-ol (cholestanol) in the nervous system of CTX patients first observed by Menkes and colleagues[354] and the high plasma concentrations of this sterol[316] are unique features of the disease. An elevated plasma cholestanol-to-cholesterol ratio has been proposed to be diagnostic[355] but is not specific because elevations in this ratio also occur in liver disease. The origins of the increased cholestanol may be from elevations in the precursor sterol 4-cholesten-3-one; hepatic microsomes prepared from CTX patients have been shown to produce three times more 4-cholesten-3-one than similar preparations from healthy controls.[356] Using pulse-labeling techniques, Salen and colleagues showed that 4-cholesten-3-one would yield

labeled cholestanol, whereas the corresponding 7α-hydroxyl intermediate was converted to bile acids.[356] An alternative pathway for the formation of cholestanol, not involving 7α-hydroxyl intermediates, was proposed implicating hepatic, rather than intestinal, 7α-dehydroxylation with the production of cholest-4,6-dien-3-one intermediate.[357,358] Evidence to support this pathway is the finding of increased levels of 7α-hydroxy-4-cholesten-3-one and cholest-4,6-diene-3-one in CTX and the observation that cholestyramine treatment, which stimulates cholesterol 7α-hydroxylase activity, increases cholestanol output, whereas the opposite response occurs during chenodeoxycholic acid feeding. The neurologic dysfunction observed in CTX appears to be a consequence of cholestanol deposition in the tissues, and because the sterol 27-hydroxylase is found in extrahepatic tissues, it is possible that some of the manifestations of the disease may be the result of nonhepatic perturbations in metabolism. Recent studies in a rat model indicate that cholestanol induces apoptosis of cerebellar neurons, and it was suggested that this could induce cerebellar ataxia in CTX patients.[359] Early diagnosis of this disorder, which is readily

FIGURE 55.4-6 Negative-ion liquid secondary ionization–mass spectrometry mass spectra comparing the urine of a normal infant with that of a patient with cerebrotendinous xanthomatosis (CTX). The presence of increased levels of bile alcohol glucuronides is indicated by the specific ions at m/z 611, 627, 643, and 659.

achieved by mass spectrometry analysis of the urine, is crucial to prevent the progressive accumulation of cholestanol and cholesterol in tissues in the long term, but suspicion of a metabolic defect is not always realized because in the early years, the patients may be relatively asymptomatic. More recently, we have found a number of infants that had deficiencies in the sterol 27-hydroxylase owing to mutations in the gene encoding this enzyme but only because of a clinical presentation of elevated liver enzymes and bilirubin, which ultimately resolved by about 6 months of age presumably because the size of the cholic acid pool expanded with compensatory synthesis via the alternative 25-hydroxylation pathway. We suggest that this may be the typical early clinical presentation of CTX even though this has never been previously documented. The earliest age of diagnosis we have made was in a 1-day-old infant, which was made possible by the fact that this infant was born to a family that had a previous child with neonatal cholestasis that we had diagnosed with sterol 27-hydroxylase defect at 8 weeks of age.

3β-Hydroxy-C27-Steroid Oxidoreductase Deficiency

This was the first metabolic defect to be described involving an early step in the bile acid biosynthetic pathway; the conversion of 7α-hydroxycholesterol is to 7α-hydroxy-4-cholesten-3-one, a reaction catalyzed by a 3β-hydroxy-C27-steroid oxidoreductase. In response to a deficiency in this enzyme, 7α-hydroxycholesterol is metabolized by the remaining reactions, and the final products of hepatic synthesis are C24 bile acids that retain the 3β-hydroxy-Δ5 structure characteristic of the enzyme substrates (Figure 55.4-7).[6] The index case was identified in a fifth child born to Saudi Arabian parents who were first cousins and was the third infant to be affected by progressive liver disease from birth; the previous infants had died within the first few years of life following similar clinical histories. Subsequently, a further infant with this defect was born to a first-cousin marriage in the kindred. The 3β-hydroxy-C27-steroid oxidoreductase is the most common of all of the bile acid synthetic defects described thus far.

Although the clinical presentation of this disorder is somewhat heterogeneous, all patients generally present with progressive jaundice, elevated transaminases, and a conjugated hyperbilirubinemia.[6,58,59] Clinical features include hepatomegaly, with or without splenomegaly, fat-soluble vitamin malabsorption, and mild steatorrhea, and in most instances, pruritus is absent. The liver histology shows a generalized hepatitis, the presence of giant cells, and evidence of cholestasis.[6,58,360–362] Although the earliest cases were identified in infants, increasingly, idiopathic late-onset chronic cholestasis has been explained by this disorder.[58,59] In such patients, liver disease is not always evident in the early presentation, and many patients often have fat-soluble vitamin malabsorption and rickets, which are corrected with vitamin supplementation. Serum liver enzymes that are often normal in the early stages of the disease later show progressive increases. Serum bile acid concentrations when measured by conventional routine methods are normal or low and incompatible with the severity of liver dysfunction. However, urinary and serum bile acid concentrations are always elevated when determined by more specific techniques.

Of significance is the finding of a high association of this disease with a normal γ-glutamyl transpeptidase (Figure 55.4-8).[58,59,363] This is also a feature of patients with other conditions of familial progressive intrahepatic cholestasis or Byler disease,[364–367] but differential diagnosis of the two disorders can be readily made on the basis of the serum primary bile acid concentration, which, in the latter, is markedly elevated. Measurement of serum bile acids can be useful in establishing a diagnosis of inborn errors in bile acid synthesis and should be included in the workup of the patient with idiopathic cholestasis.

Definitive diagnosis of the 3β-hydroxy-C27-steroid oxidoreductase deficiency presently requires mass spectrometric analysis of biologic fluids and is readily accomplished by LSIMS, formerly referred to as FAB-MS,[2,4,350] or by electrospray and tandem mass spectrometry.[368–371] LSIMS analysis of the urine permits the detection of the sulfate and glycosulfate conjugates of the 3β-hydroxy-Δ5 bile acids that are the signature metabolites of this bile acid defect (Figure 55.4-9). Additionally, sulfate conjugates of tetrahydroxy-

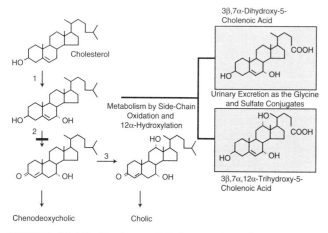

FIGURE 55.4-7 Biochemical defect in the 3β-hydroxy-C27-steroid oxidoreductase deficiency.

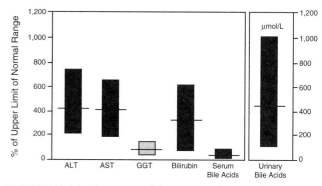

FIGURE 55.4-8 Summary of the mean and range of serum biochemistries in patients (n = 20) with the 3β-hydroxy-C27-steroid oxidoreductase deficiency. ALT = alanine transaminase; AST = aspartate transaminase; GGT = γ-glutamyl transpeptidase.

and pentahydroxy-bile alcohols with a $3\beta,7\alpha$-dihydroxy-Δ^5 and $3\beta,7\alpha,12\alpha$-trihydroxy-Δ^5 nucleus are also found in significant amounts in the serum and urine.[60]

Primary bile acids are not found in the urine but may be present in small amounts in the bile because of the action of a bacterial 3β-hydroxysteroid dehydrogenase/isomerase during the enterohepatic recycling of the atypical bile acids. This may explain the longer survival of these patients compared with patients with other defects in bile acid synthesis. Interestingly, 3β-hydroxysteroid dehydrogenase/isomerase isozymes are also involved in catalyzing analogous reactions in the pathways for steroid hormones, but steroid hormone synthesis and metabolism are unaffected in these patients. This is because the enzyme, which was recently purified, uses only intermediates that have a 3β-hydroxy-Δ^5 structure and is inactive on C_{19} and C_{21} steroids.[95]

Expression of the 3β-hydroxy-C_{27}-steroid oxidoreductase in fibroblasts affords a means of further establishing a deficiency in the activity of this enzyme. In contrast to healthy controls, patients with this defect have undetectable enzyme activity in fibroblasts, whereas the heterozygous genotypes have low or subnormal levels of activity.[102] However, this approach is somewhat redundant because molecular techniques that have led to the cloning of the *HSD3B7* gene encoding 3β-hydroxy-C_{27}-steroid oxidoreductase now permit the accurate genetic basis of the defect.[96] Using this approach to confirming the biochemical diagnosis of this enzyme deficiency in 15 patients from 13 kindreds, 12 different mutations were found to account for the disease.[97] The mechanism of cholestasis and liver injury is speculated to be the result of the failure to synthesize adequate amounts of primary bile acids that are essential to the promotion and secretion of bile and the increased production of unusual bile acids with hepatotoxic potential. The monohydroxy bile acid 3β-hydroxy-5-cholenoic acid has been shown to be markedly cholestatic in the rat and hamster,[229] and although $3\beta,7\alpha$-dihydroxy-5-cholenoic acid did not cause cholestasis in this latter species,[247] this may be explained by its metabolism to chenodeoxycholic acid. Recent studies using rat liver

membrane vesicles have demonstrated that the taurine conjugate of $3\beta,7\alpha$-dihydroxy-5-cholenoic acid inhibits adenosine triphosphate–dependent bile acid transport at the canalicular plasma membrane and is not transported across this membrane.[15,372] These findings serve to explain the failure to find significant levels of bile acids in the bile of patients with the 3β-hydroxy-C_{27}-steroid dehydrogenase/isomerase defect and substantiate our initial theory that this is a cause of cholestasis.

Δ^4-3-OXOSTEROID 5β-REDUCTASE DEFICIENCY

Application of LSIMS for urine analysis led to the discovery of a defect in the Δ^4-3-oxosteroid 5β-reductase, which catalyzes the conversion of the intermediates 7α-hydroxy-4-cholesten-3-one and $7\alpha,12\alpha$-dihydroxy-4-cholesten-3-one to the corresponding 3-oxo-5β(H) intermediates (Figure 55.4-10).[7] The defect was initially identified in monochorionic male twins born with a marked cholestasis; a previous sibling with neonatal hepatitis had died of liver failure at 4 months of age. The clinical presentation of this defect is similar to that of patients with the 3β-hydroxy-C_{27}-steroid dehydrogenase/isomerase deficiency; however, in contrast, the γ-glutamyl transpeptidase is usually elevated, and the average age at diagnosis is lower in the Δ^4-3-oxosteroid 5β-reductase. The Δ^4-3-oxosteroid 5β-reductase has since been found in a number of patients presenting with neonatal hemochromatosis.[8] Liver function tests in these infants showed elevations in serum transaminase levels, marked conjugated hyperbilirubinemia, and coagulopathy. Liver biopsies[362,373] revealed marked lobular disarray as a result of giant cell and pseudoacinar transformation of hepatocytes, hepatocellular and canalicular bile stasis, and extramedullary hematopoiesis. On electron microscopy, bile canaliculi were small and sometimes slit-like in appearance and showed few or absent microvilli containing electron-dense material.[7]

Diagnosis of this defect is possible by LSIMS and gas chromatography–mass spectrometry (GC-MS) analysis of the urine. LSIMS spectra reveal elevated amounts of bile acids with molecular weights consistent with taurine con-

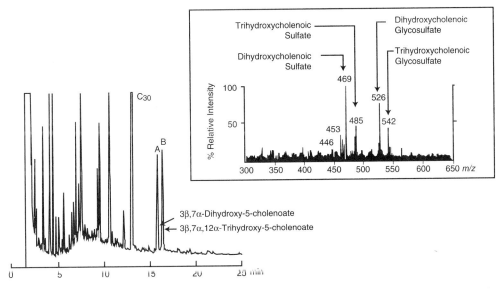

FIGURE 55.4-9 Negative-ion liquid secondary ionization–mass spectrometry mass spectrum and gas chromatography analysis of a typical urine from a patient with a 3β-hydroxy-C_{27}-steroid oxidoreductase deficiency.

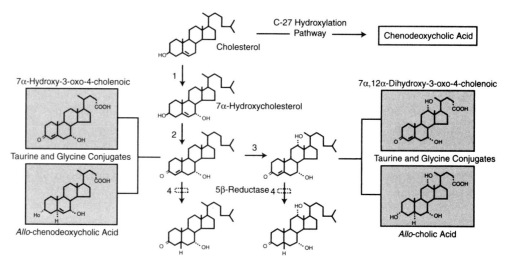

FIGURE 55.4-10 Biochemical defect in the Δ^4-3-oxosteroid 5β-reductase deficiency.

jugates of hydroxyoxocholenoic and dihydroxyoxocholenoic acids. GC-MS analysis following extraction, solvolysis, hydrolysis, and derivatization of bile acids[374] is essential to confirm the predominance of the major metabolites, 3-oxo-7α-hydroxy-4-cholenoic and 3-oxo-7α,12α-dihydroxy-4-cholenoic acids. Urinary bile acid excretion is generally elevated and consistent with a cholestatic condition. Quantitatively, the Δ^4-3-oxo bile acids comprise more than 75% of the total urinary bile acids. Gallbladder bile contains only traces (less than 2 μM) of bile acids, and because urinary excretion becomes the major route for bile acid loss, estimates of bile acid synthesis rates can be made from the daily urinary output and indicate markedly reduced total bile acid synthesis rates (less than 3 mg/d) compared with reported data for newborn infants[282] or adults.[375] In serum, relatively high concentrations of *allo*-chenodeoxycholic and *allo*-cholic acids are found, which lends support for an active hepatic Δ^4-3-oxosteroid 5α-reductase catalyzing the conversion of the Δ^4-3-oxo sterol intermediates to the corresponding 3α-hydroxy-5α(H) structures.

The Δ^4-3-oxosteroid 5β-reductase is exclusively of hepatic origin and, unlike the 3β-hydroxy-C_{27}-steroid dehydrogenase/isomerase, is not expressed in fibroblasts. Monoclonal antibodies raised against the rat cytosolic Δ^4-3-oxosteroid 5β-reductase have been used to demonstrate an absence of the 38 kD protein in a number of these patients and the formation of a truncated protein.[3] In one patient from Japan who met our previous biochemical criteria for a deficiency in this enzyme, sequence analysis of the gene revealed a single silent mutation in the coding region of the gene,[117] but the protein was normally expressed when analyzed by immunoblot of the liver homogenate using a monoclonal antibody.[376] Increased production of Δ^4-3-oxo bile acids occurs in patients with severe liver disease[121] and in infants during the first few weeks of life.[291] It is important to perform a repeat analysis of urine in the case of a suspected Δ^4-3-oxosteroid 5β-reductase deficiency because on rare occasions, a resolution of the liver disease occurs and the atypical bile acids disappear.[377] This is also the case with developmental immaturity. In general, however, it is our experience that

markedly elevated levels of 3-oxo-Δ^4 bile acids are indicative of a poor clinical prognosis.

The liver injury in this defect is presumed to be the consequence of the diminished primary bile acid synthesis and the hepatotoxicity of the accumulated Δ^4-3-oxo bile acids. The lack of canalicular secretion can be explained by the relative insolubility of oxo-bile acids, and the cholestatic effects of the taurine conjugate of 7α-dihydroxy-3-oxo-4-cholenoic acid have been demonstrated in rat canalicular plasma membrane vesicles.[15] The unique morphologic findings in these patients[373] may indicate that maturation of the canalicular membrane and the transport system for bile acid secretion may require a threshold concentration of primary bile acids in early development.

OXYSTEROL 7α-HYDROXYLASE DEFICIENCY

The recent discovery of a genetic defect in oxysterol 7α-hydroxylase[9] establishes the acidic pathway as a quantitatively important pathway for bile acid synthesis in early life. Unlike the mouse, in which this enzyme appears to be developmentally regulated,[37] or the rat, in which it is induced when there is suppression in cholesterol 7α-hydroxylase activity,[36] it would appear that in the human, the oxysterol 7α-hydroxylase may be more important than cholesterol 7α-hydroxylase for bile acid synthesis in early life. In common with the 3β-hydroxy-Δ^5 steroid-C_{27}-oxidoreductase deficiency[6] and the Δ^4-oxosteroid 5β-reductase deficiency,[7] this genetic defect presents as severe progressive cholestatic liver disease.

To date, this defect has been found in only one infant, a 10-week-old boy of parents who were first cousins, who presented with severe cholestasis, cirrhosis, and liver synthetic failure from early infancy. The patient became progressively jaundiced by 8 weeks of age and had markedly elevated serum transaminases and a normal serum γ-glutamyl transpeptidase. On examination, there was hepatosplenomegaly, and his liver biopsy revealed cholestasis, bridging fibrosis, extensive giant cell transformation, and proliferating bile ductules.[9] Oral UDCA therapy led to deterioration in liver function tests, and oral cholic acid was therapeutically ineffective. The patient subsequently underwent orthotopic liver transplant at 4½ months of age, only to succumb to a disseminated Epstein-Barr virus–related lymphoproliferative disease.

Analysis of the urine by LSIMS revealed intense ions in the spectrum at mass-to-charge ratio (m/z) 453 and m/z 510, corresponding to sulfate and glycosulfate conjugates of 3β-hydroxy-5-cholenoic and 3β-hydroxy-5-cholestenoic acids (Figure 55.4-11). These accounted for 97% and 86% of the total serum and urinary bile acids, respectively, and primary bile acids were virtually undetectable. Monohydroxy bile acids with the 3β-hydroxy-Δ^5 structure have been previously shown to be extremely cholestatic.[229,230] Their hepatotoxicity in this patient is presumed to have been exacerbated by the lack of primary bile acids necessary for the maintenance of bile flow. Because the formation of 3β-hydroxy-5-cholenoic and 3β-hydroxy-5-cholestenoic acids occurs exclusively in the acidic pathway,[378] these findings and the observation that 27-hydroxycholesterol concentrations in serum and urine were more than 4,500 times normal support a defect in the oxysterol 7α-hydroxylase enzyme (Figure 55.4-12). Analysis of the neutral sterol fraction from serum and urine failed to demonstrate any 7α-hydroxysterols.

Molecular studies of the liver tissue established the cholesterol 7α-hydroxylase gene to be normal, but there was no measurable enzyme activity or mRNA; low or undetectable cholesterol 7α-hydroxylase activity has been previously reported for the human infant.[77] It is conceivable that gene expression may have been repressed by accumulation of the vast amounts of oxysterols. Oxysterol 7α-hydroxylase mRNA was also not present in this patient's liver tissue, and analysis of the oxysterol 7α-hydroxylase gene revealed a cytosine to thymidine transition mutation in exon 5 that converts an arginine codon at position 388 to a stop codon. The patient was homozygous for this nonsense mutation, whereas both parents were heterozygous.[9] When human embryonic 293 or Chinese hamster ovary cells were transfected with the cDNA with the R388* mutation, there was no detectable 7α-hydroxylase activity, and immunoblot analysis confirmed that the mutated gene encoded a truncated and inactive protein.

Unlike the other two nuclear defects in bile acid synthesis, the oxysterol 7α-hydroxylase deficiency is particularly severe and untreatable by primary bile acid therapy. It is possible that this cause of idiopathic liver disease may go unrecognized owing to its rapid downhill course in the early months of life. The characteristic metabolites formed in the genetic defect are some of the most cholestatic bile acids known, and, clearly, oxysterol 7α-hydroxylase is crucial for protecting the liver against the toxicity of monohydroxy bile acids produced in the acidic pathway. It is probable that our failure to find additional patients with this inborn error may be because of the devastatingly severe nature of this fatal liver disease, which does not respond to oral bile acid therapy, as in the other bile acid synthetic defects.[9]

2-METHYLACYL-CoA RACEMASE DEFICIENCY

2-Methylacyl-CoA racemase is a crucial enzyme that is uniquely responsible for the racemization of (25R)THCA-CoA to its (25S) enantiomer, while also performing the same reaction on the branched-chain fatty acid (2R)pristanoyl-CoA (Figure 55.4-13). Defects in this enzyme therefore have profound effects on both the bile acid and the fatty acid pathways. Mutations in the gene encoding 2-methylacyl-CoA racemase were first reported in three adults who presented with a sensory motor neuropathy[155] and later in a 10-week-old infant who exhibited severe fat-soluble vitamin deficiencies, hematochezia, and mild cholestatic liver disease in the first months of life.[13] This patient was initially and incorrectly reported in the previous edition of this book and elsewhere as having a possible THCA-CoA oxidase deficiency.[10] The infant had the same missense mutation (S52P) as that described in two of the adult patients yet was seemingly phenotypically quite different.[13] Two of the adult patients had neurologic symptoms but were asymptomatic until the fourth decade of life, whereas the other adult was described as having the typical features of Niemann-Pick type C disease at 18 months of age and presumably had some liver dysfunction. The clinical descriptions of these adult patients,[155] in particular the early history, were too scant to draw conclusions about the

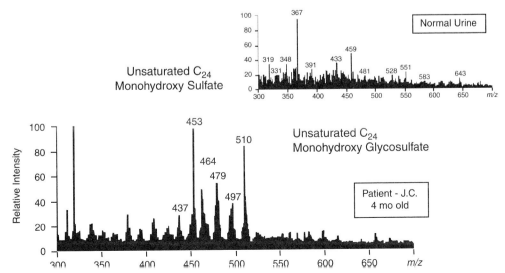

FIGURE 55.4-11 Negative-ion liquid secondary ionization–mass spectrometry mass spectra of the urine from a patient with the oxysterol 7α-hydroxylase deficiency and a normal age-matched infant. Ions characteristic of the signature metabolites of the defect are seen at m/z 453 and 510, corresponding to the sulfate and glycosulfate conjugates, respectively, of the monohydroxylated bile acid 3β-hydroxy-5-cholenoic acid.

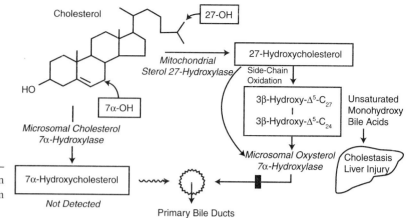

FIGURE 55.4-12 Biochemical basis for a defect in the oxysterol 7α-hydroxylase. Reproduced from Setchell KDR et al.[9]

phenotypic differences between the adult and the early presentation of the 2-methylacyl-CoA racemase. It is therefore possible that these adults could have had undocumented mild liver disease and fat-soluble vitamin absorption early in life and, if undiagnosed in infancy, would probably lead to a neuropathy owing to the tissue accumulation of phytanic and pristanic acids. Remarkable about the case of the first infant described with the 2-methylacyl-CoA racemase deficiency was the finding that the liver from a 5½-month-old sibling, who 2 years previously had died from an intracranial bleed, had been used for transplant in a child with end-stage liver disease.[13] Analysis of the urine from the recipient confirmed the same biosynthetic defect in the donor liver. Diagnosis of the defect in the infant was based on urinary, serum, and biliary bile acid analysis by FAB-MS, GC-MS, and electrospray ionization–tandem mass spectrometry, which revealed subnormal levels of primary bile acids and markedly increased concentrations of cholestanoic (C_{27}) acids, which are characteristically found as major bile acids of the alligator, other reptiles, and amphibians.[379,380] However, these cholestanoic acids were identified exclusively as the (25R)enantiomers.[13,381] The mass spectrum and GC profiles in this defect resemble closely those observed in peroxisomal disorders impacting bile acid synthesis, such as Zellweger syndrome; however, in other peroxisomopathies, both the (25S)THCA and (25R)THCA enantiomers are present, but the (25S)isomer predominates.[381] Differential diagnosis of the 2-methylacyl-CoA racemase deficiency from generalized peroxisomal disorders requires direct analysis

of the urine or serum, omitting the use of destructive alkaline hydrolysis methods.[13,381] This is best achieved by high-performance liquid chromatography electrospray ionization–tandem mass spectrometry, which permits the separation and quantification of the two enantiomers of THCA,[382] which are otherwise difficult to measure by conventional techniques of bile acid analysis. Fibroblast studies can be used to further confirm a deficiency in peroxisomal 2-methylacyl-CoA racemase.[383] Incubation of cultured fibroblasts with the stereospecific (25R)THCA and (2R)pristanoic acid, the signature metabolites of this disorder, permits reduced activity of the enzyme to be established, although DNA sequencing would be the preferred approach to confirmation.

Primary bile acid therapy with cholic acid has proven effective in normalizing liver enzymes and preventing the onset of neurologic symptoms in the infant; additionally, dietary restriction of phytanic acid and pristanic acids is likely to be necessary in the long term for such patients to prevent neurologic symptoms owing to the brain accumulation of these fatty acids.

THCA-CoA Oxidase Deficiency

A number of patients have been reported to have side-chain oxidation defects involving the THCA-CoA oxidase.[12,302–305] The clinical presentation differs among these cases, and although all impact on primary bile acid synthesis, neurologic disease was the main clinical feature.[13] Whether these are primary bile acid defects or secondary to single-enzyme defects in peroxisomal β-oxidation is

FIGURE 55.4-13 Biochemical defect in bile acid synthesis showing position of the enzyme deficiency in 2-methylacyl-CoA racemase and depicting its impact on the fatty acid and cholestanoic acid oxidation pathways. CoA = coenzyme A; THCA = 3α,7α,12α-trihydroxy-5β-cholestanoic acid.

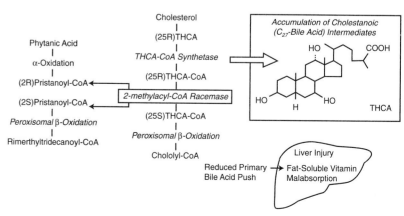

unclear. Two distinct acyl-CoA oxidases have been identified in humans,[156] whereas the rat has three isozymes.[384] The human acyl-CoA oxidase active on bile acid C_{27} cholestanoic acid intermediates has been found to be the same enzyme that catalyzes the oxidation of 2-methyl branched-chain fatty acids.[156] The cDNA of the gene encoding this human enzyme has been cloned.[161] Of the case reports in the literature of the proposed THCA-CoA oxidase deficiency, interestingly, phytanic and pristanic acids, when measured, were elevated.[12,302–305] All had ataxia as a primary feature of the disease, with its onset occurring at about $3^{1}/_{2}$ years of age. None had evidence of liver disease. It is possible, with the exception of the patient described by Clayton and colleagues,[306] that these patients had a 2-methylacyl-CoA racemase deficiency, but the analysis of the cholestanoic acids was not sufficiently detailed to permit the diastereoisomers of THCA and $3\alpha,7\alpha$-dihydroxy-5β-cholestanoic acid (DHCA) or pristanic acid to be measured, which would have helped in the differential diagnosis. In the case of the patient reported by Clayton and colleagues, we were able to obtain urine, serum, and bile for analysis by electrospray ionization–tandem mass spectrometry, and the major enantiomer of THCA in this patient was found to be the (25S) isomer, therefore excluding the 2-methylacyl-CoA racemase as an explanation for the clinical presentation.[306] It is evident that the phenotypic presentation of defects involving the peroxisomal apparatus can present with a wide diversity in symptoms that make it difficult to pinpoint the exact defect involved. In all suspected cases, analysis of peroxisomal enzymes, pristanic and phytanic acids, VLCFAs, and plasmalogens should be performed to complement detailed bile acid analysis.

BILE ACID CoA LIGASE DEFICIENCY AND DEFECTIVE AMIDATION

The final step in bile acid synthesis involves conjugation with the amino acids glycine and taurine.[23] Hepatic conjugation is extremely efficient, and negligible amounts of unconjugated bile acids typically appear in bile under normal and cholestatic conditions[385] and also when large doses of an unconjugated bile acid such as UDCA are administered.[386] Two enzymes catalyze the reactions leading to amidation of bile acids. In the first, a CoA thioester is formed by the rate-limiting bile acid–CoA ligase, after which glycine or taurine is coupled in a reaction catalyzed by a cytosolic bile acid–CoA:amino acid N-acyltransferase.

A defect in bile acid amidation, presumed to involve the bile acid–CoA ligase, was described in three patients presenting with fat and fat-soluble vitamin malabsorption.[11]

The index case was a 14-year-old boy of Laotian descent who, in the first 3 months of life, presented with conjugated hyperbilirubinemia, elevated serum transaminases, and normal γ-glutamyl transpeptidase. This child also had a form of β-thalassemia. Two other patients, a 5-year-old Saudi Arabian boy and his 8-year-old sister, who were products of a consanguineous marriage, have since been diagnosed. In early life, the boy had undergone a Kasai procedure for a mistakenly diagnosed biliary atresia. The girl was asymptomatic at the time of diagnosis, and there was little clinical history available. Liver function tests were either normal or mildly elevated at the time of diagnosis. The primary manifestation of a bile acid conjugation defect is severe fat-soluble vitamin malabsorption with rickets, and in one patient, this had led to a fracture. All had subnormal levels of vitamin E, vitamin K, 25-hydroxyvitamin D, and 1,25-dihydroxyvitamin D.

The diagnosis was based on the LSIMS analysis of the urine and serum and bile, which revealed unique negative-ion spectra featuring a major peak of mass (m/z 407) corresponding to unconjugated cholic acid (Figure 55.4-14). In addition, ions characterizing sulfate and glucuronide conjugates of dihydroxy and trihydroxy bile acids were present. There was a complete lack of the usual glycine and taurine conjugated bile acids, and this was confirmed after chromatographic separation and GC-MS. Serum and urinary bile acids were markedly elevated and comprised predominantly cholic and deoxycholic acids. Attempts to identify bile acid–CoA esters yielded negative data, suggesting that the likely point of defective bile acid amidation was rate-limiting bile acid–CoA ligase.[174,177–179] All of these patients have been lost to follow-up, making it impossible to ascertain the molecular genetics of the defect despite the fact that the cDNAs for both conjugating enzymes have been cloned.[181,188]

The clinical presentation and biochemical features of defective amidation in these patients closely parallel the presentation and features hypothesized by Hofmann and Strandvik.[387] Whereas the previously described inborn errors in bile acid synthesis present as well-defined progressive familial cholestatic liver diseases,[6,7,9] in contrast, cholestasis does not occur in this amidation defect because the synthesis of unconjugated cholic acid provides sufficient stimulus for bile flow. The fat-soluble vitamin malab-

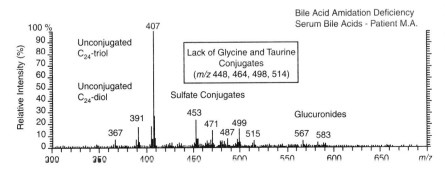

FIGURE 55.4-14 Negative-ion liquid secondary ionization–mass spectrometry mass spectrum of the serum from a patient with a defect in the bile acid-CoA ligase leading to deficient amidation of bile acids. The major ion at m/z 407 indicates the presence of unconjugated cholic acid.

sorption in these patients is postulated to be the result of reduced biliary secretion of bile acids and the inability to form mixed micelles because of rapid passive absorption of unconjugated cholic acid in the proximal small intestine.[388] Although these patients did conjugate bile acids with glucuronic and sulfuric acids, these conjugated bile acids are of little help in promoting lipid absorption.[389–391] Administration of primary conjugated bile acids should provide a therapeutic approach to correcting the fat-soluble vitamin malabsorption in this defect, and the recognition that genetic defects in bile acid synthesis are associated with fat-soluble vitamin malabsorption warrants a more concerted effort to explore this type of patient population.

SIDE-CHAIN OXIDATION DEFECT IN THE ALTERNATE 25-HYDROXYLATION PATHWAY

A speculative diagnosis of a defect in side-chain oxidation in the 25-hydroxylation pathway[144–146] was proposed by Clayton and colleagues for a 9-week-old infant presenting with familial giant cell hepatitis and severe intrahepatic cholestasis.[306] The rationale for the diagnosis was based on the finding of reduced cholic and chenodeoxycholic acids in the serum, concomitant with high concentrations of bile alcohol glucuronides, specifically 5β-cholestane-3α,7α,12α,24-tetrol, 5β-cholest-24-ene-3α,7α,12α,24-tetrol, and 5β-cholestane-3α,7α,12α,25-tetrol. These bile alcohols are not normally found in the plasma of infants with liver disease. Bile alcohol glucuronides were also identified as major metabolites in the urine.[306] Although the profile resembled that seen in CTX patients, it was concluded on the basis of the liver disease (not previously reported for CTX) that this represented a different side-chain defect and that it was possibly an oxidation defect downstream of the 25-hydroxylation step in this minor pathway for bile acid synthesis. The implications of the findings are that it could indicate that the 25-hydroxylation pathway, considered of negligible importance in adults,[146] may be an important pathway for infants. This is speculation, and further studies to prove the exact site of the defect are required before this is convincing. The patient was, however, treated with chenodeoxycholic acid and cholic acid, and this led to a normalization in serum transaminases and a suppression in the production of bile alcohols.

CHOLESTEROL 7α-HYDROXYLASE DEFICIENCY

Several patients have recently been identified with a homozygous mutation deletion in the CYP7A1 gene, and when the cDNA of this mutant was expressed in vitro in cultured HEK 293 cells, cholesterol 7α-hydroxylase was found to be inactive.[300] Bile acid synthesis was reduced, and up-regulation of the alternative sterol 27-hydroxylase pathway presumably compensated for the reduced synthesis of bile acids via absent cholesterol 7α-hydroxylase activity. Three patients carrying this mutation were found to have abnormal lipids, but, in contrast to an infant identified with a mutation in oxysterol 7α-hydroxylase,[9] there was no evidence for abnormal liver function in these patients. Instead, the clinical phenotype was one of markedly elevated total and low-density lipoprotein (LDL)

cholesterol and premature gallstones in two patients and premature coronary and peripheral vascular disease in one patient. The elevated serum cholesterol concentration was unresponsive to HMG-CoA reductase inhibitor therapy. Interestingly, individuals who were shown to be heterozygous for this mutation were found to have an above normal level of serum cholesterol. The phenotype of this deficiency in cholesterol 7α-hydroxylase differed significantly from that expressed in the CYP7A1 knockout mouse model.[37] It is possible that CYP7A1 deficiency predisposes the patient to cholesterol gallstone disease and seems to account for abnormal lipids but, surprisingly, not to liver disease. The important role of CYP7A1 in the regulation of lipids is further supported by earlier studies showing that a number of polymorphisms in the CYP7A1 gene were associated with abnormal LDL cholesterol concentrations in the general population.

SECONDARY BILE ACID DEFECTS

DISORDERS OF PEROXISOMAL FUNCTION

Genetic defects involving peroxisomes include the cerebrohepatorenal syndrome of Zellweger[307] and related diseases. Excellent reviews describe the clinical and biochemical features of these disorders[308,392–395]; consequently, the following text focuses only on the impact of these diseases on bile acid synthesis (see Chapter 55.8, "Zellweger Syndrome and Other Disorders of Peroxisomal Metabolism").

The peroxisomopathies can be broadly subdivided into two main groups. Those syndromes in which there is a generalized impairment in numerous peroxisomal functions as a consequence of a markedly reduced or undetectable number of peroxisomes include Zellweger syndrome,[307,392,396] infantile Refsum disease,[397] neonatal adrenoleukodystrophy,[398] hyperpipecolic acidemia,[399] and rhizomelic chondrodysplasia punctata,[400] and these conditions share many similarities in their clinical presentation and neurologic manifestation. These include severe hypotonia, psychomotor retardation, hepatomegaly, simian crease, craniofacial dysmorphism, and failure to thrive. Genetic diseases involving a single-enzyme defect and a normal number of peroxisomes[401–403] include pseudo-Zellweger syndrome,[403] which shows many clinical and pathologic similarities to Zellweger syndrome.

Only those disorders with a generalized impairment in peroxisomal function have been found to have abnormal bile acid synthesis reflected by an accumulation of bile acid precursors. Although both the mitochondrial and microsomal fractions were originally shown to convert THCA into cholic acid, the peroxisomal fraction was later found to have the highest capacity for this reaction.[164] For this reason, elevated levels of trihydroxycoprostanoic (THCA) and dihydroxycoprostanoic (DHCA) acids are consistently found in the biologic fluids of patients with Zellweger syndrome, neonatal adrenoleukodystrophy, pseudo-Zellweger syndrome, and infantile Refsum disease (Figure 55.4-15). Interestingly, these long-chain C_{27} bile acids are not found in rhizomelic chondrodysplasia punctata,[400] and to our knowledge, there appear to have been no studies of bile acid metabolism in hyperpipecolic acidemia[399] and acatalasemia.[404] The presence of other bile acid precursors is not uncommon, and it is possible that earlier descriptions of increased proportions of bile acid precursors in children with intrahepatic biliary atresia may have been due to the failure to recognize milder variants of Zellweger syndrome.[405,406] The in vivo and in vitro capacity of the liver to convert bile acid precursors into cholic and chenodeoxycholic acids by patients with Zellweger syndrome was studied by Kase and colleagues.[164,242,407] Tritiated 7α-hydroxy-4-cholesten-3-one was rapidly converted to DHCA and THCA but only slowly converted to cholic and chenodeoxycholic acids, with only 10% conversion after 48 hours, whereas cholic acid and chenodeoxycholic acid pool sizes and synthesis rates were markedly reduced. These data confirmed a defect in side-chain cleavage of the cholestanoic acid precursors and highlighted the important role of the peroxisome in bile acid synthesis.[408] Frequently, levels of DHCA are lower than THCA, which may be accounted for by its rapid transformation by 12α-hydroxylation to THCA.[409] Despite the reportedly low bile acid synthesis rate,[242] many studies have shown normal or increased serum levels of primary bile acids in patients with peroxisomal disorders. This may be a consequence of impaired hepatic uptake of bile acids because of generalized hepatic dysfunction.

In addition to DHCA, THCA, and varanic acid (the C-24 hydroxylated derivative of THCA), other atypical bile acids have been identified in Zellweger syndrome. C_{29} dicarboxylic acid is a major component of the serum (see Figure 55.4-15),[410,411] and although not always present, it can account for up to 40% of the total serum bile acids in Zellweger syndrome and infantile Refsum disease.[192,242,410,412–414] The biosynthetic pathway leading to the production of this unusual bile acid is uncertain. Administration of tritiated 5β-cholestane-3α,7α,12α-triol and THCA to a patient with Zellweger syndrome showed only a slow conversion to the C_{29} bile acid; however, its accumulation in serum may be accounted for by its relatively poor renal clearance and biliary excretion. Monohydroxy C_{27} bile acids also found in the serum of patients with Zellweger syndrome include 3α-hydroxy-5β-cholestanoic and 3β-hydroxy-5-cholestenoic acids.[410,415] In contrast to other cholestatic conditions, only

low concentrations of 3β-hydroxy-5-cholenoic acid have been reported in the serum and urine of three patients with Zellweger syndrome.[410]

Perhaps not surprisingly, in view of the predominance of 1β- and 6α-hydroxylation pathways in early life,[21,270] the urine of these patients usually contains large proportions of 1β- and 6α-hydroxylated tetrahydroxycholestanoic acids that are mainly conjugated with taurine.[192] These more polar metabolites arise from the accumulated THCA and DHCA, and this metabolic pathway consequently facilitates the urinary excretion of these metabolites. These specific urinary metabolites are of diagnostic significance for the Zellweger and pseudo-Zellweger syndromes and can be recognized by LSIMS from the intense ion of m/z 572 corresponding in mass to the taurine conjugated tetrahydroxycholestanoic acids.[192]

Of the well-defined single-enzyme defects, X-linked adrenoleukodystrophy,[416–418] involving the VLCFA acyl-CoA synthetase, and pseudoneonatal adrenoleukodystrophy,[419] a defect in the VLCFA-CoA oxidase, both show normal bile acid synthesis and highlight the fact that there are separate isozymes for this common reaction sequence. Pseudo-Zellweger syndrome, a defect of the thiolase,[170,412] and a deficiency in the multifunctional protein[420] are conditions that present with abnormal bile acid synthesis.[421] A number of isolated examples of patients in whom there is impaired β-oxidation of bile acids have been reported, but the exact defects were not defined. With improvements in methodologies[422] and the advantage of molecular probes to identify the enzymes and sequence genes, it is expected that further defects will be delineated.

DEFECTS IN CANALICULAR BILE ACID TRANSPORT PROTEINS

In the last decade, tremendous strides have been made in the understanding of the mechanisms behind bile formation and the transport of organic anions across the hepatocyte.[423,424] Full details of these advances are in Chapter 55.6, "Biliary Transport," and in an excellent summary by Trauner and colleagues.[425] It is outside the scope of this

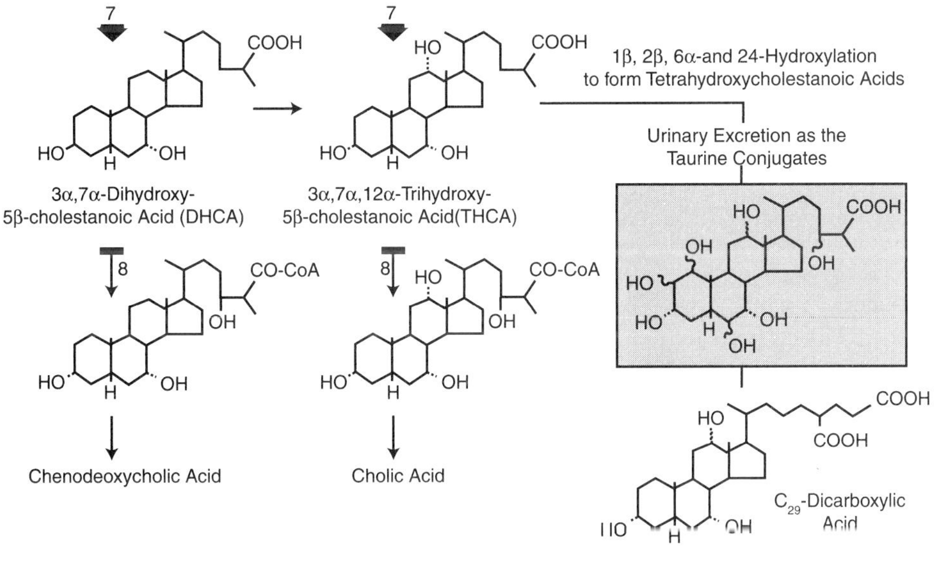

FIGURE 55.4-15 Biochemical defect in the cerebrohepatorenal syndrome of Zellweger.

3α,7α-Dihydroxy-5β-cholestanoic Acid (DHCA)

3α,7α,12α-Trihydroxy-5β-cholestanoic Acid (THCA)

1β, 2β, 6α-and 24-Hydroxylation to form Tetrahydroxycholestanoic Acids

Urinary Excretion as the Taurine Conjugates

Chenodeoxycholic Acid

Cholic Acid

C_{29}-Dicarboxylic Acid

review to detail the voluminous work on transport proteins and their role in cholestasis, and the reader is directed to an excellent summary by Trauner and colleagues.[425] Bile acids play a critical role in providing the major driving force for the promotion and secretion of bile, and defects in bile acid synthesis will inevitably cause cholestasis. In recent years, familial cholestasis has also been associated with mutations in the genes encoding the transport proteins for organic anions.[310,426,427] In the context of bile acid synthesis, patients with Byler disease (now classified as PFIC type 1) are of interest. This is an autosomal recessive familial progressive intrahepatic cholestasis[364,428] that has been shown to be due to a mutation in the *FIC1* gene encoding a P-type adenosine triphosphatase.[309] Some of the clinical features of PFIC are shared with bile acid synthetic defects, most notably the low γ-glutamyl transpeptidase.[59,367,429] However, they are easily differentiated because, unlike primary bile acid synthetic defects, patients with PFIC type 1 do synthesize primary bile acids, albeit in suboptimal levels. A striking feature of the bile from patients with PFIC type 1 is the negligible amount of chenodeoxycholic acid present, even though cholic acid is secreted, indicating impaired canalicular secretion of this dihydroxy bile acid.[430] In contrast, serum and urinary bile acids are composed of large proportions of chenodeoxycholic acid and its 6α-hydroxylated metabolite hyocholic acid.[367,429,431] 6α-Hydroxylation of bile acids is not, however, specific for PFIC type 1 because hyocholic acid can be found in biologic fluids from patients with other cholestatic diseases and is a characteristic of early development. Activation of this P-450 enzyme is presumed to occur in response to increases in intracellular chenodeoxycholic acid concentrations. Biochemical confirmation of this specific bile acid transport defect is by analysis of duodenal or biliary bile for the ratio and concentration of the primary bile acids.

RSH/SMITH-LEMLI-OPITZ SYNDROME

Since publication of the previous edition of this book, there has been an expansive literature on the RSH/Smith-Lemli-Opitz syndrome covering clinical features and variants, biochemical presentation, pre- and postnatal diagnosis, and the molecular genetics of this syndrome. It is beyond the scope of this review to detail all of these studies, and the reader is directed to the articles cited here and references therein. RSH/Smith-Lemli-Opitz syndrome is an autosomal recessive disease with an estimated frequency of 1 in 20,000 to 40,000.[4] The clinical characteristics of this syndrome are highly variable but include dysmorphism, microcephaly; poor growth; limb abnormalities; cardiac, renal, and endocrine abnormalities; cataracts; mental retardation; and early death.[311,432–434] It is considered the second-most common genetic defect in the North American white population. Biochemically, the condition is characterized by markedly reduced plasma cholesterol concentrations and elevated concentrations of 7-dehydrocholesterol and isodehydrocholesterol, and these Δ^7 sterols, which are normally not present, are the major neutral sterols of tissue, plasma, and feces.[435–437] The condition is accounted for by a defect in the 7-dehydrocholesterol Δ^7-reductase (7-DHC), an

enzyme that catalyzes the final reaction in the formation of cholesterol.[438] 7-DHC has the highest activity in the adrenal glands and the liver.[439] The defect can be reproduced in an animal model using a drug (BM 15.766), a competitive inhibitor of 7-DHC.[440] The 7-DHC gene has been cloned for the human[439,441,442] and rat[443] enzymes and is localized on chromosomes 11q13 and 7F5, respectively. It encodes a 55 kD protein,[439] and a number of missense, nonsense, and splice-site mutations have been described.[432,444] Although this is a primary defect in cholesterol biosynthesis, it impacts on bile acid synthesis because the available supply of cholesterol is reduced, and Δ^7 sterols are poor substrates for 7α-hydroxylation; consequently, bile acid synthesis is markedly reduced.[436]

DIAGNOSIS AND TREATMENT OF INBORN ERRORS IN BILE ACID SYNTHESIS

A battery of techniques is available for the measurement of bile acids in biologic fluids, and these have been compiled and extensively reviewed in the book series *The Bile Acids*[1] and elsewhere.[445–447] Technologic advances have meant that techniques such as paper and thin-layer chromatography have largely become superseded by extremely sensitive and specific assays. Immunoassays[448] are commonly used in routine laboratories because of their high sensitivity, precision, and suitability for handling large numbers of samples but presently lack the specificity for detecting specific inborn errors in bile acid metabolism. High-performance liquid chromatography is a useful tool[449,450] but, owing to its limited sensitivity, particularly with ultraviolet detection, is best suited to the analysis of the principal amidated species of biliary bile acids and has limited value in measuring the lower concentrations of bile acids in serum. Improvements in sensitivity have been achieved by pre- or postcolumn reactions,[447,449] coupling with thermospray,[450] or electrospray ionization–mass spectrometry.[451,452]

Accurate identification of inborn errors in metabolism requires techniques that afford detailed metabolic profiles, and, for the moment, GC-MS continues to be the principal confirmatory analytic tool.[446,453,454] Because of the high cost, technical difficulty, and time-consuming nature of bile acid analysis by GC-MS, the technique is outside the scope of most routine clinical laboratories. For this reason, the diagnosis of patients with inborn errors in bile acid synthesis has proven difficult and probably accounts for the low reported incidence of such metabolic defects.

Perhaps the most significant advances in mass spectrometry in recent years have been the introduction of FAB-MS and electrospray mass spectrometry, both of which are referred to by the generic term LSIMS. These techniques greatly simplified and extended the scope of mass spectrometry so that many nonvolatile compounds can be analyzed rapidly and directly in biologic samples or simple crude extracts, thereby circumventing the need for extensive and time-consuming sample pretreatments. Intact bile acid conjugates are ideally suited to LSIMS, and negative ionization mass spectra of steroid and bile acid conjugates can be generated from microliter volumes of urine and blood.[2,192,350,370,446,451–456]

In healthy individuals, urinary bile acid excretion is of negligible quantitative importance; consequently, the mass spectrum obtained is unremarkable, showing only background ions from the matrix and the presence of some steroid hormone metabolites. During cholestasis, urinary bile acid excretion increases and bile acid conjugates can be readily detected by the presence of single intense ions corresponding to the pseudomolecular ($[M-H]^-$) ions. With cholestasis, and in the absence of an inborn error in bile acid synthesis, the ions corresponding to the glyco- and tauroconjugates of the primary bile acids appear in the mass spectrum, and the intensity of the ions is proportional to the degree of cholestasis.[2] When bile acid synthesis is impaired, a unique mass spectrum is obtained, revealing ions corresponding in mass to the accumulated intermediates and/or metabolites with structural characteristics of the substrates proximal to the enzyme block. Positive identification of these bile acids generally requires GC-MS analysis after prior hydrolysis of the conjugates and preparation of volatile derivatives, and this is a time-consuming technique. Positional or stereoisomers of bile acid conjugates can be differentiated if reaction chemistry is carried out in a tandem mass spectrometer, and useful collision-dissociated spectra can be obtained.[369,457-460] The potential for rapid screening of bile acid defects has been realized with the electrospray ionization–mass spectrometry, and bile acid metabolites can be detected in dried blood spots obtained from newborns for the Guthrie test.[370] This approach allows fast throughput of samples for screening, but definitive diagnosis of suspected inborn errors in bile acid synthesis is still likely to be complemented with GC-MS and, for the moment, will be restricted to specialist laboratories. Now that many of the genes encoding the enzymes involved in bile acid synthesis have been cloned, the application of molecular techniques to sequence DNA from patients identified by mass spectrometry as having bile acid synthetic defects is an important complementary tool and should prove of value in prenatal diagnosis in these familial diseases.

Early diagnosis of inborn errors in bile acid synthesis is important because, untreated, these conditions are inevitably fatal. The reduced or total lack of synthesis of primary bile acids, coupled with the overproduction of large amounts of atypical bile acids and sterols that have intrinsic hepatotoxicity,[15,228,372] results in a clinical course leading to fibrosis, cirrhosis, and liver failure in most patients with the steroid nuclear defects.[6,7,9] The possibility of bile acid synthetic defects in older children, and even some adults with idiopathic forms of liver disease, should also be considered given that many cases of 3β-hydroxy-C_{27}-steroid oxidoreductase have been found in older children and teenagers presenting with late-onset chronic cholestasis.

We now appreciate that the inability to synthesize primary bile acids may clinically manifest as a fat-soluble vitamin malabsorption syndrome that can cause rickets in the absence of symptomatic liver disease. Again, treatment with primary bile acids is important in these conditions because it will facilitate the absorption of vitamins A, D, E, and K while also staving off cholestatic liver disease in the

longer term. The rationale for using primary bile acids, rather than UDCA, which is commonly prescribed for cholestatic liver diseases, is threefold. Primary bile acids provide a stimulus for bile flow and will generate a choleresis. Primary bile acids, unlike UDCA, down-regulate cholesterol 7α-hydroxylase, the rate-limiting enzyme for bile acid synthesis, thereby limiting further production and accumulation of hepatotoxic atypical bile acids. Also, primary bile acids will facilitate the absorption of fats and fat-soluble vitamins by providing adequate intraluminal bile acid concentrations.

The earliest experience with feeding a primary bile acid was for the treatment of CTX,[56,57] even though this is not a condition that is manifest as liver disease. Long-term treatment with chenodeoxycholic acid (750 mg/d) normalized plasma cholestanol concentrations,[56,461] markedly reduced the urinary excretion of bile alcohols,[2,57,348] and improved the clinical condition.[461-463] Similar suppression of endogenous synthesis of cholestanol and bile alcohols occurs with cholic acid and deoxycholic acid administration.[57] UDCA, which is unable to down-regulate cholesterol 7α-hydroxylase, is ineffective in CTX.[57,461] The improvement in the biochemical and clinical status of CTX patients treated with chenodeoxycholic acid is the result of marked suppression in endogenous bile acid synthesis mediated by the negative feedback on hepatic cholesterol 7α-hydroxylase and HMG-CoA reductase, the latter enzyme being rate controlling for cholesterol synthesis. Treatment of these patients may be more effective if bile acid is combined with an HMG-CoA reductase inhibitor because this combination has a greater effect in lowering plasma cholestanol.[464,465]

Oral bile acid therapy was found to be an effective means of treating patients with the 3β-hydroxy-C_{27}-steroid oxidoreductase (Figure 55.4-16) and the Δ^4-3-oxosteroid 5β-reductase deficiencies.[58,60,466] The first patient diagnosed with the 3β-hydroxy-C_{27}-steroid oxidoreductase deficiency was treated with chenodeoxycholic acid (125–250 mg/d), with remarkable results.[60] Serum liver enzymes and bilirubin normalized, and there was an improvement in clinical symptoms. However, one concern with chenodeoxycholic acid therapy, particularly for patients with liver disease, is that it can cause increases in serum transaminases and symptoms of diarrhea, as was documented when it was used for gallstone dissolution. For patients with preexisting liver disease, chenodeoyxcholic acid alone is a less desirable option. We subsequently chose to treat patients with cholic and ursodeoxycholic acids in combination or with cholic acid alone. The therapeutic dose of bile acid is somewhat empiric and has been based on the ability to significantly suppress the continued production of the atypical bile acids that are monitored by LSIMS. In general, the dose administered is in the range of 10 to 15 mg/kg body weight/d. UDCA has proven helpful for some patients with the 3β-hydroxy-C_{27}-steroid oxidase deficiency, lowering serum transaminases and improving liver histology.[59] However, it does not suppress the synthesis of atypical 3β-hydroxy-Δ^5 bile acids, which, over the long term, is important given that these bile acids are cholestatic and interfere with canalicular bile acid transport.[15,372] When UDCA was used in combination with cholic acid, it was our experience that the effectiveness of cholic acid in down-regulating endogenous bile acid synthesis was reduced, and this we believe is because UDCA during its enterohepatic recycling competitively inhibits the ileal uptake of cholic acid. Based on our experiences to date, we recommended that these patients be treated with cholic acid alone.

We have learned that it is almost impossible to completely shut down hepatic bile acid synthesis by feeding orally primary bile acids. Nevertheless, significant down-regulation occurs, sufficient to markedly reduce the signature atypical metabolites of the inborn error. Concomitant with this effect is an improvement in liver function tests, clinical symptoms, and liver histology.[373] In several patients, significant morphologic changes in the fine ultrastructure were noted. Electron micrographs of the canaliculi of patients with the Δ^4-3-oxosteroid 5β-reductase indicate significant abnormalities, including a loss of the usual microvillus structure and electron-dense material within and around the canaliculi. After bile acid therapy, electron microscopy showed a normalization in morphology with a disappearance of the electron-dense material,[373] suggesting that a threshold level of primary bile acids may be essential for normal morphologic development of canalicular structure.

The success of this therapeutic approach for patients with these two defects[58-60,466] is evident from the few treatment failures, and several patients have avoided the need for orthotopic liver transplant even though they were waitlisted for a donor liver. One notable failure was the treatment of the only patient found to have a mutation in the oxysterol 7α-hydroxylase gene.[9] Cholic acid therapy was unable to down-regulate the synthesis of the oxysterols and hepatotoxic 3β-hydroxy-Δ^5-monohydroxy bile acids, and this patient eventually underwent transplant.[9] Although cholic acid treatment should be considered potentially beneficial for patients with an oxysterol 7α-hydroxylase deficiency because it will provide a pool of primary bile acid, it is crucial to concomitantly inhibit the sterol 27-hydroxylase to protect the liver from the toxicity of the monohydroxy bile acids that are synthesized.

Oral bile acid therapy has been used to treat the liver disease associated with some of the peroxisomal disorders affecting side-chain oxidation of bile acids. Its success, however, has been hampered by the multiorgan involvement of these conditions, but it can be helpful in managing some of the symptoms of the disease. Peroxisomal proliferating drugs such as clofibrate[467,468] have proved to be of no therapeutic value. The progressive liver disease in peroxisomopathies is probably the result of the increased synthesis and accumulation of C_{27} bile acids combined with reduced primary bile acid synthesis. Infusion of tauro-THCA in rats, for example, has been shown to induce red cell hemolysis and to produce hepatic lesions showing mitochondrial disruptions similar to those found in patients with Zellweger syndrome.[469] Down-regulation in endogenous synthesis of C_{27} bile acids, as occurs with primary bile acid administration, was found to improve serum liver enzymes and bilirubin in one patient with Zellweger syndrome, even though

the patient eventually succumbed with pulmonary failure.[470] Liver histology showed a reduction in the extent of bile duct proliferation and inflammation, and a significant improvement in neurologic symptoms occurred after initiating bile acid therapy with cholic acid.[470] It is probable that cholic acid may be of greater benefit to patients with single-enzyme defects involving bile acid synthesis by preventing liver disease in the longer term. One patient with the 2-methylacyl-CoA racemase deficiency has now been on therapy for 7 years, and this has served to correct the abnormally low serum fat-soluble vitamin levels.

Finally, what can be offered to patients with a bile acid conjugation (amidation) defect?[11] In these cases, they are able to make unconjugated bile acids, mostly cholic acid, yet they fail to absorb fat-soluble vitamins. Restoring the conjugated bile acid pool seems logical, and this is possible by administration of a conjugated bile acid such as taurocholate or glycocholate. Alternatively, cholylsarcosine may also be helpful because this has been shown to improve fat absorption in a patient with short-bowel syndrome.[471] The limited availability of these primary bile acids and their conjugated forms remains a major problem that needs to be addressed for the clinic.

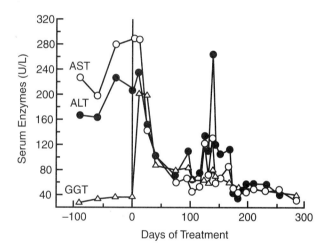

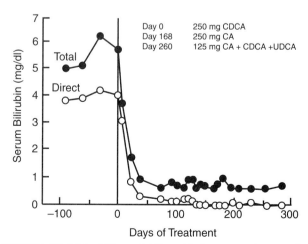

FIGURE 55.4-16   Effect of bile acid therapy on serum liver enzymes and bilirubin concentrations in a patient with a 3β-hydroxy-C_{27}-steroid oxidoreductase deficiency. ALT = alanine transaminase; AST = aspartate transaminase; GGT = γ-glutamyl transpeptidase.

SUMMARY

Inborn errors in bile acid synthesis represent a specific category of metabolic liver disease. These disorders have a significant effect on gastrointestinal physiology and function because of the key role that bile acids play in maintaining the enterohepatic circulation and in facilitating the absorption of fats and fat-soluble vitamins. At the Cincinnati Children's Hospital Medical Center, almost 4,000 cases of idiopathic liver disease have been screened in the last 15 years for bile acid synthetic defects, and more than 100 patients have been identified with defects, accounting for 2 to 3% of the cases of unexplained liver disease in infants and children. Early diagnosis is important because the liver disease and fat-soluble vitamin malabsorption associated with these inborn errors can be successfully treated medically, thereby avoiding the only alternative of orthotopic liver transplant in what are otherwise progressive and fatal conditions when undiagnosed or untreated.

REFERENCES

1. Setchell KDR, Kritchevsky D, Nair PP. The bile acids: methods and applications. New York: Plenum Press; 1988.
2. Setchell KDR, Street JM. Inborn errors of bile acid synthesis. Semin Liver Dis 1987;7:85–99.
3. Russell DW, Setchell KDR. Bile acid biosynthesis. Biochemistry 1992;31:4737–49.
4. Setchell KDR, O'Connell NC. Inborn errors of bile acid metabolism. In: Suchy FJ, editor. Liver disease in children. St. Louis: Mosby-Yearbook, Inc.; 1994. p. 835–51.
5. Setchell KDR. Disorders of bile acid synthesis and metabolism. In: Walker WA, Durie PR, Hamilton JR, et al, editors. Pediatric gastrointestinal disease. Pathophysiology, diagnosis, management. Toronto/Phildelphia: BC Decker Inc.; 1996.
6. Clayton PT, Leonard JV, Lawson AM, et al. Familial giant cell hepatitis associated with synthesis of 3 beta, 7 alpha-dihydroxy-and 3 beta,7 alpha, 12 alpha-trihydroxy-5-cholenoic acids. J Clin Invest 1987;79:1031–8.
7. Setchell KDR, Suchy FJ, Welsh MB, et al. Delta 4-3-oxosteroid 5 beta-reductase deficiency described in identical twins with neonatal hepatitis. A new inborn error in bile acid synthesis. J Clin Invest 1988;82:2148–57.
8. Shneider BL, Setchell KDR, Whitington PF, et al. Delta 4-3-oxosteroid 5 beta-reductase deficiency causing neonatal liver failure and hemochromatosis. J Pediatr 1994;124:234–8.
9. Setchell KDR, Schwarz M, O'Connell NC, et al. Identification of a new inborn error in bile acid synthesis: mutation of the oxysterol 7alpha-hydroxylase gene causes severe neonatal liver disease. J Clin Invest 1998;102:1690–703.
10. Setchell KDR, O'Connell NC, Squires RH, Heubi JE. Congenital defects in bile acid synthesis cause a spectrum of diseases manifest as severe cholestasis, neurological disease, and fat-soluble vitamin malabsorption. In: Northfield TC, Ahmed H, Jazwari R, Zentler-Munro P, editors. Bile acids in hepatobiliary disease. Dordrecht: Kluwer Academic Publishers; 1999. p. 55–63.
11. Setchell KDR, Heubi JE, O'Connell NC, et al. Identification of a unique inborn error in bile acid conjugation involving a deficiency in amidation. In: Paumgartner G, Stiehl A, Gerok W, editors. Bile acids in hepatobiliary diseases: basic research and clinical application. Dordrecht/Boston/London: Kluwer Academic Publishers; 1997. p. 43–7.
12. Clayton PT, Johnson AW, Mills KA, et al. Ataxia associated with increased plasma concentrations of pristanic acid, phytanic acid and C_{27} bile acids but normal fibroblast branched-chain fatty acid oxidation. J Inherit Metab Dis 1996;19:761–8.
13. Setchell KDR, Heubi JE, Bove KE, et al. Liver disease caused by failure to racemize trihydroxycholestanoic acid: gene mutation and effect of bile acid therapy. Gastroenterology 2003;124:217–32.
14. Boyer JL. New concepts of mechanisms of hepatocyte bile formation. Physiol Rev 1980;60:303–26.
15. Stieger B, Zhang J, O'Neill B, et al. Transport of taurine conjugates of 7alpha-hydroxy-3-oxo-4-cholenoic acid and 3beta,7alpha-dihydroxy-5-cholenoic acid in rat liver plasma membrane vesicles. In: Van Berge-Henegouwen GP, Van Hock B, De Groote J, et al, editors. Cholestatic liver diseases. Dordrecht/Boston/London: Kluwer Academic Press; 1994. p. 82–7.
16. Klyne W. The chemistry of the steroids. London: Methuen and Co., Ltd.; 1957.
17. Haslewood GAD. The biological importance of bile salts. Amsterdam: North Holland Publishing Co.; 1978.
18. Elliott WH. Allo bile acids. In: Nair PP, Kritchevsky D, editors. The bile acids: chemistry, physiology and metabolism. New York: Plenum Press; 1971. p. 47–93.
19. Bjorkhem I. Mechanism of bile acid biosynthesis in mammalian liver. In: Danielsson H, Sjovall J, editors. Sterols and bile acids. Amsterdam: BV Elsevier Science Publishers; 1985. p. 231–77.
20. Lester R, St. Pyrek J, Little JM, Adcock EW. Diversity of bile acids in the fetus and newborn infant. J Pediatr Gastroenterol Nutr 1983;2:355–64.
21. Setchell KDR, Dumaswala R, Colombo C, Ronchi M. Hepatic bile acid metabolism during early development revealed from the analysis of human fetal gallbladder bile. J Biol Chem 1988;263:16637–44.
22. Hofmann AF, Sjovall J, Kurz G, et al. A proposed nomenclature for bile acids. J Lipid Res 1992;33:599–604.
23. Sjovall J. Dietary glycine and taurine conjugation in man. Proc Soc Exp Biol Med 1959;100:676–8.
24. Back P, Spaczynski K, Gerok W. Bile-salt glucuronides in urine. Hoppe Seylers Z Physiol Chem 1974;355:749–52.
25. Shattuck KE, Radominska-Pyrek A, Zimniak P, et al. Metabolism of 24-norlithocholic acid in the rat: formation of hydroxyl- and carboxyl-linked glucuronides and effect on bile flow. Hepatology 1986;6:869–73.
26. Palmer RH. The formation of bile acid sulfates: a new pathway of bile acid metabolism in humans. Proc Natl Acad Sci U S A 1967;58:1047–50.
27. Matern H, Matern S. Formation of bile acid glucosides and dolichyl phosphoglucose by microsomal glucosyltransferases in liver, kidney and intestine of man. Biochim Biophys Acta 1987;921:1–6.
28. Marschall HU, Egestad B, Matern H, et al. Evidence for bile acid glucosides as normal constituents in human urine. FEBS Lett 1987;213:411–4.
29. Marschall HU, Egestad B, Matern H, et al. N-Acetylglucosaminides. A new type of bile acid conjugate in man. J Biol Chem 1989;264:12989–93.
30. Sweeny DJ, Barnes S, Heggie GD, Diasio RB. Metabolism of 5-fluorouracil to an N-cholyl-2-fluoro-beta-alanine conjugate: previously unrecognized role for bile acids in drug conjugation. Proc Natl Acad Sci U S A 1987;84:5439–43.
31. LaRusso NF, Korman MG, Hoffman NE, Hofmann AF. Dynamics of the enterohepatic circulation of bile acids. Postprandial serum concentrations of conjugates of cholic acid in health,

cholecystectomized patients, and patients with bile acid malabsorption. N Engl J Med 1974;291:689–92.

32. Setchell KDR, Street JM, Sjovall J. Fecal bile acids. In: Setchell KDR, Kritchevsky D, Nair PP, editors. The bile acids: methods and applications. New York: Plenum Press; 1988. p. 441–570.

33. Axelson M, Sjovall J. Potential bile acid precursors in plasma—possible indicators of biosynthetic pathways to cholic and chenodeoxycholic acids in man. J Steroid Biochem 1990; 36:631–40.

34. Axelson M, Shoda J, Sjovall J, et al. Cholesterol is converted to 7 alpha-hydroxy-3-oxo-4-cholestenoic acid in liver mitochondria. Evidence for a mitochondrial sterol 7 alpha-hydroxylase. J Biol Chem 1992;267:1701–4.

35. Javitt NB. Bile acid synthesis from cholesterol: regulatory and auxiliary pathways. FASEB J 1994;8:1308–11.

36. Vlahcevic ZR, Stravitz RT, Heuman DM, et al. Quantitative estimations of the contribution of different bile acid pathways to total bile acid synthesis in the rat. Gastroenterology 1997;113:1949–57.

37. Schwarz M, Lund EG, Setchell KDR, et al. Disruption of cholesterol 7alpha-hydroxylase gene in mice. II. Bile acid deficiency is overcome by induction of oxysterol 7alpha-hydroxylase. J Biol Chem 1996;271:18024–31.

38. Babiker A, Andersson O, Lindblom D, et al. Elimination of cholesterol as cholestenoic acid in human lung by sterol 27-hydroxylase: evidence that most of this steroid in the circulation is of pulmonary origin. J Lipid Res 1999;40:1417–25.

39. Bjorkhem I, Andersson O, Diczfalusy U, et al. Atherosclerosis and sterol 27-hydroxylase: evidence for a role of this enzyme in elimination of cholesterol from human macrophages. Proc Natl Acad Sci U S A 1994;91:8592–6.

40. Reiss AB, Martin KO, Javitt NB, et al. Sterol 27-hydroxylase: high levels of activity in vascular endothelium. J Lipid Res 1994;35:1026–30.

41. Stapleton G, Steel M, Richardson M, et al. A novel cytochrome P450 expressed primarily in brain. J Biol Chem 1995;270:29739–45.

42. Zhang J, Akwa Y, Baulieu EE, Sjovall J. 7 Alpha-hydroxylation of 27-hydroxycholesterol in rat brain microsomes. C R Acad Sci III 1995;318:345–9.

43. Babiker A, Andersson O, Lund E, et al. Elimination of cholesterol in macrophages and endothelial cells by the sterol 27-hydroxylase mechanism. Comparison with high density lipoprotein-mediated reverse cholesterol transport. J Biol Chem 1997;272:26253–61.

44. Lund E, Andersson O, Zhang J, et al. Importance of a novel oxidative mechanism for elimination of intracellular cholesterol in humans. Arterioscler Thromb Vasc Biol 1996;16:208–12.

45. Zhang J, Larsson O, Sjovall J. 7 alpha-Hydroxylation of 25-hydroxycholesterol and 27-hydroxycholesterol in human fibroblasts. Biochim Biophys Acta 1995;1256:353–9.

46. Danielsson H, Einarsson K. Further studies on the formation of the bile acids in the guinea pig. Acta Chem Scand 1964; 18:831–2.

47. Myant NB, Mitropoulos KA. Cholesterol 7 alpha-hydroxylase. J Lipid Res 1977;18:135–53.

48. Pandak WM, Li YC, Chiang JY, et al. Regulation of cholesterol 7 alpha-hydroxylase mRNA and transcriptional activity by taurocholate and cholesterol in the chronic biliary diverted rat. J Biol Chem 1991;266:3416–21.

49. Danielsson H, Einarsson K, Johansson G. Effect of biliary drainage on individual reactions in the conversion of cholesterol to taurochlic acid. Bile acids and steroids 180. Eur J Biochem 1967;2:44–9.

50. Vlahcevic ZR, Heuman DM, Hylemon PB. Regulation of bile acid synthesis. Hepatology 1991;13:590–600.

51. Shefer S, Nguyen LB, Salen G, et al. Regulation of cholesterol 7 alpha-hydroxylase by hepatic 7 alpha-hydroxylated bile acid flux and newly synthesized cholesterol supply. J Biol Chem 1991;266:2693–6.

52. Heuman DM, Vlahcevic ZR, Bailey ML, Hylemon PB. Regulation of bile acid synthesis. II. Effect of bile acid feeding on enzymes regulating hepatic cholesterol and bile acid synthesis in the rat. Hepatology 1988;8:892–7.

53. Thomason JC, Vars HM. Biliary excretion of cholic acid and cholesterol in hyper-, hypo- and euthyroid rats. Proc Soc Exp Biol Med 1953;83:246–8.

54. Eriksson S. Biliary excretion of bile acids and cholesterol in bile fistula rats; bile acids and steroids. Proc Soc Exp Biol Med 1957;94:578–82.

55. Bergstrom S, Danielsson H. On the regulation of bile acid formation in the rat liver. Acta Physiol Scand 1958;43:1–7.

56. Salen G, Meriwether TW, Nicolau G. Chenodeoxycholic acid inhibits increased cholesterol and cholestanol synthesis in patients with cerebrotendinous xanthomatosis. Biochem Med 1975;14:57–74.

57. Koopman BJ, Wolthers BG, van der Molen JC, Waterreus RJ. Bile acid therapies applied to patients suffering from cerebrotendinous xanthomatosis. Clin Chim Acta 1985;152:115–22.

58. Setchell KDR, Flick R, Watkins JB, Piccoli DA. Chronic hepatitis in a 10 yr old due to an inborn error in bile acid synthesis—diagnosis and treatment with oral bile acid. Gastroenterology 1990;98:A578.

59. Jacquemin E, Setchell KD, O'Connell NC, et al. A new cause of progressive intrahepatic cholestasis: 3 beta-hydroxy-C27-steroid dehydrogenase/isomerase deficiency. J Pediatr 1994;125:379–84.

60. Ichimiya H, Egestad B, Nazer H, et al. Bile acids and bile alcohols in a child with hepatic 3 beta-hydroxy-delta 5-C27-steroid dehydrogenase deficiency: effects of chenodeoxycholic acid treatment. J Lipid Res 1991;32:829–41.

61. Goldstein JL, Brown MS. Regulation of the mevalonate pathway. Nature 1990;343:425–30.

62. Danielsson H. Relationship between diurnal variations in biosynthesis of cholesterol and bile acids. Steroids 1972;20: 63–72.

63. Mitropoulos KA, Balasubramaniam S, Gibbons GF, Reeves BE. Diurnal variation in the activity of cholesterol 7-hydroxylase in the livers of fed and fasted rats. FEBS Lett 1972;27:203–6.

64. Duane WC, Levitt DG, Mueller SM, Behrens JC. Regulation of bile acid synthesis in man. Presence of a diurnal rhythm. J Clin Invest 1983;72:1930–6.

65. Pooler PA, Duane WC. Effects of bile acid administration on bile acid synthesis and its circadian rhythm in man. Hepatology 1988;8:1140–6.

66. Shefer S, Hauser S, Bekersky I, Mosbach EH. Biochemical site of regulation of bile acid biosynthesis in the rat. J Lipid Res 1970;11:404–11.

67. Andersson S, Bostrom H, Danielsson H, Wikvall K. Purification from rabbit and rat liver of cytochromes P-450 involved in bile acid biosynthesis. Methods Enzymol 1985; 111:364–77.

68. Noshiro M, Nishimoto M, Morohashi K, Okuda K. Molecular cloning of cDNA for cholesterol 7 alpha-hydroxylase from rat liver microsomes. Nucleotide sequence and expression. FEBS Lett 1989;257:97–100.

69. Noshiro M, Okuda K. Molecular cloning and sequence analysis of cDNA encoding human cholesterol 7 alpha-hydroxylase. FEBS Lett 1990;268:137–40.

70. Jelinek DF, Andersson S, Slaughter CA, Russell DW. Cloning and regulation of cholesterol 7 alpha-hydroxylase, the rate-limiting enzyme in bile acid biosynthesis. J Biol Chem 1990;265:8190–7.

71. Pandak WM, Heuman DM, Redford K, et al. Hormonal regulation of cholesterol 7alpha-hydroxylase specific activity, mRNA levels, and transcriptional activity in vivo in the rat. J Lipid Res 1997;38:2483–91.

72. Goodart SA, Huynh C, Chen W, et al. Expression of the human cholesterol 7alpha-hydroxylase gene in transgenic mice. Biochem Biophys Res Commun 1999;266:454–9.

73. Crestani M, Sadeghpour A, Stroup D, et al. Transcriptional activation of the cholesterol 7alpha-hydroxylase gene (CYP7A) by nuclear hormone receptors. J Lipid Res 1998;39:2192–200.

74. Rudling M, Parini P, Angelin B. Growth hormone and bile acid synthesis. Key role for the activity of hepatic microsomal cholesterol 7alpha-hydroxylase in the rat. J Clin Invest 1997;99:2239–45.

75. Arnon R, Yoshimura T, Reiss A, et al. Cholesterol 7-hydroxylase knockout mouse: a model for monohydroxy bile acid-related neonatal cholestasis. Gastroenterology 1998;115:1223–8.

76. Ishibashi S, Schwarz M, Frykman PK, et al. Disruption of cholesterol 7alpha-hydroxylase gene in mice. I. Postnatal lethality reversed by bile acid and vitamin supplementation. J Biol Chem 1996;271:18017–23.

77. Gustafsson J. Bile acid biosynthesis during development: hydroxylation of C27-sterols in human fetal liver. J Lipid Res 1986;27:801–6.

78. Collins JC, Altman RP, Martin KO, Javitt NB. Bile acid synthesis in fetal and neonatal life: expression of cholesterol 7alpha-hydroxylase and 27-hydroxycholesterol-7alpha-hydroxylase activities. Pediatr Res 1994;35:126A.

79. Gustafsson JA. Seeking ligands for lonely orphan receptors. Science 1999;284:1285–6.

80. Russell DW. Nuclear orphan receptors control cholesterol catabolism. Cell 1999;97:539–42.

81. Kliewer SA, Lehmann JM, Willson TM. Orphan nuclear receptors: shifting endocrinology into reverse. Science 1999;284:757–60.

82. Setchell KDR, Rodrigues CMP, Clerici C, et al. Bile acid concentrations in human and rat liver tissue and in hepatocyte nuclei. Gastroenterology 1997;112:226–35.

83. Peet DJ, Turley SD, Ma W, et al. Cholesterol and bile acid metabolism are impaired in mice lacking the nuclear oxysterol receptor LXR alpha. Cell 1998;93:693–704.

84. Nitta M, Ku S, Brown C, et al. CPF: an orphan nuclear receptor that regulates liver-specific expression of the human cholesterol 7alpha-hydroxylase gene. Proc Natl Acad Sci U S A 1999;96:6660–5.

85. Janowski BA, Willy PJ, Devi TR, et al. An oxysterol signalling pathway mediated by the nuclear receptor LXR alpha. Nature 1996;383:728–31.

86. Forman BM, Ruan B, Chen J, et al. The orphan nuclear receptor LXRalpha is positively and negatively regulated by distinct products of mevalonate metabolism. Proc Natl Acad Sci U S A 1997;94:10588–93.

87. Lehmann JM, McKee DD, Watson MA, et al. The human orphan nuclear receptor PXR is activated by compounds that regulate CYP3A4 gene expression and cause drug interactions. J Clin Invest 1998;102:1016–23.

88. Makishima M, Okamoto AY, Repa JJ, et al. Identification of a nuclear receptor for bile acids. Science 1999;284:1362–5.

89. Sinal CJ, Tohkin M, Miyata M, et al. Targeted disruption of the nuclear receptor FXR/BAR impairs bile acid and lipid homeostasis. Cell 2000;102:731–44.

90. Parks DJ, Blanchard SG, Bledsoe RK, et al. Bile acids: natural ligands for an orphan nuclear receptor. Science 1999;284:1365–8.

91. Wang H, Chen J, Hollister K, et al. Endogenous bile acids are ligands for the nuclear receptor FXR/BAR. Mol Cell 1999;3:543–53.

92. Green K, Samuelsson B. Mechanisms of bile acid biosynthesis studies with 3alpha-H3 and 4beta-H3-cholesterol. J Biol Chem 1964;239:2804–8.

93. Bjorkhem I. On the mechanism of the enzymatic conversion of cholest-5-ene-3-beta, 7-alpha-diol into 7-alpha-hydroxy-cholest-4-en-3-one. Eur J Biochem 1969;8:337–44.

94. Wikvall K. Purification and properties of a 3 beta-hydroxy-delta 5-C27-steroid oxidoreductase from rabbit liver microsomes. J Biol Chem 1981;256:3376–80.

95. Furster C, Zhang J, Toll A. Purification of a 3beta-hydroxy-delta5-C27-steroid dehydrogenase from pig liver microsomes active in major and alternative pathways of bile acid biosynthesis. J Biol Chem 1996;271:20903–7.

96. Schwarz M, Wright AC, Davis DL, et al. Expression cloning of 3β-hydroxy-Δ^5-C$_{27}$-steroid oxidoreductase gene of bile acid synthesis and its mutation in progressive intrahepatic cholestasis. J Clin Invest 2000;79:1031–8.

97. Cheng JB, Jacquemin E, Gerhardt M, et al. Molecular genetics of 3β-hydroxy-Δ^5-C$_{27}$-steroid oxidoreductase deficiency in 16 patients with loss of bile acid synthesis and liver disease. J Clin Endocrinol Metab 2003;88:1833–41.

98. The VL, Lachance Y, Labrie C, et al. Full length cDNA structure and deduced amino acid sequence of human 3 beta-hydroxy-5-ene steroid dehydrogenase. Mol Endocrinol 1989;3:1310–2.

99. Zhao HF, Simard J, Labrie C, et al. Molecular cloning, cDNA structure and predicted amino acid sequence of bovine 3 beta-hydroxy-5-ene steroid dehydrogenase/delta 5-delta 4 isomerase. FEBS Lett 1989;259:153–7.

100. Zhao HF, Labrie C, Simard J, et al. Characterization of rat 3 beta-hydroxysteroid dehydrogenase/delta 5-delta 4 isomerase cDNAs and differential tissue-specific expression of the corresponding mRNAs in steroidogenic and peripheral tissues. J Biol Chem 1991;266:583–93.

101. Lorence MC, Murry BA, Trant JM, Mason JI. Human 3 beta-hydroxysteroid dehydrogenase/delta 5—4isomerase from placenta: expression in nonsteroidogenic cells of a protein that catalyzes the dehydrogenation/isomerization of C21 and C19 steroids. Endocrinology 1990;126:2493–8.

102. Buchmann MS, Kvittingen EA, Nazer H, et al. Lack of 3 beta-hydroxy-delta 5-C27-steroid dehydrogenase/isomerase in fibroblasts from a child with urinary excretion of 3 beta-hydroxy-delta 5-bile acids. A new inborn error of metabolism. J Clin Invest 1990;86:2034–7.

103. Ishida H, Noshiro M, Okuda K, Coon MJ. Purification and characterization of 7 alpha-hydroxy-4-cholesten-3-one 12 alpha-hydroxylase. J Biol Chem 1992;267:21319–23.

104. Eggertsen G, Olin M, Andersson U, et al. Molecular cloning and expression of rabbit sterol 12alpha-hydroxylase. J Biol Chem 1996;271:32269–75.

105. Gafvels M, Olin M, Chowdhary BP, et al. Structure and chromosomal assignment of the sterol 12alpha-hydroxylase gene (CYP8B1) in human and mouse: eukaryotic cytochrome P-450 gene devoid of introns. Genomics 1999;56:184–96.

106. Mitropoulos KA, Suzuki M, Myant NB, Danielsson H. Effects of thyroidectomy and thyroxine treatment on the activity of 12alpha-hydroxylase and of some components of microsomal electron transfer chains in rat liver. FEBS Lett 1968;1:13–5.

107. Bjorkhem I, Danielsson H, Gustafsson J. On the effect of thyroid hormone on 26-hydroxylation of C 27-steroids in rat liver. FEBS Lett 1973;31:20–2.

108. Vlahcevic ZR, Eggertsen G, Bjorkhem I, et al. Regulation of sterol 12α-hydroxylase and cholic acid biosynthesis in the rat. Gastroenterology 2000;118:599–607.

109. Danielsson H. Influence of dietary bile acids on formation of bile acids in rat. Steroids 1973;22:667–76.

110. Ahlberg J, Angelin B, Bjorkhem I, et al. Effects of treatment with chenodeoxycholic acid on liver microsomal metabolism of steroids in man. J Lab Clin Med 1980;95:188–94.

111. Angelin B, Bjorkhem I, Einarsson K, Ewerth S. Cholestyramine treatment reduces postprandial but not fasting serum bile acid levels in humans. Gastroenterology 1982;83:1097–101.

112. Johansson G. Effect of cholestyramine and diet on hydroxylations in the biosynthesis and metabolism of bile acids. Eur J Biochem 1970;17:292–5.

113. Bjorkhem I, Eriksson M, Einarsson K. Evidence for a lack of regulatory importance of the 12 alpha-hydroxylase in formation of bile acids in man: an in vivo study. J Lipid Res 1983;24:1451–6.

114. Berseus O. Conversion of cholesterol to bile acids in rat: purification and properties of a delta-4-3-ketosteroid 5-beta-reductase and a 3-alpha-hydroxysteroid dehydrogenase. Eur J Biochem 1967;2:493–502.

115. Berseus O, Bjorkhem I. Enzymatic conversion of a delta-4-3-ketosteroid into a 3-alpha-hydroxy-5-beta steroid: mechanism and stereochemistry of hydrogen transfer from NADPH. Bile acids and steroids 190. Eur J Biochem 1967;2:503–7.

116. Okuda A, Okuda K. Purification and characterization of delta 4-3-ketosteroid 5 beta-reductase. J Biol Chem 1984;259:7519–24.

117. Kondo KH, Kai MH, Setoguchi Y, et al. Cloning and expression of cDNA of human delta 4-3-oxosteroid 5 beta-reductase and substrate specificity of the expressed enzyme. Eur J Biochem 1994;219:357–63.

118. Onishi Y, Noshiro M, Shimosato T, Okuda K. delta 4-3-Oxosteroid 5 beta-reductase. Structure and function. Biol Chem Hoppe Seyler 1991;372:1039–49.

119. Onishi Y, Noshiro M, Shimosato T, Okuda K. Molecular cloning and sequence analysis of cDNA encoding delta 4-3-ketosteroid 5 beta-reductase of rat liver. FEBS Lett 1991;283:215–8.

120. Axelson M, Bjorkhem I, Reihner E, Einarsson K. The plasma level of 7 alpha-hydroxy-4-cholesten-3-one reflects the activity of hepatic cholesterol 7 alpha-hydroxylase in man. FEBS Lett 1991;284:216–8.

121. Clayton PT, Patel E, Lawson AM, et al. 3-Oxo-delta 4 bile acids in liver disease [letter]. Lancet 1988;i:1283–4.

122. Penning TM, Abrams WR, Pawlowski JE. Affinity labeling of 3 alpha-hydroxysteroid dehydrogenase with 3 alpha-bromoacetoxyandrosterone and 11 alpha-bromoacetoxyprogesterone. Isolation and sequence of active site peptides containing reactive cysteines; sequence confirmation using nucleotide sequence from a cDNA clone. J Biol Chem 1991;266:8826–34.

123. Cheng KC, White PC, Qin KN. Molecular cloning and expression of rat liver 3 alpha-hydroxysteroid dehydrogenase. Mol Endocrinol 1991;5:823–8.

124. Pawlowski JE, Huizinga M, Penning TM. Cloning and sequencing of the cDNA for rat liver 3 alpha-hydroxysteroid/dihydrodiol dehydrogenase. J Biol Chem 1991;266:8820–5.

125. Stolz A, Rahimi-Kiani M, Ameis D, et al. Molecular structure of rat hepatic 3 alpha-hydroxysteroid dehydrogenase. A member of the oxidoreductase gene family. J Biol Chem 1991;266:15253–7.

126. Stolz A, Takikawa H, Sugiyama Y, et al. 3 alpha-Hydroxysteroid dehydrogenase activity of the Y′ bile acid binders in rat liver cytosol. Identification, kinetics, and physiologic significance. J Clin Invest 1987;79:427–34.

127. Takikawa H, Stolz A, Kaplowitz N. Cyclical oxidation-reduction of the C3 position on bile acids catalyzed by rat hepatic 3 alpha-hydroxysteroid dehydrogenase. I. Studies with the purified enzyme, isolated rat hepatocytes, and inhibition by indomethacin. J Clin Invest 1987;80:852–60.

128. Su P, Rennert H, Shayiq RM, et al. A cDNA encoding a rat mitochondrial cytochrome P450 catalyzing both the 26-hydroxylation of cholesterol and 25-hydroxylation of vitamin D3: gonadotropic regulation of the cognate mRNA in ovaries. DNA Cell Biol 1990;9:657–67.

129. Wikvall K. Hydroxylations in biosynthesis of bile acids. Isolation of a cytochrome P-450 from rabbit liver mitochondria catalyzing 26-hydroxylation of C27-steroids. J Biol Chem 1984;259:3800–4.

130. Akiyoshi-Shibata M, Usui E, Sakaki T, et al. Expression of rat liver vitamin D3 25-hydroxylase cDNA in Saccharomyces cerevisiae. FEBS Lett 1991;280:367–70.

131. Bjorkhem I, Gustafsson J. Omega-hydroxylation of steroid side-chain in biosynthesis of bile acids. Eur J Biochem 1973;36:201–12.

132. Bjorkhem I, Gustafsson J. Mitochondrial omega-hydroxylation of cholesterol side chain. J Biol Chem 1974;249:2528–35.

133. Okuda K, Weber P, Ullrich V. Photochemical action spectrum of the co-inhibited 5beta-cholestane-3alpha, 7alpha, 12alpha-triol 26-hydroxylase system. Biochem Biophys Res Commun 1977;74:1071–6.

134. Dahlback H, Holmberg I. Oxidation of 5 beta-cholestane-3 alpha,7 alpha, 12 alpha-triol into 3 alpha,7 alpha,12 alpha-trihydroxy-5 beta-cholestanoic acid by cytochrome P-450(26) from rabbit liver mitochondria. Biochem Biophys Res Commun 1990;167:391–5.

135. Cronholm T, Johansson G. Oxidation of 5 beta-cholestane-3alpha, 7alpha, 12alpha-triol by rat liver microsomes. Eur J Biochem 1970;16:373–81.

136. Andersson S, Davis DL, Dahlback H, et al. Cloning, structure, and expression of the mitochondrial cytochrome P-450 sterol 26-hydroxylase, a bile acid biosynthetic enzyme. J Biol Chem 1989;264:8222–9.

137. Skrede S, Bjorkhem I, Kvittingen EA, et al. Demonstration of 26-hydroxylation of C27-steroids in human skin fibroblasts, and a deficiency of this activity in cerebrotendinous xanthomatosis. J Clin Invest 1986;78:729–35.

138. Usui E, Noshiro M, Okuda K. Molecular cloning of cDNA for vitamin D3 25-hydroxylase from rat liver mitochondria. FEBS Lett 1990;262:135–8.

139. Cali JJ, Russell DW. Characterization of human sterol 27-hydroxylase. A mitochondrial cytochrome P-450 that catalyzes multiple oxidation reaction in bile acid biosynthesis. J Biol Chem 1991;266:7774–8.

140. Araya Z, Sjoberg H, Wikvall K. Different effects on the expression of CYP7 and CYP27 in rabbit liver by cholic acid and cholestyramine. Biochem Biophys Res Commun 1995;216:868–73.

141. Xu G, Salen G, Shefer S, et al. Increasing dietary cholesterol induces different regulation of classic and alternative bile acid synthesis. J Clin Invest 1999;103:89–95.

142. Rao YP, Vlahcevic ZR, Stravitz RT, et al. Down-regulation of the rat hepatic sterol 27-hydroxylase gene by bile acids in transfected primary hepatocytes: possible role of hepatic nuclear factor 1alpha. J Steroid Biochem Mol Biol 1999;70:1–14.

143. Rosen H, Reshef A, Maeda N, et al. Markedly reduced bile acid synthesis but maintained levels of cholesterol and vitamin D metabolites in mice with disrupted sterol 27-hydroxylase gene. J Biol Chem 1998;273:14805–12.

144. Shefer S, Cheng FW, Dayal B, et al. A 25-hydroxylation pathway of cholic acid biosynthesis in man and rat. J Clin Invest 1976;57:897–903.

145. Duane WC, Bjorkhem I, Hamilton JN, Mueller SM. Quantitative importance of the 25-hydroxylation pathway for bile acid biosynthesis in the rat. Hepatology 1988;8:613–8.

146. Duane WC, Pooler PA, Hamilton JN. Bile acid synthesis in man. In vivo activity of the 25-hydroxylation pathway. J Clin Invest 1988;82:82–5.

147. Masui T, Herman R, Staple E. The oxidation of 5-beta-cholestane-3-alpha, 7-alpha, 12-alpha, 26-tetraol to 5-beta-cholestane-3-alpha, 7-alpha, 12-alpha-triol-26-oic acid via 5-beta-cholestane-3-alpha, 7-alpha, 12-alpha-triol-26-al by rat liver. Biochim Biophys Acta 1966;117:266–8.

148. Okuda K, Takigawa N. The dehydrogenation of 5 beta-cholestane-3-alpha, 7-alpha, 12-alpha, 26-tetrol by rat liver. Biochim Biophys Acta 1969;176:873–9.

149. Okuda K, Takigawa N. Separation of 5-beta-cholestane-3-alpha,7-alpha,12-alpha,26-tetrol oxidoreductase, and acetaldehyde-NAD oxidoreductase from the soluble fraction of rat liver by gel filtration. Biochim Biophys Res Commun 1968;33:788–93.

150. Okuda K, Takigawa N. Rat liver 5 beta-cholestane-3 alpha,7 alpha,12 alpha,26-tetrol dehydrogenase as a liver alcohol dehydrogenase. Biochim Biophys Acta 1970;220:141–8.

151. Okuda K, Higuchi E, Fukuba R. Horse liver 3,7,12-trihydroxy-5-cholestan-26-al dehydrogenase as a liver aldehyde dehydrogenase. Biochim Biophys Acta 1973;293:15–25.

152. Bjorkhem I. Mechanism of degradation of the steroid side chain in the formation of bile acids. J Lipid Res 1992;33:455–71.

153. Prydz K, Kase BF, Bjorkhem I, Pedersen JI. Subcellular localization of 3 alpha, 7 alpha-dihydroxy- and 3 alpha,7 alpha,12 alpha-trihydroxy-5 beta-cholestanoyl-coenzyme A ligase(s) in rat liver. J Lipid Res 1988;29:997–1004.

154. Schepers L, Casteels M, Verheyden K, et al. Subcellular distribution and characteristics of trihydroxycoprostanoyl-CoA synthetase in rat liver. Biochem J 1989;257:221–9.

155. Ferdinandusse S, Denis S, Clayton PT, et al. Mutations in the gene encoding peroxisomal 2-methyl-acyl racemase cause adult-onset sensory motor neuropathy. Nat Genet 2000;24:188–91.

156. Vanhove GF, Van Veldhoven PP, Fransen M, et al. The CoA esters of 2-methyl-branched chain fatty acids and of the bile acid intermediates di- and trihydroxycoprostanic acids are oxidized by one single peroxisomal branched chain acyl-CoA oxidase in human liver and kidney. J Biol Chem 1993;268:10335–44.

157. Masui T, Staple E. The formation of bile acids from cholesterol. The conversion of 5-beta-cholestane-3-alpha,7-alpha-triol-26-oic acid to cholic acid via 5-beta-cholestane-3-alpha,7-alpha,12-alpha, 24-xi-tetraol-26-oic acid I by rat liver. J Biol Chem 1966;241:3889–93.

158. Gustafsson J. Biosynthesis of cholic acid in rat liver. 24-Hydroxylation of 3alpha, 7alpha, 12alpha-trihydroxy-5beta-cholestanoic acid. J Biol Chem 1975;250:8243–7.

159. Baumgart E, Vanhooren JC, Fransen M, et al. Molecular cloning and further characterization of rat peroxisomal trihydroxy-coprostanoyl-CoA oxidase. Biochem J 1996;320:115–21.

160. Baumgart E, Vanhooren JC, Fransen M, et al. Mammalian peroxisomal acyl-CoA oxidases. II. Molecular characterization of rat trihydroxycoprostanoyl-CoA oxidase. Ann N Y Acad Sci 1996;804:676–7.

161. Baumgart E, Vanhooren JC, Fransen M, et al. Molecular characterization of the human peroxisomal branched-chain acyl-CoA oxidase: cDNA cloning, chromosomal assignment, tissue distribution, and evidence for the absence of the protein in Zellweger syndrome. Proc Natl Acad Sci U S A 1996;93:13748–53.

162. Pedersen JI, Eggertsen G, Hellman U, et al. Molecular cloning and expression of cDNA encoding 3alpha,7alpha,12alpha-trihydroxy-5beta-chole stanoyl-CoA oxidase from rabbit liver. J Biol Chem 1997;272:18481–9.

163. Schepers L, Van Veldhoven PP, Casteels M, et al. Presence of three acyl-CoA oxidases in rat liver peroxisomes. An inducible fatty acyl-CoA oxidase, a noninducible fatty acyl-CoA oxidase, and a noninducible trihydroxycoprostanoyl-CoA oxidase. J Biol Chem 1990;265:5242–6.

164. Kase F, Bjorkhem I, Pedersen JI. Formation of cholic acid from 3 alpha, 7 alpha, 12 alpha-trihydroxy-5 beta-cholestanoic acid by rat liver peroxisomes. J Lipid Res 1983;24:1560–7.

165. Dieuaide-Noubhani M, Novikov D, Vandekerckhove J, et al. Identification and characterization of the 2-enoyl-CoA hydratases involved in peroxisomal beta-oxidation in rat liver. Biochem J 1997;321:253–9.

166. Jiang LL, Kurosawa T, Sato M, et al. Physiological role of D-3-hydroxyacyl-CoA dehydratase/D-3-hydroxyacyl- CoA dehydrogenase bifunctional protein. J Biochem (Tokyo) 1997; 121:506–13.

167. Kurosawa T, Sato M, Yoshimura T, et al. Stereospecific formation of (24R,25R)-3 alpha,7 alpha,12 alpha,24-tetrahydroxy-5 beta-cholestan-26-oic acid catalyzed with a peroxisomal bifunctional D-3-hydroxyacyl-CoA dehydratase/D-3-hydroxy-acyl-CoA dehydrogenase. Biol Pharm Bull 1997;20:295–7.

168. Dieuaide-Noubhani M, Asselberghs S, Mannaerts GP, Van Veldhoven PP. Evidence that multifunctional protein 2, and not multifunctional protein 1, is involved in the peroxisomal beta-oxidation of pristanic acid. Biochem J 1997;325:367–73.

169. Kannenberg F, Ellinghaus P, Assmann G, Seedorf U. Aberrant oxidation of the cholesterol side chain in bile acid synthesis of sterol carrier protein-2/sterol carrier protein-x knockout mice. J Biol Chem 1999;274:35455–60.

170. Schram AW, Goldfischer S, van Roermund CW, et al. Human peroxisomal 3-oxoacyl-coenzyme A thiolase deficiency. Proc Natl Acad Sci U S A 1987;84:2494–6.

171. Antonenkov VD, Van Veldhoven PP, Waelkens E, Mannaerts GP. Substrate specificities of 3-oxoacyl-CoA thiolase A and sterol carrier protein 2/3-oxoacyl-CoA thiolase purified from normal rat liver peroxisomes. Sterol carrier protein 2/3-oxoacyl-CoA thiolase is involved in the metabolism of 2-methyl-branched fatty acids and bile acid intermediates. J Biol Chem 1997;272:26023–31.

172. Kase BF, Prydz K, Bjorkhem I, Pedersen JI. Conjugation of cholic acid with taurine and glycine by rat liver peroxisomes. Biochem Biophys Res Commun 1986;138:167–73.

173. Kase BF, Bjorkhem I. Peroxisomal bile acid-CoA:amino-acid N-acyltransferase in rat liver. J Biol Chem 1989;264:9220–3.

174. Killenberg PG. Measurement and subcellular distribution of choloyl-CoA synthetase and bile acid-CoA:amino acid N-acyltransferase activities in rat liver. J Lipid Res 1978;19:24–31.

175. Lim WC, Jordan TW. Subcellular distribution of hepatic bile acid-conjugating enzymes. Biochem J 1981;197:611–8.

176. Schersten T. The synthesis of taurocholic and glycocholic acids by preparations of human liver. I. Distribution of activity between subcellular fractions. Biochim Biophys Acta 1967;141:144–54.

177. Bremer J, Gloor V. Studies on the conjugation of cholic acid with taurine in cell subfractions. Acta Chem Scand 1955; 9:689–98.

178. Wheeler JB, Shaw DR, Barnes S. Purification and characterization of a rat liver bile acid coenzyme A ligase from rat liver microsomes. Arch Biochem Biophys 1997;348:15–24.

179. Vessey DA, Zakim D. Characterization of microsomal choloyl-coenzyme A synthetase. Biochem J 1977;163:357–62.

180. Kwakye JB, Johnson MR, Barnes S, et al. Identification of bile acid-CoA:amino acid N-acyltransferase in rat kidney. Biochem J 1991;280:821–4.

181. Falany CN, Xie X, Wheeler JB, et al. Molecular cloning and expression of rat liver bile acid CoA ligase. J Lipid Res 2002;43:2062–72.

182. Mallonee DH, Adams JL, Hylemon PB. The bile-acid-inducible baiB gene from Eubacterium sp. strain VPI 12708 encodes a bile acid-coenzyme A ligase. J Bacteriol 1992;174:2065–71.

183. Killenberg PG. Bile acid-CoA:amino acid N-acyltransferase. Methods Enzymol 1981;77:308–13.

184. Johnson MR, Barnes S, Kwakye JB, Diasio RB. Purification and characterization of bile acid-CoA:amino acid N-acyltransferase from human liver. J Biol Chem 1991;266:10227–33.

185. Kirkpatrick RB, Green MD, Hagey LR, et al. Effect of side chain length on bile acid conjugation: glucuronidation, sulfation and coenzyme A formation of nor-bile acids and their natural C24 homologs by human and rat liver fractions. Hepatology 1988;8:353–7.

186. Czuba B, Vessey DA. The effect of bile acid structure on the activity of bile acid- CoA:glycine/taurine-N-acetyltransferase. J Biol Chem 1982;257:8761–5.

187. Falany CN, Johnson MR, Barnes S, Diasio RB. Glycine and taurine conjugation of bile acids by a single enzyme. Molecular cloning and expression of human liver bile acid CoA:amino acid N-acyltransferase. J Biol Chem 1994;269:19375–9.

188. Falany CN, Fortinberry H, Leiter EH, Barnes S. Cloning, expression, and chromosomal localization of mouse liver bile acid CoA:amino acid N-acyltransferase. J Lipid Res 1997;38:1139–48.

189. Furutani M, Arii S, Higashitsuji H, et al. Reduced expression of kan-1 (encoding putative bile acid-CoA-amino acid N-acyltransferase) mRNA in livers of rats after partial hepatectomy and during sepsis. Biochem J 1995;311:203–8.

190. O'Maille ER, Richards TG, Short AH. Acute taurine depletion and maximal rates of hepatic conjugation and secretion of cholic acid in the dog. J Physiol (Lond) 1965;180:67–79.

191. O'Byrne J, Hunt MC, Rai DK, et al. The human bile acid-CoA:amino acid N-acyltransferase functions in the conjugation of fatty acids to glycine. J Biol Chem 2003;278:34237–44.

192. Lawson AM, Madigan MJ, Shortland D, Clayton PT. Rapid diagnosis of Zellweger syndrome and infantile Refsum's disease by fast atom bombardment–mass spectrometry of urine bile salts. Clin Chim Acta 1986;161:221–31.

193. Hardison WG. Hepatic taurine concentration and dietary taurine as regulators of bile acid conjugation with taurine. Gastroenterology 1978;75:71–5.

194. Sturman JA, Gaull GE. Taurine in the brain and liver of the developing human and monkey. J Neurochem 1975;25:831–5.

195. Stegink LD, Reynolds WA, Pitkin RM, Cruikshank DP. Placental transfer of taurine in the rhesus monkey. Am J Clin Nutr 1981;34:2685–92.

196. Hagey LR, Schteingart CD, Rossi SS, et al. An N-acyl glycyltaurine conjugate of deoxycholic acid in the biliary bile acids of the rabbit. J Lipid Res 1998;39:2119–24.

197. Back P. Bile acid glucuronides, II[1]. Isolation and identification of a chenodeoxycholic acid glucuronide from human plasma in intrahepatic cholestasis. Hoppe Seylers Z Physiol Chem 1976;357:213–7.

198. Alme B, Sjovall J. Analysis of bile acid glucuronides in urine. Identification of 3 alpha, 6 alpha, 12 alpha-trihydroxy-5 beta-cholanoic acid. J Steroid Biochem 1980;13:907–16.

199. Radominska-Pyrek A, Zimniak P, Chari M, et al. Glucuronides of monohydroxylated bile acids: specificity of microsomal glucuronyltransferase for the glucuronidation site, C-3 configuration, and side chain length. J Lipid Res 1986;27:89–101.

200. Radominska-Pyrek A, Zimniak P, Irshaid YM, et al. Glucuronidation of 6 alpha-hydroxy bile acids by human liver microsomes. J Clin Invest 1987;80:234–41.

201. Marschall HU, Matern H, Wietholtz H, et al. Bile acid N-acetylglucosaminidation. In vivo and in vitro evidence for a selective conjugation reaction of 7 beta-hydroxylated bile acids in humans. J Clin Invest 1992;89:1981–7.

202. Malet-Martino MC, Bernadou J, Martino R, Armand JP. 19F NMR spectrometry evidence for bile acid conjugates of alpha-fluoro-beta-alanine as the main biliary metabolites of antineoplastic fluoropyrimidines in humans. Drug Metab Dispos 1988;16:78–84.

203. Sweeny DJ, Barnes S, Diasio RB. Formation of conjugates of 2-fluoro-beta-alanine and bile acids during the metabolism of 5-fluorouracil and 5-fluoro-2-deoxyuridine in the isolated perfused rat liver. Cancer Res 1988;48:2010–4.

204. Scholmerich J, Becher MS, Schmidt K, et al. Influence of hydroxylation and conjugation of bile salts on their membrane-damaging properties—studies on isolated hepatocytes and lipid membrane vesicles. Hepatology 1984;4:661–6.

205. Hofmann AF, Roda A. Physicochemical properties of bile acids and their relationship to biological properties: an overview of the problem. J Lipid Res 1984;25:1477–89.

206. Chen LJ, Bolt RJ, Admirand WH. Enzymatic sulfation of bile salts. Partial purification and characterization of an enzyme from rat liver that catalyzes the sulfation of bile salts. Biochim Biophys Acta 1977;480:219–27.

207. Loof L, Hjerten S. Partial purification of a human liver sulphotransferase active towards bile salts. Biochim Biophys Acta 1980;617:192–204.

208. Barnes S, Burhol PG, Zander R, et al. Enzymatic sulfation of glycochenodeoxycholic acid by tissue fractions from adult hamsters. J Lipid Res 1979;20:952–9.

209. Watkins JB, Goldstein E, Coryer R, et al. Sulfation of bile acids in the fetus. In: Presig R, Bircher J, editors. The liver: quantitative aspects of structure and function. Gstaad: Edito Cantor Aulendorf; 1979. p. 249–54.

210. Summerfield JA, Gollan JL, Billing BH. Synthesis of bile acid monosulphates by the isolated perfused rat kidney. Biochem J 1976;156:339–45.

211. Summerfield JA, Cullen J, Barnes S, Billing BH. Evidence for renal control of urinary excretion of bile acids and bile acid sulphates in the cholestatic syndrome. Clin Sci Mol Med 1977;52:51–65.

212. Setchell KDR, Balistreri WF, Lin Q, et al. Metabolism of ursodeoxycholic acid in normal subjects and in patients with cholestatic liver disease: biotransformation by conjugation and urinary excretion. In: Paumgartner G, Stiehl A, Gerok W, editors. Bile acids and the hepatobiliary system. From basic science to clinical practice. Dordrecht/Boston/London: Kluwer Academic Publishers; 1993. p. 245–9.

213. Fournel-Gigleux S, Sutherland L, Sabolovic N, et al. Stable expression of two human UDP-glucuronosyltransferase cDNAs in V79 cell cultures. Mol Pharmacol 1991;39:177–83.

214. Little JM, St. Pyrek J, Lester R. Hepatic metabolism of 3 alpha-hydroxy-5 beta-etianic acid (3 alpha-hydroxy-5 beta-androstan-17 beta-carboxylic acid) in the adult rat. J Clin Invest 1983;71:73–80.

215. Parquet M, Pessah M, Sacquet E, Salvat C, Raizman A. Effective glucuronidation of 6 alpha-hydroxylated bile acids by human hepatic and renal microsomes. Eur J Biochem 1988; 171:329–34.

216. Matern H, Matern S, Gerok W. Formation of bile acid glucosides by a sugar nucleotide-independent glucosyltransferase isolated from human liver microsomes. Proc Natl Acad Sci U S A 1984;81:7036–40.

217. Marschall HU, Green G, Egestad B, Sjovall J. Isolation of bile acid glucosides and N-acetylglucosaminides from human urine by ion-exchange chromatography and reversed-phase high-performance liquid chromatography. J Chromatogr 1988;452:459–68.

218. Wietholtz H, Marschall HU, Reuschenbach R, et al. Urinary excretion of bile acid glucosides and glucuronides in extrahepatic cholestasis. Hepatology 1991;13:656–62.

219. Marschall HU, Griffiths WJ, Gotze U, et al. The major metabolites of ursodeoxycholic acid in human urine are conjugated with N-acetylglucosamine. Hepatology 1994;20:845–53.

220. Vlahcevic ZR, Schwartz CC, Gustafsson J, et al. Biosynthesis of bile acids in man. Multiple pathways to cholic acid and chenodeoxycholic acid. J Biol Chem 1980;255:2925–33.

221. Swell L, Gustafsson J, Schwartz CC, et al. An in vivo evaluation of the quantitative significance of several potential pathways to cholic and chenodeoxycholic acids from cholesterol in man. J Lipid Res 1980;21:455–66.

222. Yamasaki K. Alternative biogenetic pathways of C24-bile acids with special reference to chenodeoxycholic acid. Kawasaki Med J 1978;4:227–64.

223. Anderson KE, Kok E, Javitt NB. Bile acid synthesis in man: metabolism of 7-hydroxycholesterol- 14 C and 26-hydroxy-cholesterol-3 H. J Clin Invest 1972;51:112–7.

224. Zhang J, Akwa Y, el-Etr M, et al. Metabolism of 27-, 25- and 24-hydroxycholesterol in rat glial cells and neurons. Biochem J 1997;322:175–84.

225. Zhang J, Dricu A, Sjovall J. Studies on the relationships between 7 alpha-hydroxylation and the ability of 25- and 27-hydroxy-cholesterol to suppress the activity of HMG-CoA reductase. Biochim Biophys Acta 1997;1344:241–9.

226. Axelson M, Larsson O, Zhang J, et al. Structural specificity in the suppression of HMG-CoA reductase in human fibroblasts by intermediates in bile acid biosynthesis. J Lipid Res 1995;36:290–8.

227. Hall R, Kok E, Javitt NB. Bile acid synthesis: down-regulation by monohydroxy bile acids. FASEB J 1988;2:152–6.

228. Emerman S, Javitt NB. Metabolism of taurolithocholic acid in the hamster. J Biol Chem 1967;242:661–4.

229. Javitt NB, Emerman S. Effect of sodium taurolithocholate on bile flow and bile acid exeretion. J Clin Invest 1968;47: 1002–14.

230. Mathis U, Karlaganis G, Preisig R. Monohydroxy bile salt sulfates: tauro-3 beta-hydroxy-5-cholenoate-3-sulfate induces intrahepatic cholestasis in rats. Gastroenterology 1983;85:674–81.

231. Toll A, Shoda J, Axelson M, et al. 7 alpha-Hydroxylation of 26-hydroxycholesterol, 3 beta-hydroxy-5-cholestenoic acid and 3 beta-hydroxy-5-cholenoic acid by cytochrome P-450 in pig liver microsomes. FEBS Lett 1992;296:73–6.

232. Toll A, Wikvall K, Sudjana-Sugiaman E, et al. 7 alpha Hydroxylation of 25-hydroxycholesterol in liver microsomes. Evidence that the enzyme involved is different from cholesterol 7 alpha-hydroxylase. Eur J Biochem 1994;224:309–16.

233. Bjorkhem I, Nyberg B, Einarsson K. 7 alpha-Hydroxylation of 27-hydroxycholesterol in human liver microsomes. Biochim Biophys Acta 1992;1128:73–6.

234. Wu Z, Martin KO, Javitt NB, Chiang JY. Structure and functions of human oxysterol 7alpha-hydroxylase cDNAs and gene CYP7B1. J Lipid Res 1999;40:2195–203.

235. Schwarz M, Lund EG, Lathe R, et al. Identification and characterization of a mouse oxysterol 7alpha-hydroxylase cDNA. J Biol Chem 1997;272:23995–4001.

236. Schwarz M, Russell DW, Dietschy JM, Turley SD. Alternate pathways of bile acid synthesis in the cholesterol 7α-hydroxylase knockout mouse are not upregulated by either cholesterol or cholestyramine feeding. J Lipid Res 2001;42: 1594–603.

237. Li-Hawkins J, Lund EG, Lathe R, et al. Disruption of the oxysterol 7α-hydroxylase gene in mice. J Biol Chem 2000;275: 16536–42.

238. Li-Hawkins J, Lund EG, Bronson AD, Russell DW. Expression cloning of an oxysterol 7α-hydroxylase selective for 24-hydroxycholesterol. J Biol Chem 2000;275:16543–9.

239. Lund EG, Guileyardo JM, Russell DW. cDNA cloning of cholesterol 24-hydroxylase, a regulator of cholesterol homeostasis in the brain. Proc Natl Acad Sci U S A 1999;96:7238–43.

240. Hanson RF, Staples AB, Williams GC. Metabolism of 5 beta-cholestane-3 alpha, 7 alpha, 12 alpha, 26-tetrol and 5 beta-cholestane-3 alpha, 7 alpha, 12 alpha, 25-tetrol into cholic acid in normal human subjects. J Lipid Res 1979;20:489–93.

241. Hanson RF, Williams GC. Metabolism of 3alpha, 7alpha, 12alpha-trihydroxy-5beta-cholestan-26-oic acid in normal subjects with an intact enterohepatic circulation. J Lipid Res 1977;18:656–9.

242. Kase BF, Pedersen JI, Strandvik B, Bjorkhem I. In vivo and vitro studies on formation of bile acids in patients with Zellweger syndrome. Evidence that peroxisomes are of importance in the normal biosynthesis of both cholic and chenodeoxycholic acid. J Clin Invest 1985;76:2393–402.

243. Wachtel N, Emerman S, Javitt NB. Metabolism of cholest-5-ene-3 beta, 26-diol in the rat and hamster. J Biol Chem 1968;243:5207–12.

244. Krisans SK, Thompson SL, Pena LA, et al. Bile acid synthesis in rat liver peroxisomes: metabolism of 26-hydroxycholesterol to 3 beta-hydroxy-5-cholenoic acid. J Lipid Res 1985;26: 1324–32.

245. Mitropoulos KA, Myant NB. The formation of lithocholic acid, chenodeoxycholic acid and alpha- and beta-muricholic acids from cholesterol incubated with rat-liver mitochondria. Biochem J 1967;103:472–9.

246. Kok E, Burstein S, Javitt NB, et al. Bile acid synthesis. Metabolism of 3 beta-hydroxy-5-cholenoic acid in the hamster. J Biol Chem 1981;256:6155–9.

247. Kulkarni B, Javitt NB. Chenodeoxycholic acid synthesis in the hamster: a metabolic pathway via 3 beta, 7 alpha-dihydroxy-5-cholen-24-oic acid. Steroids 1982;40:581–9.

248. Karavolas HJ, Elliott WH, Hsia SL, et al. Bile acids. XXII. Allocholic acid, a metabolite of 5alpha-cholestan-3beta-ol in the rat. J Biol Chem 1965;240:1568–77.

249. Hofmann AF, Mosbach EH. Identification of allodeoxycholic acid as the major component of gallstones induced in the rabbit by 5alpha-cholestan-3beta-ol. J Biol Chem 1964;239:2813–21.

250. Shefer S, Hauser S, Mosbach EH. 7-alpha-Hydroxylation of cholestanol by rat liver microsomes. J Lipid Res 1968; 9:328–33.

251. Bjorkhem I, Gustafsson J. On the conversion of cholestanol into allocholic acid in rat liver. Eur J Biochem 1971;18:207–13.

252. Ali SS, Elliott WH. Bile acids. LI. Formation of 12alpha-hydroxyl derivatives and companions from 5 alpha-sterols by rabbit liver microsomes. J Lipid Res 1976;17:386–92.

253. Mui MM, Elliott WH. Bile acids. XXXII. Allocholic acid, a metabolite of allochenodeoxycholic acid in bile fistula rats. J Biol Chem 1971;246:302–4.

254. Blaskiewicz RJ, O'Neil GJ Jr, Elliott WH. Bile acids. XLI. Hepatic microsomal 12 alpha-hydroxylation of allochenodeoxycholate to allocholate. Proc Soc Exp Biol Med 1974;146:92–5.

255. Bjorkhem I, Einarsson K. Formation and metabolism of 7 alpha-hydroxy-5-alpha-cholestan-3-one and 7 alpha, 12 alpha-dihydroxy-5-alpha-cholestan-3-one in rat liver. Eur J Biochem 1970;13:174–9.

256. Hylemon PB. Metabolism of bile acids in intestinal microflora. In: Danielsson H, Sjovall J, editors. Sterols and bile acids. Amsterdam: Elsevier Science; 1985. p. 331–43.

257. Ye HQ, Mallonee DH, Wells JE, et al. The bile acid-inducible baiF gene from Eubacterium sp. strain VPI 12708 encodes a bile acid-coenzyme A hydrolase. J Lipid Res 1999;40:17–23.

258. Back P, Walter K. Developmental pattern of bile acid metabolism as revealed by bile acid analysis of meconium. Gastroenterology 1980;78:671–6.

259. Shoda J, Mahara R, Osuga T, et al. Similarity of unusual bile acids in human umbilical cord blood and amniotic fluid from newborns and in sera and urine from adult patients with cholestatic liver diseases. J Lipid Res 1988;29:847–58.

260. Nakagawa M, Setchell KDR. Bile acid metabolism in early life: studies of amniotic fluid. J Lipid Res 1990;31:1089–98.

261. Setchell KDR, Lawson AM, Blackstock EJ, Murphy GM. Diurnal changes in serum unconjugated bile acids in normal man. Gut 1982;23:637–42.

262. Lewis B, Tabaqchali S, Panveliwalla D, Wootton ID. Serum-bile-acids in the stagnant-loop syndrome. Lancet 1969;i:219–20.

263. Setchell KDR, Harrison DL, Gilbert JM, Mupthy GM. Serum unconjugated bile acids: qualitative and quantitative profiles in ileal resection and bacterial overgrowth. Clin Chim Acta 1985;152:297–306.

264. Bartholomew TC, Summerfield JA, Billing BH, et al. Bile acid profiles of human serum and skin interstitial fluid and their relationship to pruritus studied by gas chromatography-mass spectrometry. Clin Sci 1982;63:65–73.

265. Encrantz JC, Sjovall J. On the bile acids in duodenal contents of infants and children. Clin Chim Acta 1959;4:793–9.

266. Poley JR, Dower JC, Owen CA, Stickler GB. Bile acids in infants and children. J Lab Clin Med 1964;63:838–46.

267. Bongiovanni AM. Bile acid content of gallbladder of infants, children and adults. J Clin Endocrinol Metab 1965;25:678–85.

268. Tohma M, Mahara R, Takeshita H, et al. Synthesis of the 1 beta-hydroxylated bile acids and identification of 1 beta,3 alpha,7 alpha-trihydroxy- and 1 beta,3 alpha,7 alpha,12 alpha-tetrahydroxy-5 beta-cholan-24-oic acids in human meconium. Chem Pharm Bull (Tokyo) 1985;33:3071–3.

269. Sharp HL, Peller J, Carey JB, Krist W. Primary and secondary bile acids in meconium. Pediatr Res 1971;5:274–9.

270. Colombo C, Zuliani G, Ronchi M, et al. Biliary bile acid composition of the human fetus in early gestation. Pediatr Res 1987;21:197–200.

271. Dumaswala R, Setchell KDR, Zimmer-Nechemias L, et al. Identification of 3 alpha,4 beta,7 alpha-trihydroxy-5 beta-cholanoic acid in human bile: reflection of a new pathway in bile acid metabolism in humans. J Lipid Res 1989;30:847–56.

272. Haber LR, Vaupshas V, Vitullo BB, et al. Bile acid conjugation in organ culture of human fetal liver. Gastroenterology 1978;74:1214–23.

273. Gustafsson J, Andersson S, Sjovall J. Bile acid metabolism during development: metabolism of taurodeoxycholic acid in human fetal liver. Biol Neonate 1985;47:26–31.

274. Gustafsson J, Anderson S, Sjovall J. Bile acid metabolism during development: metabolism of lithocholic acid in human fetal liver. Pediatr Res 1987;21:99–103.

275. Danielsson H, Rutter WJ. The metabolism of bile acids in the developing rat liver. Biochemistry 1968;7:346–52.

276. Smallwood RA, Lester R, Plasecki GJ, et al. Fetal bile salt metabolism. II. Hepatic excretion of endogenous bile salt and of a taurocholate load. J Clin Invest 1972;51:1388–97.

277. Little JM, Smallwood RA, Lester R, et al. Bile-salt metabolism in the primate fetus. Gastroenterology 1975;69:1315–20.

278. Subbiah MT, Marai L, Dinh DM, Penner JW. Sterol and bile acid metabolism during development. 1. Studies on the gallbladder and intestinal bile acids of newborn and fetal rabbit. Steroids 1977;29:83–92.

279. Sewell RB, Hardy KJ, Smallwood RA, Hoffman NE. Fetal bile salt metabolism: placental transfer of taurocholate in sheep. Am J Physiol 1980;239:G354–7.

280. Suchy FJ, Balistreri WF, Breslin JS, et al. Absence of an acinar gradient for bile acid uptake in developing rat liver. Pediatr Res 1987;21:417–21.

281. Whitehouse MW, Cottrell MC, Briggs T, Staple E. Catabolism in vitro of cholesterol: some comparative aspects. Arch Biochem Biophys 1962;98:305–11.

282. Watkins JB, Ingall D, Szczepanik P, et al. Bile-salt metabolism in the newborn. Measurement of pool size and synthesis by stable isotope technic. N Engl J Med 1973;288:431–4.

283. Watkins JB, Szczepanik P, Gould JB, et al. Bile salt metabolism in the human premature infant. Preliminary observations of pool size and synthesis rate following prenatal administration of dexamethasone and phenobarbital. Gastroenterology 1975;69:706–13.

284. Heubi JE, Balistreri WF, Suchy FJ. Bile salt metabolism in the first year of life. J Lab Clin Med 1982;100:127–36.

285. Watkins JB, Jarvenpaa AL, Szczepanik-Van Leeuwen P, et al. Feeding the low-birth weight infant: V. Effects of taurine, cholesterol, and human milk on bile acid kinetics. Gastroenterology 1983;85:793–800.

286. Kimura A, Suzuki M, Murai T, et al. Perinatal bile acid metabolism: analysis of urinary bile acids in pregnant women and newborns. J Lipid Res 1997;38:1954–62.

287. Alme B, Bremmelgaard A, Sjovall J, Thomassen P. Analysis of metabolic profiles of bile acids in urine using a lipophilic anion exchanger and computerized gas-liquid chromatography-mass spectrometry. J Lipid Res 1977;18:339–62.

288. Bremmelgaard A, Sjovall J. Bile acid profiles in urine of patients with liver diseases. Eur J Clin Invest 1979;9:341–8.

289. Strandvik B, Wikstrom SA. Tetrahydroxylated bile acids in healthy human newborns. Eur J Clin Invest 1982;12:301–5.

290. Bremmelgaard A, Sjovall J. Hydroxylation of cholic, chenodeoxycholic, and deoxycholic acids in patients with intrahepatic cholestasis. J Lipid Res 1980;21:1072–81.

291. Wahlen E, Egestad B, Strandvik B, Sjoovall J. Ketonic bile acids in urine of infants during the neonatal period. J Lipid Res 1989;30:1847–57.

292. Dumaswala R, Setchell KD, Moyer MS, Suchy FJ. An anion exchanger mediates bile acid transport across the placental microvillous membrane. Am J Physiol 1993;264:G1016–23.

293. Stiehl A. Bile salt sulphates in cholestasis. Eur J Clin Invest 1974;4:59–63.

294. Makino I, Shinozaki K, Nakagawa S, Mashimo K. Measurement of sulfated and nonsulfated bile acids in human serum and urine. J Lipid Res 1974;15:132–8.

295. Stiehl A, Raedsch R, Rudolph G, et al. Biliary and urinary excretion of sulfated, glucuronidated and tetrahydroxylated bile acids in cirrhotic patients. Hepatology 1985;5:492–5.

296. Deleze G, Paumgartner G, Karlaganis G, et al. Bile acid pattern in human amniotic fluid. Eur J Clin Invest 1978;8:41–5.

297. St Pyrek J, Sterzycki R, Lester R, Adcock E. Constituents of human meconium: II. Identification of steroidal acids with 21 and 22 carbon atoms. Lipids 1982;17:241–9.

298. St. Pyrek J, Lester R, Adcock EW, Sanghvi AT. Constituents of human meconium—I. Identification of 3-hydroxy-etianic acids. J Steroid Biochem 1983;18:341–51.

299. Street JM, Balistreri WF, Setchell KDR. Bile acid metabolism in the perinatal period—excretion of conventional and atypical bile acids in meconium. Gastroenterology 1986;90:1773.

300. Pullinger CR, Eng C, Salen G, et al. Human cholesterol 7α-hydroxylase (CYP7A1) deficiency has a hypercholesterolemic phenotype. J Clin Invest 2002;110:109–17.

301. Van Bogaert L, Scherer HJ, Epstein E. Une forme cerebrale de la cholesterinose generalisee. Paris: Masson et Cie; 1937.

302. Christensen E, Van Eldere J, Brandt NJ, et al. A new peroxisomal disorder: di- and trihydroxycholestanaemia due to a presumed trihydroxycholestanoyl-CoA oxidase deficiency. J Inherit Metab Dis 1990;13:363–6.

303. ten Brink HJ, Wanders RJ, Christensen E, et al. Heterogeneity in di/trihydroxycholestanoic acidaemia. Ann Clin Biochem 1994;31:195–7.

304. Przyrembel H, Wanders RJ, van Roermund CW, et al. Di- and tri-hydroxycholestanoic acidaemia with hepatic failure. J Inherit Metab Dis 1990;13:367–70.

305. Wanders RJ, Casteels M, Mannaerts GP, et al. Accumulation and impaired in vivo metabolism of di- and trihydroxycholestanoic acid in two patients. Clin Chim Acta 1991;202:123–32.

306. Clayton PT, Casteels M, Mieli-Vergani G, Lawson AM. Familial giant cell hepatitis with low bile acid concentrations and increased urinary excretion of specific bile alcohols: a new inborn error of bile acid synthesis? Pediatr Res 1995;37:424–31.

307. Bowen P, Lee CSN, Zellweger H, Lindenberg R. A familial syndrome of multiple congenital defects. Bull Johns Hopkins Hosp 1964;114:402–14.

308. Lazarow PB, Moser HW. Disorders of peroxisome biogenesis. In: Scriver CR, Beaudet AL, Sly WS, editors. The metabolic basis of inherited disease. New York: McGraw-Hill; 1989. p. 1479–509.

309. Bull LN, van Eijk MJT, Pawlikowska L, et al. A gene encoding a P-type ATPase mutated in two forms of hereditary cholestasis. Nat Genet 1998;18:219–24.

310. De Vree JML, Jacquemin E, Sturm E, et al. Mutations in the MDR3 gene cause progressive familial intrahepatic cholestasis. Proc Natl Acad Sci U S A 1998;95:282–7.

311. Smith DW, Lemli L, Opitz JM. A newly recognized syndrome of multiple congenital anomalies. J Pediatr 1964;64:210–7.

312. Clayton PT. Inborn errors of bile acid metabolism. J Inherit Metab Dis 1991;14:478–96.

313. Salen G, Shefer S, Cheng FW, et al. Cholic acid biosynthesis: the enzymatic defect in cerebrotendinous xanthomatosis. J Clin Invest 1979;63:38–44.

314. Setoguchi T, Salen G, Tint GS, Mosbach EH. A biochemical abnormality in cerebrotendinous xanthomatosis. Impairment of bile acid biosynthesis associated with incomplete degradation of the cholesterol side chain. J Clin Invest 1974;53:1393–401.

315. Salen G, Grundy SM. The metabolism of cholestanol, cholesterol, and bile acids in cerebrotendinous xanthomatosis. J Clin Invest 1973;52:2822–35.

316. Salen G. Cholestanol deposition in cerebrotendinous xanthomatosis. A possible mechanism. Ann Intern Med 1971;75:843–51.

317. Salen G, Shefer S, Tint GS, et al. Biosynthesis of bile acids in cerebrotendinous xanthomatosis. Relationship of bile acid

318. Oftebro H, Bjorkhem I, Skrede S, et al. Cerebrotendinous xanthomatosis: a defect in mitochondrial 26-hydroxylation required for normal biosynthesis of cholic acid. J Clin Invest 1980;65:1418–30.

319. Javitt NB, Kok E, Cohen B, Burstein S. Cerebrotendinous xanthomatosis: reduced serum 26-hydroxycholesterol. J Lipid Res 1982;23:627–30.

320. Salen G, Shefer S, Mosbach EH, et al. Metabolism of potential precursors of chenodeoxycholic acid in cerebrotendinous xanthomatosis (CTX). J Lipid Res 1979;20:22–30.

321. Bjorkhem I, Oftebro H, Skrede S, Pedersen JI. Assay of intermediates in bile acid biosynthesis using isotope dilution–mass spectrometry: hepatic levels in the normal state and in cerebrotendinous xanthomatosis. J Lipid Res 1981;22:191–200.

322. Oftebro H, Bjorkhem I, Stormer FC, Pedersen JI. Cerebrotendinous xanthomatosis: defective liver mitochondrial hydroxylation of chenodeoxycholic acid precursors. J Lipid Res 1981;22:632–40.

323. Watts GF, Mitchell WD, Bending JJ, et al. Cerebrotendinous xanthomatosis: a family study of sterol 27-hydroxylase mutations and pharmacotherapy. QJM 1996;89:55–63.

324. Chen W, Kubota S, Nishimura Y, et al. Genetic analysis of a Japanese cerebrotendinous xanthomatosis family: identification of a novel mutation in the adrenodoxin binding region of the CYP27 gene. Biochim Biophys Acta 1996;1317:119–26.

325. Garuti R, Lelli N, Barozzini M, et al. Cerebrotendinous xanthomatosis caused by two new mutations of the sterol-27-hydroxylase gene that disrupt mRNA splicing. J Lipid Res 1996;37:1459–67.

326. Cali JJ, Hsieh CL, Francke U, Russell DW. Mutations in the bile acid biosynthetic enzyme sterol 27-hydroxylase underlie cerebrotendinous xanthomatosis. J Biol Chem 1991;266:7779–83.

327. Kim KS, Kubota S, Kuriyama M, et al. Identification of new mutations in sterol 27-hydroxylase gene in Japanese patients with cerebrotendinous xanthomatosis (CTX). J Lipid Res 1994;35:1031–9.

328. Leitersdorf E, Safadi R, Meiner V, et al. Cerebrotendinous xanthomatosis in the Israeli Druze: molecular genetics and phenotypic characteristics. Am J Hum Genet 1994;55:907–15.

329. Reshef A, Meiner V, Berginer VM, Leitersdorf E. Molecular genetics of cerebrotendinous xanthomatosis in Jews of north African origin. J Lipid Res 1994;35:478–83.

330. Meiner V, Marais DA, Reshef A, et al. Premature termination codon at the sterol 27-hydroxylase gene causes cerebrotendinous xanthomatosis in an Afrikaner family. Hum Mol Genet 1994;3:193–4.

331. Verrips A, Steenbergen-Spanjers GC, Luyten JA, et al. Two new mutations in the sterol 27-hydroxylase gene in two families lead to cerebrotendinous xanthomatosis. Hum Genet 1996;98:735–7.

332. Segev H, Reshef A, Clavey V, et al. Premature termination codon at the sterol 27-hydroxylase gene causes cerebrotendinous xanthomatosis in a French family. Hum Genet 1995;95:238–40.

333. Garuti R, Lelli N, Barozzini M, et al. Partial deletion of the gene encoding sterol 27-hydroxylase in a subject with cerebrotendinous xanthomatosis. J Lipid Res 1996;37:662–72.

334. Wakamatsu N, Hayashi M, Kawai H, et al. Mutations producing premature termination of translation and an amino acid substitution in the sterol 27-hydroxylase gene cause cerebrotendinous xanthomatosis associated with parkinsonism. J Neurol Neurosurg Psychiatry 1999;67:195–8.

335. Shiga K, Fukuyama R, Kimura S, et al. Mutation of the sterol

27-hydroxylase gene (*CYP27*) results in truncation of mRNA expressed in leucocytes in a Japanese family with cerebrotendinous xanthomatosis. J Neurol Neurosurg Psychiatry 1999;67:675–7.

336. Chen W, Kubota S, Seyama Y. Alternative pre-mRNA splicing of the sterol 27-hydroxylase gene (*CYP27*) caused by a G to A mutation at the last nucleotide of exon 6 in a patient with cerebrotendinous xanthomatosis (CTX). J Lipid Res 1998; 39:509–17.

337. Chen W, Kubota S, Teramoto T, et al. Genetic analysis enables definite and rapid diagnosis of cerebrotendinous xanthomatosis. Neurology 1998;51:865–7.

338. Verrips A, Steenbergen-Spanjers GC, Luyten JA, et al. Exon skipping in the sterol 27-hydroxylase gene leads to cerebrotendinous xanthomatosis. Hum Genet 1997;100:284–6.

339. Chen W, Kubota S, Teramoto T, et al. Silent nucleotide substitution in the sterol 27-hydroxylase gene (*CYP27*) leads to alternative pre-mRNA splicing by activating a cryptic 5' splice site at the mutant codon in cerebrotendinous xanthomatosis patients. Biochemistry 1998;37:4420–8.

340. Okuyama E, Tomita S, Takeuchi H, Ichikawa Y. A novel mutation in the cytochrome P450(27) (*CYP27*) gene caused cerebrotendinous xanthomatosis in a Japanese family. J Lipid Res 1996;37:631–9.

341. Nagai Y, Hirano M, Mori T, et al. Japanese triplets with cerebrotendinous xanthomatosis are homozygous for a mutant gene coding for the sterol 27-hydroxylase (Arg441Trp). Neurology 1996;46:571–4.

342. Chen W, Kubota S, Kim KS, et al. Novel homozygous and compound heterozygous mutations of sterol 27-hydroxylase gene (*CYP27*) cause cerebrotendinous xanthomatosis in three Japanese patients from two unrelated families. J Lipid Res 1997;38:870–9.

343. Chen W, Kubota S, Ujike H, et al. A novel Arg362Ser mutation in the sterol 27-hydroxylase gene (*CYP27*): its effects on pre-mRNA splicing and enzyme activity. Biochemistry 1998; 37:15050–6.

344. Ahmed MS, Afsar S, Hentati A, et al. A novel mutation in the sterol 27-hydroxylase gene of a Pakistani family with autosomal recessive cerebrotendinous xanthomatosis. Neurology 1997;48:258–60.

345. Shefer S, Dayal B, Tint GS, et al. Identification of pentahydroxy bile alcohols in cerebrotendinous xanthomatosis: characterization of 5beta-cholestane-3alpha, 7alpha, 12alpha, 24xi, 25-pentol and 5beta-cholestane-3alpha, 7alpha, 12alpha, 23xi, 25-pentol. J Lipid Res 1975;16:280–6.

346. Hoshita T, Yasuhara M, Kihira K, Kuramoto T. Identification of (23S)-5beta-cholestane-3alpha, 7alpha, 12alpha, 23, 25-pentol in cerebrotendinous xanthomatosis. Steroids 1976;27:657–64.

347. Hoshita T, Yasuhara M, Une M, et al. Occurrence of bile alcohol glucuronides in bile of patients with cerebrotendinous xanthomatosis. J Lipid Res 1980;21:1015–21.

348. Wolthers BG, Volmer M, van der Molen J, et al. Diagnosis of cerebrotendinous xanthomatosis (CTX) and effect of chenodeoxycholic acid therapy by analysis of urine using capillary gas chromatography. Clin Chim Acta 1983;131:53–65.

349. Karlaganis G, Karlaganis V, Sjovall J. Bile alcohol glucuronides in urine: secondary metabolites of intermediates formed in the formation of bile acids from cholesterol? In: Paumgartner G, Stiehl A, Gerok K, editors. Bile acids and cholesterol in health and disease. Lancaster (UK): MTP Press, Ltd.; 1983. p. 119–27.

350. Egestad B, Pettersson P, Skrede S, Sjovall J. Fast atom bombardment mass spectrometry in the diagnosis of cerebrotendinous xanthomatosis. Scand J Clin Lab Invest 1985;45:443–6.

351. Shimazu K, Kuwabara M, Yoshii M, et al. Bile alcohol profiles in bile, urine, and feces of a patient with cerebrotendinous xanthomatosis. J Biochem (Tokyo) 1986;99:477–83.

352. Hoshita T. Bile alcohols and primitive bile acids. In: Danielsson H, Sjovall J, editors. Sterols and bile acids. Amsterdam: Elsevier; 1985. p. 279–300.

353. Yasuhara M, Kuramoto T, Hoshita T, et al. Identifications of 5 beta-cholestane-3 alpha, 7 alpha, 12 alpha, 23 beta-tetrol, 5 beta-cholestane-3 alpha, 7 alpha, 12 alpha, 24 alpha-tetrol, and 5 beta-cholestane-3 alpha, 7 alpha, 12 alpha, 24 beta-tetrol in cerebrotendinous xanthomatosis. Steroids 1978;31:333–45.

354. Menkes JH, Schimschock JR, Swanson PD. Cerebrotendinous xanthomatosis. The storage of cholestanol within the nervous system. Arch Neurol 1968;19:47–53.

355. Koopman BJ, van der Molen JC, Wolthers BG, et al. Capillary gas chromatographic determination of cholestanol/cholesterol ratio in biological fluids. Its potential usefulness for the follow-up of some liver diseases and its lack of specificity in diagnosing CTX (cerebrotendinous xanthomatosis). Clin Chim Acta 1984;137:305–15.

356. Salen G, Shefer S, Tint GS. Transformation of 4-cholesten-3-one and 7 alpha-hydroxy-4-cholesten-3-one into cholestanol and bile acids in cerebrotendinous xanthomatosis. Gastroenterology 1984;87:276–83.

357. Skrede S, Bjorkhem I, Buchmann MS, et al. A novel pathway for biosynthesis of cholestanol with 7 alpha-hydroxylated C27-steroids as intermediates, and its importance for the accumulation of cholestanol in cerebrotendinous xanthomatosis. J Clin Invest 1985;75:448–55.

358. Skrede S, Buchmann MS, Bjorkhem I. Hepatic 7 alpha-dehydroxylation of bile acid intermediates, and its significance for the pathogenesis of cerebrotendinous xanthomatosis. J Lipid Res 1988;29:157–64.

359. Inoue K, Kubota S, Seyama Y. Cholestanol induces apoptosis of cerebellar neuronal cells. Biochem Biophys Res Commun 1999;256:198–203.

360. Witzleben CL, Piccoli DA, Setchell K. A new category of causes of intrahepatic cholestasis. Pediatr Pathol 1992;12:269–74.

361. Horslen SP, Lawson AM, Malone M, Clayton PT. 3 beta-Hydroxy-delta 5-C27-steroid dehydrogenase deficiency; effect of chenodeoxycholic acid therapy on liver histology. J Inherit Metab Dis 1992;15:38–46.

362. Bove KE, Daugherty CC, Tyson W, et al. Bile acid synthetic defects and liver disease. Pediatr Dev Pathol 2000;3:1–16.

363. Setchell KDR. Inborn errors of bile acid synthesis: a new category of metabolic liver disease. In: Van Berge Henegouwen GP, Van Hoek B, De Groote J, et al, editors. Cholestatic liver diseases: new strategies for prevention and treatment of hepatobiliary and cholestatic liver diseases. Dordrecht/Boston/London: Kluwer Academic Publishers; 1994. p. 164–7.

364. Clayton RJ, Iber FL, Ruebner BH, McKusick VA. Byler disease. Fatal familial intrahepatic cholestasis in an Amish kindred. Am J Dis Child 1969;117:112–24.

365. Maggiore G, Bernard O, Riely CA, et al. Normal serum gamma-glutamyl-transpeptidase activity identifies groups of infants with idiopathic cholestasis with poor prognosis. J Pediatr 1987;111:251–2.

366. Chobert MN, Bernard O, Bulle F, et al. High hepatic gamma-glutamyltransferase (gamma-GT) activity with normal serum gamma-GT in children with progressive idiopathic cholestasis. J Hepatol 1989;8:22–5.

367. Whitington PF, Freese DK, Alonso EM, et al. Progressive familial intrahepatic cholestasis (Byler's disease). In: Lentze M, Reichen J, editors. Pediatric cholestasis: novel approaches to treatment. Boston: Kluwer Academic Publishers; 1991. p. 165–80.

368. Lemonde HA, Johnson AW, Clayton PT. The identification of unusual bile acid metabolites by tandem mass spectrometry: use of low-energy collision-induced dissociation to produce informative spectra. Rapid Commun Mass Spectrom 1999; 13:1159–64.

369. Libert R, Hermans D, Draye JP, et al. Bile acids and conjugates identified in metabolic disorders by fast atom bombardment and tandem mass spectrometry. Clin Chem 1991;37:2102–10.

370. Mushtaq I, Logan S, Morris M, et al. Screening of newborn infants for cholestatic hepatobiliary disease with tandem mass spectrometry. BMJ 1999;319:471–7.

371. Mills KA, Mushtaq I, Johnson AW, et al. A method for the quantitation of conjugated bile acids in dried blood spots using electrospray ionization-mass spectrometry. Pediatr Res 1998;43:361–8.

372. Stieger B, Zhang J, O'Neill B, et al. Differential interaction of bile acids from patients with inborn errors of bile acid synthesis with hepatocellular bile acid transporters. Eur J Biochem 1997;244:39–44.

373. Daugherty CC, Setchell KD, Heubi JE, Balistreri WF. Resolution of liver biopsy alterations in three siblings with bile acid treatment of an inborn error of bile acid metabolism (delta 4-3-oxosteroid 5 beta-reductase deficiency). Hepatology 1993;18:1096–101.

374. Setchell KDR, Matsui A. Serum bile acid analysis. Clin Chim Acta 1983;127:1–17.

375. Hofmann AF, Cummings SA. Measurement of bile acid and cholesterol kinetics in man by isotope dilution: principles and applications. In: Barbara L, Dowling RH, Hofmann AF, Roda E, editors. Bile acids in gastroenterology. Lancaster (UK): MTP Press; 1982. p. 75–7.

376. Sumazaki R, Nakamura N, Shoda J, et al. Gene analysis in delta 4-3-oxosteroid 5 beta-reductase deficiency [letter]. Lancet 1997;349:329.

377. Setchell KDR, O'Connell NC. Inborn errors of bile acid biosynthesis: update on biochemical aspects. In: Hofmann AF, Paumgartner G, Stiehl A, editors. Bile acids in gastroenterology. Basic and clinical advances. Dordrecht/Boston/London: Kluwer Academic Publishers; 1995. p. 129–36.

378. Axelson M, Mork B, Sjovall J. Occurrence of 3 beta-hydroxy-5-cholestenoic acid, 3 beta,7 alpha-dihydroxy-5-cholestenoic acid, and 7 alpha-hydroxy-3-oxo-4-cholestenoic acid as normal constituents in human blood. J Lipid Res 1988;29:629–41.

379. Kuramoto T, Kikuchi H, Sanemori H, Hoshita T. Bile salts of anura. Chem Pharm Bull (Tokyo) 1973;21:952–9.

380. Haslewood GA. Bile salt evolution. J Lipid Res 1967;8:535–50.

381. Setchell KDR, Heubi JE, O'Connell NC, et al. Neonatal liver disease in two siblings caused by a failure to racemize (25R)trihydroxy-cholestanoic acid due to a gene mutation in 2-methylacyl-CoA racemase—effectiveness of cholic acid therapy in preventing liver and neurological disease. In: Paumgartner G, Keppler D, Leuschner U, Stiehl A, editors. Bile acids: from genomics to disease and therapy. Kluwer Academic Publishers; Boston: 2003. p. 206–13.

382. Ferdinandusse S, Overmars H, Denis S, et al. Plasma analysis of di- and trihydroxycholestanoic diastereoisomers in peroxisomal α-methylacyly-CoA racemase deficiency. J Lipid Res 2001;42:137–41.

383. Van Veldhoven PP, Meyhi E, Squires J, et al. Fibroblast studies documenting a case of peroxisomal 2-methylacyl-CoA racemase deficiency; possible link between racemase deficiency and malabsorption and vitamin K deficiency. Eur J Clin Invest 2001;31:714–22.

384. Van Veldhoven PP, Vanhove G, Assselberghs S, et al. Substrate specificities of rat liver peroxisomal acyl-CoA oxidases: palmitoyl-CoA oxidase (inducible acyl-CoA oxidase), pristanoyl-CoA oxidase (non-inducible acyl-CoA oxidase), and trihydroxycoprostanoyl-CoA oxidase. J Biol Chem 1992; 267:20065–74.

385. Matoba N, Une M, Hoshita T. Identification of unconjugated bile acids in human bile. J Lipid Res 1986;27:1154–62.

386. Crosignani A, Podda M, Battezzati PM, et al. Changes in bile acid composition in patients with primary biliary cirrhosis induced by ursodeoxycholic acid administration. Hepatology 1991;14:1000–7.

387. Hofmann AF, Strandvik B. Defective bile acid amidation: predicted features of a new inborn error of metabolism. Lancet 1988;ii:311–3.

388. Hofmann AF. Pharmacology of ursodeoxycholic acid, an enterohepatic drug. Scand J Gastroenterol Suppl 1994;204:1–15.

389. De Witt EH, Lack L. Effects of sulfation patterns on intestinal transport of bile salt sulfate esters. Am J Physiol 1980; 238:G34–9.

390. Lack L. Properties and biological significance of the ileal bile salt transport system. Environ Health Perspect 1979;33:79–90.

391. Low-Beer TS, Tyor MP, Lack L. Effects of sulfation of taurolithocholic and glycolithocholic acids on their intestinal transport. Gastroenterology 1969;56:721–6.

392. Kelley RI. Review: the cerebrohepatorenal syndrome of Zellweger, morphologic and metabolic aspects. Am J Med Genet 1983;16:503–17.

393. Kaiser E, Kramar R. Clinical biochemistry of peroxisomal disorders. Clin Chim Acta 1988;173:57–80.

394. Wanders R, van Roermund C, Schutgens R, et al. The inborn errors of peroxisomal β-oxidation: a review. J Inherit Metab Dis 1990;13:4–36.

395. van den Bosch H, Schutgens RB, Wanders RJ, Tager JM. Biochemistry of peroxisomes. Annu Rev Biochem 1992;61:157–97.

396. Goldfischer S, Moore CL, Johnson AB, et al. Peroxisomal and mitochondrial defects in the cerebro-hepato-renal syndrome. Science 1973;182:62–4.

397. Poll-The BT, Saudubray JM, Ogier H, et al. Infantile Refsum's disease: biochemical findings suggesting multiple peroxisomal dysfunction. J Inherit Metab Dis 1986;9:169–74.

398. Goldfischer S, Collins J, Rapin I, et al. Peroxisomal defects in neonatal-onset and X-linked adrenoleukodystrophies. Science 1985;227:67–70.

399. Burton BK, Reed SP, Remy WT. Hyperpipecolic acidemia: clinical and biochemical observations in two male siblings. J Pediatr 1981;99:729–34.

400. Heymans HS, Oorthuys JW, Nelck G, et al. Rhizomelic chondrodysplasia punctata: another peroxisomal disorder [letter]. N Engl J Med 1985;313:187–8.

401. Moser HW, Moser AE, Singh I, O'Neill BP. Adrenoleukodystrophy: survey of 303 cases: biochemistry, diagnosis, and therapy. Ann Neurol 1984;16:628–41.

402. Aebi HE, Wyss SR. Acatalasemia. In: Stanbury JB, Wyngaarden JB, Fredrickson DS, editors. The metabolic basis of inherited disease. New York: McGraw-Hill; 1978. p. 1792–802.

403. Goldfischer S, Collins J, Rapin I, et al. Pseudo-Zellweger syndrome: deficiencies in several peroxisomal oxidative activities. J Pediatr 1986;108:25–32.

404. Schutgens RB, Heymans HS, Wanders RJ, et al. Peroxisomal disorders: a newly recognised group of genetic diseases. Eur J Pediatr 1986;144:430–40.

405. Hanson RF, Isenberg JN, Williams GC, et al. The metabolism of 3alpha, 7alpha, 12alpha-trihydroxy-5beta-cholestan-26-oic acid in two siblings with cholestasis due to intrahepatic bile

duct anomalies. An apparent inborn error of cholic acid synthesis. J Clin Invest 1975;56:577–87.

406. Eyssen H, Parmentier G, Compernolle F, et al. Trihydroxycoprostanic acid in the duodenal fluid of two children with intrahepatic bile duct anomalies. Biochim Biophys Acta 1972;273:212–21.

407. Kase BF, Bjorkhem I, Haga P, Pedersen JI. Defective peroxisomal cleavage of the C27-steroid side chain in the cerebro-hepatorenal syndrome of Zellweger. J Clin Invest 1985;75:427–35.

408. Bjorkhem I, Kase BF, Pedersen JI. Role of peroxisomes in the biosynthesis of bile acids. Scand J Clin Lab Invest Suppl 1985;177:23–31.

409. Hanson RF. The formation and metabolism of 3,7-dihydroxy-5-cholestan-26-oic acid in man. J Clin Invest 1971;50:2051–5.

410. Parmentier GG, Janssen GA, Eggermont EA, Eyssen HJ. C27 bile acids in infants with coprostanic acidemia and occurrence of a 3 alpha,7 alpha,12 alpha-tridhydroxy-5 beta-C29 dicarboxylic bile acid as a major component in their serum. Eur J Biochem 1979;102:173–83.

411. Janssen G, Toppet S, Parmentier G. Structure of the side chain of the C29 dicarboxylic bile acid occurring in infants with coprostanic acidemia. J Lipid Res 1982;23:456–65.

412. Eyssen H, Eggermont E, van Eldere J, et al. Bile acid abnormalities and the diagnosis of cerebro-hepato-renal syndrome (Zellweger syndrome). Acta Paediatr Scand 1985;74:539–44.

413. Deleze G, Bjorkhem I, Karlaganis G. Bile acids and bile alcohols in two patients with Zellweger (cerebro-hepato-renal) syndrome. J Pediatr Gastroenterol Nutr 1986;5:701–10.

414. Clayton PT, Lake BD, Hall NA, et al. Plasma bile acids in patients with peroxisomal dysfunction syndromes: analysis by capillary gas chromatography-mass spectrometry. Eur J Pediatr 1987;146:166–73.

415. Janssen G, Parmentier G. A further study of the bile acids in infants with coprostanic acidemia. Steroids 1981;37:81–9.

416. Hashmi M, Stanley W, Singh I. Lignoceroyl-CoASH ligase: enzyme defect in fatty acid beta-oxidation system in X-linked childhood adrenoleukodystrophy. FEBS Lett 1986;196:247–50.

417. Lazo O, Contreras M, Hashmi M, et al. Peroxisomal lignoceroyl-CoA ligase deficiency in childhood adrenoleukodystrophy and adrenomyeloneuropathy. Proc Natl Acad Sci U S A 1988;85:7647–51.

418. Wanders RJ, van Roermund CW, van Wijland MJ, et al. Direct demonstration that the deficient oxidation of very long chain fatty acids in X-linked adrenoleukodystrophy is due to an impaired ability of peroxisomes to activate very long chain fatty acids. Biochem Biophys Res Commun 1988;153:618–24.

419. Poll-The BT, Roels F, Ogier H, et al. A new peroxisomal disorder with enlarged peroxisomes and a specific deficiency of acyl-CoA oxidase (pseudo-neonatal adrenoleukodystrophy). Am J Hum Genet 1988;42:422–34.

420. Watkins PA, Chen WW, Harris CJ, et al. Peroxisomal bifunctional enzyme deficiency. J Clin Invest 1989;83:771–7.

421. Novikov D, Dieuaide-Noubhani M, Vermeesch JR, et al. The human peroxisomal multifunctional protein involved in bile acid synthesis: activity measurement, deficiency in Zellweger syndrome and chromosome mapping. Biochim Biophys Acta 1997;1360:229–40.

422. Vreken P, van Rooij A, Denis S, et al. Sensitive analysis of serum 3alpha, 7alpha, 12alpha,24-tetrahydroxy-5beta-cholestan-26-oic acid diastereomers using gas chromatography-mass spectrometry and its application in peroxisomal D-bifunctional protein deficiency. J Lipid Res 1998;39:2452–8.

423. Nathanson MH, Boyer JL. Mechanisms and regulation of bile secretion. Hepatology 1991;14:551–66.

424. Boyer JL. Bile duct epithelium: frontiers in transport physiology. Am J Physiol 1996;270:G1–5.

425. Trauner M, Meier PJ, Boyer JL. Molecular pathogenesis of cholestasis. N Engl J Med 1998;339:1217–27.

426. Deleuze JF, Jacquemin E, Dubuisson C, et al. Defect of multidrug-resistance 3 gene expression in a subtype of progressive familial intrahepatic cholestasis. Hepatology 1996;23:904–8.

427. Bull LN, Carlton VE, Stricker NL, et al. Genetic and morphological findings in progressive familial intrahepatic cholestasis (Byler disease [PFIC-1] and Byler syndrome): evidence for heterogeneity. Hepatology 1997;26:155–64.

428. Linarelli LG, Williams CN, Phillips MJ. Byler's disease: fatal intrahepatic cholestasis. J Pediatr 1972;81:484–92.

429. Tazawa Y, Yamada M, Nakagawa M, et al. Bile acid profiles in siblings with progressive intrahepatic cholestasis: absence of biliary chenodeoxycholate. J Pediatr Gastroenterol Nutr 1985;4:32–7.

430. Jacquemin E, Dumont M, Bernard O, et al. Evidence for defective primary bile acid secretion in children with progressive familial intrahepatic cholestasis (Byler disease). Eur J Pediatr 1994;153:424–8.

431. Stellaard F, Watkins JB, Szczepanik-van Leeuwen P, Alagille D. Hyocholic acid, an unusual bile acid in Byler's disease. Gastroenterology 1979;77:A42.

432. Kelley RI. A new face for an old syndrome [editorial]. Am J Med Genet 1997;65:251–6.

433. Opitz JM. RSH (so-called Smith-Lemli-Opitz) syndrome. Curr Opin Pediatr 1999;11:353–62.

434. Ryan AK, Bartlett K, Clayton P, et al. Smith-Lemli-Opitz syndrome: a variable clinical and biochemical phenotype. J Med Genet 1998;35:558–65.

435. Irons M, Elias ER, Salen G, et al. Defective cholesterol biosynthesis in Smith-Lemli-Opitz syndrome [letter]. Lancet 1993;341:1414.

436. Tint GS, Irons M, Elias ER, et al. Defective cholesterol biosynthesis associated with the Smith-Lemli- Opitz syndrome. N Engl J Med 1994;330:107–13.

437. Tint GS, Seller M, Hughes-Benzie R, et al. Markedly increased tissue concentrations of 7-dehydrocholesterol combined with low levels of cholesterol are characteristic of the Smith-Lemli-Opitz syndrome. J Lipid Res 1995;36:89–95.

438. Rilling HC, Chayet LT. Biosynthesis of cholesterol. In: Danielsson H, Sjovall J, editors. Sterols and bile acids. Amsterdam: Elsevier Science Publishing BV; 1985. p. 1–39.

439. Moebius FF, Fitzky BU, Lee JN, et al. Molecular cloning and expression of the human delta7-sterol reductase. Proc Natl Acad Sci U S A 1998;95:1899–902.

440. Xu G, Salen G, Shefer S, et al. Reproducing abnormal cholesterol biosynthesis as seen in the Smith-Lemli-Opitz syndrome by inhibiting the conversion of 7-dehydrocholesterol to cholesterol in rats. J Clin Invest 1995;95:76–81.

441. Wassif CA, Maslen C, Kachilele-Linjewile S, et al. Mutations in the human sterol delta7-reductase gene at 11q12-13 cause Smith-Lemli-Opitz syndrome. Am J Hum Genet 1998;63:55–62.

442. Waterham HR, Wijburg FA, Hennekam RC, et al. Smith-Lemli-Opitz syndrome is caused by mutations in the 7-dehydrocholesterol reductase gene. Am J Hum Genet 1998;63:329–38.

443. Bae SH, Lee JN, Fitzky BU, et al. Cholesterol biosynthesis from lanosterol. Molecular cloning, tissue distribution, expression, chromosomal localization, and regulation of rat 7-dehydrocholesterol reductase, a Smith-Lemli-Opitz syndrome-related protein. J Biol Chem 1999;274:14624–31.

444. Fitzky BU, Witsch-Baumgartner M, Erdel M, et al. Mutations in the delta7-sterol reductase gene in patients with the Smith-

Lemli-Opitz syndrome. Proc Natl Acad Sci U S A 1998;
95:8181–6.

445. Street JM, Trafford DJ, Makin HL. The quantitative estimation of bile acids and their conjugates in human biological fluids. J Lipid Res 1983;24:491–511.

446. Setchell KDR, Lawson AM. The bile acids. In: Lawson AM, editor. Clinical biochemistry principles, methods, applications. Volume 1: mass spectrometry. Berlin: Walter de Gruyter; 1988. p. 54–125.

447. Street JM, Setchell KD. Chromatographic methods for bile acid analysis. Biomed Chromatogr 1988;2:229–41.

448. Roda A, Roda E, Festi D, Colombo C. Immunological methods for serum bile acid analysis. In: Setchell KDR, Kritchevsky D, Nair PP, editors. The bile acids. Volume 4: Methods and applications. New York: Plenum Press; 1988. p. 269–314.

449. Nambara T, Goto J. High-performance liquid chromatography. In: Setchell KDR, Kritchevsky D, Nair PP, editors. The bile acids. Volume 4: Methods and applications. New York: Plenum Press; 1988. p. 43–64.

450. Setchell KDR, Vestal CH. Thermospray ionization liquid chromatography-mass spectrometry: a new and highly specific technique for the analysis of bile acids. J Lipid Res 1989;30:1459–69.

451. Roda A, Gioacchini AM, Cerre C, Baraldini M. High-performance liquid chromatographic-electrospray mass spectrometric analysis of bile acids in biological fluids. J Chromatogr B Biomed Appl 1995;665:281–94.

452. Ikegawa S, Murao N, Motoyama T, et al. Separation and detection of bile acid 3-glucuronides in human urine by liquid chromatography/electrospray ionization-mass spectrometry. Biomed Chromatogr 1996;10:313–7.

453. Lawson AM, Setchell KDR. Mass spectrometry of bile acids. In: Setchell KDR, Kritchevsky D, Nair PP, editors. The bile acids. Volume 4: Methods and applications. New York: Plenum Press; 1988. p. 167–268.

454. Sjovall J, Lawson AM, Setchell KDR. Mass spectrometry of bile acids. In: Law JH, Rilling HC, editors. Methods in enzymology. London: Academic Press; 1985. p. 63–113.

455. Evans JE, Ghosh A, Evans BA, Natowicz MR. Screening techniques for the detection of inborn errors of bile acid metabolism by direct injection and micro-high performance liquid chromatography-continuous flow/fast atom bombardment mass spectrometry. Biol Mass Spectrom 1993;22:331–7.

456. Meng LJ, Griffiths WJ, Nazer H, et al. High levels of (24S)-24-hydroxycholesterol 3-sulfate, 24-glucuronide in the serum and urine of children with severe cholestatic liver disease. J Lipid Res 1997;38:926–34.

457. Zhang J, Griffiths WJ, Bergman T, Sjovall J. Derivatization of bile acids with taurine for analysis by fast atom bombard-

ment mass spectrometry with collision-induced fragmentation. J Lipid Res 1993;34:1895–900.

458. Griffiths WJ, Egestad B, Sjovall J. Charge-remote fragmentation of taurine-conjugated bile acids. Rapid Commun Mass Spectrom 1991;5:391–4.

459. Eckers C, New AP, East PB, Haskins NJ. The use of tandem mass spectrometry for the differentiation of bile acid isomers and for the identification of bile acids in biological extracts. Rapid Commun Mass Spectrom 1990;4:449–53.

460. Stroobant V, de Hoffmann E, Libert R, Van Hoof F. Fast-atom bombardment mass spectrometry and low energy collision-induced tandem mass spectrometry of tauroconjugated bile acid anions. J Am Soc Mass Spectrom 1995;6:588–96.

461. Berginer VM, Salen G, Shefer S. Long-term treatment of cerebrotendinous xanthomatosis with chenodeoxycholic acid. N Engl J Med 1984;311:1649–52.

462. van Heijst AF, Wevers RA, Tangerman A, et al. Chronic diarrhoea as a dominating symptom in two children with cerebrotendinous xanthomatosis. Acta Paediatr 1996;85:932–6.

463. van Heijst AF, Verrips A, Wevers RA, et al. Treatment and follow-up of children with cerebrotendinous xanthomatosis. Eur J Pediatr 1998;157:313–6.

464. Lewis B, Mitchell WD, Marenah CB, et al. Cerebrotendinous xanthomatosis: biochemical response to inhibition of cholesterol synthesis. BMJ 1983;287:21–2.

465. Verrips A, Wevers RA, Van Engelen BG, et al. Effect of simvastatin in addition to chenodeoxycholic acid in patients with cerebrotendinous xanthomatosis. Metabolism 1999;48:233–8.

466. Clayton PT, Mills KA, Johnson AW, et al. Delta 4-3-oxosteroid 5 beta-reductase deficiency: failure of ursodeoxycholic acid treatment and response to chenodeoxycholic acid plus cholic acid. Gut 1996;38:623–8.

467. Lazarow PB, Black V, Shio H, et al. Zellweger syndrome: biochemical and morphological studies on two patients treated with clofibrate. Pediatr Res 1985;19:1356–64.

468. Bjorkhem I, Blomstrand S, Glaumann H, Strandvik B. Unsuccessful attempts to induce peroxisomes in two cases of Zellweger disease by treatment with clofibrate. Pediatr Res 1985;19:590–3.

469. Mathis RK, Watkins JB, Szczepanik-Van Leeuwen P, Lott IT. Liver in the cerebro-hepato-renal syndrome: defective bile acid synthesis and abnormal mitochondria. Gastroenterology 1980;79:1311–7.

470. Setchell KDR, Bragetti P, Zimmer-Nechemias L, et al. Oral bile acid treatment and the patient with Zellweger syndrome. Hepatology 1992;15:198–207.

471. Gruy-Kapral C, Little KH, Fordtran JS, et al. Conjugated bile acid replacement therapy for short-bowel syndrome. Gastroenterology 1999;116:15–21.

5. Bilirubin Metabolism

Glenn R. Gourley, MD

Many diseases are associated with elevations of the serum bilirubin level. This chapter focuses on conditions in which hyperbilirubinemia results from a primary abnormality in the metabolism of bilirubin, whereas other liver disease is absent (Tables 55.5-1 and 55.5-2). These conditions must be distinguished from many other conditions in which hyperbilirubinemia is a secondary phenomenon caused by such things as primary liver disease, hematologic abnormalities, or infection. To understand and remember these primary defects in the metabolism of bilirubin, it is helpful to approach them from the viewpoint of the normal route by which bilirubin is metabolized and cleared from the circulation. Thus, this chapter begins by presenting the three hepatic steps necessary for clearance of bilirubin: (1) hepatocyte uptake of bilirubin from the sinusoid, (2) enzymatic conjugation of bilirubin within the endoplasmic reticulum of the hepatocyte, and (3) secretion of bilirubin conjugates out of the hepatocyte via the canalicular membrane. Defects in these metabolic steps result in the disorders described in this chapter. Recent reviews exist.[1-3]

BILIRUBIN MEASUREMENT

Serum bilirubin measurements are very common, being made in 61% of term newborns.[4] The two components of total serum bilirubin routinely measured in the clinical laboratory are conjugated bilirubin ("direct" reacting in van den Bergh test in which color develops directly without adding methanol) and unconjugated bilirubin ("indirect"). Together these components comprise the total bilirubin. Although the terms direct and conjugated bilirubin are often used as synonyms, this is not always quantitatively correct because the direct fraction includes both conjugated bilirubin and delta bilirubin.[5] Delta bilirubin results spontaneously when the conjugated bilirubin is elevated and a covalent bond is formed with albumin. Delta bilirubin is metabolized with albumin (half-life approximately 22 days), thus potentially prolonging jaundice when other liver function tests are improving. Serum bilirubin measurement has long been known to have significant interlaboratory variability,[6,7] and a variety of methods exist.[5,8,9] The Jendrassik-Grof procedure is very popular, although it is not without problems.[10] Two newer methods use high-performance liquid chromatography (HPLC)[11] and multilayered slides.[12] Analysis with HPLC is the acknowledged "gold standard" but too costly for a routine clinical laboratory.[5] Analysis with automated multilayered slide technology (Kodak Ektachem/Vitros, Johnson & Johnson Clinical Diagnostics, Rochester, NY) is currently used in some clinical laboratories and allows measurement of specific conjugated and unconjugated bilirubin fractions

TABLE 55.5-1   COMPARISON OF DISORDERS OF UNCONJUGATED HYPERBILIRUBINEMIA

	GILBERT SYNDROME	CRIGLER-NAJJAR TYPE 1	CRIGLER-NAJJAR TYPE 2
Prevalence	3%	Rare	Rare
Inheritance	Autosomal dominant or recessive	Autosomal recessive	Autosomal recessive, rarely dominant
Genetic defect	*UGT1A1* gene	*UGT1A1* gene	*UGT1A1* gene
Hepatocyte defect site	Microsomes ± plasma membrane	Microsomes	Microsomes
Deficient hepatocyte function	Glucuronidation ± uptake	Glucuronidation	Glucuronidation
BUGT activity	5–53% of controls	Severely decreased	2–23% of controls
Hepatocyte uptake	Decreased in 20–30%	Normal	Normal
Serum total bilirubin level (mg/dL)	0.8–4.3	15–45	8–25
Serum bilirubin decrease with phenobarbital (%)	70	0	77
HPLC serum bilirubin composition:			
Fraction (Normal %)			
Unconjugated (92.6)	98.8	~ 100	99.1
Diglucuronide (6.2)	1.1	0	0.6
Monoglucuronide (0.5)	0	0	0
Bile bilirubin conjugates:			
Fraction (Normal %)			
Diglucuronide (~ 80)	60	0 to trace	5–10
Monoglucuronide (~ 15)	30	Predominant if measurable	90–95
Other routine liver function tests	Normal	Normal	Normal
Prognosis	Benign	Kernicterus common	Occasional kernicterus

BUGT = bilirubin uridine diphosphate glucuronosyltransferase; HPLC = high-performance liquid chromatography.

TABLE 55.5-2   COMPARISON OF DISORDERS OF CONJUGATED HYPERBILIRUBINEMIA

	ROTOR SYNDROME	DUBIN-JOHNSON SYNDROME
Prevalence	Rare	Rare
Inheritance	Autosomal recessive	Autosomal recessive
Genetic defect	Unknown	MRP2 (cMOAT) gene
ABCC2		
Hepatocyte defect site	GST	Apical canalicular membrane
Deficient hepatocyte function	Intracellular binding of bilirubin and conjugates	Canalicular secretion of bilirubin conjugates
Brown-black liver	No	Yes
Serum total bilirubin level (mg/dL)	2–7	1.5–6.0
Serum conjugated bilirubin (%)	> 50	> 50
Other routine liver function tests	Normal	Normal
Oral cholecystogram	Usually visualizes	Usually does not visualize
^{99m}Tc- HIDA cholescintigraphy		
Liver	Poor to no visualization	Intense, prolonged visualization
Gallbladder	Poor to no visualization	Delayed or nonvisualization
Sulfobromophthalein clearance test	Serum sulfobromophthalein levels elevated (delayed clearance)	Serum sulfobromophthalein levels normal at 45 min but elevated at 90–120 min
Indocyanine green clearance test	Delayed clearance	Normal
Response to estrogens or pregnancy	No change	Increased jaundice
Total urinary coproporphyrin excretion (isomers I + III)	2.5–5 times increased	Normal
Urinary coproporphyrin isomer I composition (%) (normal = 25%)	Usually < 80% of total	> 80% of total
Prognosis	Benign (asymptomatic)	Benign (occasional abdominal complaints; probably incidental)

ABCC2 = ATP-binding cassette, subfamily C (CFTR/MRP), member 2 (cMOAT); cMOAT = canalicular multispecific organic anion transporter; GST = glutathione S-transferase; MRP2 = multidrug resistance–associated protein 2; ^{99m} Tc-HIDA = technetium 99m hepatobiliary iminodiacetic acid.

without inclusion of delta bilirubin. Noninvasive point of care methods for transcutaneous bilirubin measurement continue to develop. At present, two such methods are available in the United States: BiliCheck (Respironics, Pittsburgh, PA)[13] and Jaundice Meter (Minolta/Air Shields, Air-Shields Vickers, Hatboro, PA).[14]

BILIRUBIN CLEARANCE

HEPATOCYTE UPTAKE

The architecture of the liver is important for hepatic uptake of bilirubin. Cords of hepatocytes are arranged radially so that adjacent sinusoids border all hepatocytes and allow uptake of bilirubin by individual hepatocytes. Portal venous pressure rather than arterial pressure generates slow sinusoidal flow of blood. Albumin-bound bilirubin from the plasma passes into the tissue fluid space (space of Disse) between the endothelium and the hepatocyte. This is facilitated by the lack of basal laminae, which are found in other organ capillary systems.[15,16] The pores of the endothelium allow direct contact with the plasma membrane of the hepatocyte.

A schematic illustration of hepatic bilirubin metabolism is shown in Figure 55.5-1. Bilirubin dissociates from albumin[17] and can enter the hepatocyte via a membrane receptor-carrier. Carrier-facilitated transport into the hepatocyte has been demonstrated for organic anions such as bilirubin, sulfobromophthalein (Bromsulfphthalein), and indocyanine green.[18] Recently, bilirubin has also been shown to be able to pass through membranes by simple passive diffusion.[19] Bilirubin, sulfobromophthalein, and indocyanine green are believed to share the same hepato-

cyte receptor-carrier because they exhibit competitive inhibition when injected simultaneously. Subsequent intrahepatic metabolism of these anions is quite different and therefore cannot explain their competitive inhibition: bilirubin undergoes microsomal glucuronidation, sulfobromophthalein undergoes cytosolic conjugation with glutathione, and indocyanine green is excreted directly without biotransformation. Rat hepatocyte data suggest that the receptor-carrier is a dimeric protein with a subunit molecular weight of 55,000.[20–22] Additional supportive data regarding this receptor-carrier include antibody studies showing the expected plasma membrane location[21] and demonstrating blockage of uptake.[22]

Differences in protein binding inside and outside the hepatocyte necessitate carrier-mediated transport of bilirubin. Outside the hepatocyte, bilirubin is bound to albumin (affinity constant ~ 10^8; concentration 0.6 mM).[23] Inside the hepatocyte, bilirubin is bound to glutathione S-transferase B (GST; also known as ligandin or the Y protein; affinity constant ~ 10^6; concentration 0.04 mM).[24,25] GST consists of a family of proteins that can function both as enzymes and as intracellular binding proteins for nonsubstrate ligands such as bilirubin.[26] GST binds both bilirubin and bilirubin conjugates and decreases reflux from the hepatocyte back into plasma.[27]

CONJUGATION

Inside the hepatocyte, bilirubin enters the endoplasmic reticulum (microsomes), where it is conjugated with glucuronic acid.[28] Uridine diphosphate glucuronic acid (UDPGA) is the glucuronic acid donor. Conjugation disrupts the intracellular hydrogen bonding (Figure 55.5-2A) by forming an ester linkage with one or both of the propionic acid side chains on the

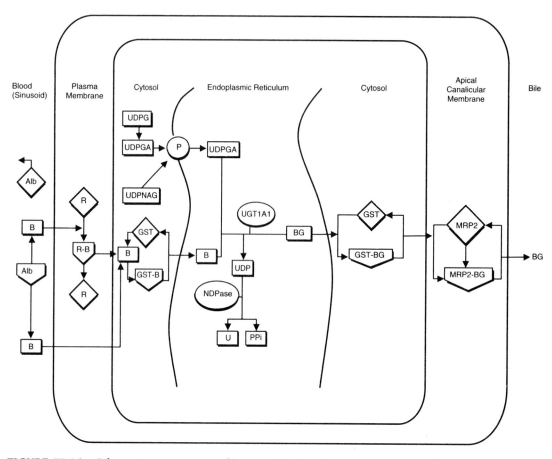

FIGURE 55.5-1   Schematic representation of hepatic bilirubin (B) metabolism. Alb = albumin; BG = bilirubin glucuronides (mono- and di-); GST = glutathione *S*-transferase (ligandin); MRP2 = multidrug resistance–associated protein 2; NDPase = nucleoside diphosphatase; P = permease; PPi = inorganic pyrophosphate; R = membrane carrier; U = uridine; UDPG = uridine diphosphate glucose; UDPGA = uridine diphosphate glucuronic acid; UDPNAG = uridine diphosphate *N*-acetylglucosamine; UGT1A1 = bilirubin uridine diphosphate glucuronosyltransferase 1A1, the isoform responsible for bilirubin conjugation.

B and C pyrrole rings of bilirubin (Figure 55.5-2B). Bilirubin uridine diphosphate glucuronosyltransferase (BUGT; Online Mendelian Inheritance in Man [OMIM] *191740; < http://www.ncbi.nlm.nih.gov/Omim/>) is the enzyme responsible for this esterification. Other glucuronosyltransferase isoforms catalyze the conjugation of thyroxine, steroids, bile acids, and xenobiotics.[29–33] The lipid environment of BUGT is important in determining enzyme activity. In vitro assays of BUGT can use different methods to perturb this lipid environment and thus greatly affect measured BUGT activity. A permease has been hypothesized to facilitate the transport of UDPGA from the cytosol across the lipid layers to the interior of the endoplasmic reticulum, where BUGT is located. The existence of a permease has been proposed because UDPGA is the preferred donor for bilirubin conjugation, despite the observation that uridine diphosphate glucose (UDPG) is present in the cytosol at higher concentrations.[34] Uridine diphosphate *N*-acetylglucosamine can increase in vitro BUGT activity threefold and is therefore considered to be a physiologic regulator of BUGT.[35] It is speculated that the mechanism for this involves facilitation of the permease UDPGA transporter.[36] Following conjugation, UDP can be converted to uridine and inorganic pyrophosphate by

a nucleoside diphosphatase in the interior of the endo-plasmic reticulum,[37] thus preventing the reverse reaction.

The specific isoform responsible for bilirubin conjugation is UGT1A1 (trivial name HUG-Br1, EC 2.4.1.17).[38] This is part of the UDP glycosyltransferase superfamily of enzymes encoded by the *UGT1* gene complex on chromosome 2 (Figure 55.5-3).[39] The *UGT1* gene encodes several isoforms and has a complex structure consisting of four common exons (2–5) and 13 variable exons encoding different isoforms.[40] During transcription, messenger ribonucleic acid from each variable exon 1 is spliced to exon 2 and the intervening ribonucleic acid is excised. The variable exons impart substrate specificity, whereas the common exons determine the UDPGA binding site and the membrane spanning region of the enzyme. More than 30 different *UGT1* mutant alleles have been described that cause Gilbert syndrome (GS) and Crigler-Najjar syndrome types I and II.[41] UGT1A1 catalyzes the formation of both bilirubin mono- and diglucuronides.[42–46] In normal human adults, bilirubin conjugates are excreted in the bile mainly as bilirubin diglucuronides (~ 80%) (Figure 55.5-4) with lesser amounts of bilirubin monoglucuronides (~ 15%) and very small amounts of unconjugated bilirubin and other bilirubin conjugates (eg, glucose, xylose, and mixed diesters).[47–52]

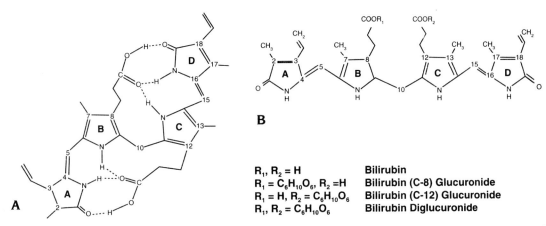

FIGURE 55.5-2 4Z,15Z-bilirubin IX-α depicted with standard carbon atom numbering demonstrating (A) normal internal hydrogen bonding and (B) conjugation sites. Substitutions (R_1 and R_2) indicate mono- and diglucuronides, which interrupt the internal hydrogen bonding, thus increasing the solubility of the bilirubin conjugates.

SECRETION OF BILIRUBIN CONJUGATES

Following conjugation, bilirubin conjugates are excreted against a concentration gradient from the hepatocyte through the canalicular membrane into the bile. Data from purified rat liver canalicular membrane vesicles indicate that bilirubin diglucuronide transport through the canalicular membrane is carrier mediated, electrogenic, and stimulated by bicarbonate.[53] Similar data suggest that bilirubin glucuronides are transported across the canalicular membrane by both adenosine triphosphate (ATP)-dependent and membrane potential–dependent transport systems, and in the normal rat, these systems are additive.[54] The ATP-dependent transporter responsible for bilirubin glucuronide passage from the hepatocyte through the canalicular membrane is canalicular multispecific organic anion transporter (cMOAT). cMOAT is a member of the ATP-binding cassette (ABC) transporter superfamily and is homologous to the multidrug resistance–associated protein 2 (MRP2).[55,56] cMOAT/MRP2 is involved with ATP-dependent transport across the apical canalicular membrane of a variety of endogenous compounds and xenobiotics,[57] including both bilirubin mono- and diglucuronide.[58] cMOAT/MRP2 has previously been described as the non–bile acid organic anion transporter, the glutathione S-conjugate export pump, or the leukotriene export pump.[59] Genetic mutations that alter these ABC transporters cause diseases, which include cystic fibrosis, hyperinsulinemia, adrenoleukodystrophy, multidrug resistance,[60] and, as is discussed later in this chapter, Dubin-Johnson syndrome (DJS). This mechanism can be saturated with increasing amounts of bilirubin or bilirubin conjugates.[61–63] Many other organic anions (eg, sulfobromophthalein, indocyanine green) are believed to share this same canalicular membrane excretion mechanism.[64] Simultaneous infusions of sulfobromophthalein and indocyanine green will decrease the maximal canalicular excretion of bilirubin and vice versa.[65,66] Bile salts do not use the same canalicular excretion mechanisms. In DJS, biliary excretion of conjugated bilirubin and sulfobromophthalein is decreased, although bile salt excretion is not impaired.[67] However, infusion of bile salts does increase the maximal excretion of bilirubin conjugates so that bile salt and bilirubin conjugate excretion by the canalicular membrane are not completely independent.[68] A similar effect is also seen with phenobarbital.[69] Conversely, the maximal excretion of bilirubin conjugates can be decreased by cholestatic agents such as estrogens and anabolic steroids.[70,71]

GILBERT SYNDROME

CLINICAL PRESENTATION

GS (OMIM #143500) was first described in 1901 by Gilbert and Lereboullet.[72] GS is a hereditary, chronic or

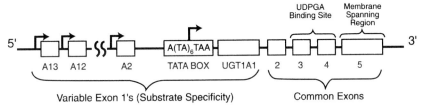

FIGURE 55.5-3 The human uridine diphosphate glucuronosyltransferase-1 (*UGT1*) gene. During transcription messenger ribonucleic acid from each variable, exon 1 (A1–A13) is spliced to exon 2, and the intervening ribonucleic acid is excised, resulting in a variety of isoforms. The variable exons impart substrate specificity, whereas the common exons determine the uridine diphosphate glucuronic acid (UDPGA) binding site and the membrane spanning region of the enzyme. The *UGT1A1* gene that results from this splicing encodes bilirubin glucuronosyltransferase.

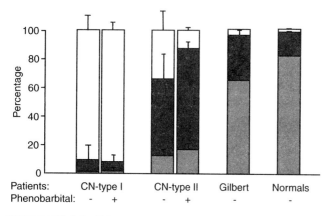

FIGURE 55.5-4   Bile pigment composition in bile from normal ($n = 8$), Crigler-Najjar (CN) syndrome type I ($n = 3$), CN type II ($n = 3$), and Gilbert syndrome ($n = 16$) patients, receiving (+) or not receiving (–) phenobarbital. Relative bile pigment composition is indicated in the vertical columns as a percentage of the total ± SD. Shading: white = unconjugated bilirubin; intermediate = bilirubin monoconjugate; dark = bilirubin diconjugate. Reproduced with permission from Sinaasappel M and Jansen PL.[49]

recurrent, mild unconjugated hyperbilirubinemia with otherwise normal liver function tests.[2,73,74] The serum unconjugated bilirubin level usually ranges from 1 to 4 mg/dL (17 µmol/L = 1 mg/dL). Often patients are first identified by an elevated serum bilirubin on routine blood chemistry or mild jaundice (perhaps only scleral icterus) during a period of fasting associated with viral illness or religious activities[75] or anorexia nervosa.[76] Icteric plasma from a blood donor may suggest GS.[77] Alternatively, hyperbilirubinemia post-transplant of an apparently healthy donor liver may be a sign that the donor had GS.[78–81] GS is generally associated with no negative implications for health or longevity, despite the large variety of symptoms reported by GS patients.[82,83] These symptoms include vertigo, headache, fatigue, abdominal pain, nausea, diarrhea, constipation, and loss of appetite. The possible relationship of these symptoms to GS has been evaluated in a group of 2,395 Swedish subjects.[84] The only symptom that was more common in the GS group was diarrhea in male subjects aged 57 to 67 years. The authors suggested that this was most likely type 1 error because of the large number of comparisons made and concluded that there was no higher prevalence of symptoms associated with GS. There are limited reports suggesting that GS is a risk factor for chronic fatigue syndrome.[85,86]

Large surveys of normal individuals found approximately 3% of the population with serum bilirubin levels greater than 1.0 mg/dL.[87,88] Although one survey noted a bimodal distribution of serum bilirubin concentrations with antimodes of 1.4 mg/dL in male patients and 0.7 mg/dL in female patients,[87] other studies have not observed this. If these levels were used to define the upper limit of normal for serum bilirubin concentration, the incidence of GS would be approximately 6% of the population, and the sex distribution would be close to 1:1. If 1.4 mg/dL is used as the upper limit of serum bilirubin concentration

for both sexes, then there is a strong male predominance (approximately 4:1). This finding might be related to the observation that female subjects clear bilirubin better than male subjects.[89] GS may be inherited in either an autosomal dominant[90–93] or recessive[94] fashion.

GS is rarely diagnosed before puberty, although it is a congenital disorder. Hormonal changes of puberty have been suggested as one explanation. Steroid hormones can suppress hepatic bilirubin clearance.[71] Increased estrogen levels of pregnancy are associated with impaired clearance of exogenous bilirubin.[95] Gonadectomy has been shown to alter BUGT activity.[96] Odell speculated that some infants with nonhemolytic neonatal jaundice are manifesting GS.[97] Use of genetic markers (see below) has allowed investigation of the role that GS plays in neonatal jaundice. Individuals carrying such markers have been shown to have a more rapid rise in their jaundice levels during the first 2 days of life,[98] a predisposition to prolonged or severe neonatal hyperbilirubinemia,[99–101] and variably increased jaundice when the GS polymorphism is coinherited with hematologic abnormalities such as glucose-6-phosphatase dehydrogenase (G6PD) deficiency,[102,103] β-thalassemia,[102,104,105] hereditary spherocytosis,[106] ABO incompatibility,[107] and sickle cell disease.[108] Kaplan and colleagues have shown that infants with G6PD deficiency do not have an increased incidence of hyperbilirubinemia (compared with G6PD normals) unless they also carry the UGT1A1 promoter polymorphism[103]; homozygotes for this polymorphism have a significantly higher incidence of hyperbilirubinemia than do heterozygotes (Figure 55.5-5). Thus, numerous studies indicate that GS, as detected by *UGT1A1* analysis, is one of the many factors related to neonatal jaundice. GS may also be a factor related to the jaundice associated with pyloric stenosis.[109] GS is associated with an increased incidence and/or earlier diagnosis of gallstones when coinherited with hematologic abnormalities such as congenital dyserythropoietic anemia,[110] thalassemia,[111] or hereditary spherocytosis.[112]

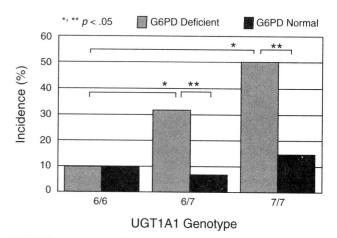

FIGURE 55.5-5   Incidence (percentage) of hyperbilirubinemia (serum total bilirubin ≥ 257 µmol/L) in glucose-6-phosphatase dehydrogenase (G6PD)-deficient neonates and normal controls, stratified for the three genotypes of the bilirubin uridine diphosphate glucuronosyltransferase 1A1 (UGT1A1) promoter. Reproduced with permission from Kaplan M et al.[103]

PATHOPHYSIOLOGY

GS is a heterogeneous group of disorders sharing a significant (≥ 50%) decrease in hepatic BUGT activity.[113–116] There are at least four subtypes of GS based on the plasma clearance of sulfobromophthalein and indocyanine green, which share the same hepatocyte uptake receptor-carrier.[117,118] In GS type I, clearance of sulfobromophthalein and indocyanine green is normal. In GS type II, sulfobromophthalein clearance is delayed, but indocyanine green clearance is normal. Because sulfobromophthalein uptake is normal in type II, delayed clearance must be related to subsequent intrahepatic metabolism or canalicular excretion.[119] In GS type III, clearance of both sulfobromophthalein and indocyanine green is delayed. The delay in the initial rate of disappearance from the plasma suggests a defect in uptake at the hepatocyte plasma membrane.[119] In GS type IV, indocyanine green uptake is delayed, but sulfobromophthalein uptake is normal. Thus, GS may include delayed uptake of bilirubin into the hepatocyte, delayed biotransformation, or both abnormalities.[52,120–122] Immunohistochemical staining for BUGT shows a clear reduction throughout the hepatic lobule in specimens from individuals with GS when compared with normals.[123]

The elucidation of the structure of the *UGT1* gene that encodes human bilirubin, phenol, and other UDP-glucuronosyltransferase isozymes[39] led to the discovery of *UGT1A1* mutations or polymorphisms associated with GS.[124] In white populations, the homozygous finding of an additional TA repeat in the promoter region or so-called TATA box (ie, [TA]$_7$TAA, rather than [TA]$_6$TAA) of the *UGT1A1* gene has been shown to be a necessary, although not sufficient, condition for GS.[125–127] This homozygous polymorphism occurs in 10 to 13% of whites.[125,128] Approximately 42% are heterozygous for the (TA)$_7$, and these individuals have significantly higher serum bilirubin levels than individuals with the wild-type six repeats ([TA]$_6$).[125] Hepatic UDP glucuronosyltransferase activity appears to be inversely related to the number of TA repeats in whites.[129] In Asian populations, the (TA)$_7$TAA mutation is relatively rare,[130] but several different *UGT1A1* mutations have been associated with GS.[93,131,132] These Asian mutations involve exons of the *UGT1A1* gene rather than the previously described promoter region. One of the most common mutations in Asians, a Gly71Arg mutation in exon 1, has also linked GS and severe or prolonged neonatal hyperbilirubinemia.[100,101,133] It has recently been reported that although within whites, the promoter TA repeat number and bilirubin level are strongly positively correlated, in other ethnic groups (eg, Africans, where two other variants [TA]$_5$ and [TA]$_8$ have been identified), there is a negative correlation.[134] Thus, the ethnic implications of these genetic polymorphisms of the *UGT1A1* gene require further analysis.

Despite the universal BUGT decrease in GS, the correlation is poor between measured hepatic enzyme activity and serum bilirubin concentration.[135] This may be due to the increased bilirubin production associated with the decreased red cell half-life seen in up to 40% of patients with GS.[97,177] Although some conditions with increased bilirubin production (eg, sickle cell disease) result in BUGT induction, this is not the case in GS.[136] Even phenobarbital produces little BUGT induction in GS.[114] Hepatic BUGT activity in GS significantly overlaps with that seen in Crigler-Najjar type II (CNII),[116] although activity in GS is usually higher. If an individual has one allele producing nonfunctional UGT1A1 (Crigler-Najjar) and the other structurally normal allele possesses the GS promoter polymorphism, the resulting hyperbilirubinemia would be expected to be more severe than that found in GS but less severe than that found in Crigler-Najjar I (CNI).[137]

Consistent with the decreased hepatic BUGT activity, bile from GS individuals contains decreased bilirubin diglucuronides and increased bilirubin monoglucuronides compared with normals (see Figure 55.5-4).[49,52,116,138] This finding is similar to biliary bile pigment profiles seen in infants.[139] Phenobarbital normalizes the bile pigment profile in duodenal fluid,[52] lowers plasma bilirubin levels, and increases hepatic clearance of bilirubin.[140,141] Clofibrate and glutethimide also normalize serum bilirubin levels but do not normalize the distribution of bilirubin conjugates in duodenal bile.[142] In animals, clofibrate is an inducer of BUGT but does not affect sulfobromophthalein uptake or GST.[143]

A characteristic but poorly understood finding in GS is the exaggerated rise in serum bilirubin associated with fasting.[144–147] Normal individuals can double their serum bilirubin level when fasting, but in GS, a more pronounced increase occurs. Because indocyanine green clearance is not affected, this is not related to decreased hepatic blood flow.[145] Fasting reduces BUGT activity[147] and increases heme oxygenase (the enzyme responsible for bilirubin production) activity,[148] but these effects are not believed to explain the fasting hyperbilirubinemia of GS.[140,149] Intraluminal noncalorie food bulk can blunt the bilirubin rise.[150]

DIAGNOSIS AND TREATMENT

Generally, a diagnosis of GS can be made when there is a mild fluctuating unconjugated hyperbilirubinemia; otherwise, liver function tests are normal, and there is no hemolysis. Hemolysis can add confusion because it can result in similar findings, and it is not unusual in GS. Hence, other diagnostic tests are sometimes helpful.

One diagnostic test used with GS involves measuring the rise in serum bilirubin following intravenous administration of nicotinic acid.[151] Nicotinic acid is usually administered to adults in a dose of 50 mg over 30 seconds,[152–154] although similar results were seen with 300 mg injections.[155] Nonconjugated serum bilirubin is then measured every 30 to 60 minutes for the next 4 to 5 hours. Nicotinic acid produces a rise in serum unconjugated bilirubin in both normals and those with GS. However, in GS, the bilirubin rise is higher, and clearance is delayed longer.[151,155–158] Nicotinic acid causes increased osmotic fragility and hemolysis of red blood cells with splenic sequestration. Induced splenic heme oxygenase rapidly converts heme to bilirubin.[157] Nicotinic acid–induced hemolysis produces a rise in serum iron that is similar in healthy controls and those with GS.[158] Hence, the prolonged serum bilirubin levels are related to delayed hepatic clearance of bilirubin. Nicotinic acid infusion can be a better diagnostic method for GS than a 400 kcal fast because delayed bilirubin clearance can be seen after nicotinic acid in GS subjects who otherwise had normal serum bilirubin levels.[152] The nicotinic acid test cannot differentiate GS from chronic liver disease.[159]

Rifampin, given to fasting or nonfasting adults in one oral dose of 900 mg, increases total serum bilirubin levels in normal subjects and subjects with GS, although there is an exaggerated rise in those with GS (fasting: > 1.9 mg/dL rise in bilirubin concentration 2 to 6 hours after rifampin; nonfasting: > 1.5 mg/dL rise 4 to 6 hours after rifampin).[160] This exaggerated rise in serum bilirubin enabled differentiation of 10 normal subjects and 15 GS patients with high sensitivity and specificity. This finding could not be explained by hemolysis, although haptoglobin levels were significantly lower in GS patients, compatible with baseline hemolysis.

Alkaline methanolysis and thin-layer chromatography have been used to diagnose GS by accurately separating and measuring total serum bilirubin as conjugated and unconjugated fractions.[161,162] In GS, only approximately 6% of the total serum bilirubin was conjugated compared with approximately 17% in normal subjects or those with chronic hemolysis and 28% in those with chronic persistent hepatitis. Fasting increased the serum total bilirubin level but did not change the percentage of conjugates in GS. An overlap of only three individuals was seen among the 77 subjects with GS and 60 normal subjects.[162] Other studies support these findings.[163] HPLC of serum showed similar findings with significantly decreased bilirubin monoglucuronides (1.1% vs 6.2% in normals) and increased unconjugated bilirubin (98.8 vs 92.6 in normals).[164]

Monaghan and colleagues have suggested GS genetic screening for the UGT1A1 TA repeat as a simple, useful additional test in the investigation of very prolonged neonatal jaundice in North American, African, and European populations and for the Gly71Arg mutation in Asians.[99] Although genetic testing may be helpful in individual patients, the screening value of such a genetic test cannot be fully determined until accurate data regarding the prevalence and penetrance of the GS genotype are known.[165] Thus, genetic testing for GS cannot be routinely recommended.[165]

GS is generally believed to have no significant negative health implications. Drug metabolism studies have revealed no major dangers,[163,166] although there appears to be an increased incidence of slow acetylators,[167,168] lorazepam clearance is 20 to 40% decreased,[169] and drug-mediated toxicity is a concern.[170] Concurrent genetic deficiencies in other xenobiotic pathways may put individuals with GS at increased risk of drug toxicity to such compounds as acetaminophen[171,172] or CPT-11 irinotecan, a cancer chemotherapeutic agent metabolized by UGT1A1.[173] No specific treatment is necessary for GS, although phenobarbital has been shown to lower serum bilirubin levels.[174] If the well-documented antioxidant effect of bilirubin[175] provides a biologic advantage,[176] then the mild hyperbilirubinemia of GS might actually be a significant benefit against such things as ischemic heart disease,[177–179] in which free radicals are involved in pathogenesis. Schizophrenic patients with

GS have significant enlargement of many components of their cerebrospinal fluid spaces compared with schizophrenic patients without GS and normal controls, although the significance of this remains unknown.[180]

CRIGLER-NAJJAR SYNDROME

CLINICAL PRESENTATION
Crigler and Najjar, in 1952, reported seven infants with congenital familial nonhemolytic jaundice who developed severe unconjugated hyperbilirubinemia shortly after birth and died from kernicterus within months.[181] These infants were from three related families. Serum bilirubin levels reached 25 to 35 mg/dL despite a lack of hemolytic disease and otherwise normal liver function tests. Liver histology showed only deposition of bile pigments. Many subsequent reports have documented kernicterus as the main risk for patients with the Crigler-Najjar syndrome.[182] An excellent review of the neurologic perspectives of Crigler-Najjar syndrome has recently been published.[183] Although some patients survive into the second decade with normal development,[184] the possibility of developing late kernicterus is always a concern, even in adulthood.[185–188] Serum bilirubin levels vary from approximately 15 to 45 mg/dL. A Web site addressing many aspects of Crigler-Najjar syndrome has been developed (<www.crigler-najjar.com>).

Arias and colleagues, in 1969, reported a second, more frequent type of severe nonhemolytic hyperbilirubinemia.[189] The previous syndrome was termed CNI (OMIM #218800), whereas the new findings were termed CNII or Arias syndrome (OMIM #606785).[189] In CNII, hyperbilirubinemia is less severe, varying from approximately 8 to 25 mg/dL. Hence, kernicterus, although reported,[190,191] is less common in CNII.

PATHOPHYSIOLOGY
Both CNI and CNII are generally inherited in an autosomal recessive manner, although one case of autosomal dominant inheritance of CNII has been reported.[192] CNI and CNII result from mutations to the UGT gene complex,[40] of which more than 50 different mutations have been described.[193] Patients with one normal allele demonstrate normal metabolism of bilirubin.[194] The genetic details determine the severity of clinical disease. In CNI, there is a complete absence of functional UGT1A1, whereas in CNII, UGT1A1 activity is markedly reduced.[195] In CNI, 18 of 23 described mutations of the UGT1 gene are found in the common exons 2 to 5 and thus affect many UGT1 enzymes.[40,196] Intronic mutations causing CNI have also been reported.[197] However, in CNII, four of nine known mutations are found in exon 1A1. There is some overlap in classification of mild CNII and GS (eg, Gly71Arg), which relates to differences in definitions based on serum bilirubin levels.[40] The TATA box TA_7 repeat mutation seen in GS can be seen along with other mutations resulting in either CNI or CNII.[198] Thus, various homozygous, heterozygous, or compound heterozygous mutations of the UGT1A1 gene can lead to varying degrees of reduction in hepatic bilirubin UGT activity and thus to varying degrees of clinical

hyperbilirubinemia, including severe CNI, intermediate CNII, and milder GS.[199]

In both CNI and CNII, assays of liver tissue from affected patients demonstrate negligible or very low BUGT activity.[49,50,116,186,189,200,201] Thus, liver biopsy is not helpful in differentiating these two disorders. This inability to conjugate bilirubin results in a profound block in bilirubin excretion. Study of the resected livers from four patients with CNI undergoing liver transplant showed that there was heterogeneity of the ability to glucuronidate various substrates other than bilirubin.[202] There is considerable overlap of hepatic BUGT activity between CNII and GS (see Table 55.5-1).[116] Consistent with the presumed autosomal inheritance of CNI, family studies have shown partial deficiencies in the glucuronidation of salicylate and menthol among siblings, parents, and grandparents.[203,204]

CNI and CNII are differentiated by the response to drugs that stimulate hyperplasia of the endoplasmic reticulum. In CNII, phenobarbital or diphenylhydantoin caused a significant decline in the serum bilirubin level, increased hepatic clearance of radiolabeled bilirubin,[141,189,190,205–208] and increased biliary levels of bilirubin diglucuronides (see Figure 55.5-4).[49,191] In a study of five CNII patients, phenobarbital caused a decrease in serum bilirubin ranging from 2.1 to 12.1 mg/dL (27–72%) with pre- and postphenobarbital serum bilirubin levels ranging from 7.8 to 16.9 and 4.7 to 10.1 mg/dL, respectively.[49] Summarizing data from seven earlier studies[141,189,190,205–208] regarding the response of CNII patients to oral phenobarbital treatment revealed that 11 female patients and 13 male patients had a total serum bilirubin of 15.7 ± 13.8 (mean ± SD) prior to phenobarbital. After phenobarbital (90–390 mg/d or alternatively 4 mg/kg/d), the serum bilirubin decreased 12.0 ± 4.0 mg/dL (77 ± 13%). The lowest total serum bilirubin following phenobarbital therapy was 5.9 mg/dL. Drugs have no significant effect on serum bilirubin or biliary bilirubin conjugates in CNI (see Figure 55.5-4).[49,185] Thus, response to phenobarbital is the accepted criterion by which CNI and CNII are differentiated.[209] Bile analysis has also been suggested as another method to differentiate CNI and CNII.[49] In CNI, bile contains insignificant bilirubin conjugates (< 10%), and unconjugated bilirubin predominates. In CNII, bile contains predominantly bilirubin monoglucuronides (> 60%).[116]

Two cousins with Crigler-Najjar syndrome have been described, which raises the possibility of a new variant of this syndrome (CNIII).[210] This new variant resembled CNI with no biliary excretion of bilirubin mono- or diglucuronide, but there was excretion of mono- and diglucoside conjugates of bilirubin. It has been speculated that type III patients lack the long proposed permease,[36] which has been hypothesized to transport UDP-glucuronic acid to the luminal side of the endoplasmic reticulum, where BUGT is located. This absence is suggested to result in UDP-glucose being used for bilirubin conjugation.

DIAGNOSIS AND TREATMENT
Evaluation for Crigler-Najjar syndrome invariably begins during the first few days of life, when serum bilirubin levels exceed 20 mg/dL. The conjugated fraction will not be elevated except possibly for the factitious elevation, which is sometimes seen when the total serum bilirubin is very high.[211] Evaluation of such infants should eliminate the more common causes of jaundice, including hemolysis, hypothyroidism, and infection. Formula feedings will help identify those infants with jaundice related to human milk. During these early days of life, Crigler-Najjar patients will require prompt and intense phototherapy and possibly exchange transfusion to avoid kernicterus and bilirubin encephalopathy.[212] Jaundice will be persistent and problematic. At present, there is no widely available simple clinical test to confirm a diagnosis of Crigler-Najjar syndrome. Crigler-Najjar syndrome can be excluded by finding significant amounts of bilirubin conjugates in neonatal stools. This HPLC analysis must be done on stools collected prior to establishment of sufficient intestinal bacterial flora to convert all bilirubin conjugates to urobilinoids.[182] HPLC analysis of duodenal bile will show that in CNI, there are negligible bilirubin di- or monoglucuronides, whereas in CNII, these conjugates are present but in low concentration.[40,49] However, this bile analysis led to misdiagnosis in six of nine infants examined during the first 3 months of life.[213] Bile can easily be collected with a pediatric Enterotest capsule (HDC Corporation, San Jose, CA).[138] This approach can potentially avoid a liver biopsy for confirmation of negligible BUGT activity using an in vitro assay. The ratio of serum bilirubin conjugates (as determined by alkaline methanolysis with thin-layer chromatography or HPLC) to total bilirubin, although abnormally low, does not allow differentiation of Crigler-Najjar patients from those with GS.[162] Deoxyribonucleic acid (DNA) analysis can be very helpful in establishing the correct diagnosis, although this is not routinely available.[214]

A world registry of patients with CNI aimed at developing management guidelines has been published.[215] Phenobarbital (4 mg/kd/d in infants) should be used when there is concern about CN. Within 48 hours, CNII patients can demonstrate a significant decrease in the serum bilirubin levels (as detailed above) and an increased biliary excretion of bilirubin di- and monoglucuronide,[50,191] whereas CNI patients will show no significant response. Occasionally, CNII patients do not respond to the first trial of phenobarbital therapy, but subsequent trials months later will demonstrate the significant decrease in serum bilirubin level.[209] Doses of phenobarbital as low as 0.6 mg/kg/d have been reported to completely normalize serum bilirubin in one patient. However, despite the decrease in serum bilirubin in response to phenobarbital, CNII patients will usually continue to manifest a significant hyperbilirubinemia (approximately 5–15 mg/dL). Phototherapy for 6 to 12 hours daily has been the primary modality to keep serum bilirubin levels below 20 mg/dL during the first several months of life[216] because CNI patients can excrete all bilirubin photoisomers.[217] CNI patients will require lifelong treatment with phototherapy until more definitive therapy such as liver transplant. Phototherapy has been found to be least intrusive when given at night, and improvements have been made in effectiveness and comfort.[218] Although phototherapy is very helpful in infancy, in adolescence, social inconvenience and compliance problems can bring increased risk of kernicterus.[215]

Oral administration of agents that bind bilirubin can be helpful. Options include agar, cholestyramine, and calcium phosphate.[219–222] These agents block the enterohepatic circulation by binding to bilirubin, which has reached the intestinal lumen owing to phototherapy or through direct intestinal permeation.[223] Agar varies significantly in bilirubin binding affinity among various preparations and batches.[186,219,224] Cholestyramine prompts concerns about cost, taste, and bile salt depletion and fat malabsorption. Plasmapheresis can be very helpful after the first year of life as it has been shown to rapidly decrease serum bilirubin levels.[186,225] Peritoneal dialysis and exchange transfusion have not been helpful in this setting.[185] Repeated intramuscular injections of tin-protoporphyrin, a heme oxygenase inhibitor that blocks bilirubin formation, have been used in a CNI patient, with data suggesting a decreased need for phototherapy.[226] Two patients with CNI were treated with tin-mesoporphyrin to block bilirubin formation, daily phototherapy, and intermittent plasmapheresis over a 400-day period.[227] They developed an iron deficiency anemia believed to be due to the porphyrin therapy,[228] but tin-mesoporphyrin (2–4 μmol/kg)[229] is suggested to offer a promising, although still experimental, additional therapy for controlling episodes of acute, severe jaundice. Drugs that bind to albumin and can potentially displace bilirubin should be avoided at all times.[230]

Auxiliary liver transplant would be feasible for CNI patients because their liver function is normal, except for bilirubin glucuronidation. This option has only recently become clinically available.[231–233] Thus, more commonly, orthotopic liver transplant,[234–241] including living-related liver transplant,[242] represents the only true cure for the hyperbilirubinemia of CNI. The timing of transplant should precede irreversible neurologic injury. When infants are small, sleeping under a phototherapy unit plus the medical measures noted above can be effective in managing hyperbilirubinemia and avoiding kernicterus. However, there is always the risk of intercurrent illness, which can precipitate worrisome hyperbilirubinemia. As children grow, phototherapy and other medical therapies may decrease in effectiveness. Thus, the risk of kernicterus must be balanced against the risks associated with liver transplant, including lifelong immunosuppression. This can be a very difficult decision. The effectiveness and ease of medical management of hyperbilirubinemia are important considerations, as are the long-term success and complication rate of the specific transplant center involved. Bilirubin levels must be followed and extreme hyperbilirubinemia avoided at any age because the development of kernicterus is not restricted to the neonatal period. Transplant of other BUGT-containing tissues (eg, segments of small intestine,[243,244] kidneys[245]) remains experimental. Successful cloning of the gene responsible for bilirubin glucuronosyltransferase activity offers the hope of future gene therapy to correct this deficiency.[246–250] Gene therapy,[251–254] encapsulated hepatocytes,[255] and gene repair have shown success in lowering serum bilirubin levels in Gunn rats,[256] the congenitally

jaundiced model for CNI.[257] In a 10-year-old girl with CNI, isolated hepatocytes equivalent to approximately 5% of the normal host hepatocyte mass were infused through the portal vein, survived for more than 11 months, and lowered serum bilirubin levels from approximately 25 mg/dL to 10 to 15 mg/dL while still receiving 6 to 8 hours of phototherapy per day.[258] More recent isolated hepatocyte transplant for the correction of another inborn error of metabolism (ornithine transcarbamylase deficiency) resulted in temporary improvement, which was lost after 11 days presumably because of rejection of the transplanted cells because of insufficient immunosuppression.[259] Isolated hepatocyte transplant remains experimental.[257]

ROTOR SYNDROME

CLINICAL PRESENTATION

Rotor syndrome (RS; OMIM *237450) is a familial disorder, first described in 1948, that involves chronic elevation of both the conjugated and unconjugated serum bilirubin fractions.[260,261] Fractionation of the serum total bilirubin shows that half or more is conjugated, and total bilirubin levels range from 2 to 7 mg/dL but occasionally may reach 20 mg/dL.[262] Liver functions tests are otherwise normal, and there is no evidence of hemolysis. Both light and electron microscopy reveal normal liver histology. Oral cholecystograms reveal normal gallbladder opacification. This disorder can present in early childhood[263] or in infancy if associated with other hematologic diseases[264] and manifests no gender predisposition. Family studies suggest an autosomal recessive mode of inheritance.[260,261,265]

PATHOPHYSIOLOGY

The primary abnormality in RS is a deficiency in the intracellular storage capacity of the liver for binding anions.[266,267] This can be demonstrated by constant infusions of sulfobromophthalein and indocyanine green.[268] Patients with RS demonstrate a delayed plasma clearance of both sulfobromophthalein and indocyanine green, and heterozygotes show delayed sulfobromophthalein clearance with values intermediate between normal subjects and those with homozygous RS.[266] GST serves as an intracellular carrier protein of certain organic molecules, acting as an intracellular equivalent to albumin in blood plasma.[269] Patients with RS have been shown to have a deficiency of hepatic GST,[270,271] resulting in impaired uptake of bilirubin within the cytosol. This appears to be due to mutations in the hGSTA1-1 gene.[271] In addition, because bilirubin conjugates are bound to GST while awaiting excretion from the hepatocyte via the canalicular membrane,[272] deficient intracellular storage would result in leakage of bilirubin conjugates back into the circulation, with subsequent serum elevations of both conjugated and unconjugated bilirubin.

Urinary excretion of coproporphyrin is important in RS. In normal healthy individuals, only the I and III isomers of coproporphyrin are excreted in the urine. In RS, total urinary coproporphyrin excretion (isomers I + III) is markedly increased, and, usually, isomer I comprises less than 80% of the total. Heterozygotes demonstrate urinary coproporphyrin values, which are intermediate between normal subjects and homozygotes.[273] Urinary excretion of coproporphyrin is believed to be increased because biliary excretion of coproporphyrin is impaired, similar to findings in other liver diseases.[274]

DIAGNOSIS AND TREATMENT

In all individuals with elevation of both conjugated and unconjugated serum bilirubin fractions along with otherwise normal liver function tests, a diagnosis of RS should be considered. The diagnosis can be confirmed by measuring urinary coproporphyrin levels, which are 2.5 to 5 times higher than normal levels.[273] Of the total urinary coproporphyrin isomers (I + III), isomer I constitutes less than 80% of the total in RS.[275] Technetium 99m hepatobiliary iminodiacetic acid cholescintigraphy has also been shown to be useful to diagnose RS and demonstrates poor to no visualization of the liver.[276,277]

Patients with RS require no specific therapy and are asymptomatic. Although jaundice is a lifelong finding, it is not associated with morbidity or mortality.

DUBIN-JOHNSON SYNDROME

CLINICAL PRESENTATION

DJS (OMIM #237500) was first described in 1954[278] and involves elevation of both the conjugated and unconjugated serum bilirubin fractions.[279] Fractionation of the serum total bilirubin shows that half or more is conjugated, and total bilirubin levels usually range from 1.5 to 6 mg/dL, although they have been reported to be as high as 25 mg/dL during intercurrent illness.[280] Patients with DJS report vague abdominal complaints, although this is not believed to reflect serious pathology. Hepatomegaly is sometimes seen, but liver function tests are otherwise normal, including bile acids,[281] and there is no evidence of hemolysis.[278,279,282] Although this syndrome occurs in both sexes, males predominate and present at an earlier age. It occurs in all races; however, Iranian Jews have an increased incidence.[283,284] It is usually diagnosed after puberty, although cases have also been reported in neonates,[285–288] at which time, cholestasis can be significant.[287,289–292] DJS is inherited as an autosomal recessive trait, with heterozygotes manifesting normal serum bilirubin levels.[283,293,294] This syndrome is far more common than RS, and jaundice can be worsened by pregnancy and oral contraceptives.[295] Often patients with DJS do not visualize the gallbladder with an oral cholecystogram.[279]

Brown to black discoloration of the liver is a striking characteristic of this syndrome. This pigment is located in the lysosomes.[296] The exact identity of this pigment is still uncertain. Once thought to be lipofuscin, more recent data provide conflicting evidence for a relationship to melanin[297–299] or polymerized epinephrine or other metabolites,[300,301] which accumulate in the lysosomes. It is hypothesized that these pigments accumulate in the liver because of impaired secretion of various metabolites from the hepatocyte into the bile.[301] This pigment has been shown to disappear from the liver during acute viral hepatitis, with subsequent reappearance.[302] Other than this striking pigmentation, the liver histology is normal.

PATHOPHYSIOLOGY

The primary defect in DJS is deficient hepatic excretion of non–bile salt organic anions at the apical canalicular membrane by the ABC transporter originally known as cMOAT (OMIM 601107)[303,304] but now also called MRP2.[305,306] The gene encoding this protein is designated ABCC2. cMOAT/MRP2 is encoded by a single-copy gene located on chromosome 10q24.[307] Mutations of this gene have been shown to produce a highly defective cMOAT/MRP2, which is nonfunctional or absent from the apical membrane and associated with DJS.[60,303,304,308–311] Similar findings made in the homologous cMOAT/MRP2 gene of two rat models of hyperbilirubinemia (GY/TR⁻ and Eisai) have been very helpful in understanding DJS in humans.[60,312]

Although hepatic sulfobromophthalein clearance tests are no longer performed, they clearly demonstrate the effect of deficient transport via the canalicular membrane, which is characteristic of DJS.[313] Initially, the clearance rate of intravenously administered sulfobromophthalein from the circulation is rapid and results in sulfobromophthalein retention that is often normal at 45 minutes. However, a subsequent rise in serum sulfobromophthalein concentration occurs at 90 and 120 minutes because the conjugated sulfobromophthalein cannot be excreted and thus refluxes out of the hepatocyte back into the circulation.[313–316] Data suggest that sulfobromophthalein hepatic storage is normal, but there is a 90% decrease in the sulfobromophthalein excretory transport maximum.[295,315] Other substances (eg, indocyanine green, rose bengal, and dibromosulfophthalein) have also been shown to have a decreased excretory transport maximum, although these substances do not require hepatic biotransformation and do not show the late rise in plasma levels during clearance tests.[317] Hence, in DJS, deficient excretion of bilirubin glucuronides at the canalicular membrane, in the presence of otherwise normal intrahepatic metabolism, results in reflux of conjugated bilirubin back into the circulation.

Urinary excretion of coproporphyrins is important in patients with DJS.[318,319] DJS patients have an increase in the urinary excretion of coproporphyrin I with a concomitant decrease in the excretion of coproporphyrin III. This results in a total coproporphyrin excretion (I + III) that is normal or only slightly increased but that consists of greater than 80% coproporphyrin I (normal 25%).[319–322] In heterozygotes, the coproporphyrin I-to-III ratios are intermediate between normal subjects and homozygotes,[319,321,322] although there is some overlap between them. The explanation for these findings regarding urinary coproporphyrin excretion is unclear, and several pathogenic mechanisms have been suggested.[319] Fecal coproporphyrin levels are normal.[319] Healthy neonates have been shown to have impressive elevations of urinary coproporphyrin levels, with more than 80% isomer I on the first 2 days of life[323]; however, by day 10, levels fell to overlap normal adult values.

DIAGNOSIS AND TREATMENT

A diagnosis of DJS should be considered in all individuals with an elevation of conjugated bilirubin in the serum along with otherwise normal liver function tests. Measurement of urinary coproporphyrin isomers I and III can confirm the diagnosis. The total coproporphyrin level will be approximately normal, but more than 80% will be isomer I. This finding is pathognomonic for DJS when congenital erythropoietic porphyria[324] or arsenic poisoning[325] has been excluded. Although an oral cholecystogram may fail to visualize the gallbladder, ultrasound examination will show a normal biliary tree. Cholescintigraphy demonstrates prolonged intense visualization of the liver with delayed appearance of the gallbladder and only faint or nonvisualization of the biliary ducts.[277,326,327] Computed tomography of the liver has shown increased attenuation in one report.[328] Because cMOAT/MRP2 transport of leukotrienes into bile is defection in DJS, there is increased excretion of leukotriene metabolites into urine, and this has been suggested to be a new approach to the noninvasive diagnosis of this disease.[329]

No specific therapy is needed for patients with DJS. Although jaundice is a lifelong finding, it is not associated with morbidity or mortality. Avoidance of oral contraceptives has been recommended[330] because this can increase jaundice. Anticipatory guidance regarding pregnancy[295] is appropriate. Increased fetal wastage has been reported in one study.[331] In one case report of neonatal DJS with severe cholestasis, phenobarbital significantly decreased serum levels of bilirubin and bile acids,[289] although chronic phenobarbital therapy is not recommended.[1]

ACKNOWLEDGMENTS

The invaluable technical assistance of Lisa Shields and Bill Kreamer is gratefully acknowledged.

REFERENCES

1. Berk PD, Noyer C. The familial conjugated hyperbilirubinemias. Semin Liver Dis 1994;14:386–94.
2. Berk PD, Noyer C. The familial unconjugated hyperbilirubinemias. Semin Liver Dis 1994;14:356–85.
3. Nowicki MJ, Poley JR. The hereditary hyperbilirubinaemiass. Baillieres Clin Gastroenterol 1998;12:355–67.
4. Newman TB, Easterling MJ, Goldman ES, Stevenson DK. Laboratory evaluation of jaundice in newborns—frequency, cost and yield. Am J Dis Child 1990;144:364–8.
5. Rutledge JC, Ou CN. Bilirubin and the laboratory. Advances in the 1980's, considerations for the 1990's. Pediatr Clin North Am 1989;36:189–97.
6. Vreman HJ, Verter J, Oh W, et al. Interlaboratory variability of bilirubin measurements. Clin Chem 1996;42:869–73.
7. Sirota L, Nussinavitch M, Landman J, Dulitzky F. Breast milk jaundice in preterm infants. Clin Pediatr 1988;27:195–7.
8. Rosenthal P, Keefe MT, Henton D, et al. Total and direct-reacting bilirubin values by automated methods compared with liquid chromatography and with manual methods for determining delta bilirubin. Clin Chem 1990;36:788–91.
9. Westwood A. The analysis of bilirubin in serum. Ann Clin Biochem 1991;28:119–30.
10. Schlebusch H, Axer K, Schneider C, et al. Comparison of five routine methods with the candidate reference method for the determination of bilirubin in neonatal serum. J Clin Chem Clin Biochem 1990;28:203–10.
11. Blanckaert N, Kabra PM, Farina FA. Measurement of bilirubin and its monoconjugates and diconjugates in human serum by alkaline methanolysis and high-performance liquid chromatography. J Lab Clin Med 1980;96:198–212.
12. Wu TW, Dappen GM, Powers DM. The Kodak EKTACHEM clinical chemisty slide for measurement of bilirubin in newborns: principles and performance. Clin Chem 1982;28:2366–72.
13. Bhutani VK, Gourley GR, Adler S, et al. Noninvasive measurement of total serum bilirubin in a multiracial predischarge newborn population to assess the risk of severe hyperbilirubinemia. Pediatrics 2000;106:e17.
14. Robertson A, Kazmierczak S, Vos P. Improved transcutaneous bilirubinometry: comparison of SpectR(X) BiliCheck and Minolta Jaundice Meter JM-102 for estimating total serum bilirubin in a normal newborn population. J Perinatol 2002;22:12–4.
15. Vracko R. Basal lamina scaffold. Anatomy and significance for maintenance of orderly tissue structure. Am J Pathol 1974;77:314–38.
16. Schaffner F, Popper H. Capillarization of hepatic sinusoids in man. Gastroenterology 1963;44:239–42.
17. Bloomer JR, Berk PD, Vergalla J, Berlin NI. Influence of albumin on the hepatic uptake of unconjugated bilirubin. Clin Sci Mol Med 1973;45:505–16.
18. Scharschmidt BF, Waggoner JG, Berk PD. Hepatic organic anion uptake in the rat. J Clin Invest 1975;56:1280–92.
19. Zucker SD, Goessling W, Hoppin AG. Unconjugated bilirubin exhibits spontaneous diffusion through model lipid bilayers and native hepatocyte membranes. J Biol Chem 1999;274:10852–62.
20. Wolkoff AW, Chung CT. Identification, purification and partial characterization of an organic anion binding protein from rat liver plasma membrane. J Clin Invest 1980;65:1152–61.
21. Wolkoff AW, Sosiak A, Greenblutt HC, et al. Immunologic studies on an organic anion-binding protein isolated from rat liver cell plasma membrane. J Clin Invest 1985;76:454–9.
22. Stremmel W, Gerber M, Glezerov V, et al. Physiochemical and immunohistological studies of a sulfobromophthalein- and bilirubin-binding protein from rat liver plasma membranes. J Clin Invest 1983;71:1796–805.
23. Jacobsen J. Binding of bilirubin to human serum albumin-determination of the dissociation constants. FEBS Lett 1969;5:112–4.
24. Wolkoff AW, Weisiger RA, Jakoby WB. The multiple roles of the glutathione transferases (ligandin). Prog Liver Dis 1979;6:213–24.
25. Wolkoff AW, Goresky CA, Sellin J, et al. Role of ligandin in transfer of bilirubin from plasma into liver. Am J Physiol 1979;236:E638–48.
26. Boyer TD. The glutathione S-transferases: an update. Hepatology 1989;9:486–96.
27. Madlon-Kay DJ. The clinical significance of ABO blood group incompatibility. Arch Fam Med 1993;2:285–7.
28. Dutton GJ. The biosynthesis of glucuronides. In: Dutton GJ, editor. Glucuronic acid, free and combined: chemistry, biochemistry, pharmacology and medicine. London: Academic Press; 1966. p. 186–299.
29. Burchell B. Substrate specificity and properties of uridine diphosphate glucuronyltransferase purified to apparent homogeneity from phenobarbital-treated rat liver. Biochem J 1978;173:749–57.

30. Bock KW, Josting D, Lilienblum W, Pfeil H. Purification of rat liver microsomal UDP-glucuronyltransferase. Separation of two enzyme forms inducible by 3-methylcholanthrene or phenobarbital. Eur J Pediatr 1979;98:19–26.

31. Falany CN, Tephly TR. Separation, purification and characterization of three isozymes of UDP-glucuronyltransferase from rat liver microsomes. Arch Biochem Biophys 1983;227:248–58.

32. Matern H, Matern S, Gerok W. Isolation and characterization of rat liver microsomal UDP-glucuronosyltransferase activity toward chenodeoxycholic acid and testosterone as a single form of enzyme. J Biol Chem 1982;257:7422–9.

33. Roy Chowdhury N, Gross F, Moscioni AD, et al. Isolation of multiple normal and functionally defective forms of uridine diphosphate-glucuronosyl-transferase from inbred Gunn rats. J Clin Invest 1987;79:327–34.

34. Senafi SB, Clarke DJ, Burchell B. Investigation of the substrate specificity of a cloned expressed human bilirubin UDP-glucuronosyltransferase: UDP-sugar specificity and involvement in steroid and xenobiotic glucuronidation. Biochem J 1994;303:233–40.

35. Grupp-Phelan J, Taylor JA, Liu LL, Davis RL. Early newborn hospital discharge and readmission for mild and severe jaundice. Arch Pediatr Adolesc Med 1999;153:1283–8.

36. Berry C, Hallinan T. Summary of a novel, three-component regulatory model for uridine diphosphate glucuronyltransferase. Biochem Soc Trans 1976;4:650–2.

37. Kuriyama T. Studies on microsomal nucleoside diphosphatase of rat hepatocytes. Its purification, intramembranous location and turnover. J Biol Chem 1972;247:2979–88.

38. Bosma PJ, Seppen J, Goldhoorn B, et al. Bilirubin UDP-glucuronosyltransferase 1 is the only relevant bilirubin glucuronidating isoform in man [published erratum appears in J Biol Chem 1994;269:2542]. J Biol Chem 1994;269:17960–4.

39. Ritter JK, Chen F, Sheen Y, et al. A novel complex locus UGT1 encodes human bilirubin, phenol, and other UDP-glucuronosyltransferase isozymes with identical carboxyl termini. J Biol Chem 1992;267:3257–61.

40. Clarke DJ, Moghrabi N, Monaghan G, et al. Genetic defects of the UDP-glucuronosyltransferase-1 (UGT1) gene that cause familial non-haemolytic unconjugated hyperbilirubinaemias. Clin Chim Acta 1997;266:63–74.

41. Mackenzie PI, Owens IS, Burchell B, et al. The UDP glycosyltransferase gene superfamily: recommmended nomenclature update based on evolutionary divergence. Pharmacogenetics 1997;7:255–69.

42. Blanckaert N, Gollan J, Schmid R. Bilirubin diglucuronide synthesis by a UDP-glucuronic acid-dependent enzyme system in rat liver microsomes. Proc Natl Acad Sci U S A 1979;76:23037–41.

43. Gordon ER, Meier PJ, Goresky CA, Boyer JL. Mechanism and subcellular site of bilirubin diglucuronide formation in rat liver. J Biol Chem 1984;259:5500–6.

44. Hauser SC, Ziurys JC, Gollan JL. Regulation of bilirubin glucuronide synthesis in primate (Macaca fascicularis) liver-kinetic analysis of microsomal bilirubin uridine diphosphate glucuronyltransferase. Gastroenterology 1986;91:287–96.

45. Burchell B, Blanckaert N. Bilirubin mono- and diglucuronide formation by purified rat liver microsomal bilirubin UDP-glucuronyltransferase. Biochem J 1984;223:461–5.

46. Chowdhury NR, Arias IM, Lederstein M, Chowdury JR. Substrates and products of purified rat liver bilirubin UDP-glucuronsyltransferase. Hepatology 1986;6:123–8.

47. Fevery J, Van Damme B, Mechiel R, et al. Bilirubin conjugates in bile of man and rat in the normal state and in liver disease. J Clin Invest 1972;51:2482–92.

48. Gordon ER, Goresky CA, Chan TH, Perlin AS. The isolation and characterization of bilirubin diglucuronide, the major bilirubin conjugate in dog and human bile. Biochem J 1976;155:477–86.

49. Sinaasappel M, Jansen PL. The differential diagnosis of Crigler-Najjar disease, types 1 and 2, by bile pigment analysis. Gastroenterology 1991;100:783–9.

50. Fevery J, Blanckaert N, Heirwegh KPM, et al. Unconjugated bilirubin and an increased proportion of bilirubin monoconjugates in the bile of patients with Gilbert's syndrome and Crigler-Najjar disease. J Clin Invest 1977;60:970–9.

51. Fevery J, Blanckaert N, Leroy P, et al. Analysis of bilirubins in biological fluids by extraction and thin-layer chromatography of the intact tetrapyrrole: application to bile of patients with Gilbert's syndrome, hemolysis, or cholelithiasis. Hepatology 1983;3:177–83.

52. Goresky CA, Gordon ER, Shaffer EA, et al. Definition of a conjugation dysfunction in Gilbert's syndrome: studies of the handling of bilirubin loads and of the pattern of bilirubin conjugates secreted in bile. Clin Sci 1978;55:63–71.

53. Adachi Y, Kobayashi H, Kurumi Y, et al. Bilirubin diglucuronide transport by rat liver canalicular membrane vesicles: stimulation by biocarbonate ion. Hepatology 1991;14:1251–8.

54. Nishida T, Gatmaitan Z, Roy-Chowdhry J, Arias IM. Two distinct mechanisms for bilirubin glucuronide transport by rat bile canalicular membrane vesicles. Demonstration of defective ATP-dependent transport in rats (TR-) with inherited conjugated hyperbilirubinemia. J Clin Invest 1992;90:2130–5.

55. Paulusma CC, Oude ER. The canalicular multispecific organic anion transporter and conjugated hyperbilirubinemia in rat and man. J Mol Med 1997;75:420–8.

56. Keppler D, Konig J. Hepatic canalicular membrane 5: expression and localization of the conjugate export pump encoded by the MRP2 (cMRP/cMOAT) gene in liver. FASEB J 1997;11:509–16.

57. Paulusma CC, Bosma PJ, Zaman GJ, et al. Congenital jaundice in rats with a mutation in a multidrug resistance-associated protein gene. Science 1996;271:1126–8.

58. Kamisako T, Leier I, Cui Y, et al. Transport of monoglucuronosyl and bisglucuronosyl bilirubin by recombinant human and rat multidrug resistance protein 2. Hepatology 1999;30:485–90.

59. Keppler D, Leier I, Jedlitschky G, et al. The function of the multidrug resistance proteins (MRP and cMRP) in drug conjugate transport and hepatobiliary excretion. Adv Enzyme Regul 1996;36:17–29.

60. Wada M, Toh S, Taniguchi K, et al. Mutations in the canilicular multispecific organic anion transporter (cMOAT) gene, a novel ABC transporter, in patients with hyperbilirubinemia II/Dubin-Johnson syndrome. Hum Mol Genet 1998;7:203–7.

61. Erlinger S. Physiology of bile flow. Prog Liver Dis 1975;4:63–82.

62. Weinbren K, Billing BH. Hepatic clearance of bilirubin as an index of cellular function in the regenerating rat liver. Br J Exp Pathol 1956;37:199–204.

63. Natzschka JC, Odell GB. The influence of albumin on the distribution and excretion of bilirubin in jaundiced rats. Pediatrics 1966;37:51–61.

64. Albert S, Mosher M, Shanske A, Arias IM. Multiplicity of hepatic excretory mechanisms for organic anions. J Gen Physiol 1969;53:238–47.

65. Hargreaves T, Lathe GH. Inhibitory aspects of bile secretion. Nature 1963;200:1172–6.

66. Clarenburg R, Kao CC. Shared and separate pathways for biliary excretion of bilirubin and BSP in rats for biliary excretion of bilirubin and BSP in rats. Am J Physiol 1973;225:192–200.

67. Schoenfield LJ, McGill DB, Hunton DB, et al. Studies of chronic idiopathic jaundice (Dubin-Johnson syndrome). I. Demonstration of hepatic excretory defect. Gastroenterology 1963;44:101–11.

68. Goresky CA, Haddad HH, Kluger WS, et al. The enhancement of maximal bilirubin excretion with taurocholate-induced increments in bile flow. Can J Physiol Pharmacol 1974;52: 389–403.

69. Roberts RJ, Plaa GS. Effect of phenobarbital on the excretion of an exogenous bilirubin load. Biochem Pharmacol 1967; 16:827–35.

70. Gallagher TF, Mueller MN, Kappas A. Estrogen pharmacology. IV. Studies on the structural basis for estrogen-induced impairment of liver function. Medicine 1966;45:471–9.

71. Zimmerman HJ. Hormonal derivatives and other drugs used to treat endocrine disease. Hepatotoxicity. The adverse effects of drug and other chemicals on the liver. New York: Appleton, Crofts; 1978. p. 436–67.

72. Gilbert A, Lereboullet P. La cholemie simple familiale. Semain Med 1901;21:241–3.

73. Odell GB, Gourley GR. Hereditary hyperbilirubinemia. In: Lebenthal E, editor. The textbook of gastroenterology and nutrition in infancy. New York: Raven Press; 1989. p. 949–67.

74. Watson KJ, Gollan JL. Gilbert's syndrome. Baillieres Clin Gastroenterol 1989;3:337–55.

75. Ashraf W, van Someren N, Quigley EM, et al. Gilbert's syndrome and Ramadan: exacerbation of unconjugated hyperbilirubinemia by religious fasting. J Clin Gastroenterol 1994;19:122–4.

76. Maruo Y, Wada S, Yamamota K, et al. A case of anorexia nervosa with hyperbilirubinaemia in a patient homozygous for a mutation in the bilirubin UDP-glucuronosyltransferase gene. Eur J Pediatr 1999;158:547–9.

77. Naiman JL, Sugasawara EJ, Benkosky SL, Mailhot EA. Icteric plasma suggests Gilbert's syndrome in the blood donor. Transfusion 1996;36:974–8.

78. Lachaux A, Aboufadel A, Chambon M, et al. Gilbert's syndrome: a possible cause of hyperbilirubinemia after orthotopic liver transplantation. Transplant Proc 1996;28:2846.

79. Jansen PL, Bosma PJ, Bakker C, et al. Persistent unconjugated hyperbilirubinemia after liver transplantation due to an abnormal bilirubin UDP-glucuronosyltransferase gene promoter sequence in the donor. J Hepatol 1997;27:1–5.

80. Gates LKJ, Wiesner RH, Krom RA, et al. Etiology and incidence of unconjugated hyperbilirubinemia after orthotopic liver transplantation. Am J Gastroenterol 1994;89:1541–3.

81. Arnold JC, Otto G, Kraus T, et al. Gilbert's syndrome—a possible cause of hyperbilirubinemia after orthotopic liver transplantations. J Hepatol 1992;14:404.

82. Wilding P, Rollason JG, Robinson D. Patterns of change for various biochemical constituents detected in well population screening. Clin Chim Acta 1972;41:375–87.

83. Sieg A, Schlierf G, Stiehl A, Kommerell B. Die prävalenz des Gilbert-Syndroms in Deutschland. Dtsch Med Wochenschr 1987;112:1206–8.

84. Olsson R, Bliding Å, Jagenburg R, et al. Gilbert's syndrome—does it exist? Acta Med Scand 1988;244:485–90.

85. Cleary KJ, White PD. Gilbert's and chronic fatigue syndromes in men. Lancet 1993;341:842.

86. Valesini G, Conti F, Priori R, Balsano F. Gilbert's syndrome and chronic fatigue syndrome. Lancet 1993;341:1162–3.

87. Owens D, Evans J. Population studies on Gilbert's syndrome. J Med Genet 1975;12:152–6.

88. Bailey A, Robinson D, Dawson AM. Does Gilbert's disease exist? Lancet 1977;i:931–3.

89. Berk PD, Howe RB, Bloomer JR, Berlin NI. Studies of bilirubin kinetics in normal adults. J Clin Invest 1969;48:2176–90.

90. Alwall N, Laurell CB, Nilsby I. Studies on hereditary in cases of "nonhemolytic bilirubinemia without direct van den Bergh reaction" (hereditary, nonhemolytic bilirubinemia). Acta Med Scand 1946;124:114–25.

91. Foulk WT, Butt HR, Owen CA, et al. Constitutional hepatic dysfunction (Gilbert's disease): its natural history and related syndromes. Medicine 1959;38:25–46.

92. Powell LW, Hemingway E, Billing BH, Sherlock S. Idiopathic unconjugated hyperbilirubinemia (Gilbert's syndrome). A study of 42 families. N Engl J Med 1967;277:1108–12.

93. Aono S, Adachi Y, Uyama E, et al. Analysis of genes for bilirubin UDP-glucuronosyltransferase in Gilbert's syndrome. Lancet 1995;345:958–9.

94. Bosma P, Chowdhury JR, Jansen PH. Genetic inheritance of Gilbert's syndrome. Lancet 1995;346:314–5.

95. Soffer LJ. Bilirubin excretion as a test for liver function during normal pregnancy. Bull Johns Hopkins Hosp 1933;52:365–75.

96. Muraca M, Fevery J. Influence of sex and sex steroids on bilirubin uridine diphosphate-glucuronsyltransferase activity of rat liver. Gastroenterology 1984;87:308–13.

97. Odell GB. The estrogenation of the newborn. Neonatal hyperbilirubinemia. New York: Grune & Stratton; 1980. p. 39–41.

98. Bancroft JD, Kreamer B, Gourley GR. Gilbert syndrome accelerates development of neonatal jaundice. J Pediatr 1998; 132:656–60.

99. Monaghan G, McLellan A, McGeehan A, et al. Gilbert's syndrome is a contributory factor in prolonged unconjugated hyperbilirubinemia of the newborn. J Pediatr 1999;134:441–6.

100. Akaba K, Kimura T, Sasaki A, et al. Neonatal hyperbilirubinemia and a common mutation of the bilirubin uridine diphosphate-glucuronosyltransferase gene in Japanese. J Hum Genet 1999;44:22–5.

101. Maruo Y, Nishizawa K, Sato H, et al. Prolonged unconjugated hyperbilirubinemia associated with breast milk and mutations of the bilirubin uridine diphosphate-glucuronosyltransferase gene. Pediatrics 2000;106(5):e59.

102. Sampietro M, Lupica L, Perrero L, et al. The expression of uridine diphosphate glucuronosyltransferase gene is a major determinant of bilirubin level in heterozygous beta-thalassaemia and in glucose-6-phosphate dehydrogenase deficiency. Br J Haematol 1997;99:437–9.

103. Kaplan M, Renbaum P, Levy-Lahad E, et al. Gilbert syndrome and glucose-6-phosphate dehydrogenase deficiency: a dose-dependent genetic interaction crucial to neonatal hyperbilirubinemia. Proc Natl Acad Sci U S A 1997;94:12128–32.

104. Galanello R, Cipollina MD, Dessi C, et al. Co-inherited Gilbert's syndrome: a factor determining hyperbilirubinemia in homozygous beta-thalassemia. Haematologica 1999;84:103–5.

105. Galanello R, Perseu L, Melis MA, et al. Hyperbilirubinaemia in heterozygous beta-thalassaemia is related to co-inherited Gilbert's syndrome. Br J Haematol 1997;99:433–6.

106. Sharma S, Vukelja SJ, Kadakia S. Gilbert's syndrome co-existing with and masking hereditary spherocytosis. Ann Hematol 1997;74:287–9.

107. Kaplan M, Hammerman C, Renbaum P, et al. Gilbert's syndrome and hyperbilirubinaemia in ABO-incompatible neonates. Lancet 2000;356:652–3.

108. Borker A, Udall J, Warrier R. Coexisting Gilbert's syndrome and sickle cell disease. South Med J 2002;95:939–40.

109. Trioche P, Chalas J, Francoual J, et al. Jaundice with hypertrophic pyloric stenosis as an early manifestation of Gilbert syndrome. Arch Dis Child 1999;81:301–3.

110. Perrotta S, Miraglia del Giudice E, Carbone R, et al. Gilbert's syndrome accounts for the phenotypic variability of congenital dyserythropoietic anemia type II (CDA-II). J Pediatr 2000;136:556–9.

111. Galanello R, Piras S, Barella S, et al. Cholelithiasis and Gilbert's syndrome in homozygous beta-thalassaemia. Br J Haematol 2001;115:926–8.

112. Miraglia del Giudice E, Perrotta S, et al. Coinheritance of Gilbert syndrome increases the risk for developing gallstones in patients with hereditary spherocytosis. Blood 1999;94:2259–62.

113. Black M, Billing BH. Hepatic bilirubin UDP-glucuronyl transferase activity in liver disease. N Engl J Med 1969;280:1266–71.

114. Felsher BF, Craig JR, Carpio N. Hepatic bilirubin glucuronidation in Gilbert's syndrome. J Lab Clin Med 1973;81:829–37.

115. Auclair C, Hakim J, Boivin H, et al. Bilirubin and paranitrophenol glucuronyl transferase activities of the liver in patients with Gilbert's syndrome. An attempt at a biochemical breakdown of the Gilbert's syndrome. Enzyme 1976;21:97–107.

116. Adachi Y, Yamashita M, Nanno T, Yamamoto T. Proportion of conjugated bilirubin in bile in relation to hepatic bilirubin UDP-glucuronyltransferase activity. Clin Biochem 1990;23:131–4.

117. Martin JF, Vierling JM, Wolkoff AW, et al. Abnormal hepatic transport of indocyanine green in Gilbert's syndrome. Gastroenterology 1976;70:385–91.

118. Ohkubo H, Okuda K, Jida S. A constitutional unconjugated hyperbilirubinemia combined with indocyanine green intolerance: a new functional disorder. Hepatology 1981;1:319–24.

119. Berk PD, Blaschke TF, Waggoner JG. Defective bromosulfophthalein clearance in patients with constitutional hepatic dysfunction (Gilbert's syndrome). Gastroenterology 1972;63:472–81.

120. Billing BH, Williams R, Richards TG. Defects in hepatic transport of bilirubin in congenital hyperbilirubinemia: an analysis of plasma bilirubin disappearance curves. Clin Sci 1964;27:245–57.

121. Berk PD, Bloomer JR, Hower RB, Berlin NI. Constitutional hepatic dysfunction (Gilbert's syndrome): a new definition based on kinetic studies with unconjugated radiobilirubin. Am J Med 1970;49:296–305.

122. Okoliesanyi L, Ghidini O, Orlando R, et al. An evaluation of bilirubin kinetics with respect to the diagnosis of Gilbert's syndrome. Clin Sci Mol Med 1978;54:539–47.

123. Debinski HS, Lee CS, Dhillon AP, et al. UDP-glucuronosyltransferase in Gilbert's syndrome. Pathology 1996;28:238–41.

124. Jansen PL, Bosma PJ, Chowdhury JR. Molecular biology of bilirubin metabolism. Prog Liver Dis 1995;13:125–50.

125. Bosma PJ, Chowdhury JR, Bakker C, et al. The genetic basis of the reduced expression of bilirubin UDP-glucuronosyltransferase 1 in Gilbert's syndrome. N Engl J Med 1995;333:1171–5.

126. Sampietro M, Lupica L, Perrero L, et al. TATA-box mutant in the promoter of the uridine diphosphate glucuronosyltransferase gene in Italian patients with Gilbert's syndrome. Ital J Gastroenterol Hepatol 1998;30:194–8.

127. Monaghan G, Ryan M, Seddon R, et al. Genetic variation in bilirubin UPD-glucuronosyltransferase gene promoter and Gilbert's syndrome. Lancet 1996;347:578–81.

128. Borlak J, Thum T, Landt O, et al. Molecular diagnosis of a familial nonhemolytic hyperbilirubinemia (Gilbert's syndrome) in healthy subjects. Hepatology 2000;32:792–5.

129. Raijmakers MTM, Jansen PLM, Steegers EA, Peters WHM.

130. Ando Y, Chida M, Nakayama K, et al. The UGT1A1*28 allele is relatively rare in a Japanese population. Pharmacogenetics 1998;8:357–60.

131. Koiwai O, Nishizawa M, Hasada K, et al. Gilbert's syndrome is caused by a heterozygous missense mutation in the gene for bilirubin UDP-glucuronosyltransferase. Hum Mol Genet 1995;4:1183–6.

132. Maruo Y, Sato H, Yamano T, et al. Gilbert syndrome caused by a homozygous missense mutation (Tyr486Asp) of bilirubin UDP-glucuronosyltransferase gene. J Pediatr 1998;132:1045–7.

133. Hsieh S-Y, Wu Y-H, Lin D-Y, et al. Correlation of mutational analysis to clinical features in Taiwanese patients with Gilbert's syndrome. Am J Gastroenterol 2001;96:1188–93.

134. Beutler E, Gelbart T, Demina A. Racial variability in the UDP-glucuronosyltransferase 1 (UGT1A1) promoter: a balanced polymorphism for regulation of bilirubin metabolism? Proc Natl Acad Sci U S A 1998;95:8170–4.

135. Metreau JM, Yvart J, Dhumeaux D, Berthelot P. Role of bilirubin overproduction in revealing Gilbert's syndrome: is dyserythropoiesis an important factor? Gut 1978;19:838–43.

136. Maddrey WC, Cukier JO, Maglalang AC, et al. Hepatic bilirubin UDP-glucuronyltransferase in patients with sickle cell anemia. Gastroenterology 1978;74:193–5.

137. Kadakol A, Sappal BS, Ghosh SS, et al. Interaction of coding region mutations and the Gilbert-type promoter abnormality of the UGT1A1 gene causes moderate degrees of unconjugated hyperbilirubinaemia and may lead to neonatal kernicterus. J Med Genet 2001;38:244–9.

138. Gourley GR, Siegel FL, Odell GB. A rapid method for collection and analysis of bile pigments in humans. Gastroenterology 1984;86:1322A.

139. Onishi S, Itoh S, Kawade N, et al. An accurate and sensitive analysis by high-pressure liquid chromatography of conjugated and unconjugated bilirubin IX-α in various biological fluids. Biochem J 1980;185:281–4.

140. Blaschke TF, Berk PD, Rodkey FL, et al. Drugs and the liver. I. Effects of glutethimide and phenobarbital on hepatic bilirubin clearance, plasma bilirubin turnover and carbon monoxide production in man. Biochem Pharmacol 1974;23:2795–806.

141. Black M, Fevery J, Parker D, et al. Effect of phenobarbitone on plasma [^{14}C] bilirubin clearance in patients with unconjugated hyperbilirubinemia. Clin Sci Mol Med 1974;46:1–17.

142. Kutz K, Kandler H, Gugler R, Fevery J. Effect of clofibrate on metabolism of bilirubin, bromosulphophthalein and indocyanine green and on the biliary lipid composition in Gilbert's syndrome. Clin Sci 1984;66:389–97.

143. Foliot A, Drocourt JL, Etienne JP, et al. Increase in the hepatic glucuronidation of bilirubin in clofibrate-treated rats. Biochem Pharmacol 1977;26:547–9.

144. Felsher BF, Richard D, Redeker AG. The reciprocoal relation between caloric intake and the degree of hyperbilirubinemia in Gilbert's syndrome. N Engl J Med 1970;283:170–2.

145. Bloomer JR, Barrett PV, Rodkey FL, Berlin NI. Studies of the mechanisms of fasting hyperbilirubinemia. Gastroenterology 1971;61:479–87.

146. Whitmer DI, Gollan JL. Mechanisms and significance of fasting and dietary hyperbilirubinemia. Semin Liver Dis 1983;3:42–51.

147. Owens D, Sherlock S. Diagnosis of Gilbert's syndrome: role of reduced caloric intake test. BMJ 1973;3:559–63.

148. Bakken AF, Thaler MM, Schmid R. Metabolic regulation of heme catabolism and bilirubin production I. Hormonal control of hepatic heme oxygenase activity. J Clin Invest 1972; 51:530–6.

149. Kirshenbaum G, Shames DM, Schmid R. An expanded model of bilirubin kinetics; effect of feeding, fasting and phenobarbital in Gilbert's syndrome. J Pharmacokinet Biopharm 1976;4: 115–55.

150. Ricci GL, Ricci RR. Effect of an intraluminal food-bulk on low calorie induced hyperbilirubinemia. Clin Sci 1984;66:493–6.

151. Fromke VL, Miller D. Constitutional hepatic dysfunction (CHD; Gilbert's snydrome): a review with special reference to a characteristic increase and prolongation of the hyperbilirubinemic response to nicotinic acid. Medicine 1972;51:451–64.

152. Rollinghoff W, Paumgartner G, Preisig R. Nicotinic acid test in the diagnosis of Gilbert's syndrome: correlation with the bilirubin clearance. Gut 1981;22:663–8.

153. Gentile S, Orzes N, Persico M, et al. Comparison of nicotinic acid and caloric restriction induced hyperbilirubinemia in the diagnosis of Gilbert's syndrome. J Hepatol 1985;1:537–45.

154. Gentile S, Rubba P, Persico M, et al. Improvement of the nicotinic acid test in the diagnosis of Gilbert's syndrome by pretreatment with indomethacin. Hepatogastroenterology 1985;33:267–9.

155. Gentile S, Marmo R, Persico M, et al. Dissociation between vascular and metabolic effects of nicotinic acid in Gilbert's syndrome. Clin Physiol 1990;10:171–8.

156. Davidson AR, Rojas Bueno A, Thompson RPH, Williams R. Reduced caloric intake test and nicotinic acid provocation test in the diagnosis of Gilbert's syndrome. BMJ 1975;2:480.

157. Ohkubo H, Musha H, Okuda K. Stuides on nicotinic acid interaction with bilirubin metabolism. Dig Dis Sci 1979;24:700–4.

158. Gentile S, Tiribelli C, Persico M, et al. Dose dependence of nicotinic acid-induced hyperbilirubinemia and its dissociation from hemolysis in Gilbert's syndrome. J Lab Clin Med 1986; 107:166–71.

159. Dickey W, McAleer JJ, Callender ME. The nicotinic acid provocation test and unconjugated hyperbilirubinaemia. Ulster Med J 1991;60:49–52.

160. Murthy GD, Byron D, Shoemaker D, et al. The utility of rifampin in diagnosing Gilbert's syndrome. Am J Gastroenterol 2001;96:1150–4.

161. Sieg A, Stiehl A, Raedsch R, et al. Gilbert's syndrome: diagnosis by typical serum bilirubin pattern. Clin Chim Acta 1986; 154:41–7.

162. Sieg A, Konig R, Ullrich D, Fevery J. Subfractionation of serum bilirubins by alkaline methanolysis and thin-layer chromatography. An aid in the differential diagnosis of icteric diseases. J Hepatol 1990;11:159–64.

163. Ullrich D, Sieg A, Blume R, et al. Normal pathways for glucuronidation, sulphation and oxidation of paracetamol in Gilbert's syndrome. Eur J Clin Invest 1987;17:237–40.

164. Adachi Y, Katoh H, Fuchi I, Yamamoto T. Serum bilirubin fractions in healthy subjects and patients with unconjugated hyperbilirubinemia. Clin Biochem 1990;23:247–51.

165. Rudenski AS, Halsall DJ. Genetic testing for Gilbert's syndrome: how useful is it in determining the cause of jaundice? Clin Chem 1998;44:1604–9.

166. Berk PB, Isola LM. Specific defects in hepatic storage and clearance of bilirubin. In: Ostrow JD, editor. Bile pigments and jaundice: molecular, metabolic and medical aspects. New York: Marcel Dekker; 1986. p. 279–316.

167. Evans DA. Survey of the human acetylator polymorphism in spontaneous disorders. J Med Genet 1984;21:243–53.

168. Siegmund W, Fengler JD, Franke G, et al. N-Acetylation and debrisoquine hydroxylation polymorphisms in patients with Gilbert's syndrome. Br J Clin Pharmacol 1991;32:467–72.

169. Herman RJ, Chaudhary A, Szakacs CB. Disposition of lorazepam in Gilbert's syndrome: effects of fasting, feeding, and enterohepatic circulation. J Clin Pharmacol 1994;34:978–84.

170. Burchell B, Soars M, Monaghan G, et al. Drug-mediated toxicity caused by genetic deficiency of UDP-glucuronosyltransferases. Toxicol Lett 2000;112–113:333–40.

171. de Morais SM, Uetrecht JP, Wells PG. Decreased glucuronidation and increased bioactivation of acetaminophen in Gilbert's syndrome. Gastroenterology 1992;102:577–86.

172. Esteban A, Perez-Mateo M. Gilbert's disease: a risk factor for paracetamol overdosage? J Hepatol 1993;18:257–8.

173. Wasserman E, Myara A, Lokiec F, et al. Severe CPT-11 toxicity in patients with Gilbert's syndrome: two case reports. Ann Oncol 1997;8:1049–51.

174. Black M, Sherlock S. Treatment of Gilbert's syndrome with phenobarbitone. Lancet 1970;i:1359–61.

175. Stocker R, McDonagh AF, Glazer AN, Ames BN. Antioxidant activities of bile pigments: biliverdin and bilirubin. Method Enzymol 1990;186:301–9.

176. McDonagh AF. Is bilirubin good for you? Clin Perinatol 1990; 17:359–69.

177. Breimer LH, Wannamethee G, Ebrahim S, Shaper AG. Serum bilirubin and risk of ischemic heart disease in middle-aged British men. Clin Chem 1995;41:1504–8.

178. Schwertner HA, Jackson WG, Tolan G. Association of low serum concentration of bilirubin with increased risk of coronary artery disease. Clin Chem 1994;40:18–23.

179. Vitek L, Jirsa M, Brodanova M, et al. Gilbert syndrome and ischemic heart disease: a protective effect of elevated bilirubin levels. Atherosclerosis 2002;160:449–56.

180. Miyaoka T, Seno H, Itoga M, et al. Structural brain changes in schizophrenia associated with idiopathic unconjugated hyperbilirubinemia (Gilbert's syndrome): a planimetric CT study. Schizophr Res 2000;52:291–3.

181. Crigler JF, Najjar VA. Congenital familial nonhemolytic jaundice with kernicterus. Pediatrics 1952;10:169–80.

182. Gourley GR. Bilirubin metabolism and kernicterus. Adv Pediatr 1997;44:173–229.

183. Shevell MI, Majnemer A, Schiff D. Neurologic perspectives of Crigler-Najjar syndrome type I. J Child Neurol 1998;13:265–9.

184. Childs B, Najjar VA. Familial nonhemolytic jaundice with kernicterus. A report of two cases without neurologic damage. Pediatrics 1956;18:369–77.

185. Blumenschein SD, Kallen RJ, Storey B, et al. Familial nonhemolytic jaundice with late onset of neurologic damage. Pediatrics 1968;42:786–92.

186. Blaschke TF, Berke PD, Scharschmidt BF, et al. Crigler-Najjar syndrome: an unusual course with development of neurological damage at age eighteen. Pediatr Res 1974;8:573–90.

187. Labrune PH, Myara A, Francoual J, et al. Cerebellar symptoms as the presenting manifestations of bilirubin encephalopathy in children with Crigler-Najjar type I disease. Pediatrics 1992;89:768–70.

188. Chalasani N, Chowdhury NR, Chowdhury JR, Boyer TD. Kernicterus in an adult who is heterozygous for Crigler-Najjar syndrome and homozygous for Gilbert-type genetic defect. Gastroenterology 1997;112:2099–103.

189. Arias IM, Gartner LM, Cohen M, et al. Chronic nonhemolytic unconjugated hyperbilirubinemia with glucuronyl transferase deficiency. Am J Med 1969;47:395–409.

190. Gollan JL, Huang SM, Billing B, Sherlock S. Prolonged survival

in 3 brothers with severe type II Crigler-Najjar syndrome: ultrastructural and metabolic studies. Gastroenterology 1975;68:1543–55.

191. Gordon ER, Shaffer EA, Sass-Kortsak A. Bilirubin secretion and conjugation in the Crigler-Najjar syndrome type II. Gastroenterology 1976;70:761–5.

192. Koiwai O, Aono S, Adachi Y, et al. Crigler-Najjar syndrome type II is inherited both as a dominant and as a recessive trait. Hum Mol Genet 1996;5:645–7.

193. Kadakol A, Ghosh SS, Sappal BS, et al. Genetic lesions of bilirubin uridine-diphosphoglucuronate glucuronosyltransferase (UGT1A1) causing Crigler-Najjar and Gilbert syndromes: correlation of genotype to phenotype. Hum Mutat 2000;16:297–306.

194. Burchell B, Coughtrie MW, Jansen PL. Function and regulation of UDP-glucuronosyltransferase genes in health and liver disease: report of the Seventh International Workshop on Glucuronidation, September 1993, Pitlochry, Scotland. Hepatology 1994;20:1622–30.

195. Seppen J, Bosma PJ, Goldhoorn BG, et al. Discrimination between Crigler-Najjar type I and II by expression of mutant bilirubin uridine diphosphate-glucuronosyltransferase. J Clin Invest 1994;94:2385–91.

196. Labrune P, Myara A, Hadchouel M, et al. Genetic heterogeneity of Crigler-Najjar syndrome type I: a study of 14 cases. Hum Genet 1994;94:693–7.

197. Gantla S, Bakker CT, Deocharan B, et al. Splice-site mutations: a novel genetic mechanism of Crigler-Najjar syndrome type 1. Am J Hum Genet 1998;62:585–92.

198. Ciotti M, Chen F, Rubaltelli FF, Owens IS. Coding defect and a TATA box mutation at the bilirubin UDP-glucuronosyltransferase gene cause Crigler-Najjar type I disease. Biochim Biophys Acta 1998;1407:40–50.

199. Strassburg CP, Manns MP. Jaundice, genes and promoters. J Hepatol 2000;33:476–9.

200. Szabo L, Kovács Z, Ebrey PB. Crigler-Najjar syndrome. Acta Paediatr Hung 1962;3:49–70.

201. Duhamel G, Blanckaert N, Metreau JM, et al. An unusual case of Crigler-Najjar disease in the adult. Classification into types I and II revisited. J Hepatol 1985;1:47–53.

202. van Es HHG, Goldhoorn BG, Paul-Abrahamse M, et al. Immunochemical analysis of uridine diphosphate-glucuronosyltransferase in four patients with Crigler-Najjar syndrome type I. J Clin Invest 1990;85:1199–205.

203. Childs B, Sidbury JB, Migeon CJ. Glucuronic acid conjugation by patients with familial nonhemolytic jaundice and their relatives. Pediatrics 1959;23:903–13.

204. Szabo L, Ebrey P. Studies on the inheritance of Crigler-Najjar's syndrome by the menthol test. Acta Paediatr Hung 1963;4:153–9.

205. Ertel IJ, Newton WA Jr. Therapy in congenital hyperbilirubinemia: phenobarbital and diethylnicotinamide. Pediatrics 1969;44:43–8.

206. Crigler JF, Gold NI. Effect of phenobarbital on bilirubin metabolism in an infant with congenital, nonhemolytic, unconjugated hyperbilirubinemia, and kernicterus. J Clin Invest 1969;48:42–55.

207. Yaffe SJ, Levy G, Matsuzawa T, Baliah T. Enhancement of glucuronide-conjugating capacity in a hyperbilirubinemic infant due to apparent enzyme induction by phenobarbital. N Engl J Med 1966;275:1461–6.

208. Kreek MJ, Sleisenger MH. Reduction of serum-unconjugated bilirubin with phenobarbitone in adult nonhaemolytic unconjugated hyperbilirubinaemia. Lancet 1968;ii:73–8.

209. Rubaltelli FF, Novello A, Zancan L, et al. Serum and bile bilirubin pigments in the differential diagnosis of Crigler-Najjar disease. Pediatrics 1994;94:553–6.

210. Odell GB, Whitington PF. Crigler-Najjar syndrome, type III: a new variant of hereditary non-hemolytic, non-conjugated hyperbilirubinemia. Hepatology 1990;12:871.

211. Mair B, Klempner LB. Abnormally high values for direct bilirubin in the serum of newborns as measured with the DuPont aca. Am J Clin Pathol 1987;87:642–4.

212. Odell GB, Schutta HS. Bilirubin encephalopathy. In: McCandless DW, editor. Cerebral energy metabolism and metabolic encephalopathy. New York: Plenum Publishing Corp; 1985. p. 229–61.

213. Lee WS, McKiernan PJ, Beath SV, et al. Bile bilirubin pigment analysis in disorders of bilirubin metabolism in early infancy. Arch Dis Child 2002;85:38–42.

214. Moghrabi N, Clarke DJ, Burchell B, Boxer M. Cosegregation of intragenic markers with a novel mutation that causes Crigler-Najjar syndrome type I: implication in carrier detection and prenatal diagnosis. Am J Hum Genet 1993;53:722–9.

215. van der Veere CN, Sinaasappel M, McDonagh AF, et al. Current therapy for Crigler-Najjar syndrome type 1: report of a world registry. Hepatology 1996;24:311–5.

216. Gorodischer R, Levy G, Krasner J, Jaffe SJ. Congenital nonobstructive, nonhemolytic jaundice. Effect of phototherapy. N Engl J Med 1970;282:375–80.

217. Agati G, Fusi F, Pratesi S, et al. Bilirubin photoisomerization products in serum and urine from a Crigler-Najjar type I patient treated by phototherapy. J Photochem Photobiol B Biol 1998;47:181–9.

218. Job H, Hart G, Lealman G. Improvements in long term phototherapy for patients with Crigler-Najjar syndrome type I. Phys Med Biol 1996;41:2549–56.

219. Odell GB, Gutcher GR, Whitington PF, Yang G. Enteral administration of agar as an effective adjunct to phototherapy of neonatal hyperbilirubinemia. Pediatr Res 1983;17:810–4.

220. Arrowsmith WA, Payne RB, Littlewood JM. Comparison of treatments for congenital nonobstructive nonhaemolytic hyperbilirubinemia. Arch Dis Child 1975;50:197–201.

221. van der Veere CN, Jansen PL, Sinaasappel M, et al. Oral calcium phosphate: a new therapy for Crigler-Najjar disease? Gastroenterology 1997;112:455–62.

222. Nicolopolous D, Hadjigeorgiou E, Malamitsi A, et al. Combined treatment of neonatal jaundice with cholestyramine and phototherapy. J Pediatr 1978;93:684–8.

223. Kotal P, van der Veere CN, Sinaasappel M, et al. Intestinal excretion of unconjugated bilirubin in man and rats with inherited unconjugated hyperbilirubinemia. Pediatr Res 1997;42:195–200.

224. Kemper K, Horwitz RI, McCarthy P. Decreased neonatal serum bilirubin with plain agar: a meta-analysis. Pediatrics 1988;82:631–8.

225. Sherker AH, Heathcote J. Acute hepatitis in Crigler-Najjar syndrome. Am J Gastroenterol 1987;82:883–5.

226. Rubaltelli FF, Guerrini P, Reddi E, Jori G. Tin-protoporphyrin in the management of children with Crigler-Najjar disease. Pediatrics 1989;84:728–31.

227. Galbraith RA, Drummond GS, Kappas A. Suppression of bilirubin production in the Crigler-Najjar type I syndrome: studies with the heme oxygenase inhibitor tin-mesoporphyrin. Pediatrics 1992;89:175–82.

228. Kappas A, Drummond GS, Galbraith RA. Prolonged clinical use of a heme oxygenase inhibitor: hematological evidence for an inducible but reversible iron-deficiency state. Pediatrics 1993;91:537–9.

229. Rubaltelli FF. Current drug treatment options in neonatal hyperbilirubinaemia and the prevention of kernicterus. Drugs 1998;56:23–30.

230. Prager MC, Johnson KL, Ascher NL, Roberts JP. Anesthetic care of patients with Crigler-Najjar syndrome. Anesth Analg 1992;74:162–4.

231. Whitington PF, Emond JC, Heffron T, Thistlethwaite JR. Orthotopic auxiliary liver transplantation for Crigler-Najjar syndrome type 1. Lancet 1993;342:779–80.

232. Rela M, Muiesan P, Andreani P, et al. Auxiliary liver transplantation for metabolic diseases. Transplant Proc 1997;29:444–5.

233. Rela M, Muiesan P, Vilca-Melendez H, et al. Auxiliary partial orthotopic liver transplantation for Crigler-Najjar syndrome type I. Ann Surg 1999;229:565–9.

234. Kaufman SS, Wood RP, Shaw BW Jr, et al. Orthotopic liver transplantation for type 1 Crigler-Najjar syndrome. Hepatology 1986;6:1259–62.

235. Shevell MI, Bernard B, Adelson JW, et al. Crigler-Najjar syndrome type I: treatment by home phototherapy followed by orthotopic hepatic transplantation. J Pediatr 1987;110:429–31.

236. Sokal EM, Silva ES, Hermans D, et al. Orthotopic liver transplantation for Crigler-Najjar type I disease in six children. Transplantation 1995;60:1095–8.

237. McDiarmid SV, Millis MJ, Olthoff KM, So SK. Indications for pediatric liver transplantation. Pediatr Transplant 1998;2:106–16.

238. Rela M, Muiesan P, Heaton ND, et al. Orthotopic liver transplantation for hepatic-based metabolic disorders. Transpl Int 1995;8:41–4.

239. Mowat AP. Orthotopic liver transplantation in liver-based metabolic disorders. Eur J Pediatr 1992;151 Suppl 1:S32–8.

240. Gridelli B, Lucianetti A, Gatti S, et al. Orthotopic liver transplantation for Crigler-Najjar type I syndrome. Transplant Proc 1997;29:440–1.

241. Pratschke J, Steinmuller T, Bechstein WO, et al. Orthotopic liver transplantation for hepatic associated metabolic disorders. Clin Transplant 1998;12:228–32.

242. Al Shurafa H, Wali S, Chehab MS, et al. Living-related liver transplantation for Crigler-Najjar syndrome in Saudi Arabia. Clin Transplant 2002;16:222–6.

243. Jaffe BM, Burgos AA, Martinez-Noack M. The use of jejunal transplants to treat a genetic enzyme deficiency. Ann Surg 1996;223:649–56.

244. Medley MM, Hooker RL, Rabinowitz S, et al. Correction of congenital indirect hyperbilirubinemia by small intestinal transplantation. Am J Surg 1995;169:20–7.

245. Kokudo N, Takahashi S, Sugitani K, et al. Supplement of liver enzyme by intestinal and kidney transplants in congenitally enzyme-deficient rat. Microsurgery 1999;19:103–7.

246. Ritter JK, Crawford JM, Owens IS. Cloning of two human liver bilirubin UDP-glucuronosyltransferase cDNAs with expression in COS-1 cells. J Biol Chem 1991;266:1043–7.

247. Kim BH, Takahashi M, Tada K, et al. Cell and gene therapy for inherited deficiency of bilirubin glucuronidation. J Perinatol 1996;16:S67–72.

248. Brierley CH, Burchell B. Human UDP-glucuronosyl transferases: chemical defence, jaundice and gene therapy. Bioessays 1993;15:749–54.

249. Raper SE. Hepatocyte transplantation and gene therapy. Clin Transplant 1995;9:249–54.

250. Roy-Chowdhury N, Kadakol A, Sappal BS, et al. Gene therapy for inherited hyperbilirubinemias. J Perinatol 2001;21:S114–8.

251. Tada K, Chowdhury NR, Neufeld D, et al. Long-term reduction of serum bilirubin levels in Gunn rats by retroviral gene transfer in vivo. Liver Transplant Surg 1998;4:78–88.

252. Askari F, Hitomi E, Thiney M, Wilson JM. Retrovirus-mediated expression of HUG Br1 in Crigler-Najjar syndrome type I human fibroblasts and correction of the genetic defect in Gunn rat hepatocytes. Gene Ther 1995;2:203–8.

253. Li Q, Murphree SS, Willer SS, et al. Gene therapy with bilirubin-UDP-glucuronosyltransferase in the Gunn rat model of Crigler-Najjar syndrome type 1. Hum Gene Ther 1998;9:497–505.

254. Thummala NR, Ghosh SS, Lee SW, et al. A non-immunogenic adenoviral vector, coexpressing CTLA4Ig and bilirubin-uridine-diphosphoglucuronateglucuronosyltransferase, permits long-term, repeatable transgene expression in the Gunn rat model of Crigler-Najjar sysndrome. Gene Ther 2002;9:981–90.

255. Bruni S, Chang TM. Encapsulated hepatocytes for controlling hyperbilirubinemia in Gunn rats. Int J Artif Organs 1991;14:239–41.

256. Kren BT, Parashar B, Bandyopadhyay P, et al. Correction of the UDP-glucuronosyltransferase gene defect in the Gunn rat model of Crigler-Najjar syndrome type I with a chimeric oligonucleotide. Proc Natl Acad Sci U S A 1999;96:10349–54.

257. Chowdhury JR, Kondapalli R, Chowdhury NR. Gunn rat: a model for inherited deficiency of bilirubin glucuronidation. Adv Vet Sci Comp Med 1993;37:149–73.

258. Fox IJ, Chowdhury JR, Kaufman SS, et al. Treatment of the Crigler-Najjar syndrome type I with hepatocyte transplantation. N Engl J Med 1998;338:1422–6.

259. Horslen SP, McCowan TC, Goertzen TC, et al. Isolated hepatocyte transplantation in an infant with a severe urea cycle disorder. Pediatrics 2003;111:1262–7.

260. Rotor AB, Manahan L, Florentin A. Familial nonhemolytic jaundice with direct van den Bergh reaction. Acta Med Phil 1948;5:37–49.

261. Namihisa T, Yamaguchi K. The constitutional hyperbilirubinemia in Japan: studies on 139 cases reported during the period 1963-1969. Gastroenterol Jpn 1973;8:311–21.

262. Wolkoff AW. Inheritable disorders manifested by conjugated hyperbilirubinemia. Semin Liver Dis 1983;3:65–72.

263. Vest MF, Kaufmann JH, Fritz E. Chronic nonhaemolytic jaundice with conjugated bilirubin in the serum and normal histology: a case study. Arch Dis Child 1960;36:600–4.

264. Fretzayas A, Koukoutsakis P, Moustaki M, et al. Coinheritance of Rotor syndrome, G-6-PD deficiency and heterozygous beta thalassemia: a possible genetic interaction. J Pediatr Gastroenterol Nutr 2001;33:211–3.

265. Pascasio FM, de la Fuenta D. Rotor-Manahan-Florentin syndrome: clinical and genetic studies. Phil J Int Med 1969;7:151–7.

266. Wolpert E, Pascasio FM, Wolkoff AW. Abnormal sulfobromophthalein metabolism in Rotor's syndrome and obligate heterozygotes. N Engl J Med 1977;296:1099–101.

267. Dhumeaux D, Berthelot P. Chronic hyperbilirubinemia associated with hepatic uptake and storage impairment. Gastroenterology 1975;69:988–93.

268. Wheeler HO, Meltzer JI, Bradley SE. Biliary transport and hepatic storage of sulfobromophthalein sodium in the unanesthetized dog, in normal man, and in patients with hepatic disease. J Clin Invest 1960;39:1131–44.

269. Tipping E, Ketterer B. The role of intracellular proteins in the transport and metabolism of lipophilic compounds. In: Blaver G, Sund H, editors. Transport by proteins. Berlin: Walter de Gruyter & Co.; 1978. p. 369.

270. Adachi Y, Yamamoto T. Partial defect in hepatic glutathione S-transferase activity in a case of Rotor's syndrome. Gastroenterology 1987;22:34–8.

271. Abei M, Matsuzaki Y, Tanaka N, et al. Defective hepatic glu-

tathione s-transferase in Rotor's syndrome. Am J Gastroenterol 1995;90:681–2.

272. Wolkoff AW, Ketley JN, Waggoner JG, et al. Hepatic accumulation and intracellular binding of conjugated bilirubin. J Clin Invest 1978;61:142–9.

273. Wolkoff AW, Wolpert E, Pascasio FN, Arias IM. Rotor's syndrome. A distinct inheritable pathophysiologic entity. Am J Med 1976;60:173–9.

274. Aziz MA, Schwartz S, Watson CJ. Studies on coproporphyrin VIII. Reinvestigation of the isomer distribution in jaundice and liver diseases. J Lab Clin Med 1964;63:596–604.

275. Shimizu Y, Naruto H, Ida S, Kohakura M. Urinary coproporphyrin isomers in Rotor's syndrome: a study in eight families. Hepatology 1981;1:173–8.

276. Fretzayas AM, Garoufi AI, Moutsouris CX, Karpathios TE. Cholescintigraphy in the diagnosis of Rotor syndrome. J Nucl Med 1994;35:1048–50.

277. Bar-Meir S, Baron J, Seligson U, et al. 99mTc-HIDA cholescintigraphy in Dubin-Johnson and Rotor syndromes. Radiology 1982;142:743–6.

278. Dubin IN, Johnson FB. Chronic idiopathic jaundice with unidentified pigment in liver cells: a new clinicopathologic entity with a report of 12 cases. Medicine 1954;33:155–97.

279. Dubin IN. Chronic idiopathic jaundice. A review of fifty cases. Am J Med 1958;24:268–92.

280. Gustein SL, Alpert L, Arias IM. Studies of hepatic excretory function. IV. Biliary excretion of sulfobromophthalein sodium in a patient with Dubin-Johnson syndrome and a biliary fistula. Isr J Med Sci 1968;4:36–40.

281. Javitt NB, Kondo T, Kuchiba K. Bile acid excretion in Dubin-Johnson syndrome. Gastroenterology 1978;75:931–2.

282. Sprinz H, Nelson RS. Persistent nonhemolytic hyperbilirubinemia associated with lipochrome-like pigment in liver cells: report of four cases. Ann Intern Med 1954;41:952–62.

283. Shani M, Seligsohn V, Gilon E, et al. Dubin-Johnson syndrome in Israel. I. Clinical, laboratory and genetic aspects of 101 cases. Q J Med 1970;39:549–67.

284. Zlotogora J. Hereditary disorders among Iranian Jews. Am J Med Genet 1995;58:32–7.

285. Kondo T, Yagi R. Dubin-Johnson syndrome in a neonate. N Engl J Med 1975;292:1028–9.

286. Nakata F, Oyanagi K, Fujiwara M, et al. Dubin-Johnson syndrome in a neonate. Eur J Pediatr 1979;132:299–301.

287. Haimi-Cohen Y, Merlob P, Marcus-Eidlits T, Amir J. Dubin-Johnson syndrome as a cause of neonatal jaundice: the importance of coproporphyrins investigation. Clin Pediatr 1998;37:511–3.

288. Tsai WH, Teng RJ, Chu JS, et al. Neonatal Dubin-Johnson syndrome. J Pediatr Gastroenterol Nutr 1994;18:253–4.

289. Kimura A, Ushijima K, Kage M, et al. Neonatal Dubin-Johnson syndrome with severe cholestasis: effective phenobarbital therapy. Acta Paediatr Scand 1991;80:381–5.

290. Shieh CC, Chang MH, Chen CL. Dubin-Johnson syndrome presenting with neonatal cholestasis. Arch Dis Child 1990;65:898–9.

291. Haimi-Cohen Y, Amir J, Merlob P. Neonatal and infantile Dubin-Johnson syndrome. Pediatr Radiol 1998;28:900.

292. Kimura A, Yuge K, Kosai KI, et al. Neonatal cholestasis in two siblings: a variant of Dubin-Johnson syndrome? J Paediatr Child Health 1995;31:557–60.

293. Kondo T, Kuchiba K, Ohtsuka Y, et al. Clinical and genetic studies on Dubin-Johnson syndrome in a cluster area in Japan. Jpn J Hum Genet 1974;18:378–92.

294. Edwards RH. Inheritance of the Dubin-Johnson-Sprinz syndrome. Gastroenterology 1975;63:734–49.

295. Cohen L, Lewis C, Arias IM. Pregnancy, oral contraceptives and chronic familial jaundice with predominantly conjugated hyperbilirubinemia (Dubin-Johnson syndrome). Gastroenterology 1972;62:1182–90.

296. Muscatello U, Mussini I, Agnolucci MT. Dubin-Johnson syndrome: an electron microscopic study of the liver cell. Acta Hepatosplenol 1967;14:162–70.

297. Ehrlich JC, Novikoff AB, Platt R, et al. Hepatocellular lipofuscin and the pigment of chronic idiopathic jaundice. Bull N Y Acad Med 1960;36:488–91.

298. Swartz HM, Sarna T, Varma RR. On the nature and excretion of the hepatic pigment in the Dubin-Johnson syndrome. Gastroenterology 1979;76:958–64.

299. Swartz HM, Chen K, Roth JA. Further evidence that the pigment in the Dubin-Johnson syndrome is not melanin. Pigment Cell Res 1987;1:69–75.

300. Arias IM, Blumberg W. The pigment in Dubin-Johnson syndrome. Gastroenterology 1979;77:820–1.

301. Kitamura T, Alroy J, Gatmaitan Z, et al. Defective biliary excretion of epinephrine metabolites in mutant (TR-) rats: relation to the pathogenesis of black liver in the Dubin-Johnson syndrome and Corriedale sheep with an analogous excretory defect. Hepatology 1992;15:1154–9.

302. Hunter FM, Sparks RD, Flinner RL. Hepatitis with resulting mobilization of hepatic pigment in a patient with Dubin-Johnson syndrome. Gastroenterology 1964;47:631–5.

303. Paulusma CC, Kool M, Bosma PJ, et al. A mutation in the human canalicular multispecific organic anion transporter gene causes the Dubin-Johnson syndrome. Hepatology 1997;25:1539–42.

304. Toh S, Wada M, Uchiumi T, et al. Genomic structure of the canalicular multispecific organic anion-transporter gene (MRP2/cMOAT) and mutations in the ATP-binding-cassette region in Dubin-Johnson syndrome. Am J Hum Genet 1999; 64:739–46.

305. Borst P, Evers R, Kool M, Wijnholds J. A family of drug transporters: the multidrug resistance-associated proteins. J Natl Cancer Inst 2000;92:1295–302.

306. Kruh GD, Zeng H, Rea PA, et al. MRP subfamily transporters and resistance to anticancer agents. J Bioenerg Biomembr 2001;33:493–501.

307. van Kuijck MA, Kool M, Merkx GF, et al. Assignment of the canalicular multispecific organic anion transporter gene (CMOAT) to human chromosome 10q24 and mouse chromosome 19D2 by fluorescent in situ hybridization. Cytogenet Cell Genet 1997;77:285–7.

308. Kajihara S, Hisatomi A, Mizuta T, et al. A splice mutation in the human canalicular multispecific organic anion transporter gene causes Dubin-Johnson syndrome. Biochem Biophys Res Commun 1998;253:454–7.

309. Keitel V, Kartenbeck J, Nies AT, et al. Impaired protein maturation of the conjugate export pump multidrug resistance protein 2 as a consequence of a deletion mutation in Dubin-Johnson syndrome. Hepatology 2002;32:1317–28.

310. Keppler D, Konig J. Hepatic secretion of conjugated drugs and endogenous substances. Semin Liver Dis 2000;20:265–72.

311. Mor-Cohen R, Zivelin A, Rosenberg N, et al. Identification and functional analysis of two novel mutations in the multidrug resistance protein 2 gene in Israeli patients with Dubin-Johnson syndrome. J Biol Chem 2001;276:36923–30.

312. Elferink RO, Groen AK. Genetic defects in hepatobiliary transport. Biochim Biophys Acta 2002;1586:129–45.

313. Mendema E, DeFraiure WH, Nieweg HO, et al. Familial chronic idiopathic jaundice. Am J Med 1960;28:42–50.

314. Charbonnier A, Brisbois P. Etude chromatographique de la BSP au cours de l'epreuve clinique d'epuration plasmatique de ce colorant. Rev Int Hepatol 1960;10:1163–213.

315. Shani M, Gilon E, Ben-Ezzer J, Sheba C. Sulfobromophthalein tolerance test in patients with Dubin-Johnson syndrome and their relatives. Gastroenterology 1970;59:842–7.

316. Abe H, Okuda K. Biliary excretion of conjugated sulfobromophthalein (BSP) in constitutional conjugated hyperbilirubinemias. Digestion 1975;13:272–83.

317. Erlinger S, Dhumeaux D, Desjeux JF, Benhamou JP. Hepatic handling of unconjugated dyes in the Dubin-Johnson syndrome. Gastroenterology 1973;64:106–10.

318. Koskelo P, Toivonen I, Aldercreutz H. Urinary coproporphyrin isomer distribution in Dubin-Johnson syndrome. Clin Chem 1967;13:1006–9.

319. Frank M, Doss M, de Carvalho DG. Diagnostic and pathogenetic implications of urinary coproporphyrin excretion in the Dubin-Johnson syndrome. Hepatogastroenterology 1990; 37:147–51.

320. Ben-Ezzer J, Seligson U, Shani M, et al. Abnormal excretion of the isomers of urinary coproporphyrin by patients with Dubin-Johnson syndrome in Israel. Clin Sci 1971;40:17–30.

321. Wolkoff AW, Cohen LE, Arias IM. Inheritance of the Dubin-Johnson syndrome. N Engl J Med 1973;288:113–7.

322. Kondo T, Kuchiba K, Shimizu Y. Coporporphyrin isomers in Dubin-Johnson syndrome. Gastroenterology 1976;70:1117–20.

323. Rocchi E, Balli F, Gibertini P, et al. Coproporphyrin excretion in healthy newborn babies. J Pediatr Gastroenterol Nutr 1984;3:402–7.

324. Kappas A, Sassa S, Anderson KE. In: Standbury JB, Wyngaarden JB, Fredrickson DS, et al, editors. The metabolic basis of inherited disease. New York: McGraw-Hill; 1983. p. 1299–384.

325. Garcia-Vargas GG, Del Razo LM, Cebrian ME, et al. Altered urinary porphyrin excretion in a human population chronically exposed to arsenic in Mexico. Hum Exp Toxicol 1994;13:839–47.

326. Kladchareon N, Suwannakul P, Bauchum V. Dubin-Johnson syndrome: report of two siblings with Tc-99 m IODIDA cholescintigraphic findings. J Med Assoc Thai 1988;71:640–2.

327. Pinós T, Constansa JM, Palacin A, Figueras C. A new diagnostic approach to the Dubin-Johnson syndrome. Am J Gastroenterol 1990;85:91–3.

328. Shimizu T, Tawa T, Maruyama T, et al. A case of infantile Dubin-Johnson syndrome with high CT attenuation in the liver. Pediatr Rediol 1997;27:345–7.

329. Mayatepek E, Lehmann WD. Defective hepatobiliary leukotriene elimination in patients with the Dubin-Johnson syndrome. Clin Chim Acta 1996;249:37–46.

330. Lindberg MC. Hepatobiliary complications of oral contraceptives. J Gen Intern Med 1992;7:199–209.

331. Di Zoglio JD, Cardillo E. Dubin-Johnson syndrome and pregnancy. Obstet Gynecol 1973;42:560–3.

6. Biliary Transport

Benjamin L. Shneider, MD

Cholestasis, which is a major manifestation of a wide range of pediatric liver diseases, is ultimately the result of specific or nonspecific abnormalities in biliary transport. These abnormalities can be the result of genetic defects in specific hepatic-based transporters or can be part of a series of molecular responses to a pathophysiologic process. Examples of the former include genetically determined defects in the expression of the canalicular bile acid transporter or the canalicular phospholipid flippase. An example of the latter is the cascade of responses that follow gram-negative sepsis. This chapter describes the current knowledge of disorders of biliary transport and how pathologic changes in these systems lead to pediatric liver disease. Current understandings of the natural history of, diagnostic approaches to, and treatment of these newly described diseases are reviewed.

BILIARY TRANSPORT

Bile flow is dependent on a series of vectorial transport proteins that are arrayed on the basolateral and canalicular membranes of hepatocytes (Figure 55.6-1). In addition, bile flow also requires an ordered hepatocellular processing of bile components. Transport processes in the intestine, kidney, pancreas bile duct, and gallbladder have significant effects on bile formation. This highly complex process is subject to a number of levels of regulation and consists of a diversity of genetically distinct elements. Bile itself consists of multiple individual components, including bile salts, bilirubin, phospholipids, cholesterol, and a large variety of endogenous and xenobiotic organic compounds. Vectorial flow of each of these components may be under separate genetic and regulatory controls. As such, it is not surprising that a wide variety of cholestatic liver diseases may exist, each with a separate genetic basis and each with distinct clinical characteristics and therapeutic approaches. A brief review of hepatocyte transport of bilirubin, bile acids, and organic anions is presented here (see Chapter 5.1, "Bile Formation and Cholestasis," for a comprehensive review of bile formation), especially as it pertains to the biliary transport disorders listed below. The interested reader is also directed to recent comprehensive reviews of biliary transport and analyses of modifications of bile by bile ductular epithelium.[1–5] Given the interrelation of disease and physiology in this rapidly developing field, details of the discovery of the various transporters are described in the following sections related to specific biliary transport diseases.

Highly efficient mechanisms for the basolateral extraction of bile components from serum into hepatocytes have developed partly in an effort to minimize the concentrations of these potentially toxic compounds in the systemic circulation. At least three different transporters have been shown to be potentially involved in basolateral transport of bile acids. The first and potentially most physiologically significant of these is the Na^+-dependent taurocholate cotransporting polypeptide (NTCP). This 48 kD protein is a hepatocyte-specific integral membrane protein.[6,7] It was the first of the bile acid–specific transport proteins to be cloned. Its discovery revolutionized the current approach to studying the physiology and pathophysiology of bile formation. In addition to NTCP, two other proteins have been shown to transport bile salts: the organic anion transport protein (OATP[8]) and microsomal epoxide hydrolase.[9] The physiologic significance of these latter two proteins in hepatic extraction of bile salts is currently not clear. OATP may be more important in hepatic extraction of organic anions such as bilirubin.[10]

The mechanisms involved in the transcellular movement of bile components from the basolateral to the canalicular membrane are not well understood. It is not certain whether this process involves specific binding proteins or specialized vesicles. Intracellular binding proteins for bile components have been described, although their physiologic necessity is not known. Bile acids have been shown to bind to dihydrodiol dehydrogenase, whereas bilirubin binds to ligandin.[11] Several lines of investigation have suggested that bile components are associated with or found within intracellular vesicles. As such, it is possible that molecular motor systems using

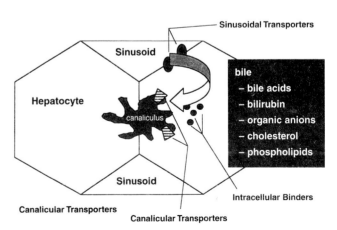

FIGURE 55.6-1 Diagram of mechanisms of bile flow. Cartoon depiction of hepatocyte couplet with vectorial flow of bile from sinusoidal blood to bile canaliculus via basolateral and canalicular transporters.

microfilaments and/or microtubules may play a role in promoting transcellular bile flow. These processes have been very difficult to assess using currently available experimental methods. Like the biliary transport proteins, it is very likely that studies of naturally occurring defects in these proteins will clarify this field. Bile acid conjugation is an additional intracellular event that influences bile flow. Conjugated bile acids are more water soluble and thus are more easily excreted.

Canalicular transport of bile components is generally recognized to be rate limiting for bile flow, and, as such, these transporters have been under active investigation by a number of laboratories. In addition, impairment of the function of any of these transport proteins has the potential to lead to the hepatocellular accumulation of toxic compounds and therefore directly lead to liver disease. A variety of studies indicated that many of these transport processes were adenosine triphosphate (ATP) dependent; thus, the ATP-binding cassette (ABC) proteins became likely candidates as transporters. A combination of basic laboratory investigations, animal models, and genetic analysis of cholestatic liver diseases (see individual sections below) ultimately identified three important ABC proteins as canalicular biliary transport proteins (Table 55.6-1). Specific and genetically distinct proteins have been identified that mediate ATP-dependent transport of bile acids (bile salt export pump [BSEP]/sister of P-glycoprotein [SPGP]), organic anions (multidrug resistance–associated protein 2 [MRP2]/canalicular multispecific organic anion transporter [cMOAT]), and phospholipids (multidrug resistance protein 3 [MDR3]) from the hepatocyte into the bile canaliculus. ATP hydrolysis is critical for each of these transport functions because the transport process takes place against a very steep con-centration gradient (ie, concentrations in bile are much greater than within the hepatocyte).

NOMENCLATURE

The nomenclature that currently exists in the field of biliary transport disorders is complex, confusing, and likely to undergo significant change. In this chapter, older terminology, in particular that uses progressive familial intrahepatic cholestasis (PFIC), is generally replaced by specific reference to the defective gene or protein. This has only recently become possible because the molecular identification of the defects involved in the various forms of PFIC have been elucidated.[1–3] The future utility of these historical designations may no longer be apparent. Many of the patients who have these diseases do not have other family members who are affected by the disease; thus, the familial portion of the designation becomes limiting. As the full range of the clinical phenotype of these various disorders becomes known, a more specific and helpful system of nomenclature may be devised.

DEFECTS IN CANALICULAR BILE ACID TRANSPORT

The pivotal role of canalicular transport of bile acids in the formation of bile has made this transport process a focus of active investigation in the pathophysiology of pediatric cholestatic liver disease. In spite of the fact that it has been expected that a defect in canalicular transport of bile acids would lead to severe cholestatic liver disease, discovery of this abnormality had been very difficult. Technical problems in the analysis of canalicular transport processes have been in large part responsible for delays in these discover-

TABLE 55.6-1   SUMMARY OF BILIARY TRANSPORT DISEASES

DISEASE	SPGP/BSEP DEFICIENCY	MDR3 DEFICIENCY	DUBIN-JOHNSON SYNDROME	BYLER DISEASE
PFIC designation	PFIC2	PFIC3	None	PFIC1
Common name	BSEP	MDR3	MRP/cMOAT	FIC1
Defective transport gene	ABCB11	ABCB4	ABCC2	ATP8B1
Chromosomal localization	2q24	7q21	10q24	18q21-q22
mRNA size (kb)	5.5	4.1	6.5–9.5	7.0
Protein size (kD)	170	170	200	145
Tissue distribution	Liver	Liver	Liver >> intestine	Intestine > liver
Transporter substrate	Bile acids	Phospholipids	Organic anions	Aminophospholipids?
Animal model	Mouse knockout[27]	Mouse mdr2 knockout[31]	Rat TR− or Eisai[58]	Mouse Byler equivalent[83]
Alanine aminotransferase level	++	++	nl	+
Bilirubin level	+ -> +++	+ -> +++	++	++ -> nl -> +++
Cholesterol and γ-GTP levels	nl	++	nl	nl
Serum bile acid level	+++	++	nl	+++
Histologic findings	Giant cell transformation	Ductular prolifer Portal fibrosis/cirrhosis	Melanin-like pigment in hepatocytes	Bland intracanalicular cholestasis; diminished canalicular γ-GTP
Special diagnostic tests	Biliary bile acids	Lipoprotein X; biliary phospholipids	Urine coproporphyrin I	Electron microscopy
Treatment	Liver transplant; biliary diversion?	Liver transplant	None	Partial biliary diversion; ileal bypass
Key references	17, 20	42	54, 61	66, 70, 78

BSEP = bile salt export pump; cMOAT = canalicular multispecific organic anion transporter; GTP = glutamyl transpeptidase; MDR = multidrug resistance; mRNA = messenger ribonucleic acid; MRP = multidrug resistance–associated protein; PFIC = progressive familial intrahepatic cholestasis; SPGP = sister of P-glycoprotein.

ies. Efflux transport processes, by their very nature, are much more complex to study than uptake mechanisms.[12] Accurate analysis of efflux is critically dependent on uniform loading of either cells or vesicles, which can be nearly impossible to perform. The alternative of examining reverse transport into cells or vesicles is subject to a number of artifacts. Isolation of relatively purified inside-out canalicular membrane vesicles permitted more exact analysis of canalicular transport via uptake.[13] It was not until recently that it was determined that the primary driving force for canalicular transport of bile acids was related to the hydrolysis of ATP.[14–16] This finding suggested that the canalicular bile acid transporter might belong to a superfamily of proteins referred to as ABC transporters. These transport proteins include a number of critically important proteins that, when defective, lead to a range of diseases, including cystic fibrosis, Wilson disease, adrenoleukodystrophy, Tangier disease, and Dubin-Johnson syndrome. The ABC transporters are integral membrane proteins, which typically have two cytoplasmic consensus sequences for ATP binding. Degenerate oligonucleotide primers were designed for these binding domains, and reverse transcriptase–polymerase chain reactions were used to clone the rat canalicular bile acid transporter.[17] The cloned gene was very similar to a previously cloned pig gene referred to as the SPGP.[18] Expression of the protein product of the SPGP complementary deoxyribonucleic acid (DNA) in two separate systems, Xenopus laevis oocytes and Sf9 insect cells, resulted in augmentation and acquisition, respectively, of ATP-dependent taurocholic acid transport activity. Northern blotting and immunoelectron microscopy indicate that the expression of this gene is hepatocyte specific and is localized to the canalicular membrane. Overall, these studies therefore indicated that the SPGP was a canalicular BSEP.

The clinical relevance of the discovery of BSEP became apparent as a result of genetic studies that were conducted nearly simultaneously. Homozygosity linkage studies mapped the genetic defect in a subset of Saudi Arabian patients with progressive familial cholestasis to chromosome 2q24.[19] Further refinement of the PFIC2 locus was performed using a larger group of patients with progressive familial cholestasis and ultimately led to the identification of the human correlate of BSEP as the defective gene in PFIC2.[20] Ten different mutations in BSEP were initially described (Figure 55.6-2). Four were nonsense mutations leading to a truncated protein, whereas the remaining six were missense mutations involving amino acid residues in key portions of the predicted bile acid transporter structure.

The clinical presentations of defects in BSEP are being defined, although the full range of presentations is not yet well understood.[20–24] Cholestasis often is manifest by pruritus and jaundice early in life, typically before 1 year of age. The inability of infants to scratch may translate into irritability as a first feature of this disorder. Biochemical findings are consistent with progressive intrahepatic cholestasis and include markedly elevated serum bile salts. There are typically variable elevations in serum bilirubin and aminotransferase levels with normal γ-glutamyl transpeptidase and normal cholesterol levels (see Table 55.6-1). Liver biopsies performed in the first 2 years of life are notable for giant cell hepatitis and cholestasis. The electron microscopic appearance of bile is reported to be distinct from that seen in familial intrahepatic cholestasis type 1 (FIC1) disease (see below). Immunohistochemical analysis of hepatic γ-glutamyl transpeptidase has been preliminarily reported to reveal strong staining at the bile canaliculus in contrast to the diminished staining observed in FIC1 disease (see below).[25] Some defects in BSEP lead to absent expression of its protein, which potentially can be demonstrated by immunohistochemistry.[26] Prospective and/or blinded analysis of these findings will be needed to confirm them as potential diagnostic criteria. Given the key role of BSEP in bile formation, it is not surprising that the clinical progression of liver disease in these patients is relatively rapid. Interestingly, a BSEP knockout mouse is

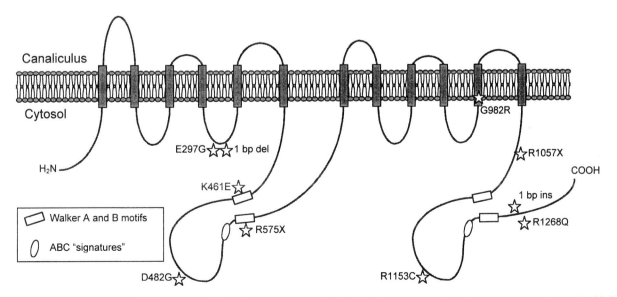

FIGURE 55.6-2 Diagram of defects in the bile salt excretory protein. Model of canalicular bile salt transporter protein embedded within the cell membrane. Specific mutations are indicated by the stars. Reproduced with permission from Thompson R.[20]

not characterized by progressive liver disease, suggesting that alterative transport mechanisms exist.[27] Because BSEP is liver specific, it is also not surprising that liver transplant appears to be curative.[17,20] A subset of patients may have mutations in BSEP that lead to a partially active protein.[23,28] These patients may have a more moderate disease course and could potentially be amenable to nontransplant surgical interventions such as partial biliary diversion or ileal bypass (see below).[29]

The diagnosis of a defect in *BSEP* should be suspected in any infant or young child with cholestasis who has normal γ-glutamyl transpeptidase and cholesterol levels. Biliary bile salt levels have been reported to be very low; unfortunately, biliary bile is often not available for routine clinical analysis. Differentiation of this disease from FIC1 disease may be problematic. It has been assumed that defects in *BSEP* have significantly more rapid progression to decompensated liver disease than seen in FIC1 disease. Careful genotype and phenotype studies are under way, and preliminary reports indicate that this assumption may not have been entirely accurate.[29] The ultrastructural appearance of canalicular bile in patients who are not receiving ursodeoxycholic acid may also be diagnostically useful.[30] Ultimately, some form of molecular diagnostic study, either analysis of hepatic protein or messenger ribonucleic acid (mRNA) expression or genomic sequencing of the *BSEP* gene, may be required to confirm a suspected diagnosis. Accuracy in assigning an appropriate diagnosis may be imperative because defects in *BSEP* appear to respond well to liver transplant, whereas FIC1 disease may not and may require a more specialized surgical approach (see below).

DEFECTS IN CANALICULAR PHOSPHOLIPID TRANSPORT

Phospholipid excretion into bile was presumed to be a passive process until the recent discovery of a P-glycoprotein, which mediates ATP-dependent phospholipid transport into bile.[31] This transport protein was somewhat serendipitously discovered in an effort to further understand the multidrug resistance proteins. One member of this class, *MDR3* (*mdr2* in mice), had been cloned and was found to be expressed in human liver, although its function was unknown.[32] Preliminary attempts to express this gene product in cell lines were uninformative with regard to its function[33]; therefore, the gene was "knocked out" of mice by homozygous targeted disruption. The resulting homozygous *mdr2⁻/⁻* mice have provided great insights into the physiology of bile formation and formed the basis for the understanding of a new class of cholestatic liver diseases.[31] Elevated bilirubin, alkaline phosphatase, and alanine aminotransferase were detected in the serum of these mice. Bile duct proliferation with a mixed portal infiltrate associated with loss of bile canalicular microvilli was observed in the homozygote knockout mice. Biliary bile flow and bile acid output by these mice were normal. Phospholipid, cholesterol, and glutathione secretion were all markedly reduced in bile with a graded reduction in phos-

pholipid only in heterozygote mice. The *mdr2* gene product was therefore presumed to be involved in canalicular excretion of phospholipid.

Further analysis of the *mdr2* knockout mice provided additional insights into the function and importance of this P-glycoprotein. Long-term histopathologic studies of the *mdr2⁻/⁻* mice demonstrated a novel progression from a nonsuppurative inflammatory cholangitis to metastatic hepatocarcinogenesis.[34] MDR3, the human homologue of the mouse *mdr2* gene, was introduced as a transgene into *mdr2⁻/⁻* mice.[35] Fibroblasts from the transgenic mice and not the knockout mice were able to transfer phospholipid from the inner hemileaflet to extracellular acceptor liposomes. This apparent phospholipid flippase activity was found to be an ATP-dependent phenomenon that could be observed using hepatic canalicular membrane.[36] Ultrarapid cryofixation of the liver from *mdr2⁻/⁻* mice with subsequent analysis by electron microscopy elegantly confirmed the suspected function of the mdr2 protein to be a phospholipid flippase (Figure 55.6-3).[37] In normal bile canaliculi, phospholipid accumulation on the outer hemileaflet of the canaliculus leads to the formation of vesicles that ultimately bud off into the canalicular lumen. These vesicles primarily contain cholesterol and phospholipid. These vesicles are targeted to plasma as opposed to bile in cholestasis and result in the formation of the characteristic lipoprotein X that is seen in obstructive liver disease, especially when it is secondary to bile duct obstruction.[38] *Mdr2⁻/⁻* mice do not accumulate lipoprotein X in the face of extrahepatic bile duct obstruction. Absence of phospholipid flippase function results in bile characterized by significant concentrations of unmicellized bile salts. This bile therefore has high detergent capacity and is toxic to the canalicular membrane and therefore the liver. Interestingly, *mdr2⁻/⁻* mice can be functionally rescued by either hepatic-specific transgenic expression of the human homologue MDR3 or by hepatocyte transplant.[39,40]

The comprehensive characterization of the *mdr2⁻/⁻* mouse and the elucidation of the function of the *mdr2* gene product laid the groundwork for identification of human disease related to abnormal expression of the human homologue MDR3. The first preliminary description of a defect in this gene product included two children who initially presented with pruritus and hepatosplenomegaly. The *MDR3* mRNA could not be detected by Northern blotting in one of these patients, and phospholipid levels in bile were markedly reduced in the second.[41] Neither of these suggestive findings could definitively demonstrate a genetic abnormality in *MDR3*.

A subsequent report definitively established defects in *MDR3* as a cause of cholestatic liver disease in two children.[42] As in the previous report, both children presented with jaundice and hepatosplenomegaly. Like the *mdr2⁻/⁻* mice, both children had elevated alanine aminotransferase and γ-glutamyl transpeptidase levels. Serum bile acid levels were markedly elevated in both children. Portal inflammation with bile duct proliferation and fibrosis was present despite a patent and normal extrahepatic biliary tree. Neither child was responsive to ursodeoxycholic acid therapy,

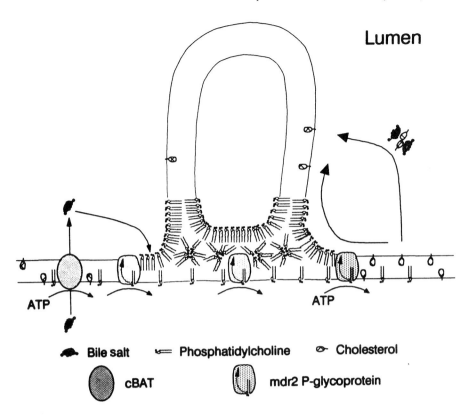

Lumen

FIGURE 55.6-3 Diagram of function of the multidrug resistance 2 (mdr2) protein. In this model, the mdr2 (equivalent to human MDR3) protein is shown to function as a phospholipid flippase. Adenosine triphosphate (ATP) hydrolysis leads to the "flipping" of phospholipid from the inner to the outer hemileaflet of the lipid bilayer. Accumulation of phospholipid on the outer hemileaflet leads to the formation of vesicles, which contain cholesterol and phospholipid. cBAT = canalicular bite acid transporter (also known as BSEP). Reproduced with permission of Crawford AR et al.[37]

and complications of end-stage liver disease led to liver transplant at the ages of 3.5 and 9.0 years. Immunohistochemical analysis of the explanted liver from both children revealed an absence of staining for the MDR3 protein using a specific polyclonal antibody.[43] Reverse transcriptase–polymerase chain reaction analysis of the MDR3 mRNA sequence in both patients identified homozygous defects that lead to premature stop codons and presumably truncated, unstable, and nonfunctional phospholipid flippase proteins. In one patient, the specific defect permitted genomic analysis of the proband and his family. The patient was found to be homozygous for the mutation at the genomic level, whereas his parents were both heterozygotes. His unaffected sister was homozygous for the wild-type gene.

The full range of the phenotypic expression of defects in the MDR3 gene is not known and is under investigation at this time. Cholestasis of pregnancy was prevalent in one of the families of the children reported to have an MDR3 nonsense mutation. There appears to be an association between heterozygosity for this defect and the propensity for the development of cholestasis of pregnancy.[44–46] A similar phenomenon has been observed with fatty liver of pregnancy and heterozygosity for fatty acid oxidation defects.[47] MDR3 defects have been reported in children with neonatal cholestasis, in children and adults with intrahepatic cholelithiasis, and in adults with chronic hepatitis and biliary cirrhosis.[48–52] Therefore, defects in MDR3 should be considered in any child or adult with high γ-glutamyl transpeptidase levels and cholestasis or biliary cirrhosis of unknown etiology. Supporting clinical, biochemical, and histologic features would include onset in early childhood, significant pruritus, absent serum lipoprotein X, a normal extrahepatic biliary tree, and histologic findings, including bile duct proliferation, portal inflammation, and biliary fibrosis and cirrhosis (see Table 55.6-1). When available, analysis of phospholipid in bile can also support this diagnosis. Immunohistochemical analysis of a percutaneous liver biopsy might someday be a useful screening assay. Ultimately, analysis of genomic DNA and/or liver mRNA will be required to establish a specific genetic defect.

There are important clinical implications of a diagnosis of an MDR3 defect. At present, in its severe form, this appears to be a progressive and unremitting disease, which leads to end-stage liver disease within the first two decades of life, typically in the first decade. Neither ursodeoxycholic acid nor partial biliary diversion or ileal bypass appears to be effective in amelioriating either the pruritus or progression of this disease. Animal models of this disease indicate a potential risk for the development of liver cancer, although this has yet to be described in humans. The tissue distribution of the MDR3 protein appears to be liver specific, and, as such, liver transplant should be and has been curative.[43] Interestingly, animal studies have shown that the functional defect and presumably the disease can be ameliorated by both transgenic expression of a normal MDR3 gene or by hepatocyte transplant.[42,53] There appears to be a subset of patients with presumably partial defects in MDR3 that are responsive to high-dose ursodeoxycholic acid.[51] Therefore, a trial of ursodeoxycholic acid is warranted in children with cryptogenic and nonobstructive liver disease characterized by high serum γ-glutamyl transpeptidase levels.

DEFECTS IN CANALICULAR ORGANIC ANION TRANSPORT

Dubin-Johnson syndrome was described in the 1950s and has been presumed to be the result of a defect in canalicular bilirubin transport.[54] Transport studies had indicated that a variety of organic anions, including conjugated bilirubin, were transported into the bile canaliculus by an ATP-dependent mechanism.[55] The identification of the specific protein involved in this transport process was aided by a naturally occurring rat species with chronic conjugated hyperbilirubinemia, the TR⁻ rat.[56,57] Presuming that the canalicular organic anion transporter was homologous to a previously cloned human MRP1, Paulusma and colleagues screened a rat liver complementary DNA library for related gene products.[58] One of the novel isolated genes was highly expressed in liver and ultimately found to be mutated in the TR⁻ rat. Immunoblot analysis revealed that this new protein, MRP2 (which is also referred to as cMOAT), was absent from canalicular membrane vesicles prepared from the TR⁻ rat. Subsequent studies demonstrated a different defect in the same gene product in the Eisai hyperbilirubinemic rat.[59] The role of defects of the *MRP2* gene in Dubin-Johnson syndrome was initially complicated by the finding of absent immunostaining for MRP2 at the bile canaliculus but unexpected strong staining at the lateral or basolateral membrane of the hepatocyte.[60]

Dubin-Johnson syndrome is characterized by benign direct hyperbilirubinemia. Diagnosis is made on the finding of mild direct hyperbilirubinemia, with an absence of evidence of hepatocellular or canalicular injury. Urine typically contains an elevated percentage of coproporphyrin isomer I. Liver biopsy reveals no significant changes in hepatic architecture and characteristic melanin-like pigment in hepatocytes. When performed, the sulfobromphthalein test reveals normal hepatic uptake, delayed canalicular excretion, and a secondary peak owing to presumed reflux of dye into plasma. A number of mutations have now been described in the *MRP2/cMOAT* gene in patients with well-characterized Dubin-Johnson syndrome.[61–64] The initial confusion about the persistent basolateral staining for the transporter in these patients has been clarified with the current identification of six *MRP* genes. MRP2-specific antibodies reveal no immunologically recognizable protein in the liver from Dubin-Johnson syndrome patients.[65] The originally described basolateral staining was, in fact, cross-recognition with MRP3.

FIC1 DISEASE (BYLER DISEASE)

Byler disease has been viewed by many as the prototype for a genetic form of biliary transport disorder, yet unlike the other transport defects, its exact molecular pathophysiology remains elusive. Byler disease was first described in the 1960s as a cholestatic disease that affected members of the Amish community who were direct descendants of Jacob Byler and Nancy Kaufmann.[66,67] The disease appears to consist of two phases; the first cholestatic jaundice phase occurs in infancy. The jaundice associated with the first phase typically resolves, although the hallmark pruritus persists. The second phase of the disease includes end-stage liver disease with associated recurrent jaundice and typically becomes manifest at the end of the first decade or some time into the second decade of life. Early investigations into the pathophysiology of this disease included in vivo analysis of bile acid clearance in a patient with Byler disease.[68] Kinetic analysis of these studies pointed to a defect in hepatic excretion of bile salts, and, as such, Byler disease has always been presumed to be the result of defective biliary transport. Subsequent examination of the composition of bile in a separate set of patients supported the concept of a defect in canalicular excretion of bile salts.[69]

The clinical syndrome of Byler disease is characteristic and ultimately permitted genetic studies of a relatively homogeneous patient population. All patients have severe and, if untreated, relatively unremitting pruritus. This is in contrast to benign recurrent intrahepatic cholestasis, where the pruritus is episodic.[70] The pruritus in Byler disease is associated with markedly elevated serum bile salt levels. The biochemical pattern of the cholestasis in Byler disease is quite characteristic and includes relatively normal transaminase levels, variable bilirubin levels depending on the phase of the disease, and normal cholesterol and γ-glutamyl transpeptidase levels. In many ways, the biochemical markers are quite similar to those seen in defects in *BSEP* disease. Severe and sometimes disabling diarrhea and malabsorption may also be present. This appears to be the result of more than simple cholestasis because it may persist after successful liver transplant.[71] Wheezing and elevated sweat chloride levels have been described in some patients with Byler disease.[72,73]

The histologic findings in Byler disease have been carefully documented.[30,74] Prospective correlation of histology with genotyping is needed. Therefore, at present, it is difficult to assess whether the histologic findings that are described are relevant for PFIC in a general sense or to genetically proven Byler disease. It appears that Byler disease leads to a histologically bland form of intracanalicular cholestasis.[30] Histologic findings are clearly dependent on the age of the patient at the time of the biopsy. Early on, minimal giant cell hepatitis with mild portal inflammation is present. Bile duct paucity is not a characteristic finding, although the bile ducts themselves may be small. Over time, fibrosis in the biopsy may progress, and bile duct proliferation may be noted. A characteristic appearance of the bile on electron microscopic analysis (Figure 55.6-4) includes a coarsely particulate and amorphous granular biliary material.[30,75] Immunohistochemical analysis of liver from children with FIC1 deficiency has revealed diminished expression of γ-glutamyl transpeptidase at the bile canaliculus.[25] The specificity of these histologic and ultrastructural findings will need to be reassessed and correlated with genetic abnormalities in the *FIC1* gene (see below).

The approach to the identification of the cause of Byler disease used a genome screening technique referred to as searching for share segment.[76,77] This approach is based on the assumption that there is a common founder mutation in a population and that this mutation is the basis of a well-characterized disease in a relatively closed community. Byler disease, as described in the Amish community, a priori appeared to fit these criteria quite well. Initially, analysis revealed that the Byler locus was found at chromosome 18q21-q22. Interestingly, this is the same locus that was identified for benign recurrent intrahepatic cholestasis. At the time of this discovery, interesting speculation took place as to the relationship between Byler disease and benign recurrent intrahepatic cholestasis. Possibilities included linked genes, a common regulatory gene, or different mutations with different functional consequences. Ultimately, more refining linkage analysis and complementary DNA library screening led to the identification of a defect in a gene labeled *FIC1* as the cause of both Byler disease and benign recurrent intrahepatic cholestasis.[78] Subsequent clinical studies have revealed that there is a clinical spectrum of disease between benign recurrent intrahepatic cholestasis and Byler disease and the designation of all of these disorders because FIC1 disease is more accurate.[79]

The current challenge is to determine the function of FIC1 and how different mutations lead to the diseases recognized as either benign recurrent intrahepatic cholestasis or Byler disease. Cloning of FIC1 led to the discovery that this gene product has a wide tissue distribution, including mRNA expression in the pancreas, small intestine, stomach, bladder, heart, placenta, lung, liver, and kidney.[78] Surprisingly, expression appears to be greatest in the pancreas and intestine. Immunohistochemistry reveals that it is expressed on the apical surface of many of these cells.[80,81] The range of tissues that express FIC1 might explain many of the systemic manifestations, including wheezing, elevated sweat chloride, and diarrhea. Recent investigations have revealed expression in bile duct epithelium, and this may be as relevant for the hepatic manifestations of the disease.[81] Computer-assisted homology analysis indicates that *FIC1* may be related to a previously cloned bovine adenosine triphosphatase II gene, which appears to have aminophospholipid transporting activity.[82] This type of transport function is critical for perpetuation of the physiologically important assymmetry of phosphatidylserine distribution within the lipid bilayer of a variety of cells. The exact interaction between FIC1 and bile acid transporters is yet to be determined. A mouse model of Byler disease is characterized by abnormal regulation of ileal bile acid transport.[83] Analysis of human ileum indicated that the ileal bile acid transporter (apical sodium dependent bile acid transporter = *SLC10A2*) is relatively overexpressed in children with absent FIC1 expression.[84] This suggests that FIC1 disease may, in part, be the result of a gain of function defect in the ileal bile acid transporter. In rats, indirect immunofluorescence and Western blotting indicate that the FIC1 protein is expressed on the canalicular surface of hepatocytes and the brush border membrane of enterocytes.[80,81] Expression in the intestine appears to be along the entire length of the small intestine. Presumably, abnormalities in FIC1 function alter the assymmetric distribution of phospholipids in the hepatic canalicular and intestinal brush border membrane and secondarily affect the normal function of critical solute trans-

porters. The common link in these abnormalities may be a defect in the activity of the farnesoid X receptor (FXR). The FXR plays a key role in the regulation of genes involved in bile acid biosynthesis and transport.[85,86] Absence of FIC1 in the ileum of patients and in cell lines treated with FIC1 antisense oligonucleotides is associated with a reduction in FXR expression.[84] In cell lines FXR does not translocate into the nucleus when FIC1 is not expressed.[84] These studies suggest that FIC1 activity alters signal transduction pathways involved in FXR nuclear translocation.

Mutational analysis of FIC1 disease patients has revealed specific and distinct homozygous defects in patients of Amish and European origin.[78,87,88] Severe mutations have the potential to disrupt key ATP-binding sites in the FIC1 molecule. In contrast, the defects that have been identified in patients with benign recurrent intrahepatic cholestasis appear to involve less critical residues. As such, the defect in benign recurrent intrahepatic cholestasis may only partially affect FIC1 function and thus might lead to a milder phenotype. A wide variety of distinct mutations have been described in patients with either Byler disease or benign recurrent intrahepatic cholestasis (BRIC), including 13 missense mutations, 1 nonsense mutation, 3 small deletions, 1 large genomic deletion, and 5 splice-site defects.[87] A number of compound heterozygote states have been detected, most of which lead to a phenotype most consistent with BRIC. Homozygosity for one of these defective alleles (G308V) is associated with classic Byler disease, whereas compound heterozygosity of the same allele leads to BRIC. This defect has been introduced into a mouse model of this disease, which is currently under study.[89] Careful analysis of the clinical course of these patients appears to indicate that a spectrum of disease

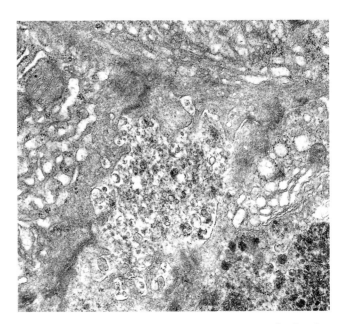

FIGURE 55.6-4 Electron microscopic appearance of Byler disease bile. Coarsely granular bile is seen in a patient with Byler disease (osmium tetroxide/uranyl acetate/lead citrate; ×31,625 original magnification). Courtesy of A. S. Knisely, Institute of Liver Studies, London, UK.

exists between BRIC and Byler disease. Clinical variability has been observed between patients with the same FIC1 genotype, suggesting that environmental influences and/or variable penetrance may exist for this disease.

Correct diagnosis of FIC1 disease has potentially very important clinical and therapeutic consequences. This diagnosis should certainly been considered in the setting of a patient with cholestasis characterized by severe pruritus who has markedly elevated serum bile salts with relatively normal cholesterol and γ-glutamyl transpeptidase. Being a member of the Amish community is highly suggestive but not diagnostic of this disorder.[90] Alternative defective genes have recently been described in Amish children. These children have compound defects involving tight junction proteins and bile acid conjugation enzymes. The slower clinical progression of FIC1 disease may help distinguish it from defects in BSEP. The characteristic electron microscopic appearance of bile (with the patient off ursodeoxycholic acid therapy) is highly suggestive of this diagnosis.[30] Immunohistochemical analysis of γ-glutamyl transpeptidase in liver may also be suggestive of a defect in FIC1.[25] Molecular analysis is now available on a research basis and should be sought out to help confirm a defect in PFIC1. Absence of intestinal FIC1 expression at the level of either protein or mRNA may be a shortcut to this diagnosis in patients with defects that lead to an unstable or absent mRNA or protein.[84]

The clinical consequences of a correct diagnosis are related to the appropriate choice of therapy. It has become apparent from clinical experience and basic investigations that FIC1 has a wide distribution of tissue expression, and FIC1 disease, as such, is a systemic disease. Liver transplant is therefore not necessarily curative, unlike the clinical experience in cases of BSEP and MDR3 deficiencies. Persistent diarrhea, graft steatosis, growth failure, and pancreatitis have all been observed after liver transplant in children with FIC1 disease.[71] Instead, surgical approaches that use depletion of the bile salt pool seem to be effective and involve significantly less risk than liver transplant. These methods include partial biliary diversion and partial ileal bypass.[91–98] Both techniques lead to wasting of bile salts and presumed depletion of toxic bile salts, although this explanation is not completely clear. Interruption of the enterohepatic circulation may ameliorate some of the problems associated with the gain of function in the ileal bile acid transporter. Both treatments have been shown to markedly improve pruritus and to stabilize or even improve both the biochemical and histologic manifestations of the disease. Clearly, at this time, these surgical approaches are the treatment of choice for compensated FIC1 disease. Better understanding of the pathophysiology of FIC1 disease might lead to alternative medical approaches, potentially including specific and highly potent bile acid–binding resins or bile acid transport inhibitors.

DISORDERS OF BILIARY TRANSPORT IN SYSTEMIC DISEASE

Jaundice and cholestasis are well-recognized features of conditions that nonspecifically affect the liver. Examples include gram-negative sepsis, administration of parenteral hyperalimentation, drug toxicity, and liver regeneration. The specific effects of these various conditions on transporters involved in bile formation can explain the development of cholestasis and might lead to specific interventions to prevent liver injury. The best understood example is the effect of gram-negative sepsis. The association between jaundice and cholestasis[99] and gram-negative sepsis has been recognized for a long time.[100,101] The molecular basis of this is now beginning to be understood. Gram-negative sepsis is associated with circulation of endotoxin, which leads to the formation of tumor necrosis factor-α and a range of inflammatory cytokines (eg, interleukins 1 and 6). Via specific interactions with cis elements in the promoter of the basolateral bile acid transporter, NTCP is down-regulated.[99,102–104] Canalicular transport of bile acids and organic anions also appears to be impaired by sepsis and is mediated by down-regulation in MRP2/cMOAT and BSEP.[105–107] The molecular effects of the administration of parenteral hyperalimentation, drug toxicities, and hepatic regeneration are currently under investigation.

CLINICAL APPROACH TO COMPLEX FORMS OF CHOLESTASIS

In the current era, the clinician is faced with an evolving and complex series of potential diagnostic and therapeutic approaches for children and adults with nontypical forms of cholestasis. An algorithmic approach to the evaluation of these nonstandard forms of cholestatic liver disease is suggested in Figure 55.6-5. The presence of pruritus and/or significantly elevated serum bile acid levels in combination with measurement of serum γ-glutamyl transpeptidase may be useful in the initial categorization of the potential molecular process underlying the particular cholestatic condition. Supplemental assays including electron microscopy, biliary bile acid and biliary phospholipid analysis, serum lipoprotein X measurement, and urine coproporphyrin analysis may support a potential molecular diagnosis. In the current era, molecular diagnostics should be strongly considered part of the comprehensive evaluation of the patient with complex cholestasis. Given the divergent potential treatments for these distinct disorders, this degree of sophisticated diagnostic testing appears warranted.

FUTURE DIRECTIONS

Our current understanding of biliary transport defects is clearly in its infancy. A variety of areas of investigation will need to be explored. New molecular mechanisms of cholestasis and genetic defects leading to biliary transport disorders are yet to be discovered. The full range of the clinical phenotypes of the currently described disorders needs to be discerned. The role of partially functioning transporters or heterozygote states in commonly occurring but poorly understood cholestatic conditions, like that seen during parenteral hyperalimentation, will need to be investigated.

Bile excretion by the liver is a critical function, and, as such, its underlying molecular mechanisms are complex.

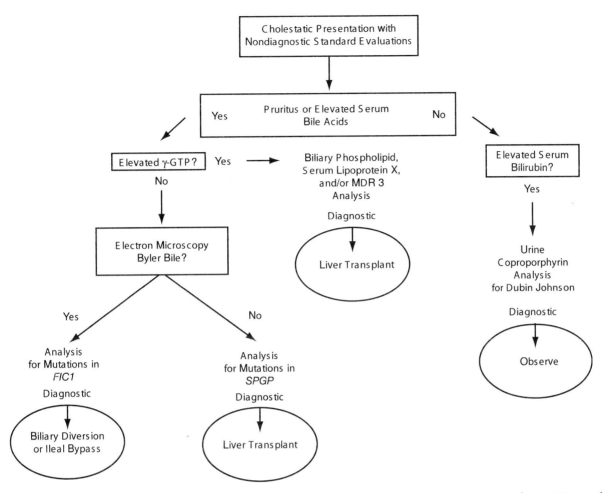

FIGURE 55.6-5   Diagnostic and therapeutic algorithm for complex cholestasis. GTP = γ-glutamyl transpeptidase; MDR = multidrug resistance; *SPGP* = sister of P-glycoprotein.

Significant achievements have been made in understanding the process of bile excretion, but a great deal remains undiscovered. Examples of areas of ongoing research include the exact pathways involved in the intracellular translocation of components of bile from the basolateral membrane to the bile canaliculus, the role of the cytoskeleton in canalicular function, the mechanisms of regulation of canalicular transport proteins, and the functional consequences of bile duct transport processes on the formation of bile. It is expected that molecular defects in each of these important pathways and mechanisms of regulation of bile formation may lead to cholestatic liver disease.

A number of cholestatic phenotypes exist for which a molecular mechanism remains elusive. A third locus for low γ-glutamyl transpeptidase cholestasis appears to exist.[108] Aagenaes syndrome is another form of inherited cholestasis that consists of periods of severe pruritus but has the additional finding of lower extremity lymphedema.[109] A syndrome of arthrogryposis, renal tubular acidosis, and cholestasis with normal γ-glutamyl transpeptidase levels has been reported in 11 kindreds, and the molecular defect has recently been described.[110,111] Rotor syndrome, like Dubin-Johnson syndrome, is characterized by persistent direct hyperbilirubinemia with no significant intrahepatic liver injury.[112] Distinguishing features include

the absence of hepatic pigmentation and the urinary pattern of coproporphyrins. Neonatal sclerosing cholangitis is a relatively rare form of neonatal cholestasis and has been linked to a new and unique genetic locus (R. Thompson, personal communication, 1999).[113] Genetic, molecular, and physiologic studies of these syndromes are likely to expand our knowledge of disorders of biliary transport.

The current clinical presentations of the various disorders of biliary transport that have been described in this chapter probably do not represent the full spectrum of the clinical phenotypes that may exist. As the molecular etiology of a disease is discovered, the clinical spectrum of the disease in question changes significantly, and, in some ways, the definition of the original disease comes into question. Two recent noteworthy examples are cystic fibrosis and Alagille syndrome.[114–116] Abnormalities in the *CFTR* gene have recently been described in patients with absent vas deferens or chronic pancreatitis who do not have the usual clinical features that are characteristic of cystic fibrosis.[117–119] Similarly, isolated cardiac anomalies have been described in patients with mutations in the *JAGGED1* gene, yet these patients do not meet the standard defining criteria for a diagnosis of Alagille syndrome.[120,121] It will therefore be very important to examine the level of expression and genotype of the various newly described transport genes in a spectrum of pediatric liver diseases in which the etiology is currently unknown.

In a related area of investigation, it will be important to carry out similar investigations of the level of expression and genotype of transporter genes in what are currently felt to be relatively well-understood disorders. Many cholestatic liver diseases have well-described phenotypes and are labeled with well-entrenched names, but have basic etiologies that are not well understood. Primary sclerosing cholangitis, total parenteral hyperalimentation, and drug-related cholestasis are potential examples. Many of the features of primary sclerosing cholangitis, especially the intrahepatic form, are akin to defects in *MDR3*. Predisposition to the development of cholestasis during total parenteral hyperalimentation may, in some cases, be related to heterozygote status for defects in one of the biliary transport genes. Alternatively, patients might be homozygotes or compound heterozygotes for mutations that lead to partial inactivation of the transporter. Similarly, drug-related cholestasis might be the result of partially dysfunctional genotypes, especially those that involve the *MRP2/cMOAT* gene. The recent description of cholestasis of pregnancy being related to heterozygote status for a defect in the *MDR3* gene is a good example of the potential implications of this process.[44]

SUMMARY

A new era in the understanding of cholestatic liver disease in children has been ushered in by the discovery of a variety of gene products that play a key role in the formation of bile. Defects in the canalicular transporters for bile acids, organic anions, and phospholipids all lead to distinct forms of cholestatic liver disease, whose onset is during early childhood. Liver transplant at present remains the best long-term approach to the treatment of defects in bile acid or phospholipid excretion. Byler disease is distinct from these disorders and involves a defect in a gene whose exact function in bile formation remains a subject of intense investigation. Clinical and laboratory studies indicate that Byler disease is a systemic disease, and, as such, liver transplant may not be curative. Partial biliary diversion or ileal bypass may be more appropriate means of treatment of this disease. Our understanding of biliary transport disorders is in its infancy, and the future holds great promise for further understanding of the mechanisms of and optimal treatment for cholestatic liver disease in children.

REFERENCES

1. Elferink R, Groen A. Genetic defects in hepatobiliary transport. Biochim Biophys Acta 2002;1586:129–45.
2. Meier P, Stieger B. Bile salt transporters. Annu Rev Physiol 2002;64:635–61.
3. Muller M, Jansen PLM. The secretory function of the liver: new aspects of hepatobiliary transport. J Hepatol 1998;28:344–54.
4. Trauner M, Boyer J. Bile salt transporters: molecular characterization, function, and regulation. Physiol Rev 2003;83:633–71.
5. Boyer JL. Bile duct epithelium: frontiers in transport physiology. Am J Physiol 1996;270:G1–5.
6. Hagenbuch B, Stieger B, Foguet M, et al. Functional expression cloning and characterization of the hepatocyte Na+/bile acid cotransport system. Proc Natl Acad Sci U S A 1991;88:10629–33.
7. Hagenbuch B, Meier PJ. Molecular cloning, chromosomal localization, and functional characterization of a human liver Na+/bile acid cotransporter. J Clin Invest 1994;93:1326–31.
8. Jacquemin E, Hagenbuch B, Stieger B, et al. Expression cloning of a rat liver Na(+)-independent organic anion transporter. Proc Natl Acad Sci U S A 1994;91:133–7.
9. von Dippe P, Amoui M, Stellwagen RH, Levy D. The functional expression of sodium-dependent bile acid transport in Madin-Darby canine kidney cells transfected with the cDNA for microsomal epoxide hydrolase. J Biol Chem 1996;271:18176–80.
10. Reichel C, Gao B, van Montfoort J, et al. Localization and function of the organic anion-transporting polypeptide OATP2 in rat liver. Gastroenterology 1999;117:688–95.
11. Stolz A, Hammond L, Lou H, et al. cDNA cloning and expression of the human hepatic bile acid-binding protein. A member of the monomeric reductase gene family. J Biol Chem 1993;268:10448–57.
12. Shneider BL, Moyer MS. Characterization of endogenous carrier-mediated taurocholate efflux from Xenopus laevis oocytes. J Biol Chem 1993;268:6985–8.
13. Inoue M, Kinne R, Tran T, et al. Rat liver canalicular membrane vesicles: isolation and topological characterization. J Biol Chem 1983;258:5183–8.
14. Adachi Y, Kobayashi H, Kurumi Y, et al. ATP-dependent taurocholate transport by rat liver canalicular membrane veiscles. Hepatology 1991;14:655–9.
15. Muller M, Ishikawa T, Berger U, et al. ATP-dependent transport of taurocholate across the hepatocyte canalicular membrane mediated by a 110-kDa glycoprotein binding ATP and bile salt. J Biol Chem 1991;266:18920–6.
16. Nishida T, Gatmaitan Z, Che M, Arias IM. Rat liver canalicular membrane vesicles contain an ATP-dependent bile acid transport system. Proc Natl Acad Sci U S A 1991;88:6590–4.
17. Gerloff T, Stieger B, Hagenbuch B, et al. The sister of P-glycoprotein represents the canalicular bile salt export pump of the mammalian liver. J Biol Chem 1998;273:10046–50.
18. Childs S, Yeh RL, Georges E, Ling V. Identification of a sister gene to P-glycoprotein. Cancer Res 1995;55:2029–34.
19. Strautnieks S, Kagalwalla A, Tanner S, et al. Identification of a locus for progressive familial cholestasis PFIC2 on chromosome 2q24. Am J Hum Genet 1997;61:630–3.
20. Strautnieks SS, Bull LN, Knisely AS, et al. A gene encoding a liver-specific ABC transporter is mutated in progressive familial intrahepatic cholestasis. Nat Genet 1998;20:233–8.
21. Jansen P, Strautnieks S, Jacquemin E, et al. Hepatocanalicular bile salt excretory pump deficiency in patients with progressive familial intrahepatic cholestasis. Gastroenterology 1999;117:1370–9.
22. Chen H, Chang P, Hsu H, et al. FIC1 and BSEP defects in Taiwanese patients with chronic intrahepatic cholestasis with low gamma-glutamyltranspeptidase levels. J Pediatr 2002;140:119–24.
23. Wang L, Soroka C, Boyer J. The role of bile salt export pump mutations in progressive familial intrahepatic cholestasis type II. J Clin Invest 2002;110:965–72.
24. Eloranta M, Hakli T, Hiltunen M, et al. Association of single nucleotide polymorphisms of the bile salt export pump gene with intrahepatic cholestasis of pregnancy. Scand J Gastroenterol 2003;38:648–52.

25. Hanigan M, Bull L, Strautnieks S, et al. Low serum concentrations of γ-GT activity in progressive familial intrahepatic cholestasis: evidence for different mechanisms in PFIC, type 1 (FIC1 disease) and in PFIC, type 2 (BSEP disease) [abstract]. Hepatology 2002;36:310A.

26. Jansen P, Hooiveld G, Jacquemin E, et al. The canalicular bile salt exporting protein is not expressed in patients with progressive familial cholestasis type 2 [abstract]. Hepatology 1998;28:498A.

27. Wang R, Salem M, Yousef IM, et al. Targeted inactivation of sister of P-glycoprotein gene (sPgp) in mice results in nonprogressive but persistent intrahepatic cholestasis. Proc Natl Acad Sci U S A 2001;98:2011–6.

28. Plass J, Mol O, Heegsma J, et al. Effect of PFIC2 mutations on function and sorting of the bile salt export pump. Hepatology 2003;36:310A.

29. Bull L, Freimer N, Czubkowski P, et al. Clinical and biochemical features of FIC1 (ATP8B1) and BSEP (ABCB11) disease. Hepatology 2003;36:310A.

30. Bull LN, Varlton VEH, Stricker NL, et al. Genetic and morphological findings in progressive familial intrahepatic cholestasis (Byler disease [PFIC-1] and Byler syndrome): evidence for heterogeneity. Hepatology 1997;26:155–64.

31. Smit JJM, Schinkel AH, Oude Elferink RPJ, et al. Homozygous disruption of the murine mdr2 P-glycoprotein gene leads to a complete absence of phospholipid from bile and to liver disease. Cell 1993;75:451–62.

32. Van der Bliek AM, Baas F, Houte de Lange TT, et al. The human mdr3 gene encodes a novel P-glycoprotein homologue and gives rise to alternatively spliced mRNAs in liver. EMBO J 1987;6:3325–31.

33. Schinkel AH, Roelofs MEM, Borst P. Characterization of the human MDR3 P-glycoprotein and its recognition by P-glycoprotein-specific monoclonal antibodies. Cancer Res 1991;51:2628–35.

34. Mauad TH, van Nieuwkerk CMJ, Dingemans KP, et al. Mice with homozygous disruption of the mdr2 P-glycoprotein gene. A novel animal model for studies of nonsuppurative inflammatory cholangitis and hepatocarcinogenesis. Am J Pathol 1994;145:1237–45.

35. Smith AJ, Timmermans-Hereijgers JLPM, Roelofsen B, et al. The human MDR3 P-glycoprotein promotes translocation of phosphatidylcholine through the plasma membrane of fibroblasts from transgenic mice. FEBS Lett 1994;354:263–6.

36. Nies AT, Gatmaitan Z, Arias IM. ATP-dependent phosphatidylcholine translocation in rat liver canalicular plasma membrane vesicles. J Lipid Res 1996;37:1125–36.

37. Crawford AR, Smith AJ, Hatch VC, et al. Hepatic secretion of phospholipid vesicles in the mouse critically depends on mdr2 or MDR3 P-glycoprotein expression. J Clin Invest 1997;100:2562–7.

38. Oude Elferink RPJ, Ottenhoff R, van Marle J, et al. Class III P-glycoproteins mediate the formation of lipoprotein X in the mouse. J Clin Invest 1998;102:1749–57.

39. Smith AJ, de Vree ML, Ottenhoff R, et al. Hepatocyte-specific expression of the human MDR3 P-glycoprotein gene restores the biliary phosphatidylchol in excretion absent in Mdr2 (−/−) mice. Hepatology 1998;28:530–6.

40. De Vree J, Ottenhoff R, Bosma P, et al. Correction of liver disease by hepatocyte transplantation in a mouse model of progressive familial intrahepatic cholestasis. Gastroenterology 2000;119:1720–30.

41. Deleuze JF, Jacquemin E, Dubuisson C, et al. Defect of multidrug-resistance 3 gene expression in a subtype of progressive familial intrahepatic cholestasis. Hepatology 1996;23:904–8.

42. De Vree JM, Jacquemin E, Sturm E, et al. Mutations in the MDR3 gene cause progressive familial intrahepatic cholestasis. Proc Natl Acad Sci U S A 1998;95:282–7.

43. Smit JJM, Schinkel AH, Mol CA, et al. The tissue distribution of the human MDR3 P-glycoprotein. Lab Invest 1994;71:638–49.

44. Jacquemin E, Cresteil D, Manouvrier S, et al. Heterozygous non-sense mutation of the MDR3 gene in familial intrahepatic cholestasis of pregnancy. Lancet 1999;353:210–1.

45. Dixon P, Weerasekera N, Linton K, et al. Heterozygous MDR3 missense mutation associated with intrahepatic cholestasis of pregnancy: evidence for a defect in protein trafficking. Hum Mol Genet 2000;9:1209–17.

46. Gendrot C, Bacq Y, Brechot M, et al. A second heterozygous MDR3 nonsense mutation associated with intrahepatic cholestasis of pregnancy. J Med Genet 2003;40:e32.

47. Treem W, Rinaldo P, Hale D, et al. Acute fatty liver of pregnancy and long-chain 3-hydroxyacyl-coenzyme A dehydrogenase deficiency. Hepatology 1994;19:339–45.

48. Jacquemin E, De Vree J, Cresteil D, et al. The wide spectrum of multidrug resistance 3 deficiency: from neonatal cholestasis to cirrhosis of adulthood. Gastroenterology 2001;120:1448–58.

49. Chen H, Chang P, Hsu H, et al. Progressive familial intrahepatic cholestasis with high gamma-glutamyltranspeptidase levels in Taiwanese infants: role of MDR3 gene defect? Pediatr Res 2001;50:50–5.

50. Rosmorduc O, Hermelin B, Poupon R. MDR3 gene defect in adults with symptomatic intrahepatic and gallbladder cholesterol cholelithiasis. Gastroenterology 2001;120:1459–67.

51. Jacquemin E. Role of multidrug resistance 3 deficiency in pediatric and adult liver disease: one gene for three diseases. Semin Liver Dis 2001;21:551–62.

52. Lucena JF, Herrero JI, Quiroga J, et al. A multidrug resistance 3 gene mutation causing cholelithiasis, cholestasis of pregnancy, and adulthood biliary cirrhosis. Gastroenterology 2003;124:1037–42.

53. de Vree JML, Ottenhoff R, Smith AJ, et al. Rapid correction of Mdr2 deficiency by transplantation of MDR3 transgenic hepatocytes [abstract]. Hepatology 1998;28:387A.

54. Dubin IN, Johnson FB. Chronic idiopathic jaundice with unidentified pigment in liver cells: new clinico-pathologic entity with report of 12 cases. Medicine 1954;33:155–97.

55. Oude Elferink RP, Ottenhoff R, Liefting WG, et al. ATP-dependent efflux fo GSSG and GS-conjugates from isolated rat hepatocytes. Am J Physiol 1990;258:G699–706.

56. Jansen PLM, Peters WH, Lamers WH. Hereditary chronic conjugated hyperbilirubinemia in mutant rats caused by defective hepatic anion transport. Hepatology 1985;5:573–9.

57. Kitamura T, Jansen P, Hardenbrook C, et al. Defective ATP-dependent bile canalicular transport of organic anions in mutant (TR⁻) rats with conjugated hyperbilirubinemia. Proc Natl Acad Sci U S Am 1990;87:3557–61.

58. Paulusma CC, Bosma PJ, Zaman GJR, et al. Congenital jaundice in rats with a mutation in a multidrug resistance-associated protein gene. Science 1996;271:1126–8.

59. Ito K, Suzuki H, Hirohashi T, et al. Molecular cloning of canalicular multispecific organic anion transporter defective in EHBR. Am J Physiol 1997;35:G16–22.

60. Kartenbeck J, Leuschner U, Mayer R, Keppler D. Absence of the canalicular isoform of the MRP-gene encoded conjugate export pump from the hepatocytes in Dubin-Johnson syndrome. Hepatology 1996;23:1061–6.

61. Paulusma CC, Kool M, Bosma PJ, et al. A mutation in the human canalicular multispecific organic anion transporter gene causes the Dubin-Johnson syndrome. Hepatology 1997;25:1539–42.

62. Kajihara S, Hisatomi A, Mizuta T, et al. A splice mutation in the human canalicular multispecific organic anion transporter gene causes Dubin-Johnson syndrome. Biochem Biophys Res Commun 1998;253:454–7.

63. Wada M, Toh S, Taniguchi K, et al. Mutations in the canalicular multispecific organic anion transporter (cMOAT) gene, a novel ABC transporter, in patients with hyperbilirubinemia II/Dubin-Johnson syndrome. Hum Mol Genet 1998;7:203–7.

64. Toh S, Wada M, Uchiumi T, et al. Genomic structure of the canalicular multispecific organic anion-transporter gene (MPR2/cMOAT) and mutations in the ATP-binding-cassette region in Dubin-Johnson syndrome. Am J Hum Genet 1999;64:739–46.

65. Konig J, Rost D, Cui Y, Keppler D. Characterization of the human multidrug resistance protein isoform MRP3 localized to the basolateral hepatocyte membrane. Hepatology 1999;29:1156–63.

66. Clayton RJ, Iber FL, Ruebner BH, McKusick VA. Byler disease. Fatal familial intrahepatic cholestasis in an Amish kindred. J Pediatr 1965;67:1025–8.

67. Clayton RJ, Iber FL, Ruebner BH, McKusick VA. Byler disease: fatal familial intrahepatic cholestasis in an Amish kindred. Am J Dis Child 1969;117:112–26.

68. Williams CN, Kaye R, Baker L, et al. Progressive familial cholestatic cirrhosis and bile acid metabolism. J Pediatr 1972;81:493–500.

69. Jacquemin E, Dumont M, Bernard O, et al. Evidence for defective primary bile acid secretion in children with progressive familial intrahepatic cholestasis (Byler disease). Eur J Pediatr 1994;153:424–8.

70. Summerskill WHJ, Walshe JM. Benign recurrent intrahepatic "obstructive" jaundice. Lancet 1959;ii:686–90.

71. Lykavieris P, van Mil S, Cresteil D, et al. Progressive familial intrahepatic cholestasis type 1 and extrahepatic features: no catch-up of stature growth, exacerbation of diarrhea, and appearance of liver steatosis after liver transplantation. J Hepatol 2003;39:447–52.

72. Whitington PF, Freese DK, Alonso EM, et al. Clinical and biochemical findings in progressive familial intrahepatic cholestasis. J Pediatr Gastroenterol Nutr 1994;18:134–41.

73. Bourke B, Goggin N, Walsh D, et al. Byler-like familial cholestasis in an extended kindred. Arch Dis Child 1996;75:223–7.

74. Alonso EM, Snover DC, Montag A, et al. Histologic and pathology of the liver in progressive familial intrahepatic cholestasis. J Pediatr Gastroenterol Nutr 1994;18:128–33.

75. Linarelli LG, Williams CN, Phillips MJ. Byler's disease: fatal intrahepatic cholestasis. J Pediatr 1972;81:484–92.

76. Houwen RHJ, Baharloo S, Blankenship K, et al. Genome screening by searching for shared segments: mapping a gene for benign recurrent intrahepatic cholestasis. Nat Genet 1994;8:380–6.

77. Carlton VEH, Knisely AS, Freimer NB. Mapping of a locus for progressive familial intrahepatic cholestasis (Byler disease) to 18q21-q22, the benign recurrent intrahepatic cholestasis region. Hum Mol Genet 1995;4:1049–53.

78. Bull LN, van Eijk MJT, Pawlikowska L, et al. Identification of a P-type ATPase mutated in two forms of hereditary cholestasis. Nat Genet 1998;18:219–24.

79. van Mil SW, Klomp LW, Bull LN, Houwen RH. FIC1 disease: a spectrum of intrahepatic cholestatic disorders. Semin Liver Dis 2001;21:535–44.

80. Ujhazy P, Ortiz D, Misra S, et al. Familial intrahepatic cholestasis 1: studies of localization and function. Hepatology 2001;34:768–75.

81. Eppens EF, van Mil SW, de Vree JM, et al. FIC1, the protein affected in two forms of hereditary cholestasis, is localized in the cholangiocyte and the canalicular membrane of the hepatocyte. J Hepatol 2001;35:436–43.

82. Tang X, Halleck MS, Schlegel RA, Williamson P. A subamily of P-type ATPases with aminophospholipid transporting activity. Science 1996;272:1495–7.

83. Pawlikowska L, Ottenhoff R, Looije N, et al. FIC1 mutant mice have a defect in the regulation of intestinal bile salt absorption. Hepatology 2001;34:240A.

84. Shneider B, Ananthanarayanan M, Emre S, et al. Progressive familial intrahepatic cholestasis, type 1, is associated with decreased farnesoid X receptor activity. Gastroenterology 2004;126:756–64.

85. Makishima M, Okamoto A, Repa J, et al. Identification of a nuclear receptor for bile acids. Science 1999;284:1362–5.

86. Lu T, Makishima M, Repa J, et al. Molecular basis for feedback regulation of bile acid synthesis by nuclear receptors. Mol Cell 2000;6:507–15.

87. Klomp L, Bull L, Jujin J, et al. Characterization of multiple different mutations in FIC1 associated with hereditary cholestasis. Hepatology 1999;30:407A.

88. Vargas J, Strautnieks S, Byrne J, et al. Large-scale screening and identification of mutations in ATP8B1 (FIC1) in patients with hereditary cholestasis. Hepatology 2002;36:309A.

89. Oude Elferink R, Pawlikowska L, Looije N, et al. Defective regulation of ASBT activity in FIC1 mutant mice. Hepatology 2002;36:334A.

90. Carlton VE, Harris BZ, Puffenberger EG, et al. Complex inheritance of familial hypercholanemia with associated mutations in TJP2 and BAAT. Nat Genet 2003;34:91–6.

91. Whitington PF, Whitington GL. Partial external diversion of bile for the treatment of intractable pruritus associated with intrahepatic cholestasis. Gastroenterology 1988;95:130–6.

92. Rebhandl W, Felberbauer FX, Turnbull J, et al. Biliary diversion by use of the appendix (cholecystoappendicostomy) in progressive familial intrahepatic cholestasis. J Pediatr Gastroenterol Nutr 1999;28:217–9.

93. Ng V, Ryckman F, Porta G, et al. Long-term outcome after partial external biliary diversion for intractable pruritus in patients with intrahepatic cholestasis. J Pediatr Gastroenterol Nutr 2000;30:152–6.

94. Melter M, Rodeck B, Kardorff R, et al. Progressive familial intrahepatic cholestasis: partial biliary diversion normalizes serum lipids and improves growth in noncirrhotic patients. Am J Gastroenterol 2000;95:3522–8.

95. Ismail H, Kalicinski P, Markiewicz M, et al. Treatment of progressive familial intrahepatic cholestasis: liver transplantation or partial external biliary diversion. Pediatr Transplant 1999;3:219–24.

96. Hollands CM, Rivera-Pedrogo J, Gonzalez-Vallina R, et al. Ileal exclusion for Byler's disease: an alternative surgical approach with promising early results for pruritus. J Pediatr Surg 1998;33:220–4.

97. Felberbauer FX, Amann G, Rebhandl W, Huber WD. Follow-up after partial external biliary diversion in familial cholestasis of infancy. J Pediatr Gastroenterol Nutr 2000;31:322.

98. Emond JC, Whitington PF. Selective surgical management of progressive intrahepatic cholestasis (Byler's disease). J Pediatr Surg 1995;30:1635–41.

99. Moseley RH, Wang W, Takeda H, et al. Endotoxin and tumor necrosis factor α inhibition of sinusoidal and canalicular bile acid transport—functional and molecular studies. Hepatology 1993;18:136A.

100. Bernstein J, Brown A. Sepsis and jaundice in early infancy. Pediatrics 1962;28:873–82.
101. Zimmerman H, Fang M, Utili R, et al. Jaundice due to bacterial infection. Gastroenterology 1979;77:362–74.
102. Green RM, Beier D, Gollan JL. Regulation of hepatocyte bile salt transporters by endotoxin and inflammatory cytokines in rodents. Gastroenterology 1996;111:193–8.
103. Moseley RH, Wang W, Takeda H, et al. Effect of endotoxin on bile acid transport in rat liver—a potential model for sepsis-associated cholestasis. Am J Physiol 1996;271:G137–46.
104. Trauner M, Arrese M, Soroka C, et al. The rat canalicular conjugate export pump (Mrp2) is down-regulated in intrahepatic and obstructive cholestasis. Gastroenterology 1997;113:255–64.
105. Roelofsen H, Van der Veere CN, Ottenhoff R, et al. Decreased bilirubin transport in perfused liver of endotoxemic rats. Gastroenterology 1994;107:1075–84.
106. Bolder U, Ton-Nu HT, Schteingart CD, et al. Hepatocyte transport of bile acids and organic anions in endotoxemic rats: impaired uptake and secretion. Gastroenterology 1997;112:214–25.
107. Vos TA, Hooiveld GJEJ, Koning H, et al. Up-regulation of the multidrug resistance genes, Mrp1 and Mrp2, and down-regulation of the organic anion transporter, Mrp2 and the bile salt transporter, sPgp, in endotoxemic rat liver. Hepatology 1998;28:1637–44.
108. Strautnieks S, Byrne J, Knisely A, et al. There must be a third locus for low GGT PFIC. Hepatology 2001;34:240A.
109. Aagenaes O. Hereditary cholestasis with lymphoedema (Aagenes syndrome, cholestasis-lymphoedema syndrome). Scand J Gastroenterol 1998;33:335–45.
110. Eastham KM, McKiernan PJ, Milford DV, et al. ARC syndrome: an expanding range of phenotypes. Arch Dis Child 2001;85:415–20.
111. Gissen P, Johnson C, Morgan N, et al. Mutations in VPS33B, encoding a regulator of SNARE-dependent membrane fusion, cause arthrogryposis-renal dysfunction-cholestasis (ARC) syndrome. Nat Genet 2004;36:400–4.
112. Wolkoff AW, Wolpert E, Pascasio FN, et al. Rotor's syndrome, a distinct inheritable pathophysiologic entity. Am J Med 1976;60:173–9.
113. Baker AJ, Portmann B, Westaby D, et al. Neonatal sclerosing cholangitis in two siblings: a category of progressive intrahepatic cholestasis. J Pediatr Gastroenterol Nutr 1993;17:317–22.
114. Riordan JR, Rommens JM, Kerem B, et al. Identification of the cystic fibrosis gene: cloning and characterization of complementary DNA. Science 1989;245:1066–73.
115. Oda T, Elkahloun AG, Pike BL, et al. Mutations in the human JAGGED1 gene are responsible for Alagille syndrome. Nat Genet 1997;16:235–42.
116. Li L, Krantz ID, Deng Y, et al. Alagille syndrome is caused by mutations in human JAGGED1, which encodes a ligand for Notch1. Nat Genet 1997;16:243–51.
117. Chillon M, Casals T, Mercier B, et al. Mutations in the cystic fibrosis gene in patients with congenital absence of the vas deferens. N Engl J Med 1995;332:1475–80.
118. Sharer N, Schwarz M, Malone G, et al. Mutations of the cystic fibrosis gene in patients with chronic pancreatitis. N Engl J Med 1998;339:645–52.
119. Cohn JA, Friedman KJ, Noone PG, et al. Relation between mutations of the cystic fibrosis gene and idiopathic pancreatitis. N Engl J Med 1998;339:653–8.
120. Alagille D. Alagille syndrome today. Clin Invest Med 1996;19:325–30.
121. Krantz ID, Smith R, Colliton RP, et al. Jagged1 mutations in patients ascertained with isolated congenital heart defects. Am J Med Genet 1999;84:56–60.

7. α_1-Antitrypsin Deficiency

David H. Perlmutter, MD

The classic form of α_1-antitrypsin (α_1-AT) deficiency, homozygous for the mutant α_1-ATZ allele, is associated with premature development of pulmonary emphysema and, in some cases, chronic liver disease. This deficiency is the most common metabolic cause of emphysema in adults and liver disease in children and is the most common metabolic disease for which children undergo liver transplant (United Network for Organ Sharing Data Request Service, personal communication, 2000). In the most extensively studied population (the Swedish population), the incidence of the deficiency is approximately 1 in 1,639 live births.[1] Data from eight separate studies suggest that the prevalence of α_1-AT deficiency in the United States is 1 in approximately 2,000 individuals.[2] It especially affects whites of northern European ancestry.[3,4]

α_1-AT is an approximately 55 kD secretory glycoprotein that inhibits destructive neutrophil proteases, including elastase, cathepsin G, and proteinase 3. Plasma α_1-AT is predominantly derived from the liver and increases three- to fivefold during the host response to tissue injury or inflammation. It is the archetype of a family of structurally related circulating serine protease inhibitors termed serpins.

In the deficient state, there is ~ 85 to 90% reduction in serum concentrations of α_1-AT. A single amino acid substitution results in an abnormally folded protein that is unable to traverse the secretory pathway. This α_1-ATZ protein is retained in the endoplasmic reticulum (ER) rather than secreted into the blood and body fluids.

Although it does not occur until adulthood, many α_1-AT–deficient individuals develop destructive lung disease and emphysema. Most of the data in the literature indicate that emphysema results from a decreased number of α_1-AT molecules within the lower respiratory tract, allowing unregulated elastolytic attack on the connective tissue matrix of the lung.[5,6] Oxidative inactivation of residual α_1-AT as a result of cigarette smoking accelerates lung injury.[7] Moreover, the elastase-antielastase theory for the pathogenesis of emphysema is based on the concept that oxidative inactivation of α_1-AT as a result of cigarette smoking plays a key role in the emphysema of α_1-AT–sufficient individuals, the vast majority of emphysema patients.[5,8]

It has been more difficult to explain the pathogenesis of liver injury in this deficiency. The results of transgenic animal experiments have provided strong evidence that liver disease does not result from a deficiency in antielastase activity.[9,10] Most of the data in the literature corroborate the concept that liver injury in α_1-AT deficiency results from the hepatotoxic effects of retention of the aggregated mutant α_1-ATZ molecule in the ER of liver cells. Nationwide prospective screening studies done by Sveger in Sweden have shown that only 10 to 15% of the deficient population develop clinically significant liver disease over the first 20 years of life.[1,11] These data indicate that other genetic traits and/or environmental factors predispose a subgroup of deficient individuals to liver injury.

The diagnosis of α_1-AT deficiency is based on the altered migration of the abnormal α_1-ATZ molecule in serum specimens subjected to isoelectric-focusing gel analysis. Treatment of liver disease associated with α_1-AT deficiency is mostly supportive. Liver replacement therapy has been used successfully for severe liver injury. Although clinical efficacy has not been demonstrated, many patients with emphysema owing to α_1-AT deficiency are currently being treated by intravenous or intratracheal aerosol administration of purified plasma α_1-AT. An increasing number of patients with severe emphysema have undergone lung transplant. Several new pharmacologic and genetic strategies for prophylaxis of both liver and lung disease are currently under development for clinical application.

STRUCTURE OF α_1-ANTITRYPSIN

α_1-AT is encoded by a single approximately 12.2 kb gene on human chromosome 14q31-32.3.[12–15] There is a sequence-related gene 12 kb downstream from this gene.[14,16–18] Because there is no evidence that the sequence-related gene is expressed, it is considered a pseudogene. The genes for three other members of the serpin family, α_1-antichymotrypsin, protein C inhibitor, and corticosteroid-binding globulin, are also closely linked on chromosome 14.[15,19]

The α_1-AT gene (Figure 55.7-1) is organized in seven exons and six introns.[12,20] The first three exons and a short 5′ segment of the fourth exon code for 5′ untranslated regions of the α_1-AT messenger ribonucleic acid (mRNA). The first two exons and a short 5′ segment of the third exon are included in the primary transcript in macrophages but not in hepatocytes, accounting for a slightly longer mRNA. There are, in fact, two mRNA species in macrophages, depending on alternative post-transcriptional splicing pathways involving one of the first two most 5′ exons.[20,21] Most of the fourth exon and the remaining three exons encode the protein sequence of α_1-AT. There is a 72-base sequence that constitutes the 24–amino acid amino-terminal signal sequence. There are three sites for asparagine-linked carbohydrate attachment: residues 46, 83, and 247. All three are used for post-translational glycosylation. The active

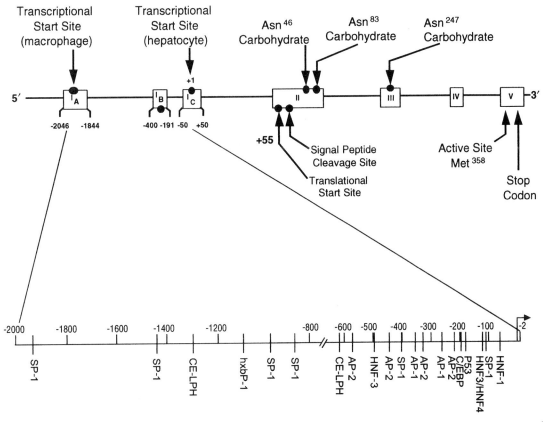

FIGURE 55.7-1 Schematic representation of the structure of the α₁-antitrypsin gene (not to scale) and map of potential regulatory elements based on its sequence.

site, so-called P₁ residue, Met 358, is encoded within the seventh exon (exon V).

The α₁-AT protein is a single-chain, approximately 52 to 55 kD polypeptide with 394 amino acids and three asparagine-linked complex carbohydrate side chains.[22] There are two major isoforms in serum, depending on the presence of a biantennary or triantennary configuration for the carbohydrate side chains.[23] X-ray crystallography studies have shown that α₁-AT has a globular shape and a highly ordered internal domain composed of two central β sheets surrounded by a small β sheet and nine α helices.[24,25] The dominant structure is the five-stranded β-pleated sheet termed the A sheet (Figure 55.7-2).

α₁-AT is the archetype of a family of structurally related proteins called serpins that includes antithrombin III, α₁-antichymotrypsin, C1 inhibitor, α₂-antiplasmin, protein C inhibitor, heparin cofactor II, plasminogen activator inhibitors I and II, protease nexin I, ovalbumin, angiotensinogen, corticosteroid-binding globulin, and thyroid-binding globulin.[25,26] These proteins share about 25 to 40% primary structural homology with higher degrees of regional homology in functional domains. Most serpins function as suicide inhibitors by forming equimolar complexes with a specific target protease. Other serpins are not inhibitory. For instance, corticosteroid and thyroid hormone–binding globulins, which are thought to represent carriers for corticosteroid and thyroid hormone, respectively, form complexes with, but do not inactivate, their hormone ligands.

A comparison of α₁-AT with other members of the serpin supergene family has generated several important concepts about the structure and function of α₁-AT. For instance, the reactive site P1 residue of α₁-AT is localized to a canonical loop that rises above the gap in the center of the A sheet (see Figure 55.7-2).[27,28] This loop may provide a certain degree of flexibility to the functional activity of the inhibitor. The reactive loop conformation of serpins is also thought to make them susceptible to proteolytic cleavage by thiolenzymes and metalloenzymes. The P1 residue itself is the most important determinant of functional specificity for each serpin molecule. This concept was dramatically confirmed by the discovery of α₁-AT Pittsburgh, a variant in which the P1 residue of α₁-AT, Met 358, is replaced by Arg 358. In this variant, α₁-AT functions as a thrombin inhibitor, and severe bleeding diathesis results.[29]

The carboxyl-terminal fragment of α₁-AT and the other serpins also bears important structural and functional characteristics. There is a much higher degree of sequence homology among serpins in the carboxyl terminus. A small fragment at this terminus is cleaved during formation of the inhibitory complex with serine protease. This carboxyl-terminal fragment possesses chemotactic activity.[30,31] Moreover, this fragment bears the receptor-binding domain for cell surface binding, internalization of α₁-AT elastase and other serpin-enzyme complexes, and activating a signal transduction pathway for up-regulation of α₁-AT gene expression.[32,33]

PROTEASE INHIBITOR SYSTEM FOR CLASSIFICATION OF STRUCTURAL VARIANTS OF α_1-ANTITRYPSIN

Variants of α_1-AT in humans are classified according to the protease inhibitor phenotype system as defined by agarose electrophoresis at acid pH or isoelectric focusing of plasma

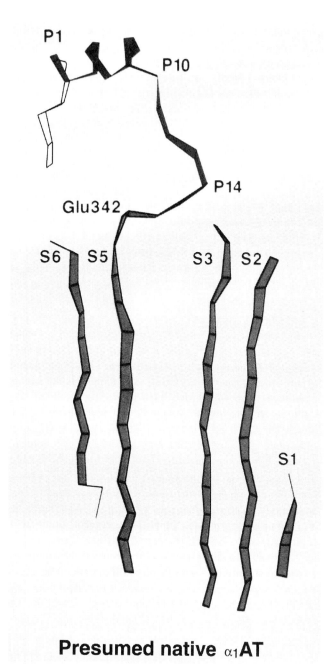

Presumed native α_1AT

FIGURE 55.7-2 Ribbon diagram of the A sheet and reactive center loop of native α_1-antitrypsin (AT). Because native α_1-AT has not been crystallized, this ribbon diagram is generated by computer models, based on the crystal structures of cleaved α_1-AT and native ovalbumin. The reactive center loop is shown in dark gray (magenta). Residues P10 and P14 are numbered from the reactive-site methionine P1. The carboxyl-terminal fragment is shown as a white ribbon. Beta-helices of the A sheet are shown as light gray (blue) ribbons and referred to as S1, S2, S3, S5, and S6 (for color figure, see CD-ROM). The Glu 342 residue that is replaced by Lys in α_1-ATZ is designated. Adapted from Carrell RW, Evans DL, Stein DE. Mobile reactive centre of serpins and the control of thrombosis. Nature 1991;353:576.

in polyacrylamide.[34] The protease inhibitor classification assigns a letter to variants according to the migration of the major isoform, in alphabetic order from anode to cathode or from low to high isoelectric point. For example, the most common normal variant migrates to an intermediate isoelectric point, designated M. Individuals with the most common severe deficiency have an α_1-AT allelic variant that migrates to a high isoelectric point, designated Z. Using restriction fragment length and direct deoxyribonucleic acid (DNA) sequence analysis together with isoelectric focusing, more than 100 allelic variants of α_1-AT have been reported.[35]

Normal Allelic Variants. The most common normal variant of α_1-AT is termed M_1 and is found in 65 to 70% of whites in the United States.[35] A restriction fragment length polymorphism may further subdivide individuals with the classic M_1 allele.[36] The normal M_3 allele, which differs from M_1 by a single-base change,[35] is found in approximately 10% of the same population. The M_2 allele, characterized by an additional base change from the M_3 sequence, occurs in 15 to 20% of the white population.[37,38] There are many rare normal allelic variants with allelic frequencies of less than 0.1%.[38–42] In each case, these variants are associated with serum concentrations of and functional activity for α_1-AT within the normal range.[1]

Null Allelic Variants. Variants in which α_1-AT is not detectable in serum are called null allelic variants (Table 55.7-1) and, when inherited with another null variant or deficiency variant, are associated with premature development of emphysema.[43] Several types of defects, including insertions and deletions, appear to be responsible for these variants. In two cases, α_1-AT Null_Isola di procida and α_1-AT Null_Reidenburg, there is deletion of all α_1-AT coding regions.[44,45] In two other cases, α_1-AT Null_Bellingham and α_1-AT Null_Granite Falls, α_1-AT mRNA is undetectable.[46–49] Three other null alleles result in truncated proteins that are degraded in the ER—Null_Mattawa, Null_Hong Kong, and Null_Clayton.[50–53] A single-base substitution has been discovered in the Null_Ludwigshafen allele.[54] A recent study suggests that this mutant α_1-AT molecule is synthesized and secreted in transfected heterologous cells, but there is a slight decrease in its rate of secretion, and it completely lacks functional activity.[55] It is not yet known whether instability or accelerated catabolism in vivo is the explanation for the inability to detect this mutant α_1-AT molecule in serum specimens.

Dysfunctional Variants. Dysfunctional variants of α_1-AT include α_1-AT_Pittsburgh.[29] There also is a decrease in serum concentration and functional activity for α_1-AT M_Mineral Springs.[56] For several variants that have been identified in compound heterozygotes, such as α_1-AT F,[57] α_1-AT Null_Newport, and α_1-AT Z_Wrexham,[58] it is not clear whether the variants result in normal, null, deficient, or dysfunctional changes.

Deficiency Variants. Several variants of α_1-AT associated with a reduction in serum concentrations of α_1-AT have been described and are called deficiency variants

TABLE 55.7-1   NULL VARIANTS OF α₁-ANTITRYPSIN

DEFECT			CLINICAL DISEASE		
			LIVER	LUNG	CELLULAR DEFECT
Null$_{Granite\ Falls}$	Single base deletion	Tyr 160	−	+	No detectable RNA
Null$_{Bellingham}$	Single base deletion	Lys 217	−	+	No detectable RNA
Null$_{Mattawa}$	Single base insertion	Phe 353	−	+	?IC degradation
Null$_{Hong\ Kong}$	Dinucleotide deletion	Leu 318	−	+	IC accumulation
Null$_{Ludwigshafen}$	Single base substitution	Isoleu 92-Asp	−	+	Dysfunctional protein (?EC degradation)
Null$_{Clayton}$	Single base insertion	Glu 363	−	+	?IC degradation
Null$_{Bolton}$	Single base deletion	Glu 363	−	+	?IC degradation
Null$_{Isola\ di\ Procida}$	Deletion	Exons II-V	−	+	Unknown
Null$_{Riedenburg}$	Deletion	Exons II-V	−	+	Unknown
Null$_{Newport}$	Single base substitution	Gly 115-Ser	−	+	Unknown
Null$_{bonny\ blue}$	Intron deletion	—	−	+	Unknown
Null$_{new\ hope}$	Two base substitutions	Gly 320-Glu Glu 342-Lys	−	+	Unknown
Null$_{Trastavere}$	Single base substitution	Trp 194-stop	−	+	Unknown
Null$_{Kowloon}$	Single base substitution	Tyr 38-stop	−	+	Unknown
Null$_{Saarbruecken}$	Single base insertion	Pro 362-stop	−	+	Unknown
Null$_{Lisbon}$	Single base substitution	Thr 68-Ile	−	+	Unknown
Null$_{West}$	Intron deletion	—	−	+	Unknown

EC = extracellular; IC = intracellular; RNA = ribonucleic acid.

(Table 55.7-2). Some of these variants, such as the S variant, are not associated with clinical disease.[12,59,60] Other deficiency variants are associated with emphysema, such as M$_{Heerlen}$,[61,62] M$_{Procida}$,[63] M$_{Malton}$,[64,65] M$_{Duarte}$,[66] M$_{Mineral\ Springs}$,[56] P$_{Lowell}$,[42] and W$_{Bethesda}$.[67] In two persons with M$_{Malton}$ and one with M$_{Duarte}$, hepatocyte α₁-AT inclusions and liver disease have been reported.[64,66,68] In one person with the deficiency variant S$_{Iiyama}$, emphysema and hepatocyte inclusions were reported, but this person did not have liver disease.[69]

FUNCTION

α₁-AT is an inhibitor of serine proteases in general, but its most important targets are neutrophil elastase, cathepsin G, and proteinase 3, proteases released by activated neutrophils. Several lines of evidence suggest that inhibition of neutrophil elastase is the major physiologic function of α₁-AT. First, individuals with α₁-AT deficiency are susceptible to premature development of emphysema, a lesion that can be induced in experimental animals by instillation of excess amounts of neutrophil elastase in the airways.[70] In fact, these observations have led to the concept that destructive lung disease may result from perturbations of the net balance of elastase and α₁-AT within the local environment of the lung.[5] Second, the kinetics of association of α₁-AT and neutrophil elastase are more favorable by several orders of magnitude than those for α₁-AT and any other serine protease.[71] Third, α₁-AT constitutes more than 90%

TABLE 55.7-2   DEFICIENCY VARIANTS OF α₁-ANTITRYPSIN

DEFECT			CLINICAL DISEASE		
			LIVER	LUNG	CELLULAR DEFECT
Z	Single base substitution M₁ (Ala 213)	Glu 342-Lys	+	+	IC accumulation
S	Single base substitution	Glu 264-Val	−	−	IC accumulation
M$_{Heerlen}$	Single base substitution	Pro 369-Leu	−	+	IC accumulation
M$_{Procida}$	Single base substitution	Leu 41-Pro	−	+	IC accumulation
M$_{Malton}$	Single base deletion	Phe 52	?	+	IC accumulation
M$_{Duarte}$	Unknown	Unknown	?+	+	Unknown
M$_{Mineral\ Springs}$	Single base substitution	Gly 57-Glu	−	+	No function; ?EC degradation
S$_{Iiyama}$	Single base substitution	Ser 53-Phe	−	+	IC accumulation
P$_{Duarte}$	Two base substitutions	Arg 101-His Asp 256-Val	?+ +	+ +	Unknown
P$_{Lowell}$	Single base substitution	Asp 256-Val	−	+	IC accumulation; reduced function
W$_{Bethesda}$	Single base substitution	Ala 336-Thre	−	+	?EC degradation
Z$_{Wrexham}$		Ser 19-Leu	?	?	Unknown
F	Single base substitution	Arg 223-Cys	−	−	Unknown
T	Single base substitution	Glu 264-Val	−	−	Unknown
I	Single base substitution	Arg 39-Cys	−	−	IC accumulation; reduced function
M$_{palermo}$	Single base deletion	Phe 51	−	−	Unknown
M$_{nichinan}$	Single base deletion and single base substitution	Phe 52 Gly 148-Arg	−	−	Unknown
Z$_{ausburg}$	Single base substitution	Glu 342-Lys	−	−	Unknown

EC = extracellular; IC = intracellular.

of the neutrophil elastase inhibitory activity in the one body fluid that has been examined, pulmonary alveolar lavage fluid.

α_1-AT acts competitively by allowing its target enzymes to bind directly to a substratelike region within the carboxyl-terminal region of the inhibitor molecule. This reaction between enzyme and inhibitor is essentially second order, and the resulting complex contains one molecule of each of the reactants. A peptide bond in the inhibitor is hydrolyzed during formation of the enzyme-inhibitor complex. However, hydrolysis of this reactive site peptide bond does not proceed to completion. An equilibrium near unity is established between complexes in which the reactive site peptide bond of α_1-AT is intact (native inhibitor) and complexes in which this peptide bond is cleaved (modified inhibitor). The complex of α_1-AT and serine protease is a covalently stabilized structure that is resistant to dissociation by denaturing compounds, including sodium dodecyl sulfate and urea. The interaction between α_1-AT and serine protease is suicidal in that the modified inhibitor is no longer able to bind and/or inactivate enzyme. Studies have now shown that the irreversible trapping of target enzyme is mediated by a profound conformational change in α_1-AT such that the cleaved reactive loop, with bound enzyme, inserts into the gap in A sheet (see Figure 55.7-2).[72] Carrell and Lomas have likened the inhibitory mechanism to a "mousetrap, with the active inhibitor circulating in a metastable, stressed-form and then springing into the stable relaxed form to lock the complex with its target protease."[72] The protease is crushed and inactivated during this structural transition.[73]

The net functional activity of α_1-AT in complex biologic fluids may be modified by several factors. First, the reactive site methionine of α_1-AT may be oxidized and thereby rendered inactive as an elastase inhibitor.[74] In vitro, α_1-AT is oxidatively inactivated by oxidants released by activated neutrophils and alveolar macrophages of cigarette smokers.[75,76] Second, the functional activity of α_1-AT may be modified by proteolytic inactivation. Several members of the metalloprotease family (including collagenase and *Pseudomonas* elastase) and the thiol protease family can cleave and inactivate α_1-AT.[77] DNA released by dying cells at sites of tissue injury or inflammation has the capacity to interfere with the protease inhibitory activity of α_1-AT. [78]

Although α_1-AT from the plasma[79] or liver[80] of individuals with α_1-AT deficiency is functionally active, there may be a decrease in its specific elastase inhibitory capacity. Ogushi and colleagues have shown that the kinetics of association with neutrophil elastase and the stability of complexes with neutrophil elastase were significantly decreased for α_1-AT from deficient plasma.[81] There was no decrease in functional activity of α_1-AT from individuals homozygous for the α_1-ATS allelic variant.

Several studies have indicated that α_1-AT protects experimental animals from the lethal effects of tumor necrosis factor.[82,83] Most of the evidence from these studies indicates that this protective effect is due to inhibition of the synthesis and release of platelet-activating factor from neutrophils,[83,84] presumably through the inhibition of neutrophil-derived proteases. A recent report has suggested that α_1-AT inhibits infectivity of human immunodeficiency virus (HIV) type 1 and its production by infected cells.[85]

α_1-Antitrypsin also appears to have functional activities that do not involve the inhibition of neutrophil proteases. The carboxyl-terminal fragment of α_1-AT, which can be generated during the formation of a complex with serine protease or during proteolytic inactivation by thiol- or metalloproteases, is a potent neutrophil chemoattractant.[30,31,86] This fragment also appears to activate mononuclear phagocytes with respect to production of cytokines, active oxygen intermediates, scavenger activity, and lipid metabolism.[87]

There are several reports of α_1-AT altering immune function through effects on lymphocytes.[88,89] However, there are inherent conflicts in some of the reports, and the data have not been duplicated. There is no evidence that the immune response is systemically altered in α_1-AT–deficient individuals.

BIOSYNTHESIS AND REGULATION OF α_1-ANTITRYPSIN

The predominant site of synthesis of plasma α_1-AT is the liver. This is most clearly shown by conversion of plasma α_1-AT to donor phenotype after orthotopic liver transplant.[90,91] It is synthesized in human hepatoma cells as a 52 kD precursor, undergoes post-translational, dolichol phosphate–linked glycosylation at three asparagine residues, and undergoes tyrosine sulfation.[92–94] It is secreted as a 55 kD native single-chain glycoprotein with a half-time for secretion of 35 to 50 minutes.

Tissue-specific expression of α_1-AT in human hepatoma cells is directed by structural elements within a 750-nucleotide region upstream of the hepatocyte transcriptional start site in exon Ic (see Figure 55.7-1). Within this region, there are structural elements that are recognized by nuclear transcription factors, including hepatocyte nuclear factor (HNF)-1α and HNF-1β (–70 to –57), C-EBP (–86 to –75), HNF-4 (–134 to –100), and HNF-3 (–195 to –185).[95]

Of these factors, HNF-1α and HNF-4 appear to be particularly important for expression of the human α_1-AT gene. Two distinct regions within the proximal element bind these two transcription factors. In fact, substitution of five nucleotides at positions –77 to –72 disrupts binding of HNF-1α and dramatically reduces expression of the human α_1-AT gene in the liver of transgenic mice.[96] Substitution of four nucleotides at positions –118 to –115 disrupts the binding of HNF-4 but does not alter expression of the human α_1-AT gene in the liver of adult transgenic mice. The latter mutation does result in a reduction in the expression of human α_1-AT in the liver during embryonic development. HNF-1α and HNF-4 have a synergistic up-regulating effect on expression of the α_1-AT gene in hepatocytes and enterocytes.[97]

Several elements in the upstream flanking region have enhancer activity. There is a strong enhancer element located approximately 200 nucleotides upstream of the transcriptional start site, but the element is not specific for hepatocyte transcription.[98] This element is identical to the binding site for transcription factor AP-1. Similar AP-1 binding sequences have been identified in the 5′ flanking region of metallothioneins I and IIa, sv40, retinol-binding protein, collagenase, and stromelysin. Transcription factor AP-1 is also thought to be one of the transcription factors that mediate the effects of phorbol esters and thus of the activation of protein kinase C.[99] It represents a complex of several different proteins, including proteins encoded by the proto-oncogenes c-*jun* and c-*fos*.[100] There is a region with weak enhancer activity at residues −488 to −356,[98] but it is not clear whether this is due to transcription factor AP-1, AP-2, SP-1, HNF-3, or another transcription factor with a consensus element in this region. There are also several regions with similarity to the recognition element for transcription factor IL-6DBP (also called H-APF-2, NF-IL-6, LAP/LIP) at −195 to −189 and −169 to −164 from the hepatocyte α₁-AT cap site and −178 to −169 from the macrophage α₁-AT cap site, which may explain the effect of interleukin (IL)-6 on α₁-AT gene expression.[21]

Plasma concentrations of α₁-AT increase three- to five-fold during the host response to inflammation and/or tissue injury.[101] The source of this additional α₁-AT has always been considered the liver; thus, α₁-AT is known as a positive hepatic acute-phase reactant. Synthesis of α₁-AT in human hepatoma cells (HepG2, Hep3B) is up-regulated by IL-6 but not by IL-1 or tumor necrosis factor.[102] Plasma concentrations of α₁-AT also increase during oral contraceptive therapy and pregnancy.[103]

α₁-AT is also synthesized and secreted in primary cultures of human blood monocytes as well as bronchoalveolar and breast milk macrophages.[104] The cellular defect in homozygous α₁-AT deficiency, the selective defect in secretion of α₁-AT, is expressed in monocytes and macrophages from deficient individuals.[105] Transcription of the α₁-AT gene in macrophages starts about 2 kb upstream from the start site used in hepatocytes.[21,22,106] Although the same polypeptide is synthesized in the two cell types, slightly longer mRNA transcripts are present in macrophages (see Figure 55.7-1), depending on alternative post-transcriptional splicing of two upstream short open reading frames.[21,22]

Expression of α₁-AT in monocytes and macrophages is profoundly influenced by products generated during inflammation, such as bacterial lipopolysaccharide[107,108] and IL-6[102] (Figure 55.7-3). Bacterial lipopolysaccharide mediates a 5- to 10-fold increase in synthesis of α₁-AT in mononuclear phagocytes, predominantly increasing the translation efficiency of α₁-AT mRNA. The translational regulation of α₁-AT by lipopolysaccharide therefore involves a mechanism analogous to that of the yeast gene *GCN4* during amino acid starvation and that of the human ferritin gene in response to iron. The analogy to yeast *GCN4* is interesting in that both macrophage α₁-AT mRNA and *GCN4* mRNA have multiple short open reading frames with initiation codons in the upstream untranslated regions.[21,22,106] These sequences have been shown to control the translation of the yeast *GCN4* gene product, both under basal conditions and in response to amino acid starvation.[109]

Synthesis of α₁-AT in liver cells and mononuclear phagocytes is also regulated by a feed-forward mechanism (Figure 55.7-4). In this regulatory loop, α₁-AT–elastase complexes mediate an increase in synthesis of α₁-AT through the interaction of a pentapeptide domain in the carboxyl-terminal tail of α₁-AT with a novel cell

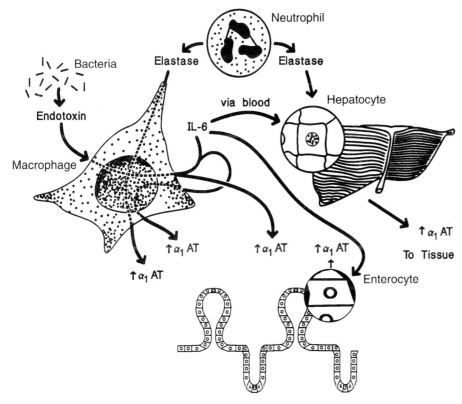

FIGURE 55.7-3 Schematic representation of the regulatory factors that affect α₁-antitrypsin (AT) expression in hepatocytes, enterocytes, and macrophages. IL-6 = interleukin-6.

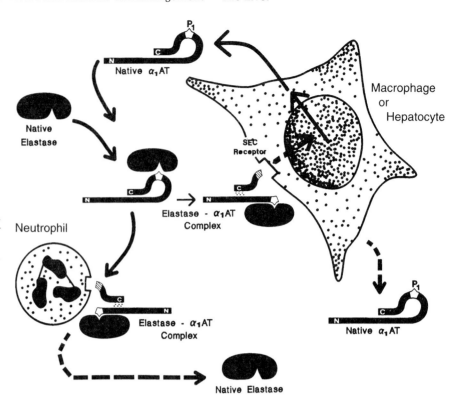

FIGURE 55.7-4 Feedback regulation of α_1-antitrypsin (AT) synthesis and neutrophil chemotactic activity mediated by the serpine-enzyme complex (SEC) receptor. Reproduced with permission from Perlmutter DH. α_1-Antitrypsin: structure, function, physiology. In: Mackiewicz A, Kusher I, Baumann H, editors. Acute phase proteins: molecular biology, biochemistry and clinical applications, Boca Raton (FL): CRC Press; 1993. p. 49–167.

surface receptor.[32,33,86,110,111] These receptor molecules are now referred to as serpin enzyme complex (SEC) receptors because they recognize the highly conserved domains of other SECs, such as antithrombin III–thrombin, α_1-antichymotrypsin–cathepsin G, and, to a lesser extent, Cl inhibitor–C1s and tissue plasminogen activator–plasminogen activator inhibitor I complexes, as well as α_1-AT–elastase complexes.[32,112] Substance P, several other tachykinins, bombesin, and the amyloid-β peptide bind to the SEC receptor through a similar pentapeptide sequence.[113] Recent studies indicate that the SEC receptor can mediate endocytosis of soluble amyloid-β peptide, but it does not recognize the aggregated form of amyloid-β peptide that is toxic to neurons and other cell types.[114] Thus, the SEC receptor may play a role in preventing amyloid-β peptide from accumulating into neurotoxic mature amyloid deposits associated with Alzheimer disease.

α_1-AT mRNA has been isolated from multiple tissues in transgenic mice,[106,115,116] but only in some cases have studies distinguished whether such α_1-AT mRNA is in ubiquitous tissue macrophages or other cell types. For instance, α_1-AT is synthesized in enterocytes and intestinal Paneth cells, as determined by studies in intestinal epithelial cell lines, ribonuclease protection assays of human intestinal RNA, and in situ hybridization analysis in cryostat sections of human intestinal mucosa.[21,117–119] Expression of α_1-AT in enterocytes increases markedly as they differentiate from crypt to villus, in response to IL-6 and during inflammation in vivo. α_1-AT is also synthesized by pulmonary epithelial cells.[120,121] Interestingly, synthesis of α_1-AT in pulmonary epithelial cells is less responsive to regulation by IL-6 than to a related cytokine, oncostatin M.[121]

CLEARANCE AND DISTRIBUTION

The half-life of α_1-AT in plasma is approximately 5 days.[122–124] It is estimated that its daily production rate is 34 mg/kg of body weight, with 33% of the intravascular pool of α_1-AT being degraded daily. Several physiologic factors may affect the rate of its catabolism. First, desialylated α_1-AT is cleared from the circulation in minutes,[124,125] probably via hepatic asialoglycoprotein receptor–mediated endocytosis. Second, α_1-AT in complex with elastase or proteolytically modified is cleared more rapidly than native α_1-AT.[126] Because its ligand specificity is similar to that required for in vivo clearance of SECs, the SEC receptor may also be involved in the clearance and catabolism of α_1-AT–elastase complexes and other SECs.[33] The low-density protein receptor–related protein can also mediate clearance and catabolism of α_1-AT–elastase complexes.[127,128] Third, the rate of α_1-AT clearance may increase during the host response to inflammation.[129] There is a slight increase in the rate of clearance of radiolabeled α_1-ATZ compared with wild-type α_1-AT when infused into normal individuals, but this difference does not account for the decrease in serum levels of α_1-AT in deficient individuals.[123,125,130]

α_1-AT diffuses into most tissues and is found in most body fluids.[5] Its concentration in lavage fluid from the lower respiratory tract is approximately equivalent to its concentration in serum.[5] It is also found in feces, and increased fecal concentrations of α_1-AT correlate with inflammatory lesions of the bowel.[131] In each case, it has been assumed that the α_1-AT is derived from serum. Local sites of synthesis, such as macrophages and epithelial cells, may also make important contributions to the α_1-AT pool in these tissues and body fluids. In fact, it has been reported that fecal α_1-AT clearance is higher in patients with homozygous α_1-AT deficiency than in normal persons.[132] Because the former have only 10 to 15% of the normal serum concentrations of α_1-AT, a local intestinal source for fecal α_1-AT is implicated. One possible explanation is that the bulk of α_1-AT in feces is derived from sloughed enterocytes. Increased fecal α_1-AT in those with homozygous α_1-AT deficiency would result from turnover or sloughing of enterocytes, with a greater amount of α_1-AT per cell owing to intracellular accumulation. Increased fecal α_1-AT in normal persons with inflammatory-related, protein-losing enteropathy would result from increased turnover or sloughing of enterocytes with a normal amount of α_1-AT per cell.

MECHANISM OF α_1-ANTITRYPSIN DEFICIENCY IN PIZZ INDIVIDUALS

The mutant α_1-ATZ molecule is characterized by a single-nucleotide substitution that results in an amino acid substitution of Lys for Glu 342.[133–135] There is a selective decrease in the secretion of α_1-AT, with the abnormal protein accumulating in the ER.[105,136] The defect is not specific for liver cells because it also affects extrahepatic sites of α_1-AT synthesis, such as macrophages[105] and transfected cell lines.[137–139] Site-directed mutagenesis studies have shown that this single amino acid substitution is sufficient to produce the cellular defect.[139] Once translocated into the lumen of the ER, the mutant α_1-AT protein is unable to traverse the remainder of the secretory pathway because it is abnormally folded.

Substitution of Glu 342 by Lys in the α_1-ATZ variant reduces the stability of the molecule in its monomeric form and increases the likelihood that it will form polymers by means of a "loop-sheet" insertion mechanism.[140] In this mechanism, the reactive center loop of one α_1-AT molecule inserts into a gap in the β-pleated A sheet of another α_1-AT molecule (see Figure 55.7-2). Lomas and colleagues were the first to notice that the site of the amino acid substitution in the α_1-ATZ variant was at the base of the reactive center loop, adjacent to the gap in the A sheet.[140] These investigators predicted that a change in the charge at this residue, as occurs with the substitution of Lys for Glu, would prevent the insertion of the reactive site loop into the gap in the A sheet during interaction with enzyme; therefore, the mutant α_1-ATZ would be susceptible to the insertion of the reactive center loop of adjacent molecules into the gap in its A sheet. This would, in turn, cause the mutant α_1-ATZ to be more susceptible to polymerization than the wild-type α_1-AT. In fact, their experiments showed that α_1-ATZ undergoes this form of polymerization to a certain extent spontaneously and to a greater extent during relatively minor perturbations, such as a rise in temperature. Presumably, an increase in body temperature during systemic inflammation would exacerbate this tendency in vivo. Polymers could also be detected by electron microscopy in the ER of hepatocytes in a liver biopsy specimen from a deficient individual.[140] Similar polymers have been found in the plasma of patients with the PIS$_{\text{Iiyama}}$ and PIM$_{\text{Malton}}$ α_1-AT variants.[141,142] The mutations in α_1-AT PIS$_{\text{Iiyama}}$ (Ser 53 to Phe)[69] and PIM$_{\text{Malton}}$ (Phe 52 deletion)[64]

affect residues that provide a ridge for the sliding movement that opens the A sheet. Thus, these mutations would be expected to interfere with the insertion of the reactive center loop into the gap in the A sheet and, therefore, to leave the gap in the A sheet available for spontaneous loop-sheet polymerization. It is indeed interesting that hepatocytic α_1-AT globules have been observed in a few patients with these two variants. Recent observations suggest that the α_1-ATS variant also undergoes loop-sheet polymerization[143] and that this may account for its retention in the ER, albeit a milder degree of retention than that for α_1-ATZ.[144] Moreover, α_1-ATS can apparently form heteropolymers with α_1-ATZ,[145] providing a potential explanation for liver disease in patients who are compound heterozygotes for the α_1-ATS and Z alleles. In a recent study, Davis and colleagues have shown that dementia in two families is associated with mutations that cause polymerization of another member of the serpin family, neuroserpin.[146] The mutations, mechanism of polymerization, and morphology of the inclusion bodies in affected neurons are remarkably similar to those that occur in the classic form of α_1-AT deficiency

The precise mechanism by which the loop-sheet insertion develops is not yet completely understood and may be more complicated than previously thought.[141,147,148] Further studies to characterize the mechanism more precisely will undoubtedly be forthcoming.

A study by Yu and colleagues compared the folding kinetics of α_1-ATZ in transverse urea gradient gels.[149] This study shows, for the first time, that α_1-ATZ folds at an extremely slow rate, unlike the wild-type α_1-AT, which folds in minutes. This folding defect leads to the accumulation of an intermediate, which has a high tendency to polymerize, presumably by the loop-sheet insertion mechanism.

By themselves, however, these data do not prove that the polymerization of α_1-ATZ results in retention within the ER. In fact, many polypeptides must assemble into oligomeric or polymeric complexes to traverse the ER and reach their destination within the cell, at the surface of the plasma membrane, or into the extracellular fluid. If viral proteins, such as the vesicular stomatitis virus G protein or influenza virus hemagglutinin, and host proteins, such as the T-cell receptor and fibrinogen, do not assemble into oligomers, they are retained and ultimately degraded in the ER.[150]

The strongest evidence that polymerization results in the retention of α_1-ATZ in the ER has been provided by studies in which the fate of α_1-ATZ is examined after the introduction of additional mutations into this molecule. For instance, Kim and colleagues introduced a mutation into the α_1-AT molecule at amino acid 51, F51L.[151] This mutation is remote from the Z mutation, E342K, but it apparently impeded loop-sheet polymerization and prevented insertion of synthetic peptide into the gap in the A sheet, implying that the mutation led to the closing of this gap. The double-mutated F51L α_1-ATZ molecule was also less prone to polymerization and folded more efficiently in vitro than α_1-ATZ. Moreover, the introduction of the F51L mutation partially corrected the intracellular retention properties of α_1-ATZ in microinjected Xenopus oocytes[152] and in yeast.[153]

However, Lin and colleagues recently found that a novel, naturally occurring variant of α_1-AT, bearing the K342Q mutation that characterizes α_1-ATZ as well as carboxyl-terminal truncation, is retained in the ER for as long, or longer, than α_1-ATZ even though it does not polymerize.[154] These results could indicate that mechanisms other than polymerization determine whether mutant α_1-AT molecules are retained in the ER. An alternative possibility is that polymerization of α_1-ATZ is not the cause of ER retention but rather its result.

Despite what is stated in one review,[155] it is still not entirely clear what proportion of the newly synthesized mutant α_1-ATZ molecules is converted to the polymeric state in the ER. In one cell culture model system, Lin and colleagues found that $17.0 \pm 0.9\%$ of α_1-ATZ is in the insoluble fraction at steady state,[154] but comparable in vivo data are not yet available. It is also not known whether polymeric molecules are degraded in the ER less rapidly than their monomeric counterparts or whether polymeric molecules, when retained in the ER, are more hepatotoxic than their monomeric counterparts. Indeed, recent studies on the effect of temperature on α_1-ATZ have indicated the high degree of complexity involved in these issues. Although Lomas and colleagues showed that a rise in temperature to 42°C increases the polymerization of purified α_1-ATZ in vitro,[140] Burrows and colleagues found that a rise in temperature to 42°C resulted in increased secretion of α_1-ATZ and decreased intracellular degradation of α_1-ATZ in a model cell culture system.[156] In contrast, lowering the temperature to 27°C resulted in diminished intracellular degradation of α_1-ATZ, without any change in the small amount of α_1-ATZ that is secreted.[156] Consistent with the well-established role that temperature plays in most biochemical processes, these results suggest that changes in temperature have the potential to affect multiple steps in the pathways by which α_1-ATZ is translocated through the secretory and degradative compartments/systems, as well as affecting the relative proportions of α_1-ATZ in the monomeric and polymeric state. On the basis of these considerations, as well as long-standing clinical experience with α_1-AT–deficient children and other children with liver disease, and in the complete absence of any epidemiologic evidence, it seems unlikely that there is a simple relationship between febrile episodes and phenotypic expression of liver disease in α_1-AT–deficient patients.

To understand how polymerization of α_1-AT or alteration in folding of monomeric α_1-AT might result in retention within the ER, one needs to consider what is now known about the biology of protein secretion. Most newly synthesized secretory proteins are translocated into the lumen of the ER. Before being transported to their final destination, these nascent secretory polypeptide chains undergo a series of post-translational modifications, including glycosylation, formation of disulfide bonds, oligomerization, and folding. Moreover, transport through the secretory pathway involves interaction with resident ER proteins, termed molecular chaperones. These interactions facilitate disulfide bond formation, assembly, and folding.

Several families of ER chaperones have been identified. One has been referred to as the polypeptide chain–binding protein family and includes several heat shock/stress proteins (HSPs), GRP78/BiP and GRP94, protein disulfide isomerase, and Erp72.[157] Several calcium-binding phosphoproteins of the ER, most notably calnexin and calreticulin, have also been implicated as having molecular chaperone activity within the ER. Calnexin is an approximately 88 kD transmembrane ER-resident phosphoprotein originally discovered in association with class I major histocompatibility complex (MHC) molecules.[158,159] It is now known to facilitate the folding and assembly of many membrane and secretory glycoproteins. This chaperone activity involves a lectinlike mechanism in which calnexin binds the innermost glucose residue of the asparagine-linked oligosaccharide side chains present on most glycoproteins. The innermost glucose residue becomes accessible almost immediately after the secretory glycoprotein has undergone the initial stages of oligosaccharide side chain trimming in the lumen of the ER, including the removal of the two outermost glucose residues by the actions of glucosidases I and II (Figure 55.7-5). Once bound to calnexin, monoglucosylated glycoproteins are retained in the ER until properly folded.[160] Once folding is complete, the glycoprotein can dissociate from calnexin for vesicular transport out of the ER. Recent studies have indicated that a unique reglucosylating enzyme, uridine diphosphate–glucose:glycoprotein glucosyltransferase (UDGGT), can transfer glucose onto unfolded or denatured deglucosylated proteins in the ER.[161,162] In fact, the binding of glycoproteins to calnexin during folding in the ER is now thought to depend on a cycle of glucosidase II activity, producing the deglucosylated form of a protein, and reglucosylation by ER–luminal UDGGT, leading to regeneration of the monoglucosylated form. The glucosyltransferase acts preferentially on unfolded or denatured proteins. Thus, the repeated cycles of binding to and dissociation from calnexin are designed to maximize the possibility that a given unfolded or denatured protein will undergo proper folding for transport out of the ER.

It is now well established that the ER possesses a machinery whereby it can degrade any mutant or unassembled polypeptides that are unable to fold properly even after interaction with the ER chaperones. This machinery has come to be called the "ER degradation pathway" or the "quality control apparatus" of the ER.[163] Although the ER degradation pathway was originally thought to involve a distinct proteolytic system, it now appears to be mediated in large part from the cytoplasmic aspect of the ER by the proteasome.

Several studies have shown that α_1-ATZ is degraded in the ER and that the proteosome is a key component of the degradation pathway.[164–166] Degradation of α_1-ATZ is markedly reduced by specific proteosome inhibitors in yeast and mammalian cells.[165,166] In a mammalian cell–free system, degradation of α_1-ATZ is, at least in part, attributable to a pathway that involves interaction with the transmembrane ER chaperone calnexin, polyubiquitination of calnexin, and targeting of the α_1-ATZ–polyubiquitinated calnexin complex by the proteosome.[166] There is also evidence for the involve-

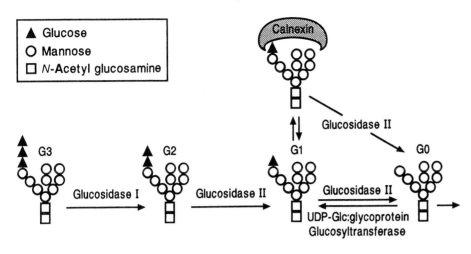

FIGURE 55.7-5 Model of glucose trimming and reglucosylation in relation to interaction with calnexin. Adapted from Hebert DN, Helenius A. Glucose trimming and reglucosylation determine glycoprotein association with calnexin in the endoplasmic reticulum. Cell 1995;81:425–33.

ment of ubiquitin-independent proteosomal and nonproteosomal pathways in degradation of α₁-ATZ in the mammalian cell–free system.[167]

As discussed below, autophagy may represent one nonproteosomal mechanism for degradation of α₁-ATZ.[168] Because this is based on the effect of chemical inhibitors of autophagy, which have other effects on cellular metabolism, definitive evidence for the role of autophagy in degradation of α₁-ATZ will require more detailed, probably genetic studies. Cabral and colleagues have recently provided evidence for a nonproteosomal degradation pathway that is sensitive to tyrosine phosphatase inhibitors.[169] In their studies, degradation of α₁-ATZ in a hepatoma cell line was not affected by proteosome inhibitors but was reduced by tyrosine phosphatase inhibitors. Although this finding was originally interpreted to suggest that there were cell type–specific differences in the role of proteosomal and nonproteosomal degradation mechanisms and that nonproteosomal degradation mechanisms were more important in hepatocytes, subsequent studies have shown that the proteosome still plays a major role in degradation of α₁-ATZ in other hepatoma cell lines.[170] This means it is more likely that nonproteosomal mechanisms, sensitive to tyrosine phosphatase inhibitors, are particularly important in specific cell lines rather than specific cell types. The relative importance of proteosomal and nonproteosomal mechanisms to the disposal of α₁-ATZ in vivo is still unknown. Despite what was stated in one review,[155] there are no data on the effect of age, inflammation, or other physiologic conditions on degradation of mutant α₁-ATZ.

The mechanism by which the proteosome gains access from the cytoplasm to α₁-ATZ on the luminal side of the ER membrane is also uncertain. Although retrograde translocation from the ER to the cytoplasm has been demonstrated for some luminal substrates of the proteosome, there is very limited evidence for retrograde translocation of α₁-ATZ. Werner and colleagues detected α₁-ATZ free in the cytosolic fraction of yeast when the proteosome was inhibited,[165] but only a small fraction of the total α₁-ATZ in the ER could be detected,[165] and there has been no other evidence for retrotranslocation. Recent studies have provided evidence for extraction of substrates through the ER membrane by the proteosome.[171] The AAA adenosine triphosphatase Cdc 48/p97 and its partners appear to play an important role in this process.[172] It is also possible that the proteasome gains access to α₁-ATZ and/or the α₁-ATZ–polyubiquitinated calnexin during the formation of autophagic vacuoles. Our recent studies have shown that retention of α₁-ATZ in the ER is associated with the induction of an autophagic response.[168] The autophagic response is thought to be a general mechanism by which intracellular organelles, or parts of organelles, are degraded. It is a highly evolutionarily conserved process that occurs in many cell types, especially during stress states, such as nutrient deprivation, and during the cellular remodeling that accompanies morphogenesis, differentiation, and senescence. Several studies have suggested that autophagic vacuoles are derived in part from subdomains of ER.[173] Autophagosomes initially form as invaginations from ribosome-free areas of the ER membrane. Together with constituents of the ER, autophagosomes engulf cytosolic constituents, including components of the ubiquitin system and the proteasome.[174,175] Thus, it is possible that degradation of α₁-ATZ is mediated by proteasomal machinery engulfed during formation of the autophagosome. Indeed, in our recent studies, an intense autophagic response was demonstrated in cell culture model systems with ER retention of mutant α₁-ATZ and in liver biopsy specimens from patients with α₁-AT deficiency.[168] Moreover, α₁-AT and calnexin were colocalized within autophagosomes as well as within the ER. Finally, degradation of α₁-ATZ in the cell culture model system is partially abrogated by inhibitors of autophagy, including wortmannin, 3-methyladenine, and LY294002. However, it is also possible that α₁-ATZ molecules taken up into autophagosomes are degraded by a nonproteasomal mechanism when the autophagosomes merge or fuse with the lyosomal pathway and that the autophagic and proteasomal pathways constitute completely independent mechanisms for degradation of α₁-ATZ.

A study by Van Leyen and colleagues suggested the possibility that a type of autophagic response termed "programmed organelle degradation" allows access of cytoplasmic proteases to both luminal and integral membrane proteins.[176] This process appears to involve the highly regulated recruitment of 15-lipoxygenase from the cytoplasm to the ER membrane, where it presumably oxygenates membrane phospholipids, in turn releasing proteins from the ER lumen and membrane. A mechanism like this could possibly account for the ER degradation pathway of some substrates.

PATHOGENESIS OF LIVER INJURY IN α_1-ANTITRYPSIN DEFICIENCY

There are several theories for the pathogenesis of liver injury in α_1-AT deficiency. According to the immune theory, liver damage results from an abnormal immune response to liver antigens.[177] This theory is based on the observation that peripheral blood lymphocytes from PIZZ infants are cytotoxic for isolated hepatocytes. However, this is probably a nonspecific effect of liver injury in that peripheral blood lymphocytes from PIMM infants with a similar degree of liver injury on the basis of idiopathic neonatal hepatitis syndrome are also cytotoxic for isolated hepatocytes. More recent studies have indicated an increase in the human leukocyte antigen (HLA)-DR3-DW25 haplotype in α_1-AT–deficient individuals with liver disease.[178] However, there is no difference in the expression of class II MHC antigen in the livers of these individuals compared with normal controls.[179] Moreover, an increase in the prevalence of a particular HLA haplotype in the affected population does not by itself imply altered immune function. In fact, because of the linkage dysequilibrium displayed by genes within the MHC, it is possible that increased susceptibility is caused by the products of unrelated but linked genes. For instance, the MHC contains genes for several HSPs,[180,181] which play an important role in the biogenesis and transport of other proteins through the secretory pathway.

The accumulation theory, in which liver damage is thought to be caused by accumulation of mutant α_1-AT molecules in the ER of liver cells, is the most widely accepted theory. Experimental results in transgenic mice are most consistent with this theory and completely exclude the possibility that liver damage is caused by "proteolytic attack" as a consequence of diminished serum α_1-AT concentrations.[26] Transgenic mice carrying the mutant Z allele of the human α_1-AT gene develop periodic acid–Schiff–positive diastase-resistant intrahepatic globules and liver injury early in life.[9,10] Because there are normal levels of α_1-AT and (presumably) other antielastases in these animals, as directed by endogenous murine genes, the liver injury cannot be attributed to proteolytic attack.

Some have argued that the histologic characteristics of the liver in the transgenic mouse model are not identical to those in humans. Detailed histologic characterization of the liver in one transgenic mouse model by Geller and colleagues has shown that there are focal areas of liver cell necrosis, microabscesses with an accumulation of neutrophils and regenerative activity in the form of multicellular liver plates, and focal nodule formation during the neonatal period.[182] Nodular clusters of altered hepatocytes that lack α_1-AT immunoreactivity are also seen during the neonatal period. With aging, there is a decrease in the number of hepatocytes containing α_1-ATZ globules; there

is also an increase in the number of nodular aggregates of α_1-AT–negative hepatocytes and development of periosinusoidal fibrosis.[183] Within 6 weeks, there are dysplastic changes in these aggregates. Adenomas occur within 1 year, and invasive hepatocellular carcinoma is seen between 1 and 2 years of age.[183] However, the relationship between the α_1-ATZ globules and inflammation or dysplasia is not yet apparent from these animal studies. The histopathology of the α_1-ATZ transgenic mice is remarkably similar to that of hepatitis B virus surface antigen–transgenic mice; this similarity is particularly interesting because hepatitis B virus is retained in the ER, or in the ER-Golgi intermediate compartment of hepatocytes, often called "ground-glass hepatocytes."[184] It is still unclear why the liver injury in this transgenic mouse model is somewhat milder and less fibrogenic than that seen in children with liver disease associated with α_1-AT deficiency. It is possible that there are strain-specific factors that condition the response to injury in the mouse model. There are certainly host-specific factors that determine the amount of liver injury in α_1-AT deficiency (see below), and the degree of inflammation and fibrosis varies widely among our patients with liver disease from α_1-AT deficiency.

Data from individuals who have null alleles of α_1-AT and therefore negligible serum levels of α_1-AT have also been used as evidence against the "proteolytic attack" theory. These individuals do not develop liver injury, at least not enough to result in clinical detection. However, only a few individuals with null alleles have been reported; each has a different allele, and based on data in PIZZ individuals showing that only 10 to 15% of these individuals develop clinically significant liver injury, it might be necessary to evaluate 7 to 10 individuals with each null allele before detecting one with liver injury.

The recognition that several other naturally occurring variant alleles of α_1-AT associated with deficiency can undergo polymerization has provided some support for the accumulation theory. The most important of these variant alleles is the compound heterozygous α_1-ATSZ phenotype. Work by Lomas and colleagues has shown that α_1-ATS and α_1-ATZ may form heteropolymers.[145] We know from the nationwide study of α_1-AT deficiency in Sweden that the incidence of liver disease among individuals with the α_1-ATSZ phenotype is similar to that of individuals with the α_1-ATZ phenotype.[1,11] We also now know that the PIM$_{Malton}$ allele undergoes polymerization, and liver injury has been reported in several patients with this allele.[64,68,141] However, there is a report of an individual with the PIS$_{Iiyama}$ allele having hepatocyte α_1-AT globules but no liver injury.[69] Moreover, a recent report by Ray and Brown has indicated that PIM$_{Heerlen}$ and PIM$_{Procidia}$ undergo aggregation and that PIM$_{Mineral Springs}$ and PINull$_{Ludwigshafen}$ may undergo aggregation, but there are no reports of liver disease in individuals carrying these alleles.[55] However, only a few patients with M$_{Malton}$, S$_{Iiyama}$, M$_{Heerlen}$, M$_{Procida}$, M$_{Mineral Springs}$, and Null$_{Ludwigshafen}$ have been identified. It is also not clear how many of these patients have been thoroughly examined for liver disease. Again, on the basis of what we know about the α_1-ATZ and α_1-ATSZ phenotypes, at least

7 to 10 individuals with each of these alleles would need to be examined to detect one with liver injury.

It has been difficult to reconcile the accumulation theory with the observations of Sveger,[11] which show that only a subset of α₁-AT–deficient individuals develop significant liver damage. We have made the prediction that a subset of the deficient population is more susceptible to liver injury by virtue of one or more additional inherited traits or environmental factors that exaggerate the intracellular accumulation of the α₁-ATZ protein or that exaggerate the cellular pathophysiologic consequence of mutant α₁-AT accumulation (Figure 55.7-6). To address this prediction experimentally, the Perlmutter laboratory transduced skin fibroblasts from deficient individuals, with or without liver disease, with amphotropic recombinant retroviral particles designed for constitutive expression of the mutant α₁-ATZ gene.[185] Human skin fibroblasts do not express the endogenous α₁-AT gene but presumably express other genes involved in the postsynthetic processing of secretory proteins. The results show that expression of the human α₁-AT gene was conferred on each fibroblast cell line. Compared with the same cell line transduced with the wild-type α₁-AT gene, there was selective intracellular retention of the mutant α₁-ATZ protein in each case. However, there was a marked delay in degradation of the mutant α₁-ATZ protein after it accumulated in the fibroblasts from deficient individuals with liver disease (susceptible hosts) compared with those without liver disease (protected hosts) (Figure 55.7-7). Thus, these data provide evidence that other factors that affect the abnormal α₁-ATZ molecule, such as a lag in ER degradation, at least in part, determine susceptibility to liver disease.

The lag in ER degradation of α₁-ATZ in susceptible hosts may involve several distinct mechanisms. In one susceptible host, the retained α₁-ATZ interacts poorly with calnexin.[185] In the liver cells of this host, there is likely to be only a very little polyubiquitinated α₁-ATZ–calnexin complex that can be recognized for proteolysis by the proteasome. In several other susceptible hosts, the retained α₁-ATZ interacts well with calnexin but is degraded slowly

(J. Teckman, D. Qu, D. H. Perlmutter, unpublished data, 1997). These hosts may have a defect in calnexin that prevents its ubiquitination or a defect in the ubiquitin system of the proteasome. Hosts with the latter defect would also be more likely to respond to a pharmacologic agent, such as interferon-γ,[186] that enhances the activity of the ubiquitin-dependent proteasomal system. This type of study, which involves complementation in human skin fibroblast cell lines, and recent studies involving yeast that have identified at least 30 putative recessive mutants and 7 complementation groups of strains defective in ER degradation of α₁-ATZ[187] are likely to lead to recognition of other mechanisms for excessive ER retention of α₁-ATZ.

There is still relatively limited information about the short- and long-term effects of ER retention of α₁-ATZ in model systems. In one report, the accumulation of α₁-ATZ in Xenopus oocytes was associated with the release of lysosomal enzymes.[188] Several recent studies have shown that ER retention of mutant α₁-ATZ provokes a rather specific cellular response with autophagy as a major feature. Autophagosomes develop in several different model cell culture systems genetically engineered to express α₁-ATZ, including human fibroblasts and murine hepatoma and rat hepatoma cell lines. Moreover, in a HeLa cell line engineered for inducible expression of α₁-ATZ, autophagosomes appear as a specific response to the expression of α₁-ATZ and its retention in the ER.[168] There is a marked increase in autophagosomes in hepatocytes in transgenic mouse models of α₁-AT deficiency and a disease-specific increase in autophagosomes in liver biopsies from patients with α₁-AT deficiency. Mutant α₁-ATZ molecules can be detected in autophagosomes by immune electron microscopy, often together with the ER molecular chaperone calnexin.

Taken together, these results have suggested that the autophagic response is induced to protect liver cells from the toxic effects of aggregated α₁-ATZ retained in the ER. We have also speculated about the role of autophagy in protecting liver cells from tumorigenesis. Several recent studies have shown that autophagic activity is decreased in tumors and that reconstitution of autophagic activity inhibits

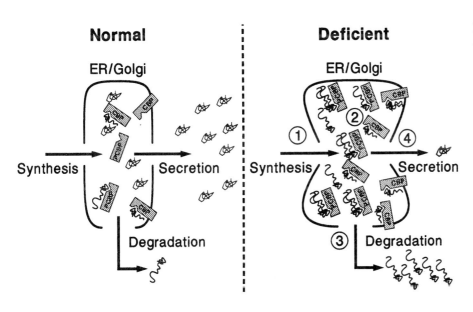

FIGURE 55.7-6 Conceptual model for liver injury in α₁-antitrypsin (AT) deficiency. CBP = calcium-binding protein; ER = endoplasmic reticulum; PCBP = polypeptide chain-binding protein. Adapted from Perlmutter DH. The cellular basis for liver injury in α₁-antitrypsin deficiency. Hepatology 1991;13:172–85.

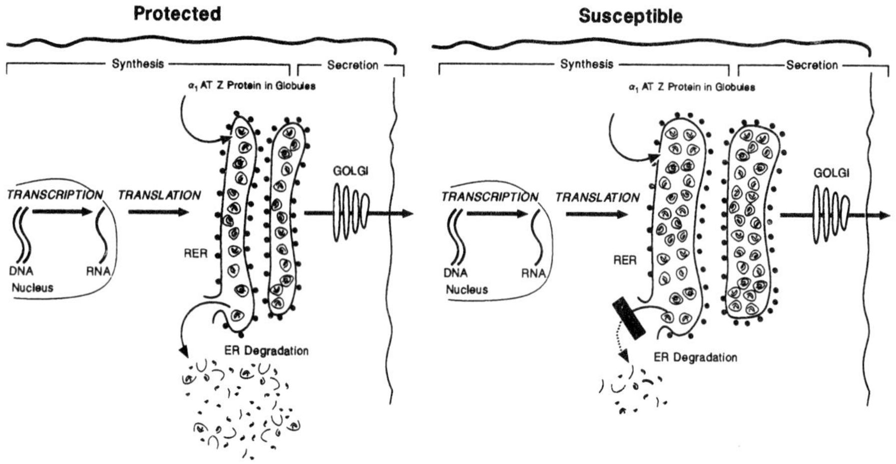

FIGURE 55.7-7 Difference in endoplasmic reticulum (ER) degradation of α_1-ATZ protein in protected and susceptible hosts. The block in ER degradation in susceptible hosts is represented by the small dark bar. Adapted from Teckman JH, Perlmutter DH. Conceptual advances in the pathogenesis and treatment of childhood metabolic liver disease. Gastroenterology 1995;108:1263–79.

tumorigenesis in vivo.[189,190] In our studies, autophagosomes are predominantly found in liver cells with dilated ER in both human and transgenic mouse liver.[168] Previous studies in transgenic mouse models of α_1-AT deficiency have shown that hepatocarcinogenesis evolves within nodular aggregates of hepatocytes that are negative for α_1-AT expression by immunofluorescent staining.[183]

It is not yet clear whether autophagy is substrate specific for α_1-ATZ or provides a more general response to aggregated proteins retained in the ER. No such cellular response has been described in studies of mutant proteins that aggregate in the cytoplasm or nucleus. Although there is some mention of autophagic vacuoles around the aggresomes that form when cystic fibrosis transmembrane regulator (CFTR) ΔF508 accumulates in the presence of proteosomal inhibitors,[191,192] the histologic pictures in cells expressing α_1-ATZ or CFTR ΔF508 are quite distinct.[168] Autophagy is not induced by tunicamycin or thapsigargin, agents that cause a generalized form of "ER stress" (N. Mitzushima, personal communication, 2002). Russell bodies, which have been described in cells retaining certain mutant immunoglobulin molecules in the ER,[193] do have many characteristics of autophagosomes. Autophagy has also been implicated in the cellular response to the mutant form of the ER membrane protein peripheral myelin protein 22, which causes a gain of function disease in Schwann cells in Charcot-Marie-Tooth disease and Dejerine-Sottas disease.[194]

Recently, we examined the autophagic response to ER retention of α_1-ATZ in vivo by testing the effect of fasting on the liver of the PiZ mouse model of α_1-AT deficiency.[195] Starvation is a well-defined physiologic stimulus of autophagy and a known environmental stressor of liver disease in children. The results show that there is a marked increase in fat accumulation and in α_1-AT–containing, ER-derived globules in the liver of the PiZ mouse induced by fasting. These changes were particularly exaggerated at 3 to 6 months of age. Three-month-old PiZ mice had a significantly decreased tolerance for fasting compared with nontransgenic C57 black mice (none of the PiZ mice tolerated a 72-hour fast even though 100% of C57BL mice survive the same duration of fasting). Although fasting induced a

marked autophagic response in wild-type mice, the autophagic response was already activated in PiZ mice to levels that were more than 50% higher than those in the liver of fasted wild-type mice, and they did not increase further during fasting. These results indicate that autophagy is constitutively activated in α_1-AT deficiency and that the liver is unable to mount an increased autophagic response to physiologic stressors. From our search of the literature, the only other condition in which there is accumulation of autophagic vacuoles under homeostatic conditions is Danon disease.[196] In contrast to α_1-AT deficiency, however, autophagosomes accumulate in Danon disease because of a genetic defect in the terminal phases of autophagy, that is, the fusion of autophagic vacuoles with lysosomes and subsequent degradation within autolysosomes.[196,197]

In the course of our ultrastructural studies of the liver of the PiZ mouse and of patients with α_1-AT deficiency, we have recently been struck by the degree of mitochondrial autophagy that is induced.[198] A comparison of the liver from four α_1-AT–deficient patients with livers from eight patients with other liver diseases and four normal livers showed a marked significant increase in mitochondrial autophagy associated with α_1-AT deficiency. Even more interesting is the observation that many mitochondria that are not surrounded by autophagic vacuolar membranes are nevertheless damaged or are in various phases of degeneration in liver cells from α_1-AT–deficient hosts. This damage is characterized by the formation of multilamellar structures within the limiting membrane, condensation of the cristae and matrix, and, in some cases, dissolution of the internal structures, often leaving only electron-dense debris compressed into a thin rim at the periphery of the mitochondrion. Although this second type of damaged mitochondria appears distinct from the mitochondria that are degenerating within autophagosomes, these mitochondria are sometimes seen in close proximity to, or even fusing with, autophagic vacuoles or lysosomes.

Mitochondrial autophagy and injury are also marked in the liver of the PiZ transgenic mouse model of α_1-AT deficiency. Immunofluorescence analysis shows the presence of activated caspase 3 in the PiZ mouse liver.[198] Because cyclosporin A (CsA) has been shown to reduce mitochondrial injury[199] and inhibit starvation-induced autophagy,[200] we examined the effect of CsA on PiZ mice and found that it significantly reduces hepatic mitochondrial injury while eliminating activated caspase 3 and improving the animals' tolerance of starvation. These results provide evidence for the novel concept that mitochondrial damage and caspase activation play a role in the mechanism of liver cell injury in α_1-AT deficiency. Although this analysis suggests that there is mitochondrial injury that is separate from the autophagic process, the possibility that autophagy plays some role in all of the mitochondrial damage that is observed cannot be completely excluded. Thus, one model of mitochondrial damage in this deficiency holds that accumulation of α_1-ATZ in the ER is in itself responsible for mitochondrial dysfunction. Indeed, there is now ample evidence in the literature for functional interactions between mitochondria and closely apposed ER cisternae.[201,202] Recent studies show that specific signals are transmitted between these two intracellular compartments[203,204] and that mitochondrial dysfunction, including release of cytochrome c and caspase 3 activation, is associated with the ER dilatation and stress induced by brefeldin A, tunicamycin, and thapsigargin.[205,206] It is not yet known, however, whether mitochondrial dysfunction in the latter cases is due to ER dilatation and/or ER stress or to independent effects on mitochondria by these experimental drugs. A second possible explanation, not necessarily incompatible with the first, envisages mitochondrial dysfunction as a result of the autophagic response to ER retention of α_1-ATZ. In this scenario, mitochondria are recognized nonspecifically by the autophagic response, which is constitutively activated to somehow remove and degrade areas of the ER that are distended by aggregated mutant protein. Although our data indicate that CsA inhibits hepatic mitochondrial injury in vivo, this benefit could reflect the drug's known effects on the mitochondrial permeability transition,[199] on autophagy,[200] or on both.

The CsA findings are also noteworthy for their therapeutic implications. They indicate that CsA can prevent mitochondrial damage even under circumstances in which α_1-ATZ continues to accumulate in the ER. Thus, they provide proof in principle for mechanism-based therapeutic approaches to liver disease in α_1-AT deficiency—pharmacologic intervention directed as distal steps in the pathobiologic pathway that leads to liver injury, such as the "mitochondrial" step, without correction of the primary defect and/or the more proximal steps in the pathobiology of this liver disease.

Other cellular response pathways could potentially be activated by ER retention of mutant proteins. Work in several laboratories has shown that a novel structure called the aggresome is formed in cells when expression of misfolded membrane proteins (such as CFTRΔF508, other mutant membrane proteins, and mutant viral proteins) exceeds the capacity of the proteasome to degrade them.[191,192,207] The aggresome is a pericentriolar membrane-free cytoplasmic inclusion containing misfolded ubiquitinated protein ensheathed in a case of vimentin and perhaps other intermediate filaments. Recent studies indicate that retention of

α_1-ATZ induces expansion of the ER, alteration in the structure of the ER and formation of autophagic vesicles but does not cause aggresome formation.[168]

The unfolded protein response is also induced by the accumulation of unfolded proteins in the ER. It results in the induction, or up-regulation, of a repertoire of genes that serve to protect the cell from damage by the denatured proteins.[208,209] This includes up-regulation of chaperones and enzymes in the phospholipid biosynthetic pathway to permit new ER membrane biogenesis and attenuation of the translation of most endogenous proteins, which could become denatured.

Two other signal transduction pathways activated by misfolded proteins in the ER have recently been characterized and may be relevant to α_1-AT deficiency. The ER overload pathway is a signaling pathway that appears to be distinct from the unfolded protein response and that involves activation of nuclear factor κB and release of active oxygen intermediates.[210] So far, this pathway has been described only in experimental conditions associated with ER overload of misfolded or unassembled membrane proteins. Recent studies in the Morimoto laboratory have shown that heat shock factor (HSF)2 may be activated by the accumulation of ubiquitinated proteins.[211] The downstream effect of HSF2 activation by ubiquitinated protein is induction of the classic heat shock response, including cytoplasmic and nuclear chaperones HSP90, HSP70, HSC70, HSP27, an ER chaperone GRP78/BiP, and mitochondrial chaperone HSP60.

It is not yet known whether one or all of these signaling pathways are induced by ER retention of α_1-ATZ or whether there is any alteration in their activation in the subgroup of α_1-AT–deficient patients who are susceptible to liver disease. Because these are considered response pathways that are designed to protect the cell, it is presumed that they must be overwhelmed by the concentration or intrinsic toxic potential of a particular mutant protein before cell injury occurs. However, the consequences of prolonged activation of these response pathways are entirely unknown and could potentially include cytotoxic and/or oncogenic effects.

LIVER DISEASE IN α₁-ANTITRYPSIN DEFICIENCY

Soon after homozygous PIZZ α_1-AT deficiency was described, an association with premature development of emphysema was discovered.[212] Eriksson noticed that some of the individuals with emphysema also had cirrhosis of the liver,[213] but an association between α_1-AT deficiency and liver disease was first clearly established in 1969 by Sharp and colleagues[214]; Sharp also noticed the distinctive histopathologic features of inclusion bodies in the ER of liver cells in these children.[215]

The most important study of liver disease in α_1-AT deficiency was conducted by Sveger, who prospectively screened 200,000 newborn infants in Sweden.[1] Sveger identified 127 deficient infants and has followed them since then. These infants were evaluated clinically at the age of 6 months. Fourteen of the 127 PIZZ infants had prolonged obstructive jaundice (group I). By clinical and laboratory criteria, 9 of these infants had severe liver disease and 5 had mild liver disease. Eight other PIZZ infants (group II) had minimal abnormalities in serum bilirubin, serum transaminases, and hepatic size. Approximately 50% of the remaining infants (group III) had abnormal serum transaminases.

Sveger collated data regarding the clinical outcome for these infants at 18 years of age. Three children from the group with prolonged obstructive jaundice (group I) died from liver disease before reaching 8 years of age. One group I child died from an unrelated cause. More than 85% of the remaining PIZZ children have persistently normal serum transaminases and no evidence of liver dysfunction.

Other studies of the incidence, prevalence, or prognosis of liver disease in α_1-AT deficiency[216–226] cannot be compared with the Sveger study[1] in that these studies involve PIZZ populations in which there is a bias in ascertainment (ie, the studies include only children referred to a specialty clinic). One issue not addressed by the Sveger study is whether 18-year-old patients with α_1-AT deficiency have persistent subclinical histologic abnormalities, despite the lack of clinical or biochemical evidence of liver injury, and whether liver disease will eventually become clinically evident during adulthood.

Liver involvement is often first noticed at 1 to 2 months of age because of persistent jaundice. Conjugated bilirubin levels in the blood and serum transaminase levels are mildly to moderately elevated. Blood levels of alkaline phosphatase and γ-glutamyl transpeptidase may also be elevated. The liver may be enlarged. There is a tendency for some of the affected infants to be small for gestational age. Affected infants are usually admitted to the hospital with a diagnosis of neonatal hepatitis syndrome and are subjected to a detailed diagnostic evaluation.[214,215,227] In fact, homozygous PiZZ α_1-AT deficiency appears to be the most common metabolic disease causing neonatal hepatitis syndrome.[216,228]

Infants may also be initially evaluated for α_1-AT deficiency because of an episode of gastrointestinal bleeding, bleeding from the umbilical stump, and/or bruising.[229] Occasionally, the deficiency is identified because of hepatosplenomegaly, ascites, and liver synthetic dysfunction in early infancy; an even smaller number have severe fulminant liver failure in infancy.[230] A few infants are recognized initially because of a cholestatic clinical syndrome characterized by pruritus and hypercholesterolemia. The clinical picture in these infants resembles extrahepatic biliary atresia, but histologic examination shows a paucity of intrahepatic bile ducts. Despite what is stated in one review,[155] many infants with homozygous PiZZ α_1-AT deficiency are completely asymptomatic and often go undetected. Even when detected in the Swedish screening study, only approximately 50% of the asymptomatic infants had elevated transaminases.[1,231]

Liver disease associated with α_1-AT deficiency may also be first discovered in late childhood or early adolescence, when the affected individual has abdominal distention from hepatosplenomegaly and/or ascites or has upper intestinal bleeding caused by esophageal variceal hemorrhage. Some of these patients have a history of unexplained prolonged obstructive jaundice during the neonatal period. In others, there is no evidence of any previous liver injury, even when the neonatal history is carefully reviewed.

α_1-AT deficiency should be considered in the differential diagnosis of any adult who presents with chronic hepatitis, cirrhosis, portal hypertension, or hepatocellular carcinoma of unknown origin. An autopsy study in Sweden shows a much higher risk of cirrhosis in adults with α_1-AT deficiency than was previously suspected and shows that this deficiency has a strong association with primary liver cancer.[232]

It is still not clear which clinical manifestations or abnormal laboratory test results can be used to predict a poor prognosis for individuals with liver disease associated with α_1-AT deficiency. One study suggested that persistent hyperbilirubinemia, hard hepatomegaly, early development of splenomegaly, and progressive prolongation of prothrombin time were indicators of poor prognosis.[223] In another study, elevated transaminase levels, prolonged prothrombin time, and a lower trypsin inhibitor capacity correlated with worse prognosis.[227] However, in my experience, some children with liver disease associated with α_1-AT deficiency can lead relatively normal lives for years after the development of hepatosplenomegaly and mild prolongation of prothrombin time. Volpert and colleagues reviewed 44 patients with α_1-AT deficiency seen at St. Louis Children's Hospital since 1984 when a registry was established.[233] Seventeen of these patients had cirrhosis and/or portal hypertension. Nine of these have had a prolonged, relatively uneventful course for at least 4 years after diagnosis. Of these patients, two eventually underwent liver transplant, but seven have led relatively healthy lives for up to 22 years after diagnosis. These nine patients could be distinguished only from the remaining eight patients by overall life functioning and not by any single clinical or biochemical characteristic. Thus, the prediction of poor prognosis for liver disease associated with α_1-AT deficiency and the timing of liver transplant depend more on the overall functioning of the affected child than on the histology or laboratory data.

There is currently no evidence that the heterozygous α_1-AT MZ phenotype causes liver disease in children by itself. It is not clear whether heterozygous MZ adults are predisposed to liver injury. Early studies of liver biopsy collections suggested that there was a relationship between heterozygosity and development of liver disease.[234] A retrospective study of liver transplant recipients at the Mayo Clinic showed that they had a higher prevalence of heterozygosity for α_1-ATZ in a group of these patients without another explanation for liver disease.[235] However, these studies are biased in ascertainment and do not include concurrent prospective controls. A cross-sectional study of patients with α_1-AT deficiency in a referral-based Austrian university hospital who were re-examined with the most sophisticated and sensitive assays available suggests that liver disease in heterozygotes can be accounted for, to a great extent, by infections with hepatitis B or C virus or by autoimmune disease.[236] Although there is an overall impression that heterozygotes for α_1-ATZ are susceptible to liver disease, the literature does not provide convincing evidence that liver injury can be explained by the α_1-AT MZ heterozygous state alone.

Liver disease has been described for several other allelic variants of α_1-AT. Children with compound heterozygosity type PISZ are affected by liver injury in a manner similar to that of PIZZ children.[1,11] There are several reports of liver disease in α_1-AT deficiency-type PIM$_{Malton}$.[64,68] This is a particularly interesting association because the abnormal PIM$_{Malton}$ α_1-AT molecule has been shown to undergo polymerization and retention within the ER.[141] Liver disease has been detected in single patients with several other α_1-AT allelic variants, such as PIM$_{Duarte}$,[66] PIW,[237] and PIFZ,[238] but it is not clear whether other causes of liver injury for which there are more sophisticated diagnostic assays (such as hepatitis C infection and autoimmune hepatitis) have been completely excluded in these cases.

The distinctive histologic feature of homozygous PIZZ α_1-AT deficiency—periodic acid–Schiff–positive diastase-resistant globules in the ER of hepatocytes—substantiates the diagnosis (Figure 55.7-8). According to some observers, these globules are not as easy to detect in the first few months of life.[239,240] The presence of these inclusions should not be interpreted as diagnostic of α_1-AT deficiency; similar structures are occasionally observed in PIMM individuals with other liver diseases.[241] The inclusions are eosinophilic, round to oval, and 1 to 40 μm in diameter. They are most prominent in periportal hepatocytes but may also be seen in Kupffer cells and cells of biliary ductular lineage.[242] There may be evidence of variable degrees of hepatocellular necrosis, inflammatory cell infiltration, periportal fibrosis, and/or cirrhosis. There is often evidence of bile duct epithelial cell destruction, and there is occasionally a paucity of intrahepatic bile ducts. Our recent study has shown that there may also be an intense

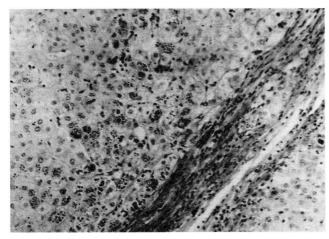

FIGURE 55.7-8 Hepatic histology in homozygous PIZZ α_1-antitrypsin (AT) deficiency. Micrograph of liver biopsy specimen in α_1-AT deficiency (periodic acid–Schiff [PAS]/diastase stain; ×40 original magnification), demonstrating the PAS+, diastase-resistant globules.

autophagic reaction detected by electron microscopic examination of liver biopsies, with a full array of nascent and degradative-type autophagic vacuoles.[168]

Diagnosis is established by a serum α_1-AT phenotype determination in isoelectric focusing or by agarose electrophoresis at acid pH (Figure 55.7-9). The phenotype should be determined in all cases of neonatal hepatitis or unexplained chronic liver disease in older children, adolescents, and adults. It is particularly important in the neonatal period because it may be very difficult to distinguish patients with α_1-AT deficiency from those with biliary atresia. Moreover, it is not uncommon for neonates with a PIZZ phenotype to have no biliary excretion on scintigraphic studies.[243] There is one report of α_1-AT deficiency and biliary atresia in a single patient.[244] We have had several patients with homozygous PIZZ α_1-AT deficiency and cholestasis and no biliary excretion of technetium-labeled mebrofenin, but with more prolonged observation in each of these cases, cholestasis remitted, so that it was then obvious that the patient did not have biliary atresia.

When used with isoelectric focusing, serum concentrations of α_1-AT may be helpful in distinguishing individuals who are homozygous for the Z allele from SZ compound heterozygotes, both of whom may develop liver disease. In some cases, phenotype determinations of parents and/or other relatives are also necessary to ensure the distinction between ZZ and SZ allotypes, a distinction that is important for genetic counseling. Serum concentrations of α_1-AT are occasionally misleading. For instance, concentrations may increase during the host response to inflammation, even in homozygous PIZZ individuals, giving a falsely reassuring impression.

LUNG DISEASE IN α_1-ANTITRYPSIN DEFICIENCY

The incidence and prevalence of emphysema in α_1-AT deficiency have not been studied prospectively. Autopsy studies suggest that 60 to 65% of people with homozygous PIZZ α_1-AT deficiency develop clinically significant lung injury. However, there are PIZZ smokers who do not have any symptoms of lung disease or evidence of pulmonary function abnormalities until the seventh or eighth decade of life.[245]

The typical person with lung disease is a male cigarette smoker. Onset of dyspnea is insidious in the third to fourth decade of life. About 50% of affected persons develop cough and recurrent lung infections. The disease progresses to a severe limitation of airflow. A reduction in the forced expiratory volume, increase in total lung capacity, and reduction in diffusing capacity occur. Chest radiography demonstrates hyperinflation with marked lucency at the lung bases.[246] Histopathologic studies demonstrate panacinar emphysema, which is more prominent in the lower lung.[246,247]

It is rare for emphysema to affect an α_1-AT–deficient patient during childhood. A number of patients have been described in the literature, but an alternative explanation can be offered in each of these cases. In the most convincing case, emphysema developed several years after a porta

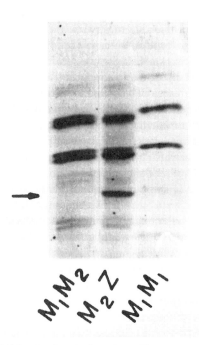

FIGURE 55.7-9 Isoelectric focusing of human serum samples for diagnosis of α_1-AT deficiency. Sera from a normal M_1M_2 individual, an M_2Z heterozygote, and a normal M_1M_1 individual were subjected to isoelectric focusing, with the anode at top and cathode at bottom. Migration of the Z allele is indicated by the arrow. The gel was provided by J. A. Pierce, St. Louis, MO. Reproduced with permission from Perlmutter DH. Alpha-1-antitrypsin deficiency. In: Snape WJ, editor. Consultations in gastroenterology. Philadelphia: WB Saunders; 1996. p. 793.

caval shunt procedure was done.[248] In three early cases, there were problems with the phenotypic diagnosis of α_1-AT deficiency.[249–251] In a more recent report, two patients had pulmonary abnormalities that could have been attributed to severe systemic illness associated with end-stage liver disease.[252] In a number of infants with α_1-AT deficiency, pulmonary function testing suggested a subtle degree of hyperinflation.[253] However, another study detected no significant difference between the pulmonary function of PIZZ children aged 13 to 17 years and that of an age-matched control group.[254] These data indicate that it is extremely rare for α_1-AT deficiency to cause emphysema in individuals less than 25 years of age.

The destructive effect of cigarette smoking on the outcome of lung disease in α_1-AT deficiency has been demonstrated in many studies. Actuarial studies suggest that cigarette smoking reduces median survival by over 20 years in deficient persons.[255] The rate of decline in forced expiratory volume is four times greater in α_1-AT–deficient persons who smoke than in α_1-AT–deficient persons who do not smoke.[256]

There is still very limited information about the incidence of liver disease in α_1-AT–deficient individuals with emphysema. In one study of 22 PIZZ patients with emphysema, there was an elevated transaminase level in 10 patients and cholestasis in 1 patient.[257] Liver biopsies were not done in this study, and such biopsies may be necessary to accurately determine the extent of liver injury in α_1-AT–deficient patients with emphysema.

TREATMENT

The most important principle in the treatment of α_1-AT deficiency is avoidance of cigarette smoking. Cigarette smoking markedly accelerates the destructive lung disease associated with α_1-AT deficiency, reduces the quality of life, and significantly shortens longevity.[255,256,258] These facts need to be presented to the families of affected pediatric patients in an unambiguous manner. Although it is not usually an issue that arises in the pediatric gastrointestinal and liver clinic, it may be necessary to carefully monitor the smoking habits of the family and, during interval visits, to re-emphasize the important effect of smoking on outcomes for deficient individuals.

There is no specific therapy for liver disease associated with α_1-AT deficiency. Therefore, clinical care largely involves supportive management of symptoms owing to liver dysfunction and prevention of complications. Although the use of ursodeoxycholic acid and colchicine has been mentioned in the literature, there is no evidence for biochemical or clinical efficacy for either drug.

Progressive liver dysfunction and liver failure in children have been treated by orthotopic liver transplant, with survival rates in one study approaching 90% at 1 year and 80% at 5 years.[259] A more recent study put 10-year actuarial survival at 68%.[260] Nevertheless, a number of PIZZ individuals with severe liver disease (even cirrhosis and/or portal hypertension) may have a relatively low rate of disease progression and may lead a relatively normal life for extended periods of time. With the availability of transplant techniques with living related donors, it may be possible to manage these patients expectantly for some time. Children with α_1-AT deficiency and mild liver dysfunction (elevated transaminases and/or hepatomegaly) and without functional impairment may never need liver transplant surgery.

Most α_1-AT–deficient children with liver disease are not candidates for alternative surgical interventions. However, there are rare specific clinical situations in which a portacaval or splenorenal shunt might be considered (such as in a child with only mild liver synthetic dysfunction and mild parenchymal liver injury but severe portal hypertension). Several children with severe liver disease and α_1-AT deficiency have survived 10 to 15 years after shunt surgery before requiring orthotopic liver transplant.[261] Moreover, previous hepatobiliary surgery is not a statistically significant risk factor for poor outcome of subsequent orthotopic liver transplant.[262]

Trials of pharmacologic therapy for α_1-AT deficiency have been conducted. Patients have been given the synthetic androgens danazol or stanazolol because of the dramatic effects of the same agents in patients with hereditary angioedema,[263] which is a deficiency of the homologous serine proteinase inhibitor C1 inhibitor, and because danazol was initially found to increase serum levels of α_1-AT in PIZZ persons.[264] However, further evaluation has demonstrated that danazol increases serum levels of α_1-AT in only 50% of deficient persons, and the magnitude of the effect is small.[265] Moreover, it was not clear from any of the studies whether the effect of androgens occurred at the level of synthesis and might also be associated with increased accumulation of α_1-ATZ in the ER, with potential hepatotoxic consequences.

Several studies have shown that a class of compounds called chemical chaperones can reverse the cellular mislocalization or misfolding of mutant plasma membrane, lysosomal, nuclear, and cytoplasmic proteins (including CFTRΔF508, prion proteins, mutant aquaporin molecules associated with nephrogenic diabetes insipidus, and mutant galactosidase A associated with Fabry disease).[266] These compounds include glycerol, trimethylamine oxide, deuterated water, and 4-phenylbutyric acid (PBA). Burrows and others recently found that glycerol and PBA mediate a marked increase in secretion of α_1-ATZ in a model cell culture system.[156] Moreover, oral administration of PBA was well tolerated by PiZ mice (transgenic for the human α_1-ATZ gene) and consistently mediated an increase in blood levels of human α_1-AT, reaching 20 to 50% of the levels present in PiM mice and normal humans. The synthesis or intracellular degradation of α_1-ATZ was not affected by PBA. The α_1-ATZ secreted in the presence of PBA was functionally active in that it could form an inhibitory complex with neutrophil elastase. Because PBA has been used safely for years in children with urea cycle disorders as an ammonia scavenger, and because clinical studies have suggested that only partial correction is needed for prevention of both liver and lung injury in α_1-AT deficiency, PBA constitutes a candidate for chemoprophylaxis of target organ injury in α_1-AT deficiency.

It also now appears that several iminosugar compounds may be potentially useful for chemoprophylaxis of liver and lung disease in α_1-AT deficiency. These compounds are designed to interfere with oligosaccharide side chain trimming of glycoproteins and are now being examimed as potential therapeutic agents for viral hepatitis and other types of infections.[267,268] We have examined several of these compounds initially to determine the effect of inhibiting glucose or mannose trimming from the carbohydrate side chain of mutant α_1-ATZ on its fate in the ER but found to our surprise that one glucosidase inhibitor, castanospermine, and two α-mannosidase I inhibitors, kifunensine and deoxymannojirimicin, actually mediate increased secretion of α_1-ATZ.[269] The α_1-ATZ that is secreted in the presence of these drugs is partially functionally active. Kifunensine and deoxymannojirimicin are less attractive candidates for chemoprophylactic trials because they delay degradation of α_1-ATZ in addition to increasing its secretion and therefore have the potential to exacerbate susceptibility to liver disease. However, CST has no effect on the degradation of α_1-ATZ and, therefore, may be targeted for development of a chemoprophylactic agent. The mechanism of action of castanospermine on α_1-ATZ secretion is unknown. An interesting hypothesis for the mechanism of action of kifunensine and deoxymannojirimicin has mutant α_1-ATZ interacting with ERGIC-53 for transport from the ER to the Golgi complex when mannose trimming is inhibited.

Novoradovskaya and others have suggested that inhibition of ER degradation of α_1-ATZ by proteasome inhibitor lactacystin and by protein synthesis inhibitor cyclohex-imide is associated with increased secretion of α_1-ATZ.[270] Burrows and others have been unable to confirm this result.[156] Moreover, there are now several lines of evidence indicating that there is no simple relationship between ER degradation of α_1-ATZ and its secretion such that perturbations that delay degradation are automatically accompanied by increased secretion. Some physiologic and pharmacologic perturbations are associated with delayed degradation without any change in secretion. Other perturbations increase secretion without any change in degradation. Increased temperature is associated with both delayed degradation and increased secretion.[156]

Some patients with α_1-AT deficiency and emphysema are currently receiving replacement therapy with purified or recombinant plasma α_1-AT either by intravenous or intratracheal aerosol administration.[271] This therapy is associated with an improvement in serum concentrations of α_1-AT and in neutrophil elastase inhibitory capacity in bronchoalveolar lavage fluid, without significant side effects. Although an initial study suggested that there is a slower decline in forced expiratory volume in patients on replacement therapy, this occurred only in a subgroup of patients, and the study was not randomized.[272]

Protein replacement therapy is designed only for individuals with established and progressive emphysema. It is not being considered for individuals with liver disease because there is no information to support the notion that deficient serum levels of α_1-AT are mechanistically related to liver injury.

A number of patients with severe emphysema from α_1-AT deficiency have undergone lung transplant in the past 10 years. The latest data from the St. Louis International Lung Transplant Registry show that 91 patients with emphysema and α_1-AT deficiency underwent single or bilateral lung transplant by 1993. Actuarial survival for patients in this category who underwent transplant between 1987 and 1994 is approximately 50% for 5 years. Lung function and exercise tolerance are significantly improved.[273]

Replacement of α_1-AT by somatic gene therapy has also been discussed in the literature.[271] This strategy is potentially less expensive than replacement therapy with purified protein and would alleviate the need for intravenous or inhalation therapy. Again, this form of therapy would be useful only in ameliorating emphysema because liver disease associated with α_1-AT deficiency is not caused by deficient levels of α_1-AT in the serum or tissue. Before clinical trials involving gene therapy are conducted, it would be helpful to know that replacement therapy with purified α_1-AT, as it is currently applied, is effective in ameliorating emphysema in this deficiency. Also, there are still major issues that need to be addressed before gene therapy becomes a realistic alternative.[274] Several novel types of gene therapy, such as repair of mRNA by trans-splicing ribozymes[275] and chimeric RNA/DNA oligonucleotides,[276] are theoretically attractive alternative strategies for liver disease in α_1-AT deficiency because they would prevent the synthesis of mutant α_1-ATZ protein and ER retention. In fact, a chimeric RNA/DNA oligonucleotide based on the sequence of coagulation factor IX in complex with lactose (so that it could be taken up by asialoglycoprotein receptor–mediated endocytosis) was delivered to hepatocytes with surprisingly high efficiency after intravenous administration.[276] However, efficiency has been much lower for other mutant proteins.

Recent studies have shown that transplanted hepatocytes can repopulate the diseased liver in several mouse models,[277,278] including a mouse model of a childhood metabolic liver disease termed hereditary tyrosinemia. Replication of the transplanted hepatocytes occurs only when there is injury and/or regeneration in the liver. The results provide evidence that it may be possible to use hepatocyte transplant techniques to treat hereditary tyrosinemia and perhaps other metabolic liver diseases in which the defect is cell autonomous. For instance, α_1-AT deficiency involves a cell-autonomous defect and would be an excellent candidate for this strategy.

Alternative strategies for at least partial correction of α_1-AT deficiency may result from a more detailed understanding of the fate of the α_1-ATZ molecule in the ER. First, delivery of synthetic peptides to the ER to insert into the gap in the A sheet or into a particular hydrophobic pocket of the α_1-AT molecule[279] and prevent polymerization of α_1-AT might result in the release of the mutant α_1-ATZ molecules into the extracellular fluid and might prevent its accumulation in the ER. Although it is not yet entirely clear, there is some evidence from studies on the assembly of class I MHC molecules that synthetic peptides may be delivered to the ER from the extracellular medium of cultured cells.[280] There is also evidence that certain molecules may be transported retrograde to the ER by receptor-mediated endocytosis.[281,282] Second, elucidation of the biochemical mechanism by which abnormally folded α_1-AT undergoes intracellular degradation might allow pharmacologic manipulation of this degradative system, such as enhancing proteasomal activity with interferon-γ in the subpopulation of PIZZ individuals predisposed to liver injury. Third, a competitive antagonist of binding or signal transduction by α_1-AT–proteinase complexes at the SEC receptor might prevent increases in intracellular accumulation of α_1-AT during augmentation of α_1-AT levels with protein replacement or gene replacement therapies.

GENETIC COUNSELING

Restriction fragment length polymorphisms detected with synthetic oligonucleotide probes[283,284] and family studies[285] allow prenatal diagnosis of α_1-AT deficiency. Nevertheless, it is not clear how prenatal diagnosis for this deficiency should be used and how families should be counseled regarding the diagnosis. Data from the Sveger study indicate that 70 to 75% of persons with α_1-AT deficiency do not have evidence of liver disease at the age of 18 years and that nonsmoking PIZZ persons may not develop emphysema or even pulmonary function abnormalities until 60 to 70 years of age.[11] These data could support a counseling strategy in which amniocentesis and abortion are discouraged. The only other data on this subject suggest a 78% chance that a second PIZZ child will have serious liver disease if the older sibling had serious liver disease.[224] However, this study was

retrospective and was influenced by bias in the ascertainment of patients. The issue will not be resolved until it is studied prospectively.[1,11]

SCREENING FOR α_1-ANTITRYPSIN DEFICIENCY

Several recent studies have suggested that population screening for α_1-AT deficiency would be efficacious. First, there is now evidence that knowledge of and counseling in the consequences of α_1-AT deficiency are associated with a reduced rate of smoking among affected adolescents.[286,287] Second, although there was some evidence for adverse psychological effects from knowledge of the deficiency by affected families,[288] more recent studies have indicated that there were no significant negative psychosocial consequences in early adulthood from neonatal screening for α_1-AT deficiency in Sweden.[289] These data should give new momentum to the reconsideration of screening programs for α_1-AT deficiency.

ACKNOWLEDGMENT

I am indebted to the family of Sean Welek and to the support of National Institutes of Health grants HL37784, DK52526 and DK61760.

REFERENCES

1. Sveger T. Liver disease in α_1-antitrypsin deficiency detected by screening of 200,000 infants. N Engl J Med 1976;294:1316–21.
2. Silverman EK, Miletich JP, Pierce JA, et al. α_1-Antitrypsin deficiency. High prevalence in the St. Louis area determined by direct population screening. Am Rev Respir Dis 1989;140:961–6.
3. Fagerhol MK. Serum Pi types in Norwegians. Acta Pathol Microbiol Scand 1967;70:421–6.
4. Pierce JA, Eradio B, Dew TA. Antitrypsin phenotypes in St. Louis. JAMA 1975;231:609–12.
5. Gadek JE, Fells GA, Zimmerman RL, et al. Antielastases of the human alveolar structure: implications for the protease-antiprotease theory of emphysema. J Clin Invest 1981;68:889–98.
6. Perlmutter DH, Pierce JA. The alpha-1-antitrypsin gene and emphysema. Am J Physiol 1989;257(4 Pt 1):L147–62.
7. Janoff A. Elastases and emphysema: current assessment of the protease-antiprotease hypothesis. Am Rev Respir Dis 1985;132:417–33.
8. Crystal RG. Alpha-1-antitrypsin deficiency, emphysema and liver disease: genetic basis and strategies for therapy. J Clin Invest 1990;95:1343–52.
9. Carlson JA, Rogers BB, Sifers RN, et al. Accumulation of PiZ antitrypsin causes liver damage in transgenic mice. J Clin Invest 1989;83:1183–90.
10. Dycaico JM, Grant SG, Felts K, et al. Neonatal hepatitis induced by alpha-1-antitrypsin: a transgenic mouse model. Science 1988;242:1409–12.
11. Sveger T. The natural history of liver disease in alpha-1-antitrypsin deficient children. Acta Paediatr Scand 1995;77:847–51.
12. Long GL, Chandra T, Woo SL, et al. Complete sequence of the cDNA for human α_1-antitrypsin and the gene for the S variant. Biochemistry 1984;23:4828–37.
13. Pearson SJ, Tetri P, George DL, Francke U. Activation of human α_1-antitrypsin gene in rat hepatoma x human fetal liver cell

hybrids depends on presence of human chromosome 14. Somat Cell Mol Genet 1983;9:567–92.

14. Lai EC, Kao FT, Law ML, Woo SL. Assignment of the α_1-antitrypsin gene and sequence-regulated gene to human chromosome 14 by molecular hybridization. Am J Hum Genet 1983;35:385–92.

15. Rabin M, Watson M, Kidd V, et al. Regional location of α_1-anti-chymotrypsin and α_1-antitrypsin genes on human chromosome 14. Somat Cell Mol Genet 1986;12:209–14.

16. Hofker MH, Nelen M, Klasen EC, et al. Cloning and characterization of an alpha-1-antitrypsin-like gene 12 kb downstream of the genuine alpha-1-antitrypsin gene. Biochem Biophys Res Commun 1988;155:634–42.

17. Kelsey GD, Parker M, Povey S. The human alpha-1-antitrypsin-related sequence gene: isolation and investigation of its sequence. Ann Hum Genet 1988;52:151–60.

18. Sefton L, Kelsey G, Kearney P, et al. A physical map of human PI and AACT genes. Genomics 1990;7:382–8.

19. Seralini GE, Berube D, Gagne R, Hammond GL. The human corticosteroid binding globulin gene is located on chromosome 14q31-q32.1 near two other serine protease inhibitor genes. Hum Genet 1990;86:73–5.

20. Perlino E, Cortese R, Ciliberto G. The human α_1-antitrypsin gene is transcribed from two different promoters in macrophages and hepatocytes. EMBO J 1987;6:2767–71.

21. Hafeez W, Ciliberto G, Perlmutter DH. Constitutive and modulated expression of the human α_1-antitrypsin gene: different transcriptional initiation sites used in three different cell types. J Clin Invest 1992;89:1214–22.

22. Carrell RW, Jeppson JO, Laurell CB, et al. Structure and variation of human alpha-1-antitrypsin. Nature 1982;298:329–34.

23. Vaughan L, Lorier MA, Carrell RW. Alpha-1-antitrypsin microheterogeneity: isolation and physiological significance of isoforms. Biochim Biophys Acta 1982;701:339–45.

24. Loebermann H, Tokuoka R, Deisenhofer J, Huber R. Human alpha-1-proteinase inhibitor: crystal structure analysis of two crystal modifications, molecular model and preliminary analysis of the implications for function. J Mol Biol 1984; 177:531–57.

25. Huber R, Carrell RW. Implications of the three-dimensional structure of alpha-1-antitrypsin for structure and function of serpins. Biochemistry 1990;28:8951–66.

26. Teckman JH, Qu D, Perlmutter DH. Molecular pathogenesis of liver disease in α_1-antitrypsin deficiency. Hepatology 1996; 24:1504–16.

27. Elliott PR, Lomas DA, Carrell RW, Abrahams JP. Inhibitory conformation of the reactive loop of α_1-antitrypsin. Nat Struct Biol 1996;3:676–81.

28. Elliott PR, Abrahams J-P, Lomas DA. Wild-type α_1-antitrypsin is in the cannonical inhibitory conformation. J Mol Biol 1998; 275:419–25.

29. Owen MC, Brennan SO, Lewis JH, Carrell RW. Mutation of antitrypsin to antithrombin: alpha-1-antitrypsin Pittsburgh (358 Met-Arg), a fatal bleeding disorder. N Engl J Med 1983; 309:694–8.

30. Banda MJ, Rice AG, Griffin GL, Senior RM. Alpha-1-proteinase inhibitor is a neutrophil chemoattractant after proteolytic inactivation by macrophage elastase. J Biol Chem 1998;263: 4481–4.

31. Banda MJ, Rice AG, Griffin GL, Senior RM. The inhibitory complex of human alpha-1-proteinase inhibitor and human leukocyte elastase is a neutrophil chemoattractant. J Exp Med 1998;167:1608–15.

32. Perlmutter DH, Glover GI, Rivetna M, et al. Identification of a serpin-enzyme complex (SEC) receptor on human hepatoma cells and human monocytes. Proc Natl Acad Sci U S A 1990;87:3753–7.

33. Perlmutter DH, Joslin G, Nelson P, et al. Endocytosis and degradation of alpha-1-antitrypsin-proteinase complexes is mediated by the SEC receptor. J Biol Chem 1990;265:16713–16.

34. Pierce JA, Eradio BG. Improved identification of antitrypsin phenotypes through isoelectric focusing with dithioerythritol. J Lab Clin Med 1979;94:826–31.

35. Barker A, et al. α_1-Antitrypsin deficiency: memorandum from a WHO meeting. Bull World Health Organ 1997;75:397–415.

36. Nukiwa T, Brantly M, Ogushi F, et al. Characterization of the M1 (ala 213) type of α_1-antitrypsin, a newly recognized common "normal" α_1-antitrypsin haplotype. Biochemistry 1987; 26:5259–67.

37. Kueppers F, Christopherson MJ. α_1-Antitrypsin: further genetic heterogeneity revealed by isoelectric focusing. Am J Hum Genet 1978;30:359–65.

38. Dykes D, Miller S, Polesky H. Distribution of α_1-antitrypsin variants in a US white population. Hum Hered 1984;34: 308–10.

39. Graham A, Hayes K, Weidinger S, et al. Characterization of alpha-1-antitrypsin M3 gene, a normal variant. Hum Genet 1990;85:381–2.

40. Jeppsson J-O, Laurell C-B. The amino acid substitutions of human alpha-1-antitrypsin M_3, X and Z. FEBS Lett 1988;231:327–30.

41. Brennan SO, Carrell RW. Alpha-1-antitrypsin Christchurch, 363Glu-Lys: mutation at the P'5 position does not affect inhibitory activity. Biochem Biophys Acta 1986;573:13–9.

42. Holmes MD, Brantly ML, Crystal RG. Molecular analysis of the heterogeneity among the P-family of alpha-1-antitrypsin alleles. Am Rev Respir Dis 1990;142:1185–92.

43. Talamo RC, Langley CE, Reed CE, Makino S. Alpha-1-antitrypsin deficiency: a variant with no detectable alpha-1-antitrypsin. Science 1973;181:70–1.

44. Takahashi H, Crystal RG. Alpha-1-antitrypsin null isola di procida: alpha-1-antitrypsin deficiency allele caused by deletion of all alpha-1-antitrypsin coding exons. Am J Hum Genet 1990;47:403–13.

45. Poller W, Faber JP, Weidinger S, Olek K. DNA polymorphisms associated with a new alpha-1-antitrypsin PIQ0 variant (PIQ0riedenberg). Hum Genet 1991;86:522–4.

46. Garver RI, Mornex JF, Nukiwa T, et al. Alpha-1-antitrypsin deficiency and emphysema caused by homozygous inheritance of on-expressing alpha-1-antitrypsin genes. N Engl J Med 1986;314:762–6.

47. Satoh K, Nukiwa T, Brantly M, et al. Emphysema associated with complete absence of alpha-1-antitrypsin in serum and the homozygous inheritance of stop codon in an alpha-1-antitrypsin coding exon. Am J Hum Genet 1988;42:77–83.

48. Holmes M, Curiel D, Brantly M, Crystal RG. Characterization of the intracellular mechanism causing the alpha-1-antitrypsin Null$_{granite\ falls}$ deficiency state. Am Rev Respir Dis 1989;140: 1662–7.

49. Nukiwa T, Takahashi H, Brantly M, et al. Alpha-1-antitrypsin Null$_{Granite\ Falls}$ a nonexpressing alpha-1-antitrypsin gene associated with a frameshift stop mutation in a coding exon. J Biol Chem 1987;262:11999–2004.

50. Curiel D, Brantly M, Curiel E, et al. Alpha-1-antitrypsin deficiency caused by the alpha-1-antitryspin null Mattawa gene: an insertion mutation rendering the alpha-1-antitrypsin gene incapable of producing alpha-1-antitrypsin. J Clin Invest 1989;83:1144–52.

51. Muensch H, Gaidulis L, Kueppers F, et al. Complete absence of

serum alpha-1-antitrypsin in conjunction with an apparently normal gene structure. Am J Hum Genet 1986;38:898–907.

52. Sifers RN, Brashears-Macatee S, Kidd VJ, et al. A frameshift mutation results in a truncated alpha-1-antitrypsin that is retained within the rough endoplasmic reticulum. J Biol Chem 1988;263:7330–5.

53. Brantly M, Lee JH, Hildesheim J, et al. α_1-Antitrypsin gene mutation hot spot associated with the formation of a retained and degraded null variant. Am J Respir Cell Mol Biol 1997;16:224–31.

54. Frazier GC, Siewertsen MA, Hofker MH, et al. A null deficiency allele of alpha-1-antitrypsin, QO Ludwigshafen, with altered tertiary structure. J Clin Invest 1990;86:1878–84.

55. Ray S, Brown JL. Comparison of the properties of rare variants of α_1-proteinase inhibitor expressed in COS-1 cells and assessment of their potential as risk factors in human disease. Biochim Biophys Acta 2003. [In press]

56. Curiel DT, Vogelmeier C, Hubbard RC, et al. Molecular basis of alpha-1-antitrypsin deficiency and emphysema associated with alpha-1-antitrypsin M Mineral Springs allele. Mol Cell Biol 1990;10:47–56.

57. Okayama H, Brantly M, Holmes M, Crystal RG. Characterization of the molecular basis of the alpha-1-antitrypsin F allele. Am J Hum Genet 1991;48:1154–8.

58. Graham A, Kalsheker NA, Bamforth FJ, et al. Molecular characterization of two alpha-1-antitrypsin deficiency variants: proteinase inhibitor (Pi) Null newport (Gly^{165}-Ser) and (Pi) Z Wrexham (Ser^{-19}-Leu). Hum Genet 1990;85:537–40.

59. Carrell RW. Alpha-1-antitrypsin molecular pathology, leukocytes and tissue damage. J Clin Invest 1986;77:1427–31

60. Curiel D, Chytil A, Courtney M, Crystal RG. Serum alpha-1-antitrypsin deficiency associated with the common S-type (Glu^{364}-Val) mutation results from intracellular degradation of alpha-1-antitrypsin prior to secretion. J Biol Chem 1989;264:10477–86.

61. Hofker MH, et al. A Pro-Leu substitution in codon 369 in the alpha-1-antitrypsin deficiency variant PiM$_{heerlen}$ [abstract]. Am J Hum Genet 1987;41:A220.

62. Kramps JA, et al. PiM$_{heerlen}$ a PiM allele resulting in very low alpha-1-antitrypsin serum levels. Hum Genet 1981;59:104–7.

63. Takahashi H, et al. Characterization of the gene and protein of the alpha-1-antitrypsin "deficiency" allele M procida. J Biol Chem 1988;263:15528–34.

64. Curiel DT, et al. Molecular basis of the liver and lung disease associated with α_1-antitrypsin deficiency allele M$_{malton}$. J Biol Chem 1989;264:13938–45.

65. Sproule BJ, et al. Pulmonary function associated with the M Malton deficient variant of alpha-1-antitrypsin. Am Rev Respir Dis 1983;127:237–40.

66. Crowley JJ, et al. Fatal liver disease associated with α_1-antitrypsin deficiency PIM/PIM$_{duarte}$. Gastroenterology 1987;93:2–4.

67. Holmes MD, et al. Alpha-1-antitrypsin W$_{Bethesda}$: molecular basis of an unusual alpha-1-antitrypsin deficiency variant. Biochem Biophys Res Commun 1990;170:1013–22.

68. Reid CL, et al. Diffuse hepatocellular dysplasia and carcinoma associated with the M$_{malton}$ variant of α_1-antitrypsin. Gastroenterology 1987;93:181–7.

69. Seyama K, et al. S$_{Iiyama}$ serine 53 (TCC) to phenylalanine 53 (TTC): a new alpha-1-antitrypsin deficient variant with mutation on a predicted conserved residue of the serpin backbone. J Biol Chem 1991;266:12627–32.

70. Senior RM, et al. The induction of pulmonary emphysema with human leukocyte elastase. Am Rev Respir Dis 1977;116:469–75.

71. Travis J, Salveson GS. Human plasma proteinase inhibitors. Annu Rev Biochem 1983;52:655–709.

72. Carrell RW, Lomas DA. Conformational disease. Lancet 1997;350:134–8.

73. Huntington JA, Read RJ, Carrell RW. Structure of a serpin-protease complex shows inhibition by deformation. Nature 2000;407:923–6.

74. Carp H, Janoff A. Possible mechanisms of emphysema in smokers: in vitro suppression of serum elastase inhibitory capacity by fresh cigarette smoke and its prevention by antioxidants. Am Rev Respir Dis 1978;118:617–21.

75. Ossanna PJ, et al. Oxidative regulation of neutrophil elastase-alpha-1-proteinase inhibitor interactions. J Clin Invest 1986;72:1939–51.

76. Hubbard RC, et al. Oxidants spontaneously released by alveolar macrophages of cigarette smokers can inactivate the active site of α_1-antitrypsin, rendering it ineffective as an inhibitor of neutrophil elastase. J Clin Invest 1987;80:1289–95.

77. Mast AE, et al. Kinetics and physiologic relevance of the inactivation of α_1-proteinase inhibitor, α_1-antichymotrypsin, and antithrombin III by matrix metalloproteinases-1 (tissue collagenase), -1 (72-kDa gelatinase/type IV collagenase), and -3 (stromelysin). J Biol Chem 1991;266:15810–6.

78. Duranton J, et al. DNA strongly impairs the inhibition of cathepsin G by α_1-antichymotrypsin and α_1-proteinase inhibitor. J Biol Chem 2000;275:3787–92.

79. Miller RR, et al. Comparison of the chemical, physical and survival properties of normal and Z-variant α_1-antitrypsin. J Biol Chem 1976;251:4751–7.

80. Bathurst IC, et al. Structural and functional characterization of the abnormal Z α_1-antitrypsin isolated from human liver. FEBS Lett 1984;177:179–83.

81. Ogushi F, et al. Z-type α_1-antitrypsin is less competent than M1-type α_1-antitrypsin as an inhibitor of neutrophil elastase. J Clin Invest 1987;89:1366–74.

82. Libert C, Van Molle W, Brouckaert P, Fiers W. α_1-Antitrypsin inhibits the lethal response to TNF in mice. J Immunol 1996;157:5126–9.

83. Van Molle W, Libert C, Fiers W, Brouckaert P. α_1-Acid glycoprotein and α_1-antitrypsin inhibit TNF-induced, but not anti-Fas-induced apoptosis of hepatocytes in mice. J Immunol 1997;159:3555–64.

84. Camussi G, Tetta C, Bussolino F, Baglioni C. Synthesis and release of platelet-activating factor is inhibited by plasma α_1-proteinase inhibitor or α_1-antichymotrypsin and is stimulated by proteinases. J Exp Med 1988;168:1293–306.

85. Shapiro L, Pott GB, Ralston AH. Alpha-1-antitrypsin inhibits human immunodeficiency virus type I. FASEB J 2001;15:115–22.

86. Joslin G, et al. The serpin-enzyme complex (SEC) receptor mediates the neutrophil chemotactic effect of α_1-antitrypsin-elastases complexes and amyloid-β peptide. J Clin Invest 1992;90:1150–4.

87. Morago F, Joncidaus Kiene S. Activation of primary human monocytes by the oxidized form of α_1-antitrypsin. J Biol Chem 2000;275:7693–700.

88. Wilson-Cox D. Alpha-1-antitrypsin deficiency. In: Scriber CB, Beaudet AL, Aly QA, Valle D, editors. The metabolic basis of inherited disease. New York: McGraw-Hill; 1989. p. 2409–37.

89. Breit SN, et al. The role of alpha-1-antitrypsin deficiency in the pathogenesis of immune disorders. Clin Immun Immunopathol 1985;35:363–80.

90. Hood JM, et al. Liver transplantation for advanced liver disease with α_1-antitrypsin deficiency. N Engl J Med 1980;302:272–6.

91. Alper CA, et al. Studies of hepatic synthesis in vivo of plasma proteins including orosomucoid, transferrin, alpha-1-antitrypsin, C8, and factor B. Clin Immunol Immunopathol 1980;16:84–8.

92. Lodish HF, et al. Hepatoma secretory proteins migrate from rough endoplasmic reticulum to Golgi at characteristic rates. Nature 1983;304:80–3.

93. Lodish HF, Kong N. Glucose removal from N-linked oligosaccharides is required for efficient maturation of certain secretory glycoproteins from the rough endoplasmic reticulum to the Golgi complex. J Cell Biol 1984;98:1720–9.

94. Liu M-C, et al. Tyrosine sulfation of proteins from human hepatoma cell line HepG2. Proc Natl Acad Sci U S A 1985;82:7160–4.

95. DeSimone V, Cortese R. Transcription factors and liver-specific genes. J Biol Biophys Acta 1992;1132:119–26.

96. Tripodi M, et al. Disruption of the LF-A1 and LF-B1, binding sites in the human alpha-1-antitrypsin gene, has a differential effect during development in transgenic mice. EMBO J 1991;10:3177–82.

97. Hu C, Perlmutter DH. Regulation of α_1-antitrypsin gene expression in human intestinal epithelial cell line Caco2 by HNF1a and HNF4. Am J Physiol 1999;276:G1181–94.

98. Monaci P, Nicosia A, Cortese R. Two different liver-specific factors stimulate in vitro transcription from the human α_1-antitrypsin promoter. EMBO J 1991;10:1435–43.

99. Bohmann D, et al. Human proto-oncogene c-jun encodes a DNA binding protein with structural and functional properties of transcription factor AP-1. Science 1987;238:1386–92.

100. Franza BR, et al. The Fos complex and Fos-related antigens recognize sequence elements that contain AP-1 binding sites. Science 1988;239:1150–3.

101. Dickson I, Alper CA. Changes in serum proteinase inhibitor levels following bone surgery. Clin Chim Acta 1974;54:381–5.

102. Perlmutter DH, May LT, Sehgal PB. Interferon β_2/interleukin-6 modulates synthesis of α_1-antitrypsin in human mononuclear phagocytes and in human hepatoma cells. J Clin Invest 1989;264:9485–90.

103. Laurell CB, Rannevik G. A comparison of plasma protein changes induced by danazol, pregnancy and estrogens. J Clin Endocrinol Metab 1979;49:719–25.

104. Perlmutter DH, et al. Expression of the α_1-proteinase inhibitor gene in humanmonocytes and macrophages. Proc Natl Acad Sci U S A 1985;82:795–9.

105. Perlmutter DH, et al. The cellular defect in α_1-proteinase inhibitor deficiency is expressed in human monocytes and in Xenopus oocytes injected with human liver mRNA. Proc Natl Acad Sci U S A 1985;82:6918–21.

106. Kelsey GD, et al. Species- and tissue-specific expression of human alpha-1-antitrypsin in transgenic mice. Genes Dev 1987;1:161–71.

107. Barbey-Morel C, et al. Lipopolysaccharide modulates the expression of α_1-proteinase inhibitor and other serine proteinase inhibitors in human monocytes and macrophages. J Exp Med 1987;166:1041–54.

108. Perlmutter DH, Punsal PI. Distinct and additive effects of elastase and endotoxin on α_1-proteinase inhibitor and other serine proteinase inhibitor expression in macrophages. J Biol Chem 1988;263:16499–503.

109. Mueller PP, Hinnebusch AG. Multiple upstream AUG codons mediate translational control of GCN4. Cell 1986;45:201–7.

110. Perlmutter DH, Travis J, Punsal PI. Elastase regulates the synthesis of its inhibitors, α_1-proteinase inhibitor, and exaggerates the defect in homozygous PIZZ α_1-proteinase inhibitor deficiency. J Clin Invest 1988;81:1774–8.

111. Joslin G, et al. The SEC receptor recognizes a pentapeptide neodomain of α_1-antitrypsin-protease complexes. J Biol Chem 1991;266:11281–8.

112. Joslin G, et al. Cross-competition for binding of α_1-antitrypsin (α-1-AT)-elastase complexes to the serpin-enzyme complex receptor by other serpin-enzyme complexes and by proteolytically modified α-1-AT. J Biol Chem 1993;268:1886–93.

113. Joslin G, et al. Amyloid-β peptide, substance P and bombesin bind to the serpin-enzyme complex receptor. J Biol Chem 1991;266:21897–902.

114. Boland K, et al. The serpin-enzyme complex receptor recognizes soluble, nontoxic amyloid-β peptide but not aggregated, cytotoxic amyloid-β peptide. J Biol Chem 1996;271:18032–44.

115. Sifers RN, et al. Tissue-specific expression of the human α_1-antitrypsin gene in transgenic mice. Nucleic Acid Res 1987;15:1459–75.

116. Carlson JA, et al. Multiple tissues express alpha-1-antitrypsin in transgenic mice and man. J Clin Invest 1988;82:26–36.

117. Perlmutter DH, Alpers DH, Daniels JD. Expression of the α_1-antitrypsin gene in a human intestinal epithelial cell line. J Biol Chem 1989;264:9485–90.

118. Molmenti EP, Perlmutter DH, Rubin DC. Cell-specific expression of α_1-antitrypsin in human intestinal epithelium. J Clin Invest 1993;92:2022–34.

119. Molmenti EP, Ziambaras T, Perlmutter DH. Evidence for an acute phase response in human intestinal epithelial cells. J Biol Chem 1993;268:14116–24.

120. Venembre P, et al. Secretion of α_1-antitrypsin by alveolar epithelial cells. FEBS Lett 1994;346:171–4.

121. Cichy J, Potempa J, Travis J. Biosynthesis of α_1-proteinase inhibitor by human lung-derived epithelial cells. J Biol Chem 1997;272:8250–5.

122. Makino S, Reed CE. Distribution and elimination of exogenous alpha-1-antitrypsin. J Lab Clin Med 1970;75:742–6.

123. Laurell C-B, Nosslin B, Jeppsson J-O. Catabolic rate of α_1-antitrypsin of Pl type M and Z in man. Clin Sci Mol Med 1977;52:457–61.

124. Jones EA, et al. Metabolism of intact and desialylated α_1-antitrypsin. Clin Sci Mol Med 1978;55:139–48.

125. Jeppsson J-O, et al. Catabolic rate of Pl types S, and M Malton and of asialylated M-protein in man. Clin Sci Mol Med 1978;55:103–7.

126. Mast AE, Enghild JJ, Pizzo SV, Salvesen G. Analysis of the plasma elimination kinetics and conformational stabilities of native, proteinase-complexed, and reactive site cleaved serpins: comparison of alpha 1-proteinase inhibitor, alpha1-antichymotrypsin, antithrombin III, alpha 2-antiplasmin, angiotensinogen, and ovalbumin. Biochemistry 1991;30:1723–30.

127. Poller W, Willnow TE, Hilpert J, Herz J. Differential recognition of α_1-antitrypsin-elastase and α_1-antichymotrypsin-cathespin G complexes by the low density lipoprotein receptor-related protein. J Biol Chem 1995;270:2841–5.

128. Kounnas MZ, Church FC, Argraves WS, Strickland DK. Cellular internalization and degradation of antithrombin-III-thrombin, heparin cofactor II-thrombin, and α_1-antitrypsin-trypsin complexes is mediated by the low density lipoprotein receptor-related protein. J Biol Chem 1996;271:6523–9.

129. Koj A, Regoeczi E. Effect of experimental inflammation on the synthesis and distribution of antithrombin III and α_1-antitrypsin in rabbits. Br J Exp Pathol 1978;59:473–81.

130. Glaser CB, et al. Plasma survival studies in rat of the normal and homozygote deficient forms of α_1-antitrypsin. Biochim Biophys Acta 1977;495:87–95.

131. Thomas DW, Sinatra FR, Merritt RJ. Random fecal alpha-1-antitrypsin concentration in children with gastrointestinal disease. Gastroenterology 1981;80:776–82.

132. Grill B, et al. Increased intestinal clearance of alpha-1-antitrypsin in patient with alpha-1-antitrypsin deficiency. J Pediatr Gastroenterol Nutr 1983;2:95–8.

133. Kidd VJ, Walker RB, Itakura K, Woo SLC. α_1-Antitrypsin deficiency detection by direct analysis of the mutation of the gene. Nature 1983;304:230–4.

134. Jeppsson J-O. Amino acid substitution Glu-Lys in alpha1-antitrypsin PiZ. FEBS Lett 1976;65:195–7.

135. Owen MC, Carrell RW. α_1-Antitrypsin: sequence of the Z variant tryptic peptide. FEBS Lett 1976;79:247–9.

136. Foreman RC, Judah JD, Colman A. Xenopus oocytes can synthesize but do not secrete the Z variant of human α_1-antitrypsin. FEBS Lett 1984;169:84–8.

137. McCracken AA, Kruse KB, Brown JL. Molecular basis for defective secretion of variants having altered potential for salt bridge formation between amino acids 240 and 242. Mol Cell Biol 1989;9:1408–14.

138. Sifers RN, Hardick CP, Woo SLC. Disruption of the 240-342 salt bridge is not responsible for the defect of the PIZ alpha1-antitrypsin variant. J Biol Chem 1989;264:2997–3001.

139. Wu Y, Foreman RC. The effect of amino acid substitutions at position 342 on the secretion of human α_1-antitrypsin from Xenopus oocytes. FEBS Lett 1990;268:21–3.

140. Lomas DA, Evans DL, Finch JJ, Carrell RW. The mechanism of Z α_1-antitrypsin accumulation in the liver. Nature 1992;357:5–7.

141. Lomas DA, et al. α_1-Antitrypsin M_{Malton} (Phe[52 deleted]) forms loop-sheet polymers in vivo: evidence for the C-sheet mechanism of polymerization. J Biol Chem 1995;270:16864–74.

142. Lomas DA, et al. α_1-Antitrypsin S_{Iiyama} (SER53ÆPhe): further evidence for intracellular loop-sheet polymerization. J Biol Chem 1993;268:15333–5.

143. Elliott PR, et al. Structural explanation for the deficiency of S α_1-antitrypsin. Nat Struct Biol 1996;3:910–1.

144. Teckman JH, Perlmutter DH. The endoplasmic reticulum degradation pathway for mutant secretory proteins α_1-antitrypsin Z and S is distinct from that for an unassembled membrane protein. J Biol Chem 1996;271:13215–20.

145. Mahadeva R, et al. Heteropolymerization of S, I, and Z α_1-antitrypsin and liver cirrhosis. J Clin Invest 1999;103:999–1006.

146. Davis RL, et al. Familial dementia caused by polymerization of mutant neuroserpin. Nature 1999;401:376–9.

147. Dafforn TR, et al. A kinetic mechanism for the polymerization of α_1-antitrypsin. J Biol Chem 1999;274:9548–55.

148. James EL, Whisstock JC, Gore MG, Bottomley SP. Probing the unfolding pathway of α_1-antitrypsin. J Biol Chem 1999;274:9482–8.

149. Yu M-H, Lee KN, Kim J. The Z type variation of human α_1-antitrypsin causes a protein folding defect. Nat Struct Biol 1995;2:363–7.

150. Hurtley SM, Helenius A. Protein oligomerization in the endoplasmic reticulum. Annu Rev Cell Biol 1989;5:277–307.

151. Kim J, Lee KN, Yi G-S, Yu M-H. A thermostable mutation located at the hydrophobic core of α_1-antitrypsin suppresses the folding defect of the Z-type variant. J Biol Chem 1995;270:8597–601.

152. Sidhar SK, Lomas DA, Carrell RW, Foreman RC. Mutations which impede loop-sheet polymerization enhance the secretion of human α_1-antitrypsin deficiency variants. J Biol Chem 1995;270:8393–6.

153. Kang HA, Lee KN, Yu M-H. Folding and stability of the Z and S_{Iiyama} genetic variants of human α_1-antitrypsin. J Biol Chem 1997;272:510–6.

154. Lin L, Schmidt B, Teckman J, Perlmutter DH. A naturally occurring nonpolymerogenic mutant of α_1-antitrypsin characterized by prolonged retention in the endoplasmic reticulum. J Biol Chem 2001;276:33893–98.

155. Carrell RW, Lomas DA. Alpha-1-antitrypsin deficiency—a model for conformational diseases. N Engl J Med 2002;346:45–53.

156. Burrows JAJ, Willis LK, Perlmutter DH. Chemical chaperones mediate increased secretion of mutant α_1-antitrypsin (α_1-AT) Z. A potential pharmacological strategy for prevention of liver injury and emphysema in α_1-AT deficiency. Proc Natl Acad Sci U S A 2000;97:1796–801.

157. Rothman JE, Wieland FT. Protein sorting by transport vesicles. Science 1996;272:227–34.

158. Helenius A, Trombetta ES, Hebert DN, Simons JF. Calnexin, calreticulin and the folding of glycoproteins. Trends Cell Biol 1997;7:193–200.

159. Ou W-J, Cameron PH, Thomas DY, Bergeron JJM. Association of folding intermediates of glycoproteins with calnexin during protein maturation. Nature 1993;364:771–6.

160. Zapun A, et al. Conformation-independent binding of monoglucosylated ribonuclease B to calnexin. Cell 1997;88:29–38.

161. Sousa MC, Ferrero-Garcia MA, Parodi AJ. Recognition of the oligosaccharide and protein moieties of glycoproteins by the UDP-glucose:glycoprotein glucosyltransferase. Biochemistry 1992;31:97–105.

162. Hebert DN, Foellmer B, Helenius A. Glucose trimming and reglucosylation determine glycoprotein association with calnexin in the endoplasmic reticulum. Cell 1995;81:425–53.

163. Bonifacino JS, et al. Pre-Golgi degradation of newly synthesized T-cell antigen receptor chains: intrinsic sensitivity and the role of subunit assembly. J Cell Biol 1989;109:73–83.

164. McCracken AA, Brodsky JL. Assembly of ER-associated protein degradation in vitro: dependence on cytosol, calnexin and ATP. J Cell Biol 1996;132:291–8.

165. Werner ED, Brodsky JL, McCracken AA. Proteasome-dependent endoplasmic reticulum-associated protein degradation: an unconventional route to a familiar fate. Proc Natl Acad Sci U S A 1996;93:13797–801.

166. Qu D, Teckman JH, Omura S, Perlmutter DH. Degradation of mutant secretory protein, α_1-antitrypsin Z, in the endoplasmic reticulum requires proteasome activity. J Biol Chem 1996;271:22791–5.

167. Teckman JH, Gilmore R, Perlmutter DH. The role of ubiquitin in proteasomal degradation of mutant α_1-antitrypsin Z in the endoplasmic reticulum. Am J Physiol 2000;278:G39–48.

168. Teckman JH, Perlmutter DH. Retention of the mutant secretory protein α_1-antitrypsin Z in the endoplasmic reticulum induces autophagy. Am J Physiol 2000;279:G961–74.

169. Cabral CM, Choudhury P, Liu Y, Sifers RN. Processing by endoplasmic reticulum mannosidases partitions a secretion-impaired glycoprotein into distinct disposal pathways. J Biol Chem 2000;275:25015–22.

170. Teckman JH, Burrows J, Hidvegi T, et al. The proteasome participates in degradation of mutant α_1-antitrypsin Z in the endoplasmic reticulum of hepatoma-derived hepatocytes. J Biol Chem 2001;48:44865–72.

171. Mayer T, Braun T, Jentsch S. Role of the proteasome in membrane extraction of a short-lived ER-transmembrane protein. EMBO J 1998;17:3251–7.

172. Ye Y, Meyer HH, Rapoport TA. The AAA ATPase Cdc48/p97 and

its partners transport proteins from the ER into the cytosol. Nature 2001;414:652–6.

173. Dunn WA. Studies on the mechanism of autophagy: formation of the autophagic vacuole. J Cell Biol 1991;110:1923–33.

174. Kopitz J, Kisen GO, Gordon PB, et al. Nonselective autophagy of cytosolicenzymes by isolated rat hepatocytes. J Cell Biol 1990;111:94153.

175. Lenk SE, Dunn WA, Trausch JS, et al. Ubiquitin-activating enzyme, E1, is associated with maturation of autophagic vacuoles. J Cell Biol 1992;118:301–8.

176. Van Leyen K, Duvoisin R, Engelhardt H, Wiedmann M. A function for lipoxygenase in programmed organelle degradation. Nature 1998;395:392–5.

177. Povey S. Genetics of α₁-antitrypsin deficiency in relation to neonatal liver disease. Mol Biol Med 1990;7:161–2.

178. Dougherty DG, et al. HLA phenotype and gene polymorphism in juvenile liver disease associated with α₁-antitrypsin deficiency. Hepatology 1990;12:218–23.

179. Lobo-Yeo A, et al. Class I and class II major histocompatibility complex antigen expression on hepatocytes: a study in children with liver disease. Hepatology 1990;12:223–32.

180. Sargent CA, et al. Human major histocompatibility complex contains genes for the major heat shock protein HSP 70. Proc Natl Acad Sci U S A 1989;86:1968–77.

181. Albertella MR, et al. Localisation of eight additional genes in the human major histocompatibility complex, including the gene encoding the casein kinase II beta subunit, and DNA sequence analysis of the class III region. DNA Seq 1996;7:9–12.

182. Geller SA, et al. Histopathology of α₁-antitrypsin liver disease in a transgenic mouse model. Hepatology 1990;12:40–7.

183. Geller SA, et al. Hepatocarcinogenesis is the sequel to hepatitis in Z #2 α₁-antitrypsin transgenic mice: histopathological and DNA ploidy studies. Hepatology 1994;19:389–97.

184. Chisari FV. Hepatitis B virus transgenic mice: insights into the virus and the disease. Hepatology 1995;22:1317–25.

185. Wu Y, et al. A lag in intracellular degradation of mutant α₁-antitrypsin correlates with the liver disease phenotype in homozygous PiZZ α₁-antitrypsin deficiency. Proc Natl Acad Sci U S A 1994;91:9014–8.

186. Gaczynska M, Rock KL, Goldber AL. Gamma-interferon and expression of MHC genes regulate peptide hydrolysis by proteasomes. Nature 1993;365:264–7.

187. McCracken AA, et al. Yeast mutants deficient in ER-associated degradation of the Z variant of alpha-1-protease inhibitor. Genetics 1996;144:1355–62.

188. Bathurst IC, et al. Human Z alpha-1-antitrypsin accumulates intracellularly and stimulates lysosomal activity when synthesized in the *Xenopus* oocyte. FEBS Lett 1985;183:304–8.

189. Kisen GO, Tessitore L, Costelli P, et al. Reduced autophagic activity in primary rat hepatocellular carcinoma and ascites hepatoma cells. Carcinogenesis 1993;14:2501–5.

190. Liang XH, Jackson S, Seaman M, et al. Induction of autophagy and inhibition of tumorigenesis by beclin 1. Nature 1999; 402:672–6.

191. Johnston JA, Ward CL, Kopito RR. Aggresomes: a cellular response to misfolded proteins. J Cell Biol 1998;7:1883–98.

192. Kopito RR. Aggresomes, inclusion bodies and protein aggression. Trends Cell Biol 2000;10:524–7.

193. Kopito RR, Sitia R. Aggresomes and Russell bodies. Symptoms of cellular indigestion? EMBO J 2000;3:225–31.

194. Dickson JM, Bergeron JJM, Shames I, et al. Association of calnexin with mutant peripheral myelin protein-22 ex vivo: a basis for "gain-of-function" ER diseases. Proc Natl Acad Sci U S A 2002;99:9852–7.

195. Teckman JH, An JK, Loethen S, Perlmutter DH. Effect of fasting on liver in a mouse model of α₁-antitrypsin deficiency: constitutive activation of the autophagic response. Am J Physiol 2002;283:G1156–65.

196. Nishino I, Fu J, Tanji K, et al. Primary LAMP-2 deficiency causes X-linked vacuolar cardiomyopathy and myopathy (Danon disease). Nature 2000;406:906–10.

197. Tanka Y, Guhde G, Suter A, et al. Accumulation of autophagic vacuoles and cardiomyopathy in LAMP-2-deficient mice. Nature 2000;406:902–6.

198. Teckman JH, An JK, Loethen S, Perlmutter DH. Mitochondrial autophagy and injury in the liver in alpha-1-antitrypsin deficiency. Am J Physiol. [In press]

199. Lemasters JJ, Nieminen AL, Qian T, et al. The mitochondrial permeability transition in cell death: a common mechanism in necrosis, apoptosis and autophagy. Biochim Biophys Acta 1998;1366:177–96.

200. Elmore SP, Qian T, Grisson DF, Lemasters JJ. The mitochondrial permeability transition initiates autophagy in rat hepatocytes. FASEB J 2001;15:2286–7.

201. Perkins G, Renken C, Martone ME, et al. Electron tomography of neuronal mitochondria: three-dimensional structure and organization of cristae and membrane contacts. J Struct Biol 1997;119:260–72.

202. Achleitner G, Gaigg B, Krasser A, et al. Association between the endoplasmic reticulum and mitochondria of yeast facilitates intraorganelle transport of phospholipids through membrane contact. Eur J Biochem 1999;264:545–53.

203. Wang HJ, Guay G, Pogan L, et al. Calcium regulates the association between mitochondria and a smooth subdomain of the endoplasmic reticulum. J Cell Biol 2000;150:1489–97.

204. Arnaudeau S, Kelley WL, Walsh JV, Demaurex N. Mitochondria recycle Ca2+ to the endoplasmic reticulum and prevent the depletion of neighboring endoplasmic reticulum regions. J Biol Chem 2001;276:29430–9.

205. Hacki J, Egger L, Conus S, et al. Apoptotic crosstalk between the endoplasmic reticulum and mitochondria controlled by Bcl-2. Oncogene 2000;19:2286–95.

206. Wei MC, Zong WX, Cheng EH-Y, et al. Proapoptotic BAX and BAK: a requisite gateway to mitochondrial dysfunction and death. Science 2001;292:727–30.

207. Anton LC, et al. Intracellular localization of proteasomal degradation of a viral antigen. J Cell Biol 1999;146:113–24.

208. Kaufman RL. Orchestrating the unfolded protein response in health and disease. J Clin Invest 2002;110:1389–98.

209. Ron D. Translational control in the endoplasmic reticulum stress response. J Clin Invest 2002;110:1383–8.

210. Pahl HL, Baeuerle PA. Endoplasmic-reticulum-induced signal transduction and gene expression. Trends Cell Biol 1997;7: 50–5.

211. Mathew A, Mathur SK, Morimoto RI. Heat shock response and protein degradation: regulation of HSF2 by the ubiquitin-proteasome pathway. Mol Cell Biol 1998;18:5091–8.

212. Laurell C-B, Eriksson J. The electrophoretic β₁-globulin pattern of serum in α₁-antitrypsin deficiency. Scand J Clin Lab Invest 1963;15:132–40.

213. Eriksson S. Studies in α₁ antitrypsin deficiency. Acta Med Scand Suppl 1965;432:1–85.

214. Sharp HL, et al. Cirrhosis associated with alpha-1-antitrypsin deficiency: a previously unrecognized inherited disorder. J Lab Clin Med 1969;73:934–9.

215. Sharp HL. Alpha-1-antitrypsin deficiency. Hosp Pract 1971; 6:83–96.

216. Moroz SP, et al. Liver disease associated with alpha-1-

antitrypsin deficiency in childhood. J Pediatr 1976;88: 19–25.

217. Hadchouel M, Gautier M. Histopathologic study of the liver in the early cholestatic phase of alpha-1-antitrypsin deficiency. J Pediatr 1976;89:211–5.

218. Odievre M, et al. Alpha-1-antitrypsin deficiency and liver disease in children: phenotypes, manifestations and prognosis. Pediatrics 1976;57:226–31.

219. McPhie JL, Binnie S, Brunt PW. α_1-Antitrypsin deficiency and infantile liver disease. Arch Dis Child 1976;51:584–8.

220. Hirschberger M, Stickler GB. Neonatal hepatitis and alpha-1-antitrypsin deficiency: the prognosis in five patients. Mayo Clin Proc 1977;52:241–5.

221. Nemeth A, Strandvik B. Natural history of children with alpha-1-antitrypsin deficiency and neonatal cholestasis. Acta Paediatr Scand 1982;71:993–9.

222. Nemeth A, Strandvik B. Liver disease in children with alpha-1-antitrypsin deficiency without neonatal cholestasis. Acta Paediatr Scand 1982;71:1001–5.

223. Nebbia G, et al. Early assessment of evolution of liver disease associated with α_1-antitrypsin deficiency in childhood. J Pediatr 1983;102:661–5.

224. Psacharopoulos HT, et al. Outcome of liver disease associated with α_1-antitrypsin deficiency (PiZ). Arch Dis Child 1983;58:882–7.

225. Udall JN, et al. Liver disease in α_1-antitrypsin deficiency: a retrospective analysis of the influence of early breast- vs bottle-feeding. JAMA 1985;253:2679–82.

226. Ghishan FK, Greene HL. Liver disease in children with PiZZ α_1-antitrypsin deficiency. Hepatology 1988;8:307–10.

227. Ibarguen E, Gross CR, Savik SK, Sharp HL. Liver disease in α_1-antitrypsin deficiency: prognostic indicators. J Pediatr 1990;117:864–70.

228. Cottrall K, Cook PJL, Mowat AP. Neonatal hepatitis syndrome and alpha-1-antitrypsin deficiency: an epidemiological study in Southeast England. Postgrad Med J 1974;50:376–80.

229. Hope PL, Hall MA, Millward-Sadler GH, Normand IC. Alpha-1-antitrypsin deficiency presenting as a bleeding diathesis in the newborn. Arch Dis Child 1982;57:68–70.

230. Ghishan FR, Gray GF, Greene HL. α_1-Antitrypsin deficiency presenting with ascites and cirrhosis in the neonatal period. Gastroenterology 1983;85:435–8.

231. Laurell CB, Sveger T. MARS screening of newborn Swedish infants for α_1-antitrypsin deficiency. Am J Hum Genet 1975; 27:213–7.

232. Eriksson S, Carlson J, Velez R. Risk of cirrhosis and primary liver cancer in alpha-1-antitrypsin deficiency. N Engl J Med 1986;314:736–9.

233. Volpert D, Molleston JP, Perlmutter DH. Alpha-1-antitrypsin deficiency-associated liver disease may progress slowly in some children. J Pediatr Gastroenterol Nutr 2001;32:265–9.

234. Hodges JR, Millward Sadler GH, Barbatis C, Wright R. Heterozygous MZ α_1-antitrypsin deficiency in adults with chronic active hepatitis and cryptogenic cirrhosis. N Engl J Med 1981;304:357–60.

235. Graziadei IW, et al. Increased risk of chronic liver failure in adults with heterozygous α_1-antitrypsin deficiency. Hepatology 1998;28:1058–63.

236. Propst T, et al. High prevalence of viral infections in adults with homozygous and heterozygous α_1-antitrypsin deficiency and chronic liver disease. Ann Intern Med 1992;117:641–5.

237. Clark P, Chong AYH. Rare alpha-1-antitrypsin allele PI$_w$ and a history of infant liver disease. Am J Med Genet 1992;45: 674–6.

238. Kelly CP, et al. Heterozygous FZ α_1-antitrypsin deficiency asso-

ciated with severe emphysema and hepatic disease: case report and family study. Thorax 1989;44:758–9.

239. Ghishan FK, Greene HL. Inborn errors of metabolism that lead to permanent liver injury. In: Zakim D, Boyer TD, editors. Hepatology: a textbook of liver disease. Philadelphia: WB Saunders; 1982. p. 1351.

240. Mowat AP. Hepatitis and cholestasis in infancy: intrahepatic disorders. In: Mowat AP, editor. Liver disorders in childhood. London: Butterworths & Co; 1982. p. 50.

241. Qizibash A, Yong-Pong O. Alpha-1-antitrypsin liver disease: differential diagnosis of PAS-positive diastase-resistant globules in liver cells. Am J Clin Pathol 1983;79:697–702.

242. Yunis EJ, Agostini RM, Glew RH. Fine structural observations of the liver in α_1-antitrypsin deficiency. Am J Clin Pathol 1976;82:265–86.

243. Johnson K, Alton HM, Chapman S. Evaluation of mebrofenin hepatoscintigraphy in neonatal-onset jaundice. Pediatr Radiol 1998;28:937–41.

244. Nord KS, Saad S, Joshi VV, McLoughlin LC. Concurrence of α_1-antitrypsin deficiency and biliary atresia. J Pediatr 1987;416–8

245. Silverman EK, et al. A family study of the variability of pulmonary function in alpha-1-antitrypsin deficiency. Am Rev Respir Dis 1990;142:1015–21.

246. Guenter CA, et al. The pattern of lung disease associated with alpha-1-antitrypsin deficiency. Arch Intern Med 1968;122: 254–9.

247. Thurlbeck WM, et al. Chronic obstructive disease: a comparison between clinical, roentgenologic, functional and morphologic criteria in chronic bronchitis, emphysema, asthma and bronchiectasis. Medicine 1970;49:81–98.

248. Glasgow JFT, et al. Alpha$_1$ antitrypsin deficiency in association with both cirrhosis and chronic obstructive lung disease in two sibs. Am J Med 1973;54:181–94.

249. Talamo RC, et al. Symptomatic pulmonary emphysema in childhood associated with hereditary alpha-1-antitrypsin and elastase inhibitor deficiency. J Pediatr 1971;79:20–6.

250. Houstek J, et al. Alpha1-antitrypsin deficiency in a child with chronic lung disease. Chest 1973;64:773–6.

251. Dunand P, Cropp GJA, Middleton E Jr. Severe obstructive lung disease in a 14-year-old girl with alpha-1 antitrypsin deficiency. J Allergy Clin Immunol 1975;57:615–22.

252. Wagener JS, Sobonya RE, Taussig LM, Lemen RJ. Unusual abnormalities in adolescent siblings with α_1-antitrypsin deficiency. Chest 1983;83:464–8.

253. Hird MF, et al. Hyperinflation in children with liver disease due to α_1-antitrypsin deficiency. Pediatr Pulmonol 1991;11:212–6.

254. Wiebicke W, Niggermann B, Fischer A. Pulmonary function in children with homozygous alpha-1-protease inhibitory deficiency. Eur J Pediatr 1996;155:603–7.

255. Larsson C. Natural history and life expectancy in severe alpha-1-antitryspin deficiency, PiZ. Acta Med Scand 1978;204:345–51.

256. Janus ED, Phillips NT, Carrell RW. Smoking, lung function and alpha-1-antitrypsin deficiency. Lancet 1985;i:152–4.

257. Schonfeld JV, et al. Liver function in patients with pulmonary emphysema due to severe alpha-1-antitrypsin deficiency (PIZZ). Digestion 1996;57:165–9.

258. Tobin MJ, Cook PJL, Hutchison DCS. Alpha-1-antitrypsin deficiency: the clinical and physiological features of pulmonary emphysema in subjects homozygous for P$_1$ type Z. Br J Dis Chest 1983;77:14–27.

259. Casavilla F, et al. Liver transplantation for neonatal hepatitis as compared to the other two leading indications for liver transplantation in children. Hepatology 1994;21:1035–9.

260. Kayler LK, et al. Long-term survival after liver transplantation

in children with metabolic disorders. Pediatr Transplant 2002;6:295–300.

261. Starzl TE, et al. Liver disease in alpha-1-antitrypsin deficiency: prognostic indicators. J Pediatr 1990;117:864–70.

262. Cuervas-Mons V, et al. Does previous abdominal surgery alter the outcome of pediatric patients subjected to orthotopic liver transplantation? Gastroenterology 1986;90:853–7.

263. Gelfand JA, et al. Treatment of hereditary angioedema with danazol: reversal of clinical and biochemical abnormalities. N Engl J Med 1976;195:1444–8.

264. Gadek JE, et al. Danazol-induced augmentation of serum alpha-1-antitrypsin levels in individuals with marked deficiency of this anti-protease. J Clin Invest 1980;66:82–7.

265. Wewers MD, et al. Evaluation of danazol therapy for patients with PiZZ alpha-1-antitrypsin deficiency. Am Rev Respir Dis 1986;134:476–80.

266. Perlmutter DH. Chemical chaperones: a pharmacological strategy for disorders of protein folding and trafficking. Pediatr Res 2002;52:832–6.

267. Jacobs GS. Glycosylation inhibitors in biology and medicine. Curr Opin Struct Biol 1995;5:605–11.

268. Zitzmann N, Mehta AS, Carrouee S, et al. Imino sugars inhibit the formation and secretion of bovine viral diarrhea virus, a pestvirus model of hepatitis C virus: implications for the development of broad spectrum antihepatitis virus agents. Proc Natl Acad Sci U S A 1999;96:11878–82.

269. Marcus NY, Perlmutter DH. Glucosidase and mannosidase inhibitors mediate increased secretion of mutant α_1-antitrypsin Z. J Biol Chem 2000;275:1987–92.

270. Novoradovskaya N, et al. Inhibition of intracellular degradation increases secretion of a mutant form of alpha1-antitrypsin associated with profound deficiency. J Clin Invest 1998;101:2693–701.

271. Crystal RG. Alpha-1-antitrypsin deficiency, emphysema and liver disease: genetic basis and strategies for therapy. J Clin Invest 1990;95:1343–52.

272. Alpha-1-Antitrypsin Deficiency Registry Study Group. Survival and FEV_1 decline in individuals with severe deficiency of α_1-antitrypsin. Am J Respir Crit Care Med 1998;158:49–59.

273. Trulock EP. Lung transplantation for α_1-antitrypsin deficiency emphysema. Chest 1996;110:284S–94S.

274. Anderson WF. Human gene therapy. Nature 1998;392:25–30.

275. Lan N, et al. Ribozyme-mediated repair of sickle β-globin mRNAs in erythrocyte precursors. Science 1998;280:1593–6.

276. Kren BT, Bandyopadhyay P, Steer CJ. In vivo site-directed mutagenesis of the factor IX gene by chimeric RNA/DNA oligonucleotides. Nat Med 1998;4:285–90.

277. Rhim JA, Sandgen EP, Degen JL, Brinster RL. Replacement of disease mouse liver by hepatic cell transplantation. Science 1994;263:1149–52.

278. Overturf K, et al. Hepatocytes corrected by gene therapy are selected in vivo in a murine model of hereditary tyrosinaemia type I. Nat Genet 1996;12:266–73.

279. Mahadeva R, Dafforn TR, Carrell RW, Lomas DA. 6-Mer peptide selectively anneals to a pathogenic serpin conformation and blocks polymerization. J Biol Chem 2002;277:6771–4.

280. Day PM, et al. Direct delivery of exogenous MHC class I molecule-binding oligopeptides to the endoplasmic reticulum of viable cells. Proc Natl Acad Sci U S A 1997;94:8064–9.

281. Johannes L, Goud B. Surfing on a retrograde wave: how does Shiga toxin reach the endoplasmic reticulum? Trends Cell Biol 1998;8:158–62.

282. Lord JM, Roberts LM. Toxin entry: retrograde transport through the secretory pathway. J Cell Biol 1998;140:733–6.

283. Kidd VJ, et al. Prenatal diagnosis of alpha-1-antitrypsin deficiency by direct analysis of the mutation site in the gene. N Engl J Med 1984;310:639–42.

284. Cox DW, Mansfield T. Prenatal diagnosis of alpha-1-antitrypsin deficiency and estimates of fetal risk for disease. J Med Genet 1987;24:52–9.

285. Nukiwa T, et al. Evaluation of "at risk" alpha-1-antitrypsin genotype SZ with synthetic oligonucleotide gene probes. J Clin Invest 1986;77:528–37.

286. Thelin T, Sveger T, McNeil TF. Primary prevention in a high-risk group: smoking habits in adolescents with homozygous alpha-1-antitrypsin deficiency. Acta Paediatr 1996;85:1207–12.

287. Wall M, et al. Long-term follow-up of a cohort of children with alpha-1-antitrypsin deficiency. J Pediatr 1990;116:248–51.

288. McNeil TF, Sveger T, Thelin T. Psychosocial effects of screening for somatic risk: the Swedish α_1-antitrypsin experience. Thorax 1988;43:505–7.

289. Sveger T, Thelin T, McNeil TF. Young adults with α_1-antitrypsin deficiency identified neonatally: their health, knowledge about and adaptation to the high-risk condition. Acta Paediatr 1997;86:37–40.

8. Zellweger Syndrome and Other Disorders of Peroxisomal Metabolism

Richard I. Kelley, MD, PhD

Gerald V. Raymond, MD

Paul A. Watkins, MD, PhD

Zellweger syndrome and an expanding spectrum of related peroxisomal diseases have emerged in the last 20 years as major identifiable causes of liver disease in the pediatric population. Because of the wide range of associated nonhepatic abnormalities in these disorders and the often initially silent nature of the progressive liver disease, many patients with peroxisomal diseases come to the attention of the gastroenterologist from a number of different hospital clinics, where they may have been followed for many months or years. Thus, a thorough understanding of the full spectrum of clinical and metabolic characteristics of peroxisomal disorders is essential for practicing gastroenterologists.

The cerebrohepatorenal syndrome of Zellweger is by far the best known genetic disorder of peroxisomal metabolism. Although Zellweger syndrome was first described as an autosomal recessive, multiple anomaly syndrome in 1964,[1] the discovery in 1973 that hepatic and renal cells of patients with Zellweger syndrome were devoid of recognizable peroxisomes and had dysfunctional mitochondria refocused attention on Zellweger syndrome as a possible metabolic disorder.[2] As a result, Zellweger syndrome emerged as the prototypic "metabolic malformation syndrome" and spawned the development of a new field of biochemical genetics. Indeed, more than a dozen clinical disorders have been identified or redescribed as diseases of the peroxisome. In some, such as classic Zellweger syndrome and neonatal adrenoleukodystrophy (ALD), the entire peroxisome and most of its associated biochemical functions appear to be lost or severely deficient. In others, such as X-linked ALD and several disorders of bile acid biosynthesis, only a single peroxisomal protein appears to be deficient. The different patterns of biochemical abnormalities manifest by these diverse syndromes are now understood to be caused by, principally, several different defects of peroxisomal protein importation and a variety of single enzymatic deficiencies. Overall, the discovery and biochemical characterization of these peroxisomal experiments of nature have fundamentally changed our understanding of the role of the peroxisome in human metabolism. In this chapter, the principal metabolic functions of the peroxisomes and the major clinical disorders associated with an apparent primary deficiency of peroxisomal metabolism are reviewed. Guides to the diagnosis and treatment of the peroxisomal disorders are also presented.

STRUCTURE AND FUNCTION OF NORMAL PEROXISOMES

TISSUE DISTRIBUTION AND CHARACTERISTICS OF PEROXISOMES

Peroxisomes are ubiquitous subcellular organelles defined by de Duve as small (0.1–1.0 µm), dense, subcellular particles bounded by a single membrane and containing the enzymatic machinery for the evolution and consumption of hydrogen peroxide.[3] Similar peroxidative organelles in plants contain the important glyoxylate cycle and related carbohydrate pathways and are known as glyoxysomes. The term *microbodies* is commonly used to refer to both organelles.[4,5]

Although large (0.5–1.5 µm) and more conspicuous peroxisomes were first identified only in hepatocytes (Figure 55.8-1) and renal proximal tubule cells, essentially all mammalian cells except erythrocytes have since been found to contain peroxisomes. These organelles range in size from smaller (0.1–0.2 µm) microperoxisomes in the brain to the larger structures found in liver and kidney. Hepatocytes and renal tubule cells have the greatest abundance of peroxisomes, which may constitute as much as 1% of the cell mass, whereas the collective volume of peroxisomes in muscle, fibroblasts, and neuronal tissue is at least an order of magnitude less.[6,7] The number of peroxisomes per cell can range from fewer than 100 to more than 1,000. In most tissues, peroxisomes appear as round or ovoid organelles with a finely granular matrix, bounded by a single membrane and stainable by a catalase-detecting reaction with diaminobenzidine. Although by electron microscopy the single peroxisomal membrane appears trilaminar, it is notably thinner than the trilaminar single membrane of lysosomes and lacks the clear zone subjacent to the lysosomal membrane. The larger peroxisomes of some species include a dense, crystalline-like "nucleoid" core containing urate oxidase. Species that lack urate oxidase, such as humans and birds, also lack peroxisomal cores. An important characteristic of hepatic peroxisomes of some species, especially rats and mice, is proliferation induced by a variety of natural and xenobiotic compounds, such as *trans*–unsaturated fatty acids, clofibrate, and thyroxine.[8,9] The proliferative action of these compounds is mediated by peroxisome proliferator-activated receptors

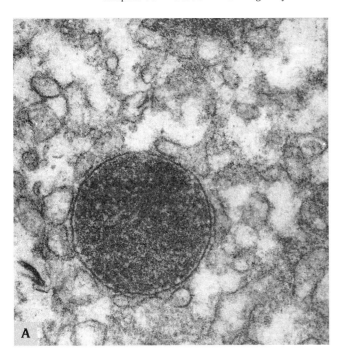
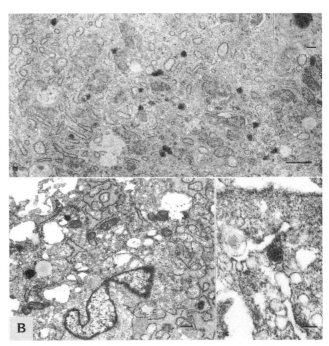

FIGURE 55.8-1 *A*, Electron micrograph of a normal human liver peroxisome showing a heterogeneous matrix surrounded by a single membrane. Human peroxisomes lack the dense "nucleoids" present in the peroxisomes of most other vertebrate species. *B*, Electron micrographs of fibroblasts incubated in a medium for the demonstration of peroxisomal catalase by the deposition of an electron-dense reaction product. *Bottom*, Normal human fibroblast containing several peroxisomes with variable staining (*inset*: magnification to show heterogeneous distribution of catalase staining). *Top*, Electron-dense small peroxisomes in the cytoplasm of fibroblasts from a patient with Zellweger syndrome. Courtesy of Sydney Goldfischer, MD.

(PPARs), which are closely related to steroid hormone receptors.[10–13] However, although peroxisomal proliferation is associated with hepatic neoplasia in rats,[14] there is little evidence for drug-mediated peroxisomal proliferation or hypolipidemic drug-mediated carcinogenesis in humans despite the presence of PPARs in human tissues.[13]

Peroxisomes appear to be independent organelles with a biogenesis separate from other subcellular organelles and compartments.[15,16] Extensive investigation of peroxisome biogenesis has refuted early hypotheses that these organelles arise from budding of the endoplasmic reticulum (ER). Gould and colleagues have proposed that there are two coexisting pathways of peroxisome biogenesis: one involving growth and division of preexisting peroxisomes and the other beginning with a preperoxisomal membrane vesicle.[16] Both models require uptake of lipid and membrane proteins as well as matrix proteins, followed by fission once a critical size is reached. Extensive genetic studies using yeast mutants, Chinese hamster ovary cell mutants, and skin fibroblasts from patients with peroxisomal biogenesis disorders have revealed the existence of at least 23 genes involved in peroxisome biogenesis.[15] The genes are referred to as *PEX* genes and their protein products as peroxins. Deficiency or mutation in 11 of the *PEX* genes is now known to result in human peroxisomal biogenesis disorders. Unlike mitochondria, there is no evidence for specific peroxisomal deoxyribonucleic acid (DNA) encoding the synthesis of peroxisomal proteins. All peroxins, as well as other membrane and matrix proteins, are encoded by nuclear genes and are synthesized on free polyribosomes.

Matrix proteins are targeted to peroxisomes primarily by one of two peptidyl targeting signals. The majority of matrix proteins have been found to contain peroxisome targeting signal (PTS) 1, a carboxy-terminal tripeptide with a suggested consensus of (S/A/C)-(K/R/H)-L-COOH.[17] Fewer matrix proteins are targeted to the organelle by PTS2, found near but not at the amino terminus, which has a consensus sequence of (R/K)-(L/V/I)-X$_5$-(Q/H)-(L/A).[16] The receptors for PTS1 and PTS2 proteins are encoded by the *PEX5* and *PEX7* genes, respectively.[18,19] The currently accepted model of peroxisomal matrix protein import involves numerous peroxins located in both the cytoplasm and the peroxisomal membrane.[16] After a newly synthesized matrix protein binds to its receptor in the cytoplasm, the complex is transported to the surface of the peroxisome, where it interacts with docking proteins and the import machinery. The matrix protein is imported into the peroxisome, and the receptor is returned to the cytoplasm via recycling factors. Although several peroxins have been implicated in the import of peroxisomal membrane proteins, this process remains less well characterized than matrix protein import.

Peroxisomes are mostly randomly distributed in hepatocytes but may occur closely juxtaposed to the ER, from which peroxisomes were once thought to arise by budding. In some cells, peroxisomes are seen surrounding glycogen or triglyceride deposits.[20] The close association of peroxisomes with ER is denoted structurally by a dense thickening (the "marginal plate") of the segment of the peroxisomal membrane paralleling the ER.[21,22] Moreover, in tissues with a high rate of fatty acid β-oxidation, there is a nonrandom association of peroxisomes with mitochondria, usually separated by an intercalated bilayer of ER.[20] An extreme structural specialization of peroxisomes occurs in the cells of sebaceous glands, wherein the peroxisomal compartment exits as an extensive filamentous network believed to subserve the synthesis of the unusual waxes and ether-lipids of sebum.[23] Coreless, filamentous tails and interperoxisomal connections have also been found by careful serial sectioning of rat liver[24] and may be common, if variable, features of the peroxisomal space.

METABOLIC PATHWAYS OF THE PEROXISOME

Once thought to be vestigial, the vertebrate peroxisome is now known to contain a remarkable variety of highly specialized and essential enzymatic systems for the synthesis and catabolism of, largely, lipids and amino acids (Table 55.8-1).[5] From a clinical-biochemical standpoint, the most important of these functions are (1) β-oxidation of very-long-chain fatty acids (VLCFAs) and 2-methyl branched-chain fatty acids; (2) synthesis of sterols and bile acids; (3) synthesis of plasmalogens; (4) α-oxidation of phytanic acid, a 3-methyl branched-chain fatty acid; (5) oxidase-mediated metabolism of amino acids; and (6) catalatic and peroxidatic decomposition of hydrogen peroxide. In addition, peroxisomes appear to have a role in the synthesis of cholesterol and, in some species, in the synthesis of highly specialized biochemicals such as waxy esters and pheromones.[25] For some processes, such as β-oxidation of fatty acids, a complete pathway exists in the peroxisome, whereas for others, such as bile acid or plasmalogen synthesis, only a portion of the pathway is unique to the peroxisome.

MAJOR METABOLIC FUNCTIONS OF THE PEROXISOME

Peroxisomal Fatty Acid β-Oxidation. Although fatty acid β-oxidation was first recognized as a function of peroxisomes (more exactly, glyoxysomes) of germinating seedlings in 1969,[26] not until 1978 was a complete ensemble of β-oxidative enzymes functionally similar to those of mitochondria found in mammalian peroxisomes (Figure 55.8-2).[27] However, despite identical stereochemistry and evolutionary homology of most of the peroxisomal β-oxidation enzymes and their counterparts in mitochondria,[28] the rate-limiting enzymes and substrate specificities

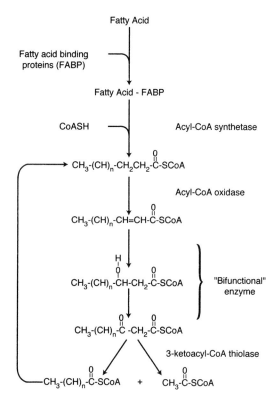

FIGURE 55.8-2 Peroxisomal pathway for β-oxidation of fatty acids. Medium-chain, long-chain, and very-long-chain fatty acids are shortened by two carbons for each cycle of β-oxidation down to an 8- or 6-carbon fatty acid. The acetate units and remnant fatty acids leave the peroxisome as carnitine esters via the action of acetylcarnitine and octanoylcarnitine transferases.

of β-oxidation in the two organelles are distinctly different. Recently, additional enzymes comprising a second, complete peroxisomal β-oxidation pathway have been identified in mammals.[29] Whereas the original peroxisomal β-oxidation pathway follows L-isomer enzymology and oxidizes straight-chain saturated fatty acids, the second, the D-specific peroxisomal pathway, catalyzes the oxidation of branched-chain fatty acids, including oxidation of the branched sterol side chain required for the synthesis of bile acids.[30] There is compelling evidence for interaction and crossover between the L- and D-specific pathways because the degradation of straight-chain VLCFAs requires enzymes from both pathways.[31]

There is considerable similarity between the enzymes and the enzymatic reactions of the two peroxisomal β-oxidation pathways. The first step in both pathways is carried out by an acyl coenzyme A (CoA) oxidase that consumes molecular oxygen and generates hydrogen peroxide. The straight-chain oxidase has broad specificity for all but short-chain (C_4–C_8) fatty acids.[32] In contrast, at least four separate acyl-CoA dehydrogenases—short-, medium-, long-, and very-long-chain acyl-CoA dehydrogenases—catalyze the degradation of straight-chain fatty acids in mitochondria. Deficiency of the straight-chain acyl-CoA oxidase in humans leads to the accumulation of VLCFAs and a distinct clinical disorder.[33,34] Known substrates for the branched-chain acyl-CoA oxidase are 2-methylacyl CoAs and include pristanic acid, a product of phytanic acid

TABLE 55.8-1   MAJOR METABOLIC FUNCTIONS OF THE PEROXISOME

β-Oxidation of very-long-chain fatty acids
β-Oxidation of branched-chain fatty acids
β-Oxidation of dicarboxylic acids
α-Oxidation of phytanic acid
Synthesis of ether lipids (eg, plasmalogens)
Synthesis of sterol precursors and bile acids
Synthesis of waxy esters
Amino acid transamination
Oxidation of D- and L-amino acids
Oxidation of L-α-hydroxy acids
Oxidative catabolism of polyamines
Catabolism of purines
Catalatic and peroxidatic decomposition of hydrogen peroxide

oxidation,[35] and precursors of bile acids.[36] The second and third reactions of both peroxisomal pathways are carried out by monomeric, multifunctional proteins that contain both enoyl-CoA hydratase and 3-hydroxyacyl-CoA dehydrogenase activities.[37] In contrast, two separate proteins in mitochondria catalyze these steps. The originally identified "bifunctional enzyme," now known as either multifunctional enzyme (MFE) 1 or L-bifunctional protein (L-BP), is L-specific. However, human deficiency of the more recently described D-specific enzyme, referred to as either MFE2 or D-bifunctional protein (D-BP), causes a failure in the oxidation of VLCFAs and branched-chain fatty acids. MFE2 was found to be identical to 17β-hydroxysteroid dehydrogenase type 4 and has a domain at its carboxy terminus that resembles sterol carrier protein (SCP) 2, an important intracellular sterol and lipid-binding and transport protein.[38] The terminal β-oxidation reactions for both peroxisomal pathways are catalyzed by a 3-ketoacyl CoA thiolase, as in the mitochondrial β-oxidation system. The thiolase of the L-specific peroxisomal pathway is one of the few known PTS2-containing proteins. The thiolase of the D-specific pathway resides in the amino-terminal domain of SCPX, a 58 kD protein that is cleaved to form the two smaller functional proteins.[39]

Several other enzymes and proteins are involved in peroxisomal β-oxidation, and deficiencies of two of these are known to cause human disease. Clinically, the most important of these is the ALD protein, ALDP, a peroxisomal transmembrane transporter protein.[40] Mutations in the *ABCD1* gene that encodes ALDP lead to the accumulation of VLCFAs and the most common peroxisomal disease, X-linked ALD. Despite extensive investigation since the discovery of ALDP in 1993, the exact function of this protein remains unknown.

More recently, the importance of 2-methylacyl CoA racemase in peroxisomal β-oxidation of 2-methyl branched-chain compounds such as pristanic acid and bile acid precursors has been recognized. Only one of the two naturally occurring stereoisomers of pristanic acid or bile acid precursors, the *S*-conformers, are substrates for branched-chain acyl CoA oxidase.[41,42] Peroxisomal racemase converts compounds with an *R*-conformation at the 2-carbon to the corresponding *S*-conformer, allowing subsequent metabolism to occur. Four patients with deficiency of 2-methylacyl CoA racemase have now been identified.

From a physiologic standpoint, mitochondria are most important in the conversion of dietary fatty acids—palmitate, oleate, linoleate, and stearate—into acetyl CoA for energy metabolism, ketogenesis, and various synthetic pathways. Peroxisomes, on the other hand, appear to specialize in the β-oxidation of VLCFAs (more than 22 carbons),[43] certain unsaturated fatty acids,[44,45] dicarboxylic acids,[46] branched-chain fatty acids,[47] and a variety of xenobiotic acids, such as phenyl-substituted fatty acids.[48] The end products of β-oxidation—acetyl CoA in mitochondria versus acetylcarnitine and octanoylcarnitine in peroxisomes—as well as the fate of the extracted reducing equivalents—coupled to adenosine triphosphate (ATP) synthesis in mitochondria versus lost to hydrogen peroxide and

its exergonic reactions in peroxisomes—also differ. Lastly, the total capacity of peroxisomal, but not mitochondrial, β-oxidation can be substantially amplified in some species by exposure to preferred substrates or drugs, such as clofibrate and related hypolipidemic drugs,[8,9] which also cause peroxisomal proliferation. The deficiency of this highly specialized system for β-oxidation is responsible for several of the clinically most important biochemical markers for peroxisomal disease, such as increased levels of VLCFAs.

Phytanic Acid Oxidation. Phytanic acid (3,7,11,15-tetramethylhexadecanoic acid) is a 3-methyl branched-chain fatty acid produced by oxidation of the free phytol

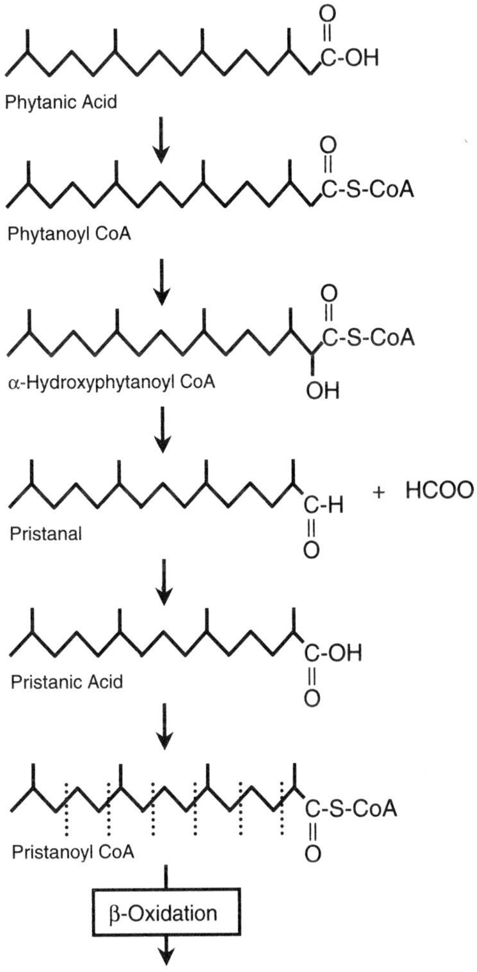

FIGURE 55.8-3 Sequence of α-oxidation of phytanic acid to pristanic acid and subsequent β-oxidation of pristanic acid to acetate and propionate units. α-Oxidation of phytanic acid, once thought to be coenzyme A (CoA) independent, requires activation of phytanate to a CoA intermediate, similar to β-oxidation in both mitochondria and peroxisomes. Pristanic acid, after reactivation to its CoA derivative, undergoes three cycles of β-oxidation in peroxisomes, alternately yielding propionyl CoA and acetyl CoA. The product of peroxisomal metabolism, 4,8-dimethylnonanoyl CoA, undergoes further degradation by mitochondrial β-oxidation. Not shown in this scheme is α-methylacyl CoA racemase, which is indispensible for converting any 2R-methylacyl CoAs to their 2s conformation.

chain of chlorophyll (Figure 55.8-3). Free phytol is concentrated in green vegetables, vegetable fats, and animal fats. However, phytanic acid formed by the action of phytol-metabolizing rumen bacteria and subsequently stored in animal and fish fats is the primary source of phytanic acid in human nutrition.[49,50] Once absorbed, dietary phytanic acid must undergo further α-oxidation in peroxisomes to remove the terminal carboxyl carbon to form pristanic acid (2,6,10,14-tetramethylpentadecanoic acid), a 2-methyl branched-chain fatty acid that is sequentially catabolized by the peroxisomal and mitochondrial β-oxidative systems.[35] Terminal Ω-oxidation activates a small portion of phytanic acid for β-oxidation from the omega end.[51]

Although it was originally thought that α-oxidation of phytanic acid began with a direct α-hydroxylation of the free acid by phytanic acid oxidase, more recent studies have established that a CoA derivative must be formed first.[52] Hydroxylation of the α-carbon by phytanoyl CoA α-hydroxylase (PAHX) yields L-2-hydroxyphytanoyl CoA, which is subsequently cleaved to formyl CoA and the aldehyde pristanal by 2-hydroxyphytanoyl CoA lyase.[53–56] Oxidation of pristanal to pristanic acid requires an aldehyde dehydrogenase, and early studies suggested that this dehydrogenase was identical to the microsomal enzyme defective in the mental retardation–ichthyosis disorder Sjögren-Larsson syndrome.[57] Most investigators now believe that a peroxisomal rather than a microsomal aldehyde dehydrogenase is responsible for the formation of pristanic acid, which, after activation to its CoA thioester, undergoes three rounds of peroxisomal β-oxidation (D-pathway) before transfer to mitochondria for further β-oxidation cycles.[35] As noted previously, pristanic acid β-oxidation requires the participation of α-methylacyl CoA racemase to convert R-pristanoyl CoA to S-pristanoyl CoA. Refsum disease has now been shown to be caused by mutations in PAHX.[58–60] Failure to import enzymes of both the α- and β-oxidation pathways in disorders of peroxisome biogenesis such as Zellweger syndrome results in the decreased ability to catabolize both phytanic acid and pristanic acid and the characteristic elevation of both phytol derivatives. Because phytanyl CoA α-hydroxylase is targeted to peroxisomes by PTS2, patients with rhizomelic chondrodysplasia punctata (RCDP) have impaired phytanic acid oxidation but normal pristanic acid oxidation.[61]

Cholesterol Biosynthesis. Hypocholesterolemia was one of the first relatively consistent biochemical abnormalities found in patients with Zellweger syndrome, suggesting that peroxisomes have a role in cholesterol biosynthesis. Sterols are synthesized by a complex series of reactions beginning with 3-hydroxy-3-methylglutaryl (HMG)-CoA and ending with the 30-carbon precursor of all other sterols, lanosterol (4,4,14-trimethylcholesta-8(9),24-dien-3β-ol). The first reaction in this complex biosynthetic pathway, the reduction of HMG-CoA to the 6-carbon acid alcohol mevalonic acid, is catalyzed by HMG-CoA reductase, which is generally accepted as the principal rate-determining step of cholesterol biosynthesis.[62] Cholesterol, a 27-carbon, monounsaturated sterol, is synthesized from

lanosterol by a series of oxidations, reductions, and demethylations. Although all steps of cholesterol synthesis in mammals were once thought to take place in the ER, studies by Krisans and colleagues have established that the second enzyme of the pathway, mevalonate kinase, and at least two other enzymes required for the conversion of mevalonate phosphate to farnesyl pyrophosphate—mevalonate phosphate kinase and farnesyl diphosphate synthase—are exclusively or largely localized to peroxisomes.[63–65] SCP2, an apparent carrier protein for intracellular sterol transport, also appears to be targeted to and processed by peroxisomes.[66] In contrast, various subcellular localization studies have shown that synthesis of squalene, a nonsterol precursor of lanosterol, by squalene synthase occurs exclusively in the ER.[67] Peroxisomes also contain a form of HMG-CoA reductase that is structurally and functionally distinct from the HMG-CoA reductase in the ER.[68,69] Because the HMG-CoA reductase of the ER is clearly the apparent rate-limiting enzyme for cholesterol biosynthesis, the role of the peroxisomal isozyme is unknown at this time. In addition, although there is evidence from one laboratory that peroxisomes contain all of the enzymes necessary for the conversion of lanosterol to cholesterol,[70] the relative role of these and other peroxisomal enzymes in overall cholesterol biosynthesis and homeostasis is unclear. Nevertheless, observations that patients with Zellweger syndrome have markedly depressed serum cholesterol levels[71] and that Zellweger fibroblasts in vitro have depressed rates of cholesterol synthesis[72] suggest an important role for peroxisomes in cholesterol biosynthesis. However, not all laboratories have found that Zellweger fibroblasts have decreased rates of cholesterol synthesis. Also important to consider is that because the earlier enzymatic steps of cholesterol biosynthesis also participate in the synthesis of all isoprenoid compounds, peroxisomes must also have an important role in the synthesis of dolichols and coenzyme Q, among the many diverse products of isoprenoid biosynthesis.

Bile Acid Synthesis. Bile acids are synthesized from cholesterol by a complex series of cytochrome P-450–dependent ring hydroxylations of the cholesterol steroid nucleus, followed by a final β-oxidative cleavage of a propionate group from the C_{20}–C_{27} branched side chain of cholesterol (Figure 55.8-4). Normally, only the final end products of bile acid synthesis, cholic acid and chenodeoxycholic acid, are present in bile or other body fluids in any significant amount. However, in 1972, Eyssen and colleagues reported that the duodenal fluid of infants with a Zellweger-like syndrome contained unusually large amounts of the bile acid intermediates dihydroxycholestanoic acid (DHCA) and trihydroxycholestanoic acid (THCA).[73] Until then, DHCA and THCA had been known to be abundant acids only in the bile of certain primitive vertebrates, such as the alligator. In addition, significant levels of a previously unknown C_{29}-dicarboxylic bile acid were found in the blood of patients with Zellweger syndrome.[74] The finding of increased levels of DHCA and THCA in Zellweger syndrome and the discov-

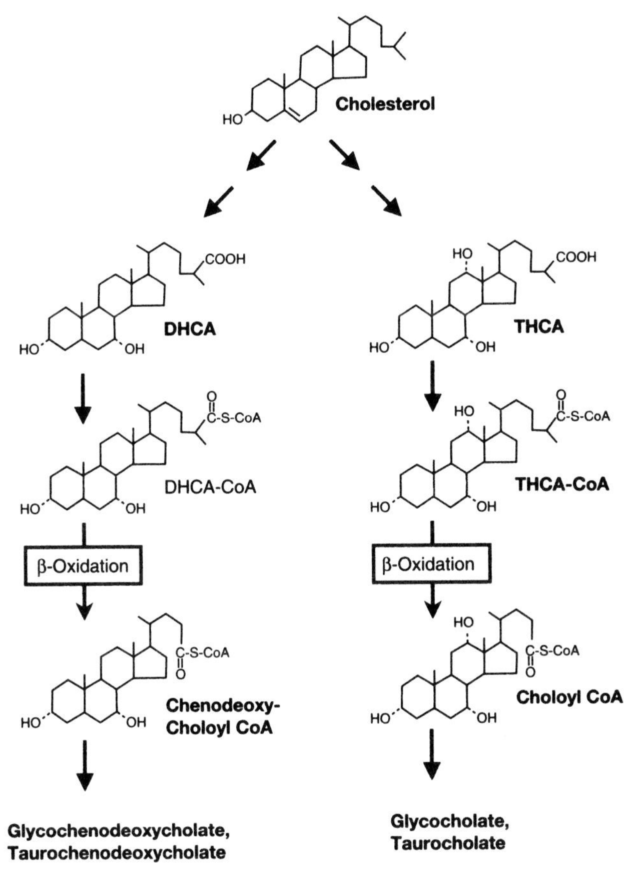

FIGURE 55.8-4 Conversion of cholesterol to bile acids via β-oxidation of the C_{22}–C_{27} side chain. After activation to their coenyzme A (CoA) derivatives, dihydroxycholestanoic acid (DHCA) and trihydroxycholestanoic acid (THCA) undergo one cycle of peroxisomal β-oxidation, yielding propionyl CoA and the CoA derivatives of chenodeoxycholic acid and cholic acid. DHCA-CoA and THCA-CoA can be conjugated to glycine or taurine by the peroxisomal enzyme bile acyl CoA:amino acid transferase. The levels of both DHCA and THCA are markedly increased in most patients with a peroxisome biogenesis disorder, such as Zellweger syndrome.

ery that hepatocytes of Zellweger syndrome are devoid of peroxisomes focused attention on the role of peroxisomes in the conversion of DHCA and THCA to their respective C_{24} bile acids, chenodeoxycholic acid and cholic acid.[36,74] Studies of the bile acids of patients with deficiency of the D-specific peroxisomal MFE2[30] also suggested involvement of peroxisomes in cholesterol side-chain cleavage.

Although bile acid ring hydroxylations take place primarily in the microsomal compartment, experimental evidence is compelling that cleavage of the cholesterol side chain, the final step in the synthesis of bile acids, occurs exclusively in the peroxisome. This conclusion has been reached both from careful subcellular fractionation studies in rat liver[36] and from the evidence that essentially all patients with Zellweger syndrome and related peroxisomal biogenesis disorders have increased levels of THCA, DHCA, and C_{29}-dicarboxylic bile acids.[75] The specific subcellular site of activation of DHCA and THCA to their CoA derivatives has not been resolved because enzymes capable of catalyzing this reaction are found both in microsomes and peroxisomes.[76,77]

Naturally occurring THCA and DHCA are mixtures of R- and S-stereoisomers, but only the latter can be chain-shortened by the peroxisomal β-oxidation machinery.[41] Once inside peroxisomes, the CoA derivatives of R-THCA and R-DHCA must be converted to their respective S-conformers by peroxisomal α-methylacyl CoA racemase. S-C27-CoA derivatives undergo side-chain shortening via the D-specific peroxisomal β-oxidation pathway, converting DHCA-CoA and THCA-CoA to chenodeoxycholyl CoA and cholyl CoA, respectively.[29,78] These C_{24}-CoA compounds are substrates for the peroxisomal PTS1-containing enzyme, bile acyl CoA:amino acid N-acyltransferase, yielding glycine and taurine conjugates of the primary bile acids.[79] The mechanism by which these compounds exit the peroxisome is not understood. As discussed in Chapter 55.4, "Disorders of the Bile Acid Synthesis," in addition to peroxisomal diseases, abnormal bile acid synthesis is characteristic of a number of genetic defects of microsomal oxidases and dehydrogenases, most of which are associated with progressive congenital or postnatal liver disease.

Ether-Lipid Biosynthesis. In contrast to conventional phospholipids, which contain two fatty acyl groups ester-linked to a glycerophosphoryl backbone, plasmalogens are phospholipids with one acyl group *ester*-linked to the second carbon and an unusual, α-unsaturated long-chain alcohol *ether*-linked to the first carbon. Plasmalogens are major components of membrane structural phospholipids in all cells and constitute up to 90% of ethanolamine phospholipids in myelin.[80] Platelet activating factor (alkyl-, acetyl-glycerophosphorylcholine) also is an ether-lipid, the only one known to have a specific biochemical function.[81]

The first two steps of ether-lipid biosynthesis (Figure 55.8-5) have been shown to take place in the peroxisome.[82] Esterification of fatty acyl CoA to the sn-1 position of dihydroxyacetone phosphate (DHAP) is first catalyzed by DHAP acyltransferase,[83] a PTS1-containing protein. Subsequently, the PTS2 protein alkyl-DHAP synthase catalyzes the replacement of the sn-1 acyl group with a fatty alcohol.[83] The product of these initial reactions, 1-alkyl-glycerol-3-phosphate, is then transferred to the ER, where α,-β desaturation of the alcohol occurs and where enzymes for normal ester-lipid biosynthesis complete the formation of plasmalogens. There is also evidence that acyl CoA reductase, which catalyzes the synthesis of the long-chain alcohols incorporated into plasmalogens, is a peroxisomal enzyme and derives its reducing equivalents from reduced nicotinamide adenine dinucleotide phosphate generated through the action of a peroxisomal form of isocitrate dehydrogenase.[84]

Catabolism of Pipecolic Acid and Other Amino Acids. Pipecolic acid (2-piperidinecarboxylic acid), a cyclic imino acid and homolog of proline, is synthesized in animals via a minor pathway of lysine catabolism and then further oxidized sequentially to α-aminoadipic acid and glutaric acid (Figure 55.8-6).[85] The initial and probable rate-limiting step in the catabolism of L-pipecolic acid is catalyzed by a flavin adenine dinucleotide–dependent, L-pipecolic acid oxidase,[86] a PTS1 protein that has now been purified and

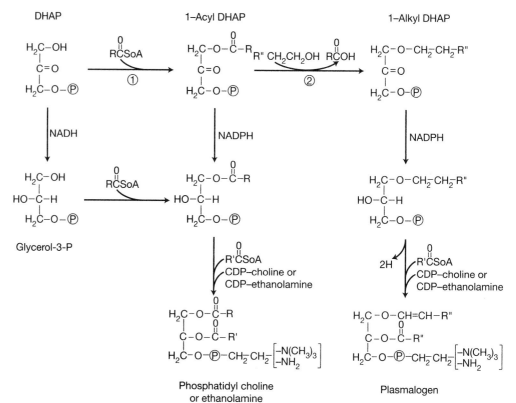

FIGURE 55.8-5 Pathway for biosynthesis of glycerol-ether lipids. Dihydroxyacetone phosphate (DHAP) acyltransferase and alkyl DHAP synthase, which catalyze the first two steps (labeled 1 and 2) in the synthesis of plasmalogens, are located in the peroxisome, whereas other reactions illustrated here take place in microsomes or mitochondria or both. CDP = cytidine diphosphate; CoA = coenzyme A; NADH = reduced nicotinamide adenine dinucleotide; NADPH = reduced nicotinamide adenine dinucleotide phosphate.

enzymatically and molecularly characterized.[87,88] Whereas both D and L forms of pipecolic acid occur in nature, only the L-isomer appears to be synthesized in animals, and only L-pipecolic acid accumulates to any significant degree in patients with peroxisomal biogenesis disorders.[89]

Although L-pipecolic acid has been shown experimentally to meet most criteria for an endogenously synthesized central nervous system (CNS) neurotransmitter and to have strong inhibitory effects on selected CNS neurons,[90] it is not clear what, if any, physiologic role pipecolic acid plays in the CNS. The rates of synthesis and oxidation of pipecolic acid, their tissue distribution, and even their subcellular localization appear to vary considerably among different vertebrate animals.[91] In most mammals, formation of pipecolic acid contributes to less than 1% of lysine degradation in the liver,[92] where the alternative saccharopine pathway of lysine metabolism (see Figure 55.8-6) appears to predominate. In contrast, conversion to L-pipecolic acid may be the major catabolic fate of L-lysine in rat brain.[93] More interesting is that whereas the peroxisome is the site of L-pipecolic acid oxidation to L-α-aminoadipic acid in humans and other primates,[94,95] only mitochondria appear to contain this activity in rabbits and rats.[95] Such differences in subcellular enzyme localization are unusual but not unprecedented and may reflect evolutionary flexibility of enzyme targeting mediated by cellular gene-splicing strategies. Interestingly, D-pipecolic acid, which is not abnormally elevated in Zellweger syndrome, appears to be oxidized only in peroxisomes in the rat and other animals.[96]

Metabolism of Hydrogen Peroxide. In mitochondria, the oxidation of a substrate by a nicotinamide adenine din-ucleotide– or flavin adenine dinucleotide–dependent dehydrogenase is followed by transfer of the extracted electrons to the electron transport (respiratory) chain and then eventually to oxygen to form water. In contrast, reducing equivalents in the peroxisome are transferred directly to molecular oxygen through the action of one of the flavin-dependent peroxisomal oxidases to form hydrogen peroxide.[5] The large amounts of hydrogen peroxide generated by the many different peroxisomal oxidases would be cytotoxic without mechanisms for its safe decomposition within the peroxisome. Catalase, which is one of the most abundant proteins in liver,[97] serves this function and decomposes hydrogen peroxide by either a *catalatic* mechanism:

$$2 H_2O_2 \rightarrow 2 H_2O + O_2$$

or a *peroxidatic* process:

$$H_2O_2 + RH_2 \rightarrow R + 2 H_2O$$

Most oxidase-generated hydrogen peroxide appears to be degraded in situ by the peroxidatic mechanism.[98] Although the absolute level of catalase activity in Zellweger syndrome cells is normal, most of the enzyme is found in the cytoplasmic compartment and not in the particulate (ie, peroxisome containing) fraction.[99]

The hydrogen peroxide–generating reactions of peroxisomal oxidases are highly exergonic and, unlike mitochondrial dehydrogenation reactions, are unconstrained by respiratory control and the synthesis of ATP. This exothermic nature of peroxisomal respiration may contribute to the heat-producing capacity of specialized tissues such as brown fat, in which cold adaptation causes a marked proliferation of peroxisomes.[100]

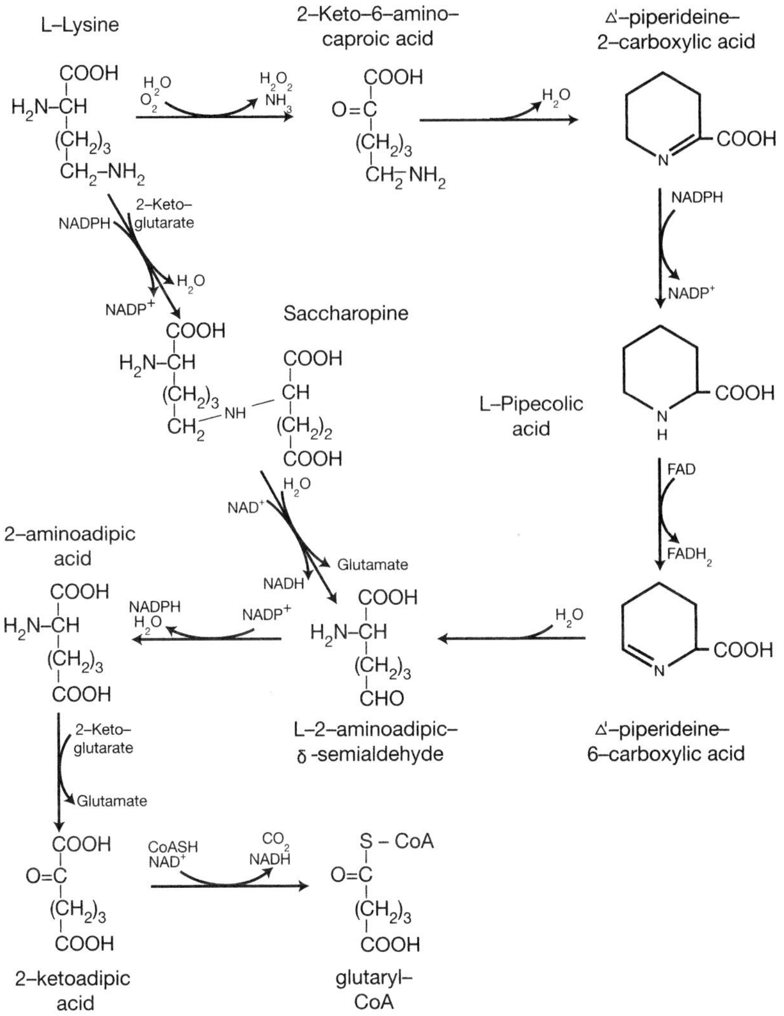

FIGURE 55.8-6   Biosynthesis of pipecolic acid and its relationship to the dual pathways for lysine catabolism to glutaryl coenzyme A (CoA). Glutaryl CoA is further catabolized both in peroxisomes and mitochondria. NADPH = reduced nicotinamide adenine dinucleotide phosphate.

PEROXISOMAL DISEASES

DISORDERS OF PEROXISOMAL BIOGENESIS

The nomenclature of the three syndromes now classified as disorders of peroxisomal biogenesis—Zellweger syndrome, infantile Refsum disease, and neonatal ALD—reflects more the type of specialists who first described the patients than the characteristic biochemistry or pathology of these overlapping syndromes (Table 55.8-2). Indeed, evidence has appeared that, for example, patients with the clinical diagnosis of infantile Refsum disease have mutations in one of at least three different genes, all of which can also be associated with the other two clinical phenotypes of generalized peroxisomal disease.[101] Altogether, 11 different complementation groups for disorders of peroxisomal biogenesis have been defined,[16,102,103] and, among these, mutations in 10 different *PEX* genes affecting PTS1-mediated peroxisomal assembly and enzyme import have been associated with one or more of these clinical syndromes. Two of the original complementation groups, numbers 1 and 4, now associated with mutations in *PEX1* and *PEX6*, respectively, include patients of all three clinical phenotypes and account for more than 80% of patients with a disorder of peroxisomal biogenesis. Mutations in *PEX7*, which encodes the receptor for proteins containing the second peroxisomal

enzyme import system PTS2, have been linked to the clinically quite different disorder RCDP.[61] These remarkable advances in our understanding of the molecular basis of peroxisomal diseases may eventually lead to a better understanding of the biochemical pathology and possibly even to therapy of these disorders. Despite our current understanding that Zellweger syndrome, infantile Refsum disease, and neonatal ALD can all be caused by different mutations in a single gene, and despite their often overlapping clinical and biochemical features, because much of the existing clinical literature views these three syndromes as separate clinical entities, they are discussed here individually.

Zellweger Syndrome.   Zellweger syndrome was first delineated in 1967 as a multiple congenital anomaly syndrome by Passarge and McAdams, who suggested the descriptive term "cerebrohepatorenal" syndrome.[104] Subsequently, Opitz presented a comprehensive study of the pathology of Zellweger syndrome,[105] whereas later review articles discussed the complexity of the associated biochemical abnormalities.[71,75]

The majority of patients with Zellweger syndrome are identified as newborns or young infants, based on a relatively stereotypic phenotype (Table 55.8-3) and a variety of anatomic and histologic abnormalities (Table 55.8-1).

TABLE 55.8-2   CLASSIFICATION OF PEROXISOMAL
                 DISEASES

DISORDERS OF PEROXISOMAL BIOGENESIS
  Zellweger cerebrohepatorenal syndrome
  Neonatal adrenoleukodystrophy
  Infantile Refsum disease
  Hyperpipecolic acidemia
  Rhizomelic chondrodysplasia punctata

DEFICIENCY OF A SINGLE PEROXISOMAL ENZYME OR PROTEIN
  Acyl CoA oxidase deficiency
    ("pseudo–neonatal adrenoleukodystrophy")
  Peroxisomal multifunctional enzyme 2 deficiency
  X-linked adrenoleukodystrophy
  CADDS (contiguous *ABCD1 DXS1357E* deletion syndrome)
  α-Methylacyl CoA racemase deficiency
  Dihydroxyacetone phosphate acyltransferase deficiency
  Alkyl-dihydroxyacetonephosphate synthase deficiency
  Hyperoxaluria type I (alanine:glyoxylate aminotransferase deficiency)
  Refsum disease (phytanyl CoA α-hydroxylase deficiency)
  Glutaryl CoA oxidase deficiency
  Acatalasemia

TABLE 55.8-4   ANATOMIC AND HISTOLOGIC
                 ABNORMALITIES IN ZELLWEGER
                 SYNDROME

Neurologic	Cerebral/cerebellar neuronal migration defects Microgyria, pachygyria, olivary dysplasia Septo-optic dysplasia, agenesis corpus callosum Dysmyelination, demyelination
Hepatic	Fibrosis progressing to cirrhosis Intrahepatic biliary dysgenesis and stasis Absent peroxisomes, abnormal mitochondria Iron storage (early); lipid storage (late)
Renal	Cortical glomerulocystic disease Hydronephrosis, persistent fetal lobulation
Skeletal	Chondrodysplasia punctata (nonrhizomelic) Osteoporosis, retarded skeletal maturation Bell-shaped chest (secondary to hypotonia)
Other	Pancreatic islet cell hyperplasia Thymic hypoplasia; Di George sequence

During infancy, the abnormalities that most suggest the diagnosis of Zellweger syndrome are the characteristic facial appearance (Figure 55.8-7), profound hypotonia, and absent neonatal reflexes. A typical infant with Zellweger syndrome has a high forehead with a widely open metopic suture, wide-spaced appearing and upslanting palpebral fissures, underdeveloped supraorbital ridges, triangular mouth, and apparently low-set, abnormally shaped ears. The appearance is sometimes reminiscent of Down syndrome. However, because most of the craniofacial and other dysmorphic characteristics of Zellweger syndrome are individually relatively nonspecific, the diagnosis of Zellweger syndrome is often missed at birth. Hepatocellular disease is usually less apparent during the first 3 months than later

TABLE 55.8-3   MAJOR CLINICAL CHARACTERISTICS
                 OF ZELLWEGER SYNDROME

Craniofacial	Midface hypoplasia resemblance to Down syndrome Hypertelorism, narrow papebral fissures Inner epicanthal folds, anteverted nares High narrow forehead, large fontanels, micrognathia
Skeletal	Clinodactyly, camptodactyly Equinovarus deformity, joint contractures
Neurologic	Severe hypotonia; absent Moro reflex, suck, grasp Complex seizure disorder (often neonatal) Profound psychomotor retardation Degenerative neurologic disease
Sensory	Optic atrophy, pigmentary retinopathy Cataracts, glaucoma, Brushfield spots Blindness (often congenital), nystagmus Sensorineural deafness
Hepatic	Hepatomegaly ± splenomegaly Prolonged or persistent jaundice Signs of portal hypertension Coagulopathy, biliary cirrhosis
Other	Cryptorchidism, hypospadias Patent ductus arteriosis, septal defects Single palmar creases

but may be evident as direct hyperbilirubinemia, hypertransaminasemia, coagulopathy, or hepatomegaly alone.[106,107] Other important and somewhat more specific clues to the diagnosis of Zellweger syndrome are glomerulocystic kidney disease,[108] abnormal calcification of the patella and other apophyseal cartilage (chondrodysplasia punctata),[109] cerebral dysgenesis,[110,111] and pigmentary retinopathy.[112] Structural abnormalities of the heart, mostly septal defects and conotruncal malformations, are also not uncommon. Seizures, which occur in over 70% of patients, are often difficult to treat. Indeed, a severe neonatal seizure disorder is one of the more common clinical problems that alone suggests the diagnosis of Zellweger syndrome. Because of the severity of the cerebral malformations, most infants with Zellweger syndrome achieve no developmental milestones and die within a few weeks or months of birth from seizures, apnea, aspiration, or pneumonia. Those patients who survive the first 6 months may show a slight degree of neurologic development and improved muscular tone but often eventually succumb to the complications of their severe neurologic disease. Rare patients in whom Zellweger syndrome has been diagnosed in the neonatal period have survived for more than 3 years.[113] Detailed compilations of the clinical characteristics of patients with Zellweger syndrome have been published by Heymans[114] and Wilson and colleagues.[115] Despite the tremendous expansion in our understanding of the biochemical and molecular bases of Zellweger syndrome and its related disorders, none of their malformative or degenerative characteristics has a clearly understood biochemical pathogenesis.

Although glomerulocystic disease of the kidney in Zellweger syndrome can be anatomically quite severe, renal glomerular or tubular insufficiency, apart from mild generalized aminoaciduria and proteinuria, is not common.[108] Similarly, the diagnostically important chondrodysplasia punctata affects mostly apophyseal cartilage, such as the patella, and does not itself cause dwarfing.[109] Other unexplained abnormalities with less obvious clinical consequences include islet cell hyperplasia, thymic hypoplasia, and siderosis.[104]

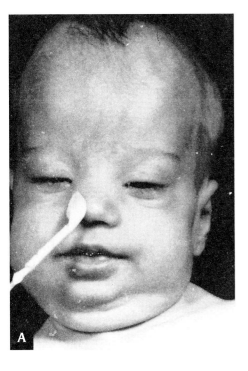
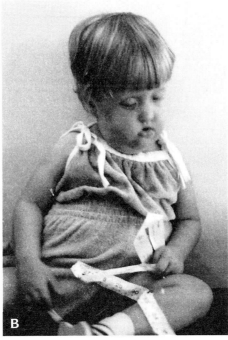

FIGURE 55.8-7 Facial appearance of two patients with Zellweger syndrome. A, At birth; B, at 3 years. Note in B the postural evidence of severe hypotonia.

The CNS disease of Zellweger syndrome is notable for the coexistence of congenital developmental abnormalities and acquired degenerative changes.[111,116-118] The most common CNS malformations are cerebral and cerebellar heterotopias, centrosylvian pachygyria and polymicrogyria, and olivary hypoplasia. Partial agenesis of the corpus callosum, hypoplasia of the cerebellar vermis, and septo-optic dysplasia are also common. Another unusual characteristic of patients with Zellweger syndrome is increased brain water and correspondingly increased brain weight. In addition to these abnormalities, most of which can be attributed to defective neuronal migration, myelin synthesis is qualitatively abnormal, and in longer-surviving individuals, a demyelinating process occurs.[116,118-120] When active demyelination is present (most commonly in the centrum semiovale, corpus callosum, occipital white matter, and cerebellum), macrophages with vacuolar lipid inclusions and "angulate" lysosomes are found. These storage macrophages are essentially the same as those found in the degenerating white matter of patients with X-linked ALD.[116,118,121] The recognition of an ALD-like white matter disease in Zellweger syndrome led to the discovery that patients with Zellweger syndrome, like those with X-linked ALD, have increased concentrations of VLCFAs, both in the CNS and systemically.[122-124]

Severe liver disease is almost universal in patients with Zellweger syndrome who survive the neonatal period.[106,107,125-128] Although the liver disease is often minimal during the first few months of life and may even appear to be absent, some combination of lobular disarray, focal hepatocytic necrosis, portal fibrosis or cirrhosis, intracellular and intracanalicular cholestasis, and increased iron storage can usually be found on biopsy. Foamy, lipid-filled hepatocytes, biliary dysgenesis, multinucleated giant cells, and focal areas of parenchymal collapse are also found, but less commonly (Figure 55.8-8). By electron microscopy and histochemistry (for the marker enzyme catalase), peroxi-

somes have been undetectable in the liver of almost all patients with classic Zellweger syndrome.[2,127] Abnormally shaped and dark-staining mitochondria with tubular cristae and paracrystalline inclusions, as well as scattered lipid-storage macrophages with angulate lysosomes, are also often found (Figure 55.8-9).[126] The chemical composition of the lamellar lipid material causing the distortion of lysosomes is not known but is suspected to consist of condensations of VLCFAs. Except for scattered cellular necrosis, the histology of individual hepatocytes is surprisingly normal, particularly in older infants, despite the progression of fibrosis and cirrhosis. By the age of 6 months, advanced cirrhosis and its many sequelae may dominate the clinical picture. Rapid progression from giant cell transformation without fibrosis to hepatocyte necrosis to cirrhosis in 3 to 4 months has been documented by serial biopsy in several patients. The cause of cirrhosis in Zellweger syndrome is not known, but increased levels of compounds such as hydrogen peroxide and unsaturated VLCFAs, which have aberrant metabolism in a peroxisome-deficient liver, have been proposed as hepatotoxins.

Another complication of liver disease in Zellweger syndrome and its related disorders is fat malabsorption and its multiple metabolic consequences, such as deficiencies of fat-soluble vitamins and nutritional failure to thrive. The cause of the malabsorption is often attributed to both the primary deficiency of bile acids and to the biliary abnormalities that follow the progressive cholestatic liver disease. These problems are not uncommon and, in milder forms of the disease, may even be the mode of presentation.[129,130]

Two biochemical abnormalities may have special importance in the evolution—and treatment—of the hepatic disease in Zellweger syndrome. First, the many abnormal species of bile acid that accumulate in the liver and other tissues of patients with Zellweger syndrome may cause injury to the liver. For this reason, there have

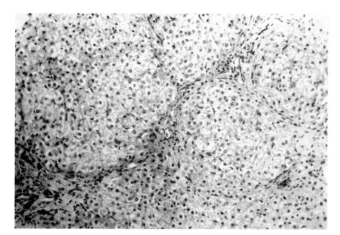

FIGURE 55.8-8   Liver histology in Zellweger syndrome showing lobular disorganization and early bridging fibrosis. Courtesy of H. Moser, MD.

been attempts to ameliorate possible bile acid toxicity by administration of bile acid supplements such as ursodeoxycholic acid, with some evidence of benefit.[131] Another more recently recognized abnormality is an almost universal severe deficiency of docosahexaenoic acid (DHA) and other related essential polyunsaturated fatty acids.[132,133] The cause of DHA deficiency in peroxisomal biogenesis disorders is reduced retroconversion of the precursor, $C_{24:6}$, to DHA via one cycle of peroxisomal β-oxidation.[134,135] Accordingly, many surviving patients

with Zellweger syndrome and related disorders have been treated with supplements of DHA.[133] A third deficiency that may have a role in the degenerative pathology of Zellweger syndrome is the severely depressed level of plasmalogens, which, some have speculated, have important antioxidant properties in cell membranes.[136]

In addition to a variety of diagnostically useful anatomic and histologic abnormalities, several laboratory tests are now available for diagnosis of defective peroxisomal metabolism; these are listed in Table 55.8-5 and discussed in more detail in following sections. All of these peroxisomal abnormalities can usually be demonstrated in an infant with Zellweger syndrome, and their documentation in the proper clinical setting usually obviates the need to demonstrate absent peroxisomes by liver biopsy. Other less specific but relatively common biochemical abnormalities are also listed in Table 55.8-5. Once biochemical studies have established that a patient with a Zellweger phenotype has abnormalities in multiple peroxisomal biochemical pathways, complementation analysis and now mutational studies can be undertaken to identify the specific genetic lesion.

Infantile Refsum Disease. Infantile Refsum disease was first described in 1982 by Scotto and colleagues as a syndrome of developmental retardation, pigmentary retinopathy, sensorineural hearing loss, and mildly to moderately increased plasma levels of phytanic acid.[137] Although infantile Refsum disease differs clinically from Zellweger syndrome, early fibroblast complementation studies indicated

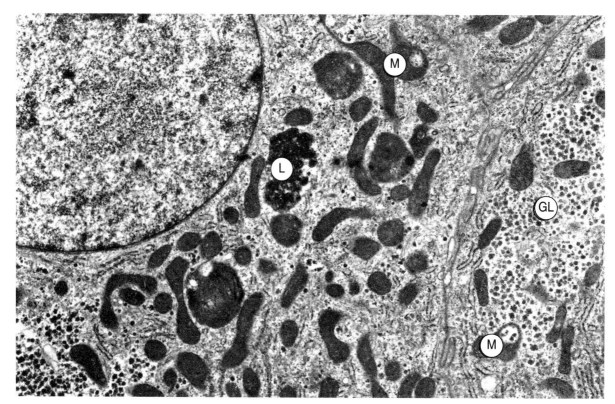

FIGURE 55.8-9   Liver ultrastructure in Zellweger syndrome. Mitochondria (M) with bizarre shapes and dense matrices are seen, together with normal lysosomes (L) and glycogen (GL). The mitochondrial abnormalities are most likely secondary phenomena because many patients with Zellweger syndrome have normal-appearing mitochondria. Courtesy of Sydney Goldfischer, MD.

TABLE 55.8-5   LABORATORY ABNORMALITES COMMON IN ZELLWEGER SYNDROME

ABNORMALITIES OF PEROXISOMAL METABOLISM

Increased levels of
  Very-long-chain fatty acids (p, u, t)
  Di- and trihydroxycholestanoic acids (p, u)
  Pipecolic and hydroxypipecolic acids (p, u)
  Phytanic and pristanic acids (p, t)
  Dicarboxylic and epoxydicarboxylic acids (p, u)
Decreased levels of
  Plasmalogens, platelet activating factor (p, t)
  Phytanic acid β-oxidation (t)
  Peroxisomal fatty acid β-oxidation (t)
  Particulate catalase (t)
  Normal bile acids (p, u)
  Docosahexaenoic and related acids (p, t)

SECONDARY OR UNEXPLAINED BIOCHEMICAL ABNORMALITIES

Increased levels of
  Serum transaminases, bilirubin
  Serum iron and iron saturation (early months)
  Cerebrospinal fluid protein (variable, late)
  Threonine (p, u)
  Urinary amino acids (generalized aminoaciduria)
  4-Hydroxyphenyllactate (u)
Decreased levels of
  Cholesterol (p)
  Prothrombin, other coagulation factors (p)

p = plasma; t = tissues/fibroblasts; u = urine.

that infantile Refsum disease is actually a mild form of Zellweger syndrome,[102,103] as originally suggested by Poulos and colleagues[138] and now fully confirmed by mutational studies of the involved *PEX* genes.[101,139]

The first patients with infantile Refsum disease described in the literature lacked the characteristic facial appearance of Zellweger syndrome, except for mild craniofacial abnormalities such as epicanthal folds, anteverted nares, and midfacial hypoplasia. Unlike patients with classic Zellweger syndrome, who rarely achieve any psychomotor development, those with infantile Refsum disease have learned to walk and even have acquired some language.[139,140] Similarly, hypotonia is less severe in infantile Refsum disease, and a few patients have shown improving or normal muscle tone and brisk deep tendon reflexes beyond infancy. However, because pigmentary retinopathy, macular degeneration, and sensorineural hearing loss are progressive conditions, the majority of patients with infantile Refsum disease become blind and deaf because of their longer survival.

Liver disease is much less prominent in infantile Refsum disease than it is in Zellweger syndrome. Levels of serum transaminases and bilirubin are usually normal or only slightly increased, and hepatomegaly is less common. Nevertheless, major complications of hepatic disease, such as cerebral and gastrointestinal hemorrhages secondary to coagulopathy, have occurred.[140] Both intrinsic liver disease and malabsorption of vitamin K secondary to defective bile acid synthesis probably contribute to the coagulopathy. Associated vitamin A and vitamin E deficiencies are also common and may exacerbate visual and neurologic degeneration, as likely does the associated deficiency of DHA.[141] Histologically, the livers of patients with infantile Refsum

disease do not have the lobular disorganization and biliary dysgenesis typical of Zellweger syndrome, but progressive fibrosis, apparently, is common. Morphologically recognizable peroxisomes are absent or at most represented by small numbers of catalase-positive microperoxisomes.[142] Hepatocytes and especially Kupffer cells often have inclusions of lipid vacuoles and leaflets similar to those of X-linked and neonatal ALD. In addition, unusual hepatocytic glycogen inclusions, only infrequently seen in Zellweger syndrome, appear to be relatively common in infantile Refsum disease. In one 12-year-old boy with infantile Refsum disease who came to autopsy, advanced micronodular cirrhosis was found.[143] Other important pathologic abnormalities in that patient included hypoplastic adrenal glands without degenerative changes, extensive infiltrates of lipid-storage macrophages in the lymph nodes, severe hypoplasia of the cerebellar granule layer, and severe degenerative changes in the retina and cochlea.

In addition to the full spectrum of peroxisomal biochemical abnormalities—increased levels of VLCFA, phytanic acid, pipecolic acid, and bile acid intermediates and depressed levels of DHA and erythrocyte plasmalogens—patients with infantile Refsum disease commonly have persistently low levels of serum cholesterol and both α- and β-lipoproteins.[140] Because plasmalogens and their precursors can be assimilated from the diet, erythrocyte plasmalogen levels, which are very low in infants with Zellweger syndrome, may increase and even normalize over a period of 6 to 12 months after birth. Nevertheless, when assayed in liver or fibroblasts, tissue levels and rates of synthesis of plasmalogens are consistently depressed.[140]

Neonatal Adrenoleukodystrophy. Between 1978 and 1982, several reports were published describing a total of 11 infants and young children of both sexes who suffered from a constellation of CNS, adrenal, and biochemical abnormalities almost identical to those of childhood (X-linked) ALD.[144,145] However, the apparent autosomal recessive inheritance of the disorder, its neonatal presentation, and a variety of associated systemic abnormalities uncharacteristic of X-linked ALD suggested that this new "neonatal" ALD was a genetically distinct disorder. The observation that some infants with neonatal ALD resembled patients with Zellweger syndrome then led to the discovery of multiple defects of peroxisomal metabolism and absent or severely diminished peroxisomes on liver biopsy in a number of these patients. Several review articles have described in detail the full spectrum of clinical and biochemical abnormalities in neonatal ALD.[145-147]

As in Zellweger syndrome, most infants with the neonatal ALD phenotype are severely hypotonic at birth and develop myoclonic seizures in the newborn period or the first few weeks of life. Dysmorphic features may be limited to midfacial hypoplasia, epicanthal folds, and simian creases or be absent altogether (Figure 55.8-10). Psychomotor development is globally retarded, and few patients achieve a mental age greater than 2 years. Growth is usually moderately retarded, although some patients have had normal linear growth. In addition, nystagmus, pigmentary retinopathy, optic atrophy, limited vision, and deafness further handicap most of these children. After many months or years of slow psychomotor development, children with neonatal ALD may develop a leukodystrophy, a progressive demyelination process, and begin to lose skills and enter a phase lasting over several months or years, during which complete neurologic deterioration to a terminal vegetative state ensues. The onset of the destructive white matter loss cannot be predicted, and the course is extremely variable.

The diagnosis of neonatal ALD is sometimes unsuspected until autopsy, when the finding of demyelination and adrenal atrophy suggests the diagnosis of a form of ALD. However, in contrast to the postnatally acquired CNS defects of X-linked ALD, signs of prenatal CNS maldevelopment such as dysmyelination, polymicrogyria, and cerebral and cerebellar heterotopias, similar to those of Zellweger syndrome, are found at autopsy. In addition, infiltrates of macrophages filled with lamellar lipid inclusions are typically dispersed throughout the nervous system and the reticuloendothelial system. The principal difference between the CNS disease of neonatal ALD and that of patients classified as having Zellweger syndrome and infantile Refsum disease is the greater degree of demyelination in the children with neonatal ALD.

Unlike Zellweger syndrome, but more like infantile Refsum disease, most patients with neonatal ALD have hepatic disease that is clinically silent or very mild. Typically, only limited fibrosis or early cirrhosis is found by biopsy or at autopsy.[145,147] By electron microscopy, hepatic peroxisomes are severely reduced in both number and size but usually detectable, unlike in patients with Zellweger syndrome and most patients with infantile Refsum disease. Renal cysts and punctate cartilage calcification have been absent in neonatal ALD, an apparent distinction between neonatal ALD and Zellweger syndrome when the presence of demyelination and frank adrenal atrophy is used as a primary criterion for the diagnosis of neonatal ALD.[145,147]

Most patients with neonatal ALD manifest all of the peroxisomal biochemical abnormalities characteristic of Zellweger syndrome, although the measured activity of some enzymes, such as phytanic acid oxidase and DHAP acyltransferase, may be somewhat higher than in Zellweger syndrome. Similarly, the plasma levels of VLCFA are often lower than in Zellweger syndrome and may be limited to increases of only saturated VLCFAs.[145,147]

Hyperpipecolic Acidemia. Three separate reports have described infants with progressive neurodegenerative disease and hyperpipecolic acidemia who, for a variety of reasons, were not considered to meet criteria for the diagnosis of Zellweger syndrome.[148–150] Although these patients are often grouped separately in reviews of peroxisomal disorders, studies of cultured fibroblasts or autopsy tissues from these patients later showed that all of them also had increased levels of VLCFA.[151] Accordingly, because of apparent deficiencies of at least two metabolically unrelated peroxisomal enzyme systems, these cases should be reclassified as examples of neonatal ALD or other disorders of peroxisomal biogenesis rather than cases of isolated hyperpipecolic acidemia. Although there are several as yet unreported patients who are suspected to have isolated hyperpipecolic acidemia (R. Kelley, unpublished observations, 1989) and who differ clinically from Zellweger syndrome, infantile Refsum disease, or neonatal ALD, none has yet been proven enzymatically to have a deficiency of either D-pipecolic acid oxidase or L-pipecolic acid oxidase, both of which appear to be peroxisomal enzymes in humans.[95] Isolated marked hyperpipecolic acidemia may be an unrelated, common autosomal recessive variant because it has been reported as an associated abnormality in isolated cases of autosomal recessive Joubert syndrome and Dyggve-Melchior-Clausen dwarfism.[152,153] Thus, it remains unknown whether isolated hyperpipecolic acidemia exists as a disease or only a biochemical curiosity of no clinical significance.

DISEASES CAUSED BY DEFICIENCY OF A SINGLE PEROXISOMAL β-OXIDATION ENZYME

X-Linked Adrenoleukodystrophy. The degradation of VLCFAs begins with their apparently specific transport into peroxisomes followed by activation to CoA thioesters by a specific very-long-chain fatty (VLCF)–acyl CoA synthetase (ligase). The VLCF–acyl CoA esters are then degraded by successive cycles of β-oxidative cleavage of 2-carbon acetyl CoA units mediated by three peroxisome-

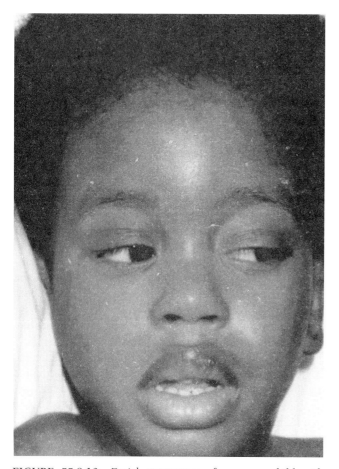

FIGURE 55.8-10 Facial appearance of a young child with neonatal adrenoleukodystrophy. Dysmorphic features are few but include a low nasal bridge and mild ptosis.

specific enzymes: acyl CoA oxidase, MFE2, and 3-ketoacyl CoA thiolase (see Figure 55.8-2). The cause of reduced VLCFA oxidation in X-linked ALD was thought for many years to be caused by an isolated deficiency of peroxisomal VLCF–acyl CoA synthetase activity.[154,155] However, in 1993, the biochemical defect in X-linked ALD was shown to be caused by mutations in the *ABCD1* gene, which encodes ALDP.[40,156] ALDP is a peroxisomal membrane protein that is a member of the large family of ATP-binding cassette transmembrane transporter proteins, of which, for example, the cystic fibrosis protein (cystic fibrosis transmembrane receptor) is also a member.[157,158] This large class of membrane proteins transports substrates as diverse as chloride ions and entire proteins. Although ALDP has been studied intensely since its discovery, its exact role in the metabolism of VLCFAs remains unclear. Studies by Yamada and colleagues suggested that ALDP was important for the correct localization of the VLCF–acyl CoA synthetase within the peroxisome.[159] However, more recent work by Heinzer and colleagues has cast doubt on this hypothesis.[160]

X-linked ALD is the most common peroxisomal disorder and is unusual in its varying presentations from early childhood to late adult years.[161] When onset is between 5 and 10 years of age, X-linked ALD usually begins with a combination of behavioral, gait, and auditory disturbances and ends fatally after several years of devastating, global neurologic degeneration, with or without adrenal insufficiency. In adults, in whom a milder form of ALD is known as adrenomyeloneuropathy, peripheral nerve dysfunction and adrenal insufficiency predominate over relatively mild CNS disturbances. Occasionally, adults with isolated Addison disease or even clinically unaffected older adults with classic biochemical findings are discovered within pedigrees of cases of typical X-linked ALD or adrenomyeloneuropathy.

In contrast to the multiple congenital abnormalities characteristic of neonatal ALD, all of the neurologic and endocrinologic problems of X-linked ALD are acquired after birth. Nevertheless, diagnostic elevations of VLCFA in plasma and other tissues in X-linked ALD are present at birth.[161] Moreover, because of its mode of inheritance, X-linked ALD is also often manifest to a milder degree clinically and biochemically by carrier female patients.[162,163] Although X-linked ALD offers an excellent opportunity to understand the mechanism by which increased levels of VLCFA affect the CNS and steroid-secreting organs, very little is known at this time about the pathogenesis of VLCFA-associated CNS degeneration or endocrine dysfunction in either neonatal or X-linked ALD.

Individuals with X-ALD may come to the attention of the gastroenterologist when in childhood they present with cyclic vomiting, which is secondary to primary adrenal insufficiency. However, in the majority of individuals, there are no abnormalities of the liver or other gastrointestinal system abnormalities.

CADDS. Corzo and colleagues recently reported three boys with an apparently new syndrome characterized by neonatal hypotonia and cholestatic liver disease.[164] They were determined to have elevated VLCFA levels and were initially felt to have either Zellweger syndrome or one of the single enzyme defects in peroxisomal β-oxidation other than X-linked ALD. However, further study showed that they lacked immunoreactive ALDP. Mutation analysis identified deletions in the 5' region of the *ABCD1* gene that extended through the promotor region and the neighboring gene, *DXS1357E*. The authors proposed the term CADDS for "contiguous *ABCD1 DXS1357E* deletion syndrome." The lack of ALDP in CADDS is noteworthy in that patients with childhood X-linked ALD typically present at 7 years of age but never < 3 years of age. In addition, liver disease is not found in patients with X-linked ALD. Liver biopsies of all three CADDS patients showed intracanalicular and ductal cholestasis. All three boys died in infancy (4–11 months), and causes of death included liver failure, gastrointestinal bleeding, and respiratory failure.

Acyl CoA Oxidase Deficiency (Pseudo–neonatal ALD). Two siblings who had severe hypotonia and myoclonic seizures in the first week of life but who lacked the dysmorphic appearance and other malformations characteristic of Zellweger syndrome were found by Poll-The and colleagues to have an apparently isolated deficiency of peroxisomal acyl CoA oxidase.[33] VLCFAs were markedly elevated in plasma and fibroblasts, but all other markers of peroxisomal dysfunction, including levels of bile acid intermediates, were normal. After a number of months of slow development, the children developed progressive sensorineural deafness, pigmentary retinopathy, and adrenal insufficiency and died in a vegetative state at age 4 years. There was no clinical or biochemical evidence of liver disease during life, and liver histology was notable only for somewhat increased peroxisomal size and lipoid deposits in hepatocytes. Cirrhosis or fibrosis, present in almost all patients with a disorder of PTS1-linked peroxisomal biogenesis, was not found. Isolated acyl CoA oxidase deficiency was documented by enzymatic assay of fibroblasts and immunologic methods[33] and, more recently, by DNA mutational analysis in the original and a second similar patient.[165] Additional patients with acyl CoA oxidase deficiency have been reported by Watkins and colleagues.[34]

Peroxisomal MFE2 Deficiency. More than 30 patients with a deficiency of peroxisomal MFE2 ("bifunctional enzyme") have now been described.[34,166,167] MFE2 is also known as D-BP. In contrast to the multisystem involvement of Zellweger syndrome, infants with MFE2 deficiency have a disorder dominated by their abnormal nervous system.[168] At birth, affected infants are severely hypotonic, macrocephalic, and neurologically depressed but usually lack hepatosplenomegaly, skeletal disease, or other important systemic abnormalities of Zellweger syndrome. However, neonatal seizures and severe psychomotor retardation are typical, and some of the infants have had dysmorphic facies reminiscent of Zellweger syndrome.[34] Although MFE2 deficiency is, in general, not a multisystem disorder like Zellweger syndrome, variable degrees of adrenal insufficiency, hepatic fibrosis, sensorineural hearing loss, pigmentary retinopathy, glomerulocystic kidney disease, and central white matter deterioration have been found. In contrast to Zellweger syndrome, however, hepatic peroxisomes are present. Despite the lesser systemic involvement, the severe CNS disease leads to the death of most MFE2-deficient patients in the first year.

Peroxisomal biochemical abnormalities in MFE2 deficiency are limited to increased tissue and plasma levels of VLCFAs and increased levels of bile acid intermediates, which MFE2 has a role in synthesizing. The absence of peroxisomal MFE2, but not peroxisomal oxidase or thiolase, was demonstrated by immunoblot analysis in the first patient identified.[166] Subsequently, more than 30 additional patients have been identified, mostly based on the clinical biochemical profile[166] and complementation analysis of cultured skin fibroblasts.[169] Of the three possible single enzyme defects of peroxisomal VLCFA β-oxidation, MFE2 deficiency is by far the most common.

Peroxisomal 3-Ketoacyl CoA Thiolase Deficiency (Pseudo–Zellweger Syndrome). Goldfischer and colleagues described a female infant who had Zellweger-like biochemical abnormalities but abundant hepatic peroxisomes and referred to this patient as having "pseudo–Zellweger syndrome."[170] As a result, a more detailed study of the enzymes of peroxisomal β-oxidation was undertaken by Schram and colleagues.[171] They reported that a single peroxisomal enzyme, 3-ketoacyl CoA thiolase, appeared to be deficient in liver tissue from this patient. Ferdinandusse and colleagues reinvestigated this case and determined that this patient with the only reported deficiency of peroxisomal 3-ketoacyl CoA thiolase actually had MFE2 deficiency.[172] The group of single peroxisomal β-oxidation enzyme deficiencies therefore appears to be limited to straight-chain acyl CoA oxidase, MFE2, and α-methylacyl CoA racemase (below) deficiency, and there is no longer evidence for the existence of peroxisomal 3-ketoacyl CoA thiolase deficiency as a distinct clinical entity.

2-Methylacyl CoA Racemase Deficiency. Ferdinandusse and colleagues reported three patients with elevations in pristanic acid and C_{27}-bile acid interediates, specifically DHCA and THCA, who were found to have a deficiency of 2-methylacyl CoA racemase.[173] This peroxisomal enzyme catalyzes the conversion of (2R)-methyl branched-chain fatty acyl CoAs to their (2S)-isomers. Only the S-conformers can undergo further β-oxidation. Two of the original patients had adult-onset neuropathy, but children with liver disease have also been reported. Setchell and colleagues described two sisters.[174] The proband was a 2-week-old girl with coagulopathy, vitamin D and E deficiencies, and mild cholestasis. A sibling who died at 5.5 months of age had had similar findings. Liver biopsy specimens showed neonatal hepatitis with giant cell transformation and hepatocyte necrosis, and peroxisomes were reduced in number. A high concentration of (25R)-THCA was found in the urine, bile, and serum and was similar to that seen in Zellweger syndrome. Serum phytanic acid was normal, whereas pristanic acid was

markedly elevated. This patient was successfully treated with cholic acid therapy.

Other Peroxisomal Syndromes with Abnormal β-Oxidation. There are a number of other peroxisomal syndromes in which abnormal peroxisomal β-oxidation has been found, but not all are necessarily genetically distinct from the known peroxisomal disease complementation groups. Rather, they may differ only in the relative severity of the measured deficiencies. In our experience, there exist cases of peroxisomal disease featuring almost any combination of normal and abnormal levels of peroxisomal metabolites. Some of these, especially those with abnormal bile acid species, have been associated with progressive cholestatic liver disease. Similarly, several syndromes have been described in which phytanic acid oxidation and one or more peroxisomal functions are impaired.[175] Again, however, whether these represent genetically distinct syndromes or variants of other peroxisomal diseases is often unclear.

Pathophysiology of Zellweger Syndrome and Other Disorders with Abnormal Peroxisomal β-Oxidation. All of the primary defects of peroxisomal β-oxidation except X-linked ALD are associated with some degree of hypotonia, abnormal reflexes, seizures, and, in some instances, neuronal migration defects. This suggests that prenatal elevations of VLCFA-CoA esters, or possibly other acyl CoA substrates of the enzymes, may be involved in the congenital CNS abnormalities. However, there is not a clear understanding of how these compounds lead to abnormalities. It has been suggested that the increased levels of bile acid intermediates or the increased levels of unsaturated or 3-hydroxy-VLCF acyl CoA compounds may be contributing to maldevelopment. Such an association is also supported by the description of a patient with only impaired phytanic acid and bile acid metabolism who had the large fontanels and other craniofacial features of classic Zellweger syndrome.[47] Similarly, the abnormal CNS development of chondrodysplasia punctata may be dependent on deficient plasmalogen synthesis, which appears to be the biochemical common ground shared by Zellweger syndrome and various forms of RCDP, described below.

D-Specific Acyl CoA (Trihydroxycoprostanyl CoA) Oxidase Deficiency. The finding of increased levels of DHCA and THCA in peroxisomal MFE2 and thiolase deficiencies,[175] but not in peroxisomal acyl CoA oxidase deficiency, first suggested the existence of a specific oxidase for the initial hydroxylation step in the β-oxidative cleavage of the cholesterol side chain. This has now been confirmed enzymatically and by the description of patients who have normal VLCF acyl CoA oxidase activity but defective oxidation of trihydroxycholestanoyl CoA.[47,176] Interestingly, these infants resembled Zellweger syndrome physically and had progressive cholestatic liver disease. In addition, the patients had elevated levels of phytanic acid, presumably secondary to elevations of its metabolite, pristanoyl CoA, which, like VLCFA-CoA, is a substrate of the D-specific acyl CoA oxidase. In contrast, in disorders of peroxisomal biogenesis and in adult Refsum disease, the elevation of phytanic acid occurs without bile acid abnormalities and is caused by a primary genetic (adult Refsum disease) or secondary (peroxisomal biogenesis disorder) deficiency of PAHX.[60]

OTHER DISORDERS OF PEROXISOMAL METABOLISM

Rhizomelic Chondrodysplasia Punctata. Although named for its severe rhizomelic dwarfism and diffuse epiphyseal and extraepiphyseal punctate calcification, RCDP is a complex, multiple congenital malformation syndrome with major nonskeletal abnormalities in the CNS (neuronal migration defect, seizures, deafness), eye (cataracts, blindness, corneal defects), and skin (ichthyosis).[177] Children with classic RCDP have severe growth retardation and profound mental deficiency, and most die before 1 year of age from respiratory insufficiency or complications of the CNS disease.

Recognizing that the punctate cartilage calcification of RCDP resembles that of Zellweger syndrome, Heymans and colleagues tested patients with RCDP for abnormalities of peroxisomal metabolism and discovered that both plasmalogen synthesis and phytanic acid oxidation were severely deficient.[178] By enzymatic assay, alkyl-DHAP synthase, the second enzyme of peroxisomal plasmalogen synthesis, and phytanic acid oxidase activity were depressed to less than 10% of normal activity. Plasma levels of phytanic acid in RCDP patients are usually higher than those of age-matched patients with Zellweger syndrome and may even reach the very high levels characteristic of adult Refsum disease in longer-surviving patients with RCDP.[179]

Because levels of intermediates of phytanic acid oxidation are not increased, the defective phytanic acid oxidation in RCDP is presumed to be limited to the initial α-hydroxylation step, as in adult Refsum disease. Plasma levels of pipecolic acid, VLCFAs, and bile acids are normal in RCDP, and liver disease and renal disease have also been absent.[179] Although one RCDP patient was reported to have reduced numbers of hepatic peroxisomes, others have had normally sized and abundant peroxisomes.[178] In addition to its multiple enzymatic deficiencies, the first clue that RCDP could be caused by a disorder of peroxisomal enzyme import distinct from that of the Zellweger syndrome group was the finding that fibroblasts of patients with RCDP contained a peroxisomal thiolase of a larger than normal molecular weight, indicating a failure of normal peroxisomal processing.[61,179] Molecular studies have now shown that, indeed, patients with RCDP have mutations in PEX7, a gene that codes for the PTS2 receptor.[61] Additional studies have shown that other PTS2-targeted enzymes, such as mevalonate kinase and phosphomevalonate kinase, are deficient in patients with RCDP.[180] Thus, RCDP is now classified with Zellweger and related peroxisomal syndromes as a disorder of peroxisomal biogenesis.

In recent years, several mild variants of RCDP have been found,[181,182] including children with normal stature who may have mild mental retardation and cataracts as only clinical problems. Others with the full RCDP biochemical phenotypes but normal stature have nevertheless had

severe progressive neurologic disease.[181] Conversely, some patients with relatively typical adult Refsum disease and very high phytanic acid levels have been found to have milder but definite abnormalities in plasmalogen biosynthesis and, by complementation analysis, have been shown to have RCDP instead.[181] These milder forms of RCDP, wherein the major pathology may be caused by accumulation of phytanic acid, will likely be more treatable than classic RCDP using dietary restriction and direct elimination (plasmapheresis) of phytanic acid.[183] Although classic RCDP is clearly a disease affecting multiple peroxisomal enzymes, Barr and colleagues reported a patient with otherwise typical RCDP who had an isolated deficiency of DHAP acyltransferase.[184] This observation suggested that the clinical phenotype in classic RCDP is caused largely by defective plasmalogen biosynthesis. Other similar patients with isolated DHAP acyltransferase deficiency have been reported.[185,186] Rare cases of isolated DHAP synthase deficiency have also been reported.[187] Although abnormalities of plasmalogen synthesis and catalase distribution in a patient with the X-linked form of chondrodysplasia punctata, also known as Conradi-Hünermann syndrome, were reported by Emami,[188] these must be secondary abnormalities because the primary defect in Conradi-Hünermann syndrome was recently found to be a deficiency of 3β-hydroxysteroid-Δ8,Δ7-isomerase, a primary enzyme of cholesterol biosynthesis located in the microsomes.[189,190]

Heredopathia Atactica Polyneuritiformis: Adult Refsum Disease. In contrast to the early onset of infantile Refsum disease, adult Refsum disease (heredopathia atactica polyneuritiformis) is usually not evident clinically until the second or third decade. The major abnormalities in adult Refsum disease, all of which are acquired and progressive, include pigmentary retinopathy, sensorineural deafness, cerebellar ataxia, polyneuritis, ichthyosis, and cardiac conduction abnormalities.[191] Although clinical hepatic disease is absent, ultrastructural changes in the liver have been found to include excessive hepatocytic deposits of lipofuscin, vacuoles containing various types of lipoid accumulations, and an apparent deficiency of rough ER.[192] Vacuolization of renal tubular cells and structural abnormalities of their mitochondria have been reported and related to mild to moderate degrees of proximal renal tubular insufficiency in adult Refsum disease. Biochemically, Refsum disease is characterized by increased levels of free and esterified phytanic acid in the blood and tissues and a corresponding absence of phytanic acid β-oxidation activity as measured in fibroblasts and other solid tissues[193] and now known to be represented by a deficiency of phytanyl CoA α-hydroxylase.[60,194] All other peroxisomal functions appear to be normal. Because of the many years of accumulation of phytanic acid before diagnosis, levels of phytanic acid in plasma at the time of diagnosis of adult Refsum disease are often greater than 1,000 μg/mL compared with typical plasma levels of 10 to 200 μg/mL in Zellweger syndrome, infantile Refsum disease, or RCDP.[136,195] Refsum disease, which is one of the rarest inborn errors of metabolism, is inherited as an autosomal recessive genetic trait.

Stabilization and even partial reversal of the complications of adult Refsum disease can be achieved by restriction of dietary phytanic acid combined with direct elimination of accumulated phytanic acid by plasmapheresis, if necessary.[193] Although phytanic acid oxidase activity segregates with mitochondria in rats,[196] the localization is clearly peroxisomal in humans[60,194]; thus, adult Refsum disease is now securely classified as a peroxisomal disorder.

Primary Hyperoxaluria: Alanine:Glyoxylate Aminotransferase Deficiency.

Primary (type I) hyperoxaluria is characterized by excessive oxalate synthesis, precipitation of calcium oxalate in the kidney, and progressive nephrocalcinosis.[197,198] Renal insufficiency usually develops during the first decade and may be followed by extrarenal calcification of the joints and, especially, myocardium. Except for some patients for whom pharmacologic doses of pyridoxine can substantially reduce the synthesis and excretion of oxalate, renal failure is inevitable. Although most of the oxalic acid in primary hyperoxaluria is produced by the liver, the liver is not subject to oxalate deposition or otherwise clinically diseased. Hepatic and peroxisomal ultrastructure is normal, apart from a mild to moderate increase in lipofuscin deposits.[199]

Danpure and colleagues have shown that type I hyperoxaluria is caused by deficient reclamation of glyoxylate, most of which is normally transaminated to glycine by alanine:glyoxylate aminotransferase (AGT).[200] A deficiency of this pyridoxine-dependent enzyme causes glyoxylate instead to be further oxidized to the metabolic end product oxalate. AGT has for many years been known to be located exclusively within the peroxisome,[201] and its deficiency appears to be the only peroxisomal defect in primary hyperoxaluria. In some cases of type I hyperoxaluria, an abnormality in the tripeptide peroxisomal targeting sequence causes AGT to relocate to the mitochondrial space.[202] Interestingly, hyperoxaluria does not occur in Zellweger syndrome, in which tissue levels, but not subcellular distribution, of AGT are normal.[203] Apparently, location of AGT in the cytoplasm does not impair its function as a transaminase. Because the AGT-deficient liver is the major source of oxalate and the kidney is the major target organ for the disease, combined kidney-liver transplant has become a standard of therapy for type I hyperoxaluria. As reviewed by Cochat and colleagues, patient survival after combined liver-kidney transplant at 5 and 10 years has been approximately 80% and 70%, respectively.[204] As anticipated, renal function in surviving transplant recipients has remained stable.

Acatalasemia.

Catalase is present in all peroxisomes at high concentrations and serves the vital function of peroxidatic and catalatic disposal of hydrogen peroxide produced by the many peroxisomal oxidases.[5] Catalase is also present in the cytosol of erythrocytes, which lack recognizable peroxisomes. Acatalasemia is a rare, autosomal recessive disorder first identified in patients with progressive oral gangrene and characterized biochemically by a complete absence of enzymatically and, in some patients, immunologically detectable catalase in erythrocytes.[205] Because the only pathology associated with human acatalasemia is oral gangrene,[206] catalase in other tissues is presumed to be at least partially active. The pathogenesis of oral gangrene in this disorder is not fully understood, and only a minority of patients have any recognizable pathology. One theory holds that erythrocyte catalase detoxifies hydrogen peroxide produced by bacteria that invade superficial mucosal capillaries.[205] In the absence of catalase, tissue destruction by bacterial hydrogen peroxide proceeds unchecked and encourages further invasion of bacteria.

DIAGNOSIS OF PEROXISOMAL DISEASES

CLINICAL PROBLEMS SUGGESTING A PEROXISOMAL DISEASE

Even though children with Zellweger syndrome, infantile Refsum disease, or neonatal ALD are almost always considered abnormal at birth, the diagnosis of a peroxisomal disorder is often delayed for many months. For example, the not uncommon neonatal history of a difficult breech delivery, severe neonatal hypotonia, and abnormal neonatal reflexes characteristic of Zellweger syndrome is often misdiagnosed as perinatal asphyxia before the later development of liver disease, pigmentary retinopathy, or degenerative neurologic disease suggests a different diagnosis. The initial clinical impression of birth injury is often reinforced by the occurrence of myoclonic seizures during the newborn period. Alternatively, the finding of a combination of salt-and-pepper retinopathy and psychomotor retardation in some of the less severely affected children may lead to a mistaken diagnosis of congenital rubella or other prenatal infection. Cockayne syndrome, Leber congenital amaurosis, and Usher syndrome are other diagnoses commonly given to the more mildly affected patients with prominent pigmentary retinopathy and an extinguished electroretinogram. Similarly, Zellweger syndrome is occasionally misdiagnosed as Alagille syndrome (arteriohepatic dysplasia), another diagnosis that combines cholestatic liver disease with dysmorphic facial features. For such children, it is usually the appearance of an unexpected abnormality for the assigned diagnosis, such as pigmentary retinopathy or frank neurologic deterioration, that leads to the ultimate diagnosis of a peroxisomal disorder. Table 55.8-6 lists some of the diagnoses most commonly considered or given to patients with disorders of peroxisomal biogenesis. The clinician should consider the possibility of an underlying peroxisomal disorder when consulted about a patient with any of these diagnoses. Conversely, it is important to recognize that children with primary defects of bile acid biosynthesis (see Chapter 55.4, "Bile Acid Synthesis and Metabolism") may present as cholestatic liver disease and seizures and be initially considered for the diagnosis of Zellweger syndrome.

A number of clinical abnormalities that are especially important clues for the diagnosis of a peroxisomal disorder are summarized in Table 55.8-7.

Gastroenterologists are not uncommonly the first to suggest the diagnosis of a peroxisomal disease when consulted about a neurologically handicapped child who has

TABLE 55.8-6   DIFFERENTIAL DIAGNOSIS OF
ZELLWEGER SYNDROME, INFANTILE
REFSUM DISEASE, AND NEONATAL
ADRENOLEUKODYSTROPHY

Down syndrome; other chromosomal disorders
Congenital hepatic fibrosis/polycystic kidneys
Congenital infection (TORCH) syndrome
Rhizomelic chondrodysplasia punctata
Smith-Lemli-Opitz syndrome
Lowe oculocerebrorenal syndrome
Usher syndrome
Leber congenital amaurosis
Cockayne syndrome
Septo-optic dysplasia (de Morsier syndrome)
Meckel syndrome (encephalosplanchnocystica)

TORCH = toxoplasmosis, other agents, rubella, cytomegalovirus, herpes simplex.

been found to have hepatomegaly, hepatic dysfunction, or simply persistently elevated serum transaminases. Gastrointestinal bleeding secondary to a coagulopathy, varices, or both is another common cause for involvement of the gastrointestinal specialist. However, more than once, evidence by liver biopsy of lipid inclusions in the Kupffer cells has been misdiagnosed as Niemann-Pick disease or another lysosomal lipidosis in a child with neonatal ALD or infantile Refsum disease who has marked VLCFA storage in macrophages. In these cases, careful electron microscopic examination of the storage material should differentiate the lipoid globules with associated birefringent lamellar lipid structures characteristic of the peroxisomal diseases from the lipid inclusions of the lysosomal sphingolipidoses. Other diverse routes have led to the diagnosis of a peroxisomal disease. The finding of either chondrodysplasia punctata (usually without rhizomelic shortening) or characteristic glomerular polycystic kidney disease in a neonate with typical neurologic signs is virtually diagnostic of Zellweger syndrome. In the older,

more mildly affected child without clinically evident renal or skeletal lesions, neurosensory defects—optic atrophy, pigmentary retinopathy, abnormal electroretinogram, and deafness—are the most common problems that should lead to the consideration of a peroxisomal disease.

In general, a patient with any two of the major diagnostic criteria listed in Table 55.8-8 should lead the clinician to serious consideration of a disorder of peroxisomal biogenesis or one of the single enzyme defects of peroxisomal β-oxidation, which can closely mimic Zellweger syndrome, infantile Refsum disease, and neonatal ALD. The two newly described entities of CADDS and α-methylacyl CoA racemase deficiency may prove to be important causes of neonatal cholestatic jaundice, and appropriate investigations should be made.

LABORATORY EVALUATION OF PATIENTS WITH PEROXISOMAL DISORDERS

Although a definitive diagnosis of a generalized peroxisomal disorder at one time required demonstration of abnormal or absent peroxisomes by liver biopsy, now the diagnosis can virtually always be established with certainty by measurement of specific peroxisomal metabolites and enzymes in plasma, erythrocytes, fibroblasts, and other tissues, as outlined in Table 55.8-9. Nevertheless, whenever the diagnosis of a peroxisomal disease is entertained for a patient who is to have a liver biopsy, a portion of the biopsy specimen should be processed for study of peroxisomal ultrastructure and specific staining. Although for many of the peroxisomal disorders discussed in this chapter, the relevant genes have been cloned and causative mutations have been found, clinical findings and biochemical studies are still the mainstay of peroxisomal diagnosis and are likely to remain so for many years, especially for the peroxisomal biogenesis disorders, which have the most distinctive and usually unequivocally diagnostic biochemical abnormalities.[101,207]

TABLE 55.8–7   CLINICAL AND PATHOLOGIC CHARACTERISTICS OF THE PEROXISOMAL DISORDERS OF INFANCY
AND EARLY CHILDHOOD

CHARACTERISTIC	ZELLWEGER SYNDROME	INFANTILE REFSUM DISEASE	NEONATAL ADRENOLEUKO-DYSTROPHY	ACYL COA OXIDASE DEFICIENCY	BIFUNCTIONAL ENZYME DEFICIENCY	3-KETOACYL COA THIOLASE DEFICIENCY	RHIZOMELIC CHONDRODYSPLASIA PUNCTATA
Abnormal facies	+++	+	+	−	±	+++	+++
Congenital hypotonia	+++	++	++	+++	+++	+++	−
Neonatal seizures	+++	+	++	+	+	++	+
Psychomotor retardation	+++	++	++	++	+++	+++	+++
Pigmentary retinopathy	++	+++	+++	++	++	+++	−
Sensorineural deafness	++	++	++	++	++	++	−
Absent or diminished hepatic peroxisomes	+++	+++	+	−	−	−	−
Hepatic fibrosis/cirrhosis	+++	+	+	−	±	±	−
Coagulopathy	+++	++	++	−	−	−	−
Adrenal lipid inclusions and/or atrophy	+	+	++	+++	+++	++	−
Polycystic kidneys	+++	±	±	−	±	+	−
Epiphyseal/apophyseal calcific stippling	++	−	−	−	−	+	+++
Growth retardation	+++	++	++	−	+	+	+++
Mean survival (yr)	0.6	> 5	3	4	1	0.9	1

− = absent; + = mild or occasional; ++ = moderate or common; +++ = severe or universal.

In general, the measurement of VLCFA levels in plasma, which is now available in several laboratories, is a good screening test for a disorder of peroxisomal biogenesis, X-linked ALD, or a single enzyme defect of peroxisomal β-oxidation.[101,207,208] The most important measurements in plasma are the absolute level of $C_{26:0}$ VLCFAs and the ratio of $C_{26:0}$ to $C_{22:0}$ VLCFAs, both of which are markedly elevated in Zellweger syndrome and related disorders. VLCFA abnormalities can even be detected in autopsy tissues preserved in formalin for many years. If RCDP or one of its variants is the diagnosis under consideration, then the measurement of plasmalogen levels in erythrocyte cell membranes, or, better, plasmalogen synthesis in cultured fibroblasts, and a plasma phytanic acid level are required. False-negative results are uncommon, and more detailed testing of plasma or fibroblasts is not usually required to diagnose Zellweger syndrome, neonatal ALD, infantile Refsum disease, RCDP, or X-linked ALD. There have been only a few cases of autopsy-confirmed neonatal ALD in which plasma levels of VLCFAs were only slightly increased, but subsequent studies in cultured fibroblasts were diagnostic of a multiple peroxisomal deficiency syndrome (R. Kelley and A. Moser, unpublished observations, 1987–1990). Also, it is important to recognize that tissue specimens obtained postmortem or from patients with severe hepatic disease or sepsis may have mild elevations of VLCFAs or pipecolic acid as secondary phenomena. As expected for a relatively newly delineated group of diseases, the clinical spectrum of peroxisomal diseases continues to widen, and new variants, particularly those with partial deficiencies, probably remain to be described.

When plasma levels of VLCFAs are increased in a patient suspected to have a peroxisomal biogenesis disorder, additional metabolite measurements are needed to help define the disorder. When all or most other basic peroxisomal metabolite measurements (pipecolic acid, plasmalogens, phytanic acid, bile acid intermediates) are abnormal, then Zellweger syndrome, infantile Refsum disease, or neonatal ALD is the diagnosis. On the other hand, if plasma levels of pipecolic acid and plasmalogen metabolism in fibroblasts are normal in a Zellweger-like patient or the nondysmorphic, severely hypotonic patient with elevated VLCFAs, then one of the isolated defects of peroxisomal β-oxidation is likely, that is, D-specific acyl CoA oxidase deficiency or MFE2 deficiency. The clinical distinction between X-linked ALD and one of the other isolated peroxisomal β-oxidation defects is usually not a

TABLE 55.8-8   MAJOR DIAGNOSTIC CRITERIA FOR A DISORDER OF PEROXISOMAL BIOGENESIS

Abnormal peroxisomal enzyme or metabolite level
Characteristic facial appearance
Evidence of cerebral dysgenesis
Hepatic fibrosis/cirrhosis, cholestasis, biliary dysgenesis
Polycystic (cortical) kidney disease
Abnormal electroretinogram, optic atrophy, pigmentary retinopathy
Sensorineural hearing loss
Punctate calcification of cartilage

TABLE 55.8-9   DIAGNOSTIC TESTS FOR PEROXISOMAL DISORDERS

Plasma	VLCFAs, phytanic acid, pipecolic acid, bile acid intermediates, essential fatty acids
Erythrocytes	Plasmalogens
Urine	Pipecolic acid; long-chain, odd-carbon, and epoxy dicarboxylic acids; bile acids
Fibroblasts, tissues	VLCFA levels, VLCFA β-oxidation, phytanic acid oxidation, plasmalogen levels and biosynthesis, DHAP acyl-transferase activity, alkyl-DHAP synthase activity, sedimentable catalase, peroxisomal size and abundance

DHAP = dihydroxyacetone phosphate; VLCFA = very-long-chain fatty acid.

question. However, the diagnosis of CADDS requires the demonstration of a lack of ALDP or a deletion in the appropriate region of the *ABCD1* gene. Despite the often severe adrenal atrophy present in patients with single β-oxidation enzyme defects, neonatal ALD, and infantile Refsum syndrome, adrenal insufficiency is usually not evident clinically but can sometimes be demonstrated by provocative tests of adrenal function.[145,147]

Because renal tubular immaturity limits pipecolic acid reabsorption (via the iminoglycine transport system) in newborns, some infants with Zellweger syndrome may have normal or near-normal plasma pipecolic acid levels but diagnostically increased urinary pipecolic acid levels.[209] Conversely, after maturation of renal imino acid transport, previously diagnostic urinary levels of pipecolic acid may revert to normal at the same time that plasma levels become markedly increased. In addition, because red cell plasmalogens may with time normalize from dietary sources, specific assay of plasmalogen synthesis in cultured fibroblasts may be necessary in some cases.[101]

Except for X-linked ALD and the associated disorder CADDS, all of the other known peroxisomal disorders are inherited as autosomal recessive traits and therefore carry a 25% recurrence risk in future pregnancies. Prenatal diagnosis of peroxisomal diseases is possible both by traditional amniocyte culture and by chorionic villus biopsy technique. Measurement of VLCFAs, plasmalogen synthesis, and phytanic acid oxidase are commonly performed and reliable.[210–212] In addition, assay of VLCFA oxidation and measurement of particulate (ie, peroxisomal) catalase versus soluble catalase can be performed on amniocytes and cultured chorionic villus cells as backup tests.[210,211] Although there is less experience with prenatal diagnosis of the single enzyme defects of peroxisomal β-oxidation, they are detectable by measurement of peroxisomal β-oxidation rates in prenatally obtained specimens. The absence of a peroxisomal β-oxidation enzyme can also be detected in some cases by indirect immunofluorescence analysis or immunoblot analysis, whereas except for acyl CoA oxidase deficiency, direct enzymatic assay of tissues would be technically difficult because of the presence of much greater quantities of homologous mitochondrial enzyme. Of course, these analyses can be normal if a defect in a peroxisomal β-oxidation enzyme does not change the amount and electrophoretic character of the enzyme.

Finally, because prenatal diagnosis of most of the peroxisomal disorders involves the determination of metabolite and enzyme activity levels that are secondarily abnormal rather than the measurement of the primary genetic defect, it is important to measure more than one diagnostic metabolite or enzyme level and also to have evidence of the feasibility of a tissue biochemical diagnosis documented by prior studies of the proband's fibroblasts or other tissues. The recent finding of genetic mutations causing most of the more common peroxisomal disorders will eventually permit confirmation of a prenatal diagnosis by molecular methods in families with known mutation.

TREATMENT OF PEROXISOMAL DISORDERS

General Measures: Zellweger Syndrome, Infantile Refsum Disease, and Neonatal ALD.

Treatment of peroxisomal disorders is mostly supportive. For the more severe disorders of peroxisomal biogenesis, neurologic deficits appear to be dictated largely by primary brain malformations and, as such, are irreversible. Even if the postnatal demyelination and CNS degeneration that occur in the disorders of peroxisomal biogenesis could be prevented, it is unlikely that any of the classically affected patients would achieve even a marginal level of function. Supportive therapy for longer-surviving children with generalized peroxisomal deficiency syndromes should address at least five main areas: nutrition, seizures and other neurologic disabilities, progressive liver disease, adrenal insufficiency, and sensory or communication deficits.

Nutrition. Growth retardation in Zellweger syndrome, infantile Refsum disease, and neonatal ALD is common but not universal. Nutritional efforts to improve growth may be beneficial if significant malabsorption exists. Most often, however, even intensive nutritional therapy does little to ameliorate the growth retardation, which appears to be intrinsic in most cases and not caused by inadequate nutrition. Nevertheless, the absorption of fat and fat-soluble vitamins should be monitored. In the more severely affected children, swallowing dysfunction and gastroesophageal reflux are common problems that require medical attention, including nasogastric or gastrostomy feeding for many, if not most, patients.

Neurologic Problems. Seizures in this group of patients are typically myoclonic and may respond poorly to traditional one- or two-drug anticonvulsant therapy. However, there are no associated contraindications to medications, and any appropriate anticonvulsant may be used. Apnea, primary or secondary to seizures, is almost universal in Zellweger syndrome and is one of the more common causes of death.

Liver Disease. Liver disease is rapidly progressive in classic Zellweger syndrome but more variably progressive in patients with milder forms of the disorders. Early in the course of Zellweger syndrome, the only therapy needed for liver disease may be pharmacologic amounts of vitamin K to ameliorate (but not usually cure) a coagulopathy and special dietary measures to minimize the complications of fat malabsorption. Later, the expected complications of cirrhosis and end-stage liver disease—variceal bleeding, ascites, hemorrhoids, rarely hepatic encephalopathy, deteriorating seizure control, multiple hepatic synthetic deficiencies, and delayed drug metabolism—may emerge and require appropriate clinical management. Variceal bleeding in children with neonatal ALD and infantile Refsum disease has been treated by endoscopic sclerosing therapy.

Adrenal Insufficiency. In X-linked ALD, clinically significant adrenal insufficiency is common and requires appropriate adrenal steroid replacement therapy. Addison disease may be the only sign of X-linked ALD in the older child. It may appear at any age in individuals with the biochemical defect but is rarely seen in heterozygous women. It is rarely seen in Zellweger syndrome but may be seen in older individuals with peroxisome assembly disorders and does respond to appropriate replacement therapy.

Sensory Deficits. For patients with neonatal ALD or infantile Refsum disease phenotypes, who occasionally may achieve a developmental level of 2 or 3 years, visual and auditory deficiencies often become important management issues. The use of hearing aids may enable some patients to make surprising gains in communication skills and interactions with others. Even the use of sign language by severely hearing- and/or speech-impaired patients is known. Seemingly poor cognitive development in these children should not automatically be attributed to their congenital and acquired CNS defects if auditory and visual deficits remain unaided.

Other Peroxisomal Disorders.

Because of its greater rarity, there is much less experience with the care of children with RCDP than the other disorders of peroxisomal biogenesis. Whereas liver disease is absent in RCDP, seizures, respiratory insufficiency, and recurrent pneumonia are common management problems. Despite excellent care, most RCDP patients die before 1 year of age from the complications of respiratory insufficiency. Growth retardation in long-term survivors is quite severe and, of course, not specifically treatable. Treatment of the single enzyme defects of peroxisomal β-oxidation varies. Patients with isolated defects of acyl CoA oxidase or MFE2 require therapy for the same range of neurologic and sensory deficits found in neonatal ALD, but significant liver disease has been absent in the few reported cases. However, as older, more mildly affected variants of these newer peroxisomal diseases are found, liver disease may yet emerge as a clinical problem.

Specific Metabolic Therapies.

In part because of the often excellent response of patients with adult Refsum disease to dietary restriction of phytanic acid, a number of attempts have been made to treat patients with Zellweger syndrome or related peroxisomal diseases by correction of one or more of the characteristic biochemical abnormalities. Specifically, diets to limit the intake of pipecolic acid, phytanic acid, and VLCFAs have been given to several patients with Zellweger syndrome or infantile Refsum disease.[115,213,214] No therapy, however, has been clearly beneficial, despite sometimes substantial improvement in the metabolite levels. In one patient with infantile Refsum disease treated with a low phytanic acid diet, phytanic acid levels normalized and VLCFA levels improved, but the abundance of hepatic lamellar lipid inclusions continued to increase.[213,214] Batyl alcohol, an octadecyl ether of glycerol that can be converted to plasmalogens in the microsomes, has also been given as a dietary supplement. Although red cell plasmalogen levels rose to normal on batyl alcohol supplements, there was no definite clinical improvement.[213,214] Other therapies without obvious benefit have included adrenal steroids and treatment with clofibrate, which in rats, but apparently not humans, increases peroxisomal numbers.[215] The deficient synthesis of DHA $(C_{22:6})$[132] in peroxisomal biogenesis disorders can be ameliorated by dietary supplementation.[216,217] A more recent report of DHA treatment of children with peroxisomal biogenesis disorders showed remarkable improvement in clinical function and diverse biochemical abnormalities, including normalization of serum transaminases.[216] DHA supplementation was even associated with improved cerebral myelinization by magnetic resonance imaging.[218] Confirmation of efficacy of this as therapy awaits completion of an ongoing placebo-controlled study (G. V. Raymond and colleagues, unpublished data, 2003). Although the low levels of cholesterol and the antioxidant protection afforded by cholesterol may explain some of the evidence for hepatic fibrosis and cirrhosis, there is as yet no experience with prolonged cholesterol supplementation in children with Zellweger syndrome.

Another area of therapy for Zellweger syndrome and related disorders of peroxisomal biogenesis being explored has been the use of bile acid supplements. Anecdotally, liver function, seizure frequency, and growth all improved in a 6-month-old boy with Zellweger syndrome who was treated with a combination of cholic acid and chenodeoxycholic acid.[131] If, as speculated, the cholestatic liver disease characteristic of Zellweger syndrome is caused by the accumulation of abnormal bile acid species, then bile acid replacement therapy may indeed be beneficial. Despite the poor results of metabolic therapies for the peroxisomal disorders, there remains the possibility that extended trials of this nature may affect the course of sensory or other neurologic deterioration in some of the more mildly affected, longer-surviving patients if treatment is begun before degenerative neurologic changes have advanced.[219,220]

A mixture of triolein ($C_{18:1}$ triglyceride) and trierucin ($C_{22:1}$ triglyceride) ("Lorenzo's oil") has been used in X-linked ALD. There is very clear evidence of improvement of levels of VLCFAs in plasma. However, there is no clinical improvement in boys affected with cerebral disease or in men with adrenomyeloneuropathy.[221] Ongoing trials are presently evaluating this therapy as a preventive therapy.[222] A striking improvement in a case of X-linked ALD was achieved following bone marrow transplant.[223] Additional experience has allowed the development of guidelines for the appropriate selection of patients.[224] Whether bone marrow transplant will be a successful long-term therapy remains to be determined.

REFERENCES

1. Bowen P, Lee CSN, Zellweger H, Lindenberg R. A familial syndrome of multiple congenital defects. Bull Johns Hopkins Hosp 1964;114:402–14.
2. Goldfischer S, Moore CL, Johnson AB, et al. Peroxisomal and mitochondrial defects in the cerebro-hepato-renal syndrome. Science 1973;182:62–4.
3. De Duve C. Evolution of the peroxisome. Ann N Y Acad Sci 1969;168:369–81.
4. Novikoff AB, Novikoff PM. Microperoxisomes. J Histochem Cytochem 1973;21:963–66.
5. Tolbert NE. Metabolic pathways in peroxisomes and glyoxysomes. Annu Rev Biochem 1981;50:133–57.
6. Bock P, Kramar R, Pavelka M. Peroxisomes and related particles in animal tissues. In: Berkeley MA, editor. Cell biology monographs. Vol 7. New York: Springer Verlag; 1980.
7. Hruban Z, Vigil EL, Slesers A, Hopkins E. Microbodies: constituent organelles of animal cells. Lab Invest 1972;27:184–91.
8. Svoboda DJ, Azarnoff DL. Response of hepatic microbodies to a hypolipidemic agent, ethyl chlorophenoxyisobutyrate (CPIB). J Cell Biol 1966;30:442–50.
9. Hawkins JM, Jones WE, Bonner FW, Gibson GG. The effect of peroxisome proliferators on microsomal, peroxisomal, and mitochondrial enzyme activities in the liver and kidney. Drug Metab Rev 1987;18:441–515.
10. Hihi AK, Michalik L, Wahli W. PPARs: transcriptional effectors of fatty acids and their derivatives. Cell Mol Life Sci 2002;59:790–8.
11. Clarke SD, Thuillier P, Baillie RA, Sha X. Peroxisome proliferator-activated receptors: a family of lipid-activated transcription factors. Am J Clin Nutr 1999;70:566–71.
12. Berger J, Moller DE. The mechanisms of action of PPARs. Annu Rev Med 2002;53:409–35.
13. Green S. PPAR: a mediator of peroxisome proliferator action. Mutat Res 1995;333:101–9.
14. Cattley RC, Miller RT, Corton JC. Peroxisome proliferators: potential role of altered hepatocyte growth and differentiation in tumor development. Prog Clin Biol Res 1995;391:295–303.
15. Purdue PE, Lazarow PB. Peroxisome biogenesis. Annu Rev Cell Dev Biol 2001;17:701–52.
16. Gould SJ, Raymond GV, Valle D. The peroxisome biogenesis disorders. In: Scriver CR, Beaudet AL, Valle D, Sly WS, editors. The metabolic and molecular bases of inherited disease. 8th ed. New York: McGraw-Hill; 2001. p. 3181–217.
17. Gould SJ, Keller GA, Hosken N, et al. A conserved tripeptide sorts proteins to peroxisomes. J Cell Biol 1989;108:1657–64.
18. Mccollum D, Monosov E, Subramani S. The pas8 mutant of pichia-pastoris exhibits the peroxisomal protein import deficiencies of Zellweger syndrome cells—the PAS8 protein binds to the COOH-terminal tripeptide peroxisomal targeting signal, and is a member of the TPR protein family. J Cell Biol 1993;121:761–74.
19. Marzioch M, Erdmann R, Veenhuis M, Kunau WH. PAS7 encodes a novel yeast member of the WD-40 protein family essential for import of 3-oxoacyl-CoA thiolase, a PTS2-containing protein, into peroxisomes. EMBO J 1994;13:4908–18.
20. Hruban Z, Rechcigl M Jr. Microbodies and related particles. Morphology, biochemistry, and physiology. Int Rev Cytol Suppl 1969;1:1–296.
21. Gorgas K, Zaar K. Peroxisomes in sebaceous glands. III. Morphological similarities of peroxisomes with smooth endo-

plasmic reticulum and Golgi stacks in the circumanal gland of the dog. Anat Embryol (Berl) 1984;169:9–20.

22. Zaar K, Volkl A, Fahimi HD. Association of isolated bovine kidney cortex peroxisomes with endoplasmic reticulum. Biochim Biophys Acta 1987;897:135–42.

23. Gorgas K. Peroxisomes in sebaceous glands. V. Complex peroxisomes in the mouse preputial gland: serial sectioning and three-dimensional reconstruction studies. Anat Embryol (Berl) 1984;169:261–70.

24. Gorgas K. Serial section analysis of mouse hepatic peroxisomes. Anat Embryol (Berl) 1985;172:21–32.

25. Kolattukudy PE, Bohnet S, Rogers L. Diesters of 3-hydroxy fatty acids produced by the uropygial glands of female mallards uniquely during the mating season. J Lipid Res 1987;28:582–8.

26. Beevers H. Glyoxysomes of castor bean endosperm and their relation to gluconeogenesis. Ann N Y Acad Sci 1969;168:313–24.

27. Lazarow PB. Rat liver peroxisomes catalyze the beta oxidation of fatty acids. J Biol Chem 1978;253:1522–8.

28. Hijikata M, Ishii N, Kagamiyama H, et al. Structural analysis of cDNA for rat peroxisomal 3-ketoacyl-CoA thiolase. J Biol Chem 1987;262:8151–8.

29. van Grunsven EG, Mooijer PA, Aubourg P, Wanders RJ. Enoyl-CoA hydratase deficiency: identification of a new type of D-bifunctional protein deficiency. Hum Mol Genet 1999;8:1509–16.

30. Une M, Konishi M, Suzuki Y, et al. Bile acid profiles in a peroxisomal D-3-hydroxyacyl-CoA dehydratase/D-3-hydroxyacyl-CoA dehydrogenase bifunctional protein deficiency. J Biochem (Tokyo) 1997;122:655–8.

31. Wanders RJA, Barth PC, Heymans HSA. Single peroxisomal enzyme deficiencies. In: Scriver CR, Beaudet AL, Sly WS, Valle D, editors. The metabolic and molecular bases of inherited disease. 8th ed. New York: McGraw-Hill; 2001. p. 3219–56.

32. Osumi T, Hashimoto T, Ui N. Purification and properties of acyl-CoA oxidase from rat liver. J Biochem (Tokyo) 1980;87:1735–46.

33. Poll-The BT, Roels F, Ogier H, et al. A new peroxisomal disorder with enlarged peroxisomes and a specific deficiency of acyl-CoA oxidase (pseudo-neonatal adrenoleukodystrophy). Am J Hum Genet 1988;42:422–34.

34. Watkins PA, McGuinness MC, Raymond GV, et al. Distinction between peroxisomal bifunctional enzyme and acyl-CoA oxidase deficiencies. Ann Neurol 1995;38:472–7.

35. Verhoeven NM, Roe DS, Kok RM, et al. Phytanic acid and pristanic acid are oxidized by sequential peroxisomal and mitochondrial reactions in cultured fibroblasts. J Lipid Res 1998;39:66–74.

36. Bjorkhem I, Kase BF, Pedersen JI. Role of peroxisomes in the biosynthesis of bile acids. Scand J Clin Lab Invest Suppl 1985;177:23–31.

37. Verhoeven NM, Wanders RJ, Poll-The BT, et al. The metabolism of phytanic acid and pristanic acid in man: a review. J Inherit Metab Dis 1998;21:697–728.

38. Leenders F, Dolez V, Begue A, et al. Structure of the gene for the human 17beta-hydroxysteroid dehydrogenase type IV. Mamm Genome 1998;9:1036–41.

39. Seedorf U, Brysch P, Engel T, et al. Sterol carrier protein X is peroxisomal 3-oxoacyl coenzyme A thiolase with intrinsic sterol carrier and lipid transfer activity. J Biol Chem 1994;269:21277–83.

40. Mosser J, Lutz Y, Stoeckel ME, et al. The gene responsible for adrenoleukodystrophy encodes a peroxisomal membrane protein. Hum Mol Genet 1994;3:265–71.

41. Pedersen JI, Veggan T, Bjorkhem I. Substrate stereospecificity in oxidation of (25S)-3 alpha,7 alpha,12 alpha-trihydroxy-5 beta-cholestanoyl-CoA by peroxisomal trihydroxy-5 beta-cholestanoyl-CoA oxidase. Biochem Biophys Res Commun 1996;224:37–42.

42. Vanveldhoven PP, Croes K, Asselberghs S, et al. Peroxisomal beta-oxidation of 2-methyl-branched acyl-CoA esters: stereospecific recognition of the 2S-methyl compounds by trihydroxycoprostanoyl-CoA oxidase and pristanoyl-CoA oxidase. FEBS Lett 1996;388:80–4.

43. Singh I, Moser AE, Goldfischer S, Moser HW. Lignoceric acid is oxidized in the peroxisome: implications for the Zellweger cerebro-hepato-renal syndrome and adrenoleukodystrophy. Proc Natl Acad Sci U S A 1984;81:4203–7.

44. Bremer J, Norum KR. Metabolism of very long-chain monounsaturated fatty acids (22:1) and the adaptation to their presence in the diet. J Lipid Res 1982;23:243–56.

45. Neat CE, Thomassen MS, Osmundsen H. Induction of peroxisomal beta-oxidation in rat liver by high-fat diets. Biochem J 1980;186:369–71.

46. Mortensen PB, Kolvraa S, Gregersen N, Rasmussen K. Cyanide-insensitive and clofibrate enhanced beta-oxidation of dodecanedioic acid in rat liver. An indication of peroxisomal beta-oxidation of N-dicarboxylic acids. Biochim Biophys Acta 1982;713:393–7.

47. Vanhove GF, Van Veldhoven PP, Fransen M, et al. The CoA esters of 2-methyl-branched chain fatty acids and of the bile acid intermediates di- and trihydroxycoprostanic acids are oxidized by one single peroxisomal branched chain acyl-CoA oxidase in human liver and kidney. J Biol Chem 1993;268:10335–44.

48. Yamada J, Ogawa S, Horie S, et al. Participation of peroxisomes in the metabolism of xenobiotic acyl compounds: comparison between peroxisomal and mitochondrial beta-oxidation of omega-phenyl fatty acids in rat liver. Biochim Biophys Acta 1987;921:292–301.

49. Masters-Thomas A, Bailes J, Billimoria JD, et al. Heredopathia atactica polyneuritiformis (Refsum's disease): 2. Estimation of phytanic acid in foods. J Hum Nutr 1980;34:251–4.

50. Steinberg D, Herndon JH Jr, Uhlendorf BW, et al. Refsum's disease: nature of the enzyme defect. Science 1967;156:1740–2.

51. Billimoria JD, Clemens ME, Gibberd FB, Whitelaw MN. Metabolism of phytanic acid in Refsum's disease. Lancet 1982;i:194–6.

52. Watkins PA, Howard AE, Mihalik SJ. Phytanic acid must be activated to phytanoyl-CoA prior to its alpha-oxidation in rat liver peroxisomes. Biochim Biophys Acta 1994;1214:288–94.

53. Verhoeven NM, Schor DS, ten Brink HJ, et al. Resolution of the phytanic acid alpha-oxidation pathway: identification of pristanal as product of the decarboxylation of 2-hydroxy-phytanoyl-CoA. Biochem Biophys Res Commun 1997;237:33–6.

54. Croes K, Casteels M, Asselberghs S, et al. Formation of a 2-methyl-branched fatty aldehyde during peroxisomal alpha-oxidation. FEBS Lett 1007;412:643–5.

55. Croes K, Van Veldhoven PP, Mannaerts GP, Casteels M. Production of formyl-CoA during peroxisomal alpha-oxidation of 3-methyl-branched fatty acids. FEBS Lett 1997;407:197–200.

56. Foulon V, Antonenkov VD, Croes K, et al. Purification, molecular cloning, and expression of 2-hydroxyphytanoyl-CoA lyase, a peroxisomal thiamine pyrophosphate-dependent enzyme that catalyzes the carbon-carbon bond cleavage during alpha-oxidation of 3-methyl-branched fatty acids. Proc Natl Acad Sci U S A 1999;96:10039–44.

57. Verhoeven NM, Jakobs C, Carney G, et al. Involvement of microsomal fatty aldehyde dehydrogenase in the alpha-oxidation of phytanic acid. FEBS Lett 1998;429:225–8.

58. Jansen GA, Ofman R, Ferdinandusse S, et al. Refsum disease is caused by mutations in the phytanoyl-CoA hydroxylase gene. Nat Genet 1997;17:190–3.

59. Jansen GA, Ferdinandusse S, Skjeldal OH, et al. Molecular basis of Refsum disease: identification of new mutations in the phytanoyl-CoA hydroxylase cDNA. J Inherit Metab Dis 1998;21:288–91.

60. Mihalik SJ, Morrell JC, Kim D, et al. Identification of PAHX, a Refsum disease gene. Nat Genet 1997;17:185–9.

61. Braverman N, Steel G, Obie C, et al. Human PEX7 encodes the peroxisomal PTS2 receptor and is responsible for rhizomelic chondrodysplasia punctata. Nat Genet 1997;15:369–76.

62. Brown MS, Goldstein JL. Multivalent feedback regulation of HMG CoA reductase, a control mechanism coordinating isoprenoid synthesis and cell growth. J Lipid Res 1980;21:505–17.

63. Krisans SK. The role of peroxisomes in cholesterol metabolism. Am J Respir Cell Mol Biol 1992;7:358–64.

64. Stamellos KD, Shackelford JE, Tanaka RD, Krisans SK. Mevalonate kinase is localized in rat liver peroxisomes. J Biol Chem 1992;267:5560–8.

65. Biardi L, Krisans SK. Compartmentalization of cholesterol biosynthesis. Conversion of mevalonate to farnesyl diphosphate occurs in the peroxisomes. J Biol Chem 1996;271:1784–8.

66. Keller GA, Scallen TJ, Clarke D, et al. Subcellular localization of sterol carrier protein-2 in rat hepatocytes—its primary localization to peroxisomes. J Cell Biol 1989;108:1353–61.

67. Stamellos KD, Shackelford JE, Shechter I, et al. Subcellular localization of squalene synthase in rat hepatic cells. Biochemical and immunochemical evidence. J Biol Chem 1993;268:12825–36.

68. Aboushadi N, Shackelford JE, Jessani N, et al. Characterization of peroxisomal 3-hydroxy-3-methylglutaryl coenzyme A reductase in UT2 cells: sterol biosynthesis, phosphorylation, degradation, and statin inhibition. Biochemistry 2000;39:237–47.

69. Keller GA, Pazirandeh M, Krisans S. 3-Hydroxy-3-methylglutaryl coenzyme A reductase localization in rat liver peroxisomes and microsomes of control and cholestyramine-treated animals: quantitative biochemical and immunoelectron microscopical analyses. J Cell Biol 1986;103:875–86.

70. Appelkvist EL, Reinhart M, Fischer R, et al. Presence of individual enzymes of cholesterol biosynthesis in rat liver peroxisomes. Arch Biochem Biophys 1990;282:318–25.

71. Kelley RI. Review: the cerebrohepatorenal syndrome of Zellweger, morphologic and metabolic aspects. Am J Med Genet 1983;16:503–17.

72. Hodge VJ, Gould SJ, Subramani S, et al. Normal cholesterol synthesis in human cells requires functional peroxisomes. Biochem Biophys Res Commun 1991;181:537–41.

73. Eyssen H, Eggermont E, van Eldere J, et al. Bile acid abnormalities and the diagnosis of cerebro-hepato-renal syndrome (Zellweger syndrome). Acta Paediatr Scand 1985;74:539–44.

74. Parmentier GG, Janssen GA, Eggermont EA, Eyssen HJ. C27 bile acids in infants with coprostanic acidemia and occurrence of a 3 alpha,7 alpha,12 alpha-tridhydroxy-5 beta-C29 dicarboxylic bile acid as a major component in their serum. Eur J Biochem 1979;102:173–83.

75. Schutgens RB, Heymans HS, Wanders RJ, et al. Peroxisomal disorders: a newly recognised group of genetic diseases. Eur J Pediatr 1986;144:430–40.

76. Simion FA, Fleischer B, Fleischer S. Subcellular distribution of cholic acid:coenzyme A ligase and deoxycholic acid:coenzyme A ligase activities in rat liver. Biochemistry 1983;22:5029–34.

77. Mihalik SJ, Steinberg SJ, Pei Z, et al. Participation of two members of the very long-chain acyl-CoA synthetase family in bile acid synthesis and recycling. J Biol Chem 2002;277:24771–9.

78. Natowicz MR, Evans JE, Kelley RI, et al. Urinary bile acids and peroxisomal bifunctional enzyme deficiency. Am J Med Genet 1996;63:356–62.

79. Kase BF, Bjorkhem I. Peroxisomal bile acid-CoA-amino-acid N-acyltransferase in rat liver. J Biol Chem 1989;264:9220–3.

80. Snyder F, editor. Ether lipids. New York: Academic Press; 1972.

81. Hanahan DJ, Demopoulos CA, Liehr J, Pinckard RN. Identification of platelet activating factor isolated from rabbit basophils as acetyl glyceryl ether phosphorylcholine. J Biol Chem 1980;255:5514–6.

82. Hajra AK, Burke CL, Jones CL. Subcellular localization of acyl coenzyme A: dihydroxyacetone phosphate acyltransferase in rat liver peroxisomes (microbodies). J Biol Chem 1979;254:10896–900.

83. Hajra AK, Horie S, Webber KO. The role of peroxisomes in glycerol ether lipid metabolism. Prog Clin Biol Res 1988;282:99–116.

84. Hayashi H, Hara M. 1-Alkenyl group of ethanolamine plasmalogen derives mainly from de novo-synthesized fatty alcohol within peroxisomes, but not extraperoxisomal fatty alcohol or fatty acid. J Biochem (Tokyo) 1997;121:978–83.

85. Rothstein M, Miller L. The conversion of lysine to pipecolic acid in the rat. J Biol Chem 1954;211:851–58.

86. Meister A, Radhakrishnan A, Buckley S. Enzymatic synthesis of L-pipecolic acid and L-proline. J Biol Chem 1957;229:789–800.

87. Mihalik SJ, McGuinness M, Watkins PA. Purification and characterization of peroxisomal L-pipecolic acid oxidase from monkey liver. J Biol Chem 1991;266:4822–30.

88. Dodt G, Kim DG, Reimann SA, et al. L-Pipecolic acid oxidase, a human enzyme essential for the degradation of L-pipecolic acid, is most similar to the monomeric sarcosine oxidases. Biochem J 2000;345:487–94.

89. Lam S, Hutzler J, Dancis J. L-Pipecolaturia in Zellweger syndrome. Biochim Biophys Acta 1986;882:254–7.

90. Takahama K, Miyata T, Hashimoto T, et al. Pipecolic acid: a new type of alpha-amino acid possessing bicuculline-sensitive action in the mammalian brain. Brain Res 1982;239:294–8.

91. Mihalik SJ, Rhead WJ. Species variation in organellar location and activity of L-pipecolic acid oxidation in mammals. J Comp Physiol [B] 1991;160:671–5.

92. Ghadimi H, Chou WS, Kesner L. Biosynthesis of saccharopine and pipecolic acid from L- and DL- 14 C-lysine by human and dog liver in vitro. Biochem Med 1971;5:56–66.

93. Chang YE. Lysine metabolism in the rat brain: the pipecolic acid-forming pathway. J Neurochem 1978;30:347–54.

94. Wanders RJ, Romeyn GJ, van Roermund CW, et al. Identification of L-pipecolate oxidase in human liver and its deficiency in the Zellweger syndrome. Biochem Biophys Res Commun 1988;154:33–8.

95. Mihalik SJ, Moser HW, Watkins PA, et al. Peroxisomal L-pipecolic acid oxidation is deficient in liver from Zellweger syndrome patients. Pediatr Res 1989;25:548–52.

96. Zaar K, Angermuller S, Volkl A, Fahimi HD. Pipecolic acid is oxidized by renal and hepatic peroxisomes. Implications for Zellweger's cerebro-hepato-renal syndrome (CHRS). Exp Cell Res 1986;164:267–71.

97. de Duve C, Baudhuin P. Peroxisomes (microbodies and related particles). Physiol Rev 1966;46:323–57.

98. Chance B, Oshino N. Kinetics and mechanisms of catalase in peroxisomes of the mitochondrial fraction. Biochem J 1971; 122:225–33.

99. Wanders RJ, Kos M, Roest B, et al. Activity of peroxisomal enzymes and intracellular distribution of catalase in Zellweger syndrome. Biochem Biophys Res Commun 1984;123: 1054–61.

100. Nedergaard J, Alexson S, Cannon B. Cold adaptation in the rat: increased brown fat peroxisomal beta-oxidation relative to maximal mitochondrial oxidative capacity. Am J Physiol 1980;239:C208–16.

101. Moser HW. Genotype-phenotype correlations in disorders of peroxisome biogenesis. Mol Genet Metab 1999;68:316–27.

102. Brul S, Westerveld A, Strijland A, et al. Genetic heterogeneity in the cerebrohepatorenal (Zellweger) syndrome and other inherited disorders with a generalized impairment of peroxisomal functions. A study using complementation analysis. J Clin Invest 1988;81:1710–5.

103. Roscher AA, Hoefler S, Hoefler G, et al. Genetic and phenotypic heterogeneity in disorders of peroxisome biogenesis—a complementation study involving cell lines from 19 patients. Pediatr Res 1989;26:67–72.

104. Passarge E, McAdams AJ. Cerebro-hepato-renal syndrome. A newly recognized hereditary disorder of multiple congenital defects, including sudanophilic leukodystrophy, cirrhosis of the liver, and polycystic kidneys. J Pediatr 1967;71:691–702.

105. Opitz JM. The Zellweger syndrome (cerebro-hepatorenal syndrome). Birth Defects Orig Artic Ser 1969;V:144–58.

106. Mooi WJ, Dingemans KP, van den Bergh Weerman MA, et al. Ultrastructure of the liver in the cerebrohepatorenal syndrome of Zellweger. Ultrastruct Pathol 1983;5:135–44.

107. Carlson BR, Weinberg AG. Giant cell transformation: cerebrohepatorenal syndrome. Arch Pathol Lab Med 1978;102:596–9.

108. Bernstein J, Brough AJ, McAdams AJ. The renal lesion in syndromes of multiple congenital malformations. Cerebrohepatorenal syndrome; Jeune asphyxiating thoracic dystrophy; tuberous sclerosis; Meckel syndrome. Birth Defects Orig Artic Ser 1974;10:35–43.

109. Poznanski AK, Nosanchuk JS, Baublis J, Holt JF. The cerebro-hepato-renal syndrome (CHRS) (Zellweger's syndrome). AJR Am J Roentgenol 1970;109:313–22.

110. Liu MC, Yu S, Suiko M. Tyramine-O-sulfate, in addition to tyrosine-O-sulfate, is produced and secreted by Hepg2 human hepatoma cells, but not by 3Y1 rat embryo fibroblasts. Biochem Int 1990;21:815–21.

111. Volpe JJ, Adams RD. Cerebro-hepato-renal syndrome of Zellweger: an inherited disorder of neuronal migration. Acta Neuropathol (Berl) 1972;20:175–98.

112. Cohen SM, Brown FR III, Martyn L, et al. Ocular histopathologic and biochemical studies of the cerebrohepatorenal syndrome (Zellweger's syndrome) and its relationship to neonatal adrenoleukodystrophy. Am J Ophthalmol 1983;96:488–501.

113. Bleeker-Wagemakers EM, Oorthuys JW, Wanders RJ, Schutgens RB. Long term survival of a patient with the cerebro-hepato-renal (Zellweger) syndrome. Clin Genet 1986;29:160–4.

114. Heymans HS. Cerebro-hepato-renal (Zellweger) syndrome. Clinical and biochemical consequences of peroxisomal dysfunction[thesis]. Amsterdam: University of Amsterdam; 1984.

115. Wilson GN, Holmes RG, Custer J, et al. Zellweger syndrome: diagnostic assays, syndrome delineation, and potential therapy. Am J Med Genet 1986;24:69–82.

116. Liu HM, Bangaru BS, Kidd J, Boggs J. Neuropathological considerations in cerebro-hepato-renal syndrome (Zellweger's syndrome). Acta Neuropathol (Berl) 1976;34:115–23.

117. Powers JM, Tummons RC, Moser AB, et al. Neuronal lipidosis and neuroaxonal dystrophy in cerebro-hepato-renal (Zellweger) syndrome. Acta Neuropathol (Berl) 1987;73:333–43.

118. Powers JM. The pathology of peroxisomal disorders with pathogenetic considerations. J Neuropathol Exp Neurol 1995; 54:710–9.

119. Vuia O, Hager H, Rupp H, Koch F. The neuropathology of a peculiar form of cerebro-renal syndrome in a child. Neuropadiatrie 1973;4:322–37.

120. Agamanolis DP, Robinson HB Jr, Timmons GD. Cerebro-hepatorenal syndrome. Report of a case with histochemical and ultrastructural observations. J Neuropathol Exp Neurol 1976;35:226–46.

121. Schaumburg HH, Powers JM, Raine CS, et al. Adrenoleukodystrophy. A clinical and pathological study of 17 cases. Arch Neurol 1975;32:577–91.

122. Moser AE, Singh I, Brown FR III, et al. The cerebrohepatorenal (Zellweger) syndrome. Increased levels and impaired degradation of very-long-chain fatty acids and their use in prenatal diagnosis. N Engl J Med 1984;310:1141–6.

123. Poulos A, Sharp P, Singh H, et al. Detection of a homologous series of C26-C38 polyenoic fatty acids in the brain of patients without peroxisomes (Zellweger's syndrome). Biochem J 1986;235:607–10.

124. Brown FR III, McAdams AJ, Cummins JW, et al. Cerebro-hepato-renal (Zellweger) syndrome and neonatal adrenoleukodystrophy: similarities in phenotype and accumulation of very long chain fatty acids. Johns Hopkins Med J 1982;151:344–51.

125. Pfeifer U. [Liver cirrhosis in cerebro-hepato-renal syndrome (Zellweger syndrome) in early childhood.] Pathologe 1979; 1:47–9.

126. Muller-Hocker J, Bise K, Endres W, Hubner G. [Morphology and diagnosis of Zellweger syndrome. A contribution to combined cytochemical-finestructural identification of peroxisomes in autopsy material and frozen liver tissue with case report.] Virchows Arch A Pathol Anat Histol 1981;393:103–14.

127. Govaerts L, Monnens L, Tegelaers W, et al. Cerebro-hepatorenal syndrome of Zellweger: clinical symptoms and relevant laboratory findings in 16 patients. Eur J Pediatr 1982; 139:125–8.

128. Challa VR, Geisinger KR, Burton BK. Pathologic alterations in the brain and liver in hyperpipecolic acidemia. J Neuropathol Exp Neurol 1983;42:627–38.

129. Mandel H, Meiron D, Schutgens RB, et al. Infantile Refsum disease: gastrointestinal presentation of a peroxisomal disorder. J Pediatr Gastroenterol Nutr 1992;14:83–5.

130. Mandel H, Berant M, Meiron D, et al. Plasma lipoproteins and monocyte-macrophages in a peroxisome-deficient system: study of a patient with infantile Refsum disease. J Inherit Metab Dis 1992;15:774–84.

131. Setchell KD, Bragetti P, Zimmer-Nechemias L, et al. Oral bile acid treatment and the patient with Zellweger syndrome. Hepatology 1992;15:198–207.

132. Martinez M. Severe deficiency of docosahexaenoic acid in peroxisomal disorders: a defect of delta 4 desaturation? Neurology 1990;40:1292–8.

133. Martinez M. Abnormal profiles of polyunsaturated fatty acids in the brain, liver, kidney and retina of patients with peroxisomal disorders. Brain Res 1992;583:171–82.

134. Su HM, Moser AB, Moser HW, Watkins PA. Peroxisomal straight-chain acyl-CoA oxidase and D-bifunctional protein are essential for the retroconversion step in docosahexaenoic acid synthesis. J Biol Chem 2001;276:38115–20.

135. Moore SA, Hurt E, Yoder E, et al. Docosahexaenoic acid synthesis in human skin fibroblasts involves peroxisomal retroconversion of tetracosahexaenoic acid. J Lipid Res 1995;36:2433–43.

136. Brosche T, Platt D. The biological significance of plasmalogens in defense against oxidative damage. Exp Gerontol 1998;33:363–9.

137. Scotto JM, Hadchouel M, Odievre M, et al. Infantile phytanic acid storage disease, a possible variant of Refsum's disease: three cases, including ultrastructural studies of the liver. J Inherit Metab Dis 1982;5:83–90.

138. Poulos A, Sharp P, Whiting M. Infantile Refsum's disease (phytanic acid storage disease): a variant of Zellweger's syndrome? Clin Genet 1984;26:579–86.

139. Poulos A, Whiting MJ. Identification of 3 alpha,7 alpha,12 alpha-trihydroxy-5 beta-cholestan-26-oic acid, an intermediate in cholic acid synthesis, in the plasma of patients with infantile Refsum's disease. J Inherit Metab Dis 1985;8:13–7.

140. Budden SS, Kennaway NG, Buist NR, et al. Dysmorphic syndrome with phytanic acid oxidase deficiency, abnormal very long chain fatty acids, and pipecolic acidemia: studies in four children. J Pediatr 1986;108:33–9.

141. Martinez M. Severe changes in polyunsaturated fatty acids in the brain, liver, kidney, and retina in patients with peroxisomal disorders. Adv Exp Med Biol 1992;318:347–59.

142. Roels F, Cornelis A, Poll-The BT, et al. Hepatic peroxisomes are deficient in infantile Refsum disease: a cytochemical study of 4 cases. Am J Med Genet 1986;25:257–71.

143. Torvik A, Torp S, Kase BF, et al. Infantile Refsum's disease: a generalized peroxisomal disorder. Case report with postmortem examination. J Neurol Sci 1988;85:39–53.

144. Ulrich J, Herschkowitz N, Heitz P, et al. Adrenoleukodystrophy. Preliminary report of a connatal case. Light- and electron microscopical, immunohistochemical and biochemical findings. Acta Neuropathol (Berl) 1978;43:77–83.

145. Kelley RI, Datta NS, Dobyns WB, et al. Neonatal adrenoleukodystrophy: new cases, biochemical studies, and differentiation from Zellweger and related peroxisomal polydystrophy syndromes. Am J Med Genet 1986;23:869–901.

146. Vamecq J, Draye JP, Van Hoof F, et al. Multiple peroxisomal enzymatic deficiency disorders. A comparative biochemical and morphologic study of Zellweger cerebrohepatorenal syndrome and neonatal adrenoleukodystrophy. Am J Pathol 1986;125:524–35.

147. Aubourg P, Scotto J, Rocchiccioli F, et al. Neonatal adrenoleukodystrophy. J Neurol Neurosurg Psychiatry 1986;49:77–86.

148. Gatfield PD, Taller E, Hinton GG, et al. Hyperpipecolatemia: a new metabolic disorder associated with neuropathy and hepatomegaly: a case study. Can Med Assoc J 1968;99:1215–33.

149. Burton BK, Reed SP, Remy WT. Hyperpipecolic acidemia: clinical and biochemical observations in two male siblings. J Pediatr 1981;99:729–34.

150. Thomas GH, Haslam RH, Batshaw ML, et al. Hyperpipecolic acidemia associated with hepatomegaly, mental retardation, optic nerve dysplasia and progressive neurological disease. Clin Genet 1975;8:376–82.

151. Wanders RJ, van Roermund CW, van Wijland MJ, et al. Peroxisomes and peroxisomal functions in hyperpipecolic acidaemia. J Inherit Metab Dis 1988;11 Suppl 2:161–4.

152. Buissonniere RF, Storni V, Robain O, Ponsot G. Joubert's syndrome. Ann Pediatr 1990;37:151–6.

153. Roesel RA, Carroll JE, Rizzo WB, et al. Dyggve-Melchior-Clausen syndrome with increased pipecolic acid in plasma and urine. J Inherit Metab Dis 1991;14:876–80.

154. Wanders RJ, van Roermund CW, van Wijland MJ, et al. Peroxisomal fatty acid beta-oxidation in relation to the accumulation of very long chain fatty acids in cultured skin fibroblasts from patients with Zellweger syndrome and other peroxisomal disorders. J Clin Invest 1987;80:1778–83.

155. Wanders RJA, van Roermund CWT, van Wijland MJA, et al. X-linked adrenoleukodystrophy: identification of the primary defect at the level of a deficient peroxisomal very long chain fatty acyl-CoA synthetase using a newly developed method for the isolation of peroxisomes from skin fibroblasts. J Inherit Metab Dis 1988;11 Suppl 2:173–7.

156. Mosser J, Douar AM, Sarde CO, et al. Putative X-linked adrenoleukodystrophy gene shares unexpected homology with ABC transporters. Nature 1993;361:726–30.

157. Klein I, Sarkadi B, Varadi A. An inventory of the human ABC proteins. Biochim Biophys Acta 1999;1461:237–62.

158. Holland IB, Blight MA. ABC-ATPases, adaptable energy generators fuelling transmembrane movement of a variety of molecules in organisms from bacteria to humans. J Mol Biol 1999;293:381–99.

159. Yamada T, Taniwaki T, Shinnoh N, et al. Adrenoleukodystrophy protein enhances association of very long-chain acyl-coenzyme A synthetase with the peroxisome. Neurology 1999;52:614–6.

160. Heinzer AK, Kemp S, Lu JF, et al. Mouse very long-chain acyl-CoA synthetase in X-linked adrenoleukodystrophy. J Biol Chem 2002;277:28765–73.

161. Moser HW, Moser AE, Singh I, O'Neill BP. Adrenoleukodystrophy: survey of 303 cases: biochemistry, diagnosis, and therapy. Ann Neurol 1984;16:628–41.

162. Moser HW, Moser AE, Trojak JE, Supplee SW. Identification of female carriers of adrenoleukodystrophy. J Pediatr 1983;103:54–9.

163. O'Neill BP, Moser HW, Saxena KM, Marmion LC. Adrenoleukodystrophy: clinical and biochemical manifestations in carriers. Neurology 1984;34:798–801.

164. Corzo D, Gibson W, Johnson K, et al. Contiguous deletion of the X-linked adrenoleukodystrophy gene (ABCD1) and DXS1357E: a novel neonatal phenotype similar to peroxisomal biogenesis disorders. Am J Hum Genet 2002;70:1520–31.

165. Fournier B, Munnich A, Saudubray JM, et al. Large DNA deletion in two peroxisomal acyl-CoA oxidase patients. Biol Cell 1993;77:116.

166. Watkins PA, Chen WW, Harris CJ, et al. Peroxisomal bifunctional enzyme deficiency. J Clin Invest 1989;83:771–7.

167. Wanders RJA, Vanroermund CWT, Brul S, et al. Bifunctional enzyme deficiency—identification of a new type of peroxisomal disorder in a patient with an impairment in peroxisomal beta-oxidation of unknown aetiology by means of complementation analysis. J Inherit Metab Dis 1992;15:385–8.

168. Kaufmann WE, Theda C, Naidu S, et al. Neuronal migration abnormality in peroxisomal bifunctional enzyme defect. Ann Neurol 1996;39:268–71.

169. McGuinness MC, Moser AB, Poll-The BT, Watkins PA. Complementation analysis of patients with intact peroxisomes and impaired peroxisomal beta-oxidation. Biochem Med Metab Biol 1993;49:228–42.

170. Goldfischer S, Collins J, Rapin I, et al. Pseudo-Zellweger syndrome: deficiencies in several peroxisomal oxidative activities. J Pediatr 1986;108:25–32.

171. Schram AW, Goldfischer S, van Roermund CW, et al. Human peroxisomal 3-oxoacyl-coenzyme A thiolase deficiency. Proc Natl Acad Sci U S A 1987;84:2494–6.

172. Ferdinandusse S, Van Grunsven EG, Oostheim W, et al. Reinvestigation of peroxisomal 3-ketoacyl-CoA thiolase deficiency: identification of the true defect at the level of d-bifunctional protein. Am J Hum Genet 2002;70:1589–93.

173. Ferdinandusse S, Denis S, Clayton PT, et al. Mutations in the gene encoding peroxisomal alpha-methylacyl-CoA racemase cause adult-onset sensory motor neuropathy. Nat Genet 2000;24:188–91.

174. Setchell KD, Heubi JE, Bove KE, O'Connell NC, et al. Liver disease caused by failure to racemize trihydroxycholestanoic acid: gene mutation and effect of bile acid therapy. Gastroenterology 2003;124:217–32.

175. Clayton PT, Lake BD, Hall NA, et al. Plasma bile acids in patients with peroxisomal dysfunction syndromes: analysis by capillary gas chromatography-mass spectrometry. Eur J Pediatr 1987;146:166–73.

176. Christensen E, Pedersen SA, Leth H, et al. A new peroxisomal beta-oxidation disorder in twin neonates: defective oxidation of both cerotic and pristanic acids. J Inherit Metab Dis 1997;20:658–64.

177. Spranger JW, Opitz JM, Bidder U. Heterogeneity of chondrodysplasia punctata. Humangenetik 1971;11:190–212.

178. Heymans HS, Oorthuys JW, Nelck G, et al. Rhizomelic chondrodysplasia punctata: another peroxisomal disorder. N Engl J Med 1985;313:187–8.

179. Hoefler G, Hoefler S, Watkins PA, et al. Biochemical abnormalities in rhizomelic chondrodysplasia punctata. J Pediatr 1988;112:726–33.

180. Wanders RJ, Romeijn GJ. Differential deficiency of mevalonate kinase and phosphomevalonate kinase in patients with distinct defects in peroxisome biogenesis: evidence for a major role of peroxisomes in cholesterol biosynthesis. Biochem Biophys Res Commun 1998;247:663–7.

181. Moser AB, Rasmussen M, Naidu S, et al. Phenotype of patients with peroxisomal disorders subdivided into sixteen complementation groups. J Pediatr 1995;127:13–22.

182. Nuoffer JM, Pfammatter JP, Spahr A, et al. Chondrodysplasia punctata with a mild clinical course. J Inherit Metab Dis 1994;17:60–6.

183. Smeitink JA, Beemer FA, Espeel M, et al. Bone dysplasia associated with phytanic acid accumulation and deficient plasmalogen synthesis: a peroxisomal entity amenable to plasmapheresis. J Inherit Metab Dis 1992;15:377–80.

184. Barr DG, Kirk JM, al Howasi M, et al. Rhizomelic chondrodysplasia punctata with isolated DHAP-AT deficiency. Arch Dis Child 1993;68:415–7.

185. Hebestreit H, Wanders RJA, Schutgens RBH, et al. Isolated dihydroxyacetonephosphate-acyl-transferase deficiency in rhizomelic chondrodysplasia punctata: clinical presentation, metabolic and histological findings. Eur J Pediatr 1996;155:1035–9.

186. Clayton PT, Eckhardt S, Wilson J, et al. Isolated dihydroxyacetonephosphate acyltransferase deficiency presenting with developmental delay. J Inherit Metab Dis 1994;17:533–40.

187. de Vet EC, Ijlst L, Oostheim W, et al. Alkyl-dihydroxyacetonephosphate synthase. Fate in peroxisome biogenesis disorders and identification of the point mutation underlying a single enzyme deficiency. J Biol Chem 1998;273:10296–301.

188. Emami S, Hanley KP, Esterly NB, et al. X-linked dominant ichthyosis with peroxisomal deficiency. An ultrastructural and ultracytochemical study of the Conradi-Hünermann syndrome and its murine homologue, the bare patches mouse. Arch Dermatol 1994;130:325–36.

189. Braverman N, Lin P, Moebius FF, et al. Mutations in the gene encoding 3 beta-hydroxysteroid-delta 8, delta 7-isomerase cause X-linked dominant Conradi-Hünermann syndrome. Nat Genet 1999;22:291–4.

190. Kelley RI, Wilcox WG, Smith M, et al. Abnormal sterol metabolism in patients with Conradi-Hünermann-Happle syndrome and sporadic lethal chondrodysplasia punctata. Am J Med Genet 1999;83:213–9.

191. Refsum S. Heredopathia atactica polyneuritiformis: a familial syndrome not hitherto described. Acta Psychiatr Neurol Scand 1946;38:1–303.

192. Kolodny E. Refsum's disease. Report of a case including electron microscopic studies of the liver. Arch Neurol 1965;12:583–96.

193. Eldjarn L, Stokke O, Try K. Alpha-oxidation of branched chain fatty acids in man and its failure in patients with Refsum's disease showing phytanic acid accumulation. Scand J Clin Lab Invest 1966;18:694–5.

194. Jansen GA, Mihalik SJ, Watkins PA, et al. Phytanoyl-CoA hydroxylase is present in human liver, located in peroxisomes, and deficient in Zellweger syndrome: direct, unequivocal evidence for the new, revised pathway of phytanic acid alpha-oxidation in humans. Biochem Biophys Res Commun 1996;229:205–10.

195. Poulos A, Sharp P, Fellenberg AJ, Danks DM. Cerebro-hepato-renal (Zellweger) syndrome, adrenoleukodystrophy, and Refsum's disease: plasma changes and skin fibroblast phytanic acid oxidase. Hum Genet 1985;70:172–7.

196. Skjeldal OH, Stokke O. The subcellular localization of phytanic acid oxidase in rat liver. Biochim Biophys Acta 1987;921:38–42.

197. Latta K, Brodehl J. Primary hyperoxaluria type I. Eur J Pediatr 1990;149:518–22.

198. Danpure CJ, Jennings PR, Fryer P, et al. Primary hyperoxaluria type 1: genotypic and phenotypic heterogeneity. J Inherit Metab Dis 1994;17:487–99.

199. Iancu TC, Danpure CJ. Primary hyperoxaluria type I: ultrastructural observations in liver biopsies. J Inherit Metab Dis 1987;10:330–8.

200. Danpure CJ, Jennings PR, Watts RW. Enzymological diagnosis of primary hyperoxaluria type 1 by measurement of hepatic alanine:glyoxylate aminotransferase activity. Lancet 1987;i:289–91.

201. Noguchi T, Takada Y. Peroxisomal localization of alanine:glyoxylate aminotransferase in human liver. Arch Biochem Biophys 1979;196:645–7.

202. Danpure CJ, Cooper PJ, Wise PJ, Jennings PR. An enzyme trafficking defect in two patients with primary hyperoxaluria type 1: peroxisomal alanine/glyoxylate aminotransferase rerouted to mitochondria. J Cell Biol 1989;108:1345–52.

203. Wanders RJ, van Roermund CW, Westra R, et al. Alanine glyoxylate aminotransferase and the urinary excretion of oxalate and glycollate in hyperoxaluria type I and the Zellweger syndrome. Clin Chim Acta 1987;165:311–9.

204. Cochat P, Gaulier JM, Koch Nogueira PC, et al. Combined liver-kidney transplantation in primary hyperoxaluria type 1. Eur J Pediatr 1999;158 Suppl 2:S75–80.

205. Eaton JW, Mouchou M. Acatalasemia. In: Scriver CV, Beaudet AL, Sly WS, Valle D, editors. The metabolic and molecular bases of inherited disease. 7th ed. New York: McGraw-Hill; 1995 p. 2371–84.

206. Takahara S. Progressive oral gangrene probably due to a lack of catalase in the blood (acatalasemia). Lancet 1952;ii:1011.

207. Moser HW. Peroxisomal disorders. Semin Pediatr Neurol 1996; 3:298–304.

208. Moser AB, Singh I, Brown FRI, et al. The cerebro-hepato-renal (Zellweger) syndrome: increased levels and impaired oxidation of very-long-chain fatty acids, and their use in prenatal diagnosis. N Engl J Med 1984;310:1141–6.

209. Kelley RI. Quantification of pipecolic acid in plasma and urine by isotope dilution gas chromatography/mass spectrometry. In: Hommes FA, editor. Techniques in diagnostic human biochemical genetics: a laboratory manual. New York: Wiley-Liss; 1991. p. 205–18.

210. Wanders RJ, Schutgens RB, van den Bosch H, et al. Prenatal diagnosis of inborn errors in peroxisomal beta-oxidation. Prenat Diagn 1991;11:253–61.

211. Schutgens RB, Schrakamp G, Wanders RJ, et al. Prenatal and perinatal diagnosis of peroxisomal disorders. J Inherit Metab Dis 1989;12 Suppl 1:118–34.

212. Danpure CJ, Rumsby G. Strategies for the prenatal diagnosis of primary hyperoxaluria type 1. Prenat Diagn 1996;16:587–98.

213. Holmes RD. Oral ether-lipid therapy in patients with peroxisomal disorders. J Inherit Metab Dis 1987;10 Suppl 2:239–41.

214. Robertson EF, Poulos A, Sharp P, et al. Treatment of infantile phytanic acid storage disease: clinical, biochemical and ultrastructural findings in two children treated for 2 years. Eur J Pediatr 1988;147:133–42.

215. Bjorkhem I, Blomstrand S, Glaumann H, Strandvik B. Unsuccessful attempts to induce peroxisomes in two cases of Zellweger disease by treatment with clofibrate. Pediatr Res 1985;19:590–3.

216. Martinez M, Vazquez E, Garcia-Silva MT, et al. Therapeutic effects of docosahexaenoic acid ethyl ester in patients with generalized peroxisomal disorders. Am J Clin Nutr 2000; 71:376S–85S.

217. Martinez M, Pineda M, Vidal R, et al. Docosahexaenoic acid—a new therapeutic approach to peroxisomal-disorder patients—experience with two cases. Neurology 1993;43:1389–97.

218. Martinez M, Vazquez E. MRI evidence that docosahexaenoic acid ethyl ester improves myelination in generalized peroxisomal disorders. Neurology 1998;51:26–32.

219. Moser AB, Borel J, Odone A, et al. A new dietary therapy for adrenoleukodystrophy: biochemical and preliminary clinical results in 36 patients. Ann Neurol 1987;21:240–9.

220. Moser HW. New approaches in peroxisomal disorders. Dev Neurosci 1987;9:1–18.

221. van Geel BM, Assies J, Haverkort EB, et al. Progression of abnormalities in adrenomyeloneuropathy and neurologically asymptomatic X-linked adrenoleukodystrophy despite treatment with "Lorenzo's oil." J Neurol Neurosurg Psychiatry 1999;67:290–9.

222. Moser HW, Raymond GV, Kohler W, et al. Evaluation of the preventive effect of gylceryl trioleate-trierucate ("Lorenzo's oil") therapy in X-linked adrenoleukodystrophy: results of two concurrent trials. In: Roels F, Baes M, De Bie S, editors. Peroxisomal disorders and regulation of genes. New York: Kluwer Academic/Plenum; 2003. [In press]

223. Aubourg P, Blanche S, Jambaque I, et al. Reversal of early neurologic and neuroradiologic manifestations of X-linked adrenoleukodystrophy by bone marrow transplantation. N Engl J Med 1990;322:1860–6.

224. Shapiro E, Krivit W, Lockman L, et al. Long-term effect of bone-marrow transplantation for childhood-onset cerebral X-linked adrenoleukodystrophy. Lancet 2000;356:713–8.

9. Lysosomal Acid Lipase Deficiencies: Wolman Disease and Cholesteryl Ester Storage Disease

Gregory A. Grabowski, MD

Kevin Bove, MD

Hong Du, PhD

HISTORICAL OVERVIEW

Abramov and colleagues described patients with severe malnutrition, hepatosplenomegaly, calcified adrenal glands, and death occurring within the first few months of life.[1] Additional patients in this family were described in 1961,[2] and the term Wolman disease was applied to such patients. These patients accumulated cholesteryl esters and triglycerides in many organs, most predominantly in the liver, spleen, adrenal glands, and lymph nodes. However, in 1946, Alexander described a patient with Niemann-Pick disease with a similar phenotype and calcification of the adrenal glands.[3] This is likely to be the earliest description of Wolman disease. During the period of 1963 to 1968, additional variants similar to but more mild than Wolman disease were described by Fredrickson, Schiff, Langeron, and Infante and their colleagues.[4–7] These individuals ranged in age from childhood to the fourth decade with hepatomegaly and increased levels of cholesteryl esters in the liver. The intestinal biopsy abnormalities in two such patients were described by Partin and Schubert; they coined the term cholesteryl ester storage disease (CESD).[8]

These two disorders represent a continuum of disease severity and are due to mutations in the locus for lysosomal acid lipase (LAL), an enzyme essential to the degradation of cholesteryl esters and triglycerides that arrive in the lysosome by receptor-mediated endocytosis. These allelic variants of LAL deficiency are termed Wolman disease and CESD. Because of the apparent rarity of the disorders, the full clinical spectra have yet to be fully described. These disorders represent a continuum of disease from the most severe variants, termed Wolman diseases, to progressively less severe involvement in CESD (Figure 55.9-1). The complete clinical spectrum, biochemistry, and pathophysiology have yet to be elucidated, although the availability of animal models should provide additional insight into the disease development and progression.[9,10] The work of Horton, Brown, and Goldstein and their colleagues has made clear the central role that LAL plays in intracellular cholesterol and lipid metabolism.[11–13] The disruption of intracellular lipid regulation leads to severe global metabolic derangements and lipodystrophy.[14]

CLINICAL/PATHOLOGIC PRESENTATION OF WOLMAN DISEASE AND CHOLESTERYL ESTER STORAGE DISEASE

WOLMAN DISEASE

The clinical course of Wolman disease has remarkable uniformity. Patients present within the first month of life with vomiting and diarrhea, hepatosplenomegaly, abdominal distention, and inanition with pyrexia and severe failure to thrive. This clinical course perpetuates itself in a downhill spiral to death by age 3 to 7 months.[15] An occasional patient survives beyond 1 year depending on the supportive medical interventions.

The first overt sign is protracted and persistent vomiting associated with abdominal distention. This occurs within

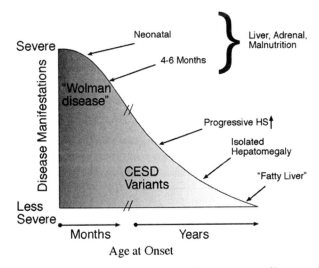

FIGURE 55.9-1 Schematic diagram of a continuum of lysosomal acid lipase deficiency states. Early-onset variants have manifestations in the first few days to weeks of postnatal life and by 4 to 6 months display characteristics of Wolman disease, including hepatosplenomegaly, adrenal enlargement and calcifications, and malnutrition. Variants with components of these signs occur from 1 to 12 years of age, and patients with cholesteryl ester storage disease (CESD), adrenal calcification, and pulmonary hypertension have been reported. At advanced ages, the only manifestation of poorly characterized "fatty liver" may represent late-onset CESD.

the first weeks of life and is accompanied by watery diarrhea, jaundice (occasionally), and low-grade fever. These are intractable to medical interventions or changes in diet and lead to severe weight loss, cachexia, and malnutrition.[1,16,17] Physical examination reveals hepatosplenomegaly with predominant liver enlargement. Enlargement of these organs can occur very soon after birth and has been noted as early as 4 days of age.[18] The first indication of Wolman disease is the abdominal radiograph showing massive enlargement and calcification of the adrenal glands.[16] The adrenal glands have punctate calcification throughout their parenchyma, are symmetrically and massively enlarged, and retain their normal shapes (Figure 55.9-2). Although not well delineated in published reports, these children also manifest adrenal cortical insufficiency (W. Krivit, personal communication, 2003).[18] Analyses of the abdomen by magnetic resonance imaging, computed tomography, or radiography also disclose massively enlarged liver and spleen with lymph node hypertrophy.[19] The latter can include the tonsils and adenoids that may be enlarged sufficiently to cause obstruction.

No specific signs or symptoms are referable to the central nervous system.[15] General deterioration is noted, with the progressive malnutrition and inanition that these children experience.[18,20] However, seizure, convulsions, and paralysis are reported occasionally in Wolman disease. These few central nervous system abnormalities are not primarily related to Wolman disease but rather are related to the malnutrition and specific nutritional deficiencies because of the severe malabsorption (see below).

No specific routine blood chemical abnormalities are present in Wolman disease patients. Anemia, abnormal liver function studies, or other chemical abnormalities referable to severe malnutrition can be present. Malabsorption of fats and other food stuffs has been documented. Specifically, triolein malabsorption is present.[20] This correlates with the infiltration of the jejunum with lipid-laden macrophages (see below). Indeed, intestinal damage may be so severe as to prevent enteral nutrition, and parenteral supplementation should be considered.[21] Because of the

adrenal calcification, it is not surprising that patients have adrenocortical insufficiency and require supplementation.[16]

Wolman disease should be considered in the differential diagnosis of any child presenting with persistent vomiting or diarrhea, failure to thrive, hepatosplenomegaly, and malabsorption within the first month of life. The presence of enlarged calcified adrenal glands should be an immediate clue to the diagnosis of Wolman disease.

CHOLESTERYL ESTER STORAGE DISEASE

In comparison with Wolman disease, CESD is a more variable and poorly delineated clinical syndrome. Although CESD is thought to be quite rare, this is an underestimate because of poor disease recognition. The clinical spectrum ranges from children diagnosed at age 3 to 4 years to adults in the fifth to sixth decade who present with variable manifestations but including isolated hepatomegaly.[22] The clinical course and progression of CESD in young children have been poorly documented. The relationship between apparent involvement early in life and the potential for significant progression to severe disease later in life remains to be elucidated. Importantly, the fulminant course is poorly documented and includes development of cirrhosis, pulmonary hypertension, onset of adrenal calcifications in adolescence, and failure to thrive.[23–25] In comparison, other patients may have a much more indolent course, with slow progression throughout their lifetimes. Except for mild hepatomegaly, these patients may go undiagnosed throughout their lives. The number of such patients and lack of follow-up information severely limit the ability of physicians to provide accurate information on disease progression to involved families.

Clearly, only the most severely involved patients are usually reported in the literature. This skews the perception of patients and physicians as to the degree of severity and progression of this disease. In particular, the presence of hepatic fibrosis may not be associated with progression to nodular cirrhosis, although both have been reported. Furthermore, the degree of variation within subpopulations

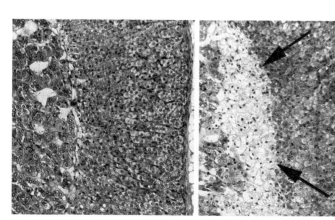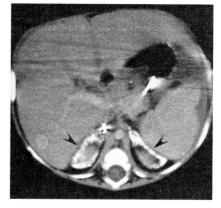

FIGURE 55.9-2   Histology and computed tomographic (CT) scan of abdomen. The zona reticularis of the lysosomal acid lipase (LAL)-deficient adrenal gland (*right*) becomes infiltrated with lipid-laden cells (*arrows*) containing birefringent material under polarized light. Normal adrenal gland is shown on the left. These are from the LAL-deficient mouse at age 4 months. The *arrows* show the calcific deposits in very enlarged adrenal glands in a human patient with Wolman's disease. The adrenal outlines are symmetric, as is the calcification. The CT scan is courtesy of William Krivit, MD, PhD.

may be significant and may or may not relate to the types of mutations that are present in these patients (see below).

Except for some hepatomegaly, there may be no specific abnormality leading the physician to the diagnosis. Specifically, malabsorption, malnutrition, and cachexia have not been reported as consistent components of CESD. Acute or chronic liver failure has occurred, as have progressive fibrosis and cirrhosis with varices.[23,24] Pulmonary hypertension has been described in one patient, but its relationship specifically to CESD is unknown.[24]

Hyperlipidemia may be the most consistent chemical abnormality in CESD patients. Some patients manifest a type IIb hyperlipoproteinemia profile, whereas others do not. Although CESD patients may have intestinal abnormalities on biopsy, abdominal pain and other indications of malabsorption, or cholelithiasis, have not been present in reported patients. Secondary abnormalities of the coagulation system may be noted and may depend on the degree of hepatic dysfunction.

Clearly, the literature is skewed toward reports of more severe CESD patients, and the disease may be much more common than such reports would suggest. The disease should be suspected in patients with uncharacterized vacuolization of the liver, hepatic steatosis involving Kupffer cells, and hepatomegaly, uncharacterized hyperlipidemia, or type II-b hyperlipidemia. Isolated hepatomegaly early in life or isolated hepatosplenomegaly may be the only finding in CESD, and the differential diagnosis of these findings should include CESD.

PATHOLOGY OF WOLMAN DISEASE AND CESD

LIVER PATHOLOGY

The liver in Wolman disease is characteristically enlarged (> twofold) and progressively increases in size during the life span of the affected infant. Grossly, the liver is yellow in color and greasy in appearance. This is very similar to that in the LAL-deficient mouse.[9] Early in the disease course, the portal and lobular architecture is normal. Later, distortion of the portal spaces occurs with development of fibrosis and, occasionally, frank cirrhosis. Lymphoid infiltration without hepatitis also can be present. Progressive hepatic fibrosis is associated with marked accumulation of a mixture of triglyceride and cholesteryl esters in the lysosomes of hepatocytes, in Kupffer cells, and in portal area macrophages that develop in clusters. The lipid in macrophages tends to be more finely vacuolated than that in hepatocytes. Appropriate lipid stains performed on unfixed frozen sections demonstrate cholesterol and triglyceride in hepatocytes and an admixture of more complex, partly insoluble lipid in the macrophages. Ultrastructural study reveals lipid accumulation, mostly in lysosomes, and increased ceroid-lipofuchsin bodies. The latter are more evident in the macrophages than in hepatocytes.

In CESD, the liver has a gross appearance that is similar to that in Wolman disease (Figure 55.9-3), except that the liver may be more orange and less greasy. Biopsy specimens

have a bright orange-yellow color and tend to float in formalin. The hepatocytes contain cytoplasmic vacuoles of variable size that can resemble nonalcoholic steatosis with septal fibrosis (Figure 55.9-4, A and B). The Kupffer cells and portal area macrophages have finely vacuolated cytoplasm and tend to occur in clusters, as in Wolman disease. Acid phosphatase activity is abnormally high in hepatocytes (Figure 55.9-4C). Lipid stains demonstrate a mixture of neutral lipid, cholesterol, cholesteryl esters, and ceroid (Figure 55.9-4D). The cholesteryl ester content of liver tissue is much higher in CESD than in Wolman disease. Because the lipid in tissues is extracted during processing into paraffin or plastic, cholesteryl ester crystals can be demonstrated only in unfixed frozen sections viewed in polarized light (Figure 55.9-4E). However, electron microscopy reveals a high content of cholesterol clefts (crystal-shaped voids) mixed with other lipids in membrane-bound vesicles (Figure 55.9-4F), presumably lysosomes where esterified lipid crystals had existed prior to processing. Septal fibrosis, periportal lymphocytic infiltration, and occasional plasma cells can develop. Portal fibrosis (see Figure 55.9-4B) and cirrhosis occur, but the fibrogenic mechanism is unknown, and progressive liver disease is not established as an inevitable outcome. Foamy macrophages, similar to the Kupffer cells, occur in the spleen, bone marrow, and lymph nodes.

ADRENAL GLANDS

In Wolman disease, the adrenal glands are two to three times normal weight (~ 13–15 g) and have a yellow color. Characteristically, the zona reticularis has broad infiltration by large vacuolated cells that are scattered in haphazard clumps throughout this zone. Areas of necrosis and calcification occur. The adrenal glands have not been well studied in CESD. The adrenal gland in the LAL-deficient mice is very similar to that in Wolman disease, but the massive enlargement and necrosis with calcification are not present (see Figure 55.9-2).

SMALL INTESTINE

Intestinal malabsorption, a primary feature of Wolman disease but not of CESD, is associated with severe infiltration of

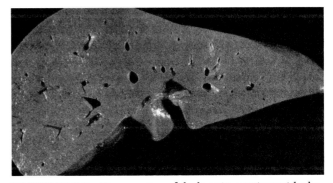

FIGURE 55.9-3 Cross-section of the liver in a patient with cholesteryl ester storage disease. The liver has an orange-yellow color that is immediately apparent on percutaneous or open liver biopsy. The color derives from the deposition of the major storage lipids and also carotene-like lipids (see CD-ROM for color image). Reproduced with permission from Dincsoy HP et al.[76]

the lamina propria by foamy lipid-laden macrophages, as well as accumulation of lipid in small intestinal epithelium. In contrast, Partin and Schubert reported that the proximal small intestinal epithelium of CESD is normal, the macrophages and the extracellular space of the lamina propria contain abundant lipids, including cholesteryl ester crystals, and macrophages at the tips of villi contain autofluorescent material, suggestive of ceroid-lipofuchsin.[8]

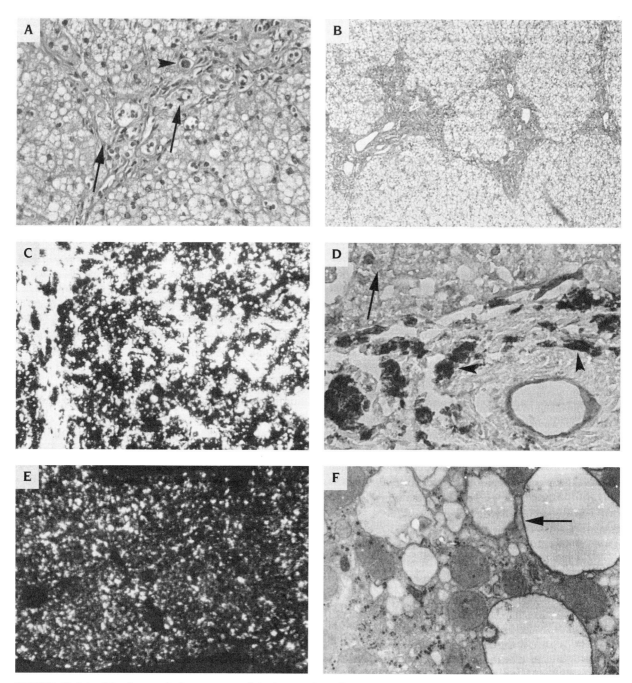

FIGURE 55.9-4   Histology and ultrastructure of the liver and small intestine in cholesteryl ester storage disease (CESD). *A*, Paraffin section of a liver biopsy in an adolescent with CESD. Hepatocyte cytoplasm is pale and vacuolated owing to lipid accumulation. Enlarged vacuolated cells in portal zone are macrophages (*arrows*). Occasional necrotic hepatocytes are present (*arrowhead*) (hematoxylin and eosin; x200 original magnification). *B*, Delicate septal fibrosis in liver from a child with CESD appears to originate in the portal zones without accompanying inflammation (hematoxylin and eosin; x200 original magnification). *C*, Acid phosphatase staining on unfixed cryostat section demonstrates massive increase of activity within hepatocytes in CESD (x200 original magnification). *D*, Nile blue sulfate lipid stain of unfixed cryostat section of liver in CESD demonstrates pale peach–colored neutral lipid in hepatocytes (*long arrow*) and dark blue-purple complex lipid mixture in portal area macrophages (*arrowheads*) (x200 original magnification) (see CD-ROM for color image). *E*, Unfixed unstained cryostat section of liver in CESD viewed in polarized light contains large numbers of anisotropic cholesteryl ester crystals. *F*, Liver cytoplasmic droplets in CESD have well-defined dense membranes (*arrow*), unlike usual hepatocyte lipid vesicles. This is consistent with the presumed lysosomal location of most of the lipid in CESD. Electron micrograph.

LIVER, ADRENAL GLANDS, SMALL INTESTINE, SPLEEN, AND OTHER TISSUES IN RODENT MODELS OF LAL DEFICIENCY

Most published descriptions of Wolman disease are based on autopsy findings in infants, whereas most reports of CESD are based on clinical findings and study of biopsy tissue obtained during childhood and adulthood. The phenotypes are distinct in many ways, but overlapping phenotypes occur, and the concept of an incompletely defined spectrum is appealing (see Figure 55.9-1). The paucity of fully studied patients with Wolman disease or CESD limits the ability to define the morphology and natural history of these two closely related disorders. The two rodent models of LAL deficiency have provided insights into its pathogenesis and progression.[9,10] The most detailed descriptions are from the knockout mice with a complete deficiency of LAL in all tissues. These mice present with a phenotype that exhibits some of the manifestations of Wolman disease and CESD.[9,14] However, the calcification of the adrenal glands of Wolman disease and the hyperlipidemia of CESD are lacking. The mouse knockout model does not have progressive hepatic cirrhosis, although some fibrotic changes are present.

The mouse model provides insight into time-dependent changes in the hepatic disease. Specifically, the liver begins as a normal organ with relatively little change in hepatic weight or consistency in the first 2 to 4 weeks of life. During the second month, vacuolization and lipid storage of the hepatocytes become evident, as does the development of discrete areas of macrophages that are engorged with neutral lipids. Although the progression of hepatocellular storage may continue, the major pathologic abnormality from 2 to 8 months of life is the proliferation of Kupffer cells and portal macrophages that become engorged with cholesteryl esters and triglycerides. These cells can account for over 50% of the liver. The hepatomegaly is progressive and may reach 25% of body weight by 8 months of age, the life span of these mice. This progressive hepatomegaly is accompanied by macrophage storage cell infiltration in the spleen, small intestine, and lymph nodes throughout the body. Although the spleen has large numbers of storage cells, splenomegaly does not become as massive as that observed for the liver. Lymph nodes can be completely replaced by macrophage storage cells. Strikingly, macrophage infiltration of the villi of the jejunum is progressive (Figure 55.9-5). This extends progressively from the proximal to the distal small intestine so that the entire small intestine becomes infiltrated by these storage cells. The histopathology of the small intestine is nearly identical to that described by Partin and Schubert in the original human cases of CESD[8] and in the autopsy cases of Wolman disease.

Concomitant with the progression of hepatomegaly and storage cell infiltration throughout the body, LAL-deficient mice develop lipodystrophy leading to a complete loss of subcutaneous white fat and brown fat. By 6 months of age, essentially all white adipose tissue has disappeared: insulin resistance and low leptin levels develop simultaneously. The LAL-deficient mice are not hyperlipidemic, probably owing to malabsorption and massive redirection of lipids to liver Kupffer cells. This is reminiscent of the "triglyceride steal syndrome." The infiltration of the adrenal glands precisely mimics that in human Wolman disease, albeit without calcification. The zona reticularis is replaced progressively by storage cells (see Figure 55.9-5). The lungs have a few interstitial cells with vacuolization but no specific abnormalities. No gross behavioral or histologic abnormalities have been noted in the central nervous system.

This mouse model indicates that the complete absence of LAL leads to a macrophage and hepatocellular disease with macrophage proliferation and storage of cholesteryl esters and triglycerides as the primary pathologic abnormality. This leads to malabsorption and malnutrition, hepatic dysfunction, and infiltration of the adrenal cortex. The absence of significant fibrosis and/or cirrhosis in the mouse model suggests that either this is not a major or consistent component of the human disease or that mice simply do not survive long enough to develop reactions to the stored lipid in the macrophages.

In addition, mice do not develop the "premature arthrosclerosis" that has been described in human CESD. Thus, the mouse model more closely resembles the human Wolman disease model, with normal to subnormal plasma lipids. In the absence of hyperlipidemia, potentially caused by malabsorption, arteriosclerosis may not develop. If the LAL deficiency is placed against the background of an apolipoprotein E deficiency, a spontaneous atherogenic model in the mouse, doubly homozygous mice for apolipoprotein E and LAL deficiency have much more rapidly progressive lesions with apolipoprotein E deficiency alone.[26] Thus, the premature arteriosclerosis in the CESD may be accentuated by the presence of dietary or other genetic abnormalities in some patients, leading to hyperlipoproteinemia and progression of arteriosclerosis.

BIOCHEMICAL PATHOLOGY OF LAL DEFICIENCY

LIPOPROTEIN AND LIPID ABNORMALITIES

Plasma triglyceride and cholesterol levels are usually normal in Wolman disease. Three cases showed elevated

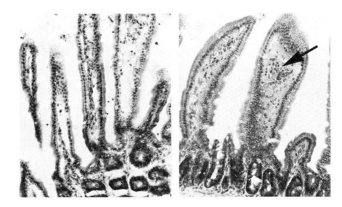

FIGURE 55.9-5 Small intestine in lysosomal acid lipase deficiency. The small intestinal villi become infiltrated with lipid-laden macrophages that contain cholesteryl esters and triglycerides. Normal and lysosomal acid lipase–deficient samples are on the left and right, respectively. The arrow shows oil red O–positive macrophages (see CD-ROM for color image).

triglycerides and very-low-density lipoprotein (LDL) cholesterol,[17,27] whereas plasma high-density lipoprotein (HDL) was decreased in others.[27–29] In comparison, CESD patients usually have hypercholesterolemia with increases of very LDL and LDL cholesterol levels. The plasma HDL in some CESD patients can be less than the 5th percentile (ie, < 20 mg/dL). In some other cases, the ratio of HDL_2-cholesterol to HDL_3 cholesterol was reversed (10:1) compared with the normal ratio (1:10).[30]

Patients with Wolman disease accumulate cholesteryl esters and triglycerides in the liver, spleen, small intestine, and adrenal glands. Compared with normal levels, the triglyceride concentrations can be 2- to 10-fold increased in the liver and 8- to 100-fold increased in the spleen. Quantitative analyses are not available for the patient's small intestine, but gross and histologic observations of the intestine from Wolman disease and CESD patients show accumulation of these lipids.[31] The mouse model of LAL deficiency showed total cholesterol increases of 43-fold in the liver, 27-fold in the spleen, and 2.5-fold in the small intestine by 8 months of age.[14]

All patients with Wolman disease have increased total cholesterol levels in the liver (~ 5- to 160-fold), spleen, small intestine, and adrenal glands (8-fold).[32] More than 98% of the accumulated total cholesterol are cholesteryl esters.[9] The fatty acid content of liver and spleen also can be increased, whereas the phospholipid and glycolipid contents are not, even at 8 months of age.[33,34]

In cases of CESD, triglyceride and cholesteryl esters were elevated in the liver. The cholesteryl ester storage in liver can be 120- to 350-fold higher than normal. Triglyceride levels have minor increases. Inconsistently elevated values were in spleen, small intestine, kidney, and lung. Analysis of acyl groups in the cholesteryl esters in the liver and small intestine of CESD patients revealed predominantly oleic and linoleic acids.[29,35–37]

INTRACELLULAR DERANGEMENTS IN LAL DEFICIENCY

LAL plays a central role in the modulation of cholesterol metabolism in all cells. The LDL receptor or other receptors on the plasma membranes of various cells can deliver LDL-bound cholesteryl esters and triglycerides to the lysosomes. Once delivered to the lysosome, the released cholesteryl esters and triglycerides are cleaved by LAL to free cholesterol and fatty acids. After LAL cleaves these lipids, they exit the lysosome and enter the cytosol. Normally, cholesterol will interact with the sterol response element binding protein system to modulate the intracellular production of cholesterol (Figure 55.9-6).[11] This system, elucidated by Goldstein and Brown over the past three decades, is a major component of modulation of neutral lipid metabolism in the body.[11] In LAL deficiency, cholesteryl esters and triglycerides cannot be cleaved; therefore, free cholesterol and fatty acids cannot leave the lysosome.[12,38] The cells detect an intracellular (cytosolic) cholesterol deficiency, and the cholesterol biosynthetic pathway is up-regulated to compensate. The increased

production of cholesterol leads to enhanced esterification of cholesterol via the cytoplasmic enzyme acyl CoA:cholesterol acyltransferase and enhances the synthesis of very LDL to export the synthesized cholesterol. Similarly, the lack of fatty acid egress from the lysosome leads to up-regulation of a series of other biosynthetic fatty acid enzymes with enhanced fatty acid synthesis. The details of this fatty acid synthetic pathway are not fully elucidated, but the control of this pathway from lysosomally derived free fatty acids appears clear.[11]

The up-regulation of these systems in LAL deficiency has led to the use of statins for the treatment of hypercholesterolemia in CESD.[39] Apolipoprotein B synthesis and the plasma lipid abnormalities are partially corrected by statins, but this may be transient. Statins may be important for the therapy of CESD in the prevention of secondary disease but do not theoretically or practically have a major effect on the lipid accumulation in the lysosomes of various tissues, although re-esterification and the pathway should be diminished.

LAL PROPERTIES

LAL is a typical lysosomal hydrolase that is synthesized in the rough endoplasmic reticulum and is cotranslationally glycosylated as it emerges into the endoplasmic reticulum lumen.[38,40] Following clipping of the leader sequence, the enzyme is modified during transit through the Golgi apparatus but without further proteolytic modification. The oligosaccharides are remodeled to attach the mannose 6-phosphate targeting signal for lysosomal sorting. The newly synthesized LAL is delivered to the lysosome by the mannose 6-phosphate receptor system. LAL is not known to require cofactors for optimal hydrolysis, and it functions as a monomer. LAL has significant similarity to other acidic lipases, for example, hepatic or gastric lipases that cleave similar substrates in the hepatocyte cytosol or stomach, respectively. Because the isolation of LAL from natural tissues has been difficult, purified LAL has been characterized using recombinant expression systems.[41] The enzyme can be produced in large quantities from appropriately designed genetic sequences from humans using insect cells, Chinese hamster ovary cells, *Pichia pastoris* and *Pombe* yeasts, and other heterologous expression systems (G. A. Grabowski and H. Du, unpublished data, 2003).[42–44] As indicated above, LAL has significant homology to other acid lipases but is clearly distinct from hormone-sensitive lipase, pancreatic lysophospholipid lipase, lecithin cholesterol acyl transferase, lipoprotein lipase, hepatic lipase, and pancreatic lipase. A significant homology exists with a shared amino acid motif, –Gly-X-Ser-X-Gly, that is common to most lipases and is an essential pentapeptide in the active site.[43,45] This pentapeptide occurs twice in LAL, and serine 153 appears to be important to catalytic activity. Several other polymorphic variants of LAL have been described, and their physiologic significance and importance are under investigation.[46]

Recombinant heterologous expression and characterization of purified human LAL have proven that the triglyceridase and cholesteryl esterase activities are present in

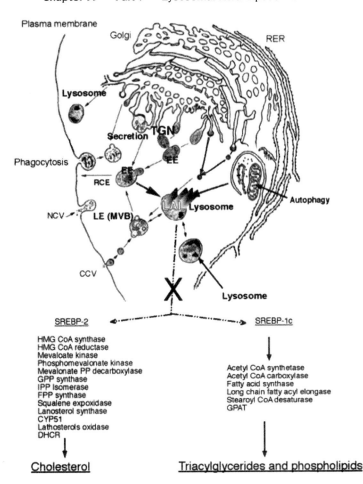

Plasma membrane

Golgi

RER

Lysosome

Secretion TGN

Phagocytosis

EE

RCE

NCV

LE (MVB)

CCV

LAL Lysosome

Autophagy

Lysosome

SREBP-2

HMG CoA synthase
HMG CoA reductase
Mevalonate kinase
Phosphomevalonate kinase
Mevalonate PP decarboxylase
GPP synthase
IPP Isomerase
FPP synthase
Squalene expoxidase
Lanosterol synthase
CYP51
Lathosterols oxidase
DHCR

Cholesterol

SREBP-1c

Acetyl CoA synthetase
Acetyl CoA carboxylase
Fatty acid synthase
Long chain fatty acyl elongase
Stearoyl CoA desaturase
GPAT

Triacylglycerides and phospholipids

FIGURE 55.9-6 Schematic of the lysosomal acid lipase (LAL) system and its connection to cellular cholesterol and fatty acid metabolism. There are several types of lysosomes within cells that can contain different substrates and/or storage materials. Material can enter the lysosome from the surface, by autophagy of intracellular organelles, and after transit through the Golgi apparatus. LAL is synthesized in the rough endoplasmic reticulum (RER) and is post-translationally modified (oligosaccharides) and targeted to the lysosome following passage through the trans-Golgi network (TGN). CCV = clatherin CV; CV = coated vesicle; EE and LE = early and late endosomes, respectively; MVB = multivesicular body; NCV = nonclatherin CV; RCE = recycled coated endosome. The egress of cholesterol or fatty acids from the lysosome feeds back to the cytoplasmic, plasma membrane, ER-controlled SREBP systems for altering translation of specific enzymes leading to the synthesis of cholesterol and/or triacylglycerides and phospholipids.

the same polypeptide sequence.[44] This also is evident from the LAL knockout mouse. More importantly, serine 153 appears to be critical to the catalytic function for both substrates.[44] Thus, the deficiencies and abnormalities of LAL in Wolman disease and CESD must be explained by a single enzyme deficiency.

How can one explain the massive accumulation of cholesteryl esters and triglycerides in Wolman disease and just cholesteryl esters in the tissues from CESD patients? From mutagenesis data, the following appears clear: complete deficiency of LAL leads to Wolman disease with subsequent accumulation of cholesteryl esters and triglycerides. Diacylglycerides and monoacylglycerides also accumulate in smaller amounts because these are also LAL substrates. The catalytic activity of human LAL has a significant preference for tri-, di-, and monoacylglyceride substrates compared with cholesteryl esters.[44] The presence of apparently small amounts of normal LAL in tissues from CESD patients may provide an explanation for the variant phenotypes. A recurrent mutation in CESD leads to abnormal splicing and production of nearly normal amounts of a LAL messenger ribonucleic acid (RNA). But the mutation allows for only ~ 1 to 3% normal levels of LAL messenger RNA in the tissues of CESD patients.[30,47–49] This small amount of LAL RNA allows for the production of low levels of normal LAL that may be sufficient to nearly normalize the preferential acylglycerol substrate cleavage. However, this is insufficient to normalize metabolism of the less efficiently cleaved sub-

strate, cholesteryl esters with their resultant accumulation in various cells. This indicates that large amounts of enzyme are not required for normalization and that low levels of LAL activity may be sufficient for prolonged survival with minor manifestations of disease.[50] LAL deficiency is very similar to other lysosomal hydrolase deficiency disorders in which small amounts of residual activity can normalize the flux of substrates through the lysosome. Higher thresholds of enzymatic activity are consistent with later-onset mild disease and, potentially, normalcy.

GENETICS AND MOLECULAR BIOLOGY

Wolman disease and CESD result from allelic mutations at the LAL locus on human chromosome 10q23.2–q23.3. The gene spans 45 kb, has 10 exons (Figure 55.9-7), and contains no unusual structures except for a large intron 3. The mutations found in Wolman disease and CESD are listed in Table 55.9-1 and represent patients from a variety of nationalities. A curious finding is the presence of mutations in intron 8 that result in abnormal splicing in either Wolman disease or CESD. This abnormal splice could eliminate intron 8 as owing to a splice junction abnormality. However, the location of the base change, either one or three bases following this donor slice, appears to affect the ability of the cell to produce normal LAL messenger RNA. The recurrent mutation in Wolman disease is a base substitution in exon 8 either one or three bases prior to the intron 8 splice donor site. These appear to be incompatible with normal splicing and lead to a deletion of exon 8. The resultant truncated unstable protein in Wolman disease has no LAL activity and is rapidly degraded. In comparison, the substitution of a base at the +1 position downstream from the spliced donor site has been found in several CESD patients. This leads to ~ 5% of normal LAL messenger RNA splicing and the production of low levels of normal LAL protein from this mutant allele. Most (95%) of the mutant RNA produces a deletion of exon 8 and a truncated protein. The major difference, then, between Wolman disease and CESD is the absence or presence, respectively, of small amounts of normal LAL in cells and, as indicated above, the preferential cleavage of triglycerides compared with cholesteryl ester.

The most common mutation, a deletion of $254\text{-}277_1$, $\Delta254\text{-}277_1$ allele, was screened for in a randomly selected population in northwestern Germany.[15] In a cohort of 1,887 people aged 20 to 70 years, the frequency of $\Delta254\text{-}277_1$ was 0.0019, giving an estimated homozygosity frequency of 1 in 300,000 or approximately 260 cases of CESD in Germany. If such calculations apply to the US population, there would be about 1,000 homozygotes for CESD. These calculations suggest that the frequency may be high enough to entertain screening of hyperlipidemic patients, particularly those with a type II-b profile, for CESD. The frequency of Wolman disease has been estimated at < 1 in 500,000 live births.[51]

DIAGNOSIS

The diagnosis of Wolman disease should be considered in any infant with persistent vomiting and hepatomegaly in the first month of life, with progressive failure to thrive, and/or with hepatosplenomegaly and malabsorption. A radiograph of the abdomen may reveal adrenal calcifica-

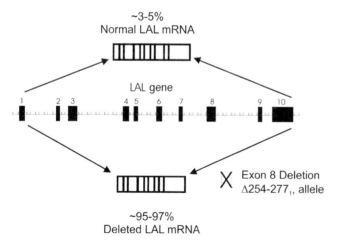

~3-5%
Normal LAL mRNA

LAL gene

1   2 3   4 5   6   7   8   9   10

X Exon 8 Deletion
$\Delta254\text{-}277_1$, allele

~95-97%
Deleted LAL mRNA

FIGURE 55.9-7 Schematic of the lysosomal acid lipase gene. The *LAL* is about 45 kb in size with 10 exons (*numbered rectangles*). Exons in the gene (*center*) are filled rectangles, and introns are represented by the thin horizontal rectangle. The spliced messenger ribonucleic acid (mRNA) is shown above and below to represent different mRNA products, resulting in a small amount of normal mRNA being formed. The majority of mutant mRNA leads to the splicing of exon 8 and a truncated translated protein.

tions (see Figure 55.9-2). The presence of adrenal calcifications can be observed in other conditions, but most occur later in life or are asymmetric. Thus, symmetric adrenal calcifications in the first few months of life may be pathognomonic of Wolman disease. Other lysosomal storage disease presenting this early in life with hepatosplenomegaly and severe failure to thrive includes the Niemann-Pick A variant with severe central nervous system involvement and inanition owing to sphingomyelinase deficiency. The severe variants of Gaucher disease type 2 have their onset in the similar time frame but with lesser degrees of hepatosplenomegaly, no malabsorption or diarrhea, and a predominant finding of rapidly developing neurologic signs with bulbar involvement. Suspect cases should have peripheral blood leukocyte LAL activities measured. The isolated deficiency of LAL is diagnostic. Contributing and supporting evidence for the diagnosis includes massive involvement of Kupffer cells on liver biopsy with or without some fibrosis and cholesterol crystals in the liver. Bone marrow biopsy may also show foam storage cells. Importantly, hypercholesterolemia and hypertriglyceridemia are not components of Wolman disease. Once the diagnosis is made by LAL enzyme assay, LAL mutations can be determined, and these may be used in further family studies or for prenatal diagnostic testing.

CESD early in life must be considered in any child with hepatosplenomegaly and hyperlipidemia. CESD may be confused with glycogen storage disease (GSD) type IA or B because that disorder also presents with hepatomegaly and hypertriglyceridemia. Lactic acidosis can be a component of GSD IA or B but is not a component of CESD. Young children with CESD generally do not have failure to thrive but can have isolated hepatomegaly, prompting liver biopsy. The presence of engorged Kupffer cells with or without some fibrotic changes and cholesterol crystal deposition is highly suggestive. The CESD liver is distinguished from other lysosomal storage diseases, that is, Gaucher disease, Niemann-Pick A or B, and Pompe disease (GSD II), by its characteristic orange color and neutral lipid storage. GSD IA or B is not lysosomal, and glycogen storage predominates, not neutral fat. The diagnosis is made by isolated LAL deficiency in any nucleated cell. Peripheral white blood cells and cultured fibroblasts are the usual and most general sources for enzyme diagnosis. Thus, in the presence of hepatomegaly and hyperlipidemia, the diagnosis of CESD should be entertained in any child. On liver biopsy, the core may be orange in color, immediately suggesting the diagnosis.

In older children or adults, the findings are nonspecific. Mild hepatosplenomegaly or mild hepatomegaly with or without significant hyperlipidemia suggests the diagnosis of CESD. Characteristic liver biopsy findings and, occasionally, bone marrow biopsy findings should prompt LAL assays. The spectrum of the adult variants of CESD may be quite broad and include a large number of asymptomatic individuals. The diagnosis should be suspected in individuals with a type II-b hyperlipidemic pattern. LAL assays may obviate the need for liver biopsy for diagnosis. Mutation

TABLE 55.9-1   WOLMAN DISEASE AND CESD MUTATIONS

ALLELE	EXON	cDNA NUMBER*	BASE CHANGE	AA NUMBER†	AA CHANGE	WD	CESD	REFERENCE
E3Δ8bp	3	159–166	del 8 bp	19	Frame shift/stop	+		42
Y22X	3	169	C→A	22	Tyr-X	+		56
R44X	3	233	C→T	44	Arg-X	+		30, 48, 57
E4skip	4	270–468	?	56	Frame shift/stop	+		30
Q64R	4	294	A→G	64	Gln-Arg		+	58
G66V	4	300	G→T	66	Gly-Val		+	59, 60
W95X	4	387	G→A	95	Trp-X	+		30
H108P	4	426	A→C	108	His-Pro		+	59, 61, 62
H108R	4	426	A→G	108	His-Arg		+	63, 64
E4Δ2bp	4	435–436	del TC	111	Frame shift/stop	+		42
S112X	5	438	del C	112	Ser-X	+		60, 65
fs112	5	437–438	del TC	112	Frame shift/stop		+	30
fs177	6	634	T→TT	177	Frame shift/stop	+		30, 66
L179P	6	639	T→C	179	Leu-Pro	+	+	66, 67
P181L	6	645	C→T	181	Pro-Leu		+	59
E7SJM	6 (intron)		a→g	205–253	del 48 aa		+	59
fs219	7	722	del T	219	Frame shift/stop	+		30, 57
G245X	7	836	G→T	245	Gly-X		+	47
T267I	7	903	C→T	267	Thr-Ile		+	58
S268C	8	906	C→G	268	Ser-Cys		+	30
L273S	8	921	T→C	273	Leu-Ser		+	59
H274Y	8	923	C→T	274	His-Tyr		+	49
Q277X	8	932	C→T	277	Gln–X	+		68
E8SJM-1	8	863–934	G→A	254–277	del 24 aa		+	30, 62, 64, 67, 69–71
E8SJM+1	8 (intron)		g→a	254–277	del 24 aa	+		47
E8SJM-3	8	863–934	C→T	254–277	del 24 aa	+		68
E10ΔAG	10	1,007–1,008	del AG	302	Frame shift/stop		+	69
Y303X	10	1,012	T→A	303	Tyr-X	+		72
E10ΔC	10	1,020	del C	306	Frame shift/stop		+	30
T316A	10	1049	A→G	316	Thr-Ala			73
E10ΔG	10	1064	del G	321	Frame shift/stop		+	57
G321W	10	1064	G→T	321	Gly-Trp		+	42
L336P	10	1110	T→C	336	Leu-Pro		+	74

CESD = cholesteryl ester storage disease; LAL = lysosomal acid lipase.

*The complementary deoxyribonucleic acid (cDNA) number is according to human LAL cDNA clone that was published by Anderson and Sando in 1991.[75]

†The amino acid (AA) number is from mature N-terminus, which is started from 22 aa from the first Met.

analysis in affected individuals may be helpful for family screening and additional diagnostic and correlative studies.

TREATMENT

Currently, there is no specific treatment for Wolman disease or CESD that is generally available. One patient with CESD had a liver transplant for chronic liver failure and was apparently well 2 years after the procedure,[52] but additional data have not been forthcoming. For Wolman disease, bone marrow or stem cell transplant has been attempted in several cases.[53,54] Because of the severity of the illness and the adrenal insufficiency, the mortality rate has been high. In one series, four of five patients succumbed to transplant complications. In the surviving patient, the bone marrow transplant appeared to be successful, with disappearance of storage macrophages in the liver, spleen, and, presumably, other tissues. The adrenal glands appear to atrophy following bone marrow transplant (W. Krivit, personal communication, 2003), and lifelong corticosteroid replacement therapy is necessary. Enzyme replacement and gene therapy studies have been conducted in the mouse knockout model with resolution of the hepatocellular and macrophage storage.[41,55] These remain investigational and provide proof of

principle for the treatment of this disease. Currently, no clinical trials are ongoing for these modes of therapy. The approaches of enzyme replacement or gene therapy for enzyme replacement should be efficacious in both Wolman disease and CESD. Prenatal diagnosis is available for families who wish to exercise this option.

Supportive therapies for Wolman disease have been inadequate, and long-term therapies with intravenous alimentation have not been reported. Because enteral nutrition may be impossible owing to the severity of involvement of the gastrointestinal tract in Wolman disease, supportive parenteral nutrition may be the only option. In CESD, adjunctive therapy with statins or other suppressors of 3-hydroxy-3-methylglutaryl CoA reductase function has been useful in suppressing very LDL and LDL with subsequent lowering of plasma lipoprotein levels. This may lead to a decreased risk of heart disease. Statins have not been shown to prevent the development of progressive hepatocellular disease or adrenal insufficiency. Because of the intestinal involvement in CESD, studies for malabsorption should be undertaken, and supplementation with vitamins A, D, E, and K may be appropriate. Other supplements should be undertaken if malabsorption is present.

REFERENCES

1. Abramov A, Schorr S, Wolman M. Generalized xanthomatosis with calcified adrenals. J Dis Child 1956;91:282–6.

2. Wolman M, Sterk VV, Gatt S, Frenkel M. Primary familial xanthomatosis with involvement and calcification of the adrenals: report of two more cases in siblings of a previously described infant. Pediatr 1961;28:742–57.

3. Alexander W. Niemann-Pick disease: report of a case showing calcification in the adrenal glands. N Z Med J 1946;45:43–5.

4. Fredrickson DS, Sloan HR, Ferrans VJ, Demosky SJ Jr. Cholesteryl ester storage disease: a most unusual manifestation of deficiency of two lysosomal enzyme activities. Trans Assoc Am Physicians 1972;85:109–19.

5. Schiff L, Schubert WK, McAdams AJ, et al. Hepatic cholesterol ester storage disease, a familial disorder. Am J Med 1968; 44:538–46.

6. Langeron A, Caroli I, Stralin H, Barbier P. Polycorie cholesterique de l'adulte. I. Etude clinique, electronique, histochimique. Presse Med 1967;75:2785–91.

7. Infante R, Polonovski J, Caroli J. Polycorie cholesterique de l'adulte. II. Etude biochemique. Presse Med 1967;75:2329–32.

8. Partin JC, Schubert WK. Small intestinal mucosa in cholesterol ester storage disease: a light and electron microscopic study. Gastroenterology 1969;57:542–58.

9. Du H, Duanmu M, Witte D, Grabowski GA. Targeted disruption of the mouse lysosomal acid lipase gene: long-term survival with massive cholesteryl ester and triglyceride storage. Hum Mol Genet 1998;7:1347–54.

10. Kuriwaki K, Yoshida H. Morphological characteristics of lipid accumulation in liver-constituting cells of acid lipase deficiency rats (Wolman's disease model rats). Pathol Int 1999;49:291–7.

11. Horton JD, Goldstein JL, Brown MS. SREBPs: activators of the complete program of cholesterol and fatty acid synthesis in the liver. J Clin Invest 2002;109:1125–31.

12. Brown MS, Sobhani MK, Brunschede GY, Goldstein JL. Restoration of a regulatory response to low density lipoprotein in acid lipase-deficient human fibroblasts. J Biol Chem 1976; 251:3277–86.

13. Goldstein JL, Dana SE, Faust JR, et al. Role of lysosomal acid lipase in the metabolism of plasma low density lipoprotein. Observations in cultured fibroblasts from a patient with cholesteryl ester storage disease. J Biol Chem 1975;250:8487–95.

14. Du H, Heur M, Duanmu M, et al. Lysosomal acid lipase-deficient mice: depletion of white and brown fat, severe hepatosplenomegaly, and shortened life span. J Lipid Res 2001;42:489–500.

15. Assmann G, Seedorf U. Acid lipase deficiency: Wolman disease and cholesteryl ester storage disease. In: Scriver CR, Beaudet AL, Valle D, Sly WS, editors. Metabolic and molecular bases of inherited diseases. New York: McGraw-Hill; 2001. p. 3551–72.

16. Crocker AC, Vawter GF, Neuhauser ED, Rosowsky A. Wolman's disease: three new patients with a recently described lipidosis. Pediatrics 1965;35:627–39.

17. Marshall WC, Ockenden BG, Fosbrooke AS, Cumings JN. Wolman's disease. A rare lipidosis with adrenal calcification. Arch Dis Child 1969;44:331–41.

18. Lough J, Fawcett J, Wiegensberg B. Wolman's disease. An electron microscopic, histochemical, and biochemical study. Arch Pathol 1970;89:103–10.

19. Hill SC, Hoeg JM, Dwyer AJ, et al. CT findings in acid lipase deficiency: Wolman disease and cholesteryl ester storage disease. J Comput Assist Tomogr 1983;7:815–8.

20. Eto Y, Kitagawa T. Wolman's disease with hypolipoproteinemia and acanthocytosis: clinical and biochemical observations. J Pediatr 1970;77:862–7.

21. Kikuchi M, Igarashi K, Noro T, et al. Evaluation of jejunal function in Wolman's disease. J Pediatr Gastroenterol Nutr 1991; 12:65–9.

22. Elleder M, Ledvinova J, Cieslar P, Kuhn R. Subclinical course of cholesterol ester storage disease (CESD) diagnosed in adulthood. Report on two cases with remarks on the nature of the liver storage process. Virchows Arch A Pathol Anat Histopathol 1990;416:357–65.

23. Beaudet AL, Ferry GD, Nichols BL Jr, Rosenberg HS. Cholesterol ester storage disease: clinical, biochemical, and pathological studies. J Pediatr 1977;90:910–4.

24. Cagle PT, Ferry GD, Beaudet AL, Hawkins EP. Pulmonary hypertension in an 18-year-old girl with cholesteryl ester storage disease (CESD). Am J Med Genet 1986;24:711–22.

25. Edelstein RA, Filling-Katz MR, Pentchev P, et al. Cholesteryl ester storage disease: a patient with massive splenomegaly and splenic abscess. Am J Gastroenterol 1988;83:687–92.

26. Heur M. Lysosomal regulation of gene expression [PhD thesis]. In: Developmental biology. Cincinnati (OH): University of Cincinnati; 2002. p. 146.

27. Schaub J, Janka GE, Christomanou H, et al. Wolman's disease: clinical, biochemical and ultrastructural studies in an unusual case without striking adrenal calcification. Eur J Pediatr 1980;135:45–53.

28. Wallis K, Gross M, Kohn R, Zaidman J. A case of Wolman's disease. Helv Paediatr Acta 1971;26:98–111.

29. Kyriakides EC, Filippone N, Paul B, et al. Lipid studies in Wolman's disease. Pediatrics 1970;46:431–6.

30. Anderson RA, Bryson GM, Parks JS. Lysosomal acid lipase mutations that determine phenotype in Wolman and cholesterol ester storage disease. Mol Genet Metab 1999;68:333–45.

31. Roytta M, Fagerlund AS, Toikkanen S, Salmi TT, et al. Wolman disease: morphological, clinical and genetic studies on the first Scandinavian cases. Clin Genet 1992;42:1–7.

32. Assmann G, Fredrickson DS, Sloan HR, et al. Accumulation of oxygenated steryl esters in Wolman's disease. J Lipid Res 1975;16:28–38.

33. Konno T, Fujii M, Watanuki T, Koizumi K. Wolman's disease: the first case in Japan. Tohoku J Exp Med 1966;90:375–89.

34. Patrick AD, Lake BD. Deficiency of an acid lipase in Wolman's disease. Nature 1969;222:1067–8.

35. Malewiak MI, Rozen R, Le Liepvre X, Griglio S. Oleate metabolism and endogenous triacylglycerol hydrolysis in isolated hepatocytes from rats fed a high-fat diet. Diabetes Metab 1988;14:270–6.

36. Kuriyama M, Yoshida H, Suzuki M, et al. Lysosomal acid lipase deficiency in rats: lipid analyses and lipase activities in liver and spleen. J Lipid Res 1990;31:1605–12.

37. Groener JE, Bax W, Poorthuis BJ. Metabolic fate of oleic acid derived from lysosomal degradation of cholesteryl oleate in human fibroblasts. J Lipid Res 1996;37:2271–9.

38. Sando GN, Ma GP, Lindsley KA, Wei YP. Intercellular transport of lysosomal acid lipase mediates lipoprotein cholesteryl ester metabolism in a human vascular endothelial cell-fibroblast coculture system. Cell Regul 1990;1:661–74.

39. Ginsberg HN, Le NA, Short MP, et al. Suppression of apolipoprotein B production during treatment of cholesteryl ester storage disease with lovastatin. Implications for regulation of apolipoprotein B synthesis. J Clin Invest 1987;80:1692–7.

40. Sando GN, Henke VL. Recognition and receptor-mediated endocytosis of the lysosomal acid lipase secreted by cultured human fibroblasts. J Lipid Res 1982;23:114–23.

41. Du H, Schiavi S, Levine M, et al. Enzyme therapy for lysosomal acid lipase deficiency in the mouse. Hum Mol Genet 2001; 10:1639–48.

42. Lohse P, Maas S, Sewell AC, et al. Molecular defects underlying Wolman disease appear to be more heterogeneous than those resulting in cholesteryl ester storage disease. J Lipid Res 1999;40:221–8.

43. Lohse P, Chahrokh-Zadeh S, Seidel D. Human lysosomal acid lipase/cholesteryl ester hydrolase and human gastric lipase: site-directed mutagenesis of Cys227 and Cys236 results in substrate-dependent reduction of enzymatic activity. J Lipid Res 1997;38:1896–905.

44. Sheriff S, Du H, Grabowski GA. Characterization of lysosomal acid lipase by site-directed mutagenesis and heterologous expression. J Biol Chem 1995;270:27766–72.

45. Roussel A, Canaan S, Egloff MP, et al. Crystal structure of human gastric lipase and model of lysosomal acid lipase, two lipolytic enzymes of medical interest. J Biol Chem 1999; 274:16995–7002.

46. Muntoni S, Wiebusch H, Funke H, et al. A missense mutation (Thr-6Pro) in the lysosomal acid lipase (LAL) gene is present with a high frequency in three different ethnic populations: impact on serum lipoprotein concentrations. Hum Genet 1996;97:265–7.

47. Aslanidis C, Ries S, Fehringer P, et al. Genetic and biochemical evidence that CESD and Wolman disease are distinguished by residual lysosomal acid lipase activity. Genomics 1996;33: 85–93.

48. Redonnet-Vernhet I, Chatelut M, Salvayre R, Levade T. A novel lysosomal acid lipase gene mutation in a patient with cholesteryl ester storage disease. Hum Mutat 1998;11:335–6.

49. Redonnet-Vernhet I, Chatelut M, Basile JP, et al. Cholesteryl ester storage disease: relationship between molecular defects and in situ activity of lysosomal acid lipase. Biochem Mol Med 1997;62:42–9.

50. Groener JE, Bax W, Stuani C, Pagani F. Difference in substrate specificity between human and mouse lysosomal acid lipase: low affinity for cholesteryl ester in mouse lysosomal acid lipase. Biochim Biophys Acta 2000;1487:155–62.

51. Meikle PJ, Hopwood JJ, Clague AE, Carey WF. Prevalence of lysosomal storage disorders. JAMA 1999;281:249–54.

52. Arterburn JN, Lee WM, Wood RP, et al. Orthotopic liver transplantation for cholesteryl ester storage disease. J Clin Gastroenterol 1991;13:482–5.

53. Krivit W, Freese D, Chan KW, Kulkarni R. Wolman's disease: a review of treatment with bone marrow transplantation and considerations for the future. Bone Marrow Transplant 1992;10 Suppl 1:97–101.

54. Krivit W, Peters C, Dusenbery K, et al. Wolman disease successfully treated by bone marrow transplantation. Bone Marrow Transplant 2000;26:567–70.

55. Du H, Heur M, Witte DP, et al. Lysosomal acid lipase deficiency: correction of lipid storage by adenovirus-mediated gene transfer in mice. Hum Gene Ther 2002;13:1361–72.

56. Fujiyama J, Sakuraba H, Kuriyama M, et al. A new mutation (LIPA Tyr22X) of lysosomal acid lipase gene in a Japanese patient with Wolman disease. Hum Mutat 1996;8:377–80.

57. Lohse P, Maas S, Elleder M, et al. Compound heterozygosity for a Wolman mutation is frequent among patients with cholesteryl ester storage disease. J Lipid Res 2000;41: 23–31.

58. Pagani F, Pariyarath R, Garcia R, et al. New lysosomal acid lipase gene mutants explain the phenotype of Wolman disease and cholesteryl ester storage disease. J Lipid Res 1998;39:1382–8.

59. Pagani F, Garcia R, Pariyarath R, et al. Expression of lysosomal acid lipase mutants detected in three patients with cholesteryl ester storage disease. Hum Mol Genet 1996;5:1611–7.

60. Zschenker O, Jung N, Rethmeier J, et al. Characterization of lysosomal acid lipase mutations in the signal peptide and mature polypeptide region causing Wolman disease. J Lipid Res 2001;42:1033–40.

61. Ries S, Buchler C, Langmann T, et al. Transcriptional regulation of lysosomal acid lipase in differentiating monocytes is mediated by transcription factors Sp1 and AP-2. J Lipid Res 1998;39:2125–34.

62. Gasche C, Aslanidis C, Kain R, et al. A novel variant of lysosomal acid lipase in cholesteryl ester storage disease associated with mild phenotype and improvement on lovastatin. J Hepatol 1997;27:744–50.

63. Pariyarath R, Pagani F, Stuani C, et al. L273S missense substitution in human lysosomal acid lipase creates a new N-glycosylation site. FEBS Lett 1996;397:79–82.

64. Ries S, Buchler C, Schindler G, et al. Different missense mutations in histidine-108 of lysosomal acid lipase cause cholesteryl ester storage disease in unrelated compound heterozygous and hemizygous individuals. Hum Mutat 1998;12:44–51.

65. Mayatepek E, Seedorf U, Wiebusch H, et al. Fatal genetic defect causing Wolman disease. J Inherit Metab Dis 1999;22:93–4.

66. Anderson RA, Byrum RS, Coates PM, Sando GN. Mutations at the lysosomal acid cholesteryl ester hydrolase gene locus in Wolman disease. Proc Natl Acad Sci U S A 1994;91:2718–22.

67. Maslen CL, Babcock D, Illingworth DR. Occurrence of a mutation associated with Wolman disease in a family with cholesteryl ester storage disease. J Inherit Metab Dis 1995;18:620–3.

68. Ries S, Aslanidis C, Fehringer P, et al. A new mutation in the gene for lysosomal acid lipase leads to Wolman disease in an African kindred. J Lipid Res 1996;37:1761–5.

69. Ameis D, Brockmann G, Knoblich R, et al. A 5′ splice-region mutation and a dinucleotide deletion in the lysosomal acid lipase gene in two patients with cholesteryl ester storage disease. J Lipid Res 1995;36:241–50.

70. Du H, Duanmu M, Rosa LR. Mouse lysosomal acid lipase: characterization of the gene and analysis of promoter activity. Gene 1998;208:285–95.

71. Muntoni S, Wiebusch H, Funke H, et al. Homozygosity for a splice junction mutation in exon 8 of the gene encoding lysosomal acid lipase in a Spanish kindred with cholesterol ester storage disease (CESD). Hum Genet 1995;95:491–4.

72. Seedorf U, Guardamagna O, Strobl W, et al. Mutation report: Wolman disease. Hum Genet 1999;105:337–41.

73. Nagano M, Iwasaki T, Hattori H, Egashira T. A novel missense mutation Thr316Ala in lysosomal acid lipase gene in Japanese population. Hum Mutat 1999;14:271.

74. Seedorf U, Wiebusch H, Muntoni S, et al. A novel variant of lysosomal acid lipase (Leu336→Pro) associated with acid lipase deficiency and cholesterol ester storage disease. Arterioscler Thromb Vasc Biol 1995;15:773–8.

75. Anderson RA, Sando GN. Cloning and expression of cDNA encoding human lysosomal acid lipase/cholesteryl ester hydrolase. Similarities to gastric and lingual lipases. J Biol Chem 1991;266:22479–84.

76. Dincsoy HP, Rolfes DB, McGraw CA, Schubert WK. Cholesterol ester storage disease and mesenteric lipodystrophy. Am J Clin Pathol 1984;81:263–9.

10. Wilson Disease

Ariel E. Feldstein, MD

Denesh K. Chitkara, MD

Randi Plescow, MD

Richard J. Grand, MD

Wilson disease is a rare autosomal recessive disorder of copper metabolism. S. A. Kinnear Wilson described the entity in 1912 and considered it to be a degenerative disorder of the central nervous system (CNS) associated with asymptomatic cirrhosis.[1] In 1921, Hall reported the hepatic symptoms and introduced the name "hepatolenticular degeneration."[2] It is generally accepted that the disorder is related to excessive accumulation of copper in the liver, CNS, kidneys, cornea, skeletal system, and other organs. The prevalence of the disorder is 1 in 30,000 persons worldwide, with a carrier frequency of 1 person in 90.[3] Wilson disease frequently presents in childhood, although the diagnosis may not be confirmed until adulthood. Early recognition of this disease and institution of appropriate therapy may be lifesaving.

PATHOPHYSIOLOGY

Wilson disease has been recognized as an entity for more than 80 years; the genetic defect has been identified, and the basic biochemical abnormalities are continuing to be elucidated. Wilson disease is a disorder of copper balance in which the biliary excretion of copper is inadequate, leading to excess accumulation in the other organs.[4] Copper is an essential trace element required in a number of enzyme systems. The main dietary sources of copper include liver, kidney, shellfish, chocolate, dried beans, peas, and unprocessed wheat. The average American diet includes 1.0 mg of copper per day.[5,6] Under normal circumstances, 50% of ingested copper is unabsorbed and lost in the feces[7] and 30% is lost through the skin.[8] A negligible amount normally is excreted in the urine. The remaining 20%, which is critically balanced for homeostasis, is normally excreted into the feces via bile.[4,5,9] Wilson disease is caused by the inability to excrete this remaining 0.2 mg of copper into bile; copper absorption from the gastrointestinal tract is normal. Studies measuring the peak copper concentration in blood after an oral dose of radiocopper have shown no difference between patients with Wilson disease and control patients.[7]

MOLECULAR GENETICS

Initial genetic linkage studies showed that the Wilson disease locus segregated with the red cell enzyme esterase D on chromosome 13.[10] Subsequent linkage analysis confined the disease locus proximally by the deoxyribonucleic acid (DNA) marker D13S31 and distally by the DNA marker D13S59.[11,12] Soon after it was confirmed that the Menkes disease gene (*MNK*) encoded a copper-binding P-type adenosine triphosphatase (ATPase) protein,[13–15] four independent groups identified the gene responsible for Wilson disease.[16–19] Three of these groups used the human Menkes disease gene as a probe,[16–18] whereas the fourth group used linkage disequilibrium and haplotype analysis.[19] The Wilson disease gene transcript encodes a transmembrane copper-transporting ATPase protein with a strong homology to the Menkes disease gene. The messenger ribonucleic acid for the Wilson disease gene is highly expressed in the liver, with limited expression in other tissues. The strong homology between the Wilson disease gene and the Menkes disease gene is interesting considering the different clinical manifestations of these two diseases. This can be better understood if both are considered to be disorders of ineffective intracellular transfer of copper.

The mechanism by which the Wilson protein, ATPase 7B, participates in copper metabolism is beginning to be understood (Figure 55.10-1). Dietary copper is absorbed in the upper intestine, where it binds to the proteins, albumin, copper histidine, and transcuprein.[20] Most of the copper is transported to the liver via the portal system and enters the hepatocyte, possibly by the cell surface transporter human copper transporter 1.[21] Once inside the hepatocyte, copper is transported by "copper chaperones," which traffic the metal within the cytoplasm. The identified copper chaperone in humans, known as human ATX homologue 1 (HAH1), functions as both a regulator of copper homeostasis and an antioxidant.[22,23] HAH1 transports copper to the Wilson ATPase 7B, which is located in the *trans*-Golgi network and, under basal conditions, also facilitates transfer of copper into ceruloplasmin.[24,25] However, an increase in cellular copper concentration has been shown to cause movement of the ATPase 7B protein to a cytoplasmic vesicle by a mechanism that appears to be reversible and independent of new protein synthesis.[24] This vesicle is hypothesized to be one of the mechanisms by which copper normally leaves the hepatocyte. Interestingly, ATPase 7B has also been found in the hepatocyte membrane and may represent a direct route to transport copper through the canalicular membrane.[25] Mutations in the ATPase 7B protein represent

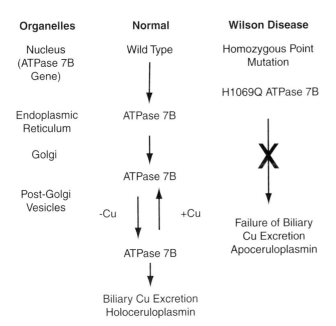

Organelles	Normal	Wilson Disease
Nucleus (ATPase 7B Gene)	Wild Type	Homozygous Point Mutation

FIGURE 55.10-1 Molecular defect in Wilson disease. Under normal conditions, adenosine triphosphatase (ATPase) 7B is a transmembrane protein that traffics from the endoplasmic reticulum to the Golgi apparatus, where it is localized under basal conditions. ATPase 7B is responsible for the movement of copper into the Golgi, where ceruloplasmin probably acquires its copper. When copper is abundant, ATPase 7B traffics to a post-Golgi compartment, where it delivers copper to biliary excretory pathways that are thought to involve transfer to lysosomes and then to bile by a canalicular membrane transporter. In Wilson disease, the mutant protein fails to leave the endoplasmic reticulum and therefore is unable to transfer copper in the Golgi or facilitate copper excretion in bile. Reproduced with permission of Lippincott, Williams and Wilkins from Schilsky M. Inherited metabolic disease. Curr Opin Gastroenterol 1999;15:200–7.

the molecular basis of Wilson disease and are thought to cause a disruption in the transport of copper from the hepatocyte. Greater than 60 disease-specific mutations already have been identified[16,18,26] that make genetic screening of Wilson disease challenging. The most common mutation of the Wilson disease gene, His 1069 Glu (H1069Q), represents 30 to 60% of the Wilson disease alleles in North American, Austrian, Russian, and Swedish samples.[26,27] Two mutations not yet described in European samples have been found in Japanese children: 2874 del C in exon 13 and Arg 778 Leu in exon 8.[28]

The ability to study Wilson disease is enhanced with the recent identification of the Long-Evans cinnamon rat as an animal model.[29] This model has been used to demonstrate correction of the defect using complementation with a wild-type ATPase 7B complementary DNA incorporated into a recombinant adenovirus.[30] Under these conditions, ceruloplasmin synthesis was restored as well.

Much attention also has been given to the role that ceruloplasmin may play in the pathogenesis of disease. Ceruloplasmin is a blue-colored, α-globulin with a molecular mass of 132 kD. The gene for ceruloplasmin is on chromosome 3. It is produced exclusively in the liver, but its role in copper metabolism is unknown. It may function

in iron transport.[20] Typically, patients with Wilson disease have low serum levels of ceruloplasmin. However, 5 to 25% of patients with Wilson disease have normal levels.[31] At times, this is secondary to an acute-phase response associated with active liver disease, but approximately 10% of patients have unexplainably normal values. Low values may be found in some heterozygotes who have no manifestations of the disease.[32]

The cause of the decreased and the occasional normal values of ceruloplasmin in Wilson disease is unknown, but available data do provide interesting clues. Both apoceruloplasmin and the number of atoms of copper per ceruloplasmin molecule are normal in Wilson disease, but the rate of holoceruloplasmin synthesis seems to be reduced.[3] Knowledge that Wilson disease results from a mutation of a copper transport protein is useful in explaining the variations observed in ceruloplasmin levels. Copper is incorporated during the biosynthesis of ceruloplasmin by transfer from the ATPase 7B located in the trans-Golgi network; ceruloplasmin is then secreted from the hepatocyte into the plasma.[33] Yet reduction of copper transport into excretory pathways still occurs, resulting in hepatic copper accumulation.[34] These mutations may also affect ATPase 7B interaction with copper chaperones or the excretion of copper across the canaliculus. In in vitro experiments, the H1069Q mutation appears to demonstrate an abnormal mechanism of protein folding that affects its ability to be expressed in the trans-Golgi network in the murine-mottled fibroblast cell line.[33]

The transfer of copper into the pathway for ceruloplasmin synthesis is altered by Wilson disease mutations, thereby causing decreased ceruloplasmin levels. Different mutations may alter copper transport to different degrees and at different cellular sites. Therefore, certain mutations may allow normal transport of copper for ceruloplasmin synthesis so that normal ceruloplasmin levels are maintained. Yet reduction of copper transport into excretory pathways still occurs, resulting in hepatic copper.

CLINICAL MANIFESTATIONS

The clinical manifestations of Wilson disease usually are related to hepatic or CNS involvement (Table 55.10-1). The presenting features are variable, and clinical disease is rarely present before patients reach 5 years of age. Most of the manifestations are related to deposition of copper in specific organs. In the series of Scheinberg and Sternlieb, the initial clinical manifestations were hepatic in 42% of patients, neurologic in 34%, psychiatric in 10%, hematologic or endocrinologic in 12%, and renal in 1% (Table 55.10-2). Approximately 25% of patients have more than one organ involved.[3] Of 50 cases reviewed by Walshe, 31 cases had hepatic and 17 had neurologic presentations.[35] In the pediatric age group, it is common for the hepatic manifestations to precede the neurologic manifestations by many years.

HEPATIC MANIFESTATIONS

Manifestations of liver disease are greatly varied. Wilson disease may present as acute self-limited hepatitis, full

TABLE 55.10-1   MANIFESTATIONS OF WILSON DISEASE

HEPATIC
Acute hepatitis
Chronic active hepatitis
Cirrhosis
Fulminant hepatic failure

CENTRAL NERVOUS SYSTEM
Neurologic
Psychiatric

OPHTHALMOLOGIC
Kayser-Fleischer ring
Sunflower cataracts

MISCELLANEOUS
Hemolytic anemia
Endocrinologic
Renal
Skeletal
Cardiac
Cholelithiasis

recovery may appear to occur, in which case, the patient is thought to have had a viral hepatitis. Many months or years may elapse before the patient again has evidence of liver disease. Patients, especially younger ones, may come to medical attention because of fulminant hepatic failure with jaundice, hypoalbuminemia, coagulation defects, ascites, hepatic encephalopathy, and, frequently, hemolysis.[36–38] Large amounts of copper are released by the liver, resulting in high serum copper levels associated with hemolytic anemia. Without a family history of hepatic or neurologic conditions, or Wilson disease itself, it is difficult to distinguish fulminant Wilson disease from fulminant hepatic failure of another cause. Patients with fulminant Wilson disease have a particularly poor outcome even if the diagnosis of Wilson disease is made. Interestingly, in one series, 16 of 21 patients with fulminant Wilson disease were female.[39] This observation of a female predominance for fulminant Wilson disease has been confirmed by others and is hypothesized to be due to the influence of sex hormones. Children and adolescents may also present with clinical features of chronic liver failure and cirrhosis with ascites, edema, hypoalbuminemia, and evidence of portal hypertension. These patients may be jaundiced. In contrast to other causes of cirrhosis, few reported cases exist of hepatocellular carcinoma evolving from Wilson disease.[40] Young patients also may come to medical attention with a clinical

and histologic picture similar to that of chronic hepatitis. The presenting symptoms and signs range from elevations in liver-derived serum enzymes to symptoms resulting from complications of portal hypertension or liver failure. In such patients, neurologic dysfunction and Kayser-Fleischer (KF) rings may not be found[31,41] and the serum ceruloplasmin level may be normal,[31] adding to the difficulty in diagnosis.

CNS INVOLVEMENT

When Wilson initially described hepatolenticular degeneration, he thought that the CNS damage was limited to the basal ganglia, especially the putamen.[1] CNS involvement is now known to be more extensive, and a wide spectrum of neurologic findings ensues. Neurologic manifestations have been reported to occur as early as 6 years of age,[3] but more typically they begin in the second to third decade of life and are usually associated with the presence of KF rings. Reports of Wilson disease without KF rings illustrate that this diagnosis should be considered in patients who exhibit the typical neurologic manifestations without other signs of disease.[42] The onset of neurologic symptoms is gradual, and severity progresses without treatment. CNS damage in Wilson disease is limited almost exclusively to the motor system, with the sensory system being spared. Common first neurologic symptoms are tremor, incoordination, dystonia, and difficulty with fine motor tasks such as dressing and writing. Later, other manifestations such as mask-like facies, drooling, dysarthria, rigidity, and gait disturbances may become apparent. The patient often becomes highly frustrated because the intellect is unchanged. Older patients are frequently misdiagnosed as having a pure psychiatric disorder or neurologic disease, such as multiple sclerosis or a disorder of the basal ganglia.[43] In pediatric patients, the first neuropsychiatric symptom of Wilson disease may be deteriorating school performance.

Computed tomographic (CT) scan of the head may be helpful in making the diagnosis (Table 55.10-3). CT findings are more likely to be abnormal in patients with neurologic involvement but also may be abnormal in patients who are asymptomatic or have only hepatic involvement. In one study of 60 patients with Wilson disease, 73% had ventricular dilatation, 63% had cortical atrophy, 55% had brainstem atrophy, 45% had basal ganglia hypodensity, and 10% had posterior fossa atrophy; in 18%, the findings were normal.[44] Other studies have shown changes in the internal capsule, thalamus, and white matter.[44,45] The CT

TABLE 55.10-2   PRESENTING SYMPTOMS OF WILSON DISEASE*

SYSTEM INVOLVED	STERNLIEB AND SCHEINBERG[3] (%)	WALSHE[35] (%)
Hepatic	42	62
Central nervous system		34
Neurologic	34	
Psychiatric	10	
Hematologic and endocrinologic	12	
Renal	1	

*More than one organ was involved in 25% of patients.

TABLE 55.10-3   FINDINGS FROM COMPUTED TOMOGRAPHY OF THE HEAD IN WILSON DISEASE

OBSERVATION	FREQUENCY (%)
Ventricular dilatation	73
Cortical atrophy	63
Brainstem atrophy	55
Basal ganglia hypodensity	45
Posterior fossa atrophy	10
Normal	18

Adapted from Williams FJB and Walshe JM.[44]

abnormalities do not represent actual copper deposition because this would be expected to show as hyperdense areas. Rather, the changes are likely to result from the damage caused by copper deposition. The hypodense areas, along with areas of generalized atrophy, are fairly characteristic of Wilson disease.[44] The severity of the CT abnormalities does not correlate with clinical symptoms[46] and is also of little prognostic value because patients with extensive involvement often do well in response to therapy.[44] Magnetic resonance imaging (MRI) supports the abnormalities seen on CT scan and may be more sensitive in identifying abnormal regions.[43–47] The hypodense areas seen on CT scan appear as regions of increased intensity on MRI, suggesting that edema may produce the abnormality seen on CT scan.[48] In one report, high signal intensity was seen in the basal ganglia, with involvement in nearly all areas of gray and white matter with generalized atrophy. MRI has also identified abnormalities in the lentiform and dentate nuclei, substantia nigra, and vermis cerebelli.[49] Both positron emission tomography and MRI spectroscopy are beginning to be used to correlate the clinical manifestations with the gross findings in Wilson disease.[50]

PSYCHIATRIC MANIFESTATIONS

Psychiatric manifestations may be dramatic in patients with Wilson disease. These include poor school performance, anxiety, depression, compulsive behavior, phobias, aggressive outbursts, neurosis, and even psychosis.[51,52] Affected patients frequently are labeled with erroneous psychiatric diagnoses before the correct diagnosis of Wilson disease is made. It is sometimes difficult to distinguish the behavioral symptoms resulting from excessive copper deposition from those secondary to the individual's reaction to having a chronic disease. This is particularly an issue in adolescent patients, and psychological intervention is often helpful.

OPHTHALMOLOGIC MANIFESTATIONS

Ophthalmologic manifestations of Wilson disease have received considerable attention because their presence may help lead to the diagnosis before any laboratory result is available. Kayser first described the "ring" in a patient thought to have multiple sclerosis,[53] and several years later, Fleischer reported an association of the ring with Wilson disease.[54] The KF ring may have a variable color, depending in part on the color of the iris. It has been described as a golden brown, brownish green, greenish yellow, bronze, or tannish green discoloration in the zone of Descemet membrane in the limbic region of the cornea (Figure 55.10-2). It can sometimes be seen with the naked eye, but a slit-lamp examination is mandatory. The rings consist of copper granules; however, they represent only a small fraction of the total corneal copper content. The bulk of copper deposition is in the stromal layer, but no color change is seen in any of the corneal layers except in Descemet membrane. Copper is initially taken up by the aqueous humor and diffuses into the cornea. Movement of water-soluble substances such as copper is a function of the evaporation of tears from the surface of the cornea. Evaporation is less at the superior poles and somewhat less at the infe-

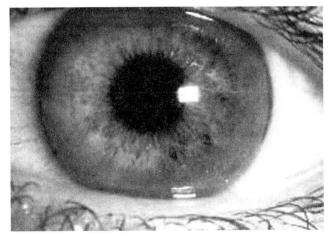

FIGURE 55.10-2 Appearance of the Kayser-Fleischer ring in a patient with Wilson disease. Note the deposition surrounding the limbus in this eye. With a darker iris, the ring may be observed only when using the slit lamp.

rior poles. Because the solvent flow is less in these areas, copper deposition is first seen there. Therefore, the rings first form superiorly and then inferiorly and finally extend laterally to complete the ring. Likewise, with treatment, the rings fade in the reverse order in which they appear.[55]

KF rings usually are present in patients with neurologic findings but frequently are present in those with only hepatic manifestations, as well as in some asymptomatic patients.[56] KF rings are not specific for Wilson disease. They have been seen in patients with chronic active hepatitis, primary biliary cirrhosis, and cryptogenic cirrhosis and in children with chronic intrahepatic cholestasis (Table 55.10-4).[55–61]

Sunflower cataracts are seen less frequently than KF rings and, when present, are accompanied by KF rings.[55] They can be seen with an ophthalmoscope as a greenish gray or golden disk in the anterior capsule of the lens, with spokes radiating toward the lens periphery.[61,62] Most of these cataracts resolve with therapy and will not affect vision.[55]

CARDIAC MANIFESTATIONS

Although Wilson disease is a multisystem disorder, few studies have evaluated the cardiac manifestations. One study of 53 patients showed electrocardiographic (ECG) abnormalities in 34%, including left ventricular hypertrophy, ST depression, T-wave inversion, premature ventricular contractions, sinoatrial block, and atrial fibrillation.[63] Thirteen percent of patients had arrhythmias, whereas 40 control patients of similar age all had normal ECG results. Of the patients with Wilson disease, 19% had mild asymp-

TABLE 55.10-4   CONDITIONS ASSOCIATED WITH KAYSER-FLEISCHER RINGS

Wilson disease
Chronic active hepatitis
Primary biliary cirrhosis
Cryptogenic cirrhosis
Intrahepatic cholestasis with cirrhosis

Adapted from references 38 to 45.

tomatic orthostatic hypotension. Response to a Valsalva maneuver (as a test for normal autonomic functioning) was abnormal in 6 of 18 patients with Wilson disease who were able to perform the maneuver.[63] Autopsy reports have shown cardiac hypertrophy, fibrosis, small vessel sclerosis, and myocardial inflammatory cell infiltrates, although gross abnormalities are not impressive. Pathologic findings did not correlate with myocardial copper content, which may be low or high. Several cases of sudden death are reported, presumably secondary to cardiac arrhythmia that may be related to Wilson disease.[64]

RENAL MANIFESTATIONS

Renal involvement is a widely recognized complication of Wilson disease. It is characterized by proximal tubular dysfunction as indicated by aminoaciduria, glycosuria, increased excretion of uric acid and calcium, and a decrease in filtration rate and effective renal blood flow.[65] There is an acidification defect that is likely a distal tubular dysfunction, in which patients are unable to acidify urine to a pH of less than 5.2 despite an acid load. Renal acidification defects can cause renal potassium wasting and recurrent hypokalemia.[66] Usually, however, patients are able to maintain normal or nearly normal plasma pH levels despite this renal tubular defect.[67–69] Renal stones are common and may predate the diagnosis of the disease. Hypercalciuria and inadequate acidification of urine may contribute to stone formation.[67] The histopathologic changes in renal biopsy specimens are not impressive. Membranoproliferative glomerulonephritis has been reported in association with Wilson disease but is more likely related to the presence of liver disease than Wilson disease itself.[70] Scheinberg and Sternlieb reported elevated copper concentrations in the kidney at autopsy in eight patients with untreated Wilson disease.[3] Rubeanic acid staining has demonstrated granules, presumed to be copper, within the tubular epithelium.[71] Renal function has been shown to improve with penicillamine therapy.[72]

SKELETAL MANIFESTATIONS

A variety of skeletal changes are observed in patients with Wilson disease. These include osteoporosis, rickets, osteomalacia, spontaneous fractures, osteochondritis dessicans, and osteoarthritis.[73] Bone demineralization is the most common abnormality seen. Renal defects causing hypercalciuria and hyperphosphaturia, with resultant hypocalcemia and hypophosphatemia, are the main cause of demineralization.[74,75] Other factors include dystonic contractures and immobilization. Chronic liver disease itself may cause skeletal abnormalities.[76] High levels of copper have been found in cartilage in some patients who underwent biopsy.[77] Pediatric patients rarely have significant skeletal changes on radiograph. Acute rhabdomyolysis has been reported as a presenting feature of Wilson disease.[78]

OTHER MANIFESTATIONS

Hemolysis is a recognized complication of Wilson disease. It may precede other clinical manifestations of the disease and be short-lived or may progress to anemia and be the first recognized abnormality of the disease.[79] Hemolysis

may occur secondary to an oxidative injury to red blood cell membranes from excess copper,[80] but the exact mechanism remains unknown.

As a consequence of hemolysis and cirrhosis, cholelithiasis may complicate Wilson disease. The stones are a mixed type, containing both cholesterol and pigment. Patients with Wilson disease should be examined for gallstones; likewise, in a child with gallstones, Wilson disease should be considered in the differential diagnosis.[81] Spontaneous splenic rupture has been reported as a presenting feature of Wilson disease.[82]

LIVER PATHOLOGY

The liver is the major organ for storage of copper. From more than 260 patients with Wilson disease analyzed by Scheinberg and Sternlieb, none of the liver specimens were normal; even a specimen from a 3.5-year-old boy was abnormal.[3] Cirrhosis has been seen in patients as young as 5 years of age.[83] Characteristic histologic findings are present but not pathognomonic. Fat deposition is one of the earliest changes seen in the liver biopsy specimen. Fine lipid droplets composed of triglycerides are dispersed throughout the cytoplasm.[3,84] As the disease progresses, these lipid droplets increase in size until hepatic steatosis is manifested. In early stages, electron microscopic study shows the mitochondria to be of varying shapes and sizes. The matrix density is increased, with vacuolated and crystalline inclusions. Inner and outer mitochondrial membranes, which are normally opposed, become separated, and the intercristal spaces expand. Peroxisomes, which are involved in cellular lipid metabolism, may become enlarged with a granular, flocculent matrix of varying density rather than with the homogeneous matrix seen in normal peroxisomes.[85] With progression of the hepatic lesion, there is collagen deposition and eventually development of fibrosis. Histologic features that are indistinguishable from those of autoimmune chronic hepatitis may develop, as well as hepatic necrosis (Figure 55.10-3).

If the diagnosis of Wilson disease is not made, and the patient survives, cirrhosis develops. Once cirrhosis is established, the fatty changes disappear, as do those changes seen in the mitochondria and peroxisomes. The electron microscopic findings are then relatively normal, except for excessive amorphous or globular copper-containing lipofuscin granules and lipid-containing lysosomes.[86]

A high copper content is found normally in the fetal and neonatal liver.[87] The cause is not known, but it is postulated that immaturity of bile excretion plays a role in this increased copper level.[88] Some of the copper binds to a sulfhydryl-rich protein, known as copper-associated or copper-binding protein, which is bound in hepatic lysosomes.[89] This lysosomal copper may be stained by orcein.[89] Between the third and sixth month postnatally, hepatic copper levels fall to within the normal adult range, and these orcein-positive granules are no longer seen in the normal liver. In children older than 6 months of age, orcein-positive granules indicative of elevated hepatic lysosomal copper are found only in abnormal conditions, including Wilson dis-

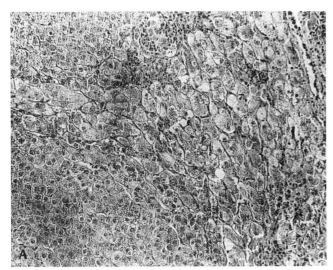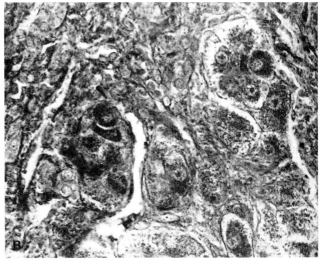

FIGURE 55.10-3   *A,* Wedge biopsy specimen from a child with Wilson disease showing a broad band of fibrous tissue at the right margin. An intense portal inflammatory response can be seen with lymphocytes spilling across the limiting plate into the lobule. Considerable hepatocellular necrosis exists with marked variations in cell size and some fat and pigment deposition. *B,* High-power view showing irregularities in cell size, hepatocellular necrosis, pigment deposition, and bile ductular proliferation. The limiting plate has been distorted, as shown by interdigitation of connective tissue and hepatocellular elements. Inflammatory cells are seen crossing the limiting plate into the lobule. Reproduced with permission from Grand RJ and Vawter GF.[122]

ease, biliary atresia, paucity of intrahepatic ducts, primary biliary cirrhosis, sclerosing or chronic cholangitis, cirrhosis, and primary hepatic tumors (Table 55.10-5). Orcein-positive granules are not seen in acute liver disease, except hepatitis B. In contrast to Wilson disease, the orcein-positive granules in other disease states are found mainly at the periphery of the liver lobules.[90] In Wilson disease, these granules are widespread in some lobules but may be completely absent in others.[90] Not all of the livers from patients with Wilson disease contain stainable copper-associated protein. In the early stages of the disease, when the liver copper concentration is highest, the copper is distributed diffusely in the cytoplasm and is absent from the lysosomes[91]; it is therefore not stainable. In the later stages of the disease, copper is redistributed to the lysosomes, and then copper may be stained by rubeanic acid and copper-associated protein by orcein.[86] However, histochemical techniques cannot confirm a diagnosis of Wilson disease, and they cannot be used to rule it out. Confirmation depends on quantitative measurement of hepatic copper content. Other disorders associated with elevated hepatic copper concentrations are listed in Table 55.10-5.

DIAGNOSIS

The diagnosis of Wilson disease may be made readily when the classic triad of hepatic disease, neurologic involvement, and KF rings is present. However, in the absence of this triad, the diagnosis begins with a high index of suspicion, especially in children. No single test can confirm the diagnosis with 100% accuracy (Table 55.10-6). Rather, the clinical and family history, physical examination, and certain key laboratory investigations collectively may establish the diagnosis. In ambiguous cases, genetic analysis may be required.

The first diagnostic test should be measurement of serum ceruloplasmin. Most children and adolescents with Wilson disease have decreased serum ceruloplasmin values, and at least 75% of those presenting with hepatic manifestations have low values.[92–94] Decreased values also may be seen in conditions associated with decreased hepatic synthetic function, such as malnutrition and severe hepatic insufficiency.[3,95] Ceruloplasmin also may be low in protein-losing enteropathy, nephrotic syndrome, and hereditary hypoceruloplasminemia.[92] Infants younger than 6 months of age normally have low serum ceruloplasmin levels.[93] Because ceruloplasmin is an acute-phase reactant, its value may be low-normal to normal in patients with Wilson disease during periods of active hepatic inflammation.[96] Its synthesis is stimulated by estrogens; hence, pregnancy (and estrogen therapy) is associated with near-normal to normal ceruloplasmin levels (Table 55.10-7).[96] Difficulty in establishing a diagnosis also occurs in 10% of heterozygotes who have low serum ceruloplasmin levels but no manifestations of Wilson disease.[96] Therefore, serum ceruloplasmin level should not be used as the sole determinant in diagnosing the disease.

TABLE 55.10-5   CONDITIONS ASSOCIATED WITH ELEVATED HEPATIC COPPER CONCENTRATION

Normal infant younger than 6 mo of age
Cholestasis syndromes
  Biliary atresia
  Paucity of intrahepatic ducts
Sclerosing cholangitis
Primary biliary cirrhosis
Indian childhood cirrhosis
Primary hepatic tumors
Wilson disease

TABLE 55.10-6   DIAGNOSIS OF WILSON DISEASE

Clinical information
Family history
Kayser-Fleischer rings
Laboratory tests
  Hematologic
  Liver function
Copper status
  Serum copper: < 20 μg/dL
  Urinary copper: > 100 μg/24 h
  Hepatic copper: > 250 μg/g dry weight of liver
  Low serum ceruloplasmin
  Radiocopper excretion abnormal
Genetic analysis

Serum or plasma copper levels should be obtained at the time of diagnosis, although it should be noted that their concentration cannot be used as a diagnostic test for Wilson disease. In classic cases of Wilson disease, the serum or plasma copper levels are decreased, in conjunction with the low ceruloplasmin values. However, in certain stages of the disease, copper levels are elevated as a consequence of the flooding of the plasma with nonceruloplasmin-bound copper released from the liver. As will be discussed below, serum copper levels are also necessary for the assessment of the patient's adherence to therapy. Total serum copper levels are readily obtained in most laboratories.

In contrast to plasma copper determination, urinary copper excretion is a useful diagnostic test. It is normally less than 40 μg/24 h. The conventional level taken as diagnostic for Wilson disease is greater than 100 μg/24 h in symptomatic patients.[97] However, recent studies have shown that basal determination may be less than 100 μg/24 h in up to 25% of patients diagnosed with Wilson disease,[94,98,99] indicating that 24-hour urinary excretion of copper greater than 40 μg/24 h may be a better threshold for diagnosis of Wilson disease and requires further investigation. Abnormal urinary copper excretion is not specific for Wilson disease because it may be elevated in patients with primary biliary cirrhosis,[100] chronic active hepatitis,[31] fulminant hepatitis, and cholestasis (Table 55.10-8).[35] The urine collections must be obtained in copper-free containers.

TABLE 55.10-7   CONDITIONS ASSOCIATED WITH ALTERED CERULOPLASMIN CONCENTRATIONS

Dᴇᴄʀᴇᴀsᴇᴅ
Malnutrition
Protein-losing enteropathy
Nephrotic syndrome
Hepatic insufficiency
Hereditary hypoceruloplasminemia
Neonates
Menkes syndrome
Wilson disease
Heterozygosity for Wilson disease

Eʟᴇᴠᴀᴛᴇᴅ
Estrogen therapy
Infection/inflammation
Pregnancy

The use of the penicillamine-stimulated copper excretion test remains controversial. Many studies have found no difference in penicillamine-induced copper excretion between Wilson disease and chronic hepatitis.[101] However, one study exclusively in children suggested that this test might be valuable. After collecting one 24-hour urine sample in a copper-free container, patients received 500 mg penicillamine at the start of, and 12 hours into, the second 24-hour urine collection. Urinary copper excretion was measured in both specimens. Although there was overlap between copper excretion in patients with Wilson disease and those with chronic hepatitis, a penicillamine-induced cupruresis (> 25 μmol/24 h) was shown to be valuable in the diagnosis of Wilson disease.[102] There is some question as to the capacity of such brief exposure to penicillamine to sensitize the patient and render allergic reactions later more likely. This remains to be resolved. Whether this test is useful for diagnosis, 24-hour urinary copper excretion is a good measurement to follow during treatment of patients with Wilson disease because it allows quantification of the success of chelation therapy.

The clinician should look for KF rings by using slit-lamp examination, but the rings are not pathognomonic for Wilson disease (see Table 55.10-4).[57,58] However, in Wilson disease, they are present in approximately 50% of patients with a hepatic presentation and 95% of those with neurologic or psychiatric symptoms. They may also be helpful when considering the possibility of nonadherence to treatment, as in a patient whose KF rings have faded and then returned.

A liver biopsy should be performed whenever possible because the quantification of hepatic copper concentration will, in most cases, establish the diagnosis in the absence of known obstructive liver disease. Microscopic and ultrastructural analyses are valuable, whereas copper staining is not. Measurements of quantitative hepatic copper concentrations are mandatory. Normal hepatic copper concentration is less than 50 μg/g of dry weight of liver.[103] Patients with Wilson disease generally have values greater than 250 μg/g of dry liver, and values may be greater than 1,000 μg/g of dry liver. Presymptomatic homozygous patients, especially young children, may not always have levels greater than 250 μg/g. Heterozygotes may have values up to 150 to 200 μg/g. A normal hepatic copper concentration rules out the diagnosis of Wilson disease, whereas an elevated value confirms the diagnosis in the proper clinical setting. Elevated values may be seen in

TABLE 55.10-8   CONDITIONS ASSOCIATED WITH ELEVATED URINARY COPPER EXCRETION

Wilson disease
Primary biliary cirrhosis
Chronic active hepatitis
Fulminant hepatic failure
Cholestasis syndromes
  Biliary atresia
  Paucity of intrahepatic ducts
Sclerosing cholangitis

other conditions (see Table 55.10-5).[104–106] These usually can be distinguished by other techniques.

If the diagnosis is still uncertain, the rate of incorporation of radiocopper into ceruloplasmin may be determined or genetic testing obtained. The radiocopper test is performed after a fast of 8 hours; a dose of 2.0 mg of radiocopper is administered orally. The concentration of radiocopper is measured in the serum at intervals of 1, 2, 4, 24, and 48 hours later. The radiocopper rises in the 1-hour and 2-hour samples and then falls. In normal individuals, the serum concentration rises again to a higher level in the 24-hour or 48-hour sample, representing incorporation into ceruloplasmin. However, in patients with Wilson disease, even those with normal ceruloplasmin levels, the secondary rise is not achieved. One needs to be cautious in interpreting these results because considerable overlap occurs with heterozygotes, especially those with low serum ceruloplasmin concentrations.[107] If the index patient's serum ceruloplasmin is relatively high, other family members also may have near-normal values yet still have Wilson disease.

Currently, genetic analysis is mostly limited to identification of first-degree relatives of newly diagnosed patients. The pedigree analysis is performed using haplotypes based on polymorphisms surrounding the Wilson disease gene and requires the identification of a patient within the family (the proband). De novo diagnosis by molecular studies remains difficult at present owing mostly to the large numbers of disease-specific mutations of ATP7B; it is done only in the context of research protocols.[108]

Asymptomatic relatives, especially siblings of patients with Wilson disease, should be screened (Table 55.10-9). They should have a careful physical examination, ophthalmologic slit-lamp examination, measurement of serum ceruloplasmin and copper concentration, hepatic transaminase levels, and 24-hour urinary copper excretion. If all of these screening tests give absolutely normal results, the diagnosis is most likely excluded, although it may be prudent to repeat them at least once several months later. However, if even one test result is abnormal, a liver biopsy should be performed and samples sent for quantitative copper determination and histologic examination. In the young pediatric age group, if the 24-hour urinary copper result is normal, it should be repeated when the child is older, at which time enough copper would have accumulated to be reflected in an elevated urinary value. Subtle evidence of Wilson disease may be reflected in the presence of hemolysis, elevated reticulocyte values, depressed haptoglobin levels, and hypercalciuria. In equivocal cases, genetic analysis can be used to establish a diagnosis. In general, any liver disease in pediatric patients should be considered to be Wilson disease until proven otherwise.

NATURAL HISTORY

Deiss and others have devised a valuable staging system that explains many of the confusing findings in Wilson disease.[109] Revisions of the scheme also are available.[3] In stage I, a progressive accumulation of copper occurs in the cytosol of the hepatocytes. The process continues until all hepatic binding sites for copper are saturated. This stage is asymptomatic and usually occurs before age 5 years. In stage II, copper in the hepatocyte is redistributed from the cytosol to the lysosomes, and, at the same time, copper is released from the liver. If this release occurs gradually, the patient remains asymptomatic. If the redistribution is rapid, hepatic necrosis may occur, and the patient may become symptomatic from liver disease. In addition, rapid release of copper into the blood may result in hemolytic anemia. This stage is often accompanied by fulminant hepatic failure, leading to liver transplant. However, if patients pass through stage II without clinical illness, they remain asymptomatic. In stage III, copper continues to be stored in the lysosomes, and varying degrees of fibrosis or cirrhosis develop. In this stage, accumulation of copper also occurs in other tissues, such as brain, cornea, kidney, or skeleton. Patients may remain asymptomatic for years if the brain deposition of copper progresses slowly. Stage IV is characterized by symptomatic CNS disease. If copper accumulation occurs rapidly, then liver disease, CNS disease, or both become apparent in a short time. Stage V occurs when treatment is begun before the patient dies from hepatic failure or irreversible brain damage. In stage V, cupruresis leads to reductions in copper accumulation, repair of tissue injury, and improvement in the clinical status of the patient.[110]

Few series of patients with Wilson disease have partially characterized the long-term prognosis of patients with this disease.[111–113] These series have suggested that the long-term outcome of these patients is mainly dependent on adherence to lifelong treatment with excellent prognosis in those patients who are compliant with effective medical therapy, even if cirrhosis is present at the time of diagnosis. However, it is important to note that none of these studies have compared the long-term survival of patients with Wilson disease with that of an age- and gender-matched population. Furthermore, there is no study assessing the quality of life of patients on long-term treatment for this condition.

TREATMENT

At the time of the discovery of Wilson disease, and for many years subsequently, early diagnosis had little clinical

TABLE 55.10-9   SCREENING OF ASYMPTOMATIC RELATIVES OF PATIENTS WITH WILSON DISEASE

MANDATORY
History and physical examination
Ophthalmologic slit-lamp examination
Serum ceruloplasmin and copper concentrations
Hepatic transaminase levels
24-Hour urinary copper excretion

ADDITIONAL
Blood smear for hemolysis
Reticulocyte count and haptoglobin
Urinary calcium level
Genetic analysis

If any of the above is abnormal, liver biopsy becomes mandatory with examination of histology and measurement of quantitative liver copper content.

significance. In 1951, Denny-Brown and Porter and Cumings[115] introduced dimercaprol (BAL) as an effective treatment for Wilson disease.[114,115] However, the daily painful intramuscular injections made BAL impractical. In 1956, Walshe drastically changed the outcome of patients with Wilson disease by showing that D-penicillamine is an effective treatment.[95] Wilson disease is fatal if untreated, but successful outcome is achieved with effective pharmacologic therapy. The US Food and Drug Administration approved D-penicillamine as effective and safe for Wilson disease in 1963. In 1968, in a landmark paper, Sternlieb and Scheinberg showed its effectiveness in presymptomatic homozygous patients.[116]

PENICILLAMINE

Penicillamine remains the chelating agent with which there has been the greatest experience. Initial therapy with trientine is emerging as an acceptable alternative. Penicillamine is a sulfur-containing amino acid that is a metabolite of penicillin; it chelates copper and then is excreted in the urine. When initiating therapy, a small dose should be used; the dose should then be gradually increased and administered orally on an empty stomach in four divided doses, 30 to 45 minutes before meals and at bedtime, or 2 or more hours after eating. In children and adolescents, the dose is 20 mg/kg of body weight; the customary adult dose is 1.0 g/d.[3] Penicillamine is better absorbed in the absence of food.[117] Patients should also receive 25 mg of pyridoxine three times a week because of the potential antipyridoxine effects of penicillamine.[118] As a consequence of treatment, urinary copper excretion may be more than 5,000 μg in a 24-hour period. However, this decreases with time; after months to years of therapy, it can be as low as 600 μg in a 24-hour period.[109] Usually, there is a dramatic improvement in symptoms within weeks of beginning therapy. If no improvement occurs, the daily dose of penicillamine may be raised to 1.5 to 2 g/d or its equivalent according to body weight, although one must consider faulty patient compliance as a possible cause of poor response. The higher dose of penicillamine is associated with an increased risk of side effects. Most patients become clinically asymptomatic, or nearly so, within months of beginning treatment, but some may not show significant functional improvement before 1 year. One concern when deciding on the correct drug for treatment is that neurologic symptoms may worsen with the initiation of penicillamine treatment. It is postulated that with treatment, large amounts of hepatic copper are mobilized and then deposited in the brain, worsening neurologic symptoms. There is also concern that treatment with penicillamine may initiate neurologic symptoms in previously asymptomatic patients with Wilson disease.[119] Such patients may not return to pretreatment baseline.[120] Trientine appears to be associated with a lower risk of this phenomenon and may be preferred as first-line therapy for neurologic Wilson disease. Perhaps gradual introduction of penicillamine prevents this occurrence. In general, neurologic manifestations improve, although dysarthria associated with mask-like facies may not disappear.[121] KF rings may disappear or fade partially. As a consequence of therapy, liver function test results improve and hepatic concentration of copper decreases.[122]

Studies have shown improvement in liver biopsy findings with decreased portal fibrosis, inflammation, and necrosis.[110,120,123] There is a report of a 10-year-old child who had advanced liver cirrhosis whose repeated liver biopsy showed practically normal results 27 months after starting penicillamine therapy. The biopsy samples were obtained by laparotomy, with multiple samples taken to decrease sampling error.[123] This report is unusual in showing virtually complete reversal of liver disease.

The patient's adherence to therapy is best assessed using sequential determinations of 24-hour urinary copper excretion. In addition, Scheinberg and Sternlieb recommend the assessment of free serum copper.[3] This is accomplished by spot determinations of total serum copper (μg/dL) and ceruloplasmin (mg/dL) concentrations. The unit designations are then ignored. A factor of 3 is multiplied by the ceruloplasmin value, and that value is subtracted from the total serum copper level. A resulting figure not greater than 20 indicates compliance.[124]

Undesirable side effects of penicillamine therapy may occur within the first 3 weeks of treatment in 20% of patients. These include fever, skin rash, lymphadenopathy, granulocytopenia, and thrombocytopenia.[125] Other reactions that may occur later include nephrotoxicity with proteinuria or even nephrotic syndrome,[126] lupus-like syndrome,[127] Goodpasture syndrome (which was fatal in three patients),[128] elastosis perforans serpiginosa,[129] and pemphigoid lesions of the mouth, vagina, and skin.[130,131] A penicillamine dermatopathy may occur in patients receiving more than 2 g of penicillamine for several months. Penicillamine interferes with crosslinking of collagen and elastin, which leads to a weakening of the subcutaneous tissue so that bleeding into the subcutaneous tissue may occur with even slight trauma.[129] If a reaction occurs, penicillamine should be stopped. The clinician may then pretreat with 20 to 30 mg of prednisone (0.5 mg/kg of body weight) daily for 2 to 3 days before reinstituting therapy. Penicillamine should be introduced in a much lower dose and gradually increased. Once penicillamine is tolerated, the prednisone may be withdrawn.[129] If the reaction was severe, the clinician may not wish to attempt this but to institute other decuprinizing agents (Table 55.10-10). The success of treatment with oral D-penicillamine may be limited by the presence of renal failure. Adding penicillamine to peritoneal dialysis solution is not beneficial.[132,133] Post-dilution hemofiltration and continuous arteriovenous hemofiltration with oral penicillamine have been effective.[134] Although there are incidental reports of connective tissue defects and cleft palate in the offspring of pregnant women taking penicillamine[135,136] and other therapeutic agents available (see below), Scheinberg and Sternlieb point out that cessation of treatment is dangerous, and such complications are extremely infrequent.[3] Population-based, case-controlled studies of birth defects in the children of women taking penicillamine for Wilson disease and other disorders, compared with in the random population, are not available.

Death has occurred as early as 8 months after discontinuation of D-penicillamine in a patient who had become asymptomatic with treatment and then was noncompliant. There are several reports of death within 1 year of stopping therapy in noncompliant patients. This raises the question of the exact mechanisms of D-penicillamine action. A patient who has been decuprinized with therapy should not die after just 8 months of copper reaccumulation (because initial copper accumulation takes more than 5 years in stage I). Sternlieb and colleagues suggest that penicillamine may form a nontoxic complex with copper.[130] When penicillamine treatment is suddenly stopped, there may be a sudden dissociation of this complex, and massive amounts of copper may be released, accounting for the rapid hepatic decompensation that occurs in suddenly noncompliant patients. The first sign of relapse after stopping penicillamine is a silent rise in serum transaminase levels.[130] The rise may be low compared with the amount of ongoing hepatic injury. Bilirubin becomes elevated later, and there is a decrease in serum albumin concentration, an elevation in free serum copper levels,[3] and an elevation in 24-hour urinary excretion of copper. The urinary copper excretion may be greater than 2,000 µg in a patient who has been noncompliant and then begins taking penicillamine again before urine collection.[130] It is rarely greater than 1,000 µg per 24 hours in patients taking penicillamine regularly.

TRIENTINE

In 1969, Walshe introduced triethylene tetramine dihydrochloride (trientine) as an alternative chelating agent to penicillamine for a patient who had developed an immune complex nephritis after 6 years of penicillamine treatment.[137] Cupruresis, as great as or greater than that achieved with penicillamine, may be achieved with trientine.[138] Most patients have complete reversal of the side effects seen with penicillamine, although at least one patient with elastosis perforans serpiginosa did not improve with trientine.[139] Two other patients with penicillamine-induced lupus did not improve on discontinuation of penicillamine and introduction of trientine. Iron deficiency anemia may develop in patients treated with trientine, especially women. This resolves with daily iron supplements.[139] Trientine is safe during pregnancy.[140] Trientine is given orally in divided doses of 1 to 1.5 g daily, 1 hour before or 2 hours after meals. In children younger than 10 years of age, 0.5 g (approximately 20 mg/kg) daily is recommended.[139] Renal complications from trientine can occur.

ZINC

Zinc, a known antagonist of copper absorption, has been introduced as a possible alternative maintenance treatment for Wilson disease in patients previously successfully treated with penicillamine. In 1946, Smith and Larson reported on the antagonistic effects of zinc on copper balance in rats.[141] A decrease in liver copper content secondary to zinc supplementation in sheep was reported in 1954.[142] Patients with sickle cell anemia treated with zinc had been observed to develop copper deficiency.[143] In

TABLE 55.10-10 TREATMENT OF WILSON DISEASE

Dietary restriction of copper
D-Penicillamine (with pyridoxine)
Triethylene tetramine (trientine)
Ammonium tetrathiomolybdate
Zinc
Liver transplant

1961, the role of zinc in producing negative copper balance in Wilson disease was first described.[144] Patients have subsequently demonstrated clinical improvement when treated with zinc alone.[145,146]

Copper is absorbed mainly in the proximal small intestine.[147] Its absorption is increased in the presence of chelating agents, a high-protein diet, anions, and L-amino acids. Fiber, bile, ascorbic acid, and zinc inhibit its absorption. Once copper crosses the intestinal brush border, it binds to metallothioneine in the cytosol of the enterocytes. Zinc, copper, cadmium, glucagon, glucocorticoids, and bacterial infections induce the synthesis of intestinal metallothioneine.[148] Metallothioneine has a higher affinity for copper than for zinc.[149] The copper that is metallothioneine bound cannot pass the serosa but is sloughed with the intestinal cells into the lumen and then excreted in the stool. Therefore, copper levels in stool are increased in patients treated with zinc.[150]

Experience is growing in the use of zinc in Wilson disease, and thus far, no treatment failures have occurred.[150,151] The adult recommended dose is 50 mg of elemental zinc taken three times a day, spacing each dose from food or liquids by at least 1 hour. Children and pregnant women should receive 25 mg per dose three times a day.[150] Treatment can be monitored by measuring 24-hour urinary copper. Because decoppering occurs in the gastrointestinal tract, urinary copper reflects body copper burden. A value greater than 125 µg per 24 hours suggests patient noncompliance. Twenty-four-hour urinary zinc levels average 3.5 mg and should be at least 2 mg when a therapeutic dose is taken.[150,152]

Because it takes 1 to 2 weeks to induce metallothioneine levels in the intestine, in addition to its slower rate of decoppering, zinc is not practical for initial treatment in symptomatic patients. As maintenance therapy, it has less toxicity than penicillamine, and there is more experience with zinc than with trientine.

Although zinc seems to be a basically safe medication, long-term effects are not known. Lymphocyte response to phytohemagglutinin, neutrophil chemotaxis, and bacterial phagocytosis were reduced in normal male subjects taking 150 mg of zinc twice a day for 6 weeks.[153] This observation has been challenged in a subsequent study because of the possibility that inducing copper deficiency in normal subjects may have been responsible for the decrease in lymphocyte function. Examining mitogenic response and levels of natural killer cell activity in patients treated with zinc for 15 years showed no evidence of decrease in lymphocyte function.[152] Zinc has been reported to reduce high-density lipoprotein cholesterol in normal male subjects.[154] Finally, an elevation in serum amylase and lipase has been reported during zinc therapy; however, it is believed to be caused by higher levels of these proteins induced by zinc rather than by pancreatic damage.[150]

TETRATHIOMOLYBDATE

A new potential therapeutic option is ammonium tetrathiomolybdate (TM). It has two anticopper mechanisms. It complexes ingested copper, thereby preventing absorption. Second, TM forms complexes with copper and albumin in blood, making the copper unavailable for cellular uptake. Most recently, it has been found that TM has antifibrotic and anti-inflammatory effects mainly through inhibition of profibrotic and proinflammatory cytokines.[155] In a trial of 33 patients with neurologic manifestations of Wilson disease treated with TM, only 1 patient had deterioration of neurologic function, with good to excellent recovery in a 1- to 6-year follow-up period.[156] This appears to be a promising alternative to penicillamine because it is associated with a low prevalence of complications. However, this medication remains experimental in the United States and is not commercially available.

ANTIOXIDANTS

Antioxidants, mainly vitamin E, may have a role as adjunctive therapy. Experimental studies have suggested that an increase in oxidative stress may play a central role in the liver injury seen in patients with Wilson disease.[157] Moreover, serum and hepatic vitamin E levels have been found to be low in patients with this condition.[158,159] Although symptomatic improvement when vitamin E was added to the treatment has been occasionally reported, further studies are still needed to better determine the possible role of this vitamin and other antioxidants in the treatment of patients with Wilson disease.

With the potential of genetic testing to establish the diagnosis of Wilson disease in presymptomatic homozygous relatives, treatment may begin at an early age. A recent retrospective review showed that 32 asymptomatic homozygous children were treated safely with penicillamine prophylaxis as early as 1.5 years of age.[125] However, the necessity for such early treatment must be balanced against the risks of increasing the total duration of exposure to penicillamine.

Liver transplant has been performed in a number of patients with Wilson disease[39] (Table 50.10-11). At least four groups of patients can be defined who should be considered for liver transplant[39]: (1) patients presenting with a clinical picture of fulminant hepatic failure, often adolescent or young patients; (2) patients with findings of severe hepatic decompensation who have not improved after several months of adequate chelation therapy; (3) patients who have been effectively treated but have developed severe progressive hepatic insufficiency acutely after stopping penicillamine; and (4) patients with progressive and/or irreversible neurologic dysfunction. Reports of Wilson disease patients surviving liver transplants have demonstrated extremely favorable outcomes, with a recent study showing a quality of life comparable to that of age- and sex-matched controls from

TABLE 55.10–11   INDICATIONS FOR ORTHOTOPIC LIVER TRANSPLANT IN WILSON DISEASE

Fulminant hepatic failure
Cirrhosis with decompensation
Progression of hepatic dysfunction despite treatment
Exacerbation after discontinuation of therapy
Progressive and irreversible neurologic disease

the general population.[160] Tests of copper status, including serum ceruloplasmin, serum copper, and 24-hour urinary copper excretion, normalize within 1 to 2 months.[39,161] Several reports have shown improvement of neurologic symptoms after transplant. Polson and colleagues described two patients: one preoperatively had continued worsening of neurologic manifestations despite penicillamine treatment and the other had continued worsening of hepatic and neurologic symptoms. In both patients, recovery of neurologic function occurred but was slow.[162] The findings that clinical and laboratory abnormalities normalize after liver transplant confirm the accepted theory that the metabolic defect of Wilson disease is localized within the liver.

Plasma exchange has been used to reduce serum copper levels and treat the hemolytic anemia associated with fulminant Wilson disease prior to liver transplant.[163] Experimental treatment for Wilson disease may involve the use of hepatocyte transplant. Using the Long-Evans cinnamon rat, hepatic disease has been prevented with infusion of normal rat hepatocytes.[164]

SUMMARY

Wilson disease should be considered in every pediatric patient with liver disease of unknown origin. Early diagnosis and institution of therapy prevent progression of disease and permit normal life expectancy. A variety of therapeutic strategies are available, but penicillamine remains the initial therapy of choice. Lifelong copper chelation or zinc therapy is mandatory.

REFERENCES

1. Wilson SAK. Progressive lenticular degeneration: a familial nervous disease associated with cirrhosis of the liver. Brain 1912;34:295–509.
2. Hall HC. La degenerescence hepatico-lenticulaire malade de Wilson-pseudo-sclerose. Paris: Mason and Cie; 1921.
3. Scheinberg IH, Sternlieb I. Wilson's disease. Philadelphia: WB Saunders; 1984.
4. Frommer DJ. Defective biliary excretion of copper in Wilson's disease. Gut 1974;15:125–9.
5. Hill GM, Brewer GJ, Prasad AS, et al. Treatment of Wilson's disease with zinc. I. Oral zinc therapy regimens. Hepatology 1987;7:522–8.
6. Holden JM, Wolf WR, Mertz W. Zinc and copper in self-selected diets. J Am Diet Assoc 1979;75:23–8.
7. Strickland GT, Beckner WM, Leu ML. Absorption of copper in homozygotes and heterozygotes for Wilson's disease and controls: isotope tracer studies with 67 Cu and 64 Cu. Clin Sci 1972;43:617–25.

8. Jacob RA, Sandstead HH, Munoz JM, et al. Whole body surface loss of trace metals in normal males. Am J Clin Nutr 1981;34:1379–83.

9. Gibbs K, Walshe JM. Biliary excretion of copper in Wilson's disease. Lancet 1980;ii:538–9.

10. Frydman M, Bonne-Tamir B, Farrer LA, et al. Assignment of the gene for Wilson disease to chromosome 13: linkage to the esterase D locus. Proc Natl Acad Sci U S A 1985;82:1819–21.

11. Bowcock AM, Farrer LA, Hebert JM, et al. Eight closely linked loci place the Wilson disease locus within 13q14-q21. Am J Hum Genet 1988;43:664–74.

12. Bowcock AM, Tomfohrde J, Weissenbach J, et al. Refining the position of Wilson disease by linkage disequilibrium with polymorphic microsatellites. Am J Hum Genet 1994;54:79–87.

13. Vulpe C, Levinson B, Whitney S, et al. Isolation of a candidate gene for Menkes disease and evidence that it encodes a copper-transporting ATPase [published erratum appears in Nat Genet 1993;3:273]. Nat Genet 1993;3:7–13.

14. Mercer JF, Livingston J, Hall B, et al. Isolation of a partial candidate gene for Menkes disease by positional cloning. Nat Genet 1993;3:20–5.

15. Chelly J, Tumer Z, Tonnesen T, et al. Isolation of a candidate gene for Menkes disease that encodes a potential heavy metal binding protein. Nat Genet 1993;3:14–9.

16. Bull PC, Thomas GR, Rommens JM, et al. The Wilson disease gene is a putative copper transporting P-type ATPase similar to the Menkes gene [published erratum appears in Nat Genet 1994;6:214]. Nat Genet 1993;5:327–37.

17. Tanzi RE, Petrukhin K, Chernov I, et al. The Wilson disease gene is a copper transporting ATPase with homology to the Menkes disease gene. Nat Genet 1993;5:344–50.

18. Petrukhin K, Fischer SG, Pirastu M, et al. Mapping, cloning and genetic characterization of the region containing the Wilson disease gene. Nat Genet 1993;5:338–43.

19. Yamaguchi Y, Heiny ME, Gitlin JD. Isolation and characterization of a human liver cDNA as a candidate gene for Wilson disease. Biochem Biophys Res Commun 1993;197:271–7.

20. Cox DW. Disorders of copper transport. Br Med Bull 1999;55:544–55.

21. Zhou B, Gitschier J. hCTR1: a human gene for copper uptake identified by complementation in yeast. Proc Natl Acad Sci U S A 1997;94:7481–6.

22. Hung IH, Casareno RL, Labesse G, et al. HAH1 is a copper-binding protein with distinct amino acid residues mediating copper homeostasis and antioxidant defense. J Biol Chem 1998;273:1749–54.

23. Klomp LW, Lin SJ, Yuan DS, et al. Identification and functional expression of HAH1, a novel human gene involved in copper homeostasis. J Biol Chem 1997;272:9221–6.

24. Hung IH, Suzuki M, Yamaguchi Y, et al. Biochemical characterization of the Wilson disease protein and functional expression in the yeast Saccharomyces cerevisiae. J Biol Chem 1997;272:21461–6.

25. Nagano K, Nakamura K, Urakami KI, et al. Intracellular distribution of the Wilson's disease gene product (ATPase7B) after in vitro and in vivo exogenous expression in hepatocytes from the LEC rat, an animal model of Wilson's disease. Hepatology 1998;27:799–807.

26. Shah AB, Chernov I, Zhang HT, et al. Identification and analysis of mutations in the Wilson disease gene (ATP7B): population frequencies, genotype-phenotype correlation, and functional analyses. Am J Hum Genet 1997;61:317–28.

27. Maier-Dobersberger T, Ferenci P, Polli C, et al. Detection of the His1069Gln mutation in Wilson disease by rapid polymerase chain reaction. Ann Intern Med 1997;127:21–6.

28. Shimizu N, Kawase C, Nakazono H, et al. A novel RNA splicing mutation in Japanese patients with Wilson disease. Biochem Biophys Res Commun 1995;217:16–20.

29. Yamaguchi Y, Heiny ME, Shimizu N, et al. Expression of the Wilson disease gene is deficient in the Long-Evans cinnamon rat. Biochem J 1994;301:1–4.

30. Terada K, Nakako T, Yang XL, et al. Restoration of holoceruloplasmin synthesis in LEC rat after infusion of recombinant adenovirus bearing WND cDNA. J Biol Chem 1998;273:1815–20.

31. Perman JA, Werlin SL, Grand RJ, Watkins JB. Laboratory measures of copper metabolism in the differentiation of chronic active hepatitis and Wilson disease in children. J Pediatr 1979;94:564–8.

32. Gibbs K, Walshe JM. A study of the caeruloplasmin concentrations found in 75 patients with Wilson's disease, their kinships and various control groups. QJM 1979;48:447–63.

33. Payne AS, Gitlin JD. Functional expression of the Menkes disease protein reveals common biochemical mechanisms among the copper-transporting P-type ATPases. J Biol Chem 1998;273:3765–70.

34. Schilsky ML, Stockert RJ, Sternlieb I. Pleiotropic effect of LEC mutation: a rodent model of Wilson's disease. Am J Physiol 1994;266:G907–13.

35. Walshe JM. Wilson's disease: a review. In: Peisach J, Aisen P, Blumberg WE, editors. The biochemistry of copper. New York: Academic Press; 1966.

36. McCullough AJ, Fleming CR, Thistle JL, et al. Diagnosis of Wilson's disease presenting as fulminant hepatic failure. Gastroenterology 1983;84:161–7.

37. Doering EJ III, Savage RA, Dittmer TE. Hemolysis, coagulation defects, and fulminant hepatic failure as a presentation of Wilson's disease. Am J Dis Child 1979;133:440–1.

38. Adler R, Mahnovski V, Heuser ET, et al. Fulminant hepatitis. A presentation of Wilson's disease. Am J Dis Child 1977;131:870–2.

39. Schilsky ML, Scheinberg IH, Sternlieb I. Liver transplantation for Wilson's disease: indications and outcome. Hepatology 1994;19:583–7.

40. Polio J, Enriquez RE, Chow A, et al. Hepatocellular carcinoma in Wilson's disease. Case report and review of the literature. J Clin Gastroenterol 1989;11:220–4.

41. Slovis TL, Dubois RS, Rodgerson DO, Silverman A. The varied manifestations of Wilson's disease. J Pediatr 1971;78:578–84.

42. Demirkiran M, Jankovic J, Lewis RA, Cox DW. Neurologic presentation of Wilson disease without Kayser-Fleischer rings. Neurology 1996;46:1040–3.

43. Starosta-Rubinstein S, Young AB, Kluin K, et al. Clinical assessment of 31 patients with Wilson's disease. Correlations with structural changes on magnetic resonance imaging. Arch Neurol 1987;44:365–70.

44. Williams FJ, Walshe JM. Wilson's disease. An analysis of the cranial computerized tomographic appearances found in 60 patients and the changes in response to treatment with chelating agents. Brain 1981;104:735–52.

45. Selekler K, Kansu T, Zileli T. Computed tomography in Wilson's disease. Arch Neurol 1981;38:727–8.

46. Harik SI, Post MJ. Computed tomography in Wilson disease. Neurology 1981;31:107–10.

47. Lawler GA, Pennock JM, Steiner RE, et al. Nuclear magnetic resonance (NMR) imaging in Wilson disease. J Comput Assist Tomogr 1983;7:1–8.

48. Aisen AM, Martel W, Gabrielsen TO, et al. Wilson disease of the brain: MR imaging. Radiology 1985;157:137–41.

49. van Wassenaer-van Hall HN, van den Heuvel AG, Algra A, et al.

Wilson disease: findings at MR imaging and CT of the brain with clinical correlation. Radiology 1996;198:531–6.

50. Buchman AL. PET scanning as a diagnostic tool in Wilson's disease. Gastroenterology 1998;114:227–8.

51. Scheinberg IH, Sternlieb I. Wilson disease and idiopathic copper toxicosis. Am J Clin Nutr 1996;63:842S–5S.

52. Goldstein NP, Ewert JC, Randall RV, Gross JB. Psychiatric aspects of Wilson's disease (hepatolenticular degeneration): results of psychometric tests during long-term therapy. Am J Psychiatry 1968;124:1555–61.

53. Kayser B. Ueber einen Fall Von angeborener grunlicher Verfarbung der Cornea. Klin Monatsbl Augenheilkd 1902;40:22–5.

54. Fleisher B. Die periphere braun-grunliche Hornhautverfarbung, Als Symptom einer eigenertigen allgemeiner Krankung. Munch Med Wochenschr 1909;56:1120–3.

55. Wiebers DO, Hollenhorst RW, Goldstein NP. The ophthalmologic manifestations of Wilson's disease. Mayo Clin Proc 1977;52:409–16.

56. Werlin SL, Grand RJ, Perman JA, Watkins JB. Diagnostic dilemmas of Wilson's disease: diagnosis and treatment. Pediatrics 1978;62:47–51.

57. Fleming CR, Dickson ER, Wahner HW, et al. Pigmented corneal rings in non-Wilsonian liver disease. Ann Intern Med 1977;86:285–8.

58. Fleming CR, Dickson ER, Hollenhorst RW, et al. Pigmented corneal rings in a patient with primary biliary cirrhosis. Gastroenterology 1975;69:220–5.

59. Rimola A, Bruguera M, Rodes J. Kayser-Fleischer-like ring in a cryptogenic cirrhosis. Arch Intern Med 1978;138:1857–8.

60. Jones EA, Rabin L, Buckley CH, et al. Progressive intrahepatic cholestasis of infancy and childhood. A clinicopathological study of patient surviving to the age of 18 years. Gastroenterology 1976;71:675–82.

61. Herron BE. Wilson's disease (hepatolenticular degeneration). Ophthalm Semin 1976;1:63–9.

62. Stevens AC, Glaser J. Image of the month. Sunflower cataract. Gastroenterology 1997;112:6.

63. Kuan P. Cardiac Wilson's disease. Chest 1987;91:579–83.

64. Factor SM, Cho S, Sternlieb I, et al. The cardiomyopathy of Wilson's disease. Myocardial alterations in nine cases. Virchows Arch 1982;397:301–11.

65. Leu ML, Strickland GT, Gutman RA. Renal function in Wilson's disease: response to penicillamine therapy. Am J Med Sci 1970;260:381–98.

66. Chu CC, Huang CC, Chu NS. Recurrent hypokalemic muscle weakness as an initial manifestation of Wilson's disease. Nephron 1996;73:477–9.

67. Wiebers DO, Wilson DM, McLeod RA, Goldstein NP. Renal stones in Wilson's disease. Am J Med 1979;67:249–54.

68. Wilson DM, Goldstein NP. Bicarbonate excretion in Wilson's disease (hepatolenticular degeneration). Mayo Clin Proc 1974;49:394–400.

69. Fulop M, Sternlieb I, Scheinberg IH. Defective urinary acidification in Wilson's disease. Ann Intern Med 1968;68:770–7.

70. Gunduz Z, Dusunsel R, Anarat A. Wilson cirrhosis associated with membranoproliferative glomerulonephritis. Nephron 1996;74:497–8.

71. Reynolds ES, Tannen R, Tyler H. The renal lesion in Wilson's disease. Am J Med 1966;40:518–27.

72. Walshe JM. Effect of penicillamine on failure of renal acidification in Wilson's disease. Lancet 1968;i:775–8.

73. Mindelzun R, Elkin M, Scheinberg IH, Sternlieb I. Skeletal changes in Wilson's disease. A radiological study. Radiology 1970;94:127–32.

74. Strickland GT, Leu ML. Wilson's disease. Clinical and laboratory maniestations in 40 patients. Medicine 1975;54:113–37.

75. Golding DN, Walshe JM. Arthropathy of Wilson's disease. Study of clinical and radiological features in 32 patients. Ann Rheum Dis 1977;36:99–111.

76. Paterson CR, Losowsky MS. The bones in chronic liver disease. Scand J Gastroenterol 1967;2:293–300.

77. Menerey KA, Eider W, Brewer GJ, et al. The arthropathy of Wilson's disease: clinical and pathologic features. J Rheumatol 1988;15:331–7.

78. Propst A, Propst T, Feichtinger H, et al. Copper-induced acute rhabdomyolysis in Wilson's disease. Gastroenterology 1995; 108:885–7.

79. Passwell J, Cohen BE, Bassat IB, et al. Hemolysis in Wilson's disease. The role of glucose-6-phosphate dehydrogenase inhibition. Isr J Med Sci 1970;6:549–54.

80. Meyer RJ, Zalusky R. The mechanisms of hemolysis in Wilson's disease: study of a case and review of the literature. Mt Sinai J Med 1977;44:530–8.

81. Rosenfield N, Grand RJ, Watkins JB, et al. Cholelithiasis and Wilson disease. J Pediatr 1978;92:210–3.

82. Ahmed A, Feller ER. Rupture of the spleen as the initial manifestation of Wilson's disease. Am J Gastroenterol 1996; 91:1454–5.

83. Dorney SF, Kamath KR, Procopis PG, Kan AE. Wilson's disease in childhood. A plea for increased awareness. Med J Aust 1986;145:538–41.

84. Sternlieb I. Mitochondrial and fatty changes in hepatocytes of patients with Wilson's disease. Gastroenterology 1968;55: 354–67.

85. Sternlieb I, Quintana N. The peroxisomes of human hepatocytes. Lab Invest 1977;36:140–9.

86. Goldfischer S, Sternlieb I. Changes in the distribution of hepatic copper in relation to the progression of Wilson's disease (hepatolenticular degeneration). Am J Pathol 1968;53:883–901.

87. Epstein O. Liver copper in health and disease. Postgrad Med J 1983;59 Suppl 4:88–94.

88. Shenker S, Dawber N, Schmid R. Bilirubin metabolism in the fetus. J Clin Invest 1964;43:32–9.

89. Nakanuma Y, Karino T, Ohta G. Orcein positive granules in the hepatocytes in chronic intrahepatic cholestasis. Morphological, histochemical and electron x-ray microanalytical examination. Virchows Arch 1979;382:21–30.

90. Sumithran E, Looi LM. Copper-binding protein in liver cells. Hum Pathol 1985;16:677–82.

91. Goldfischer S, Popper H, Sternlieb I. The significance of variations in the distribution of copper in liver disease. Am J Pathol 1980;99:715–30.

92. Edwards CQ, Williams DM, Cartwright GE. Hereditary hypoceruloplasminemia. Clin Genet 1979;15:311–6.

93. Patel AD, Bozdech M. Wilson disease. Arch Ophthalmol 2001; 119:1556–7.

94. Steindl P, Ferenci P, Dienes HP, et al. Wilson's disease in patients presenting with liver disease: a diagnostic challenge. Gastroenterology 1997;113:212–8.

95. Walshe JM. Prophylactic use of penicillamine. N Engl J Med 1968;278:795–6.

96. Brewer GJ. Diagnosis of Wilson's disease: an experience over three decades. Gut 2002;50:136.

97. Gaffney D, Walker JL, O'Donnell JG, et al. DNA-based presymptomatic diagnosis of Wilson disease. J Inherit Metab Dis 1992;15:161–70.

98. Giacchino R, Marazzi MG, Barabino A, et al. Syndromic variability of Wilson's disease in children. Clinical study of 44 cases. Ital J Gastroenterol Hepatol 1997;29:155–61.

99. Sanchez-Albisua I, Garde T, Hierro L, et al. A high index of suspicion: the key to an early diagnosis of Wilson's disease in childhood. J Pediatr Gastroenterol Nutr 1999;28:186–90.
100. Dickson ER, Fleming CR, Ludwig J. Primary biliary cirrhosis. Prog Liver Dis 1979;6:487–502.
101. Walshe JM. Wilson's disease and chronic active hepatitis. Lancet 1977;i:605–6.
102. Martins da Costa C, Baldwin D, Portmann B, et al. Value of urinary copper excretion after penicillamine challenge in the diagnosis of Wilson's disease. Hepatology 1992;15:609–15.
103. Smallwood RA, Williams HA, Rosenoer VM, Sherlock S. Liver-copper levels in liver disease: studies using neutron activation analysis. Lancet 1968;ii:1310–3.
104. Evans J, Newman S, Sherlock S. Liver copper levels in intrahepatic cholestasis of childhood. Gastroenterology 1978;75:875–8.
105. Tanner MS, Portmann B, Mowat AP, et al. Increased hepatic copper concentration in Indian childhood cirrhosis. Lancet 1979;i:1203–5.
106. Maggiore G, De Giacomo C, Sessa F, Burgio GR. Idiopathic hepatic copper toxicosis in a child. J Pediatr Gastroenterol Nutr 1987;6:980–3.
107. Sternlieb I, Scheinberg IH. The role of radiocopper in the diagnosis of Wilson's disease. Gastroenterology 1979;77:138–42.
108. Roberts EA, Schilsky ML; Division of Gastroenterology and Nutrition, Hospital for Sick Children, Toronto, Ontario, Canada. A practice guideline on Wilson disease. Hepatology 2003;37:1475–92.
109. Deiss A, Lee GR, Cartwright GE. Hemolytic anemia in Wilson's disease. Ann Intern Med 1970;73:413–8.
110. Shimizu N. Wilson disease. Nippon Rinsho 2002;60 Suppl 4:433–6.
111. Deiss A, Lynch RE, Lee GR, Cartwright GE. Long-term therapy of Wilson's disease. Ann Intern Med 1971;75:57–65.
112. Saito T. Presenting symptoms and natural history of Wilson disease. Eur J Pediatr 1987;146:261–5.
113. Schilsky ML, Scheinberg IH, Sternlieb I. Prognosis of wilsonian chronic active hepatitis. Gastroenterology 1991;100:762–7.
114. Denny-Brown D, Porter H. The effect of BAL (2,3dimercaptopropanol) on hepatolenticular degeneration. N Engl J Med 1951;245:922–5.
115. Cumings JN. The effect of BAL in hepatolenticular degeneration. Brain 1951;74:10–22.
116. Sternlieb I, Scheinberg IH. Prevention of Wilson's disease in asymptomatic patients. N Engl J Med 1968;278:352–9.
117. Bergstrom RF, Kay DR, Harkcom TM, Wagner JG. Penicillamine kinetics in normal subjects. Clin Pharmacol Ther 1981;30:404–13.
118. Jaffe IA. Antivitamin B6 effect of D-penicillamine. Ann N Y Acad Sci 1969;166:57–60.
119. Porzio S, Iorio R, Vajro P, et al. Penicillamine-related neurologic syndrome in a child affected by Wilson disease with hepatic presentation. Arch Neurol 1997;54:1166–8.
120. Brewer GJ, Yuzbasiyan-Gurkan V. Wilson disease. Medicine 1992;71:139–64.
121. Rothstein JD, Herlong HF. Neurologic manifestations of hepatic disease. Neurol Clin 1989;7:563–78.
122. Grand RJ, Vawter GF. Juvenile Wilson disease: histologic and functional studies during penicillamine therapy. J Pediatr 1975;87:1161–70.
123. Marecek Z, Heyrovsky A, Volek V. The effect of long term treatment with penicillamine on the copper content in the liver in patients with Wilson's disease. Acta Hepatogastroenterol 1975;22:292–6.
124. Stremmel W, Meyerrose KW, Niederau C, et al. Wilson disease: clinical presentation, treatment, and survival. Ann Intern Med 1991;115:720–6.
125. El-Youssef M. Wilson disease. Mayo Clin Proc 2003;78:1126–36.
126. Adams DA. Nephrotic syndrome associated with penicillamine therapy of Wilson's disease. Am J Med 1964;36:330–6.
127. Walshe JM. Penicillamine-induced SLE. Lancet 1981;ii:1416.
128. Sternlieb I, Bennett B, Scheinberg IH. D-Penicillamine induced Goodpasture's syndrome in Wilson's disease. Ann Intern Med 1975;82:673–6.
129. Pass F, Goldfischer S, Sternlieb I, Scheinberg IH. Elastosis perforans serpiginosa during penicillamine therapy for Wilson disease. Arch Dermatol 1973;108:713–5.
130. Sternlieb I, Fisher M, Scheinberg IH. Penicillamine-induced skin lesions. J Rheumatol Suppl 1981;7:149–54.
131. Scheinberg IH, Jaffe ME, Sternlieb I. The use of trientine in preventing the effects of interrupting penicillamine therapy in Wilson's disease. N Engl J Med 1987;317:209–13.
132. Rector WG Jr, Uchida T, Kanel GC, et al. Fulminant hepatic and renal failure complicating Wilson's disease. Liver 1984;4:341–7.
133. Hamlyn AN, Gollan JL, Douglas AP, Sherlock S. Fulminant Wilson's disease with haemolysis and renal failure: copper studies and assessment of dialysis regimens. BMJ 1977;2:660–2.
134. Rakela J, Kurtz SB, McCarthy JT, et al. Fulminant Wilson's disease treated with postdilution hemofiltration and orthotopic liver transplantation. Gastroenterology 1986;90:2004–7.
135. Walshe JM. Pregnancy in Wilson's disease. QJM 1977;46:73–83.
136. Rosa FW. Teratogen update: penicillamine. Teratology 1986;33:127–31.
137. Walshe JM. Copper chelation in patients with Wilson's disease. A comparison of penicillamine and triethylene tetramine dihydrochloride. QJM 1973;42:441–52.
138. Walshe JM. Management of penicillamine nephropathy in Wilson's disease: a new chelating agent. Lancet 1969;ii:1401–2.
139. Walshe JM. Treatment of Wilson's disease with trientine (triethylene tetramine) dihydrochloride. Lancet 1982;i:643–7.
140. Walshe JM. The management of pregnancy in Wilson's disease treated with trientine. QJM 1986;58:81–7.
141. Smith SE, Larson EJ. Zinc toxicity in rats: antagonist effects of the copper and liver. J Biol Chem 1946;163:29–38.
142. Dick AT. Studies on the accumulation and storage of copper in crossbred sheep. Aust J Agricult Res 1954;5:511–4.
143. Brewer GJ, Schoomaker EB, Leichtman DA, et al. The use of pharmacological doses of zinc in the treatment of sickle cell anemia. Prog Clin Biol Res 1977;14:241–58.
144. Hoogenraad TU, Van den Hamer CJ, Koevoet R, Korver EG. Oral zinc in Wilson's disease. Lancet 1978;ii:1262.
145. Hoogenraad TU, Koevoet R, de Ruyter Korver EG. Oral zinc sulphate as long-term treatment in Wilson's disease (hepatolenticular degeneration). Eur Neurol 1979;18:205–11.
146. Hoogenraad TU, Van den Hamer CJ. 3 years of continuous oral zinc therapy in 4 patients with Wilson's disease. Acta Neurol Scand 1983;67:356–64.
147. Sternlieb I. Gastrointestinal copper absorption in man. Gastroenterology 1967;52:1038–41.
148. Cousins RJ. Absorption, transport, and hepatic metabolism of copper and zinc: special reference to metallothionein and ceruloplasmin. Physiol Rev 1985;65:238–309.
149. Menard MP, McCormick CC, Cousins RJ. Regulation of intestinal metallothionein biosynthesis in rats by dietary zinc. J Nutr 1981;111:1353–61.
150. Brewer GJ, Hill GM, Prasad AS, et al. Oral zinc therapy for Wilson's disease. Ann Intern Med 1983;99:314–9.

151. Lipsky MA, Gollan JL. Treatment of Wilson's disease: in D-penicillamine we trust—what about zinc? Hepatology 1987;7:593–5.

152. Brewer GJ, Johnson V, Kaplan J. Treatment of Wilson's disease with zinc: XIV. Studies of the effect of zinc on lymphocyte function. J Lab Clin Med 1997;129:649–52.

153. Chandra RK. Excessive intake of zinc impairs immune responses. JAMA 1984;252:1443–6.

154. Black MR, Medeiros DM, Brunett E, Welke R. Zinc supplements and serum lipids in young adult white males. Am J Clin Nutr 1988;47:970–5.

155. Brewer GJ. Tetrathiomolybdate anticopper therapy for Wilson's disease inhibits angiogenesis, fibrosis and inflammation. J Cell Mol Med 2003;7:11–20.

156. Brewer GJ, Hedera P, Kluin KJ, et al. Treatment of Wilson disease with ammonium tetrathiomolybdate: III. Initial therapy in a total of 55 neurologically affected patients and follow-up with zinc therapy. Arch Neurol 2003;60:379–85.

157. Sokol RJ, Twedt D, McKim JM Jr, et al. Oxidant injury to hepatic mitochondria in patients with Wilson's disease and Bedlington terriers with copper toxicosis. Gastroenterology 1994; 107:1788–98.

158. von Herbay A, de Groot H, Hegi U, et al. Low vitamin E content in plasma of patients with alcoholic liver disease, hemochromatosis and Wilson's disease. J Hepatol 1994;20:41–6.

159. Ogihara H, Ogihara T, Miki M, et al. Plasma copper and antioxidant status in Wilson's disease. Pediatr Res 1995;37:219–26.

160. Sutcliffe RP, Maguire DD, Muiesan P, et al. Liver transplantation for Wilson's disease: long-term results and quality-of-life assessment. Transplantation 2003;75:1003–6.

161. Sokol RJ, Francis PD, Gold SH, et al. Orthotopic liver transplantation for acute fulminant Wilson disease. J Pediatr 1985;107:549–52.

162. Polson RJ, Rolles K, Calne RY, et al. Reversal of severe neurological manifestations of Wilson's disease following orthotopic liver transplantation. QJM 1987;64:685–91.

163. Kiss JE, Berman D, Van Thiel D. Effective removal of copper by plasma exchange in fulminant Wilson's disease. Transfusion 1998;38:327–31.

164. Yoshida Y, Tokusashi Y, Lee GH, Ogawa K. Intrahepatic transplantation of normal hepatocytes prevents Wilson's disease in Long-Evans cinnamon rats. Gastroenterology 1996;111: 1654–60.

CHAPTER 56

PARENTERAL NUTRITION–ASSOCIATED LIVER DISEASE

Julie E. Bines, MD, FRACP

Liver dysfunction is reported to occur in 7.4 to 84% of patients receiving parenteral nutrition (Table 56-1).[1–4] In most patients, this presents as a transient abnormality in serum liver enzyme levels that return to normal with cessation of parenteral nutrition. Cholestasis is the most common manifestation in infants and children, whereas steatosis is more common in adults.[3,4] The incidence of parenteral nutrition–associated liver disease (PNALD) in neonates receiving parenteral nutrition for more than 2 weeks has decreased from 31 to 25% over the past 10 to 15 years, although mortality related to PNALD has not significantly altered.[5] Children with short bowel syndrome requiring long-term parenteral nutrition are at increased risk for the development of complicated PNALD, and liver failure is reported in 3 to 19% of these patients.[6–8]

The etiology of PNALD is unknown. Initially, it was presumed that parenteral nutrition solutions contained a toxic substance or lacked an essential component required for normal hepatic function.[9,10] However, in animal studies, the administration of parenteral nutrition solutions results in hepatic injury but not liver failure.[11,12] The role of sepsis in the early development of PNALD has been the focus of a number of studies.[6,13–15] Current evidence suggests that the developing liver is particularly sensitive to injury resulting from a range of individual factors, such as infection and intestinal stasis, and that PNALD has a multifactorial etiology that reflects the underlying clinical indication for administration of parenteral nutrition (Table 56-2).[6,9,16]

TABLE 56-1 SPECTRUM OF HEPATOBILIARY DYSFUNCTION IN PATIENTS RECEIVING PARENTERAL NUTRITION

Abnormal liver function tests
Cholestasis
Cirrhosis
Liver failure
Hepatocellular carcinoma
Acalculous cholecystitis
Biliary sludge
Cholelithiasis, cholecystitis

RISK FACTORS FOR THE DEVELOPMENT OF PNALD

PATIENT-RELATED FACTORS

Birth Weight and Gestational Age. Low birth weight is a key predisposing factor for the development of PNALD.[9,17] PNALD was reported in 50% of infants with a birth weight < 1,000 g compared with 7% of infants weighing > 1,500 g at birth (Figure 56-1).[17] Gestational age has been identified as an independent factor for the development of PNALD in some but not all studies.[9,17–19] There is a direct relationship between the duration of parenteral nutrition administration and the prevalence of PNALD in premature infants.[17] Almost two-thirds of all infants weighing less than 2,000 g at birth develop cholestasis after 2 weeks of parenteral nutrition therapy.[17]

The increased incidence of PNALD observed in premature infants is thought to reflect the immaturity of hepatic function and the enterohepatic circulation of bile acids.[17,20–22] Normal enterohepatic circulation requires that bile acids are delivered to the intestinal lumen, reabsorbed, and then returned to the hepatocyte for recirculation. However, neonates have reduced hepatic uptake, bile acid synthesis, and the volume of the total bile salt pool.[20–23] Intraluminal concentration and intestinal reabsorption of bile acids are also reduced in premature infants.[24,25] Glutathione is required for normal bile secretion. Glutathione levels are depleted in weanling rats during administration of parenteral nutrition.[26]

Ninety percent of the normal bile acid pool consists of cholic acid, deoxycholic acid, and chenodeoxycholic acid.[27] Bacterial overgrowth of the small intestine induces intraluminal deconjugation of bile salts and increases production of potentially toxic bile acids such as lithocholic acid.[27,28] Patients with PNALD have increased serum and bile concentration of lithocholic acid.[29,30] Lithocholic acid impairs bile flow and, in animals, is associated with hepatic injury similar to the histologic changes observed in patients with PNALD.[30,31] Lithocholic acid is solubilized in the liver by sulfation. Infants have reduced hepatic sulfation and, as a result, may be at increased risk of hepatic injury owing to toxic bile acids.[32]

TABLE 56-2   FACTORS ASSOCIATED WITH DEVELOPMENT OF PARENTERAL NUTRITION–ASSOCIATED LIVER DISEASE

PATIENT FACTORS
Low birth weight
  Prematurity
Male sex
  Preexisting liver disease

DISEASE FACTORS
Gastrointestinal disease status
  Primary disease etiology
  Length of residual small intestine
  Dysmotility in remaining segment of small intestinal
  Residual intestinal disease (ie, Crohn disease)
  Length of time with diverting ileostomy or colostomy
  Small intestinal bacterial overgrowth
Sepsis
  Type of microorganism
  Source of infection

NUTRITIONAL FACTORS
Enteral nutrition
  Lack of enteral feeding
  Undigested nutrients and bacterial overgrowth
  Substrate related
  Proportion of enteral calories
  Formula composition
Parenteral nutrition
  Duration of parenteral nutrition administration
  Overfeeding
  Substrate related
  Glucose excess
  Specific amino acid excess/deficiency
  Lipid excess
  Accumulation of phytosterols
  Specific micronutrient excess/deficiency

Gender. An association between male sex and the development of PNALD was recently reported.[13] The investigators postulate that a genetic and/or hormonal effect on immune function predisposes males to infection and PNALD.

Preexisting Illness. Preexisting liver disease or a parenteral nutrition–independent risk factor for liver disease is associated with an increased incidence of PNALD.[33]

DISEASE-RELATED FACTORS

Gastrointestinal Disease. Massive small bowel resection is an important risk factor for the development of PNALD in children and adults.[6,33] Parenteral nutrition–associated cholestasis is reported in 30 to 60% of children with short bowel syndrome.[7,8] Residual small intestinal length was identified as the only independent predictor of peak serum bilirubin level in infants and children with parenteral nutrition–associated cholestasis.[34] Seventy percent of infants with < 50 cm of residual small intestine and all adults with entire small intestinal resection developed parenteral nutrition–associated cholestasis.[33,35,36] Chronic cholestasis is the precursor of complicated PNALD and liver failure.[33,37,38]

A link between gastroschisis and PNALD has been reported.[6] Infants with gastroschisis frequently develop intestinal obstruction in utero, and, following surgery,

there is a high rate of dilatation and dysmotility of the proximal intestine.

The approach to surgical management of short bowel syndrome in the neonatal period may influence the development of progression of PNALD. Although emphasis is placed on retaining the maximal length of intestine, there is a risk of enhancing exposure of the liver to intestinally derived endotoxin from retained ischemic bowel.[16] Absence of disease in the remaining small intestine is associated with improved survival in patients receiving home parenteral nutrition for intestinal failure.[33] The number of operations and the length of time with a diverting ileostomy or colostomy have been identified as risk factors for the development of PNALD.[34,37] Conversely, the absence of the ileocecal valve did not predispose patients to PNALD.[34]

As part of the adaptive process following resection, the residual small intestine becomes dilated and intestinal transit is slowed in an attempt to compensate for loss of bowel length. Intestinal stasis predisposes the patient to the proliferation of strict anaerobic and facultative anaerobic bacteria within the small intestine. Incomplete absorption of enteral feeds provides a rich source of nutrients for luminal bacteria. Sixty-four percent of infants receiving parenteral nutrition who have bacterial overgrowth later develop sepsis with the same microorganism (such as *Klebsiella*, *Escherichia coli*, enterococci, *Candida*).[38] Bacterial overgrowth is also associated with the deconjugation of bile acids and the production of potentially hepatotoxic bile acids.

Sepsis. Sepsis is associated with cholestasis in infants receiving parenteral nutrition and in infants who have never received parenteral nutrition.[3,14,17,37,39,40] Cholestasis occurs more commonly after gram-negative bacterial infections (in particular *E. coli*).[41] In patients with a normal gastrointestinal tract, cholestasis during an episode of sepsis is usually transient.[16] However, in patients with short bowel syndrome, sepsis has been closely linked to the development of parenteral nutrition–associated cholestasis and progressive PNALD.[6,16,33]

Lipopolysaccharide and peptidoglycan-polysaccharide endotoxins produced by gram-negative and gram-positive

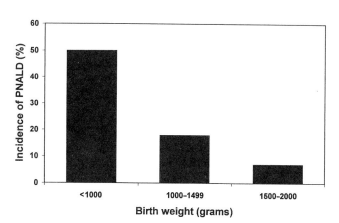

FIGURE 56-1 Relationship between the incidence of parenteral nutrition–associated liver disease (PNALD) and low birth weight. Adapted from Beale EF et al.[17]

bacteria promote the release of tumor necrosis factor (TNF)-α and interleukin-2 from Kupffer cells in rats, resulting in hepatic inflammation and fibrosis.[42] The potential role of TNF in the pathogenesis of PNALD has been a recent focus of interest.[43,44] The administration of antibodies to TNF to rats fed parenteral nutrition results in an improvement in PNALD.[44] Polymyxin B is effective against gram-negative bacteria. In rats with PNALD, polymyxin B blocked endotoxin activity and TNF production and resulted in an improvement in steatosis.[45]

Cholestasis occurred in 26% of 152 neonates who developed an infection while receiving short-term parenteral nutrition.[14] In contrast, cholestasis was not observed in any patient who did not develop an infection.[14] A close association between invasive bacterial or fungal infection and the onset of jaundice in neonates with short bowel syndrome has been observed.[6] Infection occurred before the onset of jaundice in 90% of infants and occurred earlier in cholestatic patients compared with noncholestatic patients (Figure 56-2).[6] Cholestatic patients had more episodes of infection in the first 6 months of life, although the total number of episodes was the same in both groups. Importantly, once established, cholestasis did not resolve with antibiotic therapy and continued to rise, either progressing to hepatic failure or gradually resolving.[6] These data suggest that early exposure to infection is important in the development of PNALD in infants with short bowel syndrome, in whom the liver is immature and susceptible to cholestatic injury and potentially sensitized or stressed by parenteral nutrition administration.[6]

NUTRITION-RELATED FACTORS

Enteral Nutrition. *Lack of Enteral Feeding.* A lack of enteral feeding has been reported as an important risk factor for the development of PNALD in a number of studies.[15,37,46] Enteral feeding induces hormonal stimulation of bile flow, gallbladder emptying, and hepatobiliary development.[47,48] Serum cholecystokinin, glucagon, enteroglucagon, gastrin, motilin, gastric inhibitory polypeptide, and secretin levels differ markedly between infants who are enterally fed and parenterally fed infants.[47,48] In animals with PNALD, treatment with cholecystokinin-octapeptide resulted in decreased periportal inflammation and fibrosis but no improvement in bile flow, bile acid secretion, or hepatocellular injury.[49] Human studies suggest that cholecystokinin (or cholecystokinin-octapeptide) may improve the conjugated hyperbilirubinemia associated with PNALD provided that liver failure is not established.[50,51]

Luminal nutrients aid in the maintenance of gut mucosal barrier function. In the absence of enteral nutrition, the intestine undergoes atrophy, which may increase the risk of bacterial translocation and portal sepsis.[52] In the absence of enteral feeding, intestinal motility and the enterohepatic circulation of bile acids are decreased.[53] These factors may contribute to hepatocyte stress and injury.

Enteral Nutrition Substrates. In neonates with short bowel syndrome, there is a significant relationship between the proportion of calories received enterally at 6 and

12 weeks and subsequent weaning from parenteral nutrition therapy.[6,34] The composition of the enteral feed may also contribute to the development of PNALD. Breast milk or amino acid formulas are associated with greater success at weaning from parenteral nutrition in children with short bowel syndrome.[34,54] Formula composition or excess macronutrients may increase the risk of bacterial overgrowth. Increased bacterial overgrowth and bacterial translocation were observed in mice fed a commercial liquid enteral formula compared with control animals fed chow.[55]

Parenteral Nutrition. *Duration of Parenteral Nutrition Administration.* There is a direct relationship between the duration of parenteral nutrition administration and the prevalence of PNALD in premature infants.[17] In surgical neonates, the incidence of cholestasis is reported to increase from 35% after 2 weeks of parenteral nutrition therapy to 75% after 90 days and 100% after 180 days of therapy.[41] The incidence of cholestasis is higher in infants commencing parenteral nutrition at an earlier age and in infants who have had a delay in the introduction of enteral feeds.[37] Chronic cholestasis developed in 65% of adults receiving parenteral nutrition for a median of 6 months.[33] Complicated PNALD developed in 50% of adults after receiving parenteral nutrition for 6 years.[33]

Overfeeding. Total caloric and carbohydrate overfeeding is associated with metabolic changes and alteration in bile flow and liver function.[56] In normal healthy subjects and in clinically stable patients, excessive glucose intake increases insulin concentration, resulting in a decrease in ketogenesis, an increase in glucose oxidation and lipogenesis, and a decrease in fatty acid oxidation.[57] The insulin-to-glucagon ratio is increased in the portal vein. These metabolic changes have been associated with increased levels of serum hepatic enzymes and hepatic steatosis.[57] Clinically stable adult patients fed a glucose-based parenteral nutrition solution to an average of 177% of predicted energy expenditure developed fatty infiltration and intrahepatic cholestasis on liver biopsy within 5 days of commencing parenteral nutrition.[56] Abnormal serum tests of liver function were detected by 14 days in 83% of

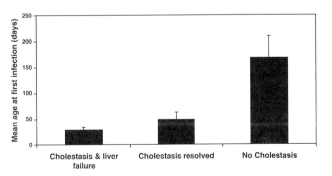

FIGURE 56-2 The effect of age at first infection on the development and severity of parenteral nutrition–associated cholestasis in neonates with intestinal resection. Adapted from Sondheimer JM, Asturias E, Cadnapaphornchai M. Infection and cholestasis in neonates with intestinal resection and long-term parenteral nutrition. J Pediatr Gastroenterol Nutr 1998;27:131–7.

patients, with abnormalities occurring in proportion to the increase in carbohydrate load.[56] Repeat liver biopsy at day 21 showed bile duct proliferation, canalicular bile plugs, centrilobular cholestasis with accumulation of bile pigment within hepatocytes, and periportal inflammation.[56] Similar abnormalities have been observed in stable infants receiving glucose-based parenteral nutrition.[58]

Acute metabolic stress may exacerbate the impact of carbohydrate overfeeding on hepatic morphology and function. With acute stress, lipolysis and fatty acid oxidation increase relative to glucose oxidation owing to the action of counterregulatory hormones, resulting in insulin resistance.[59] In the presence of excessive glucose administration, serum glucose and insulin concentrations are elevated.[59] These factors may increase the risk for hepatic injury. Pyruvate dehydrogenase is a rate-limiting step in glucose oxidation; however, during sepsis, the activity of this enzyme may be inhibited.[60] Increased glucose load during a period of inhibition of this enzyme may further add to the insult to the hepatocyte during stress.[60] Overfeeding during a stress-free period is reported to diminish the hepatic response to subsequent injury, in particular sepsis.[61] In addition, bacterial translocation from the gut is increased during periods of nonprotein overfeeding in animals.[62] Overfeeding during critical illness may further contribute to the hypermetabolic response and hepatocyte injury.

Overfeeding with lipid emulsions containing long-chain triglycerides has been associated with decreased clearance of bacteria from the reticuloendothelial cells. Although this may be clinically significant in terms of posing an increased risk of bacterial sequestration into the lung, these changes have not been associated with characteristic features of hepatocyte injury or disturbances in bile flow.[63]

Substrate-Related Mechanisms. The chemical composition of parenteral nutrition solutions has been implicated in the development of PNALD.[9,28,56] These solutions may include specific nutrient deficiency or excess/toxicity. Contaminants infused with the parenteral nutrition solution may also contribute to hepatic injury.

Glucose infusion has been associated with hepatic steatosis.[9,28] Bile flow is reduced during glucose infusion in animal studies.[64,65] Preterm infants require approximately 4 to 8 mg/kg/min of glucose to suppress hepatic glucose oxidation; however, infusions should not exceed 12.6 mg/kg/min because excess exogenous glucose that is not oxidized may be converted to glycogen or fat in the liver.[66]

Amino acid infusions have been associated with cholestatic liver disease in both human and animal studies.[19,56] A more rapid rise and higher bilirubin concentration were reported in premature infants receiving 3.6 g amino acids/kg/d compared with infants receiving 2.5 g amino acids per kilogram body weight per day.[19]

Individual amino acids have been implicated in the development of parenteral nutrition–associated cholestasis.[9,28] This may reflect immaturity of amino acid metabolism, resulting in an excess of precursor amino acids or a defect in the synthesis of amino acids or proteins. Serum methionine levels are increased in some infants receiving parenteral nutrition owing to a block in the transsulfura-

tion pathway, remethylation of homocystine, or impaired oxidation of sulfur-containing amino acids.[67] Hepatocellular injury observed in neonatal rats receiving infusions of methionine was prevented by supplementation with arginine and glycine.[68,69] Increased cystine has been related to cholestasis and morphologic alterations, including bile duct proliferation, periportal necrosis, portal fibrosis, and inflammation of portal triads.[70] Increased homocystine causes hepatocellular injury and iron deposition in animal studies.[71] Photo-oxidation of amino acid solutions may result in production of hepatotoxic metabolites.[72] The extent of cholestasis was dependent on the dose of tryptophan and degree of light protection in newborn rats receiving an intraperitoneal amino acid solution.[72]

Owing to the immaturity of amino aid metabolic pathways, some amino acids become conditionally essential in premature infants. Evidence supporting the role of a lack of taurine in the development of PNALD remains controversial.[73] Taurine is important in the conjugation of bile acids in neonates, and a lack of taurine results in bile acids becoming predominantly glycine conjugated. These bile acids are potentially hepatotoxic in the infant.[73] The benefit of taurine-supplemented parenteral nutrition to reduce the incidence of PNALD has not been confirmed.[74,75]

Carnitine is absent from most commercially available amino acid solutions. Carnitine is synthesized from methionine and lysine; however, in infants, this conversion may be limited owing to immature metabolic pathways.[76] Carnitine is required for fatty acid oxidation in the mitochondria, and carnitine deficiency is associated with hepatic steatosis. Low serum carnitine levels have been observed in infants and adults receiving parenteral nutrition; however, intravenous carnitine supplementation has not consistently improved serum and hepatic carnitine levels or features of PNALD.[77–79]

High-dose infusion of lipid emulsion is associated with impaired bilirubin excretion in adults.[79] Early lipid emulsions containing cottonseed oil were associated with the development of cholestasis and liver damage.[80] These solutions are no longer in use. Long-chain triglyceride lipid emulsions are a rich source of linoleic acid that promote the synthesis of leukotriene B_4, a proinflammatory cytokine, and may contribute to an increased inflammatory response to cytokines.[81] Commercially available long-chain triglyceride lipid emulsions were not thought to cause PNALD if administered in doses of 1 to 2 g per kilogram body weight per day.[19,56,80] However, in a recent study in intestinal failure patients receiving home parenteral nutrition, cholestasis and complicated PNALD were associated with a dose of lipid emulsion ≥ 1 g/kg/d.[33]

Clayton and colleagues have reported that the long-term use of a long-chain triglyceride lipid emulsion (Intralipid) results in the progressive accumulation of phytosterols.[82] In some patients, plasma concentrations of phytosterols were up to 25% of total plasma sterols and were even higher than in the Intralipid preparation.[82] Phytosterols are present in small amounts as contaminants of the lipid emulsion. Because they are insufficiently metabolized by the liver, it has been suggested that phytosterols accumulate in the macrophages of hepatic sinusoids and disrupt normal macrophage function.[83] Intravenous phytosterol infusion caused reduced bile flow but not liver injury in newborn piglets.[82]

Choline is absent from commericially available parenteral nutrition solutions, and low serum choline levels have been reported in adults on parenteral nutrition therapy.[84] Phosphatidylcholine is required for the synthesis of lipoproteins. Choline deficiency in rats is associated with hepatic steatosis; however, it is not known if this relationship also exists in man.[85]

Selenium and molybdenum deficiency has been reported in association with PNALD; however, the role they may play in the pathogenesis is uncertain.[86] Serum manganese levels are increased in 79% of long-term parenteral nutrition patients.[87] Manganese can be toxic to the brain and the liver. There is a significant correlation between serum manganese levels and asparate transaminase levels; however, it is unclear whether this is a primary or a secondary effect owing to delayed biliary excretion.[88]

CLINICAL MANIFESTATIONS

HEPATIC STEATOSIS
Fatty infiltration of the liver is the most common manifestation of PNALD in adults.[4] It usually occurs secondary to excessive parenteral carbohydrate intake and resolves with a reduction in parenteral carbohydrate intake. Hepatic steatosis clinically presents as hepatomegaly associated with a mild to moderate increase in serum aminotransferase levels.[4]

CHOLESTASIS
Chronic cholestasis is the primary manifestation of PNALD in infants and children and in adults with intestinal failure.[4,6,33] Persistent elevation of serum conjugated bilirubin level is the most consistent biochemical predictive marker of progressive PNALD.[16,89] Cholestasis is usually defined as a serum conjugated bilirubin level of > 1.5 mg/dL or 40% total bilirubin concentration. In infants, serum bilirubin levels may begin to rise as early as 1 to 2 weeks after initiation of parenteral nutrition therapy. Elevation of serum bile acids, either total bile acids or specific cholic acid conjugates, including lithocholate, has been reported to detect early evidence of PNALD prior to elevation of serum conjugated bilirubin level.[90,91] Total serum bile acids and conjugated bilirubin levels correlate with histologic changes in the liver and duration of exposure to parenteral nutrition in animals receiving parenteral nutrition.[92]

CIRRHOSIS AND COMPLICATED PNALD
With progression of disease, the serum alkaline phosphatase gradually increases. However, this may be difficult to interpret in infants and children because the bone isoenzyme may be elevated owing to bone disease or decreased owing to zinc deficiency. γ-Glutamyl transpeptidase or 5′-nucleotidase may also be elevated but does not add significant diagnostic benefit over serum bilirubin concentration alone in infants.[16,89] Levels of serum transaminases

and alkaline phosphatase did not correlate with the severity of liver histology in PNALD.[92]

Reduced serum albumin levels are associated with increased mortality owing to PNALD.[4] However, in patients with excessive protein loss or severe protein-energy malnutrition, hypoalbuminemia and hypoproteinemia may reflect nutritional deficit and not liver dysfunction. Similarly, nutritional vitamin K deficiency may also result in a prolonged prothrombin time.

BILIARY TRACT ABNORMALITIES
Biliary sludge and/or cholelithiasis occur in 12 to 40% of children receiving long-term parenteral nutrition.[93,94] These may occur as a result of gallbladder hypomotility, changes in the composition of bile, or altered enterohepatic circulation of bile acids. The risk of cholelithiasis is increased in children with ileal resection, ileal disease, or hemolytic anemia or in those receiving furosemide therapy. Biliary stones usually consist of both cholesterol and pigment. Acalculous cholecystitis is associated with high morbidity and mortality.[95]

HISTOPATHOLOGY

Characteristic histologic features are observed in liver biopsies of patients receiving parenteral nutrition; however, these changes are not specific or diagnostic.[9,96,97] The histologic changes progress with duration on parenteral nutrition. The initial lesion, steatosis, may occur within the first 2 weeks of parenteral nutrition administration. The degree of steatosis correlates with the amount of energy infused.[98] Cholestasis occurs predominantly in the centrilobular region and involves hepatocytes, canaliculi, and Kupffer cells (Figure 56-3). Serum conjugated bilirubin concentration may not accurately reflect the extent of cholestasis observed on liver

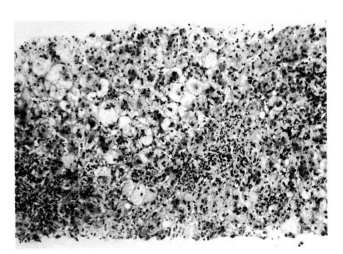

FIGURE 56-3 Light microscopy of a liver biopsy of a patient with parenteral nutrition–associated liver disease showing non-specific periportal inflammation and mild lobular disarray, with ballooning of hepatocytes, microvesicular steatosis, and focal pseudoacinar arrangement of hepatocytes. Cholestasis is present within canaliculi, hepatocytes, Kupffer cells, and occasional bile ducts. Courtesy of Antonio Perez, MD, Department of Pathology, Children's Hospital, Boston.

biopsy. Mild to moderate periportal inflammation is observed. This is usually a lymphocytic infiltrate, although neutrophils and eosinophils may also be present. With disease progression, hepatocytes become ballooned with lipofuscin granules identified in the periportal region. Kupffer cells are hyperplastic and may also have lipofuscin granules. The lobular architecture becomes disordered with periportal fibrosis observed in most patients. Bile duct proliferation and, less commonly, bridging fibrosis may occur. In infants, extramedullary hematopoiesis is common. If parenteral nutrition administration continues, steatosis and extramedullary hematopoiesis tend to improve, but cholestasis, fibrosis, and progression to cirrhosis can occur.[97] If parenteral nutrition treatment is ceased before the development of cirrhosis, many of the histologic features of liver disease improve.[97] The estimated time from onset of long-term parenteral nutrition to the development of moderate fibrosis (< 50% portal spaces involved) in children with short bowel syndrome is reported to be about 40 months.[96] After the development of fibrosis, there tends to be a more rapid progression to cirrhosis (mean duration 14 months). Hepatocellular carcinoma was reported in a 6-month-old infant dependent on long-term parenteral nutrition.[99]

MANAGEMENT

Cessation of parenteral nutrition is the most effective therapy for the management of PNALD.[4,97,99,100] However, this may not be possible in some patients, and treatment is aimed at minimizing the impact of parenteral nutrition on the liver. This includes the identification of individual risk factors and the development of a multidirected strategy to reduce the adverse impact on the liver. Meehan and Georgeson reported the prevention of liver failure in long-term parenteral nutrition patients using taurine, prevention and aggressive treatment of sepsis, strict catheter care, early parenteral nutrition cycling, "appropriate" enteral feeding, and inhibition of bacterial translocation.[101] The timing of the progression of liver disease is critical in planning which patients may require small bowel or combined liver–small bowel transplant.[4,16,89] In the absence of liver transplant, PNALD can be fatal.[6]

ENTERAL FEEDING

For patients who are unable to discontinue parenteral nutrition, small volumes of enteral nutrition have been shown to reduce the progression of PNALD.[9,102] Minimal or "trophic" enteral feeding is associated with gallbladder contraction, increased bile flow, increased gastrin and glucagon secretion, a reduction in intestinal stasis, and bacterial overgrowth.[4,102] Supplementation of enteral feeds with fish oil rich in Ω-3 long-chain polyunsaturated fatty acids has been advocated in an attempt to limit exposure to Ω-6 polyunsaturated long-chain fatty acids.[103] Excess Ω-6 polyunsaturated long-chain fatty acids have been linked to hepatic inflammation. Supplementation of feeds with Ω-3 long-chain polyunsaturated fatty acids and/or antioxidants (vitamins C and E, N-acetylcysteine) has been proposed for the prevention of PNALD.[104]

PREVENTION OF INFECTION

Meticulous catheter care and prompt and aggressive treatment of infection are important in the prevention of PNALD.[4,6,101] The supervision of central line care and nutrition therapy by a multidisciplinary nutrition support team is associated with a significant benefit in terms of the incidence and age at development of liver disease owing to parenteral nutrition.[105] Routine throat swabs have been used to predict bacteremia in infants receiving parenteral nutrition who have abnormal small intestinal flora.[106] Prompt surgical intervention with possible resection is encouraged in patients with suspected intestinal ischemia in an attempt to minimize hepatic exposure to endotoxin in the neonatal period.[16]

BACTERIAL OVERGROWTH

Bacterial overgrowth is a frequent complication of functional and mechanical disorders of the small intestine. The clinical hallmarks of bacterial overgrowth include abdominal distention, vomiting, halitosis, and loose, offensive stool. The diagnosis is established by the quantitative culture of small intestine fluid. A high fasting breath hydrogen level may also be suggestive. Treatment usually involves the use of antibiotics. Metronidazole and the oral nonabsorbable antibiotics gentamicin, kanamycin, neomycin, and polymyxin B have been studied in animals and in limited human trials.[28] Metronidazole prevents PNALD in rats; however, its role in the prevention of human disease is uncertain.[107] In infants receiving parenteral nutrition, intravenous metronidazole was associated with lower serum hepatic transaminase levels but had no effect on the incidence of hyperbilirubinemia.[108] Suppression of bacterial overgrowth may be assisted by avoiding acid-suppressing agents and carbohydrate malabsorption.[16] The use of probiotic microorganisms such as lactobacillus GG and bifidobacteria to suppress the growth of potentially harmful bacteria has been proposed, although the efficacy of probiotics for the prevention of PNALD is yet to be determined.[16,109] Patients with permanent dilatation of a loop of small intestine may benefit from surgical intervention, including resection of a stricture or stenosis or an infolding or tapering procedure.[101]

MODIFICATION TO PARENTERAL NUTRITION SOLUTION AND ADMINISTRATION

Modification of the macronutrient concentrations and balancing their composition in the parenteral nutrition solution may be required in patients with PNALD. Energy should be provided to meet individual needs for growth and activity. Infants receiving energy at 110 kcal/kg/d or greater had a higher incidence of cholestasis compared with infants receiving a lower energy intake.[3] Glucose infusions should be limited to less than or equal to 15 g/kg/d or 12.6 mg/kg/min in premature infants.[66]

Recommendations for intravenous amino acid intakes for premature infants are generally aimed at providing between 2 and 3 g/kg/d.[66] Specialized pediatric amino acid solutions have been developed with the goal of limiting the complications of amino acid imbalance owing to immature metabolism in the premature and young infant. However, the efficacy of these solutions in preventing or minimizing PNALD has not yet been established.[110,111] Supplementation of parenteral nutrition solutions with taurine has not been shown to reduce serum hepatic enzyme, bilirubin, or bile acid concentrations in premature infants receiving short-term parenteral nutrition.[73-75] Intravenous glutamine supplementation has been shown to improve gut barrier integrity, although its role in the prevention and treatment of PNALD in infants and children requires further study.[112]

Current evidence suggests that in infants and children, lipid emulsions should be limited to < 3 g/kg/d and less than 60% of total daily energy.[19,113] Lipid doses of > 1 g/kg/d were associated with cholestasis and complicated liver disease in adults with intestinal failure receiving home parenteral nutrition. However, this has not yet been confirmed in children.[33] In vitro studies suggest that exposure of lipid emulsion to ultraviolet light results in the production of potentially toxic hydroperoxidases.[114] Therefore, lipid emulsions should be protected from ultraviolet light, particularly during phototherapy. The addition of fat-soluble vitamins to the lipid emulsion may provide some protection from this effect.[115]

In the presence of progressive cholestasis and cirrhosis, modification of the micronutrient composition of the parenteral nutrition solution may include the removal of copper and manganese.[37] This underscores the importance of routine monitoring of micronutrient status in patients receiving long-term parenteral nutrition. Cycling of parenteral nutrition for up to 12 hours a day may help in limiting the progression of PNALD in patients requiring long-term parenteral nutrition.[116,117]

PHARMACOLOGIC MANAGEMENT

A number of pharmacologic agents have been proposed for the prevention and treatment of PNALD. Nonsteroidal anti-inflammatory drugs, including acetylsalicylic acid, have been shown to be beneficial in the prevention of PNALD in animal studies.[118,119]

Cholecystokinin-octapetide and the cholecystokinin analog ceruletide stimulate gallbladder contraction and prevent the development of biliary sludge and cholelithiasis in patients receiving parenteral nutrition.[49,50,120,121] The use of these agents in the prevention and treatment of PNALD is encouraging but warrants further clinical investigation.

Ursodeoxycholic acid improves bile flow and reduces serum and liver bilirubin concentrations in piglets with PNALD.[122] In humans, treatment with ursodeoxycholic acid has been associated with a reduction in markers of liver dysfunction, including serum γ-glutamyltransferase, aspartate transaminase, alanine transaminase, alkaline phosphatase, and/or serum bilirubin concentration.[123] A rebound increase in serum γ-glutamyltransferase, alkaline phosphatase, and alanine transaminase concentration was observed in children in whom ursodeoxycholic acid was discontinued in the presence of ongoing parenteral nutrition administration.[123] These patients responded to reintroduction of ursodeoxycholic acid therapy. This raises the question of whether ursodeoxycholic acid reduces serum

markers of liver dysfunction in PNALD but does not influence the progression of liver disease. Enteral administration of tauroursodeoxycholic acid was not found to be effective in the prevention of PNALD in neonates.[124]

Other pharmacologic agents, including antibiotics, cholestyramine, rifampin, and phenobarbital, have been studied in the context of management of PNALD.[28] Surgical approaches aimed at improving bile flow, including biliary irrigation, have also been associated with improvement in PNALD in some patients.[125,126]

LIVER–SMALL BOWEL TRANSPLANT

Most children requiring long-term parenteral nutrition have underlying intestinal disease, either short bowel syndrome or severe intestinal dysfunction. If transition to full enteral nutrition cannot be achieved and parenteral nutrition cannot be discontinued, over time, PNALD may progress to overt liver failure.[4] Small bowel transplant prior to progression to severe liver disease and combined liver–small bowel transplant are therapeutic options for the management of both primary gut disease and the complication of parenteral nutrition–associated liver failure. Because the morbidity and mortality associated with small bowel transplant are probably more favorable compared with combined liver–small bowel transplant, it is important that referral to a transplant center is made before the liver disease becomes irreversible.[16,89,127,128] Elevation of the total serum bilirubin level of > 3 mg/dL for over 3 months in a parenteral nutrition–dependent infant and/or early clinical features of progressive liver disease, including mild splenomegaly, dilatation of abdominal wall veins, and a deteriorating platelet count, are indications for referral.[16,89] Serum hepatic or biliary enzyme levels provide no additional predictive benefit in patients with PNALD.[16] Hypoalbuminemia, coagulopathy, and hypoglycemia during cycling of parenteral nutrition are markers of hepatic synthetic dysfunction. These are considered late features of liver disease and are associated with a poor prognosis.[16] In the setting of progressive PNALD and portal hypertension, severe bleeding may occur from stomas in patients with short bowel syndrome.

CONCLUSION

Infants and children receiving parenteral nutrition are at risk of developing PNALD. No single factor has been shown to be responsible for the development of this potentially fatal complication. Current evidence suggests that the developing liver is particularly sensitive to injury resulting from a range of individual factors, such as infection and intestinal stasis, and that PNALD has a multifactorial etiology that, in part, is determined by the underlying clinical indication for parenteral nutrition administration. Discontinuation of parenteral nutrition is the most effective treatment, but this cannot be achieved in some patients. Treatment strategies that include the identification of risk factors and the development of a multidirected approach to the prevention and treatment of PNALD are required. Although new pharmacologic and surgical approaches have been reported, the risks and benefits of these therapies still need to be assessed in randomized prospective controlled trials. Small bowel or combined liver–small bowel transplant provides a therapeutic option for long-term parenteral nutrition–dependent patients with PNALD in the presence of short bowel syndrome or severe intestinal dysfunction.

REFERENCES

1. Bell RL, Ferry GD, Smith EO, et al. Total parenteral nutrition-related cholestasis in infants. JPEN J Parenter Enteral Nutr 1985;10:356–9.

2. Cohen C, Olsen MN. Pediatric total parenteral nutrition. Liver histology. Arch Pathol Lab Med 1981;105:152.

3. Kubota A, Okada A, Nezu R, et al. Hyperbilirubinemia in neonates associated with total parenteral nutrition. JPEN J Parenter Enteral Nutr 1988:602–6.

4. Kelly DA: Liver complications of pediatric parenteral nutrition—epidemiology. Nutrition 1998;14:153–7.

5. Kubota A, Yonekura T, Hoki M, et al. Total parenteral nutrition-associated intrahepatic cholestasis in infants: 25 years' experience. J Pediatr Surg 2000;35:1049–51.

6. Sondeheimer JM, Asturias E, Cadnapaphornchai M. Infection and cholestasis in neonates with intestinal resection and longterm parenteral nutrition. J Pediatr Gastroenterol Nutr 1998;27:131–7.

7. Merritt RJ. Cholestasis associated with total parenteral nutrition. J Pediatr Gastroenterol Nutr 1986;5:9–22.

8. Caniano DA, Starr J, Ginn-Pease ME. Extensive short-bowel syndrome in neonates: outcome in the 1980's. Surgery 1998; 105:119–24.

9. Galea MH, Holloday H, Carachi R, Kapila L. Short-bowel syndrome: a collective review. J Pediatr Surg 1992;27:592–6.

10. Sax HC, Bower RH. Hepatic complications of total parenteral nutrition. JPEN J Parenter Enteral Nutr 1988;12:615–8.

11. Bucuvalas JC, Goodrich AL, Blitzer BL, Suchy FJ. Amino acids are potent inhibitors of bile acid uptake by liver plasma membrane vesicles isolated from suckling rats. Pediatr Res 1985;19:1298–304.

12. Belli DC, Fournier LA, Lepage G, et al. Total parenteral nutrition-associated cholestasis in rats. Comparison of different amino acid mixtures. JPEN J Parenter Enteral Nutr 1986;11:67–73.

13. Albers MJIJ, deGast-Bakker D-AH, van Dam NAM, et al. Male sex predisposes the newborn surgical patients to parenteral nutrition-associated cholestasis and to sepsis. Arch Surg 2002;137:789–93.

14. Wolf A, Pohlandt F. Bacterial infection: the main cause of acute cholestasis in newborn infants receiving short-term parenteral nutrition. J Pediatr Gastroenterol Nutr 1989;8:297–303.

15. Takahashi M, Sawaguchi S, Ohkawa H, et al. Hepatobiliary dysfunction in neonates associated with total parenteral nutrition. Acta Neonat Jpn 1983;19:333–41.

16. Kaufman SS. Prevention of parenteral nutrition-associated liver disease in children. Paediatr Transplant 2002;6:37–42.

17. Beale EF, Nelson RM, Bucciarelli RL, et al. Intrahepatic cholestasis associated with parenteral nutrition in premature infants. Pediatrics 1979;64:342–7.

18. Pereira GR, Sherman MS, DiGiacomo J, et al. Hyperalimentation-induced cholestasis increased frequency and severity in premature infants. Am J Dis Child 1981;135:842–5.

19. Vileisis R, Inwood RJ, Hunt CE. Prospective controlled study of parenteral nutrition associated cholestatic jaundice: effect of protein intake. J Pediatr 1980;96:893–7.

20. Balistreri WF, Heubi JE, Suchy FJ. Immaturity of the enterohepatic circulation in early life: factors predisposing to physiologic maldigestion and cholestasis. J Pediatr Gastroenterol Nutr 1983;2:346–54.

21. Back P, Walter K. Developmental pattern of bile acid metabolism as revealed by bile acid analysis of meconium. Gastroenterology 1980;78:671–6.

22. Lester R, St. Pyrek J, Little JM, Adcock EW. Diversity of bile acids in the fetus and newborn infants. J Pediatr Gastroenterol Nutr 1983;2:355–64.

23. Little JM, Richey JE, van Thiel DH, Lester R. Taurocholate pool size and distribution in the fetal rat. J Clin Invest 1979; 63:1042–9.

24. Watkins JB, Szczepanik P, Gould JB, et al. Bile salt metabolism in human premature infants: preliminary observations of pool size and synthesis rate following prenatal administration of dexamethasone and phenobarbital. Gastroenterology 1975;69:706–13.

25. de Belle RC, Vauspshas V, Vitullo BB, et al. Intestinal absorption of bile salts: immature development in the neonate. J Pediatr 1979;94:472–6.

26. Heyman MD, Tseng HC, Thaler MM. Total parenteral nutrition (TPN) decreases hepatic glutathione concentrations in weanling rats. Hepatology 1984;416:9.

27. Hofmann AF. Defective biliary secretion during total parenteral nutrition: probable mechanisms and possible solutions. J Pediatr Gastroenterol Nutr 1995;20:376–90.

28. Btaiche IF, Khalidi N. Parenteral nutrition-associated liver complications in children. Pharmacotherapy 2002;22:188–21.

29. Farrell MK, Balistreri WF, Suchy FJ. Serum sulfated lithocholate as an indicator of cholestasis during parenteral nutrition in infants and children. JPEN J Parenter Enteral Nutr 1982; 6:30–3.

30. Fouin-Fortunet H, Quernec LL, Erlinger S, et al. Hepatic alterations during total parenteral nutrition in patients with inflammatory bowel disease: a possible consequence of lithocholate toxicity. Gastroenterology 1982;82:932–7.

31. Hodes JE, Grosseld JL, Webert R, et al. Hepatic failure in infants on total parenteral nutrition (TPN) clinical and histopathologic observations. J Pediatr Surg 1982;17:463.

32. Watkins JB. Placental transport bile acid conjugation and sulphation in the fetus. J Pediatr Gastroenterol Nutr 1983;2:365.

33. Cavicchi M, Beau P, Pascal C, et al. Prevalence of liver disease and contributing factors in patients receiving home parenteral nutrition for permanent intestinal failure. Ann Intern Med 2000;132:525–32.

34. Andorsky DJ, Lund DP, Lillehei CW, et al. Nutritional and other post-operative management of neonates with short bowel syndrome correlates with clinical outcome. J Pediatr 2001; 139:27–33.

35. Ito Y, Shils ME. Liver dysfunction associated with long-term total parenteral nutrition in patients with massive bowel resection. JPEN J Parenter Enteral Nutr 1991;15:271–6.

36. Teitelbaum DH, Drongowski R, Spivak D. Rapid development of hyperbilirubinemia in infants with short bowel syndrome as a correlate to mortality: possible indication for early small bowel transplantation. Transplant Proc 1996;28:2699–700.

37. Drongowski RA, Coran AG. An analysis of factors contributing to the development of total parenteral nutrition induced cholestasis. JPEN J Parenter Enteral Nutr 1989;13:586–9.

38. Pierro A, van Saene HKF, Donnell SC, et al. Microbial translocation in neonates and infants receiving long-term parenteral nutrition. Arch Surg 1996;131:176–9.

39. Beath SV, Davies P, Papdopoulou A, et al. Parenteral nutrition-

related cholestasis in post-surgical neonates: multivariate analysis of risk factors. J Pediatr Surg 1996;31:604–6.

40. Hamilton JR, Sass-Korstak A. Jaundice associated with severe bacterial infection in young infants. J Pediatr 1963;63:121–32.

41. Ginn-Pease ME, Pantalos D, King DR. TPN-associated hyperbilirubinemia: a common problem in newborn surgical patients. J Pediatr Surg 1985;20:436–9.

42. Lichtman SN, Wang J, Schwab JH, Lemaster JJ. Comparison of peptidoglycan-polysaccharide and lipipolysaccharide stimulation of Kupffer cells to produce tumor necrosis factor and interleukin-1. Hepatology 1994;19:1013–22.

43. Jones A, Selby PJ, Viner C, et al. Tumor necrosis factor, cholestatic jaundice and chronic liver disease. Gut 1990;31:938–9.

44. Pappo I, Bercovier H, Berry E, et al. Antitumor necrosis factor antibodies reduce steatosis during total parenteral nutrition and bowel rest in the rat. JPEN J Parenter Enteral Nutr 1995; 19:80–2.

45. Pappo I, Bercovier H, Berry EM, et al. Polymyxin B reduces total parenteral nutrition-associated hepatic steatosis by its antibacterial activity and by blocking deleterious effects of lipopolysaccharide. JPEN J Parenter Enteral Nutr 1992; 16:529–32.

46. Rager R, Finegold MG. Cholestasis in immature infants: is parenteral nutrition responsible? J Pediatr 1975;86:264–5.

47. Aynsley-Green A. Plasma hormone concentrations during enteral and parenteral nutrition in the human newborn. J Pediatr Gastroenterol Nutr 1983;2 Suppl 1:108–12.

48. Lucas A, Bloom SR, Aynsley-Green A. Metabolic and endocrine consequences of depriving preterm infants of enteral nutrition. Acta Paediatr Scand 1983;72:245–9.

49. Curran TJ, Uzoaru I, Das JB, et al. The effect of cholecystokinin-octa-peptide on the hepatobiliary dysfunction caused by total parenteral nutrition. J Pediatr Surg 1995;30:242–7.

50. Teitelbaum DH, Han-Markey T, Schumacher RE. Treatment of parenteral nutrition associated cholestasis with cholecystokinin-octa-peptide. J Pediatr Surg 1995;30:1082–5.

51. Rintala RJ, Lindahl H, Pohjavuori M. Total parenteral nutrition associated cholestasis in surgical neonates may be reversed by intravenous cholecystokinin: a preliminary report. J Pediatr Surg 1995;30:827–30.

52. Johnson LR, Copeland EM, Dudrick SJ, et al. Structural and hormonal alterations in the gastrointestinal tract of parenterally fed rats. Gastroenterology 1975;68:1177–83.

53. Levinson S, Bhasker M, Gibson TR, et al. Comparison of intra-luminal and intravenous mediators of colonic response to eating. Dig Dis Sci 1985;30:33–9.

54. Bines JE, Francis D, Hill D. Reducing parenteral nutrition requirement in children with short bowel syndrome: impact of an amino acid based complete infant formula. J Pediatr Gastroenterol Nutr 1998;26:123–8.

55. Haskel Y, Udassin R, Freud HR, et al. Liquid enteral diets induce bacterial translocation by increasing cecal flora without changing intestinal motility. JPEN J Parenter Enteral Nutr 2001;25:60–4.

56. Lowry SF, Brennan MF. Abnormal liver function during parenteral nutrition: relation to infusion excess. J Surg Res 1979;26:300–7.

57. Nussbaum MS, Fischer JE. Pathogenesis of hepatic steatosis during total parenteral nutrition. In: Nyhus LM, editor. Surgery annual. Norwalk (CT): Appleton and Lange; 1991. p. 1–11.

58. Das JB, Cosentino CM, Levy MF. Early hepatobiliary dysfunction during total parenteral nutrition: an experimental study. J Pediatr Surg 1993;28:14–8.

59. Butsztein S, Elwyn DH, Askanazi J. Energy metabolism and indirect calorimetry in critically ill and injured patients. Acute Care 1988;14:91–110.

60. Vary TC, Siegel JH, Nakatani T, et al. Effects of sepsis on activity of pyruvate dehydrogenase complex in skeletal muscle and liver. Am J Physiol 1986;250:E634–40.

61. Yamazaki K, Maiz A, Moldawer LL, et al. Complications associated with overfeeding of infected animals. J Surg Res 1988; 40:152–8.

62. Yamanouchi T, Suita S, Masumoto K. Non-protein energy overloading induces bacterial translocation during total parenteral nutrition in newborn rabbits. Nutrition 1988;14:443–7.

63. Sobrado J, Moldawer LL, Pomposelli JJ, et al. Lipid emulsions and reticuloendothelial system function in healthy and burned pigs. Am J Clin Nutr 1985;42:855–63.

64. Zahari I, Shaffer EA, Gall DG. Total parenteral nutrition-associated cholestasis: acute studies in infant and adult rabbits. J Pediatr Gastroenterol Nutr 1985;4:622–7.

65. Mashima Y. Effect of caloric overload on puppy livers during parenteral nutrition. JPEN J Parenter Enteral Nutr 1979;3: 139–45.

66. Kien CL. Carbohydrates. In: Tsang RC, Lucas A, Uauy R, Zlotkin S, editors. Nutritional needs of the preterm infant: scientific basis and practical guidelines. New York: Williams and Wilkins; 1993. p. 47–63.

67. Zarif MA, Pildes RS, Szanto PM, Vidiyasagaro D. Cholestasis associated with administration of L-amino acids and dextrose solutions. Biol Neonate 1976;29:66–76.

68. Stekol JA, Szaran J. Pathological effects of excessive methionine in the diet of growing rats. J Nutr 1962;77:81–90.

69. Klavins JV, Peacocke IL. Pathology of amino acid excess III: effects of administration of excessive amounts of sulfur-containing amino acids: methionine with equimolar amounts of glycine and arginine. Br J Exp Pathol 1964;45: 533–47.

70. Klavins JV. Pathology of amino acid excess: effects of administration of excessive amounts of sulfur containing amino acids: L-cystine. Br J Exp Pathol 1963;44:516–9.

71. Klavins JV. Pathology of amino acid excess: effect of administration of excessive amounts of sulfur containing amino acids: homocystine. Br J Exp Pathol 1963;44:507–15.

72. Merritt RJ, Sinatra F, Henton D, Neustein H. Cholestatic effect of intraperitoneal administration of tryptophan to suckling rat pups. Pediatr Res 1984;18:904–7.

73. Howard D, Thompson DF. Taurine: an essential amino acid to prevent cholestasis in neonates? Ann Pharmacother 1992; 26:1390–2.

74. Heird WC, Dell RB, Helms RA, et al. Amino acid mixture designed to maintain normal plasma amino acid patterns in infants and children requiring parenteral nutrition. Pediatrics 1987;80:401–8.

75. Cooke RJ, Whittington PF, Kelts D. Effect of taurine supplementation on hepatic function during short-term parenteral nutrition in the premature infant. J Pediatr Gastroenterol Nutr 1984;3:234–8.

76. Schiff D, Chan G, Secombe D, Hohn P. Plasma carnitine levels during intravenous feeding of the neonate. J Pediatr 1979;95: 1043–6.

77. Bowyer BA, Miles JM, Haymond MW, Fleming CR. L-Carnitine therapy in home parenteral nutrition patients with abnormal liver tests and low carnitine concentration. Gastroenterology 1988;94:434–8.

78. Bonner CM, Mauer EC, Hay WW, et al. Effect of L-carnitine supplementation on fat metabolism and nutrition in premature infants. J Pediatr 1995;126:287–92.

79. Salvian AJ, Allardyce DB. Impaired bilirubin secretion during total parenteral nutrition. Surg Res 1981;28:547–55.

80. Hakansson I. Experience in long-term studies on nine intravenous fat emulsions for intravenous nutrition in dogs. Nutr Diet 1968;10:54–76.

81. Jeppesen PB, Hoy C-E, Mortensen B. Differences in essential fatty acid requirements by enteral and parenteral routes of administration in patients with fat malabsorption. Am J Clin Nutr 1999;70:78–84.

82. Clayton PT, Whitfield P, Iyer K. The role of phytosterols in the pathogenesis of liver complications of pediatric parenteral nutrition. Nutrition 1998;14:158–64.

83. Cukier C, Waitzberg DL, Logullo AF, et al. Lipid and lipid-free total parenteral nutrition: differential effects on macrophage phagocytosis in rats. Nutrition 1999;15:885–9.

84. Sheard NF, Tayek JA, Bistrian BR, et al. Plasma choline concentrations in humans fed parenterally. Am J Clin Nutr 1986; 43:219–24.

85. Zeisael SH. Dietary choline: biochemistry, physiology and pharmacology. Annu Rev Nutr 1981;1:95–121.

86. Berger HM, Den Ouden AL, Calme JJ. Pathogenesis of liver damage during parenteral nutrition: is lipofuscin a clue? Arch Dis Child 1985;60:774–6.

87. Hambridge KM, Sokol RJ, Fidanza SJ, Goodall MA. Plasma manganese concentrations in infants and children receiving parenteral nutrition. JPEN J Parenter Enteral Nutr 1989;13: 68–71.

88. Fell JM, Reynolds AP, Meadows N, et al. Manganese toxicity in children receiving long-term parenteral nutrition. Lancet 1996;347:1218–21.

89. Bueno J, Ohwada S, Kocoshis S, et al. Factors impacting the survival of children with intestinal failure referred for intestinal transplantation. J Pediatr Surg 1999;34:27–33.

90. Farrell MK, Gilster S, Balistreri WF. Serum bile acids: an early indicator of parenteral nutrition associated liver disease. Gastroenterology 1984;86:1074.

91. Kaplowitz N, Kok E, Javitt NB. Post prandial serum bile acid for the detection of hepatobiliary disease. JAMA 1973;225:292–3.

92. Demircan M, Ergun O, Avanoglu S, et al. Determination of serum bile acids routinely may prevent delay in diagnosis of total parenteral nutrition induced cholestasis. J Pediatr Surg 1999;34:565–7.

93. Roslyn JJ, Berqyuist WE, Pitt HA, et al. Increased risk of gallstones in children receiving total parenteral nutrition. Pediatrics 1983;71:784–9.

94. King DR, Ginn-Pease ME, Lloyd TV, et al. Parenteral nutrition with associated cholelithiasis: another iatrogenic disease of infants and children. J Pediatr Surg 1987;22:593–6.

95. Petersen SR, Sheldon GF. Acute acalculous cholecystitis: a complication of hyperalimentation. Am J Surg 1979;138:814–7.

96. Colomb V, Jobert A, Lacaille F, et al. Parenteral nutrition-associated liver disease in children: natural history and prognosis. J Pediatr Gastroenterol Nutr 1999;28:577.

97. Dahms BB, Halpin TC. Serial liver biopsies in parenteral nutrition-associated cholestasis of early infancy. Gastroenterology. 1981;81:136–44.

98. Sax HC, Talamini MA, Brackett K, Fischer JE. Hepatic steatosis in total parenteral nutrition: failure of fatty infiltration to correlate with abnormal serum hepatic enzyme levels. Surgery 1984;100:697–704.

99. Patterson K, Kapur SP, Chandra RS. Hepatocellular carcinoma in a noncirrhotic infant after prolonged parenteral nutrition. J Pediatr 1985;106:797–800.

100. Moss RL, Amii LA. New approaches to understanding the etiology and treatment of total nutrition associated cholestasis. Semin Pediatr Surg 1999;8:140–7.

101. Meehan JJ, Georgeson KC. Prevention of liver failure in parenteral nutrition-dependent children with short bowel syndrome. J Pediatr Surg 1997;32:473–5.

102. Berseth CL. Minimal enteral feedings. Clin Perinatol 1995; 22:195–205.

103. Chan S, McCowen KC, Bistrian BR, et al. Incidence, prognosis and etiology of end stage liver disease in patients receiving home total parenteral nutrition. Surgery 1999;126:28–34.

104. Will Y, Fischer KA, Horton RA, et al. Gamma-glutamyl transpeptidase-deficient knock out mice as a model to study the relationship between glutathione status, mitochondrial function, and cellular function. Hepatology 2000;32:740–9.

105. Beath SV, Booth IW, Murphy MS, et al. Nutritional care in candidates for small bowel transplantation. Arch Dis Child 1995;73:348.

106. Pierro A, van Saene HK, Jones MO, et al. Clinical impact of abnormal gut flora in infants receiving parenteral nutrition. Ann Surg 1998;227:547–52.

107. Lichtman SN, Keku J, Schwab JH, Sartor RB. Hepatic injury associated with small bowel bacterial overgrowth in rats is prevented by metronidazole and tetracycline. Gastroenterology 1991;100:513–9.

108. Kubota A, Okada A, Imura K, et al. The effect of metronidazole on total parenteral nutrition-associated liver dysfunction in neonates. J Pediatr Surg 1990;6:618–21.

109. Vanderhoof JA, Young RJ, Murray N, Kaufman SS. Treatment strategies for small bowel bacterial overgrowth in short bowel syndrome. J Pediatr Gastroenterol Nutr 1998;27:155–60.

110. Forchielli ML, Gura KM, Sandler R, Lo C. Aminosyn PF or Trophamine: which provide more protection from cholestasis associated with total parenteral nutrition? J Pediatr Gastroenterol Nutr 1995;21:374–82.

111. Coran AG, Drongowski RA. Studies on the toxicity and efficacy of a new amino acid solution in pediatric parenteral nutrition. JPEN J Parenter Enteral Nutr 1987;11:368–77.

112. Souba WW, Klimberg VS, Plumley DA, et al. The role of glutamine in maintaining a healthy gut and supporting the metabolic response to injury and infection. J Surg Res 1990;48: 383–91.

113. Cohen IT, Dahms B, Hays DM. Peripheral total parenteral nutrition employing a lipid emulsion (Intralipid): complications encountered in pediatric patients. J Pediatr Surg 1977;12: 837–45.

114. Neuzil J, Darlow B, Ender TE, et al. Oxidation of parenteral lipid emulsion by ambient and phototherapy lights: potential toxicity of routine parenteral feeding. J Pediatr 1995;126:785–90.

115. Silvers KM, Darlow BA, Winterbourn CC. Lipid peroxide and hydrogen peroxide formation in parenteral nutrition solutions containing multivitamins. JPEN J Parenter Enteral Nutr 2001;25:14–7.

116. Hwang T-L, Lue M-C, Chen L-L. Early use of cyclic TPN prevents further deterioration of liver functions for the TPN patients with impaired liver function. Hepatogastroenterology 2000;47:1347–50.

117. Maini B, Blackburn GL, Bistrian BR, et al. Cyclic hyperalimentation an optimal technique for the presentation of visceral protein. J Surg Res 1976;20:515–25.

118. Nussinovitch M, Zahari I, Marcus H, et al. The choleretic effect of non-steroidal anti-inflammatory drugs in total parenteral nutrition associated cholestasis. Isr J Med Sci 1996;32:1262–4.

119. Demircan M, Ugaralp S, Mutus M, et al. The effects of acetylsalicylic acid, interferon-alpha, and vitamin E in prevention

of parenteral nutrition-associated cholestasis: an experimental study. J Pediatr Gastroenterol Nutr 1999;28:291–5.

120. Sitzmann JV, Pitt HA, Steinborn PA, et al. Cholecystokinin prevents parenteral nutrition induced biliary sludge in humans. Surg Gynecol Obstet 1990;170:25–31.

121. Schwartz JB, Merritt RJ, Rosenthal P, et al. Ceruletide to treat neonatal cholestasis. Lancet 1988;i:1219–20.

122. Duerksen DR, van Averde JE, Gramlich L, et al. Intravenous ursodeoxycholic acid reduces cholestasis in parenterally fed newborn piglets. Gastroenterology 1996;11:1111–7.

123. Spagnuolo MI, Iorio R, Vegnente A, Guarino F. Ursodeoxycholic acid for the treatment of cholestasis in children on long-term parenteral nutrition: a pilot study. Gastroenterology 1996; 111:716–9.

124. Heubi JE, Wiechmann DA, Creutzinger V, et al. Tauroursodeoxy-cholic acid (TUDCA) in the prevention of total parenteral nutrition-associated liver disease. J Pediatr 2002;141:237–42.

125. Rintala R, Lindahl H, Pohjavuori M, et al. Surgical treatment of intractable cholestasis associated with total parenteral nutrition in premature infants. J Pediatr Surg 1993;28:716–9.

126. Cooper A, Ross AJ III, O'Neill JA Jr, et al. Resolution of intractable cholestasis associated with total parenteral nutrition following biliary irrigation. J Pediatr Surg 1985;20:772–4.

127. Kaufman S, Atkinson JB, Bianchi A, et al. Indications for pediatric intestinal transplantation: a position paper of the American Society of Transplanation. Pediatr Transplant 2001;5:80–7.

128. Goulet O, Lacaille F, Jan D, Ricour C. Intestinal transplantation:indications, results and strategy. Curr Opin Clin Nutr Metab Care 2000;3:329–38.

CHAPTER 57

SYSTEMIC CONDITIONS AFFECTING THE LIVER

Mounif El-Youssef, MD

Deborah K. Freese, MD

An understanding of the effects of systemic diseases on hepatobiliary function in infancy and childhood requires an understanding of liver physiology and, in particular, how that physiology changes with increasing maturity. This is described in detail in Chapter 5, "Liver Function and Dysfunction." It is particularly important to recognize that many of the cells that comprise the liver and biliary tract respond to potentially toxic insults differently at different ages and that the process of cell repair and wound healing varies with the insult to the liver and the age of the patient. The liver may be injured as a passive bystander or may actively exacerbate the systemic conditions described below.[1–19] The following discussion is organized by organ system or major categories of systemic disease and is meant to provide a clinical overview of hepatobiliary function during system illnesses.

ACUTE CARDIAC DISEASE

The pediatric hepatologist may be called on to evaluate the infant and child with cardiac disease in several situations. These include (1) the patient with acute liver injury from cardiogenic circulatory compromise, (2) the patient with chronic congestive heart failure or outflow obstruction, and (3) the patient with complex congenital anomalies in which the liver and heart are affected by associated malformations.[20–22]

Acute circulatory failure results in a typical pattern of liver injury that is a result of the unique dual blood supply to the liver and of the heterogeneity of the liver acinus. Two-thirds of the blood supply to the liver is from the portal circulation, and the remainder is from the hepatic artery. The oxygen-rich blood perfuses the liver acinus, creating a gradient of oxygenation, with the maximal concentration of oxygen delivered to the periportal zone 1 of Rappaport and the lowest concentration of oxygen to the pericentral zone 3. Blood flow to the liver is regulated locally by the concentration of adenosine, a vasodilator that is produced by endothelial cells. With poor perfusion, the local concentration of adenosine increases, and vasodilation occurs. This results in increased portal flow that compensates partially for the reduced arterial flow. Outflow resistance may

also affect oxygenation of the liver, as in acute cardiogenic shock. Thus, cells in the pericentral zone of the liver are most susceptible to perfusion-related injury.

CLINICAL PRESENTATION

The infant or child with ischemic hepatic injury is usually critically ill. Cardiac symptoms may predominate, but, occasionally, the cardiac origin may not be recognized, especially when hepatic symptoms predominate and initial attention focuses on liver dysfunction.[19] This is particularly true in cases of noncyanotic heart disease. The liver is uniformly enlarged, and the edge is round and smooth, reflecting generalized engorgement of the organ.[23,24] Jaundice, which is usually a later manifestation of liver disease, may not be apparent in the first few days after the acute event.

Concentrations of hepatic transaminases are increased up to 200 times the upper limit of the reference range. Lactic dehydrogenase is also increased and, if fractionated, is mostly of hepatic origin (Table 57-1). This increase in lactic dehydrogenase, seldom seen in viral hepatitis, may be used to distinguish ischemic hepatic injury from acute viral hepatitis.[25] The dramatic increase in aspartate aminotransferase and alanine aminotransferase reflects the predominant injury to the central zone of the liver.[26–28] Not uncommon is an association with renal hypoperfusion and increases in serum urea nitrogen and serum creatinine. Acute renal tubular necrosis may also occur. The peak concentration of the transaminases occurs in the first 3 days after the insult. The concentrations return to normal in 5 to 7 days except in patients with ongoing liver ischemia. Coagulation is significantly altered, and, typically, the prolongation of the prothrombin time, as indicated by the international normalized ratio, is not corrected by the

TABLE 57-1   THE LIVER IN HEART DISEASE

Hepatomegaly with a smooth rounded edge of the liver
Jaundice and hyperbilirubinemia
Splenomegaly with chronic cardiac insufficiency
Differential elevation of liver-derived enzymes AST > ALT
Coagulopathy unresponsive to vitamin K

ALT = alanine aminotransferase; AST = aspartate aminotransferase.

administration of vitamin K. Jaundice and the increase in bilirubin occur later, usually by the third to fifth day after the original insult. Typically, the degree of hyperbilirubinemia is mild compared with the increase in transaminases and is by no means universal.[29] Cholestasis occurs with a decrease in transaminases. Persistence of cholestasis and coagulopathy with normalizing concentrations of enzymes indicates a poor prognosis and an exhaustion of the hepatocyte mass owing to the acute ischemic event.

A pig model of cardiogenic shock showed that immediately following decreased liver perfusion, there is an increase in messenger ribonucleic acid for acute-phase proteins.[30] Expression of certain heat shock proteins was also demonstrated, with the potential for preservation of cellular integrity. The significance of this expression and its relationship to the degree of liver injury and potential for recovery are unknown.[31]

Histologically, the pericentral area shows variable degrees of parenchymal necrosis and hepatocyte loss directly related to the duration of shock. There is little inflammatory activity, and the necrotic areas are clearly defined. At this stage, cholestasis is not a prominent feature.[32] The differential diagnosis of ischemic hepatic injury is usually not a problem because cardiac signs and symptoms predominate. Patients with other conditions associated with shock and ischemic events, including septic and hypovolemic shock, may present similarly. Protracted seizures and drug-induced hepatitis must be considered as well with this constellation of biochemical and histopathologic features. Patients with severe rhabdomyolysis may present with a marked increase in aspartate aminotransferase that is out of proportion to the concentration of alanine aminotransferase. The presence of muscle pain, easy fatigability, and, occasionally, bulky muscle mass should be sought. The presence of myoglobinuria and an increase in creatinine kinase help in the differential diagnosis.

Therapy for ischemic hepatic injury is directed toward the original insult. Supportive measures include the administration of vitamin K and, if bleeding is a problem, fresh frozen plasma. The injury to zone 3 hepatocytes, the site of xenobiotic and drug metabolism, may increase the susceptibility of the liver to potentially toxic metabolites of medications administered to these patients.

PROGNOSIS

Correction of the original insult results in resolution of the hepatopathy. An ischemic event with a duration of more than 24 hours usually results in severe liver injury and may progress to liver failure. The lack of resolution of the coagulopathy together with a decrease in transaminases and deepening jaundice is ominous. In several adult and pediatric series, the most important prognostic factors for survival were the degree of shock and, most importantly, the duration of the ischemic event. A duration of circulatory disturbance of more than 24 hours is associated with significant morbidity and mortality.[33,34] The cardiac lesions that most commonly result in significant liver involvement are hypoplastic left heart syndrome and coarctation of the aorta.[24]

CHRONIC CARDIAC DISEASE

The liver is vulnerable to a chronic increase in pressure on the right side of the heart. Chronic passive congestion results in sinusoidal dilatation and engorgement, fibrosis, and, eventually, cirrhosis.[34,35]

CLINICAL MANIFESTATIONS

Clinically, the liver is enlarged and hard; the edge is usually smooth, but nodularity is apparent in the advanced stages. The increase in liver-derived enzymes is minimal or nonexistent at first. With time, a slow, mild increase in transaminase values, as well as increases in the biliary tract–derived enzymes, is seen. Presumably, the degree of fibrosis is related to the development of microthrombi in the sinusoids and in the hepatic veins. The distribution of fibrosis can be uneven, with the right and left lobes affected to different degrees.

In a series of 150 pediatric patients, the severity and duration of hypoxia correlated with the amount of connective tissue present at autopsy.[35,36] Fibrosis had asymmetrically affected the lobes of the liver. Inhomogeneous liver parenchyma was noted on computed tomography in 24 of 25 patients with congestive heart failure.[36] Other patterns noted included hepatomegaly, enlargement of the inferior vena cava, and early reflux of contrast material into the inferior vena cava. The patient may or may not be jaundiced. The degree of hyperbilirubinemia fluctuates and occasionally results in overt jaundice. In late stages, jaundice in cardiac cirrhosis indicates a poor prognosis.

HISTOLOGIC FEATURES

Bands of fibrosis and, occasionally, cirrhosis are seen. Sinusoidal engorgement and dilatation are common (Figure 57-1). With chronic congestion, zone 3 hepatocytes atrophy, and the liver grossly resembles a nutmeg because of the association of areas of engorgement and atrophy. In cases of fetal hydrops, the liver congestion is accompanied by hemosiderosis in zone 1 hepatocytes.[37]

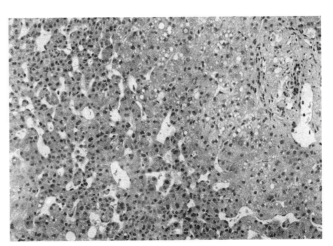

FIGURE 57-1　Venous outflow obstruction of cardiac origin. Note sinusoidal dilatation (hematoxylin and eosin; ×40 original magnification). Courtesy of Dr. L. Burgart, Mayo Clinic and Foundation

TREATMENT

For children who have a chronic increase in right-sided ventricular pressure from surgical correction of congenital heart disease, definitive correction is not always possible. With advances in medical and surgical care, more of these children are surviving into young adulthood, and cardiac cirrhosis may become the most important factor for their survival. The chronically congested liver is more susceptible to other insults. Animal studies have shown that endotoxemia with congestive heart failure can lead to fulminant hepatic failure.[35]

PROGNOSIS

Prognosis is variable because the distribution of pressure is not uniform throughout the liver, and there may be significant potential for compensated cirrhosis. Correction of the underlying cause is therapeutic in most cases.

OPEN HEART SURGERY

It is not uncommon for patients to have both congenital heart disease and congenital liver disease. The infant with a paucity of bile ducts or biliary atresia may have hemodynamically significant congenital heart disease, and the cardiac surgeon often inquires about the possibility of liver damage during open heart surgery and extracorporeal oxygenation. The infant or child with a paucity of bile ducts is usually jaundiced. The serum concentrations of biliary tract–derived enzymes are markedly increased, but the increases in transaminases are only moderate. In our experience, the prothrombin time is the best indicator of the ability of the patient to avoid fulminant hepatic failure as a result of the operation. Often the cardiac lesion is more serious than the liver lesion in patients with syndromic paucity of intrahepatic bile ducts. The same is not entirely true for the association of biliary atresia, polysplenia, dextrocardia, and congenital heart and vascular lesions. In terms of the liver, the earlier a portoenterostomy is performed, the better the hepatic outcome. If biliary drainage is accomplished and the infant is thriving, the cardiac lesion can be corrected at a later, optimal time. If biliary drainage is not accomplished, the cardiac lesion will be corrected in conjunction with liver transplant to optimize the outcomes of both operations. Once again, the prothrombin time and the degree of cholestasis and growth failure are used to determine the timing of the intervention and the degree of support required during and after the intervention.

Liver abnormalities are not uncommon after open heart surgery.[38,39] The increase in liver-derived enzymes is similar to that in ischemic hepatitis, although much smaller. Hyperbilirubinemia occurs later and is related to the duration of hypothermia and extracorporeal circulation. The infant or child with persistently low cardiac output is most susceptible to the development of liver injury. Blood transfusions during the operation add to the hyperbilirubinemia. The duration of hypoperfusion and the response to inotropic agents are important factors in the degree of liver involvement. Liver failure with encephalopathy has been reported for both adult and pediatric patients.[40–43]

CARDIAC TRANSPLANT

The liver may show evidence of being affected immediately within the first 2 weeks after cardiac transplant or not until the development of chronic liver disease. In the setting of established pulmonary hypertension, after heart transplant, the immediate insult to the liver is due to right-sided heart failure if the transplanted organ fails. This is similar to heart failure from other causes; however, the clinical case may be further complicated by acute rejection and infections. Chronic liver disease after heart transplant may be due to a lymphoproliferative disorder involving the liver or to chronic viral hepatitis acquired after transplant. The infection is due to hepatitis B and C viruses and to non-A–E hepatitis viruses, as well as to de novo infections with cytomegalovirus. Most cases of chronic hepatitis B and C are mild, and fulminant cases are rare except in cases of precore mutants of hepatitis B virus. Immunosuppression may lead to faster progression of liver fibrosis.[44]

SEPSIS

Infants and children with systemic or localized infections may have significant liver involvement.[45–48] One example is the classic description of neonatal cholestasis in the context of a urinary tract infection. Underestimation of liver dysfunction is likely because usually only jaundiced patients are evaluated. Jaundice from septicemia occurs infrequently. In an adult series of 1,150 bacteremic patients, only 7 had jaundice.[46]

The organisms implicated in the development of hepatic dysfunction include gram-negative enteric pathogens, streptococci, and staphylococci. The site of infection varies. For instance, jaundice with septicemia is one such manifestation, and hepatic abscess is known to complicate appendiceal infections. Another example is soft tissue infections leading to hepatopathy.

The onset of jaundice occurs 2 to 5 days after the infection, and the degree of direct hyperbilirubinemia varies from 5 mg/dL to more than 60 mg/dL. Hepatomegaly occurs in about 50% of the cases, and, in this instance, exclusion of hepatic abscess or cholangitis is important in the differential diagnosis.[47,48] The hepatomegaly is due to the activation of the reticuloendothelial system.[46–50]

The increases in the liver- and biliary tract–derived enzymes are only moderate compared with the degree of hyperbilirubinemia, and this dissociation is characteristic of septicemia. However, the increase in alkaline phosphatase may be significant at the onset of jaundice and during the resolution of jaundice.[46,50–52]

The recognition of the polarity of the hepatocyte has shed new light on the transport mechanisms of organic acids and bile salts. Evidence has shown that the cholestasis of septicemia is associated with abnormal regulation of the localization of the multidrug resistance protein 2. This transporter is responsible for the secretion of conjugated bilirubin at the canalicular membrane. The effect of endotoxin on this transporter results in its translocation to the inner cytoplasmic membrane. Thus, the degree of hyperbilirubinemia is out of proportion to the degree of hepatocyte damage.[53,54]

Histologically, the liver may show suppurative cholangiolitis without large duct cholangitis, in association with intrahepatic cholestasis (Figure 57-2). The lesion in the context of the clinical findings is characteristic.[48] Cholestasis alone is also common (Figure 57-3).

One important consideration is that septic patients have other confounding factors that may contribute to cholestasis. For example, some patients with multiorgan failure may have received blood products or are receiving total parenteral nutrition (TPN) and various medications. In particular, cephalosporins and biliary sludge may contribute to cholestasis. Evaluation of the patient centers on the exclusion of an hepatic abscess or ascending cholangitis. Treatment of the underlying cause is essential. There are no data on the efficacy of supportive treatment, including bile acid supplementation and early feeding, but their use is common. The prognosis is excellent after the infection is controlled.[47,50]

Characteristic features of certain infections are worth mentioning. For example, the liver may be involved in pneumococcal pneumonia.[46] The right lobe is most commonly affected, and the male-to-female ratio is 10:1.[46,47] There is swelling of hepatocytes and focal necrosis. The increase in serum transaminases may be moderate. Usually, the increase in aspartate aminotransferase is greater than the increase in alanine aminotransferase. Streptococcal infections may be associated with jaundice, and an association with scarlet fever has been described in which the liver may be tender and enlarged. Hepatomegaly and hepatitis with jaundice are not uncommon in ehrlichiosis, a tickborne infection. A history of exposure in endemic areas is helpful, and the typical rash on the palms and soles aids in the diagnosis. Hepatic involvement resolves with antibiotic therapy.[54–56]

A mild hepatitis that is often subclinical is not infrequent with varicella. The increases in serum transaminases are about three times the upper limit of the reference

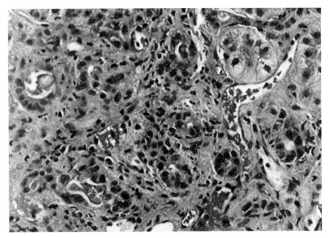

FIGURE 57-3 Cholangiolar cholestasis in the context of septicemia (hematoxylin and eosin; ×40 original magnification). Courtesy of Dr. L. Burgart, Mayo Clinic and Foundation.

range. The increase is transient, and the hepatitis usually follows a benign course.[46]

CONNECTIVE TISSUE DISEASE

Liver involvement is often considered in the child with connective tissue disease for a number of reasons: (1) the child has a new-onset disease and autoimmune hepatitis is a consideration; (2) the child has connective tissue disease and involvement of the hepatobiliary system, usually evident as increases in transaminases and alkaline phosphatase and hepatosplenomegaly; and (3) the child is receiving medications that may impair liver function and questions arise as to the potential hepatoxicity of these medications.

JUVENILE RHEUMATOID ARTHRITIS
Hepatosplenomegaly is not uncommon in juvenile rheumatoid arthritis (JRA). Approximately 10 to 15% of the children may have hepatomegaly sometime during the course of the disease. Splenomegaly is usually more prominent and occurs more frequently than hepatomegaly. The occurrence of splenomegaly with neutropenia and active systemic JRA characterizes Felty syndrome.[57] Hepatomegaly and increases in transaminases may occur with systemic JRA.[58,59] The histologic findings are nonspecific, showing Kupffer cell hyperplasia and focal hepatitis.[57–59] The occurrence of a hepatitis exacerbation is sometimes associated with improvement of the arthritis, but the mechanism is unknown.

Long-standing JRA, usually of more than 8 years, can be associated with amyloidosis.[60] The incidence is about 4% in adult series. Hepatosplenomegaly with proteinuria should increase awareness of amyloid deposition in multiple organs, but this complication is rare in pediatric patients.

Another feature is the asymptomatic increase in serum alkaline phosphatase and transaminases. The increase in alkaline phosphatase reported in the adult population is not as prevalent as in the pediatric population.[58] Some of this increase is from multiple sources, and some is from the inflamed synovium. The number of joints involved seems to

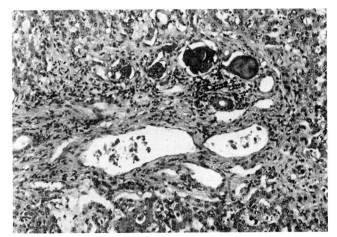

FIGURE 57-2 Cholangitis lente in the context of prolonged septicemia. Note severe cholestasis (hematoxylin and eosin; ×40 original magnification). Courtesy of Dr. L. Burgart, Mayo Clinic and Foundation.

correlate with the increase in the alkaline phosphatase. More common, however, is the increase in transaminases, which has a dose-dependent association with aspirin therapy.[61] The patient with JRA who is receiving aspirin therapy is more susceptible to the development of Reye syndrome.[61–64] One may speculate about the existence of subtle mitochondrial fatty acid oxidation genetic defects that are triggered by particular environmental factors in this population. With the discovery of more mitochondrial errors of metabolism, it is possible that concomitant administration of toxic medications may unmask these conditions.

The use of aspirin has been largely replaced by the use of nonsteroidal anti-inflammatory drugs that are less toxic to the liver. However, the potential for an idiosyncratic reaction in the form of fulminant hepatic failure is possible.[65,66] Gold toxicity manifests as cholestasis; histologically, the liver shows cholestasis and deposits of gold particles in Kupffer cells. The liver may have a brown-black pigmentation. Fulminant hepatic failure has been reported with the use of gold compounds, but the use of this treatment is uncommon in the pediatric age group.

Methotrexate is increasingly used for JRA. Two patterns of liver involvement occur. One is a mild increase in liver enzymes, about three to four times the upper limit of the reference range, that occurs in 15% of patients.[67,68] The other is progressive fibrosis that may be clinically silent. The progression to fibrosis seems to be related to a cumulative methotrexate dose of more than 1.5 g. In pediatrics, our experience and the experience of others with small series is that fibrosis is not common, even when methotrexate doses exceed 1.5 g. In adults, the toxicity of methotrexate is significantly increased with obesity and alcohol consumption.[67–71]

SYSTEMIC LUPUS ERYTHEMATOSUS

The liver is involved in up to 40% of patients with systemic lupus erythematosus (SLE). Hepatomegaly occurs in about one-third of the patients sometime during the illness. Increases in liver-derived enzymes occur in two contexts: with use of hepatotoxic medications and with use of aspirin, the most important culprit.[72–81] In addition, the use of corticosteroids may be involved with steatosis and the use of azathioprine with cholestasis.

The association of SLE and autoimmune hepatitis is well described in detail elsewhere.[73,74] The presence of autoimmune markers common to both diseases is not uncommon, and the liver lesion of SLE is indistinguishable from classic autoimmune hepatitis. This spectrum of liver disease fits into the overlap syndrome seen in adult patients who have features of autoimmune hepatitis and primary sclerosing cholangitis. The liver enzyme concentrations and the histologic changes improve rapidly with immunosuppression therapy.

The presence of a hypercoagulable state may lead to vaso-occlusive disease (VOD) of the liver or to Budd-Chiari syndrome. The association with lupus anticoagulant and anticardiolipin antibodies is well described.[78–82]

The liver may be involved in the transient abnormalities of neonatal SLE.[82,83] This occurs because of the transplacental transfer of antibodies from the mother to the fetus and is associated with anti-Ro and anti-La antibodies. The characteristic pattern is congenital heart block, dermatitis, and hematologic abnormalities. Cholestasis that resolves by 6 months of age has been described and is associated with portal fibrosis, bile duct obstruction, and inflammation. Any infant with a combination of cardiac arrhythmias and cholestasis should be evaluated for SLE, especially because the maternal disease may be asymptomatic and unrecognized.

JUVENILE DERMATOMYOSITIS

The liver is seldom involved in juvenile dermatomyositis. However, the increase in the aspartate aminotransferase from muscular origin can masquerade as hepatitis early in the disease. Hepatosplenomegaly is not uncommon in the severe form of the disease. The use of methotrexate may be associated with increases in liver-derived enzymes, and the long-term consequences are often of concern.[66,72–74] The use of nonsteroidal anti-inflammatory drugs can add to the concern for hepatotoxicity.

MISCELLANEOUS CONNECTIVE TISSUE DISEASE

The liver and spleen may be involved in mixed connective tissue disease, an overlap syndrome with features of SLE, scleroderma, and polymyositis.[82] The involvement is from generalized vasculitis, and usually there is hepatosplenomegaly. The vasculitis involves medium-size vessels, with intimal thickening and inflammation in the periportal areas.[84]

Hydrops of the gallbladder and increases in the liver enzymes occur in Kawasaki disease.[83] Hepatomegaly and increases in the liver enzymes occur in about one-third of the patients. The use of high doses of aspirin causes dose-dependent toxicity in the liver, which has occasionally led to severe hepatitis. Histologically, Kupffer cell hyperplasia, bile duct inflammation, and gallbladder wall thickening have been reported. Interestingly, hydrops of the gallbladder may respond to therapy with low doses of nonsteroidal anti-inflammatory drugs.

HEMATOLOGIC DISORDERS

SICKLE CELL DISEASE

Depending on the definition and the diagnostic methods used, the incidence of liver disease in sickle cell (SC) disease varies. If one uses abnormal concentrations of liver-derived enzymes as an indicator, liver disease may be present in up to 65% of the patients. If histologic criteria are used at autopsy, the liver is universally involved in SC disease.[84,85]

Several issues are often considered in patients with SC disease: (1) the distinction of acute crises from acute gallbladder disease, (2) the contribution of cardiac dysfunction to acute SC disease crises, (3) the chronic overload of iron and bilirubin in the liver and in other organs, and (4) the association of chronic hepatitis from contaminated blood products in patients with SC disease.

Any of the following factors lead to liver injury: (1) the increased hemolysis adds to the development of unconjugated hyperbilirubinemia[85]; (2) the increased concentrations of bilirubin and turnover lead to increased risk of pigment gallstones and acute and chronic gallbladder disease; (3) the additional transfusions increase the risk of blood-borne infections and contribute to the iron overload; iron overload with or without anemia may lead to cardiac dysfunction and secondary liver congestion; and (4) the liver may have repeated episodes of ischemic crises; the reticuloendothelial system is the first to be affected by the iron overload, and the hepatocytes are affected later. In severe cases, brown pigmentation of the hepatocytes is seen with hematoxylin and eosin stain.[84,86]

ACUTE HEPATIC CRISIS

The liver is involved in an acute hepatic crisis in about 10 to 15% of patients with SC disease.[87,88] Pain in the right upper quadrant of the abdomen, tender hepatomegaly, increases in serum transaminases, and conjugated hyperbilirubinemia develop. Fever is common. The results of coagulation studies are normal. The distinction of SC hepatopathy from acute cholecystitis may be difficult. The biliary tract–derived enzymes and serum transaminases may be equally increased. Conjugated hyperbilirubinemia is common, and concentrations may vary from 15 to 50 mg/dL. The transaminases are increased up to 10 times the upper limit of the reference range. An increase in lactic dehydrogenase is common and reflects ongoing hemolysis. Imaging of the intrahepatic and extrahepatic bile ducts is important and may help in the differential diagnosis. The difficulty arises when there is a hepatic crisis with incidental cholelithiasis. Careful observation and supportive therapy may lead to a rapid resolution of liver abnormalities, and a lack of dilated bile ducts and normal concentrations of pancreatic enzymes help in determining the course of the disease. Occasionally, a liver biopsy is indicated. The classic sinusoidal congestion, sickling, Kupffer cell hyperplasia, and erythrophagocytosis are characteristic of SC hepatopathy.

ACUTE AND CHRONIC CHOLECYSTITIS

Acute cholecystitis and choledocholithiasis in SC patients are similar to those conditions in other patients.[87,89–95] The triad of abdominal pain and tenderness in the right upper quadrant, fever, and increased serum biochemical biliary tract inflammatory markers helps in the diagnosis. Imaging studies show dilatation of the biliary tree in some patients. Others with hepatic crisis improve rapidly.

The most difficult diagnostic decisions involve conditions without a clear cause. Intrahepatic or endoscopic imaging of the biliary tree is then essential. Endoscopic imaging can be coupled with therapeutic maneuvers and may obviate the need for operative intervention. Endoscopic treatment of complications should be considered in centers with expertise in therapeutic endoscopic retrograde cholangiopancreatography.

Chronic pigment gallstones occur in 70 to 80% of patients with SC disease.[87,89–95] The incidence increases with age and is related to the increased concentrations of bilirubin from hemolysis. The consultant is often asked to consider whether an incidental cholelithiasis needs to be addressed. If the child is well and there are no significant symptoms or increases in liver enzymes, careful observation and awareness of the finding are important if pancreatitis or choledocholithiasis occurs.

CHRONIC IRON OVERLOAD

Repeated transfusions result in chronic iron overload (Table 57-2). Iron overload is most common in thalassemia.[85,96] The identification of genetic markers for hemochromatosis is challenging because the development of iron toxicity in this population is variable and occurs at a later stage in life. When thalassemia and hemochromatosis occur in the same patient, it can be difficult to determine the best method of following iron overload. There are no known reports of associated diseases (Figures 57-4 and 57-5). However, hepatitis correlated with the accumulation of more than 300 μg of iron per gram of liver tissue, presumably as a result of oxidative injury.[97] Therefore, in patients with multiple transfusions, increases in the liver enzymes may be a manifestation of iron overload, requiring measurement of ferritin and histologic confirmation with iron stains of the liver. This would also exclude other infections and vascular hepatic insults.

CHRONIC VIRAL HEPATITIS COMPLICATING IRON OVERLOAD STATES

Chronic viral hepatitis occurs in about 25 to 30% of patients with SC disease.[94,98] Screening for hepatitis C virus has reduced the risk of transfusion-associated infection. In a series of 99 patients, 23% had evidence of hepatitis C virus infection.[94] The risk of infection is related to the frequency of blood transfusions, and multiple transfusions may result in repeated infections with different genotypes. The frequency of transfusions, combined with chronic liver disease, may complicate the response to treatment. There are no reports that clarify the optimal antiviral therapy and the response to therapy for this population.

THALASSEMIA

The transfusion requirements of patients with thalassemia lead to iron overload and eventually to liver fibrosis and cirrhosis. The risk of viral infection is high in this patient population, and the patients who received transfusions before the availability of screening for hepatitis C virus have a high incidence of infection. Histologic findings in the liver are nonspecific and may show the characteristic features of hepatitis C infection.[94,98]

TABLE 57-2	CHRONIC IRON OVERLOAD

Arrhythmia
Congestive heart failure
Bronzed skin
Hepatomegaly
Splenomegaly
Diabetes
Increased susceptibility to *Yersinia* infection

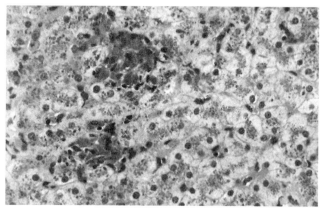

FIGURE 57-4   Severe iron overload with sickle cell disease iron content 23,000 µg/g of tissue (hematoxylin and eosin; ×40 original magnification). Courtesy of Dr. L. Burgart, Mayo Clinic and Foundation.

Infection with hepatitis C virus constitutes an important cause of morbidity in patients with β-thalassemia.[99] The patient may be infected more than once and with more than one strain of the virus. The combination of iron overload and viral burden may accelerate the progression to fibrosis.

COAGULATION DISORDERS

The use of contaminated blood products, especially before 1990, has resulted in a high incidence of hepatitis C infection in patients with hemophilia.[94,98] In this population, the liver is commonly involved, and increases in the liver-derived enzymes are not unusual. Because the patients have had multiple transfusions, infection may have occurred through more than one genotype. The results of therapeutic trials in this population are pending at this time.

BUDD-CHIARI SYNDROME

Budd-Chiari syndrome can be a manifestation of either coagulation disorders or vascular diseases affecting the liver (Table 57-3). Because coagulation disorders are associated with this syndrome, it is another example of how the liver is involved in hematologic diseases. Yet, worldwide,

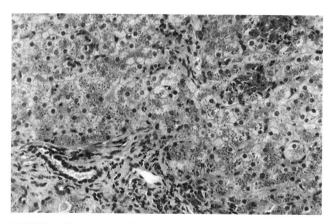

FIGURE 57-5   Severe hemosiderosis with sickle cell disease (hematoxylin and eosin; ×40 original magnification). Courtesy of Dr. L. Burgart, Mayo Clinic and Foundation.

membranous obstruction of the hepatic veins is the most frequent cause of this syndrome.[100]

The acute form is characterized by the sudden onset of abdominal pain in the right upper quadrant, tender hepatomegaly, and ascites. The acute event leads to mild increases in the liver enzymes, and in a similar fashion to cardiac congestion, the increases in enzymes reflect zone 3 involvement. Prolongation of the prothrombin time is common, but this finding may be confusing if a hypercoagulable state is present.[101,102]

Acute events may result from thrombosis of the hepatic veins as a result of protein C deficiency, antithrombin III deficiency, mutations in the genes for factor V Leiden and thrombin, polycythemia vera, primary lymphoproliferative disorders, inflammatory bowel disease, paroxysmal nocturnal hemoglobinuria, Behçet syndrome, and collagen vascular diseases, including those associated with anticardiolipin antibodies and lupus anticoagulant.

Acute obstructive lesions are usually due to tumor invasion from adrenal and renal cancers. Occasionally, patients who have hepatic tumors that have spread beyond the liver may present with acute Budd-Chiari syndrome.

Chronic Budd-Chiari syndrome is usually due to membranous obstruction of the hepatic veins, a condition common in developing countries. The lesion may be congenital or, perhaps more commonly, due to thrombosis. Thrombosis is often found histologically, but it is difficult to know whether it is a consequence of congenital occlusion. The increases in the liver-derived enzymes are mild, and coagulation is normal. Progression of the disease leads to manifestations of portal hypertension and liver failure, including ascites, hepatic encephalopathy, and variceal bleeding. Treatment of membranous occlusion is by invasive radiologic techniques. Advanced liver disease can be corrected with transplant, although recurrence of disease in the transplanted liver is possible, especially when polycythemia or primary thrombotic conditions are present.[100–120]

The diagnosis of Budd-Chiari syndrome is made with the use of several types of imaging techniques, from Doppler ultrasonography to magnetic resonance imaging. Hypertrophy of the caudate lobe is a peculiar feature found on technetium uptake because of the differential drainage of this lobe. The caudate lobe drains directly into the inferior vena cava and is enlarged because of hypertrophy from portal hypertension in Budd-Chiari syndrome.[104,118,121–124]

A dual approach is used to manage Budd-Chiari syndrome: identify the original insult and treat the present

TABLE 57-3   BUDD-CHIARI SYNDROME

Membranous obstruction of the hepatic veins
Idiopathic hypercoagulable states
Contraception
Pregnancy
Inflammatory bowel disease
Myeloproliferative disorders
Paroxysmal nocturnal hemoglobinuria
Chronic cardiac congestion
Renal and suprarenal tumor invasion
Behçet syndrome

condition. Diagnosis of hypercoagulable states should be sought and the evaluation for polycythemia pursued vigorously to prevent recurrence of vascular compromise. If the liver shows only congestion and the response to diuretic therapy is good, anticoagulation may be attempted. If a subsequent liver biopsy shows persistent congestion, only then can medical therapy be continued. If severe necrosis is present, surgical shunting is offered. If fibrosis is present, medical therapy and evaluation for liver transplant are initiated.[112–115,121]

VASCULAR DISEASES

The dual supply of blood to the liver is a fundamental difference between it and other organs.[116,117,125] Development of a liver infarct requires that occlusion to both the arterial and the venous supplies occurs simultaneously. Occasionally, occlusion of the hepatic and portal veins occurs, leading initially to loss of hepatocytes and subsequently to bridging fibrosis. After atrophy of the hepatocyte mass has occurred, compensatory hypertrophy occurs in the remaining liver tissue.[126] Depending on the location and the extent of vascular compromise and the reparative adaptation of the liver, several clinicopathologic entities may occur. In noncirrhotic portal hypertension, reactive nodular hyperplasia and idiopathic portal hypertension accompany the liver cell atrophy. The liver function is normal,[126–135] and the liver is characteristically normal in size.

Nodular hyperplasia of the liver occurs with systemic diseases (Table 57-4). The hyperplasia occurs in different forms, depending on the extent of vascular compromise. In large nodular hyperplasia, extensive areas of the liver are affected, and several large nodules are present. In regenerative nodular hyperplasia, the liver has many small nodules affecting multiple areas of the liver. Large nodules are not accompanied by portal hypertension unless they become numerous. These large lesions occur with congenital anomalies of the portal vein, such as absence of the portal vein, patent ductus venosus, or large arteriovenous shunts. A recent report of focal nodular hyperplasia mentions its association with multiple clonal chromosomal aberrations.[136] The patient presents with silent hepatomegaly owing to focal nodular hyperplasia, and the diagnosis is established by imaging studies and analysis for clonal abnormalities in the mesenchymal origin of the vascular stroma.

When the vascular supply is severely impaired, leading to significant and mainly venous injury, cirrhosis may be the end result. This leads to the loss of hepatocyte function, marginal blood supply, capillarization of sinusoids, and various degrees of cholestasis.

The involvement of hepatic arteries in systemic conditions is not uncommon. The dual supply of the liver is protective for the most part; however, arterial compromise affects the large intrahepatic bile ducts, and stricture formation secondary to biliary necrosis is a well-recognized complication of hepatic artery injury, whether surgical or thrombotic.

One report describes ischemic necrosis of bile ducts complicating Henoch-Schönlein purpura owing to hepatic vasculitis. The vasculitis affected the integrity of the biliary system and resulted in biliary cirrhosis, requiring transplant.[137]

Research into the biology of the endothelial cell has led to several conceptual advances: (1) the identification of endothelin, a potent vasoactive peptide; (2) the identification of overproduction of endothelin in the injured liver; and (3) the elucidation of the synthesis and function of nitric oxide.[13–18] The recognition that endothelin and nitric oxide are produced by endothelial cells and that they have dramatic effects on the surrounding stellate cells and on the microvasculature is shedding new light on the function of these cells in the development of portal hypertension. The recognition of the importance of the endothelial cell during ischemic liver injury and its targeting by host lymphocytes during organ rejection has become critical to our understanding of the cellular and molecular events in liver transplant and disease.[10–17]

MALIGNANCIES

LEUKEMIA

Hepatosplenomegaly is common in leukemia. About one-third of patients with leukemia have clinical and biochemical abnormalities sometime during their illness. One rare presentation of neonatal leukemia is liver failure, and biopsy results are usually needed for the diagnosis. The response to chemotherapy is dramatic. The histologic finding is leukemic infiltration of the liver by malignant cells (Figure 57-6).[138]

Increases in liver-derived enzymes occur often, especially during therapy, but the increase is transient. In our experience, several patients continued to have abnormal serum concentrations of liver enzymes while they received low-dose maintenance therapy with azathioprine. The increases in liver enzymes correlated with the metabolic activity of thiopurine methyltransferase.

Neutropenia predisposes the patient to opportunistic infections, and severe hepatitis from adenoviral infection has been reported in this population. More ominous is fungal infection, for which the only clues may be hepatomegaly, increases in liver enzymes, and fever.[139,140]

HODGKIN LYMPHOMA

The extent of liver involvement in Hodgkin disease varies with the timing of the evaluation.[141–146] Whereas the liver is clinically involved in about 5% of the patients at pre-

TABLE 57-4	NODULAR REGENERATIVE HYPERPLASIA

Juvernile rhumatoid arthritis
Systemic lupus erythematosus
Polyarteritis nodosa
Glomerulonephritis
Cryoglobulinemia
Antiphospholipid syndrome
Chronic cardiac congestion
Pulmonary hypertention
Portal vein thrombosis
Persistence of ductus venosus
Contraception

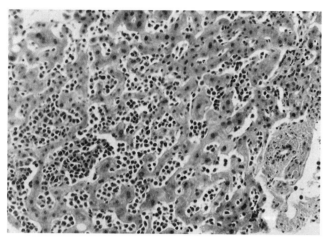

FIGURE 57-6 Liver involvement by leukemia (hematoxylin and eosin; ×40 original magnification). Courtesy of Dr. L. Burgart, Mayo Clinic and Foundation.

sentation, evidence of liver involvement is found in 50% at autopsy.

Histologic findings show either direct involvement of the liver or nonspecific inflammation and infiltration and noncaseating granulomas. Reed-Sternberg cells are found in about 25% of the cases. More commonly, nonspecific liver inflammation is found in about 50% of the cases. The detection rate of Reed-Sternberg cells is higher with laparoscopic biopsy than with percutaneous biopsy. Noncaseating granulomas, found in about 25% of the cases, are not considered to be part of the direct involvement of the liver in Hodgkin disease.

The most commonly increased biliary tract enzyme in the adult population is alkaline phosphatase, showing a correlation with disease stage. The fact that this enzyme is often elevated owing to normal bone growth in healthy children makes it a less useful indicator in pediatric patients than in adults.

Jaundice occurs with direct liver involvement. Obstructive lesions of the biliary tree are much less common. There are reports of vanishing bile duct syndrome occurring in patients with Hodgkin lymphoma. Whether this syndrome represents a variant of Hodgkin presentation or coincidental occurrence of primary sclerosing cholangitis is not clear.

LANGERHANS CELL HISTIOCYTOSIS

The liver is involved in two large groups of disorders of histiocytes. Langerhans cell histiocytosis (LCH) refers to the group that includes eosinophilic granuloma, Letterer-Siwe disease, Hand-Schüller-Christian syndrome, Hashimoto-Pritzker syndrome, and histiocytosis X.[147,148]

This group of disorders is characterized by abnormal infiltration of various tissues with phagocytic mononuclear histiocytes with particular markers. These markers indicate the dendritic lineage of the Langerhans cells that infiltrate various organs. The definitive diagnosis is determined by the presence of Birbeck granules on electron microscopy. The demonstration of T-6 antigens on the surface of cells with tissue involvement is also diagnostic. In addition, the finding of CD1a antigen on the surface of his-

tiocytes is a relatively easy way to demonstrate the cell lineage in paraffin-embedded tissue specimens. Although the presence of the CD1a marker is not 100% specific for LCH, the procedure is rapid and easy.[149]

The other group of disorders that involve histiocytes but not of the Langerhans cell type includes the familial hemophagocytic lymphohistiocytosis and the infection-associated hemophagocytic syndromes.[149–152]

Depending on the degree of organ involvement, LCH is categorized as involving either one site or multiple sites in a single system or as being multisystemic. In multisystemic LCH, patients are classified as having either organ involvement alone or organ involvement with dysfunction.[149]

Liver involvement in LCH is mostly a manifestation of multisystemic disease. The patient may have the characteristic skin lesion with diaper dermatitis, drainage from the external auditory canal, or hepatosplenomegaly. Other presentations include gastrointestinal tract bleeding and protein-losing enteropathy. The liver is almost universally involved with gut disease and is involved in up to 30% of patients with LCH. The spectrum of liver disease includes acute hepatitis, severe biliary cholestatic liver disease, and silent hepatomegaly with incidental increases in serum liver enzymes. The histologic findings vary from liver infiltration with histiocytes to destructive sclerosing cholangitis, in which the biliary enzymes are often increased, but jaundice is not prominent. The progression of the liver lesion does not parallel the response of the skin and other organs to chemotherapy. Cirrhosis may also be the presenting manifestation, especially when the disease progresses silently.[147–153] The progression to biliary cirrhosis is rapid compared with other causes of biliary cirrhosis, such as primary sclerosing cholangitis. Liver disease in LCH is progressive despite successful treatment of skin and bone lesions. After cirrhosis develops, the progression appears to be relentless.

The important point to remember is that patients with LCH require careful monitoring of liver involvement. A false sense of security should be avoided when the extrahepatic manifestations of the disease are controlled.

In a review at a single center, 75% of the neonatal patients with LCH presented with multisystemic involvement.[148] The characteristic skin lesion and the extent of the skin lesions did not correlate with systemic disease, and mortality was higher in this age group than in older children. Overall, the liver is involved in 30% of patients with LCH, but it is involved in 50% of patients with multisystemic disease. In patients with liver disease, only 25% have jaundice.[154] The others have hepatomegaly with or without increases in the liver enzymes. In a few patients, the onset of liver disease occurs well after successful treatment of skin and extrahepatic disease.

As expected, the outcome of LCH is dependent on the extent of disease at presentation. However, the progression of histiocytic infiltration of organs and the response to therapy in individual cases cannot always be predicted. A report has shown a clear association between the level of soluble interleukin-2 receptor and the extent of LCH. This association may be useful for monitoring a patient's progress and possibly monitoring the response to chemotherapy. Interestingly, there seems to be activation of the tumor necrosis factor pathway in tissues with histiocytic infiltration, and one report showed a good response to the use of tumor necrosis factor receptor:Fc-fusion protein with regression of multisystemic invasion.[149] If confirmed in more cases, this report may pave the way for treatment of disease before pathologic changes in the liver become irreversible and the only option is liver transplant.

A key feature of the management of LCH is close cooperation between hematologists and hepatologists. The patient should have frequent and focused examinations for hepatomegaly and for screening laboratory values of hepatic and biliary enzymes. The use of magnetic resonance imaging of the liver and the biliary tree seems to be promising for identifying liver disease and biliary destruction. However, changes that are detectable by this technique may be indicative of late infiltration rather than early infiltration. Therefore, histologic examination of tissue remains an important tool for confirming and analyzing liver involvement.

Liver transplant has been successful for treatment of this disease. However, a review of the transplant experience in LCH patients has shown some that there is an increased risk of lymphoproliferative disease developing post-transplant,[155] perhaps owing to an altered immune status. This speculation is based on the demonstration of increased levels of interleukin-1, tumor necrosis factor, granulocyte-macrophage colony-stimulating factor, and soluble interleukin-2 receptor. Recurrence of LCH in the transplanted organ and extrahepatic sites is reported to occur in up to 33% of the patients. Only recently has it been shown that the graft is susceptible to LCH invasion.[155] Despite chemotherapy, the disease seems to be progressive in transplants, as well as in native livers. Finally, acute rejection is nearly universal among patients who receive transplants for LCH. Patients with certain liver conditions characterized by altered immune status, such as LCH and primary sclerosing cholangitis, who undergo liver transplant may require a different immunosuppressive regimen or may develop significant morbidity later, such as post-transplant lymphoproliferative disease or exacerbation of concomitant inflammatory bowel disease.[156,157]

HEMOPHAGOCYTIC SYNDROME

Hemophagocytic syndrome (also called hemophagocytic lymphohistiocytosis), is a rare disease affecting infants and children. The hallmark of the disease is the accumulation in the reticuloendothelial system of lymphohistiocytes with features of hemophagocytosis. The diagnosis is based on a set of clinical and laboratory criteria (Table 57-5).

The liver is often involved in both infection-induced and familial hemophagocytic syndromes.[147–150] The sporadic form is a reactive proliferation of the lymphohistiocytic lineage, affecting multiple organs in reaction to a viral, bacterial, or fungal infection. The activated lymphocytes are benign, and there is evidence of hemophagocytosis. The most frequently associated infection is related to Epstein-Barr virus. The immune systems in children with hemophagocytic lymphohistiocytosis seem to lack the ability to control infections; they react with an uncontrolled inflammatory response with sustained activation of macrophages and T lymphocytes. Evidence of proliferation is present in the peripheral blood and numerous organs. Fever and hepatomegaly and other organomegaly are present. Concentrations of serum liver enzymes are abnormal in 80% of the patients. The lesion resolves with prompt resolution of the original infection in sporadic cases. The familial form is almost universally fatal without stem cell transplant.

The inheritance of the familial form is autosomal recessive. The condition occurs in the first 3 months of life and has a poor prognosis. The infant has hepatosplenomegaly, fever, and weight loss. Anemia, thrombocytopenia, hyperlipidemia, and low concentrations of fibrinogen are features of this disease as well. Neurologic involvement may also be present, manifesting as irritability, convulsions, meningitis, and altered consciousness.[158]

The liver and other organs are infiltrated with malignant histiocytes. The best area for the documentation of the diagnosis is the bone marrow because the liver lesion may show a nondiagnostic lymphocytic hepatitis without phagocytosis. Hyperlipidemia is an important feature of this condition and may help in the diagnosis. Acute fulminant hepatic failure mimicking neonatal hemochromatosis has been reported in two cases. In patients with hemophagocytic syndrome, the ferritin level may be increased, so the disease may be confused with neonatal iron storage disease. Ultrasonographic findings show hepatomegaly, thickening of the gallbladder wall, and increased periportal echogenicity. There is a report of one case successfully treated with intravenous administration of cyclosporine.[159] In one report, a deficiency in perforin, an important mediator of lymphocyte cytotoxicity, was shown to be present in familial hemophagocytic syndrome.[157]

Whereas the sporadic form occurs as a result of immunologic overactivity, as in Epstein-Barr virus–related hemophagocytic lymphohistiocytosis, the familial form is due to malignant transformation. Therefore, in the sporadic form, immunosuppression is the mainstay of therapy, whereas in the familial form, immunomodulation and immunosuppression of T-lymphocyte activation are performed in preparation for stem cell transplant as the definitive treatment.[160]

The gene encoding for perforin has been mapped to 10q22 and is mutated in familial LCH.[155] Perforin is a protein expressed in lymphocytes, macrophages, and bone marrow precursors. Its main role is the formation of pores

TABLE 57-5	CLINICAL AND LABORATORY CRITERIA FOR THE DIAGNOSIS OF HEMOPHAGOCYTIC LYMPHOHISTIOCYTOSIS

Fever and hepatosplenomegaly
Cytopenia in 2 of 3 lineages
Hypertriglyceridemia or hyperfibrinogenemia or both
Hemophagocytosis in bone marrow, spleen, or lymph nodes
Absence of malignancy

in target cells. After this occurs, the disrupted membrane of the target cell allows the entry of granzymes that trigger apoptosis. Perforin-deficient mice cannot lyse target cells and have an impaired defense against cancer and intracellular pathogens.[161] In combination with the defective aspect of antigen-presenting cells lacking perforin, this leads to several disrupted immune pathways that combine to cause the clinical manifestations of the disease.

The familial form is autosomal recessive, with an incidence estimated at 0.12 per 100,000 children.[154] Despite the classic description of sporadic cases occurring with an infection, 50 of 122 children reported to the registry for hemophagocytic lymphohistiocytosis had evidence of infection; of those, 25 had a positive family history and characteristics that were similar to those of the other 25 sporadic and nonfamilial cases.

Finally, Griscelli syndrome, a rare condition characterized by partial albinism and immunodeficiency, is also associated with perforin mutation; therefore, patients may present with hemophagocytosis with liver involvement.[162]

BONE MARROW TRANSPLANT

The liver is involved in several ways in patients undergoing bone marrow transplant. Chronologically, liver involvement occurs during the conditioning regimen; during the period of marrow ablation and pancytopenia, immediately after engraftment; and 6 months after transplant.

When malignancy recurs, the liver may be affected by the original condition that led to the transplant. The liver may become one of the sites of opportunistic infections, or it may be injured by various medications. Prolonged fasting and the use of TPN may contribute significantly to the pathophysiology of liver disease in bone marrow transplant patients.

The hepatopathy of bone marrow transplant varies from fulminant failure owing to viral infections, such as herpes simplex and adenovirus, to chronic cholestasis from graft-versus-host disease (GVHD) and prolonged nutritional support (see Table 57-4).

VENO-OCCLUSIVE DISEASE

The triad of hepatomegaly, increased liver enzymes, and ascites describes VOD owing to obstruction of the terminal hepatic venules. Originally, VOD was described in patients exposed to pyrrolizine alkaloids (Table 57-6). VOD of the liver occurs in about 20 to 25% of the patients undergoing bone marrow transplant.[152,153,157] The condition is more likely to occur with allogeneic transplants than with autologous transplants. It is more common in patients who undergo transplant for malignancies, such as leukemia, than for aplastic anemia. Preexisting liver disease, total-body irradiation, and the intensity of the conditioning regimen contribute to the endothelial injury and the development of VOD. Low levels of pseudocholinesterase, a marker of hepatic synthetic function, correlate positively with the development of liver disease, and levels of proteins C, S, and antithrombin III correlate inversely with the development of VOD.[155,163,164]

Diagnostic criteria for VOD include onset within 20 days after transplant, weight gain of 2 to 10%, hepatomegaly,

ascites, and a serum concentration of bilirubin greater than 2 mg/dL. Using these criteria, the frequency of VOD after bone marrow transplant ranges from 1 to 50%, with a mortality rate of 3 to 50%. Poor outcome is correlated with the severity of hyperbilirubinemia and the presence of multiorgan failure.[165–167]

The pathophysiologic process of VOD is presumed to be direct injury to the endothelium of the central hepatic veins. The injury is often associated with zone 3 necrosis from irradiation. The propensity of zone 3 hepatocytes to injury is multifactorial and is related to the relatively low oxygen tension in this area and the concentration of drug metabolism pathways. Glutathione depletion in this area leads to increased injury, a process that may be prevented by administration of glutamine. The combination of radiation injury and tissue hypoxia seems to involve the endothelial cells of the terminal hepatic venules and to initiate local thrombosis that potentiates congestion and hypoxia. Eventually, significant fibrosis and collagen deposition around occluded central veins lead to the clinical triad of weight gain, jaundice, and hepatomegaly that manifests between the second and sixth week after transplant. There is considerable evidence to implicate intravascular thrombosis in the early events leading to VOD.[168] The hypothesis is that reactive compounds are produced by zone 3 hepatocytes that are directly toxic to the endothelial cell. The endothelial cell injury leads to intravascular thrombosis, thereby potentiating the initial insult and leading to activation of the stellate cell. Persistent activation of the stellate cell, the principal fibrogenic cell in the liver responsible for the accumulation of collagen, is also evident from studies of autopsy cases.

VOD is characterized by fibrous intimal thickening or occlusion of hepatic venules less than 0.3 mm in diameter.[169–171] Occasionally, lesions and significant congestion are seen in larger veins (Figures 57-7 and 57-8).

Treatment for moderate and severe VOD consists of infusion of tissue plasminogen activator and transjugular intrahepatic portosystemic shunting, which may be beneficial in the early stages of the disease. In uncontrolled studies, heparin showed some efficacy.[172] Early detection is crucial. Abdominal girth measurement and twice-daily measurement of body weight are essential for the initiation of therapy. Jaundice and frank ascites are ominous signs. In about 50% of the patients, the disease resolves slowly. Fatal

TABLE 57-6   VENO-OCCLUSIVE DISEASE
                OF THE LIVER

Pyrrolidine alkaloids
Aflatoxins
Cyclophosphamide
Azathioprine and 6-thioguanine
Vincristine
Busulfan
Hypervitaminosis A
Cysteamine
Immune deficiency
Estrogens
Pregnancy

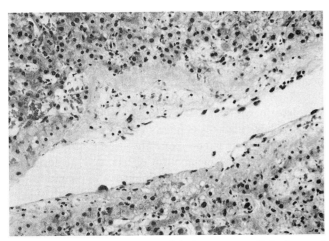

FIGURE 57-7 Veno-occlusive of the liver. Note wall thickness of hepatic venules (hematoxylin and eosin; ×40 original magnification). Courtesy of Dr. L. Burgart, Mayo Clinic and Foundation.

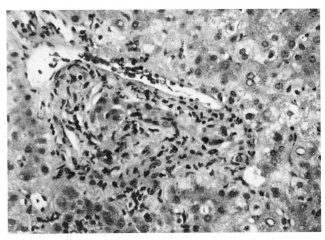

FIGURE 57-9 Graft-versus-host disease after bone marrow transplant (hematoxylin and eosin; ×40 original magnification). Courtesy of Dr. L. Burgart, Mayo Clinic and Foundation.

outcome is not uncommon, and liver transplant for VOD has been attempted.[171]

GRAFT-VERSUS-HOST DISEASE

Chronic GVHD occurs in up to 70% of the patients after bone marrow transplant. The disease most commonly affects the skin, liver, and gastrointestinal tract, but other organs and organ systems are affected as well. Isolated involvement of one organ system, such as the liver, is not uncommon. Chronic GVHD, by definition, occurs 100 days after transplant.[173,174] The disease may occur earlier, and in about one-third of the patients, it occurs after acute GVHD. The predisposing factors to GVHD include acute GVHD and the degree of human leukocyte antigen (HLA) mismatch.[173–182] The portal tracts are enlarged, and there is variable lymphocytic infiltration. Long-standing GVHD results in the vanishing bile duct syndrome and eventually may lead to cirrhosis. Treatment consists of administration of immunosuppressive medication, ursodeoxycholic acid, and thalidomide (Figures 57-9 and 57-10).

Acute GVHD may occur when an immunocompromised host receives immunocompetent T cells.[183] The condition has been described in patients after solid organ or stem cell transplant, in immunocompromised patients receiving unirradiated blood, and in newborns with hemolytic disease after exchange transfusion.[184,185] Acute GVHD, which occurs 3 to 6 weeks after the transplant, is characterized by anorexia, nausea, vomiting, and, occasionally, profuse diarrhea. A maculopapular rash is also common. Hepatocyte injury and cholestasis are common; however, severe insufficiency is rare. Histologically, the liver shows segmental destruction of small bile ducts in association with mononuclear infiltration. Rectal and skin biopsy findings may help in the diagnosis and the exclusion of hepatotoxicity and viral infections. Immunosuppression is the treatment of choice.

NUTRITIONAL DISORDERS

MALNUTRITION

The liver is affected in all forms of malnutrition.[186–189] Chronic starvation results in depletion of glycogen stores,

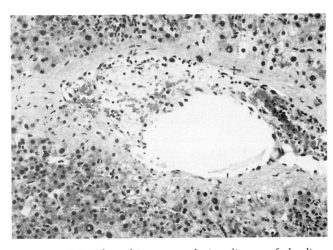

FIGURE 57-8 Idiopathic veno-occlusive disease of the liver (hematoxylin and eosin; ×40 original magnification). Courtesy of Dr. L. Burgart, Mayo Clinic and Foundation.

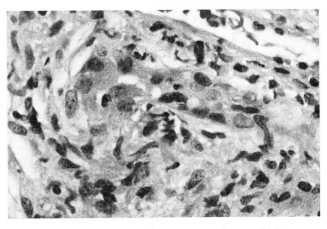

FIGURE 57-10 Hepatic graft-versus-host disease, higher magnification. Note inflammatory infiltrate (hematoxylin and eosin; ×160 original magnification). Courtesy of Dr. L. Burgart, Mayo Clinic and Foundation

reduced neoglycogenesis owing to reduced protein stores, and production of ketones as fuel for cardiac muscle and the central nervous system.

Chronic malnutrition leads to the mobilization of free fatty acids even when the intake of carbohydrates is small. The free fatty acids are mobilized from the periphery and are not oxidized effectively in the liver; eventually, fat accumulates in the hepatocytes with resultant macrovesicular steatosis. Kwashiorkor, in particular, is associated with severe steatosis, whereas marasmus is associated less often. The livers of patients in prolonged starvation have decreased numbers of peroxisomes, and their carnitine stores are depleted, which are two factors that contribute to lipid metabolic abnormalities.[188-190]

Deficiencies of trace metals, such as zinc and selenium, may contribute to liver injury. Zinc is a cofactor in several enzymatic reactions and is considered to be an antioxidant. Selenium may function as an antioxidant as well.

Among children who have undergone starvation, chronic infections and bacterial overgrowth are often present and are presumed to contribute to liver disease in some way. In developing countries, the association of parasitic infestations, such as ascariasis, that may invade the biliary tree is well known.

FATTY LIVER, OBESITY, AND NONALCOHOLIC STEATOHEPATITIS

Fatty liver occurs with obesity, diabetes mellitus (especially type 2), jejunoileal bypass, hypertriglyceridemia, and certain metabolic diseases, such as galactosemia, tyrosinemia, and hereditary fructose intolerance (Table 57-7). Mitochondrial fatty acid oxidation defects and peroxisomal disorders also cause fatty liver. Rare causes of fatty liver include cholesterol ester storage disease and neutral lipid storage disease. Fatty liver can also be a feature of drug toxicity because the drugs undergo phase I metabolism through the cytochrome P-450 enzyme system. In cases of drug toxicity, mitochondrial function is presumably affected, resulting in microvesicular steatosis. Except for the known metabolic causes of fatty liver, nonalcoholic steatohepatitis (NASH) is considered to be the most severe form of nonalcoholic fatty liver.[190-210]

The normal liver is 5% fat by weight, in the form of triglycerides, cholesterol, cholesterol esters, and fatty acids. In steatosis, the liver may be 40% fat. The metabolism of fat depends on various factors, including the presence of fed or fasting states and the hormonal conditions, such as insulin and glucagon balance, adrenergic tone, and concentrations of thyroid hormones. During the fed state, the combination of triglycerides from chylomicrons and insulin and the activation of the parasympathetic system contribute to the accumulation of lipids in the adipose tissue and liver. During the fasting state, glucagon is released in response to the sympathetic nervous system, resulting in the increased formation of free fatty acids, which are released into the circulation as fuel for muscle and the brain.

The liver is crucial not only in energy metabolism but also in hormonal homeostasis. During excessive food intake, the liver stores fats, and steatosis may develop.

During chronic starvation, fats are mobilized from the periphery, but oxidation in the liver is lacking, and steatosis is a hallmark of kwashiorkor, as previously mentioned. The same processes that occur during chronic starvation occur with prolonged use of TPN, especially if the administration of nutrients is continuous. In diabetic patients who have newly diagnosed diabetes, who are noncompliant, or whose diabetes is poorly controlled, accumulation of fat in the liver is common. The use of corticosteroids likewise affects the metabolism of fats, and steatosis is a common occurrence during prolonged administration.

Many metabolic disorders are associated with steatosis.[201-205,208,209] Classic Reye syndrome and severe steatosis occur with mitochondrial fatty acid oxidation defects. The presence of steatosis is also common in hereditary fructose intolerance, galactosemia, and tyrosinemia. Cholesterol ester storage disease produces a peculiar orange-colored liver and is also associated with steatosis. Certain medications, such as tetracycline, colchicine, and asparaginase, cause steatosis.[199]

Chronic intake of vitamin A leads to steatosis and to stellate cell hyperplasia. Long-term intake may lead to perisinusoidal fibrosis, presumably from activation of the stellate cell by accumulation of retinyl esters.[199-203]

The number of children with a body mass index (BMI) greater than the 95th percentile for age and sex has doubled since 1976.[211] About 15% of obese children have NASH, characterized by increases in serum liver enzymes that are associated with inflammatory changes and with occasional bridging fibrosis on liver biopsy. Pure macrovesicular steatosis without increases in liver enzymes is very common in obesity and reflects the accumulation of fat in the liver and in other organs.

The reason why increases in transaminases (usually four times the upper limit of the reference range) occur in certain children is unknown. Often the only clue to liver disease is an incidental finding of increased serum liver-derived enzymes on routine testing. The biliary tract–derived enzymes may be mildly increased as well. Occasionally, ultrasonography shows increased echogenic-

TABLE 57-7	CAUSES OF STEATOSIS

Malnutrition
Essential fatty acid deficiency
Celiac disease
Diabetes mellitus
Galactosemia
Hereditary fructose intolerance
Glycogen storage disease
Tyrosinemia
Homocystinuria
Mitochondrial oxidation and respiratory chain defects
Carnitine deficiency
Cholesterol ester storage disease
Abetalipoproteinemia
Cystic fibrosis
Drugs
Total parenteral nutrition
Obesity
Reye syndrome

ity of the liver parenchyma as an indicator of steatosis. However, many patients with NASH have minimal changes on ultrasonography. A more accurate, quantifiable measure of liver steatosis can be determined with magnetic resonance imaging of the liver.

All of the cases of NASH identified at the Armed Forces Institute of Pathology during a 5-year period were reviewed; 71% of the patients were obese.[199] Therefore, the association of obesity and NASH is strong in the adult population. Nevertheless, one-third of the patients were not obese. The relationship between a nonobese BMI and the development of NASH is not known, and the prevalence of NASH in the obese population is not known. Normalization of the increases in liver enzymes may occur with a decrease in the BMI. Whether this is accompanied by a decrease in the frequency of liver fibrosis in patients with NASH is unknown. Ultrasonographic echogenicity and the absence of other causes help in the determination of the diagnosis. Reports of fatty liver in adult patients followed up for 18 years showed that the group at highest risk of progression to cirrhosis is the one with fibrosis, Mallory hyaline, and significant histologic inflammation on liver biopsy.[203,204] There are no comparable data for children.

The generally benign nature of this condition and the slow progression to cirrhosis outweigh the risks involved in a biopsy. The steatosis in this condition is usually macrovesicular and occasionally microvesicular (Figures 57-11 and 57-12). There are anecdotal reports of familial NASH, although diabetes and the illicit use of alcohol are confounding variables. The familial forms seem to be associated with mild obesity. Whether there are subgroups of patients with a metabolic basis for their microvesicular steatosis is unknown.[212,213] Proposed explanations include abnormalities of lipid oxidation, chronic endotoxemia, iron overload, and concurrent infection with hepatitis C virus.

The association of type 2 diabetes and NASH is well known in adults. Whether similar changes occur in juvenile diabetes is not entirely clear.[202–208] It is well known that about 5% of patients with type 1 diabetes have associated celiac disease. Left undiagnosed, this may lead to significant malnutrition and subsequent steatosis.

SHORT-BOWEL SYNDROME

The liver is affected in short-bowel syndrome in several ways: malnutrition and vitamin and trace element deficiencies may be present,[214–216] TPN may contribute to liver injury, intra-abdominal infections may result in liver abscesses, and bacterial overgrowth may affect the development of liver inflammation and injury. The early institution of enteral feeding and the cycling of nutritional supplementation have decreased the incidence of liver injury. The recognition of the contribution of bacterial overgrowth to the malabsorption of nutrients has led to the aggressive use of antibiotics, which has a beneficial effect on the liver (see Chapter 39, "Gastrointestinal Manifestations of Immunodeficiency").

TOTAL PARENTERAL NUTRITION

TPN is the best characterized cause of nutrition-related liver disease. Cholestatic liver disease predominates in premature and young infants and steatohepatitis in older children and adolescents.[217–229] Clinical cholestasis develops in about 25% of premature infants receiving TPN.[220] The severity of the cholestasis depends on the duration of nutritional support, and cholestasis usually resolves after the cessation of parenteral support. Associated sepsis, severe lung disease, congenital heart disease, and short-bowel syndrome add to the liver insult. Amino acid and glucose concentrations may be the primary culprits in the development of liver disease, although this remains controversial. The effect of fat emulsions is not entirely clear.[220–225]

The composition of the current amino acid formula results in a serum amino acid profile that is similar to that of breastfed babies. This formulation has resulted in a decreased incidence of cholestatic liver disease. The decreased concentration of carbohydrates in the formula seems to be beneficial as well. The early institution of oral

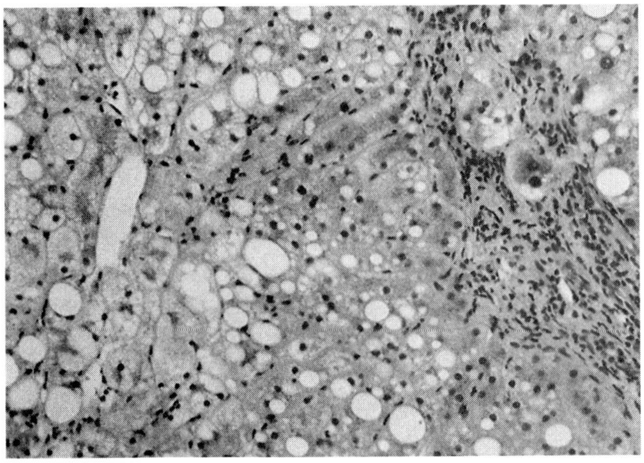

![Figure 57-11]

FIGURE 57-11 Nonalcoholic steatohepatitis (hematoxylin and eosin; ×40 original magnification). Courtesy of Dr. L. Burgart, Mayo Clinic and Foundation.

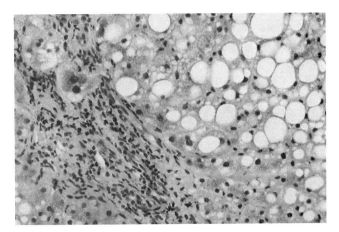

FIGURE 57-12 Nonalcoholic steatohepatitis. Note inflammatory infiltrate and macrovesicular steatosis (hematoxylin and eosin; ×100 original magnification). Courtesy of Dr. L. Burgart, Mayo Clinic and Foundation.

feeding and the cycling of TPN to nighttime feeding alone has also helped restore the natural process of gallbladder emptying and has protected the liver from injury.

The earliest biochemical abnormality is an increase in serum bile acids.[228] Hyperbilirubinemia and increases in serum alkaline phosphatase and γ-glutamyltransferase occur later. Usually, there is associated hepatomegaly. Ultrasonographic findings may show evidence of steatosis.[230] More commonly, biliary sludge and cholelithiasis can be seen, especially in premature infants who have received diuretic therapy. The development of sludge (calcium bilirubinate) occurs in 100% of infants receiving TPN for more than 6 weeks. However, gallstones develop in only a small proportion of patients. Among those patients, incidental ultrasonographic findings may be all that are documented; other patients have clear evidence of cholelithiasis and choledocholithiasis, with cholecystitis, pancreatitis, or both.

Early pathologic features consist of lobular cholestasis.[222–226] Portal inflammation and bile duct proliferation suggestive of obstruction may be present. Canalicular and cytoplasmic bile stasis, a common feature, occurs later. Giant cell transformation, indicative of a regenerative response, may occur. The lesion progresses to fibrosis and micronodular cirrhosis in a minority of patients (Figure 57-13).

The exact mechanism of TPN-related liver disease is unknown. The most important aspect of this cholestasis seems to be an exacerbation of the physiologically poor enterohepatic bile circulation already present in infants and children.

The physiologic immaturity of the enterohepatic circulation of bile is accompanied by an immaturity of the bile acid metabolism. For example, the gradient of bile acid synthesis that exists in the liver of the adult does not exist in the liver of the infant.[228] The physiologic concentration of serum bile acid in infants is clearly in the pathologic range for the adult. The result is a decreased bile acid pool, decreased circulation, increased concentration of serum bile acids, and decreased concentration of canalicular bile acid.

In animal studies, intravenous infusion of amino acids results in decreased output of bile. Infusion of large quanti-

ties of protein results in earlier and more severe cholestasis.[229] The combination of enteral starvation and parenteral nutrition results in the decrease or cessation of several hormonal stimulatory activities that are essential for proper enterohepatic circulation of bile. The lack of cholecystokinin, glucagon, insulin, and secretion affects not only cholestasis but also the formation of extrahepatic biliary sludge.

The short-bowel syndrome is associated with loss of surface area and interruption of the bile acid enterohepatic circulation. Moreover, loss of the ileocecal valve results in bacterial overgrowth, which is accompanied by increased translocation of bacteria into the bloodstream and increased incidence of septic episodes. Sepsis, especially with gramnegative enteric bacteria, can lead to dysregulation of the multidrug resistance protein 2 transport protein. The dependency of certain children on TPN for survival has led to the development of intestinal transplant as a lifesaving procedure. Occasionally, a combined liver–small bowel transplant is needed simply because of the development of end-stage liver disease from a combination of factors, including TPN.

The antioxidant role of vitamin E, selenium, and zinc in protecting the parenchyma and preventing chronic inflammation is not known.

Steatosis occurs with increased caloric intake in the form of glucose. There is a direct correlation between the amount of glucose given and the development of steatosis. The condition is usually asymptomatic, but mild increases in serum transaminases are not unusual (Figure 57-14).

HERBAL THERAPY AND THE LIVER

The use of herbal medicines has increased during the past few years. Clinicians should ask patients whether they use herbal supplements or traditional remedies because herbal therapy may be associated with liver abnormalities.

A definition of *herb* is "a plant or plant part valued for its medicinal, savory, or aromatic qualities."[231] This broad definition includes plants and trees and their products or parts as possible sources of herbal products. Herbal products are also considered to be nutritional supplements

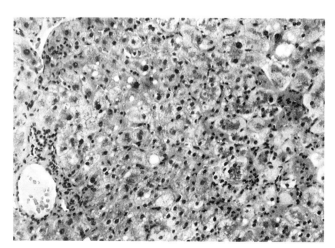

FIGURE 57-13 Total parenteral nutrition cholestasis (hematoxylin and eosin; ×40 original magnification). Courtesy of Dr. L. Burgart, Mayo Clinic and Foundation.

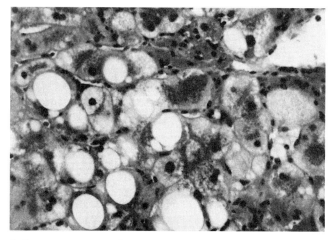

FIGURE 57-14 Total parenteral nutrition–associated steatosis (hematoxylin and eosin; ×100 original magnification). Courtesy of Dr. L. Burgart, Mayo Clinic and Foundation.

because they may contain a vitamin, an amino acid, or a trace element.

The classification of herbs and nutritional supplements as dietary supplements by the Dietary Supplement Health and Education Act of 1994 is outside the jurisdiction of many of the safety and regulatory rules that cover these categories. The purity and composition of products, as well as the consistency of dosages on labels, have varied. Some products were found to contain unlabeled compounds, and others were found to have significant heavy metal (lead) content. Table 57-8 shows the documented cases of hepatotoxicity associated with the use of herbal medicines.

CELIAC DISEASE

The liver is involved in celiac disease in several forms.[232-236] Chronic malnutrition may lead to hepatic steatosis and fatty liver that is indistinguishable from the condition in kwashiorkor. Similar mechanisms of fatty acid mobilization occur in celiac disease and kwashiorkor (see Chapter 44.1, "Celiac Disease")

A few patients with celiac disease present with increases in liver enzymes. Concentrations of serum transaminases are usually increased two to five times the upper limit of the reference range. The patient may have subtle signs of malabsorption, such as iron or folate deficiency, or only growth failure. Overt symptoms, such as diarrhea, muscle wasting, and irritability, may also be present. The increases in enzymes resolve with the elimination of gluten from the diet. The exact pathogenesis of the liver involvement in celiac disease is not known but is presumed to be autoimmune.

Histologic evaluation shows nonspecific hepatitis, chronic active hepatitis, and, rarely, cryptogenic cirrhosis. A few reports of an association with primary sclerosing cholangitis show that the liver lesion does not improve with a gluten-free diet.

Celiac disease occurs with other autoimmune diseases, such as diabetes mellitus and Hashimoto thyroiditis, and in patients with Down syndrome. The association of diabetes and celiac disease may result in both steatosis from poorly controlled diabetes and chronic malnutrition. Awareness of these associations is important in the consideration of associated liver disease.

Celiac disease has also been associated with sarcoidosis. Therefore, the liver may be secondarily affected by granulomatous changes as well.

ENDOCRINE DISEASE

HYPOPITUITARISM

The constellation of hypoglycemia, nystagmus, and cholestasis should prompt evaluation for hypopituitarism.[237,238] Hypopituitarism occurs in association with the absence of the septum pellucidum and septo-optic dysplasia. The lack of thyroid hormones and cortisol affects the bile acid–independent fraction of bile flow in the liver, with resultant cholestasis. In male infants, a micropenis may be evident. The cholestasis is similar to the cholestasis from other neonatal causes and can be

associated with acholic stools. Acholic stools occur in obstructive lesions and hepatocellular disorders such as idiopathic neonatal hepatitis and α_1-antitrypsin deficiency. Hepatomegaly may be present.

Histologic cholestasis and neonatal hepatitis have been associated with hypopituitarism. The findings are nonspecific. The jaundice is initially due to an indirect hyperbilirubinemia, and it eventually develops into a mixed hyperbilirubinemia. Treatment is aimed at the underlying disorder, and rapid correction of the cholestasis occurs with initiation of thyroid and adrenal hormone replacement therapy.

HYPOTHYROIDISM

The association of neonatal hypothyroidism and jaundice is well described.[239-242] About 20% of infants with hypothyroidism have jaundice, which is due to indirect hyperbilirubinemia and presumably to the lack of maturation of the conjugation enzymes. Abnormal bile flow may also be present.

In older children and adolescents, liver and thyroid disease are associated with autoimmune disease. The association of Hashimoto thyroiditis with hypergammaglobulinemia occurs in about 70% of the patients. The association of autoimmune chronic active hepatitis and autoimmune thyroid disease is well known. Thyroid disease may precede or follow the development of liver disease.[243]

DIABETES MELLITUS

In patients with diabetes mellitus, the liver may be involved in several ways.[243-247] The aforementioned association between celiac disease, chronic active hepatitis, and diabetes may result in chronic liver inflammation, steatosis, or even steatohepatitis, also seen in children with diabetes alone who have poor glycemic control. Poor glycemic control results in the accumulation of glycogen in the liver and hepatomegaly. The degree of hepatomegaly correlates with the amount of glycogen deposited and hence with the duration and severity of the diabetes.

There is also an association between diabetes and the development of cholelithiasis.

TABLE 57-8	HERBAL MEDICINES ASSOCIATED WITH DOCUMENTED CASES OF HEPATOTOXICITY

Soy phytoestrogens
Green tea leaf
Pyrrolizidine alkaloids and Jamaican tea preparations
Anthronoids
Protoberberine alkaloids
Germander (*Teucrium* spp)
Herbs rich in coumarin
Herbs rich in podophyllotoxin
Impila (*Callilepis laureola*) root
Kava (*Piper methysticum*) rhizome
Kombucha
Ma huang (*Ephedra* spp)
Skullcap (*Scutellaria* spp)

Adapted from Bauer BA. Herbal therapy: what a clinician needs to know to counsel patients effectively. Mayo Clin Proc 2000;75:835–41.

AUTOIMMUNE POLYGLANDULAR SYNDROME TYPE I

The association of autoimmune disease and its effect on the parathyroid glands, adrenal glands, and ovaries constitutes autoimmune polyglandular syndrome type 1,[248] which includes an association of mucocutaneous candidiasis and autoimmune hepatitis. The autoimmune hepatitis (type 2) is liver, kidney, and microsomal antibody positive. Liver disease occurs after the earlier manifestations in other organs. Hypocalcemia is common and is often exacerbated by the administration of corticosteroids for control of the liver lesion. Screening for the development of autoimmune hepatitis, with at least yearly serum liver enzyme determinations, is essential (see Chapter 48, "Systemic Endocrinopathies").

RENAL DISEASE

The association of liver and renal disease is well recognized.[249–256] Renal and hepatic disease occur concomitantly in both hepatitis C and B and in patients on dialysis. Liver abnormalities can occur in cases of glomerulonephritis and in hemolytic uremic syndrome as well. Some anomalies, such as autosomal recessive polycystic kidney disease and congenital hepatic fibrosis, affect both organs, but the degree of disease in the liver and kidney can be variable. In the infantile form of polycystic kidney disease, early renal failure predominates, whereas in Caroli disease, the liver lesion is predominant. Both entities are covered in detail elsewhere in this textbook. When hepatopathy is present in the dialysis or renal transplant patient, the liver involvement is usually attributed to viral infections, immunosuppressive medications, opportunistic infections, or iron overload.

GENETIC SYNDROMES WITH LIVER INVOLVEMENT

Liver disease is a component of many genetic syndromes (Table 57-9). Three recently reported syndromes with concomitant liver involvement are described below.

HEREDITARY FETAL GROWTH RETARDATION WITH AMINOACIDURIA, CHOLESTASIS, IRON OVERLOAD, AND LACTIC ACIDOSIS

This new genetic disease was recently described in 17 newborns from Finland. The characteristic findings are growth retardation with Fanconi-like aminoaciduria, cholestasis, and iron overload. The patients have increased serum ferritin concentrations and hypotransferrinemia. The acronym GRACILE is used to summarize the findings. Treatment in two cases with apotransferrin and exchange transfusion resulted in prolonged survival and growth. The disease locus was assigned to 2q33-37.[257]

FAMILIAL PROGRESSIVE TUBULOINTERSTITIAL NEPHROPATHY AND CHOLESTATIC LIVER DISEASE

This recently described entity is characterized by tubular nephropathy and sclerosed glomeruli with intrahepatic biliary ductular irregularities akin to primary sclerosing cholangitis. Histologically, the liver shows fibrosis with enlarged portal areas and biliary ductular proliferation. Serum concentrations of liver-derived enzymes are moderately increased.[258]

RENAL HEPATIC PANCREATIC DYSPLASIA WITH MULTIPLE CONGENITAL ANOMALIES

Syndromes of renal hepatic pancreatic dysplasias may be grouped together as dysplastic syndromes of several organs. The association of renal, hepatic, and pancreatic abnormalities is a constant feature.[259]

MISCELLANEOUS DISORDERS

AMYLOIDOSIS

Amyloid is an amorphous protein, and amyloidosis is the resultant end-organ damage from deposition of amyloid protein.[260–264] The two major amyloid proteins are designated "AL" for primary amyloid and "AA" for secondary amyloid. Primary amyloid consists of the light chain of immunoglobulin. Secondary amyloid or serum amyloid is associated with chronic inflammation. It appears to be secreted by the liver as an acute-phase reactant. Amyloid is deposited in the gastrointestinal tract, liver, and renal tissue as the result of chronic inflammation. The condition is rare in children younger than 15 years. Cystic fibrosis is the most common association, with reports of up to one-third of the patients having amyloidosis at autopsy. The association has been reported in familial Mediterranean fever, JRA, and tuberculosis as well. The association of hepatomegaly and proteinuria with a chronic inflammatory condition should prompt the search for amyloid in rectal and renal tissue. Also, a liver biopsy may be the first diagnostic test performed when a patient has silent hepatomegaly (Figures 57-15 and 57-16). There is no correlation between the degree of amyloidosis and the increases in liver enzymes.[265,266]

SARCOIDOSIS

Sarcoidosis is a multisystemic chronic granulomatous disease of unknown cause.[267–270] It is associated with Crohn disease, celiac disease, lymphoma, Addison disease, thyroiditis, and the use of various drugs. The lung is the organ involved most often. Hepatomegaly is a late phenomenon, occurring in about one-third of the patients. The differential diagnosis centers on the association of other granulomatous diseases, such as chronic drug therapy, cat-scratch disease, and immunodeficiency (Table 57-10). Long-standing sarcoidosis leads to portal hypertension, with minimal increases in liver enzymes, and eventually to fibrosis and micronodular cirrhosis. Treatment with corticosteroids and, eventually, methotrexate is advocated in reports of adult patients.

BEHÇET SYNDROME

Behçet syndrome is a multisystemic disorder characterized by ocular, mucocutaneous, articular, vascular, gastrointestinal tract, and neurologic abnormalities.[60,271–274] The clinical syndrome consists of recurrent oral, genital, and gastrointestinal tract ulcers. The association with uveitis, arthritis, and renal amyloidosis is well known. The association of

TABLE 57-9 CHARACTERISTIC FEATURES OF GENETIC DISEASES WITH LIVER INVOLVEMENT

DIAGNOSIS	AGE AT ONSET*	FEATURES
Galactosemia, tyrosinemia, neonatal iron storage disease	Neonate; infant	Jaundice, ascites, edema, coagulopathy, lethargy, sepsis, hypogylcemia, hyperammonemia, hepatitis, growth retardation, lactic acidosis, cholestasis, hypotransferrinemia
Fructosemia	Infant, with introduction of fructose	Jaundice, ascites, coagulopathy, lethargy, hypoglycemia, acidosis, hyperammonemia, phosphorus abnormalities, hepatitis
Neonatal iron storage disease	48 h	Cholestasis, coagulopathy, and liver failure (prominent); hepatitis (mild)
Inborn error of bile acid synthesis	48 h	Similar to neonatal iron storage disease; normal GGT
Ataxia telangiectasia	Infant; child	Features of ataxia telangiectasia, immunodeficiency, autoimmune markers, mild hepatitis, and steatohepatitis
SYNDROMES WITH CHOLESTASIS AND HEPATOMEGALY		
Inborn errors of bile acid metabolism	Neonatal	Mild hepatitis, normal or low GGT
Familial cholestasis	Infant; child	PFIC 1: family history features; PFIC 1 and 2: low GGT, paucity of bile ducts; PFIC 3: proliferation of bile ducts; family history of gallstones; cholestasis during pregnancy
α_1-Antitrypsin deficiency	Neonate; infant	Acholic stools, hepatomegaly
Galactosemia	As above	As above
Tyrosinemia	As above	As above
Fructosemia	As above	As above
Niemann-Pick type C	Neonate; infant	Jaundice, neurologic signs
Peroxisomal disorders	Neonate; infant	Hypotonia; low or normal GGT; varied presentations: neurologic, renal, hepatic
Adrenoleukodystrophy, Zellweger syndrome, pipecolic acidemia	Infant	As in peroxisomal disorders; hypotonia with poor sucking and retinal pigmentation, fibrosis and cirrhosis, abnormal very-long-chain fatty acids, normal GGT
Tubular nephropathy and cholestasis	Child	PSC-like with tubular nephropathy, familial pattern
Cystic fibrosis	Infant	Meconium ileus equivalent
SYNDROMES WITH HEPATOMEGALY		
Glycogenosis, types I and III; Wolman disease; familial adenomatous polyposis	Infant; 1 mo to first years	Hypoglycemia; variable clinical and metabolic features; liver with normal consistency; splenomegaly (unlike glycogenosis, type I); Wolman disease: diarrhea, vomiting, organomegaly, foam cells in the marrow, lysosomal acid lipase deficiency with storage of triglycerides and cholesterol esters, adrenal calcifications (a hallmark); familial adenomatous polyposis associated with hepatoblastoma
Glutaricaciduria, type II	Neonate	Respiratory and cardiac failure at birth with hepatomegaly
Mucopolysaccharidosis, types I and II; α-mannosidosis; fucosidosis	Neonate; infant	Progressive neurologic deterioration, splenomegaly
α_1-Antitrypsin deficiency; congenital hepatic fibrosis; glycogenosis, type IV; carbohydrate-deficient glycoprotein; fibrosis	0–6 yr	With or without splenomegaly, hard liver, portal hypertension, carbohydrate-deficient glycoprotein syndromes with intractable diarrhea and developmental delay
Cystic fibrosis, congenital hepatic fibrosis, α_1-antitrypsin deficiency, Wilson disease	Variable: 3–6 yr or later	Portal hypertension, varices, cirrhosis, typical features of biliary ectasia with fibrosis
Sialidosis, type II; mucolipidosis; Gaucher disease; mucolipidosis, type II	Early infant	Coarse features, ocular symptoms, bone changes, vacuolated lymphocytes

GGT = γ-glutamyltransferase; PFIC = progressive familial intrahepatic cholestasis; PSC = primary sclerosing cholangitis.
*Age categories: neonate, 0–4 weeks; infant, 0–12 months; child, 1 year to puberty.

hepatic vein thrombosis and Behçet syndrome was described in a report of four cases, with a review of 17 previously published cases. There was a male preponderance; the inferior vena cava was thrombosed in 90% of the patients, and the thrombosis was acute in one-third of the patients.[273]

CONCLUSION

The liver is a frequent target in systemic diseases because of its complexity and its central role in homeostasis, xenobiotic metabolism, defense against endogenous and exogenous insults, and regulation of the vascular space.

In this chapter, cellular and molecular events were linked to pathophysiologic and clinical correlates of disease. However, to cover every aspect of liver involvement in these disorders is beyond the scope of this chapter, and many subjects are covered in detail elsewhere in this textbook.

ACKNOWLEDGMENTS

We are indebted to Dr. Lawrence J. Burgart in the Department of Laboratory Medicine and Pathology, Mayo Clinic, for providing the pathology slides and to Nick A. Hegg for secretarial assistance.

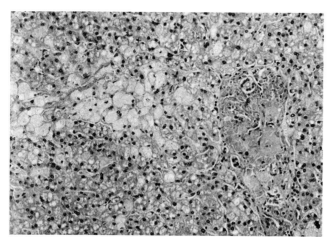

FIGURE 57-15 Amyloidosis, low power (hematoxylin and eosin). Courtesy of Dr. L. Burgart, Mayo Clinic and Foundation.

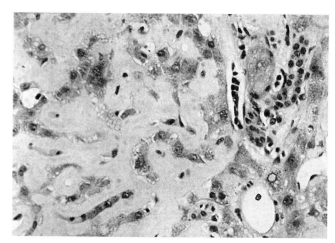

FIGURE 57-16 Amyloidosis (hematoxylin and eosin; ×100 original magnification). Courtesy of Dr. L. Burgart, Mayo Clinic and Foundation.

TABLE 57-10   GRANULOMATOUS HEPATITIS

Tuberculosis
Mycobacterial infections
Brucellosis
Typhoid fever
Listeriosis
Cat-scratch disease
Histoplasmosis
Aspergillosis
Candidiasis
Cryptococcus
Actinomycosis
Syphilis
Visceral larva migrans
Schistosomiasis
Q fever
Ehrlichiosis
Cytomegalovirus infection
Epstein-Barr infection
Erythema nodosum
Drug reaction
Systemic lupus erythematosus
Juvenile rheumatoid arthritis
Histiocytosis
Lymphoma
Sarcoidosis

REFERENCES

1. Carlton VE, Knisely AS, Freimer NB. Mapping of a locus for progressive familial intrahepatic cholestasis (Byler disease) to 18q21-q22, the benign recurrent intrahepatic cholestasis region. Hum Mol Genet 1995;4:1049–53.

2. Bull LN, van Eijk MJ, Pawlikowska L, et al. A gene encoding a P-type ATPase mutated in two forms of hereditary cholestasis. Nat Genet 1998;18:219–24.

3. Bull LN, Carlton VE, Stricker NL, et al. Genetic and morphological findings in progressive familial intrahepatic cholestasis (Byler disease [PFIC-1] and Byler syndrome): evidence for heterogeneity. Hepatology 1997;26:155–64.

4. Strautnieks SS, Kagalwalla AF, Tanner MS, et al. Identification of a locus for progressive familial intrahepatic cholestasis PFIC2 on chromosome 2q24. Am J Hum Genet 1997;61:630–3.

5. Strautnieks SS, Bull LN, Knisely AS, et al. A gene encoding a liver-specific ABC transporter is mutated in progressive familial intrahepatic cholestasis. Nat Genet 1998;20:233–8.

6. de Vree JM, Jacquemin E, Sturm E, et al. Mutations in the *MDR3* gene cause progressive familial intrahepatic cholestasis. Proc Natl Acad Sci U S A 1998;95:282–7.

7. Boland EW, Willius FA. Changes in the liver produced by chronic passive congestion: with special reference to problems of cardiac cirrhosis. Arch Intern Med 1938;62:723–39.

8. Maher JJ, McGuire RF. Extracellular matrix gene expression increases preferentially in rat lipocytes and sinusoidal endothelial cells during hepatic fibrosis in vivo. J Clin Invest 1990;86:1641–8.

9. Gressner AM. Cytokines and cellular crosstalk involved in the activation of fat-storing cells. J Hepatol 1995;22:28–36.

10. Friedman SL, Arthur MJ. Activation of cultured rat hepatic lipocytes by Kupffer cell conditioned medium: direct enhancement of matrix synthesis and stimulation of cell proliferation via induction of platelet-derived growth factor receptors. J Clin Invest 1989;84:1780–5.

11. Ramadori G, Christ B. Cytokines and the hepatic acute-phase response. Semin Liver Dis 1999;19:141–55.

12. Bissell DM, Friedman SL, Maher JJ, Roll FJ. Connective tissue biology and hepatic fibrosis: report of a conference. Hepatology 1990;11:488–98.

13. Yanagisawa M. The endothelin system: a new target for therapeutic intervention. Circulation 1994;89:1320–2.

14. Isobe H, Satoh M, Sakai H, Nawata H. Increased plasma endothelin-1 levels in patients with cirrhosis and esophageal varices. J Clin Gastroenterol 1993;17:227–30.

15. Asbert M, Gines A, Gines P, et al. Circulating levels of endothelin in cirrhosis. Gastroenterology 1993;104:1485–91.

16. Rockey DC, Fouassier L, Chung JJ, et al. Cellular localization of endothelin-1 and increased production in liver injury in the rat: potential for autocrine and paracrine effects on stellate cells. Hepatology 1998;27:472–80.

17. Mittal MK, Gupta TK, Lee FY, et al. Nitric oxide modulates hepatic vascular tone in normal rat liver. Am J Physiol 1994;267:G416–22.

18. Gupta TK, Chen L, Groszman RJ. Pathophysiology of portal hypertension. Baillieres Clin Gastroenterol 1997;11:203–19.

19. Jungermann K, Katz N. Functional specialization of different hepatocyte populations. Physiol Rev 1989;69:708–64.

20. Jacquemin E, Saliba E, Blond MH, et al. Liver dysfunction and acute cardiocirculatory failure in children. Eur J Pediatr 1992;151:731–4.

21. Papagiannis J, Kanter RJ, Effman EL, et al. Polysplenia with pulmonary arteriovenous malformations. Pediatr Cardiol 1993;14:127–9.

22. Akita H, Ohta A, Furukawa S, et al. Newborn with congenital arteriovenous fistulas of the abdominal wall complicated by a ductus arteriosus aneurysm. Pediatr Cardiol 1995;16:235–8.

23. Henrion J, De Maeght S, Schapira M, et al. Hypoxic hepatitis: a difficult diagnosis when the cardiomyopathy remains unrecognized and the course of liver enzymes follows an atypical pattern. A report of two cases. Acta Gastroenterol Belg 1998;61:385–9.

24. Mace S, Borkat G, Liebman J. Hepatic dysfunction and cardiovascular abnormalities: occurrence in infants, children, and young adults. Am J Dis Child 1985;139:60–5.

25. Weinberg AG, Bolande RP. The liver in congenital heart disease: effects of infantile coarctation of the aorta and the hypoplastic left heart syndrome in infancy. Am J Dis Child 1970;119:390–4.

26. Gibson PR, Dudley FJ. Ischemic hepatitis: clinical features, diagnosis and prognosis. Aust N Z J Med 1984;14:822–5.

27. Garland JS, Werlin SL, Rice TB. Ischemic hepatitis in children: diagnosis and clinical course. Crit Care Med 1988;16:1209–12.

28. Shiraki K. Hepatic cell necrosis in the newborn: a pathologic study of 147 cases, with particular reference to congenital heart disease. Am J Dis Child 1970;119:395–400.

29. Cohen JA, Kaplan MM. Left-sided heart failure presenting as hepatitis. Gastroenterology 1978;74:583–7.

30. Comini L, Gaia G, Curello S, et al. Right heart failure chronically stimulates heat shock protein 72 in heart and liver but not in other tissues. Cardiovasc Res 1996;31:882–90.

31. de la Monte SM, Arcidi JM, Moore GW, Hutchins GM. Midzonal necrosis as a pattern of hepatocellular injury after shock. Gastroenterology 1984;86:627–31.

32. Scheuer PJ. Liver biopsy interpretation. 4th ed. London: Baillière Tindall; 1988.

33. Arcidi JM Jr, Moore GW, Hutchins GM. Hepatic morphology in cardiac dysfunction: a clinicopathologic study of 1000 subjects at autopsy. Am J Pathol 1981;104:159–66.

34. Nouel O, Henrion J, Bernuau J, et al. Fulminant hepatic failure due to transient circulatory failure in patients with chronic heart disease. Dig Dis Sci 1980;25:49–52.

35. Katzin HM, Waller JV, Blumgart HL. "Cardiac cirrhosis" of the liver: a clinical and pathologic study. Arch Intern Med 1939;64:457–70.

36. Shibayama Y. The role of hepatic venous congestion and endotoxaemia in the production of fulminant hepatic failure secondary to congestive heart failure. J Pathol 1987;151:133–8.

37. Lefkowitch JH, Mendez L. Morphologic features of hepatic injury in cardiac disease and shock. J Hepatol 1986;2:313–27.

38. Holley HC, Koslin DB, Berland LL, Stanley RJ. Inhomogeneous enhancement of liver parenchyma secondary to passive congestion: contrast-enhanced CT. Radiology 1989;170:795–800.

39. Welling RE, Rath R, Albers JE, Glasser RS. Gastrointestinal complications after cardiac surgery. Arch Surg 1986;121:1178–80.

40. Jenkins JG, Lynn AM, Wood AE, et al. Acute hepatic failure following cardiac operation in children. J Thorac Cardiovasc Surg 1982;84:865–71.

41. Lockey E, McIntyre N, Ross DN, et al. Early jaundice after open-heart surgery. Thorax 1967;22:165–9.

42. Olsson R, Hermodsson S, Roberts D, Waldenström J. Hepatic dysfunction after open-heart surgery. Scand J Thorac Cardiovasc Surg 1984;18:217–22.

43. Kingsley DP. Hepatic damage following profound hypothermia and extracorporeal circulation in man. Thorax 1966;21:91–8.

44. Lunel F, Cadranel JF, Rosenheim M, et al. Hepatitis virus infections in heart transplant recipients: epidemiology, natural history, characteristics, and impact on survival. Gastroenterology 2000;119:1064–74.

45. Moller JH, Nakib A, Anderson RC, et al. Congenital cardiac disease associated with polyspenia: a developmental complex of bilateral "left-sidedness." Circulation 1967;36:789–99.

46. Klatskin G. Hepatitis associated with systemic infections. In: Zakim D, Boyer TD, editors. Hepatology: a textbook of liver disease. Philadelphia: WB Saunders; 1975. p. 711–3.

47. Miller DJ, Keeton DG, Webber BL, et al. Jaundice in severe bacterial infection. Gastroenterology 1976;71:94–7.

48. Fahrländer H, Huber F, Gloor F. Intrahepatic retention of bile in severe bacterial infections. Gastroenterology 1964;47:590–9.

49. Hamilton JR, Sass-Kortsak A. Jaundice associated with severe bacterial infection in young infants. J Pediatr 1963;63:121–32.

50. Moseley RH, Wang W, Takeda H, et al. Effect of endotoxin on bile acid transport in rat liver: a potential model for sepsis-associated cholestasis. Am J Physiol 1996;271:G137–46.

51. Seeler RA, Hahn K. Jaundice in urinary tract infection in infancy. Am J Dis Child 1969;118:553–8.

52. Kubitz R, Wettstein M, Warskulat U, Haussinger D. Regulation of the multidrug resistance protein 2 in the rat liver by lipopolysaccharide and dexamethasone. Gastroenterology 1999;116:401–10.

53. Franson TR, Hierholzer WJ Jr, LaBrecque DR. Frequency and characteristics of hyperbilirubinemia associated with bacteremia. Rev Infect Dis 1985;7:1–9.

54. Everett ED, Evans KA, Henry RB, McDonald G. Human ehrlichiosis in adults after tick exposure: diagnosis using polymerase chain reaction. Ann Intern Med 1994;120:730–5.

55. Yu X, Brouqui P, Dumler JS, Raoult D. Detection of *Ehrlichia chaffeensis* in human tissue by using a species-specific monoclonal antibody. J Clin Microbiol 1993;31:3284–8.

56. Moskovitz M, Fadden R, Min T. Human ehrlichiosis: a rickettsial disease associated with severe cholestasis and multisystemic disease. J Clin Gastroenterol 1991;13:86–90.

57. Thorne C, Urowitz MB, Wanless I, et al. Liver disease in Felty's syndrome. Am J Med 1982;73:35–40.

58. Rachelefsky GS, Kar NC, Coulson A, et al. Serum enzyme abnormalities in juvenile rheumatoid arthritis. Pediatrics 1976;58:730–6.

59. Kornreich H, Malouf NN, Hanson V. Acute hepatic dysfunction in juvenile rheumatoid arthritis. J Pediatr 1971;79:27–35.

60. Case records of the Massachusetts General Hospital. Weekly clinicopathological exercises: case 40-1993. A 61-year-old woman with jaundice, anemia, thrombocytopenia, and leukocytosis. N Engl J Med 1993;329:1108–15.

61. Rich RR, Johnson JS. Salicylate hepatotoxicity in patients with juvenile rheumatoid arthritis. Arthritis Rheum 1973;16:1–9.

62. Rennebohm RM, Heubi JE, Daugherty CC, Daniels SR. Reye syndrome in children receiving salicylate therapy for connective tissue disease. J Pediatr 1985;107:877–80.

63. Young RS, Torretti D, Williams RH, et al. Reye's syndrome associated with long-term aspirin therapy. JAMA 1984;251:754–6.

64. Remington PL, Shabino CL, McGee H, et al. Reye syndrome and juvenile rheumatoid arthritis in Michigan. Am J Dis Child 1985;139:870–2.

65. Smith ME, Ansell BM, Bywaters EG. Mortality and prognosis

related to the amyloidosis of Still's disease. Ann Rheum Dis 1968;27:137–45

66. Mortensen ME, Rennebohm RM. Clinical pharmacology and use of nonsteroidal anti-inflammatory drugs. Pediatr Clin North Am 1989;36:1113–39.

67. Willkens RF, Leonard PA, Clegg DO, et al. Liver histology in patients receiving low dose pulse methotrexate for the treatment of rheumatoid arthritis. Ann Rheum Dis 1990;49:591–3.

68. Giannini EH, Brewer EJ, Kuzmina N, et al. Methotrexate in resistant juvenile rheumatoid arthritis: results of the U.S.A.-U.S.S.R. double-blind, placebo-controlled trial. The Pediatric Rheumatology Collaborative Study Group and The Cooperative Children's Study Group. N Engl J Med 1992;326:1043–9.

69. Kremer JM, Lee RG, Tolman KG. Liver histology in rheumatoid arthritis patients receiving long-term methotrexate therapy: a prospective study with baseline and sequential biopsy samples. Arthritis Rheum 1989;32:121–7.

70. Graham LD, Myones BL, Rivas-Chacon RF, Pachman LM. Morbidity associated with long-term methotrexate therapy in juvenile rheumatoid arthritis. J Pediatr 1992;120:468–73.

71. Rose CD, Singsen BH, Eichenfield AH, et al. Safety and efficacy of methotrexate therapy for juvenile rheumatoid arthritis. J Pediatr 1990;117:653–9.

72. Miller MH, Urowitz MB, Gladman DD, Blendis LM. The liver in systemic lupus erythematosus. QJM 1984;53:401–9.

73. Leggett BA. The liver in systemic lupus erythematosus. J Gastroenterol Hepatol 1993;8:84–8.

74. Norris DG, Colon AR, Stickler GB. Systemic lupus erythematosus in children: the complex problems of diagnosis and treatment encountered in 101 such patients at the Mayo Clinic. Clin Pediatr (Phila) 1977;16:774–8.

75. Runyon BA, LaBrecque DR, Anuras S. The spectrum of liver disease in systemic lupus erythematosus: report of 33 histologically-proved cases and review of the literature. Am J Med 1980;69:187–94.

76. Gibson T, Myers AR. Subclinical liver disease in systemic lupus erythematosus. J Rheumatol 1981;8:752–9.

77. Matsumoto T, Yoshimine T, Shimouchi K, et al. The liver in systemic lupus erythematosus: pathologic analysis of 52 cases and review of Japanese Autopsy Registry Data. Hum Pathol 1992;23:1151–8.

78. Keshavarzian A, Rentsch R, Hodgson HJ. Clinical implications of liver biopsy findings in collagen-vascular disorders. J Clin Gastroenterol 1993;17:219–26.

79. Laxer RM, Roberts EA, Gross KR, et al. Liver disease in neonatal lupus erythematosus. J Pediatr 1990;116:238–42.

80. Rosh JR, Silverman ED, Groisman G, et al. Intrahepatic cholestasis in neonatal lupus erythematosus. J Pediatr Gastroenterol Nutr 1993;17:310–2.

81. Bernstein ML, Salusinsky-Sternbach M, Bellefleur M, Esseltine DW. Thrombotic and hemorrhagic complications in children with the lupus anticoagulant. Am J Dis Child 1984;138:1132–5.

82. Hirasaki S, Koide N, Ogawa H, et al. Mixed connective tissue disease associated with idiopathic portal hypertension and chronic thyroiditis. J Gastroenterol 1997;32:808–11.

83. Rowley AH, Shulman ST. Kawasaki syndrome. Pediatr Clin North Am 1999;46:313–29.

84. Rosenblate HJ, Eisenstein R, Holmes AW. The liver in sickle cell anemia. A clinical-pathologic study. Arch Pathol 1970;90:235–45.

85. Sheehy TW. Sickle cell hepatopathy. South Med J 1977;70:533–8.

86. Omata M, Johnson CS, Tong M, Tatter D. Pathological spectrum of liver diseases in sickle cell disease. Dig Dis Sci 1986;31:247–56.

87. Diggs LW. Sickle cell crises. Am J Clin Pathol 1965;44:1–4.

88. Yohannan MD, Arif M, Ramia S. Aetiology of icteric hepatitis and fulminant hepatic failure in children and the possible predisposition to hepatic failure by sickle cell disease. Acta Paediatr Scand 1990;79:201–5.

89. Bainbridge R, Khoury J, Mimouni F. Jaundice in neonates with sickle cell disease: a case-control study. Am J Dis Child 1988;142:569–72.

90. Descos B, Bernard O, Brunelle F, et al. Pigment gallstones of the common bile duct in infancy. Hepatology 1984;4:678–83.

91. Borgna-Pignatti C, De Stefano P, Pajno D, et al. Cholelithiasis in children with thalassemia major: an ultrasonographic study. J Pediatr 1981;99:243–4.

92. Stephens CG, Scott RB. Cholelithiasis in sickle cell anemia: surgical or medical management. Arch Intern Med 1980;140:648–51.

93. Malone BS, Werlin SL. Cholecystectomy and cholelithiasis in sickle cell anemia. Am J Dis Child 1988;142:799–800.

94. DeVault KR, Friedman LS, Westerberg S, et al. Hepatitis C in sickle cell anemia. J Clin Gastroenterol 1994;18:206–9.

95. Winter SS, Kinney TR, Ware RE. Gallbladder sludge in children with sickle cell disease. J Pediatr 1994;125:747–9.

96. Jean G, Terzoli S, Mauri R, et al. Cirrhosis associated with multiple transfusions in thalassaemia. Arch Dis Child 1984;59:67–70.

97. Jensen PD, Jensen FT, Christensen T, et al. Relationship between hepatocellular injury and transfusional iron overload prior to and during iron chelation with desferrioxamine: a study in adult patients with acquired anemias. Blood 2003;101:91–6.

98. Makris M, Preston FE. Chronic hepatitis in haemophilia. Blood Rev 1993;7:243–50.

99. Prati D. Benefits and complications of regular blood transfusion in patients with beta-thalassaemia major. Vox Sang 2000;79:129–37.

100. Simson IW. Membranous obstruction of the inferior vena cava and hepatocellular carcinoma in South Africa. Gastroenterology 1982;82:171–8.

101. Dilawari JB, Bambery P, Chawla Y, et al. Hepatic outflow obstruction (Budd-Chiari syndrome): experience with 177 patients and a review of the literature. Medicine (Baltimore) 1994;73:21–36.

102. Powell-Jackson PR, Ede RJ, Williams R. Budd-Chiari syndrome presenting as fulminant hepatic failure. Gut 1986;27:1101–5.

103. Broekmans AW, Veltkamp JJ, Bertina RM. Congenital protein C deficiency and venous thromboembolism: a study of three Dutch families. N Engl J Med 1983;309:340–4.

104. Klein AS, Cameron JL. Diagnosis and management of the Budd-Chiari syndrome. Am J Surg 1990;160:128–33.

105. Cosnes J, Robert A, Levy VG, Darnis F. Budd-Chiari syndrome in a patient with mixed connective-tissue disease. Dig Dis Sci 1980;25:467–9.

106. Kage M, Arakawa M, Kojiro M, Okuda K. Histopathology of membranous obstruction of the inferior vena cava in the Budd-Chiari syndrome. Gastroenterology 1992;102:2081–90.

107. Hoffman HD, Stockland B, von der Heyden U. Membranous obstruction of the inferior vena cava with Budd-Chiari syndrome in children: a report of nine cases. J Pediatr Gastroenterol Nutr 1987;6:878–84.

108. Mitchell MC, Boitnott JK, Kaufman S, et al. Budd-Chiari syndrome: etiology, diagnosis and management. Medicine (Baltimore) 1982;61:199–218.

109. Gentil-Kocher S, Bernard O, Brunelle F, et al. Budd-Chiari syndrome in children: report of 22 cases. J Pediatr 1988;113:30–8.

110. Rector WG Jr, Xu YH, Goldstein L, et al. Membranous obstruction of the inferior vena cava in the United States. Medicine (Baltimore) 1985;64:134–43.

111. Frank JW, Kamath PS, Stanson AW. Budd-Chiari syndrome: early intervention with angioplasty and thrombolytic therapy. Mayo Clin Proc 1994;69:877–81.

112. Lois JF, Hartzman S, McGlade CT, et al. Budd-Chiari syndrome: treatment with percutaneous transhepatic recanalization and dilation. Radiology 1989;170:791–3.

113. Lopez RR Jr, Benner KG, Hall L, et al. Expandable venous stents for treatment of the Budd-Chiari syndrome. Gastroenterology 1991;100:1435–41.

114. Bismuth H, Sherlock DJ. Portasystemic shunting versus liver transplantation for the Budd-Chiari syndrome. Ann Surg 1991;214:581–9.

115. Lang H, Oldhafer KJ, Kupsch E, et al. Liver transplantation for Budd-Chiari syndrome—palliation or cure? Transpl Int 1994;7:115–9.

116. Wanless IR, Liu JJ, Butany J. Role of thrombosis in the pathogenesis of congestive hepatic fibrosis (cardiac cirrhosis). Hepatology 1995;21:1232–7.

117. Tanaka M, Wanless IR. Pathology of the liver in Budd-Chiari syndrome: portal vein thrombosis and the histogenesis of veno-centric cirrhosis, veno-portal cirrhosis, and large regenerative nodules. Hepatology 1998;27:488–96.

118. Khuroo MS, Datta DV. Budd-Chiari syndrome following pregnancy: report of 16 cases, with roentgenologic, hemodynamic and histologic studies of the hepatic outflow tract. Am J Med 1980;68:113–21.

119. Hoyumpa AM Jr, Schiff L, Helfman EL. Budd-Chiari syndrome in women taking oral contraceptives. Am J Med 1971;50:137–40.

120. Maccini DM, Berg JC, Bell GA. Budd-Chiari syndrome and Crohn's disease: an unreported association. Dig Dis Sci 1989;34:1933–6.

121. Bolondi L, Gaiani S, Li Bassi S, et al. Diagnosis of Budd-Chiari syndrome by pulsed Doppler ultrasound. Gastroenterology 1991;100:1324–31.

122. Stark DD, Hahn PF, Trey C, et al. MRI of the Budd-Chiari syndrome. AJR Am J Roentgenol 1986;146:1141–8.

123. Meindok H, Langer B. Liver scan in Budd-Chiari syndrome. J Nucl Med 1976;17:365–8.

124. Mathieu D, Vasile N, Menu Y, et al. Budd-Chiari syndrome: dynamic CT. Radiology 1987;165:409–13.

125. Moreno-Merlo F, Wanless IR, Shimamatsu K, et al. The role of granulomatous phlebitis and thrombosis in the pathogenesis of cirrhosis and portal hypertension in sarcoidosis. Hepatology 1997;26:554–60.

126. Maddrey WC. Hepatic vein thrombosis (Budd Chiari syndrome): possible association with the use of oral contraceptives. Semin Liver Dis 1987;7:32–9.

127. Stein PE. Nodular regenerative hyperplasia of the liver. Am J Pathol 1959;35:943–53.

128. Sherlock S, Feldman CA, Moran B, Scheuer PJ. Partial nodular transformation of the liver with portal hypertension. Am J Med 1966;40:195–203.

129. Wanless IR, Godwin TA, Allen F, Feder A. Nodular regenerative hyperplasia of the liver in hematologic disorders: a possible response to obliterative portal venopathy: a morphometric study of nine cases with an hypothesis on the pathogenesis. Medicine (Baltimore) 1980;59:367–79.

130. Wanless IR, Lentz JS, Roberts EA. Partial nodular transformation of liver in an adult with persistent ductus venosus.

131. Review with hypothesis on pathogenesis. Arch Pathol Lab Med 1985;109:427–32.

131. Wanless IR, Gryfe A. Nodular transformation of the liver in hereditary hemorrhagic telangiectasia. Arch Pathol Lab Med 1986;110:331–5.

132. Terayama N, Terada T, Hoso M, Nakanuma Y. Partial nodular transformation of the liver with portal vein thrombosis: a report of two autopsy cases. J Clin Gastroenterol 1995;20:71–6.

133. Wanless IR, Mawdsley C, Adams R. On the pathogenesis of focal nodular hyperplasia of the liver. Hepatology 1985;5:1194–200.

134. Elias H, Petty D. Gross anatomy of the blood vessels and ducts within the human liver. Am J Anat 1952;90:59–111.

135. Hadengue A, Poliquin M, Vilgrain V, et al. The changing scene of hepatic vein thrombosis: recognition of asymptomatic cases. Gastroenterology 1994;106:1042–7

136. Heimann P, Ogur G, Debusscher C, et al. Multiple clonal chromosome aberrations in a case of childhood focal nodular hyperplasia of the liver. Cancer Genet Cytogenet 1995;85:138–42.

137. Viola S, Meyer M, Fabre M, et al. Ischemic necrosis of bile ducts complicating Schönlein-Henoch purpura. Gastroenterology 1999;117:211–4.

138. Choi SI, Simone JV. Acute nonlymphocytic leukemia in 171 children. Med Pediatr Oncol 1976;2:119–46.

139. Lewis JH, Patel HR, Zimmerman HJ. The spectrum of hepatic candidiasis. Hepatology 1982;2:479–87.

140. Carstensen H, Widding E, Storm K, et al. Hepatosplenic candidiasis in children with cancer: three cases in leukemic children and a literature review. Pediatr Hematol Oncol 1990;7:3–12.

141. Dich NH, Goodman ZD, Klein MA. Hepatic involvement in Hodgkin's disease: clues to histologic diagnosis. Cancer 1989;64:2121–6.

142. Kadin ME, Donaldson SS, Dorfman RF. Isolated granulomas in Hodgkin's disease. N Engl J Med 1970;283:859–61.

143. Abt AB, Kirschner RH, Belliveau RE, et al. Hepatic pathology associated with Hodgkin's disease. Cancer 1974;33:1564–71.

144. Perera DR, Greene ML, Fenster LF. Cholestasis associated with extrabiliary Hodgkin's disease: report of three cases and review of four others. Gastroenterology 1974;67:680–5.

145. Aisenberg AC, Kaplan MM, Rieder SV, Goldman JM. Serum alkaline phosphatase at the onset of Hodgkin's disease. Cancer 1970;26:318–26.

146. Gunasekaran TS, Hassall E, Dimmick JE, Chan KW. Hodgkin's disease presenting with fulminant liver disease. J Pediatr Gastroenterol Nutr 1992;15:189–93.

147. Malone M. The histiocytoses of childhood. Histopathology 1991;19:105–19.

148. Komp DM. Langerhans cell histiocytosis. N Engl J Med 1987;316:747–8.

149. Geissmann F, Lepelletier Y, Fraitag S, et al. Differentiation of Langerhans cells in Langerhans cell histiocytosis. Blood 2001;97:1241–8.

150. Heyn RM, Hamoudi A, Newton WA Jr. Pretreatment liver biopsy in 20 children with histiocytosis X: a clinicopathologic correlation. Med Pediatr Oncol 1990;18:110–8.

151. Janka GE. Familial hemophagocytic lymphohistiocytosis. Eur J Pediatr 1983;140:221–30.

152. Favara BE. Hemophagocytic lymphohistiocytosis: a hemophagocytic syndrome. Semin Diagn Pathol 1992;9:63–74.

153. Olson NY, Olson LC. Virus-associated hemophagocytic syndrome: relationship to herpes group viruses. Pediatr Infect Dis 1986;5:369–73.

154. Arico M, Danesino C, Pende D, Moretta L. Pathogenesis of haemophagocytic lymphohistiocytosis. Br J Haematol 2001; 111:761–9.

155. Rand EB, Whitington PF. Successful orthotopic liver transplantation in two patients with liver failure due to sclerosing cholangitis with Langerhans cell histiocytosis. J Pediatr Gastroenterol Nutr 1992;15:202–7.

156. Risdall RJ, McKenna RW, Nesbit ME, et al. Virus-associated hemophagocytic syndrome: a benign histiocytic proliferation distinct from malignant histiocytosis. Cancer 1979;44:993–1002.

157. Debray D, Pariente D, Urvoas E, et al. Sclerosing cholangitis in children. J Pediatr 1994;124:49–56.

158. Haddad E, Sulis ML, Jabado N, et al. Frequency and severity of central nervous system lesions in hemophagocytic lymphohistiocytosis. Blood 1997;89:794–800.

159. Squires RH Jr, Weinberg AG, Zwiener RJ, Winick N. Langerhans' cell histiocytosis presenting with hepatic dysfunction. J Pediatr Gastroenterol Nutr 1993;16:190–3.

160. Janka G, Imashuku S, Elinder G, et al. Infection- and malignancy-associated hemophagocytic syndromes: secondary hemophagocytic lymphohistiocytosis. Hematol Oncol Clin North Am 1998;12:435–44.

161. Smyth MJ, Thia KY, Cretney E, et al. Perforin is a major contributor to NK cell control of tumor metastasis. J Immunol 1999;162:6658–62.

162. Kumar M, Sackey K, Schmalstieg F, et al. Griscelli syndrome: rare neonatal syndrome of recurrent hemophagocytosis. J Pediatr Hematol Oncol 2001;23:464–8.

163. Stepp SE, Dufourcq-Lagelouse R, Le Deist F, et al. Perforin gene defects in familial hemophagocytic lymphohistiocytosis. Science 1999;286:1957–9.

164. Jones RJ, Lee KS, Beschorner WE, et al. Venoocclusive disease of the liver following bone marrow transplantation. Transplantation 1987;44:778–83.

165. Scrobohaci ML, Drouet L, Monem-Mansi A, et al. Liver veno-occlusive disease after bone marrow transplantation changes in coagulation parameters and endothelial markers. Thromb Res 1991;63:509–19.

166. Shulman HM, Gown AM, Nugent DJ. Hepatic veno-occlusive disease after bone marrow transplantation: immunohistochemical identification of the material within occluded central venules. Am J Pathol 1987;127:549–58.

167. Faioni EM, Krachmalnicoff A, Bearman SI, et al. Naturally occurring anticoagulants and bone marrow transplantation: plasma protein C predicts the development of venocclusive disease of the liver. Blood 1993;81:3458–62.

168. Bearman SI. The syndrome of hepatic veno-occlusive disease after marrow transplantation. Blood 1995;85:3005–20.

169. Carreras E, Granena A, Navasa M, et al. Transjugular liver biopsy in BMT. Bone Marrow Transplant 1993;11:21–6.

170. Rubenfeld GD, Crawford SW. Withdrawing life support from mechanically ventilated recipients of bone marrow transplants: a case for evidence-based guidelines. Ann Intern Med 1996;125:625–33.

171. Bearman SI, Anderson GL, Mori M, et al. Venoocclusive disease of the liver: development of a model for predicting fatal outcome after marrow transplantation. J Clin Oncol 1993;11:1729–36.

172. Kikuchi K, Rudolph R, Murakami C, et al. Portal vein thrombosis after hematopoietic cell transplantation: frequency, treatment and outcome. Bone Marrow Transplant 2002;29:329–33.

173. Etzioni A, Benderly A, Rosenthal E, et al. Defective humoral and cellular immune functions associated with veno-occlusive disease of the liver. J Pediatr 1987;110:549–54.

174. Snover DC, Weisdorf SA, Ramsay NK, et al. Hepatic graft versus host disease: a study of the predictive value of liver biopsy in diagnosis. Hepatology 1984;4:123–30.

175. Stechschulte DJ Jr, Fishback JL, Emami A, Bhatia P. Secondary biliary cirrhosis as a consequence of graft-versus-host disease. Gastroenterology 1990;98:223–5.

176. Yau JC, Zander AR, Srigley JR, et al. Chronic graft-versus-host disease complicated by micronodular cirrhosis and esophageal varices. Transplantation 1986;41:129–30.

177. Knapp AB, Crawford JM, Rappeport JM, Gollan JL. Cirrhosis as a consequence of graft-versus-host disease. Gastroenterology 1987;92:513–9.

178. Rhodes DF, Lee WM, Wingard JR, et al. Orthotopic liver transplantation for graft-versus-host disease following bone marrow transplantation. Gastroenterology 1990;99:536–8.

179. Gholson CF, Yau JC, LeMaistre CF, Cleary KR. Steroid-responsive chronic hepatic graft-versus-host disease without extrahepatic graft-versus-host disease. Am J Gastroenterol 1989;84:1306–9.

180. Roulet M, Laurini R, Rivier L, Calame A. Hepatic veno-occlusive disease in newborn infant of a woman drinking herbal tea. J Pediatr 1988;112:433–6.

181. McDonald GB, Sharma P, Matthews DE, et al. The clinical course of 53 patients with venocclusive disease of the liver after marrow transplantation. Transplantation 1985;39:603–8.

182. McDonald GB, Hinds MS, Fisher LD, et al. Veno-occlusive disease of the liver and multiorgan failure after bone marrow transplantation: a cohort study of 355 patients. Ann Intern Med 1993;118:255–67.

183. Mellis C, Bale PM. Familial hepatic venoocclusive disease with probable immune deficiency. J Pediatr 1976;88:236–42.

184. McDonald GB, Sharma P, Matthews DE, et al. Venocclusive disease of the liver after bone marrow transplantation: diagnosis, incidence, and predisposing factors. Hepatology 1984;4:116–22.

185. Tenore A, Berman WF, Parks JS, Bongiovanni AM. Basal and stimulated serum growth hormone concentrations in inflammatory bowel disease. J Clin Endocrinol Metab 1977;44:622–8.

186. Jelliffe DB, Jelliffe EF. Causation of kwashiorkor: toward a multifactorial consensus. Pediatrics 1992;90:110–3.

187. Golden MH, Ramdath D. Free radicals in the pathogenesis of kwashiorkor. Proc Nutr Soc 1987;46:53–68.

188. Chandra RK. Micronutrients and immune functions: an overview. Ann N Y Acad Sci 1990;587:9–16.

189. Jahoor F, Jackson AA, Golden MH. In vivo metabolism of nitrogen precursors for urea synthesis in the postprandial rat. Ann Nutr Metab 1988;32:240–4.

190. Moran JR, Ghishan FK, Halter SA, Greene HL. Steatohepatitis in obese children: a cause of chronic liver dysfunction. Am J Gastroenterol 1983;78:374–7.

191. Clain DJ, Lefkowitch JH. Fatty liver disease in morbid obesity. Gastroenterol Clin North Am 1987;16:239–52.

192. Kinugasa A, Tsunamoto K, Furukawa N, et al. Fatty liver and its fibrous changes found in simple obesity of children. J Pediatr Gastroenterol Nutr 1984;3:408–14.

193. Klain J, Fraser D, Goldstein J, et al. Liver histology abnormalities in the morbidly obese. Hepatology 1989;10:873–6.

194. Ludwig J, Viggiano TR, McGill DB, Oh BJ. Nonalcoholic steatohepatitis: Mayo Clinic experiences with a hitherto unnamed disease. Mayo Clin Proc 1980;55:434–8.

195. Nomura F, Ohnishi K, Satomura Y, et al. Liver function in moderate obesity—study in 534 moderately obese subjects among 4613 male company employees. Int J Obes 1986;10:349–54.

196. Andersen T, Christoffersen P, Gluud C. The liver in consecutive patients with morbid obesity: a clinical, morphological, and biochemical study. Int J Obes 1984;8:107–15.

197. Silber T, Randolph J, Robbins S. Long-term morbidity and mortality in morbidly obese adolescents after jejunoileal bypass. J Pediatr 1986;108:318–22.

198. Hocking MP, Duerson MC, O'Leary JP, Woodward ER.

Jejunoileal bypass for morbid obesity. Late follow-up in 100 cases. N Engl J Med 1983;308:995–9.

199. Adler M, Schaffner F. Fatty liver hepatitis and cirrhosis in obese patients. Am J Med 1979;67:811–6.

200. Drenick EJ, Simmons F, Murphy JF. Effect on hepatic morphology of treatment of obesity by fasting, reducing diets and small-bowel bypass. N Engl J Med 1970;282:829–34.

201. Palmer M, Schaffner F. Effect of weight reduction on hepatic abnormalities in overweight patients. Gastroenterology 1990;99:1408–13.

202. Yang SQ, Lin HZ, Lane MD, et al. Obesity increases sensitivity to endotoxin liver injury: implications for the pathogenesis of steatohepatitis. Proc Natl Acad Sci U S A 1997;94:2557–62.

203. Weltman MD, Farrell GC, Hall P, et al. Hepatic cytochrome P450 2E1 is increased in patients with nonalcoholic steatohepatitis. Hepatology 1998;27:128–33.

204. Loffreda S, Yang SQ, Lin HZ, et al. Leptin regulates proinflammatory immune responses. FASEB J 1998;12:57–65.

205. Tulinius MH, Holme E, Kristiansson B, et al. Mitochondrial encephalomyopathies in childhood: II. clinical manifestations and syndromes. J Pediatr 1991;119:251–9.

206. Naidu S, Moser HW. Peroxisomal disorders. Neurol Clin 1990;8:507–28.

207. Narkewicz MR, Sokol RJ, Beckwith B, et al. Liver involvement in Alpers disease. J Pediatr 1991;119:260–7.

208. DiMauro S, Bonilla E, Lombes A, et al. Mitochondrial encephalomyopathies. Neurol Clin 1990;8:483–506.

209. Boustany RN, Aprille JR, Halperin J, et al. Mitochondrial cytochrome deficiency presenting as a myopathy with hypotonia, external ophthalmoplegia, and lactic acidosis in an infant and as fatal hepatopathy in a second cousin. Ann Neurol 1983;14:462–70.

210. James OF, Day CP. Non-alcoholic steatohepatitis (NASH): a disease of emerging identity and importance. J Hepatol 1998;29:495–501.

211. Troiano RP, Flegal KM, Kuczmarski RJ, et al. Overweight prevalence and trends for children and adolescents: the National Health and Nutrition Examination Surveys, 1963 to 1991. Arch Pediatr Adolesc Med 1995;149:1085–91.

212. Hashimoto T, Fujita T, Usuda N, et al. Peroxisomal and mitochondrial fatty acid beta-oxidation in mice nullizygous for both peroxisome proliferator-activated receptor alpha and peroxisomal fatty acyl-CoA oxidase: genotype correlation with fatty liver phenotype. J Biol Chem 1999;274:19228–36.

213. Farooqi IS, Matarese G, Lord GM, et al. Beneficial effects of leptin on obesity, T cell hyporesponsiveness, and neuroendocrine/metabolic dysfunction of human congenital leptin deficiency. J Clin Invest 2002;110:1093–103.

214. Lichtman SN, Sartor RB, Keku J, Schwab JH. Hepatic inflammation in rats with experimental small intestinal bacterial overgrowth. Gastroenterology 1990;98:414–23.

215. Lichtman SN, Sartor RB. Hepatobiliary injury associated with experimental small-bowel bacterial overgrowth in rats. Immunol Res 1991;10:528–31.

216. Drenick EJ, Fisler J, Johnson D. Hepatic steatosis after intestinal bypass—prevention and reversal by metronidazole, irrespective of protein-calorie malnutrition. Gastroenterology 1982; 82:535–48.

217. Geubel AP, De Galocsy C, Alves N, et al. Liver damage caused by therapeutic vitamin A administration: estimate of dose-related toxicity in 41 cases. Gastroenterology 1991;100:1701–9.

218. Quigley EM, Marsh MN, Shaffer JL, Markin RS. Hepatobiliary complications of total parenteral nutrition. Gastroenterology 1993;104:286–301.

219. Peden VH, Witzleben CL, Skelton MA. Total parenteral nutrition. J Pediatr 1971;78:180–1.

220. Beale EF, Nelson RM, Bucciarelli RL, et al. Intrahepatic cholestasis associated with parenteral nutrition in premature infants. Pediatrics 1979;64:342–7.

221. Benjamin DR. Hepatobiliary dysfunction in infants and children associated with long-term total parenteral nutrition: a clinicopathologic study. Am J Clin Pathol 1981;76:276–83.

222. Farrell MK, Balistreri WF. Parenteral nutrition and hepatobiliary dysfunction. Clin Perinatol 1986;13:197–212.

223. Cohen C, Olsen MM. Pediatric total parenteral nutrition: liver histopathology. Arch Pathol Lab Med 1981;105:152–6.

224. Stanko RT, Nathan G, Mendelow H, Adibi SA. Development of hepatic cholestasis and fibrosis in patients with massive loss of intestine supported by prolonged parenteral nutrition. Gastroenterology 1987;92:197–202.

225. Balistreri WF, Bove KE. Hepatobiliary consequences of parenteral alimentation. Prog Liver Dis 1990;9:567–601.

226. Dosi PC, Raut AJ, Chelliah BP, et al. Perinatal factors underlying neonatal cholestasis. J Pediatr 1985;106:471–4.

227. Balistreri WF, Heubi JE, Suchy FJ. Immaturity of the enterohepatic circulation in early life: factors predisposing to "physiologic" maldigestion and cholestasis. J Pediatr Gastroenterol Nutr 1983;2:346–54.

228. Suchy FJ, Bucuvalas JC, Novak DA. Determinants of bile formation during development: ontogeny of hepatic bile acid metabolism and transport. Semin Liver Dis 1987;7:77–84.

229. Farrell MK, Balistreri WF, Suchy FJ. Serum-sulfated lithocholate as an indicator of cholestasis during parenteral nutrition in infants and children. JPEN J Parenter Enteral Nutr 1982; 6:30–3.

230. Diehl AM. Nonalcoholic steatohepatitis. Semin Liver Dis 1999; 19:221–9.

231. Merriam-Webster's collegiate dictionary. 10th ed. Springfield (MA): Merriam-Webster Inc; 1995. Herb; p. 42.

232. Mitchison HC, Record CO, Bateson MC, Cobden I. Hepatic abnormalities in coeliac disease: three cases of delayed diagnosis. Postgrad Med J 1989;65:920–2.

233. Hagander B, Berg NO, Brandt L, et al. Hepatic injury in adult coeliac disease. Lancet 1977;ii:270–2.

234. Leonardi S, Bottaro G, Patane R, Musumeci S. Hypertransaminasemia as the first symptom in infant celiac disease. J Pediatr Gastroenterol Nutr 1990;11:404–6.

235. Lindberg T, Berg NO, Borulf S, Jakobsson I. Liver damage in coeliac disease or other food intolerance in childhood. Lancet 1978;i:390–1.

236. Hay JE, Wiesner RH, Shorter RG, et al. Primary sclerosing cholangitis and celiac disease: a novel association. Ann Intern Med 1988;109:713–7.

237. Kaufman FR, Costin G, Thomas DW, et al. Neonatal cholestasis and hypopituitarism. Arch Dis Child 1984;59:787–9.

238. Leblanc A, Odievre M, Hadchouel M, et al. Neonatal cholestasis and hypoglycemia: possible role of cortisol deficiency. J Pediatr 1981;99:577–80.

239. Weldon AP, Danks DM. Congenital hypothyroidism and neonatal jaundice. Arch Dis Child 1972;47:469–71.

240. Van Steenbergen W, Fevery J, De Vos R, et al. Thyroid hormones and the hepatic handling of bilirubin: I. Effects of hypothyroidism and hyperthyroidism on the hepatic transport of bilirubin mono- and diconjugates in the Wistar rat. Hepatology 1989;9:314–21.

241. Gartner LM, Arias IM. Hormonal control of hepatic bilirubin transport and conjugation. Am J Physiol 1972;222:1091–9.

242. Layden TJ, Boyer JL. The effect of thyroid hormone on bile salt

independent bile flow and Na+, K+-ATPase activity in liver plasma membranes enriched in bile canaliculi. J Clin Invest 1976;57:1009–18.

243. Foster KJ, Griffith AH, Dewbury K, et al. Liver disease in patients with diabetes mellitus. Postgrad Med J 1980;56:767–72.

244. Mauriac P. Hepatomegalie, nanisme, obesite, dans le diabete infantile: pathogenese du syndrome. Presse Med 1946;54:826–31.

245. Goodman JI. Hepatomegaly and diabetes mellitus. Ann Intern Med 1953;39:1077–87.

246. Batman PA, Scheuer PJ. Diabetic hepatitis preceding the onset of glucose intolerance. Histopathology 1985;9:237–43.

247. Stone BG, Van Thiel DH. Diabetes mellitus and the liver. Semin Liver Dis 1985;5:8–28.

248. Neufeld M, Maclaren N, Blizzard R. Autoimmune polyglandular syndromes. Pediatr Ann 1980;9:154–62.

249. Fennell RS III, Andres JM, Pfaff WW, Richard GA. Liver dysfunction in children and adolescents during hemodialysis and after renal transplantation. Pediatrics 1981;67:855–61.

250. Johnson RJ, Gretch DR, Yamabe H, et al. Membranoproliferative glomerulonephritis associated with hepatitis C virus infection. N Engl J Med 1993;328:465–70.

251. Sechi LA, Pirisi M, Bartoli E. Membranoproliferative glomerulonephritis associated with hepatitis C infection with no evidence of liver disease. JAMA 1994;271:194.

252. Burstein DM, Rodby RA. Membranoproliferative glomerulonephritis associated with hepatitis C virus infection. J Am Soc Nephrol 1993;4:1288–93.

253. Dobrin RS, Hoyer JR, Nevins TE, et al. The association of familial liver disease, subepidermal immunoproteins, and membranoproliferative glomerulonephritis. J Pediatr 1977;90:901–9.

254. Venkataseshan VS, Lieberman K, Kim DU, et al. Hepatitis-B-associated glomerulonephritis: pathology, pathogenesis, and clinical course. Medicine (Baltimore) 1990;69:200–16.

255. Upadhyaya K, Barwick K, Fishaut M, et al. The importance of nonrenal involvement in hemolytic-uremic syndrome. Pediatrics 1980;65:115–20.

256. van Rhijn A, Donckerwolcke RA, Kuijten RH, van der Heiden C. Liver damage in the hemolytic uremic syndrome. Helv Paediatr Acta 1977;32:77–81.

257. Fellman V, Visapaa I, Vujic M, et al. Antenatal diagnosis of hereditary fetal growth retardation with aminoaciduria, cholestasis, iron overload, and lactic acidosis in the newborn infant. Acta Obstet Gynecol Scand 2002;81:398–402.

258. Neuhaus TJ, Stallmach T, Leumann E, et al. Familial progressive tubulo-interstitial nephropathy and cholestatic liver disease: a newly recognized entity? Eur J Pediatr 1997;156:723–6.

259. Witters I, Devriendt K, Spinnewijn D, et al. MCA syndrome with renal-hepatic-pancreatic dysplasia, posterior fossa cyst, symmetrical limb deficiencies, cleft palate, cardiac and müllerian duct anomalies. Am J Med Genet 2002;107:233–6.

260. Nakhleh RE, Glock M, Snover DC. Hepatic pathology of chronic granulomatous disease of childhood. Arch Pathol Lab Med 1992;116:71–5.

261. Strauss RG, Schubert WK, McAdams AJ. Amyloidosis in childhood. J Pediatr 1969;74:272–82.

262. Kyle RA, Bayrd ED. Amyloidosis: review of 236 cases. Medicine (Baltimore) 1975;54:271–99.

263. Bradstock K, Clancy R, Uther J, et al. The successful treatment of primary amyloidosis with intermittent chemotherapy. Aust N Z J Med 1978;8:176–9.

264. Fausa O, Nygaard K, Elgjo K. Amyloidosis and Crohn's disease. Scand J Gastroenterol 1977;12:657–62.

265. Gertz MA, Kyle RA. Hepatic amyloidosis (primary [AL], immunoglobulin light chain): the natural history in 80 patients. Am J Med 1988;85:73–80.

266. Paliard P, Bretagnolle M, Collet P, et al. Inferior vena cava thrombosis responsible for chronic Budd-Chiari syndrome during hepatic and digestive amyloidosis [French]. Gastroenterol Clin Biol 1983;7:919–22.

267. Pattishall EN, Strope GL, Spinola SM, Denny FW. Childhood sarcoidosis. J Pediatr 1986;108:169–77.

268. Clark SK. Sarcoidosis in children. Pediatr Dermatol 1987;4:291–9.

269. Lehmuskallio E, Hannuksela M, Halme H. The liver in sarcoidosis. Acta Med Scand 1977;202:289–93.

270. Hetherington S. Sarcoidosis in young children. Am J Dis Child 1982;136:13–5.

271. al-Dalaan A, al-Balaa S, Ali MA, et al. Budd-Chiari syndrome in association with Behçet's disease. J Rheumatol 1991;18:622–6.

272. International Study Group for Behçet's Disease. Criteria for diagnosis of Behçet's disease. Lancet 1990;335:1078–80.

273. Bismuth E, Hadengue A, Hammel P, Benhamou JP. Hepatic vein thrombosis in Behçet's disease. Hepatology 1990;11:969–74.

274. Yokogawa K, Yonekawa M, Tamai I, et al. Loss of wild-type carrier-mediated L-carnitine transport activity in hepatocytes of juvenile visceral steatosis mice. Hepatology 1999;30:997–1001.

CHAPTER 58

ACUTE LIVER FAILURE

Sanjay Bansal, MD, MRCP

Anil Dhawan, MD, FRCPCH

Acute liver failure (ALF), a clinically heterogeneous and complex multisystem disorder, is a rare but devastating sequel of an insult to the liver. The liver damage, within a few days to weeks, can cause encephalopathy and multiorgan failure. Different underlying etiologies, the age of the patient, and the duration of time over which the disease evolves contribute to the heterogeneity of this disorder. The mortality is high without liver transplant. ALF is the indication for liver transplant in about 10 to 20% of pediatric recipients in major transplant centers, with a 1-year survival rate of 60 to 75%. Auxiliary liver transplant offers the opportunity for the native liver to regenerate with the possibility of withdrawal of immunosuppression. Liver assist devices (cleansing systems and biologic systems) are being evaluated as newer treatment options. Management requires early appreciation of the severity of the illness, treatment, and prevention of complications, and if the spontaneous recovery is doubtful, emergency liver transplant before the irreversible brain damage occurs. This involves an integrated, multidisciplinary approach involving hepatologists, intensivists, and transplant surgeons; therefore, this condition should ideally be managed in a specialist center.

DEFINITION

Although the occurrence of fatal hepatitis as a consequence of epidemic hepatitis was first reported in 1946,[1] the first attempt at a formal definition was made only in 1970 by Trey and Davidson.[2] Fulminant hepatic failure (FHF) was described as "a potentially reversible condition, the consequence of severe liver injury, in which the onset of hepatic encephalopathy was within eight weeks of the first symptoms of illness, and in the absence of pre-existing liver disease."[2] In 1989, the term "late-onset hepatic failure" was used on the basis of development of hepatic encephalopathy (HE) between 8 and 24 weeks from the onset of jaundice.[3] Bernuau and Benhamou described FHF as the onset of encephalopathy within 2 weeks of the onset of jaundice (rather than other symptoms); it was subfulminant hepatic failure if encephalopathy developed between 2 and 12 weeks from the first appearance of jaundice.[4] Subsequently, O'Grady and colleagues proposed a new classification based on a retrospective study of 539 adult patients. They suggested use of the terms hyperacute, acute, and subacute failure, depending on the interval between jaun-

dice and onset of encephalopathy, less than 1 week, 1 to 4 weeks, and 5 to 12 weeks, respectively.[5] They also suggested that the lack of preexisting liver disease is not mandatory if it remained asymptomatic, for example, Wilson disease, autoimmune hepatitis, delta virus superinfection, and hepatitis B reactivation.

These definitions do not satisfactorily encompass the complexity of the condition in the pediatric population. The early stages of encephalopathy are very difficult to detect in infants and small children. Also, in children, particularly during infancy, encephalopathy may appear very late, if ever, and ALF may be the first manifestation of an underlying metabolic disease associated with a variable degree of chronic liver damage. The first pediatric definition was suggested by Bhaduri and Mieli-Vergani as "a rare multisystem disorder in which severe impairment of liver function, with or without encephalopathy, occurs in association with hepatocellular necrosis in a patient with no recognised underlying chronic liver disease."[6] This definition has addressed the issues relevant to the pediatric population.

ETIOLOGY

ALF is the final common pathway of a variety of insults to the liver. There is considerable variation in the etiologies around the world, with acute viral hepatitis and drugs accounting for the majority of cases. The frequency of ALF in all age groups in the United States is 17 cases per 100,000 population per year, but the frequency in the pediatric age group only is unknown.[7] The overall incidence of ALF complicating acute hepatitis in the United States is 0.9%, and it causes about 2,000 deaths annually, with non-A–E hepatitis being the most common cause.[8] In children, acute viral hepatitis is the most common identified cause in most of the series, but there is a lot of geographic variation, with hepatitis A being the most common cause in Asia, whereas in Europe and North America, it is seronegative hepatitis. The etiology of ALF as seen in a tertiary pediatric liver center is shown in Table 58-1.

INFECTIVE

Viruses. Infection with the hepatotropic viruses is probably the most identifiable cause of ALF. Patients usually present with icterus and markedly raised serum transaminase

TABLE 58-1   ETIOLOGIES OF ACUTE LIVER FAILURE IN NEONATES AND CHILDREN (KING'S COLLEGE HOSPITAL, 1991–2000)

ETIOLOGY	n
NEONATES (n = 31)	
Neonatal hemochromatosis	15
Hemophagocytic lymphohistiocytosis	4
Disseminated herpes simplex virus infection	5
Metabolic	4
Transplacental acetaminophen toxicity	1
Endocrine (isolated cortisol deficiency)	1
Sepsis/shock	1
CHILDREN (n = 100)	
Non-A–E hepatitis	45
Hepatitis A/B	7
Other viral infection	3
Metabolic	18
Acetaminophen toxicity	8
Other drug/toxin	5
Sepsis/hypoxia	3
Miscellaneous	11

levels. The magnitude of transaminase elevation and the rate of decline do not predict prognosis. In patients who spontaneously recover, serum bilirubin, international normalized ratio (INR), and serum transaminases gradually decline, whereas a continued rise in bilirubin levels and INR, despite declining serum transaminase levels, indicates massive hepatocyte necrosis and a poor prognosis.

The risk of developing liver failure in acute hepatitis A virus (HAV) infection is 0.1 to 0.4%.[9–12] A higher incidence of ALF is suggested when HAV infection occurs in patients with underlying chronic liver disease. Very high mortality is reported in an Italian study in which 7 of 17 children with chronic hepatitis C infection with superadded HAV infection developed ALF, and only 1 child survived.[13] The diagnosis of acute hepatitis A is made by the detection of the anti-HAV immunoglobulin (Ig)M antibody in serum. In 95% of cases, anti-HAV IgM antibody is present at the time of presentation, and the remaining 5% become positive on repeat testing.

The incidence of ALF owing to hepatitis B virus (HBV) is 1 to 4%.[8] The liver failure can present at (1) the time of acute infection, (2) reactivation of chronic HBV infection in immunocompromised patients, (3) superinfection or coinfection with hepatitis D virus, or (4) seroconversion from a hepatitis B e antigen–positive to a hepatitis B e antibody (HBeAb)-positive state. Infants born to HBeAb-positive mothers are a special group that can present with ALF around 3 weeks to 3 months of age.[14,15]

There is a theoretic risk of developing ALF after hepatitis C virus (HCV) infection, but in a large follow-up study of children with post-transfusion HCV infection, ALF was not observed.[16]

Hepatitis E virus (HEV) infection, a waterborne infection like hepatitis A and a well-recognized cause of ALF, is common in the Indian subcontinent and Africa. The risk of developing ALF in adult males is 0.6 to 2.8%, but the risk increases significantly in pregnant women, especially in the third trimester, with the case-fatality ratio of around 25%.[17] HEV infection may be responsible for up to 8% of cases, which would have been attributed to seronegative hepatitis. A history of travel to an endemic area is not always present. A study from northern India reported that 7 of 44 children with ALF had isolated HEV infection, whereas another 16 of 44 had mixed HEV and HAV infection. HEV infection is diagnosed by the presence of anti-HEV antibody in the serum.[18] Despite identification of hepatitis G (a flavivirus) virus in ALF of unknown etiology, it does not appear to cause ALF.[19] Similarly, TT virus (transfusion-transmitted virus), a single-stranded deoxyribonucleic acid (DNA) virus, was discovered in 1997 from the sera of non-A, non-B (NANB) hepatitis patients but has also not been shown conclusively to cause ALF.[20]

Non-A–E hepatitis (seronegative hepatitis) is the most common cause of ALF in the Western world. In our series, of 100 cases of ALF, 45 were due to non-A–E hepatitis.[21] Similar experience was reported from Chicago, with 26 of 42 children with ALF who were diagnosed with non-A–E hepatitis.[22] The diagnosis is one of exclusion in which other causes of ALF are eliminated with appropriate laboratory investigations and clinical examination. Non-A–E hepatitis is characterized by its propensity to cause severe hepatitis, a high fatality rate (low spontaneous remission) without liver transplant, and its association with bone marrow failure in up to 10% of patients.[23] Bone marrow failure can develop even a few weeks after the onset of symptoms of ALF.

Other Hepatotropic Viruses. Herpes simplex virus, cytomegalovirus, Epstein-Barr virus, and varicella-zoster virus, members of the herpesvirus family, can cause severe hepatic necrosis, particularly in immunocompromised patients and neonates. Herpes simplex infection–induced ALF in the neonatal period has a very high case-fatality ratio. The diagnosis is suspected in an unwell neonate with or without a vesicular lesion along with remarkably raised serum transaminases and coagulopathy. Maternal history suggestive of herpes simplex infection and/or positive serology is helpful in establishing the diagnosis. Viral studies (immunofluorescence or polymerase chain reaction) of vesicular fluid are diagnostic. Association of cytomegalovirus with ALF is not reported, although Epstein-Barr virus has been, rarely, associated with ALF.[24]

Parvovirus B19 infection can cause severe hepatitis, ALF, and, rarely, bone marrow failure in children. A retrospective study of 6 patients with ALF with peritransplant aplastic anemia owing to presumed NANB hepatitis showed the presence of parvovirus B19 DNA in 4 of 6 explanted livers, but all 6 patients had IgG antibodies against parvovirus.[25] In our experience, parvovirus infection as the cause of ALF was recognized in 2 of 8 children who had bone marrow aplasia with ALF.[23]

Echovirus (type 20) and coxsackieviruses have been reported to cause ALF, especially in neonates.[26,27] In an adult study, Toga virus–like particles were isolated in explanted livers in 7 of 18 patients who had liver transplant for ALF owing to NANB hepatitis but none in 26 explanted livers available for study after liver transplant owing to other causes. ALF, characterized by severe hemorrhagic necrosis on histology, developed 7 days after transplant in 5 patients, all in the NANB group with Toga virus–like particles in native liver. Further analysis revealed no identifiable epidemiologic factors between these and the other NANB hepatitis–induced ALF patients.[28]

Nonviral Infections. Nonviral infective agents have been implicated in the pathogenesis of ALF, although rarely. Acute liver dysfunction is well recognized in severe sepsis. Bacterial infections, especially gram-negative infections (*Salmonella, Shigella, Escherichia coli,* and *Pseudomonas*), miliary tuberculosis, brucellosis, and Q fever (owing to *Coxiella burnetii*), have been reported to cause ALF. Spirochetal infections, particularly leptospirosis, can present with severe hepatitis or ALF. The clinical picture is predominated by high fever and renal failure. In endemic areas, there have been reports of ALF following plasmodium falciparum infection.[29]

Hepatic dysfunction in sepsis is the result of decreased hepatic perfusion, hypoxia, and lactic acidosis. Bacterial cell wall products (endotoxin and lipoteichoic acid) and cytokines (tumor necrosis factor, interleukin-1β, and interferons) induce the production of nitric oxide. The elevated levels of inducible nitric oxide are toxic to liver cells.[30]

DRUGS AND TOXINS

Drugs and toxins are well known to cause liver failure in children. In general, the risk factors for drug-induced hepatotoxicity are age (very young or adolescents), abnormal renal function, concurrent use of other hepatotoxic agents, drug interactions, and preexisting liver diseases. Drug-induced hepatoxicity can be a dose-dependent response, an idiosyncratic reaction, or a synergistic reaction (Table 58-2).

Estimates of the risk of developing ALF as a result of an idiosyncratic reaction range from 0.001% for nonsteroidal anti-inflammatory drugs to 1% for the isoniazid-rifampicin combination. Drug toxicity produces a distinctive pattern of liver injury. The most common liver injury pattern owing to drugs is hepatitic (hepatocellular necrosis), accounting for about 90% of cases. Others could be cholestatic (biliary damage), mixed (both hepatitic and cholestatic), or steatosis.[31] Sodium valproate is known to unmask underlying mitochondrial cytopathies; hence, detailed investigations to exclude mitochondrial hepatopathies should be undertaken before injury is ascribed to sodium valproate. Use of antiretroviral drugs has also been associated with ALF. Ecstasy (3,4-methylene-dioxymethamphetamine), a synthetic amphetamine, has been associated with a range of clinical syndromes ranging

---

TABLE 58-2   CAUSES OF ACUTE LIVER FAILURE

INFECTIVE	Synergistic drug interactions
Viral	Isoniazid + rifampicin
Viral hepatitis	Trimethoprim + sulfamethoxazole
A, B, B + D, E	Barbiturates + acetaminophen
Non-A–E hepatitis (seronegative hepatitis)	Amoxycillin + clavulinic acid
Adenovirus, Epstein-Barr virus, cytomegalovirus	TOXINS
Echovirus	*Amanita phalloides* (mushroom poisoning)
Varicella, measles	Herbal medicines
Yellow fever	Carbon tetrachloride
Rarely, Lassa, Ebola, Marburg virus, dengue, Toga virus	Yellow phosphorus
Bacterial	Industrial solvents
Salmonellosis	Chlorobenzenes
Tuberculosis	METABOLIC
Septicemia	Galactosemia
Others	Tyrosinemia
Malaria	Hereditary fructose intolerance
Bartonella	Neonatal hemochromatosis
Leptospirosis	Niemann-Pick disease type C
DRUGS	Wilson disease
Dose dependent	Mitochondrial cytopathies
Acetaminophen	Congenital disorders of glycosylation
Halothane	Acute fatty liver of pregnancy
Idiosyncratic reaction	AUTOIMMUNE
Isoniazid	Type 1 autoimmune hepatitis
Nonsteroidal anti-inflammatory drugs	Type 2 autoimmune hepatitis
Phenytoin	Giant cell hepatitis with Coombs-positive hemolytic anemia
Sodium valproate	VASCULAR/ISCHEMIC
Carbamazepine	Budd-Chiari syndrome
Ecstasy	Acute circulatory failure
Troglitazone	Heat stroke
Antibiotics (penicillin, erythromycin, tetracyclines, sulfonamides, quinolones)	Acute cardiac failure
Allopurinol	Cardiomyopathies
Propylthiouracil	INFILTRATIVE
Amiodarone	Leukemia
Ketoconazole	Lymphoma
Antiretroviral drugs	Hemophagocytic lymphohistiocytosis

from asymptomatic hepatic liver function tests or subacute liver failure to rapidly progressive ALF.[32]

Acetaminophen, the most common drug associated with ALF, is safe when used in therapeutic doses in healthy individuals. It is normally a dose-dependent hepatotoxic agent. The hepatocyte necrosis is caused by accumulation of the N-acetylparabenzoquine amide, which is a toxic intermediate compound.[33] When cytochrome P-450 enzymes are induced either owing to drugs such as antiepilepsy drugs or chronic alcohol consumption, hepatic glutathione stores are depleted. Consequently, even therapeutic doses of acetaminophen can lead to accumulation of N-acetylparabenzoquine amide, causing ALF. Inadvertent administration of higher doses of acetaminophen can lead to ALF in children. A detailed history of exposure to acetaminophen is helpful. In 1995, a series of young children were reported with ALF without any identifiable cause but with minimal jaundice. All of these children had a history of exposure to acetaminophen, although in therapeutic doses. Fifty percent of these patients survived, and the histopathology was characterized by a varying degree of centrilobular necrosis, which is a characteristic lesion of acetaminophen toxicity, suggesting the possible role of toxicity owing to therapeutic doses of acetaminophen in the development of ALF.[34] Serum acetaminophen levels after 4 hours of ingestion are useful in identifying high-risk patients but are not informative in patients in whom toxicity is secondary to chronic administration.

Mushroom (*Amanita phalloides*) poisoning leading to ALF is mainly reported from Europe (France and eastern Europe), the west coast of the United States, and South Africa. Cases of poisoning peak in autumn, when mushrooms are plentiful. α-Amantin is a heat-stable toxin that is not destroyed by cooking. The usual presentation is severe diarrhea with or without vomiting commencing about 5 or more hours after ingestion. Liver failure is usually followed 3 to 4 days later. Other hepatotoxins include carbon tetrachloride, herbal medicines, and aflatoxins.

AUTOIMMUNE HEPATITIS

Autoimmune hepatitis can present as ALF, most of these patients being liver-kidney microsomal antibody positive. The diagnosis may be difficult because some cases may not show an antibody response at presentation. Some reports have suggested a good response to steroids and azathioprine or cyclosporine.[35,36] In our experience, children with autoimmune hepatitis presenting with ALF along with encephalopathy do not respond to any form of immunosuppression and need urgent liver transplant.

METABOLIC DISEASES

Inherited disorders of metabolism merit special attention as a differential diagnosis while investigating ALF in pediatric patients, in particular newborn babies. Although all of these patients have variable degrees of liver damage before clinical presentation as ALF, overt signs and stigmata of chronic liver disease are usually absent. A high index of suspicion is important because urgent intervention such as dietary manipulation or disease-specific treatment may be

lifesaving. Conditions that are common to the neonatal age group are listed in Table 58-3.

Galactosemia is usually associated with hypoglycemia and gram-negative septicemia. Immediate exclusion of galactose (from the diet and the medications) usually provides a quick recovery, but some cases do progress to liver failure. Tyrosinemia presents with severe coagulopathy, mild jaundice, and rickets. Hereditary fructose intolerance is rare, but a history of administration of fructose, as in fruits, sugar, or honey, may coincide with clinical symptoms.

Neonatal hemochromatosis (NH) is a disorder of iron handling of antenatal onset with excess iron deposition in the nonreticuloendothelial system. Liver failure usually presents in the first few days of life, but liver disease is generally present at birth. Maternal viral infection in the antenatal period or metabolic disease in the fetus is suggested as an underlying cause. Although an underlying genetic basis for NH has been suspected, no test is available for predictive analysis in at-risk pregnancies. In a systematic study of the mode of transmission of this disorder in a total of 40 infants born to 27 families, four pedigrees showed clear evidence of maternal infection associated with NH. One pedigree showed transmission of maternal antinuclear factor and ribonucleoprotein antibodies to the affected infants, and two families with possible matrilineal inheritance of disease in maternal half-siblings, but the large subgroup of the affected pedigrees points to the inheritance of an autosomal recessive trait. This included 14 pedigrees with affected and unaffected infants and a single pedigree in which all four affected infants were the sole offspring of consanguineous but otherwise healthy parents.[37] It can occur sporadically or recurrently, without an overt cause, in siblings. The diagnosis should be considered in every case of neonatal liver failure. Elevation of ferritin as a diagnostic test is sensitive but not specific because elevation of ferritin is commonly observed in sick babies. Hypersaturation of transferrin with relative hypotransferrinemia may be a valuable finding. Magnetic resonance imaging of the liver or pancreas to demonstrate iron is not usually rewarding, but a punch biopsy specimen of buccal mucosa is a useful diagnostic tool. Documentation of iron in salivary glands in buccal mucosa is diagnostic of NH. To ensure the presence of salivary glands in the buccal mucosal biopsy specimen, a frozen section examination is advisable. Most of the time, the biopsy can be performed safely after correction of coagulopathy with blood products. Iron chelation and antioxidant cocktail therapy (Table 58-4) for NH

TABLE 58-3   CAUSES OF NEONATAL LIVER FAILURE

Perinatal herpes simplex virus infection
Neonatal hemochromatosis
Galactosemia
Tyrosinemia
Hemophagocytic lymphohistiocytosis
Septicemia
Mitochondrial cytopathies
Congenital disorders of glycosylation
Severe birth asphyxia

has shown variable results.[38,39] Recently, successful fetal outcome following antenatal intravenous immunoglobulin therapy of pregnant mothers considered to have a high risk of carrying an affected fetus has been reported. In six pregnancies in five mothers, intravenous immunoglobulin was administered weekly at a dose of 1 g/kg body weight from the eighteenth week until the end of gestation. Four pregnancies progressed to term; one had spontaneous delivery at 36 weeks, and one had an induced birth at 32 weeks. All six were live births and were medically stable, with evidence of liver involvement. Four of six required an antioxidant or a chelation cocktail.[40]

Wilson disease, an autosomal recessive disorder, may present as ALF in an older child. The acute hepatic presentation is characterized by the presence of liver failure, Coombs-negative hemolytic anemia, and low alkaline phosphatase. Demonstration of Kayser-Fleischer rings is diagnostic of Wilson disease in a patient who presents with ALF. Serum ceruloplasmin is usually but not invariably low, and serum free copper concentration can be increased or normal. A serum alkaline phosphatase to total bilirubin ratio of < 2.0 has also been suggested as a diagnostic tool to discriminate Wilson disease from other causes of ALF.

MITOCHONDRIAL DISORDERS

In recent years, mitochondrial respiratory chain disorders have been implicated in the etiology of ALF in children.[41–43] This group of disorders encompasses a wide variety of diseases, including Pearson syndrome, mitochondrial DNA depletion syndrome, nuclear DNA defect, Alpers disease, and intestinal pseudo-obstruction with liver disease. Presenting symptoms could be hypoglycemia, vomiting, coagulopathy, acidosis, and increased lactate with or without neurologic symptoms. The presence of high serum lactate in the mother and a history of sibling deaths are suggestive of this condition. Diagnosis involves quantitative assessment of the respiratory chain enzyme complexes in the affected tissues (muscle, liver, skin fibroblast culture). Isolated hepatic involvement with successful liver transplant has been reported; however, the follow-up of these patients is not long enough to rule out future neurologic deterioration. Rarely, fatty acid oxidation defects and inborn errors of bile acid synthesis, especially Δ^4-3-oxosteroid 5β-reductase enzyme deficiency, can present as ALF.[44,45]

TABLE 58-4   DISEASE-SPECIFIC THERAPIES

Acetaminophen toxicity: N-acetylcysteine (100 mg/kg/d) until INR is < 1.5
Hereditary tyrosinemia: NTBC[93]
Neonatal hemochromatosis: iron chelation and antioxidant cocktail
    N-Acetylcysteine (100 mg/kg/d IV infusion)
    Selenium (3 μg/kg/d IV)
    Desferrioxamine (30 mg/kg/d IV)
    Prostaglandin E₁ (0.4–0.6 μg/kg/h IV)
    Vitamin E (25 U/kg/d IV/PO)
Mushroom poisoning: benzylpenicillin (1,000,000 U/kg/d) or thiotic acid (300 mg/kg/d)

INR = international normalized ratio; IV = intravenously; NTBC = 2-(2-nitro-4-trifluoromethylbenzoyl) 1,3-cyclohexanedione; PO = orally

VASCULAR/ISCHEMIC CAUSES

Any condition causing obstruction of hepatic venous outflow (eg, Budd Chiari syndrome, veno-occlusive disease, cardiomyopathies, and acute heart failure) can present with ALF. A detailed cardiovascular examination, including an echocardiogram, is essential to exclude cardiac causes. Diagnostic clues include soft hepatomegaly and ascites.

MALIGNANCIES

Hemophagocytic lymphohistiocytosis is a spectrum of inherited and acquired conditions with disturbed immunoregulation and encompasses two main conditions that have common clinical and pathobiologic characteristics: familial (primary) hemophagocytic lymphohistiocytosis and secondary hemophagocytic lymphohistiocytosis. Familial hemophagocytic lymphohistiocytosis is an invariably fatal inherited disease seen mostly in infancy and early childhood,[46] but secondary hemophagocytic lymphohistiocytosis can affect people at any age and may subside spontaneously. The annual childhood incidence of familial hemophagocytic lymphohistiocytosis has been estimated (in Sweden) at 1.2 cases per 1,000,000, corresponding to 1 in 50,000 births.[47] Clinical presentations include fever, hepatosplenomegaly, and pancytopenia. There is reduced cytotoxic T- and natural killer cell activity, as well as a widespread accumulation of T lymphocytes and macrophages, some of which may engage in hemophagocytosis.[46–48] Biochemically, it is characterized by high serum triglycerides and low fibrinogen. Usually, patients with hemophagocytic lymphohistiocytosis bleed disproportionately from venepuncture sites because of the coagulation abnormalities present.

A varied form of hematologic malignancies (eg, leukemia[49] or lymphoma) can present with ALF. Diagnostic clues include high fever, hepatosplenomegaly, high alkaline phosphatase, high lactate dehydrogenase, and abnormalities on peripheral blood film. Bone marrow examination is diagnostic.

PATHOPHYSIOLOGY OF THE CLINICAL SYNDROME

ALF is a syndrome of multiorgan involvement. Most patients are jaundiced at presentation, except those with hyperacute liver failure, in whom jaundice follows encephalopathy. Peripheral stigmata of liver cell failure may be seen occasionally. A rapid decrease in liver span is usually seen, but patients with hematologic malignancies or cardiac failure have hepatomegaly.

ENCEPHALOPATHY

The pathogenesis of encephalopathy is not clearly understood and probably is multifactorial. The most widely studied factor is ammonia (Figure 58-1). Ammonia is produced from the breakdown of proteins, amino acids, purines, and pyrimidines. Half of the ammonia in the intestine is produced by bacteria; the remainder is from the breakdown of dietary protein and glutamine. Ammonia is cleared in the liver by urea cycle enzymes. In brain, urea cycle enzymes

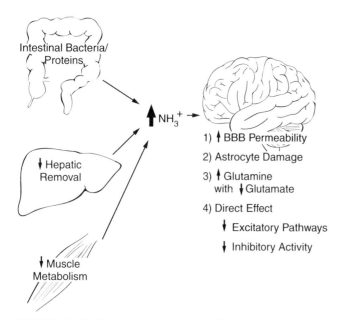

FIGURE 58-1 Summary of the role of ammonia in hepatic encephalopathy.

are absent; hence, ammonia is cleared by the formation of glutamine by enzyme glutamate synthetase. High concentration of glutamine in brain has been demonstrated by magnetic resonance spectroscopy.[50] Ammonia has a direct effect on the neural membranes and also causes postsynaptic inhibition.[50] Although the role of hyperammonemia in HE appears logical, 10% of patients with HE have normal serum ammonia levels.

γ-Aminobutyric acid (GABA), a principal inhibitory neurotransmitter in the brain, is increased in ALF.[51] GABA can act directly or in synergy with the benzodiazepine receptors. In addition to elevated blood levels, increased GABA receptor density and increased sensitivity have been shown in animal studies.

Intestinal decarboxylation of amino acids in the colon lead to the formation of β-phenylethanolamine, tyramine, and octopamine. These products inhibit dopamine- and catecholamine-mediated cerebral transmission by acting as false neurotransmitters.[52] There is also an imbalance in the ratio of plasma and intracerebral branched-chain and aromatic amino acids. Other toxins, such as mercaptans, phenols, fatty acids, and middle-molecular-weight substances, have all been implicated as causative agents. These toxins suppress neural energy metabolism and alter blood-brain barrier permeability.

Encephalopathy of variable degree is often present in patients with ALF, but early encephalopathy is difficult to recognize in children. Traditionally, the encephalopathy is believed to progress over four stages in adults. The symptomatology of stages 3 and 4 is similar in adults and children, but the following modifications could be applied to pediatric patients:

• Stage 1: Mild confusion/anxiety, disturbed or reversal of sleep rhythm, shortened attention span, slowing of ability to perform mental tasks (simple addition or sub-

traction). In young children, irritability, altered sleep pattern, unexplained bursts of excessive crying.
• Stage 2: Drowsiness, confusion, mood swings with personality changes, inappropriate behavior, intermittent disorientation of time and place, gross deficit in ability to perform mental tasks. In young children, excessive sleepiness, inability to interact with or recognize parents, lack of interest in favorite toys or activities.
• Stage 3: Pronounced confusion, delirious but arousable, persistent disorientation of time and place, hyperreflexia with a positive Babinski sign.
• Stage 4: Comatose with or without decerebrate or decorticate posturing, response to pain present (IVa) or no response to pain (IVb).

Electroencephalographic changes present in HE, although not very specific, may be useful in diagnosis and in assessment of treatment. These changes occur very early, even before the onset of psychological or biochemical disturbances. Initially, there is slowing of the alpha rhythm down to the delta range. Altering stimuli such as opening eyes may fail to reduce the background rhythmic activity. Usually, changes start in the frontal or central region and then progress posteriorly. In deeper coma, there is generalized slowing, and synchronous low-amplitude waves are recorded. It is still unclear whether routine electroencephalographic monitoring provides any advantage over clinical assessment alone except in patients who are ventilated and paralyzed, in whom it may reveal seizure activity.

INTRACRANIAL HYPERTENSION AND CEREBRAL EDEMA

Intracranial hypertension is uncommon in stages 1 and 2 but is invariably present in grade 4 encephalopathy. Raised intracerebral pressure can lead to brainstem herniation, which is the most common cause of death observed on autopsy in 80% of fatal cases.[53] Increased intracranial hypertension more commonly occurs in hyperacute liver failure (70%) rather than ALF (55%). The pathophysiology and clinical events related to it could be divided into three phases:

• Phase 1: Episodic increase in intracranial pressure (ICP) either spontaneously or in response to stimuli involved in the routine care of the patient. An intact Cushing reflex at this stage can maintain cerebral perfusion by increasing mean arterial pressure. Although the cerebral oxygenation is preserved at this stage but life-threatening, brainstem herniation can occur.
• Phase 2: At this stage, mean arterial pressure does not increase with further surges in ICP, leading to neuronal hypoxic injury.
• Phase 3: This phase is dominated by poor cerebral perfusion either owing to very high ICP or low mean arterial pressure, leading to hypoxic brain injury.

Factors responsible for encephalopathy cause cerebral edema, leading to an increase in ICP. This increase in ICP can lead to a cycle of poor cerebral perfusion, anoxic injury, and further worsening of cerebral edema. The clinical features vary depending on the severity of intracranial hypertension. The factors and mechanisms that may lead to increased ICP are shown in Figure 58-2.

The mechanism leading to increased ICP could be broadly considered under two headings: the direct toxicity of neuronal cells and vasogenic. The neuronal toxicity leads to osmotic imbalance and an increase in intracellular water, whereas disruption of the blood-brain barrier leading to plasma seepage into the cerebrospinal fluid is of vasogenic origin. Circulating endotoxin from superimposed infections,[54] fluid overload, hypoglycemia,[55] and gastrointestinal bleeding all add to further worsening of intracranial hypertension (Table 58-5).

RENAL FAILURE

Renal failure occurs in about 55% of all ALF patients referred to specialist centers.[56] A variable degree of renal dysfunction is invariably present in patients with acetaminophen-related ALF. In the pediatric population, the incidence of renal failure is lower (10–15%) than in the adult population.[57] Functional renal failure (hepatorenal syndrome) usually progresses to tubular damage as the encephalopathy advances. Avid sodium retention (urinary sodium < 20 mmol/L) and normal urine sediment may help to differentiate between functional renal failure and tubular damage. The hepatorenal syndrome recovers rapidly after liver transplant, whereas established tubular damage requires prolonged renal replacement therapy.

Renal failure could be due either to the direct toxic effect on kidneys, as in acetaminophen overdose, or to a complex mechanism such as hepatorenal syndrome or acute tubular necrosis secondary to complications of ALF (sepsis, bleeding, and/or hypotension). In hepatorenal syndrome, there is a hyperdynamic circulation with a decrease in renal perfusion pressure, leading to activation of the sympathetic nervous system and rendering the kidneys more susceptible to decreases in the renal perfusion pressure and increased synthesis of several vasoactive mediators such as renin, angiotensin, adrenaline, eicosanoids, and endothelins.[58] These vasoactive mediators not only cause vasoconstriction leading to a rise in renal vascular resistance but also a decrease in glomerular capillary ultra-

TABLE 58-5	FACTORS WORSENING INTRACRANIAL PRESSURE

Hypotension
Hypoxia
Hypoglycemia
Sepsis
Electrolyte disturbances (hyperkalemia)
Gastrointestinal bleeding

filtration coefficient leading to a fall in the glomerular filtration rate over and above that caused by the vasoconstrictors alone.

Blood urea estimation is unreliable as a marker of renal dysfunction because gastrointestinal hemorrhage may increase urea disproportionately. Serum creatinine is a better indicator of kidney function.

METABOLIC DERANGEMENTS

Hypoglycemia is present in 40% of patients with ALF. This is due to increased plasma insulin levels owing to reduced hepatic uptake and reduced gluconeogenesis. The classic signs and symptoms of hypoglycemia are often masked, and regular blood glucose monitoring is mandatory because hypoglycemia can worsen HE and cause rapid neurologic deterioration.

Acid-base imbalance is common. Metabolic acidosis is present in about 30% of patients with acetaminophen-induced ALF and is a bad prognostic marker, with greater than 90% mortality if the arterial pH is less than 7.3 on or after the second day of overdose in adequately hydrated patients. This acidosis is independent of renal function and usually precedes the onset of encephalopathy, whereas in ALF owing to other etiologies, metabolic acidosis is present in only 5% of cases, occurs late in the disease process, and is associated with a poor outcome. Lactic acidosis develops in about 50% of patients, reaching grade 3 or 4 encephalopathy, and is related to inadequate tissue perfusion owing to hypotension or hypoxemia resulting from the impaired oxygen extraction owing to microvascular shunting of blood from actively respiring tissue. Sometimes respiratory alkalosis can be present owing to hyperventilation, probably related to direct stimulation of respiratory center by unknown toxic agents. Respiratory acidosis can be caused by pulmonary complications or by respiratory depression in association with increased ICP.

Hypokalemia is common and is due to excessive urinary potassium loss with inadequate replacement. Hyponatremia may be dilutional owing to excessive antidiuretic hormone secretion, or it may represent a true sodium-depleted state in patients who are vomiting. Hypophosphatemia is most commonly associated with acetaminophen-induced ALF when renal function is preserved. Other electrolyte disturbances include hypocalcemia and hypomagnesemia.

HEMODYNAMIC ABNORMALITIES

The early hemodynamic changes in ALF patients reflect a state of hyperdynamic circulation with decreased systemic peripheral vascular resistance and increased cardiac out-

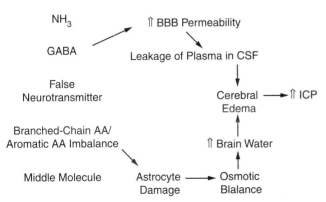

FIGURE 58-2 Schematic diagram of the pathophysiology of cerebral edema. AA = amino acid; BBB = blood-brain barrier; CSF = cerebrospinal fluid; GABA = γ-aminobutyric acid; ICP = intracranial pressure; NH₃ = ammonia.

put. These changes are similar to the one seen in systemic inflammatory response syndrome.[59] Profound vasodilatation, probably mediated by increased prostaglandin or nitric oxide, causes hypovolemia. Invasive monitoring is required to determine the adequacy of intravascular volume and appropriate fluid regimens. As the disease progresses, it can lead to circulatory failure either due to falling cardiac output or the inability to maintain an adequate mean arterial pressure despite inotropic support or depression of brainstem function as a result of cerebral edema. Cardiac arrhythmias of most types may occur in the later stages and are usually caused by electrolyte disturbances (eg, hypo- or hyperkalemia, acidosis, hypoxia, or cardiac irritation by a central venous catheter).

PULMONARY COMPLICATIONS

Pulmonary complications are common and are usually present in about 50% of patients. Aspiration of gastric contents is a significant early complication, particularly in encephalopathic patients who are vomiting; hence, early elective ventilation to protect the airway is critical in these patients. Other complications include atelectasis, infection, intrapulmonary hemorrhage, respiratory depression, or pulmonary edema. In a series of 100 patients with FHF, 52 had radiologic changes and 37 of 52 had pulmonary edema.[60]

COAGULOPATHY

The liver synthesizes not only the coagulation factors (except factor VIII) but also inhibitors of coagulation and factors involved in the fibrinolytic system. ALF is characterized by decreased synthesis of clotting factors (factors II, V, VII, IX, and X), accelerated fibrinolysis, and impaired hepatic clearance of activated clotting factors and fibrin degradation products. The prothrombin time expressed as an INR is markedly elevated and is used as an indicator of the severity of the liver damage. Factors V and VII have the shortest half-lives of all of the coagulation factors and are theoretically more sensitive markers than INR of hepatic synthetic function. Significant disseminated intravascular coagulation is unusual in ALF. Thrombocytopenia may develop rapidly, and a platelet count of less than $100 \times 10^9/L$ has been reported in about two-thirds of the patients. Causes include increased immune-mediated platelet destruction and decreased hepatic synthesis of factors necessary for platelet maturation and release into the peripheral blood. Also, abnormalities of platelet morphology and function have been reported.

Clinically, significant bleeding tends to be less severe compared with the degree of INR prolongation, although the risk of hemorrhage correlates with thrombocytopenia. Common sites of internal hemorrhage include the gastrointestinal tract, nasopharynx, lungs, and retroperitoneum. Intracranial hemorrhage is uncommon. The incidence of gastrointestinal hemorrhage has declined since the use of histamine$_2$ blockers in the management of ALF. A mild degree of hemophagocytosis (hemophagocytic lymphohistiocytosis) is commonly observed and contributes to coagulation abnormalities. The presence of significant disseminated intravascular coagulation usually indicates sepsis or secondary hemophagocytic lymphohistiocytosis.

INFECTIONS

Patients with ALF are at increased risk of bacterial infections because of poor host defenses. There is impaired Kupffer cell and polymorphonuclear function and reduced levels of factors such as fibronectin, opsonins, and chemoattractants, including components of the complement system. The additional predisposing factors are poor respiratory effort and cough reflex and the presence of an endotracheal tube, urinary catheters, and central venous and arterial lines.

Infection can lead to development and progression of multiorgan failure. An active uncontrolled infection also can render potential candidates disqualified for emergency liver transplant. It is very difficult to detect infection in the setting of ALF because there is a poor correlation between infection and normal indicators of infection, such as leukocyte count and fever. The risk factors for infections include coexisting renal failure, cholestasis, treatment with thiopental, and liver transplant. The presence of encephalopathy (grade 2 or above) has been shown to be associated with bacterial infection in about 80% of cases and fungal infections in about 32% of cases.[61] The sources of positive cultures include blood, urine, sputum, and catheter tips. More than two-thirds of bacterial infections are due to gram-positive bacteria, usually *Staphylococcus aureus*, but streptococci or gram-negative organisms such as coliforms are also isolated. *Candida* spp are the most common fungal infections. These are often unrecognized and ominous. Deterioration of HE after initial improvement, a markedly raised leukocyte count, pyrexia unresponsive to antibiotics, and established renal failure are strong indicators of fungal infection.

ACUTE PANCREATITIS

Mild elevation of serum amylase is not uncommon, but clinically significant pancreatitis is unusual. It should be suspected in patients who complain of abdominal pain or have hypocalcemia. Etiologic factors include causative virus, hemorrhage into or around the pancreas, sodium valproate–related ALF, or shock.

ADRENAL HYPORESPONSIVENESS

In a recent adult study, 62% of patients with ALF had a poor response to a short synacthen test and showed significant improvement of hemodynamic parameters after administration of replacement therapy with hydrocortisone.[62] No pediatric data are available, but corticosteroid replacement could be considered in patients with intractable hypotension unresponsive to conventional therapy.

PROGNOSIS

The prognosis of ALF varies greatly with the underlying etiology. In an adult series from King's College Hospital, London, 50% of patients survived following acetaminophen overdose, whereas the survival rate was only 12.5% following halothane-induced ALF—66% for hepatitis A and 39% for hepatitis B.[63]

Prothrombin time is the best indicator of survival.[64] Bhaduri and Mieli-Vergani have shown that the maximum INR reached during the course of illness was the most sensitive predictor of the outcome, with 73% of children with an INR less than 4 surviving compared with only 4 of 24 (16.6%) with an INR greater than 4.[6]

Factor V concentration has been used as a prognostic marker, especially in association with encephalopathy (Clichy criteria). In children, a factor V concentration of less than 25% of normal suggests a poor outcome, and in many French centers, this criterion is used for listing for liver transplant.[65]

Liver biopsy is rarely helpful in ALF and is usually contraindicated because of the presence of coagulopathy. However, it can be done using a transjugular approach. Hepatic parenchymal necrosis of more than 50% is associated with a reduced survival,[66] but the potential for sampling error is considerable. A biopsy taken from an area of complete collapse will show very few viable hepatocytes, indicating a poor prognosis. On the other hand, a biopsy specimen taken from a regenerative nodule may falsely give a good prognosis (Figure 58-3). These limitations and difficulty in performing a liver biopsy in patients with ALF have limited its value as a prognostic test.

A small liver or, more particularly, a rapidly shrinking liver is an indictor of a poor prognosis. Computed tomographic volumetry of the liver has been used to assess both the size of the liver and its functional reserve.[66]

Fulminant Wilson disease is invariably fatal, and emergency liver transplant is the only effective treatment.[67,68] Predicting the outcome of decompensated Wilson disease presenting as ALF is usually difficult. In our experience, a prognostic score has been useful in identifying the patients who carry a high risk of mortality without liver transplant (Table 58-6). It incorporates bilirubin, INR, aspartate transaminase, white blood cell count, and albumin at presentation. A score of 11 or more indicates high mortality, with 93% sensitivity and 96% specificity.

Survival depends on the ability of the liver to recover from the ensuing insult, but it is very difficult to predict the potential of recovery. There are no single criteria that can predict the outcome with absolute certainty and be universally applicable for all patients with ALF with different etiologies. However, prediction of a low level of survival (chance of < 20%) is clinically useful to decide to list the patient for orthotopic liver transplant (OLT), which has a 1-year survival rate of 75%.[69]

MANAGEMENT

An initial contact with a specialist center at diagnosis should be made to establish a management plan. Depending on the local facilities and expertise, the timing of referral to hepatology and liver transplant centers may vary, but an early transfer is always recommended. Liver transplant has undoubtedly improved the survival of this group of patients, but better intensive care monitoring and early and better management of complications can sometimes avoid transplant or death. Also, monitoring of these patients is a continuous process of assessing the clinical status so that a child who is not considered for liver transplant initially may change his/her status. Likewise, a child who has been

listed for liver transplant may show signs of unexpected improvement, hence not requiring transplant operation, or may develop complications that contraindicate it.

INITIAL ASSESSMENT
A careful and detailed history should include the mode of onset of illness, family history of liver disease, consanguinity, and exposure to drugs and toxins. Clinical examination

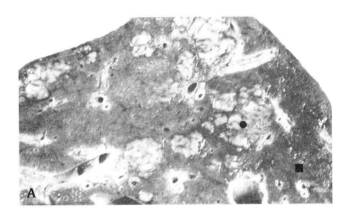
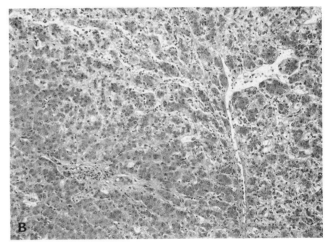
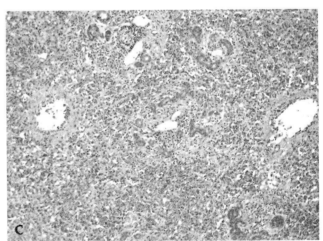

FIGURE 58-3   A, Macroscopic appearance of areas of collapse (■) and regeneration (●) in an explanted liver. Microscopic appearances from these areas show regenerating hepatic parenchyma (B) or collapse (C) (hematoxylin and eosin; ×100 original magnification). Courtesy of Professor Bernard Portmann, King's College Hospital.

TABLE 58-6   WILSON DISEASE INDEX

SCORE	BILIRUBIN (μMOL/L)	INR	AST (IU/L)	WBC (10⁹/L)	ALBUMIN (G/L)
0	0–100	0–1.2	0–100	0–6.7	> 45
1	101–150	1.3–1.6	101–150	6.8–8.3	34–44
2	151–200	1.7–1.9	151–200	8.4–10.3	25–33
3	201–300	2.0–2.4	201–300	10.4–15.3	21–24
4	> 300	> 2.5	> 300	> 15.4	0–20

AST = aspartate transaminase; INR = international normalized ratio; WBC = white blood cell count.

could give diagnostic clues such as the presence of any herpetic vesicles, signs of underlying chronic liver disease, and the presence of Kayser-Fleischer rings on slit lamp examination. All children with ALF require elaborate investigations to establish the underlying cause (Tables 58-7 and 58-8).

GENERAL MEASURES

All children with ALF should be nursed in a quiet environment with as little stimulation as possible to minimize acute increase in the ICP. Children with encephalopathy or an INR greater than 4 (without encephalopathy) should be admitted to an intensive care unit for continuous monitoring. Sedation is contraindicated unless the patient is to be mechanically ventilated because of the possibility of aggravating the encephalopathy or precipitating respiratory failure.

Monitoring of nonventilated ALF patients should include the following:

* Continuous oxygen saturation monitoring
* 6-hourly urine output
* 6-hourly vital signs including blood pressure, neurologic observations, and blood glucose estimation
* 12-hourly electrolyte and coagulation studies (INR)
* Daily full blood count along with surveillance blood and urine cultures

In addition, patients on assisted ventilation have an arterial line for invasive blood pressure monitoring and frequent blood sampling. Blood gas analysis is performed every 4 hours, and electrolytes and prothrombin time are measured every 8 hours. Sedation in these ventilated patients is maintained by a morphine and midazolam infusion in our unit. The use of benzodiazepines for sedation in ALF is only recommended once a decision has been taken to ventilate the patient (management of specific complications is discussed later). Controlled trials in adults have failed to substantiate any beneficial effect of corticosteroids, interferon, insulin and glucose, prostaglandin E₁, bowel decontamination, and charcoal hemoperfusion in patients with ALF. The use of enemas and cathartics in patients who are not constipated is usually counterproductive, not only by increasing their nursing need but also by triggering surges of ICP. Hypoglycemia should be avoided by use of intravenous glucose infusion or by ensuring adequate enteral intake. Total fluid intake is restricted to two-thirds maintenance if there is no evidence of dehydration, with the idea of decreasing the possibility of development of cerebral edema. The idea of protein restriction to limit the possibility of HE has now been disregarded, and adequate calories should be provided. Oral or nasogastric feeding is usually well tolerated. Prophylactic broad-spectrum antibi-

TABLE 58-7   DIAGNOSTIC TESTS OF THE CAUSES OF ACUTE LIVER FAILURE

CAUSE	TEST
Hepatitis A infection	Anti-HAV antibody (IgM)
Hepatitis B infection	
Acute infection/seroconversion	Anti–core antibody (IgM)/HBV profile
Increased replication	Full HBV profile
Hepatitis D infection	Anti-HDV antibody (IgM)
Parvovirus, adenovirus, EBV	Viral serology/antigen tests, PCR
Seronegative hepatitis	Diagnosis of exclusion (all tests)
Acetaminophen	History, drug level in blood
Mushroom poisoning	History, diarrhea
Autoimmune hepatitis	Autoantibodies, immunoglobulins
Wilson disease	Urinary copper, Kayser-Fleischer rings, Coombs-negative hemolytic anemia
Galactosemia	Galactose-1-phosphate uridyl transferase level in blood
Tyrosinemia	Urinary succinylacetone
Neonatal hemochromatosis	Buccal mucosal biopsy, raised ferritin, high transferrin saturation
Hemophagocytic lymphohistiocytosis	Bone marrow aspiration (typical cells)
Mitochondrial hepatopathies	Muscle and liver biopsies for quantitative assay of respiratory chain enzyme
Veno-occlusive disease	Doppler ultrasonography/venography
Malignancies	Imaging (CT/MRI) and histology
Idiosyncratic drug reactions	History, eosinophil count

CT = computed tomography; EBV = Epstein-Barr virus; HAV = hepatitis A virus; HBV = hepatitis B virus; HDV = hepatitis D virus; IgM = immunoglobulin M; MRI = magnetic resonance imaging; PCR = polymerase chain reaction.

TABLE 58-8   INVESTIGATIONS IN INFANTS AND CHILDREN WITH ACUTE LIVER FAILURE

Biochemical tests
  Liver function tests (total and direct bilirubin, AST, ALT, GGT, ALP, albumin)
  Blood sugar
  Serum electrolytes
  Serum calcium, phosphorus
  Serum magnesium
  Uric acid
  Cholesterol
  Triglyceride
  Amylase
  α_1-Antitrypsin phenotype
  Galactose-1-phosphate uridyl transferase (in infants and neonates)
  Serum copper and ceruloplasmin (in children > 3 yr old)
  Serum amino acids
  Plasma acylcarnitines
  Blood gas analysis
Hematologic tests
  Full blood count
  Reticulocyte count
  Prothrombin time or INR
  Blood for grouping and crossmatching
  Direct Coombs test
  Bone marrow examination (in seronegative hepatitis or if hematologic malignancy or HLH is suspected)
Ultrasound scan of abdomen, especially liver, portal and hepatic veins, inferior vena cava, biliary system, and spleen
Microbiologic tests
  Bacterial cultures: blood, urine, stool, throat swab, sputum, skin lesion if present, ascitic fluid if present
  Viral culture of urine and skin lesion if present

Serologic tests
  Viral hepatitis: anti-HAV IgM antibody, HBsAg, HBcAg, hepatitis D antigen and antibody, anti–hepatitis C antibody, anti–hepatitis E antibody
  Cytomegalovirus
  Epstein-Barr virus
  Human immunodeficiency virus (HIV)
  Measles
  Varicella
  Herpes simplex virus
  Adenovirus
  Echovirus
  Others: toxoplasmosis, leptospirosis, and listeriosis
Immunologic tests
  Immunoglobulins(IgG, IgA, and IgM)
  Tissue antibodies (anti-SMA, GPC, mitochondrial, liver-kidney microsomal and antinuclear antibodies)
  Complement C3 and C4
Ascitic fluid or cerebrospinal fluid cytospin for evidence of hemophagocytosis
Urine
  Toxicology
  Chemical analysis, osmolality, and electrolytes
  Organic acids
  Succinyl acetone
  24-h urinary copper prepenicillamine and postpenicillamine (2 doses of 500 mg 12 h apart)
  (5 mL of serum and aliquot of initial urine for possible subsequent investigations)
Tissue studies
  Buccal mucosal biopsy
  Muscle biopsy
  Skin fibroblast culture
  Transjugular liver biopsy

ALP = alkaline phosphatase; ALT = alanine transaminase; AST = aspartate transaminase; GGT = γ-glutamyl transferase; GPC = gastric parietal cell; HAV = hepatitis A virus; HBcAg = hepatitis B core antigen; HBsAg = hepatitis B surface antigen; HLH = hemophagocytic lymphohistiocytosis; INR = international normalized ratio; SMA = smooth muscle antibody.

otics[70] and antifungals[71] significantly reduce the incidence of infective episodes. In neonatal liver failure, intravenous acyclovir should be commenced.

MANAGEMENT OF SPECIFIC COMPLICATIONS

NEUROLOGIC COMPLICATIONS

The most important neurologic complications are HE and cerebral edema. Management options for the treatment of HE are limited. Ammonia-lowering measures such as dietary protein restriction, bowel decontamination, or lactulose are of limited or no value in rapidly advancing encephalopathy. The use of branched-chain amino acids, flumazenil, and extracorporeal circuits has only shown transient improvement in encephalopathy, without any survival benefit in larger studies.

Cerebral edema has been documented at the time of postmortem in about 30 to 40% of all patients with fatal ALF. Typical features of raised ICP include systemic hypertension, hypertonia, hyperreflexia, decerebration, hyperventilation, dysconjugate eye movements, or squint. In infants, the anterior fontanel may be tense. If uncontrolled, the clinical features progress to loss of pupillary reflexes and, ultimately, impairment of brainstem reflexes. Despite severely increased ICP, papilledema is a rare sign. Systemic hypertension is a good surrogate marker for increased ICP in the initial stages but is absent in later stages.

To date, the opinion is divided toward the risk-to-benefit ratio of using ICP monitoring devices for early detection of increased ICP. Proponents of the use of ICP monitors argue that these devices allow early and accurate detection of changes in ICP, especially in ventilated and sedated patients, in whom the clinical signs are usually masked. It also helps in accurate monitoring of ICP during interventions such as central line insertions, tracheal suctioning, and hemodialysis or hemodiafiltration. Keays and colleagues have shown that ICP monitoring identified rises in ICP unaccompanied by clinical signs, and, as a consequence, treatment was given to the monitored patients more often than the nonmonitored group. The duration of survival from the onset of grade 4 encephalopathy was significantly greater in the ICP-monitored group, although the overall survival rate was unchanged. Monitoring also provided important prognostic information because the peak ICP was higher in nonsurvivors than in survivors.[72] The group that was not enthusiastic about invasive ICP monitoring argued that the procedure is associated with a high incidence of intracranial bleeding and is never proven to improve patient survival. Epidural transducers are associated with a lower complication rate (3.8%) compared with subdural devices that carry a 22% risk of intracranial complications.[8,73] High ICP at the time of insertion of the device has been shown to be a major risk factor for the development of intracranial hemorrhage. Our practice is to insert a subdural bolt in children older than 2 years who have clinical signs of increased ICP and are awaiting liver transplant.

The aim of ICP monitoring is to maintain cerebral perfusion pressure (mean arterial blood pressure – ICP) at more than 50 mm Hg. If the cerebral perfusion pressure falls below 50 mm Hg, the adequacy of sedation and paralysis should be checked, along with $PaCO_2$ levels (in ventilated patients, $PaCO_2$ should be kept between 4 and 4.5 kPa). If the $PaCO_2$ is more than 4.5 kPa, then hyperventilation may be helpful. Excessive hyperventilation should be avoided because it may paradoxically compromise the cerebral perfusion pressure. A care pathway for the management of raised intracranial pressure is shown in Figure 58-4.

Mannitol remains the mainstay of treatment for increased ICP because of its property as an osmotic diuretic. It has also been suggested that a therapeutic response is due to the increase in cerebral blood flow, and the rapidity of action of mannitol is more consistent with this function. A rapid bolus of 0.5 g/kg as a 20% solution over a 15-minute period is recommended, and the dose can be repeated if the serum osmolarity is less than 320 mOsm/L. In anuric patients, a diuresis is simulated by ultrafitrating three times the administered volume over the next half hour.

Uncontrolled studies have shown sodium thiopental to be an effective agent in controlling mannitol-resistant cerebral edema.[74] A bolus dose of 2 to 4 mg/kg over 15 minutes is followed by a slow intravenous infusion of between 1 and 2 mg/kg/h. There has been no controlled trial of the use of sodium thiopental in lowering ICP. Major concerns are hemodynamic instability and increased incidence of infective complications following its administration. Hypothermia (core body temperature of 32°C) has been shown to be effective in the management of severe intracranial hypertension with lowering of ICP and improvement of cerebral perfusion pressure in adults.[75] Subclinical seizure activity also has been suggested as a contributing factor for the development of cerebral edema. In a study of 42 adult patients, Ellis and colleagues demonstrated a significant reduction in the seizure activity in the group treated with phenytoin infusion. Incidence of cerebral edema was also significantly less in the phenytoin-treated group compared with the control group.[76]

In severe unresponsive cerebral edema, the emphasis of management shifts toward preservation of cerebral perfusion pressure, increased oxygen delivery to the brain, and manipulation of the neuronal microcirculation to promote cerebral oxygen extraction. In this situation, inotropic agents can be used to increase the mean arterial pressure, consequently improving cerebral perfusion pressure. Normally, at this stage, spontaneous recovery is unlikely without liver transplant.

Hepatectomy with a portacaval shunt has been shown to stabilize the patients hemodynamically with reduction of ICP up to 48 hours followed by successful liver transplant. N-Acetylcysteine has been shown to increase the cerebral blood flow and cerebral metabolic rate, thereby improving the microcirculatory stability.

INFECTIONS

Bacterial and fungal infections have been documented in about 82 and 34% of patients with ALF, respectively.[61] About 60% of deaths in ALF have been attributed to sepsis.[77] Prophylactic intravenous antibiotics have been shown to reduce the incidence of culture-positive bacterial infection from 61.3 to 32.1%. The respiratory tract is the most common site (47%), followed by the urinary tract (23%).[77] A high index of suspicion, along with early and frequent bacteriologic investigations, is necessary for early diagnosis. Gram-positive bacteria are the most common organism isolated in about 70% of cases, 35% of these isolates being S. aureus.[77]

Topical antifungal prophylaxis has been used in combination with intravenous antibiotics. The efficacy of systemic antifungals as prophylaxis has not been studied systematically. Systemic fungal infection is very difficult to diagnose, but renal failure, severe cholestasis, previous or concomitant thiopental therapy, concomitant immunosuppressive therapy, and worsening coagulopathy are the high-risk factors. The choice of systemic antifungal agents is determined by the local experience. In our unit, fluconazole is the preferred agent because Candida spp. account for most of the fungal infections.

HEMODYNAMIC INSTABILITY

Circulatory failure is a common mode of death in patients with ALF, often complicating sepsis or multiorgan failure. Invasive hemodynamic monitoring may provide early evidence of circulatory failure. Despite the presence of edema, frequently these patients have intravascular volume depletion and need an appropriate combination of colloids, crystalloids, or blood products. In the presence of persistent hypotension despite normal filling, pressure vasopressors such as noradrenaline and adrenaline are inotropic agents of choice. N-Acetylcysteine has been shown to improve the

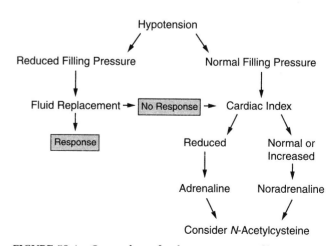

FIGURE 58-4   Care pathway for the management of hypotension.

parameters of oxygen metabolism. A combination of prostacycline and N-acetylcysteine has been found to be more beneficial for oxygen metabolism than either drug alone. In our experience, newer monitoring devices such as pulse contour cardiac output (PiCCO) and lithium dilutional cardiac output (LiDCO) monitoring, which can measure various body water compartments, are good devices to rationalize fluid management and the choice of vasopressors. The PiCCO method is a combination of transpulmonary thermodilution technique and arterial pulse contour analysis. It requires a central venous line and an arterial thermodilution catheter placed in either a femoral or an axillary artery. A bolus of cold saline is injected in the central venous line, and the thermodilution is detected from the special arterial catheter. It measures cardiac ouput (by thermodilution), continuous cardiac output using the pulse contour method, intrathoracic blood volume, and extravascular lung water.[78] LiDCO monitoring involves a bolus indicator dilutional technique for measuring cardiac output using isotonic lithium chloride as an injectate.[79] A care pathway for the management of hypotension is shown in Figure 58-5.

RENAL FAILURE

Renal failure with severe oliguria often develops in ALF, especially in later stages. Although the mechanism of renal failure is not clear, it is essential to correct intravascular hypovolemia. Recent studies have shown that low-dose dopamine is not only ineffective[80] but can have deleterious effects,[81] especially in the setting of profound vasodilatation, which is seen typically in ALF. Extracorporeal renal support was required in 75% of cases with acetaminophen-induced ALF and in 30% of patients with other etiologies of ALF. Hemodiafiltration and hemodialysis should be instituted when the urine output is less than 1 mL/kg/h. Continuous filtration or dialysis systems are associated with less hemodynamic instability and consequently less risk of aggravating latent or established encephalopathy than intermittent hemodialysis. In spite of the presence of coagulopathy, heparin requirements have been shown to be increased. Recently, prostacycline infusion at a rate of 5 ng/kg/min has been found to be superior to heparin anticoagulation with respect to functional duration of the filters and the hemorrhagic complications.[82]

COAGULOPATHY

Bleeding diathesis, although always present in ALF, differs in severity from patient to patient. Normally, disseminated intravascular coagulation is not a feature of ALF but is usually an indicator of sepsis. The possible advantage of reduced bleeding by repletion of coagulation factors with fresh frozen plasma has not been established by clinical studies. Because coagulopathy is a very good tool for assessment of prognosis and monitoring of disease progression, correction of coagulopathy is indicated only if the patient is already listed for transplant or prior to an invasive procedure such as insertion of a central line or ICP monitors. This also carries a further disadvantage of volume overload and hyperviscosity. There has been a poor

correlation between the severity of prolongation of prothrombin time and bleeding tendencies, but associated thrombocytopenia is an important risk factor for hemorrhage; hence, the platelet count should be maintained above 50×10^9/dL.

The most common site of bleeding is the gastrointestinal tract. Prophylactic ranitidine (histamine$_2$ blocker) or proton pump inhibitors have been shown to decrease the incidence of gastric bleeding.[83] A study comparing antacid with histamine$_2$ blockers showed equal efficacy if the gastric pH was kept above 3.5 by frequent administration of antacid. There is increased risk of gastric colonization with use of histamine$_2$ blockers or proton pump inhibitors. Sucralfate has the potential advantage of reducing gastric colonization and pulmonary infection by maintaining gastric acidity, but its efficacy in ALF has not been assessed.

VENTILATORY MANAGEMENT

Ventilatory support in the form of mechanical ventilation is instituted when grade 3 encephalopathy develops or when patients in grade 1 or 2 encephalopathy require sedation. Inducing agents such as suxamethonium and fentanyl are generally safe. Sedation could be maintained with a combination of an opiate such as morphine or fentanyl and a hypnotic such as midazolam. There are no special ventilatory requirements in patients with ALF; however, a peak end-expiratory pressure above 8 cm of water should be avoided because it may increase ICP.

Initially, adult respiratory distress syndrome (ARDS) is unusual, and ventilation is easy. The most severe ventilatory problems arise when liver function is improving or the patient had liver transplant when there is a chance of developing ARDS. In patients with unresponsive ARDS, nitric oxide inhalation or intravenous prostacycline may be tried, although their role has not been properly assessed in ALF.

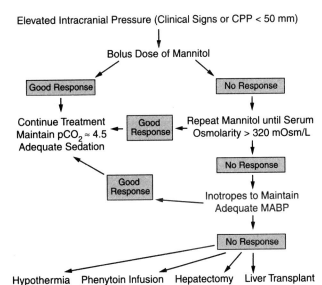

FIGURE 58-5 Care pathway for the management of raised intracranial pressure. CPP = cerebral perfusion pressure; MABP = mean arterial blood pressure; pCO$_2$ = carbon dioxide partial pressure.

LIVER ASSIST DEVICES

In ALF, pathophysiologic changes are due to impairment of synthetic, detoxifying, and biotransformatory activity resulting from the loss of functioning hepatocytes and Kupffer cells. The severity and duration of these changes also depend on the rate and extent of liver regeneration. There has been increasing interest in the possibility of providing an extracorporeal liver support system either as a bridge to liver transplant or, ideally, to obviate the need for it by supporting liver function while the native liver regenerates. Liver support devices could be either cleansing devices or a bioartificial liver support system (Table 58-9). Cleansing devices perform only the detoxifying function of the liver, whereas bioartificial liver support systems have a theoretic advantage of providing the synthetic and detoxifying properties.

Charcoal hemoperfusion was extensively assessed in an initial study of 76 adults and suggested an increase in survival in patients with grade 3 HE,[84] but a subsequent controlled trial did not show any significant difference in outcome.[63]

Recently developed cleansing devices such as Biologic-DT and the molecular adsorbent recirculating system (MARS) attempt to remove protein-bound toxins by perfusion over resins or albumin. The MARS uses an albumin-impregnated dialysis membrane and dialysate containing 5% human albumin solution. This dialysate is perfused to remove water-soluble toxins, including ammonia. Preliminary studies in adults showed a survival rate of 69%, with hemodynamic stabilization, improvement in mental status, and HE.[85] More information is required before this device can be recommended universally.

The bioartificial liver support system uses bioreactors containing hepatocytes in columns. Of three bioartificial liver support devices, the bioartificial liver and the Berlin Extracorporeal Liver Support System use primary porcine hepatocytes, whereas the extracorporeal liver assist device uses the hepatoblastoma cell line. Anticoagulated whole blood or plasma is passed through a device, allowing metabolic transfer between perfusate and hepatocytes. Although preliminary results were encouraging, a controlled pilot study of the ELAD did not show any significant benefit.[86] The bioartificial liver system has shown statistical improvement in the level of consciousness, an increase in ICP, and an increase in cerebral perfusion pressure.[87] These devices appear to be promising, but pediatric experience is limited and anecdotal.

LIVER TRANSPLANT

Liver transplant is the only proven treatment that has improved the outcome of ALF. Taking into account all age

TABLE 58-9   TYPES OF LIVER ASSIST DEVICES

CLEANSING DEVICES	BIOARTIFICIAL LIVER SUPPORT SYSTEMS
Charcoal hemoperfusion	Bioartificial liver
Biologic-DT	Extracorporeal liver assist device
Plasmapheresis	Berlin Extracorporeal Liver Support System
Molecular adsorbent recirculating system	

groups, ALF accounts for 5 to 7% of all liver transplants in the United States[88] and about 11% in Europe.[89] Reports from Europe and the United States have shown that about 45 to 50% of cases with ALF undergo liver transplant, whereas in 13 to 27% of cases, it was contraindicated at the time of admission. About 6 to 18% of cases were removed from the waiting list because of development of a contraindication or the improvement in the clinical and prognostic status or died before a donor liver became available.[8]

Because of the scarcity of donor organs, optimal use of donor livers is essential. This entails proper selection of the patients as well as timing of the operation. In adults, the King's College Hospital criteria have been extensively used for listing for liver transplant (Tables 58-10 and 58-11).[64]

Contraindications for liver transplant are fixed and dilated pupils, uncontrolled sepsis, and severe respiratory failure (ARDS). Relative contraindications are accelerating inotropic requirements, infection under treatment, cerebral perfusion pressure of less than 40 mm Hg for more than 2 hours, and a history of progressive or severe neurologic problems in which the ultimate neurologic outcome may not be acceptable.

After successful transplant, cerebral edema can persist for 12 hours, and cerebral autoregulation is restored within 48 hours. In contrast, the hemodynamic and the neurologic parameters improve during the anhepatic phase of the operation. Extending this advantage, there have been reports of using a two-stage procedure in very unstable patients with hepatectomy followed by liver transplant as soon as the donor liver is available. The longest time of the anhepatic phase preceding OLT has been 48 hours in our experience. Ringe and Pichlmayr reported the largest series of this two-stage procedure, but only 59% of patients received liver transplant[90]

AUXILIARY LIVER TRANSPLANT

The rationale behind this technique is that the allograft provides liver function while the native liver regenerates.

TABLE 58-10   INDICATORS OF A POOR PROGNOSIS IN ACETAMINOPHEN-INDUCED ACUTE LIVER FAILURE

PARAMETER	SENSITIVITY (%)	SPECIFICITY (%)	POSITIVE PREDICTIVE VALUE (%)
Arterial pH < 7.3	49	99	81
All 3 of the following:	45	94	67
Prothrombin time > 100 s or INR > 6.5			
Creatinine > 300 μmol/L (2.3 mg/dL)			
Grade 3–4 encephalopathy			

INR = international normalized ratio.

TABLE 58-11   INDICATORS OF A POOR PROGNOSIS IN NONACETAMINOPHEN ETIOLOGIES OF ACUTE LIVER FAILURE

PARAMETER	SENSITIVITY (%)	SPECIFICITY (%)	POSITIVE PREDICTIVE VALUE (%)
Prothrombin time > 100 s or INR > 6.7	34	100	46
Any 3 of the following:	93	90	92
Unfavorable etiology (seronegative hepatitis or drug reaction)			
Age < 10 yr or > 40 yr			
Acute or subacute categories			
Serum bilirubin > 300 μmol/L (2.3 mg/dL)			
Prothrombin time > 50 s or INR > 3.5			

INR = international normalized ratio.

Once the native liver shows signs of recovery, immunosuppression can be weaned and eventually stopped. Auxiliary liver transplant could be heterotopic (the donor graft is placed alongside the native liver in the right upper quadrant) or orthotopic (part of the native liver is resected and replaced with a reduced-size graft), replacing the right lobe, left lobe, or left lateral segment. Auxiliary partial OLT is preferred over heterotopic. In our center, all patients who undergo auxiliary liver transplant undergo elective liver biopsies at day 7, 6 months, and 1 year, along with computed tomographic volumetry (to assess the volume of native liver and graft) and radionucleotide scan (disopropyl iminodiacetic acid to assess the relative function of the native liver and the graft). Once the native liver has returned to normal morphology and function, immunosuppression is gradually weaned off. The donor liver is supposed to atrophy with time. In our experience, 12 of 14 children who had auxiliary liver transplant survived, and 7 of them have been able to stop immunosuppression after a median post-transplant interval of 9 months (M. Rela, unpublished data, 2003).

Because auxiliary partial OLT is technically demanding, the choice of this operation is ideally left to the local surgical team. There have been no universally accepted indications for auxiliary liver transplant in the setting of ALF.

HEPATOCYTE TRANSPLANT

Taking the success of auxiliary liver transplant further, hepatocyte transplant has been tried in experimental animals with improved survival. In a small number of clinical studies, variable improvement in encephalopathy, coagulopathy, and hyperammonemia has been reported. The procedure has shown some encouraging results as a bridge to transplant, and in one child, liver transplant was avoided; however, the technique remains experimental.[91,92]

CONCLUSION

ALF is a multisystem disorder with a very high mortality rate. In children, seronegative hepatitis is the most common cause of ALF in Western countries. Despite improvement in intensive care support, liver transplant is the only effective treatment. Liver assist devices and hepatocyte transplant hold a great potential of providing a bridge to transplant or avoiding it while the native liver regenerates. The condition should ideally be managed in a liver center with facilities for liver transplant.

REFERENCES

1. Lucke B, Mallory T. Fulminant form of epidemic hepatitis. Am J Pathol 1946;22:867–945.
2. Trey C, Davidson CS. The management of fulminant hepatic failure. Prog Liver Dis 1970;3:282–98.
3. Gimson AE, O'Grady J, Ede RJ, et al. Late onset hepatic failure: clinical, serological and histological features. Hepatology 1986;6:288–94.
4. Bernuau J, Benhamou JP. Classifying acute liver failure. Lancet 1993;342:252–3.
5. O'Grady JG, Schalm SW, Williams R. Acute liver failure: redefining the syndromes [published erratum appears in Lancet 1993;342:1000]. Lancet 1993;342:273–5.
6. Bhaduri BR, Mieli-Vergani G. Fulminant hepatic failure: pediatric aspects. Semin Liver Dis 1996;16:349–55.
7. Sussman NB. Fulminant hepatic failure. In: Zakim D, Boyer TD, editors. Hepatology. Philadelphia: WB Saunders; 2003. p. 618–50.
8. O'Grady JG. Acute liver failure. In: O'Grady JG, Lake JR, Howdle PD, editors. Comprehensive clinical hepatology. London: Mosby; 2000. p. 30.1–20.
9. Vinholt SF, Davern TJ, Obaid SA, et al. Viral hepatitis-related acute liver failure. Am J Gastroenterol 2003;98:448–53.
10. Mathiesen LR, Skinoj P, Nielsen JO, et al. Hepatitis type A, B, and non-A non-B in fulminant hepatitis. Gut 1980;21:72–7.
11. Willner IR, Uhl MD, Howard SC, et al. Serious hepatitis A: an analysis of patients hospitalized during an urban epidemic in the United States. Ann Intern Med 1998;128:111–4.
12. Shah U, Habib Z, Kleinman RE. Liver failure attributable to hepatitis A virus infection in a developing country. Pediatrics 2000;105:436–8.
13. Vento S, Garofano T, Renzini C, et al. Fulminant hepatitis associated with hepatitis A virus superinfection in patients with chronic hepatitis C. N Engl J Med 1998;338:286–90.
14. Cacciola I, Cerenzia G, Pollicino T, et al. Genomic heterogeneity of hepatitis B virus (HBV) and outcome of perinatal HBV infection. J Hepatol 2002;36:426–32.
15. Beath SV, Boxall EH, Watson RM, et al. Fulminant hepatitis B in infants born to anti-HBe hepatitis B carrier mothers. BMJ 1992;304:1169–70.
16. Alter HJ, Purcell RH, Shih JW, et al. Detection of antibody to hepatitis C virus in prospectively followed transfusion recipients with acute and chronic non-A, non-B hepatitis. N Engl J Med 1989;321:1494–500.
17. Krawczynski K, Kamili S, Aggarwal R. Global epidemiology and medical aspects of hepatitis E. Forum (Genova) 2001;11:166–79.
18. Arora NK, Nanda SK, Gulati S, et al. Acute viral hepatitis types E, A, and B singly and in combination in acute liver failure in children in north India. J Med Virol 1996;48:215–21.

19. Hadziyannis SJ. Fulminant hepatitis and the new G/GBV-C flavivirus. J Viral Hepatitis 1998;5:15–9.

20. Iriyama M, Kimura H, Nishikawa K, et al. The prevalence of TT virus (TTV) infection and its relationship to hepatitis in children. Med Microbiol Immunol (Berl) 1999;188:83–9.

21. Aw MM, Dhawan A. Acute liver failure. Indian J Pediatr 2002; 69:87–91.

22. Whittington PF, Soriano HE, Alonsoinant EM. Hepatic failure in children. In: Suchy FJ, Sokol RJ, Balistreri WF, editors. Liver disease in children. Philadelphia: Lippincott Williams & Wilkins; 2001. p. 63–88.

23. Tung J, Hadzic N, Layton M, et al. Bone marrow failure in children with acute liver failure. J Pediatr Gastroenterol Nutr 2000;31:557–61.

24. Palanduz A, Yildirmak Y, Telhan L, et al. Fulminant hepatic failure and autoimmune hemolytic anemia associated with Epstein-Barr virus infection. J Infection 2002;45:96–8.

25. Langnas AN, Markin RS, Cattral MS, Naides SJ. Parvovirus B19 as a possible causative agent of fulminant liver failure and associated aplastic anemia. Hepatology 1995;22:1661–5.

26. Verboon-Maciolek MA, Swanink CM, Krediet TG, et al. Severe neonatal echovirus 20 infection characterized by hepatic failure. Pediatr Infect Dis J 1997;16:524–7.

27. Archer JS. Acute liver failure in pregnancy. A case report. J Reprod Med 2001;46:137–40.

28. Fagan EA, Ellis DS, Tovey GM, et al. Toga virus-like particles in acute liver failure attributed to sporadic non-A, non-B hepatitis and recurrence after liver transplantation. J Med Virol 1992;38:71–7.

29. Joshi YK, Tandon BN, Acharya SK, et al. Acute hepatic failure due to Plasmodium falciparum liver injury. Liver 1986;6:357–60.

30. Rhodes A, Wendon JA. Hepatobiliary dysfunction in the critically ill. In: O'Grady JG, Lake JR, Howdle PD, editors. Comprehensive clinical hepatology. London: Mosby; 2000. p. 31.1 –14.

31. Zimmerman HJ. Drug-induced liver disease. Clin Liver Dis 2000;4:73–96.

32. Jones AL, Simpson KJ. Review article: mechanisms and management of hepatotoxicity in Ecstasy (MDMA) and amphetamine intoxications. Aliment Pharmacol Ther 1999;13:129–33.

33. Davis M. Protective agents for acetaminophen overdose. Semin Liver Dis 1986;6:138–47.

34. Alonso EM, Sokol RJ, Hart J, et al. Fulminant hepatitis associated with centrilobular hepatic necrosis in young children. J Pediatr 1995;127:888–94.

35. Viruet EJ, Torres EA. Steroid therapy in fulminant hepatic failure secondary to autoimmune hepatitis. Puerto Rico Health Sci J 1998;17:297–300.

36. Launay V, Gottrand F, Michaud L, et al. [Autoimmune hepatitis treated with cyclosporin revealed by acute hepatocellular failure]. Arch Pediatr 1997;4:40–3.

37. Kelly AL, Lunt PW, Rodrigues F, et al. Classification and genetic features of neonatal haemochromatosis: a study of 27 affected pedigrees and molecular analysis of genes implicated in iron metabolism. J Med Genet 2001;38:599–610.

38. Sigurdsson L, Reyes J, Kocoshis SA, et al. Neonatal hemochromatosis: outcomes of pharmacologic and surgical therapies. J Pediatr Gastroenterol Nutr 1998;26:85–9.

39. Flynn DM, Mohan N, McKiernan P, et al. Progress in treatment and outcome for children with neonatal haemochromatosis. Arch Dis Childhood Fetal Neonatal Ed 2003;88:F124–7.

40. Whitington PF. Immunomodulatory therapy during pregnancy prevents recurrent lethal neonatal haemochromatosis. Hepatology 2002;36(4 Pt 2):336A.

41. Bakker HD, Scholte HR, Dingemans KP, et al. Depletion of mitochondrial deoxyribonucleic acid in a family with fatal neonatal liver disease. J Pediatr 1996;128(5 Pt 1):683–7.

42. Mazzella M, Cerone R, Bonacci W, et al. Severe complex I deficiency in a case of neonatal-onset lactic acidosis and fatal liver failure. Acta Paediatr 1997;86:326–9.

43. Morris AA, Taanman JW, Blake J, et al. Liver failure associated with mitochondrial DNA depletion. J Hepatol 1998;28:556–63.

44. Shneider BL, Setchell KD, Whitington PF, et al. Delta 4-3-oxosteroid 5 beta-reductase deficiency causing neonatal liver failure and hemochromatosis. J Pediatr 1994;124:234–8.

45. Odaib AA, Shneider BL, Bennett MJ, et al. A defect in the transport of long-chain fatty acids associated with acute liver failure. N Engl J Med 1998;339:1752–7.

46. Arico M, Allen M, Brusa S, et al. Haemophagocytic lymphohistiocytosis: proposal of a diagnostic algorithm based on perforin expression. Br J Haematol 2002;119:180–8.

47. Henter JI, Elinder G, Ost A. Diagnostic guidelines for hemophagocytic lymphohistiocytosis. The FHL Study Group of the Histiocyte Society. Semin Oncol 1991;18:29–33.

48. Egeler RM, Shapiro R, Loechelt B, Filipovich A. Characteristic immune abnormalities in hemophagocytic lymphohistiocytosis. J Pediatr Hematol Oncol 1996;18:340–5.

49. Devictor D, Tahiri C, Fabre M, et al. Early pre-B acute lymphoblastic leukemia presenting as fulminant liver failure. J Pediatr Gastroenterol Nutr 1996;22:103–6.

50. Laubenberger J, Haussinger D, Bayer S, et al. Proton magnetic resonance spectroscopy of the brain in symptomatic and asymptomatic patients with liver cirrhosis. Gastroenterology 1997;112:1610–6.

51. Levy LJ, Leek J, Losowsky MS. Evidence for gamma-aminobutyric acid as the inhibitor of gamma-aminobutyric acid binding in the plasma of humans with liver disease and hepatic encephalopathy. Clin Sci (Lond) 1987;73:531–4.

52. Fischer JE, Baldessarini RJ. False neurotransmitters and hepatic failure. Lancet 1971;ii:75–80.

53. Blei AT, Larsen FS. Pathophysiology of cerebral edema in fulminant hepatic failure. J Hepatol 1999;31:771–6.

54. McClung HJ, Sloan HR, Powers P, et al. Early changes in the permeability of the blood-brain barrier produced by toxins associated with liver failure. Pediatr Res 1990;28:227–31.

55. Vilstrup H, Iversen J, Tygstrup N. Glucoregulation in acute liver failure. Eur J Clin Invest 1986;16:193–7.

56. Ring-Larsen H, Palazzo U. Renal failure in fulminant hepatic failure and terminal cirrhosis: a comparison between incidence, types, and prognosis. Gut 1981;22:585–91.

57. Ellis D, Avner ED, Starzl TE. Renal failure in children with hepatic failure undergoing liver transplantation. J Pediatr 1986;108:393–8.

58. Moore K, Wendon J, Frazer M, et al. Plasma endothelin immunoreactivity in liver disease and the hepatorenal syndrome. N Engl J Med 1992;327:1774–8.

59. Rolando N, Wade J, Davalos M, et al. The systemic inflammatory response syndrome in acute liver failure. Hepatology 2000;32(4 Pt 1):734–9.

60. Trewby PN, Warren R, Contini S, et al. Incidence and pathophysiology of pulmonary edema in fulminant hepatic failure. Gastroenterology 1978;74(5 Pt 1):859–65.

61. Rolando N, Philpott-Howard J, Williams R. Bacterial and fungal infection in acute liver failure. Semin Liver Dis 1996;16: 389–402.

62. Harry R, Auzinger G, Wendon J. The clinical importance of adrenal insufficiency in acute hepatic dysfunction. Hepatology 2002;36:395–402.

63. O'Grady JG, Gimson AE, O'Brien CJ, et al. Controlled trials of

charcoal hemoperfusion and prognostic factors in fulminant hepatic failure. Gastroenterology 1988;94(5 Pt 1):1186–92.

64. O'Grady JG, Alexander GJ, Hayllar KM, Williams R. Early indicators of prognosis in fulminant hepatic failure. Gastroenterology 1989;97:439–45.

65. Devictor D, Desplanques L, Debray D, et al. Emergency liver transplantation for fulminant liver failure in infants and children. Hepatology 1992;16:1156–62.

66. Shakil AO, Jones BC, Lee RG, et al. Prognostic value of abdominal CT scanning and hepatic histopathology in patients with acute liver failure. Dig Dis Sci 2000;45:334–9.

67. Rela M, Heaton ND, Vougas V, et al. Orthotopic liver transplantation for hepatic complications of Wilson's disease. Br J Surg 1993;80:909–11.

68. Schilsky ML, Scheinberg IH, Sternlieb I. Liver transplantation for Wilson's disease: indications and outcome. Hepatology 1994;19:583–7.

69. Ascher NL, Lake JR, Emond JC, Roberts JP. Liver transplantation for fulminant hepatic failure. Arch Surg 1993:128:677–82.

70. Rolando N, Wade JJ, Stangou A, et al. Prospective study comparing the efficacy of prophylactic parenteral antimicrobials, with or without enteral decontamination, in patients with acute liver failure. Liver Transplant Surg 1996;2(1):8–13.

71. Rolando N, Harvey F, Brahm J, et al. Fungal infection: a common, unrecognised complication of acute liver failure. J Hepatol 1991;12:1–9.

72. Keays RT, Alexander GJ, Williams R. The safety and value of extradural intracranial pressure monitors in fulminant hepatic failure. J Hepatol 1993;18:205–9.

73. Blei AT, Olafsson S, Webster S, Levy R. Complications of intracranial pressure monitoring in fulminant hepatic failure. Lancet 1993;341:157–8.

74. Forbes A, Alexander GJ, O'Grady JG, et al. Thiopental infusion in the treatment of intracranial hypertension complicating fulminant hepatic failure. Hepatology 1989;10:306–10.

75. Jalan R, Damink SW, Deutz NE, et al. Moderate hypothermia for uncontrolled intracranial hypertension in acute liver failure. Lancet 1999;354:1164–8.

76. Ellis AJ, Wendon JA, Williams R. Subclinical seizure activity and prophylactic phenytoin infusion in acute liver failure: a controlled clinical trial. Hepatology 2000;32:536–41.

77. Rolando N, Harvey F, Brahm J, et al. Prospective study of bacterial infection in acute liver failure: an analysis of fifty patients. Hepatology 1990;11:49–53.

78. Godje O, Friedl R, Hannekum A. Accuracy of beat-to-beat cardiac output monitoring by pulse contour analysis in hemodynamical unstable patients. Med Sci Monit 2001;7:1344–50.

79. Jonas MM, Tanser SJ. Lithium dilution measurement of cardiac output and arterial pulse waveform analysis: an indicator

80. Kellum JA, Decker M. Use of dopamine in acute renal failure: a meta-analysis. Crit Care Med 2001;29:1526–31.

81. Power DA, Duggan J, Brady HR. Renal-dose (low-dose) dopamine for the treatment of sepsis-related and other forms of acute renal failure: ineffective and probably dangerous. Clin Exp Pharmacol Physiol Suppl 1999;26:S23–8.

82. Kozek-Langenecker SA, Spiss CK, Gamsjager T, et al. Anticoagulation with prostaglandins and unfractionated heparin during continuous venovenous haemofiltration: a randomized controlled trial. Wien Klin Wochenschr 2002;114:96–101.

83. MacDougall BR, Bailey RJ, Williams R. H2-receptor antagonists and antacids in the prevention of acute gastrointestinal haemorrhage in fulminant hepatic failure. Two controlled trials. Lancet 1977;i:617–9.

84. Gimson AE, Braude S, Mellon PJ, et al. Earlier charcoal haemoperfusion in fulminant hepatic failure. Lancet 1982;ii:681–3.

85. Stange J, Hassanein TI, Mehta R, et al. The molecular adsorbents recycling system as a liver support system based on albumin dialysis: a summary of preclinical investigations, prospective, randomized, controlled clinical trial, and clinical experience from 19 centers. Artif Organs 2002;26:103–10.

86. Ellis AJ, Hughes RD, Wendon JA, et al. Pilot-controlled trial of the extracorporeal liver assist device in acute liver failure. Hepatology 1996;24:1446–51.

87. Chen SC, Mullon C, Kahaku E, et al. Treatment of severe liver failure with a bioartificial liver. Ann N Y Acad Sci 1997; 831:350–60.

88. Belle SH, Beringer KC, Detre KM. Liver transplantation in the United States: results from the National Pitt-UNOS Liver Transplant Registry. United Network for Organ Sharing. Clin Transpl 1994;19–35.

89. Bismuth H, Samuel D, Castaing D, et al. Liver transplantation in Europe for patients with acute liver failure. Semin Liver Dis 1996;16:415–25.

90. Ringe B, Pichlmayr R. Total hepatectomy and liver transplantation: a life-saving procedure in patients with severe hepatic trauma. Br J Surg 1995;82:837–9.

91. Strom SC, Fisher RA, Thompson MT, et al. Hepatocyte transplantation as a bridge to orthotopic liver transplantation in terminal liver failure. Transplantation 1997;63:559–69.

92. Soriano HE, Wood RP, Kang DC. Hepatocellular transplantation in children with fulminant liver failure. Hepatology 1997; 26:239A.

93. Holme E, Lindstedt S. Tyrosinaemia type I and NTBC (2-(2-nitro-4-trifluoromethylbenzoyl)-1,3-cyclohexanedione). J Inherit Metab Dis 1998;21:507–17.

CHAPTER 59

TREATMENT OF END-STAGE LIVER DISEASE

Suzanne V. McDiarmid, MB, CHB

The challenges of treating children with end-stage liver disease are considerable. As liver function deteriorates, a cascade of complications ensues, involving every major organ system. The pivotal role of the liver as the body's biochemical "brain" becomes even more evident as liver function is lost. As well, the liver is positioned at the interface of the splanchnic and systemic circulations and has a profound influence on hemodynamics.

The many diverse causes of chronic liver disease in children are discussed elsewhere, but all share a similar final common pathway as chronic liver failure evolves. Although the spectrum of complications resulting from chronic liver disease is similar in children and adults, children are more vulnerable to the profound effects of the failing liver on growth, development, and nutrition. As well, the management of portal hypertension and bleeding varices is made more technically difficult in small children because therapeutic interventions are often limited by the diminutive size of the patient and their vasculature.

The success of liver transplant over the last two decades has given the pediatric hepatologist a new perspective on managing end-stage liver disease. Because many of these children are transplant candidates, medical care has changed dramatically from the pre-1980s philosophy of supportive, palliative treatment preceding inevitable death to anticipatory management that will maintain the child in the best possible condition until transplant. One of the most effective means that the pediatric hepatologist has to ensure survival after liver transplant is to prevent the child from becoming critically ill before transplant. Keeping this in mind, this chapter reviews the management of the major complications of end-stage liver disease in children.

NUTRITIONAL SUPPORT

Cholestatic liver diseases are the most important etiology of end-stage liver disease in children. Biliary atresia is the most common, followed by the intrahepatic cholestasis syndromes. Irrespective of the cause of cholestasis, all share an increased risk of malnutrition. Because most of

these children are candidates for liver transplant and malnutrition is a known factor that adversely affects morbidity and mortality after transplant (Figure 59-1),[1-3] early recognition and timely intervention are essential.

The cause of malnutrition is multifactorial (Table 59-1).[4,5] Fat malabsorption is inevitable because of the dependence of long-chain fatty acids, the most important component of dietary fat, on the micellar action of bile acids in the intestinal lumen for absorption.[6] Compounding the risk, most children afflicted with cholestatic liver disease are infants, with high caloric requirements for growth and development. As well, increased intra-abdominal pressure, either secondary to ascites or organomegaly, is a frequent complication causing early satiety, diminished oral intake,

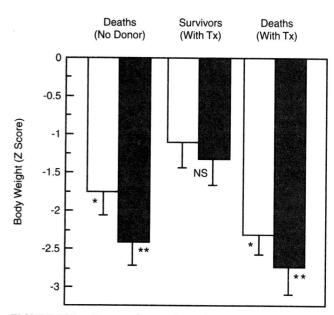

FIGURE 59-1   Z-scores for weight at the time of referral and at the time of transplant or death without a donor in three outcome groups of children with end-stage liver disease accepted for liver transplant. Open bars are scores at referral; black bars are scores at transplant or death. Deaths (no donor), $n = 8$; survivors, $n = 23$. Deaths (with transplant [Tx]), $n = 6$; $p < .05$ for deaths. *$p < .02$ versus survivors; **$p < .02$ versus survivors. NS = not significant. Reproduced with permission from Shepherd RW et al.[1]

TABLE 59-1	FACTORS CONTRIBUTING TO MALNUTRITION IN END-STAGE LIVER DISEASE

Fat malabsorption 2° to cholestasis
  Diminished oral intake 2° to ↑ abdominal girth
  Ascites
  Organomegaly
↑ Abdominal pressure → ↑ emesis
Peripheral resistance to anabolic effects of growth hormone
Anorexia 2° to chronic disease
↑ Catabolic rate
  Intercurrent infection
  Complications

and an increased risk of postprandial emesis. These infants are often debilitated by the anorexia of chronic disease, which is further exacerbated when the complications of end-stage liver disease supervene. Oral intake further decreases at a time when catabolic stresses are increased, resulting in a widening discrepancy between caloric requirement and intake. As the cycle of cholestasis-induced malabsorption and inadequate calorie and protein intake intensifies, these small children rapidly decompensate to clinically evident protein-energy malnutrition. First, subcutaneous tissue stores are depleted (evidenced by decreasing triceps skinfold thickness), followed by loss of muscle mass (measured by decreases in midarm circumference). Eventually, if left untreated, these severely cholestatic infants will present emaciated, hypotonic, dehydrated, and in need of emergency medical care.

Important metabolic and endocrine derangements are associated with chronic liver disease, further intensifying protein-energy malnutrition. Peripheral insulin resistance causing increased gluconeogenesis depletes muscle protein stores. The ratio of aromatic amino acids to branched-chain amino acids (BCAAs) (leucine, isoleucine, valine) in the peripheral blood increases, secondary to increased use of BCAAs by peripheral muscle.[7] BCAAs have important anticatabolic effects and a role in optimizing nitrogen use. As well, caloric requirements are increased above normal estimates for age, as demonstrated by studies in which children failed to show improvement in nutritional status, unless they received in excess of 1.5 to 2 times the estimated caloric requirements for age.[4,8]

Of particular importance in children are the now well-described abnormalities in the growth hormone (GH) and insulin growth factor (IGF) axis in cholestatic liver disease.[9,10] GH mediates most of its anabolic effects through IGF-1. The IGF-binding proteins (IGFBPs), especially IGFBP-3, regulate the transport of IGF to the tissues. Although IGF-1 and IGFBP-3 are produced in a variety of tissues, the most important site of synthesis is the hepatocyte for IGF-1 and the Kupffer cell for IGFBP-3. In children without liver disease but with protein-energy malnutrition, IGF-1 levels fall, suggesting an important link between nutritional status and growth.[11] In children with cholestatic liver disease, including both biliary atresia and Alagille syndrome, several authors have shown that not only are GH levels increased above normal, but IGF-1 lev-

els are decreased, suggesting peripheral resistance to GH. In a study of children with chronic liver disease, short stature, and increased GH levels, Bucuvalas showed that the expected effects of high GH levels, lypolysis, and decreased insulin sensitivity did not occur.[12] As well, several authors have shown that despite adequate protein calorie intake, GH supplementation of children with biliary atresia or Alagille syndrome had no beneficial effect on growth, anthropometric measurements, or body composition.[10,13] In addition, circulating IGF-1 and IGFBP-3 levels were unaffected.[14] This resistance to exogenous GH in the face of low levels of IGF-1 raises the possibility that these growth-retarded children may benefit from IGF-1 treatment.[10,14]

The assessment of nutritional status in children with chronic liver disease is complicated by the effects of fluid retention, ascites, and often massive hepatosplenomegaly, making changes in weight, or weight-for-height ratios, unreliable. Although height z-scores are more useful, a falloff in linear growth is a relatively late consequence of malnutrition. To accurately assess the earlier stages of protein-energy malnutrition and to follow the effects of nutritional interventions, anthropometric measurements are essential. Midarm circumference correlates with lean body mass (protein stores) and triceps or subscapular skinfold thickness with body adipose stores. More sophisticated estimates of body cell mass measure total-body potassium content. Because more than 90% of body potassium is intracellular, its measurement is not affected by fluid shifts between the intra- and extracellular compartments.[15] These principles are well demonstrated by a study that evaluated 56 children with chronic liver disease. Mean height z-scores were decreased, whereas mean weight and mean weight-for-height z-scores were close to normal.[16] Moreover, triceps skinfold z-scores were the most depressed, compared with either height or weight z-scores. Midarm circumference was also depressed but not as markedly as triceps skinfold thickness, suggesting that lean body mass was not as severely depleted as body adipose tissue reserves. This study demonstrates the important principle that children with chronic liver disease have evidence of both chronic malnutrition, as evidenced by stunted growth (decreased height z-scores), as well as acute malnutrition, characterized by depressed adipose reserves and lean body mass.

Improving nutritional status in children with chronic liver disease is challenging (Table 59-2).[17,18] Anorexia, increased abdominal girth, and intervening complications often severely limit the child's voluntary enteral intake. As well, the sodium and fluid restrictions required to manage ascites may sabotage efforts to increase caloric intake. Specialized formulas high in medium-chain triglycerides, which are not dependent on bile for absorption, are useful adjuvants. Caloric density may be further increased by the addition of medium-chain triglyceride and glucose.

However, these measures are often insufficient, necessitating supplemental nasogastic or jejunal feeds[19] or, failing this, parenteral nutritional support. Nocturnal drip feedings appear to be the best tolerated and can allow high caloric intakes without the rise in serum ammonia that might be anticipated with the increased protein intake.[8,20]

TABLE 59-2   ESCALATING LEVELS
                       OF NUTRITIONAL SUPPORT

Change to specialized formula
  Low Na
  Enriched MCT content
Supplement vitamins A, D, K, and E
↑ Caloric density of voluntary enteral formula intake
  24.27 cal/oz
  Addition of MCT oil or polycose
Supplement voluntary enteral intake
  Continuous nocturnal NG or NJ feeds
Parenteral nutritional support
  If fails to grow on maximum enteral feed or unable to tolerate ↑
    enteral feeds
  Intralipid supplementation only
  Intralipid + glucose/amino acid solutions + parenteral vitamins

MCT = medium-chain triglyceride; NG = nasogastric; NJ = nasojejunal.

The usefulness of supplementing enteral feeds with BCAA remains somewhat controversial. In one randomized study, infants receiving BCAA supplementation showed an increase in total-body potassium and improved anthropometric measurements compared with control infants fed an isocaloric formula.[15]

Supplemental enteral feeds fail in many infants because of the inability to tolerate the volumes required. Emesis and increased stool output often negate the hoped for benefits, and parenteral nutrition is the only remaining option. However, parenteral nutrition should not be viewed as a last resort but rather instituted at the first signs of failure of enteral support. Calories provided can be increased easily and weight-for-height z-scores improved[21] by using concentrated glucose solutions supplemented with intravenous lipids.[22] In addition, free water and sodium can be carefully controlled and trace element and vitamin deficiencies more effectively treated.[17,23] Although central venous catheter sepsis is always a concern, careful training of caregivers can greatly decrease this risk.[24]

FAT-SOLUBLE VITAMIN SUPPLEMENTATION (VITAMINS A, D, E, AND K)

Supplementation of the fat-soluble vitamins A, D, E, and K is especially important in children with cholestatic liver disease.[25] The decrease in intraluminal bile acids leading to malabsorption of fat, and therefore the fat-soluble vitamins, is the mechanism of these deficiencies.[26] Vitamin K deficiency, manifested by coagulopathy, is treated with oral vitamin K_1 (Mephyton, Merck & Co, Inc, West Point, PA) at a dose of 5 to 10 mg/d. Vitamin K_1 is virtually nontoxic, compared with vitamin K_3, which, although water soluble, is associated with hemolysis in large doses. The vitamin K–dependent coagulation factors are II, VII, IX, and X. Vitamin K deficiency decreases factor VII levels first so that monitoring prothrombin time is the most useful measure to assess the response to vitamin K therapy. However, as end-stage liver disease becomes more severe, decreased production of all of the coagulation factors produced in the liver occurs, even when vitamin K supplementation is adequate, with consequent prolongation of both prothrombin time and partial thromboplastin time. Occasionally, severely cholestatic children will be unable to adequately absorb oral vitamin K supplements, but the prothrombin time often normalizes after intramuscular vitamin K.

Vitamin E deficiency is a particular concern in children because of vitamin E's role in central nervous system development. Infants who develop cholestasis in the first weeks of life will have low vitamin E levels by about 4 months of age.[27] The first signs of vitamin E deficiency are a symmetric decrease in peripheral stretch reflexes. Left untreated, vitamin E deficiency will progress to cerebellar ataxia, posterior column dysfunction, and peripheral neuropathy.[28] Early recognition is therefore essential but is made more difficult by the unreliability of monitoring only serum vitamin E levels. Normal serum vitamin E levels range between 5 and 15 mg/dL. However, the most accurate evaluation of vitamin E status is the ratio of serum vitamin E to total serum lipids. In children < 12 years of age, the vitamin E–to–total serum lipid (sum of fasting cholesterol, triglycerides, and phospholipids) ratio should be > 0.6 mg/g.[29] No fully water-soluble vitamin E supplement is currently available, making effective vitamin E supplementation often difficult. The free form of vitamin E, available as an over-the-counter preparation, is most often used, but doses as high as 400 to 800 IU/d may be needed. The response to therapy is best evaluated by sequential neurologic evaluations and monitoring of serum vitamin E–to–total lipid ratios.

In those children who do not respond to supplementation of vitamin E by traditional methods, oral administration of a water-soluble form of vitamin E–α-tocopheryl polyethylene glycol–1,000 succinate (α-TPGS) has been found to correct biochemical vitamin E deficiency in doses of 15 to 25 IU/kg/d. In truly refractory cases, an admixture of all fat-soluble vitamins with TPGS may be more beneficial than administration of the supplement alone.

The familiar consequences of vitamin D deficiency—rickets and osteoporosis—can be avoided by early vitamin D supplementation. Although the liver is the site of 25-hydroxylation of vitamin D—a key step in the initiation of activation of vitamin D—malabsorption is the most important cause of vitamin D deficiency in cholestatic children.[30] 25-Hydroxyvitamin D is the major circulating form of vitamin D and, in normal children, has a serum concentration of between 25 and 30 ng/mL.[31] Orally administered 25-hydroxyvitamin D (Caderol, Orggnon Inc, West Orange, NJ) is superior to vitamin D_2 (Drisdol, Sanofi Pharmaceuticals, New York, NY). A dose of 25 to 50 μg/d or 5 to 7 μg/kg/d is adequate. Serum 25-hydroxy levels should be measured and maintained within the normal range. The 1,25-hydroxy form of vitamin D (Rocaltrol, Roche, Nutley, NJ) may be used in a dose of 0.1 to 0.2 μg/kg/d but is not superior to the 25-hydroxy form because kidney conversion of 25-hydroxy to 1,25-hydroxyvitamin D remains intact.

Vitamin A deficiency, characterized by conjunctival and corneal dryness (xerosis) and night blindness, occurs when serum levels fall below 100 to 200 mg/L. Vitamin A can be supplemented with a water-miscible form, such as Aquasol A, at a dose of 5,000 to 15,000 IU/d. Vitamin A serum concentrations should be monitored both before and during therapy to avoid vitamin A toxicity.

PORTAL HYPERTENSION

Variceal bleeding as a consequence of portal hypertension is one of the most dramatic and life-threatening complications seen in pediatric liver disease. Aggressive management begins with cardiovascular resuscitation and requires knowledge of the full range of medical, pharmacologic, and surgical therapies available (Figure 59-2).

The pathophysiology of portal hypertension is described in detail in Chapter 5.2, "Fibrogenesis and Cirrhosis." In brief, the level of portal vein obstruction can be presinusoidal, sinusodial, or postsinusoidal.[32] Presinusoidal portal hypertension can be extrahepatic or intrahepatic. Extrahepatic portal vein obstruction used to be the most frequently recognized cause of portal hypertension in children and was most often secondary to instrumentation of the umbilical vein in neonates, omphalitis, congenital malformations,

blunt trauma, or intra-abdominal infections. Intrahepatic presinusoidal portal hypertension is associated with congenital hepatic fibrosis and schistosomiasis and is relatively less common than extrahepatic or other intrahepatic postsinusoidal causes of portal hypertension in children. Cirrhosis, now the most common cause of portal hypertension in children, results in complex derangements of portal flow within the liver at all three levels but particularly within the sinusoids (reflected by an increased wedge hepatic pressure) and in the postsinusoidal space. Budd-Chiari syndrome, webs in the suprahepatic vena cava, veno-occlusive disease, and cardiac disease are some of the causes of postsinusoidal portal hypertension. The critical difference affecting management of the three levels of portal vein obstruction is that liver functional reserve is almost always normal with extrahepatic and presinusoidal obstruction but may be profoundly impaired in children with sinusoidal and postsinusoidal obstruction secondary to cirrhosis. In such children, coexistent ascites and coagulopathy make the management of variceal bleeding even more challenging.

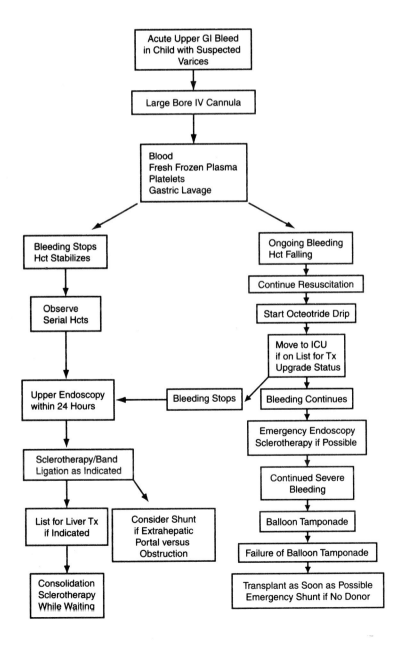

FIGURE 59-2 A management algorithm for the child with suspected bleeding. GI = gastrointestinal; Hcts = hematocrits; ICU = intensive care unit; IV = intravenous; Tx = transplant.

DEFINITION, DIAGNOSIS, AND PREDICTION OF VARICEAL BLEEDING

Portal hypertension is defined as portal vein pressure > 5 mm Hg or a portal vein to hepatic vein gradient of > 10 mm Hg.[33]

Portal hypertension can frequently be diagnosed by physical examination. The spleen is usually palpable and sometimes massively enlarged, although it must be remembered that in biliary atresia, one of the most common causes of portal hypertension in children, there may be associated asplenia, polysplenia, or situs inversus, making this physical sign not always reliable. Ascites is generally only present when portal hypertension is at the sinusoidal level. The four main portal to systemic vein collateral systems that become prominent in portal hypertension can all be readily examined. Increased pressure in the paraumbilical venous network is manifested by engorged superficial abdominal wall veins radiating from the umbilicus—the caput medusa. With overfilling of the perirectal collateral venous system, hemorrhoids appear. When abdominal organs become adherent to the abdominal wall, the collaterals formed result in visible varices seen within the stomas[34] sometimes used in biliary drainage procedures or seen in old laparotomy scars.

Esophageal varices are best examined by endoscopy. Newer, less invasive radiologic techniques are being increasingly used. In a recent study, magnetic resonance angiography had a sensitivity of 100% and a specificity of 93% compared with endoscopy for detecting collateral vessels in children with biliary atresia after portoenterostomy.[35] In a study of 50 children, intravenous computed tomography (CT) using a helical CT scanner identified changes in the esophageal and gastric vasculature earlier than endoscopy.[36]

The size of the liver is generally not especially helpful. In older children with cirrhosis, the liver is frequently small and shrunken, whereas in younger children with biliary atresia, the liver may be moderately enlarged, hard, and with an irregular edge. In children with Budd-Chiari syndrome or congenital hepatic fibrosis, the liver may be massively enlarged and firm.

Ultrasonography, particularly when enhanced by duplex sonography, is very useful in the evaluation of portal hypertension.[37] In extrahepatic causes of portal vein obstruction, the characteristic absence of the portal vein signal is replaced by the findings of multiple dilated collateral veins (cavernous transformation). The echogenicity of the liver itself is normal. Not only can the presence or absence of the portal vein be determined, but the direction of flow can also be assessed. Hepatofugal flow (ie, away from the liver) is associated with severe portal hypertension. The ultrasonographer can also provide details of increased flow in the portal collateral circulation and may be able to demonstrate findings such as enlarged coronary veins or paraesophageal veins. Evaluation of the splenic vein is also important, particularly to look for splenic aneurysms, which are found in 8 to 14.7% of patients with portal hypertension.[38,39] Once portal hypertension is suspected on clinical or ultrasound findings, elective upper endoscopy can give useful information. The size of the varices and the presence or absence of portal hypertensive gastropathy help determine the medical management.

As variceal bleeding is the most serious complication of portal hypertension, with a 30 to 50% mortality and a high risk of rebleeding,[40] several studies have addressed the issue of whether the risk of bleeding can be predicted (Table 59-3). Although most of this information is obtained from adult patients, several observations also relevant to children can be made. First, variceal bleeding rarely occurs if the portal vein to hepatic vein gradient is < 12 mm Hg.[41,42] However, in patients with a portal vein to hepatic vein gradient > 12 mm Hg, only about one-third will bleed. Second, the risk of bleeding is related to the cause of portal vein obstruction. In the Bicêtre experience of 389 children with portal hypertension, 80% of children with extrahepatic portal vein obstruction bled compared with 46% of children with congenital fibrosis and 32% of children with cirrhosis. Moreover, 41% of children with portal vein obstruction bled before the age of 3 years. Children with Budd-Chiari syndrome had a very low incidence of variceal bleeding (Figure 59-3).[43] Third, the endoscopic appearance of the varices provides some estimate of the risk of bleeding.[44,45] Large, tense varices that do not flatten with insufflation of air are more likely to bleed than small, decompressed varices. Although large varices bleed more easily, the size of the varices is not related to the measured portal hypertension.[46] Varices with congestion of the overlying or surrounding mucosa, particularly those with characteristic red spots and red wale markings ("whip-like" discolorations from dilated venules), and gastric varices are also associated with increased risk of bleeding.[43]

In children, the risk of bleeding may change over time. In those with extrahepatic portal vein obstruction, the development of a decompressing collateral circulation may actually decrease the risk as children get older. However, in the Bicêtre study, almost half of the children studied serially showed a progression in the severity of varices over time, and more than one-third of these had a bleeding episode.[43] Finally, the severity of underlying cirrhosis increases not only the risk of bleeding[45] but also the mortality after variceal hemorrhage. In a study of 134 children with biliary atresia, children after a first esophageal variceal bleed, the relative risk of death or transplant was 12.0 if the total bilirubin was more than 10 mg/dL compared with 7.2 if the bilirubin was 4 to 10 mg/dL and 0.6 if the bilirubin was less than 4 mg/dL compared with a same-aged child without a variceal bleed.[47]

MANAGEMENT OF ACUTE VARICEAL BLEEDING

Hematemesis or melena as a result of variceal bleeding is often massive, and the child may present to an emergency

TABLE 59-3   FACTORS PREDICTING VARICEAL BLEEDING

Portal vein–hepatic vein gradient > 12 mm Hg
Large, tense varices
Red wale marks, red spots on varices
Severity of underlying liver disease

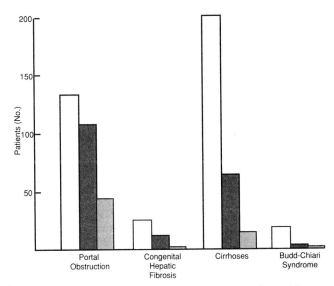

FIGURE 59-3   Relationship between the etiology of portal hypertension and risk of gastrointestinal bleeding in 380 children investigated for portal hypertension. For each etiologic group, the total number of children studied; number of children who experienced one episode of bleeding; number of children who bled before age 3 years. Reproduced with permission from Bernard O et al.[43]

room in cardiovascular shock. Immediate placement of a large-bore intravenous cannula or, if necessary, intraosseous needle in children < 2 to 3 years of age is essential so that large volumes of fluid and blood can be rapidly delivered. Children with known poor liver function should be assumed to be coagulopathic, and clotting factor supplementation should be instituted immediately. Many children will also have thrombocytopenia secondary to hypersplenism, and platelet transfusions are indicated. However, gastrointestinal bleeding in children with portal hypertension may not always be so dramatic. Small variceal bleeds or bleeding from portal hypertensive gastropathy can be much more subtle, with only small to moderate amounts of blood loss, a slow decline in hematocrit, and no overt cardiovascular decompensation. However, the propensity for these children to develop more severe bleeding must not be underestimated, and all should be admitted and carefully observed to better optimize therapy (see Figure 59-2).

Gastric lavage with saline via a nasogastric tube may be helpful in determining the extent and duration of bleeding. Perhaps the most important use of gastric lavage is to help clear the stomach of blood to allow better visualization of the mucosa at the time of endoscopy. Contraindications to gastric lavage include children in whom the procedure may increase bleeding (known large varices or intractable coagulapathy) or induce esophageal perforation (recent sclerotherapy with possible esophageal ulcerations). The choice of lavage solution is probably not particularly important. Room temperature saline is the most physiologic; iced saline lavage has not been shown to be more efficacious. Once the patient is fully resuscitated and stabilized, upper endoscopy should be performed, primarily to confirm the site and cause of bleeding and to determine if treatment is

indicated. Other etiologies of upper gastrointestinal bleeding will alter management, such as portal hypertensive gastropathy, gastric or duodenal ulcers, or Mallory-Weiss tears. If variceal bleeding is confirmed, therapeutic sclerotherapy or variceal ligation may be attempted, although this is frequently technically very difficult if bleeding is still active.

In the child who continues to have uncontrollable bleeding, balloon tamponade may be the only method that can stabilize the patient until a more definitive procedure, such as liver transplant or a portosystemic shunt, can be undertaken. The Linton tube is used for small children or if bleeding gastric varices are present, and the Sengstaken-Blakemore tube is used for larger children. The length of the esophageal balloon limits the use of the Sengstaken-Blakemore tube to children weighing over 40 kg. Both are highly effective and can stop esophageal and or gastric variceal bleeding in up to 90% of patients.[48] However, experience is required to minimize the considerable risks associated with balloon tamponade, such as aspiration, esophageal rupture and ulcers, and airway obstruction. Correct positioning of the tube must be confirmed radiographically to avoid inflating the gastric balloon in the esophagus. The volume of air inflated into the gastric and esophageal balloons varies with the child's size and must be enough to create adequate pressure to compress the bleeding sites but without causing ischemic injury to the esophageal or gastric mucosa. Pressure in the esophageal balloon should be 15 to 40 mm Hg. The gastric balloon should be inflated to 30 mL and can be incrementally increased to about 200 to 300 mL depending on the size of the child. It is recommended that the appearance of the gastric balloon in relation to the size of the stomach is checked radiographically after each incremental change in volume to avoid the risk of overinflation.

Children should be intubated and sedated to minimize the risk of aspiration. The balloons can be safely left inflated only for 12 to 24 hours. As such, balloon tamponade can be viewed only as a temporizing measure.

PREVENTION OF REBLEEDING AND PROPHYLAXIS OF FIRST VARICEAL BLEEDING

Several modalities, alone or in combination, have been investigated to control variceal bleeding. These include sclerotherapy, variceal ligation, vasoactive drugs, and portosystemic shunts. Most large controlled trials have been performed in adults, and the results have generated considerable controversy over the effectiveness of each modality.[49–53] Common principles, also relevant to pediatrics, are discussed below.

Sclerotherapy and Variceal Ligation.   Obliteration of esophageal varices may be achieved by endoscopic injection of sclerosing substances or by ligation of varices, commonly using elastic bands. Prevention of rebleeding, which occurs in up to 50% of patients and incurs a mortality of 20 to 70% if untreated, is the goal of aggressive attempts to obliterate varices.[53,54]

Sclerotherapy is a well-established modality to control variceal bleeding in children and has decreased the need for shunt surgery.[55,56] After a first variceal bleed, elective sclerotherapy, usually requiring repetition, can successfully eradicate esophageal varices in up to 90% of patients with a low incidence of rebleeding and recurrent varices. Because rebleeding often occurs within 2 to 6 weeks of the initial bleeding episode, the first sclerotherapy should be scheduled early. The short-term benefits of reducing rebleeding episodes are not to be underestimated and are particularly important while the child awaits liver transplant. Sclerotherapy or endoscopic variceal ligation should now be considered the first line of treatment for variceal bleeding. In a study comparing outcomes in children treated with a surgical shunt versus sclerotherapy, the low rate of rebleeding after sclerotherapy led the authors to conclude that the more invasive shunt surgery could usually be avoided.[57] Although some controlled trials in adults have shown that sclerotherapy reduces long-term mortality,[58] it must be remembered that sclerotherapy does nothing to decrease portal hypertension itself but only redirects blood away from the esophageal collateral circulation to other collaterals. Until the child undergoes a definitive procedure that actually decreases or eliminates portal hypertension (ie, shunt operation or liver transplant), the patient remains at risk of life-threatening variceal bleeding, often from newly formed gastric varices. Portal hypertensive gastropathy with increased bleeding risk may also be exacerbated by esophageal variceal obliteration.[59]

No consensus as to the value of prophylactic sclerotherapy has been reached. A randomized controlled trial of 100 children with esophageal varices showed that prophylactic sclerotherapy compared to observation resulted in a significant reduction in variceal bleeding in the treatment group but more congestive hypertensive gastropathy. Importantly, there was no difference in survival between the two groups.[60] In another pediatric series, 42% of children bled after prophylactic sclerotherapy.[57] In some adult studies, use of a scoring system that predicts a high risk of variceal hemorrhage has been used to justify prophylactic sclerotherapy. There is conflicting evidence as to whether the incidence of bleeding is reduced or the survival improved.[45,61]

Sclerotherapy still requires considerable operator skill, particularly in small children. Although techniques and choice of sclerosant vary among endoscopists, convincing evidence that one is better than another is lacking. Paravariceal injection of sclerosant is favored by some and intravariceal injection by others. Sclerosants used include ethanol, morrhuate, ethanolamine, and tetradecyl. We use ethanolamine 5% or diluted 1:1 with ethanol. To decrease complications, it is important to avoid a large volume of sclerosant on any single injection and to limit the number of injections, even if of relatively small volume, performed at any one time. We recommend 1 mL or less of sclerosant per site and no more than 5 to 6 mL per session in children < 10 years of age. Both practices decrease the risk of esophageal ulceration and the eventual development of esophageal strictures, perforation, and systemic absorption of sclerosant.

In recent years, the newer technique of endoscopic ligation of esophageal varices with elastic bands has sup-

planted sclerotherapy for variceal obliteration in adults and is now being used in children (Figure 59-4). Variceal ligation may be a more effective modality to prevent a first variceal bleed compared with sclerotherapy. In a randomized trial of 49 children comparing endoscopic ligation with sclerotherapy for bleeding esophageal varices secondary to extrahepatic portal venous obstruction, the rebleeding rate was significantly higher in the sclerotherapy group (25% versus 4%).[62] The advantages are increased efficacy with a reduced incidence of complications, such as esophageal ulceration, perforation, stricture, systemic sclerosant, and gastroesophageal reflux.[63] The disadvantage, now mostly eliminated in adults, is the need for a large-caliber endoscope that can accommodate, within its lumen, an outer cylinder that snares the varix and an inner cylinder that deploys the bands. Because many early models could deploy only one band at a time, an overtube was often used so that multiple intubations of the esophagus were avoided. Improved endoscopes have eliminated these problems for adults, and smaller-caliber endoscopes suitable for use in pediatric patients have been developed. As well, recent technical advances in pediatric endoscopes have overcome the previous limitation of only one band being placed at a time. Successful esophageal ligation in children is increasingly being described.[64-68] A high rate of eradication is reported (72–100%) and a low risk of rebleeding (< 25%). Note that in these studies, the mean age is between 7 and 8 years. Price and colleagues performed endoscopic variceal ligation in 22 children, ranging in age from 8 months to 19 years.[69] Of 18 children who did not undergo early liver transplant, 12 had complete eradication of the varices over an average of four sessions. Rebleeding between sessions occurred but not after obliteration of varices. None of the children developed esophageal stenosis or gastroesophageal reflux. However, perforation of the cervical esophagus occurred in one

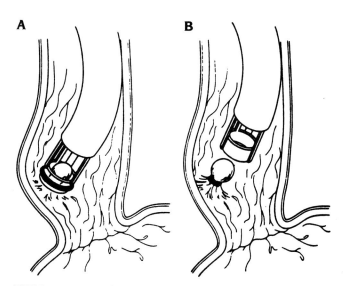

FIGURE 59-4 Endoscopic ligation of esophageal varices. The esophageal varix is drawn up into the ligation device with suction (A) and the base of the varixis ligated with an elastic band (B). From Greenfield LJ, Mulholland MW, Oldham KT, et al. Surgery, scientific principles and practice. Philadelphia: Lippincott-Raven; 1997.

child, underscoring the size limitations of the instruments needed in small children. These authors stress that the diameter of the child's esophagus should be 10 mm or more to allow for the safe passage of a 32-French instrument. They advocate limiting the technique to children over 1 year of age until endoscopic instruments can be further miniaturized. However, in a recent study using a small-diameter endoscope, 28 children, some as young as 3 months, were treated, with obliteration of varices in 26 and rebleeding in only 2.[70]

Surgical Management: Shunts, Transjugular Intrahepatic Portosystemic Shunts, and Nonshunt Procedures.

Shunts.   The success of sclerotherapy and variceal ligation in controlling variceal bleeding and the availability of liver transplant have reduced the need to perform portosystemic shunts to manage uncontrollable bleeding.[57] However, portosystemic shunts are still an important modality to treat variceal bleeding in selected cases: children with extrahepatic portal vein obstruction; children with congenital hepatic fibrosis; children with well-compensated cirrhosis, in which liver transplant may not be required for several years; children with variceal bleeding, in whom liver transplant is contraindicated; and, rarely, children awaiting liver transplant to control life-threatening variceal hemorrhage. Prophylactic shunt surgery is not advocated because previous studies showed a decreased survival and an increased risk of encephalopathy compared with no treatment.[53]

Shunt procedures, including transjugular intrahepatic portosystemic shunts (TIPS), are the only modalities that effectively reduce portal pressure and thus definitively treat the underlying cause of variceal bleeding (Figure 59-5). The major disadvantages of portosystemic shunts are hepatic decompensation caused by reduced portal blood flow and precipitation of encephalopathy. Both complications occur much more commonly with nonselective (total) shunts, that is, portocaval, mesocaval, and central splenorenal shunts (see Figure 59-5). The development of selective shunts, notably the distal splenorenal shunt first described by Warren and colleagues in 1967,[71] significantly reduces both complications as forward flow of portal venous blood to the liver is preserved. The distal splenorenal shunt and its modifications are now the preferred shunt, whenever technically possible, particularly in elective situations.[72] In a pediatric series, there was no rebleeding and no encephalopathy in the 81% of children in whom the shunt was successful.[73] In the emergency setting, surgical options are more limited, and portocaval or mesocaval shunts may be the only feasible choice. Bleeding is effectively controlled, but the mortality rate may be as high as 20 to 50%.[74,75] This is most likely related to the severity of the underlying liver disease in patients undergoing these procedures. Both portocaval and mesocaval shunts are equally effective in stopping bleeding. The side-to-side portocaval shunt and the mesocaval and portocaval H-graft shunts have the theoretical advantage of preserving at least some forward portal flow, although all have a high incidence of encephalopathy and hepatic decompensation, particularly in patients with underlying cirrhosis.

The applicability of shunt procedures to pediatric patients is constrained by the small caliber of the veins to be shunted and the subsequent risk of shunt thrombosis. In two pediatric studies,[76,77] the median ages were 9 years and 8 years, respectively, although in the latter series, children as young as 2 years were shunted. These two studies reported patency rates of 9% and 80%, respectively. In children with underlying cirrhosis, complications included ascites, hepatorenal syndrome, and encephalopathy (occurring in one patient with a nonselective shunt).

Children with extrahepatic portal vein obstruction are particularly good candidates for shunts.[78] In one experience, shunt patency was 93% in a group of 92 children with a mean age of 6.5 years.[43] Innovative shunt procedures[79] designed to restore portal blood flow include bypassing the cavernoma by an autograft (using a portion of the patient's jugular vein) placed between the superior mesenteric vein and the left portal vein (the Rex shunt). In two reports, portal decompression was achieved, with concomitant decreases in spleen size, increased white cell and platelet counts, control of bleeding, and restoration of physiologic hepatopetal flow. All shunts were patent at a median of 6 months after the procedure.[80,81]

An important consideration in placing a surgical shunt is to be certain that the shunt procedure itself does not compromise a potential liver transplant procedure required in the future.[82] Mazzaferro and colleagues showed that properly performed portosystemic shunts do not preclude successful liver transplant or have an impact

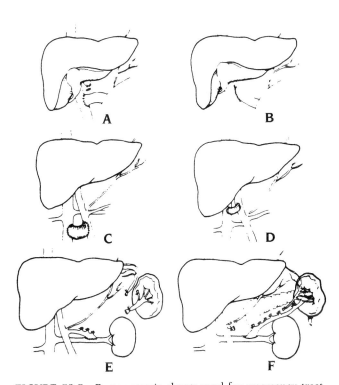

FIGURE 59-5 Portosystemic shunts used for emergency treatment of variceal bleeding: end-to-side portocaval shunt (A), side-to-side portocaval shunt (B), mesocaval interpositional H-graft (C), portocaval interpositional H-graft (D), central splenorenal shunt (E), and selective distal splenorenal shunt (Warren Shunt; F). Reproduced with permission from Terblanche J et al.[49]

on post-transplant survival.[83] A potential advantage of the mesocaval shunt, as opposed to the portocaval shunt, is that the dissection is distant from the porta hepatis and, thus, less likely to create complications for the transplant surgeon in the future.

Transjugular Intrahepatic Portosystemic Shunts.

The creation of a shunt between the intrahepatic portions of the portal vein and hepatic vein (Figure 59-6) by a minimally invasive technique avoids the risks of the major surgical procedure required for a standard shunt operation. This is a particular advantage in patients who are already severely compromised by their underlying liver disease. In brief, the procedure is performed by cannulating the right jugular vein to access the right hepatic vein. The needle is then passed through the intrahepatic portion of the hepatic vein and into the liver parenchyma to enter a branch of the portal vein. An expandable metallic stent is deployed across the hepatic parenchyma to create a shunt between the hepatic and portal vein branches. The size of the stent is increased until the gradient between the portal vein and the hepatic vein is ideally < 18 mm Hg.[84] To ensure success, the procedure requires technical expertise and a very careful appraisal of possible variations in vascular anatomy.[85] In adults, there is a 10% complication rate from the procedure itself, most often intra-abdominal bleeding.[86] The major complications are shunt occlusion or stenosis (25–75%), encephalopathy (5–35%),[87] progressive liver failure, and portal vein thrombosis. The success of the TIPS procedure in controlling bleeding (and also ascites)[88] has been widely reported in adults.[89,90] In two randomized trials, one comparing TIPS versus drug therapy[91] and another TIPS versus variceal ligation plus propranol,[92] both found that TIPS-treated patients had more complications. Although in one study, the incidence of rebleeding was less, neither study showed any difference in survival between the groups.[91] It appears to be most useful as a bridge to liver transplant and for those failing sclerotherapy or variceal ligation. A TIPS procedure is preferable to an operative shunt in the transplant candidate because it is associated with less operative complications at the time of transplant. However, migration of the stent into the suprahepatic vena cava or right atrium has been associated with major technical complications during the transplant procedure.[93]

In children, the TIPS procedure is made more complicated by the small size of the liver and the diminutive caliber of the portal and hepatic veins.[84] As well, there is more likelihood of anatomic variance, particularly of the portal vein, in some pediatric liver diseases, such as biliary atresia. Despite these technical limitations, there are now several reports describing the successful use of TIPS children,[94,95] even as an emergency procedure,[96] and in an infant.[97] In experienced hands, the overall success rate of 75 to 90% is similar to reports in adults. Hackworth and colleagues used TIPS to control variceal bleeding in 12 children (age 2 to 16 years; median age 9 years) awaiting liver transplant.[98] Ten of the 12 shunts were patent at the time of transplant at a median of 53 days after placement. None of the children rebled, and one developed encephalopathy. Heymen and colleagues described nine children (5 to 15 years in age) in whom TIPS was attempted.[99] In two children, vascular anomalies precluded successful TIPS placement. Although shunt occlusion occurred in four children, TIPS revision restored patency in three. All but one patient had successful control of bleeding. These two studies emphasize the important principles of the use of TIPS in children: size (and therefore age) is still a limiting factor, anatomic variations can preclude success, and the small caliber of the stent may increase the risk of stent occlusion.

Once in place, the patency of the TIPS stent should be monitored by ultrasonography every 3 to 4 months. In adult series, shunt stenosis or obstruction occurs in 25 to

---

FIGURE 59-6   Anatomic location of the transjugular intrahepatic portosystemic shunt. Reproduced with permission from Vargas HE and colleagues.[33]

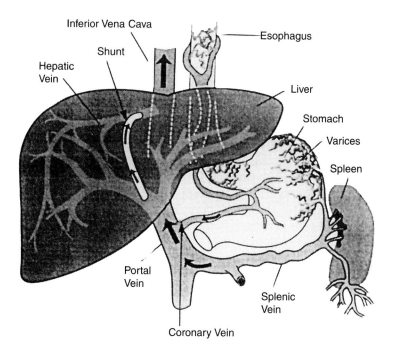

75% of patients.[89] Doppler ultrasonography has a reported sensitivity of 92% and a specificity of 72% in detecting shunt malfunction.[100]

At present, TIPS appears to be most useful in children who have failed sclerotherapy while waiting for transplant.[101] Shunt patency decreases markedly with time (48% patency at 1 year, 26% at 2 years in one study)[102]; therefore, the procedure should generally be reserved for children with refractory bleeding who will be transplanted within 6 to 12 months. Other more controversial indications include the use of TIPS to treat severe hypersplenism; however, a consistent improvement in white cell and platelet cell counts has not been demonstrated.[99]

In adult patients, TIPS placement has also been suggested for medically refractory ascites, Budd-Chiari syndrome, and veno-occlusive disease. These indications have not yet been explored adequately in pediatric patients. In addition, there is no proven role for placement of TIPS to prevent bleeding from portal hypertensive gastropathy.

The TIPS procedure is contraindicated whenever there is infection present in the liver, that is, hepatic abscess or cholangitis. Polycystic liver disease, hepatic neoplasm, right-sided heart failure, and severe hepatic failure with uncorrectable coagulopathy are also contraindications.[84]

Pharmacologic Therapy. The aim of drug therapy in the control of variceal bleeding is to reduce portal pressure either by decreasing flow into the splanchnic bed with vasoconstrictors or by decreasing the vascular resistance of the intrahepatic and portal circulation with vasodilators.[103]

Vasopressin, a potent vasoconstrictor, was the prototype drug used, and although it has been shown to increase the chance of stopping acute bleeding, no survival benefit has yet been demonstrated. The serious systemic vasoconstrictive side effects of vasopressin, including myocardial infraction, mesenteric ischemia, cerebrovascular accidents, and limb ischemia, are its major disadvantages.[104] To counteract these effects, some protocols combined vasopressin with nitroglycerin, a potent vasodilator, and the systemic vasoconstrictive properties of vasopressin were lessened.[33]

Somatostatin has proven to be a much safer alternative to vasopressin and can effectively decrease portal pressure by decreasing splanchnic blood flow and reducing the portal vein to hepatic vein pressure gradient with few systemic side effects.[105,106] However, its usefulness is limited by a very short half-life. More recently, a synthetic analog of somatostatin, octreotide, has been shown to have similar efficacy to somatostatin and vasopressin, with very few side effects and an acceptable half-life.[107–109] This agent is currently the preferred agent to treat children with acute variceal bleeding.[110] The advantage of beginning pharmacologic therapy early in the management of an acute variceal bleed is that the high technical expertise of sclerotherapy or variceal ligation is not required, and bleeding may be controlled enough to allow elective sclerotherapy. In one randomized study, octreotide alone was as effective as emergent sclerotherapy in stopping bleeding.[109] Octreotide dosing recommendations are to begin with a bolus of 1 µg/kg followed by continuous infusion of 1 µg/kg/h, with titration of both the bolus and constant

infusion up to 5 µg/kg/h. This regimen was found to be effective in stopping bleeding in 86% of patients at a mean time of 40 hours.[110]

Nonselective β-blockers have long been used for the prevention of first variceal bleeds and rebleeding. Several randomized trials in adults have confirmed that both propranolol and nadolol have a significant benefit in both the prophylaxis of variceal bleeding and prevention of rebleeding.[53] In some trials, prevention of a first variceal bleed also increased survival.[111,112] Nadolol's advantage over propranolol is that it is not metabolized by the liver and can be given once a day.[113] Nadolol was combined with isosorbide mononitrate (nitrate vasodilators also decrease portal pressure) and compared in a randomized trial with sclerotherapy to prevent variceal rebleeding. Although the probability of rebleeding was significantly decreased in the nadolol and isosorbide group, there was no survival benefit.[114] Extrapolating from the adult doses used in the study, some pediatric patients have been treated with a starting dose of 1 mg/kg/d of nadolol, with titration of the dose until the 25% reduction of heart rate is achieved. Then isosorbide nitrate is added to reach a dose over the course of 1 week of 0.5 mg/kg twice a day.

Few studies are published in children regarding the use of β-blockers in preventing first variceal bleeds. In a non-randomized study, 14 of 21 children had no episode of rebleeding when treated with propranolol. Success correlated with a reduction in heart rate of more than 25% of baseline and a dose of at least 1 mg/kg/d of propranolol.[115] In a study of 60 children with cirrhosis, propranolol (1–2 mg/kg/d) was most successful in preventing a first bleed (15.6% of children bled), whereas 53.3% of children bled if propranol was initiated after a first bleed.[116] However, the use of nonselective β-blockers can be limited by their side effects. This is particularly important in children with asthma or cystic fibrosis, in whom bronchospasm must be avoided.

More recently, several randomized trials of endoscopic treatment alone versus endoscopic treatment plus drug therapy for acute variceal bleeding, or to prevent rebleeding, have been published. Combined therapy was more effective for controlling bleeding[117] and for the prevention of rebleeding,[118] but there was no difference in survival between treatment groups. Similar studies have not yet been performed in children.

Transection and Devasculization Procedures. With the success of sclerotherapy, improved pharmacologic agents, and availability of liver transplant, esophageal transection and devascularization procedures are very infrequently necessary to control acute variceal bleeding. However, such major surgical procedures still have a place in treating exsanguinating hemorrhage uncontrollable by any other means. Three techniques are currently practiced[49]: staple gun transection of the esophagus, the extensive Sugiura procedure (devascularization of the abdominothoracic lower esophagus and upper gastric areas, followed by splenectomy, pyloromyotomy, vagotomy, and esophageal transection), and a more limited procedure combining esophagogastric devascularization with staple gun transec tion. None of these procedures have been well studied in children. However, the results in adults, particularly of the more extensive procedures, have shown a high mortality.[49] Unless contraindicated, liver transplant, even in this highly emergent situation, is most likely a better option.

ASCITES

In the child with chronic liver disease, the onset of ascites indicates that the two prerequisite conditions for ascites formation, portal hypertension and hepatic insuffiency, are worsening.[119] About 50% of patients will die within 2 years of developing ascites.[40]

The pathophysiology of ascites is discussed in detail in Chapter 5.2. In brief, intra-abdominal factors that result in a net flow of fluid (and protein) out of the mesenteric capillary bed into the peritoneal cavity are (1) decreased plasma colloid osmotic pressure, (2) increased capillary pressure, (3) increased ascitic colloid osmotic fluid pressure, and (4) decreased ascitic fluid hydrostatic pressure (Figure 59-7).[120,121] The dynamic relationship between these factors in the formation of ascites is complex. For example, hypoalbuminea (ie, decreased plasma colloid osmotic pressure) alone is not sufficient to cause ascites, and in the hepatic causes of ascites, capillary pressure increased by portal hypertension plays a key role, as supported by the observation that ascites may be ameliorated by creating portosystemic shunts.

Ascites in liver disease occurs in the context of sinusoidal and/or postsinusoidal portal hypertension and is, in part, related to obstruction of hepatic lymph flow from the sinusoids into the hepatic vein.[122] When the rate of hepatic lymph formation exceeds its drainage into the hepatic venous system, lymph accumulates in the space of Disse and then escapes into the peritoneal cavity as ascitic fluid.

Apart from the local factors leading to ascites, three theories invoke the role of systemic factors in ascites formation: (1) the underfill theory, in which decreased plasma volume increases the activity of the renin-angiotensin-aldosterone pathway, causing sodium retention[123]; (2) the overfill theory, in which renal sodium retention is the initiating event, leading to an increase in plasma volume[124]; and (3) the peripheral arterial vasodilation theory, in which the primary event is splanchnic arteriolar vasodilation secondary to portal hypertension, which causes sequestration of blood in the splanchnic bed, a decrease in circulating blood volume, and subsequent sodium and water retention.[125]

Understanding the central role of sodium retention in the pathogenesis of all three proposed mechanisms is essential for the successful management of ascites. The ability to excrete free water, independent of sodium retention, is also impaired in cirrhotic patients and may be secondary to increased plasma levels of antidiuretic hormone.[121,126]

DIAGNOSIS

Significant volumes of ascites are easily detected on physical examination. The abdominal flanks bulge with fluid, a fluid level can be percussed, the umbilicus protrudes, and a fluid wave may be detected. In addition, the liver and spleen may become ballotable, and, particularly in young children, inguinal hernias and hydroceles may develop. Common findings on a plain film of the abdomen are diffuse abdominal haziness, separation of bowel loops by fluid, and medial displacement of the bowel.

More subtle ascites is best assessed by ultrasonography, which can detect small volumes of fluid. Confirming ascites becomes important if paracentesis is being considered to diagnose spontaneous bacterial peritonitis. The ultrasound examination is also useful to differentiate free from loculated ascitic fluid.[127]

Paracentesis is usually not indicated in the initial diagnostic evaluation of ascites in the child with known liver disease. The other causes of ascites that might occur in adults with liver disease, such as malignant or tuberculous ascites, are very rare in children. It is, however, important to know the usual composition of ascitic fluid in patients with liver disease without secondary complications. The ascitic fluid is generally clear, straw colored, or bile tinged and has a protein content of < 2.5 g/dL. The cell count is < 250 cells/mm^3 and is mostly composed of lymphocytes. The glucose and lactic dehydrogenase content mirror that of plasma.[120]

MANAGEMENT

Sodium restriction and the promotion of sodium excretion are the cornerstones of ascites management (Table 59-4).[128] As the excretion of fluid passively follows that of sodium, fluid restriction is generally not necessary in the initial management plan. Dietary sodium intake should be limited to 1 to 2 mEq/kg. However, only 10 to 20% of patients, generally those with a relatively normal serum sodium and a urinary sodium of > 15 mEq/24 h, will

FIGURE 59-7   Formation of ascites. Factors favoring the net movement of fluid out of the capillary bed and into the peritoneal space. Adapted from Wyllie R, Arasu TS, Fitzgerald JF. Ascites: pathophysiology and management. J Pediatr 1980;97:167.

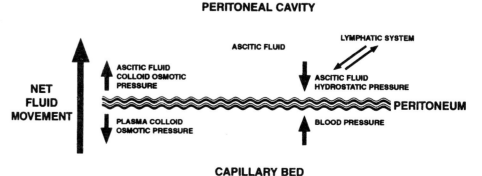

TABLE 59-4	STEPWISE MANAGEMENT OF ASCITES

Step 1. Sodium restriction: 1–2 mEq/kg/d
Step 2. Check compliance
Step 3. Spironolactone: 2–3 mg/kg/d ÷ tid
Step 4.* Spironolactone + furosemide
Step 5.* Fluid restriction
Step 6.* Intravenous albumin 1 g/kg + furosemide 1 mg/kg
  *Monitor for
    Hypovolemia
    Hyponatremia: Na < 120 mEq/mL
      → Stop diuretics
      → Continue fluid restriction
    Hypokalemia

respond to sodium restriction alone.[108] Once the urine sodium excretion falls below about 15 mEq/24 h, diuretic therapy is required.

The most logical first choice of diuretic is spironolactone because secondary hyperaldosteronism is almost always present in chronic liver disease.[129] Spironolactone is rapidly and almost completely absorbed from the gastrointestinal tract and is metabolized to a number of active compounds that competitively inhibit the binding of aldosterone to its specific receptor in the distal renal tubule and collecting system.[130]

Spironolactone therapy has proved to be safe and efficacious over many years of use. The dose should be initiated at 2 to 3 mg/kg/d per os in divided doses. At least a 3- to 4-day delay should be expected before a diuretic effect is seen.[131] If no increase in urine output occurs, the dose can be safely doubled.[120] Failure to respond to high-dose spironolactone prompts the use of a more potent second diuretic, most often furosemide. Furosemide induces not only sodium but also potassium loss in the urine so that careful monitoring of serum potassium is required. A balance between the potassium-sparing effects of spironolactone and the potassium loss induced by furosemide may obviate the need for potassium replacement when the two drugs are combined.

Hyponatremia is the electrolyte disturbance most often associated with diuretic therapy, indicating that sodium losses are exceeding water losses. Serum sodium is seldom less than 120 mEq/mL and at this level is not associated with significant complications and rarely needs to be treated. When the sodium falls below 120 mEq/mL, diuretic therapy should be suspended and fluid intake restricted.[120,128]

Monitoring 24-hour urine sodium excretion can be an important guide to therapy, particularly if ascites is failing to respond to interventions. With appropriate sodium restriction and diuretic therapy, urine sodium should certainly exceed 15 mEq/d. It has been estimated that a negative sodium balance of 120 mEq/d results in 1 L of fluid loss.[120] If the child on diuretic therapy, restricted to 1 to 2 mEq/d of sodium, still fails to diurese, water restriction of 50 to 75% of the normal daily requirement may be necessary. In patients with hypoalbuminemia, intravenous albumin infusions, which rapidly increase the intravascular colloid osmotic pressure, can be used to quickly mobilize extravascular fluid into the intravascular space. When combined with a diuretic, a brisk diuresis results. Concentrated 25% albumin can be given at a dose of 1 mg/kg intravenously followed by 0.5 to 1 mg/kg of intravenous furosemide.[120]

The most important and serious complication of aggressive diuretic therapy is hypovolemia, which occurs when water loss outstrips ascitic fluid resorption. Renal blood flow is decreased, creatinine and blood urea nitrogen are increased, and renal failure can be precipitated. Once peripheral edema has been mobilized by diuretic therapy (this occurs early in treatment), care must be taken to monitor weight, fluid balance, electrolytes, blood urea nitrogen, and creatinine. A net water loss of 200 to 300 mL/d is a useful goal,[120] but in very small children, it may be excessive. When ascites requires intensive management, such as outlined above, children should be hospitalized so that electrolyte balance, volume status, and renal function can be assessed on a daily basis. Vigorous diuretic treatment may also precipitate encephalopathy.

In children, refractory ascites is rare. Medical therapy alone is generally sufficient to reduce abdominal distention, allowing improved enteral feedings and diminished respiratory distress. However, in a recent series, if large-volume paracentesis is required, using a paracentesis needle rather than an intravascular catheter improved the efficiency of fluid removal without an increase in complications.[132] The complications of paracenteses include cardiovascular decompensation caused by rapid fluid shifts, intraperitoneal infection, and hemorrhage.

SURGICAL OPTIONS

Nowadays, the availability of liver transplant has made the surgical treatment of refractory ascites in children almost obsolete. The LeVeen shunt creates a drainage path from the intraperitoneal cavity to a jugular vein. Maintaining long-term patency is a problem, and in randomized trials, peritonovenous shunts, compared with medical therapy, did not improve survival.[133–135]

Controlling refactory ascites by decreasing portal hypertension through the creation of portosystemic shunts is a sound physiologic approach to the problem.[136] TIPS has become the most popular method. In adult studies, this procedure has been successful in controlling ascites in the majority of patients. However, mortality rates of 40 to 67% at 1 year and an incidence of encephalopathy of about 50% after TIPS have tempered enthusiasm for this approach. In one randomized trial in adults, mortality after the TIPS procedure was significantly higher compared with medical therapy alone.[137]

SPONTANEOUS BACTERIAL PERITONITIS

Spontaneous bacterial peritonitis (SBP) is defined as bacterial infection of the ascitic fluid in the absence of secondary causes, such as bowel perforation or intra-abdominal abscess. The clinical presentation of SBP can be subtle and even asymptomatic. Fever is generally present, but signs of abdominal pain and rebound tenderness are frequently absent. The child may present only with fever and irritability, the latter suggesting increasing encephalopathy. A high index of suspicion for SBP must always be maintained in any child with ascites who presents with nonspecific deterioration.[138]

Paracentesis and ascitic fluid culture are essential to the diagnosis and appropriate antibiotic therapy of SBP. Studies in adult patients have emphasized that the presence of coagulopathy is not a contraindication to paracentesis.[139] The incidence of intra-abdominal wall hematoma is surprisingly low (< 1%), and clinically evident bowel perforation is very rare when small-sized cannulas are used.

The preferred site of paracentesis is in the avascular linear alba, 2 cm directly below the umbilicus. Care must be taken that a very large spleen is not impinging on the site. The alternative location is midway along the line drawn between the umbilicus and the anterior right iliac crest. Under aseptic conditions, a 16- to 18-gauge catheter-over-the-needle is introduced, and 10 to 20 cc of fluid is withdrawn. The ascitic fluid should be directly injected into blood culture bottles at the bedside. This technique not only increases the yield of positive cultures but also decreases the time for cultures to become positive.[140,141] Examination of the cell count of the ascitic fluid is important (Table 59-5). A polymorphonuclear (PMN) count of > 500/mm³ has a sensitivity of 80% and a specificity of 98% for a positive culture. Cell counts of > 250 PMN/mm³ have a slightly increased sensitivity to 85% but a small reduction of specificity to 93%. The PMN cell count is particularly important in differentiating SBP from the more sinister causes of secondary bacterial peritonitis. With bowel perforation or intra-abdominal abscesses, the PMN count will exceed 10,000/mm³. As well, multiple organisms are cultured, the ascitic glucose concentration is decreased, and the lactate dehydrogenase concentration is increased. Differentiating primary from secondary bacterial peritonitis is crucial because secondary peritonitis is best managed by surgical intervention.[142,143]

Antibiotic therapy should be started, pending culture results, when the PMN count exceeds 500/mm³, irrespective of signs or symptoms. When the PMN count is > 250/mm³ or < 500/mm³ and there is an index of clinical suspicion, antibiotics should still be started. If withheld, retapping within 48 hours is recommended.[138]

The culture results usually yield a single gram-negative organism, with *Escherichia coli* accounting for about half of the organisms.[144] Other gram-negative enteric rods, such as *Klebsiella*, are also found. Gram-positive organisms, particularly *Streptococcus* species, are seen in about 25% of cases. Anaerobic infections are very rare. Initial antibiotic therapy should cover both the likely gram-negative

and -positive organisms. Cefotaxime alone has an 85% reported success rate. Avoiding aminoglycosides is important because many of these patients may already have some renal compromise. However, it should be remembered that cefotaxime alone will not cover *Enterococcus*, which is sometimes the offending organism. In this instance, ampicillin is the best choice Once the culture results are known, the antibiotic regimen can be tailored accordingly. An intravenous course of 10 to 14 days is recommended, although some studies have indicated that the ascitic fluid may become sterile within a few days.[145]

Spontaneous infection of ascitic fluid is most likely a result of portal hypertension leading to an increased chance of translocation of the patient's own enteric organisms into the mesenteric lymph nodes, which drain via the thoracic duct into the systemic circulation.[146] Transient bacteremia occurs, with subsequent seeding of the ascitic fluid. Also adding to the risk are the decreased complement levels in both serum and ascitic fluid, poor reticuloendothelial system function, and defective neutrophil and phagocyte function observed in patients with severe liver disease.[142,147,148]

The first occurrence of SBP portends an accelerating risk of death from liver disease and underscores the urgency for liver transplant. In adult series, mortality during the first year after SBP is as high as 79%, usually related to complications of progressive liver failure rather than the SBP itself.[149,150] Recurrence is common—70% after the first episode in some studies.[150] Although oral antibiotic prophylaxis for SBP has been advocated by some authors for adult patients with high-risk factors for SBP (eg, elevated bilirubin, prolonged prothombin time, variceal bleeding),[151] there is no good evidence to support this concept in children. Because almost all of these children are liver transplant candidates, the risk of inducing resistant bacterial strains and fungal superinfection, both of which may have serious consequences in the post-transplant period, would seem to far outweigh any benefits.

HEPATORENAL SYNDROME

The hepatorenal syndrome is defined as functional renal failure in patients with severe liver disease. Histologically, the kidneys are normal, as evidenced by recovery of function after successful liver transplant and the successful transplant of cadaveric kidneys from patients with hepatorenal syndrome.[152] Hepatorenal syndrome most often occurs in decompensated chronic liver disease but also has been described in acute liver failure.[153] Hepatorenal syndrome is sometimes precipitated by other supervening complications of end-stage liver disease, particularly spontaneous bacterial peritonitis.[154]

About 10% of adult patients with chronic liver disease develop hepatorenal syndrome, with an associated mortality of more than 70% without liver transplant. There are few published studies of the prevalence of hepatorenal syndrome in children; however, it appears to be much less common compared with adult patients,[155] although still associated with significant mortality in the pretransplant period.[156]

TABLE 59-5	PMN COUNTS ON ASCITIC FLUID
PMN COUNT	TREATMENT
< 250 mm³	No treatment
> 250 < 500 mm³	Intravenous antibiotics if clinical suspicion high or wait and retap
> 500 mm³	Intravenous antibiotics (eg, cefotaxime + ampicillin)
> 500 mm³	Rule out secondary peritonitis

PMN = polymorphonuclear.

Inherent in the diagnosis of hepatorenal syndrome is the careful exclusion of all other potential contributors to renal impairment. Most importantly, there must be no evidence of hypovolemia. This is particularly important in small children who may have unexpectedly large fluid losses from the intravascular compartment as a result of aggressive diuretic therapy for ascites, increased enteric losses from vomiting or diarrhea, or fluid shifts secondary to hypoalbuminemia. Measurement of central venous pressure can be very useful to determine intravascular fluid volume status. Importantly, intravenous fluid challenges will improve urine output in the hypovolemic child but will have no effect on the child with hepatorenal syndrome. Ongoing or recent hypovolemic shock, causing renal failure secondary to acute tubular necrosis, must be excluded.

Other important contributing factors to poor renal function that must be excluded are the effects of nephrotoxic drugs (particularly aminoglycosides and nonsteroidal anti-inflammatory drugs) and other intrinsic kidney diseases. Of the childhood diseases that cause chronic liver disease and have associated renal pathology, the most common are hereditary tyrosinemia, Alagille syndrome, and polycystic liver-kidney disease.

DIAGNOSIS AND DEFINITION

The diagnosis of hepatorenal syndrome is supported by a characteristic pattern of urine electrolyte abnormalities: urine sodium of < 10 mEq/L, a fractional excretion of sodium of < 1%, and a urine-to-plasma creatinine ratio of < 10 (Table 59-6).[157,158] Although these findings are not pathognomonic for hepatorenal syndrome and, in particular, do not differentiate hypovolemia from hepatorenal syndrome, they help to exclude unsuspected acute tubular necrosis, characterized by an increased urine sodium and increased fractional excretion of sodium, as well as other causes of intrinsic renal disease. Generally, the glomerular filtration rate (GFR) is profoundly decreased, and the child is oliguric (< 1 mL/kg/h of urine output). Significant amounts of protein or blood in the urine usually exclude the diagnosis. Type 1 hepatorenal syndrome is a rapidly progressive renal failure, often associated with a precipitating event, and has a poor prognosis, whereas type 2 is a more moderate and less precipitous loss of renal function.

It is important not to rely solely on serum creatinine as an estimate of the degree of renal impairment.[159,160] For example, a creatinine level of 0.5 mg/dL in a small child may not appear worrisome, but if such a child has reduced muscle mass, this creatinine may represent a tripling of normal creatinine for age. Moreover, the rise in serum creati-

nine is not linearly associated with falling GFR. By the time creatinine rises above normal, GFR is already reduced by about 50%. True GFR is easily measured by plasma clearance of an isotope (eg, indium = 111 diethylenetriamine pentaacetic acid) because creatinine clearance and calculated GFR both overestimate true GFR.[161] These fundamental principles are essential to diagnose impending renal failure in children and initiate appropriate corrective action.

PATHOGENESIS

The hallmark of hepatorenal syndrome is intense renal vasoconstriction with coexistent systemic vasodilation.[162] Renal blood flow, particularly to the renal cortex, is markedly reduced, despite the characteristic systemic hemodynamic changes seen in end-stage liver disease: decreased systemic vascular resistance, increased cardiac output, and decreased systemic blood pressure.[158,163] Ascites is often present, and hepatorenal syndrome is more likely to develop when ascites is resistant to diuretic therapy.[164] The mechanism of renal vasoconstriction is not yet fully understood, although several theories have been advanced. Gines and Arroyo suggest that the arterial vasodilation concept (also relevant in the mechanism of ascites generation) best explains the relationship between the opposing hemodynamic changes at the renal and systemic levels.[158] This theory proposes that portal hypertension as a result of cirrhosis causes splanchnic vascular vasodilation, with a subsequent reduction in effective systemic blood volume. The baroreceptor response is triggered, causing the activation of several systems that cause renal vasoconstriction. The splanchnic vascular system appears to be protected from the generalized vasoconstriction by the production of locally active vasodilator substances.

A variety of different mediators of renal vasoconstriction and splanchnic vasodilation have been proposed,[121] with the hope, not yet realized, that treatment could be aimed at inhibiting the causative agent.[165] The role of the renin-angiotensin axis has long been implicated in the vasoconstrictive response because cirrhotic patients are known to have high renin levels.[129] Also important is the activation of the sympathetic nervous system by the baroreceptor response to arterial hypotension. Increased sympathomimetic tone increases renal vasoconstriction and decreases GFR.[166,167] In some studies, the administration of clonidine, which decreases norepinephrine levels, has been shown to decrease renal vascular resistance.[168] Levels of antidiuretic hormone, which also cause renal vasoconstriction, are known to be elevated in cirrhotic patients.[121]

New attention is being focused on the endothelins, which are known potent vasoconstrictors that are released from many endothelial cells under conditions of stress.[169] Plasma endothelin 1 and 3 levels are two to three times higher in patients with cirrhosis and ascites, including children with biliary atresia[170] and cirrhosis,[171] compared with normal controls and are markedly increased in patients with hepatorenal syndrome.[172,173] Increased production of endothelin in the liver or splanchnic bed has been proposed. Interestingly, Nozue and colleagues reported that in eight children with cirrhosis, endothelin 1

TABLE 59-6	HEPATORENAL SYNDROME: DIAGNOSTIC CRITERIA

Oliguria: < 1 mL/kg/d
Fractorial excretion sodium < 1%
Urine-to-plasma creatinine ratio < 10
↓ Glomerular filtration rate, ↑ creatinine
Absence of hypovolemia
Other kidney pathology excluded

levels were significantly higher than in normal controls, and they correlated this with increased levels of urinary sodium acetyl-β-D glucose aminidase, a sensitive indicator of renal injury.[174] After successful liver transplant in patients with hepatorenal syndrome, endothelin 1 levels fall preceding the improvement in renal function.[175] Because endothelin levels can be elevated in a variety of stress situations that may coexist in patients with hepatorenal syndrome, their causative role in mediating renal vasoconstriction in hepatorenal syndrome remains to be determined. However, preliminary reports suggest that hepatorenal syndrome may be ameliorated by infusion of endothelin antagonists.[176]

Decreased production of renal prostaglandins, which mediate renal vasodilation, may contribute to hepatorenal syndrome. This is supported by evidence that inhibitors of prostaglandin synthetase, particularly nonsteroidal anti-inflammatory drugs, decrease GFR and renal blood flow in patients with ascites. However, treatment of hepatorenal syndrome with systemic prostaglandins has not been successful.[177]

As a mediator of the excessive vasodilation evident in systemic circulation, nitric oxide has been the best studied.[178] Nitric oxide overproduction might explain both the hyperdynamic circulation so characteristic of end-stage liver disease and the splanchnic vascular vasodilation, which results in diversion of blood away from the kidney. It has also been proposed that a local increase in the production of nitric oxide within the kidney may help protect renal perfusion by counterbalancing the renal vasoconstriction that typifies hepatorenal syndrome.[179]

A direct relationship between the liver and kidney has also been invoked to explain the changes in renal circulation seen in liver failure. The proposed mechanisms are a decrease in synthesis of a liver-associated renal vasodilator factor[180] or a hepatorenal reflex that triggers baroreceptors in the liver to increase renal sympathetic nerve activity.[181]

The hepatorenal syndrome is best treated by timely liver transplant because complete recovery can be expected.[182,183] While awaiting transplant, dialysis is the mainstay of treatment. Low-dose dopamine may increase renal blood flow but does not appear to increase GFR.[184] Peritoneovenous shunts[185] or TIPS, by reducing portal hypertension, may transiently improve renal function, but neither have shown sustained benefit.[186,187]

More recently, success has been reported in the treatment of hepatorenal syndrome in adults using terlipressin, a nonselective vasopressin analog. The mechanism of the beneficial effect on renal function is thought to be secondary to the intense splanchnic bed vasoconstriction induced, which allows improvement in systemic arterial circulation and renal blood flow. Patients who receive combined therapy with albumin infusion and terlipressin, which further improves circulatory function, have the best response. In one recent study, 77% of patients receiving albumin and terlipressin alone achieved a serum creatinine level < 1.5 mg/dL.[188] This modality may be a useful bridge until transplant. Unfortunately, at this time, terlipressin is not approved for use in the United States.

Although hepatorenal syndrome is associated with increased mortality before transplant in both adult[189] and pediatric series,[156,190] once transplanted, preexisiting hepatorenal syndrome has little effect on overall survivals.[191,192]

PULMONARY INVOLVEMENT IN LIVER DISEASE

HEPATOPULMONARY SYNDROME

The triad of hypoxemia, intrapulmonary vascular dilations, and liver disease constitutes the hepatopulmonary syndrome.[193,194] It is defined by an arterial oxygen pressure of < 70 mm Hg in room air with an alveolar/arterial gradient of > 20 mm Hg. In adults, the prevalence is between 5 and 29%,[195] with a 41% overall mortality described in hospitalized patients.[196] In children, estimates of the prevalence range from 0.5% in those with portal vein obstruction to as high as 20% in children with biliary atresia and polysplenia syndrome.[197] In other causes of childhood cirrhosis, the prevalence is between 2 and 4%.[198] Hepatopulmonary syndrome has been described in children as young as 6 months. Generally, hepatopulmonary syndrome is seen in chronic liver disease, but it has also been described in acute liver failure[199] and extrahepatic portal venous obstruction.[200] Portal hypertension is not a prerequisite for developing hepatopulmonary syndrome, although there is some evidence that the risk increases as the severity of liver disease progresses. Intrapulmonary vascular dilations may occur in patients with well-compensated chronic liver disease without demonstrating hypoxemia.[201]

There are two forms of hepatopulmonary syndrome; both are characterized by a right to left shunt within the lungs but with differing underlying mechanisms.[202] In type 1, which is more common, there is extensive dilation of the pulmonary precapillary circulation. Blood flowing through the dilated capillaries—particularly the red blood cells flowing in the central core of the stream—is less exposed to oxygen contained in the alveoli, resulting in a ventilation-perfusion mismatch. The patients with this functional shunt will be able to increase their PaO2 to some degree when breathing 100% oxygen.

About 10% of patients with hepatopulmonary syndrome will have the much more sinister type 2 form, in which anatomic arteriovenous shunts within the pulmonary circulation, and occasionally between the portopulmonary systems, can be demonstrated on pulmonary angiography.[196,203,204] These shunts may not be in close proximity to the alveoli for oxygen exchange. Patients with these fixed anatomic shunts will not be able to increase PaO2 when breathing 100% oxygen. The prognosis for type 2 hepatopulmonary syndrome is very poor.

Hepatopulmonary syndrome should be suspected if cyanosis, particularly of the lips and fingers, and digital clubbing are found on examination. Many patients with hepatopulmonary syndrome will have a plethora of spider nevi.[205] Because the pulmonary vascular dilations are more prominent at the lung bases, many patients will have increased dyspnea with standing (platypnea). Brain abscesses have been described as a complication of the intrapulmonary shunts.[206]

Arterial blood gas analysis, both in room air and in 100% oxygen, is essential and should be obtained with the patient standing. The fall in PaO_2 in moving from the recumbent to the standing position (orthodeoxia) is characteristic of hepatopulmonary syndrome. The normal response to breathing 100% oxygen is a $PaO_2 > 500$ mm Hg. Patients with hepatopulmonary syndrome breathing 100% have a moderate shunt if the PaO_2 is > 300 mm Hg but < 500 mm Hg and a severe shunt if the PaO_2 is > 100 mm Hg but < 300 mm Hg.[207]

The site and extent of the right to left shunt can be assessed by either a technetium 99m–labeled macroaggregated albumin (Tc 99m MAA) study or by a contrast echocardiogram.

The Tc 99m MAA study uses peripherally injected labeled albumin particles with a diameter of > 20 µm.[208] Because the usual pulmonary capillary diameter is 8 to 15 µm, normally all of the labeled albumin will be trapped in the lungs. In the presence of pulmonary vasodilation, the labeled albumin particles can be detected in the kidneys and brain and the degree of shunt correlated to the isotope concentration in these extrapulmonary sites. Note that this scan does not differentiate intracardiac from intrapulmonary shunting.

The best method to evaluate the shunt in hepatopulmonary syndrome is the contrast-enhanced echocardiogram,[209] making the diagnosis in 9.1% of 88 children with biliary atresia, although only 50% had symptoms.[210] In this procedure, an agitated solution of contrast is injected peripherally. When cardiopulmonary circulation is normal, microbubbles with a diameter of > 15 µm are trapped in the lungs. If an intracardiac shunt is present, the microbubbles immediately opacify the left ventricle, whereas if there is an intrapulmonary shunt, it requires three to six ventricular contractions before the microbubbles appear in the left heart. Particularly in children who may have congenital heart disease complicating chronic liver disease (eg, Alagille syndrome or biliary atresia), distinguishing the site of the shunt is essential.

The mediator of the pulmonary vascular dilation that characterizes hepatopulmonary syndrome remains speculative. In animal models, elevated levels of endothelium-derived nitric oxide were detected in the lung homogenates of animals with the clinical features of hepatopulmonary syndrome.[211,212] This finding would appear to be supported by reports documenting increased exhaled nitric oxide concentration in adults and children with hepatopulmonary syndrome.[213,214] However, without better understanding of the underlying mechanism, pharmacologic attempts to manage hepatopulmonary syndrome have not been generally successful to date.

Presently, the only definitive treatment for hepatopulmonary syndrome is liver transplant. In the past, hepatopulmonary syndrome was thought to be a contraindication to liver transplant. However, accumulated evidence documenting successful resolution of hepatopulmonary syndrome after liver transplant has reinforced the concept that in selected patients, hepatopulmonary syndrome is, in fact, best managed by liver transplant.[195,207,215,216] Patients with large anatomic shunts who are unable to increase PaO_2 over 100 mm Hg on 100% oxygen are still not suitable candidates for liver transplant.

In selecting patients for transplant, it must be determined if the patient is safe for anesthesia and if the oxygen content of the blood supplying the graft will be adequate to support early graft function. In an analysis of several studies, Krowka and colleagues noted that 30% of patients with $PaO_2 < 50\%$ in room air died after liver transplant compared with 4% of patients with $PaO_2 > 50$ mm Hg.[195] In successfully transplanted patients, complete normalization of hypoxemia occurred in 82% of transplant recipients. However, the duration of use of the mechanical ventilator and intensive care unit stay tend to be prolonged in patients with hepatopulmonary syndrome.

Encouraging evidence that hepatopulmonary syndrome is reversed by liver transplant is emerging in the pediatric experience. In seven children with hepatopulmonary syndrome undergoing liver transplant, complete reversal of the syndrome occurred in all at an average of 24 ± 10 weeks. Time to extubation in this group was 58 ± 21 hours. In one pediatric study, a PaO_2 in room air lower than 60% uniformly resulted in death after transplant,[217] and in another study, there were no survivors after liver transplant if the PaO_2 was < 200 mm Hg in 100% oxygen.[197] Egawa and colleagues categorized 21 children with hepatopulmonary syndrome into three groups, depending on their shunt ratio: mild, less than 20%; moderate, 20 to 40%; and severe, $> 40\%$.[218] An adverse significant effect on patient and graft survival was found with an increasing shunt ratio. One-year actuarial patient survivals were 80%, 66.7%, and 40% in the mild, moderate, and severe groups, respectively. Prolonged ventilator dependence, hypoxic injury to the graft, portal vein thrombosis, and intracranial thrombosis are some of the sequelae in transplanted children with severe hepatopulmonary syndrome.

PORTOPULMONARY HYPERTENSION

This phenomenon is the antithesis of hepatopulmonary syndrome and is characterized by pulmonary artery vasoconstriction (Table 59-7).[219] Why the chronically diseased liver causes two such diverse effects on pulmonary function is an unresolved conundrum. Portopulmonary hypertension has only rarely been described in children. A summary of the basic principles of the pathogenesis, diagnosis, and management is included here.[220,221]

Portopulmonary hypertension is defined as a mean pulmonary artery pressure > 25 mm Hg with a pulmonary capillary wedge pressure of < 15 mm Hg in the absence of any secondary causes of pulmonary hypertension, such as cardiac valvular disease.

On pathologic examination of the pulmonary arteries, concentric medial hypertrophy and intimal fibrosis are found.[222] The coexistence of portal hypertension appears to be a prerequisite for the development of portopulmonary hypertension.[223] In adults, the prevalence of portopulmonary hypertension in patients with portal hypertension

TABLE 59-7   COMPARISON AND CONTRAST: HEPATOPULMONARY SYNDROME AND PORTOPULMONARY HYPERTENSION

HEPATOPULMONARY SYNDROME	PORTOPULMONARY HYPERTENSION
Intrapulmonary vasodilation	Intrapulmonary vasoconstriction
Alveolar arterial gradient > 20 mm Hg	Alveolar arterial gradient usually normal
Normal mean pulmonary artery (PA) pressure	Mean PA pressure > 25 mm Hg
Perform shunt fraction study	Perform right heart catheterization
Trial of 100% O_2	Vasodilator therapy trial
Often reversible with liver treatment	May not reverse with liver transplant
Poor prognosis: PaO_2 < 300 mm Hg on 100% O_2	Poor prognosis: PA pressure > 45 mm Hg
Histology: PA normal	Histology: PA abnormal; concentric medial hypertrophy

and cirrhosis is 1 to 2%, although an 8.5% incidence was found in a recent large series of patients evaluated for liver transplant.[224] The prevalence in children is unknown.

The diagnosis may be suspected by finding abnormalities on the electrocardiogram, which are present in up to 95% of patients.[225] Right ventricular hypertrophy, right axis deviation, and right bundle branch block are common. A right heart catheterization is essential to document right heart and pulmonary pressures accurately and also allows for a trial of vasodilator therapy. Vasodilator treatment with nitric oxide, calcium channel blockers, and eprostonol has been used with varying success in adult studies.[220,226,227]

There are very few published guidelines regarding treatment of portopulmonary hypertension in children. The management of choice advocated in one article is early diagnosis followed by liver transplant as soon as possible.[228] However, experience from the adult literature recommends that patients must be carefully selected for liver transplant and that mean pulmonary artery pressure should not exceed 50 mm Hg. In one study, a mean pulmonary artery pressure of > 50 mm Hg was associated with a 100% cardiopulmonary mortality and a 50% mortality if > 35 mm Hg but < 50 mm Hg.[229] Selection of patients implies the pretransplant diagnosis of portopulmonary hypertension. However, often the diagnosis is made when anesthesia is induced at the time of transplant, thereby limiting appropriate decision making. Maintaining a high index of clinical suspicion before transplant is therefore imperative. This applies particularly to older children with cirrhosis who may wait for long periods for transplant.[230] Patients with mild to moderate pulmonary hypertension (< 40 mm Hg) will usually show resolution after liver transplant, whereas those with severe portopulmonary hypertension frequently develop progressive fatal right heart failure.

CENTRAL NERVOUS SYSTEM INVOLVEMENT

Clinically evident encephalopathy in children with chronic liver disease appears to be less common compared with adults. However, it is also possible that encephalopathy is underdiagnosed in children because its more subtle manifestations are difficult to appreciate, and there is no specific laboratory test that correlates well with encephalopathy. Irritability and lethargy are the two most common signs but may be evident in any chronically ill child. Acute changes in mental status should prompt an investigation for occult gastrointestinal bleeding (which increases

ammonia production from blood in the intestinal lumen) or an intracranial hemorrage secondary to coagulopathy. Aggressive diuretic therapy, spontaneous bacterial peritonitis, and placement of a portosystemic shunt may all precipitate the development of encephalopathy.

The pathophysiology and treatment of hepatic encephalopathy are discussed in detail in Chapter 5.3, "Normal Hepatocyte Function and Mechanisms of Dysfunction." In brief, the main principle of management is to decrease gut-derived nitrogen production by restricting dietary protein, evacuating blood from the gastrointestinal tract, and administering oral lactulose or neomycin to reduce bacterial flora in the bowel. Oral lactulose is preferred, although care must be taken not to induce hypovolemia and electrolyte disturbances from increased stool losses. Oral neomycin has some systemic absorption, which has been associated with ototoxicity; therefore, extended use should be avoided.

CHOLESTATIC LIVER DISEASES: SPECIAL ISSUES

CHOLANGITIS

Ascending infection of the biliary system is most often seen in pediatric liver disease in the context of biliary atresia with a poorly functioning Kasai portoenterostomy. The major risk factors for infection are stasis in the biliary system secondary to poor bile flow and the creation of a Roux-en-Y limb, which approximates the small intestine directly to the porta hepatis. Children with biliary atresia and recurrent episodes of cholangitis may have intrahepatic bilomas, which can be diagnosed on ultrasonography.

Although cholangitis in children with biliary atresia most often occurs when there is evidence of impaired bile flow, generally within the first year after the Kasai procedure,[231] it has also been described late after surgical repair in children with no evidence of biliary obstruction.[232] Under these circumstances, direct ascending infection through the Roux-en-Y limb occurs. However, although these children have a normal serum bilirubin, biliary stasis in the small intrahepatic bile ducts may still be a contributing factor.

Primary and secondary sclerosing cholangitis and the variants of congenital hepatic fibrosis and choledochal cysts with multiple intrahepatic biliary cysts are other intrahepatic cholestatic liver diseases of children in whom cholangitis can occur. In sclerosing cholangitis, the development of jaundice and recurrent cholangitis should prompt the radiographic examination of the biliary system, either by endoscopic retrograde cholangiopancreatography or percutaneous cholangiography, to rule out a dominant stricture that could be stented. In general, obstructive lesions to the external biliary system, such as stones in the common bile duct, cause cholangitis but do not cause chronic liver disease if treated appropriately. These disorders are discussed in Chapter 50.3, "Disorders of the Biliary Tract: Other Disorders."

Cholangitis is diagnosed in the child with cholestatic liver disease who presents with fever and elevated bilirubin and/or serum transaminases from baseline. The alkaline phosphatase or γ-glutamyltransferase will also be elevated. Abdominal pain is only variably present. The most common organisms are gram-negative enteric organisms, such as *E. coli*, *Klebsiella*, *Pseudomonas*, and *Enterococcus*. Blood cultures are frequently negative; therefore, it is important to initiate appropriate antibiotic treatment without waiting for culture results when the clinical index of suspicion is high. If the child fails to defervesce after 72 hours or has frequent recurrences, percutaneous liver biopsy with culture of the liver tissue may be indicated. A common initial antibiotic regimen is ampicillin and cefotaxime given for 10 to 14 days intravenously.

Prophylaxis of recurrent cholangitis is of variable efficacy. In one survey, 73% of physicians used antibiotic prophylaxis after the Kasai procedure.[233] Oral administration of trimethoprim-sulfamethoxazole is most conveniently used.[233] Long-term intravenous antibiotic prophylaxis in children via central venous catheters is occasionally indicated, although the risk of inducing multiply resistant bacterial organisms or fungal colonization must be considered.

There is no definitive effective treatment for recurrent cholangitis in the child with biliary atresia except liver transplant. As such, recurrent cholangitis is an indication for listing children with biliary atresia for transplant.[234] There is some evidence that children with biliary atresia who suffer recurrent episodes of cholangitis develop cirrhosis more quickly than those without cholangitis.[235]

PRURITUS

Intense pruritus can be a complication of cholestatic liver disease, causing misery to children and their caregivers alike. The well-being of the child is overwhelmed by the intense need to itch. Severely afflicted children cannot sleep, do not eat, and are constantly irritable. Although the etiology may be multifactorial, accumulation of bile acids appears to be important because pruritus is most often associated with cholestasis and is particularly problematic in progressive familial intrahepatic cholestasis syndromes. Another contributing factor appears to be increased opiate tone because opiate antagonists have some therapeutic benefit.[236,237]

Treatment is often poorly effective.[238,239] Cholestyramine is generally not helpful because there are already unusually low concentrations of bile acids in the intestinal lumen. Choleretics, such as phenobarbital, can be tried. Antihistamines are the first line of treatment but are seldom adequate alone. Ursodeoxycholic acid, by altering bile composition, will often help reduce pruritus and should be used in doses

of 25 to 30 mg/kg/d in divided doses.[240] Rifampin has also been successfully used in doses of 10 mg/kg/d.[241] Rifampin may alter bile acid composition via 6-hydroxylation of bile salts. Rifampin interacts with the nuclear receptor pregnane X and induces cyp3A, which can hydroxylate bile salts (see Chapter 5.1, "Bile Formation and Cholestasis").

Other modalities that are less well studied in children are intravenous naloxone,[242] plasmapheresis, charcoal absorption,[243] and phototherapy. The opiate antagonist approach appears to be very promising. Naloxone has been shown to be efficacious but is limited in its application by poor oral bioavailability and short half-life. Oral preparations of opiate antagonists, such as naltrexone and nalmefene, may help some patients.[244,245] A recent report suggests that dronabinol (a cannabinoid) may also be beneficial.[246]

Partial biliary diversion procedures have been successful in treating some children with progressive familial intrahepatic cholestasis syndromes and intractable pruritus.[247–249]

ACKNOWLEDGMENT

I am indebted to the expertise of Dinora Duarte in the preparation of this chapter.

REFERENCES

1. Shepherd RW, Chin SE, Cleghorn GJ, et al. Malnutrition in children with chronic liver disease accepted for liver transplantation: clinical profile and effect on outcome. J Paediatr Child Health 1991;27:295.
2. Moukarzel AA, Najm I, Vargas JV, et al. Effect of nutritional status on outcome of orthotopic liver transplantation in pediatric patients. Transplant Proc 1990;22:1560.
3. Pikul J, Sharpe MD, Lowndes R, Ghent CN. Degree of preoperative malnutrition is predictive of postoperative morbidity and mortality in liver transplant recipients. Transplantation 1994;57:469.
4. Roggero P, Cataliotti E, Ulla L, et al. Factors influencing malnutrition in children waiting for liver transplants. Am J Clin Nutr 1997;65:1852.
5. Balistreri WF, Bucuvalas JC, Ryckman FC. The effect of immunosuppression on growth and development. Liver Transplant Surg 1995;1:64.
6. Weber A, Roy CC. The malabsorption associated with chronic liver disease in children. Pediatrics 1972;50:73.
7. Weisdorf SA, Freese DK, Fath JJ, et al. Amino acid abnormalities in infants with extrahepatic biliary atresia and cirrhosis. Gastroenterol Nutr 1987;6:860.
8. Moreno LA, Gottrand F, Hoden S, et al. Improvement of nutritional status in cholestatic children with supplemental nocturnal enteral nutrition. J Pediatr Gastroenterol Nutr 1991;12:213.
9. Holt RIG, Jones J, Stone NM, et al. Sequential changes in insulin-like growth factor I (IGF-I) and IGF-binding proteins in children with end-stage liver disease before and after successful orthotopic liver transplantation. J Clin Endocrinol Metab 1996;81:160.
10. Bucuvalas JC, Horn JA, Carlsson L, et al. Growth hormone insensitivity associated with elevated circulating growth hormone-binding protein in children with Alagille syndrome and short stature. J Clin Endocrinol Metab 1993;76:1477.
11. Holt RI, Baker AJ, Jones JS, Miell JP. The insulin-like growth fac-

tor and binding protein axis in children with end-stage liver disease before and after orthotopic liver transplantation. Pediatr Transplant 1998;2:76.

12. Bucuvalas JC, Cutfield W, Horn J, et al. Resistance to the growth-promoting and metabolic effects of growth hormone in children with chronic liver disease. J Pediatr 1990; 117:397.

13. Greer R, Quirk P, Cleghorn GJ, Shepherd RW. Growth hormone resistance and somatomedins in children with end-stage liver disease awaiting transplantation. J Pediatr Gastroenterol Nutr 1998;27:148.

14. Bucuvalas JC, Horn JA, Slusher J, et al. Growth hormone insensitivity in children with biliary atresia. J Pediatr Gastroenterol Nutr 1996;23:135.

15. Chin SE, Shepherd RW, Thomas BJ, et al. Nutritional support in children with end-stage liver disease: a randomized crossover trial of a branched-chain amino acid supplement. Am J Clin Nutr 1992;56:158.

16. Sokol RJ, Stall C. Anthropometric evaluation of children with chronic liver disease. Am J Clin Nutr 1990;52:203.

17. Goulet OJ, de Ville de Goyet J, Otte JB, Ricour C. Preoperative nutritional evaluation and support for liver transplantation in children. Transplant Proc 1987;19:3249.

18. Shepherd RW. Pre- and postoperative nutritional care in liver transplantation in children. J Gastroenterol Hepatol 1996; 11:S7.

19. Duche M, Habes D, Lababidi A, et al. Percutaneous endoscopic gastrostomy for continuous feeding in children with chronic cholestasis. J Pediatr Gastroenterol Nutr 1999;29:42.

20. Charlton CP, Buchanan E, Holden CE, et al. Intensive enteral feeding in advanced cirrhosis: reversal of malnutrition without precipitation of hepatic encephalopathy. Arch Dis Child 1992;67:603.

21. Guimber D, Michaud L, Ategbo S, et al. Experience of parenteral nutrition for nutritional rescue in children with severe liver disease following failure of enteral nutrition. Pediatr Transplant 1999;3:139.

22. Druml W, Fischer M, Pidlich J, Lenz K. Fat elimination in chronic hepatic failure: long-chain vs. medium-chain triglycerides. Am J Clin Nutr 1995;61:812.

23. Greene HL, Moore ME, Phillips B, et al. Evaluation of a pediatric multiple vitamin preparation for total parenteral nutrition. Pediatrics 1986;77:539.

24. Moukarzel AA, Haddad I, Ament ME, et al. 230 patient years of experience with home long-term parenteral nutrition in childhood: natural history and life of central venous catheters. J Pediatr Surg 1994;29:1323.

25. Kaufman SS, Murray ND, Wood RP, et al. Nutritional support for the infant with extrahepatic biliary atresia. J Pediatr 1987;110:679.

26. Sokol RJ, Heubi JE, Iannaccone S, et al. Mechanism causing vitamin E deficiency during chronic childhood cholestasis. Gastroenterology 1983;85:1172.

27. Alvarez F, Cresteil D, Lemonnier F, et al. Plasma vitamin E levels in children with cholestasis. J Pediatr Gastroenterol Nutr 1984;3:390.

28. Sokol RJ. Vitamin E deficiency and neurologic disease. Annu Rev Nutr 1988;8:351.

29. Sokol RJ, Heubi JE, Iannaccone ST, et al. Vitamin E deficiency with normal serum vitamin E concentrations in children with chronic cholestasis. N Engl J Med 1984;310:1209.

30. Kooh SW, Jones G, Reilly BJ, Fraser D. Pathogenesis of rickets in chronic hepatobiliary disease in children. J Pediatr 1979;94:870.

31. Rosen JF, Chesney RW. Circulating calcitrol concentrations in health and disease. J Pediatr 1983;103:1.

32. Sherlock S. Classification and functional aspects of portal hypertension. Am J Surg 1974;127:121.

33. Vargas HE, Gerber D, Abu-Elmagd K. Management of portal hypertension-related bleeding. Surg Clin North Am 1999;79:1.

34. Fucini C, Wolff BG, Dozois RR. Bleeding from peristomal varices: perspectives on prevention and treatment. Dis Colon Rectum 1991;34:1073.

35. Kuroiwa M, Suzuki N, Hatakeyama S, et al. Magnetic resonance angiography of portal collateral pathways after hepatic portoenterostomy in biliary atresia: comparisons with endoscopic findings. J Pediatr Surg 2001;36:1012–6.

36. Gulati M, Paul SB, Arora NK, Mathur P, Berry M. Esophageal and gastric vasculature in children with extrahepatic portal hypertension: evaluation by intravenous CT portography. Clinical Imaging 2000;24:351–6.

37. Kozaiwa K, Tajiri H, Yoshimura N, et al. Utility of duplex Doppler ultrasound in evaluating portal hypertension in children. J Pediatr Gastroenterol Nutr 1995;21:215.

38. Puttini M, Aseni P, Brambilla G, Belli L. Splenic artery aneurysms in portal hypertension. J Cardiovasc Surg 1982; 23:490.

39. Boijsen E, Efsing H-O. Aneurysm of the splenic artery. Acta Radiol 1969;8:29.

40. D'Amico G, Morabito A, Pagliaro L, Marubini E. Survival and prognostic indicators in compensated and decompensated cirrhosis. Dig Dis Sci 1986;31:468.

41. Garcia-Tsao G, Groszmann RJ, Fisher RL, et al. Portal pressure, presence of gastroesophageal varices and variceal bleeding. Hepatology 1985;5:419.

42. Viallet A, Marleau D, Huet M, et al. Hemodynamic evaluation of patients with intrahepatic portal hypertension. Relationship between bleeding varices and the portohepatic gradient. Gastroenterology 1975;69:1297.

43. Bernard O, Alvarez F, Brunelle F, et al. Portal hypertension in children. Clin Gastroenterol 1985;14:33.

44. Cales P, Zabotto B, Meskens C, et al. Gastroesophageal endoscopic features in cirrhosis. Gastroenterology 1990;98:156.

45. de Franchis R, et al. Prediction of the first variceal hemorrhage in patients with cirrhosis of the liver and esophageal varices. A prospective multicenter study. N Engl J Med 1988;319:983.

46. Lebrec D, De Fleury P, Rueff B, et al. Portal hypertension, size of esophageal varices, and risk of gastrointestinal bleeding in alcoholic cirrhosis. Gastroenterology 1980;79:1139.

47. Miga D, Sokol RJ, MacKenzie T, et al. Survival after first esophageal variceal hemorrhage in patients with biliary atresia. J Pediatr 2001;139:291–6.

48. Panes J, Teres J, Bosch J, Rodes J. Efficacy of balloon tamponade in treatment of bleeding gastric and esophageal varices. Results in 151 consecutive episodes. Dig Dis Sci 1988;33:454.

49. Terblanche J, Burroughs AK, Hobbs KE. Controversies in the management of bleeding esophageal varices (1). N Engl J Med 1989;320:1393.

50. Terblanche J, Burroughs AK, Hobbs KE. Controversies in the management of bleeding esophageal varices (2). N Engl J Med 1989;320:1469.

51. Burroughs AK. The management of bleeding due to portal hypertension. Part 1. The management of acute bleeding episodes. QJM 1988;67:447.

52. Burroughs AK. The management of bleeding due to portal hypertension. Part 2. Prevention of variceal rebleeding and prevention of the first bleeding episode in patients with portal hypertension. QJM 1988;68:507.

53. D'Amico G, Pagliaro L, Bosch J. The treatment of portal hypertension: a meta-analytic review. Hepatology 1995;22:332.

54. Graham DY, Smith JL. The course of patients after variceal hemorrhage. Gastroenterology 1981;80:800.

55. Yachha SK, Sharma BC, Kumar M, Khanduri A. Endoscopic sclerotherapy for esophageal varices in children with extrahepatic portal venous obstruction: a follow-up study. J Pediatr Gastroenterol Nutr 1997;24:49.

56. Goh DW, Myers NA. Portal hypertension in children—the changing spectrum. J Pediatr Surg 1994;29:688.

57. Maksoud JG, Goncalves ME, Porta G, et al. The endoscopic and surgical management of portal hypertension in children: analysis of 123 cases. J Pediatr Surg 1991;26:178.

58. Westaby D, Macdougall BR, Williams R. Improved survival following injection sclerotherapy for esophageal varices: final analysis of a controlled trial. Hepatology 1985;5:827.

59. Yachha SK, Ghoshal UC, Gupta R, et al. Extrahepatic portal venous obstruction: role of variceal obliteration by endoscopic sclerotherapy and *Helicobacter pylori* infection. J Pediatr Gastroenterol Nutr 1996;23:20.

60. Goncalves ME, Cardoso SR, Maksoud JG. Prophylactic sclerotherpy in children with esophageal varices: long-term results of a controlled prospective randomized trial. J Pediatr Surg 2000;35:401–5.

61. Paquet KJ. Prophylactic endoscopic sclerosing treatment of the esophageal wall in varices—a prospective controlled randomized trial. Endoscopy 1982;14:4.

62. Zargar SA, Javid G, Khan BA, et al. Endoscopic ligation compared with sclerotherapy for bleeding esophageal varices in children with extrahepatic portal venous obstruction. Hepatology 2002;36:666–72.

63. Stiegmann GV, et al. Endoscopic sclerotherapy as compared with endoscopic ligation for bleeding esophageal varices. N Engl J Med 1992;326:1527.

64. Sasaki T, Hasegawa T, Nakajima K, et al. Endoscopic variceal ligation in the management of gastroesophageal varices in postoperative biliary atresia. J Pediatr Surg 1998;33:1628.

65. Cano I, Urruzuno P, Medina E, et al. Treatment of esophageal varices by endoscopic ligation in children. Eur J Pediatr 1995;5:299.

66. Reinoso MA, Sharp HL, Rank J. Endoscopic variceal ligation in pediatric patients with portal hypertension secondary to liver cirrhosis. Gastrointest Endosc 1997;46:244.

67. Ohnuma N, Takahashi H, Tanabe M, et al. Endoscopic variceal ligation using a clipping apparatus in children with portal hypertension. Endoscopy 1997;29:86.

68. Fox VL, Carr-Locke DL, Connors PJ, Leichtner AM. Endoscopic ligation of esophageal varices in children. J Pediatr Gastroenterol Nutr 1999;20:202.

69. Price MR, Sartorelli KH, Karrer FM, et al. Management of esophageal varices in children by endoscopic variceal ligation. J Pediatr Surg 1996;31:1056.

70. McKiernan PJ, Beath SV, Davison SM. A prospective study of endoscopic esophageal variceal ligation using multiband ligator. J Pediatr Gastroenterol Nutr 2002;34:207–11.

71. Warren WD, Zeppa R, Fomon JJ. Selective trans-splenic decompression of gastroesophageal varices by distal splenorenal shunt. Ann Surg 1967;166:437.

72. Mazariegos GV, Reyes J. A technique for distal splenoadrenal shunting in pediatric portal hypertension. J Am Coll Surg 1998;187:634.

73. Maksoud JG, Mies S. Distal splenorenal shunt (DSS) in children: analysis of the first 21 consecutive cases. Ann Surg 1982;195:401.

74. Rikkers LF, Jin G. Surgical management of acute variceal hemorrhage. World J Surg 1994;18:193.

75. Orloff MJ, Bell RH, Orloff MS, et al. Prospective randomized trial of emergency portacaval shunt and emergency medical therapy in unselected cirrhotic patients with bleeding varices. Hepatology 1994;20:863.

76. Evans S, Stovroff M, Heiss K, Ricketts R. Selective distal splenorenal shunts for intractable variceal bleeding in pediatric portal hypertension. J Pediatr Surg 1995;30:1115.

77. Shun A, Delaney DP, Martin HCO, et al. Portosystemic shunting for pediatric portal hypertension. J Pediatr Surg 1997;32:489.

78. Reyes J, Mazariegos GV, Bueno J, et al. The role of portosystemic shunting in children in the transplant era. J Pediatr Surg 1999;34:117.

79. D'Cruz AJ, Kamath PS, Ramachandra C, Jalihal A. Non-conventional portosystemic shunts in children with extrahepatic portal vein obstruction. Acta Paediatr Jpn 1995;37:17.

80. de Ville de Goyet J, Alberti D, Falchetti D, et al. Treatment of extrahepatic portal hypertension in children by mesenteric-to-left portal vein bypass: a new physiological procedure. Eur J Pediatr Surg 1999;165:777–81.

81. Bambini DA, Superina R, Almond PS, et al. Experience with the Rex shunt (mesenterico-left portal bypass) in children with extrahepatic portal hypertension. J Pediatr Surg 2000;35:13–9.

82. Renard TH, Andrews WS, Rollins N, et al. Use of distal splenorenal shunt in children referred for liver transplant evaluation. J Pediatr Surg 1994;29:403.

83. Mazzaferro V, Todo S, Tzakis AG, et al. Liver transplantation in patients with previous portosystemic shunt. Am J Surg 1990;160:111.

84. Heyman MB, Laberge JM. Role of transjugular intrahepatic portosystemic shunt in the treatment of portal hypertension in pediatric patients. J Pediatr Gastroenterol Nutr 1999;29:240.

85. Schultz SR, Laberge JM, Gordon RL, Warren RS. Anatomy of the portal vein bifurcation: intra- versus extrahepatic location—implications for transjugular intrahepatic portosystemic shunts. J Vasc Interven Radiol 1994;5:457.

86. Freedman AM, Sanyal AJ, Tisnado J, et al. Complications of transjugular intrahepatic portosystemic shunt: a comprehensive review. Radiographics 1993;13:1185.

87. Somberg KA, Riegler JL, Laberge JM, et al. Hepatic encephalopathy after transjugular intrahepatic portosystemic shunts: incidence and risk factors. Am J Gastroenterol 1995;90:549.

88. Somberg KA, Lake JR, Tomlanovich SJ, et al. Transjugular intrahepatic portosystemic shunts for refractory ascites: assessment of clinical and hormonal response and renal function. Hepatology 1995;21:709.

89. Laberge JM, Somberg KA, Lake JR, et al. Two-year outcome following transjugular intrahepatic portosystemic shunt for variceal bleeding: results in 90 patients. Gastroenterology 1995;108:1143.

90. Brown RSJ, Lake JR. Transjugular intrahepatic portosystemic shunt as a form of treatment for portal hypertension: indications and contraindications. Adv Intern Med 1997;42:485.

91. Escorsell A, Banares R, Garcia-Pagan JC, et al. TIPS versus drug therapy in preventing variceal rebleeding in advanced cirrhosis: a randomized controlled trial. Hepatology 2002;35:385–92.

92. Sauer P, Hansmann J, Richter GM, et al. Endoscopic variceal ligation plus propranol vs. transjugular intrahepatic portosystemic stent shunt: a long-term randomized trial. Endoscopy 2002;34:690–7.

93. Freeman RB, FitzMaurice SE, Greenfield AE, et al. Is the transjugular intrahepatic portocaval shunt procedure beneficial for liver transplant recipients? Transplantation 1994;58:297.

94. Berger H, Bugnon F, Goffette P, et al. Percutaneous transjugular intrahepatic stent shunt for treatment of intractable varicose bleeding in pediatric patients. Eur J Pediatr 1994;153:721.

95. Weinberg GD, Matalon TA, Brunner MC, et al. Bleeding stomal varices: treatment with a transjugular intrahepatic portosystemic shunt in two pediatric patients. J Vasc Interven Radiol 1995;6:233.

96. Stevenson DM, Kelly DA, Mckiernan P, et al. Emergency transjugular intrahepatic portosystemic shunt prior to liver transplantation. Pediatr Radiol 1997;27:84.

97. Cao S, Monge H, Semba C, et al. Emergency transjugular intrahepatic portosystemic shunt (TIPS) in an infant: a case report. J Pediatr Surg 1997;32:125.

98. Hackworth CA, Leef JA, Rosenblum JD, et al. Transjugular intrahepatic portosystemic shunt creation in children: initial clinical experience. Radiology 1998;206:109.

99. Heyman MB, Laberge JM, Somberg KA, et al. Transjugular intrahepatic portosystemic shunts (TIPS) in children. J Pediatr 1997;131:914.

100. Kanterman RY, Darcy MD, Middleton WD, et al. Doppler sonography findings associated with transjugular intrahepatic portosystemic shunt malfunction. AJR Am J Roentgenol 1997;168:467.

101. Johnson SP, Leyendecker JR, Joseph FB, et al. Transjugular portosystemic shunts in pediatric patients awaiting liver transplantation. Transplantation 1996;62:1178.

102. Sterling KM, Darcy MD. Stenosis of transjugular intrahepatic portosystemic shunts: presentation and management. AJR Am J Roentgenol 1997;168:239.

103. Burroughs AK. Pharmacological treatment of acute variceal bleeding. Digestion 1998;59:28.

104. Reichen J. Liver function and pharmacological considerations in pathogenesis and treatment of portal hypertension. Hepatology 1986;11:1066.

105. Avgerinos A. Approach to the management of bleeding esophageal varices: role of somatostatin. Digestion 1999;59:1.

106. Bosch J, Kravetz D, Rodes J. Effects of somatostatin on hepatic and systemic hemodynamics in patients with cirrhosis of the liver: comparison with vasopressin. Gastroenterology 1981;80:518.

107. Hadengue A. Somatostatin or octreotide in acute variceal bleeding. Digestion 1999;60:31.

108. Besson I, Ingrand P, Person B, et al. Sclerotherapy with or without octreotide for acute variceal bleeding. N Engl J Med 1995;333:555.

109. Jenkins SA, Baxter JN, Critchley M, et al. Randomized trial of octreotide for long term management of cirrhosis after variceal hemorrhage. BMJ 1997;315:1338.

110. Siafakas C, Fox VL, Nurko S. Use of octreotide for the treatment of severe gastrointestinal bleeding in children. J Pediatr Gastroenterol Nutr 1998;26:356.

111. Poynard T, Cales P, Pasta L, et al. Beta-adrenergic-antagonist drugs in the prevention of gastrointestinal bleeding in patients with cirrhosis and esophageal varices. An analysis of data and prognostic factors in 589 patients from randomized clinical trials. N Engl J Med 1991;324:1532.

112. Pascal JP, Cales P. Propranolol in the prevention of first upper gastrointestinal tract hemorrhage in patients with cirrhosis of the liver and esophageal varices. N Engl J Med 1987;317:856.

113. Bosch J, Garcia-Pagan JC, Feu F, et al New approaches in the pharmacologic treatment of portal hypertension. J Hepatol 1993;17:41.

114. Villanueva C, Balanzo J, Novella MT, et al. Nadolol plus isosorbide mononitrate compared with sclerotherapy for the prevention of variceal rebleeding. N Engl J Med 1996;334:1624.

115. Shashidhar H, Langhans N, Grand RJ. Propranolol in prevention of portal hypertensive hemorrhage in children: a pilot study. J Pediatr Gastroenterol Nutr 1999;29:17.

116. Ozsoylu S, Kocak N, Demir H, et al. Propranolol for primary and secondary prophylaxis of variceal bleeding in children with cirrhosis. Turk J Pediatr 2000;42:31–3.

117. Banares R, Albillos A, Rincon D, et al. Endoscopic treatment versus endoscopic plus pharmacologic treatment for acute variceal bleeding: a meta-analysis. Hepatology 2002;35:609–15.

118. Lo GH, Lai KH, Cheng JS, et al. Endoscopic variceal ligation plus nadolol and sucralfate compared with ligation alone for the prevention of variceal rebleeding: a prospective, randomized trial. Hepatology 2000;32:660–2.

119. Bosch J, Arroyo V, Betriu A, et al. Hepatic hemodynamics and the renin-angiotensin-aldosterone system in cirrhosis. Gastroenterology 1990;78:92.

120. Wyllie R, Arasu TS, Fitzgerald JF. Ascites: pathophysiology and management. J Pediatr 1980;97:167.

121. Ring-Larsen H, Henriksen JH. Pathogenesis of ascites formation and hepatorenal syndrome: humoral and hemodynamic factors. Semin Liver Dis 1986;6:341.

122. Witte CL, Witte MH, Dumont AE. Lymph imbalance in the genesis and perpetuation of the ascites syndrome in hepatic cirrhosis. Gastroenterology 1980;78:1059.

123. Epstein FH. Underfilling versus overflow in hepatic ascites. N Engl J Med 1999;307:1577.

124. Lieberman FL, Denison EK, Reynolds TB. The relationship of plasma volume, portal hypertension, ascites and renal sodium retention in cirrhosis: the overflow theory of ascites formation. Ann N Y Acad Sci 1990;170:202.

125. Schrier RW, Arroyo V, Bernardi M, et al. Peripheral arterial vasodilation hypothesis: a proposal for the initiation of renal sodium and water retention in cirrhosis. Hepatology 1988;8:1151.

126. Arroyo V, Claria J, Salo J, Jimenez W. Antidiuretic hormone and the pathogenesis of water retention in cirrhosis with ascites. Semin Liver Dis 1994;14:44.

127. Goldberg RB. Ultrasonic evaluation of intraperitoneal fluid. JAMA 1976;285:2427.

128. Runyon BA. Management of adult patients with ascites caused by cirrhosis. Hepatology 1998;27:264.

129. Bernardi M, Trevisani F, Gasbarrini A, Gasbarrini G. Hepatorenal disorders: role of the renin-angiotensin-aldosterone system. Semin Liver Dis 1994;14:23.

130. Funder JW. Aldosterone action. Annu Rev Physiol 1993;55:115.

131. Fogel MR, Sawhney VK, Neal EA, et al. Diuresis in the ascitic patient: a randomized controlled trial of three regimens. J Clin Gastroenterol 1981;3:73.

132. Kramer RE, Sokol RJ, Yerushalmi B, et al. Large-volume paracentesis in the management of ascites in children. J Pediatr Gastroenterol Nutr 2001;33:245–9.

133. Wong F, Blendis L. Peritoneovenous shunting in cirrhosis: its role in the management of refractory ascites in the 1990s. Am J Gastroenterol 1995;90:2086.

134. Guardiola J, Xiol X, Escriba JM, et al. Prognosis assessment of cirrhotic patients with refractory ascites treated with a peritoneovenous shunt. Am J Gastroenterol 1995;90:2097.

135. Stanley MM, Ochi S, Lee KK, et al. Peritoneovenous shunting as compared with medical treatment in patients with alcoholic cirrhosis and massive ascites. Veterans Administration cooperative study on treatment of alcoholic cirrhosis with ascites. N Engl J Med 1989;321:1632.

136. Castells A, Salo J, Planas R, et al. Impact of shunt surgery for variceal bleeding in the natural history of ascites in cirrhosis: a retrospective study. Hepatology 1994;20:584.

137. Lebrec D, Giuily N, Hadengue A, et al. Transjugular intrahepatic portosystemic shunts: comparison with paracentesis in patients with cirrhosis and refractory ascites: a randomized trial. J Hepatol 1996;25:135.

138. Gilbert JA, Kamath PS. Spontaneous bacterial peritonitis: an update. Mayo Clin Proc 1995;70:365.

139. Runyon BA. Paracentesis of ascitic fluid. A safe procedure. Arch Intern Med 1986;146:2259.

140. Runyon BA, Canawati HN, Akriviadis EA. Optimization of ascitic fluid culture technique. Gastroenterology 1988;95:1351.

141. Runyon BA, Umland ET, Merlin T. Inoculation of blood culture bottles with ascitic fluid. Improved detection of spontaneous bacterial peritonitis. Arch Intern Med 1987;147:73.

142. Guarner C, Runyon BA. Spontaneous bacterial peritonitis: pathogenesis, diagnosis, and management. Gastroenterology 1995;3:311.

143. Akriviadis EA, Runyon BA. Utility of an algorithm in differentiating spontaneous from secondary bacterial peritonitis. Gastroenterology 1990;98:127.

144. Garcia-Tsao G. Spontaneous bacterial peritonitis. Gastroenterol Clin North Am 1992;21:257.

145. Runyon BA, McHutchinson JG, Antillon MR, et al. Short-course versus long-course antibiotic treatment of spontaneous bacterial peritonitis. A randomized controlled study of 100 patients [abstract]. Gastroenterology 1991;100:1737.

146. Sorell WT, Quigley EM, Jin G, et al. Bacterial translocation in the portal-hypertensive rat: studies in basal conditions and on exposure to hemorrhagic shock. Gastroenterology 1993;104:1722.

147. Rajkovic IA, Williams R. Abnormalities of neutrophil phagocytosis, intracellular killing and metabolic activity in alcoholic cirrhosis and hepatitis. Hepatology 1999;6:252.

148. Runyon BA. Patients with deficient ascitic fluid opsonic activity are predisposed to spontaneous bacterial peritonitis. Hepatology 1988;8:632.

149. Runyon BA. Spontaneous bacterial peritonitis: an explosion of information. Hepatology1988; 8:171.

150. Tito L, Rimola A, Gines P, et al. Recurrence of spontaneous bacterial peritonitis in cirrhosis: frequency and predictive factors. Hepatology 1988;8:27.

151. Andreu M, Sola R, Sitges-Serra A, et al. Risk factors for spontaneous bacterial peritonitis in cirrhotic patients with ascites. Gastroenterology 1993;104:1133.

152. Koppel MH, Coburn JW, Matlock MM, et al. Transplantation of cadaveric kidneys from patients with hepatorenal syndrome. N Engl J Med 1969;280:1367.

153. Psacharopoulos HT, Mowat AP, Davies M, et al. Fulminant hepatic failure in childhood: an analysis of 31 cases. Arch Dis Child 1980;55:252.

154. Follo A, Llovet JM, Navasa M, et al. Renal impairment after spontaneous bacterial peritonitis in cirrhosis: incidence, clinical course predictive factors and prognosis. Hepatology 1994;20:1495.

155. Van Roey G, Moore K. The hepatorenal syndrome. Pediatr Nephrol 1996;10:100.

156. Ellis D, Avner ED, Starzl TE. Renal failure in children with hepatic failure undergoing liver transplantation. J Pediatr 1986;108:393.

157. Arroyo V, Gines P, Gerbes AL, et al. Definition and diagnostic criteria of refractory ascites and hepatorenal syndrome in cirrhosis. Hepatology 1996;23:164.

158. Gines P, Arroyo V. Hepatorenal syndrome. J Am Soc Nephrol 1999;10:1833.

159. Schwartz GJ, Brion LP, Spitzer A. The use of plasma creatinine concentration for estimating glomerular filtration rate in infants, children, and adolescents. Pediatr Clin North Am 1987;34:571.

160. Walser M, Drew HH, LaFrance ND. Creatinine measurements often yield false estimates of progression in chronic renal failure. Kidney Int 1988;34:412.

161. Shemesh O, Golbetz H, Kriss JP, Myers BD. Limitations of creatinine as a filtration marker in glomerulopathic patients. Kidney Int 1985;28:830.

162. Epstein M, Berk PD, Hollenberg NK, et al. Renal failure in the patient with cirrhosis. The role of active vasoconstriction. Am J Med 1970;49:175.

163. Bataller R, Gines P, Guevara M, Arroyo V. Hepatorenal syndrome. Semin Liver Dis 1997;17:233.

164. Gines A, Escorsell A, Gines P, et al. Incidence, predictive factors, and prognosis of the hepatorenal syndrome in cirrhosis and ascites. Gastroenterology 1993;105:229.

165. Epstein M. Hepatorenal syndrome: emerging perspectives. Semin Nephrol 1997;17:563.

166. Henriksen JH, Ring-Larsen H, Kanstrup IL, Christensen NJ. Splanchnic and renal elimination and release of catecholamines in cirrhosis. Evidence of enhanced sympathetic nervous activity in patients with decompensated cirrhosis. Gut 1984;25:1034.

167. Floras JS, Legault L, Morali GA, et al. Increased sympathetic outflow in cirrhosis and ascites: direct evidence from intraneural recordings. Ann Intern Med 1991;114:373.

168. Esler M, Dudley F, Jennings G, et al. Increased sympathetic nervous activity and the effects of its inhibition with clonidine in alcoholic cirrhosis. Ann Intern Med 1992;116:446.

169. Gerbes AL, Gulberg V, Bilzer M. Endothelin and other mediators in the pathophysiology of portal hypertension. Digestion 1998;59:8.

170. Kobayashi H, Miyano T, Horikoshi K, et al. Clinical significance of plasma endothelin levels in patients with biliary atresia. Pediatr Surg Int 1998;13:491–3.

171. Bakr AM, Abdalla AF, El-Marsafawy H, et al. Plasma endothelin-1 concentrations in children with cirrhosis and their relationship to renal function and the severity of portal hypertension. J Pediatr Gastroenterol Nutr 2002;35:149–53.

172. Moore K, Wendon J, Frazer M, et al. Plasma endothelin immunoreactivity in liver disease and the hepatorenal syndrome. N Engl J Med 1992;327:1774.

173. Moller S, Gulberg V, Henriksen JH, Gerbes AL. Endothelin-1 and endothelin-3 in cirrhosis: relations to systemic and splanchnic haemodynamics. J Hepatol 1995;23:135.

174. Nozue T, Kobayashi A, Uemasu F, et al. Plasma endothelin-1 levels of children with cirrhosis. J Pediatr Gastroenterol Nutr 1995;21:220.

175. Bachmann-Brandt S, Bittner I, Neuhaus P, et al. Plasma levels of endothelin-1 in patients with the hepatorenal syndrome after successful liver transplantation. Transplant Int 2000;13:357–62.

176. Soper CP, Latif AB, Bending MR. Amelioration of hepatorenal syndrome with selective endothelin-A antagonist. Lancet 1996;347:1842.

177. Gines A, Salmeron JM, Gines P, et al. Oral misoprostol or intravenous prostaglandin F2 do not improve renal function in patients with cirrhosis and ascites with hyponatremia or renal failure. J Hepatol 1993;17:220.

178. Groszmann RJ. Nitric oxide and hemodynamic impairment. Digestion 1998;59:6.

179. Ros J, Claria J, Jimenez W, et al. Role of nitric oxide and prostacyclin in the control of renal perfusion in experimental cirrhosis [abstract]. Hepatology 1995;22:915.

180. Alvestrand A, Bergstrom J. Glomerular hyperfiltration after protein ingestion, during glucagon infusion, and in insulin-dependent diabetes is induced by a liver hormone: deficient production of this hormone in hepatic failure causes hepatorenal syndrome. Lancet 1999;i:195.

181. Lang F, Tschernko E, Schulze E, et al. Hepatorenal reflex regulating kidney function. Hepatology 1991;14:590.

182. Iwatsuki S, Popovtzer MM, Corman JL, et al. Recovery from hepatorenal syndrome after orthotopic liver transplantation. N Engl J Med 1973;289:1155.

183. Wood RP, Ellis D, Starzl TE. The reversal of the hepatorenal syndrome in four pediatric patients following successful orthotopic liver transplantation. Ann Surg 1987;205:415.

184. Barnardo DE, Baldus WP, Maher FT. Effects of dopamine on renal function in patients with cirrhosis. Gastroenterology 1970;58:524.

185. Linas SL, Schaefer JW, Moore EE, et al. Peritoneovenous shunt in the management of hepatorenal syndrome. Kidney Int 1986;30:736.

186. Guevara M, Gines P, Bandi JC, et al. Transjugular intrahepatic portosystemic shunt in hepatorenal syndrome: effects on renal function and vasoactive systems. Hepatology 1998;28:416.

187. Brensing KA, Textor J, et al. Sustained improvement of hepatorenal syndrome after TIPS-insertion in patients with terminal liver cirrhosis not eligible for transplantation [abstract]. Gastroenterology 1996;110:1158.

188. Ortega R, Gines P, Uriz J, et al. Terlipressin therapy with and without albumin for patients with hepatorenal syndrome: results of a prospective, non randomized study. Hepatology 2002;36:941–8.

189. Gonwa TA, Poplawski S, Paulsen W, et al. Pathogenesis and outcome of hepatorenal syndrome in patients undergoing orthotopic liver transplant. Transplantation 1989;47:395.

190. Ellis D, Avner ED. Renal failure and dialysis therapy in children with hepatic failure in the perioperative period of orthotopic liver transplantation. Clin Nephrol 1986;25:295.

191. Distant DA, Gonwa TA. The kidney in liver transplantation. J Am Soc Nephrol 1993;4:129.

192. Gonwa TA, Morris CA, Goldstein RM, et al. Long-term survival and renal function following liver transplantation in patients with and without hepatorenal syndrome—experience in 300 patients. Transplantation 1991;51:428.

193. Lange PA, Stoller JK. The hepatopulmonary syndrome. Ann Intern Med 1995;122:521.

194. Scott VL, Dodson F, Kang Y. The hepatopulmonary syndrome. Surg Clin North Am 1999;79:23.

195. Krowka MJ, Porayko MK, Plevak DJ, P et al. Hepatopulmonary syndrome with progressive hypoxemia as an indication for liver transplantation: case reports and literature review. Mayo Clin Proc 1997;72:44.

196. Krowka MJ, Dickson ER, Cortese DA. Hepatopulmonary syndrome. Clinical observations and lack of therapeutic response to somatostatin analogue. Chest 1993;104:515.

197. Barbe T, Losay J, Grimon G, et al. Pulmonary arteriovenous shunting in children with liver disease. J Pediatr 1995;126:571.

198. Bernard O. Pulmonary arteriovenous shunting and pulmonary artery hypertension in children with liver disease. Pediatr Pulmonol 1999;18:88.

199. Williams A, Trewby P, Williams R, Reid L. Structural alterations to the pulmonary circulation in fulminant hepatic failure. Thorax 1979;34:447.

200. Gupta D, Vijaya DR, Gupta R, et al. Prevalence of hepatopulmonary syndrome in cirrhosis and extrahepatic portal venous obstruction. Am J Gastroenterol 2001;96:3395–6.

201. Mimidis KP, Karatza C, Spiropoulos KV, et al. Prevalence of intrapulmonary vascular dilatations in normoxaemic patients with liver cirrhosis. Scand J Gastroenterol 1998;33:988.

202. Castro M, Krowka MJ. Hepatopulmonary syndrome. A pulmonary vascular complication of liver disease. Clin Chest Med 1996;17:35.

203. Krowka MJ. Clinical management of hepatopulmonary syndrome. Semin Liver Dis 1993;13:414.

204. Krowka MJ, Cortese DA. Severe hypoxemia associated with liver disease: Mayo Clinic experience and the experimental use of almitrine bismesylate. Mayo Clin Proc 1987;62:164.

205. Rodriguez-Roisin R, Roca J, Agusti AGN, et al. Gas exchange and pulmonary vascular reactivity in patients with liver cirrhosis. Am Rev Respir Dis 1987;135:1085.

206. Molleston JP, Kaufman BA, Cohen A, et al. Brain abscess in hepatopulmonary syndrome. J Pediatr Gastroenterol Nutr 2003;29:225–6.

207. Krowka MJ, Cortese DA. Hepatopulmonary syndrome: an evolving perspective in the era of liver transplantation. Hepatology 1990;11:138.

208. Genovesi MG, Tierney DF, Taplin GV, Eisenberg H. An intravenous radionuclide method to evaluate hypoxemia caused by abnormal alveolar vessels: limitations of conventional techniques. Am Rev Respir Dis 1976;114:59.

209. Shub C, Tajik A, Seward J, Dines DE. Detecting intrapulmonary right-to-left shunt with contrast echocardiography: observations in a patient with diffuse pulmonary arteriovenous fistulas. Mayo Clin Proc 1976;51:81.

210. Sasaki T, Hasegawa T, Kimura T, et al. Development of intrapulmonary arteriovenous shunting in postoperative biliary atresia: evaluation by contrast-enhanced echocardiography. J Pediatr Surg 2000;35:1647–50.

211. Chang SW, Ohara N. Pulmonary circulatory dysfunction in rats with biliary cirrhosis. An animal model of the hepatopulmonary syndrome. Am Rev Respir Dis 1992;145:798.

212. Fallon MB, Abrams GA, Luo B, et al. The role of endothelial nitric oxide synthase in the pathogenesis of a rat model of hepatopulmonary syndrome. Gastroenterology 1997;113:606.

213. Azzolin N, Baraldi E, Carra S, et al. Exhaled nitric oxide and hepatopulmonary syndrome in a 6-year-old child. Pediatrics 1999;104:299.

214. Cremona G, Higenbottam TW, Mayoral V, et al. Elevated exhaled nitric oxide in patients with hepatopulmonary syndrome. Eur Respir J 1995;8:1883.

215. Stoller JK, Moodie D, Schiavone WA, et al. Reduction of intrapulmonary shunt and resolution of digital clubbing associated with primary biliary cirrhosis after liver transplantation. Hepatology 1990;11:54.

216. Collisson EA, Nourmand H, Fraiman MH, et al. Retrospective analysis of the results of liver transplantation for adults with severe hepatopulmonary syndrome. Liver Transplant 2002;8:925–31.

217. Hobeika J, Houssin D, Bernard O, et al. Orthotopic liver transplantation in children with chronic liver disease and severe hypoxemia. Transplantation 1994;57:224.

218. Egawa H, Kasahara M, Inomata Y, et al. Long-term outcome of living related liver transplantation for patients with intrapulmonary shunting and strategy for complications. Transplantation 1999;67:712.

219. Krowka MJ. Hepatopulmonary syndrome versus portopulmonary hypertension: distinctions and dilemmas. Hepatology 1997;25:1282.

220. Kuo PC, Plotkin JS, Gaine S, et al. Portopulmonary hyperten-

sion and the liver transplant candidate. Transplantation 1999;67:1087.

221. Rubin LJ. Primary pulmonary hypertension. Chest 1993;104:236.

222. Schraufnagel DE, Kay JM. Structural and pathologic changes in the lung vasculature in chronic liver disease. Clin Chest Med 1996;17:1.

223. Kuo PC, Plotkin JS, Johnson LB, et al. Distinctive clinical features of portopulmonary hypertension. Chest 1997;112:980.

224. Ramsay MAE, Simpson BR, Nguyen AT, et al. Severe pulmonary hypertension in liver transplant candidates. Liver Transplant Surg 1997;3:494.

225. Robalino BD, Moodie DS. Association between primary pulmonary hypertension and portal hypertension: analysis of its pathophysiology and clinical, laboratory and hemodynamic manifestations. J Am Coll Cardiol 1991;17:492.

226. Ramsay MA, Schmidt A, Hein HA, et al. Nitric oxide does not reverse pulmonary hypertension associated with end-stage liver disease: a preliminary report. Hepatology 1997;25:524.

227. Hadengue A, Benhayoun MK, Lebrec D, Benhamou JP. Pulmonary hypertension complicating portal hypertension: prevalence and relation to splanchnic hemodynamics. Gastroenterology 1991;100:520.

228. Losay J, Piot D, Bougaran J, et al. Early liver transplantation is crucial in children with liver disease and pulmonary artery hypertension. J Hepatol 1999;28:337.

229. Krowka MJ, Plevak DJ, Findlay JY, et al. Pulmonary hemodynamics and perioperative cardiopulmonary-related mortality in patients with portopulmonary hypertension undergoing liver transplantation. Liver Transplant 2000;6:451–2.

230. Plevak D, Krowka M, Rettke S, et al. Successful liver transplantation in patients with mild to moderate pulmonary hypertension. Transplant Proc 1993;25:1840.

231. Ecoffey C, Rothman E, Bernard O, et al. Bacterial cholangitis after surgery for biliary atresia. J Pediatr 1987;111:824.

232. Gottrand F, Bernard O, Hadchouel M, et al. Late cholangitis after successful surgical repair of biliary atresia. Am J Dis Child 1991;145:213.

233. Barton LL, Rathore MH. Antibiotic prophylaxis of cholangitis after the Kasai procedure. J Pediatr Gastroenterol Nutr 1990;11:559.

234. Ohkohchi N, Chiba T, Ohi R, Mori S. Long-term follow-up study of patients with cholangitis after successful Kasai operation in biliary atresia: selection of recipients for liver transplantation. J Pediatr Gastroenterol Nutr 1989;9:416.

235. Lunzmann K, Schweizer P. The influence of cholangitis on the prognosis of extrahepatic biliary atresia. Eur J Pediatr Surg 1999;9:19.

236. Summerfield JA. Naloxone modulates the perception of itch in man. Br J Clin Pharmacol 1980;10:180.

237. Terra SG, Tsunoda SM. Opioid antagonists in the treatment of pruritus from cholestatic liver disease. Ann Pharmacother 1998;32:1228.

238. Duncan JS, Kennedy HJ, Triger DR. Treatment of pruritus due to chronic obstructive liver disease. BMJ 1984;289:22.

239. Connolly CS, Kantor GS, Menduke H. Hepatobiliary pruritus: what are effective treatments? J Am Acad Dermatol 1995; 33:801.

240. Balistreri WF. Bile acid therapy in pediatric hepatobiliary disease: the role of ursodeoxycholic acid [abstract]. J Pediatr Gastroenterol Nutr 1997;24:573.

241. Cynamon HA, Andres JM, Iafrate RP. Rifampin relieves pruritus in children with cholestatic liver disease. Gastroenterology 1990;98:1013.

242. Zuckerman E, Schar M, Korula J. Naloxone for intractable pruritus. Am J Gastroenterol 1997;92:183.

243. Lauterburg BH, Taswell HF, Pineda AA, et al. Treatment of pruritus of cholestasis by plasma perfusion through USP-charcoal-coated glass beads. Lancet 1980;ii:53.

244. Bergasa NV, Alling DW, Talbot TL, et al. Oral nalmefene therapy reduces scratching activity due to the pruritus of cholestasis: a controlled study. J Am Acad Dermatol 1999;41:431.

245. Metze D, Reimann S, Luger TA. Effective treatment of pruritus with naltrexone, an orally active opiate antagonist. Ann N Y Acad Sci 1999;885:430–2.

246. Neff GW, O'Brien CB, Reddy KR, et al. Preliminary observation with dronabinol in patients with intractable pruritus secondary to cholestatic liver disease. Am J Gastroenterol 2002;8:2117–9.

247. Emond JC, Whitington PF. Selective surgical management of progressive familial intrahepatic cholestasis (Byler's disease). J Pediatr Surg 1995;30:1635.

248. Ng VL, Ryckman FC, Porta G, et al. Long-term outcome after partial external biliary diversion for intractable pruritus in patients with intrahepatic cholestasis. J Pediatr Gastroenterol Nutr 2000;30:152–6.

249. Emerick KM, Whitington PF. Partial external biliary diversion for intractable pruritus and xanthomas in Alagille syndrome. Hepatology 2002;35:1501–6.

CHAPTER 60

LIVER TRANSPLANT

Deirdre Kelly, MD, FRCP, FRCPI, FRCPCH

Successful pediatric liver transplant evolved in the 1980s and became established in the 1990s. The success of this complex procedure has led to a significant increase in the number of children undergoing liver transplant worldwide and has radically changed the prognosis of many babies and children dying of end-stage liver failure.

Liver transplant was first performed in the United States and Europe in 1963, but the first successful pediatric liver transplant was not performed until 1967, in a young girl with a malignant hepatic tumor. There were rapid advances in adult transplant throughout the 1970s, particularly after the introduction of cyclosporin A in 1978,[1] but technical difficulties and donor shortages meant that pediatric liver transplant remained hazardous. By 1986, when most adult units claimed a 1-year survival rate of 80%, average 1-year survival rates in children were only 60%.[2] Since then, there have been considerable advances in both medical and surgical management, with international 1-year survival rates from pediatric liver transplant in excess of 90% and 5- to 10-year survival rates of 80%.[3]

The improved survival rates are related to improving pre- and postoperative management in association with the development of innovative surgical techniques to expand the donor pool. These techniques have not only reduced deaths on the waiting list and improved survival overall but also have extended the range of indications for liver transplant to include semielective liver replacement, transplant for inborn errors of metabolism, and unresectable hepatic tumors. As short-term survival has improved, interest in research has focused on evaluating quality of life in long-term survivors.

By 2002, 4,252 children had undergone liver transplant in Europe,[4] with more than twice that number of children transplanted in the United States.[5] In Europe, 40% of transplants were performed in children under 2 years of age, 50% in children aged 2 to 12 years, and 10% in children aged 12 to 15 years (Figure 60-1).[4]

Despite its recorded success, liver transplant remains a complex procedure with large resource implications and a 10% mortality rate; thus, careful consideration should be given to the selection of potential recipients and the exclusion of other therapies.

INDICATIONS

Liver transplant is now accepted therapy for acute or chronic liver failure (Table 60-1; see Figure 60-1).

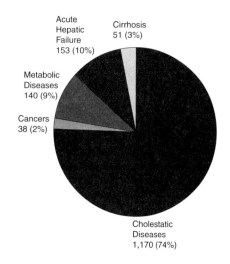

0 – 2 Years
(1,589 children)

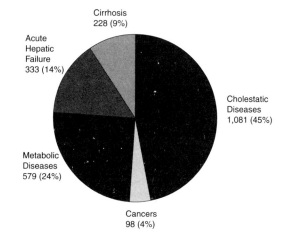

2 – 15 Years
(2,409 children)

FIGURE 60-1   Primary indications of liver transplant in 3,998 pediatric patients, 1988 to 2001. Adapted from the European Liver Transplant Registry, 2002.

TABLE 60-1 INDICATIONS FOR LIVER TRANSPLANT IN CHILDREN

CHRONIC LIVER FAILURE
Cholestatic liver disease
  Biliary atresia
  Idiopathic neonatal hepatitis
  Alagille syndrome
  Progressive familial intrahepatic cholestasis
  Nonsyndromic biliary hypoplasia
Metabolic liver disease
  α_1-Antitrypsin deficiency
  Tyrosinemia type I
  Wilson disease
  Cystic fibrosis
  Glycogen storage type IV
Chronic hepatitis
  Autoimmune
  Idiopathic
  Postviral (hepatitis B, C, other)
  Cryptogenic cirrhosis
  Fibropolycystic liver disease ± Caroli disease
  Primary immunodeficiency

ACUTE LIVER FAILURE
Fulminant hepatitis
  Autoimmune hepatitis
  Halothane anesthesia
  Acetaminophen poisoning
  Viral hepatitis (A, B, C, or NA-G)
Metabolic liver disease
  Fatty acid oxidation defects
  Neonatal hemochromatosis
  Tyrosinemia type I
  Wilson disease

INBORN ERRORS OF METABOLISM
Crigler-Najjar syndrome type I
Familial hypercholesterolemia
Organicacidemia
Urea cycle defects
Primary oxalosis

HEPATIC TUMORS
Benign tumors
Unresectable malignant tumors

CHRONIC LIVER FAILURE

CHOLESTATIC LIVER DISEASE

Chronic liver failure secondary to cholestatic liver disease is the most common indication for liver transplant in children (see Figure 60-1). Of diseases of this type, biliary atresia remains the main indication for liver transplant in children worldwide. Despite professional education on the importance of early diagnosis and management of this condition, many children continue to be referred for treatment too late to benefit from a palliative Kasai portoenterostomy. Children who have an immediately unsuccessful Kasai portoenterostomy or who develop intractable nutritional or hepatic complications[6] should be referred for urgent transplant. Approximately 60% of children with biliary atresia will have a successful Kasai portoenterostomy; in these children, cirrhosis and portal hypertension will develop at a much slower rate, and their need for liver transplant will depend on the rate of development of hepatic complications.[7]

The outcome of cholestatic liver diseases such as Alagille syndrome and progressive familial intrahepatic cholestasis is more variable. Many children will have compensated liver disease for some time or will be well maintained on supportive management. Liver transplant is indicated if decompensated cirrhosis and/or intractable portal hypertension develop, if malnutrition and growth failure are unresponsive to nutritional support, or if there is intractable pruritus that is resistant to maximum medical therapy or biliary diversion.[8]

Some infants who present with giant cell hepatitis or neonatal hepatitis of unknown etiology develop persistent cholestasis and rapid progression to cirrhosis and portal hypertension and become candidates for liver transplant in the first 2 or 3 years of life.

METABOLIC LIVER DISEASE

α_1-Antitrypsin deficiency is the most common form of inherited metabolic liver disease presenting in childhood in Europe and the United States. Although 20 to 40% of children in any population develop persistent liver disease progressing to cirrhosis, only a minority (approximately 20 to 30%) require liver transplant in childhood.[9]

Tyrosinemia type I is an autosomal recessive disorder of tyrosine metabolism, with a clinical presentation that includes both acute and chronic liver disease and multiorgan failure with cardiac, renal, and neurologic involvement. The management of this disorder has changed dramatically since the introduction of 2(2-nitro-4-trifluoromethylbenzoyl)-1,3-cyclohexenedione (NTBC), which prevents the formation of toxic metabolites and produces rapid clinical and biochemical improvement. The widespread use of this drug in tyrosinemia has altered both the natural history of the disease and the indications for transplant.[10,11] Prior to the introduction of NTBC, liver transplant was indicated for acute or chronic liver failure but, more importantly, for hepatic dysplasia or hepatocellular carcinoma. Liver transplant is now indicated only for those children who have a poor quality of life (ie, those who do not tolerate the restrictive low-protein diet and the frequent bloodletting and amino acid monitoring) or do not respond to NTBC or in whom hepatic malignancy is thought to have developed.[11] Routine monitoring of children with tyrosinemia type I being treated with NTBC includes ultrasonography, computed tomography (CT), or magnetic resonance imaging (MRI) to detect the development of nodules and/or early hepatocellular carcinoma in association with regular α-fetoprotein levels. A persistent or sustained rise of α-fetoprotein may indicate the early development of hepatocellular carcinoma, which should be confirmed by the detection of hepatic dysplasia on liver biopsy.[12,13]

Wilson disease is a rare indication for liver transplant in childhood. Early diagnosis and therapy with penicillamine should be curative, but many children will present with established cirrhosis or fulminant liver failure. Liver transplant is indicated for those children who present with advanced liver disease (Wilson score > 6) or fulminant liver failure or who have progressive hepatic disease despite penicillamine therapy or other therapy, such as trientene and zinc.[14,15]

The short-term survival for children with cystic fibrosis has improved with increased attention to nutrition and appropriate management of pulmonary disease. Liver disease develops in approximately 20% of children, mainly in boys,[16] and is becoming an increasingly common indication for liver transplant.[17] Referral for liver transplant and the timing of transplant are particularly difficult for children with cystic fibrosis. Many children present with compensated liver disease but with bleeding esophageal varices from portal hypertension.[18] In these children, management of portal hypertension by conservative means (sclerotherapy or band ligation of esophageal varices or insertion of a transhepatic portal systemic shunt) may be sufficient to control symptoms and improve quality of life for some years.[18]

Liver transplant in cystic fibrosis is indicated if there is evidence of hepatic decompensation (falling serum albumin or prolonged coagulation unresponsive to vitamin K), severe malnutrition unresponsive to nutritional therapy, or severe complications of portal hypertension that are unresponsive to medical management, such as ascites or uncontrolled variceal bleeding.[17,19] Careful assessment of pulmonary function is essential because severe lung disease (< 70% predicted lung function) may indicate the necessity for heart, lung, and liver transplant.[17,19] In some children, the choice of timing of the liver transplant may be advanced by the recognition of rapidly deteriorating pulmonary function. The management of pulmonary disease is particularly important before transplant and should include vigorous physiotherapy, intravenous antibiotics, and deoxyribonuclease.

Most children with glycogen storage disease type I should not require liver transplant and can be managed appropriately with medical and nutritional treatment. Transplant is indicated only for children who develop multiple hepatic adenomas or in whom metabolic control has affected the quality of life. Children with glycogen storage disease types III and IV are more likely to progress to cirrhosis with portal hypertension and require transplant because of hepatic dysfunction.[20]

The rare disorders of bile acid metabolism that present with persistent cholestasis may now respond to oral bile acids, reducing the need for transplant.[21,22]

CHRONIC HEPATITIS

Autoimmune Liver Disease Types I and II. Liver transplant is a rare indication for children with autoimmune liver disease type I or II, who usually respond to immunosuppression with prednisolone or azathioprine. Liver transplant is indicated for those children who have not responded to immunosuppression despite alternative therapy such as cyclosporin A, mycophenolate mofetil, or tacrolimus and for those children who present with fulminant hepatic failure.[23] Fulminant hepatic failure is more likely in children with type II autoimmune hepatitis, who have a worse prognosis and an increased requirement for liver transplant.

Chronic Hepatitis B or C. Although chronic hepatitis B or C is a major indication for transplant in adults, it is less common in children, many of whom will not develop symptomatic liver disease in childhood. Recurrence of hepatitis B or

C is likely in 90% of patients transplanted for chronic disease but not for fulminant hepatitis. Prevention or recurrence of hepatitis B is less likely with prophylactic treatment of hepatitis B immunoglobulin and/or lamivudine.

Fibropolycystic Liver Disease. Fibropolycystic liver disease is an unusual indication for liver transplant in childhood because liver function remains normal despite the development of severe portal hypertension. Liver transplant is indicated for those children in whom hepatic decompensation occurs secondary to recurrent cholangitis or portal hypertension or if hepatic enlargement affects the quality of life. Because the disease may be associated with infantile polycystic kidney disease in some children, both liver and kidney replacement may be required.[24]

Primary Immunodeficiency. As bone marrow transplant for primary immunodeficiency becomes increasingly successful, it has been recognized that many children with these diseases have associated liver disease. The most common immunodeficiency is CD40 ligand deficiency (hyperimmunoglobulin M syndrome), in which recurrent cryptosporidial infection of the gut and biliary tree lead to sclerosing cholangitis. In this group of children, it is important to consider bone marrow transplant before the development of significant liver disease or to consider combined liver and bone marrow transplant if necessary.[25]

Timing of Transplant for Chronic Liver Failure. The timing of liver transplant for children with chronic liver failure may be difficult because many children will have compensated liver disease for some years. Although it may be possible to predict biochemical decompensation by studying serial estimates of lidocaine metabolite formation and excretion,[26] this has not proved universally to be of value. The most useful guide to the timing of liver transplant is provided by a variety of parameters that include (1) a persistent rise in total bilirubin > 150 µmol/L (> 9 mg/dL), (2) prolongation of the prothrombin ratio (international normalized ratio [INR] > 1.4), and (3) a persistent fall in serum albumin to < 35 g/L.[27] Serial evaluation of nutritional parameters is a useful guide to early hepatic decompensation. Progressive reduction of fat stores (measured by triceps skinfold or subscapular skinfold) or protein stores (measured by midarm circumference or midarm muscle area) despite intensive nutritional support is a good guide to hepatic decompensation.[28] Recently, the development of the PELD Score (PELD = pediatric end-stage liver disease) has confirmed these observations.[29]

An important consideration in timing liver transplant is psychosocial development. Children with chronic liver disease may have both social and motor developmental delays that increase with time unless reversed following early liver transplant.[6,30,31]

Children with severe hepatic complications such as chronic hepatic encephalopathy, refractory ascites, intractable pruritus, or recurrent variceal bleeding despite appropriate medical management should be referred immediately for transplant. In some children, hepatopulmonary syndrome secondary to pulmonary shunting develops and is an important indication for liver transplant.[32] It is essential that transplant is performed prior to the development of severe pulmonary hypertension because this will preclude successful liver transplant.[33]

For children with chronic liver disease to benefit from transplant, it is essential that this procedure be considered before the complications of liver disease adversely impair the quality of the children's lives and before their growth and development are irreversibly retarded.

ACUTE LIVER FAILURE

Liver transplant is indicated for acute liver failure secondary to a wide range of primary etiologies (see Table 60-1). It is good practice to refer children with acute liver failure early to a specialist unit with facilities for transplant so that the child may be stabilized and sufficient time can be given to find an appropriate donor organ.

FULMINANT HEPATITIS
The management of children with fulminant hepatitis is first to assess prognosis and the necessity for liver transplant and then to prevent or treat hepatic complications while awaiting a suitable donor organ or regeneration of the native liver. The factors known to imply a poor prognosis for children with fulminant hepatitis are as follows:

1. Non–A–G hepatitis
2. Development of grade III or IV hepatic coma
3. Reduction in hepatic size in association with falling transaminases and increasing bilirubin (> 300 μmol/L or > 16 mg/dL).
4. Persistent severe coagulopathy (> 50 seconds over control; INR > 4)[34]

In infants with fulminant hepatitis, coagulopathy may be more severe than encephalopathy, and both are not required prior to listing for liver transplant.[35]

It is essential that all children who have reached grade III hepatic coma or who have a persisting coagulopathy without evidence of irreversible brain damage from cerebral edema or hypoglycemia be listed for liver transplant. It may be difficult to exclude underlying brain disease. Cerebral CT or MRI may demonstrate cerebral infarction, ischemia, or hemorrhage, whereas electroencephalography (EEG) may indicate reduced voltage of brain waves, but none of these techniques are infallible. Although intracranial pressure monitoring has been demonstrated to improve selection for liver transplant by excluding children with persistently raised intracranial pressure, it has not influenced survival.[36] The technique may be impossible in children with prolonged coagulopathy and is associated with significant morbidity unless coagulopathy can be adequately corrected without inducing cerebral edema. Measurement of cerebral blood flow is not useful because it may be reduced in hepatic failure; measurement of cerebral perfusion pressure may be a more sensitive indicator for selection. EEG may demonstrate a reduction in voltage of electrical activity and ultimately brain death, but these results

should be interpreted cautiously in ventilated patients or those treated with thiopental or other phenobarbitals because the EEG tracing may be affected by these drugs.

Acetaminophen overdose is a common indication for liver transplant in adults in the United States but is less common in pediatric practice. Of 73 children in one study who developed overdose, only 8% required liver transplant.[37] Children are more likely to require liver transplant if the overdose was taken with another drug (eg, LSD [lysergic acid diethylamide] or Ecstasy [3,4-methylenedioxymethamphetamine]) or alcohol and if they present with a persistent coagulopathy (INR > 4), metabolic acidosis (pH < 7.3), and rapid progression to hepatic coma grade III.[38]

METABOLIC LIVER DISEASE
Metabolic liver disease such as Wilson disease and tyrosinemia type I may present with acute liver failure, whereas fatty acid oxidation defects and/or mitochondrial disease occur in the neonatal period. In contrast to fulminant hepatitis, the clinical presentation is subacute, and liver failure develops in the presence of an underlying cirrhosis. Selection for liver transplant is based on response to medication and the presence of advanced liver disease or severe coagulopathy. Jaundice or encephalopathy may not be obvious.[14]

Neonatal hemochromatosis is a rare disorder of iron handling. The presentation is within days or weeks of birth, with severe coagulopathy, encephalopathy, and hypoglycemia. The diagnosis is based on the clinical features and presence of extrahepatic iron deposition. Recent experience has shown that medical management using an antioxidant "cocktail" may be beneficial for those children with a milder phenotype, particularly if the cocktail is started shortly after birth.[39,40]

INBORN ERRORS OF HEPATIC METABOLISM
A number of inborn errors of metabolism are secondary to hepatic enzyme deficiencies that do not lead to liver disease. Liver function is normal, but the enzyme deficiency leads to severe extrahepatic disease. The purpose of liver transplant in this group of diseases is to replace the missing hepatic enzyme to prevent or reverse extrahepatic disease. Selection is based on the child's quality of life, on medical management, and on the potential mortality and morbidity of the primary disease related to the risks and outcome following liver transplant.

The timing of transplant depends on the rate of progression of the disease, the quality of life of the affected child, and the development of severe irreversible extrahepatic disease.[41]

Crigler-Najjar Syndrome Type I. Crigler-Najjar syndrome type I is an autosomal recessive disease in which there is an absolute deficiency of glucuronyl transferase, which leads to high levels of unconjugated bilirubin and the eventual development of structural brain damage secondary to kernicterus. Current management includes many hours of phototherapy daily to reduce the level of unconjugated bilirubin.

Liver transplant is curative, and children should be selected for transplant prior to the development of irreversible brain damage and at a time when continuous phototherapy is affecting the quality of their life. The recent development of auxiliary liver transplant (see below), in which only part of the liver is transplanted, may be the most appropriate transplant operation for these children because it allows the possibility of gene therapy in the future.[42]

Familial Hypercholesterolemia. Children with homozygous or heterozygous familial hypercholesterolemia are prone to premature development of coronary artery disease owing to a deficiency in the number of receptors needed for the metabolism of cholesterol on hepatocytes. Liver transplant should be performed before there is irreversible coronary artery disease, but recent progress with gene therapy for this condition suggests that auxiliary liver transplant or gene therapy may be more appropriate treatment strategies at present.[42,43]

Organicacidemias. These rare disorders include propionicacidemia or methylmalonicacidemia, in which there are abnormalities in the metabolism of propionate and methylmalonate, respectively. Children with these diseases are at risk of recurrent metabolic acidosis, developmental delay, and irreversible brain damage. Liver transplant is palliative treatment for these conditions because the enzyme deficiency affects all parts of the body. Isolated case reports have indicated that orthotopic liver replacement was necessary to provide adequate enzyme supplementation, but it is possible that auxiliary liver transplant may be sufficient for mildly affected patients.[42]

Four main disorders of the urea cycle lead to neurotoxicity with accumulation of ammonia and glutamine. The defective enzymes are (1) carbamyl phosphate synthetase, (2) ornithine transcarbamylase, (3) argininosuccinic acid synthetase (deficiency causes citrullinemia), and (4) argininosuccinate lyase. Medical management of these conditions is reduction of ammonia by withdrawing dietary protein and treatment with oral sodium benzoate (0.1–0.25 g/kg/d) and/or phenylbutyrate (0.25–0.6 g/kg/d).

Liver transplant in these urea cycle defects is considered for patients in whom dietary and medical management is ineffective. Although liver transplant corrects hyperammonemia, it does not completely correct the amino acid abnormality or reverse any preexisting neurotoxicity,[44] thus indicating that transplant should be considered prior to irreversible neurotoxicity.

Primary Oxalosis. In this rare autosomal recessive disorder, there is a deficiency of the hepatic enzyme alanine–glyoxylate aminotransferase, which leads to overproduction of oxalate with deposition in the cornea, brain, cardiac muscles, bones, and kidneys, leading to renal failure and systemic oxalosis. There is considerable controversy over the best management of this condition, but it is agreed that liver transplant is required before the development of renal failure or severe systemic oxalosis. In those infants who present with renal failure, combined liver and kidney transplant is required.[45–47] Because the enzyme deficiency results in overproduction of oxalate, auxiliary liver transplant is not suitable.

HEPATIC TUMORS

With the increasing success of liver transplant, children with either benign or malignant tumors are considered for liver transplant. Benign tumors include hemangiomas or hemoangioendotheliomas, adenomas, and focal nodular hyperplasia. These tumors are selected for liver transplant only if they cause hepatic dysfunction or are associated with an unacceptable increase in liver size and hepatic resection is impractical. Persistent heart failure in hemangioendotheliomas is best treated by selective hepatic embolism.

Malignant hepatic tumors such as hepatoblastoma or hepatocellular carcinoma that are either unresectable or refractory to chemotherapy are considered for liver transplant as long as there are no extrahepatic metastases.[48] It is important to carry out a search for extrahepatic metastases that includes CT of the chest and abdomen and regular monitoring of serum α-fetoprotein. A careful assessment of cardiac function is essential to exclude the cardiotoxic effects of chemotherapeutic drugs such as daunorubicin. It is best to time the transplant between chemotherapy treatments to prevent relapse or recurrence, and elective living-related transplant is particularly helpful in this situation. Children with rhabdomyosarcomas may not be considered for transplant because of the extent of the tumor and the early presence of extrahepatic metastases.

PRETRANSPLANT EVALUATION

The pretransplant evaluation of the patient (Table 60-2) is particularly important and should include the following:

1. Assessment of the severity of the liver disease and the possibility for medical management

TABLE 60-2   PRETRANSPLANT ASSESSMENT

Nutritional status
  Height, weight, triceps skinfold, midarm muscle area, midarm
    circumference
Identification of hepatic complications
  Ascites, varices
Cardiac assessment
  Electrocardiography, echocardiography, chest radiography, cardiac
    catheterization
Respiratory function
  Oxygen saturation,* ventilation-perfusion scan,* lung function tests[†]
Neurologic and developmental assessment
  Electroencephalography, Bailey developmental scales, Stanford-Binet
    intelligence scales
Renal function
  Urea, creatinine, electrolytes, urinary protein-to-creatinine ratio,
    chromium EDTA
Serology
  Cytomegalovirus; Epstein-Barr virus; varicella-zoster virus; herpes
    simplex virus; hepatitis A, B, and C; HIV; measles
Hematology
  Full blood count, platelets, blood group
Radiology
  Ultrasonography of liver and spleen for vascular anatomy, wrist
    radiography for bone age and rickets
Dental assessment

EDTA = ethylenediaminetetraacetic acid; HIV = human immunodeficiency virus.
*If cyanosis present.
[†]In cystic fibrosis.

2. Assessment of the technical feasibility of the operation
3. Consideration of any contraindications
4. Psychological preparation of the family and child

The severity of liver disease should be assessed by evaluating the following:

1. Hepatic function. Listing for liver transplant is based on evidence of deterioration in hepatic function as indicated by albumin (> 35 g/L), coagulation time (INR > 1.4), and cholestasis, as evidenced by a rise in bilirubin (150 µmol/L, 8 mg/dL). Portal hypertension should be established by estimating the size of the spleen and portal vein by ultrasonography and by diagnosing esophageal and gastric varices by gastrointestinal endoscopy.

2. Renal function. Many children with acute or chronic liver failure will have abnormalities of renal function, including renal tubular acidosis, glomerulonephritis, acute tubular necrosis, and/or hepatorenal syndrome. Assessment of renal function is important to provide a baseline for the nephrotoxic effects of immunosuppressive drugs post-transplant and to consider the necessity for perioperative renal support.

3. Hematology. Baseline information on full blood count, platelets, and coagulopathy is obtained. Determination of blood group is essential for organ donor matching.

4. Serology. Previous evidence of varicella, measles, or infection with hepatitis A, B, or C viruses; cytomegalovirus (CMV); or Epstein-Barr virus (EBV) is important information for postoperative management. Donor grafts are matched by CMV status if possible.

5. Radiology. The rapid development of Doppler ultrasonography techniques has greatly improved the pretransplant assessment of vascular anatomy and the patency of hepatic vessels. It is unusual now to require MRI or angiography for these assessments. Evidence of retrograde flow and/or a reduction in the size of the portal vein (< 4 mm at the porta hepatis) suggest advancing portal hypertension and are indications for early transplant.[49] Children with biliary atresia have an increased incidence of abnormal vasculature, the hypovascular syndrome, which consists of an absent inferior vena cava, preduodenal or absent portal vein, azygous drainage from the liver, and polysplenia syndrome.[50] It may be associated with situs inversus, dextrocardia, or left atrial isomerism. Because these abnormalities may increase the technical risk of a liver transplant, it is important to diagnose these before transplant.[51]

6. Cardiac and respiratory assessment. Liver transplant is associated with significant hemodynamic changes during the operative and anhepatic phases. It is important, therefore, to have baseline information on both cardiac and respiratory function. Electrocardiography, echocardiography, and oxygen saturation will provide most of the necessary information. It is also important to determine the presence of congenital cardiac disease. Children with biliary atresia have an increased incidence of congenital cardiac disease, particularly atrial and ventricular septal defects, whereas peripheral pulmonary stenosis is a known feature of Alagille syndrome. Cardiomyopathy may develop secondary to tyrosinemia type I and the organicacidemias, although children with malignant tumors who have received chemotherapy need particular cardiac assessment. Cardiac catheterization is required in some cases to determine whether cardiac function is adequate to sustain the hemodynamic effect of liver transplant or if cardiac surgery is required preoperatively. If the cardiac defect is inoperable, liver transplant occasionally may be contraindicated. A small percentage of children with end-stage liver disease develop intrapulmonary shunts (hepatopulmonary syndrome). Clinical signs include cyanosis, digital clubbing, and reduced oxygen saturation. The diagnosis can be confirmed by bubble echocardiography, ventilation-perfusion scans, and/or cardiac catheterization.[32]

7. Neurodevelopmental assessment. Because the aim of liver transplant is to improve quality of life, it is important to identify any preexisting neurologic or psychological defects not only to consider whether they would be reversible post-transplant but also to evaluate the necessity for corrective management.[30,31]

8. Dental assessment. Advanced liver disease has an adverse affect on all aspects of growth and development, including dentition. Pretransplant dental problems include hypoplasia with staining of the teeth and gingival hyperplasia. Because gingival hyperplasia is a significant side effect of cyclosporine immunosuppression, it is important to establish good dental hygiene in the patient prior to transplant.[52]

CONTRAINDICATIONS FOR LIVER TRANSPLANT

With increasing experience, there are fewer contraindications to transplant. Although historically considered difficult, age < 1 year and size < 10 kg are no longer contraindications for transplant. Portal vein thrombosis increases the technical risk of the surgery, but it can now be managed with venous or prosthetic grafts. Vascular abnormalities such as the hypovascular syndrome are no longer considered contraindications. Although infection with human immunodeficiency virus (HIV) was a contraindication, the improvement in long-term prognosis with antiviral drugs means that this disease can be controlled before transplant. The following contraindications remain:

1. Severe systemic sepsis (in particular, fungal sepsis) at the time of operation. It is important that the operation be deferred until the infection has been appropriately treated.

2. Malignant hepatic tumors with confirmed extrahepatic metastases.[53]

3. Severe extrahepatic disease that is not considered reversible following liver transplant. This includes severe cardiopulmonary disease for which there is no possibility of corrective surgery or severe structural brain damage with a poor prognosis.

4. Multiorgan failure, especially owing to mitochondrial cytopathy,[54] because it has been shown that unless the

mitochondrial defect is confined to the liver, liver transplant is not curative.

5. Alpers disease and sodium valproate toxicity, related disorders in which defects in the respiratory chain have been identified in some patients. Liver transplant is contraindicated in the presence of these diseases in the same way as in the case of mitochondrial cytopathies because of the progression of neurodegeneration despite transplant.[55]

6. Recurrent disease. Hepatitis B and C have a recurrence rate of 90 to 100% post-transplant but can now be treated with antiviral agents before and after transplant.[56,57] Autoimmune liver disease recurs in 24% of cases, as does primary sclerosing cholangitis. Although liver transplant is not contraindicated for these conditions, the rate of recurrence must form part of the counseling of families. Autoimmune hemolytic anemia in association with giant cell hepatitis is a rare and fatal disease in which there is a 100% recurrence rate post-transplant, and transplant is not recommended.[58]

PREPARATION FOR LIVER TRANSPLANT

IMMUNIZATION
Most units consider live vaccines to be contraindicated after liver transplant because of the risk of dissemination secondary to immunosuppression. It is therefore better to complete normal immunizations before transplant. This includes diphtheria, tetanus, polio, Pneumovax for protection from streptococcal pneumonia, and *Haemophilus influenzae* type b vaccine for protection against *H. influenzae*. In children older than 6 months, measles, mumps, rubella, and varicella vaccinations should be offered in addition to hepatitis A and B vaccination.

MANAGEMENT OF HEPATIC COMPLICATIONS
It is important to ensure that specific hepatic complications are appropriately managed while the patient waits for transplant.

Recurrent variceal bleeding should be managed as described (see Chapter 59, "Treatment of End-Stage Liver Disease"), with sclerotherapy or esophageal varix ligation. Difficult or intractable variceal bleeding may require the insertion of a transjugular intrahepatic portal systemic shunt.[59]

Sepsis that includes ascending cholangitis and spontaneous bacterial peritonitis should be treated with broad-spectrum antibiotics, whereas in children awaiting transplant for acute liver failure, prophylactic antifungal therapy is essential.

Ascites should be managed with diuretics and restriction of salt. Intervention with hemodialysis and hemofiltration should be considered if acute renal failure or hepatorenal failure develops.[60]

NUTRITIONAL SUPPORT
The importance of nutritional support has been demonstrated with studies indicating that nutritional status at liver transplant is an important prognostic factor in survival.[61,62]

The main purpose of nutritional therapy is to prevent or reverse the malnutrition associated with liver disease and to minimize fat malabsorption and ongoing catabolism. A high-calorie protein feed (150 to 200% estimated average requirement) may be effective (Table 60-3). It is possible to provide this high-energy intake with standard feeds using calorie supplements, but a moderate liver feed that can be adapted more easily may be better for infants. Because many of the modular or supplemented feeds are unpalatable, they are best given by nocturnal nasogastric enteral feeding or continuous enteral feeding. Occasionally, enteral feeding is not tolerated owing to severe hepatic complications such as ascites and intractable variceal bleeding; in these circumstances, parenteral nutrition is necessary.[63]

PSYCHOLOGICAL PREPARATION
Liver transplant is a major undertaking for the child and family; thus, psychological counseling, information giving, and preparation of the child and family are paramount using a skilled multidisciplinary team with play therapists, psychologists, and schoolteachers. Particular care is required when counseling parents and children with inborn errors of metabolism who are not dying of liver failure. These families must be aware of the risks and complications of liver transplant and must make informed decisions with regard to potential mortality and to the necessity for long-term immunosuppression compared with medical treatment available for their children's conditions.

Parents of children who develop acute liver failure may be too stressed to fully appreciate the implications and consequences of liver transplant. In these families, counseling—in particular, counseling of the child—should continue postoperatively.

TABLE 60-3	NUTRITIONAL SUPPORT IN INFANTS AND CHILDREN UNDERGOING LIVER TRANSPLANT*	
	PREOPERATIVE	**POSTOPERATIVE**
Carbohydrate (g/kg/d)	Glucose polymer 15–20	Glucose 6–8
Protein (g/kg/d)	Low-salt protein 3–4	Whole protein 2.5–3
Fat (g/kg/d)	40–60% MCT 8	80–90% LCT 5–6
Energy intake (EAR)	120–150%	120%

Adapted from Kelly DA and Mayer ADM.[64]
EAR = estimated average requirement; LCT = long-chain triglyceride; MCT = medium-chain triglyceride.
*Best provided as a modular feed in infants and as calorie supplements in older children.

LIVER TRANSPLANT SURGERY

The organization of liver transplant is complex and involves a large multidisciplinary team. The process involves four stages: organ procurement, the donor operation, the "back-table" operation, and the recipient operation.

ORGAN PROCUREMENT

Organ donation and procurement are handled regionally or nationally, depending on geographic variation, but all countries have a national network (United Networks for Organ Sharing [UNOS] in the United States, United Kingdom Transplant Support Service Authority [UKTSSA] in the United Kingdom, and Eurotransplant in Europe). Once patients are accepted by the transplant team, they are listed and prioritized according to the severity of liver disease. All countries recognize a priority system, which allows patients with acute fulminant hepatic failure the greatest prioritization. Many countries use a system that subsequently and sequentially prioritizes patients in intensive care, in hospitals, or at home. In the United States, a scoring system (PELD) is used to prioritize patients who do not have acute fulminant hepatic failure. The majority of liver grafts are retrieved from heart-beating donors, although there are increasing donations from living-related donors. The procurement coordinator is responsible for establishing the suitability of potential cadaveric organs, for coordinating the procurement team, and for the donor operation. Liver grafts are matched by size, blood group, and (for CMV-negative children) CMV status. There are no absolute age limits, but, in general, malignancy (except localized brain tumors), uncontrolled bacterial sepsis, and HIV positivity remain absolute contraindications for acceptance as donors.[64]

The development of reduction hepatectomy has extended the size range applicable to young children, but the donor shortage has led to replacement of reduction hepatectomies with split-liver grafts.

DONOR OPERATION

It is usual to retrieve the liver from a cadaver donor as part of a multiorgan operation in which liver, kidneys, heart, lungs, small bowel, corneas, skin, and bone may also be removed. It is important to maintain appropriate hemodynamic stability and ventilation while paralyzing agents are given to prevent spinal reflexes and broad-spectrum antibiotics are used to prevent infection. The liver is evaluated to identify abnormal arterial anatomy, which is particularly important for split-liver grafting. The porta hepatis is dissected, and the common bile duct is divided. The common hepatic artery, the superior mesenteric vein, and the hepatic veins are identified. Once the cardiothoracic organs are mobilized, heparin is administered to achieve full anticoagulation, and the abdominal organs are perfused with ice-cold preservation solution and packed with ice slush to achieve rapid cooling. Liver dissection is completed once the cardiothoracic organs have been removed. The hepatic artery is resected with a patch of aorta at the origin of the celiac trunk. The portal vein is divided at the

confluence with the superior mesenteric and splenic veins. The infrahepatic vena cava is divided above the origins of the renal veins, whereas the suprahepatic vena cava is divided at the junction of the right atrium. Once the liver is removed, the hepatic artery and portal vein are flushed with preservation solution, and the bile duct is rinsed. The liver is hermetically sealed in a plastic bag, immersed in preservation solution, and transported, packed in ice.

BACK-TABLE OPERATION

The back-table operation is particularly important for reduction hepatectomies and split-liver grafting. It is usually performed at the recipient hospital at the same time as the hepatectomy of the recipient. If a whole-liver graft is being used, the back-table operation is straightforward, but in the majority of pediatric liver transplants, either a liver reduction or a split-liver graft is performed.

Some units recommend that liver reduction or splitting be performed in situ as part of the donor operation, which has the advantage that the surgery is performed in a well-perfused functioning liver, without the risk of warm ischemia. However, this increases the operating time at the donor hospital, which may compromise other donor organs. The principles of the liver reduction are based on the segmental anatomy of the liver.[65] The liver has eight segments, and although it is possible to use a single-segment liver graft for neonates, in practice, the liver is divided along the plane of the falciform ligament to produce a left lateral segmental graft (segments 2 and 3) drained by the left hepatic bile duct (Figure 60-2). The common bile duct, portal vein, and hepatic artery are all preserved with the left lateral segment. For a split-liver graft, the portal vein is preserved with the left graft, and the hepatic artery, common bile duct, and inferior vena cava are preserved with the right graft. At implant, an arterial anastomosis is required for the left split graft.[66–69] Cur-

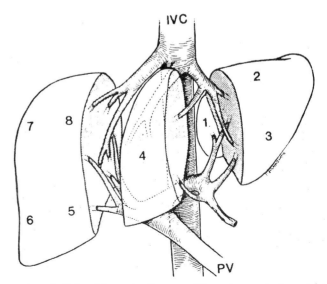

FIGURE 60-2 Schematic diagram of liver demonstrating eight segments. The left lateral segments 2 and 3 are most commonly used for reduction hepatectomy, split livers, living-related transplant, or auxiliary transplant.

rently, split-liver grafting is performed only using high-quality donor livers because of concerns related to primary graft dysfunction.

RECIPIENT OPERATION

Management of the recipient operation has been much improved by an understanding of coagulation disorders, improved monitoring, and sophisticated hemostatic techniques that have reduced transfusion requirements and allowed better hemodynamic stability. Constant monitoring of electrolytes and blood gases and coagulation is essential. Thromboelastography, if available, is helpful to assess coagulation. Adequate supplementation of bicarbonate, electrolyte solutions, coagulation products, and platelets is essential.

In adults and older children, venovenous bypass is used, in which blood is diverted from the portal and intrahepatic cable circulation to the superior vena cava, reducing portal hypertension and intestinal congestion when the portal vein is clamped. This technique also improves venous return and renal perfusion when the vena cava is clamped during the hepatectomy phase.

In patients who have had no previous abdominal operations, the hepatectomy is straightforward. The liver is mobilized, with division of adhesions and ligamentus attachments. The porta hepatis is dissected, and the bile duct, hepatic artery, and portal vein are divided. In children with biliary atresia following a Kasai portoenterostomy, the hepatic dissection is more difficult, and there is a higher risk of gastrointestinal perforation.

It is important to carry out graft implant quickly to minimize warm ischemic injury that occurs as soon as the liver graft is removed from the cold preservation fluid. If a whole graft is being implanted, the suprahepatic vena cava, infrahepatic vena cava, and portal vein are anastomosed to the equivalent recipient vessels. If a left lateral segment graft is being performed, a triangular incision is made on the anterior aspect of the recipient vena cava to anastomose the graft left hepatic vein. A similar procedure is carried out for a split-liver graft. Once the venous anastomoses are complete, the liver is flushed with a warm rinsing solution, and the venous clamps are removed. The arterial anastomosis is carried out once the liver has been perfused from the portal vein. The donor celiac artery is anastomosed to the bifurcation of the recipient hepatic and gastroduodenal or splenic arteries. A donor arterial graft may be required to act as a conduit in children with small or aberrant vessels. The biliary anastomosis is the last to be performed. In adults and larger children without biliary pathology, the donor recipient ducts may be joined together to form a duct-to-duct anastomosis. Children with biliary atresia and those weighing less than 40 kg require a choledochojejunostomy using a Roux-en-Y loop of recipient jejunum.

Once the anastomosis is completed, the operative field is examined for hemostasis, and perfusion of the liver is established. If the liver graft is too large to permit abdominal closure without compromising hepatic venous outflow, then either a Silastic patch may be inserted or the abdomen may be left open temporarily until the liver has reduced in size.

LIVING-RELATED LIVER TRANSPLANT

The shortage of suitable organ donors for young infants led to the development of living-related liver transplant.[70] This technique not only improves the supply of liver grafts for small children, it also allows optimal timing and reduces the stress of waiting for a suitable organ. In addition, the graft is obtained from a healthy individual with minimal preservation time.

The operation has received wide acceptance in Japan, where cadaveric transplant has not been possible until recently. The graft obtained from a live donor is usually a left lateral segmental graft. The liver parenchyma is divided along the line of the falciform ligament, keeping the blood supply intact. The bile duct, hepatic artery, portal vein, and hepatic vein are divided, and the graft is flushed with cold preservation fluid. Microvascular techniques are required during implant to reduce the risk of thrombosis.[71]

Although excellent results have been obtained,[72] particularly in Japan, the case for living-related transplant remains controversial because there are potential risks to the donor. Even in healthy individuals, partial hepatectomy has an appreciable morbidity, with an estimated risk of mortality of 1 in 250. It is important that donors are not only carefully evaluated for anesthetic risk, blood group compatibility, liver size, and anatomy but also that they are fully informed about the dangers of the procedure and, more importantly, the prospect of finding a cadaver graft for their child. Current organ donor shortages mean that most units will continue to offer living-related transplant.

AUXILIARY LIVER TRANSPLANT

In auxiliary liver transplant, part of the donor liver (usually segments 2 and 3) is implanted beside or in continuity with the native liver. The main purpose of this form of liver transplant is to ensure that the native liver is retained in the event of graft failure or for the future development of gene therapy. This operation is advisable for patients with metabolic liver disease secondary to hepatic enzyme deficiency in whom the liver is functioning normally but for whom liver transplant is considered because of the development of severe extrahepatic disease. Auxiliary transplant is now accepted therapy for Crigler-Najjar syndrome type I[42] and also for propionicacidemia and ornithine transcarbamalase deficiency.[73]

The role of auxiliary liver transplant in the management of fulminant hepatic failure is more controversial. The rationale for using this technique in this condition is that, with time, the native liver may regenerate. Two recent studies in adults demonstrated that the native liver regenerates in approximately half of the patients.[74,75]

POSTOPERATIVE MANAGEMENT AND COMPLICATIONS

POSTOPERATIVE MANAGEMENT

Immediate postoperative management is based on ensuring hemodynamic stability, respiratory function, and fluid balance. Most patients remain in the intensive care unit for 24 or 48 hours until liver function is satisfactory, with good hepatic artery and portal vein flow on Doppler ultrasonography. Infants with severe malnutrition owing to chronic liver disease or patients with hepatic coma secondary to fulminant hepatic failure may require a more prolonged period of intensive care.[6]

The aim of fluid management is to maintain circulating volume with crystalloid while replacing wound losses with colloid. It is important to ensure that the urine output is > 1 mL/kg/h and that central venous pressure is satisfactory (> 5–6 mm Hg). To prevent postoperative hepatic artery thrombosis, hemoglobin should be maintained between 8 and 10 g/L.[76] Immunosuppression is started immediately postoperatively, and the protocol will vary with center and experience. Standard protocols now include (1) cyclosporine microemulsion (Neoral), prednisolone, and azathioprine or (2) tacrolimus combined with low-dose steroids. Mycophenolate mofetil is a new immunosuppressive agent that may replace azathioprine in time (Table 60-4).[77,78] Recent studies that induce immunosuppression using the recently developed interleukin-2 antibodies, which selectively block the interleukin-2 receptors on T cells, reduce nephrotoxicity but are not yet in established practice.[79] Sirolimus, which is a macrolide antibiotic that prevents T-cell proliferation, is also sparing to the kidneys because it does not inhibit calcineurim. Its use in children is anecdotal.[80]

Broad-spectrum antibiotics should be prescribed for 48 hours unless there is persistent infection. Fluconazole or liposomal amphotericin is advisable in children with acute liver failure or in those who have a second laparotomy. Low-dose cotrimoxazole or trimethoprim is used for prophylaxis against Pneumocystis carinii, and oral nystatin and amphotericin are used to prevent oral and esophageal candidiasis for 6 to 12 months.

Most units use prophylaxis for CMV infection for CMV-negative recipients of a CMV-positive donor organ. Acyclovir (1,500 mg/m^2 IV) or ganciclovir (10 mg/kg IV/d) usually prevents CMV infection in the short term.[81] Although there is no proven prophylaxis for EBV, many units use either acyclovir or ganciclovir for this purpose.

Other medications include ranitidine (3 mg/kg), sucralfate (2–3 g qds), or omeprazole (10–20 mg IV bid) as prophylaxis against stress ulceration.

Because vascular thrombosis is higher in children than in adults, prophylaxis with antiplatelet drugs such as aspirin (3 mg/kg/d) and dipyridamole (25–50 mg tds) may be useful. Antihypertensive medication is usually necessary secondary to immunosuppressive treatment with steroids, tacrolimus, or cyclosporin A. Nifedipine (5–10 mg, 4 to 6 hourly) or atenolol (25–50 mg/d) may be required.[64]

Some children will require parenteral nutrition perioperatively, but the majority will begin enteral feeds between days 3 and 5. It is important to maintain adequate calories (see Table 60-3) and to encourage normal feeding.

POSTOPERATIVE COMPLICATIONS

Early postoperative complications include primary graft nonfunction, surgical complications (eg, intra-abdominal hemorrhage), vascular thrombosis, and venous outflow obstruction.

The most common cause of primary graft failure is primary nonfunctioning of the graft or thrombosis of the hepatic artery or portal vein.[82] Primary nonfunctioning of the transplanted liver occurs within 48 hours. The cause is unknown and may be related to donor factors. The presentation is with prolonged coagulation (INR > 3), raised aminotransferases (> 5,000–10,000 IU/L), a rising bilirubin, and, ultimately, a rise in serum potassium (> 6 IU/L). Primary graft function may occasionally be secondary to hyperacute rejection, the diagnosis of which can be made only by liver biopsy. The only appropriate management is retransplant.

Hepatic artery thrombosis occurs in approximately 10% of pediatric liver grafts, and its frequency has decreased considerably following the introduction of reduction hepatectomy or living-related transplant because of the increased size of the donor vessel.[83] The development of microsurgical techniques for hepatic arterial reconstruction has been additionally beneficial (Figure 60-3).[84]

Portal vein thrombosis is a less common complication, but its incidence has not been altered with reduction or split-

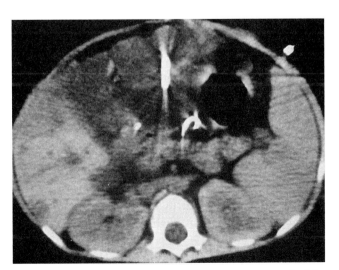

FIGURE 60-3 Hepatic artery thrombosis is a potentially life-threatening complication following liver transplant. This computed tomographic scan demonstrates a large area of infarction with abscess formation following thrombosis of the hepatic artery 7 days post-transplant. The child was successfully retransplanted.

TABLE 60-4   POSTOPERATIVE IMMUNOSUPPRESSION

| TIME OF INTRODUCTION (MO) | TROUGH LEVELS* | |
	CYCLOSPORIN A (MICROEMULSION) (5 MG/KG BD)	TACROLIMUS (0.15 MG/KG)
0–1	180–230 ng/L	10–15 ng/mL
1–3	100–160 ng/L	8–12 ng/mL
3–12	70–110 ng/L	5–8 ng/mL
>12	60–90 ng/L	3–5 ng/mL

TIME OF INTRODUCTION	IMMUNOSUPPRESSANT
3–12	Prednisolone 2 mg/kg
12	Azathioprine 2 mg/kg
—	Mycophenolate mofetil 1–3 g/d

*Whole-blood monoclonal assay.

liver techniques, although there are some advances in the management of this complication with innovative surgery.[85]

The diagnosis of hepatic artery or portal vein thrombosis is made by Doppler ultrasonography and is confirmed by angiography. Both complications may be treated by emergency thrombectomy and the use of anticoagulants or infusion of thrombolytic agents such as streptokinase. If hepatic perfusion is not adequately re-established, retransplant is required. Hepatic artery ischemia ultimately results in biliary complications, such as leaks and strictures, or hepatic abscesses.[86]

Hemorrhage from the cut surface of the liver is an occasional complication. It should be managed conservatively unless there is persistent bleeding or hemodynamic instability. Abdominal tamponade from hemorrhage may decrease blood flow and lead to renal failure.

Many factors may predispose the patient to postoperative renal failure within the first week. Patients with impaired renal function preoperatively may be further compromised by intraoperative cardiovascular instability or inotropic support. In addition, the administration of nephrotoxic immunosuppression such as cyclosporine or tacrolimus may precipitate renal failure.[64]

Oliguria (< 1 mL/kg) is common and may be managed conservatively with fluid replacement or a furosemide challenge (1–2 mg/kg IV). The development of anuria with an increase in urea, creatinine, and potassium necessitates renal dialysis or hemofiltration.

REJECTION

Acute cellular rejection may occur between 7 and 10 days postoperatively. The incidence of acute rejection varies. It is less common in infants (20%) but increases to 50 to 60% in older children and adults.[87,88] Clinical features include fever, irritability, abdominal discomfort, and, occasionally, ascites. The diagnosis is confirmed by detecting a rise in bilirubin, alkaline phosphate, γ-glutamyl transpeptidase, and aspartate and alanine transaminases. Histologic confirmation is essential. Acute rejection is indicated by demonstration of a mixed inflammatory infiltrate, including eosinophils in portal tracts. There is usually a subendothelial lymphoid infiltration of blood vessels (endotheliitis) and inflammation and infiltration of the bile ducts.[89] Most units will treat acute rejection initially by using intravenous methylprednisolone in doses varying from 20 mg/kg/d for 3 days to 45 mg/kg in total, in association with an increase in baseline immunosuppression. If there is insufficient histologic or biochemical response, treatment with methylprednisolone may be repeated, but if the rejection is unresponsive to steroids, then it is usual to convert to a more potent immunosuppressive drug such as tacrolimus or to add other agents, such as muromonab-CD3, mycophenolate mofetil, or sirolimus.[90]

Cyclosporin A (Sandimmune) has been replaced by the partially water-soluble cyclosporine microemulsion Neoral. Several studies in both adult and pediatric patients post-transplant have indicated that Neoral is very well absorbed, with a peak absorption at 2 hours and a half-life of approximately 8 to 12 hours[77,91–93] in patients immediately post-transplant and in stable patients in the long term. The incidence of side effects with Neoral is similar to the range of side effects with Sandimmune, namely, gingival hyperplasia and hirsutism, whereas the incidence of hypertension and nephrotoxicity is less. It is possible that monitoring C2 levels (2 hours after dosing) may be more effective than trough level monitoring for preventing rejection and reducing side effects.[94]

Experience with tacrolimus (FK506) is increasing, and long-term prospective therapeutic studies comparing tacrolimus and Neoral are in progress. Preliminary results with tacrolimus indicate that it is an extremely effective immunosuppressive drug in the prevention of acute rejection.[78,90] It does not cause hirsutism or gingival hyperplasia, but there has been an increase in serious neurologic side effects, lymphoproliferative disease, and hypertrophic cardiomyopathy in children taking high doses of tacrolimus.[95]

Many units consider prednisolone withdrawal at postoperative intervals ranging from 3 to 12 months, which has proved easier to accomplish using tacrolimus therapy.[96]

Chronic rejection occurs in less than 10% of children after transplant.[88] Clinical features include gradual onset of jaundice, pruritus, and pale stools, indicating biliary obstruction. The diagnosis may be confirmed by detecting biochemical changes that include a relative increase in bilirubin, alkaline phosphatase, and γ-glutamyl transpeptidase compared with aminotransferases. Liver histology demonstrates extensive damage and loss to bile ducts (vanishing bile duct syndrome with arterial obliteration and fibrosis). There may be a response to an increase in immunosuppression (eg, a change to tacrolimus[97] or the addition of mycophenolate mofetil). Nonresponse to medical management requires retransplant.[98]

BILIARY COMPLICATIONS

The range of biliary complications after transplant includes biliary leaks and strictures, which have increased with the use of reduction hepatectomies.[86] Biliary strictures may develop secondary to an anastomotic stricture related to edema of the bile ducts or hepatic artery ischemia. Biliary leaks may be secondary to leakage from the cut surface of the reduction hepatectomy or from hepatic artery ischemia. The majority of biliary leaks settle with conservative management, but large leaks that cause biliary peritonitis, biliary abscesses, or sepsis should have surgical drainage and reconstruction. The management of biliary strictures should initially be conservative, with ursodeoxycholic acid (20 mg/kg) used to allow edema to settle. Persistent strictures leading to biliary dilatation should initially be managed radiologically, using percutaneous transhepatic cholangiography. The dilated biliary tree is cannulated, and external biliary drainage is established. Once sepsis and edema of the biliary tree have reduced, biliary dilatation may be performed using balloons and biliary stents. Surgical reconstruction is required for anastomotic or recurrent biliary strictures if interventional radiology is unsuccessful.

OTHER COMPLICATIONS AND SEPSIS

Persistent drain losses may be due to preoperative ascites or secondary to rejection, sepsis, hepatic obstruction, or bacterial peritonitis. This troublesome complication leads to acidosis and coagulopathy owing to loss of bicarbonate and coagulation factors in the ascitic fluid. It is best to treat the primary cause if possible and to manage the condition conservatively with fluid restriction and diuretics.

Infection is still the most common complication following liver transplant.[6,99] Bacterial infections are most common immediately after transplant and are related to the high doses of immunosuppressive drugs and central line infections. The main bacteria identified are *Streptococcus faecalis* and *Streptococcus viridans*, *Pseudomonas aeruginosa*, and *Staphylococcus aureus*. Postoperative fungal infections are more likely in patients undergoing transplant for acute liver failure or in children undergoing laparotomies for technical complications post-transplant.[100] The most common fungal infection is with *Candida albicans*, but aspergillosis may occur in 20% of patients with fungal infections.

More recently, vancomycin-resistant enterococcus has become a significant pathogen following both liver and small bowel/liver transplant.[101] Risk factors for developing vancomycin-resistant enterococcus are recurrent central line infections treated with vancomycin therapy, but it is important to differentiate between patients who are colonized and those who have systemic infection. The mortality of patients with systemic infection is high but improved with new agents such as quinupristin and linezolide.

LATE COMPLICATIONS POST-TRANSPLANT

Late complications may occur at any time after transplant. They include CMV or EBV infection, side effects of immunosuppression, post-transplant lymphoproliferative disease (PTLD), late biliary strictures, and hepatic artery or portal vein thrombosis. Chronic rejection may occur at any time, particularly as a result of nonadherence.

Infection with CMV occurs between 5 and 6 weeks following liver transplant. The risk of CMV disease is highest in CMV-negative recipients who receive an organ from a CMV-positive donor.[81,102,103] Although prophylaxis with intravenous ganciclovir (5 mg/kg/d) and intravenous immunoglobulins is more effective than prophylaxis with ganciclovir alone, approximately 20% of patients will develop primary infection. Treatment with intravenous ganciclovir and intravenous immunoglobulin is usually effective.[104]

The development of primary infection with EBV is a significant problem in pediatric transplant. Because two-thirds of children undergoing liver transplant are likely to be EBV negative before transplant and 75% of this group will develop primary infection after transplant,[79] it is essential to diagnose primary EBV infection to reduce immunosuppression and thus prevent the development of lymphoproliferative disease.[105]

There is a well-known association between the development of primary EBV infection and the subsequent development of post-transplant lymphoproliferative disease.[105] EBV stimulates lymphocyte proliferation, which ranges from benign hyperplasia to malignant lymphoma.

The clinical features are varied and include symptoms of infections, mononucleosis (tonsillitis and lymphadenopathy), isolated lymph node involvement, and EBV infiltration in the liver, gut, and iris, ranging from isolated organ involvement to malignant lymphoma.[106]

Considerable efforts have been devoted to the early diagnosis of EBV infection and PTLD. It is now possible to measure EBV polymerase chain reaction (PCR) prospectively and to reduce immunosuppression when high levels are achieved.[106–108] Serologic confirmation of EBV infection (EBV IgM antibodies) is usually a late feature, and it may be more appropriate to measure EBV PCR sequentially. Patients who develop gut PTLD may present with diarrhea, weight loss, and gastrointestinal bleeding. The diagnosis should be confirmed histologically by biopsy of the appropriate tissue (liver, gut).[107] Characteristic histology includes polymorphic B-cell proliferation or lymphomatous features of nuclear atypia necrosis. Immunofluorescent staining of heavy- and light-chain immunoglobulins may differentiate monoclonal from polyclonal infiltrates, which has significant prognostic implications. Confirmation of EBV involvement may be obtained by using in situ hybridization techniques to demonstrate EBV-encoded small nuclear ribonucleic acid.[108] It was initially felt that the incidence of PTLD was higher with tacrolimus than with cyclosporine, but this may be due to use of inappropriately high levels of tacrolimus when the drug was initially released.[109] First-line treatment for PTLD is reduction of immunosuppression. Acyclovir (1,500 mg/m^2/d) or ganciclovir (5 mg/kg/d) may also be prescribed, but there is no clear evidence that either is effective. Use of rituximab, a monoclonal antibody, and human leukocyte antigen–matched T-cell therapy directed against EBV are under investigation and may prove effective.[110,111] As reduction of immunosuppression leads inevitably to graft rejection, balancing treatment for PTLD and rejection may be difficult. Under these circumstances (or if lymphoproliferative disease becomes overtly malignant), chemotherapy is required.[112]

Late biliary strictures may be due to hepatic artery ischemia or thrombosis and may lead to recurrent cholangitis, hepatic abscess, and the development of secondary biliary cirrhosis. Although they may be treated radiologically, as described above, retransplant may be required for the development of biliary cirrhosis.[113]

Portal vein stenosis owing to anastomotic stricture may lead to portal hypertension with varices and splenomegaly. Initial treatment is radiologic by venoplasty, but surgical reconstruction with an intrahepatic mesoportal shunt may be required.[85,114]

Gastrointestinal perforation is an infrequent complication after liver transplant. It is related to previous abdominal surgery and to malnutrition.[114,115] Some units take this potential complication so seriously that an elective laparotomy is planned at 7 and 14 days post-transplant.[116]

SURVIVAL

Current results from international centers indicate that 1-year survival following liver transplant may be in excess of 90%.[3–6] Long-term survival (5–10 years) ranges from 60 to 80%.[3,117] Preliminary results suggest that patients who undergo elective living-related transplant have a higher 1-year survival rate (94%) than those of equivalent hepatic status receiving cadaveric grafts (78%).[118]

Many different factors influence survival. Initially, age at transplant was considered a significant risk factor, and transplant was contraindicated in infants aged under 1 year and weighing less than 10 kg.[119] Reduction hepatectomy and living-related transplant have not only reduced the waiting-list mortality in this group of children[120] and extended liver transplant to this young age group,[6] they also have demonstrated that equivalent survival may be achieved in infants transplanted under the age of 1 year compared with that of older children (Figure 60-4).[121]

It has previously been demonstrated that protein malnutrition at the time of liver transplant has a significant influence on both morbidity and mortality.[61,62] The degree of malnutrition, in addition to the severity of liver disease, has been demonstrated to have a significant effect on short-term survival,[29,122,123] and a number of studies have demonstrated improved survival for children with transplants and metabolic liver disease compared with those with chronic liver disease or fulminant hepatitis (see Figure 60-4).

In general, outcome is not related to diagnosis, although children with fulminant hepatic failure are less likely to survive the initial transplant.[113] An important aspect contributing to improved survival has been the increase in surgical and medical experience,[124] particularly with the development of innovative surgery.

There has also been an improvement in the rate of retransplant for technical problems or graft failure secondary to chronic rejection.[113,125] It is clear that although the rate of retransplant has fallen with increased surgical experience, survival following retransplant is considerably less. Children receiving more than one graft have a 50% 1-year survival compared with 90% in children receiving only one graft. This may be related to the factors contributing to the necessity for retransplant, such as primary graft nonfunction, technical problems, and the development of multiorgan failure.

In some instances, survival may be affected by the recurrence of the original disease. Recurrence of hepatitis B virus (HBV) infection is 100% in patients who were positive for HBV deoxyribonucleic acid (DNA) or hepatitis B e antigen at the time of their initial operation.[126] Recurrent HBV disease is associated with chronic hepatitis or cirrhosis (79%), submassive necrosis (9%), or fibrosing cholestatic hepatitis (25%).[56,127] The recurrence rate of chronic hepatitis B post-transplant has been much reduced by therapy with the nucleoside analog lamivudine.[128]

Chronic hepatitis C is a rare indication for transplant in children, but recurrence is inevitable in those children who were infected preoperatively before screening for hepatitis C virus became available[129,130] and in those who were infected perioperatively.[131–133] The outcome for these children is varied, with the majority developing nonspecific hepatitis. However, a minority develop rapidly progressive liver failure. Treatment for hepatitis C infection has improved with the combination of interferon and ribavirin, which achieves a 45% sustained remission rate overall.[134]

It is now clear that there is recurrence of autoimmune hepatitis both immunologically and histologically post-transplant in 25% of cases. It may be more severe than the original disease,[135] and it is important to ensure that immunosuppression with steroids is continued in this group of patients. A variant of autoimmune liver disease, giant cell hepatitis with autoimmune hemolytic anemia, has also been demonstrated to recur post-transplant.[58] Recurrence of malignant hepatic tumors in children transplanted for hepatoblastoma or hepatocellular carcinoma is directly related to the presence of extrahepatic metastases at the time of surgery.[48,53]

DE NOVO AUTOIMMUNE HEPATITIS

Several studies have documented the development of autoantibodies (antinuclear antibodies, smooth muscle antibodies, and, rarely, liver-kidney antibodies) post-transplant in both children and adults in recipients without autoimmune disease pretransplant,[136,137] which is associated with a graft hepatitis and progressive fibrosis. The hepatitis resolves with steroid therapy or azathioprine.[138,139]

LONG-TERM RENAL FUNCTION

The calcineurin inhibitors cyclosporine and tacrolimus both cause nephrotoxicity, and 4 to 5% of patients develop severe

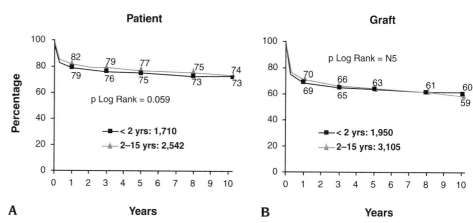

FIGURE 60-4 Patient (A) and graft (B). Survival of children following liver transplant less than and greater than 2 years at transplant, 1988 to 2001. Mean follow-up was 10 years. The survival of children older than 2 years (n = 2,542) for all indications was similar to those children under 2 years (n = 1,710) (A). There was no difference in graft survival (B). Adapted from the European Liver Transplant Registry, 2002.

chronic renal failure long term, requiring renal transplant. The use of low-dose calcineurin inhibitors or renal-sparing drugs such as mycophenolate mofetil or sirolimus for maintenance immunosuppression prevents significant renal dysfunction.[139,140] Acute postoperative hypertension is seen in 65% of children but persists long term only in 28%.[141]

HYPERLIPIDEMIA

As children survive longer, it is important to remember that both cyclosporine and sirolimus increase serum lipids, particularly cholesterol, and high levels may require transfer to tacrolimus or mycophenolate mofetil.[90]

TRANSPLANT TOLERANCE

It is now thought that 20% of adults will develop tolerance to the graft and can be withdrawn from immunosuppression.[142] Complete withdrawal of immunosuppression in children has not been documented.

QUALITY OF LIFE AFTER TRANSPLANT

It is now anticipated that children who survive liver transplant will achieve a normal lifestyle despite the necessity for continuous monitoring of immunosuppressive treatment. Children transplanted for certain metabolic liver diseases such as α_1-antitrypsin deficiency, Wilson disease, and tyrosinemia type I may have both phenotypic and functional recovery. Children with Crigler-Najjar syndrome type I have functional recovery of enzyme activity following either orthotopic or auxiliary liver transplant, whereas children with organicacidemias will have only palliation of their defect because the enzyme defect is not restricted to the liver (propionicacidemia or methylmalonicacidemia).[143] Children transplanted owing to urea cycle defects and organicacidemias may require protein restriction particularly during acute illness, reflecting the partial cure of their disease.

An important aspect in achieving normal quality of life is nutritional rehabilitation after transplant. Although early studies evaluating growth in children after liver transplant indicated that almost two-thirds did not achieve their growth potential,[144] recent studies have demonstrated that with appropriate nutritional support, 80% of survivors will achieve normal growth patterns and body habitus.[6,145] Nutritional rehabilitation begins in the first year, with a return to normal muscle and fat stores within 6 to 12 months after transplant.[6,145] Initially, weight gain may be excessive owing to the effects of steroids, increased appetite, and salt and water retention, but most children regain normal weight within 12 months, and the weight is maintained for the long term.

Linear growth may be delayed between 6 and 24 months, which is directly related to steroid dosage and preoperative stunting.[146] Children who were particularly growth retarded or stunted before transplant (height standard deviation score < –1) initially have rapid catch-up growth but may not achieve their genetic potential,[147,148] whereas children who were less stunted (height standard

deviation score > –1) have slower catch-up growth but may eventually achieve normal height.

The growth-suppressive effects of corticosteroid therapy after liver transplant have been clearly demonstrated. Centers that discontinue steroids post-transplant or institute alternate-day steroids early have reported increased catch-up growth at an earlier stage.[149]

Future growth may depend on the etiology of the pretransplant disease. For instance, 50% of children who were transplanted for the hepatic complications of Alagille syndrome and who were growth retarded before transplant did not achieve normal height.[150]

Additional factors in the etiology of post-transplant growth failure may be behavioral feeding problems and the difficulties in establishing normal feeding. Before transplant, many children will have been fed unpalatable feeds, often by nasogastric tube, and may have missed their normal developmental milestones for chewing, swallowing, and feeding. A significant proportion of these patients will have difficulty establishing normal feeding regimens post-transplant and will require nocturnal enteral feeding for 1 to 2 years.[146]

An important aspect of long-term survival is the development of puberty. A long-term study from France has demonstrated that there are no differences between the genders in attaining puberty and developing secondary sexual characteristics.[148] Girls develop menarche, and successful pregnancies have been reported for females receiving both cyclosporine and tacrolimus immunosuppression.[151]

SIDE EFFECTS OF IMMUNOSUPPRESSION
The side effects of immunosuppression are well known (Table 60-5). Hypertension is common with steroids, cyclosporine, and tacrolimus but tends to be short term and related to the intensity of immunosuppression. Growth failure and stunting related to steroids may have a significant effect on the ability to regain normal height. Hirsutism and gingival hyperplasia are recognized side effects of cyclosporine that are dose related and, although

TABLE 60-5   IMMUNOSUPPRESSIVE COMPLICATIONS POST-TRANSPLANT

Steroids
  Stunting
  Hypertension
  Cushingoid facies
  Salt and water retention
  Weight gain
Cyclosporin A
  Hirsuitism
  Gingival hyperplasia
Cyclosporin A/tacrolimus
  Nephrotoxicity
  Hypertension
  Neurotoxicity
  ? Lymphoproliferative disease
  ? Skin cancers
Tacrolimus
  Hyperglycemia
  ? Cardiomyopathy

cosmetic, have an important effect on quality of life, particularly in adolescence (Figure 60-5). There remains a long-term risk of PTLD, skin cancer, and other tumors.

PSYCHOSOCIAL DEVELOPMENT

It is of particular concern that neurodevelopmental outcomes following liver transplant should be normal. Previous studies have demonstrated that there is an initial deterioration in psychosocial development in the first year after transplant, as noted by a deterioration in social skills, language development, and eye/hand coordination,[152] pre-

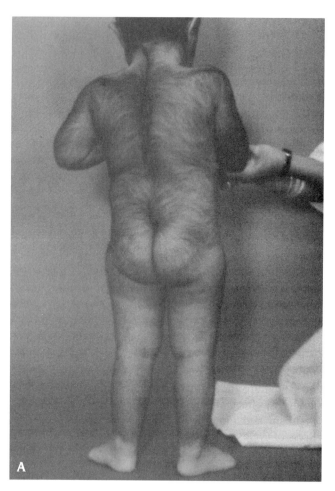

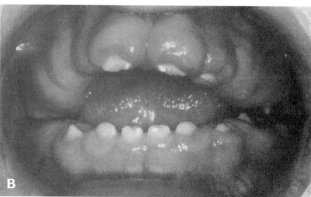

FIGURE 60-5   Quality of life of children following liver transplant is an important aspect and may be affected by cosmetic side effects such as hirsutism (*A*) or gingival hyperplasia (*B*) secondary to cyclosporine.

sumably related to the stress of the operation, the high doses of immunosuppression, and prolonged hospitalization. It is now known that most children will achieve normal psychosocial development within 1 to 2 years but that the rate of improvement is related to the age at the onset of liver disease and the age at the time of transplant.[153] Risk factors for persistent developmental delay include malnutrition at the time of transplant, length of hospital stay, and age at transplant, with younger children at particular risk of developmental delay.[31] In a longer-term study of a small group of children, 80% achieved normal height and weight measurements over a 5-year period, and all of the children attended school, but 30% had special educational needs. Psychological testing indicated that 75% of this group were functioning normally.[153–155]

The stress of liver transplant on family structure and dynamics is well known, although most parents indicate improved psychological symptoms following successful liver transplant. A longer-term study indicated that 20% of marriages dissolved and that 30% of families were considered to be functioning outside the normal range.[156]

NONCOMPLIANCE WITH THERAPY

Noncompliance with immunosuppressive therapy is less common in liver transplant recipients than in renal transplant recipients,[157,158] which may be related to the median age at renal transplant (14.3 years) compared with 2.5 years for liver transplant. It is possible that children who were grafted at a young age are more likely to accept medication through their adolescence, or there may be insufficient long-term data as yet.

SUMMARY

Liver transplant for acute or chronic liver failure or for metabolic liver disease is an effective therapy that restores good quality of life to over 80% of recipients. Considerable advances in medical and surgical expertise and immunosuppression have improved not only survival but also the quality of life for the majority of liver transplant recipients. It is essential to encourage both child and family to return to a normal life as far as possible, although continued counseling and support by a multidisciplinary team are essential. The long-term outlook for children receiving liver transplant in the twenty-first century is likely to be limited by organ donor shortages, the side effects of immunosuppressive drugs, and the potential development of post-transplant lymphoproliferative disease or other tumors. It is hoped that advances in molecular genetics will lead to effective gene therapy or hepatocyte transplant and reduce the need for solid organ transplant.[159,160]

REFERENCES

1. Starzl TE, et al. Evolution of liver transplantation. Hepatology 1982;2:614–36.
2. Shaw BW, et al. Liver transplantation therapy for children part II. J Pediatr Gastroenterol Nutr 1988;7:797–815.

3. Kelly DA. Current results and evolving indications for liver transplantation in children. J Pediatr Gastroenterol Nutr 1998;27:214–21.

4. European Liver Transplant Registry 2003. Available at: http://www.eltr.org (accessed Feb 19, 2004).

5. McDiarmid SV. The SPLIT Research Group. Studies of Pediatric liver transplantation. Update from studies in pediatric liver transplantation. Transplant Proc 2001;33:3604–5.

6. Beath SV, et al. Successful liver transplantation in babies under 1 year. BMJ 1993;307:825–8.

7. Gauthier F, et al. Urgent liver transplantation for biliary atresia. Tohoku J Exp Med 1997;181:129–38.

8. Whitington PF, et al. Clinical and biochemical findings in progressive familial intrahepatic fibrosis. J Pediatr Gastroenterol Nutr 1994;18:134–41.

9. Filipponi F, et al. Liver transplantation for end stage liver disease associated with alpha-1-antitrypsin deficiency in children. Pre-transplant natural history, timing and results of transplantation. J Hepatol 1994;20:72–8.

10. Lindstedt S, et al. Treatment of hereditary tyrosinaemia type I by inhibition of 4-hydroxyphenyl pyruvate dioxygenase. Lancet 1992;340:813–7.

11. Mohan N, McKiernan P, Precce MA, et al. Indications and outcome of liver transplantation in tyrosinaemia type I. Eur J Pediatr 1999;158 Suppl 2:349–54.

12. Macvicar D, McKiernan P, Preece MA, et al. Hepatic imaging with computed tomography of chronic tyrosinaemia type I. Br J Radiol 1990;63:605–8.

13. Manowski Z, et al. Liver cell dysplasia and early liver transplantation in hereditary tyrosinaemia. Mod Pathol 1990;36:694–701.

14. Nazer H, Ede RJ, Mowat AP, Williams R. Wilson's disease: clinical presentation and use of prognostic index. Gut 1986;27:1377–81.

15. Rela M, et al. Orthotopic liver transplantation for hepatic complications of Wilson's disease. Br J Surg 1993;80:909–11.

16. Scott-Jubb R, et al. Prevalence of liver disease in cystic fibrosis. Arch Dis Child 1991;66:698–701.

17. Milkiewicz P, et al. Transplantation for cystic fibrosis: outcome following early liver transplantation. J Pediatr Gastroenterol Nutr 2002;17:208–13.

18. Debray D, et al. Outcome of cystic fibrosis associated liver cirrhosis: management of portal hypertension. J Hepatol 1999;31:77–83.

19. Couetil JPA, et al. Combined heart/lung/ liver, double lung liver, an isolated liver transplantation for cystic fibrosis in children. Transpl Int 1997;10:33–9.

20. Sokal EM, et al. Progressive cardiac failure following orthotopic liver transplantation for type IV glycogenosis. Eur J Paediatr 1992;151:200–3.

21. Balistreri WF. Inborn errors of bile acid metabolism; clinical and therapeutic aspects. In: Hofmann AF, Paumgartner G, Stiehl A, editors. Bile acids in gastroenterology: basic and clinical advances. London: Kluwer Academic Publishers; 1995. p. 333–53.

22. Setchell KDR, O'Connell NA. Inborn errors of bile acid biosynthesis: update on biochemical aspects. In: Hofmann AF, Paumgartner G, Stiehl A, editors. Bile acids in gastroenterology: basic and clinical advances. London: Kluwer Academic Publishers; 1998. p. 129–36.

23. Gregorio GB, et al. Auto-immune hepatitis in childhood, a 20 year experience. Hepatology 1997;25:541–7.

24. Schwarz KB, Zellos A. Congenital and structural abnormalities of the liver. In: Kelly DA, editor. Diseases of the liver and biliary system in children. Oxford (UK): Blackwell Science; 1999. p. 124–40.

25. Khawaja K, et al. Bone marrow transplantation for CD40 ligand deficiency: a single center experience. Arch Dis Child 2001; 84:508–11.

26. Oellerich M, et al. Lidocaine metabolite formation as a measure of liver function in patients with cirrhosis. Ther Drug Monit 1990;12:219–26.

27. Malatack JJ, et al. Choosing a paediatric recipient of orthotopic liver transplantation. J Pediatr 1987;112:479–89.

28. Beath SV, Booth I, Kelly DA. Nutritional support in children with liver disease. Arch Dis Child 1993;69:545–27.

29. McDiarmid SV, et al. The principal investigators and institutions of the Studies of Pediatric Liver Transplantation (SPLIT) Research Group. Development of a pediatric end-stage liver disease score to predict poor outcome in children awaiting liver transplantation. Transplantation 2002;74:173–81.

30. Beath SV, et al. Quality of life after paediatric liver transplantation. Liver Transpl Surg 1995;6:429.

31. Wayman KI, et al. Neurodevelopmental outcome of young children with extrahepatic biliary atresia 1 year after liver transplantation. J Pediatr 1997;131:894–8.

32. Uemoto S, Inomata Y, Tanaka K, et al. Living related liver transplantation in children with hypoxaemia related to intrapulmonary shunting. Transpl Int 1996;9 Suppl 1:S157–9.

33. Losay J, et al. Early liver transplantation is crucial in children with liver disease and pulmonary artery hypertension. J Hepatol 1998;28:337–42.

34. Goss JA, Shackleton CR, Maggard M, et al. Liver transplantation for fulminant hepatic failure in the pediatric patient. Arch Surg 1998;133:839–46.

35. Bonatti H, et al. Liver transplantation for acute liver failure in children under 1 year of age. Transplant Proc 1997;29:434–35.

36. Lidofsky SD, et al. Intracranial pressure monitoring and liver transplantation for fulminant hepatic failure. Hepatology 1992;6:1–7.

37. Rivera-Penera T, et al. Outcome of acetaminophen overdose in pediatric patients and factors contributing to hepatotoxicity. J Pediatr 1997;130:300–4.

38. Mahadevan SBK, et al. Paracetamol hepatotoxicity in children. J Pediatr Gastroenterol Nutr 1999;28:583.

39. Shamieh I, et al. Antioxidant therapy for neonatal iron storage disease (NISD). Pediatr Res 1993;33:109A.

40. Flynn DM, et al. Progress in therapy and outcome for neonatal haemochromatosis. Arch Dis Child 2003;88:124–7.

41. Burdelski M, et al. Treatment of inherited metabolic disorders by liver transplantation. J Inherit Metab Dis 1991;14:604–18.

42. Rela M, et al. Auxiliary liver transplantation for metabolic diseases. Transplant Proc 1997;29:444–5.

43. Raper SE, Grossman M, Rader DJ, et al. Safety and feasibility of liver-directed ex vivo gene therapy for homozygous familial hypercholesterolaemia. Ann Surg 1996;223:116–26.

44. Whitington PF, et al. Liver transplantation for the treatment of urea cycle disorders. J Inherit Metab Dis 1998;21:112–8.

45. Kemper MJ, et al. Preemptive liver transplantation in primary hyperoxaluria type I: timing and preliminary results. J Nephrol 1998;11:46–8.

46. Jamieson NV. The results of combined liver/kidney transplantation for primary hyperoxaluria (PH1) 1984–1997. The European PH1 transplant registry report. European PH1 Transplantation Study Group. J Nephrol 1998;11:36–41.

47. Ellis SR, et al. Combined liver kidney transplantation for primary hyperoxaluria type I in young children. Nephrol Dial Transplant 2001;16:340–51.

48. Pimpalwar AP, et al. Strategy for hepatoblastoma management: transplant versus nontransplant surgery. J Pediatr Surg 2002; 37:240–5.

49. Badger IL, et al. Hepatic transplantation in children using reduced size allografts. Br J Surg 1989;24:77–82.

50. Lilly JR, Starzl TE. Liver transplantation in children with biliary atresia and vascular anomalies. J Pediatr Surg 1974;9:707–14.

51. Varela-Fascinetto G, et al. Biliary atresia-polysplenia syndrome: surgical and clinical relevance in liver transplantation. Ann Surg 1998;227:583–9.

52. Hosey MT, et al. Oral findings in children with liver transplants. Int J Paediatr Dent 1995;5:29–34.

53. Koneru B, et al. Liver transplantation for hepatoblastoma. Ann Surg 1991;213:118–21.

54. Thomson M, et al. Generalised mitochondrial cytopathy is an absolute contraindication to orthotopic liver transplant in childhood. J Pediatr Gastroenterol Nutr 1998;26:478–81.

55. Thomson MA, et al. Orthotopic liver transplantation is unsuccessful for valproate associated liver failure in childhood: a need for critical risk-benefit appraisal in the use of valproate. J Pediatr Gastroenterol Nutr 1995;20:451.

56. Sawyer RG, McGory RW, et al. Improved clinical outcomes with liver transplantation for hepatitis B-induced chronic liver failure using passive immunization. Ann Surg 1998;227:841–50.

57. Mutimer D, Pillay D, et al. High pre-treatment serum hepatitis B virus titre predicts failure of lamivudine prophylaxis and graft re-infection after liver transplantation. J Hepatol 1999; 30:715–21.

58. Horsmans Y, et al. Failure of ribavirin or immunosuppressive therapy to alter the course of post-infantile giant-cell hepatitis. J Hepatol 1995;22:382.

59. Johnson SP, et al. Transjugular portosystemic shunts in paediatric patients awaiting liver transplantation. Transplantation 1996;62:1178–81.

60. Ellis D, et al. Renal failure in children with hepatic failure undergoing liver transplantation. J Pediatr 1989;108:393–8.

61. Moukarzel AA, et al. Effect of nutritional status on outcome of orthotopic liver transplantation in paediatric patients. Transplant Proc 1990;22:1560–3.

62. Chin SE, et al. Survival, growth and quality of life in children after orthotopic liver transplantation: a 5 year experience. J Pediatr 1994;124:368–73.

63. Protheroe S, Kelly DA. Cholestasis and end stage liver disease. Nutritional support in paediatric gastrointestinal disease. Ballieres Clin Gastroenterol 1999;12:823–41.

64. Kelly DA, Mayer ADM. Liver transplantation. In: Kelly DA, editor. Diseases of the liver and biliary system in children. London: Blackwell Science; 1999. p. 293–312.

65. Couinaud C. Le foie. Etudes anatomiques et chirurgicale. Paris: Masson; 1957.

66. Bismuth H, Houssain D. Reduced size orthotopic liver grafts in hepatic transplantation in children. Surgery 1984;95:367–70.

67. Kalayoglu M, et al. Extended preservation of the liver for clinical transplantation. Lancet 1988;i:617–9.

68. Broelsch CE, et al. Evolution and future perspectives for reduced-size hepatic transplantation. Surg Gynaecol Obstet 1990;171:353–60.

69. De Ville de Goyet J, et al. Impact of innovative techniques on the waiting list and results in paediatric liver transplantation. Transplantation 1993;56:1130–6.

70. Broelsch CE, et al. Liver transplantation in children from living related donors. Ann Surg 1991;214:428–37.

71. Fujita S, et al. Hepatic grafts from live donors: donor morbidity for 470 cases of live donation. Transpl Int 2000;13:333–9.

72. Hayashi M, et al. Current status of living-related liver transplantation. Pediatr Transplant 1998;2:35–9.

73. Uemoto S, et al. Coexistence of a graft with the preserved native liver in auxiliary partial orthotopic liver transplantation from a living donor for ornithine transcarbamylase deficiency. Transplantation 1997;63:1026–8.

74. Pereira SP, et al. Auxiliary partial orthotopic liver transplantation for acute liver failure. J Hepatol 1997;26:1010–7.

75. Sudan DL, et al. Long-term follow up of auxiliary orthotopic liver transplantation for the treatment of fulminant hepatic failure. Surgery 1997;122:777–8.

76. Buckels JAC, et al. Low haematocrit reduces hepatic artery thrombosis after liver transplantation. Transplant Proc 1989;21:2460–1.

77. Renz JF, et al. Mycophenolate mofetil, microemulsion cyclosporine, and prednisone as primary immunosuppression for pediatric liver transplant recipients. Liver Transplant Surg 1999;5:136–43.

78. Kelly D, et al. Tacrolimus dual therapy versus cyclosporin microemulsion triple therapy in pediatric liver transplantation: results from a multicenter randomized trial. Am J Transplant 2002;3:351.

79. Ganschow R, et al. First experience with basiliximab in pediatric liver graft recipients. Pediatr Trans 2001;5:353–8.

80. Pappas PA, et al. Sirolimus in pediatric gastrointestinal transplantation: the use of sirolimus for pediatric transplant patients with tacrolimus-related cardiomyopathy. Pediatr Transplant 2000;4:45–9.

81. Davison SM, et al. Impact of cytomegalovirus and Epstein-Barr virus infection in children following liver transplantation. Gut 1993;24:S32.

82. Brant de Carvalho F, et al. Analysis of liver graft loss in infants and children below 4 years. Transplant Proc 1991;23:1451–5.

83. Rela M, et al. Hepatic artery thrombosis after liver transplantation in children under 5 years of age. Transplantation 1996; 61:1355–7.

84. Shacketon CR, et al. The impact of microsurgical hepatic arterial reconstruction on the outcome of liver transplantation for congenital biliary atresia. Am J Surg 1997;173:431–5.

85. Chardot C, et al. Portal vein complications after liver transplantation for biliary atresia. Liver Transplant Surg 1997;3:351–8.

86. Chardot C, et al. Biliary complications after paediatric liver transplantation: Birmingham's experience. Transpl Int 1995; 8:133–40.

87. Edmond JC, et al. Rejection in liver allograft recipients, clinical characterisation and management. Clin Transplant 1987;1: 143–50.

88. Murphy MS, et al. Risk factors for liver rejection: evidence to suggest enhanced allograft tolerance in infancy. Arch Dis Child 1996;75:502–6.

89. Hubscher SG, et al. Massive haemorrhagic necrosis of the liver after liver transplantation. J Clin Pathol 1989;42:360–70.

90. Egawa H, et al. FK506 conversion therapy in paediatric liver transplantation. Transplantation 1994;57:1169–73.

91. Loss GE Jr, et al. Cyclosporine versus cyclosporine microemulsion in pediatric liver transplant recipients. Transplant Proc 1998;30:1435–6.

92. Van Mourik IDM, et al. Efficacy of Neoral in the immediate postoperative period in children post liver transplantation. Liver Transplant Surg 1998;4:491–8.

93. Van Mourik IDM, et al. Comparison of pharmacokinetics of Neoral and Sandimmune in stable pediatric liver transplant recipients. Liver Transplant Surg 1999;5:107–11.

94. Keown P. Optimization of cyclosporine therapy with new ther-

apeutic drug monitoring strategies: report from the International Neoral TDM Advisory Consensus Meeting. Transplant Proc 1998;30:1645–9.

95. Chang RK, et al. Marked left ventricular hypertrophy in children on tacrolimus (FK506) after orthotopic liver transplantation. Am J Cardiol 1998;81:1277–80.

96. Abe M, et al. Successful prednisone withdrawal after living-related liver transplantation. Transplant Proc 1998;30:1441–2.

97. Sher LS, et al. Efficacy of tacrolimus as rescue therapy for chronic rejection in orthotopic liver transplantation: a report of the US. Transplantation 1997;64:258–63.

98. Nicolette LA, et al. Results of transplantation for acute and chronic hepatic allograft rejection. J Pediatr Surg 1998;33:909–12.

99. Garcia S, et al. Infection and associated risk factors in the immediate post operative period of pediatric liver transplantation: a study of 176 transplants. Clin Transplant 1998;12:190–7.

100. Gladdy RA, et al. *Candida* infection in pediatric liver transplant recipients. Liver Transplant Surg 1999;5:16–24.

101. Gray J, et al. Experience with quinupristin/dalfopristin in treatment infections with vancomycin-resistant enterococcus fecum in children. Pediatr Infect Dis J 2000;19:234–8.

102. Mellon A, et al. Cytomegalovirus infection after liver transplantation in children. J Gastroenterol Hepatol 1993;8:540–4.

103. Gane E, et al. Randomised trial of efficacy and safety of oral ganciclovir in the prevention of cytomegalovirus disease in liver transplant recipients. Lancet 1997;350:1729–33.

104. Green M, et al. Comparison of intravenous ganciclovir followed by oral acyclovir with intravenous ganciclovir alone for prevention of cytomegalovirus and Epstein-Barr virus disease and liver transplantation in children. Clin Infect Dis 1997;25:1344–9.

105. Newell KA, et al. Posttransplant lymphoproliferative disease in paediatric liver transplantation. Interplay between primary Epstein-Barr virus infection and immunosuppression. Transplantation 1996;62:370–5.

106. Robinson R, et al. Primary ocular post-transplant lymphoproliferative disease. J Paediatr Ophthalmol 1995;32:393–4.

107. Bassam S, et al. The involvement of the gastrointestinal tract in post transplant lymphoproliferative disease in pediatric liver transplantation. J Pediatr Gastroenterol Nutr 1999;28:380–5.

108. Cacciarelli TV, et al. Natural history of Epstein-Barr viral load in peripheral blood of pediatric liver transplant recipients during treatment for post transplant lymphoproliferative disorder. Transplant Proc 1999;31:488–9.

109. Cox KL, Freese DK. Tacrolimus (FK506): the pros and cons of its use as an immunosuppressant in paediatric liver transplantation. Clin Invest Med 1996;19:389–92.

110. Pinkerton CR, et al. Immunodeficiency-related lymphoproliferative disorders: prospective data from the United Kingdom Children's Cancer Study Group Registry. Br J Haematol 2002;118:456–61.

111. Haque T, et al. Complete regression of posttransplant lymphoproliferative disease using partially HLA-matched Epstein Barr virus-specific cytotoxic T cells. Transplantation 2001;72:1399–402.

112. Gross TG, et al. Treatment of post transplant lymphoproliferative disease (PTLD) following solid organ transplantation with low-dose chemotherapy. Ann Oncol 1998;9:339–40.

113. Achilleos OA, et al. Outcome of liver retransplantation in children. J Liver Transplant 1999;5:401–6.

114. De Ville de Goyet J, et al. Direct bypassing of extrahepatic portal venous obstruction in children: a new technique for combined hepatic portal revascularization and treatment of extrahepatic portal hypertension. J Pediatr Surg 1998;33:597–601.

115. Beierle EA, et al. Gastrointestinal perforation after pediatric orthotopic liver transplantation. J Pediatr Surg 1998;33:240–2.

116. Renz JF, et al. Planned exploration of pediatric liver transplant recipients reduces post-transplant morbidity and lowers length of hospitalization. Arch Surg 1997;132:950–5.

117. Sudan DL, et al. Causes of late mortality in pediatric liver transplant recipients. Ann Surg 1998;227:289–95.

118. Kuang AA, et al. Decreased mortality from technical failure improves results in pediatric liver transplantation. Arch Surg 1996;131:887–92.

119. Zitelli BJ, et al. Pediatric liver transplantation: patient evaluation and selection, infectious complications, and life-style after transplantation. Transplant Proc 1987;19:3309–16.

120. Ryckman FC, et al. Segmental orthotopic hepatic transplantation as a means to improve patient survival and waiting-list mortality. J Pediatr Surg 1991;26:422–7.

121. Van der Werf WJ, et al. Infant pediatric liver transplantation results equal those for older pediatric patients. J Pediatr Surg 1998;33:20–3.

122. Bell SH, et al. An update on liver transplantation in the United States; recipient characteristics and outcome. Clin Transplant 1995;19–33.

123. Rodeck B, et al. Liver transplantation in children with chronic end stage liver disease; factors influencing survival after transplantation. Transplantation 1996;62:1071–6.

124. Talbot D, et al. Progress in pediatric liver transplantation—the Birmingham experience. J Pediatr Surg 1997;32:710–3.

125. Newell KA, et al. An analysis of hepatic retransplantation in children. Transplantation 1998;65:1172–8.

126. O'Grady JG, et al. Hepatitis B virus reinfection after orthotopic liver transplantation. J Hepatol 1992;14:104–11.

127. Davies SE, et al. Hepatic histological findings after transplantation for chronic hepatitis B virus infection, including a unique pattern of fibrosing cholestatic hepatitis. Hepatology 1991;13:150–7.

128. Mutimer D. Long term outcome of liver transplantation for viral hepatitis: is there a need to re-evaluate patient selection? Gut 199;45:475–6.

129. Nowicki MJ, et al. The prevalence of hepatitis C virus (HC) in infants and children after liver transplantation. Dig Dis Sci 1994;39:2250–4.

130. Pastore M, et al. Role of hepatitis C virus in chronic liver disease occurring after orthotopic liver transplantation. Clinical transplantation. Arch Dis Child 1995;72:403–7.

131. Testa G, et al. Long-term outcome of patients transplanted with livers from hepatitis C-positive donors. Transplantation 1998;65:925–9.

132. Shuhart MC, et al. Histological and clinical outcome after liver transplantation for hepatitis C. Hepatology 1997;26:1646–52.

133. McDiarmid SV, et al. De novo hepatitis C in children after liver transplantation. Transplantation 1998;66:311–8.

134. Kelly DA, Bunn S. Safety, efficacy and pharmacokinetics of interferon alfa 2B plus ribavirin in children with chronic hepatitis C. Hepatology 2001;34:342A.

135. Birnbaum AH, et al. Recurrence of autoimmune hepatitis in children after liver transplantation. J Pediatr Gastroenterol Nutr 1997;25:20–5.

136. Kerkar N, et al. De-novo autoimmune hepatitis after liver transplantation. Lancet 1998;351:409–13.

137. Andries S, et al. Post transplant immune hepatitis in pediatric liver transplant recipients: incidence and maintenance therapy with azathioprine. Transplantation 2001;72:267–72.

138. Salcedo M, et al. Response to steroids in de novo autoimmune hepatitis after liver transplantation. Hepatology 2002;35:349–56.

139. Evans HM, et al. Histology of liver allografts following pediatric liver transplantation. J Pediatr Gastroenterol Nutr 2001;32:383.

140. Berg UB, et al. Renal function before and long after liver transplantation in children. Transplantation 2001;27:561–2.

141. Bartosh SM, et al. Renal outcomes in pediatric liver transplantation. Clin Transplant 1997;11:354–60.

142. Riordan SM, Williams R. Tolerance after liver transplantation: does it exist and can immunosuppression be withdrawn? J Hepatol 1999;31:1106–19.

143. Gissen P, et al. Long-term survival post early liver transplantation in organic acidemias. Hepatology 2001;34:503A.

144. Andrews WS, et al. Steroid withdrawal after pediatric liver transplantation. Transplant Proc 1994;26:159–60.

145. Holt RI, et al. Orthotopic liver transplantation reverses the adverse nutritional changes of end-stage liver disease in children. Am J Clin Nutr 1997;65:534–42.

146. Kelly DA. Post-transplant growth failure in children. Liver Transplant Surg 1997;3(5 Suppl):S32–9.

147. Sarna S, et al. Growth delay after liver transplantation in childhood: studies of underlying mechanisms. Pediatr Res 1995;38:366–72.

148. Codoner-Franch P, et al. Long-term follow up of growth in height after successful liver transplantation. J Pediatr 1994;124:368–73.

149. Andrews S, et al. 10 years of pediatric liver transplantation. J Pediatr Surg 1996;31:619–24.

150. Cardona A, et al. Liver transplantation in children with Alagille syndrome—a study of 12 cases. Transplantation 1995;60:339–42.

151. Jain A, et al. Pregnancy after liver transplantation under tacrolimus. Transplantation 1997;64:559–65.

152. Beath SV, et al. Long-term nutritional and neurodevelopmental outcome of liver transplantation in infants aged less than 12 months. J Pediatr Gastroenterol Nutr 2000;30:269–75.

153. Stewart SM, et al. Mental and motor development, social competence, and growth one year after successful pediatric liver transplantation. J Pediatr 1989;114:574.

154. Stone RD, et al. Children and families can achieve normal psychological adjustment and a good quality of life following pediatric liver transplantation: a long-term study. Transplant Proc 1997;29:1571–2.

155. Bucevalas JC, et al. Health-related quality of life in pediatric liver transplant recipients: a single-center study. Liver Transplant 2003;9:62–71.

156. Tarbell SE, Kosmach B. Parental psychosocial outcomes in pediatric liver and/or intestinal transplantation: pretransplantation and the early postoperative period. Liver Transplant Surg 1998;4:378–87.

157. Molmenti E, et al. Noncompliance after paediatric liver transplantation. Transplant Proc 1999;31:408.

158. Watson AR. Non-compliance and transfer from pediatric to adult transplant unit. Pediatr Nephrol 2000;14:469–72.

159. Vons C. Transplantation of isolated hepatocytes, is it an alternative for total liver transplantation? On the treatment of hereditary hepatic metabolic diseases. J Chirurg 2001;138:342–6.

160. Boudjema K, et al. Auxiliary liver transplantation and bioartificial bridging procedures in treatment of acute liver failure. World J Surg 2002;26:264–74.

CHAPTER 61

GALLBLADDER DISEASE

Annemarie Broderick, MB, BCh, MRCPI, MMedSc
Brian T. Sweeney, MB, BCh, Bao, MD

The role and importance of the gallbladder are summarized wittily in the following short poem:

Chemo Memo

Man's liver is a brownish blob
That does a most prodigious job.
It manufactures gall, or bile
And normally keeps some on file
Stored neatly in a pear shaped sac.
From there the liver's yields attack
The food man eats, to change its state
By methods man can't duplicate,
Or even halfway understand.
He ought to treat this outsize gland,
With due respect and loving care
To keep it in top-notch repair,
Because to get along at all
Man needs an awful lot of gall[1]

The essential functions of bile or "gall" manufactured by the liver and stored in the gallbladder are to facilitate absorption of fats and fat-soluble vitamins from the diet and to secrete heavy metals such as copper from the body. Gallstones were recognized in ancient Egypt, but it was many centuries before the functions of the gallbladder and the relationship of gallstones to disease were understood. Up until the nineteenth century, it was (mistakenly) believed that the removal of the gallbladder was incompatible with life. The first cholecystectomy was not performed until 1882 in Berlin, and it was a great success.[2]

The gallbladder is a vesicular structure, usually found under the right lobe of the liver between the porta hepatis and inferior tip of the liver lying in the gallbladder fossa. It is covered by the same peritoneal covering as the liver.[3] The liver, bile ducts, and gallbladder arise from the primitive foregut. The cranial portion develops into the hepatic parenchyma and the intrahepatic ducts, and the more caudal section evolves into the gallbladder and extrahepatic bile ducts.[4] This chapter reviews the epidemiology, genetics, pathogenesis, diagnosis, and treatment of common gallbladder diseases with particular reference to children. Gallstone disease is the most expensive gastrointestinal disease in adults in the United States today[5]; therefore, most research has concentrated on adults. The literature and clinical practice pertinent to children, extrapolating from adult studies where necessary, are reviewed.

PHYSICAL CHEMISTRY COMPOSITION OF BILE

Bile is an aqueous solution composed of bile salts, cholesterol, phospholipid, water, electrolytes, and heavy metals, as well as proteins, immunoglobulin A, vitamins, and toxins.[6] The functions of bile are myriad and in part are dependent on the function of individual components. Bile salts in the intestine act as detergents, which solubilize and aid the absorption of dietary lipids and lipid-soluble vitamins. Bile is the major route of elimination of a large number of compounds, including cholesterol, bilirubin conjugates, drugs, and heavy metals, especially copper. Cholesterol elimination from the body occurs mainly in bile either as cholesterol or as bile salts, which are products of cholesterol metabolism. Bile also contains secretory immunoglobulin A, which may play a role in prevention of infection. Bile flow resulting from the active transport of bile acids into the canalicular lumen is termed bile acid dependent, and bile flow due to the transport of glutathione and bicarbonate is bile acid independent.[7] The bicarbonate and electrolyte concentrations of human bile differ little from serum.[6,8]

A constellation of transporters, which are found on hepatocytes and cholangiocytes, modulates bile composition. Transporters allow the uptake into hepatocytes of molecules such as cholesterol and bile salts and their subsequent export into the lumen of canaliculi. These transporters are discussed in the section dealing with gallstone formation.

EPIDEMIOLOGY

In adults living in the United States, gallbladder disease is one of the most expensive digestive diseases, and annual costs of treatment were estimated to total more than $6 billion dollars in 2001.[5] Treatment of children accounts for only a fraction of this budget because gallbladder disease is uncommon in childhood. Ascertaining the true prevalence of gallbladder disease in either adults or children is difficult because most patients with gallstones are asymptomatic. Studies of hospitalizations, surgical records, and autopsy series underestimate the prevalence of gallstone disease. The introduction of ultrasonography allowed noninvasive screening for gallstone disease and therefore a more accurate estimate of prevalence. A study of gallstone prevalence in 1,570 children between the ages of 6 and 19 years in Bari, Italy, found ultrasonographic evidence of gallstones in just two asymptomatic girls, aged 13 and 18 years—a prevalence rate of 0.13%.[9] One of the two girls had a family history of gallstone disease, but the other had no recognized risk factors. In contrast, approximately 20.5 million adults in the United States are estimated to have gallstones based on extrapolation of the findings of 14,238 ultrasound examinations performed between 1988 and 1994 as part of the Third National Health and Nutrition Examination Survey (NHANES III) study.[10]

Within the United States, there are striking differences in cholesterol gallstone prevalence between ethnic groups. Native Americans have the highest rate of all groups in the United States. For example, the Pima Indians, a tribe in Arizona, were found to have a gallstone prevalence rate of 48.6%.[11] This rate was established in Pima Indians using an age- and sex-stratified random sample of 600 members of the tribe, by review of medical records, and by performing oral cholecystography in those without a history of cholecystectomy or a previous abnormal cholecystogram. In those aged 15 to 24 years, the prevalence was 5.9% in females and 0% in males. However, there was a dramatic increase in prevalence in females aged 25 to 34 years to 73.2%. In males aged 25 to 34 years, the increase was only to 4.4%. Prevalence rates in men did not approximate those of women until they were older than 55 years.[11] To investigate the reasons for this dramatic increase in gallstone prevalence in Pima Indians with age, bile composition and bile acid pool size of a group of 66 children and adolescents aged 9 to 21 years were studied. Bile cholesterol saturation increased during puberty in both genders but was 15% higher in females than in males. In males but not females, the bile acid pool increased. Hence, the metastable bile found in prepubertal children is altered by the increasing cholesterol concentration during puberty, and cholesterol precipitation and gallstone formation can occur.[12]

There are other medical conditions in children that are associated with a recognized increase in the prevalence of gallstone disease. These diseases include cystic fibrosis and hemolytic diseases, which increase the risk of pigment gallstones and are discussed in more detail later in this chapter.

As noted, the proportions of bile constituents change at puberty in both children and adolescent Pima Indians and also in white children.[13,14] Before puberty in the Pima Indians, bile cholesterol saturation (expressed as a percentage) is saturated but metastable in both girls, 116 ± 7%, and boys, 99 ± 7%. After puberty, there is a significant increase in this index, an increase that is higher in females, 156 ± 16%, than in males, 124 ± 2%. Lithogenic bile was present in 71% of females older than 19 years but only 13% of females younger than 13 years.[13] Two series have shown lower cholesterol-to-bile salt excretion ratios in white children than in adults.[15,16] Mean biliary cholesterol saturation index in 10 healthy American children with an average age of 2.3 ± 0.6 years was 0.72 ± 0.04 compared with 1.08 ± 0.09 in healthy adults[15] and 0.57 ± 0.12 in 11 Swiss children.[16] It is important to note

that in these studies of bile composition in children, bile-rich duodenal aspirates were used.

In another study, gallbladder bile composition was investigated in 18 children from whom gallbladder bile was aspirated at the time of laparotomy for nonhepatobiliary disease. Significant differences were noted between infants and children in this study. Infants displayed more dilute bile than children, but bile was more saturated with cholesterol. The cholesterol saturation index in all infants was greater than 1, whereas in almost all children, it was less than 1. Infants also had a significantly shorter nucleation time, 11.6 days, compared with children, who had a nucleation time of 28.6 days, which is similar to that of healthy adults. Total biliary lipid of infants, 3.3 ± 3.8 g/dL (mean ± SD), is significantly lower than in children, in whom the total content is 9.1 ± 3.0 g/dL. Interestingly, in all bile samples, even those supersaturated with cholesterol, cholesterol was not present in the vesicular phase.[17] It is not clear why infant gallbladder bile is so different, but potential factors are a milk-only diet and the poor concentrating ability of the gallbladder.

FORMATION AND CONTENT OF GALLSTONES

For gallstones of any type to develop, some or all of the following need to occur: alterations in the proportion of bile constituents, nucleation, changes in gallbladder motility, or infection. Infection appears to be important only for brown pigment gallstone formation. The development of each of the three major gallstone types, namely cholesterol, black pigment, and brown pigment stones, is reviewed. The location of gallstone types differs with type; cholesterol and black pigment gallstones are almost always found in the gallbladder, but brown pigment gallstones are more commonly found in the extrahepatic ducts and even in the intrahepatic ducts.[18,19] In brief, the development of cholesterol gallstones requires hypersecretion of cholesterol into bile.[20] Black pigment stones are associated with a large number of diseases, all of which elevate bilirubin concentration in bile. Brown pigment stones, which are rare in both children and in the Western world, occur in the presence of obstruction and subsequent infection.

CHOLESTEROL GALLSTONES
Cholesterol gallstones are a frequent problem in adults and, hence, extensively studied. For cholesterol gallstones to form, there must be (1) hypersecretion of cholesterol into bile, (2) decreased motility of the gallbladder, (3) increased mucin production by the gallbladder, (4) increased conversion of primary bile salts to more hydrophobic bile secondary bile salts, and (5) increased rate of formation of cholesterol crystals.[18,20] Once this pathway starts, it often leads to a self-perpetuating cycle as hypersecretion of cholesterol itself decreases gallbladder motility. This leads to a repeat of the cholesterol gallstone formation pathway, with the net result of more cholesterol gallstones.

How does cholesterol get into bile? Cholesterol is secreted into bile directly or in the altered form of bile salts, and these pathways are the routes of elimination of cholesterol from the body.[20] There are four potential fates for cholesterol in hepatocytes. Cholesterol can be (1) stored in the hepatocyte as either or both the free and the ester form, (2) returned to serum as low-density lipoproteins, (3) secreted into bile, or (4) converted into bile salts. The latter two account for cholesterol elimination and are most relevant to bile formation and composition. Cholesterol is secreted into bile via adenosine triphosphate (ATP) binding cassette (ABC) twinned sterol half-transporters ABCG5 and ABCG8.[21-23] Cholesterol conversion to bile salts starts with 7α-hydroxylase, an enzyme found only in hepatocytes, the activity of which is regulated by bile salt concentration. As illustrated in Figure 61-1, bile salts are transported into bile by the bile salt export pump known as both BSEP and ABCB11[24] and phospholipid by ABCB4, previously known as multidrug-resistance protein (MDR)[35] at the canalicular membrane.

In Figure 61-2, the physical chemical pathways of vesicle and micelle formation are illustrated. In the canalicular lumen, cholesterol and phosphatidylchloline vesicles are formed and then dissolved by bile salts to form mixed micelles. As bile ducts get bigger, bile becomes more concentrated, and more phosphatidylcholine is solubilized by bile salts.[26] The cholesterol concentration of micelles increases, and, eventually, in the gallbladder these cholesterol-rich vesicles fuse and may lead to cholesterol crystal formation. Patients with cholesterol gallstones have higher cholesterol-to-phosphatidylcholine ratios than patients without gallstones.[27] Such people are secreting cholesterol in excess of the ability of bile salts and phosphatidylcholine to form micelles; thus, the cholesterol saturation index will be greater than 1, and bile will be metastable.[18] The importance

of phosphatidylcholine secretion in prevention of cholesterol gallstone formation is illustrated by the discovery that defects in the ABCB4 (MDR3) gene are associated with symptomatic intrahepatic and gallbladder cholesterol cholithiasis. A study of six adults with recurrent cholesterol gallstones postcholecystectomy revealed mutations in ABCB4 in all six; three had homozygous missense mutations, and two were heterozygotes and one had homozygous nonsense mutations. Two of the six also displayed hepatic bile supersaturated with cholesterol and a low phospholipid concentration.[28] ABCB4 (MDR3) defects are also associated with progressive familial intrahepatic cholestasis type 3 (see Chapter 55.6, "Biliary Transport")[29] and with intrahepatic brown pigment gallstones.[19]

For the actual formation of cholesterol gallstones, nucleation or aggregation of submicroscopic cholesterol crystals must occur.[30] Both pro- and antinucleating factors are described; immunoglobulins,[31] N-aminopeptidase,[32] and fibronectin[33] have been identified as pronucleating factors and apolipoprotein A-I[34] as an antinucleating factor. Once a nucleus has formed, further cholesterol monohydrate crystals attach, as can mucin, calcium, and even unconjugated bilirubin.[18] Cholesterol stones can vary in size from a few millimeters to a few centimeters and can be solitary or multiple.

BLACK PIGMENT GALLSTONES

Black pigment stone formation requires excess bilirubin in bile.[35] Excess secretion of conjugated bilirubin into bile occurs in (1) hemolytic diseases, (2) disorders of dysfunctional erythropoiesis, and (3) diseases that cause bilirubin

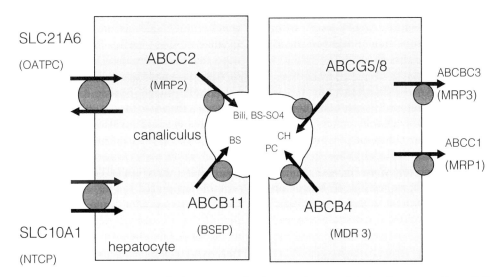

FIGURE 61-1 Transporters on the hepatocytes that have a role in modulating the composition of bile. A hepatocyte couplet is shown in this figure, and the canaliculus is in the center. The major canalicular transporters of biliary lipids are shown; the bile salt export pump (BSEP) (ABCB11) exports bile salts (BS). The half-transporters ABCG5/8 together transport cholesterol (CH). Multidrug resistance–associated protein (MRP) 2 (ABCC2) exports bilirubin conjugates (bili) and sulfated bile salts (BS-SO4). Multidrug-resistance protein (MDR) 3 P-glycoprotein (ABCB4) transports phosphatidylcholine (PC). On the basolateral surface of the hepatocytes, organic anion transporting polypeptide C (OATPC) (SLC21A6) and Na+-dependent taurocholate cotransporting polypeptide (NTCP) (SLC10A1) transport bile salts into the hepatocytes, MRP3 (ABCC3) allows monovalent bile salt efflux, and MRP1 (ABCC1) allows organic anion efflux, probably including unconjugated bilirubin. Courtesy of Dr. Richard S. Kwon, Brigham and Women's Hospital, Boston.

FIGURE 61-2 Pathway of cholesterol crystallization in bile. Cholesterol is hypersecreted into bile in the form of vesicles of cholesterol and phosphatidylcholine, as shown on the left of the diagram. As bile becomes more concentrated in bile ducts, the concentration of simple bile salt micelles also increases and the micelles preferentially extract phosphatidylcholine from vesicles, as shown in the middle column, creating thermodynamically unstable cholesterol-rich vesicles. In the gallbladder, as shown on the right, these vesicles fuse and aggregate to form a cholesterol-rich template for formation of cholesterol crystals. Reproduced with permission from Donovan JM.[20]

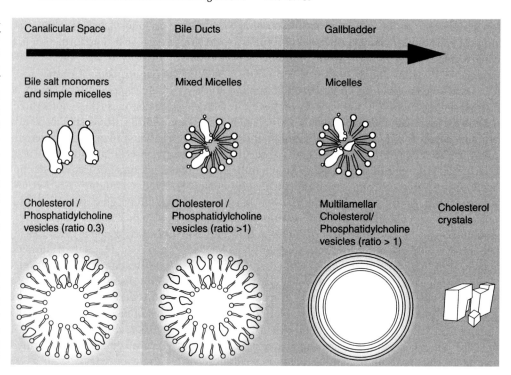

to undergo enterohepatic circulation.[36,37] When excess conjugated bilirubin is present in bile (ie, bilirubin supersaturation),[18] it can be deconjugated by β-glucuronidase or by other nonenzymatic means. This unconjugated bilirubin precipitates as an insoluble calcium salt known as calcium bilirubinate. Black pigment stones also contain calcium hydrogen bilirubinate, calcium carbonate, and calcium phosphate; small amounts of cholesterol (less than 20% by weight); and mucin in a glycoprotein matrix.[20] Free radical polymerization of calcium bilirubinate and possible oxidation in the presence of gallbladder mucin leads to the formation of black pigment gallstones.[20]

BROWN PIGMENT GALLSTONES

Brown pigment stones are laminated and contain bacterial cytoskeletons,[38] calcium bilirubinate salts, cholesterol, and fatty acids.[20] These stones can occur in the presence of cholesterol or black pigment stones, which are causing obstruction and hence infection. Intrahepatic brown pigment stones are associated with decreased expression of MDR3 and phosphatidylcholine transfer protein as well as increased 3-hydroxy-3-methylglutaryl coenzyme A reductase activity.[19]

GENETICS

Formation of cholesterol gallstones in humans is likely due to the interaction of environmental factors with genes, although none have been definitively identified in humans. Investigations in mice have led to the identification of Lith genes, which are candidate genes for cholesterol gallstone disease. The genetics of cholesterol gallstone disease is an example of a complex genetic trait, and a special investigative technique called quantitative trait locus (QTL) analysis is required.[39] Mice, which share similar hepatocyte and cholangiocyte transporter proteins to humans, are used as models for human gallstone disease. Environmental fac-

tors, especially diet, can be readily controlled in mice. To identify cholesterol gallstone genes by QTL analysis, mice strains that are gallstone resistant and others that are gallstone susceptible were identified. These mice were crossed and selectively back-crossed, and the progeny were phenotyped and genotyped. By this means, gallstone candidate genes are linked to polymorphic genetic markers, which differ between inbred mouse strains. The next step is to identify a chromosomal region that contains potential Lith genes by QTL analysis and to use the murine genome map to analyze these regions for genes, which could play a potential pathophysiologic role in cholesterol gallstone formation. Candidate genes, which colocalize with the QTLs, are studied in a specially bred mouse strain that expresses them, and the effects on cholesterol homeostasis and gallstones are investigated. Using this process, there are now nine potential Lith genes identified.[40]

The initial QTL experiments identified two potential Lith genes in mice. Abcb11 is a strong candidate gene for Lith 1[41] and Abcc2 for Lith 2.[39] Abcb11 is also known as Bsep and is a member of the ABC family. It is found on the canalicular surface of hepatocytes and actively exports monovalent bile salts. There appears to be a gain of function so that bile salt secretion rates, along with those of cholesterol, are elevated in Lith 1 congenic mice. ABCC2, also known as multidrug resistance–associated protein (MRP) 2, is an organic anion transporter also found on the canalicular membrane, which exports bilirubin and glutathione conjugates.[42] Other candidate Lith genes are involved in mucin regulation and cholesterol crystallization.[43] Human correlation of these candidate genes is actively being investigated.

For black pigment gallstones, the underlying disease (eg, sickle cell disease) leading to gallstone formation often has a genetic basis. It is interesting to note that populations with a very high rate of cholesterol gallstone disease, such as the Pima Indians, develop pigment gallstones very rarely. Brown pigment stones are formed in the setting of infection, so genetic causes are less likely to be a major factor. However, as mentioned, gene expression differs in liver tissue from those with intrahepatic brown pigment stones.[19]

DISEASES ASSOCIATED WITH GALLSTONES IN CHILDREN

CHOLESTEROL GALLSTONES

Cholesterol gallstones in children and adolescents have been associated with female gender, a positive family history, and parity. In a series of 96 patients under 25 years of age, the ratio of females to male with cholelithiasis was 4:1.[44] Unusually for a series of younger patients, only 2% of patients in this study had hemolytic disease. In another series of 50 children and adolescents with gallstones, 7 were young women who had adolescent pregnancies.[45] Three of the 50 patients in the latter study only had obesity as a risk factor for gallstones.[45] Finally, family history is significant in adults with cholesterol gallstones and in postpubertal Pima Indians.[13]

PIGMENT GALLSTONES

Black pigment gallstones are generally secondary to an identifiable risk factor. The many diseases associated with pigment gallstones in children are outlined in Table 61-1. These diseases can be categorized into three broad groupings.

Hemolytic Processes. Diseases resulting in hemolysis commonly lead to the formation of black pigment stones. An example is sickle cell disease, in which the prevalence of cholelithiasis increases with age. In an ultrasonographic study of children with major sickle hemoglobinopathies, gallstone prevalence was negligible in children younger that 6 years, but prevalence increased in the midteen years.[46] Interestingly, the severity of hemolytic disease as measured by hemoglobin levels, reticulocyte counts, and blood transfusions is not associated directly with gallstones.[46] Overall, gallstones are such a prominent feature of sickle cell disease that cholecystectomy is the most common surgical procedure performed for these patients.[47] Complication rates are equally high for both open and laparoscopic cholecystectomy in patients with sickle cell disease. Hospital stays are shorter in those who have a laparoscopic cholecystectomy, and preoperative transfusions decrease complications further.[47] Children with hereditary spherocytosis are also at increased risk of black pigment gallstone, and laparoscopic cholecystectomy for those with gallstones can be safely combined with laparoscopic splenectomy.[48] Although more common in adult populations, the presence of artificial cardiac valves can lead to red cell destruction and subsequent pigment gallstone formation in children.[49]

Enterohepatic Circulation of Bilirubin. Crohn disease, distal small intestinal resection, and cystic fibrosis

TABLE 61-1   DISEASES ASSOCIATED WITH GALLSTONES IN CHILDREN

DISEASE	GALLSTONE TYPE	PREVALENCE	AGE RANGE (YR)	REFERENCE
HEMOLYTIC PROCESSES				
Sickle cell hemoglobinopathies				
Homozygous HbSS	Pigment	26% (11/42)	2–18	46
Heterozygous HbSC	Pigment	20% (3/15)	2–18	46
β-Thalassemia anemia	Pigment	11.8% (2/17)	2–18	98
	Sludge	29.4% (5/17)	2–18	98
Hereditary spherocytosis	Pigment	3/50 children with gallstones	0–20	45
Cardiac valve replacement	Pigment	Case reports	Children and adults	52
PROBABLE ENTEROHEPATIC CIRCULATION OF BILIRUBIN				
History of abdominal surgery in infancy (especially ileal resection)	Pigment	29% < 1 yr 21% of 1–5 yr 5% of 6–21 yr	0–21	54
Cystic fibrosis	Pigment	13.2% (25/189)	3–22.5	52
Crohn disease	Pigment	Case reports	Children and adults	50
MISCELLANEOUS				
Prolonged parenteral nutrition > 4 wk	Pigment	13% (11/84)	Infants and children	53
	Sludge	3.6% (3/84)	Infants and children	53
Treatment of childhood cancer	Not reported	0.42% (16/6050)	10 yr after diagnosis of primary cancer	58
Post–heart transplant (cyclosporine immunosuppression)	Pigment and mixed type	3.2% (10/311); 8/10 transplanted < 3 mo of age	5 d to 3 yr at time of transplant	56
Down syndrome	Radiolucent gallstones (chemical analysis not reported)	4.7% (6/126)	1 mo–19 yr	57
Pregnancy	Cholesterol	7 of 50 children with gallstones	0–20	46
	Cholesterol	8/12 female patients younger than 18–26 yr with gallstones	18–26	99

HbSC = sickle cell trait (heterozygous); HbSS = sickle cell anemia (homozygous).

are examples of diseases that may result in enterohepatic circulation of excess unconjugated bilirubin from the intestine to the liver.[36,50,51] A proposed mechanism for enterohepatic circulation of unconjugated bilirubin in these disease processes is that malabsorption of bile salts from the terminal ileum leads to spillage of excess bile salts into the large intestine. These bile salts are accompanied by bilirubin conjugates, which are hydrolyzed in the large intestine by bacterial glucuronidases. The unconjugated bilirubin is further converted into either calcium salts or into urobilinoids. In the presence of large amounts of bile salts, passive nonionic diffusion of unconjugated bilirubin from the colon and return to the liver are promoted. Unconjugated bilirubin is taken up into hepatocytes, reconjugated mainly with glucuronic acid, and secreted again into canalicular bile.[36,37]

Children and adults with cystic fibrosis exhibit increased prevalence of gallstones. In a study of 189 patients (children and adults) with cystic fibrosis performed in Italy, 25 or 13.2% were found to have gallstones.[52] Gallstones have also been noted in children requiring parenteral nutrition. Those especially vulnerable are infants who have also undergone ileal resection and had multiple abdominal procedures.[53] Children with hepatobiliary disease are also at increased risk of gallstones.[54] Bile salt malabsorption leading to the interruption of the enterohepatic cycling of bile salts is the likely mechanism in the latter two diseases.

Miscellaneous.   Other risk factors for black pigment gallstones are medications, especially furosemide in infants[55] and cyclosporine in cardiac transplant patients.[56] Bronchopulmonary dysplasia, independent of furosemide use, and gram-negative sepsis are also risk factors in infancy.[54] Children with Down syndrome are at increased risk of cholelithiasis, although the etiology is not understood.[57] Survivors of childhood cancers are at increased risk, although, again, the cause of this increased risk is not known.[58]

CLINICAL FEATURES OF GALLBLADDER DISEASE

The presentation of gallbladder disease is dependent on the underlying disease process. It can be difficult to gauge the contribution of chronic acalculous cholecystitis to chronic abdominal pain. Pain in patients with acute cholecystitis or acute biliary colic is usually clearly related to the presence of gallstones. It is also not clear why most individuals with gallstones are asymptomatic for long periods, whereas others have recurrent episodes of biliary colic. It is also unclear why others can present with disease outside the gallbladder as manifestations of gallbladder disease, for example, pancreatitis or cholangitis, although stone size appears to play a role. The clinical features of gallbladder disease are reviewed systematically.

CONGENITAL ANOMALIES

These are generally asymptomatic, although they may predispose the patient to stasis and subsequent cholelithiasis.[59]

ACUTE GALLBLADDER DISEASES

Biliary Colic.   Gallstones can lead to pain, which patients describe as a steady, intense pain in the right upper quadrant or epigastrium. Some report that the pain radiates to the shoulder. Patients often vomit and classically are restless as they try to achieve a comfortable position. These episodes are usually referred to as biliary colic. Most patients have bouts of biliary colic that last for hours and can recur at random times.[60] Acute episodes of biliary colic present in a similar fashion in children, although a high index of suspicion is needed in young children. Adults can also complain of "dyspeptic" symptoms such as gas and heartburn during these episodes.

Acute Cholecystitis.   If the gallbladder is inflamed and gallstones are present during these painful episodes, this is termed acute cholecystitis. Patients with acute cholecystitis can present with fever and right upper quadrant pain and may be Murphy sign positive. They often display a leukocytosis. If there are no gallstones present but the gallbladder is inflamed, this is termed acute acalculous cholecystitis, and this generally occurs in children with other major medical problems or infections. The clinical features are reviewed further in the section discussing acute acalculous cholecystitis.

CHRONIC GALLBLADDER DISEASES

Chronic Gallstone Disease.   Biliary colic often recurs; however, the acute episodes are short in duration rather than ongoing. A myriad of gastrointestinal complaints have been attributed to the presence of gallstones, such as indigestion, abdominal discomfort, and heartburn. It is important for patients to be aware that cholecystectomy will resolve the abdominal pain associated with episodes of biliary colic but may not resolve all gastrointestinal complaints.

Chronic Acalculous Cholecystitis.   Patients with chronic acalculous cholecystitis, sometimes referred to as gallbladder dyskinesia, can present diagnostic and therapeutic challenges. These otherwise healthy children, often female, can complain of abdominal pain for months to years. The pain is often worse after eating and is localized to the right upper quadrant. Examination and routine workup are generally normal, and it is not until a hepatobiliary scintigraph scan is performed that the diagnosis is made. Excellent symptomatic relief has been reported in children with chronic alcalculous cholecystitis postcholecystectomy.[61]

Sphincter of Oddi Dysfunction.   Those with sphincter of Oddi dysfunction (SOD) have complaints similar to those of patients with gallbladder dyskinesia, but cholecystectomy will not provide relief. When SOD is present, there is effectively an obstruction at the level of the sphincter, which may be caused by fibrosis or inflammation or by elevated sphincter tone. Endoscopic retrograde cholangiopancreatography (ERCP) with manometry provides the diagnosis, and sphincterotomy is the treatment of choice. In 50 healthy adult volunteers, normal basal pressure of the sphincter of Oddi was 14.8 ± 6.3 mm Hg, and no pressure was greater than 40 mm Hg.[62] There are no comparable studies in normal children. SOD can lead to bile duct dilatation without evidence of choledocholithiasis pre- or postcholecystectomy. SOD has also been associated with acute recurrent pancreatitis and biliary colic–type pain in the absence of gallstones.

Gallstones can also lead to pancreatitis, the clinical features of which are reviewed in Chapter 64.1, "Pancreatitis: Acute and Chronic." Gallstones can also lead to obstruction of the common bile duct, causing pain, jaundice, and, if there is infection, fever.

ASSESSMENT OF FUNCTION AND IMAGING OF THE GALLBLADDER

PLAIN ABDOMINAL FILMS

Plain films are not the investigation of choice for suspected gallstones. However, radiopaque stones, which account for 10 to 15% of all stones, can be seen in the gallbladder, common bile duct, and, occasionally, even the intrahepatic ducts and may be noted when the film is taken for other purposes.[63] A rare condition called "milk of calcium cholelithiasis" is associated with dramatic findings on abdominal radiographs. In this condition, bile is primarily composed of calcium carbonate, which is normally found in bones and teeth and is radiopaque. The gallbladder is often clearly seen, filled with multiple calculi. Surgery is curative, and the etiology is unknown.[59]

ULTRASONOGRAPHY

Ultrasonography of the gallbladder and bile ducts has permitted noninvasive and safe imaging of the gallbladder, gallstones, and biliary tree to be performed. Although now firmly established as the investigation of choice, ultrasonography was regarded with some suspicion in the 1970s. Indeed, the authors of one textbook stated that:

"Neither we nor others have been convinced that this modality [ultrasonography] equals, let alone surpasses, currently available techniques."[3] Ultrasonography of the gallbladder is best performed on a patient who has fasted for 4 or more hours. Using a transducer placed on the anterior abdominal wall, the gallbladder is generally found on the undersurface of the liver between the right and left lobes. Rarely, the gallbladder can be found within the liver or underneath the left lobe.[64] Normal gallbladder size varies with fasting status and age. In infants less than 1 year of age, gallbladder length is usually between 1.5 and 3 cm. As shown in Figure 61-3, in older children, gallbladder length is usually 3 to 7 cm.[64,65] The diameter of the common bile duct varies with age. The following are the normal ranges of the common bile duct diameter: less than 1 mm in neonates, less than 2 mm in infants, less than 4 mm in children, and less than 7 mm in adolescents.[64,65] Gallbladder wall thickness increases when inflamed and is found to be greater than 3 mm in 50 to 75% of patients with acute cholecystitis.[64]

In the course of an ultrasonographic examination, the gallbladder is examined for evidence of stones, sludge, masses, distention, and pericholecystic fluid. Sludge, which is actually viscous bile, layers in the dependent part of the lumen and does not form acoustic shadows (Figure 61-4). Sludge moves slowly when the patient changes position.[64] Gallstones are usually mobile within the gallbladder lumen, unless impacted in the cystic or common bile ducts, and are brightly echogenic with posterior acoustic shadows (Figure 61-5).[65] Stones as small as 1 mm can be identified.[63] If gallstones are within the common bile duct, there is usually accompanying ductular dilatation. False-positive and -negative identification of gallstones can occur if the gallbladder is packed full of stones or nearby air-filled bowel loops create acoustic shadows.[64] Gallbladder polyps can be mistaken for gallstones, although they are not as mobile. Overall, ultrasonography

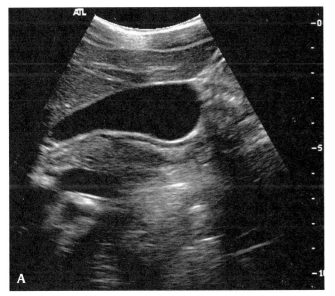
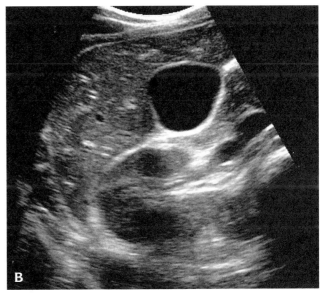

FIGURE 61-3 Ultrasonographic image of a normal gallbladder. A normal gallbladder of a healthy child is shown in two views. *A* shows the longitudinal view of the gallbladder, and *B* shows a cross-sectional view. Courtesy of Dr. Harriet J. Paltiel, Children's Hospital, Boston.

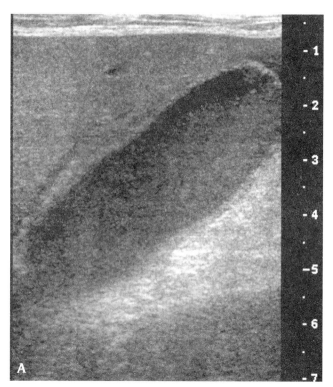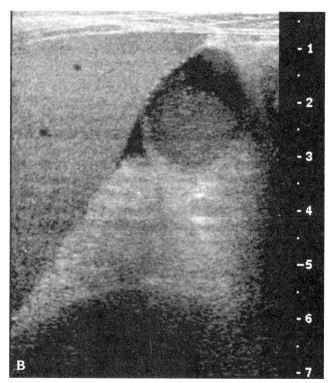

FIGURE 61-4   Ultrasonographic image of biliary sludge. *A* illustrates a child's gallbladder filled with sludge. Sludge does not form acoustic shadows (contrast this with the shadows created by gallstones in Figure 61-5). Sludge moves slowly within the gallbladder when the patient moves during the examination, and the sludge can be seen in a different position within the gallbladder in *B*. Courtesy of Dr. Harriet J. Paltiel, Children's Hospital, Boston.

has a greater than 95% sensitivity and specificity for detecting gallstones.[66]

Cholecystitis on ultrasonography is often associated with a thickened gallbladder wall (> 3 mm), an enlarged gallbladder, gallstones or sludge, and a positive Murphy sign.[64] In addition, signs of potential complications of acute cholecystitis should be sought, such as gangrene, which is suggested by irregularities in the gallbladder wall, or emphysema and perforation, which is suggested by pericholecystic fluid.[65] In chronic cholecystitis, the gallbladder may have all of the above findings or may even appear normal. In adults and very rarely in children, adenomyomatosis or strawberry gallbladder, which is due to diffuse or

focal prominence of Rokitansky-Aschoff sinuses (hyperplastic mucosa extensions into the muscular layer), can cause chronic pain.[67] Hydrops of the gallbladder, also referred to as acute alcalculous cholecystitis, is characterized on ultrasonography by a distended gallbladder without evidence of obstruction or bile duct dilatation. The bile is usually anechoic.

COMPUTED TOMOGRAPHY AND MAGNETIC RESONANCE IMAGING

Other radiologic investigations have a role in the diagnosis of specific complications. Computed tomography (CT) is used to image the pancreas, which may be inflamed sec-

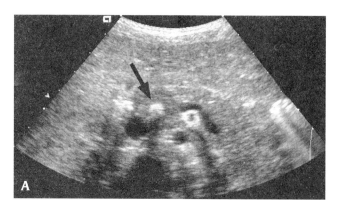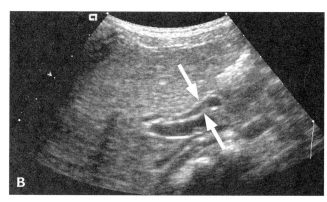

FIGURE 61-5   Ultrasonographic images of a gallstone in the common bile duct. *A*, A transverse image of the pancreas demonstrates an echogenic focus (*black arrow*) in the distal common bile duct with distal shadowing in keeping with a stone. *B* is a longitudinal oblique image of the liver hilum demonstrating dilation of the common bile duct (*between two white arrows*) down to the level of the pancreas. Courtesy of Dr. Harriet J. Paltiel, Children's Hospital, Boston.

ondary to gallstone obstruction of the pancreatic duct, and is also useful for imaging the biliary tree when complications of acute cholecystitis are suspected. It is not as reliable as ultrasonography for detection of gallstones, which may exhibit the same radiographic density as bile and therefore may not be seen on CT.[63] Magnetic resonance imaging of the pancreas and biliary tree (magnetic resonance cholangiopancreatography) is superior to CT for investigation of the anatomy of the hepatobiliary tree and the pancreatic duct. However, ERCP is still the investigation of choice to define the extrahepatic and pancreatic duct systems because there is not only excellent imaging, but therapeutic interventions, such as retrieval of impacted stones from the common bile duct and sphincterotomy, are also possible. ERCP is discussed further under surgical procedures.

RADIONUCLIDE HEPATOBILIARY SCINTIGRAPHY

Radionuclide imaging or scintigraphy plays a role in both the diagnosis of biliary disease and assessment of function. For acute cholecystitis in adults, hepatobiliary scintigraphy (HBS) has both a higher specificity and sensitivity. In a meta-analysis of 27 studies containing almost 3,000 patients, the sensitivity of HBS is 90% and the sensitivity is 97%.[66] The rates for ultrasonography diagnosis are 91% and 79%, respectively. However, the main role of HBS is when ultrasonographic findings are equivocal for acute cholecystitis. A positive test of cholecystitis by HBS is based on a lack of gallbladder visualization. An intravenously administered radioactive pharmaceutical, usually technetium 99m hepatic iminodiacetic acid, is secreted from the liver into the hepatic bile ducts but is unable to enter the gallbladder if the cystic duct is obstructed. The isotope instead enters the small intestine.[68] If the gallbladder is not seen in the first 60 minutes, there are two options: delayed imaging at 4 hours or the more popular administration of morphine. Morphine administration increases pressure at the sphincter of Oddi and forces bile into the gallbladder if the cystic duct is patent. The morphine protocol is more specific, equally sensitive, and completed within 90 minutes.[68] Despite the increased specificity of HBS, ultrasonography is still the test of choice because it allows for evaluation of gallbladder anatomy as well as other abdominal organs. Ultrasonography is also less invasive and less expensive and involves no exposure to radioactivity.

Radionuclide imaging also can play a role in the diagnosis of both acute and chronic alcalculous cholecystitis. A prospective study comparing ultrasonography and radionuclide imaging in adults with acute alcalculous cholecystitis found a sensitivity of 70% and a specificity of 100% for radionuclide scanning in association with ultrasonography.[69] Gangrene and perforation, both complications of acute acalculous cholecystitis, can be identified on HBS by spill of radionuclide into the peritoneal cavity.[68] HBS is useful for diagnosis of chronic alcalculous cholecystitis, also referred to as gallbladder dyskinesia or spasm. Cholecystokinin (CCK) is administered during the study. Poor contractility of the gallbladder in response to CCK is the hallmark of chronic acalculous cholecystitis. If the gallbladder ejection fraction is less than 35% in a patient with

a clinical history suggestive of chronic alcalculous cholecystitis, there is a greater than 90% positive predictive value.[68] False decreases can occur in patients with diabetes and celiac disease and in pregnancy, as well as in those receiving morphine and octreotide. Sphincter of Oddi spasm or bile duct dyskinesia has clinical symptoms similar to those of chronic alcalculous cholecystitis and an abnormal response to CCK—sphinchter contraction rather than dilatation. However, the best test for this condition is sphincter manometry. Finally, HBS is useful postcholecystectomy to detect bile leak complications.

MISCELLANEOUS IMAGING TECHNIQUES

The other available modalities to investigate the anatomy of the biliary tree are used much more rarely nowadays. Oral cholecystography has been superseded by ultrasonography for the detection of gallstones, and T tube cholangiography is performed infrequently in this era of laparoscopic cholecystectomies. Highly specialized interventions such as transhepatic cholangiography for investigation of strictures are still performed in the proper clinical setting.

ROLE OF ERCP

ERCP in children is not a trivial procedure because general anesthesia is generally required in young children and infants.[70] The techniques of this procedure are reviewed in detail in Chapter 67.5, "Endoscopic Retrograde Cholangiopancreatography." The roles of ERCP in gallbladder disease in children are to remove common bile duct stones in choledolithiasis, measure sphincter of Oddi pressure, and, occasionally, delineate anatomy. Children undergoing ERCP because of biliary pathology have been reported to have higher complication rates than do adults. In one reported series of 15 such children, 6 presented with pancreatitis and 1 with bleeding post-ERCP.[70] A second group emphasized the role of ERCP with sphincterotomy and stone removal in children with common bile duct stones.

ERCP is also used to perform manometry at the sphincter of Oddi to make the diagnosis of SOD. A sphincterotomy can be performed at the same time if the diagnosis is confirmed.

CHOICE OF IMAGING METHODS

The best imaging method for a child with suspected gallbladder disease depends on the suspected condition. The imaging methods of choice for a number of different gallbladder diseases are outlined in Table 61-2.

SURGICAL MANAGEMENT OF CHOLELITHIASIS

Laparoscopic cholecystectomy is currently the procedure of choice in children requiring cholecystectomy.[71] There is evidence to indicate that laparoscopic cholecystectomy patients have a shorter hospital stay and less analgesic requirements than their open cholecystectomy counterparts.[72] Open cholecystectomy is reserved for the few children in whom laparoscopic cholecystectomy is a relative contraindication or when it cannot be completed safely.

TABLE 61-2   IMAGING METHODS OF THE HEPATOBILIARY TRACT FOR DIFFERENT CLINICAL SITUATIONS

| | IMAGING METHOD OF CHOICE | | | | | |
DISEASE PROCESS	ULTRASONOGRAPHY	RADIONUCLIDE IMAGING	CT	MRI/ MRCP	ERCP	MISCELLANEOUS
Cholelithiasis	+++					
Acute cholecystitis	+++	++ (may need delayed imaging and/or intravenous morphine)				
Acute acalculous cholecystitis	++	+				
Chronic acalculous cholecystitis	+	+++ (with CCK)				
Sphincter of Oddi spasm	+	++ (with CCK)			+++ (sphincter manometry)	
Biliary leak postcholecystectomy	+	+++	+			
Bile duct obstruction	+++	++	++	+++	+++	Depending on site of obstruction, intraoperative cholangiogram or transhepatic cholangiogram may be required

CCK = cholecystokinin; CT = computed tomography; ERCP = endoscopic retrograde cholangiopancreatography; MRCP = magnetic resonance cholangiopancreatography; MRI = magnetic rseonance imaging.

Laparoscopic cholecystectomy is performed under general anesthesia with the patient in the supine position. An insufflation needle is introduced into the peritoneal cavity, with great care to prevent inadvertent visceral or vascular injury,[73] or a trochar may be introduced under direct vision to prevent damage to adjacent structures. After insufflation of the peritoneal cavity with carbon dioxide, a camera is introduced that allows the introduction of additional working ports under direct vision. Calot triangle is exposed by retracting the gallbladder up and over the liver[71] and freeing pericholecystic adhesions. Blunt dissection of the cystic duct is begun at the neck of the gallbladder, and the cystic duct–common duct junction is delineated. Clips are carefully applied to the cystic duct prior to its division before turning attention to the cystic artery, which is then clipped and ligated. The peritoneum of the gallbladder is then incised and is then freed from the gallbladder bed using hook cautery,[71] and the gallbladder is removed.

Children may also display gallstones in the common bile duct choledocholithiasis. Preoperative findings suggestive of this are listed in Table 61–3. Waldhausen and colleagues recommend routine use of intraoperative cholangiography.[74] They ultimately identified common bile duct stones in 18 of 100 patients studied and found preoperative suspicion of choledocholithiasis in 20 patients. The suspicion was based on finding one or more of the following abnormalities: ultrasonographic evidence of a dilated common or intrahepatic bile duct or identification of a specific common duct stone (6 patients), biochemical abnormalities consisting of elevated liver function tests (9 patients), elevated amylase and lipase (10 patients), or conjugated hyperbilirubinemia (2 patients). Fifteen of the 20 patients suspected preoperatively were confirmed to have evidence of

choledocholithiasis based on intraoperative cholangiography or ERCP; no stones were found in five. Three additional children in their series were found to have cholangiographic evidence of choledocholithiasis, which had not been predicted on preoperative evaluation. They concluded that intraoperative cholangiography should be performed routinely and ERCP should be reserved for patients in whom common duct stones are identified and the surgeon prefers not to perform laparoscopic or open common duct exploration. However, Newman and colleagues do not recommend routine intraoperative cholangiography but rather preoperative blood work, ultrasonography, and ERCP as indicated.[75] In their series of 117 children undergoing cholecystectomy, 14 were suspected to have common bile duct stones, of which 8 patients were confirmed at the time of ERCP. One child was found at the time of surgery to have a common bile duct stone not identified preoperatively. Therefore, 7 children were incorrectly identified in this series of 117 children (6 false-positives and 1 false-negative) as having or not having stones in the common bile duct on the basis of preoperative examination and bloodwork. These authors do not recommend routine intraoperative cholangiography because only 9 of 117 children actually had stones in the common bile duct, and 8 of these were suspected preoperatively.[75]

TABLE 61-3   PREOPERATIVE FINDINGS SUGGESTIVE OF COMMON BILE DUCT STONES

Jaundice
Elevated canalicular enzymes
Pancreatitis
Dilated common bile duct on ultrasonography
Dilated intrahepatic bile ducts on ultrasonography

Laparoscopic cholecystectomy is associated with 3 to 4 times the risk of injury to the biliary tree compared with open cholecystectomy.[76] The key factor is prevention of this serious complication by correctly identifying the cystic duct and artery. If a biliary injury is recognized intraoperatively, it is recommended to convert to an open surgical approach to repair the injury.[76] If injuries of this nature are not recognized immediately, however, they may present days or months later with the triad of fever, pain, and jaundice. ERCP can play a vital role in the diagnosis and treatment of these complications.[77] If the common bile duct or one of its major branches is transected, a hepaticojejunostomy by an experienced hepatobiliary surgeon is the standard of care.

CONTRAINDICATIONS TO LAPAROSCOPIC CHOLECYSTECTOMY

Recently, absolute contraindications for laparoscopic cholecystectomy have dramatically decreased as operative skills, experience, and equipment have developed. Hemodynamic instability, irreversible coagulopathy, and third-trimester pregnancy remain as absolute contraindications.[78] Situations that require special expertise but do not preclude laparoscopic cholecystectomy are acute gallstone pancreatitis, prior upper abdominal surgery, and second-trimester pregnancy.[79]

MEDICAL MANAGEMENT OF CHOLELITHIASIS

The advent of laparoscopic cholecystectomy has essentially eliminated medical management of gallstones. Moreover, because medical therapy targets cholesterol gallstones only, children were generally unsuitable candidates, and, indeed, no reported studies have been performed in children. Nonsurgical therapy consists of either administration of bile salts or extracorporeal shock wave lithotripsy. Ursodeoxycholic acid and chenodeoxycholic acid are two bile salts that have been used. Both of these bile salts decrease cholesterol secretion into bile so that bile becomes desaturated of cholesterol.[80] Chenodeoxycholic acid in therapeutic doses leads to diarrhea in 50% of patients and dissolved gallstones in only 14.5% of adult patients treated for 2 years.[81] Ursodeoxycholic acid treatment is associated with less diarrhea and better stone dissolution rates than chenodeoxycholic acid, up to 40% at 2 years,[80] but is rarely used for this indication now. Extracorporeal shock wave lithotripsy has been used in association with administration of bile acids to disintegrate stones. This strategy did lead to dissolution of both solitary and multiple stones in 91% of patients, but the gallbladder remains in place, and stones can therefore recur.[82]

NONGALLSTONE DISEASES OF THE GALLBLADDER

ACALCULOUS CHOLECYSTITIS

Acalculous cholecystitis, an uncommon condition in children, can be divided into two distinct clinical entities: acute, with symptoms of less than 1 month in duration, and chronic, with symptoms lasting more than 1 month.[83] Acute acalculous cholecystitis is characteristically associ-

ated with a concurrent systemic infection or recent surgery or trauma, whereas the chronic form is not. The condition appears to develop when the gallbladder either contracts or cannot empty its contents. Specific risk factors are prolonged fasting, parenteral nutrition, and sepsis. Children with acute alcalculous cholecystitis present with fever, right upper quadrant pain, and vomiting and exhibit abdominal tenderness on examination.[83,84] Leukocytosis and elevated bilirubin are also common. Ultrasonography diagnosis of acute acalculous cholecystitis requires gallbladder wall thickness greater than 3.5 mm, hydrops, sludge, and pericholecystic fluid.[83] These children often have associated illnesses such as infections like *Salmonella typhi*[85,86] or infective endocarditis[87] or a systemic disease such as Kawasaki disease.[83] A history of recent surgery or trauma is common. Treatment of acute acalculous cholecystitis involves serial examinations, gallbladder ultrasonography, and cholecystectomy when indicated by deteriorating clinical or ultrasonographic findings.[84] The histopathologic findings of gallbladders resected from children with acute acalculous cholecystitis range from edema and focal hemorrhage to gangrene.[83] For children who can be managed conservatively by active observation and antibiotic administration, the gallbladder will eventually return to normal function.

In contrast, children with chronic acalculous cholecystitis are generally female, are otherwise healthy, have a history of right upper quadrant pain that may be associated with nausea and vomiting, and have normal serum white cell counts and bilirubin.[83] The gallbladder is normal on ultrasonography, and the test of choice for diagnosis is a CCK-stimulated HBS.[60] This test measures the gallbladder ejection fraction, which is decreased with chronic acalculous cholecystitis. In adults, less than 35% is considered diagnostic; a comparable figure is not known in children.[68] Two reported series of children have shown good reduction in symptoms in children postcholecystectomy. In one study, following laparoscopic cholecystectomy, 70% of children had complete resolution of symptoms and 18% had partial relief.[61] In a second study, cholecystectomy, either laparoscopically or open, led to complete resolution of symptoms.[83]

GALLBLADDER MASSES

Gallbladder masses are, fortunately, very rare in children so are discussed only briefly.

Benign Masses of the Gallbladder. Benign masses of the gallbladder are extremely rare in children and are usually polyps.[88,89] There are four main types of polyps: cholesterol ones, which arise from infiltration of lipid-laden macrophages into lamina propria; inflammatory polyps composed of granulation and fibrous tissue; adenomyoma, which arise when adenomyomatosis is confined to the fundus of the gallbladder; and adenomas.[90] Lipomas can also be found rarely in the gallbladder.[90,91] Adenomas of the gallbladder are usually solitary and may be associated with gallstones. It is not clear if they are premalignant, like adenomas of the colon. Patients with polyps of all types can present with symptoms and signs suggestive of biliary colic, and ultrasonography may not be able to distinguish polyp type. Endoscopic ultrasonography may play a role in increasing preoperative identification of the polyp type. In a study of 182 Chinese patients aged 15 to 84 years, the sensitivity of transabdominal ultrasonography at detecting polyps was 90.1%. Of the 182 patients, 172 had polyps at the time of surgery, of which 159 were benign lesions and 13 were malignant.[91] These authors suggest surgical resection of polypoid lesions greater than 1 cm in diameter and of solitary lesions and in those older than 50 years.[91] Gallbladder polyps have been reported in three patients with Peutz-Jeghers syndrome in Germany, and conservative management is recommended unless there are symptoms suggestive of biliary colic.[92]

Malignant Tumors of the Gallbladder. Gallbladder carcinoma arises in those with a history of acute or chronic cholecystitis. It appears that chronic inflammation is necessary for this tumor to develop; it is, therefore, rare in childhood and adults under 50 years. Incidental adenocarcinoma of the gallbladder is found in 0.1 to 0.5% of adults undergoing laparoscopic cholecystectomy for gallstones and 1 to 2% of those undergoing open cholecystectomies.[93] For most patients with gallbladder cancer, however, the prognosis is poor because only 5% survive 5 years after diagnosis.[93,94] Approximately 80% of gallbladder carcinomas are adenocarcinomas and are associated with abnormal expression of *TP53*, the tumor suppressor gene.[95] Squamous cell adenocanthoma accounts for the remaining 20% of gallbladder cancers.[94] Radical cholecystectomy, ERCP placement of stents into the hepatic and common bile ducts if necessary, and palliative radiotherapy all play a role. For those found to have incidental adenocarcinomas confined to the mucosa and with lymph node metastases at the time of cholecystectomy, the cholecystectomy itself can be curative.[94]

Congenital Abnormalities of the Gallbladder. Congenital anomalies of the gallbladder are also rare, and although they may predispose the patient to inflammation and cholelithiasis, they are often found only incidentally during abdominal imaging or surgery.

Absent Gallbladder. The gallbladder can be absent, without any apparent symptoms, or can be associated with other conditions, such as extrahepatic biliary atresia. In biliary atresia, the gallbladder either fails to vacuolize from a solid state during development or postnatally becomes obstructed or obliterated. Because the mechanism of biliary atresia is unknown, the cause of the absent or "rudimentary" gallbladder also remains speculative. The gallbladder may appear to be absent in cystic fibrosis, in which recurrent attacks of cholecystitis can lead to fibrosis and/or atrophy of the gallbladder.[96]

Double Gallbladder. There are a number of forms of this anomaly. There can be a true duplicate set of gallbladders, each with its own cystic duct, which arise from an outpouching of the hepatic or common bile duct. If the pouch derives from the cystic duct, there are two gallbladders but only one cystic duct. A bilobed gallbladder appears to be similar, with two gallbladder fundi but only

one cystic duct, but this anomaly arises from a duplication of the single bud, which normally develops into the gallbladder. All of the above anomalies are rare and are usually asymptomatic.[97]

Miscellaneous. The gallbladder can be abnormally folded during development, and the appearance on cholecystograms of the folded gallbladder is that of a type of bonnet or "phrygian cap," for which the condition is named.[97] The gallbladder empties and functions normally.[2] The development of ducts can also be abnormal, and 20% of people have an aberrant insertion of the cystic duct into the common hepatic duct.[97] The cystic artery, which usually arises from the right hepatic artery, can arise aberrantly from the left. These anomalies are of great importance during cholecystectomy. Finally, the position of the gallbladder can vary; in situs inversus, the gallbladder is in a normal relationship with the liver, but the liver is now on the left side of the abdominal cavity. The gallbladder can appear to be buried in the liver or it can be excessively mobile, which increases the risk of torsion. The latter two anomalies are important for radiologic interpretation.

CONCLUSION

Gallbladder disease in children is an uncommon, although not rare, problem. Clinicians are reporting increased numbers of cholecystectomies in children. It is not yet clear if this represents a true increase in the incidence of gallstones in children or more ready access to laparoscopy. However, the current epidemic of childhood obesity is likely to lead to an increased frequency of cholesterol gallstone disease either in adolescence or early adulthood, and we will all become more familiar with this disease.

REFERENCES

1. Warsaw I. Chemo Memo. Poet's corner. JAMA 1975;231: 1260.
2. Modlin IM. The evolution of therapy in gastroenterology; a vintage of digestion. Axcan Pharma Inc; 2002.
3. Hatfield PM, Wise RE. Radiology of the gallbladder and bile ducts. Baltimore: Williams and Wilkins Company; 1976.
4. Arey LB. Developmental anatomy; a textbook and laboratory manual of embryology. Philadelphia: WB Saunders Co; 1954.
5. American Gastroenterological Association. The burden of gastrointestinal diseases. Bethesda (MD): American Gastroenterological Association; 2001. p. 41–60.
6. Boyer JL, Nathanson MH. Bile formation. In: Schiff ER, Sorrell MF, Maddrey WC, editors. Schiff's diseases of the liver. Vol. 1. 8th ed. Philadelphia: Lippincott-Raven Publishers; 1999. p. 119–46.
7. Erlinger S. New insights into the mechanisms of hepatic transport and bile secretion. J Gastroenterol Hepatol 1996;11: 575–9.
8. Waitman AM, Dyck WP, Janowitz HD. Effect of secretin and acetazolamide on the volume and electrolyte composition of hepatic bile in man. Gastroenterology 1969;56:286–94.
9. Palasciano G, Portincasa P, Vinciguerra V, et al. Gallstone prevalence and gallbladder volume in children and adolescents: an epidemiological ultrasonographic survey and relationship to body mass index. Am J Gastroenterol 1989;84:1378–82.

10. Everhart JE, Khare M, Hill M, Maurer KR. Prevalence and ethnic differences in gallbladder disease in the United States. Gastroenterology 1999;117:632–9.

11. Sampliner RE, Bennett PH, Comess LJ, et al. Gallbladder disease in Pima Indians. Demonstration of high prevalence and early onset by cholecystography. N Engl J Med 1970;283:1358–64.

12. Thistle JL, Schoenfield LJ. Lithogenic bile among young Indian women. N Engl J Med 1971;284:177–81.

13. Bennion LJ, Knowler WC, Mott DM, et al. Development of lithogenic bile during puberty in Pima Indians. N Engl J Med 1979;300:873–6.

14. Von Bergmann K, Becker M, Leiss O. Biliary cholesterol saturation in non-obese women and non-obese men before and after puberty. Eur J Clin Invest 1986;16:531–5.

15. Heubi JE, Soloway RD, Balistreri WF. Biliary lipid composition in healthy and diseased infants, children, and young adults. Gastroenterology 1982;82:1295–9.

16. Von Bergmann J, Von Bergmann K, Hadorn B, Paumgartner G. Biliary lipid composition in early childhood. Clin Chim Acta 1975;64:241–6.

17. Halpern Z, Vinograd Z, Laufer H, et al. Characteristics of gallbladder bile of infants and children. J Pediatr Gastroenterol Nutr 1996;23:147–50.

18. Carey MC. Pathogenesis of gallstones. Am J Surg 1993;165:410–9.

19. Shoda J, Oda K, Suzuki H, et al. Etiologic significance of defects in cholesterol, phospholipid, and bile acid metabolism in the liver of patients with intrahepatic calculi. Hepatology 2001;33:1194–205.

20. Donovan JM. Physical and metabolic factors in gallstone pathogenesis. Gastroenterol Clin North Am 1999;28:75–97.

21. Graf GA, Li WP, Gerard RD, et al. Coexpression of ATP-binding cassette proteins ABCG5 and ABCG8 permits their transport to the apical surface. J Clin Invest 2002;110:659–69.

22. Yu L, Hammer RE, Li-Hawkins J, et al. Disruption of Abcg5 and Abcg8 in mice reveals their crucial role in biliary cholesterol secretion. Proc Natl Acad Sci U S A 2002;99:16237–42.

23. Wittenburg H, Carey MC. Biliary cholesterol secretion by the twinned sterol half-transporters ABCG5 and ABCG8. J Clin Invest 2002;110:605–9.

24. Gerloff T, Stieger B, Hagenbuch B, et al. The sister of P-glycoprotein represents the canalicular bile salt export pump of mammalian liver. J Biol Chem 1998;273:10046–50.

25. van Helvoort A, Smith AJ, Sprong H, et al. MDR1 P-glycoprotein is a lipid translocase of broad specificity, while MDR3 P-glycoprotein specifically translocates phosphatidylcholine. Cell 1996;87:507–17.

26. Carey MC, Lamont JT. Cholesterol gallstone formation. 1. Physical chemistry of bile and biliary lipid secretion. Prog Liver Dis 1992;10:139–63.

27. Hofmann AF, Grundy SM, Lachin JM, et al. Pretreatment biliary lipid composition in white patients with radiolucent gallstones in the National Cooperative Gallstone Study. Gastroenterology 1982;83:738–52.

28. Rosmorduc O, Hermelin B, Poupon R. MDR3 gene defect in adults with symptomatic intrahepatic and gallbladder cholesterol cholelithiasis. Gastroenterology 2001;120:1459–67.

29. Jacquemin E, De Vree JML, Cresteil D, et al. The wide spectrum of multidrug resistance 3 deficiency: from neonatal cholestasis to cirrhosis of adulthood. Gastroenterology 2001;120:1448–58.

30. Holzbach R, Busch N. Nucleation and growth of cholesterol crystals. Gastroenterol Clin North Am 1991;20:67–84.

31. Harvey PR, Upadhya GA, Strasberg SM. Immunoglobulins as nucleating proteins in the gallbladder bile of patients with cholesterol gallstones. J Biol Chem 1991;266:13996–4003.

32. Offner GD, Gong D, Afdhal NH. Identification of a 130-kilodalton human biliary concanavalin A binding protein as aminopeptidase N. Gastroenterology 1994;106:755–62.

33. Chijiiwa K, Koga A, Yamasaki T, et al. Fibronectin: a possible factor promoting cholesterol monohydrate crystallization in bile. Biochim Biophys Acta 1991;1086:44–8.

34. Kibe A, Holzbach RT, LaRusso NF, Mao SJ. Inhibition of cholesterol crystal formation by apolipoproteins in supersaturated model bile. Science 1984;225:514–6.

35. Cahalane MJ, Neubrand MW, Carey MC. Physical-chemical pathogenesis of pigment gallstones. Semin Liver Dis 1988;8:317–28.

36. Brink MA, Méndez-Sánchez N, Carey MC. Bilirubin cycles enterohepatically after ileal resection in the rat. Gastroenterology 1996;110:1945–57.

37. Méndez-Sánchez N, Brink MA, Paigen B, Carey MC. Ursodeoxycholic acid and cholesterol induce enterohepatic cycling of bilirubin in rodents. Gastroenterology 1998;115:722–32.

38. Kaufman HS, Magnuson TH, Lillemoe KD, et al. The role of bacteria in gallbladder and common duct stone formation. Ann Surg 1989;209:584–91; discussion 591–2.

39. Lammert F, Carey MC, Paigen B. Chromosomal organization of candidate genes involved in cholesterol gallstone formation: a murine gallstone map. Gastroenterology 2001;120:221–38.

40. Carey MC, Paigen B. Epidemiology of the American Indians' burden and its likely genetic origins. Hepatology 2002;36:781–91.

41. Bouchard G, Nelson HM, Lammert F, et al. High-resolution maps of the murine chromosome 2 region containing the cholesterol gallstone locus, Lith1. Mamm Genome 1999;10:1070–4.

42. Muller M, Roelofsen H, Jansen PL. Secretion of organic anions by hepatocytes: involvement of homologues of the multidrug resistance protein. Semin Liver Dis 1996;16:211–20.

43. Lammert F, Wang DQ, Wittenburg H, et al. Lith genes control mucin accumulation, cholesterol crystallization, and gallstone formation in A/J and AKR/J inbred mice. Hepatology 2002;36:1145–54.

44. Dennis C, Goodman B. Cholelithiasis in persons under 25 years old. JAMA 1976;236:1731–2.

45. Reif S, Sloven DG, Lebenthal E. Gallstones in children. Characterization by age, etiology, and outcome. Am J Dis Child 1991;145:105–8.

46. Rennels MB, Dunne MG, Grossman NJ, Schwartz AD. Cholelithiasis in patients with major sickle hemoglobinopathies. Am J Dis Child 1984;138:66–7.

47. Haberkern CM, Neumayr LD, Orringer EP, et al. Cholecystectomy in sickle cell anemia patients: perioperative outcome of 364 cases from the National Preoperative Transfusion Study. Preoperative Transfusion in Sickle Cell Disease Study Group. Blood 1997;89:1533–42.

48. Caprotti R, Franciosi C, Romano F, et al. Combined laparoscopic splenectomy and cholecystectomy for the treatment of hereditary spherocytosis: is it safe and effective? Surg Laparosc Endosc Percutan Tech 1999;9:203–6.

49. Williams HJ, Johnson KW. Cholelithiasis: a complication of cardiac valve surgery in children. Pediatr Radiol 1984;14:146–7.

50. Brink MA, Slors JF, Keulemans YC, et al. Enterohepatic cycling of bilirubin: a putative mechanism for pigment gallstone formation in ileal Crohn's disease. Gastroenterology 1999;116:1420–7.

51. Broderick A, Wittenburg H, Setchell K, Carey M. In cystic fibro-

sis (CF), enterohepatic cycling of bilirubin contributes to pigment gallstone formation and chronic liver disease: studies in mice with delta F508 and G551D mutations of the cystic transmembrane conductance regulator (CFTR). Gastroenterology 2002;122:A178.

52. Colombo C, Apostolo MG, Ferrari M, et al. Analysis of risk factors for the development of liver disease associated with cystic fibrosis. J Pediatr 1994;124:393–9.

53. King DR, Ginn-Pease ME, Lloyd TV, et al. Parenteral nutrition with associated cholelithiasis: another iatrogenic disease of infants and children. J Pediatr Surg 1987;22:593–6.

54. Friesen CA, Roberts CC. Cholelithiasis. Clinical characteristics in children. Case analysis and literature review. Clin Pediatr (Phila) 1989;28:294–8.

55. Whitington PF, Black DD. Cholelithiasis in premature infants treated with parenteral nutrition and furosemide. J Pediatr 1980;97:647–9.

56. Sakopoulos AG, Gundry S, Razzouk AJ, et al. Cholelithiasis in infant and pediatric heart transplant patients. Pediatr Transplant 2002;6:231–4.

57. Toscano E, Trivellini V, Andria G. Cholelithiasis in Down's syndrome. Arch Dis Child 2001;85:242–3.

58. Mahmoud H, Schell M, Pui CH. Cholelithiasis after treatment for childhood cancer. Cancer 1991;67:1439–42.

59. Wu SS, Casas AT, Abraham SK, et al. Milk of calcium cholelithiasis in children. J Pediatr Surg 2001;36:644–7.

60. Diehl AK. Symptoms of gallstone disease. In: Sackmann M, editor. Diagnosis and management of biliary stones. Vol. 6. London: Bailliere Tindall; 1992. p. 635–57.

61. Michail S, Preud'Homme D, Christian J, et al. Laparoscopic cholecystectomy: effective treatment for chronic abdominal pain in children with acalculous biliary pain. J Pediatr Surg 2001;36:1394–6.

62. Guelrud M, Mendoza S, Rossiter G, Villegas MI. Sphincter of Oddi manometry in healthy volunteers. Dig Dis Sci 1990;35:38–46.

63. Zeman RK, Garra BS. Gallbladder imaging: the state of the art. In: Cooper AD, editor. Pathogenesis and therapy of gallstone disease. Gastroenterol Clin North Am 1991;20:127–56.

64. Carty HML, Crawford SF, Higham JB. Paediatric ultrasound. London: Greenwich Medical Media Ltd.; 2001.

65. Gubernick JA, Rosenberg HK, Ilaslan H, Kessler A. US approach to jaundice in infants and children. Radiographics 2000;20:173–95.

66. Shea JA, Berlin JA, Escarce JJ, et al. Revised estimates of diagnostic test sensitivity and specificity in suspected biliary tract disease. Arch Intern Med 1994;154:2573–81.

67. Alberti D, Callea F, Camoni G, et al. Adenomyomatosis of the gallbladder in childhood. J Pediatr Surg 1998;33:1411–2.

68. Lin EC, Kuni CC. Radionuclide imaging of hepatic and biliary disease. Semin Liver Dis 2001;21:179–94.

69. Prevot N, Mariat G, Mahul P, et al. Contribution of cholescintigraphy to the early diagnosis of acute acalculous cholecystitis in intensive-care-unit patients. Eur J Nucl Med 1999;26:1317–25.

70. Prasil P, Laberge JM, Barkun A, Flageole H. Endoscopic retrograde cholangiopancreatography in children: a surgeon's perspective. J Pediatr Surg 2001;36:733–5.

71. Davidoff AM, Branum GD, Murray EA, et al. The technique of laparoscopic cholecystectomy in children. Ann Surg 1992;215:186–91.

72. Kim PC, Wesson D, Superina R, Filler R. Laparoscopic cholecystectomy versus open cholecystectomy in children: which is better? J Pediatr Surg 1995;30:971–3.

73. Holcomb GW III. Laparoscopic cholecystectomy. Pediatr Ann 1993;22:657–62.

74. Waldhausen JH, Graham DD, Tapper D. Routine intraoperative cholangiography during laparoscopic cholecystectomy minimizes unnecessary endoscopic retrograde cholangiopancreatography in children. J Pediatr Surg 2001;36:881–4.

75. Newman KD, Powell DM, Holcomb GW III. The management of choledocholithiasis in children in the era of laparoscopic cholecystectomy. J Pediatr Surg 1997;32:1116–9.

76. Strasberg SM. Laparoscopic biliary surgery. Gastroenterol Clin North Am 1999;28:117–32, vii.

77. Siegel J, Cohen S, Kasmin F. Managment of laparoscopic cholecystectomy complications. Clin Perspect Gastroenterol 2002;Sept/Oct:287–91.

78. Bordoni L, Ginelli F, Miglierina T, et al. Laparoscopic cholecystectomy as elective approach to cholelithiasis. A six year experience of 653 patients compared to a multi-centred Italian study. Int J Surg 1999;6:97–101.

79. Curet M. Special problems in laparoscopic surgery. Previous abdominal surgery, obesity and pregnancy. Surg Clin North Am 2000;2000:1093–110.

80. Salen G, Tint GS, Shefer S. Treatment of cholesterol gallstones with litholytic bile acids. Gastroenterol Clin North Am 1991;20:171–82.

81. Schoenfield LJ, Lachin JM. Chenodiol (chenodeoxycholic acid) for dissolution of gallstones. The National Cooperative Gallstone Study, A controlled trial of efficacy and safety. Ann Intern Med 1981;95:257–82.

82. Sackmann M, Delius M, Sauerbruch T, et al. Shock-wave lithotripsy of gallbladder stones. The first 175 patients. N Engl J Med 1988;318:393–7.

83. Tsakayannis DE, Kozakewich HP, Lillehei CW. Acalculous cholecystitis in children. J Pediatr Surg 1996;31:127–30; discussion 130–1.

84. Imamoglu M, Sarihan H, Sari A, Ahmetoglu A. Acute acalculous cholecystitis in children: diagnosis and treatment. J Pediatr Surg 2002;37:36–9.

85. Winkler AP, Gleich S. Acute acalculous cholecystitis caused by *Salmonella typhi* in an 11-year-old. Pediatr Infect Dis J 1988;7:125–8.

86. Rao SD, Lewin S, Shetty B, et al. Acute acalculous cholecystitis in typhoid fever. Indian Pediatr 1992;29:1431–5.

87. Richard B, Nadal D, Meuli M, Braegger CP. Acute acalculous cholecystitis in infective endocarditis. J Pediatr Gastroenterol Nutr 1993;17:215–6.

88. Barzilai M, Lerner A. Gallbladder polyps in children: a rare condition. Pediatr Radiol 1997;27:54–6.

89. Stringel G, Beneck D, Bostwick HE. Polypoid lesions of the gallbladder in children. JSLS 1997;1:247–9.

90. Bilhartz LE. Acute acalculous cholecystitis, adenomyomatosis, cholesterolosis, and polyps of the bladder. In: Feldman M, Scharschmidt BF, Sleisenger MH, editors. Sleisinger and Fordtran's gastrointestinal and liver disease. Vol. 1. 6th ed. Philadelphia: WB Saunders Company; 1998. p. 993–1005.

91. Yang HL, Sun YG, Wang Z. Polypoid lesions of the gallbladder: diagnosis and indications for surgery. Br J Surg 1992;79:227–9.

92. Vogel T, Schumacher V, Saleh A, et al. Extraintestinal polyps in Peutz-Jeghers syndrome: presentation of four cases and review of the literature. Deutsche Peutz-Jeghers-Studiengruppe. Int J Colorectal Dis 2000;15:118–23.

93. Sheth S, Bedford A, Chopra S. Primary gallbladder cancer: recognition of risk factors and the role of prophylactic cholecystectomy. Am J Gastroenterol 2000;95:1402–10.

94. Cello JP. Tumors of the gallbladder, bile ducts, and ampulla. In: Feldman M, Scharschmidt BF, Sleisenger MH, editors. Sleisen-

ger and Fordtran's gastrointestinal and liver disease. Vol. 1. Philadelphia: WB Saunders Company; 1998. p. 1026–32.

95. Diamantis I, Karamitopoulou E, Perentes E, Zimmermann A. p53 protein immunoreactivity in extrahepatic bile duct and gallbladder cancer: correlation with tumor grade and survival. Hepatology 1995;22:774–9.

96. Mowat AP. Liver disorders in childhood. 3rd ed. Boston (MA): Butterworth-Heinemann; 1994.

97. Sherlock S, Dooley J. Cysts and congenital biliary abnormalities. In: Diseases of the liver and biliary system. 9th ed. Oxford: Blackwell Scientific Publications; 1993. p. 548–61.

98. Kalayci AG, Albayrak D, Gunes M, et al. The incidence of gallbladder stones and gallbladder function in beta-thalassemic children. Acta Radiol 1999;40:440–3.

99. Lee SS, Wasiljew BD, Lee MJ. Gallstones in women younger than thirty. J Clin Gastroenterol 1987;9:65–9.

CHAPTER 62

CONGENITAL ANOMALIES

Dominique M. Jan, MD

Congenital abnormalities of the pancreas are rare. These anomalies are more commonly discovered at endoscopy, at surgery, or by imagery. This chapter focuses on the congenital malformations of the pancreas, which could lead to clinical findings.

EMBRYOLOGY OF THE PANCREAS

Human pancreatic development has been known since the work of Streeter in 1942.[1] The pancreas forms as a result of the fusion of the two buds, which arise from the dorsal and ventral aspects of the distal foregut. Owing to craniocaudal development, the dorsal pancreas develops ahead of the ventral pancreas. The ventral bud forms the dominant pancreatic and the bile duct. The ventral pancreas rotates clockwise around the duodenal axis. The rotation of the duodenum is the result of duodenal growth. In the normal course of development, between the 8 and 12 mm stages (the fourth to sixth week), the common duct and the right portion of the ventral bud are carried dorsally around the circumference of the duodenum to lie adjacent to the dorsal pancreatic bud. This rotation is the result of duodenal growth, during which all enlargement is on the ventral side only. Thus, the dorsal pancreatic bud forms the anterior part of the head of the pancreas, the body, and the tail of the pancreas.[2] The ventral pancreatic bud forms the posterior part of the head of the pancreas and the posterior part of the uncinate process. The ventral bud is divided into right and left portions; the left portion atrophies, whereas the right portion is moved posteriorly by its connection to the bile duct. The dorsal and the ventral duct systems fuse so that most of the longer dorsal duct drains into the proximal part of the ventral duct to form the main pancreatic duct (duct of Wirsung). If the proximal portion of the dorsal duct remains, it forms an accessory duct (duct of Santorini). The fusion of the ducts occurs during the second month of development. Failure of the dorsal and ventral ducts of the fetal pancreas to fuse leads to pancreas divisum.

More recently, tissue culture and recombination experiments have shown that commitment to a pancreatic fate occurs before morphologic evidence of pancreatic development as early as embryonic day 5-8 in mice and stage 11 in chickens.[3] Experiments in mouse and chicken embryos have revealed that permissive signals secreted by adjacent mesodermal structures (notochord, aorta, and cardiac mesoderm) are important for the pancreatic program. The dorsal foregut (giving rise to the pancreas) is in close contact with the notochord. The ventral foregut is in close contact with the cardiac mesoderm (Figures 62-1 and 62-2).

Initial bud formation relies on different genes dorsally and ventrally. The expression of the homeobox gene *Hlxb9* is necessary to the dorsal bud formation.[4] The gene is active by controlling the expression of signaling molecule produced in the notochord (fibroblast growth factor 2 and activin-βB).[5] The mesenchymal tissue adjacent to the buds is important for all of the embryologic processes, expansion, branching, and differentiation.

The only gene clearly demonstrated to be causal to congenital anomalies of the pancreas formation is the gene coding for the homeodomain protein PDX1. It is expressed in the endoderm of the foregut at the regions where the ventral and the dorsal buds will form. In PDX1 null mutant mice, the ventral bud forms but fails to grow, and the dorsal bud grows but never forms a functional pancreas. Mutation in this protein has been identified in a patient with pancreas agenesis.[6]

Annular pancreas is usually sporadic, but familial descriptions have been reported with an apparent autosomal dominant transmission. Inactivation of a signaling molecule Sonic hedgehog (Shh) has been described as a potential mechanism that can lead to annular pancreas.[7] Shh is expressed in the endoderm in the regions lateral to the PDX1-expressing endoderm.

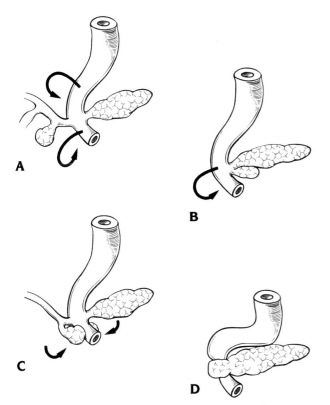

FIGURE 62-1 Embryology of the pancreas. *A*, Eight to 12 mm stage; *B*, fusion of the ducts; *C*, malrotation of the right portion of the ventral bud; *D*, annular pancreas.

Pancreas divisum, which is the most common anomaly of the pancreas, affects 5 to 6% of the population. Inappropriate fusion of the ventral and pancreatic buds has been reported in mice heterozygous for null alleles of Shh.[7]

Aberrant localization of pancreatic tissue affects 0.6 to 2% of the population.[8] The most common sites of pancreatic heterotopias are the stomach, duodenum, and Meckel diverticulum. Because inhibition of Shh leads to pancreatic ectopia in chickens, this signaling molecule may be involved in this anomaly in humans.[9]

ANNULAR PANCREAS

Annular pancreas is the complete encirclement of the second part of the duodenum in a ring-like fashion by a thin, flat band of pancreatic tissue. The annular tissue is histologically normal, containing both acini and islet cells. The anomaly may be associated with partial or complete duodenal obstruction. The annular pancreas occurs with a frequency of 1 in 20,000 births but is more commonly found in neonatal duodenal obstruction (8–21%).[10]

PATHOGENESIS

Annular pancreas may be the result of a hypertrophy of the normal pancreas tissue by failure of atrophy of the left ventral bud. The fixation of the ventral pancreas before the onset of rotation leads to formation of the annulus.[11] This theory and its chronology are supported by most of the fetal evidence reported. The ventral origin of the annulus has been confirmed immunohistochemically

Pancreatic tissue often penetrates the muscularis of the duodenum. A large duct is usually present that connects to the Wirsung duct.

Annular pancreas is associated with a number of other congenital malformations in more than 75% of children.[12] This suggests that the defect of annular pancreas is the result of an early embryologic malformation.

CLINICAL PRESENTATION

Symptomatic annular pancreas may present at any age, from birth through adult life. Approximately one-third of the cases are symptomatic during the neonatal period and half during the first year of life.[12,13] The age at presentation is determined by the degree of duodenal obstruction and by coexistent malformations.

The diagnosis of annular pancreas associated with duodenal obstruction may be suggested antenatally by polyhydramnios. The diagnosis of duodenal obstruction may be confirmed by antenatal ultrasonography.[14]

In the newborn period, the diagnosis is based on the typical appearance of a double-bubble sign of gastric and duodenal obstruction on supine and upright radiographs of the abdomen. Contrast studies are not necessary for the diagnosis unless the differential diagnosis of volvulus with malrotation is discussed.

In children beyond the neonatal period and in adults, symptoms differ because they are more likely recurrent vomiting secondary to partial duodenal obstruction and chronic gastric distention, pain as the result of mild pancreatitis, or peptic ulcers, as have also been described in patients with annular pancreas.[9] In older patients, different investigations may help the diagnosis. Upper gastrointestinal studies are useful, and ring-like smooth symmetric narrowing of the duodenum is observed in the majority of symptomatic children. Contrast-enhanced computed tomography allows direct visualization of the annular pancreas. More recently, magnetic resonance cholangiopancreatography (MRCP) has been used to visualize the pancreatic ducts and the bile duct and can demonstrate the pancreatic duct of the annular portion of the pancreas.[15] In teenagers and adults, diagnosis has also been achieved using endoscopic ultrasonography.[16]

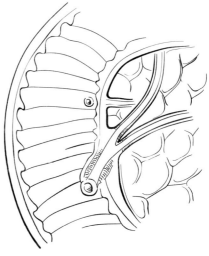

FIGURE 62-2 Normal patterns of the pancreatic ducts.

MANAGEMENT

Surgical management of annular pancreas is mostly concerned with relief of duodenal obstruction. The definitive diagnosis is made at the time of the laparotomy. Direct dissection of the annular ring is not recommended. Such attempts may be technically difficult, and the division of the annular pancreatic duct is associated with a high risk of pancreatic peritonitis or postoperative pancreatitis, fistulae, and late fibrosis. A large duodenoduodenostomy is recommended as a bypass operation. However, the morbidity is high with duodenal functional obstruction owing to the remaining dilated proximal duodenum. Duodenoplasty of the proximal duodenum and diamond-shaped duodenoduodenostomy may reduce the complication rate. The long-term prognosis is excellent.[13]

ECTOPIC PANCREATIC TISSUE

PATHOGENESIS

Ectopic pancreas is defined as the presence of pancreatic tissue lacking anatomic and vascular continuity with the main body of the pancreas. Islands of pancreatic tissue may be found in many sites and have been reported in 0.5 to 1.5% of autopsies.[17] Ectopic pancreatic tissue has been located most commonly in the pylorus, duodenum, Meckel diverticulum, and, less frequently, in the colon, appendix, gallbladder, and anomalous bronchoesophageal foregut fistulae.

Ectopic pancreatic tissue has been observed in knockout mice for homeobox gene *Cdx2*. Inhibition of Shh signaling also leads to ectopic pancreas in chickens.[18] The pathogenesis remains unclear because many theories are not demonstrated. A hypothesis regarding ectopic migration of pancreas precursor to in situ error of stem cell differentiation is still controversial. This theory is supported by the expression of PDX1, a marker of pancreatic progenitor cells, in the antral stomach, duodenum, and small bowel, the main localizations for ectopic pancreas.

CLINICAL PRESENTATION

In most cases, ectopic pancreas remains asymptomatic. It is an incidental finding during surgery for another indication. Because the ectopic pancreas may occasionally cause complications, management remains controversial. Some recommend no further investigations and management; others recommend local resection as ileal resection of the Meckel diverticulum to avoid any further bleeding.

The most common clinical findings are gastrointestinal hemorrhage secondary to mucosal ulcerations close to the pancreatic tissue,[19] pain secondary to pancreatitis and obstruction in prepyloric localization in newborns, intussusceptions, and exceptional malignant transformation of the ectopic tissue in papillary neoplasm.[20,21]

DIAGNOSIS

The diagnosis could be made endoscopically or radiographically in antral or prepyloric localizations. In other localizations, diagnosis is made at the time of surgery. A definitive diagnosis is made histologically.

MANAGEMENT

The treatment of symptomatic ectopic pancreas is surgical. Excision is indicated as Meckel diverticulectomy or antral or ileal resection.

PANCREATIC AGENESIS AND HYPOPLASIA

Complete agenesis of the pancreas is a lethal condition that has been reported in the literature. Lack of insulin leads to intrauterine growth retardation, hyperglycemia, coma, and a rapid fatal issue.[22]

Partial anatomic pancreatic agenesis is unlikely to be symptomatic because the endocrine and exocrine functions are normal. Agenesis of the dorsal pancreas has been described in diabetes and pancreatitis.[23] Magnetic resonance imaging can assist in making the diagnosis.

Agenesis of the acinar tissue occurs in Shwachman syndrome, autosomal recessive disorder with exocrine pancreas deficiency, growth retardation, skeletal anomalies, and bone marrow dysfunction.[24] The prognosis is poor until bone marrow transplant.

DUCTAL ANOMALIES

Any variation of the normal patterns of the dorsal and ventral ducts leads to a number of common ductal anomalies. Some anomalies are pure anatomic variations without any clinical significance, for example, the absence of the duct of Santorini or the absence of a connection between the accessory duct and the main duct. Two ductal anomalies have been implicated in the pathogenesis of clinical disease: the failure of the fusion of the dorsal and ventral ductal systems, which results in a ductal pattern known as pancreas divisum,[25] and the pattern of the junction with the common bile duct.

PANCREAS DIVISUM

PATHOGENESIS

The ducts remain separated, and the dorsal pancreas, which is the main drainage of the pancreas, empties into the duodenum via the smaller accessory papilla. Multiple variants of the divisum anomalies have been described anatomically or after endoscopic retrograde cholangiopancreatography (ERCP).[26] The small accessory duct leads to functional obstruction of the pancreas and pancreatitis (Figure 62-3).

CLINICAL PRESENTATION

The importance of the abnormalities lies in its presumed relationship with documented pancreatitis not attributable to alcohol, infection, or biliary tract disease. Because there is a large gap between the anatomic incidence and the frequency of these documented cases of pancreatitis, the causal relationship remains controversial. Pancreas divisum was identified in 7.4% of all children with pancreatitis and 19.2% of children with relapsing or chronic pancreatitis.[27]

DIAGNOSIS

Diagnosis of pancreas divisum depends on ERCP in children older than 3 years and/or MRCP to demonstrate the

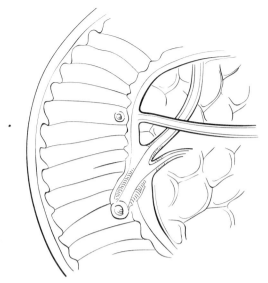

FIGURE 62-3   Ductal anomalies—pancreas divisum.

visualization of the duct of Santorini draining the pancreas. To confirm the diagnosis, the accessory papilla should be cannulated to visualize the duct of Santorini.[28]

MANAGEMENT

Because the causal relationship between pancreas divisum and pancreatitis is controversial, management is the subject of many discussions. Despite medical management of the episodes of pancreatitis, the visualization of a pancreas divisum leads to endoscopic treatment. Beneficial results could be expected by endoscopic enlargement of the accessory papilla. Surgical or endoscopic intervention is directed toward relief of ductal obstruction by a transduodenal sphincteroplasty.[29]

COMMON CHANNEL SYNDROME

PATHOGENESIS

Anomalies of the junctions of the common bile duct and the main pancreatic duct may be clinically significant. The extrahepatic bile duct is developed from the ventral pancreatic duct. Initially, the junction is extraduodenal and moves toward the duodenum wall. A failure of this progression toward the duodenum results in an abnormally long common pancreatobiliary channel. The junction remains outside the duodenum wall and is therefore not surrounded by the normal sphincter mechanism. The long common pancreatobiliary channel usually exceeds 10 mm in length compared with the normal estimated length of 5 mm in children. This may permit reflux of the pancreatic enzymes containing trypsin into the common duct, with resulting damage to the ductal wall. Occasionally, bile may reflux into the pancreatic duct as well.

Pancreaticobiliary reflux has been confirmed by dynamic MRCP after secretin stimulation.[30]

CLINICAL PRESENTATION

Reflux of ductal contents in either direction may lead to two different clinical situations: choledochal cyst and pancreati-

tis. Common channel syndrome (Figure 62-4) is identified in 75% of the children with choledochal cyst. Recurrent pancreatitis is observed in 70% of choledochal cysts even after surgical disconnection of the bile duct from the pancreatic duct. Pancreatitis without choledochal cyst is related to bile reflux in the pancreatic duct with ductal ectasia.

DIAGNOSIS

Abdominal ultrasonography is often diagnostic of choledochal cyst and is an indication for further imaging studies.

MRCP is noninvasive and can be performed in children without the use of contrast agents. It demonstrates the choledochal cyst, the common channel, and pancreatic ductal ectasia. Invasive imaging studies are mandated only if there is no clear evidence of congenital malformation and if the bile duct dilatation can be related to choledocolithiasis.

Percutaneous transhepatic cholangiography and ERCP are the most effective imaging studies to demonstrate the common channel.

In children less than 3 years of age, MRCP or percutaneous transhepatic cholangiography can be performed safely under general anesthesia. In older children, MRCP or ERCP can be discussed, but ERCP should be avoided in episodes of acute pancreatitis.

MANAGEMENT

Radical excision of the choledochal cyst and reconstruction by a Roux-en-Y hepaticoenterostomy is the treatment of choice for choledochal cyst.

Good results can be achieved with hepaticoenterostomy.[31] Postoperative complications are uncommon. Cholangitis and pancreatitis are the most frequent complications and could lead to imaging reassessment for anastomotic stricture or hepatic duct or pancreatic duct calculi. Malignancy of the biliary enteric anastomosis has been reported even many years after radical excision.[32]

Pancreaticojejunostomy and/or endoscopic sphincteroplasty may be curative in exceptional common channel syndrome without choledochal cyst but with pancreatic ductal ectasia.

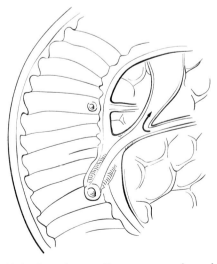

FIGURE 62-4   Ductal anomalies—common channel syndrome.

OTHER CONGENITAL ANOMALIES

CONGENITAL PANCREATIC CYSTS

Congenital pancreatic cysts are uncommon. Unilocular or multiple congenital cysts are lined by an epithelium. The presentation is variable, including asymptomatic cysts, abdominal masses, and pancreatitis. The cysts may be associated with other anomalies, such as polydactyly and anorectal malformations. Multilocular cysts may be an isolated pancreatic lesion, as well as part of von Hippel-Lindau disease, with hereditary cerebellar cysts, hemangiomas of the retina, and kidney and liver cysts.[33]

ENTERIC DUPLICATION CYSTS

Intrapancreatic or juxtapancreatic gastric or duodenal duplications with ductal communications are uncommon. Symptoms may include failure to thrive, abdominal pain, and episodes of pancreatitis. The lesion may be recognized by ultrasonography, upper gastrointestinal studies, and MRCP.

Exploration is necessary to excise the lesion and to alleviate recurrent episodes of pancreatitis. Excision of the duplication is performed close to the duodenal wall without pancreaticoduodenal resection.[34]

REFERENCES

1. Streeter GL. Developmental horizons in human embryos. Descriptions of age XI, 13 to 20 somites, and age group XII, 21 to 29 somites. Contrib Embryol 1942;30:295–300.
2. Uchid T, Takada T, Ammori BJ, et al. Three dimensional reconstruction of the ventral and dorsal pancreas: a new insight into anatomy and embryonic development. J Hepatobil Pancreat Surg 1999;6:176–80.
3. Kim SK, Hebrok M, Melton DA. Notochord to endoderm signaling is required for pancreas development. Development 1997;124:4243–52.
4. Li H, Arber S, Jessell TM, Edlund H. Selective agenesis of the dorsal pancreas in mice lacking homebox gene Hlxb9. Nat Genet 1999;23:67–70.
5. Lammert E, Cleaver O, Melton D. Induction of pancreatic differentiation by signals from blood vessels. Science 2001;294:564–7.
6. Stoffers DA, Zinkin NT, Stanojevic V, et al. Pancreatic agenesis attributable to a single nucleotide deletion in the human IPF1 gene coding sequence. Nat Genet 1997;15:106–10.
7. Hebrok M, Kim SK, St Jacques B, et al. Regulation of pancreas development by hedgehog signaling. Development 2000;127:4905–13.
8. McInnes RR, Michaud J. Development and diseases of the pancreas. Clin Genet 2002:62;14–23.
9. Kim SK, Melton DA. Pancreas development is promoted by cyclopamine, a hedgehog signaling inhibitor. Proc Natl Acad Sci U S A 1998;95:13036–41.
10. Lehman GA, O'Connor KW. Coexistence of annular pancreas and pancreas divisum: ERCP diagnosis. Gastrointest Endosc 1985;31:25–8.
11. Ikeda Y, Irving IM. Annular pancreas in a fetus and its three dimensional reconstruction. J Pediatr Surg 1984;19:160–4.
12. Kiernan PD, ReMine SG, Kiernan PC, ReMine WH. Annular pancreas. Arch Surg 1980;115:46–50.
13. Bailey PV, Tracy TF, Connors RH, et al. Congenital duodenal obstruction: a 32-year review. J Pediatr Surg 1993;28:92–5.
14. Akhtar J, Guiney EJ. Congenital duodenal obstruction. Br J Surg 1992;79:133–5.
15. Hidaka T, Hirohashi S, Uchida H, et al. Annular pancreas diagnosed by single shot MRCP. Magn Reson Imaging 1998;16:441–4.
16. Gress F, Yiengpruksawan A, Sherman S, et al. Diagnosis of annular pancreas by endoscopic ultrasound. Gastrointest Endosc 1996;44:485–9.
17. Caberval D, Kogan SJ, Levitt SB. Ectopic pancreas presenting as un umbilical mass. J Pediatr Surg 1977;12:593–5.
18. Chawengsaksophak K, James R, Hammond VE, et al. Homeosis and intestinal tumors in Cdx2 mutant mice. Nature 1997;386:84–7.
19. Schurmans J, de Baere H. Upper gastrointestinal hemorrhage caused by ectopic pancreas. Acta Clin Belg 1980;35:233–7.
20. Hickman DM, Frey CF, Carson JW. Adenocarcinoma arising in gastric heterotopic pancreas. West J Med 1981;135:57–62.
21. Ishikawa O, Ishiguro S, Ohhigashi H, et al. Solid and papillary neoplasm arising from an ectopic pancreas in the mesocolon. Am J Gastroenterol 1990;85:597–601.
22. Voldsgaard P, Kryger-Bagesen N, Lisse I. Agenesis of the pancreas. Acta Pediatr 1994;83:791–3.
23. Wilding R, Schnedl WJ, Reisinger EC, et al. Agenesis of the dorsal pancreas in a woman with diabetes mellitus and in both of her sons. Gastroenterology 1993;104:1182–6.
24. Marseglia GL, Bozzola M, Marchi A, et al. Response to long term hGH therapy in two children with Shwachman-Diamond syndrome associated with GH deficiency. Horm Res 1998;50:42–5.
25. Warshaw AL, Simeone JF, Schapiro RH, Flavin-Warshaw B. Evaluation and treatment of the dominant dorsal duct syndrome (pancreas divisum redefined). Am J Surg 1990;159:59–66.
26. Delhaye M, Engelholm L, Cremer M. Pancreas divisum: congenital anatomic variant or anomaly? Contribution of endoscopic retrograde dorsal pancreatography. Gastroenterology 1985;89:951–8.
27. Cotton PB. Congenital anomaly of pancreas divisum as a cause of obstructive pain and pancreatitis. Gut 1980;21:105–14.
28. Blustein PK, Gaskin K, Filler R, et al. ERCP in pancreatitis in children and adolescents. Pediatrics 1981;68:387–93.
29. O'Rourke RW, Harrisson MR. Pancreas divisum and stenosis of the major and minor papillae in an 8-year old girl: treatment by dual sphincteroplasty. J Pediatr Surg 1998;33:789–91.
30. Matos C, Nicaise N, Deviere J, et al. Choledocal cysts: comparison of findings at MRCP and ERCP in eight children. Radiology 1998;209:443–8.
31. Miyano T, Yamataka A, Kato Y, et al. Hepaticoenterostomy after excision of choledochal cysts in children: a 30-year experience with 180 cases. J Pediatr Surg 1996;31:1417–21.
32. Yamamoto J, Shimamura Y, Ohtani I, et al. Bile duct carcinoma arising at the anastomotic site of hepaticojejunostomy after excision of congenital biliary dilatation. Surgery 1996;119:476–9.
33. Howard JM. Congenital cysts of the pancreas. In: Beger HG, Wrashaw AI, Buchler MW, et al, editors. The pancreas. Oxford (UK): Blackwell Science; 1998. p. 1427–31.
34. Siddiqui AM, Shamberger RC, Filler R, et al. Enteric duplications of the pancreatic head: definitive management by local resection. J Pediatr Surg 1998;33:1117–21.

CHAPTER 63

TUMORS

Assad Butt, MB, BS, DCH(Lon), MRCP, CPCH

Pancreatic tumors and lesions that may mimic tumors rarely occur in childhood. They can present major diagnostic and therapeutic challenges. Pancreatic cancer in adults is the fifth leading cancer in the United States and has the poorest survival rate of the major malignancies, accounting for more than 25,000 deaths annually. In contrast, childhood pancreatic cancer represents less than 5% of all malignancies affecting children under the age of 15 years.[1,2]

Recent advances in genetics and immunohistochemistry have resulted in better understanding of the underlying pathogenetic mechanisms and biologic behavior of these lesions. Improvements in imaging techniques, including the application of newer modalities such as endoscopic ultrasonography (EUS) and magnetic resonance cholangiopancreatography (MRCP), have helped with better localization, improved noninvasive characterization, and tissue sampling of lesions.[3–5]

The World Health Organization classification of pancreatic tumors is currently one of the most widely accepted. This classification is based on the nature of the tissue of origin and relative malignant potential of the tumor (Table 63-1).[6] Although not all of the tumor subtypes have been reported in children, this classification provides a useful framework for considering the differential diagnosis and discussion of pancreatic tumors in children.[7]

PRIMARY EPITHELIAL EXOCRINE TUMORS

Benign and malignant exocrine tumors of the pancreas can be either cystic or solid and can arise from either ductal or acinar tissue. There is a spectrum of biologic behavior and tumor aggressiveness between different tumor groups.

CYSTIC TUMORS

Pancreatic cystic tumors are an important group clinically because other cystic lesions of the pancreas may mimic them. Pseudocysts are the most common cystic lesions encountered in childhood, accounting for about 75% of pancreatic cystic lesions. They occur either secondary to trauma or chronic pancreatitis resulting from other causes and are discussed in detail in Chapter 64, "Pancreatitis." Their diagnosis may be confused with cystic neoplasm and may result in inappropriate management.[8] The investigation and differential diagnosis of cystic neoplasia are considered below.

SEROUS CYSTADENOMA

Two types of serous cyst adenoma exist: serous microcystic adenoma and serous oligocystic adenoma. Both rarely occur in children.

Serous microcystic adenomas have a female predominance and are more commonly found in the pancreatic body and tail.[9] One-third of these lesions are asymptomatic and found incidentally, whereas the remainder have symptoms related to pressure of the tumor on adjacent structures.[7] The lesions are benign tumors consisting of numerous small cysts arranged around a central stellate scar. They are lined by epithelial cells and show evidence of ductular differentiation.[10] No specific tumor markers identify this lesion. Radiographs may show calcification in some patients. Computed tomography (CT) reveals a well-demarcated multiloculated cyst, on occasions demonstrating the central stellate scar.

Surgical excision of the tumors is usually unnecessary unless the patients are symptomatic. However, the histologic diagnosis must be confirmed.[7]

Serous oligocystic adenomas are benign tumors with an equal sex predominance that occur more rarely in children than the serous microcystic adenoma. The etiology is unknown; however, it is of interest that two reports in children have isolated cytomegalovirus from adjacent pancreatic tissue.[11,12]

Most tumors are located in the head and body of the pancreas and are composed of a few relatively large cysts showing evidence of ductular differentiation. Infants usually present with a palpable abdominal mass. Resection is needed if lesions are symptomatic.

MUCINOUS CYSTADENOMAS

This benign cystic pancreatic tumor is closely related to a spectrum of mucinous cystic tumors that includes mucinous cystadenocarcinoma and consequently has a definite malignant potential. There is a strong female preponderance. The majority of tumors are located in the tail of the pancreas.[9] The tumors usually consist of a solitary large unilocular cyst composed of mucin-secreting epithelial cells. Because of the malignant potential, wide surgical excision, including the associated capsule, is always recommended.[10]

TABLE 63-1   CLASSIFICATION OF PANCREATIC TUMORS

PRIMARY	EXAMPLE OF TUMOR TYPE
EPITHELIAL	
Exocrine	
Benign	Serous cystadenoma, mucinous cystadenoma (premalignant), mature cystic teratomas, papillary cystic tumor
Borderline malignant	Papillary cystic tumor
Malignant	Mucinous cystadenocarcinoma, ductal adenocarcinoma, acinar adenocarcinoma, pancreatoblastoma
Endocrine	
Benign	Insulinoma (90–95%), gastrinoma (40%), VIPoma (50%), GRFoma (67%), glucagonoma (40%), somatostatinoma (25%)
Borderline malignant	No pediatric example exists
Low-/high-grade malignant	Insulinoma (5–10%), gastrinoma (50%), VIPoma (33%), GRFoma (33%), glucagonoma (60%), somatostatinoma (75%), MEN type I (associated with gastrinoma, insulinoma, and VIPoma in decreasing frequency, respectively), islet cell carcinoma (functional or nonfunctional lesions)
NONEPITHELIAL	
Benign	Fibrous histiocytoma, juvenile hemangioendothelioma, lymphangioma, glomus tumors, myofibromatosis
Malignant	Rhabdomyosarcoma, lymphosarcoma, lymphomas
SECONDARY	
Malignant	Adenocarcinoma (local spread from stomach, intestine, biliary tract), malignant melanoma, leukemia, renal and lung tumors (hematogenous spread)
TUMOR-LIKE LESIONS	
Exocrine	Pancreatic cysts, chronic pancreatitis, ductal changes (eg, squamous metaplasia, mucinous cell hypertrophy, ductal papillary hyperplasia, adenomatoid duct hyperplasia), acinar changes (eg, focal acinar transformation), heterotopic pancreas, heterotopic spleen in pancreas, hamartomas, inflammatory pseudotumors
Endocrine	Islet cell hyperplasia, islet cell dysplasia, persistent hyperinsulinemic hypoglycemia of infancy (nesidioblastosis)

Adapted from Kloppel H et al.[6]
GRF = growth hormone releasing factor; MEN = multiple endocrine neoplasia; VIP = vasoactive intestinal polypeptide.

CYSTADENOCARCINOMA

SEROUS CYSTADENOCARCINOMA

This entity has not been reported in the pediatric literature.

MUCINOUS CYSTADENOCARCINOMA

The clinicopathologic features of this malignant tumor are similar to that of its benign counterpart, the mucinous cystadenoma. However, the tumor is invasive, tending to spread locally in the same way as ductal adenocarcinoma.

The incidence is half that of mucinous cystadenomas. The prognosis is excellent if resection is complete.[9,10]

MATURE CYSTIC TERATOMAS ("DERMOID CYSTS")

These lesions are benign extragonadal germ cell cysts derived from all three germinal layers and may include hair, teeth, cartilage, sebaceous material, and sweat glands. They are rarely found in the pancreas but can occur anywhere in the substance of the pancreas or be attached to it.[13–15] Excision is the treatment of choice.

PAPILLARY CYSTIC TUMOR

Papillary cystic tumors of the pancreas are exceptionally rare neoplasms in children. Since their original description by Frantz in 1959, more than 400 cases have been reported in the English literature (mean age 23.9 years; range 2–74 years). By 1999, approximately 90 cases were reported in children (age group < 18 years).[16] Such cases represent 8 to 17% of all pediatric pancreatic neoplasms.[17] The tumors occur most frequently in young females (91% of cases), especially adolescent girls, and there may be a preponderance in Asian and black patients.[16–18] There is no conclusive evidence for the role of sex hormones in the pathogenesis of papillary cystic tumors; however, they may have an influence on tumor growth. Patients typically present with vague gastrointestinal systems such as upper abdominal discomfort or pain caused by an enlarging and often palpable abdominal mass. Because of slow tumor growth, patients often remain asymptomatic until the tumor has enlarged considerably or is detected incidentally on ultrasound imaging for an unrelated indication. There is usually no evidence of endocrine or exocrine dysfunction, and liver function and endocrine tests are normal.[16,17,19]

The tumors are slow growing and of low malignant potential. The body and tail are more frequently affected (64%) than the head of the pancreas, with a well-circumscribed tumor mass of average diameter between 8 and 10 cm.[16] Macroscopically, the tumors are round or oval, encased by a fibrotic capsule and showing intermingling solid and overt cystic-hemorrhagic areas on the surface. Microscopically, typical features are sheets and cords of polygonal cells comprising pseudopapillary structures with fibrovascular stalks or pseudorosettes.[16] Immunohistochemically, they may express various markers, including neuron-specific enolase (91/108 cases), α_1-antitrypsin (101/132 cases), vimentin (47/65 cases), progesterone (11/31 cases), and estrogen (3/56 cases), as well as other neuropeptides.[17] Most studies have not demonstrated reactivity for pancreatic hormones; importantly, this distinguishes papillary cystic tumors from nonfunctioning endocrine tumors, which may look similar on microscopic histologic assessment.[16]

Tumor invasion of adjacent organs has been reported but is rare.[20,21] The treatment of choice is complete excision of the lesion. Overall, more than 95% of patients are cured. Long disease-free intervals have been recorded after initial resection even in patients whose tumors have either spread locally or metastasized.[21,22] More aggressive tumors are seen in older patients, tumors with a high deoxyribonucleic acid (DNA) index, aneuploidy, frequent mitotic figures, and/or nuclear atypia.[23] The origins of this tumor remain enigmatic. In a limited number of cases, chromosomal abnormalities have been found that are known to be associated with oncogenes. The chromosomal analyses have shown unbalanced translocations between chromosomes 11 and 14, loss of the X chromosome, and trisomy 3.[23] Recent studies suggest that there are abnormalities in the β-catenin or adenomatous polyposis coli (APC) gene pathways, influencing the pathways of neoplastic progression in papillary cystic tumors.[24,25] In Abraham and colleagues' study, a series of 20 papillary cystic tumors were analyzed by immunohistochemistry and molecular genetic techniques.[25] Almost all papillary cystic tumors harbored alterations in the APC–β-catenin pathway. Nuclear accumulation of β-catenin protein was present in 95% (19/20 cases), and activating β-catenin oncogene mutations were identified in 90% (18/20 cases) of the papillary cystic tumors. These findings are similar to those alterations recently identified in other nonductal pancreatic neoplasms (pancreatoblastomas and acinar carcinomas). In contrast, genetic alterations commonly found in pancreatic ductal neoplasms (ductal adenocarcinoma) were absent or detected only invariably.[25]

APPROACH TO INVESTIGATION AND DIAGNOSIS OF CYSTIC TUMORS

A precise diagnosis of all pancreatic cystic lesions is of key importance to exclude cystic pancreatic neoplasia. A more detailed discussion of non-neoplastic lesions is considered in Chapter 62, "Congenital Anomalies of the Pancreas."

Ultrasonography is the most useful initial diagnostic test and can confirm the cystic nature of the lesions. Endoluminal ultrasonography has been recently proposed for delineating small cystic lesions and obtaining tissue samples by fine-needle aspiration to aid specific diagnosis and thus help differentiate benign from potentially malignant lesions (Figure 63-1). One recent adult study suggests high sensitivity (91%), specificity (60%), and accuracy (82%) for EUS in identifying malignant or potentially malignant pancreatic cystic lesions compared with surgical histopathology.[4] The study included 34 patients (16 men, 18 women; mean age 55 years) who underwent surgery for suspected pancreatic cystic lesions based on CT and transabdominal ultrasonography. In addition to EUS, other assessments did not improve overall evaluation of the lesions. The respective sensitivity, specificity, and accuracy were (1) cyst fluid cytopathology, 27%, 100%, and 55%, and (2) carcinoembryonic antigen, 28%, 25%, and 27%. Although this approach has been applied recently to children and shows promise, it needs further evaluation.[3]

CT and/or magnetic resonance imaging (MRI) have an established role in determining the nature of a cyst and its precise relationship to the pancreatic duct and surrounding tissues.[26-30] The advent of MRCP has provided a fur-

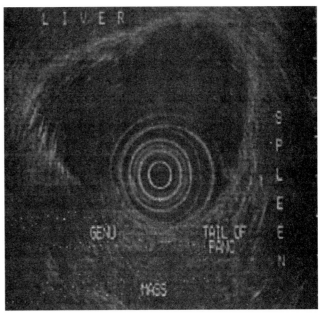

FIGURE 63-1 Papillary cystic neoplasm in a young girl as visualized via endoscopic ultrasonography. Reproduced with permission from Victor Fox, The Children's Hospital, Boston.

ther tool for evaluation. One recent study suggests that this modality has a distinct advantage over endoscopic retrograde cholangiopancreatography in the diagnosis of mucin-producing tumors of the pancreas and cystic lesions. MRCP provides a better image of the entire lesion, including the distal part that is obstructing the pancreatic duct.[5] Use of findings from multiple modalities can be helpful in formulating a differential diagnosis. Selective celiac and gastroduodenal angiography have been suggested as useful diagnostic tools in selected patients. [29]

Despite advances in imaging techniques, definitive preoperative diagnosis is not possible in many cases (Figure 63-2). In a recent multi-institutional review of 398 cases of cystadenomas and cystadenocarcinomas of the pancreas, 93% of cases required surgery to establish a definitive diagnosis.[30] The study reported cases of serous cystadenoma

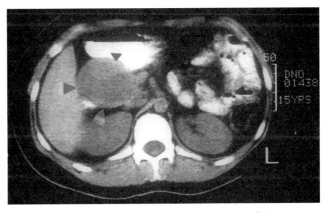

FIGURE 63-2 Appearance of a tumor in the head of the pancreas seen on an unenhanced computed tomographic scan. A definitive diagnosis of papillary cystic tumor was established postoperatively. Reproduced with permission from Professor L Spitz, The Institute of Child Health, Great Ormond Street Children's Hospital, London.

(n = 140), mucinous cystadenoma (n = 150), and mucinous cystadenocarcinomas (n = 78).[30] In approximately one-third of each group, the tumor was asymptomatic at presentation. Preoperative diagnostic accuracy was poor: 20% in cases of serous cystadenoma, 30% in cases of mucinous cyst adenoma, and 29% in those diagnosed with mucinous cystadenocarcinoma. Furthermore, even the utility of intraoperative frozen section allowed for definitive histologic diagnosis in only 50% of cases of serous and mucinous cystadenomas and 62% of cases of mucinous cystadenocarcinoma. Consequently, conservative management was warranted in only 7% of cases who had asymptomatic well-documented serous cystadenoma based on a combination of findings from spiral CT, EUS, and/or diagnostic aspiration of cyst.[30]

ADENOCARCINOMA

Adenocarcinoma of the pancreas exists in two malignant forms arising from ductal or acinar tissue. Ductal adenocarcinoma is by far the most common malignant pancreatic tumor in adults compared with acinar adenocarcinoma, which occurs in only 11%. In contrast, the incidence in children is more evenly distributed, with 53% of the carcinomas of ductal origin and 47% of acinar origin. The total number of pediatric cases reported in the English literature is very small, accounting for only 30 cases in total up to 1983.[31,32]

A combination of genetic and environmental factors most likely contributes to the pathogenesis of pancreatic adenocarcinoma. Genetic predisposition is suggested by an increased incidence in patients with hereditary pancreatitis, as well as a report of four otherwise healthy siblings of an index case of pancreatic ductal carcinoma who also developed this condition.[33]

A number of other conditions have also been linked to a potential increased risk of developing pancreatic carcinoma. These have included hamartomatous polyposis syndromes such as Peutz-Jeghers syndrome, as a direct result of functional deletion of tumor suppressor genes,[34] and celiac disease or dermatitis herpetiformis. However, an increased risk is not observed in children and adolescents with celiac disease. Epidemiologic studies have suggested an increased risk with environmental or other factors, such as men exposed to degreasing agents and women who smoke or have uterine myomas or prior oophorectomy.[35] In addition, higher social class, increased consumption of animal fat and protein, and wine consumption are potential risk factors.[35] With emergence of the field of transplant in recent years, an increased risk of developing de novo malignancies in this group should also be considered. In a series of 1,151 organ allograph recipients, 1,813 de novo malignancies were found, of which 755 involved the hepatobiliary-pancreaticoduodenal area.[36] Whereas lymphomas comprise the majority (63% of cases), pancreatic carcinomas accounted for 11% of the total.[36,37] Down syndrome shows an interesting tumor profile; whereas most solid tumors are underrepresented, pancreatic tumors are in excess.[38] Patients with cutaneous malignant melanoma have an increased risk of subsequent primary carcinoma.[39]

DUCTAL ADENOCARCINOMA

The malignant and aggressive nature of ductal adenocarcinoma relates to its ability to spread along the ducts to the capsule of the pancreas, adjacent lymph nodes, and retroperitoneal space.[31] Patients typically present with abdominal pain and weight loss. More than half of the patients present with obstructive jaundice. Additional symptoms include those of gastrointestinal bleeding, pancreatitis, and depression.[40]

The tumors are usually located in the head of the pancreas. They often generate a dense fibrotic reaction, resulting in a compact hard retroperitoneal mass. CT often demonstrates these lesions as irregular heterogeneous enhancing lesions without a visible capsule.[41] Histologically, they appear as moderately well-differentiated ductal carcinoma cells containing mucin but lacking zymogen.[7,40] Immunohistochemically, they are almost all positive for carcinoembryonic antigen.[7]

Cytogenetic studies show specific chromosomal abnormalities, including the loss of 9p, 17p, and 18q, as well as gains of 8q and 20q. Analysis of pancreatic fluid obtained at the time of endoscopic retrograde cholangiopancreatography by fluorescent in situ hybridization in 12 affected patients revealed a loss of 18q in 92%.[42] Further studies have shown that 70% of these mutations resulted in activation of oncogenes (ie, Ki-*ras*, C-*erb*B12) or in activation of tumor suppressor genes (*TP53*, *MTS1*, *Smad4*, *P16*[INK4]).[42] One study found Ki-*ras* gene mutations at codon 12 in about 90% of cases and abnormal expression of the C-*erb* B12 oncogene in nearly 20% of cases.[43] A recent report suggests that a genetic diagnosis of ductal adenocarcinoma can be made by analysis of pancreatic fluid collected endoscopically for Ki-*ras* mutation analysis of both the supernatant and sediment of pancreatic fluid.[44] Other studies have shown alterations in those factors that may promote (*bax*) or block (*bcl-2*) apoptosis.[45] Studies have also shown an important role for tumor growth factor (TGF)-β and its signaling proteins in (1) allowing for tumor cell anchorage–independent growth,[46] (2) enhancing tumorigenicity by the TGF-β signaling inhibitor *Smad7*,[47] and (3) influencing disease progression (overexpression of type 2 TGF-β receptor may be a marker that correlates with disease progression and is associated with decreased patient survival).[48] Finally, recent studies have suggested an increased expression of inducible nitric oxide synthase in human pancreatic cancer, which correlates positively with the degree of apoptosis as expressed by the apoptotic index. These findings could, in the future, provide the basis for the development of potential therapeutic strategies.[49]

Only 10 to 20% of cases are amenable to curative surgical resection. A Whipple procedure is typically performed when the tumor is confined to the head of the pancreas. In addition to removal of the tumor, en bloc resection of the distal stomach, duodenum, and common bile duct is performed. Subsequently, continuity is restored by fashioning a pancreaticojejunostomy, choledochojejunostomy, or gastrojejunostomy.[40] In general, the 3-year survival rate is approximately 2%, with a mean survival after diagnosis of 4 to 6 months.[50] The core prognosis is related to a delay in diagnosis because 85% of tumors have metastasized at the time of diagnosis.[51] Palliation with chemotherapy, either single agent or in combination, and use of external beam radiation are of value for a limited duration only. A limited experience with high linear energy transfer particle (neutron or heavy iron) radiation therapy has produced significant decreases in tumor size but no improvement in patient survival.[40] A number of patients have gained some relief from intractable peritoneal pain with celiac plexus neurolysis.[52]

ACINAR ADENOCARCINOMA

Acinar adenocarcinoma has already metastasized in most patients by the time a diagnosis is made. The tumor typically presents more commonly in males and in a reported age range from 3 to 90 years.[53,54] Symptoms at presentation are attributable to local expansion of the tumor or metastases. About 15% of patients present with a syndrome involving polyarthralgia, extrapancreatic fat necrosis, and eosinophilia.[53]

The tumor is a well-circumscribed nodular mass that occurs evenly throughout the pancreas. Ultrasonography shows a midrange echogenic mass. Dual-phase helical CT usually reveals large encapsulated lesions of lower attenuation with or without calcified and necrotic areas.[41] Histologically, acinar tumor cells are arranged in a ribbonlike configuration and contain eosinophilic cytoplasm and periodic acid–Schiff–positive zymogen granules on electron microscopy. Electron microscopic features can help distinguish acinar adenocarcinoma from islet cell tumors of the pancreas, which can look similar on routine light microscopy. In addition, immunostaining properties can distinguish between these two entities, which have also been reported to coexist as mixed acinar–islet cell carcinomas associated with insulin secretion.[55,56] Immunostaining of granules for various pancreatic enzymes is typically positive, including trypsin and lipase.

Cytogenetic studies show that these tumors typically lack those cell markers associated with ductal adenocarcinoma (ie, Ki-*ras* and *TP53*).[57] A recent study suggests that acinar adenocarcinomas are genetically distinct from their ductal counterparts, with demonstration of frequent allelic losses on chromosome 11p and alterations in the APC–β-catenin pathway.[58] It is of interest that similar genetic alterations have also been described in pancreatoblastoma (see the following section).

Treatment is directed at complete excision of the primary lesion and offers the only possible chance of cure. The prognosis is generally more favorable than that for ductal adenocarcinoma. Chemotherapy and radiotherapy are used mainly for palliation.[7]

PANCREATOBLASTOMA

Pancreatoblastoma was originally described by Becker in 1957. Subsequently, 65 pediatric cases have been reported in the literature and 4 cases in adults.[59] Although rare, it is the most common pancreatic neoplasm in childhood. It usually presents in early childhood (mean age approximately 4 years), but this tumor can occur at any age from the neonatal period to adulthood.[60] The tumor is more common in males (male-to-female ratio 1.3:1), and those of Asian descent account for approximately 50% of reported cases.[60,61] There is a reported association of pancreatoblastoma with Beckwith-Wiedemann syndrome (three reported cases).[61,62]

Clinically, most patients present with an incidental abdominal mass. Associated pain, weight loss, and obstructive jaundice are rare.[60] A number of patients have diarrhea of undetermined etiology on presentation. Cushing syndrome and the syndrome of inappropriate secretion of antidiuretic hormone (SIADH) have also been reported concurrently with pancreatoblastoma.[61]

Radiologic studies help determine tumor site and extent of disease. Ultrasonography reveals solid lobulated pancreatic masses with mixed echogenicity.[61] Fine-needle aspiration guided by ultrasonography has been useful in confirming the diagnosis.[61] CT typically reveals large firm, lobulated masses (7–8 cm in diameter) and provides more detailed information.

A review of 59 cases showed that the tumor can occur in any region of the pancreas, and typical features include hemorrhage (94% of cases), capsule formation (92% of cases), and necrosis (90% of cases).[63] All neonatal cases demonstrated cystic changes.[63] MRI, as with other pancreatic neoplasms, demonstrates high signal intensity on T_2-weighted images, with more variable intensity on T_1-weighted images.[64] Gadolinium enhancement is reported to be helpful in distinguishing pancreatoblastoma from other pancreatic tumors.[7] CT and/or MRI will usually correctly make a preoperative diagnosis of pancreatoblastoma.[65] Although a pancreatoblastoma is a malignant tumor, the course is more favorable than with pancreatic acinar cell carcinoma as a result of the presence of a surrounding capsule. Consequently, metastatic spread occurs rarely. Sites of metastases at diagnosis or at the time of recurrence are hepatic (21/69 patients), pulmonary (3/69), and bone (2/69).[59]

Serum α-fetoprotein (AFP) is elevated in nearly 80% of cases, with a median level of 1,280 ng/mL (range 30–138,000 ng/mL).[59] When elevated at diagnosis, evaluation of serum AFP levels is useful to follow the course of the disease, including monitoring for tumor recurrence. However, one reported case in the literature describes a boy with a pancreatoblastoma and a high level of AFP at diagnosis whose tumor recurred as metastatic lesions without a concomitant increase in serum AFP level above normal limits.[66] Yolk sac tumor or hepatoblastoma should also be considered in the differential diagnosis of patients with high AFP levels. One report has suggested that pancreatic AFP (yolk sac origin) can be differentiated from liver AFP (as seen with hepatoblastoma) by using lectin-affinity immunoelectrophoresis.[67]

Histologically, the tumor consists of a soft solid mass, which is usually surrounded by a fibrous capsule that becomes infiltrated in advanced cases. The tumor is composed of epithelial tissue with acinar differentiation, squamoid cell nests, and occasional endocrine cells. Rarely, cases have pronounced mesenchymal elements, including chondroid and osteoid tissue. Recent cytogenetic studies have provided insights into the possible pathogenesis of pancreatoblastomas. One report has demonstrated an association with chromosome 11p loss of heterozygosity and insulin-like growth factor 2.[68] Another suggests that pancreatoblastomas are genetically distinct from pancreatic ductal adenocarcinomas but bear a close resemblance in molecular pathogenesis to heptatoblastomas. In addition, a link is proposed between familial adenomatous polyposis and pancreatoblastoma. [69]

Treatment is by excision, often involving pancreatico-duodenectomy. If complete resection is achieved initially or after preliminary chemotherapy for reduction of tumor size, 80% achieve complete remission (21/24 cases).[61] Of 10 children who had marginally resectable tumor or partial resection, only 5 survived.[61] Because often tumors cannot be completely resected at diagnosis, preoperative chemotherapy has been employed with some success; however, there is no consensus regarding optimal chemotherapeutic regimens. In one report, a regimen including cisplatinum and doxorubicin documented good tumor response in 9 of 10 children who received the chemotherapy, with the 6 subjects remaining disease free for a median time of 28 months after initial diagnosis.[59] However, chemotherapy provides only transient benefit and must always be followed by surgery. Local radiotherapy after surgery is recommended in patients with a marginally resectable tumor or with tumor spillage during resection.[59] Prognosis is generally better in children. Overall, about 70% of patients are well at 1 year, and tumor-free survival after 5 years is approximately 30%.[7] A tumor-free follow-up of 28 years after surgery has been reported.[70]

PRIMARY EPITHELIAL ENDOCRINE TUMORS

Pancreatic endocrine tumors are a rare and diverse group of lesions that account for a greater proportion of all pancreatic tumors in children than in adults. The tumors may be either functioning or nonfunctioning. Although many of the tumors exhibit features of multihormonality, the specific clinical syndromes that are caused by these neoplasms are predominantly attributable to the systemic effects of only one of their secretory products. (Table 63-2). Advances in our ability to detect the various hormones that are secreted in excess by these tumors have resulted in major progress in our understanding and diagnosis of these challenging tumors. The diagnosis often rests more on the identification of humoral factors than on tissue biopsy. There is a wide overlap in biologic behavior and in the spectrum of benign and malignant potential of these tumors. Descriptions of gastrin-producing tumors (Zollinger-Ellison syndrome), VIPomas (vasoactive intestinal polypeptide; Verner-Morrison syndrome), and carcinoid tumors can be found in Chapter 47, "Secretory Tumors." Glucagonomas, somatostatinomas, and growth hormone–releasing factor adenomas are listed in Table 63-2

to illustrate their main biologic features but are not discussed in the text because they have not been reported in the pediatric age range.

Recent studies have shown new insights into the factors that might influence or predict the biologic behavior of these tumors. One report has suggested that assessment of tissue mitotic rate and necrosis correlates strongly with survival.[71] Other studies have suggested allelic losses on the X chromosome in foregut endocrine tumors, including pancreatic neoplasia, shown by X chromosome loss of heterozygosity.[72,73] A study using the technique of comparative genomic hybridization, which allows for the simultaneous evaluation of the entire tumor genome, has shown a variety of types of chromosomal imbalances in 96% of cases (25/26 patients). These abnormalities discriminated to some extent between sporadic foregut and midgut tumors and reveal new distinct candidate regions in the human genome that are associated with sporadic endocrine tumors.[74]

INSULINOMA

Insulinomas are the most common functioning pancreatic endocrine tumors. Benign tumors usually account for between 90 and 95% of cases. The first description of a patient with an insulinoma syndrome was in 1902, predating the discovery of insulin by Banting and Best in 1922.[75] A large review of patients with insulinoma from 1974 included 1,067 cases (mean age 45.5 years; 68% of patients in the age range of 30 to 60 years; female predominance in a ratio of 3:2).[76] The reported incidence is of 4 cases per 1 million person-years.[76]

Clinically, patients present with symptoms of hypoglycemia, including neuropsychological symptoms such as loss of consciousness, lethargy, confusion, dizziness, blurred vision, epilepsy, and coma, occurring in up to 92% of patients.[76] Amnesia is also reported in 41% of cases.[77] Irreversible central nervous system damage owing to hypoglycemia was evident in 6.8% of patients. Symptoms related to catecholamine response, such as palpitations, tachycardia, and hypertension, were also common. In addition, patients may complain of hunger, vomiting, or epigastric pain. One study documents obesity in 47% of cases.[76]

Hypoglycemia may be a feature of a number of other clinical conditions. The presence of hypoglycemic symptoms, abnormally low serum glucose, and relief of symp-

TABLE 63-2	ENDOCRINE TUMORS OF THE PANCREAS
TUMOR TYPE	**MAJOR CLINICAL FEATURE(S)**
Insulinoma	Hypoglycemia, altered mental state
Gastrinoma	Gastric acid hypersecretion, peptic ulceration, steatorrhea
GRFoma*	Achromegaly
Glucagonoma*	Hyperglycemia, mild diabetes mellitus, necrolytic erythematous migratory rash
Somatostatinoma*	Hypochlorhydria, weight loss, mild diabetes mellitus, steatorrhea, cholelithiasis
VIPoma	Severe watery diarrhea, achlorhydria, hypokalemia

*These tumors have not yet been reported in the pediatric age group

toms with glucose infusion (Whipple triad) are supportive of the diagnosis.[75] The diagnosis can be aided by inducing fasting hypoglycemia, with measurement of insulin levels. Insulin levels are typically greater than 6 µU/mL despite a serum glucose level less than 40 mg/dL.[75] In the presence of hypoglycemia, an absence of urinary ketones or elevated free fatty acids supports the diagnosis. Other supportive tests include the quantification of proinsulin, which is less than 24% of serum insulin in controlled subjects and greater than 24% in 90% of patients with insulinoma.[78,79] The classic fasting period is 72 hours because previous data suggest that all patients will become symptomatic with hypoglycemia by this time.[75] However, recent evidence suggests that with current available insulin and proinsulin assays, a 48-hour fast is sufficient for a definitive diagnosis and should now become the standard.[80]

The C-peptide suppression test has been advocated as a screening test in suspected cases. In this test, injected porcine insulin fails to suppress endogenous C-peptide levels in affected patients. Despite the various means to establish a diagnosis, there is a delay from the time of presentation of a mean of 37.4 months.[75] In unusual cases in which Munchausen syndrome by proxy is suspected, quantification of C-peptide, which is produced in equimolar concentrations with endogenous insulin but is absent in pharmaceutical insulin, and measurement of serum and urine levels of oral hypoglycemic agents should be performed.

Ninety-eight percent of insulinomas are located within the pancreas.[81] Extrapancreatic sites include the duodenum, ileum, and lungs.[82] The lesions are typically small (90% less than 2 cm in diameter), solitary (83%), and nearly equally distributed between the head, body, and tail of the pancreas.[76,83] The presence of multiple tumors should raise the suspicion of multiple endocrine neoplasia (MEN) type I, as discussed later in this chapter.

One of the major challenges in the management of insulinomas is the difficulty of preoperative localization because of their small size. In different series, 20 to 60% of tumors are not visualized prior to surgery.[84] A multi-institutional study from 1990 reported the sensitivity of localizing a tumor by various noninvasive and invasive modalities as follows: abdominal ultrasonography, 39%; CT, 33%; arteriography, 62%; and transhepatic portal venous sampling, 89%.[84] A report of 11 cases assessed by the same modalities showed similar sensitivities. In addition, newer techniques of MRI, EUS, and the arterial stimulation test with venous sampling were also reported, showing sensitivities of 30%, 50%, and 91%, respectively.[85,86] More recent experience with EUS shows promise. Evaluation of 54 endocrine tumors of the pancreas, including 29 cases of insulinomas, showed an overall sensitivity and accuracy of 93% in locating the tumor.[87] Some reports have suggested that extensive invasive investigations to achieve preoperative localization of the tumor are unnecessary because a combination of intraoperative palpation (sensitivity greater than 90%) and intraoperative ultrasonography will detect nearly all solitary lesions.[88-90]

Initial treatment of insulinoma is dietary, involving the use of frequent snacks and complex carbohydrates to pre-

vent hypoglycemia. Pharmacologic means may be used to treat hypoglycemia in patients with inoperable or metastatic disease or in those instances in which a tumor cannot be localized. Diazoxide acts by directly inhibiting beta-cell release of insulin and by increasing glycogenolysis by inhibition of cyclic adenosine monophosphate phosphodiesterase.[75,83] Diazoxide is effective in 60% of patients but has major side effects that are usually dose related, such as sodium retention, nausea, and hirsutism.[82] Other alternatives include octreotide, which is shown to be efficacious in 40 to 60% of cases, and verapamil, which reduces insulin release by calcium channel blockade.[82]

The treatment of choice is surgical removal of the tumor. Most surgeons advocate enucleation of these firm adenomas with their pseudocapsule rather than resection. In circumstances when the tumor is not localizable intraoperatively, medical treatment with possible re-exploration at a future date is favored over blind distal resection of the pancreas because 32% of lesions are located in the head of the pancreas. Tumor infiltration is indicative of a malignant state, which warrants resection rather than enucleation. Metastases occur typically to local lymph nodes or the liver. Malignant lesions are usually greater than 2.5 cm in diameter, in contrast to a typical insulinoma, which is between 0.5 and 1 cm.[90] Complications of resection can be seen in up to 55% of cases and include pancreatitis, fistula formation, pseudocyst formation, bleeding, and infection.[84] In addition to aggressive resection, malignant insulinomas have shown variable response to antihormonal chemotherapy and radiotherapy.[7,75] Postoperatively, rises in serum glucose can be seen within 20 minutes of resection in 70% of cases.[78] Consequently, intraoperative monitoring of glucose and immunoreactive insulin has been advocated to confirm that the insulinoma has been completely excised.[91] Hypoglycemia may last for up to 20 days postoperatively and therefore needs monitoring during this time.[76]

MEN TYPE I (WERMER SYNDROME)

MEN type I is a syndrome of malignant potential that involves synchronous or metachronous development of endocrine lesions in the parathyroid, pancreas, and anterior pituitary glands. Less common are associated lesions in the gastrointestinal tract, thymus, lungs, and other sites. In contrast, MEN type II involves the thyroid gland and adrenal medulla.

MEN type I is an autosomal dominant condition that can also occur sporadically. Patients may have primary hyperparathyroidism (88–97%), multiple duodenal pancreatic endocrine tumors (81–82%), and/or pituitary adenomas. Associated skin angiofibromas and collagenomas are common.[92] Of less frequent occurrence are thymic carcinoids, adrenocortical adenomas, thyroid adenomas, and subcutaneous lipomas.[93,94] Patients with MEN type I account for 17% of all patients with hyperparathyroidism, 33% of all patients with Zollinger-Ellison syndrome, 4% of patients with insulinoma, and a small fraction of patients with VIP-secreting tumors, somatostatinomas, and glucagonoma syndromes.[95]

The occurrence of MEN type I was first linked to a tumor suppressor gene (*mu*) at chromosome 11 q13 in 1988. Further studies revealed *MEN1* gene mutations in sporadic cases of gastrinoma (33%) and insulinoma (17%) and deletions of one of the MEN alleles in gastrinomas (93%) and insulinomas (50%).[96]

Pancreatic lesions are either functioning or nonfunctioning. The latter are usually numerous and are microadenomas. Of the functioning lesions, the majority are gastrinomas, followed by insulinomas and VIPomas.

Specific treatment is determined by the type of pancreatic lesion. Tumors are often multiple, especially gastrinomas, which are typically within the duodenum. Production of multiple hormones is documented in 57% of cases. However, 80% contain one predominant hormone, most commonly insulin.[97] The significant morbidity and mortality associated with these tumors and the possibility of testing for *MEN1* gene mutations have raised the issue of screening affected members and kindred. One recent study suggested that screening facilitates the identification of individuals who carry *MEN1* gene mutations and allows one to exclude nonmutant gene carriers from further investigations. This study included 45 members from 10 *MEN1* Swiss families.[98] Prospective biochemical and radiologic screening of carriers was undertaken and revealed the following abnormalities in asymptomatic *MEN1* gene carriers: nine cases of primary hyperparathyroidism, three cases of nonfunctioning pancreatic tumors, one case of gastrinoma, one case of a nonfunctioning microadenoma of the pituitary gland, and one case of macronodular adrenal hyperplasia. Earlier detection of *MEN1*-associated tumors may allow for a reduction in future morbidity and mortality. A similar approach has also been recently applied in families presenting with familial hyperparathyroidism in which genetic screening for *MEN1* mutations was carried out with the suggestion that positive genetic screening may predict disease and allow early detection and appropriate treatment before initiation of symptoms.[99]

A number of biochemical and radiologic investigations have been suggested to detect lesions associated with MEN type I. These include serum prolactin and insulin (IGF-I) for pituitary lesions, serum parathyroid hormone and total serum calcium (corrected for albumin level) for the parathyroids, and serum glucose, insulin, proinsulin, glucagon, gastrin, and plasma chromogranin A for the pancreatoduodenal tumors. In addition, a standardized meal or secretin simulation test analyzing serum polypeptides and gastrin is recommended.[100] Studies have suggested the use of fasting human pancreatic polypeptide levels as an additional screening tool. One study of 202 patients with MEN type I revealed its sensitivity to be 95% and specificity to be 88% in the detection of islet cell tumors.[101] Advances in EUS are promising for tumor localization, but other imaging modalities have been inadequate for tumor screening.[102] The risk of metastasis appears to be related to tumor size, with a 25% risk with 2 cm lesions and a 60% risk with 3 cm lesions. However, this relationship remains controversial.[103]

A recent single-institution retrospective review of 233 patients with MEN examined outcome. This revealed that 28% of patients died of causes related to MEN type I, most commonly metastatic islet cell malignancy. The remaining patients died of causes unrelated to MEN type I, most commonly coronary artery disease and nonendocrine malignancies (14% each). The overall 20-year survival of MEN type I was 64% compared with an age- and gender-matched comparison group of 81%.[104] The authors suggest that earlier diagnosis and appropriate treatment of potentially malignant tumors may lead to a reduction in premature mortality.

ISLET CELL CARCINOMA

Islet cell carcinomas arise from functional pancreatic lesions associated with hypoglycemia (see above) or the Zollinger-Ellison syndrome (Chapter 47). They are usually associated with MEN type I, which was discussed earlier. Nonfunctioning islet cell carcinomas occur more commonly in children than in adults. Diagnosis is often delayed because these tumors present as an abdominal mass with a high incidence of metastases.[7]

There is a reported association between von Hippel-Lindau (VHL) disease, a hereditary cancer syndrome, and pancreatic islet cell tumors.[105] VHL disease is caused by germline mutations of the VHL tumor suppressor gene located on chromosome 3p25. The syndrome is characterized by the development of vascular tumors of the central nervous system and retina, clear cell renal carcinomas, pheochromocytomas, endolymphatic sac tumors, and benign cysts affecting a variety of organs, in addition to pancreatic islet cell tumors.[106–107] In one report, solid pancreatic lesions were detected in 12% of patients with VHL disease.[105] Studies suggest that larger primary tumors (greater than 2–3 cm) are associated with hepatic metastases. These may be prevented by early detection and resection.[105,108] Furthermore, analysis of germline VHL mutations may help predict the occurrence of metastatic disease. Eighty percent of such patients showed mutations in exon 3 (4/5 patients) compared with 46% (18/39 patients) without metastatic disease.[108] A malignant islet cell tumor has also been reported in a 12-year-old boy with tuberous sclerosis complex.[109]

PRIMARY NONEPITHELIAL TUMORS

A variety of benign nonepithelial tumors have been reported to occur in the pancreas in childhood (see Table 63-1).[110–114]

Malignant nonepithelial tumors such as rhabdomyosarcoma and lymphoma have all been described in children, albeit rarely.[115] Primitive neuroectodermal tumors are rarely described in solid organs. A recent case series (*n* = 7 cases) shows that primitive neuroectodermal tumors can sometimes arise as primary neoplasms of the pancreas, particularly in the pediatric and adolescent population (age range 6–25 years; mean 18 years).[116] Such cases demonstrate typical translocation chromosomal abnormality, that is, (t 11; 22) (q 24; q12), and characteristic immunohistochemical staining monoclonal antibody for O13 (CD 99, p30/32 MIC2).[116]

SECONDARY TUMORS

Secondary involvement of the pancreas by tumors results most commonly from hematogenous spread and includes malignant melanoma, renal tumors, lung tumors, and leukemia. Relatively few tumors invade the pancreas directly. They are usually adenocarcinomas of the stomach, intestine, or biliary tract, which are themselves rare in childhood.

TUMOR-LIKE EXOCRINE LESIONS

The most important entity in this group is pancreatic cystic lesions, which have been discussed earlier. Other lesions that may appear tumor-like include chronic pancreatitis, ductal changes (such as squamous metaplasia, mucinous cell hypertrophy, ductal papillary hyperplasia, and adenomatoid duct hyperplasia), acinar changes (such as focal acinar transformation), heterotopic pancreas, heterotopic spleen in the pancreas, hamartomas, and inflammatory pseudotumors.[7] Inflammatory pseudotumors are an important clinical group that pose diagnostic and therapeutic challenges because of their resemblance to malignant pancreatic lesions such as sarcoma. Consequently, complete surgical excision aided by radiologic surveillance appears to offer the best chances of successful management.[117]

TUMOR-LIKE ENDOCRINE LESIONS

This group of disorders comprises the entities of islet hyperplasia/dysplasia and persistent hyperinsulinemic hypoglycemia of infancy (PHHI), formally termed nesidioblastosis.

PERSISTENT HYPERINSULINEMIC HYPOGLYCEMIA OF INFANCY

PHHI, until very recently, was an enigmatic syndrome. New advances have helped define this entity at the molecular genetic and clinical levels, permitting a rational approach to classification, diagnosis, treatment, and prognosis.[118] The autosomal recessive form of PHHI is the predominant familial type, with an estimated incidence in the white European population of 1 case per 50,000 live births. However, in populations with a high rate of consanguinity, the incidence may be as high as 1 in 2,675 live births. Sporadic PHHI accounts for 95% of all cases.[118]

Remarkable progress in this field over the last 7 years has been achieved through fundamental investigations into the regulation of insulin secretion. This process is highly complex and integrated, involving regulation by nutrients, hormones, and the autonomic nervous system. These regulatory influences impinge on the pancreatic beta cell, where insulin secretion is ultimately regulated by an adenosine triphosphate (ATP)-sensitive potassium channel (K_{ATP}) that controls the polarity of the beta-cell membrane.[119] The pancreatic K_{ATP} channel consists of two protein subunits: the sulfonylurea receptor 1 (SUR 1) and the inward rectifying potassium channel (ie, Kir 6.2), whose distinct genes are located at adjacent loci on chromosome 11 (11p15.1).[120,121] Mutations in these K_{ATP} channel genes are now known to be responsible for some forms of familial PHHI.[122–124] Furthermore, other genes that are responsible for insulin secretion but are not themselves part of the channel have also been discovered, and mutations causing autosomal dominant forms of PHHI have been described.[125,126] However, the majority of cases of PHHI (greater than 95%) are sporadic, without identifiable gene mutations. Nevertheless, one study has shown that despite the inability to detect mutations with the *SUR1* gene, all five patients with sporadic PHHI investigated had absent K_{ATP} activity in their islets, attesting to the critical role of K_{ATP} channels also in the pathogenesis of sporadic PHHI.[127]

The clinical phenotype of PHHI associated with known molecular defects is summarized in Table 63-3, including a description of their management and prognosis. The

TABLE 63-3   PERSISTENT HYPERINSULINEMIC HYPOGLYCEMIA OF INFANCY: COMPARISON OF CLINICAL PHENOTYPES ASSOCIATED WITH KNOWN MOLECULAR DEFECTS

TYPE (MOLECULAR DEFECTS)	HYPOGLYCEMIA/ HYPERINSULINEMIA	ASSOCIATED CLINICAL, BIOCHEMICAL, OR MOLECULAR FEATURES	RESPONSE TO MEDICAL MANAGEMENT	RECOMMENDED SURGICAL APPROACH	PROGNOSIS
Sporadic (?SUR1 or Kir6.2 mutations)	Moderate/severe in first days to weeks of life; macrosomic at birth	Loss of heterozygosity in microadenomatous tissue	Generally poor; may respond to somatostatin better than to diazoxide	Partial pancreatectomy (microadenoma; 30–40% cases)	Excellent
				Subtotal greater than 95% pancreatectomy (diffuse hyperplasia; 60–70% cases)	Guarded; diabetes mellitus develops in 50% of patients; hypoglycemia persists in 33%
Autosomal recessive (SUR/Kir6.2 mutations)	Severe in first days to weeks of life; macrosomic at birth	Consanguinity a feature in some populations	Poor	Subtotal pancreatectomy	Guarded

Adapted from Sperling MA and Menon RK.[118]

results of genotype-phenotype comparisons owing to mutations of the K$_{ATP}$ channel have yielded mixed results. For example, for some mutations, there is a correlation between the severity of clinical disease and demonstration of parallel severity of dysfunction of the mutant channel in in vitro functional studies. The DeltaF1388 mutation has been associated with severe disease and the H125Q mutation with mild disease. In contrast, the N188S mutation, despite a phenotype associated with severe clinical disease, shows minimal channel dysfunction in vitro.[118]

In suspected cases, a diagnosis of hyperinsulinemia must initially be established. Hyperinsulinemia is generally considered to exist if the circulating insulin concentration exceeds 5 µU/mL when the corresponding glucose concentration in the same sample is less than 2 to 2.5 mM (< 45 mg/dL). Because insulin concentrations may not always be elevated at the time of hypoglycemia, an alternative test is the measurement of IGF binding protein 1 levels at the time of hypoglycemia. The secretion of this is acutely inhibited by insulin, and patients with PHHI have serum levels that are approximately 10 to 20% of the control level values.[118] This test supplements existing indirect evidence of severe hyperinsulinemia, including a brisk glycemic response to parenteral glucagons, exceeding 30 to 45 mg/dL from a baseline hypoglycemic glucose concentration and an exogenous glucose requirement greater than 15 to 20 mg/kg/min necessary to maintain euglycemia.[118]

Initial treatment includes the administration of intravenous glucose at high rates in severe PHHI in the neonatal period. Other pharmacologic measures can also be employed. Diazoxide acts to maintain patency of the K$_{ATP}$ channel and may not respond because of the absence of functional pancreatic K$_{ATP}$ channels seen in patients with mutations in *SUR1* or *KIR 6.2* genes.[128] Calcium channel blockers, particularly the long-acting somatostatin analog octreotide, may be more effective as medical therapy, with reports of success in as many as 50% of affected infants.[129]

Failure of medical management is common and a clear indication for surgical pancreatectomy in an attempt to avoid long-term neurologic sequelae of hypoglycemia. Surgery may be guided by the type of histopathologic lesion. Focal and diffuse histopathologic lesions characterize sporadic PHHI. Focal PHHI is characterized by focal adenomatous hyperplasia of islet-like cells, with small beta-cell nuclei packed closely together. In contrast, in diffuse PHHI, the islets of Langerhans cells throughout the pancreas are irregular in size, with hypertrophied insulin-secreting cells containing large, abnormal beta-cell nuclei.[118] It has been proposed that a histologic index of beta-cell nuclear crowding may provide a reliable discrimination between the diffuse and focal adenomatous forms of sporadic PHHI, that is, focal lesions showing more nuclear crowding than diffuse—hence intraoperatively providing the ability to distinguish and potentially guide the extent of pancreatectomy necessary.[130] Further guidance to predict between the two histologic lesions has been applied preoperatively using the technique of transhepatic retrograde pancreatic venous catheterization with measurement of insulin concentration at multiple sites.[118] In diffuse hyperplasia,

uniformly high insulin concentrations without evidence of a gradient are seen. With localized lesions, a distinct gradient in insulin concentrations is observed. However, only a few centers have developed the expertise and experience to perform this catheterization procedure with a high degree of safety and success. Despite pre- and perioperative evaluations, the long-term outcome following subtotal pancreatectomy remains questionable because of persistent hypoglycemia and development of insulin-dependent diabetes in a high proportion of patients (see Table 63-3).[131]

REFERENCES

1. Kato I, Tajima K, Tominga S. Latitude and pancreatic cancer. Jpn J Clin Oncol 1985;14:403–13.
2. Sener SF, Fremgen A, Menck HR, Winchester DP. Pancreatic cancer: a report of treatment and survival trends for 100,313 patients diagnosed from 1985-1995, using the National Cancer Database. J Am Coll Surg 1999;189(1):1–7.
3. Nadler EP, Novikov A, Landzberg BR, et al. The use of endoscopic ultrasound in the diagnosis of solid pseudopapillary tumors of the pancreas in children. J Pediatr Surg 2002;37:1370–3.
4. Sedlack R, Affi A, Vazquez-Sequeiros E, et al. Utility of EUS in the evaluation of cystic pancreatic lesions. Gastrointest Endosc 2002;56:543–7.
5. Ueno E, Takada Y, Yoshida I, et al. Pancreatic diseases: evaluation with MR cholangiopancreatography. Pancreas 1998;16:418–26.
6. Kloppel H, Solcia E, Longnecker DS, et al. Histological typing of tumors of the exocrine pancreas. Berlin: Springer; 1996.
7. Johnson PR, Spitz L. Cysts and tumors of the pancreas. Semin Pediatr Surg 2000;9:209–15.
8. Ooi LL, Ho GH, Chew SP, et al. Cystic tumours of the pancreas: a diagnostic dilemma. Aust N Z J Surg 1998;68:844–6.
9. Corbally MT, McAnena OJ, Urmacher C, et al. Pancreatic cystadenoma. A clinicopathologic study. Arch Surg 1989;124:1271–4.
10. Compagno J, Oertel JE. Microcystic adenoma of the pancreas (glycogen-rich cystadenomas): a clinicopathological study of 34 cases. Am J Clin Pathol 1978;69:289–98.
11. Amir G, Hurvitz H, Neeman Z, Rosenmann E. Neonatal cytomegalovirus infection with pancreatic cystadenoma and nephrotic syndrome. Pediatr Pathol 1986;6:393–401.
12. Chang CH, Perrin EV, Hertzler J, Brough AJ. Cystadenoma of the pancreas with cytomegalovirus infection in a female infant. Arch Pathol Lab Med 1980;104:7–8.
13. Assawamatiyanont S, King AD Jr. Dermoid cysts of the pancreas. Am Surg 1977;43:503–4.
14. Iacono C, Zamboni G, Di Marcello R, et al. Dermoid cyst of the head of the pancreas area. Int J Pancreatol 1993;14:269–73.
15. Mester M, Trajber HJ, Compton CC, et al. Cystic teratomas of the pancreas. Arch Surg 1990;125:1215–8.
16. Rebhandl W, Felberbauer FX, Puig S, et al. Solid-pseudopapillary tumor of the pancreas (Frantz tumor) in children: report of four cases and review of the literature. J Surg Oncol 2001;76:289–96.
17. Wang KS, Albanese C, Dada F, Skarsgard ED. Papillary cystic neoplasm of the pancreas: a report of three pediatric cases and literature review. J Pediatr Surg 1998;33:842–5.
18. Lam KY, Lo CY, Fan ST. Pancreatic solid-cystic-papillary tumor: clinicopathologic features in eight patients from Hong Kong and review of the literature. World J Surg 1999;23:1045–50.
19. Jung SE, Kim DY, Park KW, et al. Solid and papillary epithelial neoplasm of the pancreas in children. World J Surg 1999;23:233–6.

20. Nishihara K, Nagoshi M, Tsuneyoshi M, et al. Papillary cystic tumors of the pancreas. Assessment of their malignant potential. Cancer 1993;71:82–92.

21. Matsunou H, Konishi F. Papillary-cystic neoplasm of the pancreas. A clinicopathologic study concerning the tumor aging and malignancy of nine cases. Cancer 1990;65:283–91.

22. Felan-Manolt V, Plescovic L, Pegan V. Solid papillary-cystic tumor of the pancreas. Hepatogastroenterology 1997;46:2978–82.

23. Matsubara K, Nigami H, Harigaya H, Baba K. Chromosome abnormality in solid and cystic tumor of the pancreas. Am J Gastroenterol 1997;92:1219–21.

24. Tanaka Y, Kato K, Notohara K, et al. Frequent beta-catenin mutation and cytoplasmic/nuclear accumulation in pancreatic solid-pseudopapillary neoplasm. Cancer Res 2001;61:8401–4.

25. Abraham SC, Klimstra DS, Wilentz RE, et al. Solid-pseudopapillary tumors of the pancreas are genetically distinct from pancreatic ductal adenocarcinomas and almost always harbor beta-catenin mutations. Am J Pathol 2002;160:1361–9.

26. Kawashima A, Fishman EK, Kuhlman JE, Nixon MS. CT of posterior mediastinal masses. Radiographics 1991;11:1045–67.

27. Procacci C, Biasiutti C, Carbognin G, et al. Characterization of cystic tumors of the pancreas: CT accuracy. J Comput Assist Tomogr 1999;23:906–12.

28. Ros PR, Hamrick-Turner JE, Chiechi MV, et al. Cystic masses of the pancreas. Radiographics 1992;12:673–86.

29. Mares AJ, Hirsch M. Congenital cysts of the head of the pancreas. J Pediatr Surg 1977;12:547–52.

30. Le Borgne J, de Calan L, Partensky C. Cystadenomas and cystadenocarcinomas of the pancreas: a multiinstitutional retrospective study of 398 cases. French Surgical Association. Ann Surg 1999;230:152–61.

31. Yoshimura T, Manabe T, Imamura T, et al. Flow cytometric analysis of nuclear DNA content of duct cell carcinoma of the pancreas. Cancer 1992;70:1069–74.

32. Camprodon R, Quintanilla E. Successful long-term results with resection of pancreatic carcinoma in children: favorable prognosis for an uncommon neoplasm. Surgery 1984;95:420–6.

33. MacDermott RP, Kramer P. Adenocarcinoma of the pancreas in four siblings. Gastroenterology 1973;65:137–9.

34. Wirtzfeld DA, Petrelli NJ, Rodriguez-Bigas MA. Hamartomatous polyposis syndromes: molecular genetics, neoplastic risk, and surveillance recommendations. Ann Surg Oncol 2001; 8:319–27.

35. Lin RS, Kessler II. A multifactorial model for pancreatic cancer in man. Epidemiologic evidence. JAMA 1981;245:147–52.

36. Penn I. Primary malignancies of the hepato-biliary-pancreatic system in organ allograft recipients. J Hepatobil Pancreat Surg 1998;5:157–64.

37. Askling J, Linet M, Gridley G, et al. Cancer incidence in a population-based cohort of individuals hospitalized with celiac disease or dermatitis herpetiformis. Gastroenterology 2002;123:1428–35.

38. Satge D, Sommelet D, Geneix A, et al. Tumor profile in Down syndrome. Am J Med Genet 1998;78:207–16.

39. Schenk M, Severson RK, Pawlish KS. The risk of subsequent primary carcinoma of the pancreas in patients with cutaneous malignant melanoma. Cancer 1998;82:1672–6.

40. Cello JP. Pancreatic cancer. In: Feldman M, Scharschmidt BF, Sleisenger MH, editors. Sleisenger and Fordtran's gastrointestinal and liver disease. 6th ed. Philadelphia: WB Saunders; 1998. p. 863–70.

41. Mustert BR, Stafford-Johnson DB, Francis IR. Appearance of acinar cell carcinoma of the pancreas on dual-phase CT. AJR Am J Roentgenol 1998;171:1709.

42. Fukushige S, Furukawa T, Satoh K, et al. Loss of chromosome 18q is an early event in pancreatic ductal tumorigenesis. Cancer Res 1998;58:4222–6.

43. Sakorafas GH, Tsiotou AG. Genetic basis of cancer of the pancreas: diagnostic and therapeutic applications. Eur J Surg 1994;160:529–34.

44. Ha A, Watanabe H, Yamaguchi Y, et al. Usefulness of supernatant of pancreatic juice for genetic analysis of k-ras in diagnosis of pancreatic carcinoma. Pancreas 2001;23:356–63.

45. Friess H, Lu Z, Graber HU, et al. Bax, but not Bcl-2, influences the prognosis of human pancreatic cancer. Gut 1998;43:414–21.

46. Kleeff J, Maruyama H, Friess H, et al. Smad6 suppresses TGF-beta-induced growth inhibition in COLO-357 pancreatic cancer cells and is overexpressed in pancreatic cancer. Biochem Biophys Res Commun 1999;255:268–73.

47. Kleeff J, Ishiwata T, Maruyama H, et al. The TGF-beta signaling inhibitor Smad7 enhances tumorigenicity in pancreatic cancer. Oncogene 1999;18:5363–72.

48. Wagner M, Kleeff J, Friess H, et al. Enhanced expression of the type II transforming growth factor-beta receptor is associated with decreased survival in human pancreatic cancer. Pancreas 1999;19:370–6.

49. Kong G, Kim EK, Kim WS, et al. Inducible nitric oxide synthase (INOS) immunoreactivity and its relationship to cell proliferation, apoptosis, angiogenesis, clinicopathologic characteristics, and patient survival in pancreatic cancer. Int J Pancreatol 2001;29:133–40.

50. Nagaraj H, Polk HC Jr. Pancreatic carcinoma in children. Surgery 1984;95:505.

51. Danes BS, Lynch HT. A familial aggregation of pancreatic cancer. An in vitro study. JAMA 1982;247:2798–802.

52. Sharfman WH, Walsh TD. Has the analgesic efficacy of neurolytic celiac plexus block been demonstrated in pancreatic cancer pain? Pain 1990;41:267–71.

53. Klimstra DS, Heffess CS, Oertel JE, Rosai J. Acinar cell carcinoma of the pancreas. A clinicopathologic study of 28 cases. Am J Surg Pathol 1992;16:815–37.

54. Lack EE, Cassady JR, Levey R, Vawter GF. Tumors of the exocrine pancreas in children and adolescents. A clinical and pathologic study of eight cases. Am J Surg Pathol 1983;7:319–27.

55. Ordonez NG, Mackay B. Acinar cell carcinoma of the pancreas. Ultrastruct Pathol 2000;24:227–41.

56. Shimoike T, Goto M, Nakano I, et al. Acinar-islet cell carcinoma presenting as insulinoma. J Gastroenterol 1997;32:830–5.

57. Hoorens A, Lemoine NR, McLellan E, et al. Pancreatic acinar cell carcinoma. An analysis of cell lineage markers, P53 expression, and ki-ras mutation. Am J Pathol 1993;143:685–98.

58. Abraham SC, Wu TT, Hruban RH, et al. Genetic and immunohistochemical analysis of pancreatic acinar cell carcinoma: frequent allelic loss on chromosome 11p and alterations in the APC/beta-catenin pathway. Am J Pathol 2002;160:953–62.

59. Defachelles AS, Martin De Lassalle E, Boutard P, et al. Pancreatoblastoma in childhood: clinical course and therapeutic management of seven patients. Med Pediatr Oncol 2001; 37:47–52.

60. Klimstra DS, Wenig BM, Adair CF, Heffess CS. Pancreatoblastoma. A clinicopathologic study and review of the literature. Am J Surg Pathol 1995;19:1371–89.

61. Chun Y, Kim W, Park K, et al. Pancreatoblastoma. J Pediatr Surg 1997;32:1612–5.

62. Drut R, Jones MC. Congenital pancreatoblastoma in Beckwith-Wiedemann syndrome: an emerging association. Pediatr Pathol 1988;8:331–9.

63. Kohda E, Iseki M, Ikawa H, et al. Pancreatoblastoma. Three

original cases and review of the literature. Acta Radiol 2000; 41:334–7.

64. Mergo PJ, Helmberger TK, Buetow PC, et al. Pancreatic neoplasms: MR imaging and pathologic correlation. Radiographics 1997;17:281–301.

65. Roebuck DJ, Yuen MK, Wong YC, et al. Imaging features of pancreatoblastoma. Pediatr Radiol 2001;31:501–6.

66. Frabble WJ, Still WJS, King AD Jr. Carcinoma of the pancreas, infantile type. Cancer 1971;27:667–73.

67. Tsuchida Y, Kaneko M, Fukui M, et al. Three different types of alpha-fetoprotein in the diagnosis of malignant solid tumors: use of a sensitive lectin-affinity immunoelectrophoresis. J Pediatr Surg 1989;24:350–5.

68. Kerr NJ, Chun YH, Yun K, et al. Pancreatoblastoma is associated with chromosome 11p loss of heterozygosity and IGF2 overexpression. Med Pediatr Oncol 2002;39:52–4.

69. Abraham SC, Wu TT, Klimstra DS, et al. Distinctive molecular genetic alterations in sporadic and familial adenomatous polyposis-associated pancreatoblastomas: frequent alterations in the APC/beta-catenin pathway and chromosome 11p. Am J Pathol 2001;159:1619–27.

70. Horie A. Clinicopathological features of pancreatoblastoma. Tan to Sui 1988;9:1511–9.

71. Hochwald SN, Zee S, Conlon KC, et al. Prognostic factors in pancreatic endocrine neoplasms: an analysis of 136 cases with a proposal for low-grade and intermediate-grade groups. J Clin Oncol 2002;20:2633–42.

72. Pizzi S, D'Adda T, Azzoni C, et al. Malignancy-associated allelic losses on the X-chromosome in foregut but not in midgut endocrine tumours. J Pathol 2002;196:401–7.

73. Missiaglia E, Moore PS, Williamson J, et al. Sex chromosome anomalies in pancreatic endocrine tumors. Int J Cancer 2002;98:532–8.

74. Tonnies H, Toliat MR, Ramel C, et al. Analysis of sporadic neuroendocrine tumours of the enteropancreatic system by comparative genomic hybridisation. Gut 2001;48:536–41.

75. Grant CS. Insulinoma. Baillieres Clin Gastroenterol 1996;10: 645–71.

76. Stefanini P, Carboni M, Patrassi N, Basoli A. Beta-islet cell tumors of the pancreas: results of a study on 1,067 cases. Surgery 1974;75:597–609.

77. Dizon AM, Kowalyk S, Hoogwerf BJ. Neuroglycopenic and other symptoms in patients with insulinomas. Am J Med 1999;106:307–10.

78. Proye C, Pattou F, Carnaille B, et al. Intraoperative insulin measurement during surgical management of insulinomas. World J Surg 1998;22:1218–24.

79. Vinik AI, Moatari AR. Treatment of endocrine tumors of the pancreas. Endocr Metab Clin North Am 1989;18:483–518.

80. Hirshberg B, Livi A, Bartlett DL, et al. Forty-eight-hour fast: the diagnostic test for insulinoma. J Clin Endocrinol Metab 2000;85:3222–6.

81. Grosfeld JL, Vane DW, Rescorla FJ, et al. Pancreatic tumors in childhood: analysis of 13 cases. J Pediatr Surg 1990;25: 1057–62.

82. Jensen RT, Norton JA, Feldman M, et al. Sleisenger and Fordtran's gastrointestinal and liver disease. 6th ed. Philadelphia: WB Saunders; 1998. p. 871–95.

83. Boden G. Glucagonomas and insulinomas. Gastroenterol Clin North Am 1989;18:831–45.

84. Huai JC, Zhang W, Niu HO, et al. Localization and surgical treatment of pancreatic insulinomas guided by intraoperative ultrasound. Am J Surg 1998;175:18–21.

85. Chavan A, Kirchhoff TD, Brabant G, et al. Role of the intra-

arterial calcium stimulation test in the preoperative localization of insulinomas. Eur J Radiol 2000;10:1582–6.

86. Brown CK, Bartlett DL, Doppman JL, et al. Intraarterial calcium stimulation and intraoperative ultrasonography in the localization and resection of insulinomas. Surgery 1997;122:1189–93.

87. Anderson MA, Carpenter S, Thompson NW, et al. Endoscopic ultrasound is highly accurate and directs management in patients with neuroendocrine tumors of the pancreas. Am J Gastroenterol 2000;95:2271–7.

88. Hashimoto LA, Walsh RM. Preoperative localization of insulinomas is not necessary. J Am Coll Surg 1999;189:368–73.

89. Machado MC, da Cunha JE, Jukemura J, et al. Insulinoma: diagnostic strategies and surgical treatment. a 22-year experience. Hepatogastroenterology 2001;48:854–8.

90. Simon D, Starke A, Goretzki PE, Roeher HD. Reoperative surgery for organic hyperinsulinism: indications and operative strategy. World J Surg 1998;22:666–71.

91. Amikura K, Nakamura R, Arai K, et al. Role of intraoperative insulin monitoring in surgical management of insulinoma. J Laparoendosc Adv Surg Tech A 2001;11:193–9.

92. Marx S, Spiegel AM, Skarulis MC, et al. Multiple endocrine neoplasia type 1: clinical and genetic topics. Ann Intern Med 1998;129:484–94.

93. The BT. Thymic carcinoids in multiple endocrine neoplasia type I. J Intern Med 1998;243:501–4.

94. Doherty GM, Olson JA, Frisella MM, et al. Lethality of multiple endocrine neoplasia type I. World J Surg 1998;22:581–6.

95. Brunt LM, Wells SA Jr. The multiple endocrine neoplasia syndromes. Invest Radiol 1985;20:916–27.

96. Zhuang Z, Vortmeyer AO, Pack S, et al. Somatic mutations of the MEN1 tumor suppressor gene in sporadic gastrinomas and insulinomas. Cancer Res 1997;57:4682–6.

97. Le Bodic MF, Heymann MF, Lecomte M, et al. Immunohistochemical study of 100 pancreatic tumors in 28 patients with multiple endocrine neoplasia, type I. Am J Surg Pathol 1996;20:1378–84.

98. Clerici T, Schmid C, Komminoth P, et al. 10 Swiss kindreds with multiple endocrine neoplasia type 1: assessment of screening methods. Swiss Med Wkly 2001;131:381–6.

99. Perrier ND, Villablanca A, Larsson C, et al. Genetic screening for MEN1 mutations in families presenting with familial primary hyperparathyroidism. World J Surg 2002;26:907–13.

100. Oberg K, Skosseid B. The ultimate biochemical diagnosis of endocrine pancreatic tumors in MEN type I. J Intern Med 1998;243:471–6.

101. Mutch MG, Frisella MM, DeBenedetti MK, et al. Pancreatic polypeptide is a useful plasma marker for radiographically evident pancreatic islet cell tumors in patients with multiple endocrine neoplasia type 1. Surgery 1997;122:1012–9.

102. Skogseid B, Oberg K, Akerstrom G, et al. Limited tumor involvement found at multiple endocrine neoplasia type I pancreatic exploration: can it be predicted by preoperative tumor localization? World J Surg 1998;22:673–7.

103. Lowney JK, Frisella MM, Lairmore TC, Doherty GM. Pancreatic islet cell tumor metastasis in multiple endocrine neoplasia type 1: correlation with primary tumor size. Surgery 1998; 124:1043–8.

104. Dean PG, van Heerden JA, Farley DR, et al. Are patients with multiple endocrine neoplasia type I prone to premature death? World J Surg 2000;24:1437–41.

105. Libutti SK, Choyke PL, Bartlett DL, et al. Pancreatic neuroendocrine tumors associated with von Hippel Lindau disease: diagnostic and management recommendations. Surgery 1998;124:1153–9.

106. Maher ER, Kaelin WG Jr. Von Hippel-Lindau disease. Medicine (Baltimore) 1997;76:381–91.

107. Neumann HP, Dinkel E, Brambs H, et al. Pancreatic lesions in the von Hippel-Lindau syndrome. Gastroenterology 1991; 101:465–71.

108. Libutti SK, Choyke PL, Alexander HR, et al. Clinical and genetic analysis of patients with pancreatic neuroendocrine tumors associated with von Hippel-Lindau disease. Surgery 2000;128:1022–7.

109. Verhoef S, Diemen-Steenvoorde R, Akkersdijk WL, et al. Malignant pancreatic tumour within the spectrum of tuberous sclerosis complex in childhood. Eur J Pediatr 1999;158:284–7.

110. Cubilla AL, Fitzgerald PJ. Tumors of the pancreas. Atlas of tumor pathology. Washington (DC): Armed Forces Institute of Pathology; 1984. p. 25–8.

111. Chappell JS. Case reports. benign hemangioendothelioma of the head of the pancreas treated by pancreaticoduodenectomy. J Pediatr Surg 1973;8:431–2.

112. Gregory IL. Lymphangioma of pancreas. N Y State J Med 1976; 76:289–91.

113. Miliauskas JR, Worthley C, Allen PW. Glomangiomyoma (glomus tumour) of the pancreas: a case report. Pathology 2002; 34:193–5.

114. Morrow SE, Woods GM, Garola RE, Sharp RJ. Pancreatoduodenectomy for neonatal myofibromatosis of the pancreas. J Pediatr Surg 1999;34:609–11.

115. Grosfeld JL, Clatworthy HW Jr, Hamoudi AB. Pancreatic malignancy in children. Arch Surg 1970;101:370–5.

116. Movahedi-Lankarani S, Hruban RH, Westra WH, Klimstra DS. Primitive neuroectodermal tumors of the pancreas: a report of seven cases of a rare neoplasm. Am J Surg Pathol 2002; 26:1040–7.

117. Shankar KR, Losty PD, Khine MM, et al. Pancreatic inflammatory tumour: a rare entity in childhood. J R Coll Surg Edinb 1998;43:422–3.

118. Sperling MA, Menon RK. Hyperinsulinemic hypoglycemia of infancy. recent insights into ATP-sensitive potassium channels, sulfonylurea receptors, molecular mechanisms, and treatment. Endocrinol Metab Clin North Am 1999;28:vii, 695–708i.

119. Huopio H, Shyng SL, Otonkoski T, Nichols CG. K(ATP) channels and insulin secretion disorders. Am J Physiol Endocrinol Metab 2002;283:E207–16.

120. Aguilar-Bryan L, Nichols CG, Wechsler SW, et al. Cloning of the beta cell high-affinity sulfonylurea receptor: a regulator of insulin secretion. Science 1995;268:423–6.

121. Philipson LH, Steiner DF. Pas de deux or more: the sulfonylurea receptor and K+ channels. Science 1995;268:372–3.

122. Nestorowicz A, Glaser B, Wilson BA, et al. Genetic heterogeneity in familial hyperinsulinism. Hum Mol Genet 1998;7:1119–28.

123. Thomas PM. Molecular basis for familial hyperinsulinemic hypoglycemia of infancy. Curr Opin Endocrinol Diabetes 1997;4:272.

124. Thomas PM, Cote GJ, Wohllk N, et al. Mutations in the sulfonylurea receptor gene in familial persistent hyperinsulinemic hypoglycemia of infancy. Science 1995;268:426–9.

125. Glaser B, Kesavan P, Heyman M, et al. Familial hyperinsulinism caused by an activating glucokinase mutation. N Engl J Med 1998;338:226–30.

126. Stanley CA, Lieu YK, Hsu BY, et al. Hyperinsulinism and hyperammonemia in infants with regulatory mutations of the glutamate dehydrogenase gene. N Engl J Med 1998;338:1352–7.

127. Kane C, Shepherd RM, Squires PE, et al. Loss of functional KATP channels in pancreatic beta-cells causes persistent hyperinsulinemic hypoglycemia of infancy. Nat Med 1996;2:1344–7.

128. Kane C, Lindley KJ, Johnson PR, et al. Therapy for persistent hyperinsulinemic hypoglycemia of infancy. Understanding the responsiveness of beta cells to diazoxide and somatostatin. J Clin Invest 1997;100:1888–93.

129. Thornton PS, Alter CA, Katz LE, et al. Short- and long-term use of octreotide in the treatment of congenital hyperinsulinism. J Pediatr 1993;123:637–43.

130. Sempoux C, Guiot Y, Lefevre A, et al. Neonatal hyperinsulinemic hypoglycemia: heterogeneity of the syndrome and keys for differential diagnosis. J Clin Endocrinol Metab 1998;83: 1455–61.

131. Leibowitz G, Glaser B, Higazi AA, et al. Hyperinsulinemic hypoglycemia of infancy (nesidioblastosis) in clinical remission: high incidence of diabetes mellitus and persistent beta-cell dysfunction at long-term follow-up. J Clin Endocrinol.Metab 1995;80:386–92.

CHAPTER 64

PANCREATITIS

1. *Acute and Chronic*

David C. Whitcomb, MD, PhD

Mark E. Lowe, MD, PhD

Clinical understanding and treatment of pancreatic diseases lag behind understanding and treatment of many other important diseases. This delay arises from a combination of factors making it difficult to study the pancreas, including its inaccessible location, hesitation of clinicians and researchers to use invasive testing methods, poorly understood pathophysiologic processes, and limited treatment options. However, a number of recent advances in cell biology and genetics have provided the critical tools to unravel some mysteries of pancreatic pathophysiology and have provided genetic susceptibility testing, which also allows for better classification of pancreatic diseases. In addition, high-quality abdominal imaging techniques, including magnetic resonance cholangiopancreatography (MRCP), now provide critical anatomic information with minimal risk. These advances, framed within the context of acinar and duct cell physiology, provide the foundation for future treatment and prevention of pancreatic diseases.

PATHOPHYSIOLOGY OF ACUTE PANCREATITIS

The pancreas is a gland serving three primary functions: production of a bicarbonate-rich fluid by the duct cells, which helps neutralize gastric acid entering the duodenum; synthesis of digestive enzymes within acinar cells with eventual delivery into the duodenum to help digest complex nutrients; and production of hormones by islet cells to regulate nutrient storage and use related to meals. Although each of the functions and cell types differs, their interrelationship remains critical for normal organ function.

Most of the pancreas is composed of acinar cells. The duct cells connect the acinar cells to the duodenum and flush the digestive enzymes out of the pancreas after acinar cell secretion. The islet cells function independently of the acinar cells, but the acinar cells must remain in close proximity to the islet cells to maintain normal gene expression profiles. This is accomplished through the insular-acinar portal system, in which blood vessels extend from the islets to the acinar cells so that insulin-rich fluid continually bathes the acinar cells.

ACINAR CELLS SYNTHESIZE AND STORE TRYPSINOGEN

The acinar cells synthesize and store digestive enzymes until they are stimulated to secrete the enzymes into the ducts. All of the major digestive enzymes are synthesized by all acinar cells. All enzymes, except amylase and lipase, are synthesized as proenzymes (zymogens) that require activation by cleavage of an activation peptide by trypsin. Trypsinogen (the proenzyme form of trypsin) is activated by the intestinal brush border enzyme enterokinase or by another trypsin molecule (Figure 64.1-1). Trypsinogen also slowly autoactivates, possibly because trypsinogen has some trypsin-like activity.[1] Because trypsinogen is synthesized in the same cell, is stored in the same subcellular compartment as the other enzymes, and has the potential to become active trypsin, there is always the danger of premature trypsinogen activation with subsequent activation of other digestive enzymes and digestion of the pancreas itself. Trypsin not only activates itself, it also inactivates itself through autolysis, a process that is regulated by calcium.[2–4] High calcium concentrations and pH are optimal for trypsin survival in the duodenum[5] but favor autolysis within the acinar cells when calcium concentrations are low. Thus, a number of critical mechanisms are found throughout the pancreas that protect acinar cells, the duct, and the pancreas itself from premature trypsinogen activation.

PATHOPHYSIOLOGY OF CALCIUM SIGNALING

Calcium is the most important second-messenger signaling system within the acinar cells. Activation of the acinar cell through the major receptors results in increases in intracellular calcium, which, in turn, activates protein synthesis and zymogen secretion. With physiologic stimulation, intracellular calcium levels rise and slowly oscillate within well-controlled concentrations.[6b] The process begins with opening of calcium channels on the basolateral membrane, which allows calcium to enter the cell and causes release of intracellular calcium stores. Basolateral calcium is rapidly transported through the rough endoplasmic reticulum to the apical membrane, where it initiates secretion of the zymogen granules into the duct lumen.[7] With hyperstimulation, the calcium levels rise above critical levels, followed

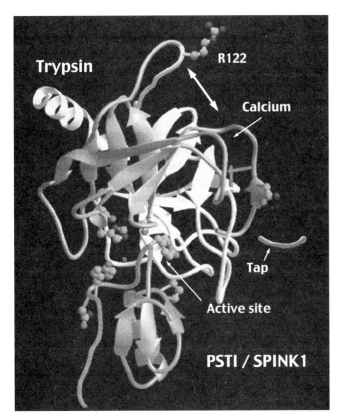

FIGURE 64.1-1   Crystallography-based model of trypsin (yellow and blue) attacking pancreatic secretory trypsin inhibitor/serine protease inhibitor, Kazal type 1 (PSTI/SPINK1-red) at the active site (*long arrow*). The critical regulatory site for trypsinogen activation is shown after cleavage of trypsinogen activation peptide (TAP). The critical regulatory region of trypsin is the flexible autolysis loop (*line with two arrowheads*) with the target amino acid residue R122 shown in the exposed conformation. The calcium binding loop is shown without calcium, which would stabilize the autolysis loop in a conformation protecting R122 from attack by another trypsin (see CD-ROM for color image).

by sustained activation of trypsin.[6b,8] The link between extracellular calcium, acinar cell stimulation, and trypsinogen activation has also been demonstrated in animal models.[9,10] Finally, exposure of the acinar cell apical membrane to bile acids (especially taurolithocholic acid 3-sulfate) causes extended calcium signals near the secretory granules, which leads to trypsin activation.[11] These observations link calcium dysregulation with acute pancreatitis.[12]

DUCT CELLS NORMALLY FLUSH SECRETED DIGESTIVE ENZYMES OUT OF THE PANCREAS

The ductal cells make up less than 5% of the total pancreatic mass but are responsible for the large volume of bicarbonate-rich pancreatic fluid. This function is critical for sweeping digestive enzymes released from the acinar cells out of the pancreas and into the duodenum. The intralobular ductules penetrate the acinus and include the centroacinar cells. Pancreatic bicarbonate secretion is derived from the centroacinar and proximal duct cells.

Duct cells are polarized cells that maintain a significant electrical membrane potential. The basolateral membrane contains ion channels and transporters that participate in

regulating chloride, bicarbonate, sodium, and potassium, as well as the sodium-potassium adenosine triphosphatase ion pump that drives secretion. The most important transporter is the sodium-2 bicarbonate cotransporter, which uses the sodium electrochemical gradient to transport bicarbonate into the cell. The apical membrane also contains channels and transporters, with the most important being the cystic fibrosis transmembrane conductance regulator (CFTR). CFTR is both a chloride and a bicarbonate channel, and the opening or closing of this channel determines duct cell fluid secretion.[13] Mutations in the CFTR reduce the fluid-secreting capacity of the pancreas, increasing the risk of having active trypsin within the pancreas for prolonged periods of time. This is especially dangerous because calcium levels within the duct lumen are elevated, thus eliminating the trypsin autolysis protective mechanism. Unregulated trypsinogen activation in the duct and failure to flush the enzymes because of mutations in the CFTR may also lead to both acute pancreatitis and chronic pancreatitis, as is seen in patients with cystic fibrosis (CF), atypical CF, or forms of CFTR-associated polygenic pancreatitis.[14,15]

OTHER PROTECTIVE MECHANISMS

The vast majority of mechanisms that are protective against acute pancreatitis center on control of trypsin. This includes preventing trypsinogen activation, inhibiting active trypsin, destroying trypsin, or sweeping trypsin out of the pancreas. Identification of specific mutations in several genes proved the importance of several of these mechanisms. As noted above, the first protective mechanism is the synthesis of trypsinogen in an inactive form (trypsinogen) with an activation site located in the target organ, which is the duodenal lumen. Several mutations in cationic trypsin gene enhance trypsin activation,[16] and these mutations increase susceptibility to acute pancreatitis.

If trypsinogen is activated within the acinar cells, it is inhibited by pancreatic secretory trypsin inhibitor (also known as serine protease inhibitor, Kazal type 1 [SPINK1]). This peptide is a specific trypsin inhibitor and an acute-phase protein.[17] Mutations in *SPINK1*, which likely reduce its ability to inhibit trypsin, are associated with pancreatitis in children, some familial pancreatitis, and various forms of tropical pancreatitis. These mutations are common, seen in 2% of most populations.[18] Although intracellular SPINK1 is a highly effective trypsin inhibitor, the number of trypsinogen molecules greatly outnumbers the number of SPINK1 molecules, so that the inhibitory capacity is limited.[1] If more trypsinogen is activated than SPINK1 can inhibit, then other mechanisms must be employed.

Studies in hereditary pancreatitis drew attention to the trypsin self-destruct mechanism.[19] The trypsin molecule has two globular domains held together by a single side chain. This side chain is critical to trypsin regulation. In the middle of the side chain is an arginine, or target amino acid for trypsin attack. Biochemical studies demonstrate that this site is sensitive to trypsin hydrolysis, and cleavage of the site is the first step in trypsin autolysis. The importance of this site and autolysis mechanism is demonstrated by patients with hereditary pancreatitis who have mutations altering the amino acid sequence at R122 (eq. R122H) and recurrent acute pancreatitis when trypsin cannot be destroyed within the acinar cells. Calcium protects trypsin from autolysis by protecting the R122 site from attack.[4,20] So trypsin autolysis only occurs in compartments with low calcium concentrations.

SUMMARY

Some of the mysteries surrounding acute pancreatitis are beginning to be solved. This allows the construction of conceptual models that help organize knowledge about pancreatic physiology, pathophysiology, and pancreatic disease.[4] Acute pancreatitis can be thought of as an event that occurs when trigger factors drive trypsinogen activation beyond the protective mechanisms. Key molecular events occur within the acinar cell in relation to loss of calcium regulation with intracellular hypercalcemia and, therefore, elimination of trypsin autolysis protective mechanisms. Trypsin that is activated outside the acinar cell in which calcium levels are already elevated must be flushed quickly out of the duct by a CFTR-dependent mechanism or inhibited, eliminated, or corraled by other means. These factors are important in understanding susceptibility to acute pancreatitis. Once initiated, the resulting immune response and a variety of complications become the primary concern.

ACUTE PANCREATITIS

Acute pancreatitis is defined clinically as the sudden onset of abdominal pain associated with a rise in digestive enzymes in the blood or urine. The mechanism appears to involve the premature activation of trypsinogen because trypsinogen activation is among the earliest biochemical changes in experimental pancreatitis. Trypsinogen activation peptide is one of the earliest markers of acute pancreatitis in humans; endoscopic retrograde cholangiopancreatography (ERCP)-associated pancreatitis can be attenuated by pretreatment with trypsin inhibitors (eg, gabexate), and mutations that enhance trypsinogen activation, diminish trypsin inactivation, or limit trypsin clearance from the ducts are associated with acute pancreatitis. Second, acute pancreatitis is associated with a vigorous immune response, which contributes to the severity of the pathologic condition. By the time acute pancreatitis is recognized clinically, the trypsinogen activation and autodigestion phase may be over, and the inflammatory consequences dominate the clinical picture.

The prevalence of acute pancreatitis in children appears to be increasing.[21-23] The reason for this observation is unclear but does not appear to be simply related to referral bias or improved methods for diagnosis.[23]

ETIOLOGY OF ACUTE PANCREATITIS

A number of factors are able to trigger an attack of acute pancreatitis. In adults, the vast majority of cases are associated with gallstones, alcohol abuse, hypercalcemia, hypertriglyceridemia, medications, and blunt trauma. This profile appears to differ in children. Recently, a number of single and multicenter studies have investigated the etiologies of acute pancreatitis in children (Table 64.1-1). Acute pancreatitis associated with severe systemic illnesses is striking, accounting for about 20% of reported cases.[23] In some cases, acute pancreatitis may be overlooked in the intensive care unit setting.[24] However, the contribution of

TABLE 64.1-1   ETIOLOGY OF PANCREATITIS IN 1,276 CHILDREN

	STUDY (SETTING)						
	BENIFLA AND WEIZMAN (REVIEW)	DEBANTO ET AL (INPATIENT [MILD])	DEBANTO ET AL (INPATIENT [SEVERE])	LOPEZ (INPATIENT)	WERLIN ET AL (D/C RECORDS)	ALVAREZ CALATAYUD ET AL (INPATIENT)	TOTAL
NUMBER	589	162	40	274	180	31	1,276
Age, mean (median)	9.2	9.4	6.9	NA	(12.5)	7.9	
Male-to-female ratio	1.2	0.9	1	NA	0.9	1.2	
ETIOLOGY							
Systemic (eg, HUS)	14	1.9	20	53	14	6.5	20.8%
Gallstone		7.4	2.5		12	16	3.1%
Structural/divisum	15	2.5	2.5	10	7.7		10.6%
Infectious (eg, viral)	10	2.5	2.5	5	8	19	7.7%
Medications	12	11.1	7.5	5	12	9.7	10.2%
Trauma	22	13	20	19	14	6.5	18.6%
Post-ERCP	3.1	0			5.5		1.2%
Familial	2	6.8	7.5	"A few"	3		2.4%
Cystic fibrosis		3.1	0	0.4	0.6	0.5	0.6%
Hypercalcemia	1	3.1	0		0		0.9%
Hypertriglyceridemia	1	0.6	2.5		1		0.8%
DKA		1.2	0	0.7	4.4		0.9%
Other		3.7	7.5	0.4	10	7	2.4%
Idiopathic	23	40.1	27.5	17	8	35	22.2%

D/C = discharge, DKA = diabetic ketoacidosis and "diabetic"; ERCP = endoscopic retrograde cholangiopancreatography; HUS = hemolytic uremic syndrome; NA = not available. Benifla and Weizman[51] is a review of 18 pre-1999 studies from the United States (n = 9), the United Kindom (n = 5), Canada, Taiwan, Hong-Kong, Switzerland, and Israel. DeBanto et al[21] is from a multicenter (n = 6) study in the midwestern United States. Lopez[22] includes outpatient (Dallas, TX), Werlin et al[23] is from a referral center in Milwaukee, WI, and Alvarez Calatayud et al[117] is from Madrid, Spain.

pancreatitis to the overall severity of these diseases cannot be calculated from these reports, and it appears that deaths owing to acute pancreatitis in children alone are now uncommon (< 2%).[21,23] Hemolytic uremic syndrome is identified as the most common of all systemic diseases, causing acute pancreatitis in children.[21,23] The mechanism of pancreatitis is unknown and likely multifactorial, noting that uremia itself is a risk factor for pancreatic injury.[25–27] Although not classified separately in most case series, acute pancreatitis after organ transplant is also common.[23]

Gallstones are an important cause of acute pancreatitis in children. Choi and colleagues reported gallstones in 16 (29%) of 56 cases in a recent report from Korea.[28] In previous studies, gallstones were often included with structural abnormalities of the pancreas and biliary system as "biliary." This etiology should not be overlooked because therapeutic ERCP may be indicated.

Structural abnormalities also increase the risk for acute pancreatitis. The most common is pancreas divisum, but other abnormalities in the pancreatic or common bile duct (eg, choledochal cysts, choledochocoeles, and partial pancreas divisum) have been identified in children with otherwise unexplained acute pancreatitis.[23]

Infectious acute pancreatitis in North America and Europe is primarily viral in etiology. This includes mumps (39% of cases of pediatric acute pancreatitis reported in a Scottish study[29]), enterovirus, Epstein-Barr virus, hepatitis A, cytomegalovirus, rubella, coxsackievirus, varicella, rubeola, measles, and influenza virus.[21,23,30–33] Children with human immunodeficiency virus (HIV) frequently develop acute pancreatitis, usually from a secondary infection such as cytomegalovirus, *Mycobacterium avium intracellulare*, *Pneumocystis carinii*, and *Cryptosporidium parvum*, as well as from HIV medications.[34,35] Bacterial infections also occasionally cause acute pancreatitis.[30] In third world countries and tropical regions, acute pancreatitis is often associated with helminth infections such as *Ascaris lumbricoides*.[36–38] These cases can be severe, complicated, and difficult to treat.[39]

A variety of mediations are associated with acute and recurrent acute pancreatitis.[31,40,41] The strongest evidence in adults includes azathioprine or 6-mercaptopurine, thiazide diuretics, sulfonamides, furosemide, estrogens, and tetracycline, with suggestive evidence for L-asparaginase, iatrogenic hypercalcemia, chlorthalidone, corticosteroids, ethacrynic acid, phenformin, and procainamide.[41] Table 64.1-2 lists medications associated with acute pancreatitis in children.[21,23] The anticonvulsant valproate is the most common medication reported in these series. Grauso-Eby and colleagues reported 4 cases (1 fatal) from their institution, plus 29 others from the literature.[42] The median age was 8.9 years (range 1–18 years), and the mean dose was 45.6 mg/kg/d (range 20–85 mg/kg/d), with approximately equal doses in fatal and nonfatal cases. Seventy-one percent were taking multiple antiepileptic drugs, and children were taking valproate for a mean of 19 months (range 1 month to 10 years).[42] However, Pellock and colleagues reviewed over 3,000 patients treated with valproate from 34 studies and found only 2 documented cases of acute pancreatitis and a similar number of cases of amlyase ele-

vations in valproate-treated versus placebo-treated patients.[43] Furthermore, in over 2,000,000 reports to the Toxic Exposure Surveillance System compiled by the American Association of Poison Control Centers, acute pancreatitis was noted in only one of the four subjects with fatal valproate ingestion.[44] These data indicate that the association of valproic acid with acute pancreatitis is idiosyncratic but remains an important cause of pancreatitis in children. The other major causes of medication-associated pancreatitis in children are L-asparaginase and prednisone.

Trauma is a common cause of acute pancreatitis in children and is responsible for nearly 20% of cases (see Table 64.1-1). In the majority of cases, the trauma is blunt and accidental (eg, bicycle handlebar), but child abuse makes up a proportion of cases.[23] A major concern in these cases is pancreatic duct transection, which may require surgical intervention.

Post-ERCP pancreatitis is reported in several series.[21,23] Newer imaging modalities such as high-resolution computed tomography (CT) and MRCP, are, therefore, replacing ERCP as a diagnostic tool. ERCP, however, remains invaluable for therapeutic interventions.

Familial pancreatitis includes hereditary pancreatitis and other forms of pancreatitis that occur in families with an incidence that is higher than expected in the population by chance alone.[45] Atypical CF with compound heterozygous CFTR mild-variable mutations or CFTR mutations plus modifying factors, such as *SPINK1* mutations, are the most common cause of familial pancreatitis in our experience (D. Whitcomb, unpublished, 2003). Note that genetic testing was not available for cationic trypsinogen gene testing before 1996,[19] and for *SPINK1* gene testing before 2000,[46,47] and the role of CFTR testing was previously unclear.[4,48,49] There is no association between α_1-antitrypsin mutations and acute pancreatitis.[50] As genetic testing and better diagnostic testing become more widely available, the percentage of children with familial or gene mutation–associated pancreatitis will rise, whereas the idiopathic category will continue to fall.[23,51]

TABLE 64.1-2 MEDICATIONS ASSOCIATED WITH ACUTE PANCREATITIS IN TWO RECENT US STUDIES

DRUG	DEBANTO (N = 202)	WERLIN (N = 180)
Acetominophen	0	1
L-Asparaginase	6	2
Azathioprine/6-mercaptopurine	0	2
Cocaine	0	1
Fosphenytoin	0	1
Furosemide	1	0
Macrodantin	1	0
Metronidazole	1	1
Pentamidine	1	0
Phenytoin	1	0
Prednisone	6	0
Valproate	8	14
Multiple (several candidate drugs)	4	0
Unknown (or not recorded)	4	0

Adapted from Wankum P and Tobias JD[24] and Choi BH et al.[28]

An evaluation of a child with acute pancreatitis should include measurement of calcium and triglyceride levels because these causes must be addressed to prevent recurrence. Pancreatitis is occasionally seen in a number of other metabolic disorders, such as diabetic ketoacidosis[21-23] and inborn errors of metabolism[52] (Table 64.1-3).

RECURRENT ACUTE PANCREATITIS

Recurrent acute pancreatitis is seen in about 10% of children after a first episode of acute pancreatitis.[23,51] Recurrent acute pancreatitis is most commonly seen in patients with structural abnormalities, idiopathic pancreatitis, or familial pancreatitis.[23,51] A careful evaluation aimed at identifying reversible causes should be undertaken. In addition to avoiding another attack of acute pancreatitis, one should consider the prevention of chronic pancreatitis through eliminating known risk factors. Theoretically, the progression to chronic pancreatitis may be slowed by the use of antioxidants (which may also reduce the frequency and severity of recurrent symptoms in hereditary pancreatitis patients[53]), but these approaches are currently unproven.

DIAGNOSIS OF ACUTE PANCREATITIS

The diagnosis of pancreatitis is currently based on the syndrome of sudden onset of typical abdominal pain plus elevation of amylase or lipase to at least three times the upper limit of normal levels.[21-23,30] The diagnosis of acute pancreatitis can be difficult because no readily available test confirms the diagnosis. Although there have been multiple attempts to determine the sensitivity and specificity of elevations in both enzymes in adults, the studies all suffer from the absence of a method to separately and absolutely document pancreatitis. It is clear that both enzymes can be normal when there is radiographic and clinical evidence of pancreatitis. Also, both enzymes can be elevated by other conditions unrelated to pancreatitis. The level of elevation is also not diagnostic, although the higher the level is above the upper reference limit, the more likely it is that there will be pancreatic inflammation. Levels just above the upper reference limits may still be secondary to pancreatitis, especially in patients presenting several days after the onset of symptoms.

Other pancreatic products, such as phospholipase A_2, trypsin, trypsinogen activation peptide, and elastase, are elevated in pancreatitis, but none have found widespread use in the clinical laboratory setting. Serum transaminases are elevated in some patients, and the combination of elevated amylase or lipase and elevated serum transaminases may be more predictive of pancreatitis than elevated amylase or lipase alone.

Diagnostic testing for acute pancreatitis begins with a high index of suspicion, such as unexplained abdominal pain or vomiting. Pain is usually epigastric, in the right upper quadrant, or in the left upper quadrant, with radiation through to the back. However, back pain can occur alone, and pain may localize to other areas of the abdomen. Nausea and vomiting are common and may be the dominant clinical features. Other less common clinical signs include fever, tachycardia, hypotension, jaundice, and abdominal signs such as guarding, rebound tenderness, and a decrease in bowel sounds.[51] Occasionally, the diagnosis is first suspected because of feeding intolerance when feeds are introduced in patients with systemic illnesses.

Transient fever or jaundice can be present. Jaundice or elevated transaminases should raise the possibility of biliary tract involvement. Rarely, patients present with ascites or an abdominal mass. Epigastric tenderness is a useful but nonspecific and unreliable sign.

CT and abdominal ultrasonography of the pancreas are primarily used to document pancreatitis, determine the severity or identify complication (eg, pseudocysts), determine if there is underlying chronic pancreatitis, or identify other causes of unexplained signs or symptoms (Figure 64.1-2). Ultrasonographic findings include enlargement of the pancreas, altered echogenicity of the pancreas, dilated main pancreatic duct, gallstones, biliary sludge, dilated common and intrahepatic bile ducts, pancreatic calcification, choledochal cysts, and fluid collections, either peripancreatic or cystic. A CT scan will show similar findings, except that abnormal attenuation is seen rather than altered echogenicity. The CT scan is usually done several days into a severe course of acute pancreatitis when the patient fails to improve. There is experimental evidence indicating that CT contrast given early in the course of acute pancreatitis may diminish already tenuous blood flow to ischemic areas of the pancreas and thereby extend the region of necrosis. Although this is difficult to prove in humans, most experts agree that there is no diagnostic utility for a CT scan in the early phases of acute pancreatitis.[23] MRCP may be helpful in defining abnormalities of the ductal system, but its utility in pediatric patients has not been carefully studied. ERCP should be reserved for patients with unexplained recurrent episodes of pancreatitis, prolonged episodes of pancreatitis when a structural defect or duct disruption is suspected, or in some cases of gallstone pancreatitis.

MEDICAL MANAGEMENT OF ACUTE PANCREATITIS

The mainstay of current treatment of acute pancreatitis in children is analgesia, intravenous fluids, pancreatic rest, and monitoring for complications.[23,30] Full attention must be paid to fluid balances because patients are usually kept without food and may lose fluids from the vascular compartment from a capillary leak syndrome and "third spacing." Fluid

---

TABLE 64.1-3   PANCREATITIS IN PATIENTS WITH INBORN ERRORS OF METABOLISM

Pancreatitis caused by hyperlipidemia
  Hereditary lipoprotein lipase deficiency
  Apolipoprotein C-II deficiency
  Familial hypertriglyceridemia and chylomicronemia
Glycogen storage disorders
Branched-chain ketoaciduria (maple syrup urine disease)
Homocystinuria owing to cystathionine β-synthase deficiency
3-Hydroxy-3-methylglutaryl-CoA lyase deficiency
Acute intermittent porphyria
Pyruvate kinase deficiency
Cystinuria
Lysinuric protein intolerance and other cationic aminoacidurias

Adapted from Simon P et al.[52]

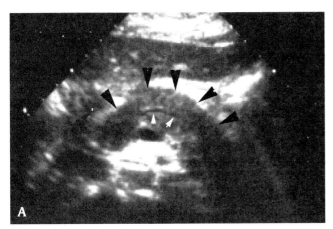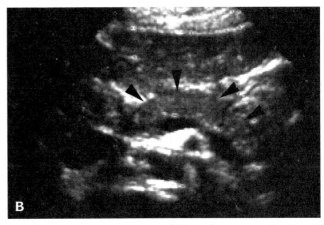

FIGURE 64.1-2   Ultrasonographic changes of pancreatitis. *A,* Sonogram of the pancreas in a 10-year-old boy who presented with epigastric pain and vomiting. He had a serum lipase 20 × upper reference limit (URL) and a serum amylase 6 × URL. The pancreas is edematous, and the main pancreatic duct is dilated. The upper edge of the pancreas is marked by *black arrowheads,* and the main pancreatic duct is indicated by *white arrowheads. B,* Sonogram of a normal pancreas. The same patient presented with periumbilical pain 2 months later. His serum lipase and amylase levels were normal. A sonogram showed a normal pancreas and did not visualize the main pancreatic duct, a normal finding in children. The *arrowheads* mark the upper edge of the pancreas.

losses are exaggerated if a nasogastric tube is used to decompress the stomach as a treatment for vomiting. Volume expansion early in the course of acute pancreatitis is important for both cardiovascular stability and preventing development of pancreatic necrosis. Meperidine 1 to 2 mg/kg intramuscularly or intravenously is used for pain control.[30] Enteral or total parenteral nutrition is often unnecessary in mild cases but should be instituted early if a severe or prolonged course is anticipated. Until recently, parenteral nutrition was considered the only option, but several studies show that adult patients with acute pancreatitis tolerate jejunal feedings with fewer complications than those given parenteral nutrition.[54] Antibiotics are usually unnecessary except for the most severe cases, especially if significant pancreatic necrosis is present.

SEVERITY OF ACUTE PANCREATITIS

Acute pancreatitis can be life threatening, although death does not appear to occur as often in children (without other systemic diseases) as it does in adults.[23] Death occurs by several mechanisms, with some occurring early and others late. The early causes of death are cardiovascular collapse and respiratory failure. The cardiovascular collapse occurs with the combination of a vascular leakage syndrome with third spacing of fluid, vomiting, and having the patient receive nothing by mouth. If recognized, this complication can be treated with fluid resuscitation, guided, when necessary, by following central venous pressure. The respiratory failure is associated with an adult respiratory distress syndrome–like situation that results from leakage of fluid into alveolar spaces and inflammation. Early recognition of this complication and management of patients at high risk within an intensive care setting can be lifesaving.

Late life-threatening complications of acute pancreatitis are related to infected pancreatic necrosis and multisystem organ failure, although pancreatic necrosis appears to be uncommon in children—1 case of 380 from 7 centers

(0.3%).[21,23] Judicious use of antibiotics and attention to nutrition may help limit these late complications.

GLOBAL ACUTE PANCREATITIS SCORING SYSTEMS

Acute pancreatitis is usually divided into mild and severe forms. Originally, mild acute pancreatitis was defined as pancreatitis limited to peripancreatic fat necrosis and interstitial edema, whereas severe pancreatitis included additional features.[55,56] Other clinically based systems also have been developed, which define mild and severe according to the absence or presence of major complications requiring prolonged treatment or specific interventions or an increased likelihood of death.[57–60] Thus, mild pancreatitis includes the majority of cases, which have minimal complications, a short clinical course requiring minimal supportive treatment, and complete recovery. It is the physician's responsibility to make a rapid assessment of the patient's condition and to predict the risk of a mild or severe clinical course. To assist the physician in this decision, a number of severity criteria have been developed, including Ranson's scores,[57,58] Glasgow score,[59] the Acute Physiology and Chronic Health Evaluation (APACHE) II score,[61,62] and Pediatric score.[21] Although these criteria add little to the assessment of the experienced physician, they remain useful in reminding one to carefully consider the major systems impacted during the more severe attacks of acute pancreatitis. In general, the signs and organic symptoms of each of these systems reflect the magnitude of the inflammatory response to acute pancreatitis rather than measure the actual amount of pancreatic injury.

Ranson's criteria were developed in adults,[57,58] and several criteria (eg, age > 55 years and fluid deficit > 6 L) are not applicable to children.[21] The Midwest Multicenter Pancreatic Study Group analyzed the criteria of the Ranson and Glasgow scores, plus additional criteria, and developed a scoring system for children.[22] The seven severity factors included age (< 7 years), weight (< 23 kg), admission white blood cell count (>18.5 x 10⁹/L), admission lactate dehydrogenase (> 2,000 IU/L), 48-hour fluid sequestration (> 75 mL/kg/48 hours), and a 48-hour rise in urea (> 5 mg/dL). If each criterion is assigned a value of 1 point, then the outcome of patients with 0 to 2 points was 8.6% severe, 1.4% death; with 2 to 4 points was 38.5% severe, 5.8% death; and with 5 to 7 points was 80% severe, 10% death.[21] The accuracy of this system was validated in three centers. Of note, young age and low weight are major risk factors. Severity was also often associated with severe systemic diseases (see Table 64.1-1, DeBanto [severe]), a pattern also noted by others.[22,23]

COMPLICATIONS OF ACUTE PANCREATITIS

A number of non–life-threatening complications of acute pancreatitis are recognized. These include both local and systemic complications (Table 64.1-4). Local complications include fluid collections, pancreatic necrosis (sterile or infected), pancreatic abscess, duct rupture, duct strictures, bleeding, and pseudocyst formation.

Pancreatic necrosis, which is a segmental pancreatic infarction, remains a major concern because it is associated with serious complications. This complication probably occurs in less than 5% of adult patients and less than 1% of children. The risk of pancreatic necrosis appears to increase with vascular leakage, as reflected by an elevated hematocrit in nearly all patients with pancreatic necrosis. The combination of intravascular volume depletion, inflammation, and high hematocrit therefore leads to blockage of pancreatic blood flow and infarction. The diagnosis is made by contrast-enhanced CT with demonstration of a segment of pancreatic gland without perfusion.

Complications of pancreatitis may require specific treatment. Pancreatic pseudocysts occur in children. Pseudocysts can be observed over time for spontaneous resorption or may require drainage. Currently, both endoscopic internal drainage and external drainage by interventional radiologists offer viable options to surgery. The chronicity, size, location, and complexity of the pseudocysts all contribute to decisions about the optimal choice for treatment. Abscesses often can be treated with external drainage and intravenous antibiotics, and only rarely is surgical drainage necessary. Surgery is usually necessary

for traumatic rupture of the duct, although endoscopic stenting across the disrupted duct is another option.

SURGICAL MANAGEMENT OF ACUTE PANCREATITIS

The role of surgery in the management of acute pancreatitis is limited to débridement of infected pancreatic necrosis and cholecystectomy to prevent recurrent gallstone pancreatitis. The differentiation of infected from sterile pancreatic necrosis should be based on fine-needle aspiration for bacteriology.[63–65] Surgery in severe pancreatitis is usually deferred for at least 2 weeks to permit proper demarcation of pancreatic and peripancreatic necrosis to occur and to provide the optimal operative conditions for necrosectomy.[65] This approach decreases the risk of bleeding and minimizes surgery-related loss of vital tissue, which can predispose the patient to surgically induced endocrine and exocrine pancreatic insufficiency.

If acute pancreatitis is caused by gallstones or biliary sludge, then a cholecystectomy should be performed to avoid recurrence of gallstone-associated acute pancreatitis. It has been recommended that cholecystectomy should be performed as soon as the patient has recovered and, ideally, during the same hospital admission in mild gallstone-associated acute pancreatitis, whereas cholecystectomy may need to be delayed after an episode of severe acute pancreatitis. Endoscopic sphincterotomy is an alternative to cholecystectomy in selected cases.

CHRONIC PANCREATITIS

Chronic pancreatitis is a syndrome of destructive, inflammatory conditions that encompasses the many sequelae of long-standing pancreatic injury.[66] Thus, acute pancreatitis is an *event*, whereas chronic pancreatitis is a *process*.[4] Histologic changes from the normal pancreatic architecture include irregular fibrosis, acinar cell loss, islet cell loss, and inflammatory cell infiltrates.[67–69] Clinical diagnosis currently depends on identifying defined clinical, functional, morphologic, and histologic features that characterize the final common pathologic pathway of a variety of pancreatic disorders.[45,66]

ETIOLOGY OF CHRONIC PANCREATITIS

In adults, chronic pancreatitis is usually associated with prolonged ingestion of large amounts of alcohol (~ 70%) or appears to be idiopathic (~ 20%).[66] In children, chronic pancreatitis is usually associated with genetic conditions such as typical or atypical CF or hereditary pancreatitis or is idiopathic. The incidence of chronic pancreatitis appears to be increasing in children, perhaps reflecting better diagnostic tools or following an apparent rise in recurrent acute pancreatitis.

Current research suggests that chronic pancreatitis is better defined as a complex process beginning with acute pancreatitis and progressing to end-stage fibrosis as the result of recurrent and chronic inflammatory processes. As with acute pancreatitis, susceptibility and the rate of progression are influenced by both genetic and environmental factors. To date, genetic susceptibility factors for chronic

TABLE 64.1-4	COMPLICATIONS OF ACUTE PANCREATITIS
LOCAL	**SYSTEMIC**
Edema	Shock
Inflammation	Pulmonary edema
Fat necrosis	Pleural effusions
Phlegmon	Acute renal failure, coagulopathy
Pancreatic necrosis	Hemoconcentration
Sterile	Bacteremia, sepsis
Infected	Distant fat necrosis
Abscess	Vascular leak syndrome
Hemorrhage	Multiorgan system failure
Fluid collections	Hypermetabolic state
Pseudocysts	Hypocalcemia
Duct rupture and strictures	Hyperglycemia
Extension to nearby organs	

pancreatitis are the same as the susceptibility factors for recurrent acute pancreatitis (ie, *PRSS1*, *SPINK1*, and *CFTR* mutations). Several genetic modifiers have been reported in abstract form, but further research must be completed before their role in chronic pancreatitis can be clearly defined.

Recently, a new classification system has been developed to organize and understand the factors associated with chronic pancreatitis (Table 64.1-5). The TIGAR-O system allows multiple factors to be assessed in a single patient either as risk factors (before chronic pancreatitis develops) or as etiologies (after pancreatitis develops). This approach also allows the clinician to identify factors that can be modified to reduce risk (eg, smoking cigarettes or drinking alcohol). The common etiologies of chronic

---

TABLE 64.1-5   ETIOLOGIC RISK FACTORS ASSOCIATED WITH CHRONIC PANCREATITIS: TIGAR-O CLASSIFICATION SYSTEM (VERSION 1.0)

TOXIC-METABOLIC
Alcoholic
Tobacco smoking
Hypercalcemia
  Hyperparathyroidism
Hyperlipidemia
Chronic renal failure
Medications
  Phenacetin abuse (possibly from chronic renal insufficiency)
Toxins
  Organotin compounds (eg, di-n-butyltin dichloride)

IDIOPATHIC
Early onset
Late onset
Tropical
  Tropical calcific pancreatitis
  Fibrocalculous pancreatic diabetes
Other

GENETIC
Autosomal dominant
  Cationic trypsinogen (codon 29 and 122 mutations)
Autosomal recessive/modifier genes
  CFTR mutations
  SPINK1 mutations
  Cationic trypsinogen (codon A16V, D22G, K23R)
  α_1-Antitrypsin deficiency (possible)

AUTOIMMUNE
Isolated autoimmune chronic pancreatitis
Syndromic autoimmune chronic pancreatitis
  Sjögren syndrome–associated chronic pancreatitis
  Inflammatory bowel disease–associated chronic pancreatitis
  Primary biliary cirrhosis–associated chronic pancreatitis

RECURRENT AND SEVERE ACUTE PANCREATITIS–ASSOCIATED
  CHRONIC PANCREATITIS
Postnecrotic (severe acute pancreatitis)
Recurrent acute pancreatitis
Vascular diseases/ischemic
Postirradiation

OBSTRUCTIVE
Pancreatic divisum
Sphincter of Oddi disorders (controversial)
Duct obstruction (eg, tumor)
Preampullary duodenal wall cysts
Post-traumatic pancreatic duct scars

Adapted from Etemad B and Whitcomb DC.[66]

---

pancreatitis in adults (eg, alcohol, hypertriglyceridemia) are reviewed elsewhere.[66]

TRYPSINOGEN MUTATIONS

Trypsinogen mutations are responsible for pancreatitis in the majority of hereditary pancreatitis kindreds. The most common mutations include the cationic trypsinogen (*PRSS1*) R122H and N29I mutations, although a variety of other mutations are occasionally seen. Recommendations for genetic testing and genetic counseling have been published.[4,70,71] Hereditary pancreatitis caused by *PRSS1* mutations usually presents as recurrent acute pancreatitis in childhood with a median age of 10 years but a range of less than 1 year to 60 years of age.[16,72–74] The chronic pancreatitis in *PRSS1* mutation–associated hereditary pancreatitis usually follows the onset of recurrent acute pancreatitis by 10 years, although only half of the patients with recurrent acute pancreatitis develop chronic pancreatitis, and the clinical course is highly variable. Occasionally, patients will present with chronic pancreatitis without a clear history of acute pancreatitis. The most important clinical clue is a family history of pancreatitis or unexplained abdominal pain lasting for 1 to 3 days in adults from previous generations, although, in some cases, no other history of pancreatitis is seen.[75] The diagnosis is confirmed by genetic testing of the *PRSS1* gene, but about 30 to 40% of smaller hereditary pancreatitis families do not have identifiable mutations in the *PRSS1* gene.[75]

CFTR-ASSOCIATED PANCREATITIS

CF is the most important cause of chronic pancreatitis in children. CF is caused by severe mutations in both CFTR gene alleles (CFTR^{sev}/CFTR^{sev}). However, over 1,200 CFTR mutations have been identified, which are organized into five or six classes depending on the effect of the mutation on CFTR expression and function.[76] Some mutations (class IV) are mild or variable (CFTR^{m-v}), and compound heterozygous genotypes (CFTR^{sev}/CFTR^{m-v}) result in total CFTR function that is a fraction of normal (eg, 5%). These genotypes are associated with atypical CF, in which some CFTR-dependent organs are spared from severe CF-associated injury, whereas others are affected.[77,78] For example, the CFTR^{sev}/CFTR^{m-v} genotypes have been associated with idiopathic chronic pancreatitis (ICP).[14,15] However, these studies also have an excess of patients who appear to be *CFTR* mutation heterozygous, whereas parents of CF patients (who are obligate *CFTR* mutation carriers) do not have an excess incidence of pancreatitis.[79]

CFTR mutation–associated pancreatitis can be divided into four mechanistic subtypes of CFTR-associated mechanisms.[4] Type 1 is CF with a CFTR^{sev}/CFTR^{sev} genotype. Type 2 is atypical cystic fibrosis with a CFTR^{sev}/CFTR^{m-v} genotype. Of specific interest are *CFTR* mutations that specifically block bicarbonate conductance but not chloride conductance.[80,81] These mutations may specifically target the pancreas over other organs because bicarbonate secretion by the pancreatic duct cells is central to pancreatic fluid secretion. Type 3 is CFTR^{sev} or CFTR^{m-v} plus a second pancreatitis modifier or susceptibility gene in a polygenetic condition such as the CFTR^{sev}/SPINK1 N34S allele. Type 4 is CFTR^{sev} or CFTR^{m-v} plus a strong environmental risk factor such as alcohol.

EARLY- AND LATE-ONSET ICP

Layer and colleagues observed that the age at onset of ICP is bimodal.[82] In early-onset ICP, calcification and exocrine and endocrine insufficiency develop more slowly than in late-onset idiopathic and alcoholic pancreatitis, but pain is more severe. In contrast, in late-onset ICP, pain is absent in 50% of patients.[82]

The etiology of early-onset ICP is being resolved. Witt and colleagues first identified the *SPINK1* N34S and other *SPINK1* mutations in children with ICP.[46] Pfützer and colleagues recently identified *SPINK1* mutations in about 25% of patients with ICP, but 87% of patients with *SPINK1* mutations developed pancreatitis before age 20 years.[47] A similar pattern was seen by Ockenga and colleagues.[83] However, 1 to 4% of representative populations have the high-risk *SPINK1* N34S allele, and the phenotype of heterozygous and homozygous genotypes is identical.[18,47] Thus, *SPINK1* mutations probably cause increased susceptibility to recurrent acute and chronic pancreatitis with homozygous mutations or as part of a polygenic condition with another genetic risk factor, such as type 3 CFTR-associated pancreatitis. Other genetic factors that increase susceptibility to pancreatitis or that modify the clinical course of recurrent acute pancreatitis toward rapid fibrosis likely will be defined in the near future.

DIAGNOSIS

The diagnosis of chronic pancreatitis can be made by histologic or morphologic criteria alone or by a combination of morphologic, functional, and clinical findings.[69,84–87] Functional abnormalities alone are not diagnostic of chronic pancreatitis because these tests do not differentiate chronic pancreatitis from pancreatic insufficiency without pancreatitis.[66] Pancreatic insufficiency should be considered as either an end stage of destructive chronic pancreatitis or as arising from an independent condition, such as Shwachman-Diamond syndrome.[88,89]

ABDOMINAL IMAGING

Four imaging procedures are commonly used for the evaluation of pancreatic disease: CT, ERCP, endoscopic ultrasonography (EUS), and magnetic resonance imaging (MRI) or MRCP. Chronic pancreatitis with calcifications also can be identified on abdominal radiography or by transabdominal ultrasonography, and, when present, the diagnosis of chronic pancreatitis can be made with 90% confidence.[90] These techniques are used as inexpensive initial screening techniques in some centers.[90] However, abdominal radiography and transabdominal ultrasonography lack the sensitivity of CT, ERCP, and EUS.[85] EUS and MRI or MRCP are less widely available and require more technical expertise, and their precise role in evaluation of chronic pancreatitis in children remains to be fully defined.[91] At some centers, MRCP[92] (especially with secretin[93]) has replaced ERCP in most cases used for diag-

nosis in children, although ERCP remains a valuable tool for therapy and in some diagnostic cases.[23] Each of these newer technologies offers significant advantages and promise over ERCP or CT, but they also have limitations.

PANCREATIC FUNCTION TESTING

Several functional tests have been developed to diagnose chronic pancreatic insufficiency. As noted above, pancreatic insufficiency is a sign of chronic pancreatitis but is not diagnostic. The pancreas has marked functional reserve, so it must be damaged severely before functional loss is clinically recognized.[94] Invasive tests of pancreatic function (eg, the "tubed" secretin test) are the gold standard for determining exocrine pancreatic function.

Pancreatic function testing serves three purposes: to diagnose exocrine pancreatic insufficiency, to aid in the evaluation of chronic pancreatitis, and to provide a basis for rational treatment.[45,95] Mechanistically, pancreatic insufficiency reflects either impaired enzyme synthesis capacity, altered release of enzymes and bicarbonate into the intestine, or intraluminal impairment of pancreatic enzyme function or mixing.[96] Pancreatic function tests are difficult to compare between centers because they often use different stimulants and measure different parameters.[96] Furthermore, few centers perform direct testing of pancreatic exocrine secretion.

Noninvasive function tests to detect pancreatic insufficiency are also used infrequently because they are insensitive and have high false-positive rates.[95] Currently, there are two noninvasive pancreatic function tests available at many centers: fecal elastase 1 (FE-1) and "functional" MRCP. The FE-1 is an excellent test for moderate to severe chronic pancreatitis in adults[97] but is less accurate in mild to moderate chronic pancreatitis.[98] FE-1 reaches normal levels by day 3 in term newborns and by 2 weeks in infants born before 28 weeks of gestation.[99] The sensitivity and specificity of FE-1 and fecal chymotrypsin have been assessed in subjects with severe and mild steatorrhea.[100] Although FE-1 had superior performance characteristics in patients with mild steatorrhea, the ability to identify patients with moderate pancreatic insufficiency without steatorrhea remains a major limitation. The possibility of having a "functional" MRCP is very attractive because both structural and functional data could be gathered in one test. A functional MRCP protocol has been published,[101] but the sensitivity and specificity compared with those of direct testing must be demonstrated because the concentration of bicarbonate compared with the volume of pancreatic fluid is a critical discriminator in exocrine pancreatic function testing.

GENETIC TESTING

Genetic testing for pancreatic diseases is becoming an important part of medical practice. The results of genetic testing are highly accurate, but positive results for the major autosomal dominant, high-penetrance mutations (eg, *PRSS1* R122H) have broad implications for the patient's future health, family, employment, and insurability.[48,71,102,103] The purpose of genetic testing can be divided into two general categories: diagnostic and predictive.[4] Diagnostic testing is done when a patient has symptoms of a disease, and a genetic test is done to determine the underlying cause(s). Examples include *CFTR* mutation testing in suspected typical or atypical cystic fibrosis or *PRSS1* (cationic trypsinogen) gene testing in suspected hereditary pancreatitis. Predictive testing is genetic testing in subjects without evidence of pancreatic disease. In general, predictive genetic testing in children is not indicated for *CFTR* or *SPINK1* mutations and is not recommended for *PRSS1* mutations unless there are first-degree relatives with a known *PRSS1* mutation, adequate genetic counseling has been offered, and the child can participate in the decision to undergo testing.[70] General guidelines are outlined in Tables 64.1-6 and 64.1-7.

Genetic testing is now commercially available for the *PRSS1* (cationic trypsinogen) R122H and N29I mutations.[66] The primary indications for cationic trypsinogen mutation testing include recurrent idiopathic acute pancreatitis, ICP, verification of a clinical suspicion in a family member of a kindred with known mutations, to help a patient understand or validate his or her condition, and to assist individuals in making lifestyle decisions (eg, reproduction, diet, smoking) based on the known risk of pancreatitis and potential pancreatic cancer.[66,71,104]

Genetic testing is also used in children with unexplained pancreatitis or episodes of pancreatitis-like pain when there is a significant concern about the possibility of hereditary pancreatitis. Identification of an established pancreatitis-associated gene mutation can be valuable in expediting an expensive and prolonged evaluation of recurrent pancreatitis in children.[45] A positive test result in a clinically unaffected person is interpreted as conferring a significant increased risk of pancreatitis, with this risk possibly diminishing with age. A negative test result in a family with a known mutation essentially eliminates the risk of this genetic form of pancreatitis. If a mutation has not been previously identified in the family, then a negative test result in an unaffected person is considered noninformative because one cannot distinguish whether the tested individual is free from genetic risk or whether he or she has inherited a different pancreatitis-predisposing gene mutation.[66] In families with hereditary pancreatitis, alcohol, emotional stress, and fatty foods are reported to precipitate pancreatitis attacks,[72] and smoking increases the risk of pancreatitis[105–107] and pancreatic cancer.[108] Testing for the purpose of encouraging mutation-positive older children to avoid these excesses is advocated by some caregivers. However, avoidance of fatty foods, alcohol, and tobacco represents excellent general medical advice and therefore provides no compelling reason for genetic testing.[71] In either case, the personal desires of older children to postpone testing or to proceed with testing to relieve their own anxieties and learn more about their own personal health must be carefully considered. Ownership of test results in children must be addressed.[66,70]

Testing for *SPINK1* mutations in individuals with early-onset chronic pancreatitis may provide important information on the predisposing causes of pancreatitis for the concerned patient.[66] However, most experts do not advocate genetic testing for *SPINK1* mutations at this time.[48,49,70] Furthermore, because less than 1% of patients with a heterozygous *SPINK1* mutation alone are likely to develop pancreatitis, the major reasons are lacking to undertake presymptomatic testing. Homozygous *SPINK1* N34S genotypes are strongly associated with chronic pancreatitis and, therefore, are likely a dominant factor in the etiology of otherwise ICP. Heterozygous *SPINK1* mutations alone are likely not disease causing[47,109] but rather act as a cofactor with other genetic mutations as part of a polygenic disorder.

There has been much interest in testing patients with ICP for *CFTR* mutations. The problem is that most panels are designed to test for the common CF-causing gene mutations, not pancreatitis-causing mutations. This area of research continues to develop, and pancreatitis-specific panels or total, low-cost CFTR gene analysis will be needed to fully interpret the CFTR genotype–pancreatitis phenotype relationship. On the other hand, pancreatitis may be the first sign of CF or atypical CF, and these children should, therefore, undergo a full evaluation for cystic fibrosis.

TABLE 64.1-6   INDICATIONS FOR GENETIC TESTING FOR *PRSS1* MUTATIONS

Recurrent (2 or more) attacks of *acute* pancreatitis for which there is no explanation (eg, anatomic anomalies, ampullary or main pancreatic strictures, trauma, viral infection, gallstones, alcohol, drugs, hyperlipidemia)

Unexplained (idiopathic) *chronic* pancreatitis

A family history of pancreatitis in a first-degree (parent, sib, child), second-degree, (aunt, uncle, niece, nephew), or third-degree (grandparent, first cousin) relative

An unexplained episode of documented pancreatitis occurring in a child who has required hospitalization and where there is significant concern that hereditary pancreatitis should be excluded

For a patient with pancreatitis eligible for an ethics committee/institutional review board–approved research protocol

Adapted from Ellis et al.[70]

TABLE 64.1-7   PREGENETIC TEST PATIENT INFORMATION FOR *PRSS1* MUTATIONS

Prior to genetic testing, patients should understand

Why the test has been suggested and provide documented informed consent

The implications of finding a pancreatitis-related mutation in the *PRSS1* gene for the health and medical care of that patient

How their genetic test result will be communicated to them and who else will be informed of their result (ie, the clinician who has requested that test, other involved pancreatic specialists, the family doctor, hospital medical records, insurance carrier)

The availability of genetic counseling after the test result is known

The pancreatic cancer risk and the possible adverse health, life insurance, and employment consequences for the patient (if not safeguarded against by state or national legislation)

The implications of a positive genetic test result for their relatives

Whether or not they wish for their test sample to be used for any research project and by what (anonymized) route this will occur

Adapted from a consensus statement of the Consensus Committees of the European Registry of Hereditary Pancreatic Diseases, the Midwest Multi-Center Pancreatic Study Group, and the International Association of Pancreatology.[70]

MODIFIER GENES

The reason that some patients with recurrent acute pancreatitis rapidly develop chronic pancreatitis whereas others do not likely involves mutations in disease-modifying genes.[4] This area of research is currently evolving, and several interesting candidate genes are under investigation and verification.

TREATMENT

The major goals in treating patients with chronic pancreatitis differ with the stage and etiology of disease. Patients with recurrent acute pancreatitis are at risk of developing chronic pancreatitis.[23,110] Efforts should be made to identify the cause of recurrent acute pancreatitis to prevent the development of chronic pancreatitis. Systematic approaches have been published,[111] and a number of risk factors can be addressed by the physician.[66] Anatomic variants can be addressed by both endoscopic and surgical interventions.

In patients with rapidly progressing chronic pancreatitis from an untreatable cause (eg, severe genetic mutations), there are two prognostic concerns. The first is development of a chronic pain syndrome, and the second is development of insulin-dependent diabetes mellitus. There are many possible etiologies of pancreatic pain.[112] The concern is that prolonged exposure of pancreatic nerves to growth factors associated with pancreatic inflammation will cause irreversible central changes so that eventual pancreatic surgery for pain will be of limited value. A second concern is the development of diabetes through destruction of the pancreatic islet cells. Although early surgical intervention with islet cell autotransplant is a consideration in these patients, the problem of islet yield, especially if delayed until chronic pancreatitis is advanced, and long-term benefit remain important issues without clear answers.

In patients with advanced chronic pancreatitis, the objectives are to treat the pancreatic insufficiency resulting from the loss of pancreatic digestive enzymes and to treat pain and diabetes mellitus if they develop. The treatment for pancreatic digestive enzyme deficiency is enzyme replacement.[113,114] The goal is to provide enzyme supplements that restore digestive function.[96] Enzymes are given with all protein- and fat-containing foods and milk products, including predigested formulas and breast milk. Microspheres, minimicrospheres, and microtablets are preferable to granules because the acid-resistant enteric coating protects the enzyme from acid degradation in the stomach and protects against the mouth and perianal excoriations that were seen previously with uncoated enzyme powders.[115,116] Enzymes should be taken about 15 minutes before each meal or snack. For prolonged meals, additional enzymes should also be taken during the meal. Parents and adolescent patients should be taught to adjust the enzyme dosage according to the anticipated amount of fat in a meal.

Generic enzymes may not be bioequivalent to proprietary enzymes.[117] Therefore, apparent treatment failures should include an investigation of the brand of enzymes that was dispensed. Another cause of failure is destruction of the digestive enzymes by gastric acid. Although enteric coating of pancreatic enzymes may protect pancreatic enzymes in the stomach, the intestine remains more acidic (1–2 pH units) in patients with *CFTR* mutations than those with other types of pancreatitis because of a loss in duodenal bicarbonate secretion.[118,119] In the past, treatment of gastric and intestinal acidity included the use of sodium bicarbonate and histamine$_2$ receptor antagonists. However, the availability, efficiency, and safety of the proton pump inhibitors have resulted in widespread use of these products. Enteric-coated products remain effective when used with proton pump inhibitors. On the other hand, patients who do not have CF and retain significant pancreatic function could theoretically benefit from a more acidic duodenal pH so that pancreatic fluid secretion is stimulated and enzymes are rapidly washed out of the pancreatic duct. In this case, gastric acid suppression would be limited, and enteric-coated enzymes are mandatory.

The dose of enzymes is usually calculated according to lipase content. A usual dose of pancreatic enzymes contains 1,000 to 2,500 U lipase/kg/meal. Adequacy of treatment is typically determined on clinical grounds. Frequent, bulky, fatty stools; excessive bloating and flatus; excessive appetite; and inadequate growth velocity are indicators of inadequate treatment. Calculation of a coefficient of fat absorption is used for clinical studies but rarely in clinical practice. Although the human FE-1 test accurately predicts exocrine pancreatic insufficiency,[120–122] it is of no value in determining the adequacy of enzyme replacements of porcine origin because the test is specific for human elastase 1.

REFERENCES

1. Rinderknecht H. Pancreatic secretory enzymes. In: Go VLW, DiMagno EP, Gardner JD, et al, editors. The pancreas: biology, pathobiology, and disease. 2nd ed. New York: Raven Press; 1993. p. 219–51.
2. Gomez JE, Birnbaum ER, Royer GP, Darnall DW. The effect of calcium ion on the urea denaturation of immobilized bovine trypsin. Biochim Biophys Acta 1977;495:177–82.
3. Colomb E, Guy O, Deprez P, et al. The two human trypsinogens: catalytic properties of the corresponding trypsins. Biochem Biophys Acta 1978;525:186–93.
4. Whitcomb DC. Value of genetic testing in management of pancreatitis. Gut 2004. [In press]
5. Rovery M. Limited proteolysis in pancreatic chymotrypsinogens and trypsinogens. Biochimie 1988;70:1131–5.
6. Raraty M, Ward J, Erdemli G, et al. Calcium-dependent enzyme activation and vacuole formation in the apical granular region of pancreatic acinar cells. Proc Natl Acad Sci U S A 2000;97:13126–31.
6b. Sutton R, Criddle D, Raraty MGT, et al. Signal transduction, calcium, and acute pancreatitis. Pancreatology 2003;3: 497–505.
7. Mogami H, Nakano K, Tepikin AV, Petersen OH. Ca²⁺ flow via tunnels in polarized cells: recharging of apical Ca2⁺ stores by focal Ca2⁺ entry through basal membrane patch. Cell 1997;88:49–55.
8. Kruger B, Albrecht E, Lerch MM. The role of intracellular calcium signaling in premature protease activation and the onset of pancreatitis. Am J Pathol 2000;157:43–50.

9. Frick TW, Fernandez-del Castillo C, Bimmler D, Warshaw AL. Elevated calcium and activation of trypsinogen in rat pancreatic acini. Gut 1997;41:339–43.

10. Mithofer K, Fernandez-del Castillo C, Frick TW, et al. Acute hypercalcemia causes acute pancreatitis and ectopic trypsinogen activation in the rat. Gastroenterology 1995; 109:239–46.

11. Voronina S, Longbottom R, Sutton R, et al. Bile acids induce calcium signals in mouse pancreatic acinar cells: implications for bile-induced pancreatic pathology. J Physiol 2002;540(Pt 1):49–55.

12. Ward JB, Petersen OH, Jenkins SA, Sutton R. Is an elevated concentration of acinar cytosolic free ionized calcium the trigger for acute pancreatitis [review]? Lancet 1995;346: 1016–9.

13. Drumm ML, Pope HA, Cliff WH, et al. Correction of the cystic fibrosis defect in vitro by retrovirus-mediated gene transfer. Cell 1990;62:1227–33.

14. Cohn JA, Friedman KJ, Noone PG, et al. Relation between mutations of the cystic fibrosis gene and idiopathic pancreatitis. N Engl J Med 1998;339:653–8.

15. Sharer N, Schwarz M, Malone G, et al. Mutations of the cystic fibrosis gene in patients with chronic pancreatitis. N Engl J Med 1998;339:645–52.

16. Whitcomb DC. Genetic predispositions to acute and chronic pancreatitis. Med Clin North Am 2000;84:531–47.

17. Ogawa M. Pancreatic secretory trypsin inhibitor as an acute phase reactant. Clin Biochem 1988;21:19–25.

18. Whitcomb DC. How to think about SPINK and pancreatitis. Am J Gastroenterol 2002;97:1085–8.

19. Whitcomb DC, Gorry MC, Preston RA, et al. Hereditary pancreatitis is caused by a mutation in the cationic trypsinogen gene. Nat Genet 1996;14:141–5.

20. Simon P, Weiss FU, Sahin-Tóth M, et al. Hereditary pancreatitis caused by a novel PRSS1 mutation (Arg-122 ->Cys) that alters autoactivation and autodegradation of cationic trypsinogen. J Biol Chem 2001;21:21.

21. DeBanto JR, Goday PS, Pedroso MR, et al. Acute pancreatitis in children. Am J Gastroenterol 2002;97:1726–31.

22. Lopez MJ. The changing incidence of acute pancreatitis in children: a single-institution perspective. J Pediatr 2002; 140:622–4.

23. Werlin SL, Kugathasan S, Frautschy BC. Pancreatitis in children. J Pediatr Gastroenterol Nutr 2003;37:591–5.

24. Wankum P, Tobias JD. Pancreatitis in the pediatric ICU patient. J Intens Care Med 2001;12:47–52.

25. Araki T, Ueda M, Ogawa K, Tsuji T. Histological pancreatitis in end-stage renal disease. Int J Pancreatol 1992;12:263–9.

26. Lerch MM, Hoppe-Seyler P, Gerok W. Origin and development of exocrine pancreatic insufficiency in experimental renal failure. Gut 1994;35:401–7.

27. Pitchumoni CS, Arguello P, Agarwal N, Yoo J. Acute pancreatitis in chronic renal failure. Am J Gastroenterol 1996; 91:2477–82.

28. Choi BH, Lim YJ, Yoon CH, et al. Acute pancreatitis associated with biliary disease in children. J Gastroenterol Hepatol 2003;18:915–21.

29. Haddock G, Coupar G, Youngson GG, et al. Acute pancreatitis in children: a 15-year review. J Pediatr Surg 1994; 29:719–22.

30. Lerner A, Branski D, Lebenthal E. Pancreatic diseases in children. Pediatr Clin North Am 1996;43:125–56.

31. Steinberg W, Tenner S. Acute pancreatitis. N Engl J Med 1994;330.1190–210.

32. Imrie CW, Ferguson JC, Sommerville RG. Coxsackie and mumpsvirus infection in a prospective study of acute pancreatitis. Gut 1977;18:53–6.

33. Arnesjo B, Eden T, Ihse I, et al. Enterovirus infections in acute pancreatitis—a possible etiological connection. Scand J Gastroenterol 1976;11:645–9.

34. Dutta SK, Ting CD, Lai LL. Study of prevalence, severity, and etiological factors associated with acute pancreatitis in patients infected with human immunodeficiency virus. Am J Gastroenterol 1997;92:2044–8.

35. Miller TL, Winter HS, Luginbuhl LM, et al. Pancreatitis in pediatric human immunodeficiency virus infection. J Pediatr 1992;120(2 Pt 1):223–7.

36. Das S. Pancreatitis in children associated with round worms. Indian Pediatr 1977;14:81–3.

37. Gilbert MG, Carbonnel ML. Pancreatitis in childhood associated with ascariasis. Pediatrics 1964;33:1964.

38. Coelho da Rocha RF, Chapcha P, Aun F. Abdominal complications of ascariasis in children. Probl Gen Surg 2001; 18:92–9.

39. Bahu Mda G, Baldisseroto M, Custodio CM, et al. Hepatobiliary and pancreatic complications of ascariasis in children: a study of seven cases. J Pediatr Gastroenterol Nutr 2001;33:271–5.

40. Somogyi L, Martin SP, Ulrich CD. Recurrent acute pancreatitis. Curr Treat Options Gastroenterol 2001;4:361–8.

41. Mallory A, Kern F. Drug-induced pancreatitis: a critical review. Gastroenterology 1980;78:813–20.

42. Grauso-Eby NL, Goldfarb O, Feldman-Winter LB, McAbee GN. Acute pancreatitis in children from valproic acid: case series and review. Pediatr Neurol 2003;28:145–8.

43. Pellock JM, Wilder BJ, Deaton R, Sommerville KW. Acute pancreatitis coincident with valproate use: a critical review. Epilepsia 2002;43:1421–4.

44. Litovitz TL, Klein-Schwartz W, White S, et al. 2000 annual report of the American Association of Poison Control Centers Toxic Exposure Surveillance System. Am J Emerg Med 2001;19:337–95.

45. Whitcomb DC. Hereditary diseases of the pancreas. In: Yamada T, Alpers DH, Laine L, et al, editors. Textbook of gastroenterology. 4th ed. Philadelphia: Lippincott, Williams and Wilkins; 2002. p. 2147–65.

46. Witt H, Luck W, Hennies HC, et al. Mutations in the gene encoding the serine protease inhibitor, Kazal type 1 are associated with chronic pancreatitis. Nat Genet 2000; 25:213–6.

47. Pfützer RH, Barmada MM, Brunskil APJ, et al. SPINK1/PSTI polymorphisms act as disease modifiers in familial and idiopathic chronic pancreatitis. Gastroenterology 2000; 119:615–23.

48. Whitcomb DC. Motion—genetic testing is useful in the diagnosis of nonhereditary pancreatic conditions: arguments for the motion. Can J Gastroenterol 2003;17:47–52.

49. Cohn JA. Motion—genetic testing is useful in the diagnosis of nonhereditary pancreatic conditions: arguments against the motion. Can J Gastroenterol 2003;17:53–5.

50. Witt H, Kage A, Luck W, Becker M. Alpha1-antitrypsin genotypes in patients with chronic pancreatitis. Scand J Gastroenterol 2002;37:356–9.

51. Benifla M, Weizman Z. Acute pancreatitis in childhood: analysis of literature data. J Clin Gastroenterol 2003;37:169–72.

52. Simon P, Weiss FU, Zimmer KP, et al. Acute and chronic pancreatitis in patients with inborn errors of metabolism. Pancreatology 2001;1:448–56.

53. Uomo G, Talamini G, Rabitti PG. Antioxidant treatment in hereditary pancreatitis. A pilot study on three young patients. Dig Liver Dis 2001;33:58–62.

54. Abou-Assi S, Craig K, O'Keefe SJ. Hypocaloric jejunal feeding is better than total parenteral nutrition in acute pancreatitis: results of a randomized comparative study. Am J Gastroenterol 2002;97:2255–62.

55. Sarles H, Adler G, Dani R, et al. The pancreatitis classification of Marseilles, Rome 1988. Scand J Gastroenterol 1989;24:641–2.

56. Sarles H. Pancreatitis: Symposium of Marseille, 1963. Basel: Karger; 1965.

57. Ranson JH, Rifkind KM, Roses DF, et al. Prognostic signs and the role of operative management in acute pancreatitis. Surg Gynecol Obstet 1974;139:69–81.

58. Ranson JH. Etiological and prognostic factors in human acute pancreatitis: a review. Am J Gastroenterol 1982;77:633–8.

59. Blamey SL, Imrie CW, O'Neill J, et al. Prognostic factors in acute pancreatitis. Gut 1984;25:1340–6.

60. Bradley EL III. A clinically based classification system for acute pancreatitis. Summary of the International Symposium on Acute Pancreatitis, Atlanta, Ga, September 11 through 13, 1992. Arch Surg 1993;128:586–90.

61. Knaus WA, Draper EA, Wagner DP, Zimmerman JE. APACHE II: a severity of disease classification system. Crit Care Med 1985;13:818–29.

62. Larvin M, McMahon MJ. APACHE-II score for assessment and monitoring of acute pancreatitis. Lancet 1989;ii:201–5.

63. Gerzof SG, Banks PA, Robbins AH, et al. Early diagnosis of pancreatic infection by computed tomography-guided aspiration. Gastroenterology 1987;93:1315–20.

64. Hiatt JR, Fink AS, King W III, Pitt HA. Percutaneous aspiration of peripancreatic fluid collections: a safe method to detect infection. Surgery 1987;101:523–30.

65. Uhl W, Warshaw A, Imrie C, et al. IAP guidelines for the surgical management of acute pancreatitis. Pancreatology 2002;2:565–73.

66. Etemad B, Whitcomb DC. Chronic pancreatitis: diagnosis, classification, and new genetic developments. Gastroenterology 2001;120:682–707.

67. Kloppel G, Maillet B. Pathology of acute and chronic pancreatitis. Pancreas 1993;8:659–70.

68. Kloppel G, Maillet B. A morphological analysis of 57 resection specimens and 9 autopsy pancreata. Pancreas 1991; 6:266–74.

69. Homma T, Harada H, Koizumi M. Diagnostic criteria for chronic pancreatitis by the Japan Pancreas Society. Pancreas 1997;15:14–5.

70. Ellis I, Lerch MM, Whitcomb DC, Committee C. Genetic testing for hereditary pancreatitis: guidelines for indications, counseling, consent and privacy issues. Pancreatology 2001;1:401–11.

71. Applebaum SE, Kant JA, Whitcomb DC, Ellis IH. Genetic testing: counseling, laboratory and regulatory issues and the EUROPAC protocol for ethical research in multicenter studies of inherited pancreatic diseases. Med Clin North Am 2000;82:575–88.

72. Sibert JR. Hereditary pancreatitis in England and Wales. J Med Genet 1978;15:189–201.

73. Sossenheimer MJ, Aston CE, Preston RA, et al. Clinical characteristics of hereditary pancreatitis in a large family based on high-risk haplotype. Am J Gastroenterol 1997; 92:1113–6.

74. Howes N, Lerch MM, Greenhalf W, et al. Clinical and genetic characteristics of hereditary pancreatitis in Europe. Clin Gastroenterol Hepatol 2004;2:252–61.

75. Applebaum-Shapiro SE, Finch R, Pfützer RH, et al. Hereditary pancreatitis in North America: the Pittsburgh-Midwest Multi-Center Pancreatic Study Group Study. Pancreatology 2001;1:43943.

76. Rowntree RK, Harris A. The phenotypic consequences of CFTR mutations. Ann Hum Genet 2003;67(Pt 5):471–85.

77. Stern RC. The diagnosis of cystic fibrosis. N Engl J Med 1997;336:48791.

78. Whitcomb DC. Hereditary and childhood disorders of the pancreas, including cystic fibrosis. In: Feldman M, Friedman LS, Sleisenger MH, editors. Sleisenger and Fortran's gastroenterology and liver diseases. 7th ed. Philadelphia: WB Saunders Company; 2002. p. 881–904.

79. Lowenfels A, Maisonneuve P, Palys B. Re: Ockenga et al—mutations of cystic fibrosis gene in patients with pancreatitis. Am J Gastroenterol 2001;96:614–5.

80. Reddy MM, Quinton PM. Control of dynamic CFTR selectivity by glutamate and ATP in epithelial cells. Nature 2003;423:756–60.

81. Choi JY, Muallem D, Kiselyov K, et al. Aberrant CFTR-dependent HCO3- transport in mutations associated with cystic fibrosis. Nature 2001;410:94–7.

82. Layer P, Yamamoto H, Kalthoff L, et al. The different courses of early- and late-onset idiopathic and alcoholic chronic pancreatitis. Gastroenterology 1994;107:1481–7.

83. Ockenga J, Vogel A, Teich N, et al. UDP glucuronosyltransferase (UGT1A7) gene polymorphisms increase the risk of chronic pancreatitis and pancreatic cancer. Gastroenterology 2003;124:1802–8.

84. Lankish PG. Progression from acute to chronic pancreatitis: a physician's view. Surg Clin North Am 1999;79:815–27.

85. Clain JE, Pearson RK. Diagnosis of chronic pancreatitis: is a gold standard necessary? Surg Clin North Am 1999; 79:829–45.

86. Ammann RW, Muellhaupt B. Progression of alcoholic acute to chronic pancreatitis. Gut 1994;35:552–6.

87. Chari ST, Singer MV. The problem of classification and staging of chronic pancreatitis: proposal based on current knowledge and its natural history. Scand J Gastroenterol 1994;29:949–60.

88. Mack DR, Forstner GG, Wilschanski M, et al. Shwachman syndrome: exocrine pancreatic dysfunction and variable phenotypic expression. Gastroenterology 1996;111: 1593–602.

89. Boocock GR, Morrison JA, Popovic M, et al. Mutations in SBDS are associated with Shwachman-Diamond syndrome. Nat Genet 2003;33:97–101.

90. DiMagno E, Layer P, Clain J. Chronic pancreatitis. In: Go V, editor. The pancreas: biology, pathophysiology and disease. New York: Raven Press, Ltd.; 1993. p. 665–706.

91. Manfredi R, Lucidi V, Gui B, et al. Idiopathic chronic pancreatitis in children: MR cholangiopancreatography after secretin administration. Radiology 2002;224:675–82.

92. Matos C, Metens T, Deviere J, et al. Pancreatic duct: morphologic and functional evaluation with dynamic MR pancreatography after secretin stimulation. Radiology 1997;203:435–41.

93. Manfredi R, Costamagna G, Brizi MG, et al. Severe chronic pancreatitis versus suspected pancreatic disease: dynamic MR cholangiopancreatography after secretin stimulation. Radiology 2000;214:849–55.

94. DiMagno EP, Go VL, Summerskill WH. Relations between

pancreatic enzyme ouputs and malabsorption in severe pancreatic insufficiency. N Engl J Med 1973;288:813–5.

95. Layer P, Rünzi M, Go VLW. Diagnosis of chronic pancreatitis. In: Howard J, Idezuki Y, Ihse I, Prinz R, editors. Surgical diseases of the pancreas. 3rd ed. Baltimore: Williams & Wilkins; 1998. p. 329–33.

96. Layer P, Keller J. Pancreatic enzymes: secretion and luminal nutrient digestion in health and disease. J Clin Gastroenterol 1999;28:3–10.

97. Loser C, Mollgaard A, Folsch UR. Faecal elastase 1: a novel, highly sensitive, and specific tubeless pancreatic function test. Gut 1996;39:580–6.

98. Amann ST, Bishop M, Curington C, Toskes PP. Fecal pancreatic elastase 1 is inaccurate in the diagnosis of chronic pancreatitis. Pancreas 1996;13:226–30.

99. Kori M, Maayan-Metzger A, Shamir R, et al. Faecal elastase 1 levels in premature and full term infants. Arch Dis Child Fetal Neonatal Ed 2003;88:F106–8.

100. Walkowiak J, Herzig KH, Strzykala K, et al. Fecal elastase-1 is superior to fecal chymotrypsin in the assessment of pancreatic involvement in cystic fibrosis. Pediatrics 2002; 110(1 Pt 1):e7.

101. Cappeliez O, Delhaye M, Deviere J, et al. Chronic pancreatitis: evaluation of pancreatic exocrine function with MR pancreatography after secretin stimulation. Radiology 2000;215:358–64.

102. Shaheen NJ, Lawrence LB, Bacon BR, et al. Insurance, employment, and psychosocial consequences of a diagnosis of hereditary hemochromatosis in subjects without end organ damage. Am J Gastroenterol 2003;98: 1175–80.

103. Applebaum SE, O'Connell JA, Aston CE, Whitcomb DC. Motivations and concerns of patients with access to genetic testing for hereditary pancreatitis. Am J Gastroenterol 2001;96:1610–7.

104. Lowenfels A, Maisonneuve P, DiMagno E, et al. Hereditary pancreatitis and the risk of pancreatic cancer. J Natl Cancer Inst 1997;89:442–6.

105. Talamini G, Bassi C, Falconi M, et al. Cigarette smoking: an independent risk factor in alcoholic pancreatitis. Pancreas 1996;12:131–7.

106. Talamini G, Bassi C, Falconi M, et al. Alcohol and smoking as risk factors in chronic pancreatitis and pancreatic cancer. Dig Dis Sci 1999;44:1301–11.

107. Lin Y, Tamakoshi A, Hayakawa T, et al. Cigarette smoking as a risk factor for chronic pancreatitis: a case-control study in Japan. Research Committee on Intractable Pancreatic Diseases. Pancreas 2000;21:109–14.

108. Lowenfels AB, Maisonneuve P, Whitcomb DC, et al. Cigarette smoking as a risk factor for pancreatic cancer in patients with hereditary pancreatitis. JAMA 2001;286169–70.

109. Threadgold J, Greenhalf W, Ellis I, et al. The N34S mutation of *SPINK1* (*PSTI*) is associated with a familial pattern of idiopathic chronic pancreatitis but does not cause the disease. Gut 2002;50:675–81.

110. Schneider A, Whitcomb DC. Hereditary pancreatitis: a model for inflammatory diseases of the pancreas. Best Pract Res Clin Gastroenterol 2002;16:347–63.

111. Somogyi L, Martin SP, Venkatesan T, Ulrich CD II. Recurrent acute pancreatitis: an algorithmic approach to identification and elimination of inciting factors. Gastroenterology 2001;120:708–17.

112. Warshaw A, Banks PA, Femandez-del Castillo C. AGA technical review: treatment of pain in chronic pancreatitis. Gastroenterology 1998;115:765–76.

113. Littlewood JM, Wolfe SP. Control of malabsorption in cystic fibrosis. Paediatr Drugs 2000;2:205–22.

114. Stern RC, Eisenberg JD, Wagener JS, et al. A comparison of the efficacy and tolerance of pancrelipase and placebo in the treatment of steatorrhea in cystic fibrosis patients with clinical exocrine pancreatic insufficiency. Am J Gastroenterol 2000;95:1932–8.

115. Borowitz D, Baker RD, Stallings V. Consensus report on nutrition for pediatric patients with cystic fibrosis. J Pediatr Gastroenterol Nutr 2002;35:246–59.

116. Stead RJ, Skypala I, Hodson ME, Batten JC. Enteric coated microspheres of pancreatin in the treatment of cystic fibrosis: comparison with a standard enteric coated preparation. Thorax 1987;42:533–7.

117. Hendeles L, Dorf A, Stecenko A, Weinberger M. Treatment failure after substitution of generic pancrelipase capsules. Correlation with in vitro lipase activity. JAMA 1990; 263:2459–61.

118. Robinson PJ, Smith AL, Sly PD. Duodenal pH in cystic fibrosis and its relationship to fat malabsorption. Dig Dis Sci 1990;35:1299–304.

119. Allen A, Flemstrom G, Garner A, Kivilaakso E. Gastroduodenal mucosal protection. Physiol Rev 1993;73:823–57.

120. Dominguez-Munoz JE, Hieronymus C, Sauerbruch T, Malfertheiner P. Fecal elastase test: evaluation of a new noninvasive pancreatic function test. Am J Gastroenterol 1995;90:1834–7.

121. Gullo L, Ventrucci M, Tomassetti P, Migliori M, Pezzilli R. Fecal elastase 1 determination in chronic pancreatitis. Dig Dis Sci 1999;44:210–3.

122. Beharry S, Ellis L, Corey M, et al. How useful is fecal pancreatic elastase 1 as a marker of exocrine pancreatic disease? J Pediatr 2002;141:84–90.

2. Juvenile Tropical Pancreatitis

C. S. Pitchumoni, MD, FRCPC, FACP, MACG, MPH
Viswanathan Mohan, MD, MRCP, PhD, DSC

Chronic pancreatitis is mostly a disease of adults secondary to 10 to 15 years of alcoholism. Although relatively rare, hereditary pancreatitis is the most common type of chronic pancreatitis in children of the developed countries of the world. In many Afro-Asian countries, a nonhereditary, nonalcoholic form of chronic calcific pancreatitis is the most common type of chronic pancreatitis in children and young adults.[1-8] Nutritional pancreatitis, tropical pancreatitis, juvenile tropical pancreatitis syndrome, tropical calculous pancreatopathy, Afro-Asian pancreatitis, and fibrocalculous pancreatic diabetes are other terms used in the literature to describe this entity.

DEFINITION

Tropical pancreatitis is a form of chronic pancreatitis characterized by recurrent abdominal pain, pancreatic calculi, and diabetes mellitus, occurring mostly among poor children and young adults of many developing nations (Figures 64.2-1 to 64.2-3). The affected individuals are generally emaciated and may show signs of malnutrition. The notable absence of other known causes of pancreatitis, the geographic prevalence of the disease in developing nations, and the scientific plausibility of pancreatic injury in malnutrition are the keys to implicating nutritional deficiency as the most likely etiologic factor for this otherwise enigmatic disease.

EPIDEMIOLOGY

Although isolated case studies have been reported in the Indian medical literature since 1930, the first clear description of this syndrome was made in 1959 by Zuidema from Indonesia.[1] This classic article described seven malnourished Indonesian patients with pancreatic lithiasis. The youngest, a 15-year-old girl, was markedly undernourished, weighing only 33.5 kg. Her main meal at home was rice, cassava (*Manihot esculenta*), and vegetables and seldom included fish, meat, or eggs. The oldest in the group was 28 years of age. None had a history of alcohol consumption. In six patients, diabetes mellitus dominated the clinical picture. Some of them had marked swelling of both parotid glands and thinning of scalp hair resembling kwashiorkor. In one case, autopsy showed fibrosed acinar tissue and stones in the duct. Zuidema subsequently reported on 45 patients from 12 to 45 years of age with the same clinicopathologic features.[1] The diabetes of the poor in Indonesia, Zuidema concluded, was a result of severe protein malnutrition.

In 1960, Shaper observed a similar syndrome in the indigenous population of Uganda, whose diet was rich in carbohydrate but low in protein and fat.[2] The youngest patient was 10 years old. Most patients had a history of moderate to severe recurrent abdominal pain, suggestive of pancreatitis. Shaper felt that the high-carbohydrate diet associated with severe protein deficiency led to increased demands for pancreatic enzymes while potentiating the effect of protein depletion.

The syndrome of chronic pancreatitis with pancreatic calculi and diabetes has subsequently been reported by different observers from many countries, such as Uganda, Nigeria, the republic of Congo, Malawi, Zambia, Ghana, the Ivory Coast, and Madagascar in Africa; Sri Lanka, Malaysia, Thailand, India, and Bangladesh in Asia; and Brazil in South America.[1] In support of the term tropical pancreatitis, the prevalence of this disease is almost restricted to latitude 30° north and south of the equator.

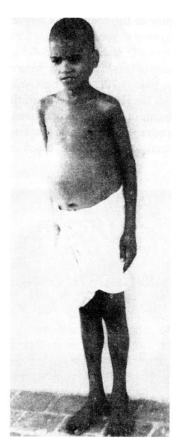

FIGURE 64.2-1   A 13-year-old boy with juvenile tropical pancreatitis. Note the emaciation and distended abdomen.

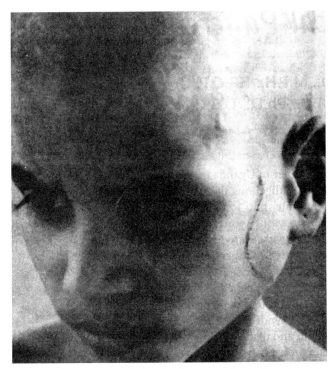

FIGURE 64.2-2   Parotid gland enlargement in the boy shown in Figure 64.2-1.

The largest series of cases of juvenile tropical pancreatitis to date is from the southwestern state of Kerala in India. This may be the result of an increased awareness and routine screening of young diabetics for pancreatic calculi with radiographic studies of the abdomen. Approximately 3,000 cases of this disease have been reported in the literature, more than 1,700 cases by GeeVarghese alone from the state of Kerala in India, where the disease was once noted to occur in endemic proportions.[5]

The true prevalence of this disease is not well established because the epidemiologic data are based exclusively on patients seen in major teaching hospitals that do not include those studied in nonteaching hospitals and outpatient clinics of private practitioners. On the other hand, the hospital data may give an erroneously high prevalence because most of the patients from villages tend to accumulate in the major teaching hospitals for treatment. The data can be further skewed because in many Afro-Asian countries, men seek medical attention more often and earlier than women. One epidemiology study in an endemic area in the state of Kerala reported a prevalence of 1 in 1,000 population.[9] In a referral diabetic center, tropical pancreatitis constituted 1% of all diabetic patients.[8] The disease currently appears to have decreased in its incidence in the state of Kerala in India, where, nearly three decades ago, it was noted to be frequent. A marked improvement in the socioeconomic status of the population in the state and an associated improvement in childhood nutrition may be reasonably assumed to be the reasons for this change in incidence.

PATHOLOGY

The pathologic changes in the pancreas and other organs in tropical pancreatitis have been well studied in material obtained at postmortem or surgery.[8,10,11] Because pancreatic biopsy is not done in the early stages of the disease, our knowledge of the pathology is limited to the late stages. The histologic changes in the pancreas are almost identical to those of alcoholic pancreatitis.

The size of the pancreas varies inversely with the duration and severity of the disease. In advanced stages of the disease, the pancreatic gland is as small as the little finger, and the surface is irregular and nodular. Uneven shrinkage and fibrous adhesions cause displacement of the pancreas from its normal location. The parenchyma may be replaced by fat and become indistinguishable from surrounding adipose tissue. The pancreas is firm, fibrous, and gritty to the touch, although the consistency of the organ may vary in different regions of the gland depending on the presence of fibrous tissue, cysts, or stones. Radiologic examination of the dissected pancreas often reveals multiple calculi, which are not noted in antemortem radiologic studies (Figure 64.2-4).

Homogeneous areas; varying degrees of fibrous, cystic dilatation of the gland; and pancreatic calculi of different shapes and sizes distributed throughout the duct system characterize the cut-section. The major pancreatic duct may be eccentrically placed as a result of uneven destruction of the glandular tissue. Areas of stenosis and dilatation of the ducts can be seen in the same gland. Incomplete pancreatic obstruction at the ampulla of Vater is noted in a large majority of carefully dissected cases, corresponding to the location of a solitary calculus ("sentinel stone") and/or larger stones.[5]

Pancreatic calculi vary in color, size, and shape. The larger stones are nearer the head, progressively diminishing in size toward the tail. The stones range in size from small sand particles to calculi 4.5 cm long, weighing up to 20 g. The shape of a stone is influenced by its location; may be smooth, rounded, or staghorn-like; and may be incarcerated in the main pancreatic duct and major branches.

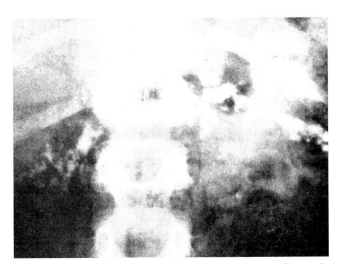

FIGURE 64.2-3   Flat plate of the pancreas in a case of juvenile topical pancreatitis. The entire main pancreatic duct and even some ductules are packed with calculi. A ductogram is seen.

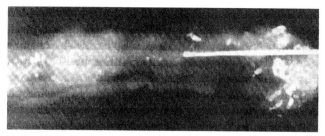

FIGURE 64.2-4 Radiologic study of the isolated postmortem pancreas. Note the numerous small radiodense areas, which are intraductal calculi. The probe is passed into the main duct to show the dilatation in relation to the shrunken pancreas.

Soft stones are formed by noncalcified protein plugs and caseous material. Sections of calcified stones show epithelial debris, fibrin, and mucinous material.

Pancreatic calculi are composed of 95.5% calcium carbonate and a small amount of calcium phosphate. Traces of magnesium, urate, and oxalate have been identified in some stones. X-ray diffraction studies of calculi have determined that calcium carbonate is found predominantly in the form of calcite and rarely in the form of vaterite.[12] Scanning electron microscopic studies and spectroscopic methods of analysis have shown that the calculi have an amorphous nidus and a cryptocrystalline periphery. The nidus is rich in iron, chromium, and nickel, and the periphery contains a number of trace elements and a preponderance of calcium.[13] These calculi are structurally and biochemically similar to stones obtained in other types of chronic pancreatitis. A nonenzymatic protein has been identified by some observers in the core of calculi. This protein, termed pancreatic stone protein (PSP), has been implicated in the pathogenesis of the disease and in calculus formation. The absence or decrease of PSP has been thought to promote nucleation of calcium carbonate and crystallization in chronic pancreatitis.[14] However, recent studies on PSP have given contradictory results, and the role of PSP in the genesis of calculi and the pathogenesis of disease is unclear.

Microscopically, the characteristic feature is diffuse fibrosis of the pancreas (Figure 64.2-5). The main duct, collecting ducts, and small ductules show marked dilatation with periductular fibrosis. Denudation of the ductular epithelium and squamous metaplasia are seen in some areas. The characteristic cellular infiltraton of the pancreas is composed of lymphocytes and plasma cells, distributed mainly around the ducts. Interlobular fibrosis is characteristic of early cases, and focal, segmental, or diffuse fibrosis is characteristic of more advanced cases. The acinar tissue shows varying degrees of atrophy and parenchymal destruction. Fibrous tissue is seen adjacent to relatively normal-looking parenchyma. As the disease advances, the islets become atrophic and are isolated and surrounded by dense fibrous tissue. In some instances, the islets appear even hypertrophied, and, as in other forms of pancreatic atrophy, a true nesidioblastosis is observed (Figure 64.2-6). Preliminary histochemical studies have identified those hyperplastic islets as B-cell nesidioblastosis. Immunohistochemistry has also shown

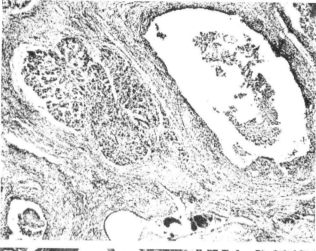

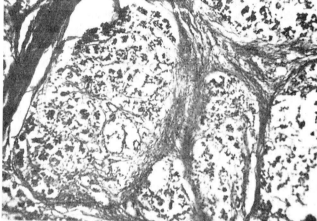

FIGURE 64.2-5 The pancreas shows extensive fibrosis, ductular dilatation, and intraductular calcium deposits. The intra- and interacinar fibrosis of the exocrine parenchyma produces the appearance of cirrhosis of the pancreas (hematoxylin and eosin).

reduced alpha cells and beta cells in the pancreas.[11,15] The vacuolation, ballooning, and glycogen infiltration of the islets characteristic of juvenile diabetes are seldom noted. The clinical significance of the islet cell hyperplasia is to be further studied.

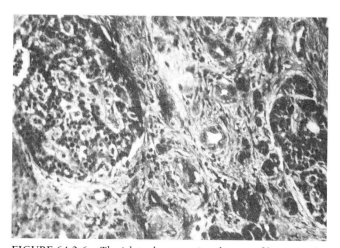

FIGURE 64.2-6 The islets show varying degrees of hypertrophy in the presence of fibrosis of the organ.

The high incidence of pancreatic carcinoma in patients of a relatively young age suggests that tropical pancreatitis is a premalignant disease similar to hereditary pancreatitis.[16,17] Other organs such as the liver and parotid glands show changes indicative of uncontrolled diabetes mellitus and/or malnutrition. The liver in the early stages shows glycogen infiltration of the cytoplasm and nuclei and fatty changes (and cirrhosis in more advanced cases). Parotid glands show hypertrophied acini, with varying degrees of round cell infiltration around the intralobular and interlobular ducts. The pathogenesis of parotid enlargement is probably a functional or compensatory hypertrophy as an adaptive mechanism to pancreatic exocrine insufficiency.[18]

ETIOLOGY AND PATHOGENESIS

The exact etiology of this disease has not yet been established. The etiologic factors proposed here are to be considered hypothetical, based on epidemiologic data, careful clinical studies, and biochemical evaluations. The hypotheses in consideration are as follows:

MALNUTRITION

The basis for considering malnutrition as a predisposing factor was the prevalence of the disease almost exclusively in the poor population groups of developing nations and the findings of malnutrition in many patients.[3-7] Protein malnutrition is known to cause pancreatic injury in experimental and clinical studies. In kwashiorkor, as well as marasmus, pancreatic structure and function are markedly altered.[17] Some of the histologic changes of the pancreas in kwashiorkor, such as atrophy of acinar cells, disorganization and loss of the acinar pattern, marked reduction in the amount of zymogen granules, vacuolization, epithelial metaplasia, cystic dilatation of the ducts, and an increase in fibrous tissue, mimic the histology of tropical pancreatitis.

A number of recent observations, however, speak against protein malnutrition as the sole or initiating factor of this disease[19]:

1. In India and Africa, the geographic prevalence of the disease does not correlate with that of kwashiorkor.
2. Protein-energy malnutrition, being prevalent in many tropical countries, is likely to be a denominator in most diseases affecting poor populations.
3. There are large pockets of malnutrition with relative infrequency or total absence of tropical pancreatitis in many parts of the world.
4. Despite some histologic similarities to tropical pancreatitis, the pathology of the pancreas in kwashiorkor is different. The latter disease seldom produces permanent pancreatic damage, and, more importantly, calculi formation is not a feature.
5. The disease currently is seen in some well-nourished children of affluent families, further complicating the malnutrition theory.

The advanced malnutrition noted in tropical pancreatitis studied three decades ago appears to be the consequence of the disease rather than its cause. It is thus clear that tropical pancreatitis is not secondary to isolated protein malnutrition, although nutritional factors as explained below cannot be excluded from its pathogenesis.

FREE RADICAL INJURY

Clinical protein-energy malnutrition is a complex syndrome complicated by deficiencies of a number of vitamins and trace elements, bacterial and viral infections and parasitic infestations, psychological stress, and hormonal and immunologic disturbances. The body's ability to scavenge the highly reactive free radicals is markedly impaired in malnutrition, whereas the endogenous and exogenous stimuli for free radical production are markedly enhanced. Chronic pancreatitis, alcoholic or tropical, has been hypothesized as one of the many diseases caused by unmitigated free radical injury.[20,21]

However, in view of the difficulties in studying free radical production and elimination in the pancreas, free radical injury as a mechanism of pancreatitis remains in the realm of hypothesis.

TRACE ELEMENTS AND VITAMIN DEFICIENCIES

Independent of their ability to scavenge free radicals, trace elements and vitamins participate in maintaining the integrity of acinar cell function and structure. Experimental studies indicate that a zinc-deficient diet results in acinar cell injury, copper deficiency induces selective and progressive atrophy of acinar cells, and selenium deficiency causes pancreatic fibrosis.[22] Vitamin A, riboflavin, folic acid, and vitamin D appear to be important for acinar cell integrity.[22] Although deficiency of these trace elements and vitamins may occur as part of the spectrum of human malnutrition, clinical pancreatic disease has not been proven to be secondary to micronutrient deficiency.

DIETARY CYANOGENS

The geographic distribution of tropical pancreatitis coincides with areas of consumption of cassava root (tapioca, *Manihot esculenta*), which is a source of carbohydrate for poor populations in parts of Nigeria, Uganda, Indonesia, Thailand, and the state of Kerala in India.[5]

Cassava root is known to contain cyanogenic glycosides: linamarin and lotaustralin.[23] Cyanide is normally detoxified in the body by conversion to thiocyanate, but this detoxification requires sulfur containing the amino acid methionine, which is deficient in cassava. A high-carbohydrate, low-protein diet was shown to cause pancreatic fibrosis in a recent experimental study, raising the possibility that the nutritional composition of the diet is important in pancreatic injury[24] rather than the source of carbohydrate or the presence or absence of cyanogen in the diet. Although tropical pancreatitis is prevalent in some parts of Africa and India where cassava is not consumed, it is not noted in some areas where cassava is consumed, as in the rural West African population.[25]

GENETIC FACTORS

Many recent studies have looked for genetic abnormalities in all forms of chronic pancreatitis following the discovery of genetic mutations in hereditary pancreatitis.[26-28]

In the normal pancreas, a number of mechanisms work synergistically, preventing the premature activation of trypsinogen to trypsin. The central mechanism of acinar cell injury is autodigestion by active trypsin. Mutations of certain genes reduce the natural ability of the body to prevent the premature activation of trypsinogen. The most important mutations studied in relation to hereditary pancreatitis and, to a lesser extent, in other forms of pancreatitis are those involving the cationic trypsinogen gene (PRSS1), serine protease inhibitor Kazal type 1 (SPINK 1), and cystic fibrosis transmembrane conductance regulator (CFTR).[29] In light of what has been learned with regard to genetic abnormalities in hereditary pancreatitis, tropical pancreatitis is being currently evaluated for possible genetic mutations. On a small cohort of tropical pancreatitis patients, the frequency of CFTR mutations was lower than that reported in idiopathic chronic pancreatitis from the West.[30]

In two recent studies, one from India and the other from Bangladesh, it was noted that tropical pancreatitis was highly associated with the SPINK 1 N34S mutation.[31,32] The high prevalence of N34S mutation in patients with and without diabetes in the Indian study suggests that these two subtypes have a similar genetic predisposition.[31,32]

In conclusion, the etiopathogenesis of this syndrome remains enigmatic, and further studies are clearly needed. Its relationship to cystic fibrosis is an area that needs to be explored.

CLINICAL FEATURES

The cardinal manifestations of juvenile tropical pancreatitis are recurrent abdominal pain in childhood, followed by diabetes mellitus and pancreatic calculi by puberty and death in the prime of life. Improvement in the management of diabetes has resulted in a longer life span not noted in earlier observations. The calculated life expectancy after the onset of abdominal pain and diabetes is 35 and 25 years, respectively.[33]

The onset of the disease is insidious in early childhood, with recurrent attacks of upper abdominal or periumbilical pain before the thirteenth year (Table 64.2-1). The history is often elicited from the patient's mother, who attests to the number of school days lost. About 5% of juvenile diabetics with pancreatic calculi do not have abdominal pain.[5] The patient usually keeps the palm on the abdomen to indicate a wide area of pain as opposed to the finger tip, as in duodenal ulcer. The pain radiates to the lower end of the sternum, the left costal margin, and along the left side or posteriorly to the lumber spine. The episodes of pain last for days, not minutes or hours. The pain is usually aggravated by small amounts of food so that the patients refuse all food by mouth. In the early stages, the bouts of pain are severe and are associated with vomiting. As years pass, painful attacks become less intense but more prolonged. In an attempt to obtain relief, patients sit up, bend forward, or walk; curl up in the lateral decubitis position; clutch the skin of the abdomen; or apply hot water bottles to the area. Recent studies have noted a change in the age at onset of the disease. Only about 12% of

TABLE 64.2-1   AGE AT ONSET OF PANCREATIC PAIN IN 100 CASES

AGE (YR)	NUMBER OF CASES
5–11	26
12–18	35
19–25	14
26–30	5
31–35	1
36–40	2
41–50	2
No pain	6
Undetermined	9
Total	100

Adapted from GeeVarghese PJ et al.[3]

patients report an onset before the age of 20 years.[7] The observed difference in the current series of cases from those reported earlier cannot be explained.[4,7]

An interval of several years may pass between the cessation of painful attacks and the onset of diabetes mellitus. Pancreatic pain totally disappears in a large number of patients either before or some years after diabetes develops, coinciding with "burning out the pancreas." It is uncommon for diabetes to precede abdominal pain.

Patients are often repeatedly treated with antihelminthics and antacids after the mistaken diagnosis of parasitic disease or peptic ulcer. Persistent abdominal pain in childhood of undetermined etiology has often led to diagnostic laparotomy. In the absence of demonstrable pancreatic calculi, there is no easily available test to establish the diagnosis of chronic pancreatitis at this stage of illness.

DIABETES MELLITUS

Most patients initially seek medical attention for diabetes mellitus, which becomes clinically manifest a few years after the onset of pancreatalgia. A pain-free period of 1 or 2 years and an apparent transient improvement in the clinical picture prior to the onset of diabetes are not unusual. The age at onset of diabetes from India is presented in Table 64.2-2.

The fasting blood glucose level ranges between 200 and 400 mg/dL, and postprandial blood glucose levels greater than 700 mg/dL are not rare. Pancreatic diabetes is characteristically brittle, with marked fluctuations of blood glu-

TABLE 64.2-2   AGE AT ONSET OF PANCREATIC DIABETES IN 100 CASES

AGE (YR)	NUMBER OF CASES
Below 13	2
14–15	3
16–20	19
21–25	10
26–30	9
31–35	7
36–40	4
41–50	2
Undetermined	44

Adapted from GeeVarghese PJ et al.[3]

cose values with or without insulin therapy. Episodes of hypoglycemia are characteristic and may complicate the administration of even small doses of insulin. This may be a reflection of depleted glycogen reserves in the liver or decreased glucagon release from the pancreas. Spontaneous hypoglycemic episodes have been recorded without insulin therapy. True insulin resistance, defined as a daily requirement of over 200 U of insulin in the absence of infection or ketosis reported earlier, is no longer seen with the use of purified and human insulins.[8] Metabolic acidosis is uncommon, but ketosis may be seen in less than 5% of cases.[7]

C-peptide assay shows partial preservation of beta cells, which is responsible for the ketosis resistance.[8] Diabetic retinopathy and nephropathy do occur and are related to the duration of diabetes.[5,8] Other complications of pancreatic diabetes include neuropathy, recurrent urinary tract infections, and pyelonephritis. The liver is palpably enlarged in 40% of diabetics, although the only liver functional abnormality may be elevation of alkaline phosphatase, indicating fatty liver.[5] Autonomic nervous system dysfunction occurs with similar frequency and severity, as in patients with non–insulin-dependent diabetes mellitus.[34]

EXOCRINE PANCREATIC INSUFFICIENCY

Overt exocrine pancreatic insufficiency characterized by steatorrhea is the least striking clinical feature, attributable to the very low consumption of fat in the diet. However, on a diet of 100 g of fat, more than 70% of patients develop biochemical steatorrhea.[7]

Clinical and biochemical evidence of obstructive jaundice is a well-recognized complication secondary to stenosis and compression of the common bile duct, which is tunnelled in the head of the pancreas. Pancreatic pseudocysts are less uncommon than in alcoholic or biliary pancreatitis.

DIAGNOSIS

The diagnosis of chronic pancreatic injury in the early stages of the disease in young children is seldom made. Abdominal pain in childhood is often ignored or attributed to psychogenic causes or, in the tropics, to parasitic infestations. Endoscopic retrograde cholangiopancreatography (ERCP) or computed tomography (CT) will be helpful in earlier detection of the disease. An ERCP characteristically shows a markedly dilated main duct with a radiopaque and lucent calculi. Sonograms and CT scans of the abdomen help in identifying the calculi and the dilated ducts. Cost and limited availability, however, make it impractical to use CT scans and ERCP for the routine diagnosis of tropical pancreatitis. There are no sensitive and specific noninvasive blood or urine tests to diagnose chronic pancreatitis. Even in the developed nations of the world, the diagnosis of chronic pancreatitis in adults or children is often elusive and made very late, only after ductal changes or calculi develop.

On the other hand, the picture of a well-established case of tropical pancreatitis is so characteristic that a diagnosis based on clinical features alone is suspect. The onset of diabetes mellitus with a present or past history of recur-

rent abdominal pain in a young individual suggests chronic pancreatitis. Extreme emaciation, bilateral parotid gland enlargement, and a distended upper abdomen are seen only in patients with established and advanced disease. A peculiar cyanotic hue of the lips has been mentioned in early reports[3,4] but is noted infrequently in the majority of patients.[7]

The diagnosis is established by demonstration of pancreatic calculi on a flat-plate radiograph of the abdomen. The most common site of pancreatic calculi on the abdominal flat plate is to the right of the first and second lumbar vertebrae. The lateral extension is up to 2 to 5 cm to the right of these vertebrae. Calculi are most numerous in the head of the pancreas. In 30% of cases, the calculi form a cast of the main duct.[5] In the lateral film, the stones are located anterior to the vertebral body but posterior to the gallbladder area.

The diagnosis of tropical pancreatitis does not depend on the demonstration of pancreatic exocrine functional abnormality. Serum amylase determination is not often useful in the diagnosis of chronic pancreatitis except in acute exacerbations. The amylase is below normal in a large number of cases. Steatorrhea is manifest only on a high-fat test diet given prior to stool fat testing. Secretin cholecystokinin stimulation tests are expensive and time consuming and are seldom performed. Limited studies done in an academic setting have shown a marked decrease in volume and enzyme output. Bicarbonate secretion is normal in some studies but markedly reduced in others. The newer diagnostic tests—bentiromide test, pancreaolauryl test, and fecal chymotrypsin assays—are likely to be of limited value except in assessing exocrine insufficiency in late stages of the disease.

MANAGEMENT

The management of tropical pancreatitis consists of alleviation of abdominal pain, treatment of diabetes, prevention of complications, and correction of nutritional problems.

The treatment of acute episodes of painful attacks is similar to the treatment of other types of pancreatitis. The measures to "put the pancreas to rest" include no feeding by mouth and the use of intravenous fluids and electrolytes. Nasogastric suction may be needed in severe cases. The treatment of pain may require repeated injections of meperidine, but there is a danger of producing narcotic addiction. The role of large doses of orally administered enzyme therapy for pain in tropical pancreatitis is not well studied. The basis of such therapy is the experimental observation that orally administered proteases suppress endogenous enzyme production through a feedback inhibition.[35,36] Enzyme therapy may not help patients with tropical pancreatitis, a disease characterized by marked dilatation of duct and ductules. Success with enzyme therapy is limited to patients with nondilated ducts with functioning acinar cells. Empiric therapy with oral antioxidants appears to be effective in the management of pain in alcoholic pancreatitis.[37] Although not well proven, in view of its simplicity, antioxidant therapy is worth a trial in all patients. Endoscopic papillotomy with the removal of stones and the clearance of dominant strictures and obstructions has shown good results in carefully chosen patients.

Unremitting pain is an indication for surgical treatment. The best procedure is the exploration of the pancreatic duct, the removal of stones, and longitudinal anastomosis of the split surface of the pancreas to the jejunum (Puestow procedure).[38] The relief of pain, even with surgery, may be temporary.

The treatment of diabetes is with dietary manipulation using oral hypoglycemic agents and insulin therapy. The dietary management of diabetes in pancreatitis is complicated.[8] The associated malnutrition, malabsorption, and tendency toward hypoglycemia deserve consideration in prescribing a suitable diet. A nutritious diet supplemented with vitamins and minerals is needed, and it is not advisable to restrict the carbohydrate content of the diet below 300 g. The diet may have to be supplemented with adequate protein intake, and pancreatic enzyme preparations are also advised to correct malabsorption.

If the diabetes is mild, oral hypoglycemic agents may be used, especially in the first few years after the onset of diabetes. Insulin therapy is required to control hyperglycemia in the large majority of cases. Often a combination of insulin and oral hypoglycemic agents is used to reduce the cost of therapy with insulin alone. Supplementary pancreatic enzyme therapy in a preliminary study was shown to reduce marked fluctuations of blood sugar.[39]

SUMMARY AND CONCLUSIONS

Juvenile tropical pancreatitis is a type of chronic pancreatitis that occurs in children and young adults of many developing nations. Although the etiology is not established, malnutrition is an important epidemiologic association. Other proposed etiologic factors include unopposed free radical injury, trace element and vitamin deficiencies, and dietary cyanogen toxicity. Many recent studies have identified genetic markers, and an association with SPINK 1 and N34S mutation has been noted. The occurrence of abdominal pain in childhood followed by the onset of diabetes in an emaciated teenager is the typical clinical picture, and the radiologic demonstration of calculi in the pancreatic duct is the hallmark of the disease. Patient management involves the control of diabetes with an oral hypoglycemic agent and/or insulin. Painful attacks of pancreatitis require the use of analgesics or surgery. Nutritional management should include a diabetic diet with adequate complex carbohydrates and frequent small meals, supplemented with oral pancreatic enzymes.

Tropical pancreatitis is an enigmatic disease that requires further study to explain its etiopathogenesis. It may be one of the preventable forms of diabetes in children in the tropics.

REFERENCES

1. Zuidema PJ. Cirrhosis and disseminated calcifications of the pancreas in patients with malnutrition. Trop Geogr Med 1959;11:70–4.
2. Shaper AG. Chronic pancreatic disease and protein malnutrition. Lancet 1960;i:1223–4.
3. GeeVarghese PJ, Pillai VK, Joseph MP, Pitchumoni CS. The diagnosis of pancreatogenous diabetes mellitus. J Assoc Phys India 1962;10:173–8.
4. GeeVarghese PJ. Pancreatic diabetes. Bombay: Popular Prakashan; 1968.
5. GeeVarghese PJ. Calcific pancreatitis. Trivandrum: St. Joseph's Press; 1986.
6. Balakrishnan V. Tropical pancreatitis: epidemiology, pathogenesis and etiology. In: Balakrishhan V, editor. Chronic pancreatitis in India. Trivandrum: St. Joseph's Press; 1987.
7. Mohan V, Chari ST, Viswanathan M, Madanagopalan N. Tropical calcific pancreatitis in Southern India. Proc R Coll Physicians Edin 1990;20:34–42.
8. Mohan V, Nagalotimath SJ, Yajnik CS, Tripathy BB. Fibrocalculous pancreatic diabetes. Diabetes Metab Rev 1998;14:153–70.
9. Balaji N. The problem of chronic calcific pancreatitis [thesis]. New Delhi: All India Institute of Medical Sciences; 1988.
10. Nagalotimath SJ. Pancreatic pathology in pancreatic calcification with diabetes. In: Podolsky S, Viswanathan M, editors. Secondary diabetes: the spectrum of the diabetic syndromes. New York: Raven Press; 1980. p. 117–45.
11. Nair B, Latha P. The pancreas in chronic calcific pancreatitis. In: Balakrishnan V, editor. Chronic pancreatitis in India. Trivandrum: St. Joseph's Press; 1987. p. 115–20.
12. Schultz AC, Moore PB, Pitchumoni CS. X-ray diffraction studies of pancreatic calculi associated with nutritional pancreatitis. Dig Dis Sci 1986;476–7.
13. Pitchumoni CS, Viswanathan KV, GeeVarghese PJ, Banks PA. Ultrastructure and elemental composition of human pancreatic calculi. Pancreas 1987;2:152–8.
14. Dagorn JC. Lithostathine. In: Go VL, Dimagno EP, Gardner JD, et al, editors. The pancreas: biology, pathobiology, and disease. New York: Raven Press; 1993. p. 253–63.
15. Govindarajan M, Mohan U, Deepa R, et al. Histopathology and immunohistochemistry of the pancreatic islets in fibrocalculous pancreatic diabetes. Diabetes Res Clin Pract 2001;51:29–38.
16. Augustine P, Ramesh H. Is tropical pancreatitis premalignant? Am J Gastroenterol 1992;87:1005–8.
17. Chari ST, Mohan U, Pitchumoni CS, et al. Risk of pancreatic carcinoma in tropical calcifying pancreatitis: an epidemiologic study. Pancreas 1994;9:62–6.
18. Blackburn WR, Vinijchaikul K. The pancreas in kwashiorkor in electron microscopic study. Lab Invest 1969;305–31.
19. GeeVarghese PJ, Pitchumoni CS, Nair R. Is protein malnutrition an initiating cause of pancreatic calcification? J Assoc Physicians India 1969;17:417–9.
20. Bonorden WR, Pariza MW. Antioxidant nutrients and protection from free radicals. In: Kotsonis FN, Mackey M, Hjelle JJ, editors. Nutritional toxicology. New York: Raven Press; 1994. p. 19–48.
21. Braganza J, Jeffrey IJM, Foster J, McCloy RF. Recalcitrant pancreatitis: eventual control by antioxidants. Pancreas 1987; 2:489–94.
22. Pitchumoni CS, Scheele GA. The interdependence of nutrition and exocrine pancreatic function. In: Go VL, Dimagno EP, editors. The pancreas: biology, pathobiology and disease. New York: Raven Press; 1993. p. 449–73.
23. McMillian D, GeeVarghese PJ. Dietary cyanide and tropical malnutrition diabetes. In: Podolsky S, Viswanathan M, editors. Secondary diabetes: the spectrum of the diabetic syndromes. New York: Raven Press; 1980. p. 239–53.
24. Sandhyamani S, Vijayakumari A, Balaraman N. Bonnet monkey

model for pancreatic changes in induced malnutrition. Pancreas 1999;18:84–95.

25. Teuscher T, Bailled P, Rosman JB, Teuscher A. Absence of diabetes in a rural West African population with a high carbohydrate/cassava diet. Lancet 1987;i:765–8.

26. Whitcomb DC, Gorry MC, Preston RA, et al. I. Hereditary pancreatitis is caused by a mutation in the cationic trypsinogen gene. Nat Genet 1996;14:141–5.

27. Creighton J, Lyall R, Wilson DI, et al. Mutations in the cationic trypsinogen gene in patients with chronic pancreatitis. Lancet 1999;354:42–3.

28. Chen JM, Montier T, Ferec C. Molecular pathology and evolutionary and physiological implications of pancreatitis-associated cationic trypsinogen mutations. Hum Genet 2001;109:245–52.

29. Witt H, Luck W, Hennies HC, et al. Mutations in the gene encoding the serine protease inhibitor, Kazal type 1 are associated with chronic pancreatitis. Nat Genet 2000;25:213–6.

30. Bhatia E, Durie P, Zielenski J, et al. Mutations in the cystic fibrosis transmembrane regulator gene in patients with tropical calcific pancreatitis. Am J Gastroenterol 2000;94:3658–9.

31. Bhatia E, Choudhari G, Sikora SS, et al. Tropical calcific pancreatitis: strong association with SPINK 1 trypsin inhibitor mutations. Gastroenterology 2002;123:1020–5.

32. Schneider A, Suman A, Rossi L, et al. SPINK 1/PSTI mutations are associated with tropical pancreatitis and type II diabetes mellitus in Bangladesh. Gastroenterology 2002;123:1026–30.

33. Mohan V, Premalatha G, Padma A, et al. Fibrocalculous pancreatic diabetes. Long term survival analysis. Diabetes Care 1996;19:1274–8.

34. Mohan V, Sastry NG, Premalatha G. Autonomic dysfunction in non-insulin-dependent diabetes mellitus and fibrocalculous pancreatic diabetes in south India. Diabet Med 1996;13:1038–43.

35. Rowell WG, Toskes PP. Pain of chronic pancreatitis: what are the management options? In: Barkin JS, Rogers AL, editors. Difficult decisions in digestive diseases. Chicago: Yearbook Medical Publishers; 1989. p. 192–7.

36. Isaksson G, Ihse I. Pain reduction by an oral pancreatic enzyme preparation in chronic pancreatitis. Dig Dis Sci 1983;28:97–102.

37. Braganza JM. The pancreas. In: Pounder RE, editor. Recent advances in gastroenterology. London: Churchill Livingstone; 1985. p. 251–80.

38. Pitchumoni CS, Varughese M. Tropical calculous pancreatitis. In: Howard J, Idezuki Y, Ihse I, Prince R, editors. Surgical diseases of the pancreas. 3rd ed. Baltimore: Williams and Wilkins; 1998. p. 411–5.

39. Mohan V, Poongothai S, Pitchumoni CS. Oral pancreatic enzyme therapy in the control of diabetes mellitus in tropical calculous pancreatitis. Int J Pancreatol 1998;24:19–22.

CHAPTER 65

EXOCRINE PANCREATIC DYSFUNCTION

1. *Cystic Fibrosis*

Kevin J. Gaskin, MD, FRACP

Cystic fibrosis (CF) is an autosomal recessively inherited disorder caused by mutations of the cystic fibrosis transmembrane conductance regulator (CFTR) gene and characterized clinically by chronic suppurative lung disease and exocrine pancreatic failure. The early postmortem descriptions of CF in the 1930s recognized both the pulmonary and pancreatic components of the disorder,[1,2] establishing it as a separate entity to "celiac syndrome" (a collective term for malabsorptive disorders of children in that era). Later, di Sant'Agnese and others demonstrated that CF patients have elevated sweat salt concentrations,[3] and this has remained the mainstay of diagnosis until the present day. The CFTR gene was discovered in the late 1980s[4–7] with the subsequent demonstration that the gene product (CFTR protein) was a cyclic adenosine monophosphate (cAMP)-stimulated Cl⁻ channel.[8] Over the same era, there were many significant advances in clinical management, including antibiotic therapy for lung disease, microspheric pancreatic enzyme replacement therapy, and nutritional therapy, all of which enhanced median survival from 10 to nearly 40 years of age over the last half-century. This chapter addresses concepts of the pathophysiology of this disease, its genetics, and associated gastrointestinal and nutritional problems. The reader is referred elsewhere for reviews of respiratory disease[9] and reproductive tract complications.[10]

ETIOLOGY

The pathophysiologic basis of CF centers on the CFTR protein and its function in absorptive and secretory epithelial tissue. The *CFTR* gene was located on chromosome 7[4] and was subsequently cloned, and the sequence of the gene and protein product were determined in 1989.[5-7] CFTR is a membrane protein, and its secondary or domain structure, proposed by Riordan and others,[6] included two membrane spanning domains (MSD1 and MSD2), two nucleotide binding domains (NBD1 and NBD2), and a regulatory domain (R), as depicted in Figure 65.1-1. The CFTR protein functions as a phosphorylation-dependent Cl⁻ channel

located in the apical membrane of epithelial cells, as evident from data showing (1) the expression of CFTR in cells that did not normally contain cAMP-dependent Cl⁻ channels and the subsequent demonstration of a Cl⁻ current activated by cAMP agonists,[11] (2) the demonstration of the similarity between Cl⁻ currents in cells expressing recombinant CFTR and in epithelial cells expressing native endogenous CFTR,[12] (3) mutations of CFTR altering Cl⁻ transport,[13] and, finally, (4) purified recombinant CFTR in planar lipid bilayers demonstrating Cl⁻ channel properties identical to those in native epithelia.[8]

CFTR is important in regulating electrolyte transport in absorptive and secretory epithelia.[14] Cholera toxin, for instance, stimulates massive chloride and subsequent fluid secretion from intestinal epithelia. The chloride secretion is mediated by a direct effect of the toxin on the cAMP-

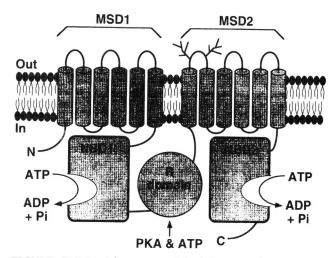

FIGURE 65.1-1 Schematic model of the cystic fibrosis transmembrane conductance regulator with membrane spanning domains (MSD1 and MSD2), nucleotide binding domains (NBD1 and NBD2), and regulatory domain (R). ADP = adenosine diphosphate; ATP = adenosine triphosphate; N = nucleotide; PKA = protein kinase A; Pi = phosphate. Reproduced with permission from Sheppard DN, Welsh MJ.[14]

dependent CFTR channel, as confirmed recently by the demonstration that the highly specific CFTR inhibitor, thiazolidinone, markedly reduces Cl⁻ secretion in response to cholera toxin stimulation.[15] As seen in Figure 65.1-2, a simple model demonstrates that Cl⁻ accumulates intracellularly following entry via the Na⁺-K⁺-Cl⁻ cotransporter in the basolateral membrane. Recycling of Na⁺ occurs by the basolateral Na⁺-K⁺ exchanger and of K⁺ through independent K⁺ channels, whereas Cl⁻ moves down its electrochemical gradient to the lumen following activation of the cAMP Cl⁻ channel in the apical luminal membrane. Na⁺ is transported paracellularly in response to the lumen negative voltage set up by Cl⁻ transport. In absorptive epithelia, for example, in the sweat duct, CFTR functions in almost a reverse fashion to the above and is involved in electrolyte and fluid absorption. In addition to its function as a cAMP-dependent Cl⁻ channel, CFTR as an ABC transporter (adenosine triphosphate [ATP] binding cassette protein) can regulate other membrane channels and the transport of drugs, amino acids, and peptides.[16] These functions are summarized in Figure 65.1-3 and include cAMP Cl⁻ channel function, facilitation of ATP release, positive regulation of outwardly rectifying Cl⁻ channels (ORCC), negative regulation of epithelial Na⁺ channels, regulation of intracellular vesicle trafficking, intracellular compartment acidification and glycoprotein processing, and modulation of renal outer medullary K⁺ channel sensitivity to sulfonylureas. Moreover, release of ATP may further enhance or regulate ORCC via purinergic receptors, and other chloride channels, including Ca⁺⁺ activated channels, appear to be regulated by external nucleotides.

Patients with CF have impaired chloride reabsorption from sweat ducts and, in general, elevated sweat chlorides greater than 60 mmol/L. Transport defects have also been demonstrated in vivo in both respiratory and pancreatic duct epithelium. In upper airway epithelium from CF subjects, the potential difference across the epithelium of 53 mV is about twice that observed in normal controls, and

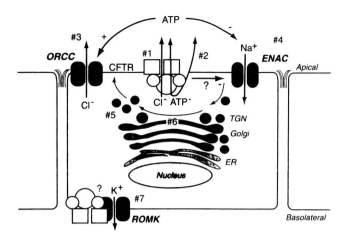

FIGURE 65.1-3 Cystic fibrosis transmembrane conductance regulator (CFTR) functions: (1) Cl⁻ channel function, (2) facilitation of adenosine triphosphate (ATP) release, (3) positive regulation of outwardly rectifying Cl⁻ channels (ORCC), (4) negative regulation of epithelial Na⁺ channels (ENAC), (5) regulation of vesicle trafficking, (6) regulation of cell acidification and protein processing, (7) modification of renal outer medullary K⁺ (ROMK) sensitivity to sulfonylureas. Reproduced with permission from Schwiebert EM et al.[16] ER = endoplasmic reticulum; TGN = trans-Golgi network.

this difference persists further down the airways, although perhaps of lesser magnitude.[17,18] Of interest, this difference in potential can be abolished by amiloride, a finding attributed to amiloride blocking the enhanced Na⁺ reabsorption in CF airway epithelium.[19] These changes in electrolyte transport help explain the impaired fluid secretion and the relative dehydration and increased viscosity of respiratory secretions in CF, the latter having previously been attributed to an abnormality of mucus.

In the normal pancreas, the major driving force for pancreatic fluid production has been attributed to secretin–stimulated ductal bicarbonate (HCO_3^-) secretion. The conventional theory proposed that duct cell chloride secretion via CFTR increased duct luminal chloride concentration. Chloride was then exchanged with intracellular HCO_3^- via an apical cell membrane Cl^--HCO_3^- exchanger, with HCO_3^- being synthesized in the cell via carbonic anhydrase action on CO_2, the latter diffusing into the cell via the basolateral membrane.[20] Because pancreatic ductal CFTR Cl⁻ secretion was impaired in CF patients, Cl⁻ was not available for exchange with HCO_3^-, thus producing the characteristically low HCO_3^- secretion defined by in vivo pancreatic function studies.[21-23] Recently, the mechanisms of both HCO_3^- production and secretion via the Cl^--HCO_3^- exchanger have been questioned on the basis that (1) there is demonstrable Na⁺ dependence of ductal HCO_3^- uptake at the basolateral cell membrane[24] and (2) there is a lack of inhibition of secretin-stimulated HCO_3^- secretion in the absence of luminal Cl⁻.[25] The current model of secretion suggests that depolarization of the cell membrane potential, owing to Cl⁻ exit via cAMP CFTR activation, stimulates HCO_3^- entry via the basolateral electrogenically driven Na⁺ HCO_3^- cotransporters and that HCO_3^- secretion into the lumen occurs predominantly via a conductive pathway. In

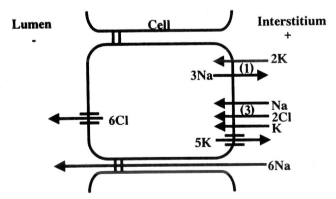

FIGURE 65.1-2 Chloride secretion via the cyclic adenosine monophosphate–activated Cl⁻ channel. Cl⁻ accumulates intracellularly via the Na⁺-K⁺-Cl⁻ cotransporter in the basolateral membrane. Na⁺ is recycled via Na⁺-K⁺-adenosine triphosphatase and K⁺ through independent K⁺ channels. Cl⁻ moves down its electrochemical gradient following activation of the Cl⁻ channel and is secreted into the lumen, and Na⁺ follows paracellularly owing to the lumen negative voltage set up by Cl⁻ transport

CF, the impaired Cl⁻ secretion and lack of cell depolarization inhibit HCO_3^- uptake and subsequent luminal HCO_3^- secretion. Although further work is required in this area, there is little question that pancreatic duct contents are relatively dehydrated and precipitate within the duct or ductule, leading to subsequent obstruction and proximal inflammation, with scarring and destruction of acinar tissue.[26] Furthermore, impaired HCO_3^- secretion may lead to polymerization and ductal precipitation of the zymogen granule–associated protein GP2, which normally undergoes a continuous exoendocytosis cycle to maintain the integrity of the zymogen granule.[27]

INCIDENCE, DIAGNOSIS, GENOTYPE

CF affects approximately 1 in 2,500 live births in white communities.[28] It is less frequent in African Americans, with a reported incidence of 1 in 15,300,[29] and is considered rare in Southeast Asians. The estimated carrier frequency of near 5% in white communities is extraordinarily high for a lethal gene and does suggest some survival advantage to mutation carriers. Quinton has postulated that carriers are protected against organisms causing toxigenic diarrheas,[30] as is evident by resistance to cholera toxin in heterozygotes of a CF mouse model.[31]

Classically, the diagnosis of CF is based on the clinical phenotype at presentation (lung disease, pancreatic insufficiency [PI]) and the presence of an elevated sweat chloride greater than 60 mmol/L. CF infants may have sweat chlorides in the borderline range of 40 to 60 mmol/L, and some normal adults could have values of up to 60 mmol/L. In addition, up to 20% of patients with milder disease and pancreatic sufficiency (PS; see later) may have sweat chloride values below 60 mmol/L, but average values even for this group are in the CF range at 85 mmol/L. In cases with borderline or even normal sweat chloride values, genotyping, nasal potential difference measurements, and quantitative pancreatic stimulation tests measuring HCO_3^- secretion are of value in determining the diagnosis.

CFTR is a large gene of 250 kb pairs containing 27 exons and encodes the CFTR protein of 1,480 amino acids. Over 1,200 mutations of the *CFTR* gene have now been described. The most common mutation, a basepair deletion in exon 10 resulting in a deletion of phenylalanine at position 508 on the CFTR protein, ΔF508, affects 66% of the CF chromosomes worldwide.[32] It is most frequent in northern Europeans (70–80%), is less frequent in southern Europeans (50–55%), and affects only a minority of Ashkenazi Jews (30%).[33] CFTR mutations have been categorized into five groups, as summarized in Figure 65.1-4, and are defined below[34]:

- Class I mutations reflect defective protein production, are associated with unstable messenger ribonucleic acid (mRNA), which is rapidly degraded, and involve nonsense, frameshift, and splice junction mutations.
- Class II mutations produce defective processing of the CFTR protein. ΔF508 is in this category, and improper folding of the molecule prevents trafficking to the apical membrane.
- Class III mutations involve defective regulation of the channel. Thus, although CFTR inserts correctly into the apical membrane, the mutation affecting the nucleotide binding fold impairs CFTR function.
- Class IV, mainly missense mutations involving organic residues in the membrane spanning part of the channel, insert normally into the apical membrane but have impaired conduction.
- Class V mutations lead to abnormal splicing of CFTR without alteration of the genomic coding sequence, leading to partial reduction of the normal CFTR protein but normal functional channels.

PANCREATIC DISEASE

In terms of exocrine pancreatic dysfunction in CF, patients are classified as having either PI or PS. PI patients have fat maldigestion and malabsorption as defined by a fecal fat > 7% of fat intake in 3- to 5-day fat balance studies.[35] In contrast, PS patients have normal fat digestion and absorp-

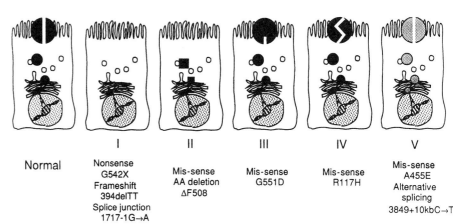

FIGURE 65.1-4 Classification of cystic fibrosis transmembrane conductance regulator (CFTR) mutations in relation to properties of CFTR protein. Class I: defective CFTR protein production: nonsense, frameshift, or aberrant splicing of messenger ribonucleic acid (mRNA); class II: defective CFTR processing: CFTR mRNA is formed, but protein fails to traffic to the cell membrane; class III: defective regulation: CFTR reaches membrane but is not stimulated by cyclic adenosine monophosphate; class IV: defective conduction: CFTR functions, but have altered properties; class V: synthesis defect: less synthesis of CFTR, but channel properties are normal.

tion, with fecal fat ≤ 7 percent of fat intake. Previously, PS patients were defined as having partial PI, partial pancreatic deficiency, or partial or normal exocrine pancreatic function.[36,37] The PS terminology reflects the fact that PS patients have sufficient endogenous pancreatic function to provide normal absorption and is based on pancreatic stimulation test studies in mainly CF patients, comparing pancreatic lipase/colipase secretion with fecal fat excretion,[38,39] as shown in Figure 65.1-5. Colipase secretion rates best delineated normal fat absorbers from those with fat malabsorption, and this is not surprising considering that the degree of lipolytic activity is dependent on the degree of colipase activity.[38] Patients with fat malabsorption had < 1% of average normal colipase activity, but those with normal absorption had a range of colipase secretion that varied from just above 1% up to within the normal control range (as depicted by clear circles in Figure 65.1-5). In large CF populations, 85 to 90% of patients are PI.[40] However, it is readily apparent in populations without newborn screening that patients may present beyond the first year of life with symptoms of malabsorption suggesting that they were PS initially and have lost pancreatic function with time. Studies of infants diagnosed by screening programs have confirmed this occurrence. At the time of neonatal diagnosis, nearly 40% were PS, but within 3 to 5 years, nearly half of these patients had developed PI.[41–43]

The occurrence of either pancreatic phenotype appears to be directly linked to the patient's genotype. In one of the first genotype–phenotype correlation studies, Kerem and colleagues demonstrated that in older CF populations, virtually all ΔF508 homozygotes and 70% of ΔF508 compound heterozygotes were PI, but over 60% of non-ΔF508 compound heterozygotes (who represented 8% of the total population) were PS, as per Table 65.1-1.[44] Subsequently, a number of non-ΔF508 mutations, including R117H and A455E, were demonstrated to be associated with the PS phenotype even if associated with a "severe" mutation (eg, ΔF508), suggesting that the mild PS mutation was dominant.[45] These findings were generally confirmed in a newborn screening population, noting that those who were

initially PS and then developed PI had two "severe" mutations, but those with persistent PS had at least one "mild" mutation.[42] In regard to the genotype classification and degree of CFTR dysfunction, as shown in Figure 65.1-4, the vast majority of patients with class I to III mutations are PI, whereas those with class IV and V mutations are PS.

Among PS patients, the phenotype can vary markedly. Some will have obvious lung disease, but others will have minimal or no lung disease. Sweat chlorides may be elevated, borderline (40–60 mmol/L), or even normal, and the latter patients may have only a single mode of presentation (eg, absence of the vas deferens in males or recurrent acute pancreatitis in previously asymptomatic adults who have been subsequently identified with double mutations).[46]

Some of this phenotype variation may be explained by gene modifiers. The R117H mutation is of interest because the polythymidine tract in intron 8 (containing 5, 7, or 9 thymidines) can alter the splicing on exon 9, such that introns with fewer thymidines lead to inefficient splicing and more severe disease.[47]

PANCREATIC INSUFFICIENCY

In postmortem studies of CF infants dying in the first 4 months of life, there is a marked lack of development of pancreatic acinar tissue.[48,49] Duct luminal volume as a proportion of the total volume exceeds that found in normal subjects, and the ratio of acinar to connective tissue diminishes with age. In premature infants dying from CF, secretory material obstructing pancreatic ducts is an early pathologic feature leading to duct dilatation and progressive atrophy of acinar tissue. Fibrosis can occur early, but in later childhood, patients with PI demonstrate cyst formation, calcification, and, on occasions, a grossly shrunken pancreas. These pathologic changes, which vary with age, have not been correlated with pancreatic function.

Clinical Features. CF infants with PI present with oily stools, and some parents will describe them graphically as looking like melted cheese, butter, or bacon fat. Undigested triglyceride is easily confirmed by stool microscopy

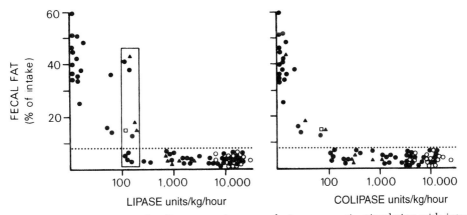

FIGURE 65.1-5 Lipase and colipase secretion rates during pancreatic stimulation with intravenous cholecystokinin and secretin in comparison with fecal fat expressed as a percentage of oral fat intake in 3- to 5-day fat balance studies. Dotted line represents 7% fat excretion. All patients with colipase < 100 U/kg/h have steatorrhea and are pancreatic insufficient, and those with colipase > 100 U/kg/h and normal fat absorption are pancreatic sufficient.

TABLE 65.1-1   ΔF508 GENOTYPING–PANCREATIC PHENOTYPE RELATIONSHIPS

GENOTYPE	PHENOTYPE	
	PI*	PS*
ΔF508/ΔF508	99	1
ΔF508/Other	72	28
Other/Other	36	64

Adapted from Kerem E et al.[44]
*Percentage of patients with pancreatic insufficiency (PI) or pancreatic sufficiency (PS) in specific genotype groups.

following staining of the specimen with oil red O or Sudan red. Up to 50% of PI patients are hypoalbuminemic with or without peripheral edema at presentation; some may have hemolysis associated with vitamin E deficiency, rectal prolapse, coagulopathy owing to vitamin K deficiency, or even raised intracranial pressure owing to vitamin A deficiency.[50,51] Macronutrient deficiency owing to severe maldigestion and malabsorption, poor feeding, or anorexia with intercurrent illness can be associated with severe failure to thrive, wasting, and even stunting. In nonscreened populations, malnutrition and hypoalbuminemia have been attributed to the lower protein content of breast milk, leading many centers to the recommendation of cessation of breastfeeding following the diagnosis of CF in infancy.

Later presentations during childhood have included patients who develop PI with oily stools and associated vitamin deficiencies, including night blindness associated with vitamin A deficiency. These older patients may have obvious chest symptoms or signs, including clubbing, and some have presented with liver disease. In a sizable proportion of patients, chest symptoms and signs predominate and are responsible for early recognition of the disease.

Diagnosis. In the context of an infant or child with a positive sweat chloride presenting with oily stools, there is little doubt that the patient is PI. However, particularly among infants from newborn screening programs, a history of oily stools may not be forthcoming. Historically, documentation of exocrine pancreatic function status has best been achieved with formal fat balance studies, with PI patients demonstrating, on average, a fecal fat excretion near 40% of fat intake, with variation from 10 to 80%.[35] Formula-fed PI infants will have fat excretions > 10% of fat intake and breastfed PI infants a fecal fat > 2 g/d.[41] In many units, fat balance studies are not undertaken owing to the natural reluctance of collectors and laboratory staff handling fecal material and the risks of contamination and cross-infection. More recently, spot stool analysis for fecal elastase 1 (FE1) has been suggested as a possible alternative, noting that FE1 was very successful in predicting the occurrence of PI.[52] However, some caution is still required with the interpretation of this test because in non-CF adults with chronic pancreatitis with moderate to severe pancreatic dysfunction but with normal fat excretion, approximately 50% registered a near-zero FE1 level, suggesting that they were PI. Moreover, with relevance to units with screening programs, FE1 has not been adequately tested in CF infants.

Treatment. Once PI is diagnosed in a CF infant, treatment should commence with oral enzyme replacement therapy (OERT). Most clinics now use the enteric-coated microspheric OERT preparations that were first marketed in the early 1980s. Prior to that time, OERT preparations consisted of dried pancreatic extract, either in powder, tablet, or capsule form. When ingested, these products were exposed to acid pepsin digestion and thus were mainly ineffective, reducing fecal fat outputs by less than 10%. The microspheric preparations were developed so that the enzyme powder was enclosed in a small bead with a pH-sensitive enteric coating, resistant to acid dissolution but readily dissolved in a pH > 6. In theory, therefore, the microspheres would dissolve only when reaching the upper small intestine. Fat balance studies on CF patients treated with these preparations have consistently shown a marked improvement in average fecal fats in older children and adolescents. Using the standard 5,000 IU capsule, patients receiving 6 to 9 capsules per day had an average fecal fat of 22%,[53] and incremental increases to 25 to 30 capsules per day produced a plateau effect, with average fecal fats between 10 and 15% per day.[54,55] In up to 50% of treated patients, fat excretion decreased to below 10% of fat intake, whereas 5 to 10% treated maintained fecal fats over 20%.[56]

Despite these improvements, during the late 1980s, additional microspheric OERT preparations were marketed containing 10,000 to 25,000 IU of lipase to aid those patients who had persistently high steatorrhea on standard-dose OERT and to reduce the number of capsules consumed by older patients in an effort to improve compliance.[57] These aims were laudable, but many patients were able to self-determine their dose of enzymes; consequently, they were consuming very large doses of lipase, often in excess of 50,000 IU/kg/d. Fat balance studies were not performed to justify these large doses, and as subsequently shown epidemiologically, the introduction of such therapy was coincidental with the emergence of a new complication of CF, namely, fibrosing colonopathy (FC).[58] This complication was a noninflammatory, colonic obstruction associated with marked intramural fibrosis, usually in the ascending or transverse colon.[59] Many patients who developed FC experienced considerable morbidity and required surgical intervention to relieve the obstruction. With doses of lipase in excess of 50,000 IU/kg/d, there is a marked risk of FC; this lessens with decreasing doses, although there is still considerable risk above 20,000 IU/kg/d.[58] Most would recommend keeping the dose below 10,000 IU/kg/d and optimally around 5,000 units/kg/d.

In patients who remain symptomatic on the standard-dose regimen, one should document the degree of steatorrhea. If it exceeds 20%, and the patient is compliant with the dose prescribed, he should be assessed for liver or biliary tract disease, giardiasis, and celiac disease. If such studies are negative, adjunctive therapy using gastric acid suppressants (eg, H_2 receptor antagonists or proton pump inhibitors) should be considered.[54] There are few patients who do not respond to such maneuvers; they may respond better to some of the acid-resistant acid lipases that are under development.

PANCREATIC SUFFICIENCY

PS patients comprise 10 to 20% of large CF clinic populations,[40] although, as indicated above, this occurrence is much higher in neonates.[41] In nonscreened populations, they usually present at a later age than PI patients[40] and may have unimodal presentations as adults, with congenital bilateral absence of the vas deferens in males at infertility clinics or recurrent acute pancreatitis. In newborn screening programs using the two-tiered immunoreactive trypsin (IRT) screening strategy, PS infants had IRT values similar to their PI counterparts.[41] However, the more recent strategy using a single IRT test and a ΔF508 mutation analysis will miss non-ΔF508 compound heterozygotes and a proportion of PS patients.[60]

Characteristically, PS patients have a mild disease with minimal pulmonary involvement and encounter nutritional, gut, or liver problems infrequently.[40] *Pseudomonas* lung colonization is reduced compared with PI patients, and the overall prognosis is vastly improved; in the United States, CF median survival of PS patients is 53 years and of PI patients 28 years. It is apparent that persistently PS patients have one or more so-called "mild" mutations, including R117H, A455E, and R347P. They demonstrate impaired Cl⁻ transport in their sweat, but it is less severe than that of PI patients because they have an average sweat chloride of 86 mmol/L compared with 104 mmol/L in the PI group; they consistently have higher pancreatic HCO_3^- secretion than their PI counterparts.[22] Mild chest disease occurs in 75% of PS patients, 39% have digital clubbing, and 30% have nasal polyps.[40] Interestingly, 4% had rectal prolapse, thus underscoring the validity of obtaining a sweat chloride in every child who presents with rectal prolapse even in the absence of gastrointestinal symptoms. Of equal importance, PS patients develop pancreatitis,[40,46,61] an entity that does not occur in PI patients who have lost their functioning acinar tissue. PS patients do not require enzyme therapy because, by definition, they have sufficient endogenous enzyme production to prevent malabsorption. Equally, they do not require fat-soluble vitamin supplementation. It is imperative for clinics to assess their patients for PS because treating a patient unnecessarily for years is a considerable burden to the child and an unnecessary financial burden to the health care system.

HEPATOBILIARY COMPLICATIONS

A variety of biliary tract and hepatic complications of CF have been described in CF patients, as summarized in Table 65.1-2. They include specific gallbladder diseases, including microgallbladder with or without atretic ducts, dilated or distended gallbladders and cholelithiasis, bile duct diseases with common duct or intrahepatic duct lithiasis, a disease resembling sclerosing cholangitis, and distal common bile duct stenosis. Liver complications include hepatosteatosis and the two forms of fibrotic liver disease considered pathognomonic of CF, namely, focal and multilobular biliary cirrhosis (FBC and MBC, respectively).

Pathologically, gallbladder hypoplasia with or without atretic cystic ducts has been recognized in early childhood.[48] The gallbladder wall contains small epithelial cysts,

often distended with eosinophilic material; there is often mucous gland metaplasia and occasionally marked mucosal hyperplasia, but no inflammatory changes. One autopsy study of older patients demonstrated that 14% had calculi.[62] Common bile duct stenosis owing to extrinsic compression of the bile duct has been identified in postmortem specimens of infants, and in one case, the patient was mistakenly diagnosed as having biliary atresia.[63] Liver disease in CF was first recognized by Anderson and was later confirmed by Farber and Bodian.[2,64,65] Farber recognized inspissated material obstructing small bile ductules,[64] and Bodian described the entity of FBC.[65] Later, di Sant'Agnese and Blanc described the severe form of liver disease, MBC.[66] Because patients with MBC also had evidence of FBC, the authors suggested that there was a progression of the focal disease with coalescence and generation of the large nodules characteristic of MBC, as seen in Figure 65.1-6. The focal scarring histologically, as shown in 65.1-7, is associated with fibrosis of portal triads with accompanying inflammatory infiltration, bile ductular hyperplasia, and eosinophilic secretions expanding bile ductules.

Postmortem studies suggest that there is a rising incidence of liver disease with age; FBC is present in 10.6 to 15.6% of infants less than 12 months of age,[48] in 19 to 50% during childhood,[65–67] and in up to 72% of adult CF patients.[68] Similarly, MBC increased from < 1% in early childhood to up to 24% in the above adult postmortem study.[68] In addition to the fibrotic changes, almost 60% of liver specimens showed hepatosteatosis, a finding hitherto unexplained.[69] Currently, the etiology of fibrotic liver disease is also enigmatic. It is likely that the underlying CFTR transport defect impairs fluid secretion from the cholangiolar epithelium,[70] contributing to inspissation of material and obstruction in bile ductules, but it is not clear why some patients develop liver disease and others do not. A distinct possibility is that a gene modifier may influence the operation of CFTR. To date, the presence of liver disease has not correlated with the severity of lung or intestinal disease; it has been described in three patients with PS and no detectable abnormalities in pulmonary function.[71]

TABLE 65.1-2   BILIARY TRACT AND LIVER COMPLICATIONS IN CYSTIC FIBROSIS PATIENTS

GALLBLADDER
Microgallbladder
Atretic cystic ducts
Distended gallbladder
Cholelithiasis

BILIARY TRACT
Ductal stones
Common bile duct stenosis
Sclerosing cholangitis
Cholangiocarcinoma

LIVER
Hepatosteatosis
Focal biliary fibrosis (cirrhosis)
Multilobular biliary cirrhosis
  ± Portal hypertension
  + Liver failure

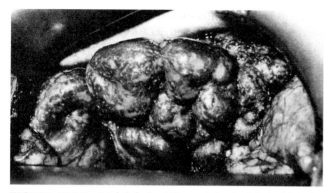

FIGURE 65.1-6   Multilobular biliary cirrhosis. Marked lobulation of the liver occurs in some patients. Focal areas of scarring are readily visible in each lobule.

It may well be that other entities, including common bile duct disease, distal stenosis, and sclerosing cholangitis, contribute to biliary tract stasis to explain the variable occurrence of liver disease.[69]

DIAGNOSIS

The diagnosis of CF liver disease can be difficult.[72] There is little debate regarding patients with multilobular cirrhosis who have peripheral signs of chronic liver disease, spider nevi, and an obvious multilobulated firm liver, with abdominal distention and signs of portal hypertension, including splenomegaly. Such patients can be recognized clinically and confirmation provided by ultrasonographic examination of the liver. The difficulty comes when attempting to diagnose milder cases who are devoid of physical signs, except perhaps hepatomegaly. Liver function tests may be completely normal, even in subjects with MBC and portal hypertension,[72–74] and ultrasound examinations may demonstrate increased echogenicity of the liver not related to fibrosis but attributable to impacted secretions or the presence of parenchymal steatosis. In addition, although liver biopsy has been touted as being necessary to determine the presence or absence of liver disease, there is considerable sampling error, and biopsies can be normal even in those with MBC.[69] Tests of liver function, including serum bile acids[75] and hepatobiliary scintigraphy,[69] also fail to distinguish between patients with and without liver disease. Ultimately, a combination of findings (clinical, imaging, and biochemical) is used to determine the onset and progression of this complication.

CLINICAL PRESENTATION

Patients with hepatosteatosis and focal biliary disease are relatively asymptomatic, although in one series, FBC patients had a higher incidence of abdominal pain.[69] Those with multilobular disease may have signs of chronic liver disease, spider nevi, liver palms, abdominal distention, and signs of portal hypertension or ascites. Some may present with esophageal variceal bleeding even prior to diagnosis of CF in late childhood and may have minimal signs of lung disease. The course of those with portal hypertension and splenomegaly is variable, but in my own unpublished series of 28 patients with portal hypertension, 10 experienced variceal bleeding over a 10-year period.

TREATMENT

Medical management of CF liver disease has centered around supportive measures to provide adequate nutrition, fatsoluble vitamin supplementation, and diuretic therapy for edema and ascites. Ursodeoxycholate therapy was introduced based on the theoretical possibility that it would enhance fluid secretion from the biliary tree. Initial studies were promising, reporting improvements in liver function tests and hepatobiliary scintigraphy,[76,77] but many of the studies contained small numbers of subjects with considerable heterogenicity in their underlying liver disease.[78,79] A recent Cochrane analysis concluded that there was insufficient evidence to justify the routine use of ursodeoxycholate therapy for CF patients and noted the urgent need for a prolonged multicentered collaborative trial with clinically relevant end points.[80]

The management of liver disease with portal hypertension is similar to that for non-CF populations. Patients with variceal bleeding should undergo variceal injection therapy or banding, and in many instances, their bleeding will be well controlled. If sclerotherapy fails, an alternative intervention has to be considered; possibly the best to date has been the use of reversed lienorenal shunts.[81] However, the latter procedure has to be considered in the context of the severity of the lung disease in individual patients. Often the decision is made to proceed based on the urgency of the situation.

Liver transplant is now a viable option for the unusual CF patient with synthetic liver failure or uncontrolled portal hypertension and recurrent variceal hemorrhaging. Data show survivals at least consistent with non-CF liver transplant patients, that is, 70 to 80% survival for the first 5 years post-transplant.[82] Of interest, the decline in pulmonary function was less than expected, a fact possibly related to the anti-inflammatory effects of the antirejection therapy used. Direct contraindication to transplant includes severe pulmonary disease (ie, forced expiratory volume in 1 second [FEV_1] < 50% predicted) and fungal or *Burkholderia cepacia* lung colonization.

NEONATAL LIVER DISEASE

Prolonged neonatal cholestasis occurs in CF infants, but most have considered it to be a rare phenomenon.[83,84] However, in one postmortem study, 10% of infants less than 3 months of age had FBC and 38% demonstrated histologic evidence of cholestasis[48] consistent with a clinical audit in which 35% manifested hepatomegaly/cholestasis in infancy.[72] At first glance, these disparate results are difficult to explain, but, certainly, the postmortem study included very ill septic infants from an era in which neonatal, postsurgical management would be regarded as suboptimal. Moreover, the patients were collected from a wide geographic area for which the true total incidence of CF was unknown. In preliminary results from a newborn screening program over a 14-year interval, 12 of 224 (5%) CF infants developed cholestasis, and 9 of these infants had meconium ileus (MI).[85] Prior to the diagnosis of CF, those presenting with cholestasis and acholia are often considered to have extrahepatic biliary atresia. It is thus imperative that the cholestatic infant has a sweat chloride

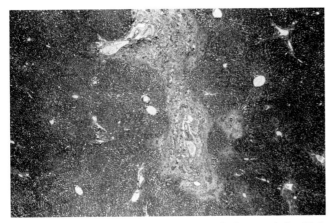

FIGURE 65.1-7 Histologic examination of a liver with focal biliary cirrhosis demonstrating fibrosis of portal triad, acute inflammatory cell infiltration, bile ductular hyperplasia, and eosinophilic secretions plugging bile ductules.

test as part of the diagnostic workup because most patients with CF do not have extrahepatic biliary atresia, although they may have prolonged jaundice for periods up to 6 months. Neonatal cholestasis in CF has been linked to MI,[85,86] but others have not found this association.[83]

GALLBLADDER OR BILIARY TRACT DISEASE

Previously, cholelithiasis was a prominent biliary tract complication of CF. With the introduction of microspheric OERT, gallstones have become virtually nonexistent, and at the Sydney clinic we have seen only 3 cases in nearly 700 patients over the last 15 years.

A few patients do experience right-sided abdominal pain unrelated to distal intestinal obstruction syndrome (DIOS); some will be tender in the right upper quadrant. Such patients may have biliary tract disease and require an ultrasound examination to exclude cholelithiasis and hepatobiliary scintigraphy to exclude distal common bile duct stenosis. Cholangiography is required to confirm the latter and may warrant surgical intervention if cholestasis ensues or the pain persists and is interfering with appetite and normal daily activity.[69]

INTESTINAL DISEASE

The gut manifestations of CF as outlined in Table 65.1-3 include esophageal, small intestinal, colonic, and rectal diseases.

ESOPHAGEAL DISEASE

There have now been several reports of esophageal disease, particularly gastroesophageal reflux (GER) and esophagitis. One unit reported that up to 25% of patients have GER[87] and another that at least 50% of those with GER will develop esophagitis.[88] Reflux is probably a multifactorial problem contributed to by the severity and treatment of lung disease, drugs that relax the lower esophageal sphincter, and physiotherapy. Delayed gastric emptying may contribute, but the most significant feature

to date is intermittent and inappropriate lower esophageal sphincter relaxation.[89]

Patients with GER may complain of heartburn, waterbrash, dysphagia, and regurgitation. Equally common are those patients whose sole symptom is anorexia; thus, patients experiencing weight loss or poor weight gain may have esophageal disease. Investigations should include a barium contrast examination and esophagogastroscopy of the esophagus and stomach, specifically looking for esophagitis, strictures, or a hiatal hernia.

Patients with esophagitis should first be treated with either H_2 receptor antagonists or proton blocking agents. Medical treatment should be prolonged for at least 6 months, and surgery should be considered only as a last resort for those unresponsive to medical therapy.

GASTRODUODENAL DISEASE

Peptic ulcer disease was considered a potentially common occurrence in CF, particularly because patients had gastric acid hypersecretion[90] and low pancreatic HCO_3^- secretion.[22] Although ulcers have been anecdotally recorded in the pre-endoscopy era, following the advent of fiberoptic endoscopy, their occurrence has been uncommon. Similarly, *Helicobacter pylori* gastritis is an unusual finding.

SMALL INTESTINAL DISEASE

CFTR has been localized to crypt[91] and villous cells[92,93] in the small intestinal mucosa, and small bowel biopsy specimens from CF patients demonstrate poor Cl^- transport in

TABLE 65.1-3   GUT MANIFESTATIONS IN PATIENTS WITH CYSTIC FIBROSIS

ESOPHAGUS
Gastroesophageal reflux
Esophagitis
Esophageal stricture
Esophageal varices (in association with portal hypertension)

GASTRODUODENUM
Peptic ulcer

SMALL INTESTINE
Neonatal meconium ileus (MI)
Complicated MI with volvulus or intestinal atresia, meconium peritonitis
Distal intestinal obstruction syndrome
Intussusception
Celiac disease
Giardiasis
Ileal adenocarcinoma

APPENDIX
Acute appendicitis ± perforation
Appendiceal abscess
Mucocele of appendix
Intussusception of appendix

COLON
Megacolon constipation
Pneumatosis intestinalis
Fibrosing colonopathy
Crohn disease
Colonic adenocarcinoma

RECTUM
Rectal prolapse

response to a number of known CFTR secretagogues.[94,95] Rectal suction biopsy specimens from CF patients demonstrate similarly impaired Cl⁻ transport,[96,97] which correlates with pancreatic phenotype, that is, samples from PI patients show undetectable transport, but those from PS patients show higher residual Cl⁻ transport. These findings have led to the proposal that the common small intestinal complications of CF, namely, neonatal MI and DIOS, result directly from impaired electrolyte and fluid secretion and subsequent inspissation of intestinal contents. This scenario is analogous to the genesis of exocrine pancreatic disease, in which poor fluid output leads to hyperconcentration of luminal contents, protein precipitation or aggregation, and subsequent ductular obstruction.[26,98] This hypothesis is supported by findings in the CF mouse model, in which intestinal complications at 12 to 40 days, including obstruction, perforation, fecal peritonitis, and the finding of large intraluminal "putty-like" masses, occur in animals in the absence of significant pancreatic pathology.[99]

In human CF patients, MI and DIOS are virtually exclusive to PI patients and are very rare in PS patients.[100] The CF consortium data furthermore demonstrated that MI occurred in patients with "severe" genotypes associated with PI but did not occur in patients with "mild" mutations associated with PS (eg, R117H).[101] These findings could argue that PI is a critical factor in the genesis of MI and DIOS, but they could equally reflect the severity of the underlying transport disorder in the pancreas and small intestine, as indicated by the correlation of rectal Cl⁻ transport with pancreatic phenotype. If so, the findings in the mouse model, which appears to have only mild exocrine pancreatic disease, could be reconciled only by the different degrees of expression of CFTR in the wild-type mouse (ie, low in the pancreas but high in the small intestine). However, to date in the small group of CF patients who are PS but have a severe genotype (eg, ΔF508/ΔF508) and poor or undetectable intestinal chloride transport, MI or DIOS has not occurred; thus, the degree of pancreatic function impairment may well contribute to the genesis of these complications.

The lack of alkalinization of intestinal contents as a result of poor pancreatic HCO_3^- secretion in PI patients can lead to protein and phospholipid precipitation in the intestinal lumen. PI patients have poor pancreatic phospholipase secretion; therefore, lecithin will accumulate in the gut lumen.[102] Although hydrolyzed by OERT to lysolecithin, OERT lacks lysolecithinase (carboxyl ester hydrolase)[103]; thus, high concentrations of lysolecithin could accumulate, which is a known hydrophobic compound capable of disrupting epithelial cells. Also, CFTR has intracellular functions that modify the production of mucus glycoproteins.[104,105] The above phenomena, including the Cl⁻ transport problems, PI and abnormal mucus production, in combination with the known impaired intestinal motility, could all contribute to the production of either MI or DIOS.

MECONIUM ILEUS

Between 10 and 20% of CF neonates will present with small intestinal obstruction owing to inspissation of meconium in the terminal ileum. This phenomenon occurs in utero, and

it remains enigmatic as to why only a small proportion of patients develop this complication. Approximately 10% of these cases will suffer perforation in utero and develop meconium peritonitis, an entity recognized by intra-abdominal calcification on abdominal radiographs. Most cases will present with signs of obstruction, including abdominal distention, bilious vomiting, and failure to pass meconium within the first 2 to 48 hours of life. The diagnosis may be suspected if there is a family history of CF but can be distinguished from other forms of neonatal gut obstruction by the lack of air fluid levels in erect or lateral decubitus plain abdominal radiographs (Figure 65.1-8) and a ground-glass appearance to the inspissated meconium. Nearly 50% of cases have complicated MI, in which, in addition to MI, they have malrotation with volvulus or intestinal atresia. Most will have an associated microcolon.

MI is almost invariably associated with CF. Of interest, in neonatally screened populations, the serum immunoreactive trypsin in MI patients can be within the normal range. It is thus important that the screening laboratory is informed of the diagnosis of MI to ensure that they proceed further to the mutational analysis, which would usually be performed only on infants with an initially high IRT value. Only rarely has MI been associated with non-CF conditions, and, to date, it has not been described with the pancreatic hypoplasia in Shwachman syndrome or other forms of childhood pancreatic diseases.

Diagnosis of MI is best achieved with nonionic contrast radiography. In uncomplicated MI, Gastrografin enemas

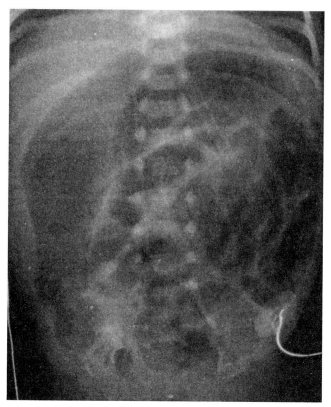

FIGURE 65.1-8 Abdominal radiograph of an infant with meconium ileus. There is marked distention of loops of small intestine without air-fluid levels. The ground-glass appearance of inspissated meconium is evident in the right iliac fossa.

can help elucidate the diagnosis, but because they are hypertonic, it may also be therapeutic in washing out the inspissated meconium. Great care is needed to avoid the perforation, dehydration, and shock associated with the use of the hypertonic enemata. Contrast radiography should be avoided in those with perforation or intra-abdominal calcification. Failure to resolve the obstruction with Gastrografin necessitates surgical intervention. The standard procedure is to milk out the inspissated material following division of the gut and to wash out the residue with saline or solutions containing N-acetylcysteine (Mucomyst). Some surgeons prefer the standard Bishop-Koop ileostomy, whereas others prefer a double-barreled ileostomy, and still others use the appendix stump.

DISTAL INTESTINAL OBSTRUCTION SYNDROME

Beyond the neonatal period, a small number of patients present with inspissation of intestinal contents in the terminal ileum, cecum, and proximal colon, a condition hitherto referred to as MI equivalent but now renamed as DIOS. Originally, this syndrome was considered to be more common in adolescents and adults, with an incidence varying from 17 to 24% in two different studies.[106,107] However, these reports were published before microspheric OERT was available, and subsequent studies have suggested a much lower overall incidence of 5%,[108] with some 7.5 cases per 1,000 patient-years occurring in the 15- to 20-year-old age group, increasing to 35.5 cases per 1,000 in the 20 to 25 year olds.

The etiology is unclear, but DIOS rarely occurs in PS patients.[100] Patients present with palpable fecal masses in the right lower quadrant, with or without abdominal pain, or with intestinal obstruction and bilious vomiting. These symptoms and signs are nonspecific and occur also in CF patients presenting with appendiceal or periappendiceal abscesses, purulent mucoceles of the appendix, intussusception, Crohn disease, or colonic strictures. A high degree of suspicion is required when dealing with DIOS, and although fevers and localized peritonism may suggest inflammatory disease, their absence does not exclude these possibilities. Indeed, DIOS can occur simultaneously with appendiceal disease and intussusception, thus adding to the complexity of the diagnosis. The diagnosis of DIOS is initially achieved with plain erect and supine abdominal radiographs. A fecal mass should be evident in the right iliac fossa, and the erect film will help to determine the presence of obstruction. If obstruction is present, one should suspect concomitant pathology such as intussusception or appendiceal disease with an acute history; one should suspect FC, or Crohn disease with a prolonged history. Ultrasound examination is useful in these circumstances and can readily identify intussusception (Figure 65.1-9), as can a computed tomographic (CT) examination (Figure 65.1-10).

In cases of intestinal obstruction or in which washout therapy has failed, Gastrografin enemas may be useful in defining colonic pathology (ie, strictures or intussusception) and relieving impaction in uncomplicated DIOS. Colonoscopy and biopsy will be required for cases in which Crohn disease is suspected radiologically.

Treatment for DIOS has been largely empiric. In simple cases of fecal impaction without obstruction, most respond to a high-dose mineral (paraffin) oil regimen, 30 to 50 mL twice daily over a 7-day period. If the patient does not evacuate, ultrasonography and a diagnostic or therapeutic examination should be performed to exclude intussusception. Thereafter, one should consider using washout therapy with the iso-osmotic colonoscopy preparation fluid Golytely, which contains polyethylene glycol for these oil-resistant cases. Patients may require up to 5 L per 2 to 4 hours to evacuate the mass, and the procedure may need repeating daily if the mass is not completely evacuated.

In DIOS cases with obstruction (ie, with distention and bilious vomiting), it is mandatory to exclude other complications. Once eliminated, washouts per rectum should be attempted, and once the obstruction is relieved, depending on nasogastric tube output, then washout therapy from above can be considered. Persistent obstruction may necessitate diagnostic laparotomy, but this situation is unusual in the absence of intussusception or appendiceal disease.

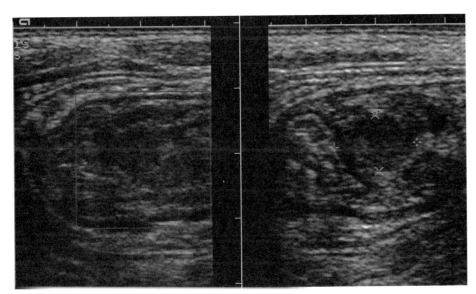

FIGURE 65.1-9 Ultrasound examination of the right lower abdomen in a patient with cystic fibrosis presenting with abdominal distention and a tender abdominal mass. The sonogram demonstrates a multilayered appearance of the intestine, representing the wall of intestine and the wall of the intussusception.

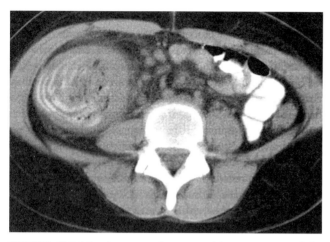

FIGURE 65.1-10   A computed tomographic examination of the abdomen of the patient in Figure 65.1-9, demonstrating the intussusception in the proximal colon.

Recurrent DIOS can be disabling for the CF patient. In such cases, novel therapies, including button placement in the appendix to allow more vigorous washouts, may be required.[109]

APPENDICEAL DISEASE

Appendiceal disease, including acute appendicitis,[110] appendiceal abscess,[111] perforation,[111] purulent mucoceles of the appendix, and intussusception of the appendix with rectal bleeding, has been described in CF patients.[112] Although less common than in the non-CF community (1 versus 7%, respectively), the diagnostic delays are of considerable concern in CF, with a high risk of perforation or abscess formation.[111] The cause for delay is unclear but may relate to the presence of a mass lesion that is mistaken for the more common DIOS or to concomitant antibiotic therapy disguising the inflammation. Fever, signs of obstruction, and localized tenderness or peritonism, with or without a tender mass in the right lower quadrant, should alert the physician to this entity, and imaging via ultrasonography or CT is essential to define such a lesion. The physical and radiologic signs may determine whether an operation is required, but the physician's suspicion will ultimately determine such action.

MISCELLANEOUS SMALL INTESTINAL DISEASES

Giardia infestation,[113] celiac disease, and Crohn disease have all been described in CF populations. Reports of giardiasis in CF are infrequent, but a recent study suggested that *Giardia* infested 28% of CF children and an even higher proportion (44%) of CF adults. These findings require confirmation but are potentially important because ongoing problems with chronic diarrhea are often misinterpreted as a failure to respond to OERT. Similarly, Crohn disease in 1 in 404 CF cases represented a prevalence approximately 11 times that observed in the non-CF control population.[114] Crohn disease should be suspected in cases presenting with abdominal pain, anemia, hypoproteinemia, and extragastrointestinal manifestations (eg, arthritis). Barium contrast imaging may demonstrate the typical segmental cobblestoned appear-

ance, and histologic examination will establish the presence of granulomatous colitis or ileitis. Treatment should be as for non-CF patients.

The coexistence of celiac disease and CF appears to be a rare occurrence.[115] However, given that in some white communities, the incidence is as high as 1 in 75, this entity may be more common than is suspected in the CF population. It should be considered in a CF patient with ongoing symptoms of malabsorption despite compliance with optimal doses of OERT. The need for small bowel biopsy should be governed by positive serum antibody screening, specifically antiendomyseal antibodies or antibodies to tissue transglutaminase. Cases with a positive diagnosis should be managed with a gluten-free diet.

LARGE INTESTINAL DISEASE

RECTAL PROLAPSE

Rectal prolapse (Figure 65.1-11) occurs in 10 to 20% of patients, usually prior to 5 years of age,[116] and may be the presenting feature of the disease.[117] It is far more common in PI patients; its occurrence has been attributed to large bulky stools in wasted patients prior to diagnosis or to ongoing malabsorption in patients following diagnosis. The entity has been described in PS patients[40]; thus, its occurrence cannot be entirely attributed to the presence of malabsorption or malnutrition, although the latter may contribute to the problem. All children presenting with isolated rectal prolapse should have a sweat chloride determination. In most cases, rectal prolapse is a self-resolving problem and requires no specific therapy other than ensuring compliance with OERT and providing laxatives if the patient is constipated. Persistent or recurrent prolapse can be disturbing to patients and their parents. Such patients respond well to pararectal triple saline injection therapy under anesthesia, with complete amelioration of their problems.

FIBROSING COLONOPATHY

This complication is a relatively new entity described in the early 1990s.[59,118] It is an intramural noninflammatory fibrosing process that affects mainly the proximal colon in CF patients up to early adolescence.[59] Pathologically and clinically, it can be associated with intestinal obstruction and may be preceded by prolonged abdominal pain with or without diarrhea and rectal bleeding. Some may also present with abdominal chylous ascites.[59,119,120]

FC may be diagnosed by imaging with contrast enemas to identify a stricture and proximal obstruction. In some, the diagnosis can be confirmed by colonoscopy and biopsy of the affected area. Surgery is required to relieve the colonic obstruction, and histologic examination of resected specimens will identify the typical elongated fibrotic stricture, which shows minimal inflammation.

Epidemiologically, the entity occurred after the introduction of high-dose lipase OERT and the consumption of large doses of enzyme in excess of 6,000 lipase units per kilogram per meal for periods exceeding 6 months.[59,119,120] Some patients were consuming greater than 50,000 lipase U/kg/d, and it is now recommended that intake does not exceed

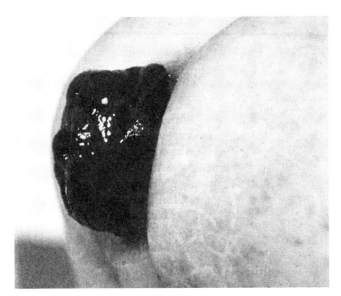

FIGURE 65.1-11 Rectal prolapse.

10,000 lipase U/kg/d or 2,500 U/kg per meal.[59,119] Since the establishment of these guidelines, the incidence of FC has substantially declined. It is important to note that although some have suggested that the entity is related to the differing copolymer content of the microspheric capsule,[121] evidence for this is tenuous because the US survey found a high odds ratio for the occurrence of FC irrespective of the capsule or microtablet used.[58]

GASTROINTESTINAL MALIGNANCY

Gastrointestinal malignancy has been described in adult patients with CF, with 24 cases reported from US and European CF clinic surveys.[122] The majority of cases were large or small intestinal adenocarcinomas, but esophageal, gastric, biliary, and pancreatic malignancies were described. In older CF patients, if confronted with unusual gut symptoms such as anemia, rectal bleeding, or non-DIOS intestinal obstruction, malignant neoplasms need consideration.

NUTRITIONAL PROBLEMS AND THEIR MANAGEMENT

Over the last two decades, nutritional problems have assumed a high priority in the management of CF. At least in part, the nutritional focus arose out of epidemiologic work at the CF Clinic, the Hospital for Sick Children, Toronto, which demonstrated that median survival of near 30 years was considerably better than the median survival of less than 20 years in other Canadian or US clinics.[123] This major difference was a surprising finding because the management of CF pulmonary disease was similar in the major clinics throughout North America. The same study emphasized the near-normal growth of the Toronto patients, except for a decline in weight of adolescent females, and, again, these results appeared superior to those previously published. Later data from Toronto demonstrated normal growth and lung function of their PS patients, and their PI males also had near-normal growth and superior lung function to their PI females, whose

weight fell off during adolescence.[40] Apparently, within this one clinic, prognosis and pulmonary function were influenced by nutritional status. Further confirmation of these findings was made following a comparative cohort study between the Boston and Toronto clinics, which demonstrated a 10-year advantage in median survival in the Toronto clinic, despite the fact that comparisons of pulmonary function tests did not demonstrate major differences at the end of adolescence.[124]

Roy and colleagues were the first to allude to a major difference in nutritional management between the Toronto and other clinics, noting that the Toronto patients had been encouraged to consume a high-fat, high-energy diet to replace fecal losses, whereas other clinics had adhered to the universally accepted low-fat diet to avoid the social inconvenience associated with ongoing malabsorption.[125] Dietary analysis demonstrated that whereas, on average, the Toronto patients consumed over 110% of the Recommended Dietary Allowance (RDA) for energy, patients at other clinics were averaging 80 to 90% of the RDA.[126] Later, CF clinics that were changing from a low- to a high-fat diet policy observed that patients consumed over 20% more of the RDA for energy and achieved normal growth, whereas those still adhering to a low-fat, low-energy diet achieved suboptimal weight gain.[127]

Because growth failure with wasting and stunting was common in most clinics, caregivers had adhered to the concept that growth failure was somehow inherent in the underlying disorder in CF. However, the Toronto data disputed this association. Moreover, if inherent in the disease, one would not expect that nutritional rehabilitation would reverse growth failure. To date, a large number of studies have shown that nutritional rehabilitation given by a variety of methods (orally, nasogastric tube, gastrostomy) not only improves weight gain and weight percentiles but also can reverse linear growth failure with achievement of previous or better growth percentiles.[55,128–130]

PATHOGENESIS OF MALNUTRITION

Protein intakes in CF children are most often very comparable to the high intakes achieved by non-CF children on Western diets of around 200% of RDA, even if a low-fat diet is used.[127] As indicated above, the major adverse effect of a low-fat diet is suboptimal energy intake and subsequent growth impairment. The patient's overall energy deficit can be influenced by other factors, including malabsorption, increased energy needs related to the underlying cellular defect, and to the occurrence of inflammatory lung disease.

Inadequate Energy Intake. Low-fat diets have been one of the main contributing factors to impaired energy intake in CF patients. Fortunately, nowadays most clinics advocate a high-energy normal fat-containing diet, with fat making up nearly 40% of the energy intake. Although, previously, patients on low-fat diets were advised to consume high-energy intakes, this was difficult on the bland high-carbohydrate diets provided. In patients on normal fat-containing diets unable to achieve required intakes for growth, the impaired intake is related to a series of interactive factors, namely, lung disease, drugs given for pulmonary disease, gastrointestinal problems (especially esophagitis), liver or biliary tract disease, long-standing DIOS, and psychoemotional problems. Many of these problems can be managed with medical therapy, but if unsuccessful, invasive nutritional intervention will be required.

Energy Losses. Energy loss occurs via the gastrointestinal tract owing to maldigestion and malabsorption of nutrients. Although 40 to 50% of patients can normalize their fat absorption on optimal regimens of microspheric OERT,[54–56,131] 60% do not, and up to 10% will continue to have fat excretions of over 20% of their fat intake. Again, after investigating such patients for the presence of other complications of CF (eg, gut or liver disease), one may have to empirically treat them with adjunctive gastric acid suppression therapy, attempting to improve the alkalinity of the small intestinal milieu and thereby improve fat digestion and absorption.[54] However, such therapy may not be successful, and larger intakes will be required to avert growth failure.

Energy Expenditure. Several studies of CF patients have demonstrated increased total and/or resting energy expenditure (TEE and REE, respectively).[132–134] In one of the first studies performed, TEE, as measured by the unique doubly labeled water technique, suggested that CF infants had an average TEE that was 25% above age-matched controls.[132] Because they were infants, they were assumed to have minimal lung disease; thus, the increased energy expenditure was attributed to the underlying disease process, in keeping with in vitro studies of CF fibroblasts demonstrating increased oxygen consumption.[135] However, the degree of lung disease in an infant population is difficult to assess; thus, the authors could not conclude that the raised TEE was not in part contributed to by suppurative lung disease. A later study of older patients suggested that REE was negatively correlated with lung function in a quadratic fashion, but this study was in part retrospective.[134] In preliminary results from another center of a large group of patients between 5 and 15 years of age with normal FEV_1 (greater than 80% predicted), PI patients averaged 107% and PS patients 100% of predicted values.[136] At the completion of that study, the latter finding was confirmed, with PI patients maintaining an 11% increase in their average REE ($p < .001$) compared with their PS counterparts, thus indicating that there is an increase in REE related to the underlying severity of the genetic mutation and it occurs independently of the effect of lung dysfunction because these patients had virtually normal lung function.[137] It is of interest that the same study detected a gender difference, with CF females maintaining an average REE of 111% versus 104% for males of their respective control values. This could well explain the noted gender differences in nutritional status and growth and the differences in survival as reported by others.[123]

Malnutrition. In light of the above discussion, it is not surprising that the CF child on a low-fat, low-energy diet consuming only 80% RDA falls well short of the near 110% required for normal growth for a PI child. Furthermore, if the child has had a series of lung infections and ongoing problems with malabsorption, the energy cost of suppuration and lung disease combined with energy losses owing to malabsorption will severely impair the chance of the child even maintaining his/her present growth let alone catching up to previous growth channels.

The consequences of malnutrition in terms of macro- and micronutrients are summarized in Table 65.1-4. Inadequate protein-energy balance is associated with wasting, stunting of linear growth, and, in older children, delayed puberty. Secondary problems occur with abdominal distention, peripheral edema, and ascites with hypoalbuminemia. Fat-soluble vitamin deficiencies can occur at any age and may vary from one age to another. Whereas vitamin A deficiency commonly presents in older children as night blindness, in young infants, it can present as benign intracranial hypertension with a distended fontanel. Vitamin E deficiency often presents as a hemolytic anemia during infancy but later as a severely debilitating neuropathy with ataxia and/or external ophthalmoplegia. Vitamin D deficiency rickets rarely occurs in the hotter subtropical climates but can certainly occur in colder temperate climates, where children are not exposed to sunlight for prolonged periods annually. Overt essential fatty deficiency, which is now seen only in infants at the time of diagnosis, is usually associated with a seborrheic skin rash. A patient on a normal diet supplemented appropriately with OERT should not develop essential fatty acid deficiency.

Malnutrition in CF infants is common where neonatal screening is not operational. Infants present with failure to thrive, wasting, short stature, and/or edema. In the presence of hypoproteinemia, the infants may have a distended fontanel and hemolysis. It is significant that such findings are rare in infants from neonatal screening programs and, if present, are usually subclinical.[41,50] Both controlled and cohort studies of neonatal screening programs demonstrate nutritional and growth advantages in screened infants, although there are limited data supporting an advantage of screening on pulmonary disease and survival.[138,139]

Clinical Evaluation and Management. A summary of a nutritional assessment program is provided in Table 65.1-5. Several other research procedures, including measurement of body cell mass, body protein, and energy expenditure, are undertaken by some units, but they do not have a routine role in the day to day management of CF patients. The major routine assessments, both initially and in follow-up, are measurement of height and weight parameters. In general, maintenance of growth at a specific percentile indicates the well-being of the subject and the adequacy of nutritional intake. Equally, a falling off from a previously held percentile may indicate the inadequacy of oral intake and/or intercurrent problems, particularly chest infection and pulmonary deterioration.

At diagnosis, the other mandatory assessment is an evaluation of pancreatic function, best achieved by a 3- to 5-day fat balance study. Fecal fat values in excess of 10% of fat intake in infants (2 g/d in breastfed infants) or in excess of

TABLE 65.1-4   MALNUTRITION IN PATIENTS WITH CYSTIC FIBROSIS

MACRONUTRIENT DEFICIENCY
Protein deficiency with hypoalbuminemia
Edema
Linear growth failure
Loss of bone matrix (osteopenia with associated low calcium intake)
Energy deficiency withweight loss
Wasting of fat and lean mass
Wasting of shoulder girdle and buttocks
Stunting of growth
Delayed puberty

MICRONUTRIENT DEFICIENCY
Fat-soluble vitamin deficiency

Vitamin A	Benign intracranial hypertension (distention of fontanel in infants)
	Night blindness
	Xerophthalmia: Bitôt spots
Vitamin D	Rickets (rare in sunny climates)
Vitamin E	Hemolytic anemia (infants)
	Peripheral neuropathy
	Ataxia with spinocerebellar tract degeneration
	External ophthalmoplegia
Vitamin K	Coagulopathy
Water-soluble vitamins	Vitamin B_{12} deficiency (rare)
Essential fatty acid deficiency	Seborrheic dermatitis
Salt depletion (hot climates)	Hyponatremia
	If severe, associated with hypochloremia, hypokalemia, and metabolic alkalosis

7% of fat intake in children over 12 months indicate PI and the necessity for OERT. Serum fat-soluble vitamin levels and albumin should be measured at diagnosis and annually thereafter. The normal range of vitamin levels for infants and young children is now available, and, in general, the CF patient should be maintained within that range.[140]

Anthropometric measurements can be repeated at 2- to 3-month clinic visits, and intermittent evaluations of fat absorption may be required in the infant or child with problematic symptoms of steatorrhea. PS patients should have their absorption evaluated at least prior to school entry if asymptomatic and maintaining normal growth or as dictated by the occurrence of symptoms of malabsorption, including failure to maintain their growth percentiles. Given that there are now reports of osteopenia with low bone mineral density in undernourished CF subjects, bone mineral density should be assessed annually in subjects with suboptimal growth.[141] It is also apparent that a large proportion of CF patients (up to 30%) over 10 years of age are glucose intolerant. Although a much smaller percentage is frankly diabetic, some clinics now recommend that a fasting blood glucose be included in the annual evaluation. It remains unclear as to how to approach patients with fasting sugars above 6 mmol/L and whether a 2-hour postprandial serum glucose would be more appropriate. Currently, patients with high fasting or 2-hour postprandial glucose should be referred for evaluation by a diabetologist.

Nutritional recommendations for CF patients are as outlined in Table 65.1-6. Energy intakes should approxi-

mate 120% of the RDA but may, of necessity, be increased in patients growing suboptimally. Fat-soluble vitamins should be given on the basis of serum results because a large proportion of subjects can maintain normal levels without supplementation. Vitamin D supplementation is rarely required in sunny climates, where the patient is exposed to ultraviolet light on a daily basis out of doors. Of note, however, those patients from hotter climates require regular salt supplementation during summer months and, to avoid salt depletion and dehydration, at least a doubling of this intake when exercise is undertaken.

SPECIFIC AREAS OF NUTRITIONAL CONCERN

Infants. Recommendations for feeding CF infants have varied over the last 30 years. Prior to microspheric OERT, enzyme replacement was given to infants in the form of enzyme powder. The latter was readily activated in the higher pH of salivary secretions, and, as a consequence, oral inflammation and ulceration were frequent problems. Moreover, the breastfeeding mother experienced excoriated nipples. Both situations, either in isolation or in combination, impaired satisfactory feeding. Consequently, semielemental formula feeds were introduced with the belief that they could be used without enzyme supplementation.[142] Fecal fat analyses purportedly showed normal fat absorption, but, at least in some instances, the analysis technique did not measure medium-chain triglycerides (MCT), and given that many of the diets had high MCT content (up to 80% of fat in the formula), fecal fats were grossly underestimated. The need of OERT to hydrolyze MCT was subsequently demonstrated using the appropriate fecal analytical techniques.[143] Subsequent to the finding that OERT was required for MCT digestion, there appeared little advantage to using semielemental formulas.

TABLE 65.1-5   NUTRITIONAL ASSESSMENT OF PATIENTS WITH CYSTIC FIBROSIS AT DIAGNOSIS

CLINICAL
Height, weight, head circumference
Skinfolds for body fat
Percentile or SD scores thereof

BIOCHEMICAL
Pancreatic function: fecal fat
Serum albumin
Serum fat-soluble vitamin levels
Coagulation screen

FOLLOW-UP
Anthropometric indices (each clinic visit)
Skinfolds (annually)
Bone mineral density (at start of puberty and thereafter as indicated)

BIOCHEMICAL
Fecal fat:
  In PS patients suspected of becoming PI
  In PI patients for adjustment of OERT
Serum albumin (annually)
Serum fat-soluble vitamins and coagulation screen (annually)
Fasting 2-hour postprandial glucose

OERT = oral enzyme replacement therapy; PI = pancreatic insufficient; PS = pancreatic sufficient.

TABLE 65.1-6   NUTRITIONAL RECOMMENDATIONS
IN CYSTIC FIBROSIS PATIENTS

ENERGY
120% RDA, with 40% as long-chain triglyceride

PROTEIN
100% RDA

FAT-SOLUBLE VITAMINS*

Vitamin A	5,000 IU/d1–3 yr of age
	10,000 IU/d > 3 yr of age
Vitamin D	500 IU/d
Vitamin E	25 IU/kg/d infants
	100–200 IU/d older children
Vitamin K	5–10 mg, once per week

SALT SUPPLEMENTATION† (hot climates)
0–6 mo: 0.5 g/d
6–12 mo: 1 g/d
1–5 yr: 2 g/d
> 5 yr: 3–5 g/d

*Fat-soluble vitamin therapy should be guided by vitamin A and E laboratory
results and vitamin K by coagulation screen. Vitamin D is not required in sunny
climates.
†Salt intakes should be doubled in hot summer months or during prolonged exercise.

In a subsequent feeding study of infants diagnosed by neonatal screening, a large group of infants achieved and maintained near-normal growth in the first 2 years of life whether breast- or standard milk formula fed.[144] Mothers provided their own choice of feeding at the time of diagnosis, and the subjects were not truly randomized to either regimen. However, in a later randomized study of nonscreened infants, those on standard milk formula achieved near-normal growth parameters.[145] There seems to be no advantage to using expensive semielemental diets in preference to breast milk or standard formula feeding in CF infants provided that the PI patient receives OERT as appropriate.

Adolescents and Adults with Growth Failure and Severe Pulmonary Disease. As respiratory disease advances in CF patients, a vicious circle occurs whereby the chest disease and its management are associated with increasing nutrient requirements in the face of severe anorexia. Weight loss, with loss of lean and muscle tissue, further impairs the likelihood of the subject responding satisfactorily to respiratory therapy, and the cycle continues. Some subjects with less severe pulmonary disease respond readily to high-energy oral supplements, including milk shakes and high-density desserts.[146] However, others with more severe disease are sufficiently anorexic to be unable to comply with these regimens. Consideration should be given in such patients to a more aggressive approach to nutritional intervention, including continuous nocturnal nasogastric tube or gastrostomy button feeds. The severity of the pulmonary disease will often preclude nightly nasogastric intubations, and permanently placed gastrostomy buttons have gained favor over the last decade. These regimens can halt weight loss and, in many instances, can be used to induce catch-up growth. However, the specific advantages of so doing have yet to be realized in terms of overall prognosis. Although initial studies indicated a slowing of the decline in lung function, they

were performed on small numbers with mostly reasonably preserved lung function at the start of the studies.[128–130] In patients with advanced lung disease, the benefits are even less obvious; in fact, they may encumber a patient unduly, interfering with the quality of life in the terminal stages of the disease. These issues need to be addressed in patients with severe disease prior to commencement of such therapy, thus preventing discomfort and the emotional challenge in a patient needing palliative therapy only. Some of these patients may be suitable candidates for receiving anabolic agents. Growth hormone can increase height and weight velocity,[147] but as they increase proportionately, patients can remain significantly wasted even after 12 months of therapy. It is also uncertain as to whether the growth changes will be sustained after cessation of the therapy. Similarly, megestrol acetate produces significant improvements in appetite and weight gain, but these are not sustained after cessation of therapy. Although further treatment could be considered, adverse events, including adrenal suppression, insulin resistance, insomnia, hyperactivity, and hypertension, have been described.[148–150]

With the advent of lung transplant, the importance of nutrition needs to be re-evaluated in pre- and post-transplant subjects. Specifically, the physicians involved need to determine whether malnutrition adversely affects transplant outcome and whether the adverse effects can be overcome with nutritional supplementation.

REFERENCES

1. Fanconi G, Uehlinger E, Knauer C. Das Coelioksyndrom bei angeborener zystisher Pankreas Fibromatose und Bronchicktasis. Wien Med Wochenschr 1936;86:753–6.
2. Anderson D. Cystic fibrosis of the pancreas and its relation to celiac disease. Am Dis Child 1938;56:344–99.
3. di Sant'Agnese P, et al. Abnormal electrolyte composition of sweat in cystic fibrosis of the pancreas. Pediatrics 1953;12:549–63.
4. Knowlton RG, et al. A polymorphic DNA marker linked to cystic fibrosis is located on chromosome 7. Nature 1985;318:380–2.
5. Kerem BS, et al. Identification of the cystic fibrosis gene: genetic analysis. Science 1989;245:1073–80.
6. Riordan JR, et al. Identification of the cystic fibrosis gene: cloning and characterization of complementary DNA. Science 1989;245:1066–72.
7. Rommens JM, et al. Identification of the cystic fibrosis gene: chromosome walking and jumping. Science 1989;245:1059–65.
8. Bear CE, et al. Purification and functional reconstitution of the cystic fibrosis transmembrane conductance regulator (CFTR). Cell 1992;68:809–18.
9. Davis PB. Clinical pathophysiology and manifestations of lung disease. In: Yankaskas JR, Knowles MR, editors. Cystic fibrosis in adults. Philadelphia: Lippincott-Raven; 1999. p. 45–67.
10. Flume PA, Yankaskas JR. Reproductive issues. In: Yankaskas JR, Knowles MR, editors. Cystic fibrosis in adults. Philadelphia: Lippincott-Raven; 1999. p. 449–64.
11. Anderson MP, et al. Generation of cAMP-activated chloride currents by expression of CFTR. Science 1991;251:679–82.
12. Hanrahan JW, Tabcharini JA, Grygorczyk R. Patch clamp studies of apical membrane chloride channels. In: Dodge JA, Brock DJH, Widdicombe JH, editors. Cystic fibrosis: current topics. New York: Wiley; 1993. p. 93–137.

13. Anderson MP, et al. Demonstration that CFTR is a chloride channel by alteration of its anion selectivity. Science 1991;253:202–5.

14. Sheppard DN, Welsh MJ. Structure and function of the CFTR chloride channel. Physiol Rev 1999;79 Suppl 1:S23–45.

15. Tonghui M, et al. Thiazolidinone CFTR inhibitor identified by high-throughput screening blocks cholera-toxin induced intestinal fluid secretion. J Clin Invest 2002;110:1651–8.

16. Schwiebert EM, et al. CFTR is a conductance regulator as well as a chloride channel. Physiol Rev 1999;79 Suppl 1:S145–66.

17. Stutts MJ, Boucher RC. Cystic fibrosis gene and functions of CFTR. Implications of dysfunctional ion transport for pulmonary pathogenesis. In: Yankaskas JR, Knowles MR, editors. Cystic fibrosis in adults. Philadelphia: Lippincott-Raven; 1999. p. 3–25.

18. Knowles MR, et al. Abnormal respiratory epithelial ion transport in cystic fibrosis. Clin Chest Med 1986;7:285–97.

19. Knowles MR, Gatzy J, Boucher RC. Increased bioelectric potential difference across respiratory epithelia in cystic fibrosis. N Engl J Med 1981;305:1489–95.

20. Case RM, Argent BE. Pancreatic duct cell secretion. Control and mechanisms of secretion. In: Go LW, editor. The pancreas: biology, pathobiology and disease. New York: Raven Press; 1993. p. 301–50.

21. Hadorn B, Johansen PG, Anderson CM. Pancreozymin secretin test of exocrine pancreatic function in cystic fibrosis and the significance of the result for the pathogenesis of the disease. Can Med J 1968;98:377–84.

22. Gaskin KJ, et al. Evidence for a primary defect in pancreatic HCO_3^- secretion in cystic fibrosis. Pediatr Res 1982;16:554–7.

23. Kopelman H, et al. Impaired chloride secretion, as well as bicarbonate secretion, underlies the fluid secretory defect in the cystic fibrosis pancreas. Gastroenterology 1988;95: 349–55.

24. Shumaker H, et al. CFTR drives Na^+-$nHCO_3^-$ cotransport in pancreatic duct cells: a basis for defective HCO_3^- secretion in CF. Am J Physiol 1999;276:C16–25.

25. Ishiguro H, Steward C, Wilson RW, Case RM. Bicarbonate secretion in interlobular ducts from guinea pig pancreas. J Physiol 1996;495:179–91.

26. Kopelman H, et al. Pancreatic fluid secretion and protein hyperconcentration in cystic fibrosis. N Engl J Med 1985;312: 329–34.

27. Freedman SD, Kern HF, Scheele GA. Coupling of ductal and acinar cell function in the exocrine pancreas: novel insights into CF. Pediatr Pulmonol 1997;14:116–7.

28. Wilcken B, Brown AR, Urwin R, Brown DA. Cystic fibrosis screening by dried blood spot trypsin assay: results in 75,000 newborn infants. J Pediatr 1983;102:383–7.

29. Macek M Jr, et al. Identification of common cystic fibrosis mutations in African-Americans with cystic fibrosis increases the detection rate to 75%. Am J Hum Genet 1997;60:1122–7.

30. Quinton PM. What is good about cystic fibrosis? Curr Biol 1994;4:742–3.

31. Gabriel SE, et al. Cystic fibrosis heterozygote resistance to cholera toxin in the cystic fibrosis mouse model. Science 1994;266:107–9.

32. Kazazian HH Jr. Population variation of common cystic fibrosis mutations: the Cystic Fibrosis Genetic Analysis Consortium. Hum Mutat 1994;4:167–77.

33. Knowles MR, Friedman KJ, Silverman LM. Genetics, diagnosis, and clinical phenotype. In: Yankaskas JR, Knowles MR, editors. Cystic fibrosis in adults. Philadelphia: Lippincott-Raven; 1999. p. 27–42.

34. Wilschanski M, et al. Correlation of sweat chloride concentration with classes of the cystic fibrosis transmembrane conductance regulator gene mutations. J Pediatr 1995;127:705–10.

35. Forstner G, et al. Digestion and absorption of nutrients in cystic fibrosis. In: Sturgess J, editor. Perspectives in cystic fibrosis: proceedings of the 8th International Congress on Cystic Fibrosis. Mississauga (ON): Imperial Press; 1980. p. 137.

36. Gibbs GE, Bostick WL, Smith PM. Incomplete pancreatic deficiency in cystic fibrosis of the pancreas. J Pediatr 1950; 37:320–5.

37. di Sant'Agnese PA. Fibrocystic disease of the pancreas with normal or partial pancreatic function. Pediatrics 1955;15:683.

38. Gaskin KJ, et al. Colipase and maximally activated pancreatic lipase in normal subjects and patients with steatorrhea. J Clin Invest 1982;69:427–34.

39. Gaskin KJ, et al. Colipase and lipase secretion in childhood onset pancreatic insufficiency: delineation of patients with steatorrhea secondary to relative colipase deficiency. Gastroenterology 1984;86:1–7.

40. Gaskin KJ, et al. Improved respiratory prognosis in CF patients with normal fat absorption. J Pediatr 1982;100:857–62.

41. Waters DL, et al. Pancreatic function in infants identified as having cystic fibrosis in a neonatal screening program. N Engl J Med 1990;322:303–8.

42. Waters D, et al. Pancreatic function and genotyping in infants with cystic fibrosis. In: Proceedings of the 11th International Cystic Fibrosis Congress; 1992; Dublin, Ireland. Dublin: Cystic Fibrosis Association; 1992. TP60.

43. Gaskin K, et al. Assessment of pancreatic function in screened infants with cystic fibrosis. Pediatr Pulmonol Suppl 1991; 7:69–71.

44. Kerem E, et al. The relation between genotype and phenotype in cystic fibrosis—analysis of the most common mutation (delta F508). N Engl J Med 1990;323:1517–22.

45. Kristidis P, et al. Genetic determination of exocrine pancreatic function in cystic fibrosis. Am J Hum Genet 1992;50:1178–84.

46. Durno C, et al. Genotype and phenotype correlations in patients with cystic fibrosis and pancreatitis. Gastroenterology 2002;123:1857–64.

47. Kiesewetter S, et al. A mutation in CFTR produces different phenotypes depending on chromosomal background. Nat Genet 1993;5:274–8.

48. Oppenheimer E, Esterly J. Cystic fibrosis of the pancreas. Arch Pathol 1973;96:149–54.

49. Imrie J, Fagan D, Sturgess J. Quantitative evaluation of the development of the exocrine pancreas in CF and control infants. Am J Pathol 1979;95:697–707.

50. Reisman J, et al. Hypoalbuminemia at initial examination in patients with cystic fibrosis. J Pediatr 1989;115:755–8.

51. Lee P, Roloff D, Howat W. Hypoproteinemia and anemia in infants with cystic fibrosis. JAMA 1974;228:585–8.

52. Beharry S, et al. How useful is fecal pancreatic elastase 1 as a marker of exocrine pancreatic disease. J Pediatr 2002;141: 84–90.

53. Weber AM, et al. Effectiveness of enteric coated Pancrease® in cystic fibrosis children under 4 years. Cystic Fibrosis Club Abstr 1979;20:18.

54. Gow R, Bradbear R, Francis P, Shepherd RW. Comparative study of varying regimens to improve steatorrhoea and creatorrhoea in cystic fibrosis. Lancet 1981;i:1071–4.

55. Gaskin KJ. Impact of nutrition in cystic fibrosis: a review. J Pediatr Gastroenterol Nutr 1988;7:S12–7.

56. Costantini D, Padoan R, Curcio L, Giunta A. The management of enzymatic therapy in cystic fibrosis patients by an individualized approach. J Pediatr Gastroenterol Nutr 1988;7:S36–9.

57. Robinson PJ, Smith AL, Sly PD. Duodenal pH in cystic fibrosis

and its relationship to fat malabsorption. Dig Dis Sci 1990;
35:1299–304.

58. FitzSimmons SC, et al. High-dose pancreatic-enzyme supplements and fibrosing colonopathy in children with cystic fibrosis. N Engl J Med 1997;336:1283–9.

59. Smyth RL, et al. Strictures of ascending colon in cystic fibrosis and high-strength pancreatic enzymes. Lancet 1994;343:85–6.

60. Wilcken B. Newborn screening for cystic fibrosis: its evolution and a review of the current situation. Screening 1993;2:43–62.

61. Shwachman H, Lebenthal E, Khaw K. Recurrent acute pancreatitis in patients with cystic fibrosis with normal pancreatic enzymes. Pediatrics 1975;55:86–94.

62. Stern RC, Rothstein FC, Doershuk CF. Treatment and prognosis of symptomatic gallbladder disease in patients with cystic fibrosis. J Pediatr Gastroenterol Nutr 1986;5:35–40.

63. Vitullo BB, et al. Intrapancreatic compression of the common bile duct in cystic fibrosis. J Pediatr 1978;93:1060–1.

64. Farber S. Pancreatic function and disease in early life. Arch Pathol 1944;37:238–50.

65. Bodian M. Fibrocystic disease of the pancreas. A congenital disorder of mucus production—mucosis. London: William Heineman Medical Books; 1952.

66. di Sant'Agnese PA, Blanc WA. A distinctive type of biliary cirrhosis of the liver associated with cystic fibrosis of the pancreas. Pediatrics 1956;18:387–409.

67. Craig JM, Haddad H, Shwachman H. The pathological changes in the liver in cystic fibrosis of the pancreas. Am J Dis Child 1957;93:357–69.

68. Vawter GF, Shwachman H. Cystic fibrosis in adults, an autopsy study. Pathol Ann 1979;14:357–82.

69. Gaskin KJ, et al. Liver disease and common-bile-duct stenosis in cystic fibrosis. N Engl J Med 1988;318:340–6.

70. Cheng S, et al. Defective intracellular transport and processing of CFTR is the molecular basis of most cystic fibrosis. Cell 1991;64:681–91.

71. Waters DL, et al. Hepatobiliary disease in pancreatic sufficient patients with cystic fibrosis. Hepatology 1995;21:963–9.

72. Roy CC, et al. Hepatobiliary disease in cystic fibrosis: a survey of current issues and concepts. J Pediatr Gastroenterol Nutr 1982;1:469–78.

73. Psacharopoulos HT, et al. Hepatic complications of cystic fibrosis. Lancet 1981;ii:78–80.

74. Feigelson J, Pecau Y, Cathelineau L, Navarro J. Additional data on hepatic function tests in cystic fibrosis. Acta Paediatr Scand 1975;64:337–44.

75. Davidson GP, et al. Immunoassay of serum conjugates of cholic acid in cystic fibrosis. J Clin Pathol 1980;33:390–4.

76. Colombo C, et al. The effects of ursodeoxycholic acid therapy in liver disease associated with cystic fibrosis. J Pediatr 1990; 117:482–9.

77. Colombo C, et al. Ursodeoxycholic acid therapy in cystic fibrosis associated liver disease: a dose-response study. Hepatology 1992;16:924–30.

78. O'Brien S, Fitzgerald MX, Hegarty JE. A controlled trial of ursodeoxycholic acid treatment in cystic fibrosis-related liver disease. Eur J Gastroenterol Hepatol 1992;4:857–63.

79. Colombo C, et al. Ursodeoxycholic acid for liver disease associated with cystic fibrosis: a double-blind multicenter trial. Hepatology 1996;23:1484–90.

80. Cheng K, Ashby D, Smyth R. Ursodeoxycholic acid for cystic fibrosis-related liver disease (Cochrane Review). In: The Cochrane Library, Issue 2. Oxford (UK): Update Software; 1999. p. 1–11.

81. Cohen D, Stephen M. Control of bleeding in extrahepatic portal hypertension—the reversed splenorenal shunt and portal-azygos disconnection. Aust Paediatr J 1984;20:147–50.

82. Mack DR, et al. Clinical denouement and mutation analysis of patients with cystic fibrosis undergoing liver transplantation for biliary cirrhosis. J Pediatr 1985;127:881–7.

83. Isenberg JN. Cystic fibrosis: its influence on the liver, biliary tree and bile salt metabolism. Semin Liver Dis 1982;2:302, 313.

84. di Sant'Agnese PA, Hubbard VS, Lowe ME. Recent developments in clinical and basic research in cystic fibrosis. Monogr Paediatr 1981;14:1–25.

85. Magoffin AK, et al. Neonatal cholestasis in CF infants from a newborn screening program [abstract]. Pediatr Pulmonol Suppl 2002;24:338.

86. Taylor WF, Qaqundah B. Neonatal jaundice associated with cystic fibrosis. Am J Dis Child 1972;123:161–72.

87. Scott RB, O'Loughlin EV, Gall DG. Gastroesophageal reflux in patients with cystic fibrosis. J Pediatr 1985;106:223–7.

88. Feigelson J, Girault F, Pecau Y. Gastro-esophageal reflux and oesophagitis in cystic fibrosis. Acta Paediatr Scand 1987; 76:989–90.

89. Cucchiara S, et al. Mechanisms of gastroesophageal reflux in cystic fibrosis. Arch Dis Child 1991;66:617–22.

90. Cox KL, Isenberg JN, Ament ME. Gastric acid hypersecretion in cystic fibrosis. J Pediatr Gastroenterol Nutr 1982;1:559–65.

91. Crawford I, et al. Immunocytochemical localization of the cystic fibrosis gene product CFTR. Proc Natl Acad Sci U S A 1991;88:9262–6.

92. O'Loughlin EV, et al. X-ray microanalysis of cell elements in normal and cystic fibrosis jejunum: evidence for chloride secretion in villi. Gastroenterology 1996;110:411–8.

93. Ameen NA, et al. A unique subset of rat and human intestinal villus cells express the cystic fibrosis transmembrane conductance regulator. Gastroenterology 1995;108:1016–23.

94. Taylor CJ, et al. Failure to induce secretion in jejunal biopsies from children with cystic fibrosis. Gut 1988;29:957–62.

95. O'Loughlin EV, et al. Abnormal epithelial transport in cystic fibrosis jejunum. Am J Physiol 1991;260(5 Pt 1):G758–63.

96. Veeze HJ, et al. Ion transport abnormalities in rectal suction biopsies from children with cystic fibrosis. Gastroenterology 1991;101:398–403.

97. Veeze HJ, et al. Determinants of mild clinical symptoms in cystic fibrosis patients. Residual chloride secretion measured in rectal biopsies in relation to genotype. J Clin Invest 1994;93: 461–6.

98. Marino CR, Gorelick FS. Scientific advances in cystic fibrosis. Gastroenterology 1992;103:681–93.

99. Snouwaert JN, et al. An animal model for cystic fibrosis made by gene targeting. Science 1992;257:1083–8.

100. Davidson AC, et al. Distal intestinal obstruction syndrome in cystic fibrosis treated by oral intestinal lavage, and a case of recurrent obstruction despite normal pancreatic function. Thorax 1987;42:538–41.

101. Hamosh A, Corey M. Correlation between genotype and phenotype in patients with cystic fibrosis: the Cystic Fibrosis Genotype-Phenotype Consortium. N Engl J Med 1993;329: 1308–13.

102. Nouri-Sorkhabi MH, Gruca MA, Kuchel PW, Gaskin KJ. Phospholipid changes in children with pancreatic sufficiency and insufficiency. Clin Chim Acta 1999;281:89–100.

103. Sternby B, Nilsson A. Carboxyl ester lipase (bile salt-stimulated lipase), colipase, lipase and phospholipase A_2 levels in pancreatic enzyme supplements. Scand J Gastroenterol 1997; 32:261–7.

104. Al-Awqati Q, Barasch J, Landry D. Chloride channels of intracellular organelles and their potential role in cystic fibrosis. J Exp Biol 1992;172:245–66.

105. Zhang Y, et al. Genotypic analysis of respiratory mucous sulfation defects in cystic fibrosis. J Clin Invest 1995;96:2997–3004.

106. Shwachman H, Kowalski M, Khaw K-T. Cystic fibrosis: a new outlook. Medicine 1977;56:129–49.

107. di Sant'Agnese PA, Davis PB. Cystic fibrosis in adults: 75 cases and a review of 232 cases in the literature. Am J Med 1979;66:121–32.

108. Andersen HO, et al. The age-related incidence of meconium ileus equivalent in a cystic fibrosis population: the impact of high-energy intake. J Pediatr Gastroenterol Nutr 1990;11: 356–60.

109. Redel CA, et al. Intestinal button implantation for obstipation and fecal impaction in children. J Pediatr Surg 1992;27:654–6.

110. Coughlin JP, et al. The spectrum of appendiceal disease in cystic fibrosis. J Pediatr Surg 1990;25:835–9.

111. Shields MD, et al. Appendicitis in cystic fibrosis. Arch Dis Child 1991;66:307–10.

112. McIntosh JC, et al. Intussusception of the appendix in a patient with cystic fibrosis. J Pediatr Gastroenterol Nutr 1990;11: 542–4.

113. Roberts DM, et al. Prevalence of giardiasis in patients with cystic fibrosis. J Pediatr 1988;112:555–9.

114. Lloyd-Still JD. Crohn's accounts for increased prevalence of inflammatory bowel disease (IBD) in CF [abstract]. Pediatr Pulmonol Suppl 1992;8:307–8.

115. Goodchild MC, Nelson R, Anderson CM. Cystic fibrosis and celiac disease: coexistence in two children. Arch Dis Child 1973;48:684–91.

116. Stern R, et al. Treatment and prognosis of rectal prolapse in cystic fibrosis. Gastroenterology 1986;82:707–10.

117. Kulczycki LL, Shwachman H. Studies in cystic fibrosis or the pancreas: occurrence of rectal prolapse. N Engl J Med 1958; 259:409–12.

118. Oades PJ, et al. High-strength pancreatic enzyme supplements and large-bowel stricture in cystic fibrosis [letter]. Lancet 1994;343:109.

119. Borowitz DS, et al. Use of pancreatic enzyme supplements for patients with cystic fibrosis in the context of fibrosing colonopathy. J Pediatr 1995;127:681–4.

120. Smyth RL, et al. Fibrosing colonopathy in cystic fibrosis: results of a case-control study. Lancet 1995;346:1247–51.

121. Van Velzen D, et al. Comparative and experimental pathology of fibrosing colonopathy. Postgrad Med J 1996;72 Suppl 2: S39–48.

122. Neglia JP, et al. The risk of cancer among patients with cystic fibrosis. N Engl J Med 1995;332:494–9.

123. Corey ML. Longitudinal studies in cystic fibrosis. In: Sturgess J, editor. Perspectives in cystic fibrosis: proceedings of the 8th International Congress on Cystic Fibrosis. Mississauga (ON): Imperial Press; 1980. p. 246.

124. Corey M, et al. A comparison of survival, growth, and pulmonary function in patients with cystic fibrosis in Boston and Toronto. J Clin Epidemiol 1988;41:583–91.

125. Roy CC, Darling P, Weber AM. A rational approach to meeting macro- and micronutrient needs in cystic fibrosis. J Pediatr Gastroenterol Nutr 1984;3 Suppl 1:S154–62.

126. Bell L, et al. Nutrient intakes of adolescents with cystic fibrosis. J Can Diet Assoc 1981;42:62–71.

127. Soutter VL, Kristidis P, Gruca MA, Gaskin KJ. Chronic undernutrition, growth retardation in cystic fibrosis. Clin Gastroenterol 1986;15:137–55.

128. Boland MP, et al. Chronic jejunostomy feeding with a non-elemental formula in undernourished patients with cystic fibrosis. Lancet 1986;i:232–4.

129. Levy LD, Durie PR, Pencharz PB, Corey M. Effects of long-term nutritional rehabilitation on body composition and clinical

130. Shepherd RW, et al. Nutritional rehabilitation in cystic fibrosis: controlled studies of effects on nutritional growth retardation, body protein turnover, and course of pulmonary disease. J Pediatr 1986;109:788–94.

131. Mitchell EA, et al. Comparative trial of viokase, pancreatin and Pancrease® pancrelipase (enteric-coated beads) in the treatment of malabsorption in cystic fibrosis. Aust Paediatr J 1982;18:114–7.

132. Shepherd RW, et al. Increased energy expenditure in young children with cystic fibrosis. Lancet 1988;i:1300–1.

133. O'Rawe A, et al. Increased energy expenditure in cystic fibrosis is associated with specific mutations. Clin Sci 1992;82:71–6.

134. Fried MD, et al. The cystic fibrosis gene and resting energy expenditure. J Pediatr 1991;119:913–6.

135. Feigal RJ, Shapiro BL. Mitochondrial calcium uptake and oxygen consumption in cystic fibrosis. Nature 1979;278:276–7.

136. Selby AM, et al. Resting energy expenditure in pancreatic sufficient and pancreatic insufficient children with cystic fibrosis. In: Proceedings of the 11th International Cystic Fibrosis Congress; 1992; Dublin, Ireland. Dublin: The Cystic Fibrosis Association; 1992. TP81.

137. Allen JR, et al. Differences in resting energy expenditure between male and female children with cystic fibrosis. J Pediatr 2003;142:15–9.

138. Waters DL, et al. Clinical outcomes from a newborn screening program for cystic fibrosis. Arch Dis Child 1999;80:F1–7.

139. Farrell PM, et al. Nutritional benefits of neonatal screening for cystic fibrosis. N Engl J Med 1997;337:997–9.

140. Karr M, et al. Age-specific reference intervals for plasma vitamins A, E and beta-carotene and for serum zinc, retinol binding protein and prealbumin for Sydney children age 9–62 months. Int J Vitam Nutr Res 1997;67:432–6.

141. Rose J, et al. Back pain and spinal deformity in cystic fibrosis. Am J Dis Child 1987;141:1313–6.

142. Gaskin KJ, Waters DL. Annotation: nutritional management of infants with cystic fibrosis. J Paediatr Child Health 1994; 30:1–2.

143. Durie PR, et al. Malabsorption of medium-chain triglycerides in infants with cystic fibrosis: correction with pancreatic enzyme supplements. J Pediatr 1980;96:862–4.

144. Holliday KE, et al. Growth of human milk-fed and formula-fed infants with cystic fibrosis. J Pediatr 1991;118:77–9.

145. Ellis L, et al. Do infants with cystic fibrosis need a protein hydrolysate formula? A prospective randomised comparative study. J Pediatr 1998;132:270–6.

146. Parsons HG, et al. Supplemental calories improve essential fatty acid deficiency in cystic fibrosis patients. Pediatr Res 1988; 24:353–6.

147. Hardin DS, et al. Growth hormone improves clinical status in pre-pubertal children with cystic fibrosis: results of a randomized controlled trial. J Pediatr 2001;139:636–42.

148. Marchand V, et al. Randomized, double-blind, placebo-controlled pilot trial of megestrol acetate in malnourished children with cystic fibrosis. J Pediatr Gastroenterol Nutr 2000;31:264–9.

149. Newkirk M, et al. Adrenal suppression in children with cystic fibrosis treated with megestrol acetate (Megace). Pediatr Pulmonol Suppl 2001;20:323.

150. Dietary reference intakes for vitamin A, vitamin K, arsenic, boron, chromium, copper, iodine, iron, manganese, molybdenum, nickel, silicon, vanadium, and zinc. Washington (DC): Food and Nutrition Board, Institute of Medicine, National Academy Press; 2001.

2. Shwachman-Diamond Syndrome

Peter R. Durie, MD, FRCPC

Johanna M. Rommens, PhD

In 1964, Shwachman and colleagues and Bodian and colleagues independently described a syndrome predominantly affecting the exocrine pancreas and bone marrow.[1,2] Subsequent reports of larger patient cohorts have demonstrated that the clinical phenotype of Shwachman-Diamond syndrome (SDS) affects additional organ systems, such as the skeleton and liver, and revealed that short stature is also a characteristic feature of the disease.[3-5] Furthermore, the SDS phenotype is extremely heterogeneous, and specific features of the disease change with advancing age.[3,5] After cystic fibrosis (CF), SDS is the most common inherited cause of exocrine pancreatic dysfunction. The disease has an estimated prevalence that is 20 times lower than that of CF, with an approximate incidence of 1 in 50,000 in the North American population. It is known to occur in diverse populations, including those with European, Indian, Chinese, Japanese, North American aboriginal, and African ancestry.

GENETICS

An autosomal mode of inheritance for SDS was initially suggested by the pedigree structure of several family reports[3,6,7] and has been confirmed in formal segregation analysis of a collection of 70 families with corrections for ascertainment considerations.[8] The same collection was then used to initiate investigation into the molecular basis of disease. A genome-wide scan and linkage analysis revealed significant association to disease with markers on chromosome 7 that spanned the centromere.[9] Data from all of the 15 families, each of whom had two or three patients, supported the linkage and confined the location of the affected gene to a 2.7 cM interval. Shared disease haplotypes, consistent with founder disease chromosomes, were identified in additional and unrelated families of common ethnic origins, permitting further refinement of the gene locus to a 1.9 cM interval at 7q11.[10]

Subsequently, an uncharacterized gene containing disease-associated mutations was identified within the 1.9 cM interval.[11] The SBDS gene (Shwachman-Bodian-Diamond syndrome) has a 1.6 kb transcript composed of 5 exons, encoding a predicted protein of 250 amino acids (Figure 65.2-1). A pseudogene (SBDSP) was identified in a locally duplicated 305 kb genomic segment with 97% nucleotide identity to the disease-causing gene. Gene conversion owing to recombination between SBDS and its pseudogene was noted to be a common event in disease alleles. Three common recurring mutations, resulting from conversion of exon 2 segments, introduce changes leading to premature protein truncation. These conversions account for 74% of alleles associated with SDS. Of the unrelated SDS individu-

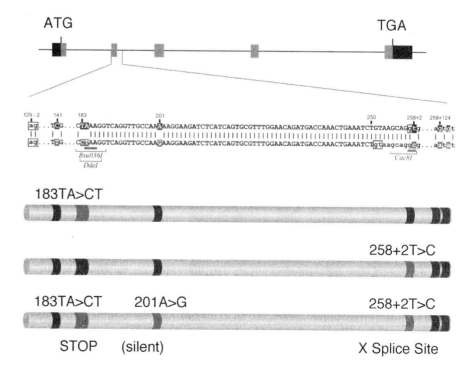

FIGURE 65.2-1 The *SBDS* gene is composed of five exons spanning 7.9 kb. A pseudogene resides in an adjoining duplicated segment. Sequence alignment of exon 2 of *SBDS* and its pseudogene *SBDPS* shows two sequence changes as well as a polymorphic change (201A→G). The most common *SBDS* mutations are derived from gene conversion events between *SBDS* and *SBDPS*. Three converted alleles are shown. These include (1) in-frame stop codon at position 184 (183 TA→CT), (2) splice site change (258+2T→C), and (3) an extended conversion mutation containing both mutant alleles and the polymorphic change.

als, 141 of 158 (89%) carried a gene conversion mutation on one allele and 60% carried conversion mutations on both alleles. Other *SBDS* mutations were identified in patients not involving gene conversion, including nucleotide substitutions leading to splicing interruption, missense changes or nonsense changes, and small deletions or insertions leading to in-frame changes or frame shifting and truncation (Table 65.2-1). These rare mutations were consistent with founder chromosome occurrence; for example, the 119delG mutation was found in two families of French Canadian descent with common haplotypes.[11]

Although the function of *SBDS* is unknown, it appears to be a member of a highly conserved family of proteins. Orthologs of *SBDS* exist in a wide variety of species, including archea, plants, and vertebrates. Ribonucleic acid (RNA) hybridization studies reveal broad but variable levels of expression in all tissues examined to date.[11] The predicted 28.8 kD protein product shows no homology to any known protein, but several lines of indirect evidence suggest that *SBDS* may be important in RNA metabolism.

CLINICAL MANIFESTATIONS

GENERAL FEATURES

Based on retrospective analysis of small patient cohorts, affected patients have lower than average weight and height at birth.[12] Although most patients have few signs and symptoms of disease in the early neonatal period, uncommon presentations include asphyxiating thoracic dystrophy, complete bone marrow failure, or severe life-threatening infections. On occasion, poor growth in infancy has raised suspicions and even accusations of parental neglect. We are aware of a tragic example of a 2-year-old girl in whom the diagnosis of SDS was established at postmortem (P. R. Durie, personal observation, 2002). This patient died of bacterial sepsis while in foster care after being removed from her biologic parents' care owing to a presumed diagnosis of "child neglect."

More commonly, patients come to medical attention in infancy or early childhood, with one or more symptoms,

which include malabsorption, malnutrition, growth failure, and recurrent infections (Table 65.2-2). Uncommonly, patients present de novo with aplastic anemia or acute myelogenous leukemia. On occasion, patients elude diagnosis until later childhood, and, rarely, the diagnosis is first established in adulthood.[13,14] As is discussed in greater detail below, a large percentage of older patients do not have severe pancreatic disease. Therefore, the absence of signs and symptoms of maldigestion does not exclude a diagnosis of SDS.

The nonspecific nature of the presenting symptoms, as well as poor awareness of the nature of the disease phenotype, can result in a delayed or even an incorrect diagnosis. The median age of diagnosis among 88 internationally ascertained patients was 1 year, with a range of 0.1 to 13 years.[5] In most case series, significantly more males than females have been diagnosed with SDS.[4,5] However, no gender differences were observed among families with more than one affected patient.[5] Given the small size of patient cohorts, the suggestion of a gender difference among isolated cases could be spurious. Alternatively, the contrasting gender differences, among singleton cases but not among multiplex patients, raises the possibility of a societal gender bias favoring clinical evaluation of males with short stature.

Although the clinical manifestations of disease are extremely heterogeneous and may change with age, all patients with SDS appear to have consistent evidence of both hematologic and exocrine pancreatic dysfunction. Other features, such as short stature, hepatic dysfunction, clinical or radiologic evidence of skeletal chondrodysplasia, and dental abnormalities, are sufficiently common to be considered primary features of the disease phenotype. Predilection to recurrent common bacterial infections, such as otitis media, as well as life-threatening deep tissue infections and sepsis, is considered to be a direct consequence of neutropenia and defective neutrophil chemotaxis. More convincing evidence is now emerging that neurologic abnormalities, learning difficulties, and psychological disorders are quite common among individuals with SDS. With further insight into disease pathobiology and evalua-

TABLE 65.2-1   MUTATIONS ASSOCIATED WITH SHWACHMAN-DIAMOND SYNDROME IN AFFECTED INDIVIDUALS FROM 158 FAMILIES

NUCLEOTIDE SEQUENCE CHANGE	AMINO ACID CHANGE	NUMBER OF ALLELES
258+2T→C*	84Cfs3	145
183-184TA→CT*	K62X	82
183-184TA→CT+258+2T→C*	K62X	8
258+1G→C*	84Cfs3	2
119delG	S41fs17	2
377G→C	R126T	2
24C→A	N8K	1
96-97insA	N34fs15	1
131A→G	E44G	1
199A→G	K67E	1
260T→G	I87S	1
291-293delTAAinsAGTTCAAGTATC	D97-K98delinsEVQVS	1
505C→T	R169C	1

Adapted from Boocock GR et al.[11]
*Gene conversion mutations accounted for 235 of 316 (74.4%) alleles associated with SDS.

TABLE 65.2-2   SPECTRUM OF CLINICAL FEATURES OF SHWACHMAN-DIAMOND SYNDROME

EXOCRINE PANCREAS	HEMATOLOGIC	SKELETAL/ DENTAL	GROWTH/ NUTRITION	LIVER	PSYCHOLOGICAL/ NEUROLOGIC
Acinar cell: dysfunction, pancreatic insufficiency, pancreatic sufficiency	Cytopenias: neutropenia, anemia, thrombocytopenia, pancytopenia ↑ Hemoglobin F Marrow aplasia Myelodysplasia Acute myelogenous leukemia	Long bones: delayed maturation, metaphyseal, dysplasia, tubulation Thorax: thoracic, dystrophy, short flared rib, costochondral thickening, clinodactyly, osteopenia Teeth: caries, dysplasia, mouth ulcer	Malnutrition (at diagnosis) Short stature	Hepatomegaly ↑ Aminotransferases Histology: portal inflammation, portal fibrosis	Low intelligence Learning difficulties Pontine leukoencephalopathy

Other: dermatologic; eczema, ichthyosis; renal: anatomic anomalies, tubular dysfunction; cardiac: endocardial fibrosis.

tion of much larger populations, it is likely that other, less common phenotypic features of SDS will be shown to be directly attributable to mutations in the *SBDS* gene.

EXOCRINE PANCREAS

Exocrine pancreatic dysfunction of varying severity appears to be a universal manifestation of SDS. Unlike CF, which is a disorder of pancreatic ductal obstruction,[15] the pancreatic defect in SDS appears to arise from a failure of pancreatic acini to develop. Histologically, the SDS exocrine pancreas shows normal ductular architecture and islets, absent or sparse acinar cells, and extensive fatty replacement (Figure 65.2-2).[2] Cross-sectional imaging may reveal a small shrunken pancreas or pancreatic enlargement owing to lipomatosis (Figure 65.2-3).[16] The suggestion that SDS is a syndrome primarily affecting acinar cells is bolstered by analysis of the results of hormonally stimulated pancreatic function studies, which reveal absent or

deficient acinar function (reduced enzyme output) but preserved ductal function.[4,17] The latter is reflected by normal output of anions (chloride and bicarbonate), cations (sodium and potassium), and fluid.

Most infants with SDS have signs and symptoms of fat maldigestion owing to pancreatic failure. Stimulated pancreatic secretions of lipolytic (lipase and colipase) and proteolytic (trypsin) enzymes fall more than 98% below the mean reference values for healthy controls.[17,18] These patients show clinical evidence of steatorrhea owing to pancreatic insufficiency based on correlative evaluation with 72-hour fecal fat balance studies.[4,18] However, cross-sectional and longitudinal evaluation of older SDS patients show that a subset of affected individuals show moderate improvement in pancreatic acinar capacity.[4,5,18] Secretions of lipolytic and proteolytic enzymes are marginally improved in these "pancreatic suffi-

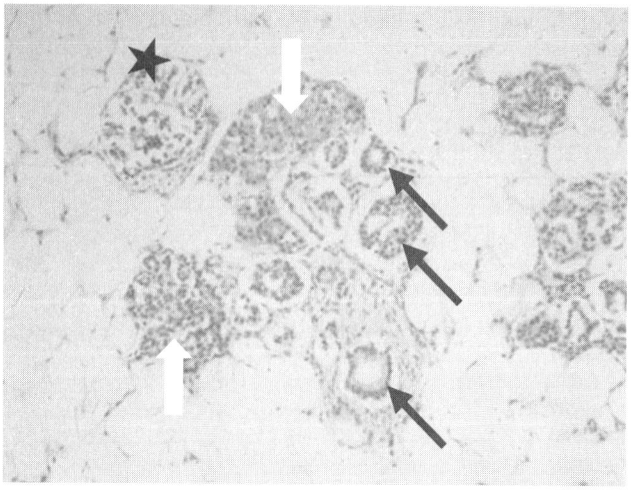

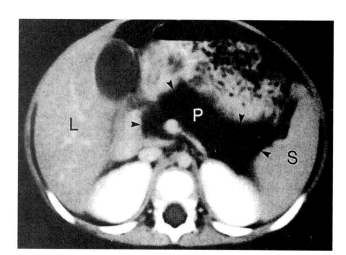

FIGURE 65.2-2   Histologic section of the pancreas from a patient with Shwachman-Diamond syndrome shows few sparse acini (*open arrows* surrounded by extensive areas of fatty replacement). Ductular architecture (*solid arrow*) and islets (*asterisk*) are normal (hematoxylin and eosin, ×50 original magnification).

FIGURE 65.2-3   Computed tomographic scan of the abdomen after intravenous contrast injection in a patient with Shwachman-Diamond syndrome. This individual presented clinically with massive hepatomegaly and intermittent neutropenia. Marked fatty infiltration of the exocrine pancreas (P) is outlined with arrowheads. This is in contrast to the soft density of the liver (L) and the spleen (S). Reproduced with permission from Wilschanski M et al.[16]

cient" patients but are sufficient to allow normal endogenous digestion of fat and protein, respectively, without the need for enzyme replacement therapy (Figure 65.2-4). Serial evaluation by 72-hour fecal fat balance studies confirms that stool fat losses, expressed as a percentage of quantified fat intake, normalize with age in this subset of patients.

Similar conclusions have been drawn from cross-sectional and longitudinal analysis of serum cationic trypsinogen concentrations.[4,5] Correlations between serum cationic trypsinogen concentrations and the results of 72-hour fecal fat balance studies (Figure 65.2-5) demonstrate that SDS patients with pancreatic insufficiency have serum enzyme concentrations of less than 6 µg/mL (lower limits of reference range 16.6 µg/mL). In contrast, those with normal fat absorption have serum trypsinogen values exceeding 6 µg/mL. Some of these patients have values within the normal reference range (16.6–45.5 µg/mL).

Taken together, these studies demonstrate that approximately 50% of affected patients will show sufficient improvement in pancreatic acinar capacity with advancing age to no longer require enzyme supplements. However, all of these patients have evidence of pancreatic dysfunction based on quantitative intubation techniques. Therefore, the absence of signs and symptoms of steatorrhea and/or normal serum trypsinogen concentrations does not exclude pancreatic acinar dysfunction or the diagnosis of SDS.

The age-related changes observed for serum trypsinogen do not hold true for other enzymes of pancreatic origin.[19]

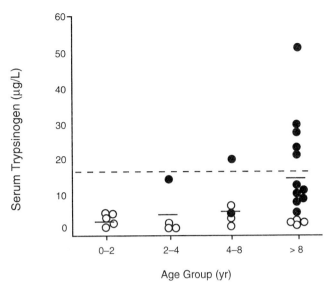

FIGURE 65.2-5 Serum cationic trypsinogen determinations grouped by age, including both pancreatic-insufficient (*open circles*) and pancreatic-sufficient (*closed circles*) patients with Shwachman-Diamond syndrome. The horizontal lines represent the mean value for each subgroup. The horizontal dashed line represents the lower reference limit (16.7 µg/mL for serum trypsinogen). Reproduced with permission from Mack DR et al.[4]

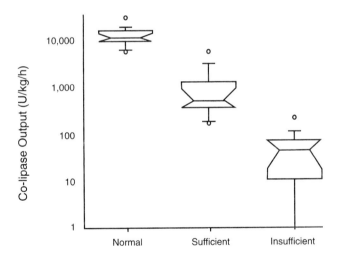

FIGURE 65.2-4 Stimulated exocrine colipase secretion controls, a pancreatic-insufficient patient, and pancreatic-sufficient patients with Shwachman-Diamond syndrome (SDS). The box plots show medians (*middle line*) and 75th (*top line*) and 25th percentiles (*bottom line*). The vertical lines extending above and below each box represent the 90th and 10th percentiles, respectively. Outliers are also shown. SDS patients with pancreatic sufficiency (based on a normal 72-hour fat balance study) have intermediate colipase secretion in comparison with healthy controls and SDS patients with pancreatic insufficiency. Similar results were obtained when total lipase and trypsin output were analyzed (data not shown). Reproduced with permission from Mack DR et al.[4]

For example, we have observed discordance between serum trypsinogen and pancreatic isoamylase determinations among patients with SDS and similarly aged healthy controls (Figure 65.2-6). In controls, serum trypsinogen concentrations were normal from birth and show no age-related alterations, whereas serum pancreatic isoamylase activities were lower at birth, rising to adult values by 3 years of age. Thereafter, serum pancreatic isoamylase activity remained unchanged with advancing age. We have concluded that the age-related differences of the two pancreatic enzymes mirror their discordant maturation rate postnatally. Pancreatic trypsin synthesis and secretion are mature after birth, whereas pancreatic isoamylase secretion is low at birth and shows gradual maturation over the first 3 years of age. In contrast to the aforementioned observations in controls, all patients with SDS had low pancreatic isoamylase activities irrespective of age, serum trypsinogen level, or their pancreatic status with regard to fat digestion. The independent age-related changes of the two enzymes, which appear to be unique to the pancreas of patients with SDS, have proven to be of great value as a clinical marker of the SDS pancreatic phenotype (see "Establishing a Clinical Diagnosis").

BONE MARROW

All patients with SDS show varying degrees of bone marrow failure. Persistent or intermittent neutropenia is virtually universal among affected patients. Some patients have a variety of other isolated cytopenias involving one or more bone marrow elements,[4,5] which may include pancytopenia and even complete bone marrow failure. The prevalence and range of hematologic abnormalities among singleton cases of SDS are similar to those seen in families with multiply affected children.[5] Furthermore, the fre-

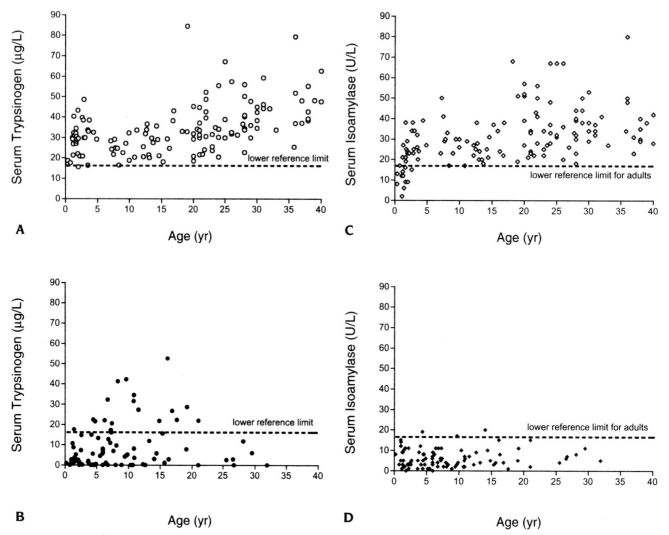

FIGURE 65.2-6 Cross-sectional serum trypsinogen levels in 23 control patients (*open circles*) and 90 patients with Shwachman-Diamond syndrome (SDS) (*closed circles*) plotted as a function of age (*A* and *B*). Twenty-two of 23 patients with SDS who were < 3 years of age showed serum trypsinogen values below the reference range, but values were within the normal range in 20% of older patients. Serum isoamylase values are plotted as a function of age in the same control patients (*open diamonds*) and patients with SDS (*closed diamonds*) (*C* and *D*). Unlike serum trypsinogen, serum isoamylase activities in control patients showed a significant age-dependent rise from birth to 3 years of age. After 3 years, intervals for pancreatic isoamylase (17–80 U/L) were similar to those previously reported for adults. All patients with SDS had low serum isoamylase activities. In 87 of 90 patients, values were below the reference range for adults. However, among patients < 3 years of age with SDS, isoamylase values tended to show overlap with values in similarly aged controls. There was no alteration of serum isoamylase with age in SDS and no association with the corresponding trypsinogen value.

quency and degree of concordance of the various bone marrow–derived cell lines in singleton cases do not differ from those observed in affected siblings.

In the largest patient cohort evaluated to date, 98% of 88 patients had chronic neutropenia, which was intermittent in 61% and persistent in the remaining patients. Iron deficiency anemia (42%) and thrombocytopenia (34%) were the next most common isolated abnormalities.[5] Abnormalities in more than one cell line were common, and pancytopenia was present in 19% of this cohort. The severity of peripheral neutropenia or other cytopenia does not appear to correlate with bone marrow cellularity. Peripheral blood counts do not necessarily predict the onset of myelodysplasia. Persistent elevation of hemoglobin F, which may reflect ineffective erythropoiesis, is present in most patients with SDS.

Neutrophil dysfunction, which is also observed in patients with SDS, almost certainly contributes to the propensity of patients with SDS to suffer from severe life-threatening bacterial infections. Chemotactic migration is significantly impaired, and some reports suggest that neutrophils from SDS patients exhibit defective bactericidal and phagocytic activity.[20–23]

The bone marrow of SDS patients shows reduced numbers of bone marrow precursors, which suggests that the bone marrow disorder is a stem cell defect.[3,24] Using long-term cultures of marrow stromal cells from SDS and unaffected subjects, Dror and Freedman demonstrated that patients with SDS also have dysfunction of the bone marrow stroma.[24] Thus, a dual bone marrow defect, namely a reduced ability of the bone marrow stroma to support and maintain effective hematopoiesis, as well as a stem cell defect, may explain the severity of the bone marrow defect in patients with SDS.

Bone marrow testing reveals a wide range of abnormalities.[3,5,25] The bone may appear normal in some patients, especially at a young age. The majority of cases show generalized hypocellularity, isolated hypoplasia of single cell lines, or generalized maturation delay or arrest. Complete bone marrow aplasia is known to occur.[26] Myelodysplasia with or without cytogenetic abnormalities is common.[5,27] The most common clonal cytogenetic abnormalities are present in chromosome 7 (eg, monosomy 7, isochromosome 7), but abnormalities are also observed in other chromosomes.[27-29] However, cytogenetic abnormalities, including those involving chromosome 7, may not be directly related to the SDS defect because similar changes are commonly observed in other bone marrow failure syndromes. The prognostic implications of finding myelodysplasia, with or without a clonal abnormality, remain uncertain.

As is the case with most bone marrow failure syndromes, patients with SDS carry a high risk of developing leukemia. The majority of individuals develop acute myelogenous leukemia, but lymphoblastic leukemia has also been reported.[30] The true prevalence of this complication is unknown. Smith and colleagues conducted a retrospective analysis of 21 patients with SDS over a 25-year period.[27] Myelodysplastic syndrome developed in 33% of patients, five of whom developed clonal chromosomal abnormalities. Twenty-five percent of these patients developed acute myeloid leukemia, which was invariably fatal in this series of patients. Males appear to carry a 10-fold greater risk of developing leukemia than affected females.[5,7,28] In general, attempts to induce remission with chemotherapeutic agents have been unsuccessful. Stem cell marrow transplant has been successful in a small number of patients. However, the success rate has been low, with an approximate 50% rate of survival (J. M. Lipton, personal communication, 2003). Also, a high complication rate, including heart and liver failure during induction, remains a concern.

INFECTIONS

The presence of neutropenia, abnormal chemotaxis, and possibly neutrophil bactericidal dysfunction function puts patients at risk of severe life-threatening infections.[20-23] The risk of infections may be exacerbated by nonspecific immunologic disorders, including dysgammaglobulinemia and T-cell dysfunction.[31] For poorly understood reasons, infants and young children appear to carry the greatest risk of morbidity and mortality from bacterial infections. Also, younger patients appeared to be particularly susceptible to upper respiratory tract infections and otitis media. In an earlier report, Shmerling and colleagues estimated that patients carried a 25% mortality rate owing to infection.[6] However, a more recent study of 25 patients from our center, who were followed for an average period of 5 years (range 0.5–20 years), showed an 8% mortality rate from infectious complications.[4] However, better survival in this cohort could be due to increased awareness of this complication. Eighty percent of these patients experienced one or more episodes of deep tissue infections, including pneu-

monia, abscess, osteomyelitis, septic arthritis, or bacterial sepsis. Recurrent fevers of unknown origin are also observed in patients with SDS.[5]

NUTRITION AND GROWTH

Short stature, which is common in patients with SDS, is considered to be a primary manifestation of the syndrome. Retrospective analysis of stature at birth shows a moderate deficiency in both height and weight in comparison with healthy newborns.[12] Patients may present with malnutrition at diagnosis.[4] Contributing factors to malnutrition include poor intake owing to recurrent infections and malassimilation of nutrients owing to pancreatic insufficiency. With adequate treatment with an appropriate diet and enzyme replacement therapy, malnutrition is rarely a long-term problem. However, short stature persists, and height and weight remain significantly below the age- and sex-adjusted values for the general population. Approximately 50% of individuals with SDS are below the 3rd percentile for height and weight.[5] Mean z-scores for height and weight are −2.2 and −1.8, below the mean for age and sex, respectively (Table 65.2-3). Cross-sectional studies of growth by age show that height relative to population norms remains the same at all ages. Weight expressed as a percentage of ideal weight for height also remains normal in childhood, but limited data show a tendency for adult patients to become relatively obese. There appear to be no differences in stature or nutritional status between patients with pancreatic sufficiency and those with pancreatic insufficiency.

SKELETON AND DENTITION

Previous small cohort studies of patients with SDS provide an incomplete picture of the skeletal aspects of the disease.[3-6,32-35] In most studies, only a subset of patients underwent radiologic evaluation, and the lack of longitudinal information failed to provide insight into the natural history of the skeletal abnormalities. Reported abnormalities included abnormal development of growth plates and metaphyses, delayed bone age, progressive deformities, and pathologic fractures. In the perinatal period, severe restrictive respiratory failure can arise as a result of asphyxiating thoracic dystrophy.

More recently, Makitie and colleagues analyzed the radiographs of 15 patients with SDS in whom the diagnosis had been confirmed by identified *SBDS* mutations on both alleles.[36] In 10 of these patients, serial radiographs were avail-

TABLE 65.2-3 GROWTH CHARACTERISTICS OF SHWACHMAN-DIAMOND SYNDROME

AGE (YR)	MEAN HEIGHT (Z-SCORE)	MEAN WEIGHT (Z-SCORE)	MEAN WEIGHT/ IDEAL WEIGHT FOR HEIGHT (%)
0–2	−2.65	−2.62	102
2–4	−2.24	−1.84	107
4–8	−1.84	−1.54	109
8–12	−2.23	−1.45	129
> 12	−2.15	−1.47	119

Adapted from Ginzberg H et al.[5]

able for longitudinal evaluation. The results of this study suggest that skeletal changes are present in all patients with SDS, but there is variable severity and localization changes with age. Typically, infants show delayed appearance of the secondary ossification centers, but epiphyseal maturation tended to improve with age. Varying degrees of widening and irregularities of the metaphyses were common in the ribs and proximal and distal femora in early childhood. With advancing age, a number of patients showed progressive thickening and irregularity of the growth plates (Figure 65.2-7). Most patients with radiologic alterations in the metaphyses showed no clinical symptoms. Some of these irregularities were associated with asymmetric growth and can progress to severe joint deformities, particularly in the proximal and distal femur, as well as the proximal tibia. Slipped femoral epiphyses and coxa vara or coxa valga deformities will require corrective surgery. Abnormal tubulation of the long bones was also observed.

This study also suggested that the right and left limbs were affected similarly, but the legs were more severely affected than the upper limbs. This report also affirmed previous observations that generalized osteopenia may be present at all ages.[3,36] There is no evidence that the osteopenic changes are related to pancreatic insufficiency or to a deficiency of vitamin D. No phenotype-genotype correlations were observed, and patients with identical *SBDS* mutations had a range of skeletal findings.

Several studies have suggested that patients with SDS are prone to oral and dental abnormalities. However, the true prevalence and severity of oral disease await careful prospective evaluation of a larger cohort of patients. Aggett and colleagues identified dental abnormalities in 10 of 21 patients with SDS.[3] Eight of these individuals had extensive caries, and three had dysplastic teeth. Other studies have also identified cases of caries and tooth dysplasia.[4,5] There have been reports of delayed loss of primary dentition and eruption of permanent teeth. Because oral diseases, including oral caries, decay, and periodontal disease, are largely preventable, further insight into the severity and extent of the problem will allow dentists to intervene more appropriately.

LIVER

Hepatomegaly is a common observation, especially in infancy.[3,5,16,37] Cross-sectional reports suggest that hepatomegaly resolves in the majority of patients by approximately 5 years of age.[3] Serum aminotransferase values are also elevated in infancy. In a larger cohort series of 88 patients, 60% had abnormal serum aminotransferase levels.[5] In most cases, values were onefold to fourfold above the upper limits of the reference range. Serial data in a subset of these patients showed a tendency for these biochemical hepatic abnormalities to resolve or improve with advancing age. Serum bilirubin levels were consistently normal. Histologic abnormalities are generally quite mild and include micro- and macrovesicular steatosis, periportal and portal inflammation and fibrosis, and, occasionally, bridging fibrosis. Progressive liver disease has not been reported in patients with SDS. There is one case report of chronic liver disease in a patient with SDS.[38] Also, affected patients have reportedly died from hepatocellular failure during induction for bone marrow transplant.

PSYCHOLOGICAL, BEHAVIORAL, AND NEUROLOGIC FEATURES

Several retrospective case studies,[4,5] clinical observations, and anecdotal expressions of concern from families suggest that individuals with SDS commonly suffer from learning and/or behavioral difficulties. At present, objective testing of patients is limited, and the prevalence and specificity of these deficits require objective prospective evaluation of a larger patient cohort. In the most extensive report to date, Kent and colleagues performed psychometric testing in affected patients, unaffected siblings, and disease controls with CF.[39] They also interviewed the patients' parents to ascertain information regarding developmental milestones, social interactions, and the impact of their child's illness on emotional and social adjustment. Psychometric testing revealed lower intelligence quotients among patients with SDS in comparison with their sibling controls and disease controls suffering from CF. Although group differences with tests of cognition and motor function were not significant, the individuals with SDS

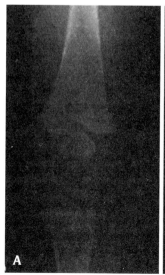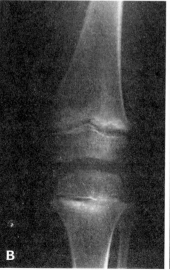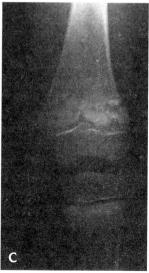

FIGURE 65.2-7 Longitudinal radiologic changes in the knee of a patient with Shwachman-Diamond syndrome. At age 5 months (A), secondary ossification centers are small. There is mild metaphyseal widening. At 4 years of age (B), secondary ossification centers are normal. The distal femoral and proximal tibial metaphyses are irregular and sclerosed. The metaphyseal changes show more severe irregularity and sclerosis at 5½ years of age (C). The femoral metaphysis is more severely affected than the tibia. Reproduced with permission from Makitie O et al.[36]

tended to have the lowest scores. In this particular report, the authors found no evidence that individuals with SDS had more behavioral difficulties than the control subjects. Interim analysis of a prospective international study that is being conducted at this center suggests that children with SDS do experience significant cognitive and retention difficulties as well as problems with emotional control.

There have been isolated case reports of specific neurologic abnormalities in both children and adults with SDS.[40,41] In three patients with SDS, focal or multifocal pontine leukoencephalopathy has been identified. Histopathologically, the pons shows lesions within pontocerebellar fibers with central necrosis, calcification, and neuroaxonal spheroids. Frequently, there are extrapontine areas of demyelination. Similar neuropathologic alterations have been recognized in patients with leukemia or lymphoma after radiotherapy or chemotherapy and in immunocompromised patients, including those with human immunodeficiency virus (HIV) or acquired immune deficiency syndrome (AIDS). It is important to note that none of the patients with SDS who developed leukoencephalopathy had evidence of malignancy, nor were they receiving immunosuppressive therapy.

OTHER FINDINGS

A variety of uncommon abnormalities have been described in patients with SDS. For example, dermatologic abnormalities, including ichthyosis and eczematous lesions, are commonly described in affected patients. There have also been reports of severe endocardial fibrosis, which led to death in a number of patients.[42]

Anatomic abnormalities of the renal system have been reported in individual cases, including double urethra and unilateral nonfunctioning kidney with urethral duplication.[3–5] Nephrocalcinosis and mixed amino acid urea have also been reported.[3–5] Although individual isolated cases of growth hormone deficiency and diabetes mellitus have been described, there is no evidence that these clinical conditions are directly associated with SDS.

ESTABLISHING A CLINICAL DIAGNOSIS

The diagnosis of SDS is established on the basis of characteristic clinical findings. There is no single disease characteristic or a simple biochemical test that is capable of definitively establishing or excluding a diagnosis of SDS. Furthermore, the existence of considerable disease heterogeneity and a lack of medical awareness of SDS make the diagnosis problematic. Other inherited causes of pancreatic exocrine dysfunction, including CF, Pearson bone marrow–pancreas syndrome, and Johansson-Blizzard syndrome, must be excluded. Similarly, transient neutropenia and bone marrow failure syndromes resembling SDS warrant serious consideration as alternative diagnoses. Pearson bone marrow–pancreas syndrome, Fanconi anemia, and Diamond-Blackfan anemia can be excluded by careful clinical assessment, bone marrow analysis, and/or specific laboratory tests.

With appropriate knowledge of the spectrum of the disease phenotype, the clinical diagnosis of SDS can be objec-

tively established or excluded with a high degree of certainty in the vast majority of patients. Two clinical features of the disease, notably exocrine pancreatic and bone marrow dysfunction, appear to be consistently observed in all patients. Therefore, objective confirmation of these two phenotypic manifestation is currently considered to be an absolute requirement for establishing a clinical diagnosis.[5,43]

Pancreatic exocrine dysfunction may be identified by one or more of the following evaluations:

1. Deficit of pancreatic enzyme secretion following quantitative pancreatic stimulation testing with intravenous cholecystokinin and secretin
2. Abnormal 72-hour fat balance study (provided intestinal mucosal disease or cholestatic liver disease is excluded) plus pancreatic imaging demonstrating a small or lipomatous pancreas
3. Low serum trypsinogen in patients under 3 years of age; low serum trypsinogen or pancreatic isoamylase in patients older than 3 years of age[19]

Bone marrow dysfunction may be established by one or more of the following evaluations:

1. Neutropenia (absolute neutrophil count < 1,500 neutrophils/mm^3). Because neutropenia can be persistent, cyclic, or intermittent, it must be documented at multiple time points (at least three times over a period of 3 months or more).
2. Anemia (hemoglobin concentration below the age-related normal range)
3. Persistent thrombocytopenia (platelet count < 150,000 platelets/mm^3)
4. Persistent pancytopenia
5. Myelodysplasia with or without clonal abnormalities

Genetic analysis may be used for diagnostic confirmation. Clinical genotyping for SDS is now available in clinical molecular diagnostic laboratories in the United States, United Kingdom, and Italy, as well as at the Hospital for Sick Children, Toronto.

Other common primary features of SDS are used to provide supportive evidence of the diagnosis of SDS. These include short stature, skeletal abnormalities, and hepatomegaly with or without elevation of serum aminotransferase levels. The absence of these features does not exclude the diagnosis of SDS. Because short stature occurs in a wide variety of other conditions and is not observed in all patients with SDS, it cannot be relied on as a feature of the disease for diagnostic purposes.

BASELINE ASSESSMENT, MONITORING, AND THERAPY

DIAGNOSTIC ASSESSMENT

The basic diagnostic evaluation of patients suspected of SDS has been outlined above. Additional baseline investigations, which are summarized in Table 65.2-4, include assessment of the status of the patient's pancreas, liver, skeleton, and bone marrow. Careful nutritional evaluation should include height, weight, anthropometry, determination of serum fat-soluble vitamin levels (A, E, 25-hydroxyvitamin D), prothrombin time, and partial thromboplastin time. Baseline bone marrow biopsy should include evaluation for evidence of cytogenetic abnormalities.

We advocate a multidisciplinary approach to the assessment, education, and treatment of the patient and family. Optimally, this should include ongoing support by a hematologist and gastroenterologist with adequate knowledge of the natural history of SDS. Depending on the family's circumstances and patient's condition, the assistance of a genetic counselor, psychologist, and/or social worker may be required. A dietitian who is familiar with nutritional care and pancreatic enzyme replacement therapy of patients with pancreatic failure should provide ongoing education and monitoring for the patient and family.

CLINICAL MONITORING AND THERAPY

The assessment should be performed every 6 to 12 months and should include weight, height, anthropometric measures, bone age, pubertal development, and review of developmental progress. A complete blood count with white cell differential and platelet count should be performed every 6 months or more frequently if indicated. We recommend that serum concentrations of vitamins A, E, and 25-hydroxyvitamin D; prothrombin time; and partial thromboplastin time be performed every 6 to 12 months.

Because a significant percentage of patients suffer from skeletal and dental disorders, anticipatory monitoring is advocated. With respect to the skeleton, we recommend radiographs of the hips and lower limbs every 1 to 2 years and, when indicated, consultation by an orthopedic surgeon with experience in chondrodysplastic disorders. Parents should be advised to seek dental evaluation at an early age, and the patient's dentist should be provided with information concerning the increased risk of oral or dental disorders in patients with SDS.

Steatorrhea may resolve with advancing age, even though pancreatic enzyme secretion remains well below normal levels. In our experience, this usually occurs within the first 4 years of life.[4] Thus, periodic reassessment for evidence of maldigestion is recommended. Monitoring can be conducted by serial measurements of serum trypsinogen concentrations. Fat absorption should be assessed using a quantitative 72-hour fecal fat analysis after the individual has discontinued enzyme supplementation for at least 24 hours. At present, there is inadequate information concerning the specificity and sensitivity of the fecal elastase 2 test for assessing pancreatic function in patients with SDS.[44]

If nutrient maldigestion is identified, pancreatic enzyme replacement therapy is required. The need for fat-soluble vitamin supplements should be determined on an individual basis. Most reports of patient cohorts indicate that patients achieve normal nutritional status with therapy. In our experience, patients with SDS respond well to enzyme therapy. The same dosing range should be used as for patients with CF.[45] There is no recommended therapy for short stature. Growth velocity is usually normal, and, with rare exceptions, growth hormone levels are normal. Pubertal progress may be delayed.

Although there is no objective evidence to support the practice, experts in bone marrow failure syndromes recommend that bone marrow aspirates, biopsies, and cytogenetic studies be performed annually. They recommend more frequent evaluation if myelodysplastic or cytogenetic abnormalities are noted. These recommendations are based on the unproven assumption that anticipatory information concerning early bone marrow changes will yield a beneficial outcome to the patient.

If a patient is experiencing repeated infections in association with severe neutropenia (absolute neutrophil count < 500/mm³), treatment with prophylactic antibiotics and/or granulocyte colony-stimulating factor (G-CSF) should be considered. There are concerns that long-term administration of G-CSF to patients with severe chronic neutropenia may increase leukemogenic risk. Although this potential risk of long-term G-CSF has not been clearly elucidated, some caregivers recommend limiting G-CSF therapy to short-term administration when a patient develops fever and/or an infection.

TABLE 65.2-4   ASSESSMENT AT DIAGNOSIS

DIAGNOSIS*
Clinical confirmation of SDS by excluding other causes of pancreatic
   dysfunction and bone marrow failure
        PLUS
Objective confirmation of pancreatic dysfunction
        AND
Bone marrow failure
BASELINE ASSESSMENT
Imaging
   Imaging of liver and pancreas (ultrasonography, CT, or MRI)
   Skeletal survey
   Bone age (older patients only)
Blood
   CBC, differential, platelets; hemoglobin electrophoresis
   Total and direct bilirubin, aminotransferases, alkaline phosphatase
   Serum vitamins A, E, D (25-hydroxyvitamin D)
   Prothrombin time, partial thromboplastin time
   Serum trypsinogen and pancreatic isoamylase
Bone marrow
   Aspirate
   Biopsy
   Cytogenetic analysis
Stool
   72-Hour fecal fat balance study

CBC = complete blood count; CT = computed tomography; MRI = magnetic resonance imaging; SDS = Shwachman-Diamond syndrome.
*Genotyping may be considered for confirming the diagnosis.

REFERENCES

1. Shwachman H, Diamond LK, Oski FA, Khaw K-T. The syndrome of pancreatic insufficiency and bone marrow dysfunction. J Pediatr 1964;65:645–63.
2. Bodian M, Sheldon W, Lighwood R. Congenital hypoplasia of the exocrine pancreas. Acta Paediatr Scand 1964;53:282–93.
3. Aggett PJ, Cavanagh NP, Matthew DJ, et al. Shwachman's syndrome. A review of 21 cases. Arch Dis Child 1980;55:331–47.
4. Mack DR, Forstner GG, Wilschanski M, et al. Shwachman syndrome: exocrine pancreatic dysfunction and variable phenotypic expression. Gastroenterology 1996;111:1593–602.

5. Ginzberg H, Shin J, Ellis L, et al. Shwachman syndrome: phenotypic manifestations of sibling sets and isolated cases in a large patient cohort are similar. J Pediatr 1999;135:81–8.

6. Shmerling DH, Prader A, Hitzig WH, et al. The syndrome of exocrine pancreatic insufficiency, neutropenia, metaphyseal dysostosis and dwarfism. Helv Paediatr Acta 1969;24:547–75.

7. Burke V, Colebatch JH, Anderson CM, Simons MJ. Association of pancreatic insufficiency and chronic neutropenia in childhood. Arch Dis Child 1967;42:147–57.

8. Ginzberg H, Shin J, Ellis L, et al. Segregation analysis in Shwachman-Diamond syndrome: evidence for recessive inheritance. Am J Hum Genet 2000;66:1413–6.

9. Goobie S, Popovic M, Morrison J, et al. Shwachman-Diamond syndrome with exocrine pancreatic dysfunction and bone marrow failure maps to the centromeric region of chromosome 7. Am J Hum Genet 2001;68:1048–54.

10. Popovic M, Goobie S, Morrison J, et al. Fine mapping of the locus for Shwachman-Diamond syndrome at 7q11, identification of shared disease haplotypes, and exclusion of TPST1 as a candidate gene. Eur J Hum Genet 2002;10:250–8.

11. Boocock GR, Morrison JA, Popovic M, et al. Mutations in SBDS are associated with Shwachman-Diamond syndrome. Nat Genet 2003;33:97–101.

12. Cipolli M, D'Orazio C, Delmarco A, et al. Shwachman's syndrome: pathomorphosis and long-term outcome. J Pediatr Gastroenterol Nutr 1999;29:265–72.

13. Hislop WS, Hayes PC, Boyd EJ. Late presentation of Shwachman's syndrome. Acta Paediatr Scand 1982;71:677–9.

14. MacMaster SA, Cummings TM. Computed tomography and ultrasonography findings for an adult with Shwachman syndrome and pancreatic lipomatosis. Can Assoc Radiol J 1993;44:301–3.

15. Stormon MO, Durie PR. Pathophysiologic basis of exocrine pancreatic dysfunction in childhood. J Pediatr Gastroenterol Nutr 2002;35:8–21.

16. Wilschanski M, van der Hoeven E, Phillips J, et al. Shwachman-Diamond syndrome presenting as hepatosplenomegaly. J Pediatr Gastroenterol Nutr 1994;19:111–3.

17. Hill RE, Durie PR, Gaskin KJ, et al. Steatorrhea and pancreatic insufficiency in Shwachman syndrome. Gastroenterology 1982;83(1 Pt 1):22–7.

18. Gaskin KJ, Durie PR, Lee L, et al. Colipase and lipase secretion in childhood-onset pancreatic insufficiency. Delineation of patients with steatorrhea secondary to relative colipase deficiency. Gastroenterology 1984;86:1–7.

19. Ip WF, Dupuis A, Ellis L, et al. Serum pancreatic enzymes define the pancreatic phenotype in patients with Shwachman-Diamond syndrome. J Pediatr 2002;141:259–65.

20. Aggett PJ, Harries JT, Harvey BA, Soothill JF. An inherited defect of neutrophil mobility in Shwachman syndrome. J Pediatr 1979;94:391–4.

21. Ruutu P, Savilahti E, Repo H, Kosunen TU. Constant defect in neutrophil locomotion but with age decreasing susceptibility to infection in Shwachman syndrome. Clin Exp Immunol 1984;57:249–55.

22. Sacchi F, Maggiore G, Marseglia G, et al. Association of neutrophil and complement defects in two twins with Shwachman syndrome. Helv Paediatr Acta 1982;37:177–81.

23. Repo H, Savilahti E, Leirisalo-Repo M. Aberrant phagocyte function in Shwachman syndrome. Clin Exp Immunol 1987;69:204–12.

24. Dror Y, Freedman MH. Shwachman-Diamond syndrome: an inherited preleukemic bone marrow failure disorder with aberrant hematopoietic progenitors and faulty marrow microenvironment. Blood 1999;91:3048–54.

25. Saunders EF, Gall G, Freedman MH. Granulopoiesis in Shwachman's syndrome (pancreatic insufficiency and bone marrow dysfunction). Pediatrics 1979;64:515–9.

26. Woods WG, Krivit W, Lubin BH, Ramsay NK. Aplastic anemia associated with the Shwachman syndrome. In vivo and in vitro observations. Am J Pediatr Hematol Oncol 1981;3:347–51.

27. Smith OP, Hann IM, Chessells JM, et al. Haematological abnormalities in Shwachman-Diamond syndrome. Br J Haematol 1996;94:279–84.

28. Dror Y, Squire J, Durie P, Freedman MH. Malignant myeloid transformation with isochromosome 7q in Shwachman-Diamond syndrome. Leukemia 1998;12:1591–5.

29. Dror Y, Durie P, Ginzberg H, et al. Clonal evolution in marrows of patients with Shwachman-Diamond syndrome: a prospective 5-year follow-up study. Exp Hematol 2002;30:659–69.

30. Strevens MJ, Lilleyman JS, Williams RB. Shwachman's syndrome and acute lymphoblastic leukaemia. BMJ 1978;2:18.

31. Dror Y, Ginzberg H, Dalal I, et al. Immune function in patients with Shwachman-Diamond syndrome. Br J Haematol 2001;114:712–7.

32. Taybi H, Mitchell AD, Friedman GD. Metaphyseal dysostosis and the associated syndrome of pancreatic insufficiency and blood disorders. Radiology 1969;93:563–71.

33. Danks DM, Haslam R, Mayne V, et al. Metaphyseal chondrodysplasia, neutropenia, and pancreatic insufficiency presenting with respiratory distress in the neonatal period. Arch Dis Child 1976;51:697–702.

34. McLennan TW, Steinbach HL. Shwachman syndrome: the broad spectrum of bony abnormalities. Radiology 1974;112:167–73.

35. Berrocal T, Simon MJ, al-Assir I, et al. Shwachman-Diamond syndrome: clinical, radiological and sonographic aspects. Pediatr Radiol 1995;25:289–92.

36. Makitie O, Ellis L, Durie P, et al. Skeletal phenotype in patients with Shwachman-Diamond syndrome and mutations in SBDS. Clin Genet 2003. [In press]

37. Brueton MJ, Mavromichalis J, Goodchild MC, Anderson CM. Hepatic dysfunction in association with pancreatic insufficiency and cyclical neutropenia. Shwachman-Diamond syndrome. Arch Dis Child 1977;52:76–8.

38. Liebman WM, Rosental E, Hirshberger M, Thaler MM. Shwachman-Diamond sydnrome and chronic liver disease. Clin Pediatr (Phila) 1979;18:695–6, 698.

39. Kent A, Murphy GH, Milla P. Psychological characteristics of children with Shwachman syndrome. Arch Dis Child 1990;65:1349–52.

40. Steinsapir KD, Vinters HV. Central pontine myelinolysis in a child with the Shwachman-Diamond syndrome. Hum Pathol 1985;16:741–3.

41. Anders KH, Becker PS, Holden JK, et al. Multifocal necrotizing leukoencephalopathy with pontine predilection in immunosuppressed patients: a clinicopathologic review of 16 cases. Hum Pathol 1993;24:897–904.

42. Savilahti E, Rapola J. Frequent myocardial lesions in Shwachman's syndrome. Eight fatal cases among 16 Finnish patients. Acta Paediatr Scand 1984;73:642–51.

43. Rothbaum R, Perrault J, Vlachos A, et al. Shwachman-Diamond syndrome: report from an international conference. J Pediatr 2002;141:266–70.

44. Beharry S, Ellis L, Corey M, et al. How useful is fecal pancreatic elastase 1 as a marker of exocrine pancreatic disease? J Pediatr 2002;141:84–90.

45. Borowitz DS, Grand RJ, Durie PR. Use of pancreatic enzyme supplements for patients with cystic fibrosis in the context of fibrosing colonopathy. Consensus Committee. J Pediatr 1995;127:681–4.

3. Other Hereditary and Acquired Disorders

Michael Wilschanski, MD

A number of rare hereditary and acquired disorders of the exocrine pancreas, apart from cystic fibrosis and Shwachman-Diamond syndrome, are discussed in this chapter.

HEREDITARY DISORDERS

PEARSON MARROW-PANCREAS SYNDROME

This syndrome was originally described in 1979 in four unrelated children with severe macrocytic anemia, variable neutropenia and thrombocytopenia, vacuolization of bone marrow precursors, and ringed sideroblasts in the bone marrow. Pancreatic insufficiency was subsequently diagnosed associated with extensive fibrosis and acinar atrophy.[1] The bone marrow changes, including cell vacuolization and the presence of ringed sideroblasts, distinguished this condition from Shwachman-Diamond syndrome. Other differences include the presence of pancreatic fibrosis rather than lipomatosis and the absence of bone lesions. It has been shown recently that this disease results from defective oxidative phosphorylation and is associated with deletions of mitochondrial deoxyribonucleic acid (DNA).[2,3] Of the respiratory chain enzymes encoded by mitochondrial DNA, complex I is the most severely affected. Genes encompassing two subunits of complex V, one subunit of complex IV, and five transfer ribonucleic acid genes are also deleted. Oxidation of reduced nicotinamide adenine dinucleotide is abnormal in lymphocytes from these patients, but respiratory chain enzyme activities are normal in muscle mitochondria. In severely affected tissues such as bone marrow, neutrophils, lymphocytes, and pancreas, the deletions are found in over 80% of cells, whereas deletions were observed in only 50% of muscle cells. Thus, expression of the phenotype in Pearson marrow-pancreas syndrome in a given tissue may require a minimum threshold number of mutated mitochondrial DNA molecules. However, in the largest series published to date, Rotig and colleagues reported that the size and location of the mitochondrial DNA rearrangements in 21 patients did not correlate with clinical severity.[4] Interestingly, some of these patients may develop visual and muscular symptoms, which are also found in Kearns-Sayre syndrome, a mitochondrial disease characterized by a large mitochondrial DNA deletion.[5]

JOHANSON-BLIZZARD SYNDROME

Johanson and Blizzard first described this syndrome whose features include pancreatic exocrine deficiency, aplasia or hypoplasia of the alae nasi, congenital deafness, hypothyroidism, developmental delay, short stature, ectodermal scalp defects, absence of permanent teeth, urogenital malformations, and imperforate anus.[6,7] More recently, other associated features were noted, including hypopituitarism,[8] diabetes mellitus,[9] growth hormone deficiency,[10] and congenital heart disease.[11] Prenatal ultrasonographic diagnosis has also recently been described.[12] The genetic defect is unknown, but the pathophysiologic basis of the pancreatic abnormality has been elucidated. Jones and colleagues performed pancreatic stimulation tests on two patients and found that the ductular output of fluid and electrolytes was preserved with decreased secretion of trypsin, colipase, and total lipase and low serum immunoreactive trypsinogen level.[13] These findings are consistent with a primary failure of pancreatic acinar development similar to that observed in patients with Shwachman-Diamond syndrome.[13] The functional exocrine disturbances are in keeping with histopathologic findings, which include absence of pancreatic acini.[14] Unlike Shwachman-Diamond syndrome, bone marrow and skeletal abnormalities are absent in Johanson-Blizzard syndrome.

JEUNE SYNDROME

This is a rare autosomal recessive disorder characterized by skeletal abnormalities of the thorax and extremities and nephronophthisis and is usually associated with respiratory distress in infancy. Karjoo and colleagues reported two families with asphyxiating thoracic dystrophy with exocrine pancreatic deficiency.[15] There is also one case report of pancreatic fibrosis.[16] Prenatal diagnosis has been reported.[17]

ISOLATED ENZYME DEFICIENCIES

The deficiencies of the pancreatic enzymes and mucosal enterokinase are very rare but have provided insight into the physiology of digestion and the sequelae resulting from their deficiency.

LIPASE DEFICIENCY

Pancreatic lipase is involved in the essential hydrolysis of long-chain dietary triglycerides to fatty acids in the intestinal lumen. The patients present with severe steatorrhea in infancy or early childhood, but despite the maldigestion of dietary fat, failure to thrive is not a feature. It has been suggested that alternative sources of lipolytic activity prevent failure to thrive.[18] Analysis of duodenal juice revealed absent or low lipase activity and, in some cases, low amylase and trypsin as well. Sheldon described this disorder in two unrelated sibships,[19] suggesting an autosomal recessive mode of inheritance. The complementary DNA encoding pancreatic lipase has been cloned[20] and the gene mapped to chromosome 10q24-q26.[21] These children respond well to exogenous pancreatic enzyme supplementation.

COLIPASE DEFICIENCY

Pancreatic colipase is a cofactor that is involved in overcoming the inhibitory effects of bile salts on pancreatic lipase. Deficiency of this enzyme has been reported in two brothers, aged 5 and 6 years, and is not associated with failure to thrive.[22]

COMBINED LIPASE–COLIPASE DEFICIENCY

Ghishan and colleagues reported a patient with < 2% of control values for lipase and colipase but normal concentrations of other pancreatic enzymes.[23] Ligumsky and colleagues reported congenital combined lipase and colipase deficiency in two brothers.[24]

AMYLASE DEFICIENCY

An abnormally low pancreatic amylase concentration below the age of 1 year may be physiologic; thus, the existence of amylase deficiency at this age may be developmentally related. Lowe and May reported a 13-year-old boy with absent amylase, diminished trypsin, and normal lipase concentrations.[25] Brock and Sjolund and their colleagues have reported familial selective deficiency of pancreatic amylase.[26,27] Because low serum pancreatic isoamylase has been observed in patients with Shwachman-Diamond syndrome who have normal fat digestion, this diagnosis should be considered in patients with isolated isoamylase deficiency.[28]

TRYPSINOGEN DEFICIENCY

There have been a few cases reported of this syndrome, which presents as severe malabsorption beginning in the neonatal period. Proteolytic enzyme activity was absent in the duodenal fluid but normalized with the addition of exogenous trypsin.[29] Normally, intestinal enterokinase activates trypsinogen, which, in turn, activates the other proenzymes. Hence, trypsinogen, chymotrypsinogen, procarboxypeptidase, and proelastase are activated to trypsin, chymotrypsin, carboxypeptidase, and elastase, respectively. Trypsinogen deficiency results in the disruption of the activation cascade because there is a lack of substrate for enterokinase. The trypsinogen gene is found on chromosome 7 and has caused renewed interest because a mutation in this gene causes hereditary pancreatitis, which is discussed elsewhere.[30]

ENTEROKINASE DEFICIENCY

Enterokinase (enteropeptidase) is an intestinal mucosal enzyme responsible for initiating the activation of pancreatic proteolytic proenzymes. It catalyzes the conversion of trypsinogen to trypsin, which, in turn, activates other proenzymes, including chymotrypsinogen, procarboxypeptidases, and proelastase.[31] The first case of congenital enterokinase deficiency was reported in 1969,[32] and

several cases have since been documented.[33] These children present in the neonatal period with diarrhea, failure to thrive, edema, and hypoproteinemia. The diagnosis was confirmed by absent trypsin activity in duodenal fluid, which then became active following exogenous addition of enterokinase. Further confirmation of an isolated enterokinase deficiency was the finding of minimal enterokinase activity in the duodenal mucosa in the presence of normal disaccharidase activities. Fat malabsorption was present despite normal amylase and lipase concentrations in unstimulated duodenal fluid because trypsin is required for the activation of colipase and phospholipase. The patients respond well to pancreatic enzyme supplementation, which generates normal duodenal proteolytic activity. This disorder has been reported in siblings, suggesting an autosomal recessive mode of inheritance. Kitamoto and colleagues have cloned the complete complementary DNA that encodes the enterokinase amino acid sequence and mapped the gene to chromosome 21q21.[34]

ACQUIRED DISORDERS

MALNUTRITION

Protein-calorie malnutrition has a significant effect on pancreatic exocrine function.[35] Studies on children with kwashiorkor have shown a generalized reduction in pancreatic size and histologic evidence of acinar atrophy. Disorganization and loss of acinar pattern were noted with little evidence of inflammation or necrosis. Acinar cells were vacuolated, and the number of zymogen granules was diminished. In more severe cases, varying degrees of fibrosis and fat accumulation were observed.[36] Functional changes in the pancreas closely resemble the structural abnormalities. Barbezat and Hansen performed pancreatic stimulation tests in children with protein-calorie malnutrition.[37] There was a reduction in enzyme output in response to hormonal stimulation, but the volume output and alkalinization of the duodenal fluid were not affected. This is consistent with the histologic observation of ductal preservation, which is the source of water and bicarbonate secretion. Prompt improvement of enzyme secretion was observed with nutritional rehabilitation, although two patients had consistently low enzyme secretion.[37]

Biochemically, acute malnutrition in children has been associated with elevated cationic trypsinogen levels, which are correlated with the severity of the malnutrition.[38] However, persistently low immunoreactive trypsin levels are found in chronically malnourished children.[39] These studies suggest that in acute malnutrition, there is abnormal pancreatic cell membrane function with leakage of zymogen into the circulation, but more chronic malnutrition is associated with extensive pancreatic acinar cell atrophy and diffuse fibrosis, thus producing low trypsinogen levels. Juvenile tropical pancreatitis and its possible association with malnutrition are discussed in Chapter 64.2, "Juvenile Tropical Pancreatitis."

SURGICAL RESECTION

Exocrine pancreatic function after surgical resection has rarely been studied in children, but even with 95% pancreatic resection for nesidioblastosis, few develop malabsorption. Studies of pancreatic lipase and colipase secretion in children have demonstrated that malabsorption occurs only when values fall below 2% and 1% of mean normal values, respectively[40]; thus, it is not surprising that large pancreatic resections may not induce malabsorption. The necessity for pancreatic enzyme supplementation in these patients can be determined by fat balance studies.

CELIAC DISEASE

Exocrine pancreatic dysfunction has been recognized in both children[41] and adults[42] with celiac disease. The degree of pancreatic impairment is variable, and its etiology is unclear. Some patients have primary pancreatic dysfunction, as evidenced by impaired release of pancreatic bicarbonate and enzymes into the duodenum in response to exogenous stimulation with intravenous cholecystokinin and secretin.[43] However, others have intact pancreatic function in response to exogenous stimulation but an impaired response to stimulation with liquid test meals.[44] This finding is consistent with impaired release of endogenous cholecystokinin and secretin, a concept supported by the demonstration of low serum secretin levels in response to duodenal perfusion of citric acid in untreated patients with celiac disease and normal levels after recovery of the intestinal lesion.[45] Impaired secretagogue release in untreated patients may explain the poor postprandial gallbladder emptying and diminished duodenal bile acid concentrations that, together with the impaired pancreatic enzyme release, contribute to the presence of fat maldigestion.

Carroccio and colleagues evaluated pancreatic function using fecal chymotrypsin levels at diagnosis of celiac disease.[46] They showed a lower weight increase in patients with initial low fecal chymotrypsin levels than in patients with normal chymotrypsin values. They suggested that there is a subset of patients who would benefit from pancreatic enzyme supplementation for a few months until pancreatic function returns to normal.[46] However, it is still unclear if indirect stool tests of pancreatic function can safely distinguish intestinal from pancreatic steatorrhea.

At the other extreme, profound, irreversible pancreatic insufficiency with acinar atrophy and fibrosis rarely occurs in celiac disease, but it has been reported.[47] The lesion may be related to chronic understimulation of the pancreas because of impaired endogenous secretagogue release and subsequent induction of pancreatic cell atrophy, which may be aggravated by malnutrition. In these cases, the coexistence of celiac disease and cystic fibrosis deserves consideration.[48] These patients may even have falsely pathologic sweat chloride concentrations owing to malnutrition, and personal experience suggests that mutation analysis and nasal potential difference measurements[49] may need to be performed.

REFERENCES

1. Pearson HA, Lobel JS, Kocoshis SA, et al. A new syndrome of refractory sideroblastic anemia with vacuolization of marrow precursors and exocrine pancreatic function. J Pediatr 1979;95:976–4.

2. Rotig A, Cormier V, Blanche S, et al. Pearson's marrow-pancreas syndrome. J Clin Invest 1990;86:1601–8.

3. Sano T, Ban K, Ichiki T, et al. Molecular and genetic analyses of two patients with Pearson's marrow-pancreas syndrome. Pediatr Res 1993;34:105–10.

4. Rotig A, Bourgeon T, Chretien D, et al. Spectrum of mitochondrial DNA rearrangements in the Pearson marrow-pancreas syndrome. Hum Mol Genet 1995;4:1327–30.

5. Becher MW, Wills MC, Noll WW, et al. Kearns-Sayre syndrome with features of Pearson's marrow-pancreas syndrome a novel 2905-base pair mitochondrial DNA deletion. Hum Pathol 1999;30:577–81.

6. Johanson AJ, Blizzard RM. A syndrome of congenital aplasia of the alae nasi, deafness, hypothyroidism, dwarfism, absent permanent teeth, and malabsorption. J Pediatr 1971;79:982–7.

7. Gershoni-Baruch R, Lerner A, Braun J, et al. Johanson-Blizzard syndrome: clinical spectrum and further delineation of the syndrome. Am J Med Genet 1990;35:546–51.

8. Kristjansoon K, Hoffman WH, Flannery DB, Cohen MJ. Johanson-Blizzard syndrome and hypopituitarism. J Pediatr 1988;113:851–3.

9. Nagashima K, Yagi H, Kuroume T. A case of Johanson-Blizzard syndrome complicated by diabetes mellitus. Clin Genet 1993;43:98–100.

10. Sandu BK, Brueton MJ. Concurrent pancreatic and growth hormone insufficiency in Johanson-Blizzard syndrome. J Pediatr Gastroenterol Nutr 1989;9:535–8.

11. Alpay F, Gul D, Lenk MK, Ogur G. Severe intrauterine growth retardation, aged facial appearance and congenital heart disease in a newborn with Johanson-Blizzard syndrome. Pediatr Cardiol 2000;21:389–90.

12. Auslander R, Nevo O, Diukman R, et al. Johanson-Blizzard syndrome: a prenatal ultrasonographic diagnosis. Ultrasound Obstet Gynecol 1999;13:450–2.

13. Jones NJ, Hofley PM, Durie PR. Pathophysiology of the pancreatic defect in Johanson-Blizzard syndrome: a disorder of acinar development. J Pediatr 1994;125:406–8.

14. Gould NS, Paton JB, Bennett AR. Johanson-Blizzard syndrome: clinical and pathological findings in 2 sibs. Am J Med Genet 1989;33:194–9.

15. Karjoo M, Koop CE, Cornfield D, Holtzapple PG. Pancreatic exocrine enzyme deficiency associated with asphyxiating thoracic dystrophy. Arch Dis Child 1973;48:143–6.

16. Georgiou-Theodoropoulos M, Agapitos M, Theodoropoulos P, Koutselnis A. Jeune syndrome associated with pancreatic fibrosis. Pediatr Pathol 1988;8:541–4.

17. den Hollander NS, Robben SG, Hoogeboom AJ, et al. Early prenatal sonographic diagnosis and follow-up of Jeune syndrome. Ultrasound Obstet Gynecol 2001;18:378–83.

18. Figarella C, De Caro A, Leupold D, Poley JR. Congenital pancreatic lipase deficiency. J Pediatr 1980;96:412–6.

19. Sheldon W. Congenital pancreatic lipase deficiency. Arch Dis Child 1964;39:268.

20. Lowe ME, Rosenblum JL, Strauss AW. Cloning and charactereization of human pancreatic lipase cDNA. J Biol Chem 1989;264:20042–8.

21. Davis RC, Diep A, Hunziker W, et al. Assignment of human pancreatic lipase gene (PNLIP) to chromosome 10q24-q26. Genomics 1991;11:1164–6.

22. Hildebrand H, Borgstrom B, Bekassy A, et al. Isolated colipase deficiency in two brothers. Gut 1982;23:243–6.

23. Ghishan FK, Moran JR, Durie PR, Greene HL. Isolated congenital lipase-colipase deficiency. Gastroenterology 1984;86:1580–2.

24. Ligumsky M, Granot E, Branski D, et al. Isolated lipase and colipase deficiency in two brothers. Gut 1990;31:1416–8.

25. Lowe CU, May CD. Selective pancreatic deficiency. Am J Dis Child 1951;83:459–64.

26. Brock A, Mortensen PB, Mortensen BB, Roge HR. Familial occurrence of diminished pancreatic amylase in serum—a silent Amy-2 allelic variant? Clin Chem 1988;34:1516–7.

27. Sjolund K, Haggmark A, Ihse I, et al. Selective deficiency of pancreatic amylase. Gut 1991;32:546–8.

28. Ip WF, Dupuis A, Ellis L, et al. Serum pancreatic enzymes define the pancreatic phenotype in patients with Shwachman-Diamond syndrome. J Pediatr 2002;141:259–65.

29. Townes PL, Bryson MF, Miller G. Further observations on trypsinogen deficiency disease: report of a second case. J Pediatr 1967;71:220–4.

30. Honey NK, Sakaguchi AY, Lalley PA, et al. Chromosomal assignments of the human genes for the serine proteases trypsin, chymotrypsin B, and elastase. Somat Cell Mol Genet 1984; 10:369–76.

31. Mann NS, Mann SK. Enterokinase. Proc Soc Exp Biol Med 1994;206:114–8.

32. Hadorn B, Tarlow MJ, Lloyd JK, Wolff OH. Intestinal enterokinase deficiency. Lancet 1969;i:812–3.

33. Ghishan FK, Lee PC, Lebenthal E, et al. Isolated congenital enterokinase deficiency: recent findings and review of the literature. Gastroenterology 1983;85:727–31.

34. Kitamoto Y, Veile RA, Donis-Keller H, Sadler JE. cDNA sequence and chromosomal localization of human enterokinase, the proteolytic activator of trypsinogen. Biochemistry 1995;34:4562–8.

35. Pitchumoni CS. Pancreas in primary malnutrition disorders. Am J Clin Nutr 1973;26:374–9.

36. Veghelyi PV, Kemeny TT, Sos J. Dietary lesions of the pancreas. Am J Dis Child 1950;79:658–65.

37. Barbezat GO, Hansen JDL. The exocrine pancreas and protein-calorie malnutrition. Pediatrics 1968;42:77–92.

38. Durie PR, et al. Elevated serum immunoreactive pancreatic cationic trypsinogen in acute malnutrition: evidence of pancreatic damage. J Pediatr 1985;106:233–8.

39. Fedail SS, Karar ZA, Harvey RF, Read AE. Serum trypsin as measure of pancreatic function in children with protein-calorie malnutrition. Lancet 1980;ii:374.

40. Gaskin KJ, Durie PR, Lee L, et al. Colipase and lipase secretion in childhood onset pancreatic insufficiency: delineation of patients. Gastroenterology 1984;86:1–7.

41. Walker-Smith J. Celiac disease. In: Walker-Smith J, Murch SH, editors. Diseases of the small intestine in childhood. 4th ed. Oxford (UK): Isis Medical Media; 1998. p. 253–4.

42. Delco F, El-Serag HB, Sonnenberg A. Celiac sprue among US military veterans: associated disorders and clinical manifestations. Dig Dis Sci 1999;44:966–72.

43. Fernandez LB, De Paula A, Prizont R, et al. Exocrine pancreatic insufficiency secondary to gluten enteropathy. Am J Gastroenterol 1970;53:564–9.

44. Regan PT, Di Magno EP. Exocrine pancreatic function in celiac sprue: a cause of treatment failure. Gastroenterology 1980;78:684–7.

45. Besterman HS, Bloom SR, Sarson DW, et al. Gut hormone profile in celiac disease. Lancet 1978;i:785–8.

46. Carroccio A, Iacono G, Lerro P, et al. Role of pancreatic impairment in growth recovery during gluten-free diet in childhood celiac disease. Gastroenterology 1997;112: 1839–44.

47. Weizman Z, Hamilton JR, Kopelman HR, et al. Treatment failure in celiac disease due to coexistent exocrine pancreatic insufficiency. Pediatrics 1987;80:924–6.

48. Valletta EA, Mastella G. Incidence of celiac disease in a cystic fibrosis population. Acta Paediatr Scand 1989;78:784–5.

49. Wilschanski M, Famini H, Strauss-Liviatan N, et al. The use of nasal potential difference measurements as a diagnostic test for questionable cystic fibrosis. Eur Respir J 2001;17: 1209–15.

CHAPTER 66

STUDY DESIGN

1. *Outcomes Research on Diagnostic and Therapeutic Procedures*

Jenifer R. Lightdale, MD, MPH
Donald Goldmann, MD

Outcomes research is the systematic study of clinical practice with a focus on clinical effectiveness and patient-centered outcomes.[1] It is designed to measure the consequences of providing medical care to determine whether and to what extent such care is beneficial. As broadly defined by the American Gastroenterological Association, outcomes research encompasses studies of (1) clinical and physiologic effects of a given medical product, procedure, or technology; (2) patient-centered end points, such as health-related quality of life (HRQOL), functional status, and patient satisfaction; and (3) medical costs relative to benefits and risks.[2] The purpose of this chapter is to provide an overview of outcomes research, highlighted by examples and pertinent studies in pediatric gastroenterology.

In recent years, outcomes research has received tremendous attention not only within the clinical research world but also from legislators and the general public. In the wake of considerable momentum over the past decade toward advancing the quality of health care, the Institute of Medicine (IOM) released its comprehensive *Crossing the Quality Chasm: A New Health System for the 21st Century* report in 2001.[3] This report highlights the importance of studying health care processes to improve medical outcomes. The IOM defines quality as "the degree to which health services for individuals and populations increase the likelihood of desired health outcomes and are consistent with current professional knowledge."[4] Outcomes research provides an important tool for amassing evidence that quality health care is being provided.

Donabedian, an early proponent of using research to advance the quality of medical care, has described a triad of (1) structure, or the characteristics of a health care setting; (2) process, or what is done to patients; and (3) outcomes, or how patients do after health care is provided.[5] His emphasis on understanding and enhancing the process of providing health care to improve outcomes can be somewhat simplistically conceptualized as "doing the right thing right."[1] Donabedian's emphasis was originally on the efficacy, effectiveness, and efficiency of health care.[6] In the past few years, this model has been expanded to incorporate safety, equity, and patient-centeredness as equally essential attributes of quality health care (Table 66.1-1).[3]

This chapter discusses these attributes of quality in the context of an introduction to outcomes research and its methodologies. Specific examples from the pediatric gastroenterology literature are used to highlight aspects of study design and their application to clinical practice. Pediatric gastroenterologists are introduced to the challenges involved in systematically evaluating their own practices with an eye to quality. Like all physicians, pediatric gastroenterologists must understand and use outcomes research to close existing gaps in the quality of care that they provide.

TABLE 66.1-1 DEFINITION OF TERMS USED IN THE EVALUATION OF MEDICAL CARE QUALITY

Efficacy	*Can* it work? (eg, in controlled trials)
Effectiveness	*Does* it work? (eg, in the real world)
Efficiency	Is it *worth* doing?
Safety	Does it *reduce risk* to patients?
Equity	Is it *nonvarying* in quality?
Patient centered	Is it *respectful* of individual patient preferences?

The first section of this chapter briefly reviews the concepts of efficacy and effectiveness, an understanding of which underlies the whole of outcomes research. In the following sections, studies of clinical outcomes, patient-centered outcomes, and health care costs are discussed. Our goal is to provide an introduction to methodology as it relates to outcomes research.

EFFICACY AND EFFECTIVENESS

Quality health care is best ensured by continual formal evaluation of the relationships between processes of providing medical care and the outcomes of those processes. Although many types of clinical research contribute to the evaluation of medical care, it is important to realize that not all clinical studies are outcomes studies. The point of distinction lies mainly in understanding the terms "efficacy" and "effectiveness."[7]

In general, efficacy studies are designed to determine if a given medical intervention can work under tightly controlled conditions. In contrast, effectiveness studies are designed to mirror daily practice and to determine if an intervention is successful in routine clinical practice. To the extent that they measure health outcomes in real-world settings, effectiveness studies are the crux of outcomes research.

Outcomes research focuses on the impact of a given medical practice on health in the real world. The data generated by outcomes research reflect changes in practice and in the natural history of the disease over time. In addition, outcomes study methodology recognizes that unpredictable and uncontrollable changes in patients' lives are important and legitimate factors in determining the ultimate effectiveness of medical care. Effectiveness studies are often less restrictive about inclusion and exclusion criteria than studies of efficacy.

Effectiveness studies, the mainstay of outcomes research, also integrate variations in clinical practice among various practitioners and in different health care settings. These characteristics of effectiveness studies are readily apparent when comparing, for example, the practices of university- or research-based health care groups with those of community-based physicians. Many outcomes studies recognize that there are physician-dependent variables in assessing the effectiveness of medical interventions.

CLINICAL OUTCOMES

In this section, we consider outcomes research that measures physiologic and clinical effects. We discuss some of the strengths and weaknesses of both experimental and observational study designs as they relate to the use of these designs in outcomes research. We also touch on the use of large administrative databases and meta-analysis as increasingly popular methodologies (Table 66.1-2).

EXPERIMENTAL STUDY DESIGN

Experimental studies are most commonly designed as clinical trials. Clinical trials aim to isolate one factor, generally an intervention, and examine its contribution to patient health by holding all other factors as constant as possible. The gold standard for experimental clinical study design is the randomized controlled trial (RCT). An RCT is a comparative study between an intervention group and a control group. The groups are as similar as possible, except the intervention group is exposed to a health care service (eg, medication, therapy) and the control group is not. Any differences in outcomes between the two groups can then be attributed to the intervention.

Participants in RCTs are randomly assigned to either the intervention or the control group. When performed correctly, the process of randomization removes the potential for bias in the allocation of participants to either group. Randomization also optimizes the chance that the two groups will be evenly matched, on average, in their known baseline characteristics (eg, age, sex, disease status), as well as any unknown factors.

Despite their many strengths, RCTs may have a limited role in clinical outcomes research. For example, if an outcome of interest is rare, an RCT may require an enormous study population to detect any differences between intervention and control groups. If the outcome takes many years to emerge, an RCT may not be feasible. It also may not be possible to randomize certain variables, such as patient preference or physician beliefs. Other limitations of applying findings from RCTs in clinical outcomes research include the fact that RCTs are usually designed to answer specific clinical questions in well-defined patient populations and may use strict exclusion criteria to create a homogeneous study sample. These characteristics of RCTs can limit their generalizability to real-world clinical practice.

However, RCTs can be designed to provide information that is relevant to clinical practice and therefore can play a role in outcomes research. One example of a well-designed prospective, double-blind, placebo-controlled RCT in the pediatric endoscopy literature evaluated the use of oral midazolam as a premedication to conscious sedation for pediatric endoscopy.[8] Although almost all pediatric gastrointestinal procedures are performed with some type of sedation, there is a lack of consensus about the use of premedications to decrease anxiety, which many children experience before the procedure.[9] In this study, Liacouras and colleagues were specifically interested in whether the use of oral midazolam prior to intravenous (IV) line placement led to less apprehension in children before, during, and after an endoscopic procedure.[8] Investigators obtained informed consent for 123 children to be randomized to receive either oral midazolam or placebo approximately 20 minutes before IV placement for endoscopy.

TABLE 66.1-2   TYPES OF OUTCOMES RESEARCH AND RELEVANT STUDY DESIGNS

EXPERIMENTAL STUDIES
Randomized controlled trials
OBSERVATIONAL STUDIES
Cohort
Case control
Cross-sectional
Case series
LARGE ADMINISTRATIVE DATABASE ANALYSIS
META-ANALYSIS

This RCT is a good example of an effectiveness trial that carefully investigated a study question while allowing real-world health care systems to function routinely. Once the oral medication (midazolam or placebo) was given, IV procedural sedation for endoscopy was administered in a routine manner. Importantly, the doses of procedural sedation were not dictated by the study design, and endoscopists were encouraged to use routine means to evaluate patients' levels of sedation. The results of this RCT strongly supported not only the safety but also the effectiveness of oral midazolam premedication for pediatric endoscopy. Such studies have the potential to change clinical practice and therefore can be considered outcomes research.

OBSERVATIONAL STUDY DESIGN

Observational studies often represent the best method for studying rare or remote conditions. In general, observational studies are easier and less expensive to perform in comparison with experimental studies. Observational studies may especially be useful when randomization schemes cannot be feasibly employed. They are also essential tools in outcomes research because they generally measure effectiveness rather than efficacy.

Nevertheless, there are many important disadvantages to observational studies that must be weighed in both critically reviewing the literature or when choosing a study design. In particular, because patients are not randomized, there is an unavoidable risk of both bias and confounding. Bias may be defined as any factor in a study that tends to produce results or conclusions that differ systematically from the truth. This includes errors in analytic methodology and errors of interpretation.[10] A confounder is a third factor in a study that may be associated with both the exposure and the outcome and may, in fact, be responsible for any observed associations between the two.[11]

In the following section, we describe four principal research designs of observational studies: cohort, case control, cross-sectional, and case series.

Cohort Studies. Cohort studies are observational studies that focus on factors related to the development of a disease of interest. They are especially useful for studying the incidence and natural history of disease. In a cohort study, a group of people (the cohort) who do not have the condition of interest at the time of enrolment is selected and observed over time. Suspected risk factors for the outcome are evaluated in all members of the cohort at enrolment and throughout the observational period.

By following all of the members of the cohort for development of the outcome, the relationship between risk factors and outcomes can be assessed. Cohort studies can also measure absolute risks of developing a new disease because rates of exposures and outcomes have been collected. Generally speaking, cohort studies are prospective in nature, meaning that a cohort is followed forward from a set point in time. However, cohort studies can also be retrospective and assemble subjects according to their history of exposure without consideration of outcomes, even though the outcomes may already have taken place.

Cohort studies have many significant advantages over other study designs for outcomes research. First, when a clinical trial cannot be conducted for either ethical or practical reasons, a cohort study may provide the best alternative method to study the question of interest. A cohort study may be useful for studying more than one risk factor and more than one outcome using the same study population. Cohort studies may simultaneously give descriptive information about several diseases or even help to tease out which risk factors are directly linked to which disease. Cohort studies are particularly relevant to outcomes research because they do not occur in tightly controlled research settings.

Cohort studies have some important disadvantages. Members of the cohort may need to be followed for a lengthy period of time before a sufficient number develop the outcome of interest. Furthermore, study resources may be spent following many people in the cohort who will not develop the outcomes of interest or may be lost to follow-up. Another limitation to cohort studies is that they may represent an impractical study design for investigating risk factors for rare diseases. This issue may especially be salient for pediatric gastroenterologists. For example, to study a disease with a known incidence of 1 in 10,000 children, 100,000 children will need to be followed to capture 10 cases of the disease. On the other hand, this issue can be minimized if a cohort is selected that is known to be at high risk of developing the disease.

Recently, several pediatric gastroenterology–oriented cohort studies have been designed that will ultimately improve our understanding of obesity in children.[12,13] For example, the ongoing Growing Up Today Study (GUTS) was established in 1996 to longitudinally follow the activity, dietary intake, and weight changes of children across all 50 United States.[12] GUTS participants were recruited from the offspring of participants from another cohort study, the Nurses Health Study II.

Another example of a recent cohort study in the pediatric endoscopy literature explored the relationship between clinical presentation and primary peptic ulcer disease in children.[14] Primary peptic ulcers are traditionally considered to be unusual in childhood.[15] It is well accepted that the rarity of this diagnosis has limited the ability of investigators to identify risk factors for childhood ulcer disease and to know when to perform endoscopy for diagnosis.[16] To investigate these questions, Roma and colleagues undertook a cohort study from 1990 to 1999, during which time they followed 2,550 children who had dyspeptic symptoms, including epigastric pain, periumbilical pain, bleeding, vomiting, and nocturnal waking.[14] All children then underwent upper gastrointestinal endoscopy with biopsies. Primary peptic ulcers were diagnosed in 2% (52 of 2,550) of the cohort and appropriately treated. Of the 52 patients with peptic ulcer on initial endoscopy, 25 (48%) became symptomatic after treatment and were re-endoscoped. Only 3 (0.12%) of these children were found to have a second ulcer.

In their primary analysis, the investigators found no significant differences between the clinical symptoms of those children with ulcers and those without. Therefore,

Roma and colleagues suggest that all children with dyspeptic symptoms be referred for upper gastrointestinal endoscopy to evaluate for ulcer disease.

This study highlights the types of information available from a cohort design. The results provide an estimate of overall disease prevalence in the population of interest. The clinical follow-up of patients with ulcers at the start of the study allows for an assessment of the effectiveness of treatment. Roma and colleagues' study represents an example of the importance of cohort studies to understanding pediatric gastrointestinal disease and disease management.

Case-Control Studies. A second observational study design method is that of case-control studies. Whereas cohort studies examine people who are initially free of the disease of interest, case-control studies compare people who already have the disease (the cases) with otherwise similar people who do not have the disease (the controls). Case-control studies start by evaluating the outcome (the presence or absence of the disease) and then look back into patients' histories to identify possible risk factors. Both cases and controls must be selected independently of exposure to the risk factors of interest. In this retrospective manner, case-control studies can be used to analyze whether identified risk factors were present more frequently in cases than in controls.

The advantages of performing case-controlled studies include the fact that they can be performed relatively quickly and inexpensively, even for diseases that are rare or that take lengthy periods of time to appear. To epidemiologists, case-control studies represent the basis of outbreak investigations, such as those conducted to determine the etiology of foodborne outbreaks of gastroenteritis. In addition, if the outcome is rare overall, case-control studies may require fewer subjects than cohort studies. They also simultaneously allow multiple risk factors to be investigated within the same study of a particular outcome. Because of these attractive features, case-control studies are often used as hypothesis-generating mechanisms for investigators exploring possible risk factors for rare diseases.

However, case-control studies do have a number of disadvantages, including that they are particularly subject to bias (eg, recall bias). Case-control studies must rely on studying cases that have already been identified. Misdiagnosed or asymptomatic cases or people who have already died either from the disease or other causes are missed by this type of study.

Case-control studies also depend on the identification of an appropriate control group. Controls should be selected from a population of individuals who would have been identified and included as cases had they also developed the disease. Selecting a control group that is comparable to a group of cases can be a surprisingly difficult task for investigators.

Recently, Lazzaroni and colleagues performed a carefully designed case-control study of primary upper gastrointestinal bleeding in infants.[17] Although significant upper gastrointestinal bleeding in otherwise healthy full-term infants has been described in case reports, the available data on the topic are limited owing to the rare occurrence of this disease.[18,19] There were three main aims to this study.[17] The first was to identify types of mucosal lesions in newborn babies with upper gastrointestinal bleeding. The second aim was to examine the safety and necessity of performing upper endoscopy in newborns with gastrointestinal bleeding, and the third was to identify risk factors associated with such bleeding.

Sixty-four of 5,180 infants (1.23%) born at the study center in Italy developed significant upper gastrointestinal bleeding within a mean of 26.5 hours of life. In 53 of 64 cases, an endoscopy was performed. Extensive demographic, prenatal, neonatal, clinical, and hematologic data were collected and analyzed for all cases and their mothers. The same data were collected for a group of 53 controls and their mothers, who were matched for age and sex to the 53 cases who underwent endoscopy. The controls were selected randomly from a population of full-term infants born in the same hospital.

All patients who underwent endoscopy were found to have mucosal lesions of either the esophagus, stomach, or duodenum. A comparison of the 53 patients who underwent endoscopy with the 53 controls revealed no significant differences in demographic or clinical characteristics, except that upper gastrointestinal bleeding was significantly more frequent in those infants whose mothers came from countries outside Europe. Therefore, the investigators concluded that the risk factors for upper gastrointestinal hemorrhages in infants remain obscure.

However, it is important to realize that this study was limited, albeit for ethical reasons, by the lack of endoscopy surveillance of the control group. A second limitation of this study lies in the selection of its control group. The study findings might have been strengthened or even different if a control group had been chosen that was matched by age and sex to all 64 cases of acute gastrointestinal bleeding—not just to those 53 patients who underwent endoscopy. Although case-control studies are important tools for outcomes research, the application of their conclusions for clinical practice may still be affected by limitations in study design.

Cross-Sectional Studies. Cross-sectional studies are based on a single examination of an entire population at a particular point in time. By surveying a whole population, cross-sectional studies assess the proportion of people with a certain disease (eg, the prevalence of the disease) and can be used to examine the relationship between the disease and other characteristics of the population under study. Cross-sectional studies are common in the medical literature and can produce valuable data about a wide range of diseases and types of risk factors. They are important for generating hypotheses for experimental designs.

However, as a descriptive research methodology, cross-sectional studies have several important limitations. In particular, because cross-sectional studies identify existing cases (prevalent cases) of a disease and do not capture the occurrence of new cases (incident cases), they are likely to overrepresent chronic diseases and underrepresent acute diseases. Also, people with certain diseases may either leave the community or be located in a place where they are not surveyed.

Cross-sectional studies may also be limited by so-called "lead time bias," whereby patients are misclassified by exposures. For example, children with symptoms of peptic disease may choose to stop drinking caffeinated beverages because of their symptoms before inclusion in the study. They would therefore be counted as nonexposed. Finally, the findings of cross-sectional studies must be interpreted cautiously; the mere fact that two variables are associated does not mean that they are causally related.

An example of a recent cross-sectional study in the pediatric endoscopic literature is an investigation into the prevalence of *Helicobacter pylori* in a population of children with chronic abdominal pain, with and without the gross endoscopic finding of nodular gastritis.[20] Endoscopic findings of nodularity are reported frequently in children[21] and have been loosely associated in the past with either acute or chronic *H. pylori* infection.[22] Nevertheless, the relationship of endoscopic nodular gastritis with *H. pylori* infection in children remains ill-defined. The investigators of this study used a cross-sectional design to examine the associations between endoscopic findings and microscopic *H. pylori* infection among children with chronic abdominal pain.[20]

Bahu and colleagues prospectively included 185 children aged 1 to 12 years who presented to two pediatric gastroenterology clinics in Brazil from 1997 to 1999 with chronic abdominal pain. To improve their diagnostic yield, the investigators chose a study population at high risk for *H. pylori*.[20]

The prevalence of endoscopic nodularity in this population was 13% (95% CI 8.5–18.7), and *H. pylori* infection was identified in 27% (95% CI 20.8–34.0) of the study population. Endoscopic nodularity was found in 44% of patients with *H. pylori* infection and in 1.5% who were *H. pylori* negative. In their discussion, the authors state that their results support a significant association between endoscopic nodular gastritis and *H. pylori* infection.[20]

However, as with all cross-sectional studies, an observed association does not prove causality. In fact, because the putative exposure (*H. pylori*) and outcome (nodularity) were assessed simultaneously, it is equally possible that the nodularity in some way predisposed the patient to infection with *H. pylori*. Additionally, it may be difficult to identify confounders in cross-sectional studies. For example, in this case, both *H. pylori* and nodularity were rare in the youngest children; therefore, age may be a confounder, and there may be no true association between *H. pylori* and nodularity.

Another issue with this particular study is that it was conducted in a high-risk study population. Therefore, the generalizability of its prevalence findings to other populations for both endoscopic nodular gastritis and *H. pylori* may be limited. Finally, there was no follow-up of the patient population, as is characteristic of a cross-sectional design. Therefore, it remains a possibility that *H. pylori*–positive children with normal mucosa will go on to develop nodularity.

Case Series. Case series are generally considered the weakest study designs in the so-called "hierarchy of evi-

dence."[23] Nonetheless, they may represent an excellent means of generating hypotheses for more robust studies to examine. A case series simply describes the presentation, and often the clinical management, of a disease in more than one patient. Patients in case series studies are generally not followed prospectively, and they are not compared with a control group. Therefore, case series are not useful for establishing a causal relationship between risk factors and disease or the clinical effectiveness of a management approach.

Case series may also be prone to selective reporting (reporting bias). Owing to small numbers and the anecdotal nature of such a report, the validity of case series findings may be difficult to establish. Similarly, a case report, as a form of case series in which only one patient is described, may suggest an association or a clinical course that is not necessarily generalizable beyond the individual case.

Nevertheless, case series and case reports are both numerous and important to medical literature. They are both used regularly to present information about patients with rare diseases and may be important for stimulating new hypotheses. In addition, a case series that describes an abnormal outcome after routine care has been administered may represent, in and of itself, a reasonable basis for re-examining that care. For example, case reports of sudden death in otherwise healthy infants receiving cisapride as a promotility agent represented sufficient basis for more outcomes studies on the use of cisapride in children with gastroesophageal reflux.[24,25]

In one recent case report, Stiffler described an 11-year-old girl with a 5-year history of persistent obscure gastrointestinal bleeding who underwent capsule endoscopy.[26] The patient described in the case report had undergone several upper gastrointestinal endoscopies, a colonoscopy, push enteroscopy, and enteroclysis prior to undergoing the capsule endoscopy—with all examinations being negative for pathology. The capsule procedure identified a small bowel narrowing with significant erosive and ulcerative changes consistent with Crohn disease.

In the discussion following the case report, Stiffler speculates that capsule endoscopy may prove to be a useful diagnostic modality in pediatric patients with gastrointestinal disease. Stiffler also explains that both pediatric gastroenterologists and their patients may prefer undergoing capsule endoscopy, which does not require sedation.

Indeed, the tactical issue of how to achieve sedation that is both safe and effective for endoscopy and colonoscopy as high-volume pediatric procedures remains a challenge for pediatric gastroenterologists. Although several studies have indicated that general anesthesia allows a safer environment for the performance of more successful traditional endoscopic procedures in children compared with conscious sedation,[27,28] others have postulated that conscious sedation can be just as safe.[29] To date, there have been no outcomes studies that have contributed to resolving this debate.[9] Instead, because most studies in the literature are based on case series at single institutions, it is difficult to compare sedation practices across investigative sites.

The decision to use one regimen over the other is generally left to the clinical judgment of individual physicians, to be made on a case-by-case basis.[9] The lack of an evidence-based approach to the question of sedation for pediatric endoscopy leaves open the real possibility that individual pediatric endoscopists may make inappropriate sedation choices for their patients.

The study of patient safety is an important subset of outcomes research. Patient safety, or the concept that patients should not experience harm from health care that is intended to help them, represents one of the major steps identified by the IOM for improving the quality of health care overall.[3] The question of sedation choice and patient safety for children undergoing endoscopic procedures is a salient example of a quality gap in health care services that will best be addressed by well-designed outcomes studies in the future.

LARGE DATABASE REVIEW STUDIES

Outcomes research may employ large administrative databases maintained by health care providers, payers, or government agencies.[30,31] There are many advantages to such databases, which are often (but not always) considered both valid and reliable. First, they are usually electronically maintained and are therefore often computer ready for analysis and inexpensive to acquire. Many databases come packaged together with computer programs for data analysis. Such databases are also often rich in demographic characteristics, as well as diagnoses of patients. Administrative databases often reflect the health care of large populations, and findings may be generalized.

However, there are also drawbacks to using large administrative databases. For instance, they can be limited in the quality and type of clinical information available. Also, because most were developed for billing or administrative purposes, they are often lacking pertinent medical information. Moreover, large institutional databases may include incorrect or incomplete datasets, especially in regard to medical and patient care information. Inconsistencies in diagnostic coding may also limit the usefulness of these databases. As an example, variation in diagnostic codes for abdominal pain in children may make it difficult to characterize the care of or evaluate the outcomes of children with this clinical problem.

Nevertheless, nationally maintained databases are becoming important tools for outcomes researchers in pediatric gastroenterology. For example, the Kids' Inpatient Database (KID) is one of several databases developed and maintained as part of the Healthcare Cost and Utilization Project, which is a federal, state, and industry partnership sponsored by the National Institutes of Health's Agency for Healthcare Research and Quality.[32] The KID pertains to children's health issues and is the only hospital administrative dataset designed specifically to assess use of hospital services by newborns, children, and adolescents.[33] It represents the only large inpatient care database for children in the United States and contains data from approximately 1.9 million hospital discharges for children across 27 states.

Importantly, the KID includes data on all patients, regardless of payer, including children covered by private insurance or Medicaid and the uninsured. This feature of the KID highlights its ability to assess the equity of care provided to chil-

dren because it includes patients who may vary greatly in personal characteristics, such as gender, ethnicity, geographic location, and socioeconomic status. According to the IOM, ensuring equitable care, or quality care that does not vary along these personal characteristic lines, is a main goal for redesigning the twenty-first century health care system.[3]

Guthery and colleagues were able to perform a population-based outcomes study using the KID to identify the principal gastrointestinal diagnoses associated with hospital use and to describe hospital use patterns associated with pediatric gastrointestinal disorders.[34] In a descriptive analysis using the KID and its associated software program, *Clinical Classification Software*,[33] Guthery and colleagues found that gastrointestinal disorders in children are a significant source of hospital resource consumption, accounting for $2.6 billion in hospital charges annually in the United States and over 1.1 million hospital days. The investigators also found that among children with principal gastrointestinal discharge diagnoses, 67.7% of discharges were from non–children's hospitals, 13.1% were from pediatric facilities, and 19.2% were from pediatric units of a general hospital. In addition, 56.7% of pediatric gastrointestinal disease discharges were from nonteaching hospitals, whereas 43.3% were from academic centers.

Guthery and colleagues concluded that care for children with gastrointestinal diseases is provided at a variety of different types of institutions, which may represent a significant source of variation in care. Further outcomes research may help to explore how this variation in care portends gaps in quality of care for children with gastrointestinal disease across the United States.

META-ANALYSIS

Meta-analysis has become an especially popular tool for outcomes research and, as a methodology, has been featured prominently in journals dedicated to the field of gastroenterology.[35–38] Meta-analysis employs specific statistical methodologies to retrospectively review and integrate available quantitative data across multiple studies. It is an especially useful method for assimilating data from multiple small studies that have found conflicting answers or statistically insignificant results for the same research question. In meta-analysis, the data of multiple independent studies on the same topic are compiled and analyzed across reports to increase overall statistical power. In essence, a meta-analysis allows the synthesis of the results of numerous tests so that an overall conclusion can be drawn.

There are some fundamental assumptions related to meta-analysis. First, it is important that all studies combined in the analysis have the same research question. Second, the separate studies included in the analysis should be independent of each other. Third, the studies should be of sufficient quality. If any of these assumptions can be challenged, then the use of meta-analysis is not appropriate.

However, there are a few important caveats to interpreting meta-analyses. In particular, there is a tendency in the medical literature to publish positive findings, which, in turn, introduces a bias into the data selection process for meta-analysis. An appropriately conducted meta-analysis will also incorporate data published only in abstract form and unpublished data collected through communication with investigators.

Additionally, to test for the possibility of publication bias, a meta-analytic study design often will include a sensitivity analysis. For instance, investigators may choose to create a type of scatter plot (a so-called "funnel plot") that allows the sample size of each study to be plotted according to its estimated effect size. In a typical funnel plot, the vertical and horizontal axes represent sample size and estimated effect size, respectively. A vertical line can then be drawn on the graph defining the pooled estimate effect size, and the points from each study included in the meta-analysis will scatter around this line. If there is no publication bias, the results from small studies plotted at the bottom of the graph should have considerable variation, whereas large studies, at the top of the graph, should show less variation in their results. Thus, the graph should look like an inverted funnel. If there is publication bias against small, nonsignificant studies or if the investigator has not included all possible studies, the graph will either not assume a funnel shape (eg, be skewed or asymmetric) or will contain gaps (Figure 66.1-1).

Another possible bias to meta-analysis is that many published studies do not contain sufficient detail that allows investigators to compare the results from one study with those of another. In fact, the main drawback of meta-analysis lies in the inequality of the study designs and end points that it measures. Strict criteria for performing meta-analysis, as well as the application and utility of this outcomes study design, are the subject of many reviews.[39–41]

In one example of meta-analysis in the pediatric gastroenterology literature, Huang and colleagues recently sought to determine whether probiotic therapy improves outcomes in children with acute infectious diarrhea.[42] Although probiotics are considered a promising adjunctive therapy for children with acute diarrhea, studies on the subject have suffered from limited study power and conflicting results.[43]

In compiling data for meta-analysis, Huang and colleagues strictly focused on clinical trials of probiotic therapy in otherwise healthy children less than 5 years old with acute-onset diarrhea in the outpatient setting.[42] The selection criteria for the meta-analysis set a priori were that each trial included must have randomized its patients into intervention and control groups. Also, each trial must have performed a direct comparison between groups and reported duration of diarrhea as an outcome variable. Of a total of 29 studies on probiotic use for diarrhea that were identified and categorized by treatment setting, population characteristics, and patient comorbidities, the investigators identified 18 that met inclusion criteria for their meta-analysis. Nine were excluded either because they lacked a control group or did not report the duration of the diarrhea. An additional two studies were excluded because they used data also published in two of the included trials.

There were two other meta-analyses published in the same year as Huang and colleagues' study that also questioned the usefulness of probiotics in the setting of pedi-

atric diarrhea. Szajewska and Mrukowicz focused on trials in children who were hospitalized and did not include abstracts or unpublished data.[44] Van Niel and colleagues used meta-analysis to look at only randomized double-blind placebo-controlled trials of probiotics in children.[45] All three meta-analyses of probiotics in children defined their outcome as the duration of the diarrhea.

As part of classic meta-analytic methodology, Huang and colleagues provided a summary table of the studies included in their analysis and concluded that probiotic therapy shortened the duration of acute diarrheal illness in children by approximately 1 day.[42] This finding was similar to both Szajewska and Mrukowicz's and Van Niel and colleagues' analyses, which detected shortened duration by 0.6 and 1.2 days, respectively.[44,45] These are three examples of well-designed, rigorously conducted outcomes studies. In their individual discussions, all three investigators appropriately questioned the real-world clinical meaning of their findings. Although probiotics may be efficacious at reducing the duration of diarrheal illness, the clinical effectiveness of this strategy that reduces symptoms by a day or less may not be convincing enough to change clinical mangement.

PATIENT-CENTERED STUDIES

In recent years, the concept that patients' perceptions of their health and satisfaction with their health are important measurable variables has emerged as a fundamental maxim. Furthermore, the more careful allotment of health care dol-

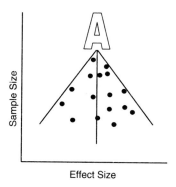

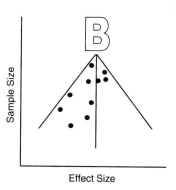

FIGURE 66.1-1   Schematic of two funnel plots for meta-analysis. Plot A shows no association between study size and effect size. Plot B depicts an asymmetric relationship, suggesting a publication bias.

lars has led to increasing demands on physicians to make informed health care decisions that truly benefit patients. In response, outcomes research has begun to focus primarily on the "patient experience"[46] of health care by extending the scope of studies beyond the end points of morbidity and mortality to include quantitative and qualitative measures of patients' perceptions of health and well-being.

Quantitative patient-centered measures may include validated instruments that are often importable across institutions and settings. Qualitative measures often rely on content analysis of open-ended patient-survey questions. The use of either type of measure in patient-centered studies may allow the evaluation of the effects of medical intervention on patients' functional status, their satisfaction, and their HRQOL.

FUNCTIONAL STATUS

Functional status is defined as a measure of the impact of health or disease condition on the ability of patients to function in various roles in society.[47] As with all patient-centered measures, it is important to recognize that the functional status of children is inherently different from that of adults. Although both may take into account the impact of health on a patient's ability to perform age-appropriate activities of daily living, as well as their moods and abilities to communicate, adult functional status may measure professional productivity, whereas pediatric functional status may be more concerned with play or school attendance.

At any age, functional status, as a measure, can be used to describe a patient at a single point in time or cumulatively over time. The latter use of functional status as a cumulative measure may allow for prediction studies of patients' likely future health gains from given treatments. A number of different pediatric instruments have been validated as measures of functional status in children with many chronic illnesses (eg, Functional Disability Inventory[48] and Functional Status II–Revised[49]). However, these instruments may not be generalizable to all patient populations.

PATIENT SATISFACTION

Patient satisfaction can be measured in terms of patients' satisfaction with health care or with their state of health or disease condition. Although the assessment of patient satisfaction has been emphasized strongly in outcomes research, it may be a difficult measure to interpret. Indeed, the IOM does not consider patient satisfaction a useful type of outcome to measure when evaluating quality of care.[3] According to the IOM, too often "it is difficult to determine what is an acceptable level of satisfaction...[because there] is generally no standard to which to compare the results."[3] Reports of actual experiences with care may provide more clinically relevant information than satisfaction ratings. For example, it may be more appropriate to ask patients whether they were informed about the specific side effects of medications on discharge than to ask whether they were satisfied with nursing care.

When evaluating patient satisfaction in children, there is generally the added complexity of using parents' reports in lieu of their children's.[50] Nevertheless, parental satisfaction continues to be considered a relevant outcome of pediatric care. As such, several instruments have recently been developed for evaluating parents' satisfaction regarding their child's care.[51]

HEALTH-RELATED QUALITY OF LIFE

HRQOL is a comprehensive term that refers to the general physical and mental health status of individuals, including their psychosocial well-being, as it is affected by illness or injury and health care interventions or policies.[52] By most definitions, HRQOL is different from functional status in that it measures psychological well-being, whereas functional status is more concerned with physical ability. However, many investigators may choose to measure functional status as a component of HRQOL.[53] In either case, the term HRQOL invokes "the capacity of an individual to perform social and domestic roles so as to meet the challenges of everyday living without emotional distress of physical disability."[54]

Although, currently, there is no gold standard for measuring HRQOL, a general consensus has emerged as to what should be measured.[50] To this end, a general framework is portrayed of a classic core set of disease-related domains that should be measured in any global assessment of HRQOL (Figure 66.1-2). For the purposes of this chapter, we assume that there are at least five domains that comprise the framework for HRQOL: (1) the state of disease, (2) associated physical symptoms, (3) functional status, (4) psychological functioning, and (5) social functioning.

Each domain of HRQOL is independently measurable and can be affected by both the disease and medical intervention. However, the complex interactions between domains must also be appreciated. Also, these domains are not mutually exclusive, and individual patients may react to their diagnosis, symptoms, and treatment in frequently unpredictable ways.

There are many obstacles to measuring pediatric HRQOL, and this area of study has been slower to develop in children, in contrast to the rapid expansion of HRQOL

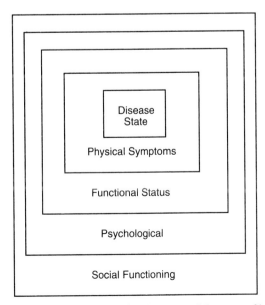

FIGURE 66.1-2 Framework for the essential domains of health-related quality of life.

research in adults.[55] Owing to inherent differences between pediatric and adult patients, most HRQOL instruments used in adult medicine are not readily applicable for use in children.[56] For example, many components of adult functional and social well-being that are measured in adult HRQOL instruments, such as economic status, job performance, and sexual satisfaction, are clearly focused on adult behaviors. Therefore, pediatric instruments, such as the Child Health Questionnaire and the Child Health and Illness Profile, have been developed to capture age-specific and -sensitive issues.[56]

Furthermore, compared with adult questionnaires, greater time and creativity are required to develop nonwritten, nonstandard means to assess HRQOL in infants and young children. Another concern that must be addressed is the incorporation and balancing of parental perceptions, which may not necessarily reflect those of their children and cannot substitute for the perspective of the child.

To date, a limited number of both general and disease-specific instruments to assess HRQOL have been developed for children.[57] Although general instruments allow physicians to assess and contrast various domains across a multiple number of disease states, they often lack the specificity required to understand the impact of a particular disease state. In contrast, disease-specific instruments are highly sensitive for a particular disease but, by definition, cannot be used to compare different disease states. Depending on research aims and feasibility, HRQOL outcomes studies in children that include a battery of both general and disease-specific instruments that measure all or some of the domains of HRQOL may be best.[58]

PATIENT-CENTERED STUDIES

In pediatric gastroenterology, there have been few patient-centered studies regarding interventional practices and procedures. Fortunately, there has been increasing interest in performing such research, and in recent years, there has been a substantial increase in the number of publications in this area.[59–61] In return, we are gaining greater understanding of the broader scope of the experiences that pediatric patients undergo related to their care. Pediatric liver transplant represents a particularly important example of an area of interest in which children with chronic gastrointestinal diseases are increasingly the focus of patient-centered research.

Liver transplant is now widely accepted as the definitive therapeutic procedure for end-stage liver disease in children.[62] Improvements in immunosuppression, surgical techniques, and postoperative management have all contributed to greater than 90% 5-year survival rates at most transplant centers, and morbidity and mortality rates are no longer sufficient indications of success.[63] Instead, increasing efforts are being made to evaluate the broader impact of this procedure on children by focusing on patient-centered measures, including physical and psychosocial functioning, growth and development, and a general perceived sense of well-being.[63,64]

On the other hand, evaluating patient-centered outcomes in children following liver transplant is a complex endeavor. For example, the measurement of HRQOL must

factor in both pre- and post-transplant status for both the patient and the family. In many instances, parents are providing living-related grafts for transplant, and their own HRQOL as donors must also be considered. Additionally, the impact of multiple underlying diagnoses and reasons for transplant must be gauged. Post-transplant, certain diseases may recur, increasing the risk of graft failure and poor HRQOL. In other cases, extrahepatic manifestations of disease may persist despite successful liver transplant.

In one study of patient-centered factors after liver transplant, Debolt and colleagues followed 65 children for up to 5 years post-transplant and measured social, behavioral, and emotional adaptation; physical function; and family stress.[65] In this highly comprehensive study, a battery of general psychometric instruments, such as the Mental Scale of the Bailey Scales of Infant Development, the Vineland Social Maturity Scales, and the Wechsler Intelligence Scale for Children-Revised, were administered to children prior to transplant and again at 1 year of follow-up. The children's scores were compared with published data from chronically ill and medically well children. This study supported previous short-term findings showing that transplant recipients had equivalent psychological and functional status compared with both comparison groups.[66]

Debolt and colleagues' findings also indicated that post-transplant, HRQOL in children is highly dependent on immunosuppressive regimens.[65] These findings supported an earlier study by Starzl and colleagues that found that across both pediatric and adult transplant survivors, 1-year post-transplant HRQOL was significantly affected by the degree of steroid dependence.[67] Other outcomes studies more interested in physiologic factors, which may be intermediate steps to HRQOL, have demonstrated the inverse relationship between steroid doses and growth in children following liver transplant.[68] In conjunction with these more clinically oriented studies, Debolt and colleagues' patient-centered results provide tremendous incentive for pediatric hepatologists to aggressively wean post-transplant immunosuppressants.

In the last few years, greater efforts have been made to design a disease-specific HRQOL instrument to assess outcomes of children with liver transplants. In one such undertaking, Andelman and colleagues reported their design and implementation of a pediatric liver transplant–specific HRQOL instrument in children and compared its utility with that of general instruments, such as those employed by Debolt and colleagues,[65] in understanding the impact of clinical management.[69] Again, overall HRQOL in children with liver transplants was found to be similar to that of national norms and control groups of children without liver transplants when assessed by either general or disease-specific instruments.

However, Andelman and colleagues' findings also indicated a greater tendency for the disease-specific instrument to detect differences between the HRQOL of children with liver transplants and that of comparison groups without liver transplants.[69] In fact, only the disease-specific instrument detected the impact of comorbid conditions and the effect of post-transplant morbidities in transplant recipients.[70] Furthermore, administration of these disease-specific age-appropriate instruments to both children with liver transplants and their parents found different responses among children compared with their parents. These findings support a growing realization that the assessment of HRQOL in children is important and must include the perspective of the child.[71]

STUDIES OF MEDICAL EFFICIENCY

As with the growing emphasis on measuring clinical effectiveness and patient-centered end points, there is increasing focus on determining the clinical efficiency or value of medical intervention to make more informed health care decisions at the individual, institutional, governmental, and societal levels. This emphasis on clinical worth that reconciles economic analyses with clinical practice has had a direct impact on all procedural specialties, including pediatric gastroenterology. In the final section of this chapter, we examine the principles of clinical economics and studies of medical costs as essential tools for evaluating efficiency.

The basic principles of health economics involve three different dimensions of analysis, which are classically represented by three axes of a cube (Figure 66.1-3).[52] In this schematic, three approaches to economic analysis are lined up along the y-axis: cost-identification, cost-benefit, and cost-effectiveness. Along the x-axis, different types of costs and benefits can be portrayed, including those that are direct costs, indirect costs, and intangible costs. Finally, the z-axis is used to display three frequently disparate perspectives: that of the patient, the provider, and the payer. An additional perspective is that of society. The societal perspective has a global impact across all of the three axes.

One important study design for determining economic outcomes is modeling. Economic modeling involves the identification of best practices by theoretically determining the costs and benefits of all possible options for a given medical problem. Similarly to meta-analysis, the methodology of modeling involves following strict a priori guidelines that begin with the performance of a comprehensive and integrative literature review. To characterize best all of the options for medical practice, modeling may also involve conducting structured discussions with recognized medical experts on the question to be studied. Ultimately, a conceptual design model should be developed that captures a majority of differences in care processes and the likely affected health outcomes. This model can be depicted as an algorithm of competing treatment paths, which, in turn, can be comparatively analyzed—often in terms of their relative costs, risks, and benefits.

TYPES OF COST ANALYES

There are several different types of cost analyses. Each can be useful in assessing medical costs, but each is also limited by specific considerations that must be understood prior to developing an analysis.

Cost-identification analysis (CIA) is the simplest means of determining health care costs. In this approach, analysts identify all of the costs involved in applying a certain medical intervention. The CIA is expressed as a ratio of cost per unit of treatment or service provided. This type of analysis is often used to compare the costs of one treatment versus another. For example, CIA can be used to calculate the cost of performing flexible sigmoidoscopy versus colonoscopy. However, it is important to recognize that CIA does not necessarily consider the outcomes or benefits, or which procedure may provide more information, in its calculation. Therefore, CIA is appropriate only if outcomes or benefits, such as information gained about the extent of disease, do not vary according to clinical approach. This approach is also known as a cost-minimization analysis.

The second type of medical cost analysis is cost-benefit analysis (CBA), which involves comparing the cost of a given medical intervention with the cost of its benefit. All other circumstances being equal, CBA determines a medical intervention of worth when economic benefits exceed costs. This type of analysis can express its results as either a ratio of benefit to costs (dollars over dollars) or as a net dollar amount (benefits minus costs). In using a CBA, costs and benefits are implicitly negative and positive, respectively. Another way to think of this is that a cost can be incurred or avoided, whereas a benefit is either gained or lost. These theoretical definitions open CBA to statistical manipulation. A medical cost may initially be classified as such and relegated to the denominator of a calculation. A medical cost can also be reclassified as a lost benefit and moved from the denominator to the numerator. Such reclassification (manipulation) can dramatically affect calculations when using ratios. Accordingly, CBAs that are presented as net costs or savings are preferable.

Regardless of how the results are presented, CBA is limited by its reliance on the ability to express costs and benefits in the same unit of measure. For instance, if both costs and benefits can be calculated in dollars, then CBA is possible. However, it is often difficult to express certain qualitative benefits (outcomes measures), such as HRQOL, in monetary units.

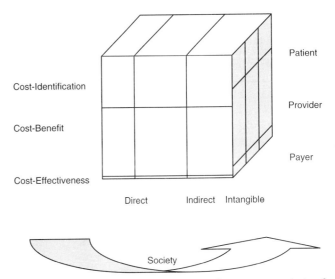

FIGURE 66.1-3   The three dimensions of economic analysis of health care. Adapted from Bombardier C and Eisenberg J.[52]

The third type of analysis is referred to as cost-effectiveness analysis (CEA). In contrast to CBA, all costs in CEA are expressed with the outcome being the denominator (dollars per outcome). This type of analysis allows costs to be expressed in terms of measured clinical or patient-centered outcomes. Accordingly, CEA is most often used to compare two different treatment options with variable or unequal end points. The option that offers less cost with the same or better outcomes is considered to be "dominant."

It is important to note that CEA is complicated by situations in which several important outcomes may result from a single medical intervention. Indeed, a CEA is expressed in terms of a single medical outcome. By definition, it excludes the incorporation of several important medical outcomes simultaneously. For example, if one were to develop a CEA for the treatment of inflammatory bowel disease in children, the results of the study might be expressed as dollars spent per prevention of remission or as dollars spent per symptom-free year of life. However, it would not be possible within the same analysis to compare the costs of remission with the costs of each symptom-free year of life.

To address this problem, analysts can rank the valued importance of the various outcomes to be measured and express the results of their analyses to each. In this weighted ranking system, the comparison of costs for each outcomes measure is called cost-utility analysis (CUA). One common strategy in CUA is to estimate people's personal preferences for different states of health and combine them into a single scale, called a quality-adjusted life-year (QALY). As a unit of "utility" that is impacted by medical intervention, QALYs are useful for measuring health improvement from health care. However, the use of QALYs has not been universally embraced because there are important ethical questions about whose values should be used to derive them.[72]

Another example of a utility-based statistical modeling technique is decision analysis, which involves analyzing decision making under conditions of uncertainty. Classically speaking, to perform a decision analysis, one needs to construct a decision model, also known as a decision tree (Figure 66.1-4). The model must include at least the following four components: (1) all possible choices that can be made in the decision making, (2) all outcomes or potential consequences of these choices, (3) the probabilities or likelihood of the outcomes of each choice, and (4) utilities or values assigned to each outcome. Utilities are often defined as a relative preference for the outcome, with 1 signaling a perfect outcome and 0 the worst possible outcome. A decision tree is then analyzed by summing the product of each probability for each outcome multiplied by its utility. The "best choice" in the decision analysis is that with the highest expected utility.

All decision analyses should include a sensitivity analysis to determine whether the "best choice" remains so if probabilities are different. There are a number of important rules to follow when performing a decision analysis. In particular, it is important to view the problem from a specific perspective (see below). Additionally, the problem must be modeled in the context of the decision and must also include an appropriate level of detail and relevance.

TYPES OF COST

Three commonly recognized types of cost may be considered in clinical economics: direct, indirect, and intangible. All three types of cost are highly dependent on the perspective of the analysis. The same cost might be classified as a direct cost from one perspective but an indirect or intangible cost when a different perspective is taken.

The most easily understood costs are direct costs, which are usually expressed in terms of actual dollars. Direct costs include all medical and nonmedical financial expenses encountered by both physicians and patients. Such costs include pharmaceutical costs, physician fees, and the costs of diagnostic interventions, among others. Other direct costs incurred include nonmedical costs related to the process of care, such as the cost of transportation to the hospital, the cost of special clothing needed because of an illness, and the cost of housing modifications to meet a patient's needs, among others.

Direct costs may be fixed or variable. Fixed costs of an intervention are not dependent on volume of treatment, whereas variable costs are incurred each time the treatment is provided. For example, when taking the perspective of a director of an endoscopy laboratory, the cost of endoscopy would have both fixed and variable components. Fixed costs might include the equipment used during the procedure, which must only be purchased once and can be used over and over. Variable costs might include costs of staffing and

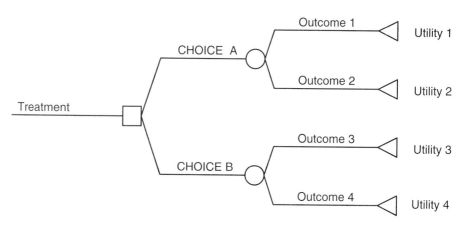

FIGURE 66.1-4   Schematic of a decision tree used in decision analysis.

disposable supplies, which vary from laboratory to laboratory based on the volume of patients undergoing procedures.

Indirect costs of health care are related to all lost opportunities in a patient's life because of illness. In general, they are the financial losses related to morbidity and mortality. For example, because of illness, adult patients may lose household income. In the case of children, indirect costs may be reflected in days away from school, which have projected financial implications for the child and for the parents. These types of costs are often difficult to calculate.

Multiple techniques have been developed for estimating the indirect costs of illness and health care in adults. Assessing the indirect costs of health care or illness in young children is more complex. Whereas the indirect cost of a complication following liver transplant in an adult may be determined by estimating the costs of time lost from the workplace, the equivalent determination in a 6-year-old child requires estimating the costs of missing part of first grade, as well as parental time lost from work.

Finally, intangible costs are those of pain, suffering, and grief. Although these costs may be very difficult to measure, they often figure prominently in decisions made by patients and physicians alike. However, few statistical techniques have been developed to determine intangible costs. Some, such as willingness-to-pay analysis, in which patients are asked to put monetary values on intangible costs, cannot be used to gain the perspective of young children, whose cognitive repertoires do not include an understanding of financial gain or loss. Therefore, although intangible costs may be among the most influential factors in the clinical decision making of pediatric gastroenterologists, they are almost uniformly absent from relevant health care cost analyses.

PERSPECTIVES OF COST

Regardless of the type of analysis and which costs are calculated, one must always be cognizant of the perspective used. In general, there are four perspectives that one might take in performing an economic analysis. These perspectives include the patient, the provider, the payer, and society. For example, indirect costs saved by spending more time following a procedure in the hospital might be important to a recuperating patient but less important to the payer, who may be more concerned with the direct costs of prolonged hospitalization. Likewise, direct out-of-pocket expenses for home nursing might be an important factor for a discharged patient recovering from a procedure but of little concern to the payer. This is true not only for adults but also for pediatric populations. Direct costs are generally incurred by parents, whereas the indirect and intangible costs might be incurred by the child and/or the parents. Factoring in all costs from the child's perspective clearly poses a unique difficulty.

Based on these definitions, a study's perspective will determine how costs and benefits are labeled and measured. For instance, early discharge following percutaneous gastrostomy tube placement can be considered at the same time a benefit to third-party payers and an incurred cost by patients and their families; parents may miss work to reha-

bilitate their children. Clearly, attention must be paid to perspective in interpreting medical cost literature. Although societal costs are generally used as a primary analysis and both CBA and CEA, it is important to keep in mind that the economic impact of an intervention will be reported very differently depending on the perspective of the study.

COST ANALYSES

Few cost analyses involving procedures in pediatric gastroenterology have appeared in the medical peer-review literature. Although limited in number, these analyses have tackled pertinent clinical controversies from the provider's perspective of costs and benefits and have contributed important clinical and economic information about current management options.

One example of a recent cost-effectiveness study in pediatric gastroenterology was published by Deutsch and Olson in 1997.[73] In this provocative modeling study, the investigators surveyed both physician practice and associated costs involved in evaluating pediatric patients with colitis-like symptoms. Using a nationwide survey, the investigators were able to demonstrate that significant regional variation in clinical practice was associated with varying costs of care but similar outcomes. At the center of Deutsch and Olson's study was the question of whether the initial evaluation of children with colitis-like symptoms (such as culture-negative diarrhea or rectal bleeding) should consist of flexible sigmoidoscopy or colonoscopy.

By using a clinical survey that identified physician reasoning at each decision-making point, the investigators designed a clinical model for each management approach with estimated costs for each scenario. This emphasis on reasoning allowed the investigators to detect that "physician desire to know the extent of disease" was the most important factor in determining which procedure was employed initially and whether colonoscopy was performed ultimately. The dominant identified strategy in this study, taking the perspective of the providers, was that early colonoscopy was most cost effective.

Deutsch and Olson's study can also be used to illustrate the importance of perspective taken in cost-analysis studies. For example, if the perspective of the payer were taken into account, a different conclusion might have been realized because the cost of colonoscopy far exceeds that of flexible sigmoidoscopy. If the perspective of the patient was used, a CUA reveals that patient-centered outcomes, such as discomfort and preparation, would need to be factored into this analysis and possibly lead to a different relative or absolute result.

In another cost-effectiveness study, Olson and colleagues compared the clinical and economic implications of several treatment strategies in children with recurrent abdominal pain.[74] In this study, the authors investigated the cost-effectiveness of five different approaches: (1) empiric symptomatic treatment for abdominal complaints in children using antisecretory therapy; (2) empiric treatment of all patients for *H. pylori* with antisecretory and antibiotic therapy; and (3) immediate referral for diagnostic endoscopy, as well as two test-and-treat strategies using

(4) noninvasive and (5) invasive (endoscopy) methods, in which treatment with antibiotics was given only for those with documented infection. In their comprehensive assessment, Olson and colleagues created a decision analytic model that incorporated both clinical and economic outcomes of these five strategies. Followed over time, costs incurred related to treatment failures, such as eventual endoscopy, were also included.

In the economic part of the analysis, the investigators assumed the perspective of payer and included only a small portion of the patients' financial burden (the direct pharmaceutical costs). Indirect and intangible costs were not included.

It is interesting to note that when a cost-minimization approach was taken to this model, empiric antisecretory therapy (arm 1) appeared to be the most economical strategy. However, the use of this type of analysis assumed equal effectiveness. Indeed, when the high rate of recurrent pain and the need for endoscopic evaluation in arms 2 to 5 of the study were taken into account, the savings achieved by initially avoiding the invasive tests in many children were lost.

In this study, the authors believed their results to be highly influenced by parents' initial willingness to have their child undergo endoscopy. They postulated that if patients and/or their parents preferred noninvasive workups, then empiric treatment would prove to be more cost-effective. However, if patients and their parents were more willing to undergo early endoscopy, this became the more cost-effective strategy. As such, the authors suggest that evaluating the cost-effectiveness of each procedural and treatment strategy is highly dependent on patient-centered factors.

REFERENCES

1. Blumenthal D, Epstein AM. Quality of health care. Part 6: the role of physicians in the future of quality management. N Engl J Med 1996;335:1328–31.
2. A primer on outcomes research for the gastroenterologist: report of the American Gastroenterological Association task force on outcomes research. Gastroenterology 1995;109:302–6.
3. Institute of Medicine. Crossing the quality chasm: a new health system for the 21st century. Washington (DC): National Academy Press; 2001.
4. Lohr KN. Developing a strategy for quality assessment. Interview by Janice C. Simmons. Internist 1990;31:17–20, 22.
5. Donabedian A. The quality of care. How can it be assessed? JAMA 1988;260:1743–8.
6. Donabedian A. The seven pillars of quality. Arch Pathol Lab Med 1990;114:1115–8.
7. Davies HT, Crombie IK. Interpreting health outcomes. J Eval Clin Pract 1997;3:187–99.
8. Liacouras CA, Mascarenhas M, Poon C, Wenner WJ. Placebo-controlled trial assessing the use of oral midazolam as a premedication to conscious sedation for pediatric endoscopy. Gastrointest Endosc 1998;47:455–60.
9. Tolia V, Peters JM, Gilger MA. Sedation for pediatric endoscopic procedures. J Pediatr Gastroenterol Nutr 2000;30:477–85.
10. Sackett D. Bias in analytic research. J Chron Dis 1979;32:51–63.
11. Blettner M, Heuer C, Razum O. Critical reading of epidemiological papers. A guide. Eur J Public Health 2001;11:97–101.
12. Berkey CS, Rockett HR, Gillman MW, Colditz GA. One-year changes in activity and in inactivity among 10- to 15-year-old boys and girls: relationship to change in body mass index. Pediatrics 2003;111:836–43.
13. Oken E, Gillman MW. Fetal origins of obesity. Obes Res 2003;11:496–506.
14. Roma E, Kafritsa Y, Panayiotou J, et al. Is peptic ulcer a common cause of upper gastrointestinal symptoms? Eur J Pediatr 2001;160:497–500.
15. Blecker U, Mehta DI, Gold BD. Pediatric gastritis and peptic ulcer disease. Indian J Pediatr 1999;66:725–33.
16. Dohil R, Hassall E. Peptic ulcer disease in children. Baillieres Best Pract Res Clin Gastroenterol 2000;14:53–73.
17. Lazzaroni M, Petrillo M, Tornaghi R, et al. Upper GI bleeding in healthy full-term infants: a case-control study. Am J Gastroenterol 2002;97:89–94.
18. Goyal A, Treem WR, Hyams JS. Severe upper gastrointestinal bleeding in healthy full-term neonates. Am J Gastroenterol 1994;89:613–6.
19. Pugh RJ, Newton RW, Piercy DM. Fatal bleeding from gastric ulceration during first day of life—possible association with social stress. Arch Dis Child 1979;54:146–8.
20. Bahu Mda G, da Silveira TR, Maguilnick I, Ulbrich-Kulczynski J. Endoscopic nodular gastritis: an endoscopic indicator of high-grade bacterial colonization and severe gastritis in children with *Helicobacter pylori*. J Pediatr Gastroenterol Nutr 2003;36:217–22.
21. Rosh JR, Kurfist LA, Benkov KJ, et al. *Helicobacter pylori* and gastric lymphonodular hyperplasia in children. Am J Gastroenterol 1992;87:135–9.
22. Mitchell HM, Bohane TD, Tobias V, et al. *Helicobacter pylori* infection in children: potential clues to pathogenesis. J Pediatr Gastroenterol Nutr 1993;16:120–5.
23. Goodacre S. Research methods: beyond the clinical trial. Ann Emerg Med 2003;42:56–65.
24. Wysowski DK, Bacsanyi J. Cisapride and fatal arrhythmia. N Engl J Med 1996;335:290–1.
25. Wysowski DK, Corken A, Gallo-Torres H, et al. Postmarketing reports of QT prolongation and ventricular arrhythmia in association with cisapride and Food and Drug Administration regulatory actions. Am J Gastroenterol 2001;96:1698–703.
26. Stiffler HL. Capsule endoscopy: a case study of an 11-year-old girl. Gastroenterol Nurs 2003;26:38–40.
27. Koh JL, Black DD, Leatherman IK, et al. Experience with an anesthesiologist interventional model for endoscopy in a pediatric hospital. J Pediatr Gastroenterol Nutr 2001;33:314–8.
28. Lamireau T, Dubreuil M, Daconceicao M. Oxygen saturation during esophagogastroduodenoscopy in children: general anesthesia versus intravenous sedation. J Pediatr Gastroenterol Nutr 1998;27:172–5.
29. Balsells F, Wyllie R, Kay M, Steffen R. Use of conscious sedation for lower and upper gastrointestinal endoscopic examinations in children, adolescents, and young adults: a twelve-year review. Gastrointest Endosc 1997;45:375–80.
30. Iezzoni LI. Assessing quality using administrative data. Ann Intern Med 1997;127:666–74.
31. Laine C. Coming to grips with large databases. Ann Intern Med 1997;127:645–7.
32. Agency for Health Care Policy and Research. Available at: http://www.ahcpr.gov/data/hcup/hcup-pkt.htm (accessed September 2003).
33. Agency for Health Care Policy and Research. Available at: http://www.ahcpr.gov/data/hcup/hcupkid.html (accessed March 15, 2004).
34. Guthery SL Hutchings C, Dean JM, Hoff C. National estimates of hospital utilization by children with gastrointestinal dis-

orders: analysis of the Kids' Inpatient Database. Gastroenterology 2003;124:A-622.

35. Rowland DY, Debanne SM. Meta-analysis, part I. Gastrointest Endosc 2002;55:612–3.

36. Rowland DY, Debanne SM. Meta-analysis, part II. Gastrointest Endosc 2002;55:772–4.

37. Sharma VK, Howden CW. Meta-analysis of randomized, controlled trials of antibiotic prophylaxis before percutaneous endoscopic gastrostomy. Am J Gastroenterol 2000;95:3133–6.

38. D'Amico G, Criscuoli V, Fili D, et al. Meta-analysis of trials for variceal bleeding. Hepatology 2002;36:1023–4; author reply 1024–5.

39. Imperiale TF. Meta-analysis: when and how. Hepatology 1999;29 Suppl:26S–31S.

40. Thacker SB. Meta-analysis. A quantitative approach to research integration. JAMA 1988;259:1685–9.

41. Bailar JC III. The promise and problems of meta-analysis. N Engl J Med 1997;337:559–61.

42. Huang JS, Bousvaros A, Lee JW, et al. Efficacy of probiotic use in acute diarrhea in children: a meta-analysis. Dig Dis Sci 2002;47:2625–34.

43. Guandalini S. The treatment of acute diarrhea in the third millennium: a pediatrician's perspective. Acta Gastroenterol Belg 2002;65:33–6.

44. Szajewska H, Mrukowicz JZ. Probiotics in the treatment and prevention of acute infectious diarrhea in infants and children: a systematic review of published randomized, double-blind, placebo-controlled trials. J Pediatr Gastroenterol Nutr 2001;33 Suppl 2:S17–25.

45. Van Niel CW, Feudtner C, Garrison MM, Christakis DA. *Lactobacillus* therapy for acute infectious diarrhea in children: a meta-analysis. Pediatrics 2002;109:678–84.

46. Rabeneck L. Why should gastroenterologists know about outcomes research? Gastrointest Endosc 1993;39:723–5.

47. Clauser SB, Bierman AS. Significance of functional status data for payment and quality. Health Care Financ Rev 2003;24:1–12.

48. Walker LS, Greene JW. The functional disability inventory: measuring a neglected dimension of child health status. J Pediatr Psychol 1991;16:39–58.

49. Stein RE, Jessop DJ. Functional status II(R). A measure of child health status. Med Care 1990;28:1041–55.

50. Pantell RH, Lewis CC. Measuring the impact of medical care on children. J Chronic Dis 1987;40 Suppl 1:99S–115S.

51. Szilagyi PG, Schor EL. The health of children. Health Serv Res 1998;33:1001–39.

52. Bombardier C, Eisenberg J. Looking into the crystal ball: can we estimate the lifetime cost of rheumatoid arthritis? J Rheumatol 1985;12:201–4.

53. Eisen GM, Farmer RG. Health-related quality of life in inflammatory bowel disease. Pharmacoeconomics 1996;10:327–35.

54. Kuchler T, Kober B, Brolsch C, et al. Quality of life after liver transplantation: can a psychosocial support program contribute? Transplant Proc 1991;23:1541–4.

55. Johanson JF. Outcomes research, practice guidelines, and disease management in clinical gastroenterology. J Clin Gastroenterol 1998;27:306–11.

56. Andelman RG, Attkisson CC, Zima BT, Rosenblatt AB. The use of psychological testing for treatment planning and outcome assessment. In: Maruish ME, editor. Mahwah (NJ): Lawrence Erlbaum Associates; 1999.

57. Ferris TG, Dougherty D, Blumenthal D, Perrin JM. A report card on quality improvement for children's health care. Pediatrics 2001;107:143–55.

58. Lohr KN. Advances in health status assessment. Overview of the conference. Med Care 1989;27 Suppl:S1–11.

59. Gremse DA, Sacks AI, Raines S. Comparison of oral sodium phosphate to polyethylene glycol-based solution for bowel preparation for colonoscopy in children. J Pediatr Gastroenterol Nutr 1996;23:586–90.

60. Kolsteren MM, Koopman HM, Schalekamp G, Mearin ML. Health-related quality of life in children with celiac disease. J Pediatr 2001;138:593–5.

61. Otley A, Smith C, Nicholas D, et al. The IMPACT questionnaire: a valid measure of health-related quality of life in pediatric inflammatory bowel disease. J Pediatr Gastroenterol Nutr 2002;35:557–63.

62. Abramson O, Rosenthal P. Current status of pediatric liver transplantation. Clin Liver Dis 2000;4:533–52.

63. Bucuvalas JC, Ryckman FC. Long-term outcome after liver transplantation in children. Pediatr Transplant 2002;6:30–6.

64. Lightdale JR, Mudge CL, Ascher NL, Rosenthal P. The role of pediatricians in the care of children with liver transplants. Arch Pediatr Adolesc Med 1998;152:797–802.

65. DeBolt AJ, Stewart SM, Kennard BD, et al. A survey of psychosocial adaptation in long-term survivors of pediatric liver transplants. Child Health Care 1995;24:79–96.

66. Zitelli BJ, Gartner JC, Malatack JJ, et al. Pediatric liver transplantation: patient evaluation and selection, infectious complications, and life-style after transplantation. Transplant Proc 1987;19:3309–16.

67. Starzl TE, Koep LJ, Schroter GP, et al. The quality of life after liver transplantation. Transplant Proc 1979;11:252–6.

68. Renz JF, Lightdale J, Mudge C, et al. Mycophenolate mofetil, microemulsion cyclosporine, and prednisone as primary immunosuppression for pediatric liver transplant recipients. Liver Transpl Surg 1999;5:136–43.

69. Andelman RL, Lightdale JR, Thornton P, et al. Measuring outcomes after pediatric liver transplantation using a disease-specific instrument. Pediatr Res 1999;45:108A.

70. Andelman RL, Lightdale J, Kruse K, et al. History of lymphoproliferative disease diminishes outcomes in children and adolescents with liver transplants. Gastroenterology 1999;116:II:A92.

71. Lightdale JR, Rosenthal P. Living related donor transplantation: the future. J Pediatr Gastroenterol Nutr 1999;28:459–60.

72. Johannesson M, O'Conor RM. Cost-utility analysis from a societal perspective. Health Policy 1997;39:241–53.

73. Deutsch DE, Olson AD. Colonoscopy or sigmoidoscopy as the initial evaluation of pediatric patients with colitis: a survey of physician behavior and a cost analysis. J Pediatr Gastroenterol Nutr 1997;25:26–31.

74. Olson AD, Fendrick AM, Deutsch D, et al. Evaluation of initial noninvasive therapy in pediatric patients presenting with suspected ulcer disease. Gastrointest Endosc 1996;44:554–61.

2. Methodology (Statistical Analysis, Test Interpretation, Basic Principles of Screening with Application for Clinical Study)

Patricia L. Hibberd, MD, PhD
Andrew B. Cooper, PhD

The ever-increasing amount of information on the screening, diagnosis, prevention, treatment, prognosis, and risk factors of pediatric gastrointestinal disease is both exciting and daunting. Fortunately, critical evaluation of the literature and use of information for evidence-based decision-making has evolved into a formal process. For example, the Cochrane Library publishes systematic reviews of studies.[1] Examples of available topics include the following:

- Enteral nutritional therapy for induction of remission in Crohn disease
- Glutamine supplementation for prevention of morbidity in preterm infants
- Feed thickener for newborn infants with gastroesophageal reflux
- Antituberculous therapy for maintenance of remission in Crohn disease
- Budesonide for maintenance of remission in Crohn disease
- Mechanical bowel preparation for elective colorectal surgery
- Interventions for treating collagenous colitis
- Cisapride treatment for gastroesophageal reflux in children

Similarly, the North American Society for Pediatric Gastroenterology, Hepatology and Nutrition (NASPGHAN) Web site provides position papers on various topics.[2] However, systematic reviews are often not available to assist with decision-making about new methods of screening or diagnosing gastrointestinal disease in pediatric patients. Therefore, this chapter focuses on a straightforward way to evaluate reports of tests to screen children for risk of developing gastrointestinal disease in the future or to determine whether disease is already present.

WHAT IS SCREENING?

Screening involves the testing of apparently healthy people to find those who are at increased risk of having a disease, either now or in the future.[3] One of the best examples of a screening program involves the screening of newborns in the United States that has been in place since the 1960s. The overall goal of screening is to reduce morbidity and mortality as a result of early detection of this increased risk, although, as recently reviewed by Khoury and colleagues,[4] concerns are increasingly being raised about population screening for genetic susceptibility to conditions that have their onset in adulthood. The most useful screening tests are for diseases that result in substantial morbidity and mortality, that have a presymptomatic phase during which time the test is positive, and for which treatment or preventive strategies are available and cost effective.

In an ideal world, screening tests would be positive for everyone at risk of developing a disease and negative for everyone who was not at risk of developing the disease. They would be safe, reliable, easy to perform, noninvasive, and inexpensive. Subjects who have a screening positive test need follow-up and may be offered a subsequent diagnostic test and/or ways to prevent disease from occurring at a later stage. One of the best ways to evaluate screening tests is to randomize subjects to receive the test or not receive the test and to compare health over time, although these studies are rarely performed, and the value of screening tests is often inferred from observational studies.

WHAT ARE DIAGNOSTIC TESTS?

Diagnostic tests are usually performed in individuals who have signs or symptoms of disease or who are at risk of having disease based on a positive screening test. Again, in an ideal world, diagnostic tests would be positive for everyone who has the disease and negative for everyone who does not have the disease (ie, the test accurately discriminates between those who do and do not have the disease). Unfortunately, there are few diagnostic tests that meet these criteria. The best way to evaluate diagnostic tests is for subjects in a defined and relevant clinical population to have both the new and a "gold standard" diagnostic test and for the results of the two tests to be read independently and compared.[5,6]

WHAT IS MEANT BY DIAGNOSTIC TEST ACCURACY?

A diagnostic test is evaluated in relationship to the truth, that is, whether or not a disease is present. Four situations are possible:

- The test may be positive, and the subject has the disease (true-positive [TP]).
- The test may be negative, and the subject does not have the disease (true-negative [TN]).
- The test may be positive, and the subject does not have the disease (false-positive [FP]).
- The test may be negative, and the subject does have the disease (false-negative [FN]).

The first step to evaluating a diagnostic test is based on how good it is at correctly identifying subjects who have the disease (sensitivity) and subjects who do not have the disease (specificity). Sensitivity is calculated as the number of TPs as a percentage of all of those with the disease [TP/(TP + FN)]. Specificity is calculated as the number of TNs as a percentage of all of those without disease [TN/(TN + FP)]. The question now is what is an acceptable level of sensitivity and specificity? This varies from test to test. For example, if the test was to diagnose a highly treatable form of cancer providing that it was caught at an early stage, then a diagnostic test that missed the diagnosis in 10% or had a sensitivity of less than 90% would likely be totally unacceptable. Similarly, to expose 5% of children to toxic chemotherapy when they did not have cancer owing to a test specificity of 95% would likely be equally unacceptable. However, sensitivity and specificity alone do not tell the whole story about the diagnostic accuracy of a test.

The next step is to take into account the population that is being tested because the sensitivity and specificity of a test depend on how common the disease is in the population being tested. To understand how this impacts on the clinical usefulness of a diagnostic test, we have made up two hypothetical populations in which the results of a serologic test for immunoglobulin G to *Helicobacter pylori* (diagnostic test) were compared with the results of a gold standard test (endoscopy, biopsy, and positive histology) (Table 66.2-1). In both situations, we assumed that the sensitivity of the test is 80% and the specificity is 90%. One hypothetical population includes consecutive asymptomatic children attending a primary care clinic, 1% of whom truly have *H. pylori*, and a second hypothetical population includes consecutive children with dyspepsia presenting to a pediatric gastrointestinal specialty clinic in a hospital, 50% of whom truly have *H. pylori*. We recognize that it would be unacceptable to perform endoscopy on healthy children, as suggested in the first example. In this example, we are drawing attention to the predictive value of a positive test (PVP) and the predictive value of a negative test (PVN). Although the relationship between test sensitivity and specificity and the prevalence of the disease is typically expressed using Bayes theorem, for practical purposes, PVP can be calculated as the odds of having the disease if the test is positive [TP/(TP + FP)], and PVN can be calculated as the odds of not having the disease if the test is negative [TN/(TN + FN)]. In this example, an asymptomatic child in population 1 has a 7% chance of having *H. pylori* based on the serologic test (very unimpressive), whereas a child with dyspepsia has an 89% chance of having *H. pylori* based on the serologic test.

WHO DECIDES WHETHER A TEST IS NEGATIVE OR POSITIVE?

Many diagnostic tests produce continuous results (eg, serum albumin). In an ideal world, patients with disease would all have test results above a certain point, and healthy subjects without disease would all have test results below a certain point. In reality, test results for those with and without disease overlap, sometimes extensively. Although it is attractive to report a diagnostic test as either positive or negative, some risks are taken when

TABLE 66.2-1   COMPARISON OF THE PERFORMANCE OF A HYPOTHETICAL SEROLOGIC TEST FOR *HELICOBACTER PYLORI* IN TWO PATIENT POPULATIONS

H. PYLORI SERUM IGG	H. PYLORI ON ENDOSCOPY		
	PRESENT	ABSENT	TOTAL
POPULATION 1*			
Positive	8 (TP)	99 (FP)	107 (TP + FP)
Negative	2 (FN)	891 (TN)	893 (FN + TN)
Total	10 (TP + FN)	990 (FP + TN)	1,000
POPULATION 2†			
Positive	400 (TP)	50 (FP)	450 (TP + FP)
Negative	100 (FN)	450 (TN)	550 (FN + TN)
Total	500 (TP + FN)	500 (FP + TN)	1,000

FN = false-negative; FP = false-positive; IGG = immunoglobulin G; TN = true-negative; TP = true-positive.
*1,000 asymptomatic children in a primary care clinic, *H. pylori* prevalence 1%: sensitivity = TP/(TP + FN) = 8/10 = 80%; specificity = TN/(TN + FP) = 891/990 = 90%; positive predictive value = TP/(TP + FP) = 8/107 = 7%; negative predictive value = TN/(TN + FN) = 891/893 = 100%.
†1,000 children with dyspepsia in a pediatric gastroenterology clinic, *H. pylori* prevalence 50%: sensitivity = TP/(TP + FN) = 400/500 = 80%; specificity = TN/(TN + FP) = 450/500 = 90%; positive predictive value = TP/(TP + FP) = 400/450 = 89%; negative predictive value = TN/(TN + FN) = 450/550 = 82%.

a cutpoint is chosen to separate normal from abnormal. Figure 66.2-1 shows a hypothetical distribution of serum albumin levels in children with and without liver disease. Let us assume that 200 children were studied, 100 with liver disease and 100 without liver disease. If the cutpoint to separate normal from abnormal is placed at 4 g/dL (see Figure 66.2-1A), in this example, 15% of subjects without liver disease will be incorrectly classified as having liver disease. In addition, 15% with liver disease will be incorrectly classified as being normal. Thus, with a cutpoint of 4 g/dL, the test specificity is 85% and the test sensitivity is also 85%. If the cutpoint is moved to 3.5 g/dL (see Figure 66.2-1B), now only 2% of subjects without liver disease will be incorrectly classified as having liver disease, but 50% with liver disease will be incorrectly classified as being normal. This time, the test specificity is improved to 98%, at the expense of loss of sensitivity, which drops to 0%. Fortunately, there is an efficient way to show the relationship between sensitivity and specificity: using receiver operating characteristic (ROC) curves. ROC curves compare the TP rate with the FP rate (see Figure 66.2-1C). The goal of the diagnostic test is to have a cutoff that has the highest TP rate and the lowest FP rate (ie, is as close to the top left as possible) and as far away as possible from the line of equality (when the TP rate is the same as the FP rate). From above, in Figure 66.2-1A, using a cutpoint of 4.0 mg/dL, the TP rate [TP/(TP + FN) – sensitivity] is 85% and the FP rate [1 – (TN/(TN + FP) or 1 – specificity] is 15%. In Figure 66.2-1B, using a cutpoint of 3.5 mg/dL, the TP rate is 50% and the FP rate is 2%. Clearly, neither cutpoint is perfect, and this raises an important question: Should a cutpoint be chosen at all and, if so, based on what?

Along with exploring the range of cutpoints, the ROC curve provides another estimate of the overall accuracy of the diagnostic test. The estimate of the area under the ROC curve (AUC), which will be between 0 and 1, is also the probability (or chance) that a random person with the disease will have a higher test value than a random person without the disease. A diagnostic test that has an AUC of 0.5 has the same accuracy as a diagnosis that is made at random (eg, by a coin toss), meaning that the test does not help sort out who does and who does not have the disease. However, just because one diagnostic test has a higher AUC (or accuracy), it does not necessarily make it a preferred test. Cost and invasiveness must also be considered in decisions about which test is preferred.

HOW DOES ONE ASSESS THE VALUE OF A DIAGNOSTIC TEST?

Authors of studies that assess the accuracy of a diagnostic test need to convince the reader that they have done everything that they can to ensure that the test results truly represent the way in which the test will work in the population studied (ie, how useful the test will be). If the test was studied in a patient population for whom the test is not relevant (eg, a new saliva enzyme-linked immunosorbent assay–based assay to detect the presence of *H. pylori* being studied in children presenting with coughs and colds), it is very difficult to make conclusions about the way in which the test will work in children presenting with dyspepsia in whom the test is likely to be relevant. Table 66.2-2 provides a checklist of points to consider while reviewing a study of a new diagnostic test and how these points affect whether the study results are likely to be valid.

Based on this checklist, a description of the study population is critically important and should include the following:

- Demographic characteristics (at least age and gender)
- Presence of comorbid conditions
- Previous tests that have been conducted (likely nondiagnostic)
- Setting of the study (eg, primary care, tertiary care, outpatient, inpatient)
- Duration of symptoms or illness prior to testing
- Spectrum of disease and nondisease in the study population

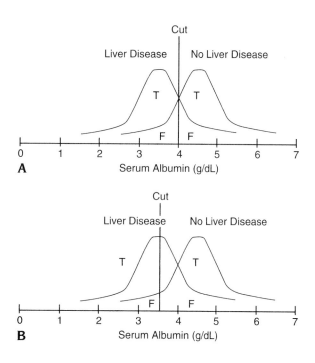

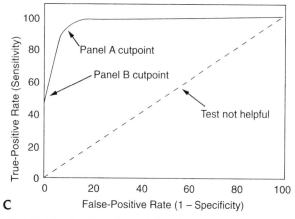

FIGURE 66.2-1 Hypothetical distribution of serum albumin levels in normal children and those with end-stage liver disease. F = false; T = true.

TABLE 66.2-2   EVALUATING STUDIES OF DIAGNOSTIC TESTS

POTENTIAL THREATS TO STUDY VALIDITY IF ANY OF THE FOLLOWING ARE PRESENT	EFFECT OF THE THREAT	BEST PRACTICES APPROACH TO MINIMIZE THE THREAT OF INVALID RESULTS
POPULATION STUDIED		
Selection of only those patients who are known to have the disease	Cannot estimate diagnostic accuracy of the test	Study population is subjects for whom the test is relevant in clinical practice (eg, all patients presenting with a symptom). Population needs to be described.
Selection of patients known to have the disease and selection of another group known to be healthy normal subjects (case-control study)	Overestimates diagnostic accuracy of the test	
Systematic or unknown reasons for excluding subjects who are part of a relevant clinical population	Over- or underestimates the diagnostic accuracy of the test depending on the reasons for excluding subjects	Consecutive patients in the relevant population are studied
Some patients studied more than once	Over- or underestimates the diagnostic accuracy of the test depending on whether overrepresented subjects have or do not have the disease being studied	Each subject is studied the same number of times (usually once or at first encounter)
COMPARISON WITH A STANDARD		
Gold standard (reference) test is not done in everyone (eg, only those with positive tests have the reference test)	Cannot estimate diagnostic accuracy of the test	Gold standard test is performed on everyone (best practices) or at least a random subset of all subjects
Gold standard test is done for only those patients with positive test and a different test is done for those with negative tests	Cannot estimate diagnostic accuracy of the test	
Gold standard test is read with knowledge of the result of the diagnostic test (or the diagnostic test is read with knowledge of the result of the gold standard test)	Overestimate the accuracy of the test, particularly if either test requires subjective interpretation	The gold standard and diagnostic tests are read independently (blinded) and, if any test requires subjective interpretation, ideally should be read by more than one independent person. Results of agreement of independent reading should be reported.
TESTING		
Way in which the gold standard and diagnostic test were performed is unclear	Cannot interpret diagnostic accuracy	Way in which the gold standard and diagnostic test were performed should be described in sufficient detail to allow reader to replicate the measurements
REPORTING OF RESULTS		
No information on whether indeterminate test results occurred and/or were included or excluded in the analysis	Potential for distortion of diagnostic accuracy	All study results should be reported (positive, negative, indeterminate), and tests of diagnostic accuracy should indicate how indeterminate values were treated and effects on measures of test accuracy

Similarly, a description of the diagnostic test should include the following:

- Precise way (adequate details) in which the test was performed to enable others to reproduce the test conditions
- Cutpoint used to categorize the test as positive or negative and explanation of why that cutpoint was chosen
- The proportion of subjects who could not have the test performed or in whom the test result was indeterminate
- Test reproducibility
- Tables summarizing the sensitivity, specificity, PVP, and PVN compared with an acceptable gold standard

THE NEXT LEVEL: STATISTICAL CONSIDERATIONS

Estimates of sensitivity, specificity, PVP, PVN, and AUC will all have uncertainty associated with them. As such,

researchers should also report the 95% confidence intervals associated with these values. The size of the confidence intervals and one's ability to compare the accuracy of a diagnostic test with either a null value or a "gold standard" test will depend on the study's sample size and design. In general, the fewer the patients studied in a study, the wider the 95% confidence intervals associated with the estimates of sensitivity, specificity, PVP, PVN, and AUC. However, most equations relating sample size to a desired power or confidence interval width rely on asymptomatic theory despite the fact that most studies rely on fewer than 50 patients.[7]

CONCLUSION

Improved, noninvasive diagnostic tests for pediatric gastrointestinal disease are urgently needed for a wide range of conditions, but despite the promise of exciting new technologies (such as genetic testing and videocapsule endoscopy), there is an even more urgent need for improved quality of diagnostic studies to evaluate these new innovations. The ethical and regulatory issues relating to diagnostic testing are discussed in the next chapter (Chapter 66.3, "Ethics and Regulatory Issues").

REFERENCES

1. Update software. The Cochrane Library. Available at: http://www.update-software.com/cochrane/ (accessed Nov 1, 2003).
2. North American Society for Pediatric Gastroenterology Hepatitis and Nutrition. Position papers. Available at: www.naspghan.org/sub/positionpapers.asp (accessed Nov 1, 2003).
3. Grimes DA, Schulz KF. Uses and abuses of screening tests. Lancet 2002;359:881–4.
4. Khoury MJ, McCabe LL, McCabe ER. Population screening in the age of genomic medicine. N Engl J Med 2003;348:50–8.
5. Jaeschke R, Guyatt GH, Sackett DL. Users' guides to the medical literature. III. How to use an article about a diagnostic test. B. What are the results and will they help me in caring for my patients? The Evidence-Based Medicine Working Group. JAMA 1994;271:703–7.
6. Jaeschke R, Guyatt G, Sackett DL. Users' guides to the medical literature. III. How to use an article about a diagnostic test. A. Are the results of the study valid? Evidence-Based Medicine Working Group. JAMA 1994;271:389–91.
7. Obuchowski NA. Sample size calculations in studies of test accuracy. Stat Methods Med Res 1998;7:371–92.

3. Ethics and Regulatory Issues

P. Pearl O'Rourke, MD

Jennifer P. Stevens, MS

Effective and safe medical care for children requires that care be appropriate to the patient's developmental and/or chronologic age.[1] Advances through research with adult subjects are not always relevant to children. Children and adults can have different manifestations of the same disease process, and age-specific differences in renal and hepatic function make it impossible to directly translate adult pharmacokinetics and pharmacodynamics to the child. In addition, children suffer unique diseases such as sudden infant death syndrome, Reye syndrome, and infantile spasms.[2]

But should children be allowed to be research subjects? Is any risk appropriate for a child? Can children truly volunteer? Can their parents "volunteer" for them? In response to such concerns, a regulatory framework that governs pediatric research has evolved.[3] Investigators working with pediatric populations must negotiate a range of federal, state, local, and institutional protections for vulnerable research participants and must also accommodate a number of methodologic challenges that are unique to pediatric research. This review summarizes the importance of pediatric research, the history of pediatric research ethics, and the fundamental regulatory requirements and provides several recommendations for pediatric research investigators.

IMPORTANCE OF PEDIATRIC RESEARCH

An often-repeated adage is that children are not small adults. Data learned from research conducted with adults may not be scalable to the child. As noted above, children have unique diseases, unique manifestations of "adult" diseases, and renal and hepatic functions that vary with developmental age. Although the focus of this chapter is children in research, it is relevant to at least note that many of the same concerns and issues are also relevant to the developing fetus. The thalidomide tragedy in the 1960s reminded the public of the importance of understanding the effects of diseases and drugs on intrauterine fetal development. Revelations about the teratogenicity of this drug generated support for a rigorous premarket drug safety screening process in the United States and continue to serve as a brutal reminder of the specific vulnerability of the developing fetus.[4]

Too often, even today, pediatric clinicians must provide clinical care without the benefit of age-appropriate, validated data.[5-7] In 2000, Conroy and colleagues demonstrated that as many as 67% of children (421/624) admit-ted to five general pediatric wards in Europe received drugs that were unlicensed for use in children or were being used off-label.[8] In this study, dosing issues (either amounts or frequency of doses) and use of the drug in an untested age group were the most common reasons for unlicensed or off-label uses. In 1998, McKinzie and colleagues reported a lower but still large rate of off-label drug use for children in a US emergency department: 179 of 521 children (34%) received off-label drug prescriptions, with the highest rate found in patients 3 to 11 years of age.[9] Turner and colleagues reported a significant association between the percentage of off-label drugs prescribed per child and the incidence of adverse events in five pediatric wards in the United Kingdom.[10]

Conducting pediatric research presents a number of unique challenges. Among these are (1) the need for multiple age cohorts to study different developmental stages, (2) small study populations owing to the limited incidence of many pediatric illnesses,[11,12] and (3) the resultant limited industry interest and financial support. There are also a number of pediatric-specific ethical issues to consider: (1) the acceptable risk to which one may expose a child, (2) under what circumstances a child may be a healthy control,[13] (3) at what age a researcher should discuss study participation with a child subject,[14,15] and (4) when and how a child participant should be remunerated.[16]

The US government created a number of initiatives to support pediatric research in the late 1990s. Briefly, these included the following: The Food and Drug Administration (FDA) Modernization Act of 1997 (FDAMA) required that the FDA extend drug testing to children.[17] The National Institutes of Health (NIH), in 1998, specified that children be included in all research barring a scientific or ethical reason for their exclusion.[18] The Children's Act of 2000 codified previous congressional decisions to increase money dedicated to pediatric research.[19]

Of interest, this support for pediatric research came at a time of growing concerns about the adequacy of protections of human research subjects in general and protections for children specifically.[3,20-25] The 1999 death of Jesse Gelsinger, an 18-year-old volunteer in a phase I gene transfer trial conducted at the University of Pennsylvania, and the 2001 death of Ellen Roche, a healthy volunteer in a lung physiology study at Johns Hopkins University, focused much of this concern. Federal assessments of these two tragedies raised issues about informed consent, coercion, reporting of adverse events, and financial conflict of interest, among others. These high-profile cases served as watershed events for many in the research safety community and prompted a number of changes in the oversight of human research.[26-29]

HISTORY OF HUMAN SUBJECT PROTECTIONS

The Nuremberg Code, which provides the foundation of the current system of human subject protections, was developed following the Nuremberg Military Tribunal convened after World War II. The Code defined 10 ethical principles for research, including, among others, the voluntariness of consent and the need to minimize risk. In the years following, other complementary guidelines and principles for the protection of human research subjects were developed at the World Medical Association Declaration of Helsinki and by the Council for International Organizations of Medical Sciences (best known as CIOMS).

In the United States, federal regulations for the protection of human subjects advanced during the 1960s and 1970s in response to several sentinel events. One of these events was Beecher's review article in 1966, which focused attention on several historic but ethically controversial published peer-reviewed studies.[30] One cited study was Krugman and colleagues' work with infectious hepatitis. The investigators intentionally exposed mentally impaired children between the ages of 3 and 10 years to hepatitis virus, arguing that the children would have been exposed to the virus at some time during their institutionalization.[31] Although parental consent was obtained at admission to the institution, there were many concerns regarding coercion, inadequate consent, and inappropriate risk to this vulnerable population. Following Beecher's article, revelations about the Tuskegee Syphilis Study became public in a 1972 *New York Times* exposé.[32] These two reports together generated a public and professional demand for a regulatory framework.

The federal government responded with a series of initiatives and regulations for the protection of human subjects. *The Belmont Report*, proposed by the National Commission for the Protection of Human Subjects of Biomedical and Behavioral Research (the National Commission) in 1979, provided landmark definitions in the ethical domains of respect for persons, beneficence, and justice and created the groundwork for the current Institutional Review Board (IRB) system of local peer review of human research protocols.[33] The National Commission's work ultimately evolved into the Common Rule, a set of federal regulations, which are described below.

The National Commission also identified additional protections for pediatric research participants. Among other recommendations, the Commission concluded that IRBs should consider the scientific significance of the pediatric protocol, that studies be conducted first in animals and adults before children, that the privacy and confidentiality of parents and children be protected, and that research with wards of the state, underage prisoners, or the mentally infirm be further restricted.[34] The National Commission drew distinctions between research of minimal risk and of greater than minimal risk for pediatric subjects and recommended seeking a child subject's assent and

parental permission for participation. These recommendations were ultimately codified in additional regulations, which are discussed below.

REQUIREMENTS FOR FEDERALLY FUNDED RESEARCH: THE COMMON RULE AND SUBPARTS OF TITLE 45 OF THE CODE OF FEDERAL REGULATIONS, PART 46

The Common Rule is the regulatory foundation for the current system of human subject protections. This rule, found at Subpart A of Title 45 of the Code of Federal Regulations, Part 46 (45 CFR 46), "Protection of Human Subjects," is called the Common Rule because it is held in "common" by 17 federal departments or agencies, including the NIH in the Department of Health and Human Services (DHHS), the largest funding agency for biomedical research.[35] Not all research is covered by the Common Rule. The Common Rule covers only human subject research that is conducted or funded by any of the 17 agencies that have accepted the rule. Research that is not conducted or supported by 1 of these 17 agencies is not subject to this rule. Despite this legal allowable "gap" in coverage, most academic institutions that receive NIH funding voluntarily extend these protections to all human subject research conducted by the institution. This extension of the Common Rule is done with a formal agreement with the federal government.

The Common Rule (subpart A of 45 CFR 46) outlines the process of required institution-level peer review of the ethics of individual research projects through a committee called an IRB. The Common Rule provides the general framework for IRB functions, organization, and operations but allows for limited institution-level interpretation in some areas.[36] Investigators are encouraged to familiarize themselves with their institution's IRB policies and procedures.

The Common Rule includes criteria for the membership of the IRB, mandating the inclusion of both scientists and laypersons with appropriate expertise. It specifies that if an IRB reviews research to be conducted with vulnerable populations (eg, children, prisoners, or pregnant women), then that IRB must have members with knowledge specific to research and ethics in those fields.[36]

The process for reviewing research protocols draws a distinction between research protocols of greater risk to subjects that require full IRB review and those of minimal risk, which can be reviewed by an accelerated review process, termed an expedited review. Per the Common Rule, research protocols can be approved only for a maximum of 1 year, at which time investigators must reapply to the IRB for continuing review and approval. The Common Rule also requires that every approved study be monitored at a level that is commensurate with the risk to subjects involved in the study. All changes to the research protocol or informed consent document must be reported to and approved by the IRB (note that sponsors may also require review and reporting of changes). For more detail regarding the Subpart A requirements for an IRB, see Table 66.3-1.[36]

In addition to the Common Rule (Subpart A), 45 CFR 46 also has three other subparts: B, C, and D. Subparts B, C, and D were codified after Subpart A and outline additional regulations for specific vulnerable subpopulations. Subpart B, codified in 1975 and revised in 2001, addresses research with pregnant women, human fetuses, and neonates; Subpart C, codified in 1978, addresses prisoners; and Subpart D, codified in 1983, addresses children. Because Subparts B, C, and D are not followed by all of the aforementioned seventeen agencies that follow Subpart A, these subparts are not considered part of the Common Rule. Researchers should note that the NIH does adhere to all subparts.

ADDITIONAL PROTECTIONS FOR CHILDREN INVOLVED AS SUBJECTS IN RESEARCH (45 CFR 46 SUBPART D)

Subpart D is of particular importance to pediatric investigators as the principal set of regulations that governs pediatric research. This subpart categorizes pediatric research, unlike adult research, into four levels of risk and benefit that trigger different levels of review, consistent with the recommendations of the National Commission (Table 66.3-2).[37] Three of the four categories can be reviewed and approved by the IRB. These include (1) research not involving greater than minimal risk, (2) research involving greater than minimal risk but presenting the potential of direct benefit to the specific child, and (3) research involving greater than minimal risk that, although not presenting the prospect of direct benefit to the specific child, is likely to produce information about the child's disease or condition. The fourth category addresses research that is greater than minimal risk, that has no prospect of direct benefit to the child, and that would not produce information about the child's disease or condition. The IRB cannot approve research in this last category; it can be approved only by the Secretary of Health and Human Services after consultation with a panel of experts.[37]

Minimal Risk in Pediatric Research. Subpart D fails to define the amount of risk that may be considered minimal for children participating in research. Some interpret minimal risk to include only those risks that a healthy child may experience in everyday activities. However, a 2002 federal advisory committee of experts to the DHHS Office of Human Research Protections interpreted minimal risk to be relative to the health condition of each specific minor. This advisory committee suggested that for a healthy child, minimal risk equated to no additional risk above and beyond the risk that a healthy child encountered on a daily basis. In contrast, chronically ill children faced substantial risk as part of their clinical care, and minimal risk for these children meant no additional risk above and beyond the risk inherent in their standard of care.[38,39]

Pediatric Assent and Parental Permission. Subpart D also amplifies the requirements of informed consent. Consistent with the National Commission's original report, subpart D requires investigators to seek parental permission rather than parental consent, drawing a distinction between the two terms to highlight that one may not consent to research conducted on another person. The IRB can require the permission of either one or both parents depending on the level of risk to the child. The permission of only one parent is adequate for research considered of minimal risk to the child participants (Section 46.404) or for research likely to yield direct benefit to the children (Section 46.405). The permission of both parents is required for pediatric research conducted under Section 46.406 or 46.407 (see Table 66.3-2) unless one parent is deceased, unknown, incompetent, or not reasonably available or when only one parent has legal responsibility for the care and custody of the child.[40] In addition, investigators must also seek the age-appropriate assent of children subjects; of note, failure to object cannot be considered an assent.[37]

TABLE 66.3-1 SUMMARY OF THE REQUIREMENTS OF INVESTIGATORS DELINEATED BY THE COMMON RULE (SUBPART A, 45 CFR 46)[36]

Requirements for IRB approval	Risk to subjects are minimized.
	Risks to subjects are reasonable in relation to anticipated benefits, if any, and the importance of the knowledge that may result.
	Subject selection is equitable. Vulnerable populations are given additional protections both in the selection of subjects and the research generally.
	An informed consent form and process are provided, or a waiver of all or part of the informed consent is approved.
	A waiver of informed consent may be obtained by an investigator from an IRB if the study involves no more than minimal risk to the subjects, if the waiver does not adversely effect the rights and welfare of the subjects, if the research cannot be conducted without the waiver, and, whenever appropriate, the subjects will be provided additional pertinent information after participation.
	Adequate provisions for data and safety monitoring are in place when appropriate.
	Adequate privacy of the subjects and confidentiality of the data are maintained.
Required elements to be provided to each subject when obtaining written informed consent	A statement that the study is research, an explanation of the purpose of the study, the length of time the subject is expected to participate, a description of the procedures, and the identification of the experimental procedures.
	A description of the risks and benefits.
	Disclosure of appropriate alternatives that might benefit the subject.
	A statement of how the confidentiality of the data will be maintained.
	A description of compensation and the procedures and treatments available for potential injury.
	Investigator contact information.
	A statement that participation is voluntary and the subject will not be penalized in any way for discontinued participation.
	Additional requirements must also be included whenever appropriate (eg, withdrawal from the research).

IRB = Institutional Review Board

TABLE 66.3-2   ALLOWABLE RESEARCH WITH MINOR SUBJECTS UNDER SUBPART D, 45 CFR 46[37]

Research not involving greater than minimal risk (Section 46.404)	These studies may be permitted if the IRB finds Adequate provisions are made for soliciting the assent of the children and the permission of their parents or guardians.
Research involving greater than minimal risk but presenting the prospect of direct benefit to the individual subjects (Section 46.405)	These studies may be permitted if the IRB finds that The risk is justified by the anticipated benefits to the subjects; The relation of the anticipated benefit to the risk is at least as favorable to the subjects as that presented by available alternative approaches.
Research involving greater than minimal risk and no prospect of direct benefit to individual subjects but likely to yield generalizable knowledge about the subject's disorder or condition (Section 46.406)	These studies may be permitted if the IRB finds that The risk represents a minor increase over minimal risk; The intervention or procedure presents experiences to subjects that are reasonably commensurate with those inherent in their actual or expected medical, dental, psychological, social, or educational situations; The intervention or procedure is likely to yield generalizable knowledge about the subjects' disorder or condition, which is of vital importance for the understanding or amelioration of the subjects' disorder or condition; Adequate provisions are made for soliciting assent of the children and permission of their parents or guardians.
Research not otherwise approvable that presents an opportunity to understand, prevent, or alleviate a serious problem affecting the health or welfare of children (Section 46.407)	Allowable only if the IRB finds that the research study meets this requirement and the Secretary of Health and Human Services, after consultation with a panel of experts, determines that The research presents a reasonable opportunity to further the understanding, prevention, or alleviation of a serious problem affecting the health or welfare of children; The research will be conducted in accordance with sound ethical principles; Adequate provisions are made for soliciting the assent of children and the permission of their parents or guardians.

IRB = Institutional Review Board.

Issues of child assent and parental permission are complex. The ethical and legal controversies surrounding parents' ability to provide permission for pediatric subjects were the focus of the 2002 *Grimes v. Kennedy Krieger Institute* case.[41] This case involved the Johns Hopkins–affiliated Kennedy Krieger Institute and its 2-year-old lead abatement study in low-income housing. The judgment of the Maryland Court of Appeals discussed issues of parental consent for the participation of children subjects and attempted to define minimal risk. The court was concerned that the parents had an inaccurate assessment of their children's risks (dust lead level reporting was delayed) and benefits (the offer of a lead-reduced household may have been coercive) in this research. Regarding minimal risk, the court initially determined so-called nontherapeutic research to have a zero-risk standard but relented to define minimal risk as "the minimal kind of risk that is inherent in any endeavor."[41] Given the judgment in the *Grimes v. Kennedy Krieger Institute* case, researchers should be aware of the fluid nature of parental permission in pediatric research.[42,43]

The issue of assent is also controversial. The American Academy of Pediatrics (AAP) recommends seeking assent from children with an intellectual age of 7 or greater.[44] Researchers working with adolescents in studies in which parental consent may be inappropriate should consider state-level laws that designate some adolescents to be "mature minors" or "emancipated minors" under specific circumstances.[15] The AAP recommends several specific elements of assent, which include (1) helping the child achieve a developmentally appropriate awareness of his or her condition, (2) explaining tests and treatment, (3)

making an appropriate assessment of the child's level of understanding, and (4) soliciting the child's willingness to participate.[15] Little research has been done in this area of pediatric consent. Tarnowski and colleagues examined forms that parents were asked to sign to grant their permission for their children to participate in research. The language in these consent documents was at the college graduate level rather than the required eighth grade reading level.[45] Susman and colleagues examined the comprehension level of children ages 7 to 20 years participating in cancer or obesity research. Several days following consent or assent, the subjects were found to be less likely to understand the purpose of the relevant research study, the procedures, and the risks involved than they were to understand other, more concrete elements of the study, such as the duration of their participation. When stratified into two age groups, 7 to 13 years and 14 to 20 years, there was no statistical difference in mean scores; age did not appear to affect the children's understanding of some elements of the research study in which they were participating.[46] These findings are similar to assessments of the readability of informed consent forms for adult subjects.[47] Issues of consent, permission, and assent require specific attention to comprehension if this process is to be meaningful.

Remuneration of Pediatric Subjects. Another concern, as in any research, is the issue of coercion or inappropriate influence to elicit a subject's assent or consent. The regulations speak to coercion broadly, but there are no specific recommendations on the issues of remuneration of pediatric or adult research subjects. Dickert and colleagues studied 32 IRBs and found that 37.5% had written guidelines for investigators about adult research subject compensation. All but one institution had "rules of thumb," suggesting that institutional approaches to adult subject remuneration varied widely.[48] In terms of remuneration of pediatric subjects, Weise and colleagues found that two-thirds of 128 participating institutions permitted payment to pediatric research subjects. Only 7% (6/84) of those who permitted remuneration had written policies. The most common method of payment was money, with gift certificates and savings bonds named as other permitted and common options.[16] Although there is little formal guidance, the AAP recommends that the families of research subjects be reimbursed for direct and indirect costs of study participation. Similarly, remuneration to child subjects should be limited to a token and should be discussed with the child only at the completion of the study.[44]

ADDITIONAL PROTECTIONS FOR PREGNANT WOMEN, HUMAN FETUSES, AND NEONATES INVOLVED IN RESEARCH (45 CFR 46 SUBPART B)

Subpart B of 45 CFR 46 addresses research with pregnant women, human fetuses, and neonates. The specific requirements of Subpart B, revised on November 13, 2001, are described in Table 66.3-3. This revision defined permissible research with fetuses, neonates of uncertain viability, and nonviable neonates, as well as requirements for paternal consent. Note that research with viable neonates, defined as newborns until 28 days of age, falls within the scope of Subpart D.[49]

Subpart B generally requires that research involving pregnant women or fetuses must be of no greater than minimal risk or should hold the possibility of direct benefit to the pregnant woman and/or fetus. Consent is required of only the mother if the research is of minimal risk or if the research is likely to yield direct benefit to either the pregnant woman alone or both the woman and the fetus. Research likely to yield direct benefit only to the fetus requires the consent of both parents.[49]

Although viable neonates are covered in Subpart D, research on neonates of uncertain viability is covered by Subpart B. Research on neonates of uncertain viability is allowed only if there is the prospect of enhancing the likelihood of survival or if the purpose of the research is important and adds no additional risk to the neonate and the information cannot be obtained in any other way. Consent is required from only one parent.[49]

Research with nonviable neonates can be approved by the IRB only if the research will not stop the respiration or heartbeat of the neonate and, similar to research with neonates of uncertain viability, the research is important and adds no additional risk to the neonate, and the information can be obtained in no other way. For research with nonviable neonates, consent must be obtained from both parents except under limited circumstances.[49]

FEDERAL REQUIREMENTS SPECIFIC TO THE FDA

The FDA has its own set of regulations that cover any research conducted on a product that is regulated by the FDA. These regulations present special considerations for human studies that involve drugs, biologics, and devices. These regulations are similar but not identical to those of the Common Rule.

Typically, a sponsor, such as a pharmaceutical, biotechnology, or medical device company, initiates the application but does not function as the investigator. Investigators are required to assume the responsibilities of conducting the research, which include (1) abiding by the investigational plan and statement, (2) protecting the rights and safety of the human subjects, and (3) controlling any drugs under investigation.[50] In some limited cases, an individual or group of individuals may serve as the sponsor-investigator.

Although the FDA requirements for informed consent and IRB review are similar to those of the Common Rule, they are not identical. Some of the differences are listed below. Note that research studies conducted under both the DHHS and FDA are subject to both sets of requirements:

- The FDA permits the use of an investigational drug, device, or biologic for a limited number of emergency uses without prior IRB approval. The emergencies qualifying for this exemption are listed in Table 66.3-4. Each of these uses must be reported in writing to the governing IRB within 5 days, and subsequent use is subject to IRB review.[51]
- The informed consent requirements may not be waived if the risk to subjects is a breach of confidentiality.[52] This is a more stringent standard for waiver criteria than that provided by the Common Rule.
- Potential subjects are required by the FDA to be informed that the agency may review the records of the study. In addition, informed consent forms must be dated and signed by the subjects.[53]

In October 2000, the Children's Health Act of 2000 (Public Law [PL] 106-310) extended Subpart D of 45 CFR 46 (pediatric research) to all health and human services agencies, including the FDA.[19] Prior to this legislation, the FDA was one of several agencies that had agreed to abide by the Common Rule (Subpart A 45 CFR 46), but as the FDA regulated rather than funded research, it did not require the same protections for children as were required by the NIH.

Pediatric drug research was a focus of the 1997 FDAMA and the FDA Pediatric Rule. The FDAMA gave pharmaceutical companies an additional 6 months of patent exclusivity for all uses of the entire active moiety if pediatric-specific trials for on- or off-label uses of those drugs were supported.[17] In 2002, the Best Pharmaceuticals for Children Act (PL 107-109) reauthorized the pediatric provisions of FDAMA.[54] Although the FDAMA produced a regulatory pathway by which sponsors could voluntarily provide these data on drugs, it did not require sponsors to generate pediatric-specific data. Concerned that many drugs would not be evaluated in the voluntary program under the FDAMA, the FDA developed the Pediatric Rule. The Pediatric Rule served as the "stick" to the FDAMA "carrot," mandating that drug companies conduct trials in children if the on-label indication was for a substantial number of children (defined as greater than 50,000 children) or if the drug or

TABLE 66.3-3   SPECIFIC RESTRICTIONS, SUBPART B 45 CFR 46[49]

Research involving pregnant women or fetuses (Section 46.204)	All of the following must be met: Preclinical animal and nonpregnant women studies have been conducted; The risk to the fetus is caused solely by the interventions or procedures that hold out the prospect of direct benefit for either woman or fetus, or the risk is no greater than minimal risk with the prospect of important biomedical knowledge; The risk is minimized for achieving the objectives of the research; The research holds the prospect of direct benefit to the woman, the fetus, or both, or the risk is no greater than minimal risk with the prospect of important biomedical knowledge; If the prospect of direct benefit is solely to the fetus, consent is required of both the mother and father, except under limited circumstances; Both mother and father are aware of potential risks to the fetus or neonate; Children who are pregnant must adhere to the restrictions under Subpart D of 45 CFR 46; No inducements will be offered to terminate the pregnancy; Individuals engaged in the research will have no part in any decision to terminate the pregnancy; Individuals engaged in the research will have no part in determining the viability of the neonate.
Research involving neonates of uncertain viability (Section 46.205(c))	All of the following must be met: Preclinical and clinical trials have been conducted to assess potential risks to the neonates; Individuals providing consent are fully informed of the risks to the neonate; Individuals involved in the research will have no part in determining the viability of the neonate; The IRB determines that (1) the research holds out the prospect of enhancing the probability of survival of the neonate or (2) the purpose of the research is the development of important biomedical knowledge that cannot be obtained any other way and there will be no additional risk to the neonate; Informed consent will be gathered from either parent.
Research involving nonviable neonates (Section 46.205(d))	All of the following must be met: Preclinical and clinical trials have been conducted to assess potential risks to the neonates; Individuals providing consent are fully informed of the risks to the neonate; Individuals involved in the research will have no part in determining the viability of the neonate; Vital functions of the neonate will not be artificially maintained; Research will not terminate the heartbeat or respiration of the neonate; There will be no added risk to the neonate resulting from the research; The purpose of the research is the development of important biomedical knowledge that cannot be obtained by other means; The informed consent of both parents must be sought, except under limited circumstances.
Research involving, after delivery, the placenta, the dead fetus, or fetal material (Section 46.206)	Research with these materials is subject to all state, federal, and local laws and regulations. If identifiable health information of living individuals is used, those individuals are considered human subjects, and all relevant regulations apply.
Research not otherwise approvable that presents an opportunity to understand, prevent, or alleviate a serious problem affecting the health or welfare of pregnant women, fetuses, or neonates (Section 46.207)	The Secretary of Health and Human Services must consult with a panel of experts to determine if the proposed research Presents a reasonable opportunity to further the understanding, prevention, or alleviation of a serious problem affecting the health or welfare of pregnant women, fetuses, or neonates; Will be conducted in accord with sound ethical principles; Will require informed consent.

IRB = Institutional Review Board.

biologic would provide "meaningful therapeutic benefit" over existing treatment.[55] In combination, the FDAMA and the Pediatric Rule resulted in an increase in the number of pediatric trials. The Pharmaceutical Research and Manufacturers of America estimated that in 2002, 194 drugs were being studied in children.[56] In 2002, however, the Pediatric Rule was struck down when the US District Court ruled that the FDA had exceeded its regulatory authority.[57] As a result, pharmaceutical companies need only comply with the voluntary provisions of the FDAMA.

TABLE 66.3-4   ALLOWABLE EMERGENCIES BY THE FDA FOR USE OF AN INVESTIGATIONAL DRUG OR BIOLOGIC WITHOUT PRIOR IRB APPROVAL[62]

Life-threatening situations necessitating use of the test article
If the subject is unable to provide consent
Insufficient time in which to obtain consent from the subject's legal representative
No available alternative method of approved or generally recognized therapy of equal or greater likelihood of saving the subject's life

FDA = US Food and Drug Administration; IRB = Institutional Review Board.

ADDITIONAL REGULATORY AREAS

NIH POLICY GUIDANCE ON THE INCLUSION OF CHILDREN IN RESEARCH

On March 6, 1998, the NIH published guidance for research conducted with children.[18] This guidance, which defines children as individuals under 21 years of age, requires that children be included in all NIH-supported research unless there are scientific or ethical reasons to exclude them. Hence, the inclusion of children in research is the rule rather than the exception. The justifications for exclusion of children in research are described in Table 66.3-5.[18]

CHILDREN'S HEALTH ACT OF 2000 (PL 106-310)

As noted above, this law extended Subpart D of 45 CFR 46 to all agencies of the DHHS. In addition, this broad piece of legislation provided several other pediatric research provisions. One of these provisions is the Pediatric Research Initiative, which authorizes $50 million in funding to support pediatric research by the NIH and to require the FDA to promote the use of clinical trials in pediatric populations. The legislation also creates a pediatric loan repayment program to be administered by the Secretary of Health and Human Services and the director of the NIH for professionals performing pediatric research.[19]

INSTITUTIONAL REQUIREMENTS AND STATE OR CASE LAW

Although federal law provides the general framework by which human subjects in research are protected, investigators should consider local requirements. State and case laws may provide specific requirements for researchers, particularly those working with vulnerable populations or working in politically charged fields. Similarly, research institutions may have more strict internal policies in place. For example, many institutions extend the requirements of the Common Rule to include all research that is conducted by its researchers rather than restrict the Common Rule to federally supported research. Institutional recruitment and remuneration policies are specific areas that vary widely across institutions.

CHALLENGES TO RESEARCHERS

There are several areas of new and innovative research in which more regulatory guidance is needed. Such research includes broad fetus to adult longitudinal studies, tissue banking, and genetic research, among others. With broad implications for the future of pediatric research and care, it remains unclear how investigators and regulators are likely to proceed in these areas.

Other challenges result from extending human subject protections to fetuses. As discussed above, fetuses are defined as a vulnerable population protected by Subpart B of 45 CFR 46.[49] In addition, in 2002, embryos and fetuses were categorized as human subjects in the charter of the recommissioned Secretary's Advisory Committee on Human Research Protections.[58] The repercussions of these determinations remain unclear.

Another area of concern is the documentation of compliance with existing protections for pediatric populations in research. Similar to studies with adult subjects, two reviews of the pediatric research literature report that in only 52 to 61% of pediatric publications was there proper documentation of appropriate ethical review in the resulting article.[59,60] Sifers and colleagues found that parental permission was documented 41.5% of the time.[61]

Current and future guidance on human subject protections is primarily provided by the DHHS Office of Human Research Protections. Investigators should familiarize themselves with changes in federal, state, and local research policy. By working with vulnerable populations, investigators have a dual responsibility: to protect minor subjects from inappropriate risk in research and to provide pediatric populations with age-specific treatment and care.

RECOMMENDATIONS TO RESEARCHERS

1. Despite difficulties in designing pediatric research, scientifically and statistically sound studies in children can and should be conducted.
2. Consider study designs that maximize benefit to the individual child subject. Minimize risk as much as possible to risk experienced in the subject's daily life.
3. When allowable by the institution, consider remuneration strategies that are age and study appropriate.
4. Consider the most appropriate way to seek a child subject's assent if possible.
5. Review institutional, case, study, and federal policies and restrictions for pediatric research.

TABLE 66.3-5   ALLOWABLE JUSTIFICATIONS FOR EXCLUSION OF CHILDREN IN NIH-FUNDED RESEARCH[18]

The research is considered to be irrelevant to children.
There are laws or regulations barring the inclusion of children to the research.
Data are already available for children elsewhere in this research area.
A separate child-specific study in this field would be more appropriate.
Insufficient data are available in adults to perform the study ethically in children.
The study is designed to collect additional data on an existing adult cohort or
Other special cases, justified by the investigator and acceptable to the review group.

NIH = National Institutes of Health.

REFERENCES

1. Future of Pediatric Education II. Organizing pediatric education to meet the needs of infants, children, adolescents and young adults in the 21st century. Pediatrics 2000;105: 163–212.

2. Hurowitz ES, Barrett MJ, Bregman D, et al. Public Health Service study of Reye's syndrome and medications. Report of the main study. JAMA 1987;257:1905–11.

3. Institute of Medicine (US). Preserving public trust: accreditation and human research participant protection programs. Washington (DC): National Academy Press; 2001.

4. Annas GJ, Sherman E. Thalidomide and the Titanic: reconstructing the technology tragedies of the twentieth century. Am J Public Health 1999;89:98–101.

5. Adcock KG, Wilson JT. Nifedipine labeling illustrates the pediatric dilemma for off-patent drugs. Pediatrics 2002;109:319–21.

6. Blumer JL. Off-label uses of drugs in children. Pediatrics 1999; 104:598–602.

7. Schirm E, Tobi H, de Jong-van den Berg LTW. Risk factors for unlicensed and off-label drug use in children outside of the hospital. Pediatrics 2003;111:291–5.

8. Conroy S, Choonara I, Impicciatore P, et al. Survey of unlicensed and off label drug use in paediatric wards in European countries. BMJ 2000;320:79–82.

9. McKinzie JP, Wright SW, Wrenn KD. Pediatric drug therapy in the emergency department; does it meet FDA-approved prescribing guidelines? Am J Emerg Med 1997;15:118–21.

10. Turner S, Nunn AJ, Fielding K, Choonara I. Adverse drug reactions to unlicensed and off-label drugs on paediatric wards: a prospective study. Acta Paediatr 1999;88:965–8.

11. Feldman BM, Giannini EH. Where's the evidence? Putting the clinical science into pediatric rheumatology. J Rheumatol 1996;23:1502–4.

12. Campbell H, Surry SAM, Royle EM. A review of randomized control trials published in Archives of Disease in Childhood 1982–96. Arch Dis Child 1998;79:192–7.

13. Freedman B, Fuks A, Weijer C. In loco parentis. Minimal risk as an ethical threshold for research upon children. Hastings Center Rep 1993;23:13–9.

14. van Stuijvenberg M, Suur MH, de Vos S, et al. Informed consent, parental awareness, and reasons for participating in a randomised controlled study. Arch Dis Child 1998;79:120–5.

15. American Academy of Pediatrics. Informed consent, parental permission, and assent in pediatric practice. Pediatrics 1995;95:314–7.

16. Weise KL, Smith ML, Maschke KJ, Copeland HL. National practice regarding payment to research subjects for participating in pediatric research. Pediatrics 2002;110:577–82.

17. Food and Drug Administration Modernization and Accountability Act of 1997, Pub. L. No. 105–115 (Nov 21, 1997).

18. NIH policy and guidance on the inclusion of children in research as participants in research involving human subjects. 1998. Office for Protections from Research Risks Report: 98–03. Available at: http://ohrp.osophs.dhhs.gov/humanrights/guidance/hsdc98-03htm (accessed April 2003).

19. Children's Health Act of 2000, Pub. L. No. 106–310 (Oct 17, 2000).

20. Blendon RJ, Altman DE, Benson JM, Brodie M. The implications of the 2000 election. N Engl J Med 2001;344:679–84.

21. Amdur RJ. Improving the protections of human research subjects. Acad Med 2000;75:718–20.

22. Snyderman R, Holmes EW. Oversight mechanisms for clinical research. Science 2000;287:595–7.

23. Sugarman J. The role of institutional support in protecting human research subjects. Acad Med 2000;75:687–92.

24. Yarborough M, Sharp R. Restoring and preserving trust in biomedical research. Acad Med 2002;77:8–14.

25. Corbie-Smith G, Thomas SB, St. George DMM. Distrust, race, and research. Arch Intern Med 2002;162:2458–63.

26. Steinbrook R. Protecting research subjects—the crisis at Johns Hopkins. N Engl J Med 2002;346:716–20.

27. Stolberg GC. The biotech death of Jesse Gelsinger. New York Times Magazine 1999;28:136–140, 149–50.

28. Weiss R. FDA seeks to penalize gene scientist. The Washington Post 2000 Dec 12;Sect. A:14.

29. Levine S. Hopkins researcher faulted in death. The Washington Post 2001 July 17;Sect. B:7.

30. Beecher HK. Ethics and clinical research. N Engl J Med 1966; 274:1354–60.

31. Krugman S, Giles JP, Hammond J. Infectious hepatitis: evidence for two distinctive clinical, epidemiological, and immunological types of infection. JAMA 1967;200:365–73.

32. Heller J. Syphilis victims in US study went untreated for 40 years. New York Times 1972 July 26;Sect. A:1.

33. National Commission for the Protection of the Human Subjects of Biomedical and Behavioral Research. The Belmont report: ethical principles and guidelines for the protection of human subjects of research. Washington (DC): US Government Printing Office; 1979.

34. National Commission for the Protection of Human Subjects. Report and recommendations: research involving children. Washington (DC): Government Printing Office; 1977.

35. Protection of Human Subjects, 45 CFR 46 (2001).

36. Protection of Human Subjects, 45 CFR 46, Subpart A (2001).

37. Protection of Human Subjects, 45 CFR 46, Subpart D (2001).

38. Final report to NHSPAC by the Children's Workgroup. National Human Subject Protections Advisory Committee, Department of Health and Human Services, 2002. Available at: http://ohrp.osophs.dhhs.gov/nhrpac/documents/nhrpac16.pdf (accessed Feb 26, 2003).

39. Protections for children in research: a report to Congress in accord with section 1003 of P.L. 106–310, Children's Health Act of 2000. Office of Human Research Protections, Department of Health and Human Services, 2001. Available at: http://ohrp.osophs.dhhs.gov/reports/ohrp5-02.pdf (accessed Feb 26, 2003).

40. Protection of Human Subjects, 45 CFR Sect. 46.408(b) (2001).

41. Grimes v. Kennedy Krieger Institute. 782 A.2d 807 (Md. 2001), reconsideration denied (Oct 11, 2001).

42. Mastroianni AC, Kahn JP. Risk and responsibility: ethics, Grimes v Kennedy Krieger, and public health involving children. Am J Public Health 2002;92:1073–6.

43. Glantz LH. Nontherapeutic research with children: Grimes v Kennedy Krieger Institute. Am J Public Health 2002;92: 1070–3.

44. American Academy of Pediatrics. Guidelines for the ethical conduct of studies to evaluate drugs in pediatric populations. Pediatrics 1995;95:286–94.

45. Tarnowski KJ, Allen DM, Mayhall C, Kelly PA. Readability of pediatric biomedical research informed consent forms. Pediatrics 1990;85:58–62.

46. Susman EJ, Dorn LD, Fletcher JC. Participation in biomedical research: the consent process as viewed by children, adolescents, young adults, and physicians. J Pediatr 1992;121:547–52.

47. Paasche-Orlow MK, Taylor HA, Brancati FL. Readability standards for informed-consent forms as compared with actual readability. N Engl J Med 2003;348:721–6.

48. Dickert N, Ezekiel E, Grady C. Paying research subjects: an analysis of current policies. Ann Intern Med 2002;136: 368–73.

49. Protection of Human Subjects, 45 CFR 46, Subpart B (2001).

50. Food and Drug. Investigational new drug application: general responsibilities of investigators. 21 CFR 312.60 (1999).

51. Food and Drug. Investigational review board: exemption from IRB requirement. 21 CFR 56.104(c) (1998).

52. Food and Drug. Investigational review board: review of research. 21 CFR 56.109 (1998).

53. Food and Drug. Protection of human subjects: informed consent: elements of informed consent. 21 CFR 50.25(a)(5) (2000).

54. Best Pharmaceuticals for Children Act, Pub. L. No. 107–109 (Jan 4, 2002).

55. FDA proposed rule of pediatric labeling. Federal Register Aug 15, 1997. Final Nov 27, 1998.

56. Steinbrook R. Testing medications in children. N Engl J Med 2002;347:1462–70.

57. Association of American Physicians & Surgeons v. FDA, 226 F.Supp.2d 204 (D.D.C. 2002).

58. Charter Secretary's Advisory Committee on Human Research Protections, Department of Health and Human Services, 2002. Available at: http://ohrp.osophs.dhhs.gov/sachrp/charter.pdf (accessed Feb 26, 2003).

59. Weil E, Nelson RM, Ross LF. Are research ethics standards satisfied in pediatric journal publications? Pediatrics 2002;110: 364–70.

60. Bauchner H, Sharfstein J. Failure to report ethical approval in child health research: review of published papers. BMJ 2001; 323:318–9.

61. Sifers SK, Puddy RW, Warren JS, Roberts MC. Reporting of demographics, methodology, and ethical procedures in journals in pediatric and child psychology. J Pediatr Psychol 2002;27:19–25.

62. Food and Drug. Protection of human subjects: informed consent: exemption from general requirements. 21 CFR 50.23(a)(1)–(4) (2000).

CHAPTER 67

GASTROINTESTINAL ENDOSCOPY

1. *Patient Preparation and General Considerations*

Victor L. Fox, MD

PATIENT AND PARENT PREPARATION

Anticipation and fear of potentially painful procedures provoke intense anxiety in children. These feelings may be compounded by a child's ability to sense parental anxiety. A detailed description of a procedure to the parents and to the patient in terms that are suitable to the child's stage of emotional and intellectual development may relieve some of this anxiety. The preoperative evaluation might also include a brief tour of the procedure facility. Adequate preoperative preparation may reduce anticipatory anxiety and increase patient and family satisfaction with the child's care. It may even have a positive impact on the amount of medication required for adequate sedation.[1] A child should be encouraged to bring attachment objects such as a favorite stuffed animal or blanket to provide comfort and security as he or she enters the strange environment of a hospital or procedure unit. The endoscopist should inquire about past problems with procedures or sedation, thus identifying medical and emotional risk factors that may guide decisions about the optimal procedure setting, type of sedation, and postprocedure monitoring.

A minor hurdle in providing controlled sedation to a child is the establishment of intravenous (IV) access. Premedication with oral[2] or intranasal midazolam[3] and dermal anesthesia using lidocaine preparations such as EMLA (Astra Pharmaceuticals, Wayne, PA) or Numby (IOMED, Inc., Salt Lake City, UT) can reduce the anxiety and pain of inserting an IV catheter. A topical lidocaine or benzocaine anesthetic applied to the posterior pharynx reduces gagging. Sprays work well with most children. Paste can be applied to the pharynx in infants using the tip of a finger or a soft-tipped applicator. Dimmed lights, soft music, comfortable room temperature, familiar objects, and a steady, soothing voice issuing reassuring comments are other environmental comforts that enhance successful sedation in children.[4] Parents are encouraged to accompany their child into the procedure room and during the initiation of sedation unless their own anxiety is too disruptive or stimulating for the child. They should then be escorted to a waiting area during the procedure. The continued presence of a parent during a procedure under sedation has no proven benefit, and distraction of the endoscopist and staff from their primary task is possible.

INFORMED CONSENT

A thoughtful discussion with the patient or guardian about the potential risks and benefits of a procedure should be the initial step in obtaining informed consent. This discussion should also identify the risks of sedation and include alternatives to the proposed procedure. The important elements of this discussion should then be acknowledged in writing. This process of informed consent enhances a sense of trust between patient and physician and provides legal documentation. Clinical investigators must clearly identify and obtain separate consent for any aspects of a procedure that are being conducted solely for the purposes of research. US federal regulations require that children and adolescents provide their "affirmative agreement" (assent) before they are enrolled in any research protocol.[5] Exceptions to this requirement are (1) children unable to provide assent because of age or cognitive abilities and (2) protocols or interventions that directly benefit the patient and are not otherwise available.

DIETARY RESTRICTIONS

Pre-endoscopy dietary restrictions reduce the potential for aspiration of gastric contents during sedation. Patients with large residual gastric fluid volumes with a low pH are at increased risk for aspiration injury.[6] Dietary guidelines are, therefore, primarily designed to minimize the volume of gastric acid at the time of sedation. High-risk patients undergoing deep sedation or general anesthesia (GA) are sometimes given acid-reducing and promotility medications to further reduce volume and elevate the pH of gastric fluid. Stomach contents may also be emptied through a nasogastric tube. Conventional recommendations for a prolonged fast prior to sedation have been challenged by two studies demonstrating the adequacy of a brief fast. Ingebo and colleagues demonstrated that the duration of fasting correlates poorly with the volume of retained gastric fluid at the time of endoscopy and that clear fluids empty rapidly from the stomach in children.[7] Schriener and colleagues found no difference in gastric volume or pH in children allowed clear liquids 2 to 3 hours before induction of anesthesia compared with conventional prolonged fasting.[8]

The following presedation dietary guidelines adapted from the American Society of Anesthesiologists[9] (ASA) are recommended by the Sedation Committee at Children's Hospital, Boston:

- Children should be offered clear liquids (this includes breast milk but not other milk or formula) up to 2 to 3 hours prior to sedation to avoid dehydration.
- Infants less than 6 months may receive formula up to 4 to 6 hours and clear liquids up to 2 hours before sedation.
- For patients older than 6 months, solids and nonclear liquids should be held for 6 to 8 hours before sedation.

SEDATION AND MONITORING

ENDOSCOPY WITH OR WITHOUT SEDATION

With the exception of limited flexible sigmoidoscopy, most endoscopic procedures of the upper and lower gastrointestinal tract are associated with periods of mild to moderate discomfort and sometimes intermittent pain. The duration and severity of discomfort and pain vary with the complexity of the procedure, patient anatomy, equipment used, and the skill of the endoscopist. A procedure may be prolonged or aborted if the patient becomes uncooperative or combative owing to discomfort. Although most endoscopists prefer the use of sedation to enhance the technical success of a procedure and minimize unpleasant recall by the patient, some will withhold sedation in selected cases to reduce additional risk, time, and cost.

Gastrointestinal endoscopy has been performed safely in children without sedation.[10,11] This practice is most often advocated for young infants, less than 6 months of age. However, it is difficult to ethically justify withholding analgesic and hypnotic medications from children who undergo potentially painful or frightening procedures regardless of age.[12] The physiologic stress and emotional trauma imposed on an unsedated child during an uncomfortable procedure are difficult to measure accurately, although they may have a negative impact on future medical encounters. Therefore, most pediatricians and parents endorse the use of sedation when it can be administered safely.

DEPTH OF SEDATION

Despite more than two decades of experience with pediatric endoscopy, controversy remains regarding the preferred depth of sedation and the level of training required to administer sedative medications.[13–15] Confusion over terminology adds to this controversy.[16,17] Levels of sedation are best viewed as a continuum of states that range from mini-

mal sedation (anxiolysis) to GA. Also, the level of sedation in a given patient may fluctuate over time. Moderate sedation, also called "conscious sedation," and deep sedation are controlled states of depressed consciousness whereby the patient maintains protective reflexes. The former describes a patient who is able to respond appropriately to physical stimulation or verbal commands, a state that is often difficult to ascertain in infants and young children. Patients under deep sedation are less arousable and respond less purposefully to pain. GA is a depressed state of consciousness in which the patient is completely unresponsive to painful stimuli and has lost protective reflexes and safe airway support. Because young children often are more anxious and less cooperative than adults, they generally require a deeper level of sedation, at times bordering on GA, to render them motionless. Some endoscopists prefer to enlist the support of an anesthesiologist or specially trained intensivist to induce the necessary level of sedation for an individual patient, while focusing their attention exclusively on the procedure. Other endoscopists will administer sedatives or supervise nurse-administered sedation.

SEDATION RISK FACTORS

A simple anesthesia risk scale used by the ASA for preoperative assessment classifies patients according to their physical status or the presence and severity of systemic disease (Table 67.1-1). ASA class I and II patients and carefully selected class III patients may be safe for IV sedation without airway intervention. Higher risk category patients require anesthesia with complete airway control.

Among ASA class I and II patients, the endoscopist must also consider other factors when choosing an optimal approach for sedation. A history of noisy breathing, nighttime snoring, or sleep apnea should alert the endoscopist to potential difficulties with airway management. Physical findings that may compromise an airway include obesity, short neck or limited neck extension, small mouth, large tongue, tonsillar hypertrophy, deformed palate, small jaw or limited jaw mobility, and generalized or pharyngeal hypotonia. Other general factors include (1) patient age; (2) the patient's prior experience with sedation; (3) expected duration, complexity, and risks of the procedure; (4) sedation, monitoring, and resuscitation skills of the endoscopist and support staff; (5) efficient use of the endoscopist's time and personnel; and (6) cost containment. Transient nonsystemic or mild systemic conditions that

TABLE 67.1-1   AMERICAN SOCIETY OF ANESTHESIOLOGISTS' PHYSICAL STATUS CLASSIFICATION

CLASS	DEFINITION
I	A normal healthy patient
II	A patient with mild systemic disease
III	A patient with severe systemic disease
IV	A patient with severe systemic disease that is a constant threat to life
V	A moribund patient who is not expected to survive without an operation

affect airway risk must also be considered. Mild upper respiratory tract congestion in an awake patient may result in airway obstruction once sedation has been administered. Therefore, elective procedures in children with mild but unresolved upper respiratory tract infection should be deferred until the congestion has cleared.

The jaw thrust maneuver, an oral airway, or a nasopharyngeal airway may be used to acutely improve a compromised airway. However, children with any airway difficulties should have an anesthesia consultation and probable airway intubation for total control.

SEDATION MONITORING

Patients who are sedated require intensive monitoring, additional skilled personnel, and immediately available resuscitation equipment. This requires that one assistant, generally a nurse who is skilled in airway management, devotes exclusive attention to patient monitoring and has no other responsibilities during the procedure.[16] A minimum of two assistants is, therefore, required when sedation is administered for endoscopy in children. One assistant supports the airway, assesses vital signs, and administers medications, whereas the other assists with biopsies or other endoscopic interventions. A third assistant may be needed occasionally to restrain an agitated child.

Essential monitoring equipment includes a transcutaneous pulse oximeter, an electrocardiogram monitor, and a blood pressure monitor, preferably an automated device. Improved technology now permits reliable expired CO_2 or capnography recording in nonintubated patients.[18,19] Although this highly accurate measurement of ventilatory function is now a standard of care for anesthetized patients, its role in monitoring nonanesthetized patients remains to be decided.[9] The endoscopy room must be equipped with a continuous source of pressurized 100% oxygen and additional suction outlets. Resuscitation equipment, including an anesthesia bag with large and small masks, medications, and equipment for airway intubation, and a defibrillator must be immediately available.

MEDICATIONS

For many years, diazepam, a benzodiazepine, and meperidine, a narcotic, were the principal medications used for endoscopy sedation. Although some centers still rely on these medications, others have converted to newer derivatives, midazolam and fentanyl, respectively. Midazolam, roughly equivalent in potency to diazepam, causes minimal pain during IV infusion and provides excellent amnesia. Midazolam alone causes minor respiratory depression but, similar to other benzodiazepines, significantly potentiates the respiratory depression of narcotics.[20] Fentanyl has 1,000 times the potency of meperidine and offers rapid onset and a short duration of action.[21,22] Less urticaria, less nausea, and fewer dysphoric reactions seem to occur with fentanyl than with meperidine.

Midazolam combined with fentanyl produces in children, as in adults, rapid-onset anxiolysis, hypnosis, amnesia, and analgesia, with a relatively brief duration of action

and a comfortable margin of safety against complete loss of consciousness. Following an initial dose, both midazolam and fentanyl are titrated using incremental doses every 3 to 5 minutes until an adequate level of sedation is achieved. Although rarely needed, reversal agents, flumazenil[23] and naloxone, are available for midazolam and fentanyl, respectively. Routine use of flumazenil for children undergoing endoscopy has not shown great benefit.[24] The recommended doses for these medications are listed in Table 67.1-2.

A newer IV sedative-hypnotic agent, propofol, has stimulated considerable interest given its rapid onset and brief duration of action with minimal side effects.[25–29] Propofol is typically used to induce a state of anesthesia. In low intermittent or continuous doses, however, it can be used to achieve deep sedation without GA. Because propofol is associated with a rapid transition to apnea and GA, specialists who are highly skilled in airway management, such as anesthesiologists or intensivists, have generally administered it to children. Yet there is growing interest among adult endoscopists for gastroenterologist-administered or supervised nurse-administered propofol.[30] Although analgesia is less important than sedation for most endoscopic procedures, propofol provides none. Therefore, narcotics or other analgesics should be added to propofol for particularly painful procedures.

The dissociative agent ketamine is another potent sedative that has been administered extensively by nonanesthesiologists to immobilize children. Ketamine possesses a number of properties that are desirable for pediatric endoscopy, including reliable deep sedation, amnesia, and analgesia without cardiopulmonary depression.[31] Enthusiasm for this drug has been tempered by concerns about nightmares and hallucinations, as well as laryngospasm. The former is less of a problem in children than in adults and can be attenuated by premedication with midazolam. The latter problem may result from heightened airway sensitivity and increased secretions.

TABLE 67.1-2   MEDICATIONS FOR SEDATION

MEDICATION	DOSE
Midazolam	Oral, rectal, or nasal presedation: 0.5 mg/kg (maximum dose 20 mg) IV initial dose 0.05 mg/kg (maximum 2.5 mg), then titrate additional doses at 3-min intervals to maximum cumulative dose 0.3 mg/kg or 15 mg, whichever is less.
Fentanyl	IV initial dose 1.0 µg/kg (maximum 50 µg), then titrate additional doses at 5-min intervals to maximum cumulative dose 5 µg/kg or 250 µg, whichever is less
Reversal agents	
Flumazenil	IV 0.01 mg/kg (maximum 0.2 mg); repeat at 1-min intervals to maximum of 0.05 mg/kg or 1.0 mg, whichever is less
Naloxone	IV 1 µg/kg, followed by 2 µg/kg if no response after 90 s, followed by 4 µg/kg if no response after additional 90 s, to a maximum cumulative dose of 400 µg

CLINICAL STUDIES

Few studies have prospectively examined the outcomes of sedation protocols for children undergoing endoscopy,[32–35] and comparison between studies is difficult owing to differences in study design. Sedation studies for endoscopy have often relied on potentially biased reporting by participants rather than use blinded observers. Nonstandardized behavioral rating scales have also been used. Sedation study methodology must incorporate blinding, validation, and reliable behavioral measures to provide useful comparative data.[36,37]

Several studies have examined the outcome of IV sedation for children undergoing endoscopy. Balsells and colleagues, at the Cleveland Clinic, reported satisfactory safety and efficacy of IV sedation in a retrospective review of 2,711 total endoscopic procedures (2,026 patients) over a period of 12 years.[38] In this group, only 96 (3.5%) procedures were performed under GA. The combined major and minor complication rate was only 0.3%, with no deaths, cardiorespiratory arrests, or aspiration events. Colonoscopy was completed to the cecum in 80% of cases. Chuang and colleagues, at the Children's Hospital of Philadelphia, reported their experience with IV sedation in 614 children undergoing upper gastrointestinal endoscopy.[35] The study included 150 infants under 1 year of age, and less than 1% of patients had incomplete procedures owing to inadequate sedation. Only 19 (3.1%) patients had prolonged oxygen desaturation that was easily corrected with supplemental oxygen, and there were no major cardiovascular or respiratory complications. Similarly, in a prospectively entered endoscopy database at Children's Hospital, Boston (V. L. Fox, unpublished data, 1994), 22 of 663 (3.3%) children undergoing upper endoscopy with IV sedation developed clinically significant oxygen desaturation sufficient to interrupt the procedure or require supplemental oxygen. Seven patients (1.7%) required supplemental oxygen postendoscopy, and two patients (0.5%) needed transient assistance with oxygen delivered by anesthesia bag and mask. No cardiopulmonary arrests or aspiration events occurred.

Gilger and colleagues detected a high incidence (79%) of cardiac dysrhythmias in a prospective study of 34 children receiving conscious sedation for endoscopy.[39] However, all of the arrhythmias were transient, and none required intervention. Sinus tachycardia was the most common, and most arrhythmias were temporally associated with transient oxygen desaturation. Twenty-two patients (65%) developed transient oxygen desaturation, and three patients (8.8%) required supplemental oxygen to correct desaturation.

Some pediatric endoscopists advocate GA for the majority of their patients. Anesthesia renders the child completely motionless and free of pain, discomfort, or memory of the events. It shifts the burden of responsibility and liability of sedation to the anesthesiologist, freeing the endoscopist to focus exclusively on the procedure. Modern pediatric anesthesia may provide superior sedation with respect to some outcome measures. Lamireau and colleagues performed a limited prospective study comparing cardiovascular and respiratory changes and operator satisfaction in two groups of 18 children (age range 3 months to 6 years) who underwent esophagogastroduodenoscopy under either IV sedation or GA.[40] Patients receiving GA desaturated less frequently, had a more stable heart rate and mean arterial pressure, and had higher operator satisfaction scores than patients receiving IV sedation. Some pediatric endoscopists fear that such deep sedation, however, may allow for serious mechanical trauma from the endoscope in an unresponsive patient, particularly during colonoscopy. Few pediatric data support this fear, although one perforation was reported in a recent study of 136 children undergoing colonoscopy under GA.[41] Stringer and colleagues prospectively evaluated 250 colonoscopies in 215 children, all performed under GA over a 3.5-year period during which they reported no colonoscopy-related complications.[42]

Squires and colleagues, at the Children's Medical Center of Dallas, prospectively evaluated the efficacy, safety, and cost of IV sedation compared with GA in 226 children undergoing endoscopy.[43] IV sedation was used in 103 and GA in 123 patients. No serious complications occurred in either group. Five (4.8%) cases with IV sedation and none with GA were incomplete owing to inadequate sedation. Procedure room time tended to be longer for children undergoing upper gastrointestinal endoscopy with IV sedation compared with GA, and no significant time difference was seen with colonoscopy. The average charge for the GA group was more than double that of the IV group.

INFECTION CONTROL

Patients and staff must be protected against infections that may be transmitted or acquired during an endoscopic procedure.[44] Although the rate of transmitted infection is estimated to be very low (1 in 1.8 million gastrointestinal endoscopic procedures[45]), the risk is always present, and most exposures are preventable by adhering to well-established protocols for equipment reprocessing.[46] Microorganisms may be spread by contact with contaminated equipment, blood, or other body fluids or tissues. Universal precautions should be practiced when handling blood or tissue samples to prevent contact with human immunodeficiency virus (HIV), hepatitis B virus, hepatitis C virus, and other serious bloodborne infections. Use of needleless injection catheters will reduce the risk of needlestick exposure during administration of IV medications. Endoscopy staff should wear protective gloves, moisture-resistant gowns, and eye protection for personal protection and to prevent cross-contamination.[47] Face shields are superior to standard eyeglasses for protection against splash contamination of eyes and other mucous membranes.

Although single-use disposable accessories have become commonplace, concerns about cost containment and the growing burden of medical waste sustain interest in reusable accessories. Once reusable equipment has been cleaned, the level of disinfection is determined by the type of item. Critical use items are devices that enter sterile tissue or vascular spaces, such as needles, biopsy forceps, and electrocautery snares. These items require sterilization, defined as a process that kills all microbial organisms, including bacterial spores. This is usually accomplished by exposure to heat or ethylene oxide gas. Although endoscope water bottles are not truly critical use items, they are easily resterilized and should be filled with sterile water to prevent waterborne microbial contamination. Semicritical items are devices that contact mucous membranes and nonintact skin, such as endoscopes. These items require high-level disinfection but not sterilization. A variety of chemical germicides are used for high-level disinfection. Glutaraldehyde has been used most commonly for disinfecting gastrointestinal endoscopes, but peracetic acid[48] and hydrogen peroxide have also been used.

There are three important steps in endoscope reprocessing: (1) mechanical cleaning, (2) disinfection, and (3) rinsing and drying. Because biologic debris may be retained inside an endoscope,[49] mechanical cleaning by hand is an essential first step. High-level disinfection may be achieved with immersion in 2% glutaraldehyde solution for a minimum of 20 minutes at a room temperature of 20°C. Then the endoscope must be rinsed free of residual germicide and dried to prevent proliferation of any residual microbes during storage. A final rinse with 70% alcohol facilitates this drying stage. Automated endoscope washers may be used, but they require vigilant surveillance for contamination. Most documented transmitted infections have resulted from a breach in disinfection protocol or a contamination of automated equipment.[50]

ANTIBIOTIC PROPHYLAXIS

Antibiotic prophylaxis (Table 67.1-3) should be used for patients with valvular heart disease, biliary obstruction, or pancreatic pseudocyst. If endoscopy-induced bacteremia or contamination occurred, subsequent infection may be life threatening. Prophylaxis is used to prevent peristomal infection for patients undergoing percutaneous endoscopic gastrostomy.[51] Because there are few data measuring the rates of endoscopy-related bacteremia and infection in children, recommendations for prophylaxis have been extrapolated from adult experience. A low rate of transient bacteremia occurs during most types of endoscopic procedures.[52] Stricture dilation and variceal sclerotherapy may result in higher rates of bacteremia. Bacteremia with colonoscopy in adult patients has been reported in the range of 4 to 5%,[53,54] and infectious sequelae are rarely reported.

There have been two prospective studies in children assessing the rate of bacteremia during endoscopy. Byrne and colleagues studied 75 patients (50 esophagogastroduodenoscopy and 25 colonoscopy).[55] They detected a single episode of bacteremia after esophagogastroduodenoscopy owing to group D *Streptococcus*. El-Baba and colleagues studied 108 patients (68 esophagogastroduodenoscopy, 29 colonoscopy, 11 sigmoidoscopy).[56] Four episodes of bacteremia immediately followed the endoscopy, and all were thought to represent skin contaminants.

Indications for antibiotic prophylaxis must take into account both the rate of bacteremia or bacterial contamination and the vulnerability to severe infectious sequelae for a particular lesion or clinical condition. The American Society for Gastrointestinal Endoscopy (ASGE)[57] and the American Heart Association (AHA)[58] have independently issued updated guidelines for antibiotic prophylaxis. The ASGE guidelines recommend prophylactic antibiotics only for patients with high-risk lesions who undergo procedures with higher rates of bacteremia or contamination. Patients with cardiovascular disease and a history of endocarditis, prosthetic cardiac valve placement, system-pulmonary shunts, complex cyanotic congenital heart disease, and synthetic vascular grafts placed less than 1 year prior, are considered to be at high risk for infectious complications. Procedures associated with a higher rate of bacteremia are esophageal stricture dilation, sclerotherapy for esophageal varices, and endoscopic retrograde cholangiopancreatography with biliary obstruction. In other situations, antibiotic prophylaxis either is not recommended or is left to the endoscopist to choose on a case by case basis. Biliary obstruction and pancreatic pseudocyst are conditions with increased risk for infectious complications following endoscopy and warrant antibiotic prophylaxis independent of endocarditis risk. Infectious sequelae are less likely to occur when adequate drainage has been established. The AHA guidelines tend to be more aggressive than the ASGE guidelines in recommending prophylaxis for moderate-risk cardiac lesions. Major changes in the AHA guidelines include a simplified clinical outcome-based stratification of endocarditis risk categories (Table 67.1-4), elimination of the follow-up dose of antibiotic for oral/dental or low-risk procedures, and elimination of erythromycin as the preferred alternative antibiotic for penicillin-allergic patients.

PROCEDURE COMPETENCE AND TRAINING

Endoscopy in children should be performed by physicians with technical and cognitive skills that are sufficient to complete the task with a high rate of success and minimal

---

TABLE 67.1-3   ANTIBIOTIC PROPHYLAXIS

ENDOCARDITIS PROPHYLAXIS
High risk
    Ampicillin 50 mg/kg (maximum 2 g) and gentamicin 1.5 mg/kg (maximum 120 mg) IV or IM 30 min before the procedure, followed by ampicillin 25 mg/kg (maximum 1 g) IV or IM or amoxicillin 25 mg/kg (maximum 1 g) PO 6 h afterward
Low risk
    Amoxicillin 50 mg/kg (maximum 2 g) PO 1 h before procedure

PENICILLIN ALLERGY
Vancomycin 20 mg/kg (maximum 1 g) IV infused slowly over 1 h beginning 1 h before procedure
Use vancomycin in place of ampicillin or amoxicillin and add gentamicin for high-risk patients

PERCUTANEOUS GASTROSTOMY
Cefazolin 25 mg/kg (maximum 1 g) IV or IM 30 minutes before the procedure

ERCP (for biliary obstruction or pancreatic pseudocyst)
Ampicillin/sulbactam 50 mg/kg (maximum 2 g) IV 30 min before the procedure or cefazolin 25 mg/kg (maximum 1 g) IV or IM 30 min before the procedure

ERCP = endoscopic retrograde cholangiopancreatography.

TABLE 67.1-4   CARDIAC CONDITIONS ASSOCIATED WITH ENDOCARDITIS

ENDOCARDITIS PROPHYLAXIS RECOMMENDED
High-risk category
 Prosthetic cardiac valves, including bioprosthetic and homograft valves
 Previous bacterial endocarditis
 Complex cyanotic congenital heart disease (eg, single-ventricle states, transposition of the great arteries, tetralogy of Fallot)
 Surgically constructed systemic pulmonary shunts or conduits
Moderate-risk category
 Most other congenital cardiac malformations (other than above and below)
 Acquired valvular dysfunction (eg, rheumatic heart disease)
 Hypertrophic cardiomyopathy
 Mitral valve prolapse with valvular regurgitation and/or thickened leaflets

ENDOCARDITIS PROPHYLAXIS NOT RECOMMENDED
Negligible-risk category (no greater risk than the general population)
Isolated secundum atrial septal defect
Surgical repair of atrial septal defect, ventricular septal defect, or patent ductus arteriosus (without residua beyond 6 mo)
Previous coronary artery bypass graft surgery
Mitral valve prolapse without valvular regurgitation
Physiologic, functional, or innocent heart murmurs
Previous Kawasaki disease without valvular dysfunction
Previous rheumatic fever without valvular dysfunction
Cardiac pacemakers (intravascular and epicardial) and implanted defibrillators

complications. The necessary skills are generally acquired through formal training programs in pediatric gastroenterology. Pediatric endoscopy is also performed by pediatric surgeons who are trained in flexible endoscopy and adult gastroenterologists who offer expertise in advanced diagnostic and therapeutic techniques.

The North American Society for Pediatric Gastroenterology and Nutrition (NASPGN) has issued revised guidelines for training in pediatric endoscopy.[59] These guidelines suggest a two-tiered program of training for basic and advanced skills and include a table of minimum threshold numbers (eg, 100 cases each for diagnostic esophagogastroduodenoscopy and diagnostic colonoscopy) that are recommended before competence can be assessed for various procedures. The threshold numbers were adapted from previous ASGE guidelines. The techniques for hemostasis of variceal and nonvariceal bleeding, dilation of strictures, and placement of enteral feeding catheters are listed under advanced training.

The ASGE has also issued updated guidelines for training in endoscopy.[60] The ASGE guidelines were revised after objective evaluation of trainee skills failed to substantiate the previously recommended threshold numbers for assessing procedure competence. Recent data indicate that much higher threshold numbers are required for the average trainee to attain competence. The current ASGE guidelines distinguish between standard and advanced types of procedures and have abandoned threshold numbers in favor of serial assessment of cognitive and technical skills for individual trainees. In contrast to NASPGN guidelines, ASGE guidelines include endoscopic hemostasis, stricture dilation, and enteral access under standard procedures.

Technical competence is defined as achieving 80 to 90% technical success with a specific skill such as intubation of the pylorus during esophagogastroduodenoscopy or intubation of the ileum during colonoscopy. Expert endoscopists are more likely to perform at a level of 95 to 100% technical success. Both the NASPGN and ASGE encourage a formal program of endoscopic training with periodic review of each trainee's progress led by a training director with advanced skills in endoscopy.

QUALITY IMPROVEMENT

Quality assurance is a term used to describe programs that identify and rectify problems leading to unacceptably poor performance or outcomes. In contrast, quality improvement is a term applied to programs that evaluate performance with the goal of continuous improvement beyond minimum standards. Endoscopy units are ideally suited to systematic data collection and multidisciplinary peer review, both core elements of a quality improvement program.[61] The procedure record and pathology reports, combined with clinical outcomes, provide a wealth of data that can be easily monitored and evaluated. Computerized reports may facilitate data collection and analysis. Once important clinical indicators are identified, an individual endoscopist or an endoscopy center can be assessed and compared with internal and external standards of care. Some examples of useful clinical indicators include (1) appropriateness of indications for specific procedures, (2) technical performance or successful procedure completion, (3) adequacy and yield of histopathology samples, (4) sedation- and procedure-related complications, and (5) beneficial clinical outcomes. Data can be used for reporting to hospital officials in charge of renewing clinical staff privileges and to agencies that issue institutional accreditation such as the Joint Commission on Accreditation of Healthcare Organizations.

REFERENCES

1. Mahajan L, Wyllie R, Steffen R, et al. The effects of a psychological preparation program on anxiety in children and adolescents undergoing gastrointestinal endoscopy. J Pediatr Gastroenterol Nutr 1998;27:161–5.
2. Liacouras CA, Mascarenhas M, Poon C, Wenner WJ. Placebo-controlled trial assessing the use of oral midazolam as a premedication to conscious sedation for pediatric endoscopy. Gastrointest Endosc 1998;47:455–60.
3. Fishbein M, Lugo RA, Woodland J, et al. Evaluation of intranasal midazolam in children undergoing esophagogastroduodenoscopy. J Pediatr Gastroenterol Nutr 1997;25:261–6.
4. Gilger MA. Conscious sedation for endoscopy in the pediatric patient. Gastroenterol Nurs 1993;16:75–9.
5. Additional Protections for Children Involved as Subjects in Research. 45 CFR 46, Subpart D (1991).
6. Cote CJ, Goudsouzian NG, Liu LM, et al. Assessment of risk factors related to the acid aspiration syndrome in pediatric patients: gastric pH and residual volume. Anesthesiology 1982;56:70–2.
7. Ingebo KR, Rayhorn NJ, Hecht RM, et al. Sedation in children: adequacy of two-hour fasting. J Pediatr 1997;131:155–0.

8. Schriener MS, Triebwasser A, Keon TP. Ingestion of liquids compared with preoperative fasting in pediatric outpatients. Anesthesiology 1990;72:593–7.

9. Practice guidelines for sedation and analgesia by non-anesthesiologists. A report by the American Society of Anesthesiologists Task Force on Sedation and Analgesia by Non-Anesthesiologists. Anesthesiology 2002;96:1004–17.

10. Hargrove CB, Ulshen MH, Shub MD. Upper gastrointestinal endoscopy in infants: diagnostic usefulness and safety. Pediatrics 1984;74:828–31.

11. Bishop P, Nowicki M, May W, et al. Unsedated upper endoscopy in children. Gastrointest Endosc 2002;55:624–30.

12. Walco GA, Cassidy RC, Schechter NL. Pain, hurt, and harm. The ethics of pain control in infants and children. N Engl J Med 1994;331:541–4.

13. Murphy MS. Sedation for invasive procedures in paediatrics. Arch Dis Child 1997;77:281–6.

14. Ament ME, Brill JE. Pediatric endoscopy, deep sedation, conscious sedation, and general anesthesia—what is best [editorial, comment]? Gastrointest Endosc 1995;41:173–5.

15. Hassall E. Should pediatric gastroenterologists be I.V. drug users? J Pediatr Gastroenterol Nutr 1993;16:370–2.

16. Committee on Drugs of the American Academy of Pediatrics. Guidelines for monitoring and management of pediatric patients during and after sedation for diagnostic and therapeutic procedures. Pediatrics 1992;89:1110–5.

17. Maxwell LG, Yaster M. The myth of conscious sedation. Arch Pediatr Adolesc Med 1996;150:665–7.

18. Vargo JJ, Zuccaro G Jr, Dumot JA, et al. Automated graphic assessment of respiratory activity is superior to pulse oximetry and visual assessment for the detection of early respiratory depression during therapeutic upper endoscopy. Gastrointest Endosc 2002;55:826–31.

19. Lightdale J, Sethna N, Heard L, et al. A pilot study of end-tidal carbon dioxide monitoring using microstream capnography in children undergoing endoscopy with conscious sedation [abstract]. Gastrointest Endosc 2002;55:AB145.

20. Yaster M, Nichols DG, Deshpande JK, Wetzel RC. Midazolam-fentanyl intravenous sedation in children: case report of respiratory arrest. Pediatrics 1990;86:463–5.

21. Singleton MA, Rosen JI, Fisher DM. Plasma concentrations of fentanyl in infants, children, and adults. Can J Anaesth 1987;34:152–5.

22. Ishido S, Kinoshita Y, Kitajima N, et al. Fentanyl for sedation during upper gastrointestinal endoscopy. Gastrointest Endosc 1992;38:689–92.

23. Shannon M, Albers G, Burkhart K, et al. Safety and efficacy of flumazenil in the reversal of benzodiazepine-induced conscious sedation. J Pediatr 1997;131:582–6.

24. Peters J, Tolia V, Simpson P, et al. Flumazenil in children after esophagogastroduodenostomy. Am J Gastroenterol 1999;94:1857–61.

25. White PF. Propofol: pharmacokinetics and pharmacodynamics. Semin Anesth 1988;7:4–20.

26. Rich J, Yaster M, Brandt J. Anterograde and retrograde memory in children anesthetized with propofol. J Clin Exp Neuropsychol 1999;21:535–46.

27. Elitsur Y, Blankenship P, Lawrence Z. Propofol sedation for endoscopic procedures in children. Endoscopy 2000;32:788–91.

28. Hammer GB, Litalien C, Wellis V, Drover DR. Determination of the median effective concentration (EC50) of propofol during oesophagogastroduodenoscopy in children. Paediatr Anaesth 2001;11:549–53.

29. Kaddu R, Bhattacharya D, Metriyakool K, et al. Propofol com-

30. Vargo JJ, Zuccaro G Jr, Dumot JA, et al. Gastroenterologist-administered propofol versus meperidine and midazolam for advanced upper endoscopy: a prospective, randomized trial. Gastroenterology 2002;123:8–16.

31. Green SM, Klooster M, Harris T, et al. Ketamine sedation for pediatric gastroenterology procedures. J Pediatr Gastroenterol Nutr 2001;32:26–33.

32. Figueroa-Colon R, Grunow JE. Randomized study of premedication for esophagogastroduodenoscopy in children and adolescents. J Pediatr Gastroenterol Nutr 1988;7:359–66.

33. Tolia V, Fleming SL, Kauffman RE. Randomized, double-blind trial of midazolam and diazepam for endoscopic sedation in children. Dev Pharmacol Ther 1990;14:141–7.

34. Bahal-O'Mara N, Nahata MC, Murray RD, et al. Efficacy of diazepam and meperidine in ambulatory pediatric patients undergoing endoscopy: a randomized, double-blind trial. J Pediatr Gastroenterol Nutr 1993;16:387–92.

35. Chuang E, Wenner WJ, Piccoli DA, et al. Intravenous sedation in pediatric upper gastrointestinal endoscopy. Gastrointest Endosc 1995;42:156–60.

36. Wilson S. A review of important elements in sedation study methodology. Pediatr Dent 1995;17:406–12.

37. Lightdale J, Scharff L, Sethna N, et al. Validation of a continuous measure of sedation in children undergoing endoscopy [abstract]. J Pediatr Gastroenterol Nutr 2002;35:438.

38. Balsells F, Wyllie R, Kay M, Steffen R. Use of conscious sedation for lower and upper gastrointestinal endoscopic examinations in children, adolescents, and young adults: a twelve-year review. Gastrointest Endosc 1997;45:375–80.

39. Gilger MA, Jeiven SJ, Barrish JO, McCarroll LR. Oxygen desaturation and cardiac dysrhythmias in children during esophagogastroduodenoscopy using conscious sedation. Gastrointest Endosc1993;39:392–5.

40. Lamireau T, Dubreuil M, Daconceicao M. Oxygen saturation during esophagogastroduodenoscopy in children: general anesthesia versus intravenous sedation. J Pediatr Gastroenterol Nutr 1998;27:172–5.

41. Dillon M, Brown S, Casey W, et al. Colonoscopy under general anesthesia in children. Pediatrics 1998;102:381–3.

42. Stringer MD, Pinfield A, Revell L, et al. A prospective audit of paediatric colonoscopy under general anaesthesia. Acta Paediatr 1999;88:199–202.

43. Squires RH, Morriss F, Schluterman S, et al. Efficacy, safety and cost of intravenous sedation versus general anesthesia in children undergoing endoscopic procedures. Gastrointest Endosc 1995;41:99–104.

44. Standards of Practice Committee of the American Society of Gastrointestinal Endoscopy. Infection control during gastrointestinal endoscopy: guidelines for clinical application. Gastrointest Endosc 1999;49:836–41.

45. Kimmey MB, Burnett DA, Carr-Locke DL, et al. Transmission of infection by gastrointestinal endoscopy. Gastrointest Endosc 1993;39:885–8.

46. American Society for Gastrointestinal Endoscopy Ad Hoc Committee on Disinfection. Reprocessing of flexible gastrointestinal endoscopes. Gastrointest Endosc 1996;43:540–6.

47. Technology Committee of the American Society for Gastrointestinal Endoscopy. Personal protective equipment. Gastrointest Endosc 1999;49:854–7.

48. Crow S. Peracetic acid sterilization: a timely development for a busy healthcare industry. Infect Control Hosp Epidemiol 1992;13:111–3.

49. Bond WW, Ott BJ, Franke KA, McCracken JE. Effective use of liquid chemical germicides on medical devices: instrument design problems. In: Block SS, editor. Disinfection, sterilization, and preservation. Philadelphia: Lea and Febiger; 1993. p. 1097–106.

50. Spach DH, Silverstein FE, Stamm WE. Transmission of infection by gastrointestinal endoscopy and bronchoscopy. Ann Intern Med 1993;118:117–28.

51. Jain NK, Larson DE, Schroeder KW, et al. Antibiotic prophylaxis for percutaneous endoscopic gastrostomy. A prospective, randomized, double-blind clinical trial. Ann Intern Med 1987;107:824–8.

52. Schembre D, Bjorkman DJ. Review article: endoscopy-related infections. Aliment Pharmacol Ther 1993;7:347–55.

53. Low DE, Shoenut JP, Kennedy JK, et al. Prospective assessment of risk of bacteremia with colonoscopy and polypectomy. Dig Dis Sci 1987;32:1239–43.

54. Shorvon PJ, Eykyn SJ, Cotton PB. Gastrointestinal instrumentation, bacteremia and endocarditis. Gut 1983;24:1078–93.

55. Byrne WJ, Euler AR, Campbell M, Eisenach KD. Bacteremia in children following upper gastrointestinal endoscopy or colonoscopy. J Pediatr Gastroenterol Nutr 1982;1:551–3.

56. El-Baba M, Tolia V, Lin CH, Dajani A. Absence of bacteremia after gastrointestinal procedures in children. Gastrointest Endosc 1996;44:378–81.

57. Standards of Practice Committee of the American Society for Gastrointestinal Endoscopy. Antibiotic prophylaxis for gastrointestinal endoscopy. Gastrointest Endosc 1995;42: 630–5.

58. Dajani AS, Tabuert KA, Wilson W, et al. Prevention of bacterial endocarditis: recommendations by the American Heart Association. JAMA 1997;277:1794–801.

59. Rudolph CD, Winter HS, and the NASPGN Executive Council, Training and Education Committee, and Contributing Authors. NASPGN guidelines for training in pediatric gastroenterology. J Pediatr Gastroenterol Nutr 1999;29 Suppl 1: S1–26.

60. Committee on Training of the American Society for Gastrointestinal Endoscopy. Principles of training in gastrointestinal endoscopy. Gastrointest Endosc 1999;49:845–53.

61. Standards of Practice Committee of the American Society for Gastrointestinal Endoscopy. Quality improvement of gastrointestinal endoscopy. Gastrointest Endosc 1999;49: 842–4.

2. Upper Gastrointestinal Endoscopy

Michela G. Schaeppi, MD

Jean-François Mougenot, MD

Dominique C. Belli, MD

In the late 1960s, endoscopic equipment saw the development of the fully flexible endoscope. This and further improvements, with smaller diameter and videoendoscopes, made it accessible to pediatrics, allowing its use in almost all ages and weights.[1-4] In 1972, a working group of the European Society of Pediatric Gastroenterology, Hepatology and Nutrition (ESPGHAN) convinced Olympus to develop the first pediatric endoscope. A new dimension was introduced 10 years later with the appearance of therapeutic endoscopy.[5] In the meantime, with advances in sedation and the development of specialized care units, it became increasingly distinct from adult endoscopy.[6-10] At present, endoscopy plays a primary role in the diagnosis and management of pediatric gastrointestinal disorders. As endoscopy has become part of the everyday life of the pediatric gastroenterologist,[11,12] guidelines for training minimums to ensure competence have been issued by the North American Society of Pediatric Gastroenterology and Nutrition,[13,14] the Joint Advisory Group, and, more recently, by the endoscopy steering group of the British Society of Paediatric Gastroenterology, Hepatology and Nutrition.

BEFORE THE PROCEDURE

An important part of the procedure actually takes place before the endoscopy itself. The need for an upper examination being established, preoperative assessment will provide information on both sides. The endoscopist will inquire about past problems with procedures or anesthesia, as well as a personal and family history, to adjust any aspect of the procedure in consequence (eg, administration of antibiotics, discontinuation of some medications). Examination of the child will reveal unusual bruises suspicious of a coagulopathy, physical attributes such as retrognathia or micrognathia, a short neck that can make intubation difficult, or a loose tooth needing to be removed. From the patients' point of view, they and their parents can address questions and concerns while benefits and potential risks are explained to them. It is essential that they are taken through all aspects of the procedure, not only for legal reasons but also to reduce their anxiety. When possible, a brief visit to the day-care unit and endoscopy suite should be proposed. The rooms are child friendly, with toys, decorations, and videotapes. In fact, good psychological preparation is known to reduce not only the stress but also the amount of sedation needed.[15] Part of this assessment can be performed by a trained nurse.

CONSENT

Over the years, informed consent has changed from an ethical notion to a legal requirement. Express consent must be obtained from at least one parent or legal guardian, ideally 24 hours before the procedure. Each unit should develop a code of practice suitable to its mode of operation; nevertheless, written should be preferred to oral consent. In some units, a leaflet is distributed containing the main information. It is the physician's duty to provide information about the nature of the procedure, its reason, and its benefits but also the risks, complications, and alternatives to the procedure. Children should be involved in the discussion, encouraging active participation in their own health care at an age-appropriate level of understanding.[16-24] An increasing number of units let adolescents sign their own consent form, although this has no legal value. The endoscopist should countersign to prove that information was provided. In case of intravenous sedation, some units allow one parent to stay during the procedure. When research biopsies are to be collected, a separate consent should be signed after approval by the institutional review board or local ethical committee.[17,25-30]

PREPARATION

The patient should fast to minimize the risk of pulmonary aspiration. Recognized as a cornerstone in safe practice, the duration of the fasting itself has not reached worldwide consensus, and every institution follows its own protocol.[31] In an attempt to rectify this, guidelines have been established,[32,33] and we recommend that gastroenterologists read those published in the country of practice. However, some general lines can be drawn: the conventional 8-hour fast applied in adult practice is suitable only for the older child. General consensus allows a last feed 4 hours prior to sedation in those 0 to 5 months old. Some institutions are more flexible and allow clear fluid, including breast milk, to be given up to 2 hours prior to sedation. In older children, feeds will be stopped 6 hours before sedation.

Adequate venous access is important not only for administration of medication but also in case quick reversal is needed. It is good practice to check patency just before the start of the procedure.

DURING THE PROCEDURE

MONITORING

At present, pediatric patients undergoing an endoscopy must have some sort of sedation. The use of the different agents available is discussed below; however, all can cause side effects and, at times, unpredictable reactions. Therefore, cardiopulmonary monitoring is essential to provide optimum safety and conditions for both the patient and the endoscopist.[34] The basic equipment includes a pulse oximeter, to monitor oxygen saturation and heart rate, a pressurized oxygen source, and a suction outlet. A ventilation bag with age-appropriate–sized masks and suction tubes should be ready and checked before the start of each procedure. Most equipment also includes a blood pressure monitoring device. In addition, an immediately accessible resuscitation trolley is an essential element. The last important factor for the comfort and safety of the patient is the room temperature, which should be adjustable and appropriate for the age to avoid hypo- or hyperthermia. The safest practice is that one person, a nurse or a physician, trained in pediatric life support is fully dedicated to the vital signs surveillance throughout the procedure.

SEDATION

Potential complications of upper endoscopy among children must not be underestimated and are related to both endoscopy methods and the medications used for sedation. The most frequent complication in endoscopy is slight to profound hypoxemia, which is mainly due to sedation, resulting in a dispute between the advocates and opponents of the need for sedation in adult cooperative patients. Unsedated upper endoscopy in children has also been documented and judged to be safe and feasible in motivated children.[35] However, 80% of these patients would choose to have sedation if upper endoscopy was to be repeated.

From a pediatric point of view, there is no doubt that children are unable to express their pain and fear. Consequently, the rationale and aims of sedation are evident in pediatrics and are shown in Table 67.2-1. At present, this attitude is shared by both American[36] and English[37] adult gastroenterologists because only 2% of physicians perform endoscopy without any medication in these countries. Furthermore, sedation must be administered to all pediatric patients, especially in infants and young children,[38] because pain is a real problem in medically and surgically treated pediatric patients, even neonates.[39]

Preparatory information and psychological preparation are mandatory before esophagogastroduodenoscopy (EGD). Indeed, they can reduce anxiety and procedural distress in both adults and children.[40] Furthermore, less sedation seems to be necessary after good psychological preparation.[41] In addition, a calm and relaxed atmosphere in the examination room is recommended. In our experience, hypnosis can also be of great help to patients who need repeated procedures.

Local anesthetic agents are widely used by adult[37] and pediatric gastroenterologists. Local anesthesia can be a good complement to intravenous sedation. Indeed, the amount of medication necessary seems to be reduced owing to the lack of pharyngeal stimulation. In our experience, this positive effect is correlated to the level of sedation depth, being more effective in the "lighter" sedation regimen. When used, local anesthesia with lidocaine, without exceeding a dose of 5 mg/kg body weight, can be recommended.

As regards pharmacologic sedation, the most important goals are maximal comfort, endoscopy amnesia, and a short-term effect drug, leading to short time of onset of sedation, length of procedure, and recovery time. The widespread use of sedation in EGD in children imposes the need for resuscitation and monitoring equipment in the endoscopy room. Standard monitoring must include an electrocardiogram, a blood pressure monitor, and a pulse oximeter. Pediatric anesthesiologists are becoming increasingly involved in this process because the risk of disaster is great when a child is sedated and scoped by the same person.

The types of sedation can be described as follows:

- Intramuscular "lytic or so-called Toronto cocktail"
- Intravenous diazepam or midazolam alone
- Intravenous diazepam or midazolam with meperidine, fentanyl, or alfentanil (± atropine)
- Intravenous propofol
- Miscellaneous drugs
- Endotracheal anesthesia

Half-life time and bolus dose of drugs used for sedation are shown in Table 67.2-2. It is important to note that half-life times are often different between children and adults.

Historically, the combination of intramuscular meperidine, promethazine, and chlorpromazine, the so-called "lytic or Toronto cocktail,"[42] was used for a large variety of pedi-

TABLE 67.2-1   AIMS OF SEDATION IN PEDIATRIC GASTROINTESTINAL ENDOSCOPY

To give maximal comfort to the child during endoscopy
To aim for amnesia of endoscopy
To facilitate quick, precise, and safe endoscopy
To use safe and short half-time agents that provide a rapid onset and effective sedation with minimal side effects

TABLE 67.2-2   HALF-LIFE TIME AND BOLUS DOSE OF DRUGS USED FOR SEDATION DURING ESOPHAGOGASTRODUODENOSCOPY

DRUG	T½ (H) CHILD 3–10 YR	T½ (H) ADULT	IV BOLUS DOSE
Diazepam	7–18	20–50	0.1–0.2 mg/kg BW
Midazolam	1.2	2–3	0.1 mg/kg BW
Meperidine	1.5–4	2–5	1–2 mg/kg BW
Fentanyl	1.1	2.5–5	1–3 µg/kg BW
Alfentanil	1.0	1.6	7.5–10 µg/kg BW
Ketamine	2.2	2.5–2.8	2 mg/kg BW
Propofol	0.5	4–7	2–3.5 mg/kg BW

BW = body weight; IV = intravenous

atric procedures. Nevertheless, the efficacy of its sedative effect is limited in EGD, and an intravenous sedation must be favored. Benzodiazepines were the most routinely used method of sedation because of their anxiolytic, sedative, amnesic, and muscle-relaxing properties. Among them, diazepam was the usual choice for many years; however, its half-life time is long, discouraging its use in newborn and young children. Moreover, diazepam has respiratory-depressing effects, especially when combined with narcotics.[43] At present, midazolam replaces diazepam because it has more sedative potency, more anterograde amnesic activity, and fewer local effects at the injection site.[44] In addition, midazolam has a short time of uptake and elimination. The effective bolus dose is of 0.1 to 0.2 mg/kg body weight. It also has a potent respiratory negative effect, which is dose dependent and enhanced by concomitant use of opioids. To shorten the total time of EGD, some adult gastroenterologists recommend reversing the effect of midazolam. However, this would not seem necessary in children because they recover rapidly after correct medication.

Opioids have also been used for many years and are synergistic with benzodiazepines.[45] They are useful in providing analgesia and sedation, as well as in decreasing the need for other drug requirement and allowing smooth recovery. Their disadvantages include nausea, vomiting, respiratory depression, hypotension, dysphoria, hallucinations, and bile duct spasm. Meperidine is a long-acting narcotic analgesic that is commonly used in pediatric EGD even if it does not represent a modern anesthesiologist approach.[46] This is explained by its large safety margin in the inexpert hands of endoscopists. Doses for intravenous sedation are a bolus of 1 to 2 mg/kg body weight and should then be titrated. Meperidine is generally used with benzodiazepine,[44,47] and 80% of patients have total amnesia after the procedure.[48] As a combination of drugs was advocated to improve the quality of sedation, other drugs were tested alone or in combination. Among them, fentanyl (1–3 µg/kg body weight) and alfentanil (7.5–10 µg/kg body weight) were studied because of their quicker effect. In a study, we compared a combination of alfentanil-midazolam with meperidine-midazolam.[38] Alfentanil-midazolam had a shorter sedation time and recovery period, with a lower risk of hypoxemia.

The recent development of propofol, a sedative-hypnotic agent, has led to an improved quality of sedation during pediatric EGD.[49] The main advantages of this drug are rapid recovery, less prolonged sedation, and a lower incidence of nausea. The dose is 1 to 3.5 mg/kg body weight as a bolus, followed by a titrated infusion of 0.1 to 0.3 mg/kg body weight/min. Propofol can be used in association with benzodiazepine.

Other drugs have been proposed: intramuscular ketamine, especially in children older than 7 years,[50] or inhaled anesthetic gas. Chloral hydrate and atropine are frequently used in addition to a standard regimen of sedation.

Finally, endotracheal anesthesia is rarely performed because effective deep intravenous sedation is satisfactory in most cases. It can be used for young children (< 2 years), for patients who undergo upper and lower endoscopy in the same session, or for interventional procedures.

ANTIBIOTIC PROPHYLAXIS

A transient bacteremia seldom occurs during a procedure and is usually cleared spontaneously by healthy patients.[51] The reported incidence ranges from 0.5 to 4.2% for diagnostic EGD.[51–55] It is important to distinguish diagnostic endoscopy from therapeutic endoscopy, which carries a higher incidence: 8.9% for variceal ligation, 11% for endoscopic retrograde cholangiopancreatography, 15.4% for variceal sclerotherapy, and 22.8% for esophageal dilation.[53,56]

The incidence might even be lower in the pediatric population as shown by the two prospective studies carried out to determine the incidence of bacteremia that identified 1 episode in 75[54] and 4 probable contaminations in 108 children.[57] Neither mucosal biopsy nor polypectomy seems to be a risk factor.[58,59] These episodes of bacteremia are asymptomatic and short-lived. The most feared complication, endocarditis, is reported in a few patients,[60,61] mainly those with risk factors.[52,54,56,62–65] Antibiotic prophylaxis has been demonstrated to be efficient and to diminish incidence by 49%.[66] Over the years, the number of patients with a cardiac implant has steadily increased, yet no evidence of any increase in the incidence of endocarditis has been reported. To answer the question of which patient should benefit from prophylaxis, guidelines have been established by several organizations.[67–74] On average, about 1 to 3% of patients undergoing endoscopy will need prophylaxis.[75] Despite these publications, inappropriate use of antibiotics reaches up to 90% of cases, with a tendency to overtreat patients,[76,77] although failure to treat is also reported.[78] The institution of a mechanism for continuous quality improvement, as simple as monthly meetings, could significantly reduce overprescription by half.[76]

Most pediatric centers use protocols following the guidelines issued by the American Heart Association (AHA) and the American Society of Gastroenterological Endoscopy (ASGE)[68,79] recommending administration of prophylactic antibiotics only in selective situations.[74] Specific clinical conditions recognized as such are cardiac lesions with high or moderate risk of bacterial endocarditis.[80–83] Durack has established a list of high, moderate, and low risks, which are summarized in Table 67.2-3.[51] Available recommendations are not standardized, with the ASGE proposing prophylaxis only in high-risk patients, whereas, recently, the AHA proposed a simplified regimen for moderate-risk patients. It consists of dropping the gentamicin and the second dose of antibiotics. The latter dose is thought to be unnecessary because prolonged serum levels above the minimal inhibitory concentration are obtained with amoxicillin.[84,85] Whereas the parenteral route is recommended in the first group, oral administration is proposed as a choice in the latter. Mitral valve prolapse is addressed specifically by Dajani, and physicians treating such a patient should refer to his publication.[70]

Other special conditions are immunocompromised, either neutropenic or immunosuppressed, children. Neutropenia, depending on the level of cells, is seen as either a high (neutrophils < 100 × 10⁹/L) or a moderate (neutrophils 100–500 × 10⁹/L) risk in Europe[73,86] but not in America and Canada.[68] An American-Canadian survey of

TABLE 67.2-3	CARDIAC INFECTION RISK LEVEL	
HIGH RISK	**MODERATE RISK**	**NEGLIGIBLE RISK**
Prosthetic valve	Congenital malformations	Isolated ASD
Surgically constructed pulmonary shunt or conduit	Acquired valvular dysfunction	Surgical repair ASD, ventricular septal defect, patent ductus arteriosus
Previous endocarditis	Hypertrophic cardiomyopathy	Pacemakers
Complex congenital cyanotic heart disease	Mitral valve prolapse with regurgitation and/or thickened leaflets	Physiologic or functional heart murmurs
		Previous Kawasaki disease or rheumatic fever without valvular dysfunction

ASD = atrial septal defect.

current practice in 15 pediatric gastroenterology centers showed that only 20% give antibiotics for upper endoscopy and 33% for lower endoscopy, yet no data on the rate of infectious complications were reported.[74] Patients carrying a central line, a ventriculoperitoneal shunt, or an orthopedic implant are also problematic patients, for which no recommendations are published. In the same study, current practice indicates that 20% will give antibiotics for upper endoscopy and 40% for lower endoscopy.[74] The final decision should be made case by case, leaving room for clinical judgment and experience.

Gram-positive bacteria are the most commonly implicated germs. Therefore, in case of cardiac risk, the recommended regimen is as follows[73,74]:

- A combination of ampicillin (50 mg/kg, maximum 2 g) and gentamicin (2 mg/kg, maximum 120 mg) intravenously or intramuscularly 30 minutes prior to the procedure. Some centers will give an additional oral dose of amoxicillin (25 mg/kg) 6 hours later or ampicillin (25 mg/kg, maximum 1 g) intravenously.
- In patients allergic to penicillin, amoxicillin is replaced by vancomycin (20 mg/kg, maximum 1g) or teicoplanin (6 mg/kg).

In addition to cardiac risks, several conditions need special attention:

1. In neutropenic patients, infections can be caused by anaerobes; as a result, metronidazole (7.5 mg/kg) is added to the above regimen.
2. In patients with central lines, prosthetic material (especially orthopedic), ventriculoperitoneal shunt, or ascites,[87] some centers recommend the use of prophylactic antibiotics.
3. During interventional procedures (stricture dilation, sclerotherapy, percutaneous endoscopic gastrostomy [PEG]), a prophylaxis is mandatory because the risk of complication following infection is higher. For example, the rate of skin infection is higher in PEG without antibiotic prophylaxis.[88]

AFTER THE PROCEDURE

MONITORING

The monitoring set during the procedure will be continued, particularly for small infants for the next 15 to 30 minutes, either in the recovery room or on the ward. If asleep, the patient is placed in the lateral position. If midazolam was used, the child stays on the ward for a minimum of 2 hours. Parents are informed that amnesia is a common effect of the drug and can last up to 8 hours. Drinks are allowed 1 hour after the end of the endoscopy; special attention is brought to the deglutition if anesthetic spray was used to avoid choking.

CLEANING THE SCOPES

Contaminated equipment can transmit infection either from one patient to another or, less commonly, to staff. Implicated germs can be either pathogenic or opportunistic in the case of the immunocompromised patient. Proper and adequate cleaning is a major concern for the patient's and staff's safety. Thus, guidelines have been formulated and modifications made in recent years by several societies.[67,89–92]

Legal Rules. Endoscopes, accessories, disinfectants, sterilizing devices, and washing machines are submitted to local laws. For example, in Europe, they must be in conformity with the European rules.

Levels of Disinfection. Three categories to which medical devices can be assigned are critical, semicritical, and noncritical. Noncritical items (eg, floors, walls, blood pressure cuffs, and furniture) come into contact with intact skin but not with mucous membranes. Semicritical items are devices that come into contact with intact mucous membranes or skin that is not intact. In general, these items should be free of all microorganisms, with the exception of small numbers of bacterial spores. The flexible scopes (gastroscope, duodenoscope, and colonoscope) are referred to as semicritical or class II. They need a high level of disinfection with mycobactericidal, viricidal, and sporicidal activity, the necessary exposure time being determined by the time it takes to inactivate 10^6 resistant non–spore-forming test microorganisms, including, for example, hepatitis B virus, human immunodeficiency virus (HIV), and *Mycobacterium tuberculosis* var. bovi. Items assigned to the critical category present a high risk of infection because they penetrate skin or mucosa or come into contact with normally sterile tissues or the vascular system. They need sterilization when possible; if not achievable, liquid chemical germicides can be used with long exposure. Accessories are defined as such; therefore, grasping forceps, polypectomy snares, injection needles, and cytology brushes should be sterilized or disposed of.

Disinfectants. Two percent glutaraldehyde is the most widely used product. At room temperature, it inactivates most bacteria in 1 minute, HIV in 2 minutes, and hepatitis B virus in less than 5 minutes.[93–98] For hepatitis C virus, the risk persists because ribonucleic acid can be present in the operating channel and on the biopsy forceps, and a longer washing time (20 minutes) is necessary.[95,96,99] The same washing time will eliminate microbacteria, in particular *M. tuberculosis*. Although this risk has not been described in digestive endoscopy, it is important to remember that some equipment can be shared with bronchoscopes, a device that can be in contact with such germs.

Glutaraldehyde creates frequent adverse reactions that can be severe. Reports of allergy, dermatitis,[100] conjunctivitis,[101] and rhinitis and asthma [102–104] in staff and colitis in patients, owing to improperly cleaned scopes, have been made.[105,106] To limit these disadvantages, procedures take place in a dedicated room, well ventilated with a minimum of 12 volumes/hour.

A suitable alternative is peracetic acid (0.2–0.35%), which has the advantage of being less of an irritant; however, it is more expensive and less stable than glutaraldehyde. It acts by releasing free oxygen and hydroxyl radicals. It has rapid activity against vegetative bacteria, mycobacteria, fungi, and viruses.[107–109] It can cause cosmetic damage to the scopes, but without functional alterations. It can be used in association with hydrogen peroxide (7.5%). It has bactericidal and viricidal activity after 5 minutes and kills spores and mycobacteria in 10 minutes.

Chloride acid and superoxide water are highly microbicidal and are used in some units. The ASGE recommends a final rinse with 70% alcohol for its drying effect on the channels.

Tap water is usable for manual washing of semicritical scopes, but sterile water is necessary for the cleaning of critical ones. For the washer or disinfectors, the water has to be of level II (< 10 opportunistic microorganisms/100 mL at 22°C and 37°C, without *Pseudomonas aeruginosa*). This quality of water is obtained by using filters (0.2–5 μm).

Biologic Controls. Hospital tap water should be controlled on a regular basis, in particular for the presence of *P. aeruginosa*. Final rinse of the scopes requires a microbiologic quality of level I: < 100 opportunistic microorganisms/100 mL at 22°C and 37°C, without *P. aeruginosa* per 100 mL.

Regular checking (once per trimester) of the scopes is necessary by swabs at the level of the canals, exits, outer sheath, and biopsy cap. This allows the identification of poor technique and the modification of clinical practice.[110] In case of contamination after glutaraldehyde sterilization, 50 mL of a sterile mixture containing Tween 80–lecithin is injected in each canal or 200 mL from a common irrigator. If the bottles of liquid lavage, the cleaning water, and the knobs are autoclaved, the vehicle responsible for the contamination is often the biopsy channel. A new washing cycle needs to be performed, including an alkaline enzymatic washing product for 15 minutes and a phase of sporicidal disinfection for 60 minutes. If the problem persists, the scope should be sent to the manufacturer, which will decide if the internal sheaths need to be changed. The remaining water in the washer or disinfectors, along with the incoming water, needs to be checked monthly.

Flexible endoscopes cannot be autoclaved. For the material that tolerates it, water vapor at a temperature of 134°C for 18 minutes should be used after a wash without glutaraldehyde.

Recently, there has been concern about Creutzfeldt-Jakcob disease (CJD) and neurodegenerative diseases in general. Their causative agent, the prion, is resistant to most physical and chemical inactivation methods; therefore, endoscopy should be reconsidered and avoided whenever possible. In pediatric endoscopic procedures with no potential risk, the above disinfection rules are estimated as sufficient by most sanitary authorities. On the contrary, the recommendation from the Gastroenterologists Working Party of the British Society of Gastroenterology Endoscopy Committee is to destroy and incinerate material used in a patient with definite disease because no safe way to guarantee prion eradication exists.[111–113] This point of view is more severe than the recommendation from infectious disease specialists suggesting that standard cleaning and high-level disinfection protocols would be adequate for reprocessing.[114] In patients suspected of CJD, no endoscopy should be scheduled before confirmation of the disease. Any patient presenting with neurologic signs or recent progressive dementia should be suspected of CJD. In patients at risk of CJD (having received extracted growth hormone or gonadotropin, a family member of a potential or confirmed case, neurosurgical intervention before 1994), the washing of the scope includes two cycles with alkaline without aldehyde for a minimum of 15 minutes before a rinse with tap water and then disinfection with glutaraldehyde. The infectivity of the variant CJD seems to affect the peripheral tissues before the brain. The protein prion (PrPsc) has been found in lymphoid tissues (tonsil, rectum,[115,116] appendix[117]). Although declared cases are rare (less than 150 people globally),[118] the endoscopy remains a risk for infection, and a supplementary chemical inactivation after the two added washes is recommended. Its efficacy on prion has not been proven. Sodium hypochlorite at 6°C or bleach can be used if it does not damage the scopes.

Cleaning of the Scopes. Manual. Because nonimmersible endoscopes have practically disappeared from practice, only the steps of cleaning and disinfection of immersible ones are addressed in this section. Disinfection is carried out at the start of the session, between cases, and at the end of the day. Scope attribution is decided before the start of the list to allow alternation and diminish waiting time and stress.

Pretreatment takes place in the endoscopy room. Still connected to the light source, air and water channels are flushed with water for at least 15 seconds to expel all organic material using a special valve supplied by the manufacturer for this purpose. The aim is to thoroughly remove all organic material and blood prior to any contact with disinfectant. Premature contact with the latter will fix the proteins, creating debris in which organisms can become imbedded and keeping them out of reach. All channels are flushed with a detergent solution, without aldehyde. The instrument is then disconnected, and caps are fitted when required (videoendoscopes). A cleaning brush is passed through the suction or biopsy channel until it comes back visually clean.

The instrument is tested for leaks and checked for faults or damage before being fully immersed in neutral or enzymatic detergent. All removable parts (water or air, suction valves, biopsy cap) are removed, the scope is washed, and the distal end, knobs, and valves are individually scrubbed with a soft toothbrush. An all-channel irrigator is put in place, and the channels are irrigated with the solution (minimum of 150 mL) for at least 5 minutes. This step is crucial because it markedly reduces microbial contamination load[119,120] and contamination of multiple-use forceps.[121] The scope and accessories are rinsed under fresh tap water and the channels are irrigated (minimum 300 mL) before air is insufflated to remove fluid residue. All of the equipment is immersed in the disinfectant for the correct contact time, depending on the level of disinfection that needs to be achieved: with 2% glutaraldehyde, according to the ASGE and the French Society of Digestive Endoscopy (FSDE), 10 to 20 minutes for intermediate level and 60 minutes for high level, and, according to the ASGE, FSDE, and the Asia-Pacific Congress of Digestive Endoscopy, 10 to 20 minutes before/after storage[92,122–125]; with peracetic acid, 5 minutes for intermediate level and 10 minutes for high (sporicidal) level.[113,124] The dilution needs to be respected and not fall below 1 to 1.5%.[114] Endoscopes and valves are rinsed with a large volume of water, 300 mL passed through the channels to avoid toxic reactions (colitis). Tap water, preferably with filter, is used when an intermediate level of disinfection is necessary and sterile water if a high level is wanted. Once more, the agent is eliminated by air insufflation. Endoscopes are connected to the light source and forced air-dried. They are then stored hanging vertically in a designated ventilated cupboard. Valves and the biopsy cap are removed and lubricated with silicone oil.

Disinfectant solution needs to be changed depending on the physicochemical stability of the product itself and the number of procedures carried out. Any cloudy solution should be renewed.

Automated Washer and Disinfectors. These machines are being used increasingly in the endoscopy suite. They need regular maintenance and control. These machines have the advantage of providing standardized disinfection and rinse, heat to optimize the process, filtered tap water, automatic record of the washing parameters, and a closed system diminishing exposure to fumes. It should be stressed that some crucial cleaning steps still need to be performed manually: the cleaning itself, the check for leaks, the alcohol rinse, and forced air drying.

Accessories. Reprocessing of these medical devices is a subject of discussion. The complexity of the material (crevices, wire coils, retractable components) and the fact that they breach mucosa classify them as critical. Therefore, they need to be sterilized or disposable. The standardized protocol for reprocessing has been shown to be reliable.[126] Recommendations are that single-use accessories are encouraged when available. Reprocessing and reuse of medical equipment intended for single use has clinical and legal implications.[127] Some working groups propose that consent should be obtained if reuse is intended.[123] However, the cost implications also raise some concerns.[128]

Some accessories that are difficult to clean can be ultrasonically (> 30 kHz) cleaned prior to disinfection or autoclaving. Sterilization should be achieved with water vapor at 134°C for a minimum of 18 minutes, the so-called "prion cycle."

Environment. Owing to common adverse reactions to glutaraldehyde, specific criteria relating to exposure levels have been established. They are defined in terms of average exposure standard and maximum exposure level, which are issued in most countries. The maximum exposure level is 0.05 ppm of glutaraldehyde in the United Kingdom and 0.2 ppm in France.

Staff. Endoscopy staff should be trained not only in the correct use of the equipment but also in case of spillage. All staff coming in contact with glutaraldehyde need to complete a health questionnaire and perform yearly lung function tests. Gloves and disposable aprons should be worn and changed regularly because they absorb the substance. Staff are also strongly advised to be vaccinated against hepatitis B.

INDICATIONS

The indications vary with age because newborn babies do not present with the same pathologies as adolescents. Table 67.2-4 shows the indications divided into three age groups.

GASTROESOPHAGEAL REFLUX

One of the major indications for EGD is gastroesophageal reflux (GER) and its complications. GER is defined by the involuntary passage of gastric content into the esophagus. The main pathophysiologic cause of GER is transient relaxation of the lower esophageal sphincter. Patients can present with dysphagia, odynophagia, hematemesis, anemia, weight loss, failure to thrive, epigastric or retrosternal pain, unexplained vomiting, spitting, or irritability depending on their age. Furthermore, abnormal anatomic conditions, such as hiatal hernia, can lead to GER. The diagnosis of hiatal hernia is made when the ascension of

TABLE 67.2-4   INDICATIONS OF ESOPHAGOGASTRODUODENOSCOPY

NEONATES AND INFANTS	TODDLERS	TEENAGERS
Vomiting	Abdominal pain	Abdominal pain
Hematemesis, melena, hematochezia	Hematemesis, melena	Dyspepsia
Apnea	Vomiting	Hematemesis, hematochezia, melena
Failure to thrive	Dysphagia, odynophagia	Weight loss
Diarrhea	Foreign body	Chronic reflux symptoms
Irritability, Sandifer syndrome	Caustic ingestion	Chronic diarrhea
	Chronic diarrhea	Iron deficiency anemia
	Chronic constipation	Caustic ingestion
	Suspected polyp	Cancer surveillance

the Z line is observed more than 2 cm above the esophageal hiatus. Although in newborns, the junction between the pale pink esophageal epithelium and the darker red gastric one takes place at the level of the diaphragmatic hiatus (pinch), with age, it has a tendency to move upward. The Z line is slightly irregular or undulating. The disappearance of multiple small linear vessels at this level helps to identify it. In moderate to severe hiatal hernia, the mucosal gastric folds slide above the diaphragmatic pinch, giving an aspect of pouch (Figures 67.2-1 and 67.2-2). With a deep breath, this becomes even more apparent as the folds move over the hiatus, particularly in retrovision.

The diagnosis of peptic esophagitis is made endoscopically. The typical lesion is a round or linear erosion with focal erythema, exudate, or ulceration usually perpendicular to the longitudinal axis. It is always localized in the lower third of the esophagus. When multiple lesions are present, they can converge and give a stellar shape. The response to treatment and prognosis depends on the gravity of the lesions seen. Thus, it is crucial to evaluate the severity of the esophagitis, which is graded from 0 to 5 (Table 67.2-5). Grade 0 corresponds to a normal esophagus; grades 1A, 1B, and 1C to reflux lesions; and above grade 2 to different severity of esophagitis. It is important to avoid confusion of grade 2 with the normal circumferential cardial redness seen in the newborn (Figures 67.2-3 and 67.2-4). This characteristic aspect is due to specific distribution of intramural veins running in the lamina propria at the level of the upper esophageal sphincter. These vessels can be seen only with the new generation of video-endoscopes.

The exact localization of the lesion is noted. The importance of biopsies remains a subject of controversy because good-quality material is difficult to obtain.[129,130] The percentage of uninterpretable biopsies can be as high as 59% for grasp and 23% for suction. With an adequate

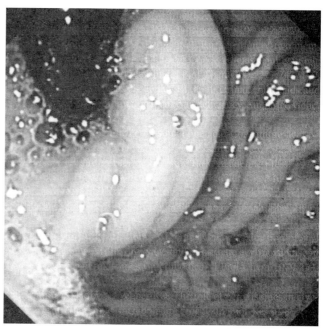

FIGURE 67.2-2   Nissen fundoplication in retroversion.

technique, good mucosal biopsies can be obtained with grasp forceps and evaluated under a microscope. Erosions and ulcerations associated with an inflammatory infiltrate are seen only in patients suffering from severe esophagitis. In fact, it is useful to take biopsies in a patient suspected of GER with a macroscopically normal esophagus. Two biopsies will be taken 2 or 3 cm above the Z line and fixed in formol.[131] The ESPGHAN has established criteria to help the correlation of histologic findings with diagnosis (Table 67.2-6). The presence of basal zone hyperplasia of the epithelium, elongated stromal papillae, and vascular ingrowth reflects reflux, whereas inflammatory infiltrate, ulceration, or modification of the epithelium confirms a microscopic esophagitis.[129,131–134]

Endoscopic examination is the only way to diagnose and establish the extent of Barrett esophagus. The typical lesion is an orange-pink spot standing out on the gray-white squamous mucosa (Figure 67.2-5).[135] Because it is frequently described in published pediatric series, it should be suspected in cases of peptic stenosis. Its existence is possible when the Z line is more than 3 cm above the superior limit of the gastric folds, with or without the presence of hiatal hernia. The use of vital colorants, such as Lugol or

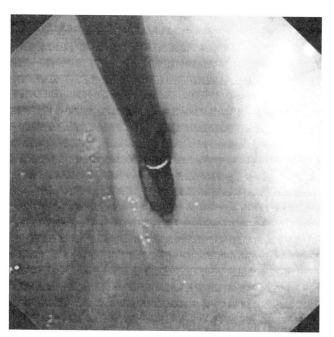

FIGURE 67.2-1   Hiatal hernia in retroversion.

TABLE 67.2-5   ESOPHAGITIS GRADE

GRADE	ASPECT
0	Normal mucosa
1	Unique or multiple, nonconfluent erythema, loss of vascular pattern or exudate appearing as red patches or stiae
2	Longitudinal noncircumferential erosions with a hemorrhagic tendency of the mucosa, with friability (bleeding to light touch: 2A) or spontaneous bleeding (2B)
3	Identical lesions with circumferential tendency
4	Ulcers, metaplasia (4A) or stricture (4B)
5	Endobrachyesophagus associated with any of the above lesions

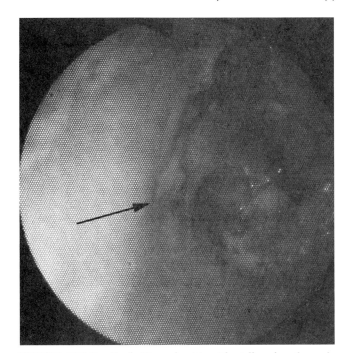

FIGURE 67.2-3   Grade II esophagitis with stellar ulcer (*arrow*).

TABLE 67.2-6   HISTOLOGIC AND DIAGNOSTIC
                 CORRELATION

GRADE	HISTOLOGY	DIAGNOSIS
0	Normal mucosa	Normal esophagus
1A	Basal zone hyperplasia	Reflux
1B	Elongated stromal papillae	
1C	Vascular ingrowth	
2	Inflammatory infiltrate of the lamina propria	Esophagitis
3	Inflammatory infiltrate of the epithelium	
4	Ulceration	
5	Aberrant columnar epithelium	

imposes a surveillance with an EGD and multiple biopsies every 2 years after 10 years of age. As a matter of fact, upper endoscopy is a crucial tool in the diagnosis and follow-up of peptic esophagitis and Barrett esophagus.[145]

UPPER DIGESTIVE HEMORRHAGE

There is little doubt that EGD has a superior yield to barium meal in localizing an upper digestive hemorrhage,[146-148] identifying the lesion in more than 80% of cases.[148,149] Ideally, endoscopy is performed in the 6 to 12 hours after stabilization of the patient. In the case of severe hemorrhage, surgeons should be informed and ready to intervene. In young individuals without signs of active bleeding, it can be delayed up to 12 hours, to a maximum of 24 hours.[148] If the patient shows an altered state of consciousness, the procedure is performed under general endotracheal anesthesia to protect the lungs. An endoscope with axial vision adapted to the age of the patient must be employed. The operating channel is often blocked by blood clots; therefore, an endoscope with an operating channel of a diameter of 2.8 mm at least should be chosen

methylene blue,[136-141] has been proposed. These methods do not help in the most important difficulty: defining the exact position of the esogastric junction. As a time-consuming method, it is not recommended. In conclusion, the diagnosis of Barrett esophagus is made with certainty only when multiple, large biopsies are taken under direct vision and a detailed histologic map is established.[142] The evaluation of the severity helps in predicting healing rate with medication.[143,144] When stenosis is present, biopsies are made only after dilatation. The risk of adenocarcinoma exists (one case was reported in an 11-year-old child[142]) and

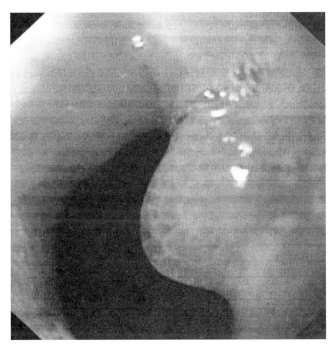

FIGURE 67.2-4   Inflammatory polyp of lower esophagus.

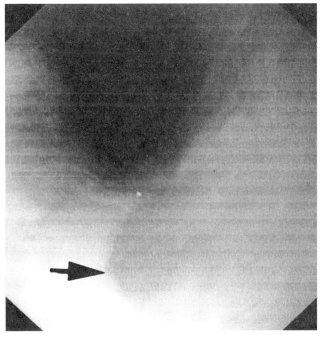

FIGURE 67.2-5   Esophageal gastric heterotopy (*arrow*).

when possible. The exploration is made with slow progression to find the origin of the blood. The instrument is advanced at least up to the genu inferius (Figures 67.2-6 through 67.2-9). Most lesions are to be found in the antrum or in the bulb. The exploration by retrovision of the fundus and the cardial regions is, however, necessary to examine these areas correctly. It might be necessary to change the patient's position to shift the blood from the great curvature. Unless the EGD takes place straight after the event, no active bleeding is normally seen. When the bleeding is still active, its cause is evident at endoscopy unless profuse bleeding obliterates the vision. When the hemorrhage has stopped, it is possible to see a stigma, generally a vessel or a clot adherent to it. In most cases, the clot only partly covers the erosion. In a few hours, the clot disappears, leaving behind a few brown spots. A hemorrhagic base indicates active bleeding within the last 48 hours. In the absence of such signs with a single lesion, it is assumed to be the cause; if multiple erosions are present, no certainty can be reached. Although common in adults, this presentation is rare in children.

At the end of the emergency EGD, three situations can be encountered: in about 70% of cases, the origin of the hemorrhage is found[148,150] or the diagnosis remains uncertain because multiple lesions have been found; finally, no mucosal lesion is seen; therefore, no diagnosis can be reached. This eventuality decreases with the delay of the endoscopy from 82% before 24 hours to 48% after 72 hours.[150] In the case of a negative endoscopy, a second procedure can be performed within 24 hours if bleeding recommences. The origin of the hemorrhage can be found in the esophagus, stomach, or duodenum depending on the age. The most frequent etiologies are shown in Table 67.2-7. Etiologies differ from one center to another and include esophagitis (Figure 67.2-10), Mallory-Weiss tears,

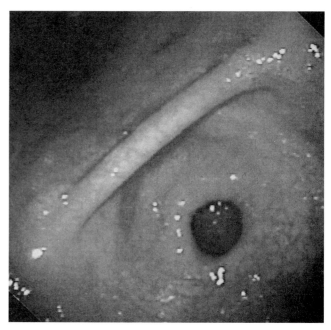

FIGURE 67.2-7 Normal aspect of cardia, angle fold, and fundus in the same view.

esophageal varices (Figure 67.2-11), gastritis (Figure 67.2-12), gastric ulcers (Figure 67.2-13), duodenitis, and duodenal ulcers (Figure 67.2-14). In addition, some specific causes are seen in newborns and infants, such as swallowed maternal blood, neonatal esogastritis, coagulopathy, vascular anomaly, and gastrointestinal duplication.[151] Some of these causes are related to *Helicobacter pylori*.[152] A nodular aspect of the antrum is highly suggestive of the presence of *H. pylori* (Figure 67.2-15).

CAUSTIC INGESTION

The ingestion of caustic substances is frequent in the pediatric age group.[153] It justifies an EGD in the 12 to 24 hours after the intake, with the exception of bleach. A thorough

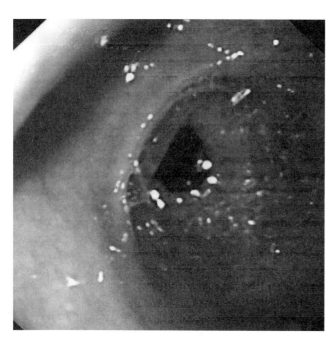

FIGURE 67.2-6 Normal aspect of lesser curvature and open pylorus.

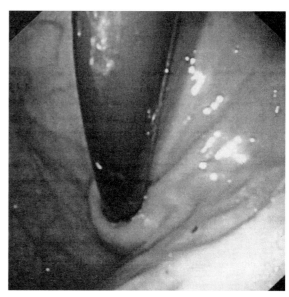

FIGURE 67.2-8 Normal retroversion of fundus of stomach.

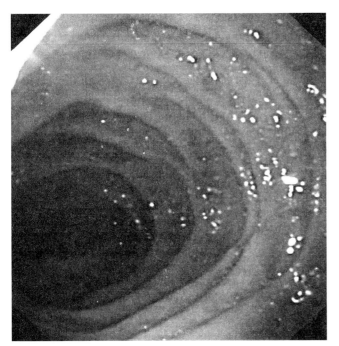

FIGURE 67.2-9 Kerckring fold in normal descending duodenum.

examination of the mouth and pharynx is not sufficient because the presence or not of lesions at this level cannot predict the gastroesophageal integrity. Half of the patients with oropharyngeal lesions have none in the esophagus, whereas around 15% of those without lesions in the top part will have an esophageal injury (J. F. Mougenot, unpublished data, 1997). Alkalis cause a deep liquefaction necrosis extending up to the muscles of the stomach and the esophagus. Acids are responsible for 15% of ingestions, causing a coagulation necrosis that will affect preferentially the stomach, the esophagus being exempt of lesions in 80% of cases (J. F. Mougenot, unpublished data, 1997).

Rigid scopes have been used in the past, but the risk of perforation is high because the instrument becomes blocked at the first proximal lesion. Flexible fibroscopes and videoendoscopes make the endoscopy safer. They can be passed down into the stomach even in the most severe cases. Fibroscopy is used to assess the extent and severity of the lesion, remembering that early examination can underestimate the injury. Early and late complications can be anticipated by the initial extent of the tissue injury. However, it has been suggested by several studies that asymptomatic children following alkali ingestion are not at risk of complications and thus do not need endoscopic examination.[154–159] In summary, the real impact of early endoscopy remains to be proven. A grading system can be used to assess mucosal injury: grade 0, normal mucosa; grade 1, hyperemia and edema; grade 2a, erosion, superficial ulceration, hemorrhage, and white membranes; grade 2b, deep or circumferential 2a lesions; grade 3, multiple ulcerations and areas of necrosis; 3b, extensive necrosis.[160]

ABDOMINAL PAIN

Subacute epigastric abdominal pain (present for more than a day and less than 3 months), with anorexia, dyspepsia, weight loss, anemia, and tiredness, that keeps the child awake or away from school needs to be investigated with an upper endoscopy. In our study of 695 consecutive endoscopies in pediatric patients, the association of an epigastric, nocturnal pain related to food intake had a predictive value on the presence of peptic disease with a sensitivity of 90% and a specificity of 37%.[161] The pathologies are shown in Figure 67.2-16. In our opinion, endoscopic examination must be reserved for abdominal pains with organic characteristics.

Recurrent chronic abdominal pains (at least 12 weeks within the preceding 12 months) are present in 10 to 15% of school-age children.[162] They represent one of the most frequent causes of specialized consultation (around 40%). In these cases, a careful clinical examination is crucial before EGD is considered because in only 20%, the investigation will be positive.[162,163] The Rome II criteria can be helpful to individualize functional abdominal pain as recurrent, periumbilical, and diurnal.[164]

DIARRHEA AND MALABSORPTION

The EGD with multiple biopsies has succeeded the suction capsule (Crosby, Kugler, Watson, Carey) introduced orally,[165] especially when investigating a malabsorption or a protein-losing enteropathy.[166] Some rules must be respected: three biopsies are taken at the genu inferius to make sure that at least one is well oriented. Some are fixed in formol, whereas others, if needed, are fixed in glutaraldehyde for electronic microscopy or frozen to allow the dosage of the brush border enzymes.

TABLE 67.2-7   ETIOLOGY OF UPPER GASTROINTESTINAL HEMORRHAGE IN CHILDREN (%)

	MOUGENOT AND BALQUET[279] (1978) (N = 62)	COX AND AMENT[149] (1979) (N = 68)	CHANG ET AL[280] (1983) (N = 27)	QUAK ET AL[281] (1990) (N = 29)	MOUTERDE ET AL[148] (1996) (N = 231)	AYOOLA ET AL[282] (1999) (N = 17)
Unknown cause	30.6	16.2	14.8	27.6	19.8	29.4
Esophagitis	4.8	14.7	11.1	17.2	30.7	0.0
Neonatal esogastritis					9.1	
Mallory-Weiss tear				3.5	9.1	
Esophagogastric varices	9.7	10.3		13.8	3.0	11.8
Gastric ulcer	16.1	17.6	33.3		5.6	
Erosive gastritis	14.6	13.2	14.8	27.6	16.2	17.6
Duodenal ulcer	24.2	20.6	29.6	10.3	6.5	5.9
Duodenitis						29.4

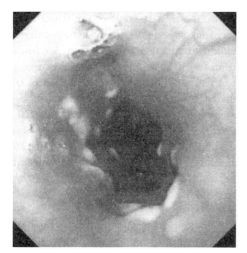

FIGURE 67.2-10   *Candida* esophagitis.

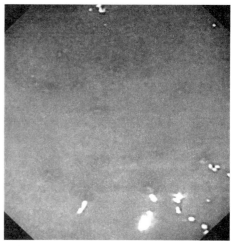

FIGURE 67.2-12   Erosive gastritis.

Some diseases can give a special aspect to duodenal mucosa and should be recognized by the pediatric gastroenterologist: in lipoprotein deficiencies (abetalipoproteinemia, hypobetalipoproteinemia, Andersen disease), a white discoloration of the duodenal mucosa and lipid droplets within the intestinal absorptive cells at biopsy are characteristic owing to the inability of the intestinal cells to export lipids as chylomicrons into the lymphatics[167,168]; a diagnosis of intestinal lymphangiectasia is highly suspect when white villae and/or spots, associated with white nodules and submucosal elevations, are seen.[169,170] Although severe intestinal villae atrophy can be diagnosed with the naked eye when duodenal folds have disappeared, biopsies are compulsory.[166]

SMALL BOWEL TRANSPLANT

Control of rejection remains the most difficult problem after intestinal transplant because the intestine seems more sus-

ceptible to rejection than any other organ. Because clinical diagnosis of graft-versus-host disease is difficult, endoscopy has become an essential tool in assessing its presence in the allograft.[171–173] An ileostomy is created at the time of the transplant to facilitate regular small bowel biopsies and histologic examination of the intestinal mucosa. The endoscopic appearance of a denuded, hemorrhagic mucosa usually correlates closely with the histologic diagnosis of severe rejection. Early changes can be too subtle to be detected with a standard endoscope, and zoom videoscope is used nowadays to look for edema, blunting of the villae, and expansion of crypt areas by a mononuclear cell infiltrate.[174]

OTHER INDICATIONS

The barium meal has a higher diagnostic yield than EGD for the diagnosis of vessel anomalies and of the esophagotracheal fistula, in which the esophageal orifice is often missed in endoscopy.

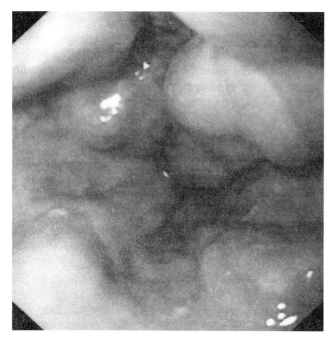

FIGURE 67.2-11   Grade II–III esophageal varices.

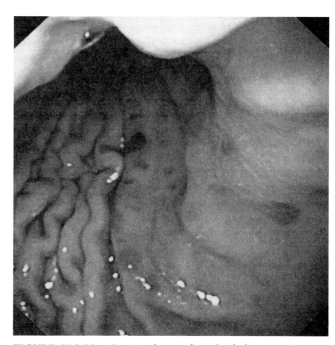

FIGURE 67.2-13   Gastric ulcer with multiple large erosions.

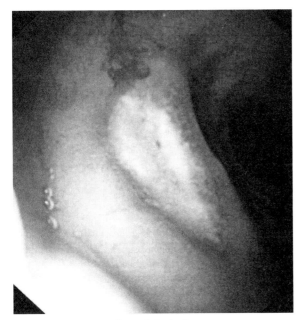

FIGURE 67.2-14   Ulcer of the bulb.

In pyloric stenosis, the first evaluation is made by ultrasonography. In case of doubt, upper endoscopy or barium meal should be performed. Indeed, small endoscopes such as GIF-N-30 (Olympus, Volketswil, Switzerland) and FG-16 X (Pentax, Walliselen, Switzerland) can be passed through a stenosis. Some authors have also proposed balloon dilation of pyloric stenosis.[175]

Despite the fact that primary gastrointestinal cancer is rare in children, EGD can be necessary in cancer surveillance. Endoscopic surveillance is warranted for polyposes syndromes with a higher risk of cancer development. Another indication for EGD can be Munchausen syndrome by proxy, which can present with a broad spectrum of manifestations, such as vomiting, abdominal pain, diarrhea, and failure to thrive.[176] Diagnosis is often delayed, and as

there is a risk of mortality due to Munchausen syndrome by proxy, invasive investigation can be mandatory. EGD in this condition has both diagnostic and legal implications.

EGD is an efficient method for follow-up of postsurgical treatment of peptic lesions.

Finally, an upper endoscopy is part of the initial evaluation in suspected inflammatory bowel diseases, and its role is also diagnostic because up to 28% of the granulomas are found only in the upper intestinal tract.[177,178] The integrity of the upper intestinal tract should no longer exclude ulcerative colitis,[177,179] and focally enhanced gastritis does not signify Crohn disease.[180]

CONTRAINDICATIONS

Absolute medical contraindications of upper endoscopy are few and include cardiovascular collapse, an unstable airway, intestinal perforation, peritonitis, and cervical traumas. On top of these pathologies, absences of consent or of competent medical personnel are also situations in which the endoscopy should be either delayed or cancelled.

Relative contraindications are the following: recent digestive surgery, bowel obstruction, coagulopathies, severe thrombocytopenia, and recent food intake. The latter needs to be corrected prior to the procedure.

The major risk with insulin-dependent diabetes is a hypoglycemic episode. The patient should be first on the endoscopy list and advised to reduce the amount of morning insulin.

In a child with hematemesis, an abdominal radiograph must be obtained to eliminate an intestinal obstruction or perforation.

INSTRUMENTATION

ENDOSCOPES

Two types of endoscopes are available that differ in the method of transmitting the image. Both systems require a fiberoptic light guide and a complex objective lens at the distal end to focus the image. The fiberoptic endoscopes use optical fibers. Imaging transmission of light is made by a bundle of glass fibers contained in a cylinder made of a material of inferior refraction index. Each fiber is made of coated glass. The coating acts as a mirror that reflects light through the fiber into the eyepiece. When the light entering the extremity of the optic fiber hits the interface between the glass with a high reflexion index and the material with a low index, it is transmitted by a series of internal reflexions up to the opposite extremity of the flexible fiber glass. A fiber alone could not do the job, but thousands put together make the transmission of an image possible. For the same image to be reproduced at the extremity as the one seen at the other extremity, the individual fibers need to occupy exactly the same position at the two ends of the scope.[181]

Videoendoscopes use advanced charge-coupled device (CCD) technology. The photo-sensible surface of the CCD is made up of a huge number of tiny image elements or pixels that gather the light. The electric charge of these pixels

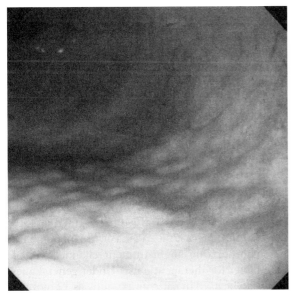

FIGURE 67.2-15   Nodular gastritis due to *Helicobacter pylori* infection.

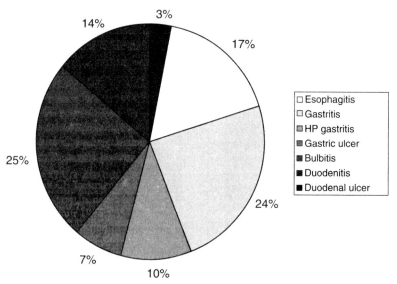

FIGURE 67.2-16 Peptic pathologies found in 695 consecutive endoscopies in a pediatric gastroenterology unit in Geneva, Switzerland. HP = *Helicobacter pylori.*

depends on the intensity and not on the color of the light. Therefore, a CCD is a black and white captor. The color image is created either by the single-plate simultaneous-color CCD chip method or the single-plate red, green, and blue (RGB) surface scanning method. In the former method, a color CCD chip built into the distal tip of the endoscope contains multicolor pixels and can simultaneously capture different color wavelengths of light: red, green, and then blue. Subsequently, the three monochrome images, specific in the intensity and position of the three colors, memorized in the microprocessor are visualized simultaneously, thus reproducing the original picture on the video monitor. In the latter method, the tip of the endoscope incorporates a monochrome CCD chip that can only provide black and white signals, with a multichrome filter added. The last generation of this type of endoscope can have a polychrome chip. This image from the filter (either RGB or a mosaic yellow-cyan-white) is passed through the video processor to modify it in the three primary colors. From a four-pixel block (one yellow, one cyan, two white), in this case, three pixels receive information about the red, four about the green, and three about the blue. The CCD converts the light into an electronic signal, which is then sent to the processing unit, where it is converted for output as a video signal for the monitor to display or to other peripherals (printer, personal computer, monitor, light source) in either RGB mode or Y-C (luminance-chrominance). With the image being directly transmitted to a color video monitor, the inspected areas can be examined fatigue free and simultaneously by several experts when required. However, the cost of the videoendoscope and accessories limits its acquisition.

All fibroscopes and videoendoscopes are waterproof, permitting appropriate washing, decontamination, and disinfection. They house an instrument channel to pass instruments (grasping forceps, polypectomy snares, injection needles, cytology brushes, extractors, retrievers, laser, guidewires, dilating balloons, bougies, diathermic snares)

and two accessory channels to insufflate air and inject and aspirate water. Through the smallest diameter of operating channel, 2 mm, fit 5 French instruments, facilitating therapeutic endoscopy in small children (injections, polypectomy). The midsize endoscopes have a 2.8 mm diameter, allowing the passage of 7 French wires. Apart from the duodenoscopes used for endoscopic retrograde cholangiopancreatography, all scopes have an axial vision.

The light source is composed of a generator of cold light (150–300 W halogen or xenon lamps), a light transmission system with automatic light adjustment to ensure sufficient brightness that maintains optimum brightness, and a high-speed rotation filter (20–30 tours/s), which is needed for the sequential RGB videoscope.

Gastroscopes with axial vision, owing to their flexibility and the amplitude of quadridimensional bending capacity (up, down, right, and left), give a full view of the upper intestinal tract from the esophagus to part 3 of the duodenum, including the cardia. An important part of the procedure is to choose the appropriate scope, depending on the size of the patient. The following rules can help in this choice: up to 15 kg, a 9 mm tip diameter can be used; from 5 to 15 kg, 8 to 9 mm; in newborns 2.5 kg to 4 kg, 5 to 8 mm; and in newborns less than 2.5 kg, only 5 mm is possible. In other words, the GIF-N30 (Olympus), the EG-1870K, and the FG-15W (both Pentax) are the only scopes usable in newborns. The GIF-XP20, GIF-XP160 (Olympus), FG-6W (Pentax), and FG-100PE (Fujinon, Wayne, NJ) are usable in term infants up to 4 years of age. Above that age, it is better to use the GIF-P30, P140, or P230. The EG-450PE5 can be used from 1 year of age. In patients older than 10 years, the GIF-XQ40, GIF-160, EG-450WR5 (Fujinon), and EG-2570K (Pentax) are preferable. The scopes incorporating an instrument channel size of 2.8 mm are better for therapeutic use. Under general anesthesia, they can be used in patients as young as 12 months old. Table 67.2-8 resumes the technical characteristics of gastroscopes that can be used in pediatrics.

TABLE 67.2-8   TECHNICAL CHARACTERISTICS OF GASTROSCOPES USED IN PEDIATRICS

ENDOSCOPES	FIELD OF VIEW (DEGREES)	OBSERVATION RANGE (MM)	WORKING LENGTH (M)	DISTAL TIP DIAMETER (MM)	BENDING CAPACITY (DEGREES)	CHANNEL DIAMETER (MM)
Fujinon						
FG series (fiberoptic)						
FG-100PE	105	5–100	1.030	9.5	U/D 210-90 R/L 100-100	2.2
EVE-400 Series (video)						
Gastroscopes						
G5-CCD 410000.0 pixels						
EG-470N5	120	2–100	1.100	5.9	U/D 210-90 R/L 100-100	2.0
EG-450P5E	120	4–100	1.100	8.2	Idem	2.2
EG-450WR5	120	4–100	1.100	9.4	Idem	2.8
EG-450WR5 optical magnification	140	6–100	1.100	9.8	Idem	2.8
Super CCD 1.2000000.0 pixels						
EG-490WR5	140	6–100	1.100	9.8	U/D 210-90 R/L 100-100	2.8
EG-490ZWR5 optical magnification	140	6–100	1.100	10.8	Idem	2.8
Duodenoscope						
ED-450XL8	120	100/15	1.250	12.5	U/D 130-90 R/L 90-110	3.2
Olympus						
EOS						
GIF N30	120	3–50	0.93	5.3	U/D 180-180 R/L 160-160	2.0
GIF-XP20	100	3–100	1.030	7.9	U/D 210-90 R/L 100-100	2.0
GIF-P30	120	3–100	1.025	9.0	Idem	2.2
GIF-XQ40	120	3–100	1.030	9.8	Idem	2.8
EVIS EXERA (video)						
Gastroscope						
GIF-XP160	120	3–100	1.030	5.9	U/D 180-90 R/L 100-100	2.0
GIF-160	140	3–100	1.030	8.6	U/D 180-90 R/L 100-100	2.8
GIF-160	140 retro	3–100	1.0300	10.9	U/D 210-90 R/L 100-100	2.8
GIF-Q160Z	140/75(télé)	8–100	1.030	10.9	U/D 210-90 R/L 100-100	2.8
Duodenoscope						
PJF-160	100/5	5–60	1.235	7.5	U/D 120-90 R/L 90-90	2.0
EVIS (video) 230 and 240						
GIF-N230	120	3–50	0.96	6.0	U/D 180-180 R/L 160-160	2.0
GIF-XP240	120	3–100	1.03	7.7	U/D 210 -90 R/L 100-100	2.2
GIF-XQ240	140	3–100	1.03	9.0	Idem	2.8
JF-240	100	5–60	1.235	12.6	U/D120-90 R/L 110-90	3.2
Pentax						
W Series						
Gastroscope						
FG-15W	95	3–50	0.925	5.3	U/D 180-180 R/L 160-160	2.0
FG-24W	105	3–100	1.050	7.8	U/D 210-120 R/L 120-120	2.4
FG-29W	100	3–100	1.050	9.8	Idem	2.8
70K Series						
EG-1870K	140	5–100	1.050	6.0	U/D 210-120 R/L 120-120	2.0
EG-2570K	140	5–100	1.050	8.7	U/D 210-120 R/L 120-120	2.4
Duodenoscope						
ED-3270K	140	5–100	1.050	13.0	R/L 110-90	3.5

FORCEPS

A range of biopsy forceps exists apart from standard models: the "crocodiles" have teeth on the edge to help in grasping the mucosa. Others have a spike in the center to facilitate the grip on the mucosa and avoid sliding.

TECHNIQUE

Endoscopy can be performed either single or two handed. In the first method, the endoscopist keeps the right hand on the shaft throughout the procedure, while the left hand is on the controls. The middle finger helps with the up/down wheel and the thumb reaches the right/left wheel. This method needs considerable practice but has the advantage of leaving the driver independent, needing less personnel. In the second method, the two hands are used to maneuver the controls, the shaft being pushed or withdrawn by a second person. The right hand is then used to move the right/left control. Easier from the start, this method can be performed more rapidly.

The help of experienced personnel is crucial. A minimum of two people, in addition to the operator, are present in the room. It is preferable that they could have met the parents and child before the endoscopy to answer questions. One will be responsible for the patient, making sure that the patient is safe and comfortable at all times. The second will assist the operator and operate the forceps when necessary.

At the start of the procedure, the patient is usually positioned on the left side, although some gastroenterologists will put the patient flat on the back. A small pillow under the head, but not the shoulder, will straighten the neck. The head is slightly flexed forward. In children with teeth, the use of a mouthguard with or without straps is recommended because bites to instruments can damage the fibers. It also helps keep the instrument on the midline. The scope is checked (suction, insufflation, and light on; zoom and brakes off) once more before lubrication is applied. Lastly, up and down movements are rehearsed to make sure that they are made in the axis of the pharynx. The room light is dimmed to allow good vision for the endoscopist. The introduction of the scope is a delicate moment owing to the extreme sensibility of the oropharynx. Two crucial rules are to be respected throughout the procedure if complications are to be avoided: never advance blindly and, if lost, come back. Four landmarks should be recognized during the procedure: cardia, angulus, pylorus, and superior duodenal angle (see Figures 67.2-6 through 67.2-8).

Three basic methods exist to intubate the esophagus:

- The safest way is under direct vision (Figure 67.2-17). The shaft is held at 30 cm and slowly introduced with the tip deflected downward up to the cricopharyngeal sphincter. In passing, the tongue, arytenoids, and vocal cords are localized to avoid impaction on the piriform fossae. If, in advancing, the teeth are seen, the shaft is twisted to put it back on the midline. Whenever landmarks are lost, withdrawal and starting again are the simplest and safest solution. The cricopharyngeal sphincter closes the entrance to the esophagus, making it difficult to locate. After a short waiting time, it will relax, allowing the intubation of the upper posterior esophagus. Insufflation of air or gentle pressure can help to relax it. In a cooperative child, swallowing will relax the upper esophageal sphincter, but it is often not obtainable in pediatrics.

- Another method uses blind manipulation. Holding the scope as before, the shaft is passed up to the back of the mouth. At this level, the tip is deflected upward and gently pushed forward. This will stretch the mucosa and allow the passage of the cricopharyngeal sphincter. Constant reorientation is necessary because the shaft easily comes out of the midline.

- An alternative method is with finger guidance. Probably the easiest for the inexperienced practitioner, it does, however, carry the risk of bites to either the scope or the fingers. The shaft is held with the right hand at about 5 cm, the mouthguard slipped over it. The shaft is pushed while the second and third fingers of the left hand are put over the tongue to help guidance. The cooperation of the patient is required as the sphincter is passed by active swallowing.

Under vision, the scope is progressively pushed forward to the lower sphincter. The Z line, the junction between the esophageal squamous mucosa and the gastric columnar, is located, usually 1 cm above the diaphragmatic hiatus. Its position in centimeters is recorded, remembering that it might be difficult to spot in newborns and infants. The diaphragmatic hiatus is situated between 12 and 40 cm from the incisors, depending on the age and size of the patient. The lower sphincter is often passed blindly owing to its contraction. The tip of the shaft is bent gently downward and to the left because the esophagus angles to the left side to avoid impaction in the fundus wall. To improve vision, air is insufflated, the lesser

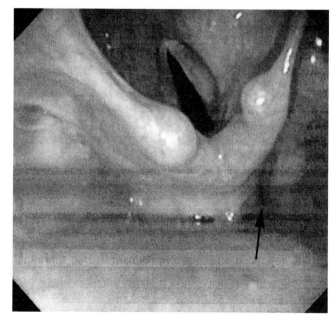

FIGURE 67.2-17   Normal laryngeal and pharyngeal structures. Upper esophageal sphincter (*arrow*).

curvature being on the right, the angulus in the distance. When liquid is present, suction is used to eliminate any risk of aspiration. At this point, most endoscopists will progress rapidly to the duodenum, careful examination of the mucosa being achieved on the way back. This method implies experience to avoid traumatic lesions (suction or rubbing) that could cause confusion afterward. Yet it has the advantage of avoiding the overinflation required for retrovision that causes discomfort. Progression is made with a clockwise (left) rotation of 90°, bending the tip upward. This double maneuver brings the pylorus into view. The bending can be quite extreme in a young child or infant because the angle is acute. To put the pylorus into the antrum axis, the tip is angled down. At this point, it helps to reduce the amount of air present in the stomach. The shaft is then advanced toward the pylorus, which will open, either spontaneously or with stimulation, by air insufflation. The intubation of the pylorus is achieved with the tip slightly bent down and right. Past the pinch, the tip tends to get impacted because the gastric loop straightens up. Withdrawal and air insufflation confer a view of the pale mucosa of the bulb, the anterior wall placed to the left and the posterior wall to the right. The superior duodenal angle is visualized before passage to the second part of the duodenum is attempted. This progression, usually carried out blindly because of the sharp angle, needs to be made with care. Pushing will bring the tip in front of the duodenal angle; it is then bent to the right and finally rotated simultaneously at 180° to the right and up (150°). Finally, to obtain an optimal view, withdrawal is normally necessary because of the paradoxical progression of the endoscope owing to the straightening of the gastric loop. Sometimes rectification of the last maneuver is needed with deflection of the tip upward and to the left. Often the Vater papilla is seen. Biopsies are taken before withdrawal. Most endoscopists will use this moment to carefully examine the duodenal, bulbic, gastric, and esophageal mucosa. Circumferential movements with air insufflation will provide well-distended mucosa in order not to miss small lesions. A retroversion maneuver in the stomach (J maneuver) is the only way to fully visualize the fundus, the lesser curvature, and the cardia. While back in the proximal part of the antrum, a 180 to 210° angulation is imposed to bring into view the angulus and the lesser curvature. Keeping the angulation, a 180° rotation around the shaft's axis will allow visualization of the greater curvature and the fundus. The withdrawal of the instrument will bring the cardia into view.

Taking biopsies is one of the main reasons for performing an endoscopy, along with visualization of the mucosa. Most gastroenterologists agree that they should be obtained even in the case of a normal mucosa.[10] The primary sites to biopsy are the distal duodenum, antrum, and esophagus. To achieve good-size specimens, some rules have to be followed. The forceps is approached at a 90° angle to the mucosa and not tangentially. The forceps protrudes no more than 3 cm from the tip of the scope to allow good control over it. This is important not only for the quality of the specimens but also to reduce the risk of per-

foration and hemorrhage. A fold biopsy is more effective because a "double" biopsy is obtained. In a limited space such as the esophagus, a good trick is to sharply bend the tip of the shaft. Firm pressure needs to be applied to the mucosa before slowly closing the forceps. Multiple specimens are taken, especially in the duodenum, so as not to miss focal villae atrophy in case of lesions. Biopsies are transferred with the help of the needle onto a piece of paper and flattened. To avoid crushing, stretching, or puncture injuries to the tissue, the back of the needle is used. The mode of fixation depends on which pathology is suspected. Clo-test (Astra Zeneca AG, Zug, Switzerland) will typically require a fresh antral biopsy, to test for the presence of *H. pylori*, by its production of urea. When cultures are needed, a small drop of saline is placed on top, and they are sent to the appropriate laboratory immediately. If special immunocytochemistry or disaccharidase levels are wanted, frozen specimens are needed. Finally, for electron microscopy, glutaraldehyde should be ready.

The whole procedure with collection of biopsies takes around 15 minutes in experienced hands.

COMPLICATIONS

Complications are uncommon during endoscopy when performed by well-trained pediatric gastroenterologists—probably less than 1%.[182] They are mainly due to the anesthesia or to the procedure itself. Endoscopy in children tends to be performed under deep sedation, making a hypoxic episode possible. On the introduction of the tube, the saturation usually drops by 5% from the basal level before quickly recuperating. However, in Bendig's series, desaturation (< 90%) was observed in 7 of 60 children.[183] Nasal oxygen is usually sufficient to correct the hypoxia. In the rare cases in which no amelioration is obtained, withdrawal of the scope is necessary. Difficulties mainly arise from inefficiency of the sedation. Aspiration is always possible, although respected fasting time reduces the risk. Allergic patients can react to the medications or to the latex. Finally, rare complications are hypotension, arrhythmia, and malignant hyperthermia.

If we now look at the complications arising from the actual procedure, they mainly consist of perforation, hematoma, air embolism and infections:

• The complications described in children owing to the actual procedure are the following: Perforation can occur, usually owing to excessive force or air insufflation on an already damaged mucosa. This mostly involves the esophagus. The majority of reported cases are due to therapeutic endoscopy and are discussed in other chapters. Mucosal tears without perforation have been described in children,[184] yet this seems to be a complication seen more frequently in the elderly presenting with hiatal hernia.[185] To minimize the risk, it is crucial to never push forward without vision. At times, it is impossible to avoid having the scope against the mucosa. In these circumstances, as long as the vessels are seen passing by in front of the camera, this means that the scope is sliding on the mucosa and that there is no danger. In contrast, if the mucosa turns white, too much pressure is being applied, and the scope needs to be withdrawn. In case of perforation, surgical referral is urgent to choose between a conservative and surgical treatment. Nevertheless, signs of perforation can appear with some delay.

- Intramural duodenal hematoma has been reported after endoscopic biopsies.[186–195] Although it is a rare complication, it seems to occur more often in children than in adults.[189] The clinical presentation mimics abdominal occlusion with severe abdominal pain and vomiting, usually starting in the 12 hours postendoscopy. Often it is associated with pancreatitis.[189,190,192,195] Spontaneous resolution is always obtained between 4 days and 2 weeks, with fasting, nasogastric suction, and fluid replacement. Total parenteral nutrition is sometimes necessary. Surgical drainage, although sometimes performed, is unnecessary and therefore contraindicated.
- Fatal massive air embolism has been reported in a 10-year-old and a 4-month-old child who had been subjected to a Kasai procedure[196,197] because of potential vessel leakage.
- Infectious complications can result from the patient's own microbial flora (autologous), from patient to patient by way of the endoscope (exogenous), or between the patient and the staff. The most frequent microorganisms depending on the mode of transmission are *Salmonella* spp, *P. aeruginosa*, *Mycobacterium* spp, and *H. pylori*.[182,198] These can be seen in cardiac-risk patients (see the antibiotic prophylaxis section); only one case of sepsis has been reported in a child without increased risk.[199] Bacteremia seems rare[52,54,57]; therefore, prophylactic antibiotics are given only to selected patients.

CAPSULE

The invention and development of more sophisticated endoscopes have allowed gastroenterologists to see further into the gut. Whereas in adults, push enteroscopy has enabled the further enhancement of possibilities and visualization of up to 90 to 120 cm beyond the ligament of Treitz,[200,201] experience in children is limited.[11] Another technique, sonde enteroscopy, in expert hands, allows us to see approximately 50 to 70% of the small bowel, the ileocecal valve being reached in only 10%.[202] Nevertheless, 30% of the small intestine could not be visualized, lying beyond our reach. Twenty years ago, Dr. Iddan had the idea of developing a video camera that would fit inside a pill.[203] Technology was not ready, and the idea was put on hold. With the turn of the millennium, engineering breakthroughs, particularly in the area of complementary metal oxide silicon, application-specific integrated circuit, and white light-emitted diode (LED) technologies, allowed all of the components of the camera to be put on a single chip, reducing both its size and power consumption. The wireless capsule endoscopy was born,[204] giving access to the so-called gut "black box."

The advantage compared with conventional upper endoscopy is that neither anesthesia nor air insufflation is necessary, making the whole procedure much more pleasant for the patient. Yet it cannot replace endoscopy for the following reasons. First, although the capsule often passes into the colon while the videotaping continues, its battery runs out before the journey through the colon is complete, not allowing a full view. However, a bowel preparation would be necessary. Furthermore, an important limitation is the inability of the device to take biopsies, although the manufacturers anticipate that improvements may permit this within the years to come. Therefore, the capsule does not replace traditional endoscopy in disorders in which a histologic diagnosis is necessary, for example, celiac and Crohn disease. Another drawback is that it may be difficult to determine the exact location of an abnormality seen. Because of these limitations, the capsule does not replace traditional endoscopy.

INDICATIONS

The main indication is obscure gastrointestinal bleeding[205] or iron deficiency anemia after a negative panendoscopy. However, it has been used to diagnose specific disorders that were otherwise difficult to establish, such as vascular abnormalities, polyposis,[206] and suspected Crohn disease.[207,208]

After animal studies demonstrated effectiveness, capsule endoscopy was used in small human prospective studies and proved to better define bleeding sites (55–76%) compared with conventional diagnostic procedures (21–30%).[209–211] When compared with barium studies, the capsule was considered diagnostic in 45% of patients versus 27%, with 31% versus 5% of the causes of obscure bleeding being found.[206] Reported diagnostic yield reaches up to 62.9%.[212] The amount of literature demonstrating its superiority in diagnosing the cause of blood loss is growing, but pediatric trials are needed.

CONTRAINDICATIONS AND COMPLICATIONS

A small risk exists that the capsule may become lodged in the intestinal strictures or diverticulae. The incidence, estimated around 1%, increases if the patient has undergone major abdominal surgery or suffers from a stenotic disorder.[213] We advise practitioners to perform a barium and follow-through prior to using the capsule to exclude stricture. Abdominal radiography should be considered in patients who do not observe passage of the capsule and whose imaging result does not indicate passage of the device into the cecum. The manufacturers themselves say that the capsule should not be used in patients with symptoms of a bowel obstruction, including nausea and vomiting and abdominal distention.

INSTRUMENTATION

The only wireless capsule endoscope available is produced by Given Imaging Ltd, Yoqneam, Israel, the M2A Capsule Endoscope, and is currently available in 33 countries worldwide. The Food and Drug Administration in the United States[214] and the Health Protection Branch of Health and Welfare in Canada recently approved its use in adults only. The capsule, measuring 11 × 26 mm, has a weight of about 4 g and contains a magnifying (1:8) color camera, four light sources, a radio transmitter, and batteries. With a 140-degree viewing angle, the capsule allows relatively complete viewing of the small intestine, but neither the velocity nor the direction can yet be controlled. Insufflation of air is unnecessary because the focal point of the lens is 1 mm. Images taken twice per second are continuously transmitted to wires placed on the body and captured on a recording device much like a Holter monitor, worn on a belt. The battery power is able to take 50,000 to 60,000 color images and lasts about 6 to 8 hours. These images are downloaded on a computer and viewed by the gastroenterologist as a video; analysis can take up to 2 hours. There is a learning curve in recognizing abnormalities even for experienced gastroenterologists because the aspect of the images is different to that acquired in a conventional way. A blood-sensing algorithm, using color pattern recognition, has recently been added to the software to help detection of intraluminal blood.

TECHNIQUE

The capsule is swallowed with a glass of water by the patient in the morning and then travels down the gut propelled by peristalsis. Neither bowel preparation nor sedation is needed, the patient having fasted 6 hours prior to the study. Although the minimal age mentioned by the manufacturer is 11 years, it has been used in younger children. The actual limitation is due to the capacity of the patient to swallow it and not the size of the capsule itself. To overcome this problem, some centers insert the capsule endoscopically in children as young as 4 years old. Patients may then perform their regular daily activities while wearing the recording device for the next 8 hours. The capsule has a mean gastric transit time of 80 minutes and a mean small intestinal transit time of 90 minutes.[204] The disposable capsule is usually passed, in the absence of any marked motility disorder, in the next 24 to 48 hours.

INTERVENTIONAL PROCEDURES

FOREIGN BODIES

Foreign body ingestion is a relatively common reason for consultation in the pediatric emergency room. More than 50% of cases are children aged 5 years or less, and most are boys. The ingestion of the foreign body is not generally voluntary, except for neurologically impaired or psychiatric patients and youngest siblings. A large variety of small objects and toys can be ingested, although coins are the most frequent (Figure 67.2-18). The vast majority of foreign bodies pass through the entire gastrointestinal tract without any problem. Indeed, only 10 to 20% will become impacted. The most frequent localization of impaction is the cervical esophagus. However, it can also occur in the medial and distal parts of the esophagus. When foreign bodies have passed through the esophagus, 95% will be spontaneously eliminated in 4 to 6 days, sometimes longer (3–4 weeks). If they pass through the esophagus, they can become lodged in the pylorus, genu inferius of the duode-

num, or ileocecal valve or on acquired or congenital stenosis. As to size, foreign bodies of a diameter of more than 20 mm or a length more than 50 mm (30 mm for infants) are particularly prone to impaction.[153] In more than 80% of cases, the foreign body is opaque, most frequently a coin.[215] The nonopaque foreign body is mainly retained food, often associated with a known history of previous repair for esophageal atresia.

Whenever a foreign body is suspected, thoracic and abdominal radiography must be performed. Every esophageal foreign body that is blocked for more than 24 hours must be removed immediately by endoscopy. Some studies have compared endoscopy, Foley catheter, and bougienage technique, especially for coin removal.[215,216] They favor Foley catheter or bougienage on a cost-effective basis.

For intragastric foreign bodies, interventional endoscopy is performed immediately only in cases of risk factors (a large foreign body with high risk of incarceration, a sharp foreign body with risk of perforation or hemorrhage, and all symptomatic ingestions). In other cases, a more conservative approach can be chosen, with an endoscopy only after 3 days to 4 weeks of nonprogression of the foreign body, depending on the experience of the center.

The special case of battery ingestion should be mentioned.[217] All types of batteries contain potassium or sodium hydrochloride and are not completely watertight. Consequently, their ingestion can lead to esophageal, gastric, or intestinal lesions such as burns or perforation, which can be lethal. Consequently, ingested batteries must be removed within 24 hours.

The endoscopic removal of foreign bodies must be performed under endotracheal anesthesia for all localizations to ensure airway protection, especially in case of an inadvertently released object.

Several devices are available: rat tooth and alligator forceps, polyp snares, retrieval nets, helical baskets, and hooded sheaths. Their specific use is related to the type of

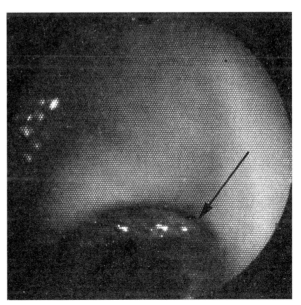

FIGURE 67.2-18   Antral foreign body (*arrow*: coin).

foreign body. It is mandatory that the removal should be carried out under view control and with optimal positioning (pointed end trailing and object close to the tip of the endoscope or in a protective device covering the end of the endoscope) to avoid unsafe removal, especially for sharp objects.

A postremoval surveillance of 12 hours is recommended.

STRICTURE DILATION

Esophageal stenosis dilatation is indicated in case of esophageal strictures, which can be secondary to several origins: congenital, postoperative, peptic, caustic, infectious, postvariceal sclerotherapy and postradiotherapy. Postoperative strictures are common complications in up to 50% of patients after surgery for esophageal atresia.[218] Peptic stenosis can also be secondary to severe GER with esophagitis, especially in neurologically handicapped children.

Since Trendelenburg in 1883, esophageal stenosis has been dilated either by antegrade or retrograde bougienage, when a gastrostomy can be used. Several types of bougie dilators are available. They develop an axial force along the esophagus, with a high risk of perforation. They are used both blindly following introduction through the mouth or on a guidewire.

An effective and safer alternative to bougienage is the balloon catheter dilation (Figure 67.2-19). Its major advantage is that it dilates uniformly the esophageal stenosis with local stationary radial forces owing to balloon inflation.[219] Indeed, a Gruentzig balloon was developed in 1981 and has been used successfully since.[220] At present, several balloon catheters are available. They can be used under radiologic control with an angiographic guidewire, with a rate of resolution of symptoms of 100% and 70% for congenital and acquired anomalies, respectively.[221]

On the other hand, other balloon devices can be used directly in the operating channel and are called the TTS system ("through the scope" system). However, the maximal dilation diameter is of 8 mm for a 2.8 mm channel and of 12 mm for a 3.5 mm channel. With this technique, the balloon can be placed across the stricture under view control. Then the balloon is inflated with a constant pressure between 3,000 and 4,500 mm Hg for 1 to 3 minutes. The benefit of this procedure is due to the fact that endoscopists can immediately visualize the effect of the dilation on the stricture. In our unit, we use larger balloon catheters (maximum 20 mm diameter), which are introduced by mouth in an antegrade approach. Simultaneously, a flexible endoscope of small size (5 mm) is introduced to control the proper passage of the structure, as well as the positioning of the balloon. Using this method, we have not experienced perforation during the last decade.[222]

This procedure can be performed under antibiotic prophylaxis, and a thoracic radiograph is obtained in case of suspicion of perforation. The reintroduction of nutrition is recommended after 24 hours if the patient remains asymptomatic. The number of dilations and their frequency depend on the type and size of the stricture. Consequently, an exact agenda cannot be recommended but will be modulated by the efficiency of the first dilation.

Note that an antisecretory medication (eg, omeprazole) can be useful after dilation to avoid relapse.

Achalasia is a special indication for balloon dilation. The treatment of this condition necessitates the use of a 35 to 40 mm balloon to reach a pressure of 500 mm Hg, to allow the rupture of the muscular layer gradually over at least two or three sessions. The results of this technique compared with conventional surgery are contradictory but are comparable to the latter in some studies.[223] The rate of esophageal perforation for achalasia is between 1.4 and 4%, with a rate of mortality around 0.5%. Recently, the injection of botulinum toxin in the lower esophageal sphincter was described as a potential alternative to balloon dilation or Heller surgery.[224,225]

BLEEDING CONTROL

Nonvariceal hemorrhage can be endoscopically treated either by thermal or nonthermal methods. Thermal coagulation includes laser, heater, monopolar, or multipolar probes. Nonthermal coagulation consists of injection of agents that can be either sclerosing or vasoconstrictive. Both seem to have the same efficacy, yet the injections are easier and cheaper and can be done with smaller endoscopes.

The two main clinical applications are active bleeding of an ulcer and a visible vessel. In active bleeding, injection of epinephrine (5–10 mL of 1:10,000) in the four angles of the lesion is the method of choice. Bleeding stops in 80 to 85% of cases.[226] Addition of a sclerosing agent, such as 1% polidocanol, is recommended in cases of visible vessels.[227] Some factors are responsible for failure: the ulcer's size (> 2 cm), hypovolemic shock, localization on the lesser curvature, and the presence of active bleeding.[228] Therapeutic endoscopy for active bleeding needs a visual control 24 hours later.

In case of severe hemorrhage, with an unsuccessful therapeutical endoscopy (5 to 8% of the adults, exceptional in children), surgery might be needed.[226]

ENDOSCOPIC THERAPY OF VARICEAL HEMORRHAGE

Variceal bleeding is the most common cause of severe gastrointestinal bleeding among children and accounts for one-third of all deaths related to cirrhosis in adults. However, the hemorrhage can be due to intra- or extrahepatic causes in childhood. Indeed, extrahepatic portal venous

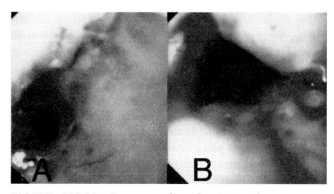

FIGURE 67.2-19 Severe esophageal stricture due to gastroesophageal reflux: *A*, before, *B*, after balloon dilation.

obstruction is a more frequent cause of bleeding in children when compared with adults. Unlike patients with cirrhosis, mainly owing to biliary atresia, those with extrahepatic portal hypertension have a better prognosis because of their liver function preservation.[229] The causes of death attributable to variceal bleeding include recurrent variceal hemorrhage, liver failure, hepatic encephalopathy, and infections. Portal hypertension is characterized by a pressure above 15 mm Hg, which leads to an impaired blood flow into the portal system. In portal hypertension, the mediastinal veins are organized in esophageal varices and in paraesophageal mediastinal veins. Esophageal varices can develop under the effect of pressure higher than 10 to 12 mm Hg.[230] However, their rupture does not seem to be due to a direct relationship between bleeding risk and exact level of portal pressure but to an imbalance between portal hypertension and resistance of the vessel wall.[231]

Endoscopic diagnosis of esophageal varices must be precise. Esophageal varices can be white or blue and are classified in four grades.[232] Grade I corresponds to varices that disappear with air insufflation, grade II corresponds to nonconfluent varices that remain identical with air insufflation, and grade III corresponds to confluent varices that cause an obstruction of the esophageal lumen (see Figure 67.2-11); the addition of red signs (cherry red spots, red wale markings, hematocystic spots, telangiectasia, varices overlying varices) leads to grade IV, with a higher and more precocious risk of bleeding. The classification of gastric varices is simpler: grade I in case of potential presence and grade II when the varices are overt, with red signs, which are easy to differentiate from gastric folds (Figure 67.2-20). Finally, the hypertensive gastropathy is secondary to the hyperkinetic syndrome owing to portal hypertension (Figure 67.2-21). It can be moderate or severe with purpuric spots, vessel ectasia, or erosions. Gastrointestinal bleeding secondary to portal hypertension is mainly due to rupture of esophageal varices. Among children, this situation represents only 15% of the causes of upper gastrointestinal hemorrhage, but it is often severe and life threatening. In specialized centers devoted to liver diseases and transplant, this percentage can be higher.

Adult guidelines for the diagnosis and treatment of gastrointestinal bleeding secondary to portal hypertension were published by the American College of Gastroenterology Practice Parameters Committee.[233] Some good reviews are available for children,[234,235] but no guidelines exist. Consequently, the optimal approach and treatment of children are still controversial, often depending on each center's competences and experience.

The diagnosis of variceal rupture is possible in up to 50% of cases.[236] The endoscopy can reveal a diffuse or localized deposit on a varice. The main localization of the variceal rupture is in the last 3 to 4 cm of the esophagus. Some endoscopic signs have a good positive predictive value for future bleeding, such as large-sized varices, cherry red spots, and varices of the cardia. Seventy-five percent of children with bleeding present with all of these signs.

To date, many modalities for treating variceal bleeding have been recommended, including pharmacologic therapy,

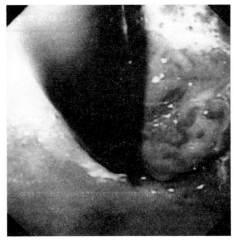

FIGURE 67.2-20   Cardial varices with red signs.

endoscopic treatment, surgical approach, and radiologic shunting. Unfortunately, none of the existing methods of treatment are optimal because the association of different therapies can be helpful.

Endoscopic Sclerotherapy. Endoscopic sclerotherapy (EST) was the first efficient endoscopic approach in both adults[237] and infants[238] to treat both acute bleeding and risk of relapse, with less morbidity and mortality when compared with surgery (Figure 67.2-22). Ideally, EST is realized after a short delay (eg, 24 hours) and under endotracheal anesthesia. The timing of EST is weekly for 3 weeks and then monthly until the total eradication of the esophageal varices. Three techniques have been used: paravariceal, intravariceal, and both para- and intravariceal injections. At present, the most common procedure is the intravariceal injection. The most popular sclerosing drug in Europe is polidocanol 1 to 2%. Note that sodium morrhuate, ethanolamine, and absolute alcohol are also used. With a mean dose of 2.5 mL of polidocanol for each injection and a total amount of 10 to 12 mL, the eradication of

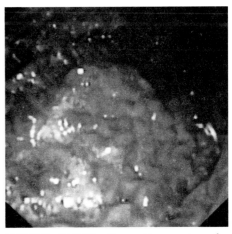

FIGURE 67.2-21   Congestive gastropathy due to severe portal hypertension in patient with cystic fibrosis.

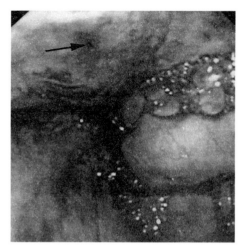

FIGURE 67.2-22 Esophageal varice after sclerotherapy with polidocanol and methylene blue. *Arrow* indicates injection point.

the varices is obtained after four to five sessions of EST. In a recent pediatric study, 95% of the patients had their varices successfully eradicated after a mean of 4.5 EST sessions.[239] The risk of a recurrence of bleeding is different among the studies depending on the realization of a liver transplant or a surgical shunt, ranging from 2[239] to 26%.[240] A rate of 10% must be considered realistic even if the rate of recurrence of varices is higher.

EST causes numerous side effects. Up to 50% of patients complain of dysphagia lasting for 2 days. Owing to the chemical properties of the sclerosing products, ulcers can appear in 17% of cases.[239] They can be responsible for precocious, severe rebleeding. Sucralfate, anti–histamine₂, or proton pump inhibitor drugs can be used to accelerate ulcer healing. Strictures are also potential complications of EST and were encountered in around 20% of cases.[239] The most serious complication of EST is perforation, which was described in up to 4% of the series[241] and in 1.4% of this recent study.[239] Its mortality is high. Perforation can also lead to esopleural or esobronchial fistulae. Infrequent complications such as sepsis,[182] bacterial peritonitis,[242] bacterial meningitis,[243–246] cerebral abscess,[245,246] and permanent paraplegia[247] have also been reported. Consequently, prophylactic antibiotics are prescribed because they have been shown to reduce bacteremia and bacterial peritonitis. The use of N-butyl-2-cyanoacrylate (Histoacryl), which coagulates instantaneously on contact with blood, is rare among pediatric patients and only related to bleeding of fundus varices. The risks of permanent obstruction of the channels of the endoscope are high. For other localization of bleeding varices, such as the duodenum or rectum, the procedure must be evaluated in each case by the operator.

Endoscopic Variceal Ligation. Endoscopic variceal ligation (EVL) was reported more recently and seen as a safe and quick procedure in adults.[248] EVL was introduced for pediatric patients only recently.[249,250] This procedure is limited in children by the size of the ligation device and by the fact that fewer bands can be applied per session owing to the small esophageal lumen. Apart from these restrictions, EVL is easy to realize, with a low complication rate. The latter is related to the mechanical strangulation of varices with little tissue inflammation and injury. The only serious complications are related to the use of an overtube: laceration, perforation, and punching injury of the esophagus. These lesions can provoke retrosternal pain or dysphagia.

Comparison of Different Modalities of Endoscopic and Medical Treatment. Most studies reported that EVL is superior to EST in terms of speediness, safety, rebleeding, and complications in adults.[237] EVL was also compared with EST in pediatric patients in a recent study.[251] No significant differences were found between EVL and EST in stopping bleeding and achieving variceal eradication. EVL eradicated varices in fewer endoscopic sessions and had significantly lower rebleeding and complication rates. However, recurrence of esophageal varices was similar in both EVL and EST groups after eradication. Consequently, both adult and pediatric data seem to favor EVL rather than EST to prevent risk of rebleeding.

Both EVL and EST are more effective when associated with vasoactive agents than alone. On the contrary, the combination of EVL and EST in the same session does not seem to be recommended because the complications increase more than the benefits.

Finally, endoscopic therapy is less effective than radiologic transjugular intrahepatic portosystemic shunt (TIPS) in terms of variceal rebleeding. However, TIPS must be considered as a rescue procedure before a liver transplant because the risk of occlusion in TIPS is high, as well as the development of encephalopathy.

PERCUTANEOUS ENDOSCOPIC GASTROSTOMY

In the early 1980s, Ponsky and Gauderer developed a PEG,[252] drastically changing the pediatric approach to enteral feeding, in particular in patients with swallowing difficulties. This minimally invasive, sutureless method is nowadays used worldwide to help provide appropriate nutritional intake

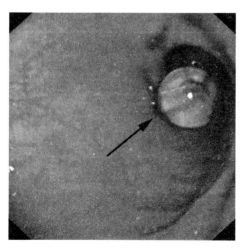

FIGURE 67.2-23 Gastrostomy button MYC-KEY type (*arrow*).

with comfort and easy care. Ethical and moral concerns were raised with the increasing number of procedures, and guidelines for indications have been drawn.[73,74]

In the pediatric population, the intervention takes place under general anesthesia on a fasted patient. The patient is at high risk of infection, and antibiotic cover is recommended by gastroenterologist societies[73,74] because it reduces the rate of both peristomal and systemic infections to less than one-quarter.[252-257] At even higher risk are patients suffering from diabetes mellitus.[258] The most commonly recommended regimen is amoxicillin or intravenous cephalosporin.

Although the risks and potential benefits of enteral access catheter placement must be weighed in each patient, certain anatomic and pathologic conditions may increase the likelihood of complications. The absolute contraindications to percutaneous feeding tube placement are uncorrectable coagulopathy and unfavorable anatomy, with inability to bring the anterior gastric wall in apposition to the abdominal one. Relative contraindications are massive ascites, peritoneal dialysis, active gastritis or peptic ulcer disease, and gastric varices. Examples of unfavorable anatomy include malrotation; interposition of the colon, spleen, or liver between the stomach and anterior abdominal wall; intrathoracic stomach; and previous gastrectomy. Hepatomegaly, severe scoliosis, and obesity are not contraindications but may impede gastric transillumination and subsequent placement of the PEG.

A portion of patients needing gastrostomy suffer from conditions associated with reflux, such as neurologic impairment, myopathies, cystic fibrosis, and chronic respiratory failure. The indication of performing a simultaneous fundoplication is still a subject of controversy[88] because it seems to bear a higher complication incidence.[259] In addition, contradictory data result from the studies performed, some showing that the PEG procedure tends to aggravate the reflux, at times antireflux treatment being necessary,[260-263] whereas some show no effect.[259,264-266] Careful evaluation of the clinic and the severity of reflux will provide the elements to decide for a prophylactic fundoplication in a case by case approach, systematic antireflux surgery being increasingly abandoned.

Three techniques have been described to insert the stoma: the "pull-through," in 1980, by its inventor[261]; the "push-pull" technique, in 1981, by Sacks and Vine[267]; and, finally, the "introducer" technique by Russell and colleagues 3 years later.[268] Only the techniques most commonly used in pediatrics are described here. Patients lie flat on their back. The abdomen is disinfected with an antiseptic solution. An endoscope is passed down to the stomach and air is insufflated to approximate the stomach to the abdominal wall. The tip of the endoscope is then applied against the anterior wall, with transillumination helping to choose the exact place for the gastrostomy. The site of choice is located at the junction of the external two-thirds of a line drawn between the umbilicus and the midportion of the left inferior costal margin. Gastric indentation is created by digital pressure on the abdominal wall to check the final stoma position. After a small incision of the skin, the

needle is passed into the gastric cavity. At this point, it is important that the endoscopist keep the stomach well inflated to avoid interposition of either the spleen, the liver, or, especially, the transverse colon. A string is then passed through the needle, to be seized by endoscopic snare or forceps and brought out through the mouth of the patient together with the gastroscope. The feeding catheter is then fixed to the oral end of the wire and is gently pulled back through the patient's mouth into the stomach and pulled out through the abdominal wall. The feeding tube ends with a stabilizer or "bumper," shaped either as a crossbar, an X, a T, or a cup, allowing it to be retained in the stomach. The maintenance of apposition of the peritoneal and serosal surfaces will create adherence. One should make sure that no excessive tension is applied to the wall by viewing it directly with the endoscope. An external retaining crossbar helps to maintain the right pressure. Daily rotation to 90° will avoid not only skin lesions but the proliferation of the gastric mucosa. Feeding through the device can start 6 hours postintervention. When the feeding tube is no longer necessary, the device is cut at the skin level. Good practice recommends performing it with endoscopic assistance to retrieve the bumper. Bowel obstruction and perforation caused by the internal part, left within the stomach to pass spontaneously, have indeed been reported in the literature.[269-271]

The feeding tube can be replaced in a second time by a button (Bard [Bard Medica, Volketswil, Switzerland], with a mushroom, or MYC-KEY [Cosanum, Schlieren, Switzerland], with a balloon as a bumper [Figure 67.2-23]). These devices, more esthetic and easier to conceal under the clothes, contain an antireflux valve that helps to avoid skin lesions. Once the gastrostomy tube or the button has been removed, the orifice will close itself in 48 hours. Delay of gastrostomy closure has rarely been observed up to 2 years later.[272]

The rates of adult morbidity and mortality are lower than those for surgical gastrostomy: 3 to 12% versus 30% for morbidity and 1 to 12% versus 16% for mortality.[273-276] Therefore, it should be preferred to surgical gastrostomy if no contraindications are present. In children, severe complications are observed in 3% of the PEG cases, including aspiration bronchopneumonopathies and migration of the bumper at the tip of the gastrostomy tube inside the abdominal wall, also called the "buried bumper syndrome." The condition resulting from excessive traction on the tube, sometimes secondary to growth of the patient, is the most common complication encountered. The button seems more likely to cause it than PEG.[272] Endoscopically, the bumper is partially or not seen, buried in the mucosa. Direct viewing will distinguish it from newly described pseudotumoral proliferative gastric mucosa, revealing an ulcerate mass or polyps. Peritonitis occurs immediately after insertion of the PEG or at the time of button change. It is due to stomal separation, tube malposition, or leakage. Rare cases of gastrocolic fistula have been reported in children, probably owing to misplacement of the colon at the time of insertion.[272,277,278] Risk factors are abdominal surgery that took place prior to insertion of the PEG and insufficient transillumination. Head supraelevation might reduce this risk by displacing the colon to the lower abdomen. Necrotizing fasciitis starting around the site and ulcers are rare complications. Two cases of hemoperitonitis have been personally encounted by one of the authors. The bleeding is caused by the lesion of parietal gastric vessel and can be fatal if the diagnosis is not made.

Less severe complications happen in 7 to 13% of the interventions, mainly represented by peristomal infections and pneumoperitonium, proving air leakage around the hole. When minor complications, such as granulation, are counted, the rate goes up to 44%.[272] When it takes place immediately after PEG insertion, simple traction on the feeding tube will abolish it by reducing the space between the stomach and the abdominal walls. Feeding through the tube should be delayed. If still present at 48 to 72 hours, laparoscopic exploration needs to be discussed. Local infections need to be taken seriously because they can lead to sepsis. Complication can also occur during replacement, the tube being not well introduced in the stomach. Endoscopic control will avoid missing such a problem. Secondary displacement of the button end has been seen. Granulation tissue sometimes grows around the site, occasionally causing oozing of blood. Treatment consists of chemically burning the tissue by topical application with silver nitrate ($AgNO_3$) sticks.

REFERENCES

1. Ashorn M, Maki M, Ruuska T, et al. Upper gastrointestinal endoscopy in recurrent abdominal pain of childhood. J Pediatr Gastroenterol Nutr 1993;16:273–7.
2. Ament ME, Christie DL. Upper gastrointestinal fiberoptic endoscopy in pediatric patients. Gastroenterology 1977;72:1244–8.
3. Rodesch P, Cadranel S, Peeters JP, et al. Colonic endoscopy in children. Acta Paediatr Belg 1976;29:181–4.
4. Cadranel S, Rodesch P, Peeters JP, et al. Fiberendoscopy of the gastrointestinal tract in children. A series of 100 examinations. Am J Dis Child 1977;131:41–5.
5. Tytgat GNJ, Classen M. The practice of therapeutic endoscopy. 2nd ed. Edinburgh: Baillière Tindall; 2000.
6. Howdle PD, Littlewood JM, Firth J, et al. Routine colonoscopy service. Arch Dis Child 1984;59:790–3.
7. Gilger MA. Gastroenterologic endoscopy in children: past, present, and future. Curr Opin Pediatr 2001;13:429–34.
8. Lobritto SJ. Endoscopic considerations in children. Gastrointest Endosc Clin N Am 2001;11:93–109.
9. Standards of Practice Committee. Modifications in endoscopic practice for pediatric patients. Gastrointest Endosc 2000;52:838–42.
10. Fox VL. Pediatric endoscopy. Gastrointest Endosc Clin N Am 2000;10:175–94.
11. Thomson M. Colonoscopy and enteroscopy. Gastrointest Endosc Clin N Am 2001;11:603–39.
12. Mougenot JF, Liguory C, Chapoy P. [Interventional digestive endoscopy in pediatrics]. Arch Fr Pédiatr 1991;48:571–9.
13. Hassall E. Requirements for training to ensure competence of endoscopists performing invasive procedures in children. Training and Education Committee of the North American Society for Pediatric Gastroenterology and Nutrition (NASPGN), the Ad Hoc Pediatric Committee of American Society for Gastrointestinal Endoscopy (ASGE), and the Executive Council of NASPGN. J Pediatr Gastroenterol Nutr 1997;24:345–7.
14. Rudolph CD, Winter HS. NASPGN guidelines for training in pediatric gastroenterology. NASPGN Executive Council, NASPGN Training and Education Committee. J Pediatr Gastroenterol Nutr 1999;29 Suppl 1:S1–26.
15. Mahajan L, Wyllie R, Steffen R, et al. The effects of a psychological preparation program on anxiety in children and adolescents undergoing gastrointestinal endoscopy. J Pediatr Gastroenterol Nutr 1998;27:161–5.
16. Adewumi A, Hector MP, King JM. Children and informed consent: a study of children's perceptions and involvement in consent to dental treatment. Br Dent J 2001;191:256–9.
17. Informed consent, parental permission, and assent in pediatric practice. Committee on Bioethics, American Academy of Pediatrics. Pediatrics 1995;95:314–7.
18. American Academy of Pediatrics Committee on Pediatric Emergency Medicine. Consent for medical services for children and adolescents. Pediatrics 1993;92:290–1.
19. Bartholome WG. Informed consent, parental permission, and assent in pediatric practice. Pediatrics 1995;96:981–2.
20. Campbell A. Infants, children, and informed consent. BMJ 1974;3:334–8.
21. King NM, Cross AW. Children as decision makers: guidelines for pediatricians. J Pediatr 1989;115:10–6.
22. Spencer GE. Children's competency to consent: an ethical dilemma. J Child Health Care 2000;4:117–22.
23. Spinetta JJ, Masera G, Jankovic M, et al. Valid informed consent and participative decision-making in children with cancer and their parents: a report of the SIOP Working Committee on psychosocial issues in pediatric oncology. Med Pediatr Oncol 2003;40:244–6.
24. Williams L, Harris A, Thompson M, et al. Consent to treatment by minors attending accident and emergency departments: guidelines. J Accid Emerg Med 1997;14:286–9.
25. Bauchner H, Sharfstein J. Failure to report ethical approval in child health research: review of published papers. BMJ 2001;323:318–9.
26. Burns JP. Research in children. Crit Care Med 2003;31 Suppl 3:S131–6.
27. Flagel DC. Children as research subjects: new guidelines for Canadian IRBs. IRB 2000;22:1–3.
28. Gill D. Guidelines for informed consent in biomedical research involving paediatric populations as research participants. Eur J Pediatr 2003;162:455–8.
29. Kodish E. Informed consent for pediatric research: is it really possible? J Pediatr 2003;142:89–90.
30. Weise KL, Smith ML, Maschke KJ, et al. National practices regarding payment to research subjects for participating in pediatric research. Pediatrics 2002;110:577–82.
31. Eriksson LI, Sandin R. Fasting guidelines in different countries. Acta Anaesthesiol Scand 1996;40:971–4.
32. Guidelines for monitoring and management of pediatric patients during and after sedation for diagnostic and therapeutic procedures: addendum. Pediatrics 2002;110:836–8.
33. American Academy of Pediatrics Committee on Drugs. Guidelines for monitoring and management of pediatric patients during and after sedation for diagnostic and therapeutic procedures. Pediatrics 1992;89:1110–5.
34. Koh JL, Black DD, Leatherman IK, et al. Experience with an anesthesiologist interventional model for endoscopy in a pediatric hospital. J Pediatr Gastroenterol Nutr 2001;33:314–8.

35. Bishop P, Nowicki M, May W, et al. Unsedated upper endoscopy in children. Gastrointest Endosc 2002;55:624–30.

36. Keeffe EB, O'Connor KW. 1989 ASGE survey of endoscopic sedation and monitoring practices. Gastrointest Endosc 1990;36 Suppl 3:S13–8.

37. Daneshmend TK, Bell GD, Logan RF. Sedation for upper gastrointestinal endoscopy: results of a nationwide survey. Gut 1991;32:12–5.

38. Belli DC, Spahr-Schopfer I, Balderrama F, et al. Sedation during gastrointestinal endoscopy in paediatric patients. Acta Endosc 1994;24:117–23.

39. Anand KJ, Sippell WG, Aynsley-Green A. Randomised trial of fentanyl anaesthesia in preterm babies undergoing surgery: effects on the stress response. Lancet 1987;i:62–6.

40. Claar RL, Walker LS, Barnard JA. Children's knowledge, anticipatory anxiety, procedural distress, and recall of esophagogastroduodenoscopy. J Pediatr Gastroenterol Nutr 2002;34:68–72.

41. Johnson JE, Morrissey JF, Leventhal H. Psychological preparation for an endoscopic examination. Gastrointest Endosc 1973;19:180–2.

42. Smith C, Rowe RD, Vlad P. Sedation of children for cardiac catheterization with ataractic mixture. Can Anaesth Soc J 1958;5:35–43.

43. Bailey PL, Andriano KP, Goldman M, et al. Variability of the respiratory response to diazepam. Anesthesiology 1986;64:460–5.

44. Martinez JL, Sutters KA, Waite S, et al. A comparison of oral diazepam versus midazolam, administered with intravenous meperidine, as premedication to sedation for pediatric endoscopy. J Pediatr Gastroenterol Nutr 2002;35:51–8.

45. Shlomo IB, Khalim HAE, Ezry I, et al. Midazolam acts synergistically with fentanyl for induction of anaesthesia. Br J Anaesth 1990;64:45–57.

46. Bianchi PG, Lazzaroni M. Preparation, premedication and surveillance. Endoscopy 1992;24:1–8.

47. Bahal-O'Mara N, Nahata MC, Murray RD, et al. Efficacy of diazepam and meperidine in ambulatory pediatric patients undergoing endoscopy: a randomized, double-blind trial. J Pediatr Gastroenterol Nutr 1993;16:387–92.

48. Nahata MC, Murray RD, Zingarelli J, et al. Efficacy and safety of a diazepam and meperidine combination for pediatric gastrointestinal procedures. J Pediatr Gastroenterol Nutr 1990;10:335–8.

49. Khoshoo V, Thoppil D, Landry L, et al. Propofol versus midazolam plus meperidine for sedation during ambulatory esophagogastroduodenoscopy. J Pediatr Gastroenterol Nutr 2003;37:146–9.

50. Law AK, Ng DK, Chan KK. Use of intramuscular ketamine for endoscopy sedation in children. Pediatr Int 2003;45:180–5.

51. Durack DT. Prevention of infective endocarditis. N Engl J Med 1995;332:38–44.

52. Botoman VA, Surawicz CM. Bacteremia with gastrointestinal endoscopic procedures. Gastrointest Endosc 1986;32:342–6.

53. Nelson DB. Infection control during gastrointestinal endoscopy. J Lab Clin Med 2003;141:159–67.

54. Byrne WJ, Euler AR, Campbell M, et al. Bacteremia in children following upper gastrointestinal endoscopy or colonoscopy. J Pediatr Gastroenterol Nutr 1982;1:551–3.

55. Pritchard TM, Foust RT, Cantely JR, et al. Prosthetic valve endocarditis due to Cardiobacterium hominis occurring after upper gastrointestinal endoscopy. Am J Med 1991;90:516–8.

56. Sontheimer J, Salm R, Friedrich G, et al. Bacteremia following operative endoscopy of the upper gastrointestinal tract. Endoscopy 1991;23:67–72.

57. el Baba M, Tolia V, Lin CH, et al. Absence of bacteremia after gastrointestinal procedures in children. Gastrointest Endosc 1996;44:378–81.

58. Shull HJ Jr, Greene BM, Allen SD, et al. Bacteremia with upper gastrointestinal endoscopy. Ann Intern Med 1975;83:212–4.

59. Low DE, Shoenut JP, Kennedy JK, et al. Prospective assessment of risk of bacteremia with colonoscopy and polypectomy. Dig Dis Sci 1987;32:1239–43.

60. Rodriguez W, Levine JS. Enterococcal endocarditis following flexible sigmoidoscopy. West J Med 1984;140:951–3.

61. Logan RF, Hastings JG. Bacterial endocarditis: a complication of gastroscopy. BMJ 1988;296:1107.

62. Goldman GD, Miller SA, Furman DS, et al. Does bacteremia occur during flexible sigmoidoscopy? Am J Gastroenterol 1985;80:621–3.

63. Norfleet RG. Infectious endocarditis after fiberoptic sigmoidoscopy. With a literature review. J Clin Gastroenterol 1991;13:448–51.

64. Rigilano J, Mahapatra R, Barnhill J, et al. Enterococcal endocarditis following sigmoidoscopy and mitral valve prolapse. Arch Intern Med 1984;144:850–1.

65. Schlaeffer F, Riesenberg K, Mikolich D, et al. Serious bacterial infections after endoscopic procedures. Arch Intern Med 1996;156:572–4.

66. Van Der Meer JT, van Wijk W, Thompson J, et al. Efficacy of antibiotic prophylaxis for prevention of native-valve endocarditis. Lancet 1992;339:135–9.

67. Infection control during gastrointestinal endoscopy: guidelines for clinical application. From the ASGE. American Society for Gastrointestinal Endoscopy. Gastrointest Endosc 1999;49:836–41.

68. Antibiotic prophylaxis for gastrointestinal endoscopy. American Society for Gastrointestinal Endoscopy. Gastrointest Endosc 1995;42:630–5.

69. Infection control during gastrointestinal endoscopy. Guidelines for clinical application. Gastrointest Endosc 1988;34 Suppl 3:37S–40S

70. Dajani AS, Taubert KA, Wilson W, et al. Prevention of bacterial endocarditis. Recommendations by the American Heart Association. JAMA 1997;277:1794–801.

71. Devlin TB. Canadian Association of Gastroenterology practice guidelines: antibiotic prophylaxis for gastrointestinal endoscopy. Can J Gastroenterol 1999;13:819–21.

72. Greff M. Guidelines of the French Society of Digestive Endoscopy (SFED): antibiotic prophylaxis in digestive endoscopy. Endoscopy 1998;30:873–5.

73. Rey JR, Axon A, Budzynska A, et al. Guidelines of the European Society of Gastrointestinal Endoscopy (E.S.G.E.) antibiotic prophylaxis for gastrointestinal endoscopy. European Society of Gastrointestinal Endoscopy. Endoscopy 1998;30:318–24.

74. Snyder J, Bratton B. Antimicrobial prophylaxis for gastrointestinal procedures: current practices in North American academic pediatric programs. J Pediatr Gastroenterol Nutr 2002;35:564–9.

75. Zuckerman GR, O'Brien J, Halsted R. Antibiotic prophylaxis in patients with infectious risk factors undergoing gastrointestinal endoscopic procedures. Gastrointest Endosc 1994;40:538–43.

76. O'Connor JB, Sondhi SS, Mullen KD, et al. A continuous quality improvement initiative reduces inappropriate prescribing of prophylactic antibiotics for endoscopic procedures. Am J Gastroenterol 1999;94:2115–21.

77. Mogadam M, Malhotra SK, Jackson RA. Pre-endoscopic antibiotics for the prevention of bacterial endocarditis: do we use them appropriately? Am J Gastroenterol 1994;89:832–4

78. Durack DT, Kaplan EL, Bisno AL. Apparent failures of endocarditis prophylaxis. Analysis of 52 cases submitted to a national registry. JAMA 1983;250:2318–22.

79. Dajani AS, Taubert KA, Wilson W, et al. Prevention of bacterial endocarditis: recommendations by the American Heart Association. Circulation 1997;96:358.

80. Steckelberg JM, Wilson WR. Risk factors for infective endocarditis. Infect Dis Clin North Am 1993;7:9–19.

81. Saiman L, Prince A, Gersony WM. Pediatric infective endocarditis in the modern era. J Pediatr 1993;122:847–53.

82. Gersony WM, Hayes CJ. Bacterial endocarditis in patients with pulmonary stenosis, aortic stenosis, or ventricular septal defect. Circulation 1977;56(1 Suppl):I84–7.

83. Practice parameters for antibiotic prophylaxis to prevent infective endocarditis or infected prosthesis during colon and rectal endoscopy. The Standards Task Force. The American Society of Colon and Rectal Surgeons. Dis Colon Rectum 2000;43:1193.

84. Dajani AS, Bawdon RE, Berry MC. Oral amoxicillin as prophylaxis for endocarditis: what is the optimal dose? Clin Infect Dis 1994;18:157–60

85. Fluckiger U, Francioli P, Blaser J, et al. Role of amoxicillin serum levels for successful prophylaxis of experimental endocarditis due to tolerant streptococci. J Infect Dis 1994;169:1397–400.

86. Mani V, Cartwright K, Dooley J, et al. Antibiotic prophylaxis in gastrointestinal endoscopy: a report by a Working Party for the British Society of Gastroenterology Endoscopy Committee. Endoscopy 1997;29:114–9.

87. Schlaeffer F, Riesenberg K, Mikolich D, et al. Serious bacterial infections after endoscopic procedures. Arch Intern Med 1996;156:572–4.

88. Gottrand F, Michaud L. Percutaneous endoscopic gastrostomy and gastro-esophageal reflux: are we correctly addressing the question? J Pediatr Gastroenterol Nutr 2002;35:22–4.

89. Guidelines on cleaning and disinfection in GI endoscopy. Update 1999. The European Society of Gastrointestinal Endoscopy. Endoscopy 2000;32:77–80.

90. Alvarado C. Reconciliation of FDA and societal guidelines for endoscope reprocessing. Gastrointest Endosc Clin N Am 2000;10:275–81.

91. Leung JW. Reprocessing of flexible endoscopes. J Gastroenterol Hepatol 2000;15 Suppl:G73–7.

92. Tandon RK, Ahuja V. Non-United States guidelines for endoscope reprocessing. Gastrointest Endosc Clin N Am 2000;10:295–318.

93. Ayliffe G. Decontamination of minimally invasive surgical endoscopes and accessories. J Hosp Infect 2000;45:263–77.

94. Hanson PJ, Gor D, Jeffries DJ, et al. Elimination of high titre HIV from fibreoptic endoscopes. Gut 1990;31:657–9.

95. Chanzy B, Duc-Bin DL, Rousset B, et al. Effectiveness of a manual disinfection procedure in eliminating hepatitis C virus from experimentally contaminated endoscopes. Gastrointest Endosc 1999;50:147–51.

96. Deva AK, Vickery K, Zou J, et al. Detection of persistent vegetative bacteria and amplified viral nucleic acid from in-use testing of gastrointestinal endoscopes. J Hosp Infect 1998;39:149–57.

97. Hanson PJ. AIDS: practising safe endoscopy. Baillieres Clin Gastroenterol 1990;4:477–94.

98. Hanson PJ, Bennett J, Jeffries DJ, et al. Enteroviruses, endoscopy and infection control: an applied study. J Hosp Infect 1994;27:61–7.

99. Charrel RN, de Chesse R, Decaudin A, et al. Evaluation of disinfectant efficacy against hepatitis C virus using a RT-PCR-based method. J Hosp Infect 2001;49:129–34.

100. Hansen KS. Occupational dermatoses in hospital cleaning women. Contact Dermatitis 1983;9:343–51.

101. Beauchamp RO Jr, St Clair MB, Fennell TR, et al. A critical review of the toxicology of glutaraldehyde. Crit Rev Toxicol 1992;22:143–74.

102. Gannon PF, Bright P, Campbell M, et al. Occupational asthma due to glutaraldehyde and formaldehyde in endoscopy and x ray departments. Thorax 1995;50:156–9.

103. McDonald JC, Keynes HL, Meredith SK. Reported incidence of occupational asthma in the United Kingdom, 1989-97. Occup Environ Med 2000;57:823–9.

104. Meredith SK, Taylor VM, McDonald JC. Occupational respiratory disease in the United Kingdom 1989: a report to the British Thoracic Society and the Society of Occupational Medicine by the SWORD project group. Br J Ind Med 1991; 48:292–8.

105. Dolce P, Gourdeau M, April N, et al. Outbreak of glutaraldehyde-induced proctocolitis. Am J Infect Control 1995;23:34–9.

106. West AB, Kuan SF, Bennick M, et al. Glutaraldehyde colitis following endoscopy: clinical and pathological features and investigation of an outbreak. Gastroenterology 1995;108: 1250–5.

107. Hernandez A, Martro E, Puzo C, et al. In-use evaluation of Perasafe® compared with Cidex® in fibreoptic bronchoscope disinfection. J Hosp Infect 2003;54:46–51.

108. Foliente RL, Kovacs BJ, Aprecio RM, et al. Efficacy of high-level disinfectants for reprocessing GI endoscopes in simulated-use testing. Gastrointest Endosc 2001;53:456–62.

109. Holton J, Shetty N, McDonald V. Efficacy of 'Nu-Cidex' (0.35% peracetic acid) against mycobacteria and cryptosporidia. J Hosp Infect 1995;31:235–7.

110. Moses FM, Lee J. Surveillance cultures to monitor quality of gastrointestinal endoscope reprocessing. Am J Gastroenterol 2003;98:77–81.

111. Axon AT, Beilenhoff U, Bramble MG, et al. Variant Creutzfeldt-Jakob disease (vCJD) and gastrointestinal endoscopy. Endoscopy 2001;33:1070–80.

112. Rey JF, Kruse A, Axon T, et al. ESGE guidelines for the prevention of endoscopic transmission of type C hepatitis and update on Creutzfeldt-Jakob disease. European Society of Gastrointestinal Endoscopy. Endoscopy 1997;29:203–4.

113. Cleaning and disinfection of equipment for gastrointestinal endoscopy. Report of a Working Party of the British Society of Gastroenterology Endoscopy Committee. Gut 1998;42: 585–93.

114. Rutala WA, Weber DJ. Creutzfeldt-Jakob disease: recommendations for disinfection and sterilization. Clin Infect Dis 2001;32:1348–56.

115. Hill AF, Butterworth RJ, Joiner S, et al. Investigation of variant Creutzfeldt-Jakob disease and other human prion diseases with tonsil biopsy samples. Lancet 1999;353:183–9.

116. Wadsworth JDF, Joiner S, Hill AF, et al. Tissue distribution of protease resistant prion protein in variant Creutzfeldt-Jakob disease using a highly sensitive immunoblotting assay. Lancet 2001;358:171–80.

117. Hilton DA, Fathers E, Edwards P, et al. Prion immunoreactivity in appendix before clinical onset of variant Creutzfeldt-Jakob disease. Lancet 1998;352:703–4.

118. Horan G, Keohane C, Molloy S, et al. Creutzfeldt-Jakob disease in Ireland: epidemiological aspects 1980-2002. Eur Neurol 2004;51:132–7.

119. Chu NS, McAlister D, Antonoplos PA. Natural bioburden levels detected on flexible gastrointestinal endoscopes after clinical use and manual cleaning. Gastrointest Endosc 1998;48: 137–42.

120. Vesley D, Melson J, Stanley P. Microbial bioburden in endoscope reprocessing and an in-use evaluation of the high-level disinfection capabilities of Cidex PA. Gastroenterol Nurs 1999; 22:63–8.

121. Kinney TP, Kozarek RA, Raltz S, et al. Contamination of single-use biopsy forceps: a prospective in vitro analysis. Gastrointest Endosc 2002;56:209–12.

122. Rutala WA. APIC guideline for selection and use of disinfectants. 1994, 1995, and 1996 APIC Guidelines Committee. Association for Professionals in Infection Control and Epidemiology, Inc. Am J Infect Control 1996;24:313–42.

123. Tandon RK. Disinfection of gastrointestinal endoscopes and accessories. J Gastroenterol Hepatol 2000;15 Suppl:G69–72.

124. Systchenko R, Marchetti B, Canard JM, et al. [Recommendations for cleaning and disinfection procedures in digestive tract endoscopy. The French Society of Digestive Endoscopy]. Gastroenterol Clin Biol 2000;24:520–9.

125. Axon A, Kruse A, Urgell R. ESGE guidelines on cleaning and disinfection. Endoscopy 1995;27:199–202.

126. Jung M, Beilenhoff U, Pietsch M, et al. Standardized reprocessing of reusable colonoscopy biopsy forceps is effective: results of a German multicenter study. Endoscopy 2003; 35:197–202.

127. Medical devices; reconditioners, rebuilders of medical devices; revocation of compliance policy guide; request for comments—FDA. Notice. Fed Reg 1998;63:67076–8.

128. Wilkinson M, Simmons N, Bramble MG, et al. Report of the Working Party of the Endoscopy Committee of the British Society of Gastroenterology on the reuse of endoscopic accessories. Gut 1998;42:304.

129. Hassall E. Macroscopic versus microscopic diagnosis of reflux esophagitis: erosions or eosinophils? J Pediatr Gastroenterol Nutr 1996;22:321–5.

130. Vandenplas Y. Reflux esophagitis: biopsy or not? J Pediatr Gastroenterol Nutr 1996;22:326–7.

131. Winter HS, Madara JL, Stafford RJ, et al. Intraepithelial eosinophils: a new diagnostic criterion for reflux esophagitis. Gastroenterology 1982;83:818–23.

132. Vandenplas Y. Reflux esophagitis in infants and children: a report from the Working Group on Gastro-Oesophageal Reflux Disease of the European Society of Paediatric Gastroenterology and Nutrition. J Pediatr Gastroenterol Nutr 1994;18:413–22.

133. Ismail-Beigi F, Horton PF, Pope CE. Histological consequences of gastroesophageal reflux in man. Gastroenterology 1970;58:163–74.

134. Knuff TE, Benjamin SB, Worsham GF, et al. Histologic evaluation of chronic gastroesophageal reflux. An evaluation of biopsy methods and diagnostic criteria. Dig Dis Sci 1984; 29:194–201.

135. Zeitoun P, Flejou JF. [Complications of gastroesophageal reflux and Barrett's esophagus]. Gastroenterol Clin Biol 1999;23: S50–60.

136. Canto MI, Setrakian S, Willis J, et al. Methylene blue-directed biopsies improve detection of intestinal metaplasia and dysplasia in Barrett's esophagus. Gastrointest Endosc 2000;51: 560–8.

137. Canto MI, Setrakian S, Petras RE, et al. Methylene blue selectively stains intestinal metaplasia in Barrett's esophagus. Gastrointest Endosc 1996;44:1–7.

138. Dave U, Shousha S, Westaby D. Methylene blue staining: is it really useful in Barrett's esophagus? Gastrointest Endosc 2001;53:333–5.

139. Gangarosa LM, Halter S, Mertz H. Methylene blue staining and endoscopic ultrasound evaluation of Barrett's esophagus with low-grade dysplasia. Dig Dis Sci 2000;45:225–9.

140. Wo JM, Ray MB, Mayfield-Stokes S, et al. Comparison of methylene blue-directed biopsies and conventional biopsies in the detection of intestinal metaplasia and dysplasia in Barrett's esophagus: a preliminary study. Gastrointest Endosc 2001; 54:294–301.

141. Wong RK, Horwhat JD, Maydonovitch CL. Sky blue or murky waters: the diagnostic utility of methylene blue. Gastrointest Endosc 2001;54:409–13.

142. Hassall E. Barrett's esophagus: new definitions and approaches in children. J Pediatr Gastroenterol Nutr 1993;16:345–64.

143. Bell NJ, Hunt RH. Role of gastric acid suppression in the treatment of gastro-oesophageal reflux disease. Gut 1992;33: 118–24.

144. Tytgat GN, Nicolai JJ, Reman FC. Efficacy of different doses of cimetidine in the treatment of reflux esophagitis. A review of three large, double-blind, controlled trials. Gastroenterology 1990;99:629–34.

145. Squires RH Jr, Colletti RB. Indications for pediatric gastrointestinal endoscopy: a medical position statement of the North American Society for Pediatric Gastroenterology and Nutrition. J Pediatr Gastroenterol Nutr 1996;23:107–10.

146. Tedesco FJ, Goldstein PD, Gleason WA, et al. Upper gastrointestinal endoscopy in the pediatric patient. Gastroenterology 1976;70:492–4.

147. Hyams JS, Leichtner AM, Schwartz AN. Recent advances in diagnosis and treatment of gastrointestinal hemorrhage in infants and children. J Pediatr 1985;106:1–9.

148. Mouterde O, Hadji S, Mallet E, et al. Les hémorragies digestives chez l'enfant: à propos de 485 endoscopies. Ann Pédiatr 1996;43:167–76.

149. Cox K, Ament ME. Upper gastrointestinal bleeding in children and adolescents. Pediatrics 1979;63:408–13.

150. Mougenot JF, Polonovski C. [Upper digestive fiberoptic endoscopy in children]. Arch Fr Pédiatr 1981;38:807–14.

151. Fox VL. Gastrointestinal bleeding in infancy and childhood. Gastroenterol Clin North Am 2000;29:37–66, v.

152. Hassall E, Dimmick JE. Unique features of *Helicobacter pylori* disease in children. Dig Dis Sci 1991;36:417–23.

153. Byrne WJ. Foreign bodies, bezoars, and caustic ingestion. Gastrointest Endosc Clin N Am 1994;4:99–119.

154. Christesen HB. Prediction of complications following unintentional caustic ingestion in children. Is endoscopy always necessary? Acta Paediatr 1995;84:1177–82.

155. Gaudreault P, Parent M, McGuigan MA, et al. Predictability of esophageal injury from signs and symptoms: a study of caustic ingestion in 378 children. Pediatrics 1983;71:767–70.

156. Gupta SK, Croffie JM, Fitzgerald JF. Is esophagogastroduodenoscopy necessary in all caustic ingestions? J Pediatr Gastroenterol Nutr 2001;32:50–3.

157. Lamireau T, Rebouissoux L, Denis D, et al. Accidental caustic ingestion in children: is endoscopy always mandatory? J Pediatr Gastroenterol Nutr 2001;33:81–4.

158. Nuutinen M, Uhari M, Karvali T, et al. Consequences of caustic ingestions in children. Acta Paediatr 1994;83:1200–5.

159. Wilsey MJ Jr, Scheimann AO, Gilger MA. The role of upper gastrointestinal endoscopy in the diagnosis and treatment of caustic ingestion, esophageal strictures, and achalasia in children. Gastrointest Endosc Clin N Am 2001;11:767–87, vii–viii.

160. Zargar SA, Kochhar R, Mehta S, et al. The role of fiberoptic endoscopy in the management of corrosive ingestion and modified endoscopic classification of burns. Gastrointest Endosc 1991;37:165–9.

161. Kernen YAM. Endoscopie haute en pratique pédiatrique: expérience genevoise [thèse]. Geneva: University of Geneva; 1999.

162. Antonson DL. Abdominal pain. Gastrointest Endosc Clin N Am 1994;4:1–21.

163. Squires RH Jr, Morriss F, Schluterman S, et al. Efficacy, safety, and cost of intravenous sedation versus general anesthesia in children undergoing endoscopic procedures. Gastrointest Endosc 1995;41:99–104.

164. Rasquin-Weber A, Hyman PE, Cucchiara S, et al. Childhood functional gastrointestinal disorders. Gut 1999;45 Suppl 2:II60–8.

165. Vukavic T, Vuckovic N, Pavkov D. Routine jejunal endoscopic biopsy in children. Eur J Pediatr 1996;155:1002–4.

166. Maksimak M, Cera PJ Jr. Mucosal biopsy. Gastrointest Endosc Clin N Am 1994;4:195–221.

167. Willemin B, Coumaros D, Zerbe S, et al. Abetalipoproteinemia. Apropos of 2 cases. Gastroenterol Clin Biol 1987;11:704–8.

168. Delpre G, Kadish U, Glantz I, et al. Endoscopic assessment in abetalipoproteinemia (Bassen-Kornzweig-syndrome). Endoscopy 1978;10:59–62.

169. Aoyagi K, Iida M, Yao T, et al. Characteristic endoscopic features of intestinal lymphangiectasia: correlation with histological findings. Hepatogastroenterology 1997;44:133–8.

170. Veldhuyzen van Zanten SJ, Bartelsman JF, Tytgat GN. Endoscopic diagnosis of primary intestinal lymphangiectasia using a high-fat meal. Endoscopy 1986;18:108–10.

171. Appleton AL, Sviland L, Pearson AD, et al. The need for endoscopic biopsy in the diagnosis of upper gastrointestinal graft-versus-host disease. J Pediatr Gastroenterol Nutr 1993;16:183–5.

172. Terdiman JP, Linker CA, Ries CA, et al. The role of endoscopic evaluation in patients with suspected intestinal graft-versus-host disease after allogeneic bone-marrow transplantation. Endoscopy 1996;28:680–5.

173. Sigurdsson L, Reyes J, Putnam PE, et al. Endoscopies in pediatric small intestinal transplant recipients: five years experience. Am J Gastroenterol 1998;93:207–11.

174. Kato T, O'Brien C, Nishida S, et al. The first case report of the use of a zoom videoendoscope for the evaluation of small bowel graft mucosa in a human after intestinal transplantation. Gastrointest Endosc 1999;50:257–61.

175. Misra SP, Dwivedi M. Long-term follow-up of patients undergoing balloon dilation for benign pyloric stenoses. Endoscopy 1996;28:552–4.

176. de Ridder L, Hoekstra JH. Manifestations of Munchausen syndrome by proxy in pediatric gastroenterology. J Pediatr Gastroenterol Nutr 2000;31:208–11.

177. Ruuska T, Vaajalahti P, Arajarvi P, et al. Prospective evaluation of upper gastrointestinal mucosal lesions in children with ulcerative colitis and Crohn's disease. J Pediatr Gastroenterol Nutr 1994;19:181–6.

178. Abdullah BA, Gupta SK, Croffie JM, et al. The role of esophagogastroduodenoscopy in the initial evaluation of childhood inflammatory bowel disease: a 7-year study. J Pediatr Gastroenterol Nutr 2002;35:636–40.

179. Tobin JM, Sinha B, Ramani P, et al. Upper gastrointestinal mucosal disease in pediatric Crohn disease and ulcerative colitis: a blinded, controlled study. J Pediatr Gastroenterol Nutr 2001;32:443–8.

180. Sharif F, McDermott M, Dillon M, et al. Focally enhanced gastritis in children with Crohn's disease and ulcerative colitis. Am J Gastroenterol 2002;97:1415–20.

181. Kawahra I, Ichikawa H. Fiberoptic instrument technology. In: Sivak MV, editor. Gastroenterologic endoscopy. Philadelphia: WB Saunders; 1987. p. 20–41.

182. Rothbaum RJ. Complications of pediatric endoscopy. Gastrointest Endosc Clin N Am 1996;6:445–9.

183. Bendig DW. Pulse oximetry and upper intestinal endoscopy in infants and children. J Pediatr Gastroenterol Nutr 1991;12:39–43.

184. Gyepes MT, Smith LE, Ament ME. Fiberoptic endoscopy and upper gastrointestinal series: comparative analysis in infants and children. AJR Am J Roentgenol 1977;128:53–6.

185. Penston JG, Boyd EJ, Wormsley KG. Mallory-Weiss tears occurring during endoscopy: a report of seven cases. Endoscopy 1992;24:262–5.

186. Alsop WR, Burt RW, Tolman KG. Intramural duodenal hematoma. Gastrointest Endosc 1985;31:32–4.

187. Ben Baruch D, Powsner E, Cohen M, et al. Intramural hematoma of duodenum following endoscopic intestinal biopsy. J Pediatr Surg 1987;22:1009–10.

188. Ghishan FK, Werner M, Vieira P, et al. Intramural duodenal hematoma: an unusual complication of endoscopic small bowel biopsy. Am J Gastroenterol 1987;82:368–70.

189. Guzman C, Bousvaros A, Buonomo C, et al. Intraduodenal hematoma complicating intestinal biopsy: case reports and review of the literature. Am J Gastroenterol 1998;93:2547–50.

190. Karjoo M, Luisiri A, Silberstein M, et al. Duodenal hematoma and acute pancreatitis after upper gastrointestinal endoscopy. Gastrointest Endosc 1994;40:493–5.

191. Middleton PH, Jones EW, Fielding JF. Intramural hematoma of the duodenum complicating peroral intestinal biopsy with a Crosby capsule. Gastroenterology 1972;63:869–71.

192. Mullinger M, Wood BJ, Kliman MR, et al. Intramural hematoma of the duodenum: an unusual complication of small bowel biopsy. J Pediatr 1971;78:323–6.

193. Ramakrishna J, Treem WR. Duodenal hematoma as a complication of endoscopic biopsy in pediatric bone marrow transplant recipients. J Pediatr Gastroenterol Nutr 1997;25:426–9.

194. Sollfrank M, Koch W, Waldner H, et al. [Intramural duodenal hematoma after endoscopic biopsy]. Rofo Fortschr Geb Rontgenstr Neuen Bildgeb Verfahr 2001;173:157–9.

195. Szajewska H, Albrecht P, Ziolkowski J, et al. Intramural duodenal hematoma: an unusual complication of duodenal biopsy sampling. J Pediatr Gastroenterol Nutr 1993;16:331–3.

196. Desmond PV, MacMahon RA. Fatal air embolism following endoscopy of a hepatic portoenterostomy. Endoscopy 1990;22:236.

197. Lowdon JD, Tidmore TL Jr. Fatal air embolism after gastrointestinal endoscopy. Anesthesiology 1988;69:622–3.

198. Spach DH, Silverstein FE, Stamm WE. Transmission of infection by gastrointestinal endoscopy and bronchoscopy. Ann Intern Med 1993;118:117–28.

199. al Zamil F, al Ballaa S, Nazer H, et al. Meningococcaemia: a life threatening complication of upper gastrointestinal endoscopy. J Infect 1994;28:73–5.

200. Davies GR, Benson MJ, Gertner DJ, et al. Diagnostic and therapeutic push type enteroscopy in clinical use. Gut 1995;37:346–52.

201. Berner JS, Mauer K, Lewis BS. Push and sonde enteroscopy for the diagnosis of obscure gastrointestinal bleeding. Am J Gastroenterol 1994;89:2139–42.

202. Lewis B, Waye JD. Total small bowel enteroscopy. Gastrointest Endosc 1987;33:435–8.

203. Meron G. The development of the swallowable video capsule (M2A). Gastrointest Endosc 2000;52:817–9.

204. Iddan G, Menon G, Glukhovsky A, et al. Wireless capsule endoscopy. Nature 2000;405:417.

205. Fireman Z, Mahajna E, Broide E, et al. Diagnosing small bowel

Crohn's disease with wireless capsule endoscopy. Gut 2003;52:390.

206. Costamagna G, Shah SK, Riccioni ME, et al. A prospective trial comparing small bowel radiographs and video capsule endoscopy for suspected small bowel disease. Gastroenterology 2002;123:999–1005.

207. Eliakim R, Fischer D, Suissa A, et al. Wireless capsule video endoscopy is a superior diagnostic tool in comparison to barium follow-through and computerized tomography in patients with suspected Crohn's disease. Eur J Gastroenterol Hepatol 2003;15:363–7.

208. Seidman EG. Wireless capsule video-endoscopy: an odyssey beyond the end of the scope. J Pediatr Gastroenterol Nutr 2002;34:333–4.

209. Ell C, Remke S, May A, et al. The first prospective controlled trial comparing wireless capsule endoscopy with push enteroscopy in chronic gastrointestinal bleeding. Endoscopy 2002;34:685–9.

210. Lewis BS, Swain P. Capsule endoscopy in the evaluation of patients with suspected small intestinal bleeding: results of a pilot study. Gastrointest Endosc 2002;56:349–53.

211. Hartmann D, Schilling D, Bolz G, et al. Capsule endoscopy versus push enteroscopy in patients with occult gastrointestinal bleeding. Z Gastroenterol 2003;41:377–82.

212. Scapa E, Jacob H, Lewkowicz S, et al. Initial experience of wireless-capsule endoscopy for evaluating occult gastrointestinal bleeding and suspected small bowel pathology. Am J Gastroenterol 2003;97:2776–9.

213. Jonnalagadda S, Prakash C. Intestinal strictures can impede wireless capsule enteroscopy. Gastrointest Endosc 2003;57:418–20.

214. Schwetz BA. Novel imaging device. JAMA 2001;286:1166.

215. Dokler ML, Bradshaw J, Mollitt DL, et al. Selective management of pediatric esophageal foreign bodies. Am Surg 1995;61:132–4.

216. Conners GP. A literature-based comparison of three methods of pediatric esophageal coin removal. Pediatr Emerg Care 1997;13:154–7.

217. Litovitz T, Schmitz BF. Ingestion of cylindrical and button batteries: an analysis of 2382 cases. Pediatrics 1992;89:747–57.

218. Schultz LR, Clatworthy HW. Esophageal strictures after anastomosis in esophageal atresia. Arch Surg 1963;87:120–3.

219. Huet F, Mougenot JF, Saleh T, et al. [Esophageal dilatation in pediatrics: study of 33 patients]. Arch Pediatr 1995;2:423–30.

220. London RL, Trotman BW, DiMarino AJ Jr, et al. Dilatation of severe esophageal strictures by an inflatable balloon catheter. Gastroenterology 1981;80:173–5.

221. Yeming W, Somme S, Chenren S, et al. Balloon catheter dilatation in children with congenital and acquired esophageal anomalies. J Pediatr Surg 2002;37:398–402.

222. La Scala GC. Le traitement par dilatateurs des lésions sténosantes bégnines de l'oesophage [thèse]. Geneva: University of Geneva; 1994.

223. Vantrappen G, Janssens J. To dilate or to operate? That is the question. Gut 1983;24:1013–9.

224. Ip KS, Cameron DJ, Catto-Smith AG, Hardikar W. Botulinum toxin for achalasia in children. J Gastroenterol Hepatol 2000;15:1100–4.

225. Pineiro-Carrero VM, Sullivan CA, Rogers PL. Etiology and treatment of achalasia in the pediatric age group. Gastrointest Endosc Clin N Am 2001;11:387–408.

226. Wara P. Endoscopic electrocoagulation of major bleeding from peptic ulcer. Acta Chir Scand 1985;151:29–35.

227. Sugawa C, Joseph AL. Endoscopic interventional management

228. Rollhauser C, Fleischer DE. Nonvariceal upper gastrointestinal bleeding: an update. Endoscopy 1997;29:91–105.

229. Mowat AP. Prevention of variceal bleeding. J Pediatr Gastroenterol Nutr 1986;5:679–81.

230. Cales P, Pascal JP. [Natural history of esophageal varices in cirrhosis (from origin to rupture)]. Gastroenterol Clin Biol 1988;12:245–54.

231. Valla D. [Esophageal varices and their rupture]. Gastroenterol Clin Biol 1986;10:571–4.

232. Prediction of the first variceal hemorrhage in patients with cirrhosis of the liver and esophageal varices. A prospective multicenter study. The North Italian Endoscopic Club for the Study and Treatment of Esophageal Varices. N Engl J Med 1988;319:983–9.

233. Grace ND. Diagnosis and treatment of gastrointestinal bleeding secondary to portal hypertension. American College of Gastroenterology Practice Parameters Committee. Am J Gastroenterol 1997;92:1081–91.

234. Ryckman FC, Alonso MH. Causes and management of portal hypertension in the pediatric population. Clin Liver Dis 2001;5:789–818.

235. McKiernan PJ. Treatment of variceal bleeding. Gastrointest Endosc Clin N Am 2001;11:789–812, viii.

236. Cales P, Oberti F. [Strategy for hemostatic treatment of hemorrhages caused by rupture of esophageal and gastric varices]. Gastroenterol Clin Biol 1995;19:B1-9.

237. Wu JC, Sung JJ. Update on treatment of variceal hemorrhage. Dig Dis 2002;20:134–44.

238. Peters JM. Management of gastrointestinal bleeding in children. Curr Treat Options Gastroenterol 2002;5:399–413.

239. Poddar U, Thapa B, Singh K. Endoscopic sclerotherapy in children: experience with 257 cases of extrahepatic portal venous obstruction. Gastrointest Endosc 2003;57:683–6.

240. Yachha SK, Sharma BC, Kumar M, et al. Endoscopic sclerotherapy for esophageal varices in children with extrahepatic portal venous obstruction: a follow-up study. J Pediatr Gastroenterol Nutr 1997;24:49–52.

241. Schuman BM, Beckman JW, Tedesco FJ, et al. Complications of endoscopic injection sclerotherapy: a review. Am J Gastroenterol 1987;82:823–30.

242. Lo GH, Lai KH, Shen MT, Chang CF. A comparison of the incidence of transient bacteremia and infectious sequelae after sclerotherapy and rubber band ligation of bleeding esophageal varices. Gastrointest Endosc 1994;40:675–9.

243. Toyoda K, Saku Y, Sadoshima S, Fujishima M. Purulent meningitis after endoscopic injection sclerotherapy for esophageal varices. Intern Med 1994;33:706–9.

244. Champigneulle B, Dollet JM, Seng G, et al. [2 cases of bacterial meningitis after sclerotherapy of esophageal varices] Gastroenterol Clin Biol 1986;10:612–3.

245. Wang WM, Chen CY, Jan CM, et al. Central nervous system infection after endoscopic injection sclerotherapy. Am J Gastroenterol 1990;85:865–7.

246. Kumar P, Mehta SK, Devi BI, et al. Pyogenic meningitis and cerebral abscesses after endoscopic injection sclerotherapy. Am J Gastroenterol 1991;86:1672–4.

247. Seidman E, Weber AM, Morin CL, et al. Spinal cord paralysis following sclerotherapy for esophageal varices. Hepatology 1984;4:950–4.

248. Laine L, Cook D. Endoscopic ligation compared with sclerotherapy for treatment of esophageal variceal bleeding. A meta-analysis. Ann Intern Med 1995;123:200–7.

249. Hassall E. Nonsurgical treatments for portal hypertension in children. Gastrointest Endosc Clin N Am 1994;4:223–58.

250. McKiernan PJ, Beath SV, Davison SM. A prospective study of endoscopic esophageal variceal ligation using a multiband ligator. J Pediatr Gastroenterol Nutr 2002;34:207–11.

251. Zargar S, Javid G, Khan B, et al. Endoscopic ligation compared with sclerotherapy for bleeding esophageal varices in children with extrahepatic portal venous obstruction. Hepatology 2002;36:666–72.

252. Ponsky JL, Gauderer MW. Percutaneous endoscopic gastrostomy: a nonoperative technique for feeding gastrostomy. Gastrointest Endosc 1981;27:9–11.

253. Sturgis TM, Yancy W, Cole JC, et al. Antibiotic prophylaxis in percutaneous endoscopic gastrostomy. Am J Gastroenterol 1996;91:2301–4.

254. Preclik G, Grune S, Leser HG, et al. Prospective, randomised, double blind trial of prophylaxis with single dose of co-amoxiclav before percutaneous endoscopic gastrostomy. BMJ 1999;319:881–4.

255. Gossner L, Keymling J, Hahn EG, et al. Antibiotic prophylaxis in percutaneous endoscopic gastrostomy (PEG): a prospective randomized clinical trial. Endoscopy 1999;31:119–24.

256. Jain NK, Larson DE, Schroeder KW, et al. Antibiotic prophylaxis for percutaneous endoscopic gastrostomy. A prospective, randomized, double-blind clinical trial. Ann Intern Med 1987;107:824–8.

257. Dormann AJ, Wigginghaus B, Risius H, et al. Antibiotic prophylaxis in percutaneous endoscopic gastrostomy (PEG)—results from a prospective randomized multicenter trial. Z Gastroenterol 2000;38:229–34.

258. Lee JH, Kim JJ, Kim YH, et al. Increased risk of peristomal wound infection after percutaneous endoscopic gastrostomy in patients with diabetes mellitus. Dig Liver Dis 2002;34:857–61.

259. Hament JM, Bax NMA, van der Zee DC, et al. Complications of percutaneous endoscopic gastrostomy with or without concomitant antireflux surgery in 96 children. J Pediatr Surg 2001;36:1412–5.

260. Langer JC, Wesson DE, Ein SH, et al. Feeding gastrostomy in neurologically impaired children: is an antireflux procedure necessary? J Pediatr Gastroenterol Nutr 1988;7:837–41.

261. Gauderer MW, Ponsky JL, Izant RJ Jr. Gastrostomy without laparotomy: a percutaneous endoscopic technique. J Pediatr Surg 1980;15:872–5.

262. Grunow JE, al Hafidh A, Tunell WP. Gastroesophageal reflux following percutaneous endoscopic gastrostomy in children. J Pediatr Surg 1989;24:42–4.

263. Heine RG, Reddihough DS, Catto-Smith AG. Gastro-oesophageal reflux and feeding problems after gastrostomy in children with severe neurological impairment. Dev Med Child Neurol 1995;37:320–9.

264. Launay V, Gottrand F, Turck D, et al. Percutaneous endoscopic gastrostomy in children: influence on gastroesophageal reflux. Pediatrics 1996;97:726–8.

265. Razeghi S, Lang T, Behrens R. Influence of percutaneous endo-scopic gastrostomy on gastroesophageal reflux: a prospective study in 68 children. J Pediatr Gastroenterol Nutr 2002;35:27–30.

266. Samuel M, Holmes K. Quantitative and qualitative analysis of gastroesophageal reflux after percutaneous endoscopic gastrostomy. J Pediatr Surg 2002;37:256–61.

267. Sacks BA, Vine HS, Palestrant AM, et al. A nonoperative technique for establishment of a gastrostomy in the dog. Invest Radiol 1983;18:485–7.

268. Russell TR, Brotman M, Norris F. Percutaneous gastrostomy. A new simplified and cost-effective technique. Am J Surg 1984;148:132–7.

269. Yaseen M, Steele MI, Grunow JE. Nonendoscopic removal of percutaneous endoscopic gastrostomy tubes: morbidity and mortality in children. Gastrointest Endosc 1996;44:235–8.

270. Mollitt DL, Dokler ML, Evans JS, et al. Complications of retained internal bolster after pediatric percutaneous endoscopic gastrostomy. J Pediatr Surg 1998;33:271–3.

271. Steinberg RM, Madhala O, Freud E, et al. Skin level division of percutaneous endoscopic gastrostomy without endoscopy retrieval: a hazardous procedure. Eur J Pediatr Surg 2002;12:127–8.

272. Segal D, Michaud L, Guimber D, et al. Late-onset complications of percutaneous endoscopic gastrostomy in children. J Pediatr Gastroenterol Nutr 2001;33:495–500

273. Nicholson FB, Korman MG, Richardson MA. Percutaneous endoscopic gastrostomy: a review of indications, complications and outcome. J Gastroenterol Hepatol 2000;15:21–5.

274. Hull MA, Rawlings J, Murray FE, et al. Audit of outcome of long-term enteral nutrition by percutaneous endoscopic gastrostomy. Lancet 1993;3:869–72.

275. Stern JS. Comparison of percutaneous endoscopic gastrostomy with surgical gastrostomy at a community hospital. Am J Gastroenterol 1986;81:1171–3.

276. Larson D, Burton D, Schroeder K, et al. Percutaneous endoscopic gastrostomy. Indications, success, complications, and mortality in 314 consecutive patients. Gastroenterology 1987;93:48–52.

277. Fernandes ET, Hollabaugh R, Hixon SD, et al. Late presentation of gastrocolic fistula after percutaneous gastrostomy. Gastrointest Endosc 1988;34:368–9.

278. Stefan MM, Holcomb GW, Ross AJ. Cologastric fistula as a complication of percutaneous endoscopic gastrostomy. JPEN J Parenter Enteral Nutr 1989;13:554–6.

279. Mougenot JF, Balquet P. Les hématèmèses de l'enfant. Approches diagnostiques actuelles. In: Sciences Flammarion, editor. Paris: Journées parisiennes de Pédiatrie; 1978. p. 243–53.

280. Chang MH, Wang TH, Hsu JY, et al. Endoscopic examination of the upper gastrointestinal tract in infancy. Gastrointest Endosc 1983;29:15–7.

281. Quak SH, Lam SK, Low PS. Upper gastrointestinal endoscopy in children. Singapore Med J 1990;31:123–6.

282. Ayoola EA, Nanda VJ, Gadour MO, et al. Upper gastrointestinal diseases in Saudi Arabian children. Trop Gastroenterol 1999;20:137–9.

3. Ileocolonoscopy and Enteroscopy

Mike Thomson, MB ChB, DCH, FCRP, FRCPCH, MD

This chapter focuses on technique and clinical application of ileocolonoscopy and enteroscopy in childhood. The impact of endoscopic investigations and therapies on specific disease processes and comparison with alternative methods are also discussed. Topics to be covered include the following:

- Patient preparation
- Bowel preparation
- Endoscopy facilities
- Monitoring and sedation or anesthetic
- Equipment
- Basic and advanced techniques in diagnostic and therapeutic ileocolonoscopy
- Indications
- Complications
- Follow-up and surveillance ileocolonoscopy
- New diagnoses
- Diagnostic comparison with noninvasive investigations
- Enteroscopy: indications, techniques, and complications

ILEOCOLONOSCOPY

Safe, informative, and effective ileocolonoscopy performed in a child-friendly environment with the minimum of distress to child and parent alike is a sine qua non for best-practice care of children and adolescents with conditions affecting the ileum and colon, such as inflammatory bowel disease, allergic colitis, and polyposis syndromes.

The care of children and adolescents differs in important ways from that of adults. This is reflected in the emphasis placed on various aspects of ileocolonoscopy, such as the frequent use of general anesthesia, the number and location of mucosal biopsies, and the routine inclusion of ileal intubation during a complete examination. The question of who should conduct the procedure continues to receive attention among pediatric gastroenterologists. It is generally accepted that a pediatrician, preferably with experience in pediatric gastroenterology, should be involved in the care of the child or adolescent and, ideally, should carry out the procedure. There can be few more satisfying experiences in medicine than making a clinical judgment and diagnosis in a child, confirming the nature and extent of the disease oneself by endoscopy, treating appropriately, and then visually demonstrating the success of such endeavours to child and parent by a follow-up procedure.

The practice of pediatric ileocolonoscopy has evolved dramatically over the past 15 to 20 years. Improvements in skill and technique have followed the advances in technology, from the advent of fiberoptic endoscopes used in pediatrics during the late 1970s[1] to the latest small-diameter, electronic videoendoscopes designed specifically for younger children.[2–8]

TRAINING

Much debate has surrounded the issue of the minimum procedure number required during training to achieve competence because a paucity of data exists to support one view or another. Guidelines issued by the North American Society of Pediatric Gastroenterology, Hepatology and Nutrition (NASPGHAN) in 1997 recommended a minimum of 50 colonoscopies. The guidelines were revised in 1999, increasing the threshold number to 100 and including numbers for therapeutic techniques such as snare polypectomy (20), stricture balloon dilation (15), and injection therapy or electrocautery (20).[9–11] It is apparent that some ongoing skill assessment is needed during training. A logbook of procedures undertaken with a trainer's assessment of skill level will undoubtedly become common practice in recognized training centers. This will shift the emphasis from "number counting" to skill assessment, which is sensible given that trainees learn at different rates. However, some minimum numbers are likely to remain.

It has previously been suggested that training on endoscopy stimulators may reduce the time needed to reach competency in endoscopy. Ferlitsch and colleagues randomly allocated beginners in adult ileocolonoscopy to either receive training on the GI-Mentor (Symbionix Ltd, Lod, Israel 71520) or no training for 3 weeks after baseline assessment.[12] They were subsequently reassessed on the endoscopy simulator, and a statistically significant difference between the two groups was seen. The Royal Free Centre for Paediatric Gastroenterology has a Symbionix GI-Mentor (Figures 67.3-1 and 67.3-2; <www.symbionix.com>), to which trainees now have access. Looking at the ileocolonoscopy skill graphs (Figure 67.3-3), it is clear that three individuals (numbered 8, 9, and 10 in the figures) exhibited much steeper learning curves and seemed more competent having completed a smaller number of procedures than the other seven. These three had had a 6-week program of training on the ileocolonoscopy simulator prior to their first "live" ileocolonoscopy. The trainees log their performance by saving it under their own identifiable code, and the trainer can assess this at any time by logging into the simulator in

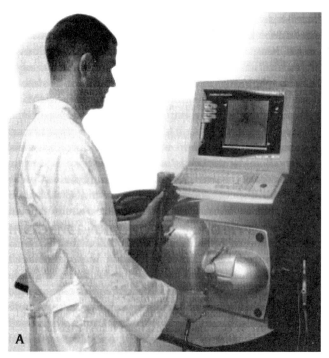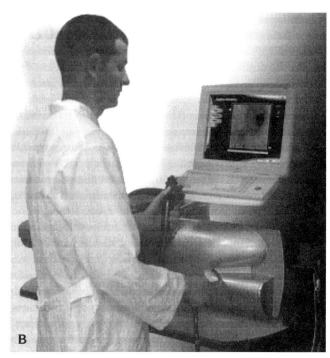

FIGURE 67.3-1   Symbionix GI-Mentor simulator for *A*, endoscopy and *B*, colonoscopy training.

trainer mode and so assess and feed back to the trainees their performance. This interactive approach is flexible and accelerates the learning process.

It is clearly preferable and more effective to learn the basic techniques on a model rather than a patient, and this approach does seem to work, at least on the basis of this preliminary experience. As these tools become more widely available, they are likely to become the first step and would seem to be the ideal introduction to training in

pediatric endoscopy and ileocolonoscopy, before actual patient procedures are undertaken.

To collate the views of all pediatric gastroenterologists, the recent World Congress on Pediatric Gastroenterology convened a working group on endoscopy, and one of its remits was to examine the issue of training.[13] This has recently been updated to coincide with the 2004 World Congress meeting in Paris but is not yet published. Three main areas requiring attention were identified: the estab-

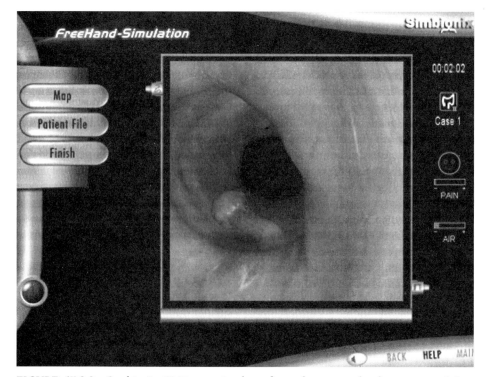

FIGURE 67.3-2   Symbionix GI-Mentor simulator for endoscopy and colonoscopy training: polyp on screen image.

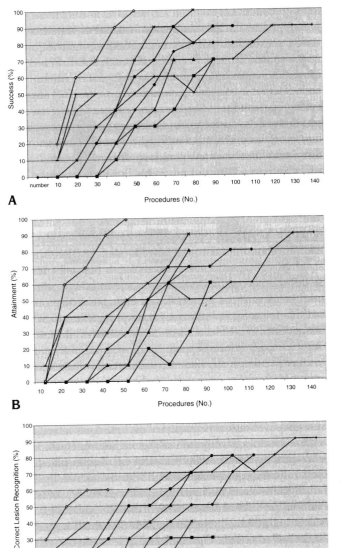

A

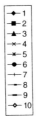

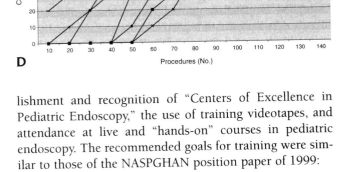

B

FIGURE 67.3-3 Trainee skill acquisition curves: *A*, transverse colon attainment; *B*, cecal intubation; *C*, ileal intubation; *D*, rates of correct lesion recognition; *E*, overall trainer's subjective assessment score. 1–7: no simulator pretraining; 8–10: simulator pretrained.

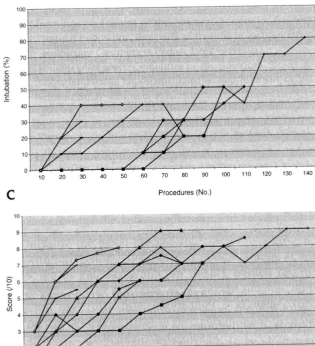

C

D

E

lishment and recognition of "Centers of Excellence in Pediatric Endoscopy," the use of training videotapes, and attendance at live and "hands-on" courses in pediatric endoscopy. The recommended goals for training were similar to those of the NASPGHAN position paper of 1999:

1. The ability to recommend endoscopic procedures based on the findings of a personal consultation and recognize indications, contraindications, and diagnostic or therapeutic alternatives for endoscopic procedures
2. To perform procedures safely, completely, and expeditiously
3. To correctly identify most endoscopic findings and perform endoscopic intervention as needed
4. To integrate endoscopic findings into a management plan
5. To understand risk factors and to recognize and manage complications
6. To recognize personal and procedural limitations and know when to request help

7. To be familiar with national organizational guidelines regarding sedation and monitoring for pediatric gastrointestinal procedures
8. To identify age- and indication-appropriate endoscopic equipment
9. The proper cleaning and maintenance of endoscopic equipment with special attention to infection control measures

Quality assurance has received little attention to date and is an issue that may begin to assume more importance, for instance, in the United Kingdom, where Clinical Governance and increased accountability are taking place. A multidiscipline body has been set up in the United Kingdom to address training issues, the Joint Advisory Group on gastrointestinal endoscopy (<www.thejag.org.uk>), and it oversees all training issues; ongoing assessment, revalidation, trainer and training center accreditation, and certification in endoscopic training are just some of the difficult issues now being dealt with effectively by this body, the view being that only through proper training can standards be improved in general. Striking differences in technical standards and appropriateness of ileocolonoscopy between centers emerged in one study in adult practice in Italy.[14] Quality improvement has been addressed by the American Society for Gastrointestinal Endoscopy.[15]

ENDOSCOPY FACILITY AND PATIENT PREPARATION

Ideally, both the child and the parents should be offered a preparatory visit to the endoscopy unit to answer questions and defuse any potential concerns and anxieties regarding the procedure and admission. Younger children undoubtedly benefit from preadmission visits and the involvement of a play therapist to enable some understanding of what is to take place and why.[16–18] Diagrams may help in explanations to older children. Preparatory videotapes are also useful for informing the patient and parent regarding what to expect. Units can benefit from devising a sample videotape specific to their own facility. A reduction in anticipatory anxiety may even reduce the amount of intravenous sedation required.[19] A child-friendly decorated endoscopy room with age-appropriate videotapes and familiar faces is important at this time of high stress. Parents may stay to watch the procedure in some units when intravenous sedation is provided. Most anesthesiologists would object to having parents present during administration of a general anesthetic, beyond the initial induction. Improved medical compliance and belief in the treatment are potential advantageous consequences of allowing parents to directly view the initial disease and its remission at follow-up ileocolonoscopy.[20] Young children often request photographs or a videotape of the ileocolonoscopy, and even older adolescents may view the procedure themselves.

A full screening is important to identify potential sedation or anesthetic risks. Although there is little correlation of mildly deranged peripheral coagulation indices with hemorrhage after mucosal biopsies, more pronounced bleeding diatheses may require forethought and appropriate blood product backup.[21] Properly informed consent should be obtained with an information sheet detailing potential complications and their incidence, and a separate consent should be signed in the event of research biopsies being requested.

Guidelines concerning antibiotic prophylaxis in children with lesions susceptible to endocarditis or in the immunocompromised child are available in the literature.[22] A low rate of bacteremia owing to bacterial translocation across the bowel wall has been demonstrated following pediatric ileocolonoscopy.[23] A combination of intravenous or intramuscular ampicillin (50 mg/kg, maximum 2 g) and gentamicin (2 mg/kg, maximum 120 mg) 30 minutes before and 6 hours after the ileocolonoscopy is generally recommended. Vancomycin (20 mg/kg slow intravenous infusion 1 hour before) can be substituted for ampicillin in those with documented penicillin allergy. It would seem reasonable to administer antibiotic prophylaxis in the rare case of percutaneous cecostomy or sigmoidostomy as for percutaneous gastrostomy insertion.

BOWEL PREPARATION

Poor bowel preparation is a major factor that may prevent or impede successful ileocolonoscopy. Although administration of regimens is not always easy, modern protocols can be remarkably effective in clearing the colon and ileum. Until 5 or 6 years ago, large volumes of oral electrolyte lavage solutions were used with variable success, coupled with the significant disadvantages of nasogastric administration and potential for fluid-electrolyte shifts in smaller children and infants. In one study, 40 mL/kg/h resulted in clear fecal effluent after a mean of 2.6 hours.[24] Subsequently, more favorable results and compliance were reported with low-volume oral agents and enemas, along with decreased oral intake.[25–28] Use of sodium phosphate preparations was associated with a transient rise in mean serum sodium and phosphate but with no change in serum calcium.[26,27] Refinements were made to these oral and enema regimens as newer preparations, which were more acceptable to children, became available; low-volume nonabsorbable polyethylene glycol preparations are becoming increasingly popular in pediatric units and are well tolerated, with no observable electrolytic disturbance.[29,30] Table 67.3-1 outlines several low-volume regimens that have been used successfully in children. The regimen employed in our unit, shown in Table 67.3-2, combines the beneficial effects of oral low-volume administration with the backup of an enema 1 to 2 hours beforehand if no clear fecal effluent is observed.[31] No clinically significant fluid shifts or electrolyte imbalances have been observed in over 2,000 colonoscopies over a 5-year period in our unit.

The benefit of an intravenous antispasmodic agent administered directly before the ileocolonoscopy has recently been demonstrated.[32] Hyoscyamine 0.5 mg was

TABLE 67.3-1   SUCCESSFUL RECENT LOW-VOLUME REGIMENS FOR THE PREPARATION OF THE BOWEL FOR ILEOCOLONOSCOPY

STUDY	REGIMEN	DIET	SUCCESS RATE
Gremse et al, 1996[27]	Oral sodium phosphate (45 mL/1.7m²) 6 pm and 6 am for am procedure	Clear liquid 24 h	18/19
da Silva et al, 1997[26]	Oral sodium phosphate (22.5 mL if < 30 kg, 45 mL if > 30 kg) pm and 5 am for am procedure	Clear liquid after first dose	10/14
Pinfield et al, 1999[30]	Sodium picosulfate with magnesium citrate (2.5 g < 2 yr, 5 g 2–5 yr, 10 g > 5 yr per dose) 24 and 18 hr preprocedure	Clear liquid for 24 h	32/32 (3 vomited)
Dahshan et al,1999[29]	Magnesium citrate and X-prep	Clear liquid for 48 h	

TABLE 67.3-2 BOWEL PREPARATION FOR CHILDREN UNDERGOING ILEOCOLONOSCOPY

Clear fluids for preceding 24 h (12 h for infants receiving no solid intake)

5 pm	Senokot	1–2 mg/kg (max 30 mg)
	Sodium picosulfate	2.5 g if < 1yr
		5 g if 1–4 yr
		10 g if > 4 yr

1 h preprocedure if no clear fecal effluent

6 am	Repeat sodium picosulfate dose
	1 h before procedure
	Phosphate enema (1/2 if < 1 yr)

given in this study of adults. An alternative could be hyoscine 20 mg adminstered intravenously. The use of such an agent given just prior to colonoscopy is determined by personal preference. Their use may facilitate ease of luminal visualization, but it also may increase the compliance of the colon, theoretically allowing a greater chance of loop formation. They are certainly of benefit in spastic colonic situations. It should be remembered that they work only for a short period of time, however—perhaps as short as 5 minutes—and they may be readministered in certain situations, such as when one needs to relax a haustral fold if a polyp is just beyond and obscured by it, or occasionally when one needs to relax a spastic ileocecal valve.

MONITORING AND SEDATION

Debate has surrounded the relative merits and safety of sedation and general anesthesia for upper gastrointestinal endoscopy and ileocolonoscopy in children for the past 5 to 10 years.[33-35] The use of sedation for endoscopy has been comprehensively reviewed recently.[35] The proponents of general anesthesia maintain that sedation is merely a financial or logistic expedient when the services of an anesthesiologist are less accessible.[33,34,36] In one US study, the cost of an endoscopy under general anesthesia was twice that under sedation.[37] It is generally agreed that children should receive, at a minimum, an analgesic in combination with a hypnotic for potentially painful or frightening procedures.[38]

It is also acknowledged that the concept of "conscious" (or "safe") sedation is not the prevailing clinical scenario in sedation in gastrointestinal endoscopy in pediatrics, and to get the requisite cooperation, and therefore a properly conducted procedure with mimimum distress to the child, deep sedation is usually necessary. It is further recognized that there are attendant safety issues of airway maintenance in this situation, and at the very least, a specific individual with appropriate advanced pediatric life support skills should be responsible for the child's cardiorespira-

tory welfare during such a procedure. The vast majority of pediatric gastrointestinal endoscopy under the age of 8 years in the United Kingdom, for instance, now occurs under general anesthesia.

When a child is sedated, resuscitation equipment should be easily accessible, and one or more people trained in pediatric advanced life support should be responsible for maintaining the airway and monitoring respiration, heart rate, blood pressure, and oxygen saturation.[39,40] Older children can sometimes benefit from conscious sedation such that they can participate in observing their ileocolonoscopy.[20] Sedation of younger children can be aided by environmental comforts such as a soothing voice or dimmed lights.[41] In all age groups, it is often necessary to use deep sedation because of the pain that can be associated with this procedure.[42] With deep sedation, it is clear that the risks are significant, including hypotension, respiratory compromise, and even respiratory arrest.[43] Combinations of benzodiazepines (midazolam in preference to diazepam) and opioids (pethidine or meperidine and fentanyl) are reported, with the occasional report of ketamine.[35,44] Table 67.3-3 lists some of the commonly used sedation regimens with the reversal agents.

Recent studies examining the safety of general anesthesia for day-case ileocolonoscopy in children refute claims that there may be more risk of perforation because the operator cannot judge the degree of discomfort as a marker of impending traction injury.[45,46] There is indeed a lack of evidence to support the contention that there is a higher complication rate with a general anesthetic than with sedation.[47] In fact, the airway is protected in a more effective and safer manner than with sedation, especially in upper endoscopy, with an improved operator satisfaction.[48]

EQUIPMENT

Most modern units employ adult and pediatric videocolonoscopes, and the general technical specifications for the pediatric instruments differ little between manufacturers (Table 67.3-4). When and in whom to use a pediatric colonoscope is mainly a matter of personal preference. We use personal judgment based on age and/or body weight. In general terms, the lower limit for the adult colonoscope is 3 to 4 years of age and/or 12 to 15 kg. The extra stiffness of the adult versions diminishes the likelihood of forming sigmoid loops, but extra care must then be taken, especially in younger children and with general anesthesia, not to advance against undue resistance, to avoid the unlikely complication of colonic perforation. The larger diameter of the adult colonoscopes can also lead to problems of

TABLE 67.3-3 SEDATION AND REVERSAL MEDICATIONS COMMONLY EMPLOYED IN PEDIATRIC ILEOCOLONOSCOPY

Midazolam: IV initial dose 0.05–0.1 mg/kg then titrate to maximum 0.3 mg/kg or 10 mg, whichever is lower[3]
   Oral dose 0.75 mg/kg or 15 mg, whichever is lower[34]
Fentanyl: IV initial dose 0.5–1.0 µg/kg, then titrate to maximum 5 µg/kg[3]
Meperidine/pethidine: IV initial dose 0.5 mg/kg, then titrate to maximum 2 mg/kg or 75 mg, whichever is lower[34]
Flumazenil: IV dose 0.02 mg/kg (maximum 0.2 mg) and repeat every minute to maximum of 0.05 mg/kg or maximum 1 mg[3]
Naloxone: IV dose 0.1 mg/kg (maximum 2 mg) and repeat every 2–3 min to maximum 10 mg[3]

TABLE 67.3-4   TECHNICAL SPECIFICATIONS OF VARIOUS PEDIATRIC COLONOSCOPES

PARAMETER	FUJINON (EC-410 MP15)	OLYMPUS (PCF 240L/I)	OLYMPUS VARIABLE STIFFNESS (CF 240AL/I)	PENTAX (EC-3440PK)
Angle of vision (deg)	140	140	140	140
Depth of field (mm)	6–100	4–100	3–100	6–100
Distal end (mm)	11	11.3	12.2	11.5
Insertion tube (mm)	11.1	11.3	12.0	11.4
Channel (mm)	2.8	3.2	3.2	3.8
Angle up/down (deg)	180/180	180/180	180/180	180/180
Angle right/left (deg)	160/160	160/160	160/160	160/160
Working length (mm)	1,520	1,330 1,680	1,330 1,680	1,500

maneuverability within the smaller colonic lumen of a young child. The variable stiffness colonoscope (see Table 67.3-4) may negotiate some of these problems. A control dial on the upper shaft of this small-diameter colonoscope (Olympus XCF-240AL/I, Olympus Corporation, Tokyo, Japan) allows an increase in the stiffness of the insertion tube when passing through the sigmoid and transverse colon to avoid looping.[49]

More recently, magnifying colonoscopes have been developed, and their value in combination with dye spray or chromoscopy in various gastrointestinal diseases has been described.[50] For instance, the decrease in the number of cryptal openings in ulcerative colitis can be observed and correlated to disease activity,[51] but this does not substitute for histologic assessment.

For insufflation, there may be some advantage awarded by the use of carbon dioxide in place of air because it is more rapidly absorbed, leading to less patient discomfort and, theoretically, less risk of perforation.[52,53]

ILEOCOLONOSCOPY BASIC TECHNIQUE

GETTING STARTED AND PATIENT POSITIONING

The patient is usually positioned in the left lateral knee to chest position, although some operators prefer the right lateral position, citing easier sigmoid negotiation. Certainly, if the procedure is not subsequently allowing easy access to the splenic flexure, then patient repositioning from one side to the supine and then to the other side may be advantageous. In general, frequent turning of the patient is conducive to easier ileocolonoscopy as a whole and is to be advocated. An assistant stands on the operator's left to administer any abdominal pressure that may subsequently be deemed necessary to control, or try to prevent, loop formation in the sigmoid or transverse colon.

PRACTICAL TIPS IN ILEOCOLONOSCOPY

One important "trick" in learning ileocolonoscopy is to grasp the concept of the lumen and the positions of a clock face. For instance, if the lumen is at 9 o'clock, then to enter this requires anticlockwise rotation combined with upward deflection of the scope tip from the "neutral" position of 12 o'clock. Similarly, a combination of upward deflection of the tip with clockwise rotation of the colonoscope will allow entry of the lumen, suggested by a dark crescent, if seen at anywhere clockwise from 12 o'clock to 6 o'clock. Obviously, one may equally use downward tip deflection combined

with the opposite rotatory control to that with upward tip deflection, and the execution and teaching of this concept are at personal discretion. With either approach, this is the most important maneuver that can be learned to assist in three-dimensional spatial orientation in the colon.

Prolonged "side viewing" of the bowel wall as it slides by should be avoided. Generally, the only place where, very temporarily, the lumen should be out of view is the occasional difficult negotiation of the splenic flexure. The patient's position may be changed throughout the procedure to facilitate removal of loops and to allow a better view of the lumen because the gravity-dependent material in the colonic lumen changes position. Relatively minimal insufflation of air is desirable in the sigmoid colon because excess air may increase the chance of sigmoid loop formation (carbon dioxide, provided by a specific commercially available delivery system attached to the colonoscope, because the insufflatory gas of choice may be preferable because it is absorbed much more quickly, decreasing pain and the very unlikely chance of perforation; see "Complications").

In handling the colonoscope, it is good practice to have a flat unimpeded surface on which to place the remainder of the colonoscope that is not yet inserted; this is particularly important because then any resistance encountered by the operator to forward advancement of the colonoscope can be attributed to colonic obstruction or loop formation within the child's colon. Hence, relatively quickly, the trainee can acquire a realization of the normal expected resistance to scope advancement. This, in turn, allows understanding of the likelihood of loop formation, without any external resistance to scope advancement, causing confusion with regard to the behavior of the colonoscope within the patient.

Generally, in ileocolonoscopy, gentle scope advancement with clear lumen visualization is desirable, and, usually, only the forefinger and thumb will be required to advance the colonoscope. If greater pressure is required, then the operator is not performing an optimum procedure, and loop formation is likely to have occurred.

RECTAL INTUBATION

Prior to any colonoscopy, it is considered good practice to perform an anal and then a rectal digital examination, the latter to avoid missing, by colonoscopy, very low-lying rectal polyps (although, where possible, retroflexion of the colonoscope in the rectum should occur prior to removal of the instrument to avoid missing lesions close to the anal margin). Adequate water-soluble lubrication, avoiding the tip of the instrument, allows easy passage into the rectum, which can occur with or without digital guidance from the operator's index finger. Posterior positioning of the tip and air insufflation will allow visualization of the rectal mucosa and the three semilunar folds, or valves of Houston, occurring on alternating sides of the lumen. Subsequently, direct visualization of the bowel lumen is mandatory, except in some circumstances at the splenic flexure. If, at any point, a maneuver results in loss of visualization of the lumen, then reversal of what the operator has just done will often return the lumen to view; if not, the gentle scope retraction combined with minor tip deflections using the wheels and minor rotation of the scope in both directions will usually result in reorientation in the lumen. Obviously, if luminal contents are blocking the view, then lens cleaning will help.

SIGMOID AND DESCENDING COLON

Gentle torquing of the shaft clockwise and anticlockwise combined with upward or downward tip deflection and scope advancement is ideal for negotiating the sigmoid colon—the so-called "torque-steering" technique. The initial sigmoid fold or valve can usually be passed by 90 to 120° of anticlockwise torsion. The different loops encountered in the sigmoid are demonstrated in Figure 67.3-4. A so-called N loop may be overcome by transabdominal pressure by an assistant on the apex of the loop pushing toward the feet (see Figure 67.3-4A). This often allows a so-called α loop to form, which can usually be tolerated as the instrument advances toward the splenic flexure (see Figure 67.3-4B). Reducing an α loop is accomplished by initial clockwise rotation and then slow removal of the colonoscope, keeping the lumen in the center of the field of vision. This may not be possible until the transverse (or even ascending) colon has been entered, in which case, it may be assisted by hooking the tip of the scope over the splenic flexure. Paradoxical movement of the tip forward may be observed as the instrument is withdrawn and the bowel "concertinas" over the colonoscope. Abdominal pressure in the left iliac fossa may be helpful. The sigmoid and descending colon are relatively featureless, with less haustral folds than more proximally in the colon.

SPLENIC FLEXURE AND TRANSVERSE COLON

Nonlooped colonoscope length used at this point might be 40 cm in older children and even 20 to 25 cm in those

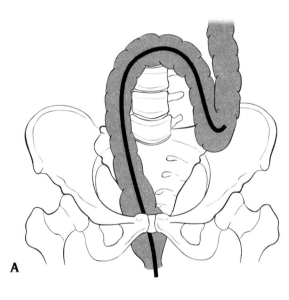

A

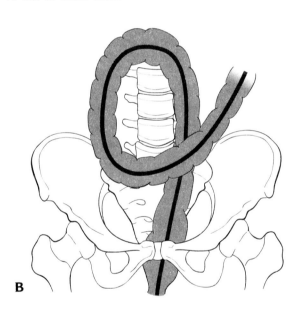

B

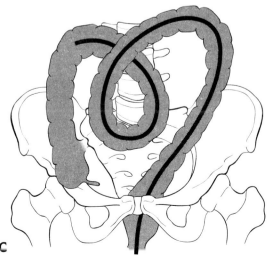

C

FIGURE 67.3-4 Diagram of colonoscope sigmoid loops that may form. *A*, an N loop in the sigmoid colon; *B*, an α loop in the sigmoid colon; *C*, a γ loop in a redundant transverse colon.

under the age of 3 to 4 years. This is valuable in determining whether a loop is present. At the splenic flexure, the spleen may then be seen as a dark blue transmural discoloration (Figure 67.3-5). When negotiating the splenic flexure, the most successful combination of tip maneuvers is that of clockwise, right, and up followed by anticlockwise after passing the flexure. Occasionally, placing the patient in the right decubitus position may assist. The transverse colon is recognized by the triangular haustral folds and is usually easily passed. Supine or right decubitus positioning may ease this. A loop in the shape of a U may occur in a dependent transverse colon, which is supported by abdominal pressure. The more difficult γ loop may occur in a redundant transverse colon (see Figure 67.3-4C). In addition, a good bit of advice is to apply gentle suction as the tip is advanced again in an attempt to concertina a potentially long dependent transverse colon over the colonoscope, thus maintaining a relatively short colonoscope and, hence, good control and maneuverability.

HEPATIC FLEXURE AND ASCENDING COLON

Nonlooped colonoscope length used at this point might be 60 cm in older children and even 40 cm in those under the age of 3 to 4 years. This is valuable in determining whether a loop is present. The hepatic flexure is also recognized by the dark, usually blue, discoloration seen through the bowel wall, and positional change to the supine or right decubitus may again facilitate identification of the lumen. The combination of right, up, and clockwise followed by anticlockwise rotation and suction down into the ascending colon once around the sharply angled hepatic flexure is usually the most effective maneuver, but various combinations, including position change and scope withdrawal, may be required. Another tip is to remember that it is easy to be too far advanced into the vault of the hepatic flexure, leading to advance into a blind end, and often slight withdrawal of the instrument may reveal the fact that one is trying to negotiate this blind-ended area. The two or three sharp folds then observed may then be most successfully negotiated by tip deflection using both up/down and left/right wheels with minimal advancement of the scope. This is most easily performed in the supine patient position, however.

Once the hepatic flexure is negotiated, the transverse colonic γ loop may be reduced with anticlockwise or clockwise rotation followed by withdrawal of the colonoscope and suction. Loop withdrawal is essentially informed guess work initially. Studies with the colon Map guider developed by Dr. Christopher Williams and Olympus, based on using a colonoscope with an inbuilt electromagnetic loop that allows accurate real-time colonoscope three-dimensional positioning by detection using an external positioning device and displayed on a screen next to the patient, have shown that even expert colonoscopists get the type of loop present wrong in half of the cases.[54-56] Once one starts to remove the loop, using rotation only initially, a tip is to gently start to remove the colonoscope and try to determine whether within-patient resistance is increasing or whether the colonoscope is trying to push your hand away from the patient as the loop unfolds. Usually, trying clockwise or anticlockwise combined with instrument withdrawal will, with experience, allow early determination of which rotation direction is likely to be successful in "delooping" the colonoscope. It is best to try to maintain good luminal vision during this procedure, but, not infrequently, the lumen is lost; however, if this loop removal technique is effective, it is then not unusual to find oneself then looking at the appendiceal orifice and hence the cecum because the scope will have naturally traveled down the ascending colon. It is important to remember that the ascending colon, which in children is of variable length, may be as short as 5 cm in some younger cases.

CECUM

Three useful ways to ensure that one has reached the cecum are as follows:

- Observing the colonoscopic illumination in the right iliac fossa (using the specific high-intensity light transillumination application available with some colonoscopes is not usually necessary in children, excepting with some obese adolescents, for whom it can be helpful when applied in a dark environment)
- Digitally indenting the abdominal wall over the right iliac fossa and observing the corresponding effect on the colonic wall with the colonoscope
- Identifying the triradiate fold, appendicele orifice, and (especially if gas bubbles or ileal effluent are being excreted from it) the typical two lips–like appearance of the ileocecal valve (Figure 67.3-6A)

A good maxim is that if there is any doubt in the operator's mind about having reached the cecum, then one is usually at the hepatic or even splenic flexure. Only about 80 cm of scope from the anus is needed when all loops are removed in an adult, and in smaller children, only 40 to 60 cm may be needed. This assumes normal anatomy of the ascending colon and cecum. Obviously, cecal strictures can confuse the picture.

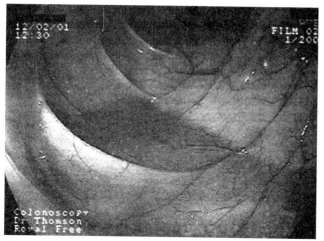

FIGURE 67.3-5   Dark shadow of spleen seen through colon at splenic flexure.

ILEAL INTUBATION AND ITS IMPORTANCE

The ileocecal valve is present approximately 1 to 4 cm distal to the appendicele orifice opening into a smooth asymmetric fold and opens perpendicular to the axis of the colon. Figure 67.3-6 shows the steps of the easiest technique for ileal intubation. Removal of any colonic loops is important to allow for a responsive scope with no paradoxical movement. Figures 67.3-6B and 67.3-7 show the valve maneuvered to the 6 o'clock position, usually after clockwise rotation of the scope and wheel-tip deflection to maintain a centered cecal view. Anticlockwise rotation can also be used but is less efficient. If too much gas is present, then the cecum may be "tented," and this should be suctioned prior to an ileal intubation attempt. Figures 67.3-6C and 67.3-8 show the insertion of the biopsy forceps such that just the tip or the first few millimeters are visibly exposed beyond the end of the scope. The scope is then inserted just beyond the fold (using the downward deflecting wheel with the scope as above already in the 6 o'clock position), and the tip is inclined downward so that the forceps gently press into the wall. Slight left inclination may be required at this point to open the valve like a pair of lips on slight withdrawal of the scope (see Figure 67.3-6C). Once the valve is opened, the scope may be passed into the ileum with further downward deflection. Often this is facilitated by small right and left deflections with an assistant pressing on the abdomen over the transverse colon to support a dependent transverse and also prevent loop formation. In the absence of ileocecal valve strictures, and with

practice, this technique will allow an ileal intubation rate of 100%. Perforation of the cecum or ileum with this technique is a theoretical concern raised by some observers unfamiliar with this technique, but this has not occurred in our experience of over 5,000 ileocolonoscopies and is extremely unlikely.

An alternative technique is "blind" intubation of the ileocecal valve. This involves the same positioning of the valve at 6 or 9 o'clock and then slowly withdrawing the scope back from just beyond the valve's fold while insufflating with air and deflecting the scope tip downward. The disadvantage of this technique is that it is not under direct vision.

ILEUM

The ileal mucosa will have the typical velvet-like appearance of small bowel, with the presence of smoother raised areas, which are Peyer patches, and, occasionally, lymphonodular hyperplasia of varying degrees. Villi are more easily seen if the lumen is flooded with water. The ileal surface is shown in greater relief with a spray of standard blue or black ink (methylene blue in a 1:20 dilution may also be used); this is also useful in showing the detail of sessile polyps in the colon. Deeper intubation of the ileum by either technique is similar to duodenal negotiation during upper gastrointestinal endoscopy, and up to 40 cm of ileum can be observed.

It is pertinent here to discuss the diagnostic need for entering the ileum in children suspected of inflammatory bowel disease. Williams and colleagues, in 1982,[7] reported

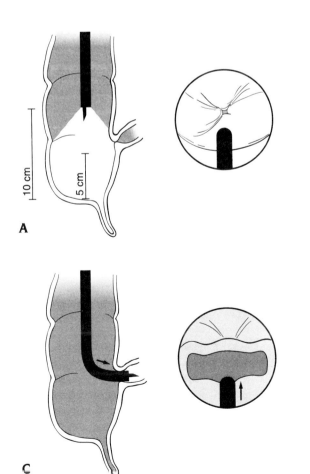

A

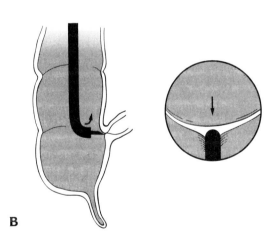

B

FIGURE 67.3-6   A, Identification of cecum with triradiate fold, appendicele orifice, and ileocecal valve. B, Ileocecal valve at 6 o'clock. C, Forceps opening up ileocecal valve with downward deflection of the colonoscope tip.

C

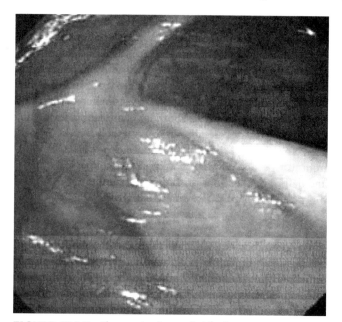

FIGURE 67.3-7   Ileocecal valve at 6 o'clock.

their experience of total ileocolonoscopy in children in which the terminal ileum was examined in 63 patients. In 6 children, ileitis detected by ileocolonoscopy was the sole finding of Crohn disease, which was previously unrecognized by radiologic contrast studies. Lipson and colleagues compared ileoscopy and barium studies, with an endoscopy specificity of 0.96 for diagnosis of Crohn disease in the terminal ileum.[57] In 14 of 46 children, ileoscopy revealed diagnosis, which would otherwise have been missed. This study also made clear that the endoscopic appearances could be completely normal, yet the diagnosis of Crohn disease could be made histologically by the presence of granulomata. Also, a pronounced lymphoid hyperplasia pattern was present radiologically in 24% of children and would have been a source of error in two cases had contrast radiographs been relied on to make the diagnosis without ileoscopy. More recently, Deere and colleagues showed that sigmoid, colonic, and rectal biopsies confirm the diagnosis of inflammatory bowel disease in only 60% of cases, and diagnosis based on morphologic criteria was possible in only 85% of cases when the cecum was reached without ileal intubation.[58] Geboes and colleagues assessed 300 patients, including adolescents and children, and found endoscopic and histologic ileal lesions in 123 and 125, respectively, of whom no colonic disease was present in 44.[59] Ileal biopsies were essential for the diagnosis in 15 patients and contributory in 53. There are, of course, other reasons apart from the principal one, that is, diagnosis of chronic inflammatory bowel disease, for entering the ileum in children. For instance, ileoscopy will facilitate diagnoses of other causes of ileitis such as infection with tuberculosis or *Yersinia*.[60] In addition, therapeutic dilation of short terminal ileal strictures by per endoscopic balloon catheter may be attempted.

SCOPE WITHDRAWAL

A more careful inspection of the colon is necessary on withdrawal of the scope, especially for the presence of polyps, which may have remained hidden behind a haustral fold during the initial insertion of the scope. Biopsies should be taken from all areas, including normal-looking mucosa to allow for accurate histologic diagnosis. Biopsy technique is similar to esophagogastroduodenoscopy, with the exception that many colonoscopic biopsy forceps have a central barb, allowing more than one biopsy to be taken each time the forceps are passed.

Lastly, before removing the scope from the anus, a retroflexion maneuver obtained by maximum upward and right or left tip deflection and slight advancement of the scope into the rectal vault, followed by rotation clockwise and anticlockwise through 180°, completes the examination. This is necessary to observe the anorectal junction and distal rectum. Distal ulcers, inflammation, or even polyps can be missed if this is not done.

ADVANCED TECHNIQUES

POLYPECTOMY

This is the most common therapeutic intervention, and the requirements for safe and effective polyp identification and removal include the following:

- Adequate sedation or general anesthetic to prevent patient movement
- Adequate bowel preparation
- Careful observation on insertion and withdrawal, changing the patient's position as needed
- Familiarity with the cauterization technique and power settings
- Availability of hemostasis techniques
- Normal or corrected coagulation indices

If bowel clearance is not good, then small or medium polyps may be missed, and feces may hamper their

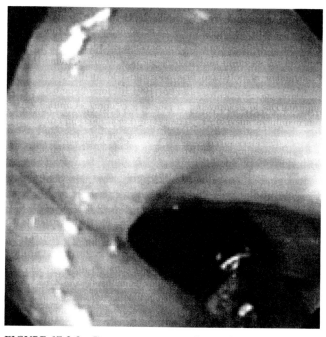

FIGURE 67.3-8   Forceps opening up ileocecal valve with downward deflection of the colonoscope tip.

removal. Sudden movement of the patient may cause premature removal of an ensnared polyp without electrocautery and lead to hemorrhage. Ensnaring the polyps may also be impeded. Delayed postpolypectomy hemorrhage is rare, but parents should be advised as to this possibility, although this is not a reason for routine overnight observation in the hospital following the procedure.

Polyps should be removed when first encountered because they may be difficult to subsequently locate. The size of a polyp and whether it is pedunculated or sessile determines the mode of removal. Those less than 5 mm in diameter may be removed by normal "cold" or monopolar or bipolar "hot" biopsy forceps (Figure 67.3-9). Monopolar forceps provide tissue for histology and cauterize surrounding tissue, whereas bipolar forceps ablate most of the tissue, making histologic interpretation more difficult.[61,62] Minisnares (15–20 mm long) may also be used for removal of small polyps by cold technique or cautery.[63] Generally, polyps greater than 5 mm require an electrocautery snare, which are available in varying sizes and shapes (eg, hexagonal, oval, crescent) (Figure 67.3-10). Most are monopolar, and the advantages of bipolar snares are not compelling.[64]

Polyps with stalks are ensnared around their neck, and if a monopolar current is employed, the colonoscope is used to angle the polyp away from the colonic wall. Otherwise, current is transmitted from the polyp to contact areas on the colonic wall with the potential for perforation (Figure 67.3-11). "Pulsed cut" (also called "blended cut and coagulation") and pure "coagulation" set at 15 to 30 watts are the favored types of current rather than pure "cut," which will not adequately cauterize the stump. The assistant slowly tightens the snare while current is applied to prevent garrotting of the polyp. Excess current may occasionally lead to transmural damage, with the potential for perforation. For larger polyps with attendant larger stalks, other methods may prevent excessive hemorrhage, for example, attachment of a metal clip to the base of the stalk,[65] prior injection of the stalk with 1:10,000 epinephrine,[46] attachment of detachable loop snares to the stalk prior to polyp removal,[66] and piecemeal removal with specially designed "endo-scissors" and "endo-forceps." This latter technique is particularly useful for large sessile polyps, in which submucosal injection of saline may divide the tissue planes and allow for endoscopic mucosal resection of the polyp (Figure 67.3-12). Rubber bands may be applied to elevate a sessile polyp prior to

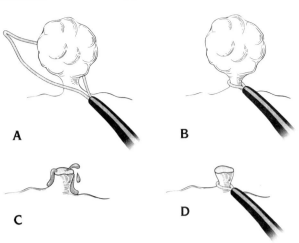

FIGURE 67.3-10 Technique of snaring larger pedunculated polyps. *A*, Polyp lassoed by snare; *B*, snare closed; care not to amputate without coagulation current; *C*, if stalk bleeds, inject base with 1:10,000 epinephrine; *D*, snare assisted coagulation of stump.

resection[67] or to the bleeding stalk postpolypectomy.[68] Techniques of endomucosal resection and polyp removal can also be aided by prior endosonographic assessment.

Retrieval also depends on size. Small polyps may be sucked up through the suction channel and caught in a suction trap. The snare itself may be used to retrieve larger polyps, or specific retrieval devices such as baskets, grasping forceps, or nets may be helpful. Without a net to gather the polyps, one may need to repeatedly remove and reinsert the scope to collect all of the polyps. Alternatively, when many large polyps are encountered and removed, it may be easier to sift the feces subsequently.

DILATION OF STRICTURES
Through-the-scope balloon dilators are appropriate for ileocolonic dilation, employing the same concept and method as for upper gastrointestinal strictures, employing radiologic screening control. Long-term symptomatic relief can be afforded in some carefully selected patients, including adolescents in reported studies.[69,70] Pressures of 35 to 50 psi in balloons of 12 to 18 mm are available. Theoretically, as for neoplastic or diverticulitis-associated strictures in adults, stent placement could be used as a last resort in inflammatory bowel disease–type strictures, but there are no reported cases of this occurring in childhood as yet.

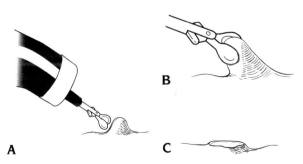

FIGURE 67.3-9 Technique for removal of small polyps using "cold" or "hot" forceps. *A*, Forceps exit scope; *B*, grasp and "tent" polyp, *C*, polyp removed, "hot" biopsy forceps with current

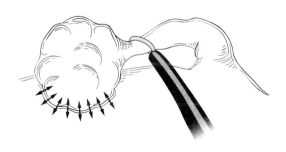

FIGURE 67.3-11 Complication of current dissipating through the colonic wall with the potential for perforation unless the polyp is drawn away from the wall.

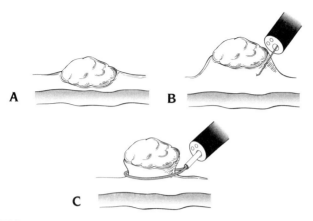

FIGURE 67.3-12 Technique of lifting a sessile polyp (*A*) away from underlying stroma prior to snare polypectomy. *B*, Saline or 1:10,000 epinephrine injected under polyp, creating a tissue plane; *C*, snare and polypectomy. Endomucosal resection may be needed.

PERCUTANEOUS ENDOSCOPIC CECOSTOMY

Percutaneous endoscopic cecostomies have been successfully placed in a number of children with intractable constipation using the same technique as for gastrostomy insertion using the pull-through technique. This approach followed reports of effective treatment of obstipation and fecal impaction in children by appendicostomy and intestinal button implantation using antegrade continence enemas, the so-called ACE procedure.[71] Intraoperative ultrasonography was used to confirm the position of the cecum just below the layers of the abdominal wall. No complications were reported in one series.[72]

A newer technique of percutaneous sigmoidostomy has recently been reported for the treatment of low left-sided refractory constipation, again employing a pull-through technique, with some success.[73]

THERAPY OF LOWER GASTROINTESTINAL BLEEDING

Interventions used to prevent bleeding during polypectomy and mentioned earlier may also be used to manage post-polypectomy bleeding. Apart from colitis and polyps, other causes of bleeding are angiodyplasias and arteriovenous malformations. Angiodysplasias are rarely reported in childhood (mean age 2–3 years) and are more easily diagnosed by selective regional angiography than by ileocolonoscopy despite occurring in the left hemicolon. In children, control of bleeding has required surgical excision.[74] Arteriovenous malformations must be subject to angiographic assessment before any endoscopic therapy is contemplated because many of these apparently innocuous-looking luminal lesions may have large vascular beds. Examples of equipment that may be used to stop a localized lesion from bleeding include heater probes,[75] bipolar cautery probe, hot biopsy forceps, neodymium:yttrium-aluminum-garnet laser set for thermal coagulation,[76] and argon plasma coagulation.

ENDOSONOGRAPHY

Endoluminal ultrasonography of the rectum has been an established technique for years; however, more recently, an echocolonoscope has allowed combined examination of the mucosa and the bowel wall. This is a forward-viewing colonoscope with the transducer (7.5 MHz) situated in the rigid tip of the scope.[77] Alternatively, an ultrasound miniprobe can be introduced via the biopsy channel (7.5 or 12.5 MHz). A fluid interface is necessary for all endosonography, and this can be achieved either with a fluid-filled balloon or filling the relevant colonic segment with water. Because this may be time-consuming, it is easier to concentrate on the region of interest rather than attempt to examine the entire colon. In adult practice, staging of cancers is the major indication for endosonography. In children and adolescents, indications for this technique might include suspicion of early invasive cancer arising from an adenoma, assessment of the extent and depth of sessile polyps to guide reception technique, assessment of colonic strictures/fistulae/anastomoses, assessment of the extent and depth of inflammatory bowel disease, assessment of the extent and depth of vascular lesions, examination of rectal and colonic portal hypertension with varices, and suspicion of lymphoma.

Inflammatory bowel disease appears as wall thickening and subsequent loss of the normal layer structure of the colon with progressive inflammation. Although theoretical differentiation between ulcerative colitis and Crohn disease is possible owing to the transmural nature of Crohn disease, it has been shown recently that active ulcerative colitis can have echotexture changes extending into the submucosa and that these changes correlate with disease activity.[78] Surgical decisions were made in one study of patients with Crohn disease[79] in which endoscopic ultrasonography was used to differentiate between superficial and transmural involvement. An ileoanal pouch was undesirable when transmural disease was identified. Perirectal and pericolonic fistulae and abscesses have been seen using the rigid rectal ultrasound probe, and this is a potential application for endoscopic ultrasonography.[80] Catheter probe–assisted endoscopic ultrasonography in inflammatory bowel disease has advantages over an echocolonoscope, which may be technically difficult to use. One study recently showed that wall thickness was twice as great in active inflammatory bowel disease, but ulcerative colitis could not be differentiated from Crohn disease.[81] Loss of wall structure correlated with disease activity score in the Crohn disease group, and wall thickness correlated with disease activity in the ulcerative colitis group. Other parameters, such as superior mesenteric artery maximum flow velocity and increased Doppler ultrasonography–demonstrated mural blood flow, are being examined as viable noninvasive substitutes for determination of post-treatment ileocecal Crohn disease activity, thus potentially avoiding the need for follow-up ileocolonoscopy, as some units advocate.

FOREIGN BODY REMOVAL

Foreign bodies in the lower gastrointestinal tract are rare in childhood. Occasionally, objects such as percutaneous endoscopic gastrostomy flanges or other ingested foreign bodies may become impacted at the ileocecal valve, necessitating endoscopic removal.[82]

REDUCTION OF INTUSSUSCEPTION AND SIGMOID VOLVULUS

Pneumatic reduction of intussusception has been described with simultaneous identification of the intussuscipiens, in one case a polyp, which was removed, and in another case, terminal ileal lymphonodular hyperplasia.[83,84] I have used air insufflation to reduce an ileocecal intussusception caused by terminal ileal Crohn disease. Reduction of sigmoid volvulus is a more common indication, particularly among patients with chronic constipation.

PER ENDOSCOPIC MANOMETRY

Per endoscopic manometry has limited application but has been studied in adults specifically identifying abnormal motor patterns and hypertension of the ileocecal valve.[85]

COMPLICATIONS OF ILEOCOLONOSCOPY

Complications, excluding those due to sedation, are summarized in Table 67.3-5. The literature to date reveals over 3,000 colonoscopies under 20 years of age reported, with 5 perforations—4 postpolypectomy and 1 in a patient with severe ulcerative colitis. Ten procedure-related minor complications are noted, including four small postpolypectomy hemorrhages, three cases of postprocedure abdominal pain with spontaneous resolution, one common peroneal nerve palsy secondary to periprocedure positioning, and two with a postprocedure fever for more than 24 hours.[1,4,5,45,46,75,86,87] This equates to a complication rate owing to the procedure itself of approximately 0.3% and, without polypectomy, of about 0.05%. This is in keeping with the British definition of "minimal" risk and the American definition of "minor risk over minimal."[88]

Perforation itself may well be relatively operator independent, occurring often in those with underlying connective tissue disease. Even enema treatment for constipation can cause perforation in patients with Ehlers-Danlos syndrome.[89] A single case of a child with serosal surface tears owing to a rigid colonoscope and a large sigmoid loop was reported in 1974.[90] Flexible pediatric colonoscopes or the new variable-stiffness colonoscopes may prevent this

TABLE 67.3-5 PROCEDURE-RELATED AND POSTPROCEDURE COMPLICATIONS IN PEDIATRIC ILEOCOLONOSCOPY

DIAGNOSTIC PROCEDURE RELATED
Vasovagal reactions
Hemorrhage
Perforation: traction serosal, direct transmural
Pancreatitis
Splenic trauma

THERAPEUTIC PROCEDURE RELATED
Perforation
Hemorrhage
Thermal injury: transmural

POSTPROCEDURE
Distention and discomfort (less if CO_2 insufflation used)
Delayed evidence of perforation or hemorrage

nowadays. Following electrocautery removal of a polyp, the stalk and the contralateral wall should be examined closely for evidence of mucosal perforation. The merits of conservative therapy of selected cases of colonic perforation have been discussed,[91] and it would seem reasonable to adopt conservative management, for instance, in the case of silent asymptomatic perforations and those with localized peritonitis without signs of sepsis who continue to improve clinically without intervention.[92] In one study in adults, only 3 of 21 patients were managed nonsurgically, and there was no difference in the morbidity or mortality between primary repair and resection and anastomosis.[93] In another, conservative management was successful in 13 of 48 patients, and 12 of the 13 were postpolypectomy perforations.[94]

In contradistinction to adults, bacteremia has not been detected in children after ileocolonoscopy.[23] In addition, modern cleaning machines seem to largely prevent the glutaraldehyde-associated colitis reported in the past.[95]

Polypectomy is the main cause of hemorrhage, and, as noted above, there are very few reported cases of this occurring in pediatrics. Hassall and colleagues noted minor bleeding, which stopped spontaneously in 2 children from 38 polypectomies in 136 children,[4] and there are no cases reported that required transfusion in children. Resnaring a bleeding stalk and maintaining pressure for 10 to 15 minutes are the first steps and, if unsuccessful, can be followed by injection of 1:10,000 epinephrine or thrombin or further electrocoagulation. Later bleeding has been reported in adults with a median delay of 37 hours in about half of one series.[96]

Splenic rupture is rarely seen and will present with hypovolemia and shoulder tip or abdominal pain within 24 hours of the ileocolonoscopy.[97] Similarly, direct trauma to the tail of the pancreas is the proposed mechanism of injury in the rare case of pancreatitis reported.[98]

Because of the rarity of complications in pediatrics, most pediatric endoscopists, when presented with such a clinical situation, will be unfamiliar with the etiology of the symptoms, and colleagues' opinions should often be sought.[99]

INDICATIONS FOR ILEOCOLONOSCOPY

The main indications, both diagnostic and therapeutic, for ileocolonoscopy in childhood and adolescence are set out in Table 67.3-6. The most common indication in the pediatric age group is, of course, suspicion of inflammatory bowel disease. As part of first-line investigation, an upper endoscopy is also indicated because up to 20% of inflammatory bowel disease cases can be differentiated into either Crohn disease or indeterminate colitis by upper gastrointestinal endoscopy.[100]

The mucosal appearances of ulcerative colitis and Crohn disease are well described and are not reiterated here.[3,101] Ileocolonoscopy of acute colitis is generally held to be a safe and reliable tool in expert hands and can help to differentiate ulcerative colitis from other pathologies and also allow prognostication.[102,103] Per rectal bleeding is also an important indication for ileocolonoscopy. With col-

TABLE 67.3-6   DIAGNOSTIC AND THERAPEUTIC
                INDICATIONS FOR ILEOCOLONOSCOPY
                IN CHILDREN AND ADOLESCENTS

DIAGNOSTIC
Suspected inflammatory bowel disease
Follow-up for assessment of efficacy of inflammatory bowel disease
  treatment
Suspected allergic colitis
Suspected colitis owing to other causes, eg, chronic granulomatous
  disease
Lower gastrointestinal hemorrhage
Chronic diarrhea
Cancer surveillance
Graft-versus-host disease
Endosonography
Manometry

THERAPEUTIC
Polypectomy
Foreign body removal
Percutaneous cecostomy
Stricture dilation
Reduction of intussusception

itis, the blood will usually be mixed in with the stool and may be associated with pain, whereas polyps are the most common cause of painless rectal bleeding.[104] Follow-up ileocolonoscopy allows assessment of treatment efficacy and can demonstrate to older children and parents these beneficial effects, promoting continued compliance.

Allergic enterocolitis usually presents in the first year to 2 years of life and may present even in the exclusively breastfed infant whose mother is ingesting antigens such as cow's milk protein.[105] A case can be made for removing the potentially offending antigen from the diet of the child or, if breastfed alone, from the mother. Ileocolonoscopy is not usually needed in such a circumstance, although it has been advocated as a diagnostic tool—the so-called "colonoscopic allergen provocation," in which, in one study in adults, 77% had a positive local visible mucosal reaction with histologic evidence of recruitment of mast cells and activation of eosinophils.[106] Simple dietary manipulation is usually sufficient to make the diagnosis in infants. Ulcerative colitis and Crohn disease are extremely rare under the age of 2 years. If appearances at ileocolonoscopy or on histology of biopsies are in keeping with such diagnoses, then it is important to think of other underlying reasons for these findings in this age group. This may include diagnoses such as enterocolitis of infancy,[107] glycogen storage disorders, chronic granulomatous disease, neutrophil chemotactic defects, and infectious enterocolitides, among others. Rare enteropathies such as tufting enteropathy may also involve the colon.

It must not be forgotten that infections such as amebic dysentery, *Campylobacter*, *Salmonella*, *Shigella*, and other common enteritides can mimic idiopathic colitis, and *Yersinia* and tuberculosis can cause ileitis that mimics Crohn disease.[51,60,108]

Enterobiasis has also been reported to cause ileal and colonic ulceration.[109] Thicker 5 µm sections stained with Ziehl-Neelsen and analysis of tissue samples by polymerase chain reaction may improve detection for tuberculosis.[60,110]

Vascular anomalies may be a rare cause of lower gastrointestinal bleeding. These lesions may have minor mucosal involvement but an extensive intra- and extramural vascular supply. Endoscopic ultrasonography with or without Doppler may help to delineate the extent of such lesions before angiography is considered or treatment is attempted. Because of the large size of some vascular lesions, simple mucosal injection, sclerosis, or heat coagulation may lead to greater bleeding. Blue rubber bleb nevus syndrome is another unusual example of vascular malformation, as is angiodysplasia, which can easily be missed if the colon is not very clean after bowel preparation.[74] Vasculitis, masquerading as inflammatory bowel disease, may have similar ileocolonic mucosal appearances. Clues to this diagnosis are the involvement of other organs and systems such as loss of beat to beat variation on electrocardiography representing atrioventricular node ischemia owing to vasculitis, perinuclear antineutrophil cytoplasmic antibody positivity, and skin lesions. Celiac axis, renal, and superior or inferior mesenteric angiograms may reveal multiple microaneurysms.

Polyps are found in 80% of instances within the rectosigmoid colon alone, reach peak incidence around 5 to 6 years, and are not usually seen in infancy.[111] Hamartomas make up the vast majority and are termed juvenile, inflammatory, or retention polyps. Approximately one-third of juvenile polyps cause anemia and often are lost by autoamputation. Even in expert hands, 10% or so of polyps can be missed at ileocolonoscopy, and the technique affording the best chance of detection is noted above. One in five rectosigmoid polyps will be accompanied by additional polyps in the proximal colon—hence the need for a full examination even if a polyp has been removed from a distal site. The recurrence rate may be 25%, but this is not well documented. Juvenile polyposis coli is often defined as the presence of more than 5 polyps, although there may be as many as 100 or more, and they may not be confined to the large bowel.[111,112] Dysplastic change with a carcinoma risk of 15% by age 35 years and 68% by 60 years is reported.[113] Adenomas can occur rarely and macroscopically are difficult to distinguish from hamartomas, dictating the need for histologic confirmation, and mixed polyps have been reported.[114,115] Familial adenomatous polyposis, an autosomal dominant disorder associated with the *APC* gene,[111] typically has hundreds or thousands of adenomas in the colon; screening in both of these conditions is dealt with in the following section. Several other syndromes may manifest with polyps and include Peutz-Jeghers, Turcot, Cronkhite-Canada, and hereditary flat adenoma syndromes.[116]

There are less than 200 cases of colonic carcinoma reported in the literature in children, and these represent less than 1% of all childhood tumors. Carcinoma has been reported in the absence of familial adenomatous polyposis or hereditary nonpolyposis colon carcinoma germline mutations.[43] Abdominal pain is the most common presenting symptom, occurring in 95% of patients,[117] and an abdominal mass is the most common finding, occurring in more than 50% of cases. Rectal bleeding is less common than in adult studies. Carcinoembryonic antigen had a specificity of 77% and a sensitivity of 68% in those under 18 years in a recent study.[118] Because this is too low to be clinically reliable, the requirement is for full ileocolonoscopy.[119]

Graft-versus-host disease (GVHD) following bone marrow, kidney, or liver transplant can have colonopathy in both acute and chronic forms. Focal apoptosis of the glandular epithelium is typical in acute GVHD,[120] and mucosal changes reminiscent of chronic idiopathic inflammatory bowel disease occur in chronic GVHD.[121]

FOLLOW-UP AND SURVEILLANCE ILEOCOLONOSCOPY

It is the practice in many units to perform a follow-up ileocolonoscopy 2 to 3 months after the start of treatment in a newly diagnosed case of inflammatory bowel disease. This practice is based on a number of premises, including evidence from studies such as those by Modigliani and colleagues, which showed that only 29% of adults with Crohn disease in clinical and biochemical remission actually achieved endoscopic remission.[122] This has a number of advantages. It allows the physician to observe the mucosal efficacy of the therapy because, in many instances, such as steroid use in colitis, the clinical improvement of the patient may not be mirrored by the mucosal improvement, which is regarded by most as the most important meter of a successful treatment regimen.[20] Ileocecal transcutaneous Doppler ultrasonography may be of benefit as a noninvasive alternative to repeat ileocolonoscopy in this situation, as noted above. In addition, the activity of mucosal inflammation may determine the long-term risk for carcinogenesis in the bowel.

NEW DIAGNOSES

Appreciation of more subtle lesions and pathology has been possible more recently as a consequence of combining high-definition videoendoscopy with sophisticated diagnostic techniques of mucosal immunology such as immunohistochemistry and gated flow cytometry. One such example is that of the histologically nonspecific colitis and ileal lymphonodular hyperplasia (Figure 67.3-13), which has been recognized recently in children with regressive autism or pervasive developmental disorder, and it is not considered to be due to any exogenous trigger, as has widely and wrongly been reported with respect to the measles, mumps, and rubella vaccine, but to be entirely independent of this or other triggers and may well be of autoimmune origin, but this is yet to be fully explored.[123,124] Nonspecific colitis appears macroscopically as granularity, loss of vascular pattern, pronounced lymphoid follicles surrounded by erythema described as the "red halo" sign (Figure 67.3-14), and aphthoid ulcers in a small proportion of cases (Figure 67.3-15). Diffuse infiltration of the lamina propria with macrophages and lymphocytes and enlarged germinal centers of lymphoid follicles containing tingible body macrophages are noted in the colon. Lymphoid follicular hyperplasia with reactive and expanded germinal centers is

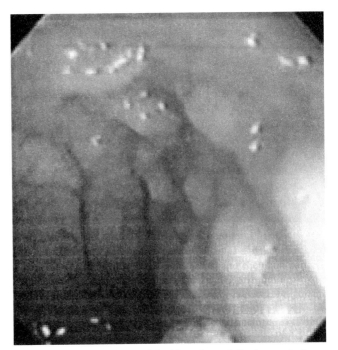

FIGURE 67.3-13   Terminal ileal lymphonodular hyperplasia.

found in the terminal ileum.[123] Further work on this observation has revealed a specific lymphocytic colitis less severe than classic inflammatory bowel disease. When compared, however, with cohorts with no histologic or clinical disease, developmentally normal children with ileal lymphonodular hyperplasia, Crohn disease, and ulcerative colitis, this group had significantly increased basement membrane thickness, mucosal $\gamma\delta$ cell density, $CD8^+$ density, and higher intraepithelial lymphocyte numbers. There were also higher CD3 and plasma cell density and greater crypt proliferation, and the disruption of epithelial but not lamina propria glycosoaminoglycans with a negative human leukocyte antigen (HLA)-DR in the

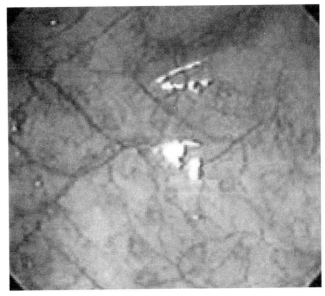

FIGURE 67.3-14   Multiple prominent lymphoid follicles in the colon surrounded by intense erythema. The so-called "halo" sign.

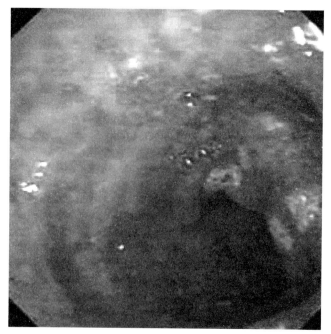

FIGURE 67.3-15   Evolution of inflamed lymphoid follicle into aphthoid ulcer.

epithelium suggested a T helper 2 response.[125] Other groups have reported similar ileocolonic lesions in patients with autism, pervasive developmental disorder of childhood, and attention-deficit/hyperactivity disorder.[126] Upper gastrointestinal pathology such as reflux esophagitis and nonspecific gastritis or duodenitis in this group of patients has also been noted recently.[127,128]

Fibrosing colonopathy has been identified in patients receiving excessive pancreatic enzyme supplements for treatment of both cystic fibrosis[129] and non–cystic fibrosis–related illness.[130]

Collagenous colitis presents with watery diarrhea, crampy abdominal pain, and a distinctive histology of the colon that includes a subepithelial collagen band and prominent chronic lamina propria inflammation with an increase in intraepithelial lymphocytes.[131] There have been only two reports of this in children, and this remains controversial.[132] Most cases occur in women over 50 years of age.

Lymphocytic (also called microscopic) colitis presents in a similar manner and is also idiopathic in origin but occurs equally between the sexes.[96] The histologic appearances are similar but without the collagen band. It is not seen commonly in children.

Diversion (also known as disuse) colitis arises in the colon, which is excluded from the fecal stream. It is time dependent, occurring with increasing frequency the longer the segment of bowel is not used, ranging from 3 to 36 months postsurgery.[133] Histology is typical of nonspecific colitis. The absence of luminal short-chain fatty acids is the most popular theory of pathogenesis because colonocytes require these for energy. Bacterial flora normally produce short-chain fatty acids from undigested carbohydrate and fiber.[134] Surgical reanastomosis is the treatment of choice, but topical fatty acids have been applied successfully when surgery is not possible.[135]

Other, more recently described disorders include autoimmune colitis, associated with autoimmune enteropathy and antienterocyte antibodies, and tufting enteropathy involving the colon.[136]

ILEOCOLONOSCOPY VERSUS OTHER DIAGNOSTIC TECHNIQUES

Although ileocolonoscopy is the gold standard for the diagnosis of pediatric inflammatory bowel disease, other noninvasive modalities may play a role in the diagnosis and assessment of treatment efficacy. Technetium hexamethylpropyleneamine oxime (Tc-HMPAO) labeling of granulocytes does not involve as much radiation burden as indium 111–tagged white cells and has been compared with ileocolonoscopy.[137] Jobling and colleagues showed that a Tc-HMPAO scan had 90% sensitivity and 75% specificity compared with biopsies at ileocolonoscopy, but this study had information from the ileum in only 12 of 39 cases—hence potentially overestimating the sensitivity and specificity of the technique.[138] The main disadvantages of the technique were lack of histologic confirmation of the disease process and lack of localization of the inflammation. More recently, the value of white cell–labeled scanning has been further questioned owing to the lack of accuracy in disease localization and sensitivity levels of approximately 75%.[139] Steroids decrease the white blood cell uptake of Tc-HMPAO by up to 50% and hence may decrease further the sensitivity of this technique. However, disease in the terminal ileum may be identified where it might otherwise have been missed because of unsuccessful endoscopic intubation of the terminal ileum.[140] Charron and colleagues showed that 6 of 106 cases of inflammatory bowel disease would have been mislabeled as ulcerative colitis or Crohn disease by technetium scan alone.[141]

Lipson and colleagues found a barium meal and follow-through to the terminal ileum to be a highly sensitive technique, especially for small bowel disease.[57] Tribl and colleagues reported a lower sensitivity of 91% but a specificity of 100%; hence, the radiologist's experience seems to be important.[142] The disadvantage of lack of histologic confirmation of the type of inflammation remains, and the diagnostic confusion owing to terminal ileal lymphonodular hyperplasia is well documented.[137] The radiation burden is also significant.

In experienced hands, ultrasonography has a sensitivity of 88% and a specificity of 93% for inflammatory bowel disease in children. Transabdominal ultrasonography assesses the bowel wall thickness in different areas, especially focusing on the terminal ileum.[143]

Spiral computed tomography (CT) may be useful in determining the nature of pericolic masses or in fistulating disease. Some authors suggest that Crohn disease can be differentiated from ulcerative colitis on the basis of finding greater colonic mural thickness in Crohn disease and greater submucosal fat deposition in ulcerative colitis, but many CT findings are nonspecific.[144] Three-dimensional CT, used to screen for carcinoma in adults, has potential application for identifying polyps in children, although the disadvantages of lacking histologic confirmation or therapeutic intervention remain. Current magnetic resonance imaging does not adequately recognize pediatric Crohn disease.[145]

The application of the novel technique of wireless capsule endoscopy (WCE) for visualization of the small bowel for occult pathology such as undiagnosed bleeding sources, mid- to small bowel polyps, and mid- to small bowel inflammatory pathologies is now well documented.[146] The use of this technique for diagnosis by direct vision of mucosal pathology in the ileum is useful (although one shortcoming is its relative contraindication in the presence of strictures) and has also been used to identify lesions in the colon; however, in the presence of good ileocolonoscopic technique and with the inability of WCE to obtain biopsies for histologic confirmation of pathology (although the next generation of capsules may have a limited biopsy facility), its application to colonic investigation remains somewhat limited to date. External steering of the capsule has recently been reported, opening up possibilities of retropulsion in the colon rather than just reliance on normal peristalsis.[147]

ENTEROSCOPY

Enteroscopy, now a standard endoscopic procedure in adult medicine and recently reviewed,[148,149] came of age because of the realization that the small bowel did indeed have specific pathology requiring not only diagnostic but also therapeutic expertise. It is of particular use in those with unexplained gastrointestinal bleeding. Pediatric enteroscopy literature is limited to Sonde-type and intraoperative-assisted push enteroscopy.[150–152] Sonde enteroscopy has largely been abandoned in favor of push enteroscopy,[153,154] given the desire for therapeutic capability. The techniques of per oral push enteroscopy and laparoscopy-assisted enteroscopy continue to evolve. In addition, newer methods of examining the small bowel are being developed and include virtual enteroscopy and WCE small bowel examination (as discussed above).[155] As noted, WCE does not allow therapeutic intervention as yet, but its diagnostic yield is certainly as good as if not better than enteroscopy for pathologies such as occult or obscure small bowel bleeding sources.[147,156]

INSTRUMENTS AND TECHNIQUE

Although a pediatric colonoscope can be used for enteroscopy, specifically designed enteroscopes up to 230 cm in length are now available. The Olympus SIF Q140 has a diameter of 10.5 mm and is 250 cm long. A push enteroscope, like a colonoscope, allows four-way tip deflection to 160 to 180 degrees. There are no enteroscopes or overtubes specifically designed for pediatric application, reflecting the lack of widespread use of this technique in children. An overtube, typically 60 to 100 cm in length with a soft Goretex tapered tip, stiffens the enteroscope within the stomach and upper duodenum, limiting looping, thereby allowing deeper advancement into the small bowel.[153] An enteroscope can be introduced 120 to 180 cm beyond the ligament of Treitz, and with laparoscopic assis-

tance, even the terminal ileum can be reached, allowing lesions such as a Meckel diverticulum to be found.[152]

Preparation for enteroscopy is the same as for upper gastrointestinal endoscopy, although the procedure may be substantially longer and more uncomfortable. Therefore, it is the practice at my unit to use general anesthesia even in adolescents. Patients are positioned left lateral or semiprone. After normal examination of the esophagus and stomach, air is removed, and minimal insufflation of the stomach allows deeper penetration into the small bowel when not using an overtube. At 60 to 80 cm in older children and adolescents, the ligament of Treitz is found, and extreme tip deflection is needed to find the lumen. The first jejunal loop is more readily identified because it is straighter and travels down to the pelvis. If using an overtube, which has been threaded over the enteroscope prior to oral insertion, this is deployed down the esophagus and into the second part of the duodenum; prepyloric deployment will not aid in deeper small bowel penetration. Some exponents use fluoroscopy to aid in overtube tip positioning.[148] When advancing the overtube, the enteroscope needs to be pulled back with clockwise rotation to straighten it, similar to the maneuver used to achieve the shortened scope position during endoscopic retrograde cholangiopancreatography. Variable-stiffness enteroscopes may soon be developed, which may remove the need for an overtube.

INDICATIONS

Table 67.3-7 details potential pediatric indications for push enteroscopy. One of few studies in children investigated the possibility of Crohn disease in children with growth retardation.[157] A number of reports demonstrate the utility of push enteroscopy in adults. In one recent series, a bleeding source was identified in 64% using push enteroscopy and an overtube.[158] Transfusion requirements can be significantly decreased in cases of angiodysplasia in the jejunum when cauterized at enteroscopy.[159,160] Nonsteroidal drugs can cause acute and chronic small bowel hemorrhage, perforation or obstruction, and an enteropathy, all diagnosed by push enteroscopy.[149,161,162]

TABLE 63.7-7   INDICATIONS FOR ENTEROSCOPY
IN CHILDREN AND ADOLESCENTS

DIAGNOSTIC
Obscure gastrointestinal bleeding (after endoscopy and ileocolonoscopy)
Iron deficiency anemia (especially if history of nonsteroidal drug use)
Extent of Crohn disease
Polyposis syndrome surveillance
Lymphoma (suspicion or follow-up post-treatment)
Lymphangiectasia
Intestinal obstruction
Graft assessment after small bowel transplant
Enteroclysis

THERAPEUTIC
Therapy of hemorrhagic lesions (eg, cauterizing angiodysplasia)
Polypectomy
Stricture dilation
Nasojejunal tube placement
Percutaneous jejunostomy tube placement

There are no data in children regarding nonsteroidal anti-inflammatory drug small bowel disease. The assessment of graft survival following small bowel transplant can be assessed by push enteroscopy. However, most often a jejunostomy is fashioned through which it is much easier to advance an enteroscope or simply use a standard endoscope. Biopsies taken for disaccharidase activity and histologic assessment are also helpful in early detection of small bowel allograft rejection.[163,164] Indeed, a zoom endoscope has recently been used to detect the early structural changes associated with graft rejection.[165]

Direct percutaneous jejunostomies can be sited using the same pull-through technique employed in percutaneous gastrostomy insertion.[166] Nasojejunal tubes can be placed accurately using a guidewire-assisted technique.[167] Finally, polypectomies can be successfully completed with a normal snare technique.

The indications for Sonde enteroscopy in children are very limited and might include a situation in which initial surgical exploration for a site of suspected small bowel bleeding is deemed undesirable.

INTRAOPERATIVE OR LAPAROSCOPY-ASSISTED ENTEROSCOPY

Intraoperative or laparoscopy-assisted enteroscopy starts with conventional enteroscopic jejunal intubation followed by surgical assistance. The endoscopist's role is relatively passive, deflecting the tip of the instrument while the surgeon, either with hands or with laparoscopic instruments, concertinas examined parts of the small bowel over the enteroscope. Both the mucosal and serosal surfaces can be examined. Very little air is insufflated into the bowel to avoid hindering the surgeon. Dimmed lights in the operating field also help to identify the position of the tip of the instrument. In experienced hands, all of the small bowel is examined in 60% of cases, taking up to 2 to 3 hours (Figure 67.3-16).[168] An enterotomy may be used to insert a sterilized enteroscope in some situations. Lesions can be marked by injection of ink or placement of a suture. Intraoperative or laparoscopy-assisted enteroscopy is the most successful technique for identifying sites of obscure gastrointestinal bleeding with diagnostic yields of between 83 and 100%.[169] Laser or bipolar coagulation can be used, and resection of lesions is recommended if intraoperative.[170] This technique has demonstrable advantages in the assessment of the extent of polyposis syndromes. "On-table" enteroscopy has a better pick-up rate for polyps at laparotomy than external transillumination and palpation.[111] When attempted in Crohn disease, up to 65% of patients have had lesions not previously identified in the small bowel by other investigations, including direct vision of the serosal surface of the bowel.[171] As previously mentioned, occult Crohn disease can be identified in children using enteroscopy.[157] Partial intestinal obstruction and Meckel diverticulum have also been identified at intraoperative enteroscopy.[150,152] Small bowel neoplasia must not be forgotten as the second most common cause of obscure gastrointestinal bleeding in younger patients, accounting for 5 to 10% of cases in young adults.[168] Exploratory

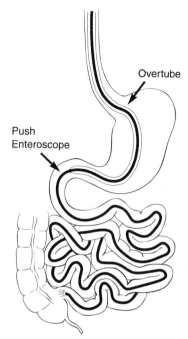

FIGURE 67.3-16   Extent of laparoscopy-assisted enteroscopy.

laparoscopy and enteroscopy are important in preventing missed diagnoses.

COMPLICATIONS

Complications are not often encountered with simple push enteroscopy, but when the overtube is employed, significant patient discomfort has been described.[153] Other, rare complications of the overtube include pharyngeal tear, Mallory-Weiss tear, gastric mucosal stripping, pancreatitis, and duodenal perforation.[158,172–174] Intraoperative enteroscopy has a 5% incidence of perforation and, in one series, a 50% incidence of mucosal laceration.[152] Prolonged ileus has been occasionally described.[173] None of these rare complications have been reported in the limited studies investigating children.

SUMMARY

Pediatric ileocolonoscopy and enteroscopy differ significantly from their adult parallels in nearly every aspect, including patient and parent management and preparation, selection criteria for sedation and general anesthetic, bowel preparation, expected diagnoses, instrument selection, imperative for terminal ileal intubation, and requirement for biopsies from macroscopically normal mucosa. The basic technique of ileocolonoscopy in children is illustrated and accompanied by discussion of advanced techniques such as endosonography, cecostomy, and therapy of lower gastrointestinal bleeding. The advantages and disadvantages of other noninvasive investigations are compared with those of ileocolonoscopy, and the former are generally held to be second best. The main aim of this chapter is to highlight those differences and to provide a workable guide for those involved or training in the discipline of pediatric ileocolonoscopy or enteroscopy.

REFERENCES

1. Gans S, Ament M, Cristie D. Pediatric endoscopy with flexible fiberscopes. J Pediatr Surg 1975;10:375–80.
2. Cotton P, Williams C. Practical gastrointestinal endoscopy. 4th ed. Oxford (UK): Blackwell Scientific; 1998.
3. Fox V. Lower gastrointestinal endoscopy. In: Walker WA, Durie PR, Hamilton JR, et al, editors. Pediatric gastrointestinal disease: pathophysiology; diagnosis; and management. 3rd ed. Hamilton (ON): BC Decker; 2000. p. 1414–28.
4. Hassall E, Barclay G, Ament M. Ileo-colonoscopy in childhood. Pediatrics 1984;73:594–9.
5. Howdle P, Littlewood J, Firth J, et al. Routine ileo-colonoscopy service. Arch Dis Child 1984;59:790–3.
6. Rossi T. Endoscopic examination of the colon in infancy and childhood. Pediatr Clin North Am 1988;35:331–56.
7. Williams C, Laage N, Campbell C, et al. Total ileo-colonoscopy in children. Arch Dis Child 1982;57:49–53.
8. Wyllie R, Kay M. Ileo-colonoscopy and therapeutic intervention in infants and children. Gastrointest Endosc Clin North Am 1994;4:143–60.
9. Fox V. Clinical competency in pediatric endoscopy. J Pediatr Gastroenterol Nutr 1998;26:200–4.
10. Hassall E. Requirements for training to ensure competence of endoscopists performing invasive procedures in children. J Pediatr Gastroenterol Nutr 1997;24:345–7.
11. Rudolph C, Winter H, NASPGN Executive Council, et al. NASPGN guidelines for training in pediatric gastroenterology. J Pediatr Gastroenterol Nutr 1999;29 Suppl 1:S1–26.
12. Ferlitsch A, Glauninger P, Gupper A, et al. Evaluation of a virtual endoscopy simulator for training in gastrointestinal endoscopy. Endoscopy 2002;34:698–702.
13. Report of the World Congress Working Group on New Endoscopic and Diagnostic Techniques. In: Report of the Working Groups 2000. World Congress of Pediatric Gastroenterology, Hepatology and Nutrition. Boston, Massachusetts, USA. August 5–9, 2000 [abstracts]. J Pediatr Gastroenterol Nutr 2000;31 Suppl 2:S1–325.
14. Minoli G, Meucci G, Prada A, et al. Quality assurance and ileo-colonoscopy. Endoscopy 1999;31:522–7.
15. Standards of Practice Committee of the American Society for Gastrointestinal Endoscopy. Quality improvement of gastrointestinal endoscopy. Gastrointest Endosc 1999;49:842–4.
16. Acharya S. Assessing the need for pre-admission visits. Paediatr Nurs 1992;4(9):20–3.
17. Glasper A, Stradling P. Preparing children for admission. Paediatr Nurs 1989;85:18–20.
18. Whiting M. Play and surgical patients. Paediatr Nurs 1993;5:11–3.
19. Mahajan L, Wyllie R, Steffen R, et al. The effects of a psychological preparation program on anxiety in children and adolescents undergoing gastrointestinal endoscopy. J Pediatr Gastroenterol Nutr 1998;27:161–5.
20. Williams C, Nicholls S. Endoscopic features of chronic inflammatory bowel disease in childhood. Baillieres Clin Gastroenterol 1994;8:121–31.
21. Ewe K. Bleeding after liver biopsy does not correlate with indices of peripheral coagulation. Dig Dis Sci 1981;26:388–93.
22. Rey J, Axon A, Budzynska A, et al. Guidelines of the European Society of Gastrointestinal Endoscopy (E.S.G.E.). Antibiotic prophylaxis for gastrointestinal endoscopy. Endoscopy 1998;30:318–24.
23. el-Baba M, Tolia V, Lin C, et al. Absence of bacteremia after gastrointestinal procedures in children. Gastrointest Endosc 1996;44:378–82.
24. Sondheimer J, Sokol R, Taylor S, et al. Safety, efficacy and tolerance of intestinal lavage in pediatric patients undergoing diagnostic ileo-colonoscopy. J Pediatr 1991;119:148–52.
25. Abubakar K, Goggin N, Gormally S, et al. Preparing the bowel for ileo-colonoscopy. Arch Dis Child 1995;73:459–61.
26. da Silva M, Briars G, Patrick M, et al. Ileo-colonoscopy preparation in children: safety, efficacy, and tolerance of high versus low-volume cleansing methods. J Pediatr Gastroenterol Nutr 1997;24:33–7.
27. Gremse D, Sacks A, Raines S. Comparison of oral sodium phosphate to polyethylene glycol-based solution for bowel preparation for ileo-colonoscopy in children. J Pediatr Gastroenterol Nutr 1996;23:586–90.
28. Trautwein A, Vinitski L, Peck S. Bowel preparation before ileo-colonoscopy in the pediatric patient: a randomized study. Gastroenterol Nurs 1996;19:137–9.
29. Dahshan A, Lin C, Peters J, et al. A randomized, prospective study to evaluate the efficacy and acceptance of three bowel preparations for ileo-colonoscopy in children. Am J Gastroenterol 1999;94:3497–501.
30. Pinfield A, Stringer M. Randomised trial of two pharmacological methods of bowel preparation for day case ileo-colonoscopy. Arch Dis Child 1999;80:181–3.
31. Chilton A, O'Sullivan M, Cox M, et al. A blinded, randomized comparison of a novel, low-dose, triple regimen with fleet phospho-soda: a study of colon cleanliness, speed and success of ileo-colonoscopy. Endoscopy 2000;32:37–41.
32. Marshall J, Patel M, Mahajan R, et al. Benefit of intravenous antispasmodic (hyoscyamine sulfate) as premedication for ileo-colonoscopy. Gastrointest Endosc 1999;49:720–6.
33. Hassall E. Should pediatric gastroenterologists be i.v. drug users? J Pediatr Gastroenterol Nutr 1993;16:370–2.
34. Murphy S. Sedation for invasive procedures in paediatrics. Arch Dis Child 1997;77:281–6.
35. Tolia V, Peters J, Gilger M. Sedation for pediatric endoscopic procedures. J Pediatr Gastroenterol Nutr 2000;30:477–85.
36. Ament M, Brill J. Pediatric endoscopy, deep sedation, conscious sedation, and general anesthesia—what is best? Gastrointest Endosc 1995;41:173–5.
37. Squires R, Morriss F, Schluterman S, et al. Efficacy, safety and cost of intravenous sedation versus general anesthesia in children undergoing endoscopic procedures. Gastrointest Endosc 1995;41:99–104.
38. Walco G, Cassidy R, Schechter N. Pain, hurt, and harm. The ethics of pain control in infants and children. N Engl J Med 1994;331:541–4.
39. Bendig D. Pulse oximetry and upper gastrointestinal endoscopy in infants and children. J Pediatr Gastroenterol Nutr 1991;12:39–43.
40. Committee on Drugs of the American Academy of Pediatrics. Guidelines for monitoring and management of pediatric patients during and after sedation for diagnostic and therapeutic procedures. Pediatrics 1992;89:1110–5.
41. Gilger M. Conscious sedation for endoscopy in the pediatric patient. Gastroenterol Nurs 1993;16:75–9.
42. Israel D, McLain B, Hassall E. Successful panileo-colonoscopy and ileoscopy in children. J Pediatr Gastroenterol Nutr 1994;19:283–9.
43. Kashiwagi H, Senba S, Konishi F, et al. Rectal cancer in a 13-year-old boy without a detectable germline mutation in FAP or HNPCC genes. J Gastroenterol 1999;34:341–4.
44. Aggarwal A, Ganguly S, Anand V, et al. Efficacy and safety of

intravenous ketamine for sedation and analgesia during pediatric endoscopic procedures. Indian Pediatr 1998;35: 1211–4.

45. Dillon M, Brown S, Casey W, et al. Ileo-colonoscopy under general anesthesia. Pediatrics 1998;102:381–3.

46. Stringer M, Pinfield A, Revell L, et al. A prospective audit of paediatric ileo-colonoscopy under general anaesthesia. Acta Paediatr 1999;88:199–202.

47. Hassall E. Who should perform pediatric endoscopic sedation? J Pediatr Gastroenterol Nutr 1994;18:114–7.

48. Lamireau T, Dubrueil M, Daconceicao M. Oxygen saturation during esophagogastroduodenoscopy in children: general anesthesia versus intravenous sedation. J Pediatr Gastroenterol Nutr 1998;27:172–5.

49. Brooker J, Saunders B, Shah S, et al. A new variable stiffness colonoscope makes ileo-colonoscopy easier: a randomised controlled trial. Gut 2000;46:801–5.

50. Tada M, Kawai K. Research with the endoscope. New techniques using magnification and chromoscopy. Clin Gastroenterol 1986;15:417–37.

51. Matsumoto T, Kuroki F, Mizuno M, et al. Application of magnifying chromoscopy for the assessment of severity in patients with mild to moderate ulcerative colitis. Gastrointest Endosc 1997;46:400–5.

52. Hussein A, Bartram C, Williams C. Carbon dioxide insufflation for more comfortable ileo-colonoscopy. Gastrointest Endosc 1984;30:68–70.

53. Stevenson G, Wilson J, Wilkinson J, et al. Pain following ileocolonoscopy: elimination with carbon dioxide. Gastrointest Endosc 1992;38:564–7.

54. Cirocco W, Rusin L. Fluoroscopy. A valuable ally during difficult ileo-colonoscopy. Surg Endosc 1996;10:1080–4.

55. Latt T, Nicholl R, Domizio P, et al. Rectal bleeding and polyps. Arch Dis Child 1993;69:144–7.

56. Williams C, Saunders B, Bell G, et al. Real-time magnetic three-dimensional imaging of flexible endoscopy. Gastrointest Endosc Clin N Am 1997;7:469–75.

57. Lipson A, Bartram CI, Williams CB, et al. Barium studies and ileoscopy compared in children with suspected Crohn's disease. Clin Radiol 1990;41:5–8.

58. Deere H, Thomson M, Murch S, et al. Histological comparison of rectosigmoid and full colonoscopic biopsies in the assessment of inflammatory bowel disease in childhood [abstract]. Gut 1998;42:A55.

59. Geboes K, Ectors N, D'Haens G, et al. Is ileoscopy with biopsy worthwhile in patients presenting with symptoms of inflammatory bowel disease? Am J Gastroenterol 1998;93:201–6.

60. Salvatore S, Thomson M. Crohn's disease or intestinal tuberculosis? Inflamm Bowel Dis Monitor 1999;1:59–61.

61. Gilbert DA, DiMarino AJ, Jensen DM, et al. Status evaluation: hot biopsy forceps. American Society for Gastrointestinal Endoscopy. Technology Assessment Committee. Gastrointest Endosc 1992;38:753–6.

62. Kimmey M, Silverstein F, Saunders D, et al. Endoscopic bipolar forceps: a potential treatment for the diminutive polyp. Gastrointest Endosc 1988;34:38–41.

63. Tappero G, Gaia E, De Guili P, et al. Cold snare excision of small colorectal polyps. Gastrointest Endosc 1992;38:310–3.

64. Technology Committee of the American Society for Gastrointestinal Endoscopy. Bipolar and multipolar accessories. Gastrointest Endosc 1996;44:779–82.

65. Iida Y, Munemoto Y, Kashara Y, et al. Endoscopic resection of large colorectal polyps using a clipping method. Dis Colon Rectum 1994;37:179–80.

66. Iishi H, Tatsuta M, Narahara H, et al. Endoscopic resection of large pedunculated colorectal polyps using a detachable snare. Gastrointest Endosc 1996;44:594–7.

67. Chaves D, Sakai P, Mester M, et al. A new endoscopic technique for the resection of flat polypoid lesions. Gastrointest Endosc 1994;40:224–6.

68. Smith R, Doull J. Treatment of colonic post-polypectomy bleeding site by endoscopic band ligation. Gastrointest Endosc 1994;40:499–500.

69. Breysem Y, Janssens J, Coremans G, et al. Endoscopic balloon dilation of colonic and ileo-colonic Crohn's strictures: long-term results. Gastrointest Endosc 1992;38:142–7.

70. Gevers A, Couckuyt H, Coremans G, et al. Efficacy and safety of hydrostatic balloon dilation of ileocolonic Crohn's strictures. A prospective long-term analysis. Acta Gastroenterol Belg 1994;57:320–2.

71. Redel C, Motil K, Bloss R, et al. Intestinal button implantation for obstipation and fecal impaction in children. J Pediatr Surg 1992;27:654–6.

72. De Peppo F, Iacobelli B, De Gennaro M, et al. Percutaneous endoscopic cecostomy for antegrade colonic irrigation in fecally incontinent children. Endoscopy 1999;31:501–3.

73. Rawat D. Percutaneous endoscopic colostomy of the left colon: a new technique for the management of intractable chronic constipation in children. J Pediatr Gastroenterol Nutr 2003; 115:162.

74. de la Torre Mondragón L, Vargas Gómez M, Mora Tiscarreno M, et al. Angiodysplasia of the colon in children. J Pediatr Surg 1995;30:72–5.

75. Holgersen L, Mossberg SM, Miller RE. Ileo-colonoscopy for rectal bleeding in childhood. J Pediatr Surg 1978;13:83–5.

76. Mathus-Vliegen E, Tytgat G. Intraoperative endoscopy: technique, indications and results. Gastrointest Endosc 1986;32: 381–4.

77. Mallery S, van Dam J. Interventional endoscopic ultrasonography: current status and future direction. J Clin Gastroenterol 1999;29:297–305.

78. Shimizu S, Tada M, Kawai K. Value of endoscopic ultrasonography in the assessment of inflammatory bowel diseases. Endoscopy 1992;24:354–8.

79. Hildebrandt U, Kraus J, Ecker K, et al. Endosonographic differentiation of mucosal and transmucosal non-specific inflammatory bowel disease. Endoscopy 1992;24:359–63.

80. Tio T, Mulder C, Wijers O, et al. Endosonography of peri-anal and peri-colorectal fistula and/or abscess in Crohn's disease. Gastrointest Endosc 1990;36:331–6.

81. Soweid A, Chak A, Katz J, et al. Catheter probe assisted endoluminal US in inflammatory bowel disease. Gastrointest Endosc 1999;50:41–6.

82. Berman J, Radhakrishnan J, Kraut J. Button gastrostomy obstructing the ileocecal valve removed by colonoscopic retrieval. J Pediatr Gastroenterol Nutr 1991;13:426–8.

83. Hasegawa T, Ueda S, Tazuke Y, et al. Colonoscopic diagnosis of lymphoid hyperplasia causing recurrent intussusception: report of a case. Surg Today 1998;28:301–4.

84. Lipschitz B, Patel Y, Kazlow P. Endoscopic reduction of an intussusception with simultaneous polypectomy in a child. J Pediatr Gastroenterol Nutr 1995;21:91–4.

85. Barberani F, Corazziari E, Tosoni M, et al. Per endoscopic manometry of the distal ileum and ileocecal junction: technique, normal patterns, and comparison with transileostomy manometry. Gastrointest Endosc 1994;40:685–91.

86. Habr Gama A. Pediatric ileo-colonoscopy. Dis Colon Rectum 1979;22:530–5.

87. Jalihal A, Misra SP, Arvind AS, Kamath PS. Colonoscopic polypectomy in children. J Pediatr Surg 1992;27:1220–2.

88. Nicholson R. Medical research with children: ethics law and practice. New York: Oxford University Press; 1986.

89. Sentongo T, Lichenstein G, Nathanson K, et al. Intestinal perforation in Ehlers-Danlos syndrome after enema treatment for constipation. J Pediatr Gastroenterol Nutr 1998;27:599–602.

90. Livstone E, Cohen G, Troncale F, et al. Diastatic serosal lacerations: an unrecognized complication of ileo-colonoscopy. Gastroenterology 1974;67:1245–7.

91. Ho H, Burchell S, Morris P, et al. Colon perforation, bilateral pneumothoraces, pneumopericardium, pneumomediastinum, and subcutaneous emphysema complicating endoscopic polypectomy: anatomic and management considerations. Am Surgeon 1996;62:770–4.

92. Damore L, Rantis P, Vernava A, et al. Colonoscopic perforations. Etiology, diagnosis, and management. Dis Colon Rectum 1996;39:1308–14.

93. Gedebou T, Wong R, Rappaport W, et al. Clinical presentation and management of iatrogenic colon perforations. Am J Surg 1996;172:454–7.

94. Orsoni P, Berdah S, Verrier C, et al. Colonic perforation due to ileo-colonoscopy: a retrospective study of 48 cases. Endoscopy 1997;29:160–4.

95. Rozen P, Somjen G, Baratz M, et al. Endoscope-induced colitis: description. Probable cause by glutaraldehyde, and prevention. Gastrointest Endosc 1994;40:547–53.

96. Jentschura D, Raute M, Winter J, et al. Complications in endoscopy of the lower gastrointestinal tract. Surg Endosc 1994;8:672–6.

97. Ong E, Bohlmer U, Wurbs D. Splenic injury as a complication of endoscopy: two case reports and a literature review. Endoscopy 1991;23:302–4.

98. Thomas A, Mitre R. Acute pancreatitis as a complication of ileo-colonoscopy. J Clin Gastroenterol 1994;19:177–8.

99. Rothbaum R. Complications of pediatric endoscopy. Gastrointest Clin North Am 1996;6:445–59.

100. Castellenita S, Murch S, Thomson M. Upper gastrointestinal involvement in children with inflammatory bowel disease: incidence, localisation and contribution to diagnosis. Arch Dis Child 2000;31:S16.

101. Griffiths A, Buller H. Inflammatory bowel disease. In: Walker WA, Durie PR, Hamilton JR, et al, editors. Pediatric gastrointestinal disease: pathophysiology; diagnosis; and management. 3rd ed. Hamilton (ON): BC Decker; 2000. p. 613–51.

102. Carbonnel F, Lavergne A, Lemann A, et al. Ileo-colonoscopy of acute colitis. A safe and reliable tool for assessment of severity. Dig Dis Sci 1994;39:1550–7.

103. Mantzaris G, Hatzis A, Archavlis E, et al. The role of ileo-colonoscopy in the differential diagnosis of acute, severe hemorrhagic colitis. Endoscopy 1995;27:645–53.

104. Perisic V. Colorectal polyps: an important cause of rectal bleeding. Arch Dis Child 1987;62:188–9.

105. Goldman H, Proujansky R. Allergic proctitis and gastroenteritis in children. Am J Surg Pathol 1986;10:75–86.

106. Bischoff S, Mayer J, Wedemeyer J, et al. Colonoscopic allergen provocation (COLAP): a new diagnostic approach for gastrointestinal food allergy. Gut 1997;40:745–53.

107. Sanderson I, Risdon R, Walker-Smith J. Intractable ulcerating enterocolitis of infancy. Arch Dis Child 1991;66:295–9.

108. Tuohy A, O'Gorman M, Bylington C, et al. Yersinia enterocolitis mimicking Crohn's disease in a toddler. Pediatrics 1999;104:36.

109. Deattie R, Wallter Smith J, Domizio P. Ileal and colonic ulceration due to enterobiasis. J Pediatr Gastroenterol Nutr 1995;21:232–4.

110. al-Quorain A, Fachartz, Satti M, et al. Abdominal tuberculosis in Saudi Arabia: a clinicopathologic study of 65 cases. Am J Gastroenterol 1993;88:75–9.

111. Hyer W, Neale K, Fell J, et al. At what age should routine screening start in children at risk of familial adenomatous polyposis? J Pediatr Gastroenterol Nutr 2000;31 Suppl 2:135.

112. Veale A, McColl I, Bussey H, Morson BC. Juvenile polyposis coli. J Med Genet 1966;3:5–16.

113. Jass J, Williams C, Bussey H, et al. Juvenile polyposis—a precancerous condition. Histopathology 1988;13:619–30.

114. Cynamon H, Milor D, Andres J. Diagnosis and management of colonic polyps in children. J Pediatr 1989;114:593–6.

115. Tolia V, Chang C. Adenomatous polyp in a four year old child. J Pediatr Gastroenterol Nutr 1990;10:262–4.

116. Winter H. Intestinal polyps. In: Walker WA, Durie PR, Hamilton JR, et al, editors. Pediatric gastrointestinal disease: pathophysiology; diagnosis; and management. 3rd ed. Hamilton (ON): BC Decker; 2000. p. 796–809.

117. Rao B, Pratt CB, Fleming IP, et al. Colon carcinoma in children and adolescents. A review of 30 cases. Cancer 1985;55:1322–6.

118. Angel C, Pratt CB, Rao BN, et al. Carcinoembryonic antigen and carbohydrate 19-9 antigen as markers for colorectal carcinoma in children and adolescents. Cancer 1992;69:1487–91.

119. Hoppin A. Other neoplasms. In: Walker WA, Durie PR, Hamilton JR, et al, editors. Pediatric gastrointestinal disease: pathophysiology; diagnosis; and management. 3rd ed. Hamilton (ON): BC Decker; 2000. p. 810–20.

120. Bombi J, Nadal A, Carreras E, et al. Assessment of histopathologic changes in the colonic biopsy in acute graft-versus-host disease. Am J Clin Pathol 1995;103:690–5.

121. Asplund S, Gramlich T. Chronic mucosal changes of the colon in graft-versus-host disease. Mod Pathol 1998;11:513–5.

122. Modigliani R, Mary J, Simon J, et al. Clinical, biochemical, and endoscopic picture of attacks in Crohn's disease: evolution on prednisolone. Gastroenterology 1990;98:811–8.

123. Wakefield A, Murch S, Anthony A, et al. Ileal-lymphoid-nodular-hyperplasia, non-specific colitis, and pervasive developmental disorder in children. Lancet 1998;351:637–41.

124. Wakefield A, Anthony A, Murch S, et al. Enterocolitis in children with developmental disorders. Am J Gastroenterol 2000;95:2285–95.

125. Furlano R, Anthony A, Day R, et al. Colonic CD8 and $\gamma\delta$ T-cell infiltration with epithelial damage in children with autism. J Pediatr 2001;138:366–72.

126. Sabra S, Bellanti J, Colon A. Ileal lymphoid nodular hyperplasia, non-specific colitis, and pervasive developmental disorder in children. Lancet 1998;352:234–5.

127. Horvath K, Papadimitriou J, Rabsztyn A, et al. Gastrointestinal abnormalities in children with autism. J Pediatr 1999;135:559–63.

128. Torrente F, Ashwood P, Heuschkel R et al. Focal enhanced gastritis in regressive autism with features distinct from Crohn's and Helicobacter pylori gastritis. Am J Gastroenterol. [In press]

129. FitzSimmons S, Burkhart G, Borowitz D, et al. High-dose pancreatic-enzyme supplements and fibrosing colonopathy in children with cystic fibrosis. N Engl J Med 1997;336:1283–9.

130. Lloyd-Still J. Colonopathy in a noncystic fibrosis patient: from excess pancreatic enzymes. J Pediatr Gastroenterol Nutr 1996;23:583–5.

131. Linstrom C. "Collagenous colitis" with watery diarrhea—a new entity? Pathol Eur 1976;11:87–9.

132. Yardley J, Lazenby A, Kornacki S. Collagenous colitis in children. Gastroenterology 1993;105:647-8.

133. Haas P, Haas G. A critical evaluation of the Hartmann's procedure. Am Surg 1988;54:380–5.

134. Rowe W, Bayless T. Colonic short-chain fatty acids: fuel from the lumen. Gastroenterology 1992;103:336–8.

135. Harig J, Soergel K, Komorowski R, et al. Treatment of diversion colitis with short chain fatty acids irrigation. N Engl J Med 1989;320:23–8.

136. Walker-Smith J, Murch S. Intractable diarrhoea. In: Diseases of the small intestine in childhood. London: Isis Medical Media; 1999. p. 290–3.

137. Chong S, Blackshaw A, Boyle S, et al. Histological diagnosis of chronic inflammatory bowel disease in childhood. Gut 1985;26:55–9.

138. Jobling J, Lindley K, Yousef Y, et al. Investigating inflammatory bowel disease—white cell scanning, radiology and ileocolonoscopy. Arch Dis Child 1996;74:22–6.

139. Cucchiara S, Celentano L, de Magistris T, et al. Ileocolonoscopy and technetium-99m white cell scan in children with suspected inflammatory bowel disease. J Pediatr 1999; 135:727–32.

140. Charron M, del Rosario J, Kocoshis S. Assessment of terminal ileal and colonic inflammation in Crohn's disease with 99mTc-WBC. Acta Pediatr 1999;88:193–8.

141. Charron M, del Rosario J, Kocoshis S. Use of the technetium-tagged white blood cells in patients with Crohn's disease and ulcerative colitis: is differential diagnosis possible? Pediatr Radiol 1998;28:871–7.

142. Tribl B, Turetscek K, Mostbeck G, et al. Conflicting results of ileoscopy and small bowel double-contrast barium examination in patients with Crohn's disease. Endoscopy 1998; 30:339–44.

143. Faure C, Belarbi N, Mougenot J, et al. Ultrasonographic assessment of inflammatory bowel disease in children: comparison with ileo-colonoscopy. J Pediatr 1997;130:147–51.

144. Philpotts L, Heiken J, Westcott M, et al. Colitis: use of CT findings in differential diagnosis. Radiology 1994;190:445–9.

145. Durno C, Sherman P, Williams T, et al. Magnetic resonance imaging to distinguish the type and severity of pediatric inflammatory bowel disease. J Pediatr Gastroenterol Nutr 2000;30:170–4.

146. Furman M, Mylonaki M, Fritshcer-Ravens A, et al. Wireless capsule endoscopy in small bowel disease in paediatrics: a study to assess the diagnostic yield. J Pediatr Gastroenterol Nutr 2003;36:544.

147. Swain P, Mosse CA, Burke P, et al. Remote propulsion of wireless capsule endoscopes. Gastrointest Endosc 2002;55:AB88.

148. Lewis B. Enteroscopy. Gastrointest Endosc Clin N Am 2000;10:101–16.

149. Morris A. Non-steroidal anti-inflammatory drug enteropathy. Gastrointest Endosc Clin N Am 1999;9:125–33.

150. Duggan C, Shamberger R, Antonioli D, et al. Intraoperative enteroscopy in the diagnosis of partial intestinal enteroscopy in infancy. Dig Dis Sci 1995;40:236–8.

151. Tada M, Misake F, Kawai K. Pediatric enteroscopy with a Sonde-type small intestine fiberscope (SSIF-type VI). Gastrointest Endosc 1983;29:44–7.

152. Turck D, Bonnevalle M, Gottrand F, et al. Intraoperative endoscopic diagnosis of heterotopic gastric mucosa in the ileum causing recurrent acute intussusception. J Pediatr Gastroenterol Nutr 1990;11:275–8.

153. Barkin J, Lewis B, Reiner D, et al. Diagnostic and therapeutic jejunoscopy with a new, longer enteroscope. Gastrointest Endosc 1996;38:55–8.

154. MacKenzie J. Push enteroscopy. Gastrointest Endosc Clin N Am 1999;9:29–36.

155. Gong F, Swain P, Mills T. Wireless endoscopy. Gastrointest Endosc 2000;51:725–9.

156. Delvaux MM, Saurin JC, Gaudin JJ, et al. Comparison of wireless endoscopic capsule and push enteroscopy in patients with obscure gastrointestinal bleeding. Results of a prospective, blinded multicenter trial. Gastrointest Endosc 2002;55: AB88.

157. Perez-Cuadrado E, Macenlle R, Iglesias J, et al. Usefulness of oral video push enteroscopy in Crohn's disease. Endoscopy 1997;29:745–47.

158. Chong J, Tagle M, Barkin J, et al. Small bowel push-type fiberoptic enteroscopy for patients with occult gastrointestinal bleeding or suspected small bowel pathology. Am J Gastroenterol 1994;89:2143–6.

159. Askin M, Lewis B, Reiner D, et al. Push enteroscopic cauterization: long-term follow-up of 83 patients with bleeding small intestine angiodysplasia. Gastrointest Endosc 1996;45: 580–3.

160. Foutch P, Sawyer R, Sanowski R. Push-enteroscopy for diagnosis of patients with gastrointestinal bleeding of obscure origin. Gastrointest Endosc 1990;36:337–41.

161. Morris A, Lee F, MacKenzie J. Small bowel enteroscopy: should jejunal biopsy be routine? Gastroenterology 1995;108:A880.

162. O'Mahoney S, Morris A, Straiton M, et al. Push enteroscopy in the investigation of small intestinal disease. QJM 1996;89: 685–90.

163. Hussanein T, Schade R, Soldevilla-Pico C, et al. Endoscopy is essential for early detection of rejection in small bowel transplant recipients. Transpl Proc 1994;26:1414–5.

164. Sigurdsson L, Reyes J, Putman P, et al. Endoscopies in pediatric small intestinal transplant recipients: five years experience. Am J Gastroenterol 1998;93:207–11.

165. Kato T, O'Brien C, Nishida S, et al. The first case report of a zoom video-endoscope for the evaluation of small bowel graft mucosa in a human after intestinal transplantation. Gastrointest Endosc 1999;50:257–61.

166. Shike M, Wallach C, Likier H. Direct percutaneous endoscopic jejunostomies. Gastrointest Endosc 1991;37:62–5.

167. Lewis B, Mauer K, Bush A. The rapid placement of jejunal feeding tube: the Seldinger technique applied to the gut. Gastrointest Endosc 1990;36:739–40.

168. Lewis B, Kornbluth A, Waye J. Small bowel tumors: the yield of enteroscopy. Gut 1991;32:763–5.

169. Lewis B, Wenger J, Waye J. Intraoperative enteroscopy versus small bowel enteroscopy in patients with obscure GI bleeding. Am J Gastroenterol 1991;86:171–4.

170. Mathus-Vliegen E. Laser treatment of intestinal vascular abnormalities. Int J Colorect Dis 1989;4:20–5.

171. Lescut D, Vanco D, Bonniere P, et al. Peri-operative endoscopy of the whole small bowel in Crohn's disease. Gut 1993;34: 3647–9.

172. Landi B, Cellier C, Fayemendy L, et al. Duodenal perforation occurring during push enteroscopy. Gastrointest Endosc 1996;43:631.

173. Whelan R, Buls J, Goldberg S, et al. Intraoperative enteroscopy: University of Minnesota experience. Am Surg 1989;55: 281–6.

174. Yang R, Laine L. Mucosal stripping: a complication of push enteroscopy. Gastrointest Endosc 1995;41:156–8.

4. Gastrointestinal Endosonography

Mini Mehra, MD

Jorge H. Vargas, MD

Gastrointestinal endosonography or endoscopic ultrasonography (EUS) is a relatively new endoscopic procedure in which a high-frequency ultrasound transducer is located on the tip of a flexible endoscope. It is unique in that it is able to obtain ultrasonographic images of the gastrointestinal tract and its surrounding structures. The arrival of EUS in the United States began in March 1980 with publication of a report by DiMagno and colleagues of a gastroscope equipped with an ultrasound probe.[1] Since the inception of EUS, it has been a novel modality looking for a purpose. Through the more than two decades since the first report, the indications for its use have increased but have not reached overall widespread use, especially in pediatrics.

EUS is not currently part of standard training programs in the United States, and few endoscopists are expert in the interpretation and performance of this modality. With further access to and improved technology of the equipment, pediatric endoscopists may develop more indications for this imaging technique.

Current indications for EUS in the adult population include evaluation of gastrointestinal submucosal lesions, cystic and solid pancreatic masses, gastrointestinal malignancy staging, and EUS-guided fine-needle aspiration (FNA).[2] In pediatrics, there has been a paucity of reports in the literature. Many of the adult indications can be applied to our patients, but, recently, there have been some small reports of other indications pertaining specifically to children, which will be outlined in this chapter.

FUNDAMENTALS OF ULTRASOUND IMAGING

Sound is a physical force that is transmitted through solid or liquid as a wave. The frequency of sound waves is measured in cycles formed per second. Their unit of measurement is a hertz. Medical imaging commonly uses frequency of waves in the 3.5 to 20 million Hz or megahertz (MHz).

Sound waves are formed by special ceramic crystals that have a piezoelectric property. The crystals vibrate to form sound waves, which are sent to tissues and reflected from the tissues back to the crystals. The incoming waves are then translated to an electrical signal, creating the ultrasound image. The transducer uses multiple crystals designed in an array to transmit and collect a series of waves to and from the tissue. Because of the multiple crystals, a two-dimensional image is created by multiple reference points that are reflections of the depth and span of the tissue being imaged.

Because sound waves travel at different speeds through different types of tissues, structures can be identified by their differences in hypo- or hyperechogenicity. Sound waves travel easily through fluid but not through air or bone. The speed of transmission is determined by the stiffness of the imaged tissue. Fat and collagen are the most reflective and therefore the brightest layers. Muscle or lean solid mass is less reflective and lighter. Interface between two tissues also creates an image owing to differing acoustic properties. Typically, lower frequencies (5–7.5 MHz) are used to image objects far away from the transducer, whereas higher frequencies (12–30 MHz) give greater detail closer to the transducer (eg, the gastrointestinal wall).

Ultrasound waves are better transmitted through a liquid medium than through an air medium. This phenomenon causes difficulties in transcutaneous ultrasonography because of areas filled with air, such as lungs and bowel. This problem is overcome within the gastrointestinal tract either by distending the gastrointestinal lumen with water or using a water-filled balloon attached to the end of the echoendoscope to improve the transmission of ultrasound waves.

EQUIPMENT AND TECHNIQUE

Current equipment available for EUS includes radial (Figure 67.4-1) and linear array (Figure 67.4-2) echoendoscopes. Both forms of echoendoscope employ regular endoscopy to guide the instrument into position before ultrasound imaging commences. More recently, catheter-based ultrasound probes (Figure 67.4-3) have been developed for use through standard endoscopes.

The original radial array echoendoscope displays a 360° cross-sectional view with gut wall layers and surrounding structures (Figure 67.4-4). The gastrointestinal wall (including the esophagus, stomach, small intestine, and rectum) has a five-layer pattern that correlates to the various histologic layers (superficial mucosa, deep mucosa, submucosa, muscularis propria, and serosa) (Figure 67.4-5). Advantages to the images in this view include the ability to compare similar images in orientation with computed tomographic (CT) cross-sectional imaging. Recent developments of this technology have included the addition of Doppler technology to detect blood flow. The smallest radial array endoscope has a 12.7 mm outer diameter (GF-UM130, Olympus America Inc., Melville, NY, USA). The disadvantages of this modality are the inability to view and guide a needle biopsy device and the inability

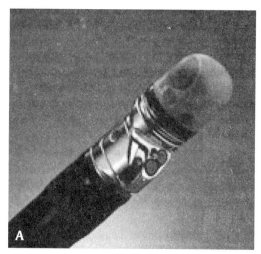
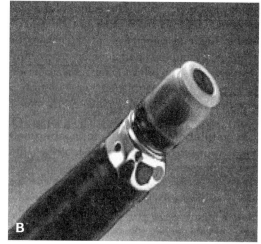

FIGURE 67.4-1   *A*, Radial ultrasound endoscope (GF-UM30P). *B*, Radial ultrasound endoscope (GF-UM130). Courtesy of Olympus Corporation (Tokyo, Japan).

to use the endoscope in small, young patients because of its large outer diameter.

The linear array echoendoscope provides a field of view in a configuration parallel to the endoscope (Figure 67.4-6). This instrument was initially developed for use with needle biopsy devices. The depth of the needle can be viewed when obtaining fluid or tissue. Along with the ability to use needle biopsy devices, the linear array echoendoscope can also facilitate use of Doppler imaging of blood vessels. A disadvantage to this type of EUS is its "forward oblique" view. For endoscopists familiar with side-viewing endoscopes, this may not be problematic, but for the average endoscopist, it can be disorienting. Another disadvantage similar to the radial array endoscope is its large outer diameter. The smallest linear array endoscope has an outer diameter of 12.1 mm (Pentax EG-3620U, Pentax Precision Instrument Corporation, Orangeburg, NY, USA).

Catheter-based ultrasound probes consist of a small-diameter transducer within a catheter sheath that can be introduced through a standard endoscope that has at least a 2.8 mm channel diameter. Catheter-based ultrasound probes using a variety of frequencies are available (5, 7.5, 12, 20, and 30 MHz). Typically, these probes are introduced into water-filled gut lumens to generate images. Probes are also available with a balloon sheath that can be filled with water to improve the image quality. Again, the disadvantage for the small pediatric patient is the need to use an endoscope that has at least a 2.8 mm channel diameter.

INDICATIONS

Because EUS is a fairly new modality and is just receiving acceptance in the adult patient population, use in the pediatric population is slow but steady. In the adult population, accepted indications for use include differential diagnosis of submucosal lesions, gastrointestinal malignancy staging, evaluation of the biliary tree, diagnosis of cystic or solid pancreatic masses, and FNA.[2] Recent case reports and retrospective publications with inclusion of some pediatric patients up to age 18 years have revealed some newer investigational indications for use of EUS in the pediatric population.

ESOPHAGUS

EUS has been used to differentiate eosinophilic esophagitis with normal controls.[3,4] Although histopathology is the gold standard method of diagnosis for this entity, findings

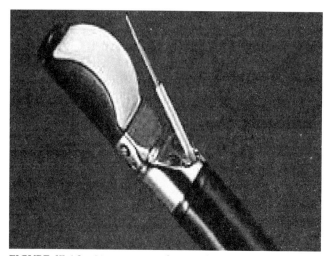

FIGURE 67.4-2   Linear array endoscope (EG3630-U). Courtesy of Pentax Precision Instrument Corporation (Orangeburg, NY, USA).

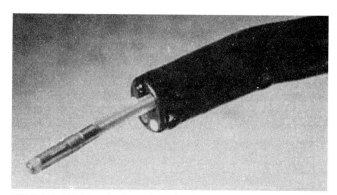

FIGURE 67.4-3   Catheter-based ultrasound probe (UM-3R). Courtesy of Olympus Corporation (Tokyo, Japan).

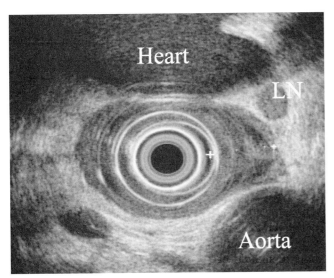

FIGURE 67.4-4 Esophageal wall layers and surrounding structures. LN = lymph node. Courtesy of J. Farrell, MD.

of esophageal wall thickening with significant expansion of the esophageal wall were noted in the subjects with eosinophilic esophagitis versus controls. Similar findings of esophageal wall thickening have been seen in subjects with gastroesophageal reflux disease[5,6]; thus, EUS only complements endoscopy and histology for the diagnosis of reflux esophagitis. Because EUS was used as an adjuvant for diagnosis of eosinophilic esophagitis and gives similar findings in patients with gastroesophageal reflux disease, this modality may be more useful as a follow-up tool in patients who are being treated for their eosinophilic esophagitis as opposed to a primary diagnostic tool.

The use of EUS in patients with congenital esophageal stenosis (CES) has been successful in a few reports for determination of the optimal treatment approach.[7–9] There are three histopathologic types of CES: tracheobronchial remnants, membranous diaphragm, and fibromuscular hypertrophy. The type of CES must be determined before

deciding on dilatation versus surgical resection. Dilatation of tracheobronchial remnants carries a higher risk of perforation and a poor success rate, with the eventual necessity of surgical resection. EUS is able to visualize cartilage associated with tracheobronchial remnants and thereby eliminates attempts at dilatation.

Many studies have used EUS in the clinical setting of portal hypertension. A specific study was undertaken to determine if variceal wall thickness correlates with the risk of variceal bleeding.[10] Using these data, along with variceal pressures, wall tension was determined to estimate the risk of bleeding. However, the researchers were unable to provide similar findings in patients with multiple varices.

An established indication for use of EUS in adults is staging of esophageal cancers and the diagnosis of mediastinal lympadenopathy. Pediatric patients may have other etiologies for mediastinal lymphadenopathy, including infectious or granulomatous disease (eg, sarcoidosis). EUS was shown to assist in the diagnosis of histoplasmosis among patients with symptoms of dysphagia and a midesophageal submucosal mass.[11] Savides and colleagues also tried to determine the cost-effectiveness of EUS versus CT scan of the chest.[11] In their institution, the cost was comparable, but the advantage of EUS was the availability to obtain tissue via FNA. They also found that EUS provided greater resolution of periesophageal lesions and a greater sensitivity of calcified lymph nodes. The real benefit of the role of EUS-guided FNA in the evaluation of pediatric mediastinal processes may be in the avoidance of more invasive and costly diagnostic procedures (eg, mediastinoscopy and thoracoscopy).

EUS has also been used for post-treatment assessment of patients with achalasia.[12] Patients with achalasia who were treated with dilation versus botulinum toxin injection underwent EUS to assess esophageal wall damage post-treatment. Transient esophageal mucosa-submucosa diameter was increased postdilation but not post–botulinum toxin injection. Also of note, the thickening normalized within 24 hours of the procedure.

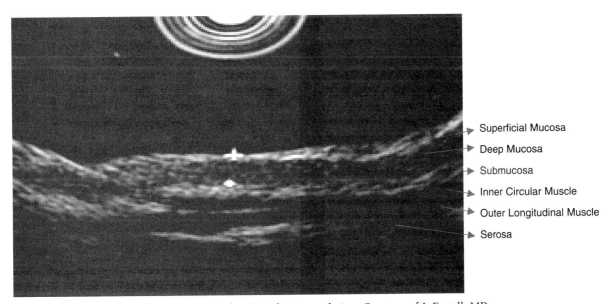

FIGURE 67.4-5 Endoscopic ultrasonography tissue layer correlation. Courtesy of J. Farrell, MD.

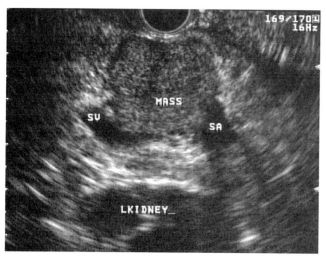

FIGURE 67.4-6   Linear array image of pancreas tail mass. Courtesy of J. Farrell, MD. SA = splenic artery; SV = splenic vein.

STOMACH

Dieulafoy lesion can occasionally be seen in the pediatric patient population. Fockens and colleagues used EUS to determine the location of this abnormal, large submucosal vessel.[13] On finding such a vessel, they performed sclerotherapy. Unfortunately, they used a rotating sector scanner that did not have Doppler capability, and with the perpendicular scanning view, needle-guided injections were difficult. Use of the linear array would most likely alleviate this problem.

Foregut duplications are a rare abnormality, but generally two-thirds are found within the first year of life. An investigational indication for EUS is defining the relationship of these duplications to their intraluminal tract.[14] Because EUS can differentiate between cystic and solid structures and is in greater proximity to the lesion, it can be a reliable tool to diagnose this entity. Also, endosonographic aspiration of the cyst can be performed to identify cells consistent with duplication. The wall layers can be identified in duplications to match the gastrointestinal tract (Figure 67.4-7).

PANCREAS/BILIARY TREE

There are a significant number of established indications for EUS use in adults in the pancreas and biliary tract. In children, reports of EUS use include diagnosis of solid pseudopapillary tumors of the pancreas (Figure 67.4-8),[15] blunt pancreatic trauma,[16] drainage of pancreatic pseudocysts (Figure 67.4-9),[17] preoperative localization of insulinomas and gastrinomas,[18] and as a screening tool prior to sphincterotomy for acute biliary pancreatitis.[19,20]

EUS-guided FNA has also been used in children for the diagnosis of solid pseudopapillary tumors of the pancreas.[15] Owing to the malignant potential of the tumor, radical resection is the mainstay of treatment in adults. The investigators postulated that surgeons reluctant to perform radical resection in children when the diagnosis is in question might be reassured by a definitive diagnosis with the assistance of EUS. EUS may also be the best modality to obtain the FNA because of the location of the mass.

Pancreatic trauma can occasionally be seen in the pediatric population. EUS has been compared with CT for diagnosis and follow-up of pancreatic trauma.[16] Several advantages were established, including mobility of the EUS equipment, lack of radiation, ability to do multiple serial examinations, and no requirement of contrast material with sensitivity equal to that of CT. Disadvantages include increased time consumption for the EUS examination and diagnosis dependent on operator expertise.

Drainage of pancreatic pseudocysts with the use of conventional endoscopy has been reported since 1981.[21] EUS-guided drainage was first described in 1996.[22] EUS plays an important role in the evaluation of pancreatic pseudocysts prior to endoscopic drainage. More recently, an EUS-guided one-step drainage procedure was used in three patients, including one pediatric patient.[17] A curved linear

FIGURE 67.4-7   Gastric duplication cyst (computed tomographic scan and endoscopic ultrasonographic images with fine-needle aspiration). Courtesy of J. Farrell, MD.

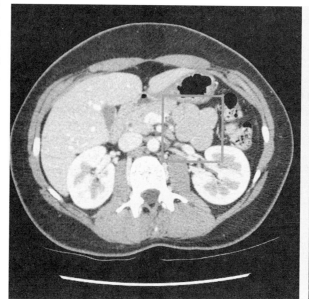
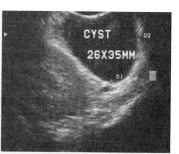
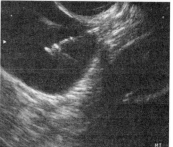

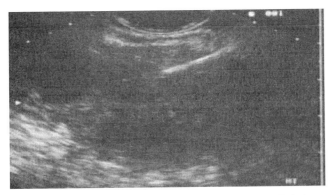

FIGURE 67.4-8 Endoscopic ultrasonography–guided fine-needle aspiration of a pancreatic mass. Courtesy of J. Farrell, MD.

array EUS with a 22-gauge needle and a 7 French drainage tube were used in this procedure. Although there were a small number of patients in this report, EUS-guided one-step drainage, with its ability to identify and avoid intra-mural vasculature, may be an advantageous procedure over a radiologic or a surgical approach.

EUS was compared with somatostatin receptor scintig-raphy (SRS), transabdominal ultrasonography, CT, and magnetic resonance imaging (MRI) for the preoperative localization of insulinomas and gastrinomas.[18] The authors found that EUS and SRS had comparable sensitivity and significantly greater sensitivity for localization of gastrino-mas than ultrasonography, CT, or MRI. EUS was the most sensitive modality for localization of insulinomas than all of the others.

Endoscopic sphincterotomy is beneficial for patients with biliary pancreatitis, but it can have serious complica-tions. The use of EUS for prescreening patients prior to sphincterotomy can reduce the complications by avoiding unnecessary cannulation of the papilla.[19]

Colon

Established indications in adults for using EUS in the lower gastrointestinal tract are primarily for staging of rectal cancer, but EUS investigational use in children has included evalua-tion of the rectal venous system in patients with portal hyper-tension,[23,24] differential diagnosis in suspected cases of inflammatory bowel disease,[25,26] and EUS evaluation of perirectal and perianal complications of Crohn disease.[27,28]

Yachha and colleagues were able to use EUS to compare children with extrahepatic portal venous obstruction and controls to determine the size, number, and location of varices.[23] They determined that EUS was able to detect the presence of rectal varices better than endoscopy. They also suggested that EUS may be useful in differentiating between portal rectopathy and inflammatory colitis.

An attempt to use EUS for differentiating Crohn disease and ulcerative colitis has been inconclusive.[27] Many stud-ies have tried to compare wall thickness and discrimina-tion between mucosal and transmural inflammation. No consistent conclusions are seen among these studies. How-ever, EUS has been used to correctly identify perirectal and perianal complications of Crohn disease better than fistula-contrast studies and CT.[20]

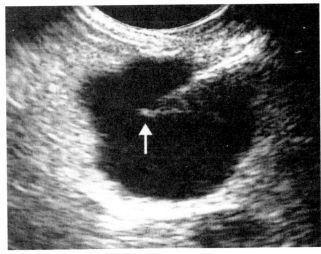

FIGURE 67.4-9 Endoscopic ultrasonography–guided fine-needle aspiration of a pancreatic cyst (*arrow*, tip of needle).

CONCLUSIONS

EUS, including EUS-guided FNA, is a new modality that has many established indications in the adult patient pop-ulation. Its pediatric indications have increased somewhat since its inception, but owing to the lack of awareness among general physicians, it may be underused. As clinical indications increase, training in this technique will also need to increase.

REFERENCES

1. DiMagno EP, Buxton JL, Regan PT, et al. Ultrasonic endoscope. Lancet 1980;i:629–31.
2. Fusaroli P, Caletti G. Endoscopic ultrasonography. Endoscopy 2003;35:127–35.
3. Fox VL, Nurko S, Teitelbaum JE, et al. High-resolution EUS in children with eosinophilic "allergic" esophagitis. Gastroin-test Endosc 2003;57:30–6.
4. Fox V, Nurko S, Furuta G. Eosinophilic esophagitis: it's not just kid's stuff. Gastrointest Endosc 2002;56:260–70.
5. Caletti GC, Ferrari A, Mattioli S, et al. Endoscopy versus endo-scopic ultrasonography in staging reflux esophagitis. Endoscopy 1994;26:794–7.
6. Kawamura O, Sekiguchi T, Kusano M, et al. Endoscopic ultra-sonographic abnormalities and lower esophageal sphincter function in reflux esophagitis. Dig Dis Sci 1995;40:598–605.
7. Takamizawa S, Tsugawa C, Mouri N, et al. Congenital esophageal stenosis: therapeutic strategy based on etiology. J Pediatr Surg 2002;37:197–201.
8. Kouchi K, Yoshida H, Matsunaga T, et al. Endosonographic evaluation in two children with esophageal stenosis. J Pedi-atr Surg 2002;37:934–6.
9. Usui N, Kamata S, Kawahara H, et al. Usefulness of endoscopic ultrasonography in the diagnosis of congenital esophageal stenosis. J Pediatr Surg 2002;37:1744–6.
10. Schiano TD, Adrain AL, Cassidy MJ, et al. Use of high-resolution endoluminal sonography to measure the radius and wall thickness of esophageal varices. Gastrointest Endosc 1996;44:425–8.
11. Savides TJ, Gress FG, Wheat LJ, et al. Dysphagia due to medi-astinal granulomas: diagnosis with endoscopic ultrasonogra-phy. Gastroenterology 1995;109:366–73.

12. Schiano TD, Fisher RS, Parkman HP, et al. Use of high-resolution endoscopic ultrasonography to assess esophageal wall damage after pneumatic dilation and botulinum toxin injection to treat achalasia. Gastrointest Endosc 1996;44:151–7.

13. Fockens P, Meenan J, van Dullemen HM, et al. Dieulafoy's disease: endosonographic detection and endosonography-guided treatment. Gastrointest Endosc 1996;44:437–42.

14. Faigel DO, Burke A, Ginsberg GG, et al. The role of endoscopic ultrasound in the evaluation and management of foregut duplications. Gastrointest Endosc 1997;45:99–103.

15. Nadler EP, Novikov A, Landzberg BR, et al. The use of endoscopic ultrasound in the diagnosis of solid pseudopapillary tumors of the pancreas in children. J Pediatr Surg 2002;37:1370–3.

16. Sugiyama M, Atomi Y, Kuroda A, et al. Endoscopic ultrasonography for diagnosing blunt pancreatic trauma. Gastrointest Endosc 1996;44:723–5.

17. Inui K, Yoshino J, Okushima K, et al. EUS-guided one-step drainage of pancreatic pseudocysts: experience in 3 patients. Gastrointest Endosc 2001;54:87–9.

18. Zimmer T, Stolzel U, Bader M, et al. Endoscopic ultrasonography and somatostatin receptor scintigraphy in the preoperative localisation of insulinomas and gastrinomas. Gut 1996;39:562–8.

19. Prat F, Edery J, Meduri B, et al. Early EUS of the bile duct before endoscopic sphincterotomy for acute biliary pancreatitis. Gastrointest Endosc 2001;54:724–9.

20. Palazzo L, Girollet PP, Salmeron M, et al. Value of endoscopic ultrasonography in the diagnosis of common bile duct stones: comparison with surgical exploration and ERCP. Gastrointest Endosc 1995;42:225–31.

21. Sahel J. Endoscopic drainage of pancreatic cysts. Endoscopy 1991;23:181–4.

22. Wiersema MJ. Endosonography-guided cystoduodenostomy with a therapeutic ultrasound endoscope. Gastrointest Endosc 1996;44:614–7.

23. Yachha SK, Dhiman RK, Gupta R, Ghoshal UC. Endosonographic evaluation of the rectum in children with extrahepatic portal venous obstruction. J Pediatr Gastroenterol Nutr 1996;23:438–41.

24. Dhiman RK, Saraswat VA, Choudhuri G, et al. Endosonographic, endoscopic, and histologic evaluation of alterations in the rectal venous system in patients with portal hypertension. Gastrointest Endosc 1999;49:218–27.

25. Soweid AM, Chak A, Katz JA, Sivak MV Jr. Catheter probe assisted endoluminal US in inflammatory bowel disease. Gastrointest Endosc 1991;50:41–6.

26. Gast P, Belaiche J. Rectal endosonography in inflammatory bowel disease: differential diagnosis and prediction of remission. Endoscopy 1999;31:158–66.

27. Lew RJ, Ginsberg GG. The role of endoscopic ultrasound in inflammatory bowel disease. Gastrointest Endosc Clin N Am 2002;12:561–71.

28. Schwartz DA, Wiersema MJ, Dudiak KM, et al. A comparison of endoscopic ultrasound, magnetic resonance imaging, and exam under anesthesia for evaluation of Crohn's perianal fistulas. Gastroenterology 2001;121:1064–72.

5. Endoscopic Retrograde Cholangiopancreatography

Claude Liguory, MD

Jean-François Mougenot, MD

Gustavo Andrade de Paulo, MD, MSc

Tell me and I forget. Teach me and I remember. Involve me and I learn.

—Benjamin Franklin (1706–1790)

Over the past 30 years, endoscopic retrograde cholangiopancreatography (ERCP) has become an integral element in the diagnostic and therapeutic tools of the gastroenterologist. It has grown from a limited procedure, performed by a few, to a mainstream modality for the diagnosis and treatment of a wide variety of benign and malignant hepatobiliary and pancreatic disorders. Since the report of the first successful cannulation of the ampulla of Vater by McCune and colleagues in 1968,[1] the role of ERCP for diagnosing and treating these diseases has evolved, providing patients with a minimally invasive method to treat problems that previously required open surgery.

ERCP is currently used for the management of bile duct stones; benign and malignant biliary obstruction; benign and malignant pancreatic neoplasms and diseases of the major and minor papilla; acute and chronic pancreatitis; bile duct injuries; pancreatic duct disruption and pseudocysts; pain syndromes considered to be of pancreatic, biliary, or sphincter of Oddi origin; certain congenital and acquired hepatic conditions affecting the biliary tract; and bleeding or infection suspected of being of hepatic, biliary, or pancreatic origin.[2–4]

Although ERCP has been widely applied in adult patients for a long time, only recently has it become an accepted modality in pediatrics. The limited use of this technique in children might be caused by multiple factors, including (1) a relatively low incidence of pancreatic and biliary diseases in childhood and a low index of clinical suspicion; (2) limited availability of pediatric instruments; (3) a lack of expertise among pediatric gastroenterologists to perform ERCP; (4) reluctance of adult gastroenterologists to study small children; (5) the impression that ERCP in children is technically more difficult to accomplish; (6) difficulty in the effective evaluation of a therapeutic result; and (7) a lack of well-defined indications and safety of ERCP in children.[5–7]

Since the first report of a successful ERCP in a 3.5-month-old child in 1976,[8] the field of pediatric ERCP has expanded dramatically, driven by the growing subspecialty of pediatric gastroenterology, refinements in design, and worldwide distribution of small-diameter duodenoscopes.[9,10]

TECHNICAL CONSIDERATIONS

ERCP is a relatively complex combined endoscopic or radiographic procedure that requires multiple skilled personnel. Our goal is to provide state-of-the-art patient care, and success depends on the combined efforts of members from the departments of surgery, medicine, pediatrics, and radiology. Hence, one weak link in this multidisciplinary venture might limit success.[11–13]

PREPROCEDURE PREPARATION

According to the Standards of Practice Committee from the American Society for Gastrointestinal Endoscopy (ASGE), "preparation for endoscopy in pediatric age patients requires attention to physiologic issues as well as emotional and psychosocial issues in both the patient and the parent or guardian."[12] The anticipation of potentially painful or noxious procedures provokes intense anxiety in children. Parental anxiety is heightened by protective feelings, wanting to shield the child against harm and unnecessary discomfort. Much of this anxiety may be relieved by providing optimal age-appropriate information and counseling to the patients and parents, with a detailed description of all aspects of the procedure.[9,12] With psychological preparation, children are less anxious and more cooperative during the procedure, requiring less sedation.[14]

DIETARY RESTRICTIONS

Dietary restrictions are necessary to minimize the risks of pulmonary aspiration of gastric contents. In pediatric patients presumed to have normal gastric emptying, the fasting interval before endoscopy should be a minimum of 2 hours for clear liquids. Guidelines for fasting after ingestion of milk and solids are diverse and related to age. Fasting from milk or solids should be for 4 hours in infants under 5 months, 6 hours in those 6 to 36 months, and 8 hours in those over 36 months of age.[12,15]

INFORMED CONSENT

Written informed consent must be obtained from the appropriately designated parent or guardian after careful explanation of the risks and benefits of the entire procedure. Adolescents might be offered the option to review and sign the consent form to acknowledge their active participation in the process.[9]

SEDATION

Premedication is not routinely used for pediatric endoscopy.[16] When necessary, oral or rectal administration of benzodiazepines might be used prior to intravenous sedation or anesthesia, improving the ease of separation from parents and of intravenous insertion.[12]

Most ERCPs are performed with the benefit of conscious sedation, deep sedation, or general anesthesia, although some experts give no sedation to selected patients.[17] The proper approach to sedation remains a major controversy among pediatric endoscopists.[9,18]

The relatively large diameter of standard duodenoscopes (eg, 11–12 mm) may cause discomfort and compress the soft-walled trachea in young children. The prone position during ERCP also compromises chest and lung excursion and may result in hypoventilation and hypoxia in a sedated child. With these considerations in mind, general anesthesia with endotracheal intubation might be appropriate for some children. Insufficient outcome data exist to make firm recommendations about the comparative adequacy, safety, and cost of sedation and general anesthesia in children undergoing ERCP (Table 67.5-1).[19]

An individual trained in pediatric monitoring and at least basic pediatric life support should be present in addition to the endoscopist for the entire duration of the procedure. Pulse oximetry and hemodynamic monitoring should be routinely used.[12]

EQUIPMENT

Fluoroscopic equipment should be suitable for children of all ages, minimizing radiation exposure.

In neonates and infants younger than 12 months, ERCP is performed with a pediatric duodenoscope, which has an insertion tube diameter of 7.5 mm, a channel of 2 mm, and an elevator (Olympus PJF–160 – Olympus, Hamburg, Germany). This endoscope, which is also preferred for children less than 2 years of age, accepts cannulas and other accessories that are 5 French or smaller. A standard diagnostic duodenoscope (insertion tube diameter approximately 11–12 mm) with a 3.2 mm operating channel may be used in most children older than 2 to 3 years. Therapeutic large-diameter (> 13 mm) endoscopes with a 4.2 mm channel are infrequently required to place 10 French stents in larger adolescents.[5,19]

ANTIMICROBIAL PROPHYLAXIS

The frequency of bacteremia associated with upper or lower gastrointestinal endoscopy with or without biopsy is low, ranging from about 2 to 5%.[20,21] In immunocompetent children, clinically relevant bacteremia is very infrequent following routine endoscopic procedures.[22] The reported risk of bacteremia with ERCP (5–6%) is similar to that for upper and lower endoscopy unless an obstructed biliary ductal system is present.[20]

Infections associated with gastrointestinal endoscopic procedures are rare, including those performed in children.[22] In a meta-analysis of antibiotic prophylaxis in ERCP, Harris and colleagues concluded that antibiotic prophylaxis prior to ERCP may reduce the incidence of bacteremia, but this has little clinical relevance. Prophylaxis does not substantially reduce the incidence of sepsis or cholangitis; thus, the routine use of antibiotic prophylaxis cannot be recommended.[23]

The American Heart Association and the ASGE have developed criteria for the use of prophylactic antibiotics for endoscopic procedures based on the associated risk of developing endocarditis. ERCP in the absence of ductal obstruction is considered to be of low risk, and routine antibiotic prophylaxis is not recommended. Evaluation should be performed on a case by case basis.[20,24,25] For endoscopic procedures associated with increased rates of transient bacteremia (ERCP with known or suspected bile duct obstruction), prophylaxis is recommended for patients at "high risk" for the development of infective endocarditis (eg, prosthetic heart valves, a previous history of endocarditis, complex cyanotic congenital heart disease, and surgically constructed systemic-pulmonary shunts). No prophylaxis is recommended for patients with those cardiac lesions and conditions at no increased risk for infective endocarditis over the general population (eg, previous coronary artery bypass, graft surgery, cardiac pacemakers and implanted defibrillators, mitral valve prolapse or previous rheumatic fever without valvular dysfunction or regurgitation). There are insufficient data to recommend routine prophylaxis for patients with cardiac lesions or conditions at intermediate risk for the development of infective endocarditis (eg, most congenital cardiac malformations, rheumatic and other acquired valvular dysfunction, even after valvular surgery, hypertrophic cardiomyopathy, and mitral valve prolapse with valvular regurgitation). The endoscopist may consider prophylaxis on a case by case basis.[24,25]

Snyder and Bratton surveyed 14 academic pediatric centers in the United States and Canada to determine the current practices of these groups with regard to antimicrobial prophylaxis in ERCP. In patients with cardiac disease at high risk for endocarditis, all centers used prophylaxis. In patients with a moderate risk, 64% of the centers used prophylaxis.[20]

The Working Party for the British Society of Gastroenterology Endoscopy Committee recommends antibiotic prophylaxis for all patients undergoing ERCP with evidence of biliary stasis or pancreatic pseudocyst. Oral ciprofloxacin or parenteral gentamicin (or parenteral quinolone, cephalosporin, or ureidopenicillin) is recommended.[26] There are no pediatric data to guide antibiotic prophylaxis for ERCP.[5,20]

PROCEDURE LENGTH

The time for total examination (from introduction of duodenoscope to withdrawal of the instrument) varies considerably according to expertise and the difficulty of the

TABLE 67.5-1   PEDIATRIC ENDOSCOPIC RETROGRADE CHOLANGIOPANCREATOGRAPHY SERIES

AUTHOR, YEAR (REF)	PATIENT	PROCEDURE (N)	SUCCESS (%)	AGE RANGE	AGE MEAN	GA (%)	INDICATIONS (%) BILIARY	INDICATIONS (%) PANCREATIC	INDICATIONS (%) PAIN	THERAPY (%)	COMPLICATIONS (%) PANCREATIC	COMPLICATIONS (%) HEMORRHAGE	COMPLICATIONS (%) PERFORATION	COMPLICATIONS (%) INFECTION
Riemann and Koch, 1978[145]	18	18	100	6–17 yr	NR	11	17	83	0	0	0	0	0	1 (death)
Cotton and Laage, 1982[29]	20	25	96	7–16 yr	NR	65	20	50	30	5	0	0	0	0
Guelrud et al, 1987[146]	23	23	96	19–150 d	67d	26	100	0	0	0	0	0	0	0
Allendorph et al, 1987[144]	39	39	92	6 mo–18 yr	12.5 yr	46	28	54	18	10	10	0	0	0
Heyman et al, 1988[28]	12	12	33	3–58 wk	11.6 wk	100	100	0	0	0	0	0	8	8
Buckley and Connon, 1990[72]	42	42	97	1–19 yr	10.5 yr	38	36	43	21	12	5	2	0	0
Guelrud et al, 1991[17]	32	32	94	16–150 d	49d	19	100	0	0	0	0	0	0	0
Putnam et al, 1991[147]	38	42	93	14 mo–19 yr	12.3 yr	32	36	64	0	0	8	0	0	0
Prite et al, 1992[148]	19	19	100	4–16 yr	11.9 yr	68	5	68	26	16.5	3	0	0	2.5
Brown et al, 1993[7]	92	121	94	4 mo–19 yr	10.9 yr	54	20	77	3	68	8	0	0	0
Brown and Goldschmiedt, 1994[76]	25	42	100	22 mo–19 yr	NR	NR	64	36	0		8	0	0	0
Eichieri et al, 1994[149]	19	19	100	1–18 yr	9.6 yr	58	58	42	0	5.3	5.3	0	0	0
Guelrud et al, 1994[105]	51	NR	98*	1–18 yr	NR	0	0	100	0	35	8	0	0	0
Derkx et al, 1994[150]	20	22	90	4–19 wk	12 wk	100	100	0	0	0	0	0	0	0
Mitchell and Wilkinson, 1994[151]	40	40	90	6–80 wk	12 wk	100	100	0	0	0	0	0	0	0
Abu-Khalaf, 1995[100]	16	16	100	2 mo–18 yr	10.5 yr	31	56	25	19	25	0	0	0	0
Ohnuma et al, 1997[152]	73	75	88	8–300 d	71 d	100	100	0	0	0	0	0	0	0
Tagge et al, 1997[13]	26	26	96†	6 mo–19 yr	10 yr	58	92	8	0	61.5	4	0	0	0
Tarnasky et al, 1998[73]	10	10	100	0.5–16.9 yr	8.8 yr	80	100	0	0	100	0	0	0	0
Graham et al, 1998[107]	17	17	94	3–16 yr	11.2 yr	88	0	100	0	53	13	0	0	0
Hsu et al, 2000[122]	22	34	100	1.5–17 yr	10.7 yr	68	0	100	0	67.6	6	0	0	2
Teng et al, 2000[68]	42	50	100	57 d–15 yr	NR	80	64	36	0	12	0	0	0	1.4
Poddar et al, 2001[6]	72	84	97	11 mo–14 yr	9 yr	0	61	28	11	30.6	7	0	0	0
Pfau et al, 2002[153]	43	53	94.3	1–18 yr	13.5 yr	60.4	47	53	0	45.2	3.8	0	1.9	0
Liguory et al, 2001 (unpublished)	51	51	92	6 mo–15 yr	8 yr	100	29.4	54.9	15.7	43.1	2	0	0	0

Adapted from Etzkorn KP et al.[18]

GA = general anesthesia; NR = not reported.

*83% success in therapeutic examinations.

†87% success in therapeutic examinations.

examination. The duration of a diagnostic examination ranges from 2 minutes to 1 hour.[17,27] In most series, the mean time is between 10 and 30 minutes.[6,17,28,29] For therapeutic ERCPs, it is difficult to define the "normal" mean time, considering the myriad of interventions available. In one study, the average time for ERCP, including both diagnostic and therapeutic studies, was 58 minutes.[12]

DIAGNOSTIC AND THERAPEUTIC INDICATIONS

Indications for diagnostic and therapeutic ERCP in pediatrics (see Table 67.5-1) are, for the most part, similar to those established for the adult population. However, the relative frequency of each indication differs because children are much more prone to congenital abnormalities and trauma than malignancy.

DIAGNOSTIC ERCP IN THE ERA OF MAGNETIC RESONANCE CHOLANGIOPANCREATOGRAPHY

Over the last two decades, several new diagnostic modalities have been developed and refined, such as ultrasonography (transabdominal and endoscopic), computed tomography (CT) (single and multislice helical), magnetic resonance imaging (MRI) and magnetic resonance cholangiopancreatography (MRCP), CT-virtual cholangiography, and laparoscopic surgery with intraoperative cholangiography. These techniques have proven useful in the diagnosis and staging of pancreatic and hepatobiliary diseases and may obviate the need for diagnostic ERCP in some cases.

MRCP is a noninvasive test for imaging the biliary and pancreatic ducts, which provides high-quality images without administration of exogenous contrast material or use of ionizing radiation.[30-36]

MRI relies on radiofrequency pulse-induced excitation of protons within a magnetic field to generate an image. Conventional MRI uses a combination of T_1- and T_2-weighted sequences to image abdominal organs (eg, liver, pancreas biliary tract, and duodenum). MRCP relies on heavily T_2-weighted sequences because fluid-containing structures have a much longer T_2 than solid tissue. Thus, stationary fluid in the biliary and pancreatic ducts serves as an intrinsic contrast medium, resulting in images similar to those obtained through ERCP.[30] Intraluminal filling defects and the nature of ductal stenoses and/or dilatation can be readily demonstrated. With current magnetic resonance scanners, images are acquired in a few seconds, virtually eliminating image degradation from motion artefacts. The entire biliary tract can be imaged in a single breath-hold of 20 seconds or less with high spatial resolution so that structures such as fourth-order intrahepatic bile ducts and small stones are detected.[35] No special preparation is required, although fasting for 2 to 4 hours is recommended to reduce gastric and duodenal fluids.[31]

Different MRCP pulse sequences have been used: steady-state free precession, two-dimensional and three-dimensional fast spin echo techniques, rapid acquisition with relaxation enhancement (RARE), and half-Fourier RARE. MRCP image sequencing differs from center to center because of rapidly evolving technology, equipment and software differences, and radiologist preferences and expertise. Currently, most centers are not equipped to perform state-of-the-art MRCP images.[30]

MRCP is a useful noninvasive alternative to diagnostic ERCP, especially when ERCP study is difficult or technically inadequate (eg, Billroth II surgical bypass, biliary-enteric anastomoses, periampullary diverticula, duodenal obstruction). It can also be used for planning surgical, endoscopic, and radiologic interventions.

The accuracy of MRCP in comparison with ERCP is very high. Adequate images can be obtained in 95 to 98% of patients.[37-39]

Currently, a limitation of MRCP is that its resolution is inferior to that of ERCP. Although MRCP detects stones as small as 2 mm, the spatial resolution of MRCP is not sufficient to detect small stones and crystals in a consistent fashion. It may not be able to detect small ampullary or distal bile duct tumors either.[35]

Absolute contraindications include the presence of a cardiac pacemaker, cerebral aneurysm clips, ocular or cochlear implants, and ocular foreign bodies. Relative contraindications include the presence of a cardiac prosthetic valve, neurostimulators, and metal prostheses. Claustrophobia accounts for 1 to 4% of failed or inadequate studies.[30,40]

In pediatrics, MRCP has been used to diagnose biliary atresia (BA) and other congenital or acquired pancreaticobiliary disorders (eg, choledochal cysts).[41-43] However, further studies are needed to support routine use of MRCP in pediatrics.[31]

DEFINING NORMAL DUCT SIZE IN PEDIATRICS

The size of a normal common bile duct (CBD) was measured in children between 7 and 16 years and varies from 2.1 to 4.9 mm, just below the entry of the cystic duct. The diameter of the pancreatic duct in the head ranges from 1.4 to 2.1 mm, and in the body from 1.1 to 1.9 mm (all measures are corrected for radiographic magnification).[29]

BILIARY INDICATIONS FOR ERCP

Indications for ERCP in children are listed in Table 67.5-2. Investigation of neonatal cholestasis is unique to pediatrics, although the role of ERCP remains controversial.[5,19] Structural causes of neonatal cholestasis include BA, choledochal cysts, choledocholithiasis, intrahepatic bile duct paucity or hypoplasia, neonatal sclerosing cholangitis, and congenital bile duct stricture.[19]

In children older than 1 year and adolescents with biliary disorders, the most frequent indications are obstructive jaundice, known or suspected choledocholithiasis, abnormal liver enzymes in children with inflammatory bowel diseases, abnormal biliary findings in abdominal ultrasonography, and therapeutic ERCP.[5]

BILIARY ATRESIA

In a child with neonatal cholestasis, symptoms and signs of BA overlap those of idiopathic neonatal hepatitis and other rare causes of cholestasis.[17,44] Early identification

TABLE 67.5-2   BILIARY INDICATIONS FOR ENDOSCOPIC RETROGRADE CHOLANGIOPANCREATOGRAPHY

DIAGNOSTIC	THERAPEUTIC
Investigation of neonatal cholestasis	Sphincterotomy
Biliary atresia	Sphincteroplasty (balloon dilation)
Choledochal cyst	Stone extraction
Choledocholithiasis	Stricture dilation
Biliary obstruction owing to parasitic infestation	Stent placement
Dilated intrahepatic bile duct	Nasobiliary drainage
Benign and malignant biliary strictures	
Primary sclerosing cholangitis	
Biliary obstruction or leaks after liver transplant	
Preoperative and postoperative evaluation (laparoscopic cholecystectomy)	
Bile plug syndrome	
Abnormal findings in other examinations	
Manometric evaluation of the sphincter of Oddi	

of BA before 8 weeks of age may be associated with better surgical results (Kasai procedure) and improved clinical outcome.[17,27,44]

BA is a localized, progressive obliteration of the extrahepatic and hilar bile ducts that uniquely presents in the first months of life. The disease occurs in approximately 1 in 8,000 to 1 in 15,000 live births, with a 1.4:1 female-to-male predominance. It accounts for 30% of all cases of cholestasis in young infants. If untreated, it leads to progressive fibrosis and, ultimately, cirrhosis and death.[44,45]

No single test or combination of tests is consistently reliable in differentiating BA from other forms of cholestasis.[27] Imaging techniques such as ultrasonography and hepatobiliary scan are useful procedures but are often inconclusive. The sensitivity and specificity of scintigraphy, with concomitant administration of phenobarbital, are about 95% and 93%, respectively. However, failure of excretion may be seen in neonatal hepatitis as well. Currently, the most reliable test, aside from exploratory laparotomy, is percutaneous liver biopsy (up to 93% accuracy).[44] However, the histologic features of giant cell transformation and bile duct proliferation can be seen in both neonatal hepatitis and early stages of BA.[17]

Duodenal intubation has been reported to exclude BA if bilirubin or bile is found in the fluid. However, 10% of infants in whom bile is not found will not have BA.[17]

The combination of several tests may improve the accuracy of the diagnosis. Discriminant analysis using clinical criteria, scintigraphic excretion scan, and liver biopsy permit accurate diagnosis of either BA or neonatal hepatitis in 80 to 94% of young infants.[17] Thus, 10 to 20% of infants might need surgical exploration to establish a diagnosis. For these children, ERCP may be of diagnostic value.[5,17,27,28,44]

ERCP is the procedure of choice for investigation of structural abnormalities or obstructive lesions of the extrahepatic bile ducts and gallbladder when the intrahepatic ducts are not dilated.[28] Three types of anatomic findings have been described in patients with BA[5,17]:

• Type 1: no visualization of the biliary tree. This is observed in about 35% of the cases. No bile is seen in the duodenum. A normal pancreatogram is obtained.

• Type 2: visualization of the distal CBD and gallbladder without visualization of the main hepatic or intrahepatic ducts (35% of the cases). No bile is seen in the duodenum, and a narrow and irregular distal CBD might be present. The pancreatic duct is normal.

• Type 3: type 3a includes visualization of the gallbladder and the complete CBD with biliary lakes at the porta hepatis; in type 3b, both hepatic ducts are seen with biliary lakes. It is present in 30% of cases. Bile can be seen in the duodenum. The pancreatic duct is normal, and a narrow distal CBD is present.

When the biliary tree is partially visualized (types 2 and 3), the diagnosis of BA is made and confirmed by surgery. When the biliary tree is not opacified and only the pancreatic duct is seen (type 1), the diagnosis is suspected, and exploratory laparotomy is indicated.

It is important to emphasize that absence of CBD opacification alone, despite several maneuvers to opacify the biliary tree, does not establish atresia.[16,27] In most situations, clinical, biochemical, and liver biopsy findings in conjunction with filling of the pancreatic duct without CBD opacification and absence of bile in the duodenum may be sufficient to establish the diagnosis of BA prior to surgical intervention.[16] Of the 310 infants with neonatal cholestasis reported in the literature and reviewed by Guelrud, the diagnosis by ERCP was incorrect in only 5 (1.6%) patients.[5]

MRCP has been used in neonates and infants for the diagnosis of BA, and the results are promising.[40] However, further studies are required.[30,43]

CHOLEDOCHAL CYSTS

Choledochal cysts are uncommon anomalies of the bile ducts, with probable congenital origin, associated with anomalous pancreaticobiliary junction in 80 to 90% of cases.[46] The incidence is higher among Japanese, being rare in Western countries, where its prevalence is estimated in 1 in 100,000 to 1 in 150,000 newborns.[47] The female-to-male predominance is 3 to 4:1. These cysts are usually found during infancy or childhood (80% of patients are younger than 10 years of age),[48] although, in some series, 30% are found in adults or among the elderly.[49,50]

The most common classification accepted nowadays was proposed by Todani and colleagues,[51] expanding the original classification of Alonso-Lej and colleagues[52] by including intrahepatic cysts and redividing the extrahepatic disease:

- Type I cysts are present in 80 to 90% of cases and are further classified according to the shape of the affected segment. A type IA cyst involves cystic dilation of the CBD, with marked dilation of part of or the entire extrahepatic biliary tree. The gallbladder commonly arises from the cyst, and the intrahepatic biliary tree is normal. Type IB cyst involves focal, segmental dilation of the CBD, usually of the most distal part of the duct. A normal segment of CBD is present between the cyst and the cystic duct. Type IC cyst involves fusiform dilation of the CBD, along with diffuse, cylindrical dilation of the common hepatic duct. The gallbladder arises from the dilated CBD, and the intrahepatic biliary system is not dilated.
- Type II cysts are present in 2% of cases and are considered true choledochal diverticula.
- Type III cyst, found in 1.5 to 5% of the patients, is a choledochocele that involves only the intraduodenal portion of the CBD. Characteristically, the papilla appears as a hemispherical cystic structure protruding into the duodenal lumen. The terminal end of the CBD is blunt and bulbous, unlike the normal tapered appearance. The cystic structure enlarges further during injection of contrast material into the distal CBD. A rounded, cystic structure filled with contrast material is noted when patients are upright.[53]
- Type IV cysts are subclassified in two groups. Type IVA cyst involves dilation of the intra- and extrahepatic bile ducts and is present in up to 20% of patients. Cholangiography shows gross cystic dilation of the extrahepatic biliary tree, with extension of the cystic dilation into the intrahepatic biliary tree. The intrahepatic dilation may affect multiple segments and be smooth and fusiform or irregular. Type IVB cysts also involve dilation of multiple segments but are confined to the extrahepatic bile duct. They are much less common than type IVA cysts. Cholangiography shows multiple segmental dilation of the CBD. The intrahepatic biliary tree is normal.
- Type V cyst (Caroli disease) involves dilation of one or several segments of the intrahepatic bile duct.[51,54]

The origin and formation of choledochal cysts have been a matter of considerable investigation and debate.[55]

The classic triad of choledochal cyst is characterized by abdominal pain, jaundice, and abdominal mass. Unusual presentations include rupture of the choledochal cyst with bile peritonitis, pancreatitis, and bleeding esophageal varices owing to biliary cirrhosis.[56] Intermittent fever, vomiting, elevation in serum transaminases and amylase, abdominal pain, and jaundice might be related to bouts of cholangitis and pancreatitis.[57]

Many complications have been associated with choledochal cysts, including cholelithiasis, choledocholithiasis, cystolithiasis, pancreatitis, intrahepatic abscesses, biliary cirrhosis, portal hypertension, and biliary carcinoma.[46]

Malignancy related to choledochal cysts is more frequent with advancing age, being reported in 23 to 40% of the cases.[58,59] These rates are extremely high if compared with biliary carcinoma in the general population (0.003–0.004%).[60] The development of cancer seems to be related to bile stasis and prolonged contact with the epithelium. It might be related to pancreatic juice reflux to the biliary tree, leading to chronic irritation and metaplasia. Most cases are detected in advanced stages, with poor prognosis. Although cyst excision eliminates the potential site for neoplasia, it does not exclude the possibility of developing cancer in the intrahepatic ducts. Long-term follow-up is always mandatory.[61]

Abdominal ultrasonography and CT are important in detecting cystic masses in close relation to the pancreatic head and hepatic hilum. CT is more accurate in depicting intrahepatic bile ducts and the distal parts of the CBD. When the cyst is round and markedly dilated, with no evidence of intrahepatic ductal dilation, its biliary origin is difficult to determine. Cystic lesions such as mesenteric, omental, ovarian, renal, adrenal, and hepatic cysts; gastrointestinal duplication; hydronephrotic kidneys; and pancreatic pseudocysts are the main differential diagnoses when a huge choledochal cyst lacks intrahepatic involvement at CT.[54] Hepatobiliary scintigraphy using technetium 99m is useful in this setting.

ERCP is the most sensitive method to define the biliary system anatomy and depict anomalous pancreaticobiliary junction and biliary malignancies.[59,62] It is invasive and operator dependent, requiring a meticulous technique. In this setting, it has been associated with a particularly high risk of pancreatitis, probably related to the fact that, in the presence of a common channel, cyst opacification often requires repetitive injections of the pancreatic duct.[62,63]

Virtual cholangiography using CT with two- or three-dimensional visualization of the biliary tract has also been used in the diagnosis of choledochal cysts. Spinzi and colleagues emphasized its advantages in depicting the entire biliary system and the capability of showing mucosal lesions.[60] However, the need for contrast administration and adequate hepatic metabolism (absorption and excretion) limits its application.

MRCP is a noninvasive method capable of examining the entire biliary tree and the pancreatic duct in two or three dimensions. The development of fast acquisition techniques for MRCP has reduced acquisition time to a few seconds and made possible the performance of dynamic studies after secretin stimulation.[63] MRCP can identify the anomalous pancreaticobiliary junction in up to 82% of the cases. It also shows good correlation with ERCP with regard to choledochal cysts and anomalous pancreaticobiliary junction diagnoses.[63–65] MRCP has established value in the diagnosis of choledocholithiasis and biliary obstruction. However, small stones and gallbladder lesions (carcinoma and mucosal hyperplasia) often associated with anomalous pancreaticobiliary junction are difficult to demonstrate.[65] Endoscopic ultrasonography can be useful in this situation.[66]

Percutaneous drainage of choledochal cysts has been reported and is supposed to help in the decompression of the biliary tree, making the surgical approach easier.[46] Dilation of the sphincter of Oddi through ERCP has also been reported, relieving symptoms.[67] The ease of stent placement provides an alternative to urgent surgery in this group of sick children.[12] However, owing to the high potential of complications, including malignant degeneration, the treatment of choice is always surgery. According to the case, a choledochojejunal anastomosis can be performed, although cyst excision and Roux-en-Y hepaticojejunostomy are preferred.[49,54]

In type III cysts (choledochocele), the incidence of cholangiocarcinoma does not appear to be as high as for type I and IV cysts. Currently, in more than 50 cases of type III cysts, no cases of cholangiocarcinoma have been reported. Thus, resection of a type III cyst may not be mandatory for control of future cancer risk. Type III cysts have been effectively treated with transduodenal sphincterotomy or sphincteroplasty. The goal of therapy is to establish effective drainage of the CBD and pancreatic duct.[45,53,68]

CHOLEDOCHOLITHIASIS

In infants and children, choledocholithiasis rarely occurs.[69–71] Perforation of the extrahepatic biliary tract with resulting biliary ascites is the more common presentation of CBD stones in infants.[69]

Although the sensitivity of abdominal ultrasonography for cholelithiasis is in excess of 95%, reported sensitivities for choledocholithiasis range from 18 to 74%. No pediatric data are available. Sensitivities of conventional CT scan range from 76 to 90%.[35]

Early studies of MRCP in choledocholithiasis noted sensitivities ranging from 81 to 92% and specificities ranging from 91 to 100%. Recent works using state-of-the-art techniques yield sensitivities of 90 to 100%, specificities of 92 to 100%, and positive predictive values of 93 to 100%. Negative predictive values range from 96 to 100%.[34] Based on these results, MRCP is being used with increasing frequency as a screening examination for the detection and exclusion of CBD stones, especially in patients with a low or moderate probability of having stones. The limitations of MRCP are as follows: (1) inferior resolution to that of ERCP; although MRCP detects stones as small as 2 mm, the spatial resolution of MRCP is not sufficient to detect small stones and crystals in a consistent fashion; (2) impacted calculi (not surrounded by bile); (3) patients with metal clips, pneumobilia, and hemobilia; (4) the latest advances are not uniformly available worldwide; (5) a lack of therapeutic options.[2,30,31,35]

ERCP is very sensitive in detecting CBD stones, although, occasionally, small stones may be missed.[2] However, with the introduction of MRCP, the focus of ERCP has shifted in many institutions from its use both as a diagnostic and therapeutic tool to its use primarily as a therapeutic procedure.[35]

Many reports in the pediatric literature confirm the ability of ERCP to treat CBD stones.[12,70–74] A variety of techniques are used, including endoscopic sphincterotomy (ES), balloon dilation of the papilla (sphincteroplasty), balloon or basket removal, and stent and nasobiliary drain placement (Figure 67.5-1).[12]

ES is a well-established procedure in adult patients with choledocholithiasis. In children, it was first reported in 1982[29] and has been performed in infants as young as 5 months old.[73,75,76] Because the long-term consequences of ES in children are unknown, endoscopic balloon dilation of the sphincter of Oddi seems to be an attractive technique.[12,73] Evidence that sphincter function returns after balloon dilation may prove to be a major advantage, particularly in a younger age group. Further evidence is required to confirm that this is the case. There must be some concern about whether balloon dilation is justifiable in patients with stones more than 8 to 10 mm in diameter because lithotripsy then seems inevitable.[77]

Biliary microlithiasis causing pancreatitis in a 14-year-old boy has also been reported.[78]

PRIMARY SCLEROSING CHOLANGITIS

Primary sclerosing cholangitis (PSC) is an inflammatory disease of the biliary tract of uncertain etiology, occurring with a prevalence of 1 to 6 in 100,000.[32] It is characterized by recurrent fever, abdominal pain, and jaundice resulting from fibrosing and inflammatory obstruction of the biliary tree.[79] At presentation, about 70% of patients report slowly progressive symptoms, such as a gradual onset of fatigue and pruritus.[32]

The diagnosis of PSC is based on a combination of the clinical features, cholestatic biochemical profile, and histologic and radiographic abnormalities.

ERCP provides an accurate and sensitive method of diagnosing PSC. The typical cholangiographic features include diffuse multifocal annular strictures, intervening segments of normal or slightly ectatic ducts, diverticular outpouchings, and short band-like strictures involving the intrahepatic and/or extrahepatic biliary tree. Pruning of the peripheral biliary tree and irregularities of the duct walls may be found.[5,32,79]

Recently, MRCP has been evaluated in patients with PSC, with high sensitivity (85%) and specificity (99%) for the diagnosis of PSC.[32]

With regard to therapy, patients with major ductal strictures are candidates for endoscopic treatment with ES and balloon dilation to relieve the obstruction and delay the progression to cirrhosis.[5,80]

CHOLANGIOPATHY ASSOCIATED WITH HIV INFECTION

Although pancreatic, hepatic, and biliary complications of human immunodeficiency virus (HIV) infection are well recognized in adults,[81–84] there have been few studies in children. Findings include cytomegalovirus infection, Kaposi sarcoma, giant cell transformation, granulomatous hepatitis, steatosis, portal inflammation, and cholestasis. Sclerosing cholangitis has been reported in children with immune deficiencies other than acquired immune deficiency syndrome (AIDS) and in HIV patients. Pancreatitis has been associated with infections with cytomegalovirus,

Cryptosporidium, Pneumocystis, and *Mycobacterium avium-intracellulare.*[85] ERCP can be safely performed on children with HIV infection. ERCP findings can direct treatment; it can also be used as a therapeutic procedure.[85]

PARASITIC INFESTATION

Ascaris lumbricoides is the most common helminth in the human gastrointestinal tract. It is estimated that more than 1 billion people in the world are infected, and the prevalence is inversely related to the level of sanitation, personal hygiene, and agricultural development.[86,87] Children are predominantly affected. Most cases have a benign course and respond well to treatment.

Most intestinal *Ascaris* infections are asymptomatic or mildly symptomatic, but classic biliary symptoms occur if the large-sized *Ascaris* worm migrates into the bile duct. Patients may present with typical biliary colic, acute cholangitis, acalculous cholecystitis, hepatic abscess, or acute pancreatitis. Biliary colic or pancreatitis is often related to a worm impacted at the ampulla.[87]

The treatment should start with conservative measures, including hydration, analgesics, antispasmodics, and antihelminthic therapy. For patients unresponsive to these, ERCP may be performed.

ERCP plays an important role both in the diagnosis of the infestation in the biliary and pancreatic ducts (serpigi-

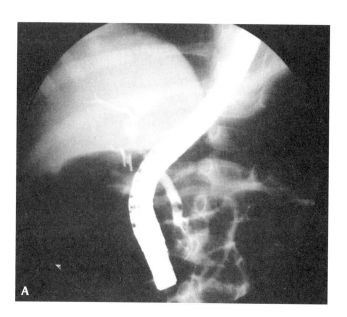

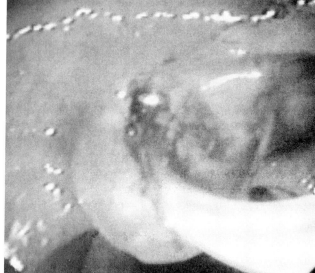

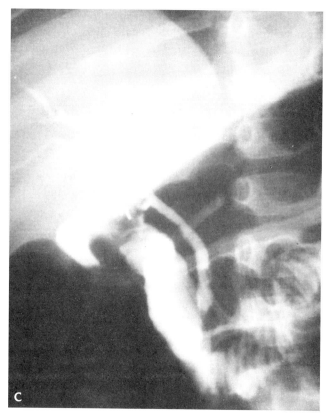

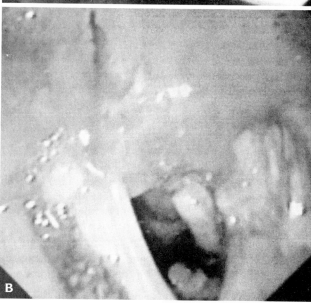

FIGURE 67.5-1 Choledocholithiasis. *A,* In a 2-year-old girl who underwent previous laparoscopic cholecystectomy, it was impossible to extract stones from the common bile duct during surgery. *B,* Endoscopic retrograde cholangiopancreatography allowed endoscopic papillotomy and stone extraction with a Dormia basket. *C,* After the procedure, opacification showed a clear common bile duct.

nous images causing filling defects) and in the treatment of this disease, removing the worms and permitting the decompression of the duct, with or without sphincterotomy. Rapid improvement of patients with pancreatic ascariasis after endoscopic removal is reported.[86, 88–90]

DUODENAL DUPLICATION CYST

Duplication cysts of the gastrointestinal tract are rare congenital anomalies that occur predominantly in males. Duodenal duplications represent only 4 to 12% of all intestinal duplications.[91,92]

Severe vomiting, relapsing pancreatitis, bowel obstruction (mimicking hypertrophic pyloric stenosis), and pain during the first 2 to 4 years of life are possible early presenting symptoms. They rarely present with gastrointestinal bleeding owing to ulceration produced by acid-secreting ectopic gastric mucosa.

Real-time ultrasonography is useful in determining a duodenal duplication cyst. A peristaltic wave is shown passing through the cystic structure.[91] ERCP provides accurate information about the exact location, size, and communication to the biliary and pancreatic tract, which is necessary for guiding the therapeutic endoscopic intervention.[92]

Duodenal duplication cysts cannot be differentiated from a choledochocele by endoscopy. However, the histologic features of a duodenal duplication cyst are quite distinct. These include the presence of a muscular lining with or without ectopic gastric or pancreatic tissue.[53]

In the past, these patients have been managed surgically.[91] In recent years, a few reports of endoscopic drainage have been published with symptomatic improvement.[91,92]

BILIARY TRACT COMPLICATIONS
AFTER LIVER TRANSPLANT

Biliary tract complications are common after orthotopic liver transplant, occurring in 13 to 35% of individuals.[93–95] Bile leaks and anastomotic strictures are the most common complications.

Leaks can occur with both duct-to-duct anastomoses and Roux-en-Y choledochojejunostomy. These can be divided into cystic duct leaks, incidental intrahepatic injury, T-tube tract leaks, and anastomotic leaks.[93]

Endoscopic treatment for bile leaks includes biliary stent placement with sphincterotomy, biliary stent placement alone, nasobiliary tube placement with sphincterotomy, and sphincterotomy alone. Excellent results are reported (up to 100% of fistula closure) after endoscopic treatment.[94]

Anastomotic strictures or stenosis can occur after choledochocholedochostomy or Roux-en-Y choledochojejunostomy and are thought to be caused by faulty surgical technique.[94] In some patients, a transient narrowing at a duct-to-duct connection appears within the first 30 to 60 days. This type of stenosis is usually caused by postoperative edema and inflammation and responds very well to balloon dilation and temporary stent placement.[93] The second type of stricture appears later, usually after 3 months. Although the narrowing responds well to initial dilation, the response is short-lived, and the relapse is predictable.[93] Dilation can be performed with either graduated bougies or bal-

loons. In all instances, a balloon larger than one of the limbs of the anastomosis should never be used. In practice, balloons between 4 and 8 mm are used. The use of a stent is quite important because it prevents edema or intramural hemorrhage, which can obstruct the anastomosis. Hence, a stent prevents any leakage of bile from the anastomosis in the event of a microscopic perforation or disruption.[93] Stents must be exchanged periodically (usually every 3–4 months) for long periods (until stricture resolution occurs). The response to endoscopic treatment is usually very good.[94]

Another type of stricture is the nonanastomotic stricture (donor duct). The causes of these strictures are less clear and are associated with occlusion of the hepatic artery, prolonged cold ischemia, rejection, and ABO blood group incompatibility.[94] By comparison with anastomotic strictures, the success rate for nonsurgical management of nonanastomotic strictures is low (58% in one series).[94]

UNEXPLAINED ABDOMINAL PAIN

Abdominal pain is a frequent cause of disability and the most common reason that a patient will seek consultation with a gastroenterologist. The perception of pain is purely subjective and is heavily influenced by psychosocial aspects. For the gastroenterologist, the differential diagnosis of abdominal pain is a common but challenging clinical problem.[96] Whereas the diagnosis of pancreatic or biliary disease in patients with "classic" clinical features is usually straightforward, patients with the sole symptom of abdominal pain might represent a "Pandora's box."

Many of these patients undergo a battery of tests, including ERCP.[97] However, the role of ERCP in patients with pain and absence of obvious obstructive disorders of the pancreatic and bile duct is less clear.[98]

In pediatrics, ERCP has been used in many patients with unexplained abdominal pain (see Table 67.5-1). However, the role of ERCP in these patients is disappointing. This is probably due to the fact that most children with unexplained pain are suffering from a functional disorder in which ERCP is clearly unlikely to demonstrate any organic problem. In such children, if investigation is really envisaged, MRCP may be a more appropriate test.[6,7,72,99,100]

PANCREATIC INDICATIONS

Pancreatic indications for diagnostic and therapeutic ERCP are listed in Table 67.5-3.

ACUTE PANCREATITIS

In adults, the two most common causes of acute pancreatitis are alcohol and gallstones. Both situations are rare in children. Other causes include drugs, infectious agents, hypertriglyceridemia, trauma, biliary tract anomalies, and pancreatic ductal obstruction.[101,102]

In patients who present with the typical findings of acute pancreatitis (elevated pancreatic enzymes, abdominal pain), ERCP has no role except when the diagnosis of acute biliary pancreatitis with concomitant cholangitis is suspected (presence of fever and abnormal liver chemistries). In most noncomplicated cases, noninvasive

TABLE 67.5-3   PANCREATIC INDICATIONS FOR
ENDOSCOPIC RETROGRADE
CHOLANGIOPANCREATOGRAPHY

DIAGNOSTIC
Unexplained persistent acute pancreatitis
Recurrent pancreatitis
    Congenital disorders
        Biliary anomalies (choledochal cyst or anomalous
            pancreaticobiliary union)
        Pancreatic anomalies (pancreas divisum, annular pancreas,
            short pancreas, pancreatocele)
        Duodenal anomalies (duodenal or gastric duplication cysts,
            duodenal diverticulum)
        Cystic fibrosis
        Hyperlipidemia/hypercalcemia
    Acquired disorders
        Parasitic infestation (Ascaris)
        Sphincter of Oddi dysfunction
        Pancreatic trauma
        Medications
Chronic pancreatitis
Pancreatic mass
Preoperative evaluation

THERAPEUTIC
Pancreatic sphincterotomy
Dilation of pancreatic stricture
Stone removal
Stent placement
Pseudocyst drainage
Nasopancreatic drainage

imaging studies such as abdominal ultrasonography and CT can define the extent of the disease, diagnose and quantify necrosis, and determine whether pseudocysts are present. MRCP is also a promising test.[2]

In patients with severe biliary pancreatitis, trials comparing early ERCP versus delayed ERCP show a benefit of early intervention, at least in a subset of patients.[2,103]

Indications for ERCP in acute biliary pancreatitis should be as follows[103]:

• Before cholecystectomy: in the presence of concomitant cholangitis, obstructive jaundice, or severe disease or in patients who suffer an in-hospital exacerbation
• After cholecystectomy: in patients with unsuccessful laparoscopic or open CBD exploration or patients with smoldering disease (± sphincter dysfunction or ductal disruption)

Anecdotal reports of therapeutic ERCP in acute biliary pancreatitis in children have been published.[104] However, no consistent data exist on the role of ERCP in acute pancreatitis in children.

RECURRENT PANCREATITIS

Recurrent pancreatitis is characterized by episodes of acute pancreatitis, manifested by unexplained recurrent bouts of abdominal pain, with intervening asymptomatic intervals of varying duration. It is rarely recognized in children because the index of clinical suspicion is low.[105] Diagnosis is often missed for several months or years. Patients are symptomatically treated during an acute attack and discharged.

Recurrent pancreatitis can be divided into two groups, depending on whether the cause is nonobstructive or obstructive.[105] Nonobstructive causes include hereditary factors, cystic fibrosis, hyperlipidemia, trauma, medication, and hypercalcemia. Obstructive causes include choledochal cysts, pancreas divisum, duodenal diverticulum, duodenal duplication, parasitic infestation, and anomalous pancreaticobiliary junction.

MRCP is a promising, noninvasive method of identifying and ruling out structural abnormalities as a cause of acute pancreatitis in children with early-stage pancreatitis.[106] However, currently, it is ERCP that offers the definition of the CBD and pancreatic ductal system that is necessary to make decisions in the management of these children. Whatever the underlying cause of pancreatitis, the possibility that there may be an anatomic abnormality amenable to endoscopic therapy or surgery should always be considered.[102,105,107] ERCP has been found useful in the identification of treatable causes in 40 to 75% of children with recurrent pancreatitis.[5]

Endoscopic therapy in recurrent pancreatitis includes standard biliary sphincterotomy, dual sphincterotomy of the pancreatic duct sphincter and the CBD sphincter, minor papilla sphincterotomy, pancreatic stone extraction, pancreatic endoprosthesis insertion, cystogastrostomy or cystoduodenostomy (Figure 67.5-2).

Pancreas Divisum.   Pancreas divisum is a congenital anomaly caused by failure of fusion of the dorsal and ventral endodermal buds during gestation. Each duct drains via its own separate orifice, the major papilla of Vater for the ventral duct of Wirsung, and the minor accessory papilla for the dorsal duct of Santorini.[108] It is the most common congenital variant of pancreatic ductal anatomy and has been found in approximately 5 to 14% of autopsy series and 0.3 to 8% of ERCP studies.[105,108,109] However, when patients with unexplained recurrent pancreatitis are studied, the incidence is 25%.[105]

The exact prevalence of pancreas divisum in children is unknown. In 272 cases of successful ERCP performed in children, pancreas divisum was found in 9 (3.3%).[108] In children with recurrent pancreatitis, the incidence ranges between 7 and 22%.[105] The clinical significance of pancreas divisum is controversial. For many authors, it is related to recurrent pancreatitis, arguing that the minor papilla could be too small to allow adequate drainage.[108,110,111] However, others have considered it to be a coincidental finding by reviewing large series of ERCP.[112]

The treatment of pancreas divisum used to be surgical (minor papilla sphincterotomy). In recent years, endoscopic therapy has been directed to decompress the dorsal duct by insertion of endoprosthesis, dilation of the minor papilla, or sphincterotomy of the minor papilla with or without stent insertion. Overall, improvement is seen in 70 to 90% of the cases.[110,113–116]

Guelrud and colleagues treated three children with pancreas divisum by ES of the minor papilla. In one, a pancreatic stent was placed for 2 weeks. Two were asymptomatic during follow-up of 10 to 17 months, and one had recurrent episodes of abdominal pain without enzyme elevation. Similar results were seen in three other patients treated surgically in the same series.[105]

Other Congenital Anomalies. Annular pancreas, short pancreas, cystic dilation of the pancreatic duct (pancreatocele), duodenal or gastric duplication, and duodenal diverticulum have been reported to be associated with recurrent pancreatitis. ERCP might be useful in the diagnostic evaluation of these entities, especially when less invasive tests, such as CT and MRCP, are inconclusive.[106]

Anomalous Pancreaticobiliary Junction. Anomalous pancreaticobiliary junction is a congenital malformation defined as a communication of the CBD with the pancreatic duct to form a long common channel outside the duodenal wall and therefore not under the influence of the sphincter of Oddi. During an ERCP, anomalous pancreaticobiliary junction is considered to be present when the common channel measures more than 15 mm or when its extraduodenal portion is more than 6 mm long.[117,118] This anomaly has been implicated as a cause of choledochal cyst, bile duct and gallbladder carcinoma, and recurrent pancreatitis.[117]

According to the classification of Kimura and colleagues,[119] there are two types of anomalous pancreaticobiliary junction:

* Type BP: when the common bile duct appears to join the pancreatic duct
* Type PB: when the pancreatic duct appears to join the CBD

Guelrud and colleagues have proposed a third type, the "long Y," in which there is only a long common channel without CBD dilation.[118] It seems that recurrent pancreatitis is more directly associated with the PB type than the BP type.[118]

One case of balloon dilation as an alternative to surgical biliodigestive anastomosis in a child with a long common channel, choledochal cyst, and multiple biliary stenoses has been reported.[120]

Sphincter of Oddi Dysfunction. Sphincter of Oddi dysfunction is an abnormality in the contractility of this sphincter. It is a benign, noncalculous obstruction to flow of bile or pancreatic juice through the pancreaticobiliary junction. Its pathogenesis is unknown.[98,121]

Sphincter of Oddi dysfunction may be manifested clinically by pancreaticobiliary pain, pancreatitis, or cholestasis. The pain is usually epigastric or in the right upper quadrant, may be disabling, and lasts for 30 minutes to several hours. It may radiate to the back or shoulder and be accompanied by nausea and vomiting. Although typically observed in middle-aged women, it may occur in pediatric or adult patients of any age.[98] It can involve abnormalities of the biliary sphincter, pancreatic sphincter, or both. Three types of suspected biliary SOD are reported:

* Biliary type I: patients with biliary-type pain, abnormal aspartate aminotransferase or alkaline phosphatase (> 2× normal documented on two or more occasions),

delayed drainage of ERCP contrast from the biliary tree (> 45 minutes), and dilated CBD (> 12 mm in diameter). The frequency of abnormal manometry ranges between 75% and 95%, and the probability of pain relief by sphincterotomy is between 90% and 95%. Although manometry may be useful in documenting sphincter of Oddi dysfunction, it is not an essential diagnostic study before endoscopic or surgical sphincter ablation.

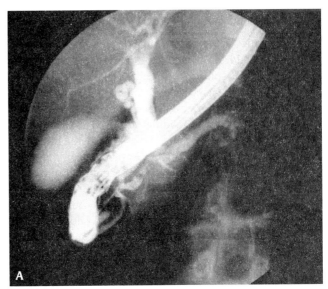
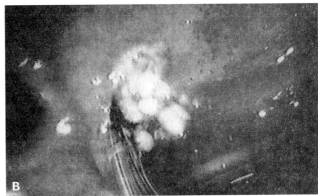
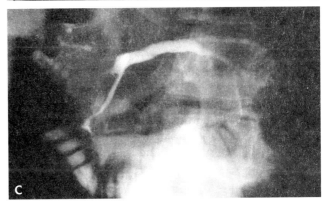

FIGURE 67.5-2   Recurrent pancreatitis. *A*, Recurrent pancreatitis in a 11-year-old girl. Endoscopic retrograde cholangiopancreatography showed a dilated main pancreatic duct with multiple filling defects owing to proteinaceous plugs. The common bile duct was also dilated. *B*, Stones were extracted after pancreatic duct sphincterotomy. *C*, Postoperative opacification showed a Wirsung duct clear of stone.

- Biliary type II: patients with biliary-type pain but only one or two of the above criteria. Manometry is abnormal in 55 to 65% of patients. If manometry is abnormal, about 85% of patients will experience pain relief by sphincterotomy. If manometry is normal, only 35% will benefit from sphincterotomy.
- Biliary Type III: patients with only biliary-type pain and no other abnormality. Manometry is abnormal in 25 to 60% of patients. If abnormal, 55 to 65% will improve with sphincterotomy. If manometry is normal, less than 10% will improve after sphincterotomy.

Manometry is the only available method to measure sphincter of Oddi motor activity directly.[98] ERCP has been used to perform sphincter of Oddi manometry in adults and children with suspected SOD. Because of the difficulties involved in performing manometry on healthy children, values obtained for adults are used as normal for children. Basal sphincter pressure is considered abnormal if it is greater than 35 mm Hg.[117] However, given that there are no normal control data in children, minimal published experience, and inherent technical difficulties with the test, no recommendation can be made regarding the clinical application or reliability of this test in children.[19]

Pediatric patients, like adults, can have pancreatitis secondary to sphincter of Oddi dysfunction. In general, they do not respond as well to endoscopic treatment, for which the complication rate tends to be higher than that for adults.[122]

CHRONIC PANCREATITIS

Chronic pancreatitis is a chronic inflammatory condition characterized by fibrosis, destruction of exocrine tissue, and, eventually, destruction of exocrine and endocrine tissue. Both parenchymal and ductular tissue may be involved. Fibrosis may be accentuated in focal areas, causing sphincter of Oddi or main duct strictures, or it may be diffuse throughout the gland, including small ducts. Three subgroups of chronic pancreatitis are delineated[123–126]:

1. Chronic calcified pancreatitis. This is the largest subgroup, and it is characterized by sporadic parenchymal fibrosis associated with intraductal protein plugs, intraductal stones, and ductal injury.
2. Chronic obstructive pancreatitis. This results from obstruction of the main pancreatic duct and is characterized by uniform ductal dilatation and atrophy, with eventual replacement of acinar cells by fibrous tissue.
3. Chronic inflammatory pancreatitis. This subgroup is characterized by fibrosis, mononuclear cell infiltration, and atrophy. It is associated with autoimmune diseases such as Sjögren syndrome and PSC of the liver.

New etiologies for chronic pancreatitis have been recently defined: autoimmune pancreatitis, eosinophilic pancreatitis, genetic pancreatitis (mutation in the trypsinogen cationic gene responsible for familial pancreatitis, with autosomal dominant inheritance, or recessive mutations in the *SPINK1* gene [serine protease inhibitor Kazal type 1] or in the *CFTR* gene [cystic fibrosis transmembrane conductance regulator], observed with high frequencies in patients with "idiopathic" pancreatitis). Before performing invasive tests such as ERCP, searching for these entities is mandatory if the first bout of pancreatitis occurs before the age of 20 years.[127,128]

Abdominal pain is the most serious clinical problem in chronic pancreatitis and the most common indication for surgery. In an exacerbation of acute inflammation, the characteristics of pain are similar to those experienced during prior episodes of acute pancreatitis. Some patients have evidence of chronic pancreatitis, including intraductal calcification, ductal dilatation, and pseudocyst in the absence of pain.

The later stages of chronic pancreatitis are characterized by spontaneous remission of abdominal pain and the appearance of signs of full-blown insufficiency of both the exocrine and endocrine pancreas. Before the disease reaches this stage, treatment is aimed at producing stable remission of painful symptoms (that respond poorly to medical treatment), prevention of complications (cystic lesions, stenosis of the main bile duct), and halting or slowing the progression of the disease. These objectives are particularly important when the disease appears early in life because it can interfere with the psychophysical development of the child. In a growing child, suspension of oral feedings prescribed during acute attacks or refusal to eat owing to fear of pain can have effects that are much more serious than in adults.[129]

In the treatment of chronic pancreatitis, endoscopy can be proposed in certain circumstances. Endoscopic treatment is useful in treating local complications such as pancreatic pseudocysts and biliary strictures. Endotherapy is also effective in treating postsurgical complications such as pancreatic leakage after pancreaticojejunostomy. However, the main indication is to control painful chronic pancreatitis resistant to medical treatment or recurrent attacks of acute pancreatitis, which frequently appear in the course of chronic pancreatitis. This goal can be achieved by endoscopic drainage procedures in cases of outflow obstruction caused by pancreatic ductal stones, strictures of the main pancreatic duct, or a compressing pseudocyst, all resulting in upstream dilation. These drainage procedures include pancreatic sphincterotomy, stone extraction, balloon dilation of strictures, usually followed by stent insertion, and pseudocyst drainage.[130,131] Most endoscopic studies have concluded that pain diminishes in a majority of patients after endoscopic therapy, particularly in those patients with a dominant duct stricture and upstream dilation.[124,126]

Because of the experience gained in adults and a greater understanding of the mechanisms underlying the pain experienced by children, endoscopic approaches are now being used to treat pediatric patients as well.[129,132] The pain experienced by children with chronic idiopathic pancreatitis appears to be more commonly caused by the transient occlusion of the sphincter of Oddi by protein plugs. In these cases, the most effective approach to restore the flow within the duct is to reduce the resistance to the passage of these plugs by sphincterotomy.[129]

In a study involving 22 children with pancreatitis (6 acute, 6 recurrent, and 10 chronic) treated endoscopically, Hsu and colleagues observed significant improvement in all 6 outcome parameters analyzed, especially improvement in the frequency and severity of pain, a decrease in health care encounters (emergency department visit, clinic visit, and hospital admission), and improvement in general conditions.[122] In an early stage, patients without diffuse ductal changes in the pancreatogram had the most significant clinical improvement.

PSEUDOCYSTS

Pancreatic pseudocysts are nonepithelium-lined fluid collections that result from transient or persistent pancreatic duct disruption. They are common consequences of acute and chronic pancreatitis. Most of the pseudocysts resolve spontaneously. In the setting of chronic pancreatitis, symptomatic pseudocysts are commonly seen in association with pancreatic stones and strictures. Symptomatic, large (> 4 cm), or persistent (beyond 6 weeks) pseudocysts are unlikely to resolve and are at risk of complications. There has been increased interest in nonoperative management of pseudocysts.[5,19,124]

Pseudocysts that connect with the main pancreatic duct and are accessible to guidewire passage and those that abut the stomach or duodenum are addressed by transductal or transmural pseudocyst entry and stent placement.[124]

In adults, successful endoscopic treatment with pseudocyst resolution has been reported in about 80 to 90% of cases within 1 to 2 months. A 15% recurrence rate has been reported. Complication rates are approximately 20%, with a 1% mortality, indicating that this is one of the more dangerous endoscopic therapies.[5,124] Pediatric experience is limited to a few case reports and insufficient to comment on either the efficacy or safety of this procedure in children.[7,19,105,132]

PANCREATIC TRAUMA

Injuries to the pancreas from blunt abdominal trauma in children are rare. Most are minor and are best treated conservatively. The mainstay for treatment of major ductal injuries has been prompt surgical resection.

Diagnostic imaging modalities are the key to the accurate classification of these injuries and planning appropriate treatment. CT has been the major imaging modality in blunt abdominal trauma for children, but it has shortcomings in the diagnosis of pancreatic ductal injury. MRCP is a promising test in these patients.[133]

ERCP has been shown recently to be superior to CT in the diagnosis of pancreatic trauma, allowing the possibility of stent placement (Figure 67.5-3).[134] In reported pediatric cases, clinical improvement is rapid, with complete resolution of clinical and biochemical pancreatitis, resumption of a normal diet, and discharge from hospital.[135]

CONTRAINDICATIONS

Contraindications to ERCP include unstable cardiovascular, pulmonary, or neurologic conditions or suspected bowel perforation. Esophageal stricture is a relative contraindication. Coagulopathies should be corrected before ERCP

whenever possible, especially if a therapeutic procedure is envisaged. Aspirin, nonsteroidal anti-inflammatory drugs, and medications that interfere with platelet function should be avoided before and immediately after the procedure.[19]

COMPLICATIONS

ERCP has evolved from a diagnostic test into a primarily therapeutic procedure for a variety of biliary and pancreatic disorders. Many short-term complications are associated with the examination, mainly pancreatitis, hemorrhage, perforation, cholangitis, and cholecystitis, and are related to the anesthesia. Short-term complications are reported to occur after 5 to 10% of ERCPs with or without sphincterotomy (see Table 67.5-1).[136,137]

In children, the major risks and complications of ERCP are the same as in adults. The relative risk for these complications in children is not well established because of the small number of patients in pediatric series.[19]

In a large pediatric ERCP series, the overall complication rate was 11.6%. Pancreatitis occurred in 3.3% (see Table 67.5-1).[7] Hemorrhage and perforation have rarely been reported after ERCP in children.[28,72,138] Rates are likely to be similar to those reported in adults: 0.7 to 2% for hemorrhage and 0.3 to 0.6% for perforation.[139,140] In Guelrud's experience with 184 neonates and young infants, minor complication without clinical significance occurred in 24 (13%) patients. In 220 ERCPs in children older than 1 year, this author observed 1.8% of complications in diagnostic examinations and 10.7% in therapeutic ERCPs.[5]

The long-term complications of ES or use of stents in pediatric patients are unknown.[19]

COMPETENCE IN PEDIATRIC ERCP

Endoscopic competence is difficult to define and almost impossible to quantitate. Strictly defined, "competence" is the ability to carry out a set of tasks or a role adequately or effectively.[141] Competency in diagnostic and therapeutic endoscopy implies a demonstration of appropriate clinical judgment in patient selection and adequate cognitive and technical skills to complete a procedure safely and successfully. Deep knowledge of appropriate indications and contraindications, potential risks, and benefits is also mandatory. The endoscopist must be prepared to manage or to enlist the help of others to manage complications or adverse outcomes expeditiously in an appropriate medical facility.[142]

According to the ASGE, endoscopic competence includes objectives that trained endoscopists will be able to[143]

- Recommend endoscopic procedures based on findings of a personal consultation and in consideration of specific indications, contraindications, and diagnostic or therapeutic alternatives
- Perform specific procedures safely, completely, and expeditiously
- Correctly interpret most endoscopic findings and undertake endoscopic interventions when indicated

- Integrate endoscopic findings or therapy into patient management plans
- Understand risk factors and recognize and manage complications
- Recognize personal and procedural limits and know when to request help

Competency in pediatric endoscopy requires a specialized knowledge of gastrointestinal diseases affecting children. Such knowledge is conventionally gained through formal training in pediatric gastroenterology. However, other physicians experienced in the care of children or adults with gastrointestinal disease may

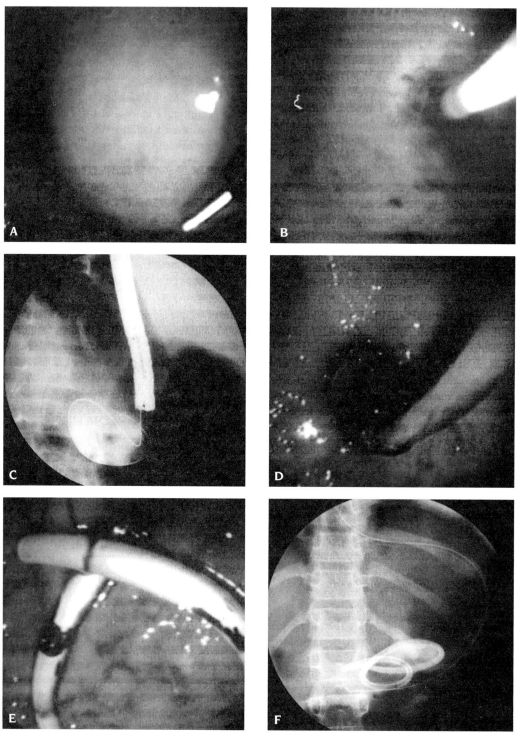

FIGURE 67.5-3 Pancreatic trauma. *A*, Traumatic pseudocyst with obvious bulging into the gastric lumen. *B*, Diathermic needle puncture of the gastric wall toward the cyst's center. *C*, Opacification of the cystic cavity and guidewire placement. *D*, Balloon dilation of the cystic opening. *E*, Insertion of a pigtail stent to maintain the patency of the cystogastrostomy. *F*, Pigtail stent allowing communication between the cystic cavity and the stomach.

acquire suitable cognitive skills to achieve competence in pediatric endoscopy.[142]

CONCLUSIONS

ERCP is a safe and valuable diagnostic and therapeutic procedure in children with presumptive pancreaticobiliary disease. Considerable experience with this endoscopic procedure is a prerequisite before undertaking cannulation in this young age group. It is anticipated that ERCP and its associated endoscopic therapy will find increasing use in the pediatric population, not only for diagnosis and preoperative delineation of the pancreaticobiliary tract but, in many instances, as a substitute for traditional operative therapy.[144] The performance of endoscopy in children assumes an adequate knowledge and understanding of pediatrics. To provide appropriate care for each child, a team approach is often required, including the pediatrician or pediatric gastroenterologist, the surgeon, and the adult endoscopist.[7,12,76]

REFERENCES

1. McCune WS, Shorb PE, Moscovitz H. Endoscopic cannulation of the ampulla of Vater: a preliminary report. Ann Surg 1968; 167:752–6.
2. Cohen S, Bacon BR, Berlin JA, et al. National Institutes of Health State-of-the-Science Conference statement: ERCP for diagnosis and therapy, January 14–16, 2002. Gastrointest Endosc 2002;56:803–9.
3. Kimmey MB, Freeman ML. Preface. Gastrointest Endosc 2002;56(6 Suppl 2):S153.
4. Carr-Locke DL. Overview of the role of ERCP in the management of diseases of the biliary tract and the pancreas. Gastrointest Endosc 2002;56(6 Suppl 2):S157–60.
5. Guelrud M. Endoscopic retrograde cholangiopancreatography. Gastrointest Endosc Clin N Am 2001;11:585–601.
6. Poddar U, Thapa BR, Bhasin DK, et al. Endoscopic retrograde cholangiopancreatography in the management of pancreaticobiliary disorders in children. J Gastroenterol Hepatol 2001;16:927–31.
7. Brown CW, Werlin SL, Geenen JE, et al. The diagnostic and therapeutic role of endoscopic retrograde cholangiopancreatography in children. J Pediatr Gastroenterol Nutr 1993;17:19–23.
8. Waye JD. Endoscopic retrograde cholangiopancreatography in the infant. J Am Gastroenterol 1976;65:461–3.
9. Fox VL. Pediatric endoscopy. Gastroint Endosc Clin N Am 2000;10:175–94.
10. Mougenot JF, Dupont C, Liguory C. Advances in upper gastrointestinal endoscopy. In: Buts JP, Sokal EM, editors. Management of digestive and liver disorders in infants and children. Amsterdam: Elsevier Science; 1993. p. 39–55.
11. Lehman GA. What are the determinants of success in utilization of ERCP in the setting of pancreatic and biliary diseases? Gastrointest Endosc 2002;56(6 Suppl 2):S291–3.
12. American Society for Gastrointestinal Endoscopy. Modifications in endoscopic practice for pediatric patients. Gastrointest Endosc 2000;52:838–42.
13. Tagge EP, Tarnasky PR, Chandler J, et al. Multidisciplinary approach to the treatment of pediatric pancreaticobiliary disorders. J Pediatr Surg 1997;32:158–64; discussion 164–5.
14. Mahajan L, Wyllie R, Steffen R, et al. The effects of a psycho-
logical preparation program on anxiety in children and adolescents undergoing gastrointestinal endoscopy. J Pediatr Gastroenterol Nutr 1998;27:161–5.
15. American Academy of Pediatrics, Committee on Drugs. Guidelines for monitoring and management of pediatric patients during and after sedation for diagnostic and therapeutic procedures. Pediatrics 1992;89(6 Pt 1):1110–5.
16. Chuang E, Zimmerman A, Neiswender KM, Liacouras CA. Sedation in pediatric endoscopy. Gastrointest Endosc Clin N Am 2001;11:569–84.
17. Guelrud M, Jaen D, Mendoza S, et al. ERCP in the diagnosis of extrahepatic biliary atresia. Gastrointest Endosc 1991; 37:522–6.
18. Etzkorn KP, Diab F, Brown RD, et al. Endoscopic retrograde cholangiopancreatography under general anesthesia: indications and results. Gastrointest Endosc 1998;47:363–7.
19. Fox VL, Werlin SL, Heyman MB. Endoscopic retrograde cholangiopancreatography in children. J Pediatr Gastroenterol Nutr 2000;30:335–42.
20. Snyder JD, Bratton B. Antimicrobial prophylaxis for gastrointestinal procedures: current practices in North American academic pediatric programs. J Pediatr Gastroenterol Nutr 2002;35:564–9.
21. Snyder JD, Bratton B. Antibiotic prophylaxis for endoscopic procedures: what is the standard in North America for children? J Pediatr Gastroenter Nutr 1998;27:482.
22. el-Baba M, Tolia V, Lin CH, Dajani AS. Absence of bacteremia after gastrointestinal procedures in children. Gastrointest Endosc 1996;44:378–81.
23. Harris A, Chan AC, Torres-Viera C, et al. Meta-analysis of antibiotic prophylaxis in endoscopic retrograde cholangiopancreatography (ERCP). Endoscopy 1999;31:718–24.
24. American Society for Gastrointestinal Endoscopy. Infection control during gastrointestinal endoscopy: guidelines for clinical application. From the ASGE. Gastrointest Endosc 1999;49:836–41.
25. Dajani AS, Taubert KA, Wilson W, et al. Prevention of bacterial endocarditis. Recommendations by the American Heart Association. JAMA 1997;277:1794–801.
26. Mani V, Cartwright K, Dooley J, et al. Antibiotic prophylaxis in gastrointestinal endoscopy: a report by a Working Party for the British Society of Gastroenterology Endoscopy Committee. Endoscopy 1997;29:114–9.
27. Ohnuma N, Takahashi T, Tanabe M, et al. The role of ERCP in biliary atresia. Gastrointest Endosc 1997;45:365–70.
28. Heyman MB, Shapiro HA, Thaler MM. Endoscopic retrograde cholangiography in the diagnosis of biliary malformations in infants. Gastrointest Endosc 1988;34:449–53.
29. Cotton PB, Laage NJ. Endoscopic retrograde cholangiopancreatography in children. Arch Dis Child 1982;57:131–6.
30. Carr-Locke DL, Conn MI, Faigel DO, et al. Technology status evaluation: magnetic resonance cholangiopancreatography: November 1998. From the ASGE. Gastrointest Endosc 1999; 49:858–61.
31. Prasad SR, Sahani D, Saini S. Clinical applications of magnetic resonance cholangiopancreatography. J Clin Gastroenterol 2001;33:362–6.
32. Textor HJ, Flacke S, Pauleit D, et al. Three-dimensional magnetic resonance cholangiopancreatography with respiratory triggering in the diagnosis of primary sclerosing cholangitis: comparison with endoscopic retrograde cholangiography. Endoscopy 2002;34:984–90.
33. Manfredi R, Costamagna G, Brizi MG, et al. Severe chronic pancreatitis versus suspected pancreatic disease: dynamic MR

cholangiopancreatography after secretin stimulation. Radiology 2000;214:849–55.

34. Manfredi R, Lucidi V, Gui B, et al. Idiopathic chronic pancreatitis in children: MR cholangiopancreatography after secretin administration. Radiology 2002;224:675–82.

35. Fulcher AS. MRCP and ERCP in the diagnosis of common bile duct stones. Gastrointest Endosc 2002;56(6 Suppl 2):5178–82.

36. Takehara Y. Can MRCP replace ERCP? J Magn Reson Imaging 1998;8:517–34.

37. Lee MG, Lee HJ, Kim MH, et al. Extrahepatic biliary diseases: 3D MR cholangiopancreatography compared with endoscopic retrograde cholangiopancreatography. Radiology 1997;202:663–9.

38. Soto JA, Barish MA, Yucel EK, et al. Magnetic resonance cholangiography: comparison with endoscopic retrograde cholangiopancreatography. Gastroenterology 1996;110:589–97.

39. Hintze RE, Adler A, Veltzke W, et al. Clinical significance of magnetic resonance cholangiopancreatography (MRCP) compared to endoscopic retrograde cholangiopancreatography (ERCP). Endoscopy 1997;29:182–7.

40. Takehara Y. MR pancreatography: technique and applications. Top Magn Reson Imaging 1996;8:290–301.

41. Guibaud L, Lachaud A, Touraine R, et al. MR cholangiography in neonates and infants: feasibility and preliminary applications. AJR Am J Roentgenol 1998;170:27–31.

42. Hirohashi S, Hirohashi R, Uchida H, et al. Pancreatitis: evaluation with MR cholangiopancreatography in children. Radiology 1997;203:411–5.

43. Miyazaki T, Yamashita Y, Tang Y, et al. Single-shot MR cholangiopancreatography of neonates, infants, and young children. AJR Am J Roentgenol 1998;170:33–7.

44. Schreiber RA, Kleinman RE. Biliary atresia. J Pediatr Gastroenterol Nutr 2002;35(Suppl 1):S11–6.

45. Lipsett PA, Segev DL, Colombani PM. Biliary atresia and biliary cysts. Baillieres Clin Gastroenterol 1997;11:619–41.

46. Savader SJ, Benenati JF, Venbrux AC, et al. Choledochal cysts: classification and cholangiographic appearance. AJR Am J Roentgenol 1991;156:327–31.

47. Tan KC, Howard ER. Choledochal cyst: a 14-year surgical experience with 36 patients. Br J Surg 1988;75:892–5.

48. Kepczyk T, Angueira CE, Kadakia SC, et al. Choledochal cyst mimicking a pancreatic pseudocyst. J Clin Gastroenterol 1995;20:139–41.

49. Yamaguchi M. Congenital choledochal cyst. Analysis of 1,433 patients in the Japanese literature. Am J Surg 1980;140:653–7.

50. Aleksic M, Ulrich B, Lutzeler J. Problems in diagnosis and surgical therapy of choledochus cysts. A case report. Langenbecks Arch Chir 1996;381:258–62.

51. Todani T, Watanabe Y, Narusue M, et al. Congenital bile duct cysts: classification, operative procedures, and review of thirty-seven cases including cancer arising from choledochal cyst. Am J Surg 1977;134:263–9.

52. Alonso-Lej F, Rever WB Jr, Pessogno DJ. Congenital choledochal cysts with a report of two and an analysis of 94 cases. Surg Gynecol Obstet 1959;108:1–30.

53. Venu RP, Geenen JE, Hogan WJ, et al. Role of endoscopic retrograde cholangiopancreatography in the diagnosis and treatment of choledochocele. Gastroenterology 1984;87:1144–9.

54. Kim OH, Chung HJ, Choi BG. Imaging of the choledochal cyst. Radiographics 1995;15:69–88.

55. Wang HP, Wu MS, Lin CC, et al. Pancreaticobiliary diseases associated with anomalous pancreaticobiliary ductal union. Gastrointest Endosc 1998;48:184–9.

56. Stringel G, Filler RM. Fictitious pancreatitis in choledochal cyst. J Pediatr Surg 1982;17:359–61.

57. Kaneko K, Ando H, Ito T, et al. Protein plugs cause symptoms in patients with choledochal cysts. Am J Gastroenterol 1997;92:1018–21.

58. Todani T, Tabuchi K, Watanabe Y, et al. Carcinoma arising in the wall of congenital bile duct cysts. Cancer 1979;44:1134–41.

59. Yoshida H, Itai Y, Minami M, et al. Biliary malignancies occurring in choledochal cysts. Radiology 1989;173:389–92.

60. Spinzi G, Martegani A, Belloni G, et al. Computed tomography-virtual cholangiography and choledochal cyst. Gastrointest Endosc 1999;50:857–9.

61. Yoshikane H, Hashimoto S, Hidano H, et al. Multiple early bile duct carcinoma associated with congenital choledochal cyst. J Gastroenterol 1998;33:454–7.

62. Swisher SG, Cates JA, Hunt KK, et al. Pancreatitis associated with adult choledochal cysts. Pancreas 1994;9:633–7.

63. Matos C, Nicaise N, Deviere J, et al. Choledochal cysts: comparison of findings at MR cholangiopancreatography and endoscopic retrograde cholangiopancreatography in eight patients. Radiology 1998;209:443–8.

64. Dohke M, Watanabe Y, Okumura A, et al. Anomalies and anatomic variants of the biliary tree revealed by MR cholangiopancreatography. AJR Am J Roentgenol 1999;173:1251–4.

65. Sugiyama M, Baba M, Atomi Y, et al. Diagnosis of anomalous pancreaticobiliary junction: value of magnetic resonance cholangiopancreatography. Surgery 1998;123:391–7.

66. Sugiyama M, Atomi Y. Endoscopic ultrasonography for diagnosing anomalous pancreaticobiliary junction. Gastrointest Endosc 1997;45:261–7.

67. Siegel EG, Folsch UR. Primary sclerosing cholangitis mimicking choledocal cyst type 1 in a young patient. Endoscopy 1999;31:200–3.

68. Teng R, Yokohata K, Utsunomiya N, et al. Endoscopic retrograde cholangiopancreatography in infants and children. J Gastroenterol 2000;35:39–42.

69. Man DW, Spitz L. Choledocholithiasis in infancy. J Pediatr Surg 1985;20:65–8.

70. Guelrud M, Mendoza S, Jaen D, et al. ERCP and endoscopic sphincterotomy in infants and children with jaundice due to common bile duct stones. Gastrointest Endosc 1992;38:450–3.

71. Guelrud M, Rincones VZ, Jaen D, et al. Endoscopic sphincterotomy and laparoscopic cholecystectomy in a jaundiced infant. Gastrointest Endosc 1994;40:99–102.

72. Buckley A, Connon JJ. The role of ERCP in children and adolescents. Gastrointest Endosc 1990;36:369–72.

73. Tarnasky PR, Tagge EP, Hebra A, et al. Minimally invasive therapy for choledocholithiasis in children. Gastrointest Endosc 1998;47:189–92.

74. Wesdorp I, Bosman D, de Graaff A, et al. Clinical presentations and predisposing factors of cholelithiasis and sludge in children. J Pediatr Gastroenterol Nutr 2000;31:411–7.

75. Guelrud M, Mendoza S, Zager A, et al. Biliary stenting in an infant with malignant obstructive jaundice. Gastrointest Endosc 1989;35:259–61.

76. Brown KO, Goldschmiedt M. Endoscopic therapy of biliary and pancreatic disorders in children. Endoscopy 1994;26:719–23.

77. Westaby D. Endoscopic balloon dilatation of biliary sphincter for removing bile duct stones. Lancet 1997;349:1114–5.

78. Julia V, Soares-Oliveira M, Lambruschini N, et al. Biliary microlithiasis: a cause of idiopathic pancreatitis in childhood. J Pediatr Gastroenterol Nutri 2001;32:596–7.

79. Marotta PJ, LaRusso NF, Wiesner RH. Sclerosing cholangitis. Baillieres Clin Gastroenterol 1997;11:781–800.

80. Stoker J, Lameris JS, Robben SG, et al. Primary sclerosing cholangitis in a child treated by nonsurgical balloon dilatation and stenting. J Pediatr Gastroenterol Nutri 1993;17:303–6.

81. Cello JP. AIDS-Related biliary tract disease. Gastrointest Endosc Clin N Am 1998;8:963.

82. Evrard S, Van Laethem JL, Urbain D, et al. Chronic pancreatic alterations in AIDS patients. Pancreas 1999;19:335–8.

83. Barthet M, Chauveau E, Bonnet E, et al. Pancreatic ductal changes in HIV-infected patients. Gastrointest Endosc 1997;45:59–63.

84. Farman J, Brunetti J, Baer JW, et al. AIDS-related cholangiopancreatographic changes. Abdom Imaging 1994;19:417–22.

85. Yabut B, Werlin SL, Havens P, et al. Endoscopic retrograde cholangiopancreatography in children with HIV infection. J Pediatr Gastroenterol Nutr 1996;23:624–7.

86. Bahu Mda G, Baldisseroto M, Custodio CM, et al. Hepatobiliary and pancreatic complications of ascariasis in children: a study of seven cases. J Pediatr Gastroenterol Nutr 2001;33:271–5.

87. Leung JW, Yu AS. Hepatolithiasis and biliary parasites. Baillieres Clin Gastroenterol 1997;11:681–706.

88. Khuroo MS, Zargar SA, Mahajan R. Hepatobiliary and pancreatic ascariasis in India. Lancet 1990;335:1503–6.

89. Khuroo MS, Zargar SA, Yattoo GN, et al. Ascaris-induced acute pancreatitis. Br J Surg 1992;79:1335–8.

90. Misra SP, Dwivedi M. Endoscopy-assisted emergency treatment of gastroduodenal and pancreatobiliary ascariasis. Endoscopy 1996;28:629–32.

91. al Traif I, Khan MH. Endoscopic drainage of a duodenal duplication cyst. Gastrointest Endosc 1992;38:64–5.

92. Lang T, Berquist W, Rich E, et al. Treatment of recurrent pancreatitis by endoscopic drainage of a duodenal duplication. J Pediatr Gastroenterol Nutr 1994;18:494–6.

93. Ostroff JW. Post-transplant biliary problems. Gastrointest Endosc Clin N Am 2001;11:163–83.

94. Rerknimitr R, Sherman S, Fogel EL, et al. Biliary tract complications after orthotopic liver transplantation with choledochocholedochostomy anastomosis: endoscopic findings and results of therapy. Gastrointest Endosc 2002;55:224–31.

95. Theilmann L, Kuppers B, Kadmon M, et al. Biliary tract strictures after orthotopic liver transplantation: diagnosis and management. Endoscopy 1994;26:517–22.

96. Kalloo AN. Overview of differential diagnoses of abdominal pain. Gastrointest Endosc 2002;56(6 Suppl 2):S255–7.

97. Pasricha PJ. There is no role for ERCP in unexplained abdominal pain of pancreatic or biliary origin. Gastrointest Endosc 2002;56(6 Suppl 2):S267–72.

98. Sherman S. What is the role of ERCP in the setting of abdominal pain of pancreatic or biliary origin (suspected sphincter of Oddi dysfunction)? Gastrointest Endosc 2002;56(6 Suppl 2):S258–66.

99. Prasil P, Laberge JM, Barkun A, Flageole H. Endoscopic retrograde cholangiopancreatography in children: a surgeon's perspective. J Pediatr Surg 2001;36:733–5.

100. Abu-Khalaf A. The role of endoscopic retrograde cholangiopancreatography in small children and adolescents. Surg Laparosc Endosc 1995;5:296–300.

101. Banks PA. Epidemiology, natural history, and predictors of disease outcome in acute and chronic pancreatitis. Gastrointest Endosc 2002;56(6 Suppl 2):S226–30.

102. Blustein PK, Gaskin K, Filler R, et al. Endoscopic retrograde cholangiopancreatography in pancreatitis in children and adolescents. Pediatrics 1981;68:387–93.

103. Kozarek R. Role of ERCP in acute pancreatitis. Gastrointest Endosc 2002;56(6 Suppl 2):S231–6.

104. Zachariassen G, Saffar DF, Mortensen J. Acute pancreatitis in children caused by gallstones. Ugeskr Laeger 1999;161:6061–2.

105. Guelrud M, Mujica C, Jaen D, et al. The role of ERCP in the diagnosis and treatment of idiopathic recurrent pancreatitis in children and adolescents. Gastrointest Endosc 1994;40:428–36.

106. Shimizu T, Suzuki R, Yamashiro Y, et al. Magnetic resonance cholangiopancreatography in assessing the cause of acute pancreatitis in children. Pancreas 2001;22:196–9.

107. Graham KS, Ingram JD, Steinberg SE, et al. ERCP in the management of pediatric pancreatitis. Gastrointest Endosc 1998; 47:492–5.

108. Guelrud M. The incidence of pancreas divisum in children. Gastrointest Endosc 1996;43:83–4.

109. O'Connor KW, Lehman GA. An improved technique for accessory papilla cannulation in pancreas divisum. Gastrointest Endosc 1985;31:13–7.

110. Liguory C, Lefebvre JF, Canard JM, et al. Pancreas divisum: clinical and therapeutic study in man. A propos of 87 cases. Gastroenterol Clin Biol 1986;10:820–5.

111. Sahel J. Pancreas divisum: a new cause of recurrent pancreatitis? Gastroenterol Clin Biol 1986;10:817–9.

112. Delhaye M, Engelholm L, Cremer M. Pancreas divisum: congenital anatomic variant or anomaly? Contribution of endoscopic retrograde dorsal pancreatography. Gastroenterology 1985;89:951–8.

113. McCarthy J, Geenen JE, Hogan WJ. Preliminary experience with endoscopic stent placement in benign pancreatic diseases. Gastrointest Endosc 1988;34:16–8.

114. Lans JI, Geenen JE, Johanson JF, Hogan WJ. Endoscopic therapy in patients with pancreas divisum and acute pancreatitis: a prospective, randomized, controlled clinical trial. Gastrointest Endosc 1992;38:430–4.

115. Soehendra N, Kempeneers I, Nam VC, Grimm H. Endoscopic dilatation and papillotomy of the accessory papilla and internal drainage in pancreas divisum. Endoscopy 1986;18:129–32.

116. Lehman GA, Sherman S, Nisi R, Hawes RH. Pancreas divisum: results of minor papilla sphincterotomy. Gastrointest Endosc 1993;39:1–8.

117. Guelrud M, Morera C, Rodriguez M, et al. Sphincter of Oddi dysfunction in children with recurrent pancreatitis and anomalous pancreaticobiliary union: an etiologic concept. Gastrointest Endosc 1999;50:194–9.

118. Guelrud M, Morera C, Rodriguez M, et al. Normal and anomalous pancreaticobiliary union in children and adolescents. Gastrointest Endosc 1999;50:189–93.

119. Kimura K, Ohto M, Saisho H, et al. Association of gallbladder carcinoma and anomalous pancreaticobiliary ductal union. Gastroenterology 1985;89:1258–65.

120. Sebesta C, Schmid A, Kier P, et al. ERCP and balloon dilation is a valuable alternative to surgical biliodigestive anastomosis in the long common channel syndrome in childhood. Endoscopy 1995;27:709–10.

121. Toouli J. Biliary motility disorders. Baillieres Clin Gastroenterol 1997;11:725–40.

122. Hsu RK, Draganov P, Leung JW, et al. Therapeutic ERCP in the management of pancreatitis in children. Gastrointest Endosc 2000;51(4 Pt 1):396–400.

123. Banks PA. Acute and chronic pancreatitis. In: Feldman M, Scharschmidt BF, Sleisenger MH, editors. Sleisenger & Fordtran's gastrointestinal and liver disease: pathophysiology, diagnosis, management. Vol 1. 6th ed. Philadelphia: WB Saunders; 1998. p. 809–62.

124. Lehman GA. Role of ERCP and other endoscopic modalities in chronic pancreatitis. Gastrointest Endosc 2002;56(6 Suppl 2): S237–40.

125. Sarles H, Adler G, Dani R, et al. The pancreatitis classification of Marseilles-Rome 1988. Scand J Gastroenterol 1989;24:641–2.

126. Eisen GM, Zubarik R. Disease-specific outcomes assessment for chronic pancreatitis. Gastrointest Endosc Clin N Am 1999;9:717–30, ix.

127. Witt H, Hennies HC, Becker M. SPINK1 mutations in chronic pancreatitis. Gastroenterology 2001;120:1060–1.

128. Etemad B, Whitcomb DC. Chronic pancreatitis: diagnosis, classification, and new genetic developments. Gastroenterology 2001;120:682–707.

129. Perrelli L, Nanni L, Costamagna G, Muitgnani M. Endoscopic treatment of chronic idiopathic pancreatitis in children. J Pediatr Surg 1996;31:1396–400.

130. Liguory C, Lefebvre JF, de Paulo GA. Endoscopic treatment of calcifying chronic pancreatitis: trick or treatment? In: Fujita R, Nakazawa S, editors. Recent advances in gastroenterology. Tokyo: Springer-Verlag; 1998. p. 63–71.

131. Liguory C, Silva MB, de Paulo GA. O papel da Endoscopias pancreatites Crônicas. In: Sociedade Brasiliera de Endoscopia Digestiva, editor. Endoscopia digestiva. 3a. Edição ed. Rio de Janeiros: Medsi Edotora e Cientifica Ltda.; 2000. p. 505–26.

132. Kozarek RA, Christie D, Barclay G. Endoscopic therapy of pancreatitis in the pediatric population. Gastrointest Endosc 1993;39:665–9.

133. Fulcher AS, Turner MA, Yelon JA, et al. Magnetic resonance cholangiopancreatography (MRCP) in the assessment of pancreatic duct trauma and its sequelae: preliminary findings. J Trauma 2000;48:1001–7.

134. Kim HS, Lee DK, Kim IW, et al. The role of endoscopic retrograde pancreatography in the treatment of traumatic pancreatic duct injury. Gastrointest Endosc 2001;54:49–55.

135. Canty TG Sr, Weinman D. Treatment of pancreatic duct disruption in children by an endoscopically placed stent. J Pediatr Surg 2001;36:345–8.

136. Freeman ML. Adverse outcomes of ERCP. Gastrointest Endosc 2002;56(6 Suppl 2):S273–82.

137. Loperfido S, Angelini G, Benedetti G, et al. Major early complications from diagnostic and therapeutic ERCP: a prospective multicenter study. Gastrointest Endosc 1998;48:1–10.

138. Wilkinson ML, Mieli-Vergani G, Ball C, et al. Endoscopic retrograde cholangiopancreatography in infantile cholestasis. Arch Dis Child 1991;66:121–3.

139. Freeman ML, Nelson DB, Sherman S, et al. Complications of endoscopic biliary sphincterotomy. N Engl J Med 1996;335:909–18.

140. Aliperti G. Complications related to diagnostic and therapeutic endoscopic retrograde cholangiopancreatography. Gastrointest Endosc Clin N Am 1996;6:379–407.

141. Bond JH. Evaluation of trainee competence. Gastrointest Endosc Clin N Am 1995;5:337–46.

142. Fox VL. Clinical competency in pediatric endoscopy. J Pediatr Gastroenterol Nutr 1998;26:200–4.

143. American Society for Gastrointestinal Endoscopy. Maintaining competency in endoscopic skills. Gastrointest Endosc 1995;42:620–1.

144. Allendorph M, Werlin SL, Geenen JE, et al. Endoscopic retrograde cholangiopancreatography in children. J Pediatr 1987;110:206–11.

145. Riemann JF, Koch H. Endoscopy of the biliary tract and the pancreas in children. Endoscopy 1978;10:166–72.

146. Guelrud M, Jaen D, Torres P, et al. Endoscopic cholangiopancreatography in the infant: evaluation of a new prototype pediatric duodenoscope. Gastrointest Endosc 1987;33:4–8.

147. Putnam PE, Kocoshis SA, Orenstein SR, Schade RR. Pediatric endoscopic retrograde cholangiopancreatography. Am J Gastroenterol 1991;86:824–30.

148. Dite P, Vacek E, Stefan H, et al. Endoscopic retrograde cholangiopancreatography in childhood. Hepatogastroenterology 1992;39:291–3.

149. Richieri JP, Chapoy P, Bertolino JG, et al. Endoscopic retrograde cholangiopancreatography in children and adolescents. Gastroenterol Clin Biol 1994;18:21–5.

150. Derkx HH, Huibregtse K, Taminiau JA. The role of endoscopic retrograde cholangiopancreatography in cholestatic infants. Endoscopy 1994;26:7248.

151. Mitchell SA, Wilkinson ML. The role of ERCP in the diagnosis of neonatal conjugated hyperbilirubinemia. Gastrointest Endosc 1994;40:55.

152. Ohnuma N, Takahashi H, Tanabe M, et al. Endoscopic retrograde cholangiopancreatography (ERCP) in biliary tract disease of infants less than one year old. Tohoku J Exp Med 1997;181:67–74.

153. Pfau PR, Chelimsky GG, Kinnard MF, et al. Endoscopic retrograde cholangiopancreatography in children and adolescents. J Pediatr Gastroenterol Nutr 2002;35:619–23.

CHAPTER 68

LIVER BIOPSY INTERPRETATION

A. S. Knisely, MD

Diagnosis in a liver biopsy specimen resembles diagnosis in a patient. The specimen, or the patient, is interrogated using a standard set of questions, or histochemical techniques. An inventory is made of the findings, or the responses, that differ from expected norms. Both the histopathologist and the clinician conclude their data-taking with a synthesis, an attempt to identify a diagnosis that accounts for any abnormalities recognized. Both the clinician and the histopathologist continue their inquiries when they believe that a better diagnosis is yet to be achieved.

Two points are particularly important in interpreting liver biopsy findings. First, the histopathologist must not work in isolation. Help from clinical colleagues is essential if the histopathologist is best to serve the patient. Second, the histopathologist must not lose information. For that as well, teamwork is essential.

This chapter outlines how to ensure, between the clinician and the histopathologist, that information is not lost as a liver biopsy specimen is obtained and processed. It lists a set of studies likely to permit a first-line diagnosis, while permitting referral, if necessary, of biopsy material in consultation, and gives examples of how each study can prove useful. The question of when biopsy is in order is raised. The chapter ends by discussing several clinical settings frequently encountered in pediatric patients in which biopsy may prove useful, as well as what biopsy may find. It does not pretend, however, to match the comprehensive accounts of liver biopsy interpretation[1] and the pathology of the liver[2] available elsewhere, to which the reader is referred.

MATTERS TO BE SETTLED BEFORE THE BIOPSY PROCEDURE

Much more can now be won from a sample of liver tissue than only morphologic data. For many, even most, purposes, formalin fixation is adequate. But genetic or proteomic information specific to the liver, such as how genomic deoxyribonucleic acid (DNA) is processed into messenger ribonucleic acid (RNA) and beyond, is lost when liver is not snap-frozen immediately on biopsy.

Formalin-fixed liver can be used only for routine microscopy and for a limited range of immunohistochemical and in situ hybridization studies. Snap-frozen liver can be used for quantitative analysis of constituents, microbiologic evaluation, molecular diagnosis, transmission electron microscopy (after thawing in proper fixative), or specialized immunohistochemical studies. It can also be used for all of the studies possible with routinely formalin-fixed liver (again, after thawing in proper fixative). A 2 cm core biopsy specimen provides ample tissue for routine processing and for freezing.

In all but rare settings, liver biopsy is an elective procedure. Referral units that specialize in liver disease routinely ensure that a Dewar flask of liquid nitrogen is brought to the bedside, the ultrasonography suite, or the operating room to receive and to snap-freeze a sample of liver as soon as it is obtained. The tissue can be placed in an embedding compound within a mold, placed inside a vial or capsule, or (perhaps giving easiest access) laid on a labeled piece of aluminum foil, which is then folded to yield a packet. For reasons presented above, immediate snap-freezing of liver tissue must be regarded as the standard of optimal care.

Pediatric gastroenterology and hepatology services have recently extended outside predominantly academic hospitals as specialty trainees take up careers in the wider community. Appropriate support from histopathology services (snap-freezing; storage and shipment at –80°C) should be in place before pediatric liver biopsy is undertaken. If liver biopsy is contemplated where snap-freezing is not available, the possible need for rebiopsy, with attendant risk, must be balanced against any inconvenience of patient transfer to a venue where liver biopsy tissue can be correctly preserved.

HANDLING THE BIOPSY CORE

A biopsy specimen intended for routine histopathologic study should be immersed in formalin as soon as it is obtained. Contact with saline solution or wicking away of fluids into a towel or gauze produces a variety of artifacts and alters immunohistochemical reactivity. Tissue should be processed in mesh cassettes rather than on biopsy sponges, which distort anatomic relationships.

Biopsy specimens often are presented to the histopathologist as "ribbons," with large numbers of sections closely packed on a single slide. Liver biopsy specimens should be handled differently, with a ribbon divided into individual, serial sections, each mounted on the proper sequentially numbered slide. Even after trimming the block, 12 pairs of such sections at 4 μ or 5 μ extend only some 200 μ into the biopsy core (1,000 μ thick before fixation and dehydration), conserving tissue against future work. At the Institute of Liver Studies, our practice is that alternate pairs are held on slides as unstained sections, early and late pairs are stained with hematoxylin and eosin (HE), and pairs in the bracketed interval are stained with diastase and periodic acid–Schiff (DPAS) technique, for iron, with orcein, and for reticulin. Abnormalities can be tracked through the core; lesions such as granulomata can be further evaluated where they occur, and with unstained sections on hand, a delay in additional studies is minimal.

Regulators in different venues require retention of glass slides and tissue blocks for different times. The pediatric gastroenterologist or hepatologist working in a facility with care of adults as its primary concern may wish to ensure that pediatric materials are held longer than the minimum time prescribed or even indefinitely.

THE NORMAL LIVER: A REFRESHER

Blood enters the liver at its hilum, through the portal vein and hepatic artery. It passes from portal tracts (Figure 68-1A) along the sinusoids within the lobule into centrilobular venules (Figure 68-1B) and leaves the liver for the inferior vena cava via the hepatic veins. The line of junction and demarcation between portal tract and lobule is known as the limiting plate. Hepatocytes extract various substances from the plasma that bathes their sides and bases. They return others to it; blood passing over hepatocytes is sequentially modified from the portal tract to the centrilobular venule.

Hepatocytes are disposed between sinusoids in cords one cell thick. Their dimensions are similar throughout the lobule. Although they exhibit zonal differences in function, on light microscopy they tend to look alike. They are

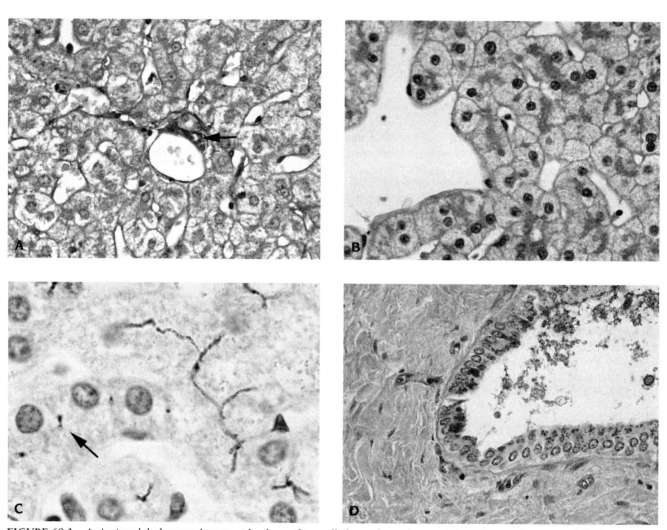

FIGURE 68-1 *A,* An interlobular portal tract, with a large, thin-walled portal venule containing a few erythrocytes; a bile duct circumscribed by basement membrane and lined by cholangiocytes (two nuclei are visible); and a small, thick-walled arteriole (*arrow*). Normal liver. Diastase and periodic acid–Schiff technique with hematoxylin counterstain (DPAS); ×400 original magnification. *B,* A centrilobular venule, with sinusoids and hepatocyte cords of the adjacent lobule. Some of the cords are two cells thick. Lysosomes, whose contents tend to mark with eosin, are clustered at the hepatocytes' canalicular poles. Normal liver (hematoxylin and eosin; ×400 original magnification). *C,* Canaliculi in transverse (*arrow*) and longitudinal section. A hepatocyte may contribute to several canaliculi, as shown. Normal liver. Hematoxylin and antibody against canalicular multispecific organic anion transporter (immunoperoxidase technique); ×1,000 original magnification. *D,* Droplets of mucin are found within columnar cholangiocytes of a septal bile duct, and scant mucus is seen in the ductal lumen. Normal liver (DPAS; ×400 original magnification).

cuboidal or polygonal and uniform in size. They have one or two nuclei, which are generally round in profile and may contain a chromocenter. Hepatocytes may be euploid or polyploid. Their cytoplasm is finely granular and uniform, although pigment may be seen at the aspect most remote from the sinusoid, the canalicular pole.

Portions of two or three hepatocytes may meet at the canaliculus, which is separated by tight junctions from the basolateral aspects of the hepatocytes that form it (Figure 68-1C). An individual hepatocyte participates in forming several canaliculi. Hepatocytes secrete various substances across the canalicular membrane into the bile. This travels from canaliculi into interlobular bile ducts, then into trabecular or septal bile ducts, and finally into segmental or lobar ducts, moving into the hilum in the direction opposite to that taken by the blood. The cholangiocytes of interlobular bile ducts are cuboidal and serous (see Figure 68-1A). Those of larger bile ducts are columnar and mucinous (Figure 68-1D). Large ducts toward the hilum also gradually acquire a mural secretory gland apparatus. Bile passing down canaliculi and ducts is sequentially modified in its transit, and bile at its exit from the liver is a very different fluid from bile within the canaliculus.

Endothelial cells with one set of characteristics line vessels within portal tracts and centrilobular venules. Those that line the sinusoids have different characteristics; they are discontinuous or fenestrated, allowing hepatocytes direct access to plasma. Within the sinusoids are the macrophages known as Kupffer cells. Nerves accompany vessels into the hilum; they enter the lobule in the space of Disse, which lies between sinusoidal basement membrane and hepatocellular basolateral membrane. This space also contains stellate cells, which are contractile and fibrogenic and which store vitamin A. Small numbers of leukocytes, principally small lymphocytes and macrophages, are normally found in portal tracts.

Liver biopsy relies on the axiom that parenchymal disease uniformly involves lobules throughout the liver. This is not true, but as an approximation, it is true enough to be useful. One should bear in mind, however, that neither percutaneous nor transvenous liver biopsy will routinely sample central or hilar structures. Processes that affect them must be studied by specifically directed biopsy.

WHAT ROUTINELY STAINED SECTIONS WILL AND WILL NOT SHOW

NUCLEIC ACIDS AND PROTEINS WITHIN NUCLEUS AND CYTOPLASM: HE

The purple-blue dye, hematoxylin, binds with electronegative substances (ie, nucleic acids or carbonates and phosphates found in mineralized tissues). It marks the DNA of nuclei and the RNA of rough endoplasmic reticulum. The orange-red dye, eosin, binds with electropositive substances (proteins). It marks much of the cytoplasm of most cells, as well as the bulk of interstitial or intercellular material. Shifts in degrees of eosinophilia or hematoxylinophilia signal various metabolic changes (eg, the move from purple-

red to orange-red, associated with loss of RNA, that indicates both maturation in erythrocytes and cell death in hepatocytes). HE-stained sections are the mainstay of histopathologic diagnosis.

GLYCOSYLATED SUBSTANCES: DPAS

Diastase digestion removes complex sugars from tissue sections; glycoproteins remain. The aldehyde moieties in these, after oxidation with periodic acid, take up the fuchsin chromophore in Schiff reagent and become magenta. Proteins not coupled with sugars are marked only very palely. DPAS-stained sections, with a hematoxylin (nuclear) counterstain, demonstrate cell outlines and basement membranes excellently. These stand out all the more because the hemoglobin of erythrocytes, which sometimes can obscure tissue details, effectively does not mark. Collections of glycoprotein within cytoplasm (mucin [see Figure 68-1D], the phagocytosed material within Kupffer cells, secondary lysosomes in hepatocytes, and some, but not all, materials accumulated in storage disorders [Figure 68-2A]) also stand out. DPAS staining is valuable in identifying residua of some structures; basement membranes of bile ducts can persist after cholangiocytes are gone. It also permits screening for fungal forms, whose cell walls take the stain.

IRON: PRUSSIAN BLUE REACTION

Acid pretreatment converts iron complexed as ferritin (or, after partial digestion within lysosomes, as hemosiderin) to its ferric form, which reacts with potassium ferrocyanide to yield bright, crisp Prussian blue. A counterstain such as nuclear fast red is often used to make it easier to identify where in the tissue stainable iron lies (Figure 68-2B). To demonstrate iron may have prognostic implications, as in hepatitis C virus infection, or permit diagnosis of a metabolic disorder, as in hemochromatosis. Because hepatocytes and Kupffer cells or macrophages may contain granular brown material other than hemosiderin (Dubin-Johnson pigment, lipofuscin, malarial pigment), to demonstrate that particular deposits do not contain iron also can be useful.

MATERIALS RICH IN SULFHYDRYLS: ORCEIN

The purple-black dyestuff, orcein, originally extracted from lichen, complexes with sulfhydryl groups. These abound in elastin (Figure 68-3A), in the surface antigen of hepatitis B virus (Figure 68-3, B and C), and in metallothioneins (see Figure 68-3A). Synthesis of metallothioneins is induced by cytosolic accumulation of several transition metals; the most clinically important is copper. Subclinical cholestasis, without hyperbilirubinemia, is associated with impaired excretion of copper into bile. Metallothioneins bind copper and sequester it within the cytosol. Over time, they accumulate in partly degenerated form in secondary lysosomes—"cuprisomes."[3] These are particularly prominent in periportal hepatocytes. Orcein staining highlights vessels by picking out elastic tissue within their walls. It shows (when elastic tissue is present) that a scar has matured.[4] By demonstrating copper-associated protein,

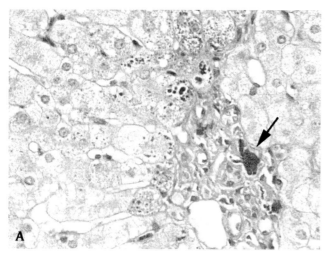 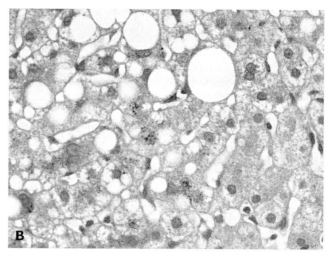

FIGURE 68-2   *A*, Granules and globules of the glycoprotein α₁-antitrypsin have accumulated within cytoplasm of periportal hepato-cytes. Portal tract macrophages (*arrow*) contain lipofuscin pigment; the two substances stain alike. α₁-Antitrypsin storage disorder (dias-tase and periodic acid–Schiff; ×400 original magnification). *B*, Finely granular dark reaction product marks hemosiderin, principally within lysosomes (note a tendency toward pericanalicular accumulation). The large and small optically clear vacuoles represent the lacunae left after elution of neutral lipid during specimen processing (Perls' Prussian blue and nuclear fast red technique; ×400 origi-nal magnification).

orcein staining can support an impression, garnered from HE-stained sections, that a cholangiopathy is present even when bilirubinostasis is not apparent, or that cholestasis is likely of long standing.

Type III Collagen: Reticulin

Abnormalities in the architecture of the liver, including the sometimes subtle changes of shrinkage or swelling of hepa-tocytes associated with perturbed vascular supply, are eas-ily assessed in sections stained for basement membrane collagen ("reticulin," in which collagen type III predomi-nates[5,6]) using a silver impregnation technique. Parenchy-mal loss with stromal collapse is marked by apposition of reticulin fibers (Figure 68-4A). Hyperplasia of hepatocytes (broadened hepatocyte cords that are two cells rather than one cell thick) is marked by splaying apart of reticulin fibers (Figure 68-4B). Hepatocellular malignancy is marked by a deficiency of reticulin fibers. The fibrosis owing to inflammation or injury is generally accompanied by an increase in reticulin within the fibrous tissue. Assess-ment of the extent of fibrosis is an important aspect of biopsy diagnosis.

Substances Lost in Processing

The formaldehyde in formalin (an aqueous solution of formaldehyde) stabilizes tissues, as a fixative, by cross-linking them. Formaldehyde cross-links proteins and nucleic acids more efficiently than it cross-links neutral lipids or simple sugars. As a liver biopsy specimen moves from formalin through alcohol into xylene and on to paraffin, the tissue is brought into contact with polar and nonpolar solvents. Most stains are applied in aqueous solution, so to permit staining, sections mounted on slides are again passed through xylene and then through alcohol into water. Once sections are stained, because coverslips are secured with adhesives dissolved in non-

polar media, the sections are exposed to alcohol and then again to xylene. Water, alcohol, and xylene leach many small molecules, such as sugars or bilirubin, and neutral lipid from the tissue (see Figures 68-2B and 68-5, A and B). These then cannot be stained, and statements that they ever were present rely on inference.

If such substances must be specifically demonstrated, fixation in absolute alcohol or other selected substances rather than in formalin can lessen tissue exposure to polar solvents and can partly conserve small molecules through subsequent handling. Postfixation in osmium tetroxide (osmication) after initial exposure to formalin can cross-link and stabilize neutral lipid against elution, permitting routine processing into paraffin thereafter. Osmication affords histologic detail superior to that available in sec-tions of frozen tissue (from which lipid is not lost) that are stained with oil red O or Sudan black.

PITFALLS OF ONTOGENY

Postnatal patterns of hepatocellular and bile duct growth in prematurely born infants may differ from those in infants born at term.[7] Standards for the former are not well defined. Caution in interpreting biopsy findings is in order.

The liver is the principal site of fetal hematopoiesis, which can persist into the first postnatal weeks. Foci of erythropoiesis in the lobule and of granulopoiesis in portal tracts should not be confused with inflammation in biopsy specimens from neonates.

Copper-associated protein is normally present in the first several tiers of periportal hepatocytes of infants born at term; it may persist for several weeks or months. The same is true for hemosiderin, which may extend into mid-zonal or even centrilobular hepatocytes. To see either, which would mark disease in older children, can be disre-garded in early infancy.

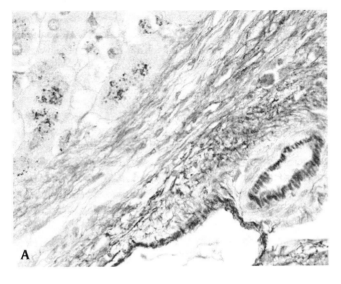

FIGURE 68-3 *A*, Granular dark material, upper left, within hepatocytes represents copper-associated protein. The corrugated, dense elastic lamina of a portal tract artery and individual elastic fibrils within looser portal tract connective tissue also mark. Familial intrahepatic cholestasis 1 at hepatectomy (orcein; ×400 original magnification). *B*, Most hepatocytes have finely granular, eosinophilic cytoplasm; that of several hepatocytes is uniformly pale (*arrows*), resembling frosted glass. A shrunken, densely eosinophilic hepatocyte at the center is undergoing cell death. Chronic hepatitis B virus infection (hematoxylin and eosin; ×400 original magnification). *C*, The cytoplasm of "ground-glass" hepatocytes like those in *B* marks when the change is due to accumulation of hepatitis B surface antigen. Chronic hepatitis B virus infection (orcein; ×400 original magnification).

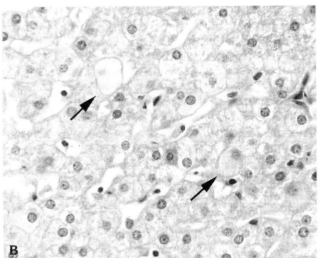

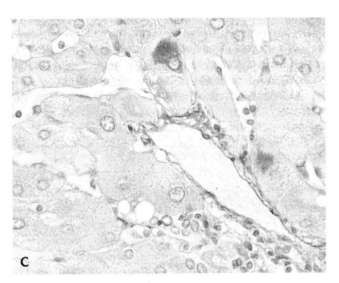

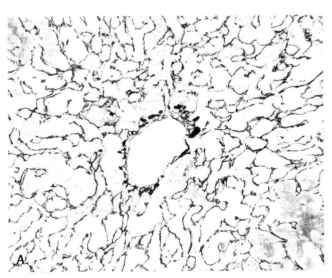

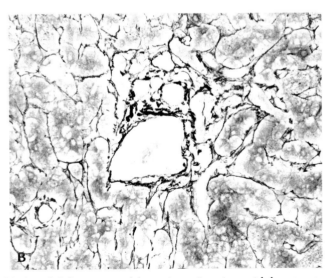

FIGURE 68-4 *A*, Silver impregnation marks reticulin fibers brown-black and defines sinusoidal margins at junctions with hepatocyte cords. They are relatively closely apposed around this centrilobular venule (reticulin; ×400 original magnification). *B*, Same patient as in *A*; acetaminophen (paracetamol) overdose with zonal hepatocyte loss. Hepatocyte cords are wider, and reticulin fibers lie farther apart, in this periportal zone than in centrilobular liver (compare with *A*). Loss of hepatocytes (*A*) and regenerative hyperplasia of hepatocytes (*B*) underlie the differences (reticulin; ×400 original magnification).

FIGURE 68-5 *A*, Accumulated glycogen within hepatocyte cytoplasm can be demonstrated histochemically. Glycogen storage disease, type I (periodic acid–Schiff technique with hematoxylin counterstain; ×200 original magnification). *B*, Diastase pretreatment of sections eliminates glycogen and, with it, histochemical reactivity (same patient as in *A*). Hepatocellular enlargement is apparent. Glycogen storage disease, type I (diastase and periodic acid–Schiff; ×200 original magnification). *C*, No particular significance inheres in slight enlargement of nuclei, with displacement of chromatin to the periphery by accumulated glycogen, as seen here in periportal hepatocytes (hematoxylin and eosin; ×400 original magnification).

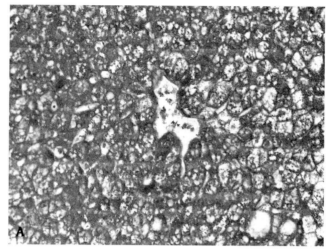
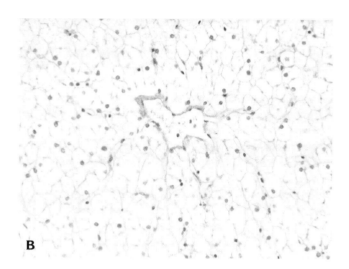
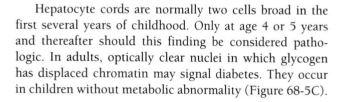
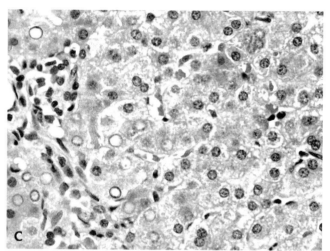

Hepatocyte cords are normally two cells broad in the first several years of childhood. Only at age 4 or 5 years and thereafter should this finding be considered pathologic. In adults, optically clear nuclei in which glycogen has displaced chromatin may signal diabetes. They occur in children without metabolic abnormality (Figure 68-5C).

WHEN IS LIVER BIOPSY IN ORDER?

Leaving aside masses within the liver, most of which continue to require direct examination of tissue for definitive diagnosis, advances in microbiology, clinical biochemistry, clinical immunology, imaging studies, and molecular genetics have made the morphologic study of the liver less and less necessary. This is as it should be; liver biopsy is invasive and carries a small but real risk to the patient.

Specialized metabolic or molecular analysis techniques may be accessible, however, at several centers worldwide at most, with no guarantee that clinically useful results ever will be supplied. Even routinely conducted assays may be seldom done, with uncomfortable delays in receiving results. The techniques used in biopsy diagnosis, in contrast, are very widely employed, with (possibly nondefinitive) results available in only a few hours. Historical experience with evaluation of disease in liver biopsy materials also is extensive.

In addition, even if noninvasive studies strongly suggest a particular diagnosis, how badly a particular disease has damaged the liver often can be determined only at biopsy. This information can be useful in assessing prognosis or, with follow-up biopsy, in evaluating response to therapy.

Biopsy is thus generally used at present to aid in selecting among a small number of likely diagnoses and to guide further work, to corroborate a provisional diagnosis already arrived at on clinical grounds, and to determine the extent of the disease or, over time, the progress of the disease. Satisfactory interpretation often depends on understanding what questions a particular biopsy is hoped to answer.

FREQUENTLY ENCOUNTERED CLINICAL SETTINGS

CONJUGATED HYPERBILIRUBINEMIA IN INFANCY
Inflammation of the extrahepatic biliary tract with perinatal onset may lead to fibrosis that occludes or obliterates the lumen of the common bile duct (extrahepatic biliary atresia [EHBA]). This process may involve the gallbladder. EHBA is manifest as conjugated hyperbilirubinemia with elevated serum concentrations of γ-glutamyl transpeptidase (GGT) activity (high-GGT cholestasis). EHBA can be palliated by hepatic portoenterostomy. The results of such

surgery are better the earlier it is performed. When imaging study results (failure to identify a normal gallbladder on ultrasonography; in some centers, failure to opacify the biliary tract on percutaneous or endoscopic cholangiography) are ambiguous, the histopathologist thus may be asked to identify changes in the liver that suggest distal biliary tract obstruction.

These changes include edema of portal tracts, fibrosis of portal tracts, an increase in the number of bile duct profiles seen, and the presence of bile plugs in the lumina of principal bile ducts, that is, of bile ducts within portal tracts rather than of recruited ductules at portal tract margins (Figure 68-6). The cholangiocytes of bile duct epithelium are irregularly arrayed, and intraepithelial leukocytes may be found, but this is the nonspecific case in any cholangiopathy. Granulocytes may be seen in portal tracts, but this also is nonspecific and may reflect not inflammation but the postnatal persistence of hematopoiesis. The lobular changes of "neonatal hepatitis" (edema of hepatocytes, with giant cell change and intrahepatocytic bile pigment; rosetting of hepatocytes around dilated canalicular lumina that contain bile plugs; necrosis of occasional hepatocytes; and clusters of hematopoietic elements, usually erythroid [Figure 68-7, A and B]) may be minimal or quite pronounced. Their extent cannot be used definitively to exclude EHBA: florid "neonatal hepatitis" and EHBA may coexist.[8]

High-GGT cholestasis can reflect, beside EHBA, syndromic and nonsyndromic paucity of interlobular bile ducts (PIB); α_1-antitrypsin (A1AT) storage disorder (A1ATSD); neonatal sclerosing cholangitis (NSC); mutation in *ABCB4*, which encodes multiple drug resistance 3 (MDR3), a "flippase" that shifts phospholipid from inner leaflet to outer leaflet of the canalicular membrane (MDR3 disease)[9]; and a long list of rarer entities, as well as infective disorders or defects in intermediary metabolism. These infective dis-

orders or defects in intermediary metabolism are generally identified by microbiologic studies, serologic work, or screening of urine and serum for unusual substances. High-GGT cholestasis also can accompany the nonspecific and highly unsatisfactory diagnosis of "neonatal hepatitis" (see above). Intralobular cholestasis and steatosis tend to mark defects of intermediary metabolism, and the latter is not a feature of EHBA. "Neonatal hepatitis" lacks the portal tract changes of EHBA (see Figure 68-7B).

PIB, A1ATSD, NSC, and MDR3 disease may pass through a phase of bile duct proliferation, with evident injury to cholangiocytes. Features that reliably permit the diagnosis of NSC on histopathologic examination have not yet been identified. NSC must be considered a diagnosis made on cholangiography.[10] MDR3 disease also has no well-defined, specific histopathologic features. To demonstrate a lack of phospholipid in bile, or to identify mutation in *ABCB4*, is necessary for diagnosis.[9]

In only A1ATSD, however, do the degree of portal tract edema and the extent of bile duct proliferation, with bile plugging, sometimes mimic those found in EHBA. Fine granules of A1AT that mark in DPAS-stained sections may be seen in periportal hepatocytes of infants several months old. In infants approximately 6 to 10 weeks old, when the urgency in diagnosing features of distal biliary tract obstruction is greatest, bile pigment and secondary lysosomes, which physiologically contain hemosiderin and metallothioneins, are easily confused on DPAS staining with the minimal quantities of stored A1AT that may be present at that age in A1ATSD. An inconstant but useful feature of A1ATSD is steatosis of periportal hepatocytes.[11] Its presence can shift EHBA down the differential diagnosis rank table.

Issues of definition tend to confound discussions of PIB. The criteria for assigning the diagnosis depend classically on finding fewer than five bile duct profiles in six interlobular portal tracts.[12,13] These criteria, however, were

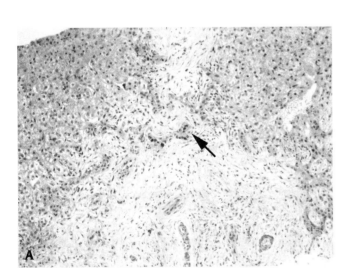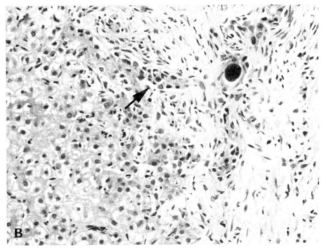

FIGURE 68-6 *A,* In distal biliary tract obstruction, a portal tract is expanded by loose, pale fibrous tissue, suggesting edema. Bile plugs are present in centrally located duct lumina (*arrow*). Extrahepatic biliary atresia (EHBA); biopsy at presentation (hematoxylin and eosin (HE); ×100 original magnification). *B,* Hepatocytes at the limiting plate have adopted a cholangiolar phenotype (the ductular reaction), and bile plugs are seen both in principal bile ducts and a newly recruited ductule (*arrow*). Hepatocyte disarray is generally slight in distal biliary tract obstruction, as seen here, but brisk giant cell change and necrosis also may be found. EHBA; biopsy at presentation (HE; ×200 original magnification).

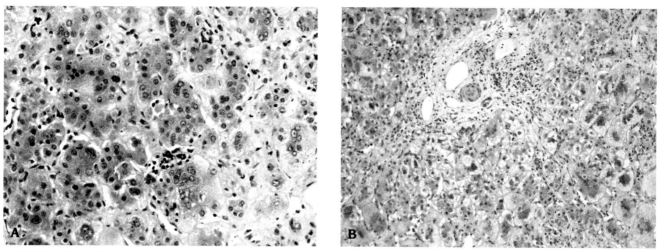

FIGURE 68-7   *A*, Typical "neonatal hepatitis" includes giant cell change and edema, with bile pigment in hepatocytes and canaliculi, as well as lobular hematopoiesis (*arrow*). Compare with *B*, in which such changes are lacking. Biopsy at presentation. Hematoxylin and eosin [HE]; ×200 original magnification. *B*, Portal tracts in usual "neonatal hepatitis" are compact, with, at most, slight ductular reaction. Cholestasis is restricted to the lobule. Compare with *A*, in which the portal tract is expanded and contains bile plugs. Biopsy at presentation (HE; ×100 original magnification).

set before the development of immunohistochemical techniques for marking bile ducts, so that strict use requires examination of HE- or DPAS-stained sections only. Finding six interlobular portal tracts seen in full cross-section can itself be difficult in slender, short needle biopsy specimens of liver. Inflammation or hematopoiesis that blurs structural detail makes identifying bile ducts harder. Personal experience suggests that immunostaining for bile duct cytokeratins often picks out bile ducts that cannot be discerned in routinely stained sections (Figure 68-8A).

Bile ducts identifiable only on immunostaining, however, generally are threadlike, with as few as one or two cholangiocytes seen (Figure 68-8B). They appear hypoplastic—a hypoplasia to be distinguished from hypoplasia of the intrahepatic biliary tree, as PIB is some-

times termed. This appearance is frequent in the setting of intralobular cholestasis, perhaps because stimuli to normal development are lacking when hepatocellular bile secretion lags. But hypoplasia of a bile duct is distinct from absence of a bile duct; hypoplastic ducts may grow and cholestasis resolve. To diagnose PIB, because of its potentially adverse prognosis, seems to require that even minute ducts be absent from more than one of six interlobular portal tracts. Whoever interprets the findings on microscopy when PIB is at issue would be prudent to specify in any report what criteria and techniques were used.

The distal biliary tract is not generally malformed in infants with either syndromic or nonsyndromic PIB. Larger bile ducts are not identifiably lacking. Peripheral larger bile ducts began as interlobular ducts and with growth were

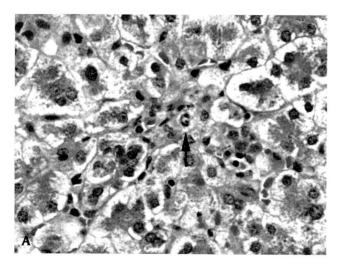
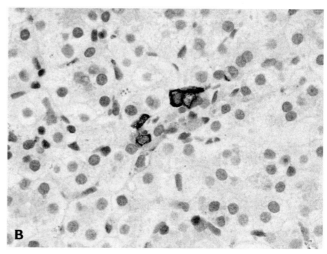

FIGURE 68-8   *A*, An interlobular portal tract in an infant with conjugated hyperbilirubinemia; compare with Figure 68-1A. An arrow indicates the hepatic arteriole. No bile duct can be discerned. Suspected paucity of interlobular bile ducts. Hematoxylin and eosin; ×400 original magnification. *B*, The same portal tract (compare with *A*), several micra distant, proves on immunohistochemical study to contain cells that express cytokeratin 19, which is usually found in cholangiocytes (hematoxylin and antibody against cytokeratin 19 [immunoperoxidase technique]; ×400 original magnification).

remodeled into trabecular or septal ducts. This suggests that bile duct morphogenesis in utero is unremarkable in such infants. Perinatal shifts in bile secretion, with alterations in bile composition,[14] may underlie perinatal development of a cholangiopathy. Septal and interlobular cholangiocytes differ in form (see Figure 68-1). Susceptibility to injury by more caustic bile may also differ between trabecular or septal ducts and interlobular ducts (the smallest, most recently formed, most peripheral ducts).

As mentioned, injured bile ducts may proliferate before they are lost. In EHBA, a vigorous increase in the number of bile ducts is initially the rule, but after several years, end-stage liver disease is characterized by bile duct disappearance.[15] This is generally ascribed to bile duct injury by bile. Such injury seems markedly accelerated in some instances of PIB. Of note is that newly laid down liver in early infancy is at the periphery of both the biliary tree and the liver itself and that newly formed interlobular ducts can be expected to predominate there. In addition, the right lobe of the infant liver grows more briskly after birth than does the left lobe.[16] Routine percutaneous biopsy is most likely to sample liver beneath the capsule in the right lobe, the youngest region. The pace of liver growth slows in later infancy, however (liver weight 75 g at term birth, 150 g at 3 months, 300 g at 1 year[17]). Follow-up biopsy, after duct loss has come to predominate over duct neogenesis, may be useful in assessing whether PIB is present. Histopathologic study cannot distinguish between syndromic PIB (associated with JAG1 mutation[18]) and nonsyndromic PIB.

Some instances of conjugated hyperbilirubinemia in infancy are marked by a failure of GGT activity to rise. This may be due to severe hepatocellular injury, in which case, low GGT is nonspecific.[19] It may be due to any number of heritable disorders of synthesis of bile acids or their precursor molecules.[20-22] In such a setting, low GGT is likely due to an absence from bile of the bile acids that usually elute canalicular membrane GGT into bile, whence it can reflux into plasma. Finally, it may be due to one of several heritable disorders (arthrogryposis-renal dysfunction-cholestasis syndrome [ARC][23]; mutation in ATP8B1, which encodes familial intrahepatic cholestasis 1 [FIC1], a protein of undefined function[24]; or mutation in ABCB11, which encodes bile salt export protein [BSEP], the pump that transports bile salts from hepatocytes into bile).[25]

The etiology of ARC is not clear; it seems, however, that deficient expression of GGT at the canaliculus may underlie the failure of GGT activity to rise.[26] The same appears true for FIC1 disease.[27] With BSEP disease, although GGT is normally expressed, a lack of bile acids within bile—as with primary disorders of bile acid synthesis—may be responsible for failure to elute GGT and, accordingly, for the failure of GGT activity to rise.[27] The renal, neuromuscular, and skeletal manifestations of ARC permit its distinction from FIC1 disease and BSEP disease. FIC1 disease and BSEP disease, however, may be difficult to differentiate from one another. Changes of cholate stasis, with hepatocellular injury generally ascribed to retained bile acids, are usually less pronounced in FIC1 disease than in BSEP disease. The former tends to manifest

as bland intracanalicular cholestasis (Figure 68-9A) and the latter as giant cell hepatitis (Figure 68-9B). Transmission electron microscopy in FIC1 disease tends to find loose, coarsely granular bile within canaliculi (Figure 68-9C), which is not usually the case in BSEP disease (Figure 68-9D).[28,29] Criteria for histopathologic diagnosis of these two recently distinguished disorders are under study.

PREDOMINANTLY HEPATOCELLULAR INJURY (TRANSAMINITIS) IN CHILDHOOD

Damage to hepatocytes and damage to the biliary tract overlap, but two patterns of clinical biochemistry findings can be broadly defined. The first, which is more usual when damage to hepatocytes predominates, is characterized most prominently by elevations in serum concentrations of transaminase activities (the hepatitic pattern). The second, which is more usual when damage to the biliary tract predominates, is characterized most prominently by elevations in serum concentrations of bilirubin and of alkaline phosphatase and GGT activities (the cholestatic pattern). These two patterns also overlap: injury to hepatocytes induces cholestasis, and cholestasis leads to injury to hepatocytes.

On liver biopsy in patients whose clinical biochemistry test results fit the hepatitic pattern, increased numbers of leukocytes are found in portal tracts and in the lobule. Regardless of the speed of clinical onset of disease, whether slow (chronic) or abrupt (acute), most of the leukocytes are the mononuclear forms (lymphocytes, macrophages, and plasma cells) that, rather than granulocytes, characterize chronic inflammation elsewhere in the body. Acute hepatitis and chronic hepatitis are thus differentiated from one another by criteria other than the composition of the inflammatory infiltrate found.

In acute hepatitis, inflammation is predominantly within the lobule; in chronic hepatitis, it is within the portal tracts. Hepatocellular injury is more pronounced in acute hepatitis than in chronic hepatitis, with edema, necrosis of individual hepatocytes (Figure 68-10A), and both hepatocellular and canalicular cholestasis (Figure 68-10B). Macrophages enlarge and become more numerous; their cytoplasm contains ingested debris (see Figure 68-10B). Loss of hepatocytes may be associated with approximation of reticulin fibers to one another (stromal collapse, bridging) (Figure 68-10C). Acute hepatitis may be due to viral infection, toxin or drug ingestion, or autoimmune disease. It may resolve entirely, be so severe that liver transplant is necessary for survival, or evolve into a chronic hepatitis, with varying degrees of scarring and persistent inflammation.

In chronic hepatitis, the extent of inflammation and of injury to hepatocytes is assessed under the general heading of "necroinflammatory activity." Points considered are the distribution of inflammation and the extent of injury to hepatocytes. When inflammation is not restricted to the portal tracts but spills across the limiting plate into the lobule (Figure 68-11), interface hepatitis is present. The proportions of portal tracts involved by interface hepatitis, the extent of their circumference at which the limiting plate is blurred or effaced, and the depth and intensity to which

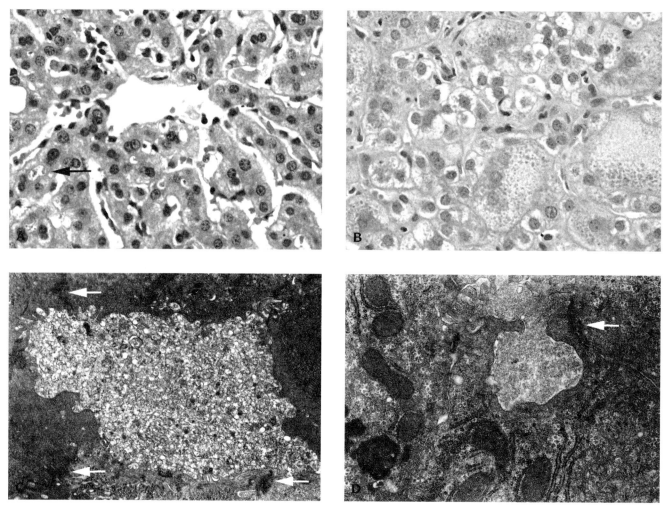

FIGURE 68-9   *A,* Small hepatocytes, varying only slightly in size, with compact cytoplasm border canaliculi containing bile plugs (*arrow*). Kupffer cells also contain bile pigment, but cholestasis within hepatocytes is not apparent. Familial intrahepatic cholestasis 1 (FIC1) disease (hematoxylin and eosin [HE]; ×400 original magnification). *B,* Giant cell change, with bile pigment in cytoplasm, is seen. Edema and variation in hepatocyte size are usual. Bile salt export protein (BSEP) disease (HE; ×400 original magnification). *C,* Circular profiles suggesting coarse granularity occupy the lumen of a canaliculus (tight junctions, *arrows*). FIC1 disease (osmium tetroxide, uranyl acetate, and lead citrate; ×16,500 original magnification). *D,* A canaliculus (tight junction, *arrow*) contains amorphous bile. Microvilli are lacking. BSEP disease (osmium tetroxide, uranyl acetate, and lead citrate; ×20,750 original magnification).

inflammation incurs into the lobule are evaluated. Changes in the appearance of hepatocytes, as listed for acute hepatitis (above), also are weighed. This assessment of injury at the moment of biopsy is called "grading." The damage to the liver caused by hepatitis is manifest as parenchymal loss, scarring, and parenchymal regeneration. If the insult to the liver is not eliminated, cirrhosis ensues. Evaluation of how far along the path to cirrhosis this damage has progressed is called "staging."

Several systems have been developed for numeric grading of the severity of chronic hepatitis and for staging associated scarring.[30–32] They are most useful when comparing instances of a particular disorder with one another and can be misleading when used too rigidly. Even the worst injury owing to hepatitis C virus infection, for example, falls short of what can be found in a florid autoimmune hepatitis. That, in turn, falls short of the devastation seen in non-A, non-B hepatitis with fulminant hepatic failure. Yet each of these varying degrees of necroinflammatory activity warrants designation as "severe"—of its kind.

This deficiency in across the board grading of necroinflammatory activity in chronic hepatitis has been expressly recognized for the changes seen in association with fatty change of hepatocytes (steatohepatitis), for which a specific grading system has been proposed.[33] It has been implicitly recognized in the lack of demand for numeric grading of necroinflammatory activity in neonatal hepatitis. Experience and access to clinical information that will help identify the etiology of a chronic hepatitis are needed for proper flexibility in choosing and applying a grading system for a particular biopsy specimen. Reliance on a numeric score alone is convenient, but the clinical practitioner should ensure, through discussions with colleagues in histopathology and, when possible, through review of findings on microscopy, that as little ambiguity as possible inheres in what, in the setting of a particular etiologic diagnosis, that score is meant to convey.

Morphologically defined chronic hepatitis has causes or associations that include viral infection, autoimmune

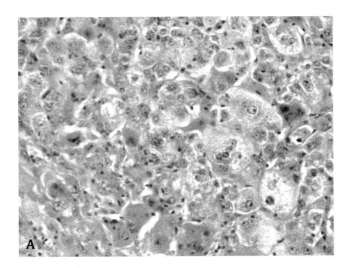

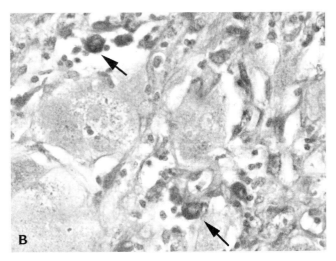

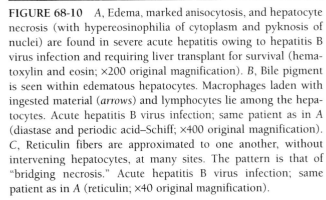

FIGURE 68-10 *A*, Edema, marked anisocytosis, and hepatocyte necrosis (with hypereosinophilia of cytoplasm and pyknosis of nuclei) are found in severe acute hepatitis owing to hepatitis B virus infection and requiring liver transplant for survival (hematoxylin and eosin; ×200 original magnification). *B*, Bile pigment is seen within edematous hepatocytes. Macrophages laden with ingested material (*arrows*) and lymphocytes lie among the hepatocytes. Acute hepatitis B virus infection; same patient as in *A* (diastase and periodic acid–Schiff; ×400 original magnification). *C*, Reticulin fibers are approximated to one another, without intervening hepatocytes, at many sites. The pattern is that of "bridging necrosis." Acute hepatitis B virus infection; same patient as in *A* (reticulin; ×40 original magnification).

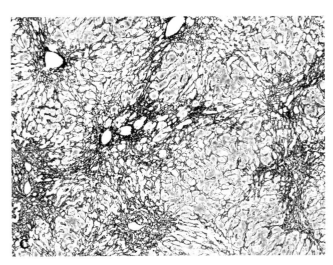

disease, toxin exposure, Wilson disease, and fatty change. A wide variety of viruses can infect the liver, with hepatitis B virus and hepatitis C virus being the most frequently encountered at biopsy. Serologic and molecular-biologic studies generally provide diagnosis; as discussed above, biopsy is used to evaluate the extent of injury and for clues to prognosis. Hepatitis B virus infection may be manifest as "ground-glass" inclusions in hepatocyte cytoplasm (see Figure 68-3B); these mark on orcein staining (see Figure 68-3C). Hepatitis C virus infection is associated with expansion of portal tracts by lymphoid aggregates or even follicles, with germinal centers (Figure 68-12A), as well as with steatosis of hepatocytes (Figure 68-12B).

Autoimmune hepatitis is necessarily a serologically assigned diagnosis, but biopsy has a place in evaluating the severity and progression of disease.[34] Some features are more common in autoimmune hepatitis than in other forms of chronic hepatitis. These include plasma cell infiltrates that extend into the lobule (Figure 68-13A) and a tendency to centrilobular injury (Figure 68-13B). Toxin or drug ingestion may trigger an autoimmune hepatitis, and the histopathologic features of toxin- or drug-associated hepatitis overlap somewhat with those of autoimmune hepatitis. Prominence of neutrophils and eosinophils among inflammatory cells may suggest that injury is drug induced.

Wilson disease results from mutation in *ATP7B*, which encodes a hepatic copper-transporting enzyme.[35] It is effectively a pediatric disorder. Wilson disease may come to attention in the second decade with acute hepatic failure superimposed on cirrhosis or be identified earlier during the evaluation of transaminitis. In later stages of disease, copper-associated protein abounds within hepatocytes, but its distribution within the liver is patchy (Figure 68-14A). Cytosolic copper cannot readily be demonstrated histochemically. However, it may be present when cuprisomal copper is not, and to quantitate copper in liver tissue is still important in confirming a clinical diagnosis. Earlier stages are marked by steatosis of hepatocytes, a generally mild chronic hepatitis, and portal tract fibrosis, with relatively scant stainable copper (Figure 68-14B). Steatosis and hepatitis in a child thus should prompt evaluation for Wilson disease.

Steatohepatitis is characterized by steatosis of hepatocytes, portal tract fibrosis with perisinusoidal extension, centrilobular fibrosis, neutrophils within the lobule, hepatocyte ballooning with Mallory hyalin, activation of Kupffer cells, and lipogranulomata formed in response to rupture of fat-laden hepatocytes (Figure 68-15).[33] Not all of these need to be present before the diagnosis can be made. These changes are not distinguishable from those induced by ingestion of alcohol to excess. Steatohepatitis associated with obesity is increasingly reported in children.[36]

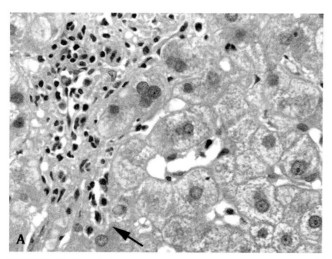 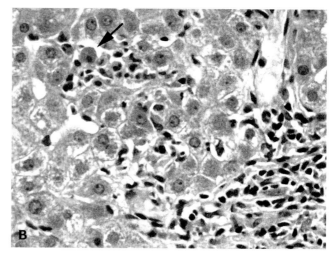

FIGURE 68-11 *A,* A portal tract contains an inflammatory infiltrate. It traverses and blurs the limiting plate, extending a short distance into the lobule. Mononuclear leukocytes are seen within hepatocytes (*arrow*). Hepatocellular anisocytosis is slight. Chronic hepatitis with mild activity; hepatitis C virus infection (hematoxylin and eosin [HE]; ×400 original magnification). *B,* A portal tract contains an inflammatory infiltrate. The present infiltrate extends more deeply into parenchyma and is more dense than that in *A.* It is associated with necrosis of a hepatocyte (*arrow*). Hepatocellular anisocytosis is pronounced. Chronic hepatitis with moderate activity; autoimmune hepatitis (HE; ×400 original magnification).

PREDOMINANTLY BILIARY TRACT INJURY (CHOLESTATIC PATTERN) IN CHILDHOOD

The changes seen in distal biliary tract obstruction (extrahepatic cholestasis), in several heritable forms of intrahepatic cholestasis, and in hepatitis with secondary cholestasis are touched on above; the changes seen in sepsis are addressed below, with other post-transplant complications. Drugs, including both endogenous and exogenous hormones, can trigger intrahepatic cholestasis that both clinically and at biopsy resembles heritable cholestasis. Such acute-onset cholestasis and its pharmacogenetics are under study. Various spectra of susceptibility to drug-induced cholestasis, with implications for prophylaxis and treatment, may at some point be defined mutationally.

Damage to large and small bile ducts in childhood may itself be a heritable condition, as in NSC[37,38] and cirhin disease (North American Indian childhood cirrhosis).[39] It may be associated with neoplasia, as in Langerhans cell histiocytosis, or with immunodeficiency and its complications.[40] More frequently encountered are the changes seen in association with inflammatory bowel disease, which are generally called primary sclerosing cholangitis. These include an obliterative atrophy of septal or trabecular ducts, which are found rarely in needle biopsy specimens, and proliferative changes in interlobular bile ducts (Figure 68-16A) proximal to sites of large duct scarring. These changes may be associated with mixed or predominantly lymphocytic inflammation and with some degree of interface hepatitis. Frank cholestasis is not generally seen,

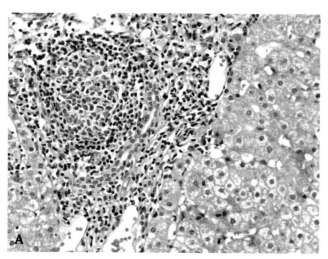 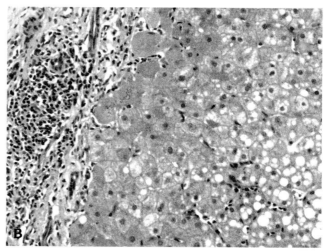

FIGURE 68-12 *A,* A germinal center lies within a portal tract. A bile duct appears draped along the germinal center's border; it is not the focus of inflammation. Slight interface activity is present. Hepatitis C virus infection (hematoxylin and eosin [HE]; ×200 original magnification). *B,* A portal tract contains a lymphoid aggregate. Slight interface activity and lobular inflammation are found. Macrovesicular steatosis of hepatocytes is seen. Hepatitis C virus infection (HE; ×200 original magnification).

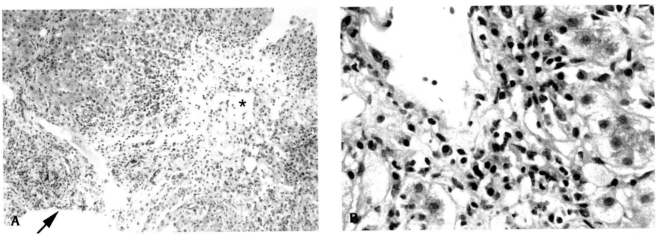

FIGURE 68-13   *A*, Brisk mononuclear leukocyte inflammation extends from the portal tract (*arrow*) to the central vein (*asterisk*), a pattern of injury leading to bridging necrosis and fibrosis. Autoimmune hepatitis (hematoxylin and eosin [HE]; ×100 original magnification). *B*, Plasma cells are conspicuous, with lymphocytes and scattered eosinophils, in a centrilobular infiltrate. Autoimmune hepatitis (HE; ×400 original magnification).

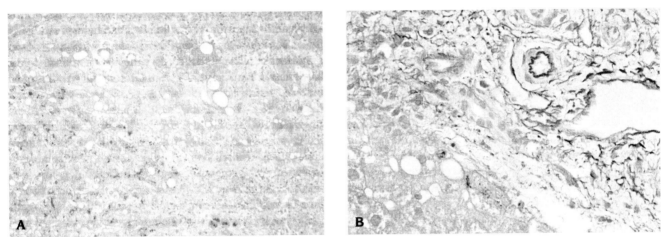

FIGURE 68-14   *A*, A nodule of hepatocytes (note the curved margin) contains substantial deposits of copper-associated protein; elsewhere in the section, none is demonstrated. Steatosis can be identified. Wilson disease at hepatectomy, age 14 years (orcein; ×100 original magnification). *B*, Small quantities of copper-associated protein are seen in hepatocytes at the limiting plate. Steatosis can be identified. Wilson disease at presentation, age 5 years (orcein; ×400 original magnification).

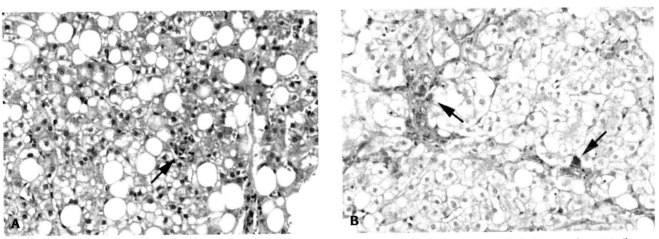

FIGURE 68-15   *A*, Nearly all hepatocytes exhibit steatosis. A small granuloma is present (*arrow*). Nonalcoholic steatohepatitis (hematoxylin and eosin; ×200 original magnification). *B*, "Turnover" pigment arising from necrosis of hepatocytes is seen in Kupffer cells and portal tract macrophages (*arrows*). Fine perisinusoidal fibrosis can be appreciated. Nonalcoholic steatohepatitis; same patient as in *A* (diastase and periodic acid–Schiff; ×200 original magnification).

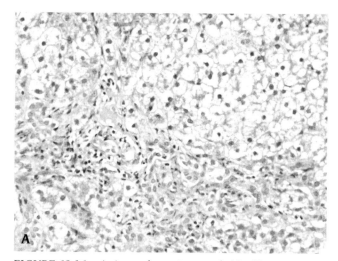
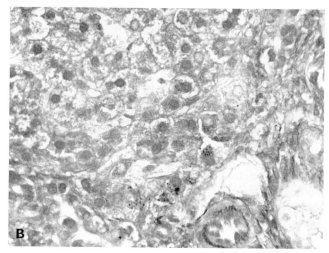

FIGURE 68-16   A, A portal tract is expanded by fibrosis and by increased numbers of bile duct profiles. Cholestasis is not seen. A scant acute and chronic pericholangitis is present. Cholangiopathy of inflammatory bowel disease (hematoxylin and eosin; ×200 original magnification). B, Copper-associated protein in small quantities is present in periportal hepatocytes. Cholangiopathy of inflammatory bowel disease; same patient as in A (orcein; ×400 original magnification).

although the hepatocellular edema of cholate stasis may be found. Copper-associated protein in periportal hepatocytes (Figure 68-16B) may mark the subclinical cholestasis of cholangiopathy and should be sought. If small duct cholangiopathy is found at biopsy and large duct cholangiopathy cannot be documented on imaging study, MDR3 disease[9] should be considered. Some patients in whom features of cholangiopathy clinically dominate features of hepatitis also have autoantibodies.[40,41] These may be considered instances of "overlap" or of an autoimmune sclerosing cholangitis. This diagnosis is made predominantly on serologic grounds.

PORTAL HYPERTENSION

Some children without apparent metabolic disorder and without clinical biochemistry evidence of hepatic injury are noted to have stigmata of portal hypertension or hepatomegaly. Evaluation of portal hypertension constitutes an indication for liver biopsy. Two conditions identified from time to time in this setting are congenital hepatic fibrosis and portal vein thrombosis. In the former, portal tracts are expanded by fibrosis and contain increased numbers of bile ducts. The profiles and locations of bile ducts are unusual. They appear dilated and often lie at the limiting plate rather than within the collagenous stroma of the portal tract (Figure 68-17A). These changes suggest persistence of a stage in fetal liver development and are one manifestation of the ductal plate malformation.[42] Portal vein branches may appear hypoplastic. Extrahepatic and intrahepatic portal vein thrombosis (hepatoportal sclerosis) sometimes follows umbilical vein catheterization, but it may have no identifiable antecedent. Portal venules of unusually small caliber (Figure 68-17B) or parenchymal atrophy, particularly of centrilobular regions, may suggest that diagnosis.[43]

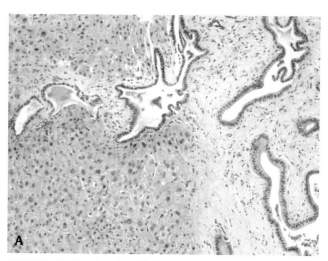
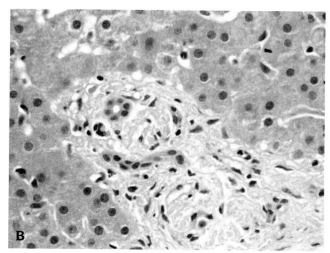

FIGURE 68-17   A, Dilated bile ducts in increased numbers are seen in and at the margins of a fibrotic portal tract. The profiles of the ducts are irregular. Congenital hepatic fibrosis (hematoxylin and eosin [HE]; ×100 original magnification). B, An interlobular portal tract lacks a portal venule of appropriate size (compare with Figure 68-1A) and exhibits slight fibrosis. History of portal vein thrombosis (HE; ×400 original magnification).

POST-TRANSPLANT COMPLICATIONS

Allograft livers are susceptible in adult and pediatric patients alike to rejection; to problems of vascular supply or drainage; to problems of biliary drainage; to infection, sometimes facilitated by immunosuppression; to involvement of the allograft by the original disorder; and to post-transplant de novo "autoimmune" hepatitis. Children who receive hepatic allografts are more likely to experience problems owing to technical aspects of surgery, to infection, and to de novo "autoimmune" hepatitis.

Rejection of allograft livers (leaving aside hyperacute rejection) takes two forms: acute and chronic. In acute rejection,[44] biopsy finds lymphocytic endotheliitis of portal and centrilobular venules, lymphocytic cholangitis, and portal tract inflammation, with lymphocytes and eosinophils (Figure 68-18A). Macrophages and neutrophils may be present as well. Centrilobular injury may extend into the parenchyma, with hepatocyte loss and hemorrhage. Intralobular cholestasis and hepatocellular edema often are seen (Figure 68-18B). Acute rejection is most frequently diagnosed on biopsy in the first weeks after liver transplant, but it can occur at any time if immunosuppression is withdrawn. Intercurrent viral infection may also precipitate acute rejection.[45] A consensus grading scheme for assessing the severity of acute rejection is available.[46] Its utility is probably greater in clinical trials than in day-to-day patient management.

Chronic rejection is characterized by loss of interlobular bile ducts and by a foam cell obliterative arteriopathy affecting larger vessels. Only bile duct injury can generally be assessed in needle biopsy specimens. Bile duct damage, with attenuation and disordered polarity of cholangiocytes (Figure 68-18C), precedes duct loss. A consensus staging scheme for assigning the diagnosis of chronic rejection is available.[47]

Global ischemic injury to the hepatic allograft may result in geographic-pattern infarction, with irregularly distributed regions of sparing and necrosis. Core needle biopsy thus cannot reliably assess the extent of injury. A late sequela of hepatic artery thrombosis can be incomplete biliary tract obstruction owing to scarring and stricture. The ductular reaction (recruitment of periportal hepatocytes to the small cholangiocyte phenotype) is found in both distal biliary tract stricture and acute rejection.[44,48] If edema of portal tracts and substantial numbers of neutrophils are particularly prominent, stricture should be considered.

Bacterial, fungal, and viral infections can damage the allograft liver. When sepsis is among the clinically considered reasons for allograft dysfunction (most commonly soon after transplant), bile plugs in the lumina of newly recruited cholangioles at the margin of the portal tract[49]

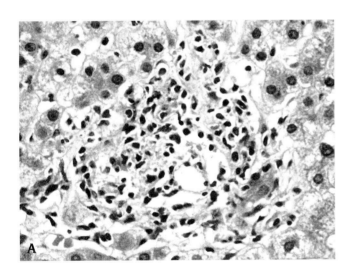

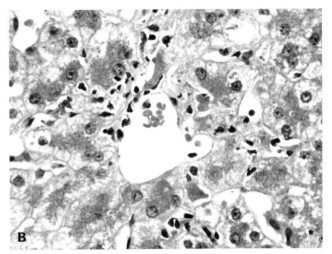

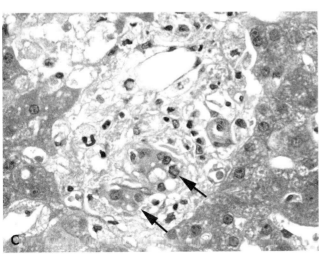

FIGURE 68-18 *A,* Mixed inflammation, with lymphocytes and occasional eosinophils, obscures the structures of an interlobular portal tract. Endotheliitis and cholangitis are apparent. Cellular rejection; adolescent noncompliance with immunosuppression after orthotopic liver transplant (hematoxylin and eosin [HE]; ×400 original magnification). *B,* Patchy centrilobular lymphocytic endotheliitis and cholestasis are present. Centrilobular inflammation is often less conspicuous than portal tract inflammation; same patient as in *A.* Cellular rejection (HE; ×400 original magnification). *C,* An interlobular portal tract is effectively free of inflammation, but cholangiocytes (*arrows*) vary in size and nuclear contour and have lost polarity (compare with Figure 68-17B). Treatment-refractory rejection; the patient went on to paucity of interlobular bile ducts and cholestatic allograft liver failure (chronic rejection) (HE; ×400 original magnification).

may support that diagnosis. Ascending cholangitis is an additional consideration, particularly when, as in EHBA, a limb of bowel has replaced the extrahepatic biliary tract. Fungal infection may complicate ischemic injury to the bile ducts, but it only very rarely involves the liver sampled by core needle biopsy.

Viral pathogens of particular note in pediatric liver transplant recipients include adenovirus, herpes simplex or varicella-zoster virus, cytomegalovirus, and Epstein-Barr virus. Adenovirus, herpes simplex, and varicella-zoster viruses produce pock-like foci of coagulative necrosis randomly distributed within the lobule; adenovirus can also directly involve the biliary tract.[50] Cytomegalovirus causes characteristic inclusions within endothelial cells, cholangiocytes, and hepatocytes, leading in the lobule to microabscess or microgranuloma formation. Epstein-Barr virus infection may lead to post-transplant lymphoproliferative disorder, more frequently so when primary infection occurs at the time of transplant or thereafter.[51] Immunosuppression predisposes the patient to development and progression of Epstein-Barr virus–associated disease. Post-transplant lymphoproliferative disorder may range from a mononucleosis-like syndrome to frank lymphoma. Features distinguishing the portal tract infiltrates of post-transplant lymphoproliferative disorder from those of acute cellular rejection include B-cell rather than T-cell predominance, immunoblastic or plasmacytoid features, and numerous—rather than occasional—cells containing Epstein-Barr virus sequences on in situ hybridization.[52,53]

Some patients who undergo liver transplant for disorders other than an autoimmune hepatitis develop allograft injury characterized by transaminitis, histopathologic findings more characteristic of autoimmune hepatitis than of either acute or chronic rejection, and circulating antinuclear or anti–smooth muscle antibodies. This pattern of disease, called de novo autoimmune hepatitis, appears more frequently in children than in adults and is not generally manifest soon after transplant.[54–56] To see a plasma cell component in an allograft liver biopsy specimen should prompt consideration of this diagnosis.

REFERENCES

1. Scheuer PJ, Lefkowitch JH. Liver biopsy interpretation. 6th ed. New York: WB Saunders; 2000.
2. MacSween RNM, Burt AD, Portmann BC, et al, editors. Pathology of the liver. 4th ed. New York: Churchill Livingstone; 2002.
3. Klein D, Lichtmannegger J, Heinzmann U, et al. Association of copper to metallothionein in hepatic lysosomes of Long-Evans cinnamon (LEC) rats during the development of hepatitis. Eur J Clin Invest 1998;28:302–10.
4. Scheuer PJ, Maggi G. Hepatic fibrosis and collapse: histological distinction by orcein staining. Histopathology 1980;4:487–9.
5. Biempica L, Morecki R, Wu CH, et al. Immunocytochemical localization of type B collagen: a component of basement membrane in human liver. Am J Pathol 1980;98:591–60.
6. Grimaud JA, Druguet M, Peyrol S, et al. Collagen immunotyping in human liver: light and electron microscope study. J Histochem Cytochem 1980;28:1145–56.
7. Kahn E, Markowitz J, Aiges H, Daum F. Human ontogeny of the bile duct to portal space ratio. Hepatology 1989;10:21–3.
8. Landing BH. Considerations of the pathogenesis of neonatal hepatitis, biliary atresia and choledochal cyst—the concept of infantile obstructive cholangiopathy. Prog Pediatr Surg 1974;6:113–39.
9. Jacquemin E, de Vree JML, Cresteil D, et al. The wide spectrum of multidrug resistance 3 deficiency: from neonatal cholestasis to cirrhosis of adulthood. Gastroenterology 2001;120:1448–58.
10. Amedée-Manesme O, Bernard O, et al. Sclerosing cholangitis with neonatal onset. J Pediatr 1987;111:225–9.
11. Amarapurkar A, Somers S, Knisely AS, Portmann BC. Steatosis of periportal hepatocytes is associated with alpha-1-antitrypsin storage disorder at presentation in infancy [abstract]. Lab Invest 2002;82:309A–10A.
12. Witzleben CL. Bile duct paucity ("intrahepatic atresia"). Perspect Pediatr Pathol 1982;7:185–201.
13. Hadchouel M. Paucity of interlobular bile ducts. Semin Diagn Pathol 1992;9:24–30.
14. Suchy FJ, Bucuvalas JC, Novak DA. Determinants of bile formation during development: ontogeny of hepatic bile acid metabolism and transport. Semin Liver Dis 1987;7:77–84.
15. Landing BH, Wells TR, Ramicone E. Time course of the intrahepatic lesion of extrahepatic biliary atresia: a morphometric study. Pediatr Pathol 1985;4:309–19.
16. Emery JL. Involution of the left liver in the newborn and its relationship to physiologic icterus. Arch Dis Child 1953;28:463–5.
17. Kayser K. Height and weight in human beings: autopsy report. Munich: Verlag für Angewandte Wissenschaften; 1987.
18. Krantz ID, Piccoli DA, Spinner NB. Clinical and molecular genetics of Alagille syndrome. Curr Opin Pediatr 1999;11:558–64.
19. Kajiwara E, Akagi K, Tsuji H, et al. Low activity of gamma-glutamyl transpeptidase in serum of acute intrahepatic cholestasis. Enzyme 1991;45:39–46.
20. Bove KE. Liver disease caused by disorders of bile acid synthesis. Clin Liver Dis 2000;4:831–48.
21. Clayton PT, Verrips A, Sistermans E, et al. Mutations in the sterol 27-hydroxylase gene (CYP27A) cause hepatitis of infancy as well as cerebrotendinous xanthomatosis. J Inherit Metab Dis 2002;25:501–13.
22. Setchell KDR, Heubi JE, Bove KE, et al. Liver disease caused by failure to racemize trihydroxycholestanoic acid: gene mutation and effect of bile acid therapy. Gastroenterology 2003;124:217–32.
23. Eastham KM, McKiernan PJ, Milford DV, et al. ARC syndrome: an expanding range of phenotypes. Arch Dis Child 2001;85:415–20.
24. Bull LN, van Eijk MJT, Pawlikowska L, et al. A gene encoding a P-type ATPase mutated in two forms of hereditary cholestasis. Nat Genet 1998;18:219–23.
25. Strautnieks SS, Bull LN, Knisely AS, et al. A gene encoding a liver-specific ABC transporter is mutated in progressive familial intrahepatic cholestasis. Nat Genet 1998;20:233–8.
26. Hanigan MH, Barbar M, Cullinane C, et al. Decreased expression of gamma-glutamyl transpeptidase at the bile canaliculus in arthrogryposis-renal dysfunction-cholestasis syndrome [abstract]. Lab Invest 2003;83:301A.
27. Hanigan MH, Bull LN, Strautnieks SS, et al. Low serum concentrations of γGT activity in progressive familial intrahepatic cholestasis: evidence for two different mechanisms in PFIC, type 1 (FIC1 disease) and in PFIC, type 2 (BSEP disease) [abstract]. Hepatology 2002;36:310A.
28. Bull LN, Carlton VEH, Stricker NL, et al. Genetic and morpho-

logic findings in progressive familial intrahepatic cholestasis (Byler disease [PFIC-1] and Byler syndrome): evidence for heterogeneity. Hepatology 1997;26:155–64.

29. Chen HL, Chang PS, Hsu HC, et al. *FIC1* and *BSEP* defects in Taiwanese patients with chronic intrahepatic cholestasis with low gamma-glutamyltranspeptidase levels. J Pediatr 2002;140:119–24.

30. Ishak K, Baptista A, Bianchi L, et al. Histological grading and staging of chronic hepatitis. J Hepatol 1995;22:696–9

31. Batts KP, Ludwig J. Chronic hepatitis: an update on terminology and reporting. Am J Surg Pathol 1995;19:1409–17.

32. Bedossa P, Poynard T. An algorithm for the grading of activity in chronic hepatitis C. Hepatology 1996;24:289–93

33. Brunt EM, Janney CG, Di Bisceglie AM, et al. Nonalcoholic steatohepatitis: a proposal for grading and staging the histological lesions. Am J Gastroenterol 1999;94:2467–74.

34. Review of criteria for diagnosis of autoimmune hepatitis. J Hepatol 1999;31:929–38.

35. Loudianos G, Gitlin JD. Wilson's disease. Semin Liver Dis 2000;20:353–64.

36. Roberts EA. Nonalcoholic steatohepatitis in children. Curr Gastroenterol Rep 2003;5:253–9.

37. Baker AJ, Portmann B, Westaby D, et al. Neonatal sclerosing cholangitis in two siblings: a category of progressive intrahepatic cholestasis. J Pediatr Gastroenterol Nutr 1993;17:317–22.

38. Baala L, Hadj-Rabia S, Hamel-Teillac D, et al. Homozygosity mapping of a locus for a novel syndromic ichthyosis to chromosome 3q27-q28. J Invest Dermatol 2002;119:70–76.

39. Chagnon P, Michaud J, Mitchell G, et al. A missense mutation (R565W) in cirhin (*FLJ14728*) in North American Indian childhood cirrhosis. Am J Hum Genet 2002;71:1443–9.

40. Mieli-Vergani G, Vergani D. Sclerosing cholangitis in the paediatric patient. Best Pract Res Clin Gastroenterol 2001;15:681–90.

41. Gregorio GV, Portmann B, Karani J, et al. Autoimmune hepatitis/sclerosing cholangitis overlap syndrome in childhood: a 16-year prospective study. Hepatology 2001;33:544–53.

42. Jørgensen MJ. The ductal plate malformation: a study of the intrahepatic bile-duct lesion in infantile polycystic disease and congenital hepatic fibrosis. Acta Pathol Microbiol Scand Suppl 1977;257:1–88.

43. Okuda K, Kono K, Ohnishi K, et al. Clinical study of eighty-six cases of idiopathic portal hypertension and comparison with cirrhosis with splenomegaly. Gastroenterology 1984;86:600–10.

44. Snover DC, Sibley RK, Freese DK, et al. Orthotopic liver transplantation: a pathological study of 63 serial liver biopsies from 17 patients with special reference to the diagnostic features and natural history of rejection. Hepatology 1984;4:1212–22.

45. Cakaloglu Y, Devlin J, O'Grady J. Importance of concomitant viral infection during late acute liver allograft rejection. Transplantation 1995;59:40–5.

46. Banff schema for grading liver allograft rejection: an international consensus document. Hepatology 1997;25:658–6.

47. Update of the International Banff Schema for Liver Allograft Rejection: working recommendations for the histopathologic staging and reporting of chronic rejection. Hepatology 2000;31:792–9.

48. Ludwig J, Batts KP, MacCarty RL. Ischemic cholangitis in hepatic allografts. Mayo Clin Proc 1992;67:519–26.

49. Lefkowitch JH. Bile ductular cholestasis: an ominous histopathologic sign related to sepsis and "cholangitis lenta." Hum Pathol 1982;13:19–24.

50. Bründler MA, Rodriguez-Baez N, Jaffe R, et al. Adenovirus ascending cholangiohepatitis. Pediatr Dev Pathol 2003;6:156–9.

51. Walker RC, Marshall WF, Strickler JG, et al. Pretransplantation assessment of the risk of lymphoproliferative disorder. Clin Infect Dis 1995;20:1346–53.

52. Randhawa PS, Jaffe R, Demetris AJ, et al. Expression of Epstein-Barr virus-encoded small RNA (by the EBER-1 gene) in liver specimens from transplant recipients with post-transplantation lymphoproliferative disease. N Engl J Med 1992;327:1710–4.

53. Hübscher SG, Williams A, Davison SM, et al. Epstein-Barr virus in inflammatory diseases of the liver and liver allografts: an in situ hybridization study. Hepatology 1994;20:899–907.

54. Kerkar N, Hadzic N, Davies ET, et al. De-novo autoimmune hepatitis after liver transplantation. Lancet 1998;351:409–13.

55. Hernandez HM, Kovarik P, Whitington PF, Alonso EM. Autoimmune hepatitis as a late complication of liver transplantation. J Pediatr Gastroenterol Nutr 2001;32:131–6.

56. Heneghan MA, Portmann BC, Norris SM, et al. Graft dysfunction mimicking autoimmune hepatitis following liver transplantation in adults. Hepatology 2001;34:464–70.

CHAPTER 69

INTESTINAL BIOPSY

Alan David Phillips, BA, PhD, FRCPCH
Virpi V. Smith, PhD

SMALL INTESTINAL BIOPSY

Small intestinal mucosal biopsy is a routine procedure in specialty centers in which considerable experience and expertise in the technique itself and in the interpretation of biopsy findings are available. Therefore, safety, minimal disturbance to the child, and reliable results are all appropriately combined. The occasional small intestinal biopsy performed by inexperienced hands may lead to a disturbed child and often yields inconclusive results.

The introduction of the techniques of proximal small intestinal mucosal biopsy to pediatric practice by Sakula and Shiner in 1957[1] was a major advance, and access to tissue samples in children has led to a burgeoning of knowledge of intestinal pathology. It has also led to a better understanding of how the intestine functions normally. Variations on the biopsy capsule format have been produced and include a smaller porthole size to provide safer tissue sampling in children and double portholes[2] to improve sampling of potentially patchy lesions.[3] It is dangerous to use the adult capsule in small children because the size of the tissue biopsy specimen may be too large and may occasionally lead to perforation. Use of the pediatric capsule is safe in the experience of most observers, although a small risk of complications still exists. However, the use of the suction biopsy capsule has been superseded in most centers by endoscopic grab biopsy, which can provide tissue samples of similar quality and size.[4,5] It is possible to combine the two techniques.[6] Endoscopic sampling gives multiple biopsy specimens of adequate quality from one region, and it is possible to use a narrow-bore endoscope to give access to patients of low weight (> 1.8 kg). In addition, endoscopy provides a surface view of the upper gastrointestinal (GI) tract, with the option to biopsy esophageal and gastric regions during the procedure, although it is usually performed under a general anesthetic. Suction biopsy, in contrast, is usually performed in a sedated patient and has no facility for a macroscopic view (thereby requiring screening to position the capsule before taking a sample). Both require sterilization after use, and suction biopsy provides a cheaper route to intestinal sampling. Historically, suction biopsies have been performed toward the duodenojejunal flexure. Small intestinal endoscopic biopsies may be performed more proximally, around the second part of the duodenum,

although distal duodenal sampling is perfectly feasible, and it is important to be aware that morphologic features may not be identical in the two regions (eg, in villous height, degree of lamina propria cellularity).

TECHNIQUE OF SMALL INTESTINAL BIOPSY

Suction Biopsy. The child should fast overnight, although small amounts of water may be given as required. Infants may have a 10 pm and sometimes a 2 am feeding if necessary. On the morning of the biopsy, the child is sedated. The Royal Free Hospital (London, UK) no longer performs suction biopsies, and all intestinal mucosal biopsies are taken via endoscopy. Historically, the following oral regimen for sedation was used: trimeprazine, chloral hydrate, and metoclopramide in an appropriate dose for age. If the child becomes highly restless or distressed during the procedure, intravenous diazepam may be given at a maximum dose of 0.5 mg/kg. This should be done only when there is no risk to the child because of heavy sedation and when resuscitation equipment is immediately available. Grossly enlarged tonsils and any compromise to the upper airways are clear contraindications to its use. Once the child is appropriately sedated, the capsule is passed. This is done in the small child by placing a tongue depressor in the mouth and placing the capsule at the back of the tongue. The depressor is withdrawn, the chin is held up, and the child swallows. The tubing is then gently advanced until the capsule is in the stomach. Resistance is often felt at the cardioesophageal junction. The child is then placed on his right side, and the capsule is further advanced. It should then fall toward the pylorus. The next step depends on whether a flexible or a more rigid tubing is being used and whether there is to be fluoroscopic screening (the preferred technique) or if progress is to be assessed by plain radiography of the abdomen. In addition, if a nonradiopaque tube is used, radiopaque material needs to be injected down the tubing before the position of the capsule can be checked radiologically. Using a flexible tubing and a plain radiograph of the abdomen is a time-consuming procedure, but it does have the virtue of providing an exact record (a radiograph) of the exact site of the biopsy. However, the more rapid technique of using a radiopaque relatively rigid tube and positioning the capsule under fluoroscopic control is preferred. Such a semirigid catheter is the metal, braided angiocardiographic catheter, which successfully transmits torque. It is also helpful to inject some air into the stomach via the capsule. A practical advantage of this technique is its usual speed, which makes the procedure preferable from the child's point of view. Care should be taken to monitor the fluoroscopy time. This should not exceed 2 minutes and usually is far shorter.

Metoclopramide introduced into the tubing in the dose of 2.5 mg for infants younger than 2 years and 5 mg for those older than 2 years usually speeds the passage of the capsule when there is a holdup at the pylorus. Alternatively, cisapride (0.2–0.3 mg/kg) can be given as a single dose via the capsule tubing. Using either procedure, once the capsule is positioned in the fourth part of the duodenum, the duodenojejunal flexure, or the first loop of the jejunum, it is "fired" by suction with a 20 mL syringe and then withdrawn. Ideally, biopsy specimens should be taken from a constant standard site. To ensure that the tube is not blocked (if radiopaque material or metoclopramide syrup has been injected down the tube), it is helpful to inject 2 mL of water followed by 2 mL of air before firing the capsule.

Ideally, some duodenal juice should be obtained either by free drainage before the capsule is fired or at the time of firing. The juice should be examined immediately by light microscopic study, under phase-contrast or high-contrast conditions, for the presence of *Giardia lamblia* and should be sent for culture if bacterial overgrowth or infection (eg, enteropathogenic *Escherichia coli* [EPEC]) is considered a diagnostic possibility.

Endoscopic Biopsy. The majority of centers now perform the small bowel biopsy during upper GI endoscopy. This has led to increased awareness of coexistent gastric and esophageal pathology, such as reflux esophagitis in many infants with cow's milk–sensitive enteropathy (CMSE). Position statements on the role of endoscopy in the investigation of conditions such as esophagitis have been published by both the North American Society for Pediatric Gastroenterology and Nutrition (NASPGN)[7] and the European Society of Pediatric Gastroenterology, Hepatology and Nutrition (ESPGHAN)[8]; however, this chapter concerns only the role of endoscopic small intestinal biopsy in the diagnosis of enteropathy. When pediatric endoscopy was first performed, concerns were expressed about the quality of tissue obtained by endoscopic grab biopsy compared with capsule biopsy. This does not appear to be a problem with modern equipment, and several studies have confirmed that endoscopic biopsies are perfectly satisfactory for diagnostic purposes provided that tissue handling is performed correctly (see below).

The techniques of upper GI endoscopy are considered in detail in Chapter 67, "Gastrointestinal Endoscopy." As for capsule biopsy, it is appropriate to consider sedative premedication for the young child or an apprehensive older child. There has been recent discussion about the relative merits of deep intravenous sedation and general anesthesia in pediatric endoscopy.[9] Although some gastroenterologists use little or no sedation for their adult patients, this is not appropriate in pediatrics. The level of sedation achieved using intravenous benzodiazepines, together with narcotic analgesics such as pethidine, may overlap with general anesthesia, and it is mandatory that an appropriately qualified specialist has continuing responsibility for supervising the safety of the sedated patient throughout and after the procedure. Thus, in addition to continuous monitoring of oxygen saturation, there is an absolute requirement for functional resuscitation equipment and the ready availability of reversal agents such as naloxone and flumazenil. Some centers use a qualified anesthetist in this role, although in other centers, a member of the pediatric gastroenterology team assumes this responsibility. It is thus desirable for pediatric gastroenterologists in training to have undergone certified training in intubation and airway maintenance. Several countries now run registered courses in pediatric advanced lifesaving techniques.

The advent of video endoscopy, which has largely superseded the old fiberoptic instruments, has increased the potential diagnostic efficacy of endoscopy, and recognition of subtle lesions has been enhanced. It is thus easier to detect patchy small bowel lesions, such as CMSE. It is also possible, using very small-diameter "neonatal" endoscopes, to perform examinations in very small infants of less than 2 kg. There is an inevitable trade-off in terms of the quality of biopsy obtained if small biopsy forceps are used, and the choice of forceps is a matter of personal or departmental choice. Diagnostic ability is always enhanced by appropriate tissue handling (see below). Conversely, the largest samples may be rendered diagnostically uninformative by mishandling. Simply dropping a small intestinal biopsy into formalin runs the risk of causing a contraction of the longitudinal muscle layer, making subsequent orientation difficult. Although this may not affect diagnosis of celiac disease, it may make secure diagnosis of subtle enteropathy impossible.

Sample Handling. Once the capsule or endoscopic biopsy forceps has been withdrawn, the biopsy specimens should be rapidly removed from the capsule onto a gloved finger using a blunt seeker. The samples are opened out carefully so that the mucosal surface is facing downward (this can be checked using a dissecting microscope or hand lens if required). A piece of dry black card is then applied gently to the serosal surface for a few seconds, resulting in the sample adhering to the card. The card and sample, with the mucosal surface now facing upward, are placed into cold (4°C) normal saline. The black card optimizes the contrast of the specimen for study and photography. Under the dissecting microscope, the appearance of the mucosa can be assessed, but fixation must be prompt so that tissue autolysis is minimized. If using suction biopsy, it is not easy to repeat the procedure, so samples for which fixation with formalin is to be avoided, for example, electron microscopic study, disaccharidase assay, and immunohistochemical study, should be taken. Using endoscopy, it is a simple process to take additional grasp biopsy samples for any other requirements.

The specimens, still on the black card, are then placed in 10% phosphate-buffered formalin and processed for histologic examination. Routinely, 10 to 20 serial sections are cut, mounted on a single glass slide, and stained with hematoxylin and eosin (HE) and with periodic acid–Schiff (PAS) stain.

Hygiene Precautions. It is good practice when handling the biopsy capsule or endoscopic forceps after firing to wear surgical gloves. It is also advisable to wear safety spectacles or a visor to avoid face splashes with tissue and/or fluids. The endoscope is cleaned in 2% activated glutaraldehyde solution in an automatic, self-contained system. The biopsy capsule should be cleaned thoroughly after use and disinfected for at least 10 minutes in 0.5% chlorhexidine gluconate (weight per volume) in 70% alcohol, followed by a minimum of 1 hour in 2% activated glutaraldehyde solution, rinsed thoroughly in water, and allowed to dry. Great care should be taken when handling glutaraldehyde, and individual exposure must be kept to a minimum by using appropriate personal protection equipment and adequate ventilation.

MORPHOLOGIC AND OTHER OBSERVATIONS OF SMALL INTESTINAL BIOPSY SPECIMENS

Dissecting Microscopy. The value of initial examination of biopsy samples with the dissecting microscope has been confirmed by many workers, both in adult medicine and pediatrics.[10,11] The following points illustrate the value of this method:

1. It facilitates the orientation of biopsy specimens to optimize histologic sectioning.
2. It allows a study to be made of the three-dimensional arrangements of mucosal architecture.
3. The entire biopsy specimen may be examined, which is particularly important in pediatrics because patchy mucosal lesions often occur (Figure 69-1).

4. Any gross artifactual damage can be recognized along with the adequacy, or otherwise, of the sample, so that a repeat biopsy can be considered while the patient remains sedated or anesthetized.
5. It allows rapid diagnosis of the presence or absence of a flat mucosa.
6. It allows parents to see the mucosa themselves (eg, a flat mucosa [Figure 69-2] and therefore reinforces the need for a gluten-free diet, particularly in postgluten challenges, when symptoms may not arise.
7. It offers the opportunity to take small samples of the specimen for other procedures (eg, electron microscopy, disaccharidase assay), although this is not necessary with endoscopy.

The drawbacks of the method are that if due care is not taken, fixation may be postponed, giving rise to the possibility of autolytic changes, and the severity of an abnormality other than a flat mucosa can be underestimated.

Some authors have considered that this method of examination adds little to histologic diagnosis and that its only value lies in the rapid recognition of a flat mucosa.[12] They instead advocate serial sectioning for histologic study of the whole biopsy specimen. However, such an approach is idealistic because it is not practical in most hospitals, whereas dissecting microscopic study is simple and straightforward and can easily be performed routinely.

In normal, healthy adults, the small intestinal mucosa is characterized principally by finger-like villi, with some leaf-like villi, but in children, the villi tend to be broader. The term "tongue-like" is used to describe such villi, and when they are extremely wide, the term "ridge-like" villi is used. The latter appearance is frequently seen in children in the first 5 years of life (Figure 69-3).[13] The appearance of leaf-like, tongue-like, or thin ridge-like villi on a proximal small

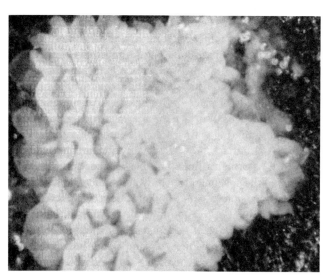

FIGURE 69-1   Dissecting microscopic study: patchy appearance showing ridgelike villi on the left side with low, closely packed ridges on the right (male infant, 13 months, postenteritis syndrome).

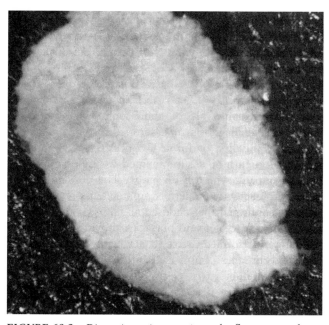

FIGURE 69-2   Dissecting microscopic study: flat mucosa showing visible crypt openings (female infant, 13 months, untreated celiac disease).

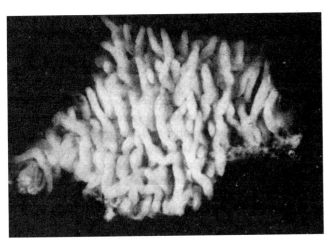

FIGURE 69-3 Dissecting microscopic study: normal appearance of tall, thin, ridgelike villi interspersed with leaflike villi (male infant, 5 months, intermittent diarrhea).

intestinal biopsy is accepted as a normal finding in children. Wright and others found that in childhood controls, the epithelial cell transit time in the crypts was 40% less than in adult controls, and the corrected mitotic index was 20% greater.[14] Thus, in early childhood, the mucosal surface area is reduced, and epithelial cell turnover is greater than in adults. The explanation for these observations is unknown. Because the changes are found in infants of 26 or more weeks gestation who have not been fed,[15] they cannot result from the ingestion of food and bacteria after birth. However, in utero ingestion of amniotic fluid or gastric acid secretions per se may play a role.

Abnormal appearances seen under the dissecting microscope are broadly grouped under two headings: a flat mucosa and a ridged or convoluted mucosa. In both types of mucosa, the normal villous architecture is lost. Mild villous shortening can be difficult to appreciate on dissecting microscopy. Patchy changes in architecture also can be seen with the dissecting microscope.[3]

Proximal intestinal isolated lymphoid follicles can be readily identified by dissecting microscopic study and are more frequent in children between 1 and 2 years old, being uncommon in children older than 6 years of age. Dilated lacteals also may be visible, but they are not indicative of lymphangiectasia in the absence of other clinical features. Endoscopy allows the clear visualization of ileal Peyer patches, which can therefore be selectively biopsied.[16]

Light Microscopy. Terminology. Small intestinal biopsy sections are routinely examined with the light microscope after the sections have been stained with HE. Current histologic terminology is unsatisfactory. The earliest reports divided pathologic small intestinal mucosa into subtotal and partial villous atrophy. The former category was characterized by a flat mucosa with thickening of the glandular layer beneath an atrophic epithelium, and the latter was characterized by a less abnormal mucosa. Some authors have further qualified partial villous atrophy with the terms "mild" and "severe." Others have used the term total villous atrophy to describe a flat mucosa. In fact, the

mucosa described as either total or subtotal villous atrophy is not a truly atrophic mucosa in that it is not thinner than normal. Currently, most pathologists avoid the terms referred to above and use the term crypt hyperplastic villous atrophy to describe lesions in which villi are shortened and crypts are lengthened. This is the most frequently observed abnormality of the small intestinal mucosa (Figure 69-4). When villous height and crypt depth are approximately equal, this is termed a mild or minor abnormality (Figure 69-4B); a moderate abnormality involves crypt depth greater than villous height (Figure 69-4C), and a flat mucosa (Figure 69-4D) is a severe abnormality. Just as observed under the dissecting microscope, a patchy histologic abnormality may be seen (ie, a patchy enteropathy; Figure 69-5).[3]

It should be recognized that it is possible to find villous atrophy without marked crypt hyperplasia.[17] This may be referred to as crypt hypoplastic villous atrophy; however, crypt dimensions are normal. Thus, a more accurate description is crypt normoplastic villous atrophy. This produces a thin mucosa, and lesions of variable severity are seen (Figure 69-6). It is also possible to see villous hyperplasia with crypt hyperplasia.[18]

Parameters of Analysis. Many parameters of mucosal structure may be appreciated on light microscopic examination. However, classification of the appearance has mainly centered on villous height and crypt depth.

Histologic Normality. A clear idea of what is "normal" is required to evaluate the appearance of the small intestinal mucosa. This is not necessarily easy to determine in childhood because it is not ethical to perform biopsies on healthy children. However, observation of the morphologic features of biopsy specimens in the following situations expands the knowledge of the morphologic features of normal small intestinal mucosa: (1) biopsy specimens from children thought to have GI disease but whose specimens turn out to be normal, (2) control biopsy specimens from children on a gluten-free diet with celiac disease in remission, and (3) postmortem studies of the small intestine from children dying without evidence of GI disease (see Figure 69-4).

It is important to study other aspects of the mucosa along with villous height and crypt depth because these can give specific diagnoses. Aspects to be studied include the following:

- *Organisms.* Look for the presence of luminal, surface-attached, and intramucosal organisms (eg, *G. lamblia, Cryptosporidium,* enteropathogenic *E. coli,* and microsporidiosis).
- *Epithelial cells.* Assess the state of the epithelium, in particular the enterocyte, for cell height and degree of vacuolation. The latter finding can indicate abetalipoproteinemia and hypobetalipoproteinemia if extensive vacuolation of villous epithelium is seen in an otherwise normal mucosa. However, this should not be confused with the lesser degree of vacuolation seen in the enteropathies of celiac disease and the postenteritis syndrome. This is usually confined to the villous tip or

to a small number of surface exposed cells in severe enteropathies.[19] Crypt epithelium should be studied for the number of mitotic figures to give an indication of cell production, and the number of goblet cells should be assessed. In some cases of autoimmune enteropathy, a complete absence of goblet cells has been noted.[20] Paneth and endocrine cells also form part of the epithelium, but these are not useful for routine diagnostic pur-

poses. Paneth cell dysplasia can be seen in conditions of increased epithelial cell turnover, and the number of endocrine cells is increased in celiac disease. This can be appreciated by studying histologic sections under fluorescence microscopy because these cells autofluoresce.

- *Intraepithelial cells.* Note the presence and number of migratory, intraepithelial cells, such as lymphocytes, eosinophils, neutrophils, and mast cells. Quantifying

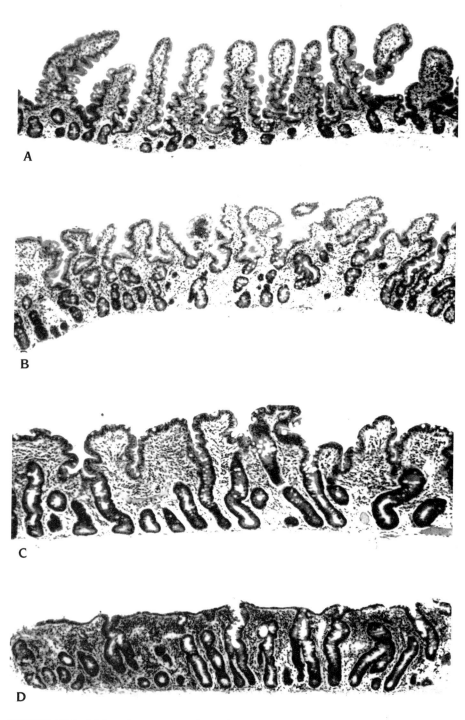

FIGURE 69-4   Light microscopic study: *A*, histologically normal small intestinal mucosa (female infant, 12 months, failure to thrive); *B*, minor enteropathy (female infant, 5 months, chronic diarrhea with failure to thrive); *C*, moderate enteropathy (boy, 6 years 9 months, celiac disease—postgluten challenge); *D*, severe enteropathy (girl, 6 years 10 months, untreated celiac disease) (hematoxylin and eosin; ×60 original magnification).

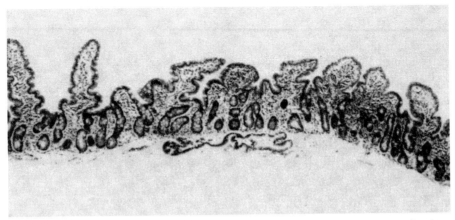

FIGURE 69-5   Light microscopic study: patchy enteropathy (girl, 2 years 2 months, diarrhea postcolectomy) (hematoxylin and eosin; ×60 original magnification).

the density of lymphocytes within the small intestinal villus or surface epithelium (number of lymphocytes per 100 epithelial cells) is of value for routine diagnostic use.[21] Children with normal histologic features (controls) have a mean value of 23,[22] which is similar to that described in adults.[23] Raised counts of intraepithelial lymphocytes (IELs) are found in children and adults with celiac disease, adults with untreated dermatitis herpetiformis or tropical sprue, and some cases of children with unexplained failure to thrive,[21] giardiasis,[21] cryptosporidiosis,[24] or CMSE.[22] IEL counts return to the normal range in cases of celiac disease when the patient is placed on a gluten-free diet, and they become lower than normal in patients with CMSE on a milk-free diet.[22] The absolute number of IEL may not alter with changes in morphologic features[25]; however, IEL density is not directly related to mucosal surface area.[26] Intraepithelial eosinophils have been reported to be increased in CMSE,[17] and intraepithelial neutrophils are seen in inflammatory bowel disease[27]

and in EPEC infections[27] but may also occasionally be noticed in active celiac disease.

• *Lamina propria cellularity*. Study the lamina propria for the degree and nature of cellular infiltrate and the appearance of lacteals. This is usually done subjectively, but more reports are making use of readily available computer-based image analysis systems that provide a means of objective analysis. Recognition of basic cell types can be performed on HE-stained sections, but it is important to use immunohistochemical techniques to investigate cell phenotype (eg, lymphocyte subclass; see below) and for secretion of specific cytokines. Mucosal mast cells are best studied using Carnoy solution as a fixative[28,29] and chloroacetoesterase reaction for staining so that they can be clearly seen,[30] although this has limited diagnostic usefulness. Using this technique, Sanderson and others have demonstrated that a higher mast cell density exists in the ileum than in the colon.[31]

• *PAS staining*. This allows the preservation of the brush border to be visualized and demonstrates mucus-

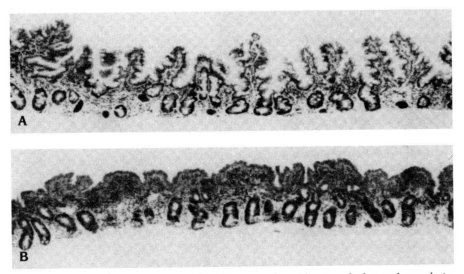

FIGURE 69-6   Light microscopic study: villous atrophy without marked crypt hyperplasia. *A,* Mild enteropathy (female infant, 1 year 7 months, cow's milk protein intolerance). *B,* Moderate enteropathy (male infant, 11 months, cow's milk protein intolerance) (hematoxylin and eosin, ×75 original magnification for both)

containing goblet cells. The presence of PAS-positive material in the apical cytoplasm of upper crypt and low villous epithelial cells indicates microvillous atrophy,[32] although this should not be confused with the granular epithelial staining seen in enteropathies, where it reflects an increased presence of lysosomal bodies. PAS-positive inspissated mucus in crypt lumina suggests cystic fibrosis.[33]

Electron Microscopy. Transmission electron microscopy and scanning electron microscopy have been used to study the morphologic characteristics of small intestinal biopsy tissue taken from children[34] and adults. It is important to consider whether electron microscopy will be of diagnostic value in advance of the biopsy so that glutaraldehyde fixation (2–3% glutaraldehyde in 0.1 M phosphate or cacodylate buffer is suitable) can be used to preserve the tissue samples and optimize interpretation. Ultrastructural studies are now routine in cases of protracted diarrhea. Disorders such as microvillous atrophy (Figure 69-7),[32] attaching and effacing *E. coli* (Figure 69-8),[35] and cryptosporidiosis (Figure 69-9)[24] are diagnostic possibilities. Small intestinal biopsy specimens from patients with acquired immune deficiency syndrome (AIDS) should also be studied by electron microscopic examination because many infectious agents are beyond the resolution of the light microscope (eg, microsporidiosis).

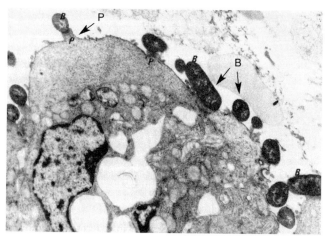

FIGURE 69-8   Electron microscopic study: enteropathogenic enteritis caused by *Escherichia coli* (male infant, 8 months). *E. coli* 0128 (B) attached to apical surface of epithelium in association with microvillous effacement and pedestal formation (P) (×18,000 original magnification).

Biochemistry. A mucosal sample should be taken and frozen for biochemical studies[36] in cases in which primary or secondary disaccharidase deficiencies are diagnostic possibilities. Although enzyme levels can be appreciated on histochemical study of frozen tissue sections[37] or on duodenal juice, the usual practice is to analyze tissue homogenates.[36,38] Breath tests can be used to indicate disaccharide malabsorption,[39] but this is not the same as disaccharidase deficiency. Other techniques are possible and may be required to diagnose rare disorders, such as the use of brush border membrane vesicles to diagnose defective sodium-proton transport.[40]

Immunohistochemistry. Conventional staining techniques give information about intestinal architecture and cellularity without shedding much light on the precise nature of the inflammatory response. All lymphocytes look similar on HE staining, and it is impossible to see whether

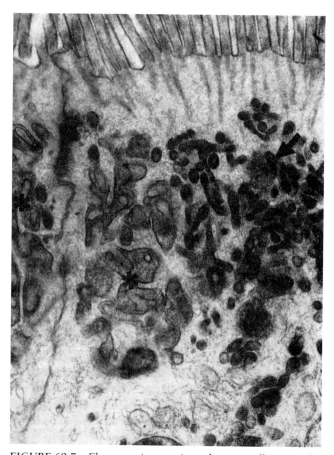

FIGURE 69-7   Electron microscopic study: microvillous atrophy (female infant, 14 months). Increased presence of secretory granules with membrane-bound inclusions containing microvillus-like projections (×40,000 original magnification).

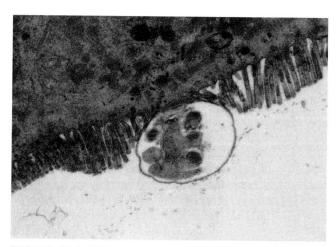

FIGURE 69-9   Electron microscopic study: cryptosporidiosis (male infant, 13 months). Cryptosporidial schizont adhering to the epithelial surface. Notice displacement of microvilli at site of attachment (×18,000 original magnification).

a lymphocyte infiltration represents oligoclonal expansion or a polyclonal response, whether an IEL has a particular T-cell receptor type,[41] or whether evidence exists of epithelial or endothelial inflammatory activation. Special techniques are required to understand disease mechanisms rather than simply describe appearances.

Immunohistochemical analysis may give highly important information in the diagnosis of enteropathy and study of disease mechanism. It is a relatively simple technique to perform, yet it is powerful because of the range of available antibodies that can give precise information on cell lineage, activation status, and functional protein expression. However, access to the full range of diagnostic markers requires the use of snap-frozen tissue because formalin fixation crosslinks tissue proteins and may alter tertiary structure enough to prevent antibody recognition. An important practical point is that any child with an unusual enteropathy should have biopsies snap-frozen at endoscopy in addition to those taken into formalin (ideally, a further biopsy should be taken into glutaraldehyde for possible electron microscopic studies). This is now accepted good practice for any infant with unexplained intractable diarrhea. The widespread use of endoscopic biopsy has removed the problems arising with capsule biopsy of balancing the need for proper histologic assessment and obtaining enough tissue for snap-freezing. Although immunohistochemistry may be considered a research tool for the majority of small bowel enteropathies, it is an important diagnostic aid for conditions such as autoimmune enteropathy, when activated mucosal lymphocytes may be seen in conjunction with class II major histocompatibility complex (MHC) expression (human leukocyte antigen [HLA]-DR) on the surface epithelium.[42] The detection of high numbers of T cells within the epithelium favors the diagnosis of celiac disease in a child with positive serology, even if the mucosa shows only subtle abnormalities otherwise.

Immunohistochemistry has been particularly useful in celiac disease, allowing the recognition of the primary role of lamina propria CD4 cells in the pathogenesis of this condition.[43,44] Immunohistochemical analysis may extend to the detection of secreted molecules such as cytokines, and most of the major immunoregulatory molecules can be demonstrated in this way.

Molecular Biology. Using molecular biologic techniques, it is possible to detect the presence of messenger ribonucleic acid (mRNA) for specific proteins. If whole biopsy specimens are homogenized, specific mRNA can be detected by Northern blotting or reverse transcriptase polymerase chain reaction. Such techniques allow detection and semiquantitative estimation of such small amounts of mRNA but do not allow localization within tissue. The technique is also dependent on expertise, and some centers have found difficulty in differentiating diseased tissue from controls because many cytokines are produced at low levels in healthy intestines and thus may be amplified to apparently similar levels. In contrast, it is possible to localize specific mRNA within individual cells using in situ hybridization, which is technically

more difficult but which may also be combined on the same slide with tissue for immunohistochemical study. These techniques are still largely reserved for research, although detection of viral or bacterial pathogens such as cytomegalovirus or mycobacteria may be efficiently achieved.

In general, in situ hybridization requires the use of frozen tissue, although mRNA for some molecules may be detected in formalin-fixed tissue after proteolytic digestion to unmask ribonucleic acid sequences.[45] The use of in situ hybridization in studying intestinal function has been demonstrated best in animal work. The development of class II MHC molecules (required for antigen presentation to T lymphocytes) in mouse small intestinal epithelium was shown to be dependent on the introduction of a complex diet at weaning.[46] The expression of the Na-glucose cotransporter gene was maximal at the crypt-villus junction in rabbits, although the actual enzyme activity was greatest at the villus tip.[47]

The advent of laser capture microdissection now allows molecular biologic analysis of collections of individual cells so that transcriptional activity of discrete cell populations can be achieved.[48] Combined with knockout mouse technology, this has allowed functional genomic analysis of intestinal stem cells,[49] and these techniques promise important advances in understanding gut function.

Lymphocyte Isolation. In addition to the staining techniques available, it is possible to obtain individual inflammatory cells from whole biopsy samples. Epithelial cells and intraepithelial lymphocyte populations can be extracted initially by separation from the rest of the biopsy using ethylenediaminetetraacetic acid (EDTA). Lamina propria lymphocytes may then be obtained by digestion of the remaining tissue with collagenase. If necessary, the lymphocyte subpopulations may be separated further by density gradient centrifugation followed by magnetic bead extraction. Once separated, the inflammatory cells may be categorized on the basis of their surface markers by fluorescent-activated cell sorter analysis,[50] which may also be employed to demonstrate spontaneous cytokine secretion (Figure 69-10). Other techniques include measuring supernatant levels after the cells are stimulated and the use of the enzyme-linked immunospot.[51]

In Vitro Organ Culture Techniques. Although it is not possible to maintain the viability of biopsy tissue for any great length of time, individual explants (approximately 2 mm² pieces) will maintain morphologic features for 24 to 48 hours under appropriate culture conditions. Cultured small intestinal explants from celiac patients show improvement in morphologic features if cultured in the absence of gluten,[52] whereas the addition of gliadin fragments upregulates the expression of HLA-DR on epithelial cells in vitro.[53] Short-term culture (8 hours) is of particular value in experimental studies of microbial pathogenesis.[54]

ROLE OF SMALL INTESTINAL BIOPSY IN DIAGNOSIS

Currently a single, investigative, small intestinal biopsy has two main roles that are of value in making a diagnosis in clinical pediatrics. The first is to demonstrate the presence or absence of a proximal small intestinal enteropathy.[55] Enteropathy may be defined as an abnormality of the small intestinal mucosa that can be demonstrated with the light microscope. The second is to provide samples of small intestinal mucosa for other diagnostic purposes (eg, for disaccharidase assay).

Arranged small intestinal biopsies are sometimes required before a final diagnosis can be made. Such situations include organized dietary challenges with pre- and postchallenge biopsies (eg, in celiac disease or dietary loading), in which diagnostic features may be more easily distinguished (eg, lipoproteinemias, lymphangiectasia).

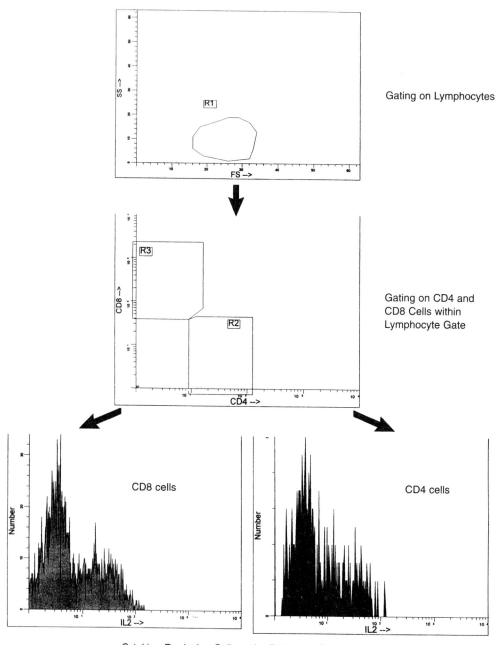

FIGURE 69-10   Fluorescent-activated cell sorter analysis (FACS). Use of flow cytometric (FACS) analysis to determine cytokine production at the single-cell level by mucosal lymphocytes. Intraepithelial lymphocytes may be studied separately from lamina propria lymphocytes, by separation of the entire epithelial compartment using ethylenediaminetetraacetic acid. Lamina propria lymphocytes are separated following collagenase digestion. The lymphocytes are first identified by "gating" on cells of appropriate size and density among the total population. Within that gate, cells expressing CD4 (T helper cells) or CD8 (cytotoxic/suppressor cells) can then be identified using monoclonal antibodies tagged with fluorescent markers—a whole panel of other cell lineage markers can be used if cell numbers and research budgets are adequate. Finally, the proportion of CD4 and CD8 cells spontaneously producing cytokines (here interleukin-2) can be identified.

The current ESPGHAN recommendations for the diagnosis of celiac disease suggest that dietary challenges are not necessary in older patients and that the demonstration of a flat mucosa with a good clinical response to gluten elimination affords a satisfactory diagnosis. However, young children under 2 years of age may require dietary challenge to confirm the diagnosis in view of other possible explanations for enteropathy in this age group.[56]

Those disorders in which small intestinal biopsy has a role in diagnosis may be placed into groups. First, there is a group of disorders for which biopsy is invariably of value in making a diagnosis (Table 69-1). These include disorders in which a proximal small intestinal enteropathy is a diagnostic prerequisite or in which there is a specific enzyme deficiency.

The demonstration of an enteropathy is an absolute requirement for the diagnosis of celiac disease, but it is not specific for this disorder. A flat small intestinal mucosa is characteristic of celiac disease, but there are other causes of a flat mucosa in childhood, and, on occasion, lesser degrees of mucosal abnormality may be found in children with celiac disease.

The enterocyte in abetalipoproteinemia cannot synthesize betalipoprotein, and, as a result, chylomicron formation is impaired. Thus, absorbed dietary fat is not properly mobilized from the enterocyte. As a result, the cytoplasm of those cells lining the upper half or two-thirds of the villi appears vacuolated in ordinary HE-stained sections. These cells can be shown to contain fat through the use of special stains on frozen sections. A similar appearance is seen in hypobetalipoproteinemia.

Children with agammaglobulinemia lack plasma cells in the lamina propria, but the mucosal architecture may range from a flat mucosa to a completely normal one.

In the enteropathy associated with multisystem autoimmune disease and the presence of circulating autoantibodies (autoimmune enteropathy) (Figure 69-11), the mucosa is severely abnormal at the time of diagnosis, sometimes with a flat mucosa. The demonstration of an enteropathy in the presence of circulating autoantibodies against the enterocyte in a child who has chronic diarrhea is essential for diagnosis of this syndrome. It is very important to do in-depth immunologic studies in these children to help identify therapeutic options.[20]

Microvillous atrophy can be diagnosed only by the demonstration of characteristic microvillous inclusions and an increase in secretory granules on electron microscopic examination of a small or large intestinal mucosal

biopsy specimen.[32,57,58] An abnormal accumulation of PAS-positive material occurs within the apical cytoplasm of epithelial cells and corresponds to the increase in secretory granules seen on electron microscopic study.[32,57]

The presence of adhering bacteria can be seen on light microscopy; however, the resolution of transmission electron microscopy is required to recognize the microvillous loss and pedestal formation of the attaching and effacing lesion, which is typical of classic EPEC infections (see Figure 69-8).[35] EPEC infections are capable of causing severe protracted diarrhea and much morbidity and mortality. The recognition of an enteropathy with the presence of attaching- and effacing lesion–forming bacteria indicates that antibiotic therapy would be appropriate.[59] This is important because nonclassic serotypes of E. coli, so-called atypical E. coli, also can cause an attaching and effacing lesion,[60] and routine stool microbiologic study would not identify them.

Children who have either of the two primary disaccharide intolerances, namely congenital alactasia and sucrase-isomaltase deficiency, have normal small intestinal morphologic features, but the characteristic enzyme deficiencies are present on disaccharidase assay.

Second, when the lesion is nonuniform (ie, patchy) or when there is penetration of the mucosa by a parasite, biopsy may provide a specific diagnosis, but in this group of disorders, the absence of abnormality (ie, a normal mucosa) does not exclude the diagnosis (Table 69-2). It is possible in parasitic situations and infections with attaching and effacing E. coli that a more distal site of the intestine is affected, and the diagnosis is made on stool microbiology.

The trophozoite of G. lamblia is often found in the duodenal juice of children with giardiasis but also may be found on section of small intestinal biopsy specimens. Similarly, in children with strongyloidiasis, larvae of Strongyloides stercoralis may be found in juice and on section of the mucosal biopsy specimens. Cryptosporidial schizonts may just be visible by light microscopic study, but the characteristic morphologic features are readily identifiable by electron microscopic examination.

Small intestinal lymphangiectasia may be diagnosed by biopsy of the small intestinal mucosa, but because the lesion is often patchy, it can be missed on a single biopsy; multiple biopsies may be indicated.

Small intestinal lymphoma are rarely diagnosed by biopsy if the lesion has invaded the mucosa.

Children with hypogammaglobulinemia may be found to have hyperplastic lymphoid follicles on small intestinal biopsy, as well as a diminished number of plasma cells and variable morphologic abnormalities. G. lamblia is often found in the duodenal juice of such children.

Third, in another group of disorders in which the lesion may also be patchy, the demonstration of an enteropathy is nonspecific (Table 69-3). However, the finding of mucosal abnormality is diagnostically useful in such patients because it indicates the presence of disease in the small intestine. Some disorders in this group (eg, CMSE) may be diagnosed by serial biopsy related to dietary protein withdrawal and challenge, although no pathologic fea

TABLE 69-1 DISORDERS IN WHICH BIOPSY IS VALUABLE

MORPHOLOGIC FEATURES	
ABNORMAL	**NORMAL**
Celiac disease	Congenital alactasia
Agammaglobulinemia	Abetalipoproteinemia
Autoimmune enteropathy	Sucrase-isomaltase deficiency
Microvillous atrophy	
Attaching-effacing Escherichia coli	

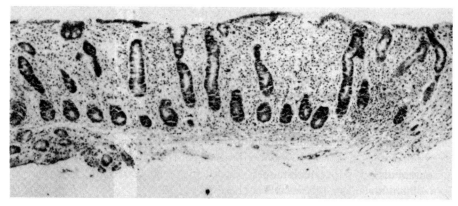

FIGURE 69-11 Light microscopic study: autoimmune enteropathy (male infant, 14 months), severe enteropathy (hematoxylin and eosin; ×120 original magnification). Reproduced with permission from Unsworth J, Hutchins P, Mitchell J, et al. Flat small intestinal musosa and autoantibodies against the gut epithelium. J Pediatr Gastroenterol Nutr 1982;1:503–13.

tures are specific for this disorder. It is unusual to perform challenges in CMSE, and diagnosis rests on a clinical response to an elimination diet with a return to normal histologic features before the reintroduction of cow's milk, when it is considered that the disease has resolved. AIDS must be added to the list of nonspecific abnormalities.

Finally, for completeness, a group of disorders in which small intestinal biopsy specimen is characteristically normal is listed in Table 69-4.

To conclude this section on the role of small intestinal biopsy in diagnosis, it is important to briefly review the diagnostic approach to a child thought to have small intestinal disease. This is summarized in Table 69-5.

The emphasis is not on demonstrating malabsorption (eg, steatorrhea or xylose malabsorption), as formerly was the case, but on pinpointing an anatomic abnormality of the small intestine, a structural abnormality of the small intestinal mucosa (ie, an enteropathy), or a specific infectious etiologic agent. Thus, barium studies, small intestinal biopsy, and stool examination are particularly important investigative tools. Hematologic investigations, such as a full blood count and serum folate levels, provide important evidence of a deficiency state that may need to be treated immediately or followed up as a marker of response to treatment. Radiologic studies are particularly important for diagnosing Crohn disease and congenital anatomic lesions of the small intestine.

LARGE INTESTINAL BIOPSY

Large intestinal pathology can be investigated using a variety of different types of biopsies of the bowel. For mucosal disease, mucosal biopsies taken during fiberoptic colonoscopy are employed. Suction rectal biopsies are suitable for the diagnosis of aganglionosis (Hirschsprung disease), but for other enteric neuromuscular diseases, full-thickness or seromuscular biopsies are required.

MUCOSAL BIOPSY TAKEN AT FIBEROPTIC COLONOSCOPY

Since its introduction in the early 1960s, the value of fiberoptic colonoscopy as a diagnostic procedure in adult patients has become well established. It is now clear that this is also a very useful technique in pediatric practice. One of its most useful aspects is in the provision of multiple large intestinal mucosal biopsies. The ileum can be entered in over three-quarters of cases with an experienced endoscopist,[61] affording an opportunity to assess the intactness of the mucosa and to study ileal histology. The availability of pediatric colonoscopy is restricted to pediatric gastroenterologic centers and is dependent on the availability of endoscopy skills. When these are available, this approach has largely overtaken the need for barium enema examination in the investigation of rectal bleeding and suspected chronic inflammatory bowel disease.[62]

The value of histologic assessment following full colonoscopy has been evaluated in the investigation of children when first presenting with inflammatory bowel disease.[61] Diagnosis of inflammatory bowel disease on morphologic criteria is possible in 85% of cases. Although sigmoid colonic and rectal biopsies can also confirm the diagnosis of inflammatory bowel disease in 65% of cases, over one-third would have been assigned to the wrong diagnostic category on the left-sided findings alone. This is particularly relevant in pediatric patients whose right colon is often affected without involvement of the rectosigmoid. Limited examination will also miss ileocecal Crohn disease and may miss multiple polyps. However, when colonoscopy is not available, rigid sigmoidoscopy must be used to obtain colonic and rectal biopsies.

The principal purpose of obtaining intestinal colonic biopsies in this context is for the diagnosis of chronic inflammatory bowel disease and Crohn disease in particular.

TABLE 69-2	DISORDERS IN WHICH BIOPSY MAY BE VALUABLE DIAGNOSTICALLY

Giardiasis
Strongyloidiasis
Small intestinal lymphangiectasia
Small intestinal lymphoma
Hypogammaglobulinemia

TABLE 69-3	DISORDERS IN WHICH BIOPSY RESULTS MAY BE ABNORMAL BUT ABNORMALITY IS NONSPECIFIC

Postenteritis syndrome	Tropical sprue
Cow's milk protein intolerance	Radiation enteritis
Transient-gluten intolerance	Drug-induced lesion,
Soy protein intolerance	eg, by methotrexate
Intractable diarrhea syndrome	Protein-energy malnutrition
	AIDS

TABLE 69-4   DISORDERS IN WHICH BIOPSY FINDINGS ARE NORMAL

Cirrhosis
Hepatitis
Exocrine pancreatic insufficiency
Toddler's diarrhea

However, there are other reasons, and Table 69-6 lists the indications for fiberoptic colonoscopy in children. The technique of colonoscopy is detailed in Chapter 67, "Gastrointestinal Endoscopy," and is not detailed here. An important diagnostic benefit from colonoscopy is the recognition of microscopic colitides that are apparent not on gross observation but only following histologic assessment of biopsies.

In recent years, rectal suction biopsy containing sufficient submucosa has replaced full-thickness biopsy for the diagnosis of Hirschsprung disease. This cannot be taken at routine colonoscopy and requires a special biopsy apparatus.[63] Full-thickness rectal biopsy or laparoscopic colonic seromuscular biopsies may still be required for the diagnosis of disorders involving the myenteric plexus or muscularis propria.[64–66]

DISORDERS DIAGNOSED BY LARGE INTESTINAL BIOPSY IN CHILDHOOD

These disorders may be broadly grouped into inflammatory disorders and motility disorders. A general schematic approach to assessment of mucosal biopsies is recommended.[67] Questions to be asked are (1) if the tissue is normal or abnormal and (2) if changes suggest chronic inflammatory bowel disease whether they favor Crohn disease or ulcerative colitis. Alternatively, it is important to ask if the inflammation suggests an acute infective etiology or another form of inflammation, such as chronic granulomatous disease,[68,69] allergic colitis, tufting enteropathy involving the large bowel,[70] or intractable enterocolitis of infancy.[71]

In mucosal disease, the diagnostically important features to be assessed are the overall architecture, the cellularity of the lamina propria, the presence of a polymorphic neutrophilic or eosinophilic infiltrate, and epithelial changes. The histologic diagnosis of chronic inflammatory bowel disease in children specifically has been reported.[72,73] The principal features of histologic diagnosis are outlined below.

Mucosal Inflammatory Disorders. *Ulcerative Colitis.*
This is a chronic intermittent disease that affects the large bowel mucosa. It is possible to make a suggested histopathologic diagnosis from biopsies taken at the initial presentation. Confident biopsy diagnoses can certainly be made in established disease. Sequential biopsies form part of the diagnostic workup and also monitor activity after treatment; symptomatic improvement may not be accompanied by endoscopic or histologic mucosal healing.[74] Ulcerative colitis usually commences in the rectum and may extend to involve the rest of the colon. Often inflammation may be absent or patchy in the rectum or sigmoid, particularly in the pediatric population.[75] Both the clinical picture and the histopathology may be considered in terms of three phases: active, resolving, and in remission (quiescent).[76]

TABLE 69–5   DIAGNOSTIC APPROACH TO CHILDREN THOUGHT TO HAVE SMALL INTESTINAL DISEASE

Initial assessment
  Detailed case history
  Physical examination
  Analysis of centile charts for height and weight
Initial investigations
  Full blood count and erythrocyte sedimentation rate in older child
    (? Crohn disease)
  Serum and red cell folate
  Antigliadin and antiendomesial antibodies
  Stool culture for bacteria
  Stool electron microscopy for viruses
  Stool examination for *Giardia lamblia* and *Cryptosporidium*
  Stool-reducing substances
Next stage
  Small intestinal biopsy
  Duodenal juice examination for *G. lamblia*
  Bacterial culture for bacteria (anerobic and aerobic as indicated)
  Barium follow-through
  Gut autoantibodies
  Response to elimination diet

Active Phase. The most specific feature is loss of crypt architecture with crypt distortion and branching (Figure 69-12). Polymorphonuclear neutrophils are present within the crypt epithelium, and there may be crypt abscesses (Figure 69-13). The epithelium shows varying amounts of degeneration and regeneration. There is mucin depletion and increased mitotic activity. The lamina propria shows capillary congestion and edema; it contains a heavy mixed inflammatory cell infiltrate. This is diffuse throughout the lamina propria and is composed of plasma cells, lymphocytes, and neutrophils. Eosinophils are also found and may be prominent, although the significance of this in relation to the natural history is not fully clear. Inflammatory cells may also be found in the submucosa; this may be associated with severe ulceration.

Resolving Phase. An important feature of ulcerative colitis is the fact that the biopsy appearances vary with time. In the resolving phase, the crypts remain distorted and branched; the surface may take on a villous appearance. Goblet cells reappear in the crypts but may be elongated. Inflammation in the lamina propria is reduced and may become focal; there is then a possibility of confusion with other disease, such as Crohn disease. There are few polymorphs at this stage.

TABLE 69-6   INDICATIONS FOR PROCEEDING TO FIBEROPTIC COLONOSCOPY IN THE PEDIATRIC PATIENT

Unexplained rectal bleeding
Bloody diarrhea in the absence of stool pathogens
  (with or without abdominal pain)
Abdominal pain associated with weight loss (with or without diarrhea)
Other features suggesting a diagnosis of chronic inflammatory bowel
  disease (eg, strictures, fistulae, disease activity extent as a guide
  to therapy)
Surveillance for malignancy (long-standing ulcerative colitis, polyposis
  coli, Peutz-Jehgers syndrome, Gardner syndrome)
Polypectomy

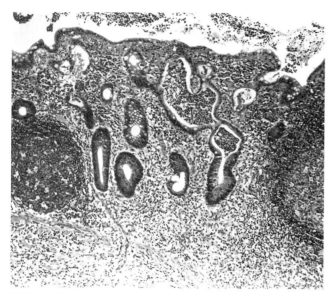

FIGURE 69-12 Chronic ulcerative colitis, active phase. Crypts are distorted and show mucus depletion; several contain neutrophils resulting in crypt abscesses. There is diffuse inflammation of the mucosa. Lymphoid follicles are also present (hematoxylin and eosin; ×100 original magnification).

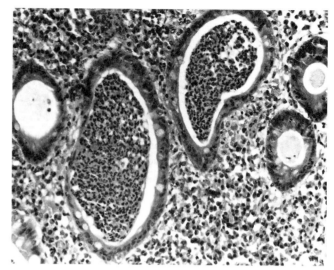

FIGURE 69-13 Chronic ulcerative colitis, active phase. High-power view showing crypt distortion, mucus depletion, and crypt abscesses. There is diffuse inflammation in the lamina propria (hematoxylin and eosin; ×250 original magnification).

Remission Phase. Here the crypts are atrophied and distorted. There is a gap between the muscularis mucosae and the crypt bases. Goblet cells are present, but there may be Paneth cell metaplasia and increased numbers of crypt endocrine cells.[77-79] There is no active inflammation; neutrophils are therefore absent.

Inflammatory Polyps (Pseudopolyps). These consist of granulation tissue, a mixture of glands and granulation tissue, or a tag of virtually normal mucosa. They are a frequent finding and indicate prior severe mucosal ulceration with irregular healing. Biopsy allows them to be distinguished from neoplastic polyps (adenomas).

Fulminant Acute Dilatation. This has been recorded in up to 13% of patients with ulcerative colitis in the early adult literature[80,81] but is probably much lower in pediatric practice today. The rectum is relatively spared, and the transverse colon is most severely affected. There are several misleading features in biopsies in this condition: inflammation may be transmural, and there may be fissuring ulceration; the crypt architecture is often intact, and inflammation may be mild.

Follicular Proctitis. Prominent lymphoid follicles are present, and there is an accompanying diffuse infiltrate of plasma cells and neutrophils. These features cause thickening of the mucosa. The crypt architecture is irregular. The differential diagnosis in this condition includes lymphoid polyps, malignant lymphoma, and lymphomatous polyposis.

Crohn Disease. Crohn disease may affect any part of the GI tract,[82-86] but most commonly it presents as regional ileitis,[87] ileocolitis, colitis, or perianal disease. It is characterized by its focal distribution and, unlike ulcerative colitis, often involves the full thickness of the bowel wall. The endoscopic appearances form an important part of the diagnosis in Crohn disease. The features include tiny aphthoid ulcers,[88] serpiginous ulceration, edema, linear ulcer-

ation ("cobblestoning"),[89,90] and, occasionally, inflammatory polyps. Areas of normal mucosa appear between abnormal areas and are thus termed skip lesions. Anal lesions consist of painless fissures, ulcers, fistulae, skin tags, and perianal abscesses.[91]

The crypt architecture and goblet cell population are usually preserved despite considerable inflammation (Figure 69-14).[92,93] However, there may be some crypt distortion close to areas of ulceration; such distortion may also occur in the early healing phase.[94] The inflammatory cell component consists of a mixture of lymphocytes, plasma cells, and polymorphs; their density varies across the biopsy.[95] Neutrophils are less conspicuous and more focal than in ulcerative colitis or infectious colitis, but crypt

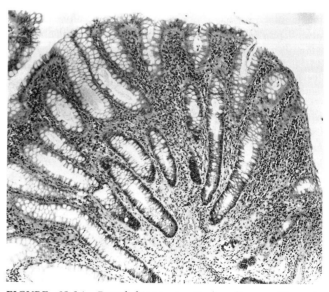

FIGURE 69-14 Rectal biopsy in Crohn disease. There is chronic inflammation in the lamina propria, but crypt architecture is well preserved (hematoxylin and eosin; ×100 original magnification).

abscesses may be found.[96] Small aggregates of lymphocytes occur adjacent to crypt bases.[97] Granulomas are also found; these are composed of collections of epithelioid histiocytes, multinucleate giant cells, and, frequently, a cuff of lymphocytes (Figure 69-15).

Granulomas occur throughout the bowel wall in Crohn disease and may be seen in both inflamed mucosa and endoscopically normal mucosa.[72,73,98] Microgranulomas consisting of clusters of histiocytes and small numbers of inflammatory cells also occur.[98] Confluent granulomas with florid central necrosis suggest a diagnosis of tuberculosis; however, a small focus of central necrosis may be seen in granulomas in Crohn disease.

The incidence of granulomas in biopsies is variable, and published figures in adults range from 0 to nearly 30%.[99–105] In the pediatric population with Crohn disease, epithelioid granulomas have been reported to be present in 36%[71] and 44%.[61] This is clearly an underestimate and is a question of sampling because in an analysis of 17 operative specimens from children with Crohn disease, 14 had noncaseating granulomas (82%) (see Figure 69-15).

Other features of biopsies in Crohn disease include aphthoid ulcers; these are seen as small areas of ulceration immediately over a lymphoid follicle.[97] Fissuring ulcers also occur; they penetrate down through the submucosa and are characteristic of Crohn disease. Fibrosing stenoses may also be found.[102] The muscularis mucosa may appear thickened.[103]

Biopsies in Crohn disease should include a portion of the superficial submucosa: this will often show "disproportionate inflammation"[94] with a mixed inflammatory cell infiltrate. This reflects the transmural nature of the inflammatory process in the disease. Granulomas in the submucosa are helpful in the diagnosis. The following features are considered to be the most helpful in the diagnosis of Crohn disease when granulomas are absent: the patchy nature of the inflammation, relatively little crypt distortion or goblet cell depletion, and the presence of basal lymphoid aggregates. Unfortunately, aphthoid ulceration and fissures are rare in biopsies.

No studies have yet been able to correlate specific features with disease activity.[104] As already mentioned, granulomas may occur in normal-appearing mucosa. Fibrosis in the submucosa and splitting up of the muscularis mucosae indicate long-standing disease. Granulomas have been claimed to indicate a favorable prognosis,[105,106] but not all studies are in agreement with this.[107,108] Ulceration and fissuring have been claimed to be indicative of a poor prognosis.[109] Overall, there appears to be no universally accepted prognostic microscopic feature.[94,110]

Infective Colitis. Infective colitis may be classified etiologically into bacterial, viral, protozoal, and fungal infections and infestation by helminths. The bacterial diarrheas cause the vast majority of diagnostic problems. *Salmonella* species, *Shigella* species, enteroinvasive *Escherichia coli*, and *Campylobacter* species may also produce similar histopathologic appearances, which have been termed infective biopsy pattern (Figure 69-16). It is important to be familiar with these histologic features so that patients with infectious disease are not mislabeled as having ulcerative colitis or Crohn disease. History of foreign travel is important to suggest more exotic infections; other clues may be the presence of numerous eosinophils or granulomas.

It is not usually possible from a biopsy to distinguish among the main causes of bacterial colitis.

Examination of the biopsy specimen indicates that the mucosa is widened by edema. Clusters of polymorphs are present throughout the biopsy but particularly in the more superficial portion and often adjacent to dilated capillaries or next to crypts. Polymorphs may be present between the crypt epithelial cells, and although crypt abscesses occur, they are less common than in active ulcerative colitis or Crohn disease.[111] Clusters of polymorphs also infiltrate

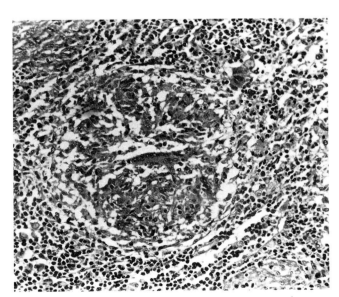

FIGURE 69-15 Crohn disease. A noncaseating granuloma in the submucosa (hematoxylin and eosin; × 250original magnification).

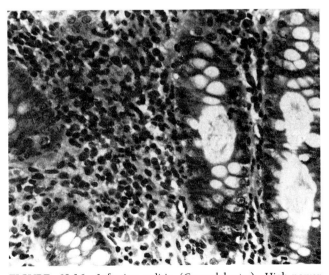

FIGURE 69-16 Infective colitis (*Campylobacter*). High-power view of a rectal biopsy showing patchy inflammation with neutrophil polymorphs in the lamina propria. One crypt is infiltrated by neutrophils (hematoxylin and eosin; ×400 original magnification).

between the cells of the surface epithelium. Although plasma cells and lymphocytes may be increased, this is often masked by edema, and polymorphonuclear neutrophils dominate the picture (see Figure 69-16).

The crypt pattern is regular, although the superficial crypt epithelium may show degenerative changes, and there is dilatation of luminal parts of the crypts (crypt "withering").[112,113] Mucin depletion and flattening of epithelial cells are also seen. Crypt destruction may be marked by a multinucleate giant cell. Other less specific abnormalities include luminal pus, margination of polymorphs, and capillary microthrombi.[114]

The above description represents a characteristic pattern and is most common in biopsies taken at the onset of symptoms or within the first 7 days.[112]

Differential Diagnosis of the Major Inflammatory Bowel Disease Entities.

No single specific histologic feature is invariably present in one condition or absent from the others.[67] The concept of a spectrum of histologic appearances in chronic inflammatory bowel disease in childhood is useful and convenient for practical assessment.[72] This is particularly true in the early histologic appearance of children with Crohn disease when the definitive criteria may not be present. From the point of view of histologic assessment, particularly of mucosal biopsies, which are small in size, the histopathologist is faced with an apparent range of inflammatory changes falling within a continuous spectrum. This approach is not intended to imply that inflammatory bowel disease is generally a continuous spectrum of a single disease but reflects the difficulty of making a confident diagnosis by extrapolation from a very restricted sample of the organ in question. Although some findings may be highly suggestive of a particular diagnosis, in one study of children at first presentation of their illness, approximately one-third showed morphologic features suggestive of both conditions[61]—in particular, diffuse active chronic coloproctitis with crypt distortion suggestive of ulcerative colitis but also with granulomas and/or ileal disease too excessive for a backwash ileitis. It is not yet clear if these children will have a different natural history.

Key features of the various disorders are the following:

- *Ulcerative colitis.* There is crypt distortion, villous surface, goblet cell depletion, prominent crypt abscesses, and diffuse predominantly plasma cell infiltrate of the lamina propria.
- *Crohn disease.* Granulomas are present (25–28% of biopsies). Crypts remain well aligned with little mucin depletion despite a moderate inflammatory cell infiltrate. The infiltrate is often patchy. Basal lymphoid aggregates are helpful. Crypt abscesses and cryptitis are less constant than in ulcerative or infective colitis. There are microgranulomas (focal collections of inflammatory cells including histiocytes) and definite patchy inflammation.
- *Indeterminate colitis.* Although this term was first used in the histologic assessment of colectomy specimens, it

has now gained general acceptance for mucosal biopsies.[67,72,115] It is used when features of chronic inflammatory bowel disease are present, but distinction as to type is not possible.
- *Infective colitis.* Crypts remain aligned but show degeneration. Polymorphs are the most conspicuous inflammatory cells; they cluster in the lamina propria and migrate between crypt epithelial cells, particularly in the superficial mucosa. Plasma cell infiltrate is light to moderate. Edema is prominent.

Other Recognized Abnormalities.

The most common abnormality under this heading is a cellular infiltrate in the lamina propria with regular crypt architecture and variable goblet cell depletion. In some biopsies, a focal polymorph infiltrate in the lamina propria may be seen. A mild increase in plasma cells and lymphocytes may be an accompanying feature. The changes can be interpreted only after consideration of the clinical data (eg, Crohn disease may be suggested if there is evidence of disease at another site).[94] Some specific features that can easily be overlooked include the following:

1. *Microgranulomas in Crohn disease.*
2. *Spirochetosis.* This represents infection of colorectal epithelium by spirochetes that belong to the genus *Borrelia.* Histologically, this is seen as a basophilic fringe along the apical border of surface epithelial cells. It is not clear whether infection produces symptoms.
3. *Amoebae. Entamoeba histolytica* may cause large intestinal infection, which may closely resemble chronic inflammatory bowel disease in childhood.[116] Ulcers occur, which may result in perforation of the bowel wall. Amoebae are found on or just beneath the surface of ulcers, but in severe cases, they enter the inflamed bowel wall and may be seen within blood vessels. Diastase-PAS is a useful staining method for demonstrating them in histologic preparations.
4. *Cytomegalovirus.* This viral infection may occur in immunosuppressed children both in disease states such as AIDS or following organ or bone marrow transplant. Inclusions occur in endothelial cells, fibroblasts, and macrophages. More rarely, they are found in epithelial cells. Immunocytochemistry and polymerase chain reaction will increase the sensitivity of viral detection within the tissue.
5. *Chronic granulomatous disease.* This rare disorder is characterized by recurrent infections with catalase-positive organisms; the patients' neutrophils are unable to kill the organisms. Gastrointestinal involvement is well recognized; there may be narrowing of the gastric antrum owing to local granulomas, and perianal fistulae may occur. Clinically, the disease may mimic Crohn disease or tuberculosis, especially when there is ileal involvement with intestinal obstruction.[117,118] Histologically, the appearances consist of paucity of neutrophils and the presence of mainly eosinophilic inflammatory infiltrate, eosinophilic crypt abscesses, and pigmented (often reddish crystalline inclusions) macrophages in

the lamina propria of the mucosa.[68,69] Granulomas, if present, are exuberant

6. *Allergic colitis.* One manifestation of food protein allergies, in particular with cow's milk protein intolerance, is diarrhea and abdominal pain; perianal disease and constipation have also recently been reported.[119] Changes may be seen in the esophagus and duodenum and also within the colon. On endoscopy, the mucosa may appear edematous; histology shows intact architecture but large numbers of eosinophils in the lamina propria. Eosinophils may also show degranulation or infiltrate the crypt and surface epithelium.

7. *Microscopic colitis.* Histologic assessment allows separation into collagenous (a thickened [> 10 μm] collagenous band under the surface epithelium) and lymphocytic (increased intraepithelial lymphocytes) variants. Both are more common in adults and are associated with watery chronic diarrhea. This condition stresses the importance of performing biopsies in the absence of overt endoscopic abnormalities.

8. *Autism-associated colitis.* A number of children with autism and nonspecific GI symptoms have been described in whom there have been changes on endoscopy and on histology. This has included prominent lymphoid hyperplasia within the ileum and very focal active inflammation with more widespread chronic inflammation within the colon and rectum. The features are not thought typical for inflammatory bowel disease, but the findings have met with some controversy.[120]

9. *Intractable ulcerating enterocolitis of infancy.* This form of familial disorder was first described over a decade ago by Sanderson and colleagues.[71] The onset of disease is within the first few months from birth, and the condition responds poorly to immunosuppressive therapy requiring colectomies. Histologic appearances include deep well-circumscribed ulcers, which penetrate into the submucosa and reach even the muscularis propria. The mucosa between the ulcers shows only a mild increase in chronic inflammatory cells. The condition is associated with Epstein-Barr virus–related lymphoid proliferations, and patients can develop B-cell lymphomas (A. D. Ramsay, personal communication, July 2003).

DISORDERS OF MOTILITY

These are due to abnormalities in the enteric nervous system or defects in the enteric musculature, resulting in functional intestinal obstruction. Of these, Hirschsprung disease is the most common, with an incidence of about 1 in 4,500 live births. The condition results from congenital aganglionosis (absent enteric nervous system) of a variable length of distal bowel but can affect the entire colon and extend to involve the small intestine and beyond.[121]

Care should be taken with the use of the term intestinal neuronal dysplasia because it means different things to different people.[122]

Other neural disorders include hypoganglionosis and hyperganglionosis. The latter may be seen proximal to the aganglionic segment in some patients with Hirschsprung disease.[123] Only aganglionosis can be diagnosed on a suc-tion rectal biopsy. For the diagnosis of hypo- or hyperganglionosis, the myenteric plexus must be examined.[124]

Suction Rectal Biopsy. *The Biopsy.* Ideally, three biopsies should be obtained 2 to 5 cm above the pectinate line and should include macroscopically obvious submucosa. The middle biopsy is processed into paraffin wax for 150 HE-stained 3 to 4 μm–thick serial sections to allow identification of any neurons present. A large number of sections must be examined to ensure that no neurons are missed even if the biopsy is taken from the physiologically hypoganglionic segment of the lower rectum.[125]

The other two are snap-frozen and cryostat sectioned alternately for HE (5–7 μm thick) and "spares" (10–12 μm thick). Two of the spares that include the most submucosa are incubated for acetylcholinesterase (AChE) activity by the standard method[126] or if the result is required urgently by the rapid method.[127]

In the case of an obstructed neonate, there is an urgency to confirm or exclude the diagnosis of Hirschsprung disease. The biopsies are usually taken not far from the dentate line. In this instance, the biopsies are snap-frozen, and serial cryostat sections are cut immediately and stained for HE. If no neurons are identified and the sections contain mucosa, muscularis mucosa, and submucosa, adjacent sections are cut and incubated for AChE activity initially using the rapid method. If the result is ambivalent, the standard method is applied on further sections. The remainder of the biopsy is fixed and processed into paraffin wax, and, subsequently, serial sections (as above) are cut and stained for HE.

Histologically normal rectal biopsy contains clusters of neurons in the submucosa in contrast to one from a patient with Hirschsprung disease, which has no neurons but has enlarged submucosal nerve trunks. However, biopsies taken from the physiologically hypoganglionic lower rectum close to the anal canal also have large nerves, particularly in association with large blood vessels. In this situation, one must not attempt to make the diagnosis of Hirschsprung disease. Of course, if an obvious neuron is found, then the diagnosis can be excluded. It is always wise to state, "Hirschsprung disease is excluded at the level examined" because the biopsy may have been taken above the aganglionic segment. Is not possible to know accurately how far from the anal verge the biopsy comes. On occasion, surgeons claim that the biopsy was performed at least 5 cm from the dentate line, but on histology, the biopsy contains anal skin instead of rectal mucosa.

AChE Activity. AChE-positive fibers are sparse and fine in the muscularis mucosae and lamina propria of the mucosa in normal rectum. There are, however, variations within normal limits. In Hirschsprung disease, at any age, there is an obvious increase in thick, knotted, crossing AChE-positive fibers in the muscularis mucosae and thick nerves in the submucosa, with no neurons present. With experience, it is possible to distinguish neurons from nerves on the AChE preparation, but it is safer to rely on the HE to do this. In an older baby with Hirschsprung disease, there is also an increase in the lamina propria in thick

AChE-positive fibers, which run not only vertically but also horizontally.

If no obvious neurons are found in the HE-stained cryostat section and the AChE pattern is not typical of Hirschsprung disease, it is vital to examine the 150 serial paraffin sections to be certain that the specimen is indeed aganglionic.

In rare cases of total colonic aganglionosis, AChE preparation may not be helpful. In these patients, there is no increase in AChE-positive fibers, and thick submucosal nerve trunks may also be absent. As many as possible serial HE-stained paraffin sections must be examined to identify any neurons present.

Age of the Patient.   In the newborn, the submucosal ganglia appear as small clusters of immature neurons, which are less easy to recognize than the larger neurons in an older baby or a child on an HE-stained section. Not differentiating the hematoxylin before the eosin helps, and if no neurons are seen, examination of the AChE pattern in the muscularis mucosae allows correct diagnosis.

Intestinal Ganglioneuromatosis.   One serious condition one should be aware of is transmural intestinal ganglioneuromatosis. These appearances can be evident in the submucosa even in a suction rectal biopsy and consist of profound proliferations of neural tissue (neurons, supporting cells, and nerves) that appear as thickened nerve trunks embedded with mature nerve cells. If there is a suspicion of ganglioneuromatosis, this warrants further investigations to exclude multiple endocrine neoplasia type IIB (MEN IIB). This involves germline M918T and/or A883 F mutation analysis of the *RET* proto-oncogene.[128] Children with intestinal ganglioneuromatosis and the above-mentioned molecular diagnosis of MEN IIB inevitably develop medullary thyroid carcinoma. In our experience, monitoring the calcitonin concentrations and scanning for adrenal and thyroid masses are not sufficient because microscopic medullary thyroid carcinoma can be present without raised calcitonin concentrations, even with pentagastrin stimulation or without identifiable masses on imaging. A prophylactic thyroidectomy is recommended, as well as continued surveillance of the adrenal glands for evidence of pheochromocytoma.

Full-Thickness Intestinal and Seromuscular Biopsies.
Identification of other intestinal neuromuscular disorders cannot be made on suction rectal biopsies. These require larger full-thickness bowel samples taken at the time of raising a stoma. However, seromuscular biopsies, if well oriented and of sufficient size, may be helpful in some myopathic disorders (fibrosis and/or abnormal contractile protein profile),[129] especially when using special stains and immunohistochemistry and acquired inflammatory conditions (ganglionitis or leiomyositis).[64,65,130]

Caution should be exercised when interpreting AChE preparations of biopsies sometimes taken from stoma sites, particularly from ileostomy sites. Small bowel normally has many AChE-positive fibers in the lamina propria, and AChE preparations on biopsies taken proximal to the splenic flexure may also be unreliable.[131]

HE-stained frozen sections of intraoperative seromuscular biopsies are used for positioning the stoma.

REFERENCES

1. Sakula J, Shiner M. Coeliac disease with atrophy of the small intestine mucosa. Lancet 1957;273:876–7.
2. Kilby A. Pediatric small intestinal biopsy capsule with two ports. Gut 1976;17:158–9.
3. Manuel PD, Walker-Smith JA, France NE. Patchy enteropathy. Gut 1979;20:211–5.
4. Granot E, Goodman-Weill M, Pizov G, Sherman Y. Histological comparison of suction capsule and endoscopic small intestinal mucosal biopsies in children. J Pediatr Gastroenterol Nutr 1993;16:397–401.
5. Thomson M, Kitchen P, Jones A, et al. Are endoscopic biopsies as good as suction biopsies for diagnosis of enteropathy? J Pediatr Gastroenterol Nutr 1999;29:438–41.
6. Sullivan PB, Phillips MB, Neale G. Endoscopic capsule biopsy of the small intestine. J Pediatr Gastroenterol Nutr 1988;7:544–7.
7. Squires R, Colletti R. Indications for pediatric gastrointestinal endoscopy: a medical position statement of the North American Society for Pediatric Gastroenterology and Nutrition. J Pediatr Gastroenterol Nutr 1996;23:107–10.
8. Vandenplas Y. Reflux esophagitis in infants and children: a report from the working group on gastro-esophageal reflux disease of the European Society of Pediatric Gastroenterology and Nutrition. J Pediatr Gastroenterol Nutr 1994;18:413–22.
9. Murphy MS. Sedation for invasive procedures in pediatrics. Arch Dis Child 1997;77:281–4.
10. Holmes R, Hourihane DO, Booth CC. Dissecting microscope appearances of jejunal biopsy specimens from patients with idiopathic steatorrhoea. Lancet 1961;i:81–3.
11. Walker-Smith JA. Dissecting microscope appearance of small bowel mucosa in children. Arch Dis Child 1967;42:626.
12. Rubin CE, Dobbins WO. Peroral biopsy of the small intestine: a review of its diagnostic usefulness. Gastroenterology 1965;49:676–97.
13. Walker-Smith JA. Variation of small intestinal morphology with age. Arch Dis Child 1972;47:80–3.
14. Wright NA, Watson A, Morley A, et al. Cell kinetics in flat (avillous) mucosa of human small intestine. Gut 1973;14:701–10.
15. Ferguson A, Maxwell JD, Carr KE. Progressive changes in the small intestinal villous pattern with increasing length of gestation. J Pathol 1969;99:87–91.
16. MacDonald TT, Spencer J, Viney JL, et al. Selective biopsy of human Peyer's patches during ileal endoscopy. Gastroenterology 1987;93:1356–62.
17. Maluenda C, Phillips AD, Briddon A, Walker-Smith JA. Quantitative analysis of small intestinal mucosa in cow's milk sensitive enteropathy. J Pediatr Gastroenterol Nutr 1984;3:349–56.
18. Lee FD, Toner PG. Biopsy pathology of the small intestine. London: Chapman and Hall; 1980. p. 69–81.
19. Variend S, Placzek M, Raafat F, Walker-Smith JA. Small intestinal mucosal fat in childhood enteropathies. J Clin Pathol 1984;37:373–7.
20. Murch SH, Fertleman CR, Rodrigues C, et al. Autoimmune enteropathy with distinct mucosal features in T cell activation deficiency: the contribution of T cells to the mucosal lesion. J Pediatr Gastroenterol Nutr 1999;28:393–9
21. Ferguson A. Intraepithelial lymphocytes of the small intestine. Gut 1977;18:921–37.
22. Phillips AD, Rice SJ, France NE, Walker-Smith JA. Small intesti-

nal intraepithelial lymphocyte levels in cow's milk protein intolerance. Gut 1979;20:509–12.

23. Ferguson A, Murray D. Quantitation of intraepithelial lymphocytes in human jejunum. Gut 1971;12:988–94.

24. Phillips AD, Thomas AG, Walker-Smith JA. Cryptosporidium, chronic diarrhoea and the proximal small intestinal mucosa. Gut 1992;33:1057–61.

25. Marsh MN. Studies of intestinal lymphoid tissue. III. Quantitative analyses of epithelial lymphocytes in the small intestine of human control subjects and of patients with celiac sprue. Gastroenterology 1980;79:481–92.

26. Phillips AD. Epithelial lymphocytes in celiac sprue. Gastroenterology 1981;80:1085–7.

27. Lewis DC, Walker-Smith JA, Phillips AD. Polymorphonuclear neutrophil leucocytes in childhood Crohn's disease: a morphological study. J Pediatr Gastroenterol Nutr 1987;6:430–8.

28. Enerbach L. Mast cell in rat gastrointestinal. Acta Pathol Microbiol Scand 1966;80:289.

29. Strobel S, Miller HPR, Ferguson A. Human intestinal mast cells: evaluation of fixation and staining techniques. J Clin Pathol 1981;34:851–8.

30. Leder LD. The chloracetoesterase reaction: a useful means of histological diagnosis of haematological disorders from paraffin sections of skin. Am J Dermatopathol 1979;1:39–42.

31. Sanderson IR, Slavin G, Walker-Smith JA. Density of mucosal mast cells in the lamina propria of the colon and terminal ileum of children. J Clin Pathol 1985;38:771–3.

32. Phillips AD, Jenkins P, Raafat F, Walker-Smith JA. Congenital microvillous atrophy: specific diagnostic features. Arch Dis Child 1985;60:135–40.

33. Heuschkel R, Phillips AD, Meadows NJ, Walker-Smith JA. Cystic fibrosis diagnosed by small bowel biopsy. Illus Case Rep Gastroenterol 1995;1:123–7.

34. Phillips AD, France NE, Walker-Smith JA. The structure of the enterocyte in relation to its position on the villus in childhood: an electron microscopical study. Histopathology 1979;3:117–30.

35. Ulshen MH, Rollo JL. Pathogenesis of *Escherichia coli* gastroenteritis in man—another mechanism. N Engl J Med 1980; 302:99–101.

36. Dahlqvist A. Assay of intestinal disaccharidases. Enzymol Biol Clin 1970;11:52–66.

37. Phillips AD, Smith MW, Walker-Smith JA. Selective alteration of brush-border hydrolases in intestinal diseases in childhood. Clin Sci 1988;74:193–200.

38. Phillips AD, Avigad S, Sacks J, Rice SJ, et al. Microvillous surface area in secondary disaccharidase deficiency. Gut 1980;21:44–8.

39. Davidson GP, Robb TA. Detection of primary and secondary sucrose malabsorption in children by means of the breath hydrogen technique. Med J Aust 1983;2:29–32

40. Booth IW, Stange G, Murer H, et al. Defective jejunal brush-border Na+/H+ exchange: a cause of congenital secretory diarrhoea. Lancet 1985;i:1066–9.

41. Spencer J, Isaacson PG, Diss TC, MacDonald TT. Expression of disulfide-linked and non-disulfide-linked forms of the T cell receptor γδ heterodimer in human intestinal intraepithelial lymphocytes. Eur J Immunol 1989;19:1335–8.

42. Walker-Smith JA, Murch SH. Intractable diarrhoea. In: Diseases of the small intestine in childhood. 4th ed. Oxford (UK): Oxford Isis Medical Media; 1999. p. 281–98.

43. Brandtzaeg P. Immunologic basis for celiac disease, inflammatory bowel disease and type B chronic gastritis. Curr Opin Gastroenterol 1991;7:450.

44. Walker-Smith JA, Murch SH. Coeliac disease. In: Diseases of the small intestine in childhood. 4th ed. Oxford (UK): Oxford Isis Medical Media; 1999. p. 235–77.

45. Harper SJ, Pringle JH, Gillies A, et al. Simultaneous in situ hybridisation of native mRNA and immunoglobulin detection by conventional immunofluorescence in paraffin wax embedded specimens. J Clin Pathol 1992;45:114–9.

46. Sanderson IR, Ouellette AJ, Carter EA, Harmatz PR. Ontogeny of Ia messenger RNA in the mouse small intestinal epithelium is modulated by age of weaning and diet. Gastroenterology 1993;105:974–80.

47. Freeman TC, Collins AJ, Heavens RP, Tivey DR. Genetic regulation of enterocyte function: a quantitative in situ hybridisation study of lactase-phlorizin hydrolase and Na(+)-glucose cotransporter mRNAs in rabbit small intestine. Eur J Physiol 1993;422:570–6.

48. Lechner S, Müller-Ladner U, Renke B, et al. Gene expression pattern of laser microdissected colonic crypts of adenomas with low grade dysplasia. Gut 2003;52:1148–53.

49. Stappenbeck TS, Mills JC, Gordon JI. Molecular features of adult mouse small intestinal epithelial progenitors. Proc Natl Acad Sci U S A 2003;100:1004–9.

50. Perez-Machado MA, Thomson MA, Walker-Smith JA, Murch SH. Constitutively decreased Th3 suppressor cells may allow low-dose sensitisation in CMSE. J Pediatr Gastroenterol Nutr 1999;29:564.

51. Hauer AC, Bajaj-Elliott M, Williams CB, et al. An analysis of interferon gamma, IL-4, IL-5 and IL-10 production by ELISPOT and quantitative reverse transcriptase-PCR in human Peyer's patches. Cytokine 1998;10:627–34.

52. Trier JS, Browning TH. Epithelial-cell renewal in cultured duodenal biopsies in celiac sprue. N Engl J Med 1970;283:1245–50.

53. Fais S, Maiuri L, Pallone F, et al. Gliadin induced changes in the expression of MHC-class II antigens by human small intestinal epithelium. Organ culture studies with coeliac disease mucosa. Gut 1992;33:472–5.

54. Hicks S, Frankel G, Kaper JB, et al. Role of intimin and bundle forming pili in enteropathogenic *Escherichia coli* adhesion to pediatric intestine in vitro. Infect Immun 1998;66:1570–8.

55. Thomas A, Phillips AD, Walker-Smith JA. The value of proximal small intestinal biopsy in the differential diagnosis of chronic diarrhoea. Arch Dis Child 1992;67:741–3.

56. Walker-Smith JA, Guandalini S, Schmitz J, et al. Revised criteria for diagnosis of coeliac disease. Arch Dis Child 1990;65: 909–11.

57. Phillips AD, Schmitz J. Familial microvillous atrophy: a clinicopathological survey of 23 cases. J Pediatr Gastroenterol Nutr 1992;14:380–96.

58. Cutz E, Rhoads JM, Drumm B, et al. Microvillous inclusion disease: an inherited defect of brush-border assembly and differentiation. N Engl J Med 1989;320:646–51.

59. Hill SM, Phillips AD, Walker-Smith JA. Enteropathogenic *E coli* and life-threatening chronic diarrhoea. Gut 1991;32:154–8.

60. Knutton S, Phillips AD, Smith HR, et al. Screening for enteropathogenic *Escherichia coli* in infants with diarrhoea by the fluorescent-actin staining test. Infect Immun 1991;59:365–71.

61. Deere HMR, Casson D, Thomson M, et al. Histological comparison of recto-sigmoid and full colonoscopic biopsies in the assessment of inflammatory bowel disease in childhood. Gut 1998;42:A55.

62. Chong SKF, Bartram C, Campbell GA. Chronic inflammatory bowel disease in childhood. BMJ 1982;284:1–3.

63. Noblet HR. A rectal suction biopsy tube for use in the diagnosis of Hirschsprung's disease. J Pediatr Surg 1969;4:406–9.

64. Schäppi MG, Smith VV, Milla PJ, Lindley KJ. Eosinophilic

myenteric ganglionitis is associated with functional intestinal obstruction. Gut 2003;52:752-5.

65. Ruuska TH, Karikoski R, Smith VV, Milla PJ. Acquired myopathic intestinal pseudo-obstruction may be due to autoimmune enteric leiomyositis. Gastroenterology 2002;122:1133–9.

66. Smith VV, Milla PJ. Histological phenotypes of enteric smooth muscle disease causing functional intestinal obstruction in childhood. Histopathology 1997;31:112–22.

67. Jenkins D, Balsitis M, Gallivan S, et al. Guidelines for the initial biopsy diagnosis of suspected chronic idiopathic inflammatory bowel disease. J Clin Pathol 1997;59:93–105.

68. Schäppi MG, Smith VV, Goldblatt D, et al. Colitis in chronic granulomatous disease. Arch Dis Child 2001;84:147–51.

69. Schäppi MG, Klein NJ, Lindley KJ, et al. The nature of colitis in chronic granulomatous disease. J Pediatr Gastroenterol Nutr 2003;36:623–31.

70. Shah NF, Schappi M, Long S, et al. Tufting enteropathy also affects the colon. J Pediatr Gastroenterol Nutr 1999;28:569.

71. Sanderson IR, Risdon RA, Walker-Smith JA. Intractable ulcerating enterocolitis of infancy. Arch Dis Child 1991;66:295–9.

72. Chong SKF, Blackshaw AJ, Boyle S, et al. Histological diagnosis of chronic inflammatory bowel disease in childhood. Gut 1985;26:55–9.

73. Domizio P. Pathology of chronic inflammatory bowel disease in children. Ballieres Clin Gastroenterol 1994;8:35–63.

74. Beattie RM, Nicholls SW, Domizio P, et al. Endoscopic assessment of the colonic response to corticosteroids in children with ulcerative colitis. J Pediatr Gastroenterol Nutr 1996;22:373–9.

75. Markowitz J, Kahn E, Grancher K, et al. Atypical rectosigmoid histology in children with newly diagnosed ulcerative colitis. Am J Gastroenterol 1993;88:2034–7.

76. Morson BC, Dawson IMP. Gastrointestinal pathology. 2nd ed. Oxford (UK): Blackwell; 1979.

77. Watson AJ, Roy AD. Paneth cells in the large intestine in ulcerative colitis. J Pathol Bacteriol 1960;80:309–16.

78. Skinner JM, Whitehead R, Pins J. Argentaffin cells in ulcerative colitis. Gut 1971;12:636–8.

79. Gledhill A, Enticott ME, Howe S. Variation in the argyrophil cell population of the rectum in ulcerative colitis and adenocarcinoma. J Pathol 1986;149:287–91.

80. Edwards FC, Truelove SC. The course and prognosis of ulcerative colitis, parts III and IV. Gut 1964;5:1–22.

81. Jalan KN, Sircus W, Card WI, et al. An experience of ulcerative colitis. 1. Toxic dilatation in 55 cases. Gastroenterology 1969;57:68–82.

82. Basu MK. Oral manifestations of Crohn's disease: studies in the pathogenesis. Proc R Soc Med. 1976;69:765–6.

83. Dunne WT, Cooke WT, Allan RN. Enzymatic and morphometric evidence for Crohn's disease as a diffuse lesion of the gastrointestinal tract. Gut 1977;18:290–4.

84. Lenaerts C, Roy CC, Vaillancourt M, et al. High incidence of upper gastrointestinal tract involvement in children with Crohn's disease. Pediatrics 1989;83:777–81.

85. Schmidt-Sommerfeld E, Kirschner BS, Stephens JK. Endoscopic and histologic findings in the upper gastrointestinal tract of children with Crohn's disease. J Pediatr Gastroenterol Nutr 1990;11:448–54.

86. Cameron DJ. Upper and lower gastrointestinal endoscopy in children and adolescents with Crohn's disease: a prospective study. J Gastroenterol Hepatol 1991;6:355–8.

87. Higgins BC, Allan RN. Crohn's disease of the distal ileum. Gut 1980;21:933–40.

88. Morson BC. The early histological lesion of Crohn's disease. Proc R Soc Med 1972;65:71–2.

89. Geboes M, Vantrappen G. The value of colonoscopy in the diagnosis of Crohn's disease. Gastrointest Endosc 1975;22:18–23.

90. Waye JD. Endoscopy in inflammatory bowel disease. Clin Gastroenterol 1980;9:297–306.

91. Palder SB, Shandling B, Bilik R, et al. Perianal complications of paediatric Crohn's disease. J Pediatr Surg 1991;26:513–5.

92. Cook MG, Dixon MF. An analysis of the reliability of detection and diagnostic value of various pathological features in Crohn's disease and ulcerative colitis. Gut 1973;14:255–62.

93. Yardley JH, Donowitz M. Colorectal biopsy in inflammatory bowel disease. In: Yardley JH, Morson BC, Abell MR, editors. The gastrointestinal tract. International Academy of Pathology monograph. Baltimore: Williams & Wilkins; 1997. p. 50.

94. Talbot IC, Price AB. Biopsy pathology in colorectal disease. London: Chapman & Hall; 1987.

95. Hamilton SR, Bassey HJR, Morson BC. En face histological technique to demonstrate mucosal inflammatory lesions in macroscopically uninvolved colon of Crohn's disease resection specimens. Lab Invest 1980;42:121.

96. Morson BC. Rectal biopsy in inflammatory bowel disease. N Engl J Med 1972;287:1337–9.

97. McGovern VJ, Goulston SJM. Crohn's disease of the colon. Gut 1968;9:164–79.

98. Rotterdam H, Korelitz BI, Sommers SC. Microgranulomas in grossly normal rectal mucosa in Crohn's disease. Am J Clin Pathol 1977;67:550–4.

99. Surawicz CM, Meisel JL, Ylvisaker T, et al. Rectal biopsy in the diagnosis of Crohn's disease: value of multiple biopsies and serial sectioning. Gastroenterology 1981;81:66–71.

100. Anderson FH, Bogoch A. Biopsies of the large bowel in regional enteritis. Can Med Assoc J 1968;98:150–3.

101. Petri M, Poulsen SS, Christensen K, Jarnum S. The incidence of granulomas in serial sections of rectal biopsies from patients with Crohn's disease. Acta Pathol Micro Immunol Scand A 1982;90:145–7.

102. Kahn E, Markowitz J, Blomquist K, Daum F. The morphologic relationship of sinus and fistula formation to intestinal stenoses in children with Crohn's disease. Am J Gastroenterol 1993;88:1395–8.

103. Lee EY, Stenson WF, DeSchryver-Kecskemeti K. Thickening of the muscularis mucosae in Crohn's disease. Mod Pathol 1991;4:87–90.

104. Gomes P, du Boulay C, Smith CL, Holdstock G. Relationship between disease activity indices and colonoscopic findings in patients with colonic inflammatory disease. Gut 1986;27:92–5.

105. Glass RG, Baker WNW. Role of the granuloma in recurrent Crohn's disease. Gut 1976;17:75–7.

106. Chambers TJ, Morson BC. The granuloma in Crohn's disease. Gut 1979;20:269–74.

107. Wilson JAP, et al. Relationship of granulomas to clinical parameters in Crohn's disease. Gastroenterology 1980;78:1292.

108. Wolfson DM, Sachar DB, Cohen A, et al. Granulomas do not affect postoperative recurrence rates in Crohn's disease. Gastroenterology 1982;83:405–9.

109. Ward M, Webb JN. Rectal biopsy as a prognostic guide in Crohn's disease. J Clin Pathol 1977;30:126–31.

110. Kotanagi H, Kramer K, Fazio VW, Petras RE. Do microscopic abnormalities at resection margins correlate with increased anastomotic recurrence in Crohn's disease? Retrospective analysis of 100 cases. Dis Colon Rectum 1991;34:909–16.

111. Anand BS, Malhotra V, Bhattacharya SK, et al. Rectal histology in acute bacillary dysentery. Gastroenterology 1986;90:654–60.

112. Kumar NB, Nostrant JJ, Appleman HD. The histopathologic spectrum of acute self-limited colitis (acute infectious-type colitis). Am J Surg Pathol 1982;6:523–9.

113. Surawicz CM, Belic L. Rectal biopsy helps to distinguish acute self-limited colitis from idiopathic inflammatory bowel disease. Gastroenterology 1984;86:104–13.

114. Mathan MM, Mathan VI. Local Schwartzman reaction in the rectal mucosa in acute diarrhoea. J Pathol 1985;146:179–87.

115. Price AB. Indeterminate colitis—broadening the perspective. Curr Diagn Pathol 1996;3:35–44.

116. Sanderson IR, Walker-Smith JA. Indigenous amoebiasis: an important differential diagnosis of chronic inflammatory bowel disease. BMJ 1984;289:823–4.

117. Isaacs D, Wright VM, Shaw DG, et al. Chronic granulomatous disease mimicking Crohn's disease. J Pediatr Gastroenterol Nutr 1985;4:498–501.

118. Harris BH, Boles ET. Intestinal lesions in chronic granulomatous disease of childhood. J Pediatr Surg 1973;8:955.

119. Iacono G, Cavataio F, Montalto G , et al. Intolerance of cow's milk and chronic constipation in children. N Engl J Med 1998;339:1100–44.

120. Wakefield A, Murch SH, Anthony A, et al. Ileal-lymphoid-nodular hyperplasia, non-specific colitis, and pervasive developmental disorder in children. Lancet 1998;351:637–41.

121. Senyuz OF, Buyukunal C, Danismend N, et al. Extensive intestinal aganglionosis. J Pediatr Surg 1989;24:453–6.

122. Lake BD. Intestinal neuronal dysplasia. Why does it only occur in parts of Europe? Virchows Arch 1995;426:537–9.

123. Meier-Ruge W. Hirschsprung's disease: its aetiology, pathogenesis and differential diagnosis. In: Grundman E, Firsten YM, editors. Current topics in pathology. Vol. 59. Berlin: Springer-Verlag; 1974. p. 131.

124. Smith VV. Intestinal neuronal density in childhood: a baseline for the objective assessment of hypo- and hyperganglionosis. Pediatr Pathol 1993;13:225–37.

125. Aldridge RT, Campbell PE. Ganglion cells distribution in the normal rectum and anal canal: a basis for the diagnosis of Hirschsprung's disease by a rectal biopsy. J Pediatr Surg 1968;3:475–89.

126. Lake BD, Puri P, Nixon HH, Claireaux AE. Hirschsprung's disease: an appraisal of histochemically demonstrated acetyl cholinesterase (AChE) activity in suction rectal biopsy specimens as an aid to diagnosis. Arch Pathol Lab Med 1978;102:244–7.

127. Filipe MI, Lake BD, editors. Appendix 5. In: Histochemistry in pathology. 2nd ed. Edinburgh: Churchill Livingstone; 1990. p. 463–4.

128. Smith VV, Eng C, Milla PJ. Intestinal ganglioneuromatosis and multiple endocrine neoplasia type 2B: implications for treatment. Gut 1999;45:143–6.

129. Smith VV, Milla PJ. Histological phenotypes of enteric smooth muscle disease causing functional intestinal obstruction in childhood. Histopathology 1997;31:112–22.

130. Smith VV, Gregson N, Foggensteiner L, et al. Acquired intestinal aganglionosis and circulating auto-antibodies without neoplasia or other neural involvement. Gastroenterology 1997;112:1366–71.

131. Meier-Ruge W. Hirschsprung's disease: its aetiology, pathogenesis and differential diagnosis. Curr Top Pathol 1974;59:131–79.

CHAPTER 70

GASTROINTESTINAL MANOMETRY: METHODOLOGY AND INDICATIONS

Samuel Nurko, MD, MPH

One of the most important functions of the gastrointestinal tract is to provide energy and nutrition. To accomplish this, the gastrointestinal tract has evolved not only specific functions for digestion and absorption but also complex mechanisms to allow for the ingestion of nutrients, their transport through different specialized areas, and the expulsion of unused portions at times when it is socially acceptable. The main result of this movement is the aboral transport or "propulsion" of gastrointestinal contents, and it results from the complex interaction between the muscles, the myenteric plexus, the peripheral nervous system. and the brain (see Chapter 4, "Motility").

Each area of the gastrointestinal tract has a specific pattern of motility. These patterns have been characterized for the esophagus, antroduodenum, jejunum and ileum, sphincter of Oddi (SO), colon, and anorectum. It has been shown that alterations in those patterns will produce functional dysfunction and clinical symptoms. By studying these alterations, it is often possible to determine if the problem that the patient has is related to motility dysfunction and if the dysfunction is occurring in the muscle or the intrinsic or extrinsic nerves.

When the symptoms of the patient suggest a motility disorder, careful exclusion of anatomic, mucosal, or metabolic disorders needs to be accomplished before motility studies are undertaken (Table 70-1).[1-3] The exclusion of an anatomic lesion is the initial and most important step, and the usual techniques that are used for this purpose are mainly radiologic or occasionally endoscopic and are reviewed in different chapters in this book.

Once a decision has been made that the problem is related to gastrointestinal motility dysfunction, transit through different segments can be evaluated, and the specific contractile or electrical activity may be studied (see Table 70-1). Research that is used to study transit includes mainly scintigraphic methods, although other techniques, such as different markers or ultrasonography, have been used. These techniques are discussed in other sections of this book. The main focus of this chapter is on tests that have been designed to study the myoelectric and motor phenomena of the gastrointestinal tract.[1]

GASTROINTESTINAL MANOMETRY

Gastrointestinal manometry has evolved during the past years and has changed from being a research technique to becoming a useful diagnostic tool.[1] The role of gastrointestinal manometry has been defined more clearly for

TABLE 70-1   APPROACH TO THE PATIENT WITH SUSPECTED MOTILITY DISORDER

1. Exclude anatomic problems (*the most important initial step, and it should be undertaken in all patients*)
   Radiography
       Plain films, upper gastrointestinal series with small bowel follow-through, barium enema, endoscopy
2. Exclude mucosal or metabolic disorders
       Endoscopy and biopsy, laboratory tests (metabolic, endocrine, etc)
3. Evaluate transit (*provides actual information on how effective the motility is*)
   pH probe/impedance
   Scintigraphy
       Gastric emptying
       Esophageal emptying
       Gallbladder emptying
       Small bowel–colon transit
   Barium
       Videofluoroscopy barium swallow
       Esophageal emptying
   Other studies to evaluate transit
       Marker-perfusion studies
       Oroanal transit—color markers, radiopaque markers
       Orocecal transit—lactulose breath test
       Colonic transit—radiopaque markers
       Ultrasonography
       Breath tests
4. Evaluate contractile activity (*provides information on contractile activity and allows the detection of problems in smooth muscle, intrinsic or extrinsic nerves*)
   Gastrointestinal manometry
5. Evaluate electrical activity (*provides information on the myoelectrical activity*)
   Electrogastrography, electromyography
6. Establish etiology and other associated problems
   Is this a primary or a secondary motility problem?
       Exclude systemic illness (endocrine, connective tissue disease, metabolic, etc)
       Associated abnormalities (autonomic dysfunction, muscle/nerve abnormalities, etc)

anorectal and esophageal manometry, and it has become better defined for small bowel and colonic motility.[1] In general, the manometric evaluation may detect aberrations that may be clinically insignificant,[4,5] and care needs to be exerted to avoid overinterpretation.[5] It is also important to remember that a dichotomy frequently exists between the use of manometry as an investigation technique or as a useful clinical test.

There are two main methods to perform gastrointestinal manometry. One requires the use of water perfusion with low-compliance systems, and the other uses miniature strain gauge pressure transducers mounted within thin catheters.[1] Most laboratories have water-perfused systems, in which the catheter is connected indirectly to a physiograph or computer by a series of transducers. The pressure is recorded from a predetermined opening in the catheters. The catheter is perfused with a pneumohydraulic pump at a predetermined rate, and pressure changes in the orifices are transmitted to pressure transducers with the use of low-compliance capillary tubing. The hydraulic capillary infusion system achieves high-fidelity recording of intraluminal pressure at infusion rates that go from 0.1 to 0.4 mL/min per port. Some disadvantages are that the system may not accurately reflect when measuring transient high-pressure events, the size of the catheters, and the amount of perfusate that can represent a large fluid bolus in small children and premature infants.

Solid-state catheters have strain gauge pressure transducers incorporated into specially designed catheters. The information is captured by digital recording systems and is later downloaded into computers for analysis. The main advantage of the solid-state catheter is that it does not have the risks associated with the perfusion, as well as the fact that it allows the performance of prolonged ambulatory studies. The main limitations have been the cost and the fact that it requires a minimum-size catheter, so these catheters cannot be used in small infants or children.

Independently of the method used, gastrointestinal manometry provides direct evidence about the contractile events of the organ that is being studied. Even though the study of gastrointestinal motility in children is similar to the study in adults, the performance of those studies in the pediatric population has certain important characteristics that make this more challenging. The first is related to the developmental aspects, the second to a paucity of studies in normal controls, and the third to technical difficulties.

The developmental aspects of gastrointestinal motility have been discussed in detail in previous chapters, but it must be remembered that any manometric findings need to be placed in that context before a study is considered abnormal.[1,6]

The lack of normal controls has been another important limiting factor for the establishment of normal motility patterns in children. This lack of control information can make the interpretation difficult and subjective and, as mentioned, may lead to overinterpretation.

Finally, there are special technical aspects that are unique to the performance of gastrointestinal manometry in children. Some are related to the size of the catheters,

the amount of fluid delivered with the perfused systems, or the lack of cooperation that may be found in younger children.[1] The size of the catheters can be a limiting factor because the standard manometric catheters have a diameter of 4.5 to 5 mm. The recent development of silicone extrusion tubing has allowed the creation of very small catheters that may include sleeves.[6,7] Studies have shown that manometric channels with diameters of 0.35 mm have acceptable fidelity and pressure increase rates with perfusion rates as low as 0.02 mL/min.[6] Multilumen catheter assemblies that measure less than 2 mm have been developed,[6] including the use of sleeves.[6–8]

APPROACH TO THE PATIENT

It is important to remember that for manometric studies to be successful, there must be a certain degree of patient cooperation. The understanding and degree of cooperation will vary according to the developmental age and previous experiences of the child. Results and patterns are difficult to interpret when there is crying or movement artifact, which can obscure pressure tracings.[1] Age and developmentally appropriate techniques should be used. The parents should be allowed to stay during the tests, and they can be an important resource for the child. The interaction between the parents and the children can be observed and can be important in understanding the child's symptoms.[1]

Young children may require sedation for the performance of the studies.[1] Medications that have been employed principally include chloral hydrate and midazolam. There are limited data on their effect on motility function. Studies have found no difference in esophageal or rectal manometry with chloral hydrate[9] or midazolam.[10]

SPECIFIC GASTROINTESTINAL MANOMETRY STUDIES

Recently, a pediatric task force of the American Motility Society (AMS) established minimum standards for the performance of manometric studies in children.[1] Standards for esophageal, antroduodenal, colonic, and anorectal manometry were published.[1]

ESOPHAGEAL MANOMETRY

Esophageal manometry is the gold standard for the diagnosis of primary motor disorders of the esophagus (Table 70-2).[4,11,12] It is most frequently performed in children with dysphagia who have no evidence of anatomic obstruction, and the clinical use of esophageal manometry is in defining the contractile characteristics of the esophagus.[1]

There are three functional regions of the esophagus: the upper esophageal sphincter (UES), the esophageal body, and the lower esophageal sphincter (LES). Both sphincter regions have a resting tone and relax in response to swallowing or other stimuli, and the body has contractions that propagate (Figure 70-1).

The UES is striated muscle that is maintained closed between swallows by tonic stimulation of the somatic nerves. It exhibits marked radial and axial asymmetry, with

TABLE 70-2 INDICATIONS FOR MANOMETRY STUDIES

Esophageal manometry
- Esophageal dysfunction that is not explained by anatomic or well-defined problems
- Dysphagia, odynophagia
- Diagnosis of achalasia and other primary esophageal motor disorders
- To support the diagnosis of connective tissue diseases or other systemic illness
- Evaluation of patients with achalasia post-treatment and recurrent symptoms
- Noncardiac chest pain
- Patients with gastroesophageal reflux in whom the diagnosis is not clear (to exclude primary motility disorders)
- Before a fundoplication when a severe motility disorder is suspected
- To localize lower esophageal sphincter before pH probe placement in patients with abnormal anatomy (eg, hiatal hernia)

Anorectal manometry
- To diagnose a nonrelaxing internal anal sphincter
- To diagnose pelvic floor dyssynergia
- To evaluate postoperative patients with Hirschsprung disease who have obstructive symptoms and to evaluate the effect of botulinum toxin
- To evaluate patients with fecal incontinence
- To evaluate postoperative patients after imperforate anus repair
- To decide if the patient is a candidate for biofeedback therapy

Antroduodenal manometry
- To establish the presence of pseudo-obstruction
- To classify pseudo-obstruction into myopathic or neuropathic forms
- To exclude a motility problem as the basis of the patients' symptoms; showing normal findings in children with "apparent intestinal failure"
- Evaluation of unexplained nausea and vomiting
- To distinguish between rumination and vomiting
- To exclude generalized motility dysfunction in patients with dysmotility elsewhere (eg, before colectomy)
- Indicated in patients with pseudo-obstruction being considered for intestinal transplant
- May be useful to predict outcome after feeding or after drug use in patients with pseudo-obstruction
- May suggest unexpected obstruction

Colonic motility manometry
- In the evaluation of selected patients with intractable constipation because it can be helpful to differentiate functional fecal retention from colonic pseudo-obstruction[78]
- Evaluation of children with pseudo-obstruction to establish presence of colonic involvement and to characterize the relationship between motor activity and persistent symptoms
- To establish the pathophysiology of persistent symptoms in selected children with Hirschsprung disease, imperforate anus, and other colorectal problems
- To assess colonic motor activity prior to intestinal transplant

Adapted from DiLorenzo C et al.[1]

greater values anteriorly and posteriorly than laterally.[4] It measures 0.5 to 1 cm at birth and increases in length to 3 cm in the adult.[13] UES relaxation occurs with swallowing. The manometric study of the UES has been difficult because the brisk movement of the larynx and sphincter is discordant with the movement of the intraluminal recording device. With the use of systems that can record changes greater than 400 mm Hg/s or sleeve devices, accurate measurements have become more feasible.[4] In adults, there is a wide range of reported UES pressure measurements, from 40 to 193 mm Hg, depending on the method used.[4] The information in normal children is very limited. It was reported to vary from 18 to 44 cm H_2O in one study.[14]

The esophageal body varies in length depending on the age of the patient. It is composed of striated and smooth muscle. In adults, approximately the upper 5% is exclusively striated muscle, the middle 35 to 40% is mixed, and the distal 50 to 60% is entirely smooth muscle.[15] No similar information is available in children. The resting pressure is usually lower than the gastric pressure and varies with respiration. Different types of esophageal contractions can occur in the esophageal body. *Primary peristalsis* is the one that occurs after swallowing. It is an orderly and progressive series of peristaltic contractions that begins in the pharynx and advances aborally (see Figure 70-1).[4,13] *Secondary peristalsis* can be elicited in response to luminal distention with air, liquid, or a balloon. *Tertiary contractions* consist of random, spontaneous, usually simultaneous, nonperistaltic contractions.

During primary peristalsis, the contractions usually progress at a speed of 2 to 4 cm/s, and there is a closely coordinated process between the UES and the LES. The mechanical effect is a stripping wave that milks the esophagus clean from the proximal to the distal end.[4] In general, a pressure complex in the distal esophagus with an amplitude < 35 mm Hg is considered hypotensive,[4,16] whereas contractions > 180 mm Hg are considered hypertensive.[4,16] Based on simultaneous manometric and videofluoroscopic studies, a cutoff of 30 mm Hg is now used to separate effective from ineffective peristalsis.[15,17] Failed peristalsis can occur in 4 to 15% of swallows in normal adult volunteers.[16] The typical duration of peristaltic contractions is around 4 seconds,[16] and double-peak contractions can occasionally occur in normal controls.[16] No similar information is available in healthy children.

The LES is tonically contracted and found at the distal end of the esophageal body (see Figure 70-1). LES pressure varies depending on the individuals and the methods used. Wide ranges have been reported. For example, Hillemeier and colleagues reported a mean LES pressure of 22.4 ± 4.7 mm Hg,[18] Cucchiara and colleagues reported 15 ± 2 mm

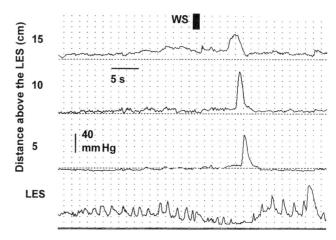

FIGURE 70-1 Normal esophageal manometry. The tracing shows the normal response to a wet swallow (WS). A peristaltic wave traveling aborally from 15 cm above the lower esophageal sphincter (LES) to the lower esophagus can be observed. Also, a normal LES relaxation after swallowing can be noted.

Hg,[19] and Moroz and colleagues reported 29.1 ± 2.4 mm Hg.[20] In adults, LES pressure varies from 10 to 45 mm Hg.[15] The LES is also asymmetric, with maximal pressures in the left lateral aspect. LES relaxation usually occurs with swallowing (see Figure 70-1), although it has been shown that it can also occur transiently when no swallowing is occurring.[15] An increased amount of transient relaxations has been reported both in adults and children with gastroesophageal reflux (GER).[15,19] The measurement of LES pressure is always performed relative to intragastric pressure. LES relaxation needs to be coordinated for more than 90% of wet swallows and complete with a drop to intragastric pressure. Different methods that have been used to measure basal sphincter pressure include either the midrespiratory or end-expiratory points. The midexpiratory pressure is the mean pressure at the midpoint of amplitude of the phasic respiratory component, whereas the end-expiratory pressure is when the tonic component is used alone.[4]

The manometry catheter is usually placed nasally, although, if necessary, it can also be placed orally, particularly in premature infants. In older children, nasal topical anesthesia with topical cocaine or viscous lidocaine is frequently used. Medications known to affect gastrointestinal motility (eg, prokinetics, anticholinergics, narcotics) are held for 48 hours before the procedure, and children are asked to fast for 4 to 6 hours, depending on the age and the need for sedation.

There is no standardized protocol to perform esophageal manometry in children. Adding to the difficulties is the fact that esophageal length varies with age, making the adoption of a standard catheter that can provide all of the information impossible. The pediatric task force of the AMS recommended the use of the slow pull-through technique.[1] Usually, detailed analyses of the LES and of the esophageal body are then done.[1] Even though UES measurements can be obtained, it is not clear that manometric findings are sensitive enough to have a clear impact on patient management.[4]

The responses to swallowing are observed. If possible, a swallowing marker is used, although, particularly in young children, careful observation and manual recording are employed. It is preferable to do "wet" swallows of water at room temperature (approximately 1 mL in infants and 3 to 5 mL in older children).[1] It has been shown that swallows with water give a more consistent peristaltic response than those that occur only with saliva.[16] In a typical study, 10 wet swallows are evaluated.

In young children, it is difficult to obtain swallows, and different techniques have been employed. Gently blowing air in the child's face (the Santmeyer reflex) may induce swallowing in young infants and neurologically abnormal children.[21]

In some centers, sleeve catheters are used to assess the LES. The sleeves are more accurate because they straddle the sphincter over 3 to 5 cm. Esophageal peristalsis is then measured by positioning the catheter at different segments of the esophageal body and using wet swallows. The amplitude, duration, and peristaltic characteristics of the contractions are measured.[16]

The UES is evaluated at the end. Techniques to measure it are the same as for the LES, although the recording speed may need to be increased. The UES relaxes to baseline, and the relationship between pharyngeal contractions and UES relaxation is determined. The clinical utility of UES/pharyngeal measurements is the least established.

Developmental Aspects. Recent advances with the use of microperfusion techniques and catheter size have allowed the study of even small premature babies.[6,8,22] It has been shown that in premature infants 26 to 33 weeks gestational age, esophageal pressure waves triggered by dry swallows were predominantly peristaltic (84%) in propagation sequence.[6] Swallow-unrelated pressure waves were usually nonperistaltic, and the researchers concluded that in infants 26 weeks or older, the control of swallow-induced peristalsis is fully developed.[6] All had tonic LES contraction with a mean resting pressure of 13.6 ± 4.2 mm Hg (range 5.0 ± 4.1 to 20.0 ± 4.8 mm Hg). In all infants, the LES relaxed in response to pharyngeal swallows. The duration of LES relaxation was 5.8 ± 3 seconds, and transient LES relaxations occurred an average of 2.6 ± 1.6 times per study. Those patterns are similar to the ones described in older premature infants.[23] Premature infants > 33 weeks of age had a mean LES pressure of 20.5 ± 1.7 mm Hg preprandially and 13.7 ± 1.3 mm Hg postprandially. It has also been shown that the patterns of LES relaxation were similar to those seen in healthy adults.[8]

Clinical Significance. Esophageal motility is mandatory for the diagnosis of primary motility disorders (Table 70-3) (see Chapter 26, "Other Motor Disorders").[1,2,4]

Esophageal motility remains the study of choice to make the diagnosis of achalasia.[1] Four manometric findings are characteristic of achalasia, as shown in Table 70-3 (see Figure 26-3 of Chapter 26).[24,25] The absence of peristalsis is the hallmark of the disease. Even though most patients with achalasia have incomplete or absent LES relaxation, the LES may occasionally show complete relaxation.[25] Manometry also provides quantitative information about the severity of the achalasia and the response to treatment.[1]

Esophageal manometry allows the diagnosis of diffuse esophageal spasm, nutcracker esophagus, or nonspecific esophageal motility disorders. The term nonspecific esophageal motility disorders has been used to describe manometric findings that are abnormal but not diagnostic of any established motility disorder.[26] Manometric features include apersistaltic, repetitive, or multipeaked contractions; low-amplitude contractions; intermittent segmental contractions; and prolonged contraction duration.[27]

Esophageal manometry is indicated to assess esophageal function in children and adolescents with dysphagia, odynophagia, and chest pain of noncardiac origin.[1]

Esophageal manometry can also be used to locate the LES for pH probe placement, particularly in patients with abnormal anatomy, such as a hiatal hernia.

Manometry has no role in the diagnosis of GER, and the exact role of esophageal motility in the preoperative evaluation of children is not clear. The only clear role it has

TABLE 70-3   DIAGNOSIS OF PRIMARY ESOPHAGEAL
MOTOR DISORDERS

Achalasia* (four manometric findings are characteristic of achalasia[24,25])
  Increased LES pressure
  Absence of esophageal peristalsis (the hallmark of the disease; see Figure 70-3)
  Incomplete or abnormal LES relaxation
  Elevated intraesophageal pressure compared with intragastric pressure

Diffuse esophageal spasm[†]
  Repetitive, simultaneous (nonperistaltic) contractions, at least 20% of wet swallows
  Periods of normal peristaltic sequences
  Alterations in the contraction waves (repetitive, increased duration and amplitude), although there are patients who can have normal amplitude
  A normal LES in most patients, although incomplete LES relaxation or a hypertensive sphincter has been described[166-168]

Nutcracker esophagus[‡]
  Increased distal peristaltic amplitude (180 mm Hg)
  Increased distal peristaltic duration (> 6 s)

Nonspecific esophageal motor diosrders[§26,27]
  Low-amplitude contractions (< 30 mm Hg)
  Triple-peaked waves, spontaneous isolated contractions, retrograde contractions
  Prolonged contractions (> 6 s)
  Aperistalsis or nontransmitted contractions (during > 20% of wet swallows)
  Simultaneous contractions (> 30% of wet swallows)

LES = lower esophageal sphincter.
*To make the diagnosis of achalasia, absence of esophageal body peristalsis is necessary; other criteria are often fulfilled but are not required.
[†]Primary finding is uncoordinated motility.
[‡]Primary finding is increased distal peristaltic amplitude.
[§]Abnormal manometric patterns that do not fit a defined entity.

in the diagnosis and medical management of GER is when there is uncertainty about the correct diagnosis and a primary motility problem such as achalasia is suspected.[4] In general, when used in the preoperative evaluation of patients with GER, it has not been shown to predict outcome.[4] The role that preoperative esophageal peristalsis plays in the development of dysphagia after fundoplication has been controversial.[28] Studies comparing preoperative patients with or without esophageal dysmotility have shown no difference in the prevalence of dysphagia after the operation.[28] At present, it can be concluded that insufficient data exist to evaluate the benefit of the routine preoperative assessment of peristaltic function.[4] However, it may have a role when there are severe preoperative dysphagia or atypical symptoms or when severe dysmotility is suspected. In children, the latter problem is commonly found in patients with scleroderma or tracheoesophageal fistulas,[29,30] in which a fundoplication may create a functional obstruction in a dysmotil esophagus.

Manometry may be useful in the diagnosis of connective tissue diseases, in which it may confirm the clinical suspicion.[1,15] Of all of the collagen vascular disorders, scleroderma shows the most marked esophageal abnormalities.[31,32] The manometric findings are quite suggestive of the diagnosis, although not pathognomonic, because severe reflux esophagitis can have the same manometric appearance.[32] The characteristic esophageal

manometric findings are (1) an incompetent LES, (2) low-amplitude esophageal contractions in the smooth portion of the esophagus, and (3) later alterations in the striated muscle section.[31-33] Even though the esophageal motor abnormalities of scleroderma have been well characterized, other connective tissue diseases also have motor alterations,[33] particularly in patients with systemic lupus erythematosus and those with mixed connective tissue diseases.[33]

Esophageal manometry is useful in the evaluation of noncardiac chest pain.[1] Manometry should not be routinely used as the initial test[15] but may be useful when other tests have not provided an explanation. Manometric abnormalities are prevalent in patients with chest pain, dysphagia, or both. Achalasia or diffuse esophageal spasm accounts for the minority,[15] and most patients fall under the category of "nonspecific disorders." In a recent report of esophageal manometric findings in 154 children, the authors described the findings in 45 children with chest pain or dysphagia not associated with GER.[26] Esophageal manometry was described as abnormal in 30 (67%). Among those, a variety of motility disorders were diagnosed in 17 patients (achalasia in 12, pseudo-obstruction in 3, diffuse esophageal spasm in 1, and dysmotility after tracheoesophageal fistula repair in 1), whereas nonspecific esophageal motor disorders were diagnosed in 13 patients (8% from the initial 154). Those children had a higher incidence of food impaction.[26]

Recently, technical advances with solid-state catheters and digital recording devices have allowed the performance of prolonged monitoring of esophageal pressure.[34] There are no control values for children, and the number of controls in adults is limited. The manometry is performed with a solid-state catheter that has pressure transducers and usually one or two pH electrodes, allowing the correlation of symptoms with both motor events and reflux. Most software does not allow the measurement of continuous LES pressure. The primary indication is for the evaluation of patients with noncardiac chest pain[34,35] because it allows the demonstration of associated esophageal events (either motor or reflux related) with the pain.[34] Preliminary reports in children have shown that it is a technique that may be useful.[36,37]

The role that provocative tests play during esophageal manometry in children has not been established, so their use is not recommended.

The future for the study of esophageal physiology may be promising. The advent of mutlichannel intraluminal impedance combined with manometry has allowed the simultaneous evaluation of esophageal contractions and bolus transit.[17] Recent publications have established normal reference values for adults,[17] and there is still no information available for children. The results in adults have already shown that the manometric evidence of ineffective peristalsis may underestimate the true bolus clearance and that the combined impedance with manometry may be a more sensitive technique to assess esophageal function.[17] More information is needed before any firm conclusions can be established.

Indications. The primary indication continues to be in the evaluation of children with esophageal dysfunction that is not explained by anatomic or well-defined problems (see Table 70-2).[1,2]

Esophageal manometry is indicated when a primary motility disorder is suspected and to support the diagnosis of connective tissue diseases or other systemic illness. Manometry may be indicated in the evaluation of patients with achalasia post-treatment who develop recurrent symptoms when there is doubt about the physiopathology. Manometry is not indicated in the routine evaluation of GER, but it should be performed in those patients with GER in whom the diagnosis is not clear, as well as before a fundoplication when a severe motility disorder is suspected. It is also used to localize the LES before placement of a pH probe in patients with abnormal anatomy (eg, hiatal hernia). Esophageal manometry, particularly 24-hour recording, is indicated in the evaluation of children with noncardiac chest pain who have no diagnosis and have not responded to antireflux therapy.

ANTRODUODENAL MANOMETRY

Antroduodenal manometry measures the intraluminal pressure of the antrum and duodenum.[1,7,38,39] Antroduodenal motility has been clearly established as an important research tool, and even though it is being gradually introduced into clinical practice, the exact role that it plays in the evaluation of children and adults has not been firmly established. Manometric data are not necessary for patient management when there is a known underlying cause of dysmotility (see Table 70-2).[1]

Clinically, manometry provides useful information regarding contraction patterns in the region. In children, its utility has been mostly hampered by the lack of data that establish patterns in normal controls because it is not ethically possible to perform those tests in healthy children.[38] Therefore, reported controls have been derived by different authors from patients referred for antroduodenal motility who later were considered as not having upper gastrointestinal motility problems.[40] These difficulties in interpretation can be illustrated in reports in which abnormal manometric patterns occurred with equal frequency in healthy and symptomatic adults.[41] Therefore, definition of what constitutes a significant abnormality remains controversial. Because of this lack of controls in children, great care needs to be exercised in the interpretation of the studies to avoid overinterpretation of the findings.[5]

Small bowel motility can be performed with solid-state pressure transducers, impedance sensors, or perfused catheters.[1] The patient stops medications that can affect motility for at least 48 hours before the test. The catheter is introduced nasally or through an existing gastrostomy or jejunostomy. The catheter requires postpyloric placement and can be introduced either endoscopically or fluoroscopically, and, ideally, it is advanced beyond the angle of Treitz. Most importantly, however, the transducers need to be positioned across the antroduodenal junction.[42] The configuration of the catheters varies, but the minimum recommended recording ports include one in the antrum and three small bowel recording sites.[1] The distance for the duodenal/jejunal ports varies depending on the age of the patients, with a range that goes from 3 to 10 cm between ports. In most children, a distance of 3 cm is sufficient. The position of the catheter needs to be checked frequently during the performance of the test to ensure the correct position across the antroduodenal junction. It has been suggested that, on average, a stationary study requires an average five adjustments of tube location in the postprandial period to ensure accurate antral recordings.[3] At times, it is necessary to reconfirm placement during the test with radiography or fluoroscopy.

When perfused studies are performed, a close follow-up of the patient is necessary to avoid fluid overload, particularly in small children.[43] With the regular perfusion equipment available in most laboratories, steel capillary or other tubes that control the rate of flow are used, and the usual perfusion rates vary from 0.1 to 0.4 mL/min per port. If six ports are being used, and the test lasts 6 hours, a large amount of fluid is being administered. This could produce volume overload or, theoretically, hyponatremia. Even though in adult laboratories, the catheter is perfused with distilled water, in children, many centers use 0.2 to 0.5 normal saline or oral hydration solutions[1,2] to avoid hyponatremia. To be able to study premature and young infants, the system has been adapted by some investigators to decrease the perfusion rate to 0.01 to 0.02 mL/min.[7,44]

It is preferable to avoid anesthesia and sedation. The effects of benzodiazepines on motility recordings have not been evaluated,[42] but in some centers, it has been suggested that sedation with midazolam (2–5 mg) followed by reversal with intravenous flumazenil (0.2–0.4 mg) does not result in any appreciable change in motility recordings. The use of sedation or general anesthesia is usually necessary in children, particularly when the catheters are being placed endoscopically. To avoid the possible effects of the sedation or anesthesia, in most centers, the study is performed the day after the catheter has been placed.

The optimum duration of the test is not known. Even though most centers use 3 to 4 hours of fasting followed by 2 hours postprandially,[42,45] some authors have advocated the use of prolonged ambulatory studies. The pediatric task force of the AMS recommends at least 3 hours of fasting (or two migrating motor complexes [MMCs]) and at least 1 postprandial hour.[1] Soffer and Thongsawat have shown that prolonged tests, including sleep periods, enhance the diagnostic accuracy of the test.[45] Most of the improvement came from extra information gained by longer fasting periods. Because of frequent catheter displacement, ambulatory tests cannot be used reliably to assess postprandial antral activity.[3,42] Therefore, if the objective is to assess postprandial antral function, a stationary manometry is necessary.[3,42]

The analysis is usually performed by visual inspection.[1] Antroduodenal manometry provides identification of certain "patterns" and limited quantitative features.[42] At times, it may be possible to administer provocative medications and analyze the responses.

During fasting, the stomach and small bowel show a cyclic pattern, known as the MMC.[40] This cyclic activity is usually divided into three phases. Phase III is the most characteristic and consists of regular rhythmic peristaltic contractions that start proximally and migrate down to the ileum. Phase III shows regular contractions that in the antrum occur at a rate of 2 to 3/min and in the small bowel at 11 to 12/min (Figure 70-2). The velocity of propagation of phase III decreases significantly, whereas the duration increases significantly with increasing distance from the mouth. Phase III is followed by a period of quiescence (phase I) that is interrupted by irregular motor activity (phase II). During phase I, contractions are not recorded. During phase II, the contractions vary in amplitude and periodicity. Phase I seems to be the most predominant in the antrum, whereas phase II is predominant in both the duodenum and the jejunum. In adults, phase I lasts from 12 to 20 minutes, phase II lasts from 30 to 130 minutes, and phase III lasts from 3 to 15 minutes.[3,42,46,47] There is also a large variation in cycle duration between individuals and within the same individual when studied on separate days.[42] There are no established standards for normal duration of the cycle in children, but in the series reported in the literature, the duration seems to be similar,[46] although it has been suggested that the cycle may be shorter.[40,48,49]

In one study of 18 children aged 2 to 12 years without upper gastrointestinal symptoms in whom antroduodenal manometry was performed, the authors found a phase III in 14 of the children during fasting, and it was induced in the other 4 children by erythromycin. Phase III propagation velocity increased with age, and the cycle length showed no age-dependent variation. Phase III occupied around 3%, phase I around 10%, and phase II around 87%.[40] These authors concluded that antroduodenal motility findings in those children were similar to those found in adults.[40]

After the ingestion of nutrients, the fasting pattern is interrupted by what has been denominated the fed pattern (Figure 70-3). The fed pattern is characterized by an irregular occurrence of contractions with various amplitudes.

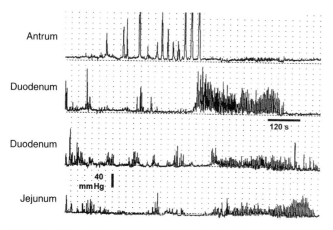

FIGURE 70-2 Normal fasting antroduodenal manometry. A normal phase III front originating in the antrum and migrating aborally along the duodenum into the jejunum can be observed. During phase III, the antrum contracts at a frequency of 3/min, whereas the small bowel contracts at a frequency of 11 to 12/min. Phase III is followed by a period of quiescence (phase I) and is preceded by intermittent irregular contractions (phase II).

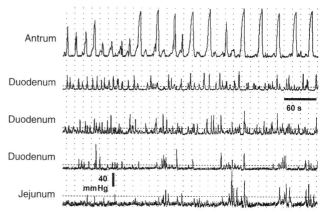

FIGURE 70-3 Normal postprandial pattern in a small bowel manometry. There are irregular persistent phasic contractions in the antrum and small bowel.

After solid meals, strong, repetitive contractions are often induced in the antrum, and the duodenal response looks similar to that of phase II, although the amplitude and frequency of contractions are greater in the fed state.[1]

An antral motility index has been used to calculate both the frequency and the amplitude of contractions. The following formula has been commonly used:

Motility index = ln (amplitude × number of contractions + 1)

with a normal value being 13.67 to 15.65 (5–95th percentile).[42,50] For this calculation to be useful and comparable, it must include 2 hours, assessed by pneumohydraulic perfusion manometry of the prepyloric antrum, and it must quantitate contractions 1 to 2 cm proximal to the pylorus.

The characteristics of the fed pattern vary with the type, composition, and amount of nutrients. For example, liquid nutrients decrease the amplitude of antral contractions and generate an irregular movement in the small bowel, whereas solid food produces high-amplitude contractions in the antrum and a pattern similar to that of liquids in the small bowel. In adults, the meal has been standardized to be at least 400 kcal to ensure a postprandial response of 2 hours duration.[42,51] The solid or liquid meal should be balanced and typical of an average US diet, with 20 to 25% fat, 20 to 25% protein, and 50 to 55% carbohydrate.[42] It has recently been shown that the caloric value of the meal regulates the duration of the fed pattern over a wide range of calories and that for caloric loads up to 1,100 kcal, there does not seem to be a maximum duration of postprandial motor activity. In children, no studies address this question, and there is no standardization, but most authors have used 5 to 10 mL/kg,[52] 20 cal/kg,[53] or 400 to 600 kcal. The AMS task force recommends that the type and size of the meal should be adjusted according to the patient's age and preference (at least 10 kcal/kg or 400 kcal; > 30% kcal from lipids).[1] The task force recommends administering the meal by mouth or intragastrically if possible.[1]

Development. Because of the recent technical advances described above, there is now a fair amount of information regarding normal patterns and age-dependent maturation in preterm infants and full-term neonates.[7,43] Duodenal motility patterns differ in preterm and term infants. Gastric and duodenal MMCs are present after the 32 to 35 weeks of gestation. Approximately two-thirds of phase III activity starts in the duodenum, and its duration is similar to that in older children and adults. In contrast, premature infants with a postconceptual age less than 32 weeks do not have phase III activity, and there are no cyclic changes in the motility patterns. They show mostly sporadic and nonmigrating clusters of contractions. The number and amplitude of duodenal contractions increase significantly between 29 and 32 weeks, and there seems to be a gradual maturation of these parameters. With maturation, the frequency of these clusters decreases until a mature pattern is observed. As they develop phase IIIs, they differ from adults, with a slower migration velocity, a shorter interval between contractions, and a smaller peak amplitude of the contractions.

In premature and full-term infants, antral motor activity was similar to that in the fasting state. Antral motility consisted of isolated single contractions and clustered phasic contractions. There were no differences in the occurrence of antral activity, and the only differences observed were in duodenal activity. The proportion of antral clusters that were temporally associated with duodenal activity was also significantly lower in preterm infants than in term infants. After feeding, motor activity changes in both full-term and premature infants. It has been shown that in term infants, there is usually a mature response (similar to the one observed in adults), whereas only a third of preterm infants have a mature response. In the term infant, the number of antral waves, the duration of antral clusters, and the antral motility index decreased by one-third; the duodenal motility index and cluster activity increased significantly. This divergent response was also seen in premature infants.[43] In a study of premature infants, the conversion from fasted to fed patterns depended on caloric strength. The threshold concentration was about 22 cal/dL when 5 mL/kg of milk was given.

In infants, phase III does not appear right after feeding. There may be differences in the response depending on the nutrient. For example, in one study with healthy neonates, phase III appeared within 3 hours after breast milk in 10 of 12 breastfed infants but in 2 of 12 infants who were formula-fed.[54] The study of the fed patterns of antropyloric motility measured with the use of high-resolution manometric microperfusion techniques has indicated that the neuroregulatory mechanisms responsible for the coordination of motility and gastric emptying are well developed by 30 weeks gestation.[7]

It has been suggested that antroduodenal motility may be useful to establish feeding readiness in premature infants[44,55] or the best way to feed them.[56] It has been shown that in premature infants, continuous infusions produce better responses and tolerance than bolus feedings and that full-strength formula triggers adult-like motor activity.

Clinical Significance. Antroduodenal motility has been used to study the physiopathology of gastrointestinal motility disorders. Different patterns also allow the classification

into neuropathic (Figure 70-4) or myopathic abnormalities (Figure 70-5).[1] They are defined based on qualitative abnormalities.[1] In general, most authors consider findings abnormal if there is abnormal propagation or configuration of the MMC, uncoordinated intestinal bursts of phasic pressure activity sustained over 30 minutes, uncoordinated intestinal pressure activity, and failure of the meal to produce a fed pattern (see Figures 70-4 to 70-6).

Based on these abnormalities, the following patterns can be seen:

1. *Antral hypomotility.* A reduced motility index of postprandial distal antral contractions is significantly correlated with the impaired gastric emptying of solids from the stomach (see Figure 70-6).[50,57]
2. *Myopathic disorders.* These disorders are characterized by low-amplitude contractions < 20 mm Hg[58] and, on average, are < 10 mm Hg. However, it is important to remember that amplitude measurements with a point sensor depend on luminal diameter and may be low because of a nonspecific dilatation (see Figure 70-5).[42]
3. *Neuropathic disorders.* These disorders have been associated with antral hypomotility, absence of phase III activity, abnormal propagation of MMC, bursts and sustained uncoordinated pressure activity (hypercontracility), and a lack of a fed response (see Figure 70-4).[59]
4. *Mechanical obstruction.* Even though mechanical obstruction needs to be diagnosed by other means, if undetected, it may be suggested by manometry. Two patterns suggestive of obstruction have been described: postprandial clustered contractions (> 30 minutes duration) separated by quiescence or simultaneous prolonged (> 8 seconds) or summated contractions.[42,60]

In an attempt to define normal fasting antroduodenal patterns in children, Tomamasa and colleagues compared the results obtained in 95 patients with symptoms suggesting a gastrointestinal motility disorder with 20 children

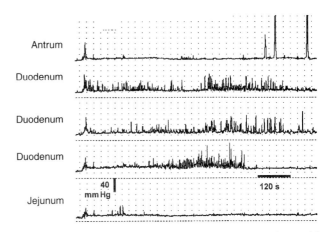

FIGURE 70-4 Antroduodenal manometry in a patient with neuropathy. The tracing shows abnormalities in the phase III of the migrating motor complex. Some uncoordinated clusters, as well as isolated irregular phasic contractions, can be observed. Throughout the study, there was no organized activity, and irregular phasic contractions were seen. No phase III could be observed, even after provocative medications.

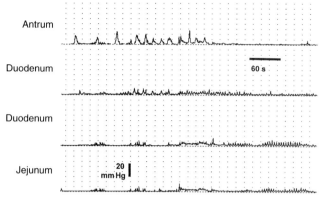

FIGURE 70-5   Antroduodenal manometry in a patient with visceral myopathy. The tracing shows the normal propagation of the interdigestive motor complex, although the amplitude is much lower than normal (see Figure 70-2).

without upper gastrointestinal disease.[38] They concluded that the following five manometric features have a clear association with pediatric gastrointestinal motility disorders: (1) absence of phase III of the MMC, (2) abnormal migration of phase III, (3) short intervals between phase III episodes, (4) persistent low-amplitude contractions, and (5) sustained tonic-phasic contractions. They mention that short or prolonged phase III, low amplitude of phase III in a single recording site, and clusters of contractions or prolonged propagating contractions during phase II were not more frequent in patients than in controls.

The presence of phase III activity appears to be a marker of neuromuscular integrity,[1,38,40,42,61] and it has been reported that the absence of phase III activity is abnormal (see Figure 70-4).[42] One-third to half of the activity front may commence distal to the stomach.[42,62,63] Hence, the absence of the antral component of phase III is not necessarily abnormal.[42,62]

In stationary studies, 66 to 75% of adult patients will have at least one duodenal/jejunal phase III activity during the 3-hour study.[42] Because even some normal adult subjects may have no phase III activity during stationary studies, this finding may have limitations in the interpretation of suspected neuropathic disorders.[41,45,64] Data from 24-hour ambulatory studies show that normal adult volunteers have at least one or more MMCs per 24 hours.[45,47,65] Therefore, the most definitive evidence of normal enteric neuromotor function can be obtained from prolonged studies.[45] In a study comparing the accuracy of short versus long manometry, the two analyses agreed in 81 of 91 cases. In 7 of 10 cases, a study was diagnosed as abnormal in the short recording but was considered normal after review of the long recording, whereas the opposite occurred in the remaining 3 cases.[45] There is no similar information in children, but it has been suggested that children have a shorter MMC cycle duration than do adults.[48,49]

If no spontaneous phase III activity is observed, intravenous erythromycin has been administered.[1,66] Erythromycin, at doses that are 10 to 20% of those used for its antibiotic properties, acts as a motilin receptor agonist.[66–68] In one study, erythromycin induced phase III activity when

given to patients with functional gastrointestinal symptoms. It induced phase III in 18 of 20 children who had phase III activity during fasting, as opposed to 1 of 15 who did not. A dose of 3 mg/kg induced a higher antral motility index when compared with 1 mg/kg, although both doses were equally efficacious in inducing phase III. The lower dose was associated with less side effects.[66] In another study, the effect of erythromycin 3 mg/kg/h was compared among 10 controls, 7 patients with functional dyspepsia, and 6 patients with pseudo-obstruction.[68] In controls, erythromycin induced a premature activity front occurring 15 ± 3 minutes after starting the infusion. The propagation and duration did not differ from the spontaneous activity front. In patients with functional dyspepsia, erythromycin induced various patterns, such as a premature antroduodenal activity front, antral phase III–like patterns with short duodenal bursts, or prolonged phasic antral waves without duodenal activity. In patients with neurogenic pseudo-obstruction, rare or absent antral activity was present with uncoordinated or absent activity, and no contractions were elicited in those with myopathic pseudo-obstruction.[68] It has therefore been suggested that in children who have a normal MMC during fasting, erythromycin produces normal phase III, whereas it is abnormal in all patients with abnormal fasting motility. Therefore, some authors have suggested that in children, a 1-hour infusion of erythromycin could replace the 4-hour fasting portion of the test as a way to establish if there is presence or absence of phase III.[49] This observation has not been validated, and the disadvantage of a shorter test would be the inability to evaluate other aspects of fasting motility. The AMS task force recommended the use of erythromycin 1 mg/kg over 30 minutes if no MMC is recorded during fasting.[1]

The administration of erythromycin to full-term neonates induces phase III activity.[67,69] However, it induces a response only in premature infants older than 32 weeks.[70]

The usefulness of antroduodenal manometry to directing therapy has not been definitely established in adults. In children, it has been suggested that absent MMCs are an indicator of a poor response to enteral feeding[53] or to cis-

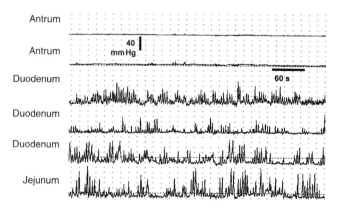

FIGURE 70-6   Antroduodenal manometry in a patient with antral hypomotility. The tracing shows normal postprandial activity in the small bowel and absent response in the antrum. This pattern is frequently seen in patients with gastroparesis.

apride.[71] Antroduodenal manometry may also be useful to study the effects of medications that may have a role in the treatment of children and adults with motility disturbances, such as octreotide.[72,73] Octreotide has been shown to induce phase III activity in the small bowel[72] and has varying effects on the antrum.

It has been suggested, however, that one of the most important contributions of the test may be in showing normal physiology in those patients with apparent intestinal failure (see Table 70-2).[1,5,38,40] Fell and colleagues tried to assess if antroduodenal manometry in the first 2 years of life helped define a neuropathic or myopathic etiology or clinical outcome in cases of pseudo-obstruction.[74] They studied 14 children histologically (5 with myopathy, 4 with neuropathy, and 5 unclassified) and manometrically. They found four abnormalities in the manometry: no detectable motor activity in 4 children, low-amplitude phase III activity in 5 children, poorly formed phase III activity in 3 children, and well-formed cyclic phase III activity with abnormal propagation in 2 children. The seven children with a low-amplitude phase III motility index < 10 pka/min had poor outcomes (death or dependence on total parenteral nutrition). The authors concluded that manometry was useful not only as an aid in diagnosing the etiology of pseudo-obstruction presenting in infancy but also in predicting outcome.[74]

Indications. Antroduodenal manometry is indicated when patients have unexplained upper gastrointestinal problems, such as nausea and vomiting or other symptoms suggestive of upper gastrointestinal dysmotility (see Table 70-2). Its main use had been in confirming or excluding the diagnosis of pseudo-obstruction or a motility disorder, and it helps to establish if the dysmotility is neuropathic or myopathic. Most importantly, a normal study may indicate that motor dysfunction is not the cause of the symptoms.[1,42] It is also used to decide if there is generalized dysmotility in patients with dysmotility elsewhere (eg, chronic constipation when surgery is contemplated, severe reflux with evidence of distal dysmotility when a fundoplication is being considered, or after a failed fundoplication that requires reintervention).[1]

It may be useful to distinguish between rumination and vomiting.[1] Some studies have also suggested that antroduodenal motility may be useful in patients with abnormal motility to predict outcome after drugs or ability to tolerate enteral feedings. It is also indicated in patients with pseudo-obstruction being considered for intestinal transplant and may suggest an unexpected obstruction.[1]

COLONIC MANOMETRY

Measurement of colonic intraluminal pressure has been performed for many years but has been confined mostly to the distal colon (anorectosigmoid segments). The study of colonic motility of more proximal segments is a technique that has recently been introduced.[75] Even though colonic intraluminal measurements alone do not have a clear role in clinical practice, the test has been shown to be useful in the evaluation of the pediatric patient with intractable constipation.[1] In adults, colonic motility does not seem to discriminate subgroups of chronic constipation more

accurately than transit and pelvic floor tests. It may be helpful in confirming a diagnosis of slow-transit constipation (colonic inertia) in patients considered candidates for surgical treatment.

In humans, there is no interdigestive cyclic motor activity. The characteristics of colonic motility are the presence of irregular alterations of quiescence with nonpropagating and propagating contractions. In humans, colonic propagated events are basically of two types, arbitrarily defined on the basis of their amplitude: low-amplitude propagated contractions (LAPCs) and high-amplitude propagated contractions (HAPCs). LAPCs have been poorly investigated and are propagated waves of 5 to 40 mm Hg. Their exact physiologic significance is still unknown but may be involved in the transport of colonic contents and the occurrence of flatus.[75] In the fasting state, the motor activity is represented mostly by low-amplitude (5–50 mm Hg), nonpropulsive, segmental contractions; peristaltic movements seldom occur.[75] Some contractions last more than 30 seconds and are considered tonic; others are shorter and are considered phasic. Segmental nonpropagating contractions are rare in infants but are more common in toddlers.[76]

HAPCs have been defined as contractions of at least 80 to 100 mm Hg, lasting 10 seconds and propagating for at least 30 cm.[75,77] HAPCs can reach amplitudes > 200 mm Hg. HAPCs originate in the proximal colon and migrate distally > 95% of the time, usually stopping in the distal sigmoid colon (Figure 70-7).[75]

Food ingestion has an important influence on colonic motility.[75] The response lasts 2 to 3 hours and is mostly composed of segmental contractions; it is also accompanied by an increase in colonic smooth muscle tone and can also have HAPCs, which have also been described in pediatric patients.[1,78–80] The colonic response to eating is influenced by the caloric content and meal composition. Fat and carbohydrate represent an important stimulant, whereas protein may have an inhibitory effect.[75]

Another cyclic activity that can be found during colonic manometry occurs distal to the rectosigmoid junc-

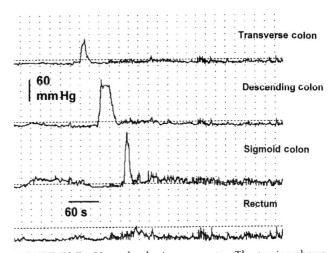

FIGURE 70-7 Normal colonic manometry. The tracing shows the presence of a high-amplitude propagating contraction that is originating in the transverse colon, advancing aborally along the large bowel, and stopping in the sigmoid colon.

tion and has been labeled the rectal motor complex.[75] This lasts an average of 10 minutes and has contractions with a mean frequency of two to four per minute and a wave amplitude of > 5 mm Hg. It occurs in adults every 90 to 300 minutes during the day and every 50 to 90 minutes at night.[75] Its physiologic role is unknown, although it is accompanied by a rise in anal canal pressure and probably represents a mechanism to preserve fecal continence, particularly during sleep.

It has been suggested that colon preparation alters colonic motility. Unfortunately, studies of colonic motility are difficult to perform in unprepared colons, so most data are available from studies in which the colon has been cleaned.[77] Usually, the patient's colon is cleaned with the use of a balanced electrolyte solution. In most studies performed in children, this is administered by a nasogastric tube. Usually, no enemas are given, no colonic preparation is given the day of the study, and medications that can influence motility are stopped at least 48 hours before the study.

The spacing of the recording ports varies, but they are generally separated by 10 to 15 cm. The catheter is placed with the use of colonoscopy. In general, a guidewire is placed into the transverse/hepatic flexure, and the colonoscope is withdrawn, leaving the guidewire in position. The motility catheter is then fed over the wire. The position of the tube is checked fluoroscopically.[49,77,79,80] The catheter can also be dragged with the colonoscope during the colonoscopy and placed directly in the desired location.

The colonoscopy is performed using either general anesthesia or intravenous sedation. When intravenous sedation is used, and only benzodiazepines are used, the motility study may be done on the same day, after the child has recovered from the sedation (mean of 3.5 hours).[77] However, the influence that the sedation or the colonoscopy may have on motility is not known. Therefore, in many cases, the catheter is placed on one day, and the study is performed on the next day.

A fasting recording is done for 2 hours, and then the patient is fed. There is no standardization of the meal. In adults, a 350 kcal meal did not stimulate colonic motility, but a 1,000 kcal meal did. In one pediatric study, patients received a combined liquid and solid meal (≥ 20 kcal/kg, with fat providing > 30% of the energy).[79] In another study, 240 mL of whole milk or formula was used in those enterally fed, and in those who were dependent on total parenteral nutrition, they gave the maximum amount of milk that the patients were able to tolerate without symptoms.[80] Usually, a motility index is calculated by measuring the area under the pressure for at least 30 to 60 minutes before and 30 to 60 minutes after the completion of the meal. HAPCs are excluded from the analysis.[77] It has been shown that meals stimulate colonic motility in healthy subjects.[79,80]

Clinical Significance.
Constipated adults with slow-transit constipation have an impairment of colonic propagated activity, principally related to a decrease or an absence in HAPCs. The enteric neural program controlling colonic propagation and its ability to contract in response to exogenous stimulation may still be preserved in some patients, as shown by the elicitation of HAPCs after intraluminal instillation of bisacodyl. Patients may also have an abnormal response to eating,[75] which may be blunted or absent.

The patterns of colonic motility in healthy children have not been established. Most information comes from studies in which children referred for evaluation of neuropathy, constipation, or nonulcer dyspepsia have been studied.[76,77,79,80] From those studies, it has been suggested that in children, HAPCs also increase after meals. These authors have described that in the postprandial period, one HAPC is usually followed by others 3 to 4 minutes later.[76,77,79,80] In a study of 32 children with a median age of 5.5 years (15 with functional fecal retention, 10 with nonulcer dyspepsia, and 7 with Munchausen syndrome by proxy), it was suggested that there was an inverse correlation between the number of HAPCs and age (before and after administration of a meal) and that colonic contractions different from HAPCs increase with age.[77] The authors found at least one HAPC in 28 of 32 subjects, and the 4 subjects without it were > 8 years. HAPCs were also more frequent in the fasting period in those ≥ 4 years when compared with those who were older (8/13 vs 3/19). There were also differences in the number of HAPCs within 30 minutes of the meal (13/13 age 4 years vs 12/19 > 4 years), whereas there were no differences in the second 30-minute interval.

It has been suggested that colonic manometry offers a tool to differentiate children with different causes of constipation and to differentiate between myopathy and neuropathy.[1,80] In one study, it was suggested that children with neuropathy could be differentiated from those with functional fecal retention (see Figure 70-7) by a lack of HAPCs and a lack of increase in the postprandial motility index (Figure 70-8).[79] Di Lorenzo and colleagues have also suggested that in young children, the lack of HAPCs is a sensitive marker of disease, but these data require further validation.[77,79,80]

Intracolonic bisacodyl has been administered to try to shorten the duration of the motility study in ill children or in

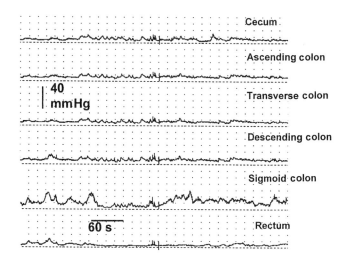

FIGURE 70-8 Abnormal colonic manometry. No high-amplitude propagating contractions (HAPCs) or changes in the motility index were seen in this patient with a colonic neuropathy. No HAPCs were seen even after the administration of bisacodyl.

those who cannot eat.[78] It has been shown that the HAPCs induced after bisacodyl were similar in amplitude, duration, propagation velocity, and sites of origin and extinction to naturally occurring HAPCs.[78] They found that the effect of intrarectal bisacodyl was similar to that of intracecal bisacodyl, except for a delay of 10 minutes in onset.[78] In their study of 28 patients with functional fecal retention, 22 had spontaneous HAPCs, whereas the 28 patients had HAPCs induced by bisacodyl. From 9 with pseudo-obstruction, none had spontaneous HAPCs, whereas 2 had HAPCs after bisacodyl. The interpretation of HAPCs in those 2 children is difficult because it raises the possibility that those children did not have pseudo-obstruction.

The use of colonic motility in children has also been found to be useful in the understanding of postoperative problems in patients with Hirschsprung disease[81] and imperforate anus.[82] It has also been suggested that colonic motility may help in the detection of abnormal colonic segments that may require surgical resection, but these findings need further validation.[81]

Indications. The information obtained from colonic motility still needs to be considered within the context of there being no normal controls in children and many unanswered questions about normal colonic function, the effects of colonic preparation on the results, and so on.[1]

Colonic motility is indicated in the evaluation of selected patients with intractable constipation because it can be helpful to differentiate functional fecal retention from colonic pseudo-obstruction.[1,78] It is also indicated in the evaluation of children with pseudo-obstruction to assess for the presence of colonic involvement and to characterize the relationship between motor abnormalities and symptoms, particularly when a colectomy is being considered. The test is also indicated to determine the relationship between motor activity and persistent symptoms following surgery for Hirschsprung disease and other colorectal problems. Colonic motility should also be performed to assess colonic motor activity prior to intestinal transplant.[1]

ANORECTAL MANOMETRY

Anorectal manometry is used for the evaluation of children with defecation abnormalities (see Table 70-2)[1,2] and probably represents one of the most frequently performed motility tests in children. The main indication is for the exclusion of Hirschsprung disease,[1,2,83] but it also has an important role in the evaluation of children with fecal incontinence from various etiologies such as myelomeningocele or imperforate anus.[2]

Anorectal physiology has been studied because it has a vital role in maintaining continence. Normal continence and defecation are complex functions. Continence is maintained by the interaction of several mechanisms, including stool consistency, delivery of colonic contents to the rectum, rectal capacity, anorectal sensation, sphincteric function, and muscles and nerves of the pelvic floor. Intra-anal pressure is a combination of both internal and external anal sphincter interaction, with the former providing about

75 to 85% of the total pressure.[84] In adults, the proximal anal canal pressures are lower in the anterior quadrant, and, distally, the pressures are lower in the posterior quadrant. The internal anal sphincter (IAS) is smooth muscle and is in a state of continuous contraction.[85] The external anal sphincter (EAS) and the muscles of the pelvic floor also maintain continuous tone. When a fecal bolus enters the rectum, there is a reflex relaxation of the IAS (rectoanal inhibitory reflex [RAIR]) (Figure 70-9) and transient contraction of the EAS.[85] This relaxation is limited, and the sphincter reacquires its tone as the rectum accommodates to the distention. The relaxation of the IAS occurs independently of the spine and is lost when there is a lack of inhibitory ganglion cells (as in Hirschsprung disease) (Figure 70-10).[86] This relaxation enables the rectal contents to come into contact with the upper anal canal ("sampling reflex"), and normal people can discriminate among solids, liquids, or gas. The transient simultaneous contraction of the EAS allows time for the IAS to recuperate, avoiding incontinence. Further rectal distention with increasing volumes results in nonrecovery of the IAS. If it is socially acceptable, the person has a bowel movement; if not, the conscious contraction of the EAS and rectal compliance allow for postponement until it is socially acceptable.

Different techniques have been used to perform anorectal manometry. In children, the most common method used is with water-perfused catheters that have side holes at different levels of the longitudinal and radial axis.[1,86–89] A balloon is attached to the distal segment and inflated to produce rectal distention.[88] Usually, it is made of latex, and care should be taken when the test is performed in children who may be allergic to it. Solid-state catheters have also been used, but they are much more expensive. Another technique involves the use of a double-balloon device, but its use in pediatrics is limited, particularly because the size is too large for smaller children. The recent advent of micromanometric techniques with the use of sleeve sensors has allowed the accurate study of anal sphincters even in the very low birth weight patient.[90]

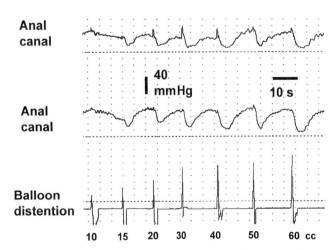

FIGURE 70-9 Normal anorectal manometry. The tracing shows the response of the internal anal sphincter to balloon distention. A normal sphincter relaxation after balloon distention can be observed. The relaxation follows a dose-response curve.

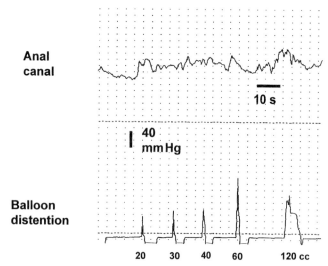

FIGURE 70-10 Anorectal manometry in a patient with Hirschsprung disease. Tracing in which balloon distention does not induce the rectoanal inhibitory reflex, even after large balloon volumes were used. This patient was later proven to have Hirschsprung disease.

In older patients, a phosphate enema is usually given the night before the manometry, and medications known to change anorectal function are stopped 48 hours before the test (eg, opiates, prokinetics, anticholinergics). If the patient is severely impacted, a cleanout is performed 2 to 3 days before the test. Children receive nothing by mouth for 4 to 6 hours before the procedure (depending on the age) if they will be sedated or when the primary indication for the test is to exclude Hirschsprung disease in case a rectal biopsy is needed.

During anorectal manometry in pediatric patients, a slow pull-through is performed in which the manometric assembly is pulled until a high-pressure zone is identified (intra-anal pressure). The probe is then positioned at the level of the maximum pressure, which is usually 1 to 2 cm above the anal verge. The balloon is then inflated to elicit the RAIR (see Figure 70-9).[1,86,88] The characteristics of the relaxation are studied. The minimum amount of air required to elicit a relaxation is determined (threshold of relaxation). The amount of relaxation is influenced not only by the volume but also by the speed of the inflated balloon, as well as by rectal resting volume and compliance. It is important to use large balloon volumes in patients with megarectum because a lack of sphincter relaxation may result from an inadequate distention of the rectal wall. The volume necessary for constant relaxation, which is the minimal amount of air that is necessary to produce a complete sustained relaxation of both the IAS and the EAS, is determined by adding air progressively until either there is constant relaxation or the patient has reached the critical volume (see below).[85]

Besides measuring the resting pressure of the anal canal, the patient is also asked to squeeze at each station. The squeeze pressure is then measured as the maximum pressure obtained above anal resting pressure.[1,88]

During manometric testing, some sensory information is obtained.[1] The most common technique is with the use of balloon distention. In cooperative children, the threshold required to perceive the distention is established (smallest volume of balloon distention) (threshold of sensation).[88,91,92] The threshold of sensation is usually determined with the use of a rectal balloon that is inflated with a handheld syringe. The air is rapidly injected and immediately withdrawn. The type of inflation (speed, phasic vs continuous), the size and shape of the balloon, or the distance of the balloon to the anal verge can affect the threshold. Critical volume has been defined as the minimum amount of air that produces a lasting urge to defecate[85,88] and the sensation of pain, which is defined as the maximum tolerable volume, although the clinical significance of those measurements is not clear.[85]

Compliance is measured as the ratio of pressure to volume at several distending volumes. Measurements are usually inaccurate and not reproducible unless a barostat is being used. Decreased compliance may be associated with an increase in stool frequency, rapid transit of stool in the rectum, and increased risk of fecal incontinence.[85] On the other hand, increased compliance may be found in patients with megarectum. There is a paucity of information on its use in pediatrics.

The study of defecation dynamics may be important (Figure 70-11).[1] This is done with the use of either electromyographic (EMG) surface electrodes or with the manometric assembly. Patients are asked to bear down, and the responses of the sphincters are recorded. Pelvic floor dyssynergia (anismus) is present when there is failure of relaxation or even an increase in pressure while attempting to defecate (Figure 70-12).[88,91,93] There has been some controversy as to whether this observed pattern is sufficient for the diagnosis. In one study, when the manometry indicated dyssynergia, the defecography was in agreement only 36% of the time, whereas when manometry was normal, defecography was normal in 88%.[94] No similar information is available in children.

Development. Studies of the developmental maturation of the rectoanal reflex have produced inconsistent results.

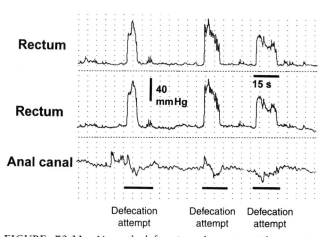

FIGURE 70-11 Normal defecation dynamics. The tracing shows the pressure changes in the rectum and anal canal when a normal child is trying to defecate. Note an increase in rectal pressure with a decrease in anal pressure.

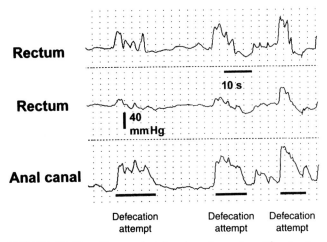

FIGURE 70-12 Abnormal defecation dynamics. The tracing shows the pressure changes in the rectum and anal canal when a child with anismus is trying to defecate. Note an increase in rectal pressure with a simultaneous increase in anal pressure.

The advent of micromanometric techniques and the use of sleeve sensors have allowed the accurate study of different sphincters even in the very low birth weight patient.[8,23,90]

Initial studies in premature infants have suggested that they do not have a RAIR. Some have shown that the RAIR may be physiologically absent up to 12 days of life in newborns, particularly if they are sick.[95] Ito and colleagues reported that the RAIR does not appear before a maturational age of 39 weeks.[96] Recently, however, other authors have found that the RAIR may be present in the first hours even in otherwise healthy premature infants,[86,89,97,98] although in three normal infants, there was absence relaxation at birth. On repeat manometries a few weeks later, the RAIR was preset, suggesting that there may be a maturational response. In a study of neonates, the range of anal resting tone was between 16 and 72 mm Hg.[86] The magnitude of anal tone was inversely correlated with weight but not gestational age. The amplitude of the RAIR in premature infants did not correlate with maturational age but correlated inversely with weight.[86]

A study of the anal inhibitory reflex in premature infants using micromanometric techniques and a sleeve has recently been published.[90] The authors studied 22 healthy neonates with a mean conceptual age of 32 weeks (30–38 weeks). They showed that the mean intra-anal pressure was 40 mm Hg (range 7–65 mm Hg), and they were able to induce a RAIR in 21 of 22 infants. The infant in which the RAIR was not present had a very low sphincter pressure (7 mm Hg), which made the determination of the reflex impossible. Resting anal pressure correlated significantly with postmenstrual age. The authors also found that gestational age, postnatal age, and time from birth to passage of the first stool did not correlate with any parameter of anorectal function. They asserted that air insufflation is the preferred method to produce the RAIR in children less than 34 weeks gestational age.[90]

Clinical Significance. Normal values for anorectal manometry in adults have been published.[85,99] The length of

the anal canal was reported to range from 2.2 to 4.0 ± 1.0 cm in women and from 2.8 to 4.0 ± 1.0 in men. Anal resting tone varied from 49 ± 3 to 58 ± 3 mm Hg in women and from 49 ± 3 to 66 ± 6 mm Hg in men. Maximum squeeze ranged from 90 ± 9 to 159 ± 45 mm Hg in women and from 218 ± 18 to 238 ± 38 in men. The threshold for IAS relaxation varied from 14 ± 1 to 25 ± 2 mL, and the threshold for sensation varied from 12 ± 1 to 17 ± 9 mL.[99]

No similar comprehensive information is available for children. Values for normal controls have been published by different authors. The mean normal anal resting pressure in children ranges from 57 ± 10 mm Hg[88] to 67 ± 12 mm Hg.[100] The maximum squeeze pressure ranges from 118 ± 42 mm Hg[88] to 140 ± 52 mm Hg,[100] anal length is around 3.3 ± 0.8 cm,[100] the threshold to produce relaxation (RAIR) ranges from 5 ± 1 mL[88] to 11 ± 5 mL,[100] the threshold of rectal sensation ranges from 5 ± 2 mL[88] to 14 ± 7 mL,[100] the volume of constant relaxation is 104 ± 49 mL,[100] and the critical volume is 101 ± 39 mL.[100]

The main indication for anorectal manometry in pediatrics is to exclude the presence of a nonrelaxing IAS (see Table 70-2).[1] The finding of sphincteric relaxation (RAIR) excludes Hirschsprung disease (see Figure 70-9), particularly in older children,[101] and avoids the performance of more invasive testing such as a biopsy.[86] On the other hand, the lack of sphincteric relaxation strongly indicates the presence of Hirschsprung disease (see Figure 70-10), but a confirmatory biopsy is necessary.[86,100] In those patients in whom there are no technical difficulties and who have a nonrelaxing IAS with normal biopsies, a diagnosis of IAS achalasia needs to be considered.[102] The accuracy for the diagnosis of Hirschsprung disease by manometry varies with the age of the patients.[101,103] Anorectal manometry seems to be more accurate in older children,[104,105] for whom recent studies have suggested an accuracy of 90 to 100%. Most authors report that the accuracy in neonates is lower.[86,96,101,104–106]

A recent study of 59 patients (2–90 days) reported a sensitivity, specificity, positive predictive value, and negative predictive value of anorectal manometry for the diagnosis of Hirschsprung disease of 0.91, 0.56, 0.84, and 0.92, respectively.[103] In other studies, the overall accuracy, sensitivity, specificity, and positive and negative predictive values were 90%, 0.79, 0.97, 0.94, and 0.88, respectively, whereas in neonates, it was 90%, 0.86, 1, 1, 0.75, and in infants, it was 94%, 0.9, 1, 1, and 0.89, respectively.[106]

In the largest study of 229 manometries, there were 10 false-positive and 8 false-negative results, indicating an overall 7.8% error rate.[101] However, in a group of 38 neonates (including 7 premature infants), 26% had an inaccurate diagnosis. In 6 newborns with Hirschsprung disease, the manometry was normal, whereas in 4 normal newborns, there was no RAIR.[101] The numbers are even more inaccurate in premature infants. In that series, the diagnosis was incorrect in 71.4% of premature infants, in whom the authors found 2 children with proven Hirschsprung disease but 3 false-negative and 2 false-positive manometric findings.[101] In 39 children from 1 to 6 months of age (8 with Hirschsprung disease), there were

2 false-positive cases and 1 false-negative case, with a 7.7% error rate. From 41 children 6 months to 2 years of age (8 with Hirschsprung disease), there were 2 false-negative cases and 1 false-positive case, with a 7.3% error rate. In 47 children from 2 to 5 years of age (1 with Hirschsprung disease), there was 1 false-positive case, for an error rate of 2%. In 64 children from 5 to 15 years (2 with Hirschsprung disease), there was 1 false-negative case, for an error rate of 1.5%. This and other studies confirm the impression that accuracy increases as age increases.

Studies specifically performed looking at the experience in neonates have confirmed those observations. In some studies, it has been reported that manometry has led to the wrong diagnosis in up to 26% of neonates,[86,96,101] and it is generally reported that the diagnostic accuracy at that age varies from 70 to 80%.[86,104,105] Recently, a study in which 64 newborns (6 premature infants) with meconium delay or obstruction in whom repeated manometries were performed weekly for the first month of life was reported. There were 5 children with Hirschsprung disease in whom repeated manometries did not show a RAIR. There were, however, 3 newborns in whom the initial manometry did not show the RAIR, but when the study was repeated a few weeks later, it showed normal relaxation.[89] The opposite has been shown by other authors[106]: the manometry performed in the first 10 days of life may also give false-negative results (normal RAIR). In one report of 26 children with Hirschsprung disease, 3 initially had normal manometries that, when repeated later because of the persistence of symptoms, did not show a RAIR, and histology subsequently diagnosed Hirschsprung disease.[107] Therefore, anorectal manometry in the newborn may show more false-positive and false-negative results.

The false-negative results during anorectal manometry probably represent artifacts, such as movements of the probe, passage of flatus or feces, or relaxation of the EAS.[101] To avoid technical mistakes, it is necessary to have an empty rectum and correct position of the probe and to watch closely for movement (which could produce an artificial relaxation).

The false-positive manometries could be explained by different factors. First, there could be immaturity of the ganglion cells, particularly in premature infants and neonates. Other factors could include the following: some children have a high relaxation threshold, there could be technical errors in which the relaxation zone may be missed, and, finally, the presence of feces in the anorectum could interfere.[101]

Before a patient who has a nonrelaxing IAS and obstructive symptoms with normal biopsies is categorized as having a false-positive manometry, one has to decide if the patient suffers from IAS achalasia, or ultrashort-segment Hirschprung disease.[102,108–110] Anorectal manometry is the only way to diagnose this entity. In IAS achalasia, there is a nonrelaxing IAS, but the biopsies show normal ganglion cells and normal acetylcholinesterase.[102,108–110]

Another important use of anorectal manometry in children with constipation, after Hirschsprung disease has been excluded, is to detect those who have pelvic floor dyssynergia (see Table 70-2 and Figures 70-11 and 70-12).[92] Pelvic floor dyssynergia has been found in 30 to 53% of patients with constipation who have undergone manometry. The significance of this finding has been controversial, but it has been suggested that it may be associated with lower recovery rates.[91,111,112] Attempts to normalize defecation dynamics have been undertaken with biofeedback therapy.[93,113–115] In multiple open-label studies, biofeedback was shown to be effective, but the results of recent randomized trials have not demonstrated long-term efficacy.[93,113–115]

Changes in resting and squeeze pressure, as well as abnormal sensation, have been found inconsistently in patients with constipation by different authors and do not seem to have any major clinical implications.[1,88,111,116–118] Abnormal sensation has also been described in children with constipation,[88,92,112] and it is not known if the abnormality represents a primary problem or if it is secondary to the megarectum.

Manometry is useful in the evaluation of patients who have undergone surgery for Hirschsprung disease and continue to have incontinence or obstructive symptoms (see Table 70-2).[1] The presence of the RAIR in postoperative patients has been variable and in most studies does not seem to be correlated with outcome.[119–121] In a long-term follow-up study of adults, there was a positive correlation between functional outcome and anal resting pressure.[122] It has recently been suggested that those with obstructive symptoms and a high-pressure, nonrelaxing sphincter may benefit from procedures designed to decrease sphincter pressure. IAS myectomy[123] or, recently, botulinum toxin injection has been used.[102,124] Anorectal manometry is therefore a technique that allows detection of the nonrelaxing sphincter and may be useful to decide if the patient is a candidate for botulinum toxin or to evaluate patients after it has been applied.

The utility of anorectal manometry in diagnosing neuronal intestinal dysplasia is controversial.[125,126] The first difficulty arises because there is no consensus regarding the histologic diagnosis.[126] However, even in those reports in which a diagnosis of neuronal intestinal dysplasia has been made, the anorectal manometry has not been able to discriminate abnormal from normal cases.[125,127,128]

Anorectal manometry has been shown to allow some discrimination between patients with or without fecal incontinence (see Table 70-2).[1,129–132] In a study of 350 patients, 178 of whom were incontinent by history, it was found that squeeze pressure had the greatest sensitivity (60%) and specificity (78%) if a cutoff value of 60 mm Hg was used.[129] The measurement of the resting anal canal pressure was less sensitive and specific. In another study comparing 302 patients with fecal incontinence and 65 controls, it was found that by taking the mean – 2 SD for controls as the cutoff, the sensitivity of the maximum squeeze pressure to predict incontinence was 92% and the specificity was 97%. Basal anal resting tone had a sensitivity of only 37%.[130] An abnormal sensation has also been reported in patients with fecal incontinence,[131] and it has been suggested that the most important component of biofeedback training for fecal incontinence is an improved ability to detect rectal distention.

In patients with imperforate anus, anorectal manometry is a useful technique to evaluate the state of intrarectal pressure and sensation, as well as of the voluntary muscles.[1,131,133–135] Some studies have found that patients with a repaired imperforate anus have significant abnormalities in anorectal function.[131,134,135] It has been shown that patients with more incontinence have lower squeeze pressures and sensation abnormalities.[131,133] In postoperative patients with fecal incontinence, the measurement of intra-anal pressure is important, particularly when a reoperation is being considered. Also, a manometric evaluation may allow the detection of abnormalities that may be amenable to biofeedback training.[2,131,135,136]

Indications. The main indication is in the evaluation of children with constipation to exclude the presence of a nonrelaxing IAS (see Table 70-2).[1] Hirschsprung disease also has to be considered in older patients (including adults) with intractable constipation.[137] It is indicated in the evaluation of patients with fecal incontinence to evaluate sphincter function and weakness, as well as sensation.[1] In patients with imperforate anus repair or neurogenic problems, it may be useful to decide if the patient is a candidate for biofeedback.[1] It is also indicated in the evaluation of children with Hirschsprung disease who have postoperative obstructive symptoms to determine if they are candidates for botulinum toxin or after botulinum toxin has been applied and the symptoms recur (see Table 70-2).[1]

The study of defecation dynamics is also important, although the use of biofeedback in children has not been shown to be effective.[1,113]

Other Tests to Evaluate Anorectal Function. EMG of the pelvic muscles can be performed using either a needle electrode, a surface electrode, or an anal plug. This test allows the identification of areas of injury, establishes if the muscle contracts or relaxes, and identifies evidence of denervation-reinnervation. The needle electrodes that are used study the activity of a large number of motor units (concentric) or a single fiber. This requires the insertion of the needle in the perineum into the sphincter muscle, so it is painful, and its utility in children is limited. In children, it is most useful in the evaluation of postoperative patients of imperforate anus, in which it may be used to show the presence or absence of striated muscle around the anal opening. It is also useful in the establishment of nerve damage from spinal lesions. Because of its invasiveness and its limited usefulness, needle EMG is not routinely used in pediatrics. On the other hand, superficial EMG electrodes can be useful, particularly to evaluate for the presence of pelvic floor dyssynergia.[88,91] This causes less discomfort to the patient. It has also been shown that the number of motor units recruited during squeeze correlates with squeeze pressure. Therefore, surface electrodes have been successfully used in the assessment of defecation dynamics and squeeze pressure and can also be used to provide biofeedback training.[113]

Other tests, such as balloon expulsion and pudendal nerve terminal motor latency, have not been shown to have a clinical role in the evaluation of children.

OTHER STUDIES TO EVALUATE GASTROINTESTINAL NEUROMUSCULAR FUNCTION

ELECTROGASTROGRAPHY

Electrogastrography (EGG) is a technique in which the electrical activity generated by gastric smooth muscles is measured.[138–140] It is a noninvasive method of assessing the gastric myoelectrical activity that controls gastric motility.[140–144] This is now done by using surface cutaneous electrodes placed on the abdomen overlying the stomach.[138,141,142] Because of its noninvasive nature, it represents an attractive tool for the diagnosis of gastric motility problems in children.[138,139,141–143]

The cutaneous EGG usually uses three to four electrodes that are placed on the abdominal wall close to the antral region to reduce interference and to obtain a high signal-to-noise ratio.[138,144] Ideally, the electrodes are placed either with ultrasound or fluoroscopic guidance to identify the gastric contour.[140–144] In adults, it has been advocated that a standard configuration can be used without the need for imaging studies.[138,140,144] The first electrode is set above the antrum (located 1 to 3 cm right of the midline, between the xiphoid process and the umbilicus), the second 45° and 3 to 6 cm above and left of the first electrode (based on the size of the subject), and the third (reference) at the left flank, horizontal to the first electrode. In an effort to establish if it is possible to accurately place the electrodes without the use of ultrasonography in neonates, Patterson and colleagues compared the results obtained by both ultrasonography or blind placement of the skin electrodes and found no differences.[142] In another study in premature infants, the first electrode was located immediately below the left costal margin in the midclavicular line.[141] The third electrode was located between the umbilicus and the xiphoid process and the second electrode between the first and third electrodes.

The duration of an EGG recording session may vary depending on the center or the working diagnosis.[138,140,144] Most commonly, the test is performed with 1-hour fasting, then a standardized meal is given, and the activity is recorded for another 1 to 2 hours postprandially.[138,140–144] It has been suggested that for the major EGG parameters, 30 minutes in the fasting state is sufficient to produce reliable results, and in the postprandial period, recordings from 30 to 60 minutes adequately represent the change after meal ingestion.[140] The recordings are analyzed by computer using specialized software, and usually the fast Fourier transform is used to detect the dominant frequencies.[42,138,139,141,143]

The major EGG parameters that are analyzed include the following: the dominant frequency, the dominant power, the percentage of normal slow waves, the percentage of gastric dysrhythmias, and, in some centers, the dominant frequency instability coefficient (DFIC).[138,139,141,143]

Many studies have documented that the dominant frequency of the cutaneous EGG corresponds to the basal gastric rhythm or frequency of the gastric slow wave.[138,140,144] It is thought that the electrical activity reflects the gastric slow wave generated by the stomach's pacemaker, the interstitial cells of Cajal of the greater curvature.[55,140,143] The normal gastric slow-wave frequency is about 3 cycles per minute (cpm) (normal range 2–4 cpm).[138] The computer also determines the "power" for each of the signal frequencies. Power is a reflection of both the amplitude and the regularity of the EGG.[140,144] It has been shown that the EGG amplitude does not always correlate with the force of the gastric contractions,[144] and the absolute value is influenced by electrode placement, skin/fat thickness (distance between stomach and skin), and movement of the stomach.[140,144] Therefore, only relative changes are considered by comparing in the same individual the change of the power after a meal.[138,140,144] This can be calculated from the ratio of the postprandial power of the dominant frequency to the preprandial power of the dominant frequency.[139,143,144] Usually, the postprandial-to-fasting power ratio value is more than 1.[55,144] It has been suggested that a diminished or absent increase in the power ratio correlates to delayed gastric emptying and antral hypomotility.[144]

The percentage of normal slow waves reflects the regularity of the EGG.[140] It is defined as the percentage of time during which 2 to 4 cpm slow waves are present across the entire recording. Studies suggest that most healthy individuals display a value above 70% in fasting and postprandial states.[140]

A dysrhythmic index (percentage of dysrhythmic time during the recording) is usually reported.[138] It measures the percentage of time during the recording in which 2 to 4 cpm slow waves are absent. It has been suggested that abnormal rhythms of gastric myoelectrical activity may be detected. They are classified as tachygastria (rapid) usually > 4 cpm, bradygastria (slow) < 2 cycles/min; bradytachyarrhythmia (mixed), or absent activity.[139,143,144] Antral hypomotility has been associated with both brady- or tachyarrhythmia.[139,144] Values for a 1-hour recording in both fasting and fed states have been reported in 10 asymptomatic children and in 14 children with dyspepsia.[145] The fasting dysrhythmic index was 1.6% (range 1.6–33.3) in the controls versus 33.3% (range 10–48) in the dyspeptic patients. The fed dysrhythmic index was 2.7% (range 1.6–5.5) in controls and 15% (range 11–66) in patients.[145]

The DFIC specifies the stability of the gastric electrical peak visible on the running spectra plot and calculated as the percentage ratio of the frequency standard deviation to mean gastric frequency.[138] The DFIC reflects subtle changes in gastric slow waves.

In children, the validation of the technique is limited, but the use of EGG is growing. One of the biggest problems so far has been the fact that there is almost no information about the normal EGG patterns in healthy children, including a lack of information on developmental aspects.

A study in 114 normal children (6–12 years) found in the preprandial state a dominant frequency of 3.0 cpm (2.1–3.5), a DFIC of 26% (6.7–54.5), normal slow waves of 81.5% (59.3–100), bradygastria of 3.7% (0–22.2), and tachygastria of 9.4% (0–38.7).[146] The dominant frequency postprandially was 3.0 cpm (2.1–3.7), the DFIC was 30% (11–67; $p < .05$), normal slow waves were 76.9% (54.4–97.2), bradygastria was 4.9% (0–29.3), and tachygastria was 11.8 (0–35). The EGG power increased postprandially to a power ratio of 3.6 (0.8–19.7). The researchers found no age differences or effects of age, gender, and body mass index.[146]

In another study of 24 normal boys ranging from 1 to 11 years (mean 6 years), Cheng and Tam found that the percentage of bradygastria was higher in younger children, accounting for 34% of the recording.[147] The normal 3 cpm increased with age, whereas the bradygastria decreased. They suggested that by the end of the first decade, the EGG patterns are similar to those in the adult,

A recent study of 50 healthy volunteers ranging in age from 6 to 18 years described a mean dominant frequency of 2.9 ± 0.4 cpm preprandially and 3.1 ± 0.35 postprandially, with $80\% \pm 13\%$ of test time spent in the normogastric range (2–4 cpm) before and $85\% \pm 11\%$ after the test meal.[143] The authors concluded that there was a postprandial increase in rhythmicity and amplitude of the gastric slow waves and that key normative values are not dependent on age, gender, or body mass index.[143]

Development. Different authors have found that both preterm and newborn infants have a low percentage of gastric slow waves.[148,149] Chen and colleagues studied EGG in five different groups: premature infants, newborns, infants 2 to 6 months, children 4 to 11 years, and adults.[149] Children and adults showed similar activity.[149] Infants showed a percentage of normal slow wave that was significantly lower than that in adults but higher than in newborn and premature infants. The percentage of 2 to 4 cpm slow waves was $26 \pm 4\%$ in premature infants, $30 \pm 4\%$ in full-term infants, 70 ± 6 in 2- to 6-month-old infants, $85 \pm 3\%$ in children 4 to 11 years, and $89 \pm 2\%$ in adults.[149] As in other studies, both newborns and premature infants showed an absence or a decrease in normal slow waves.[148–150] The biggest limitation of the study is the small number of patients. Koch and colleagues also showed that in premature infants and newborns, there were no significant differences in activity after gavage feeding.[150] Bradygastria, 3 cpm, and tachygastria comprised 49%, 17%, and 29% of the preprandial recording and 51%, 15%, and 27% of the postprandial EGG.[150]

The developmental maturation of the gastric slow waves has recently been analyzed in a longitudinal study of 19 preterm infants followed from birth to 6 months. It was shown that the percentage of 2 to 4 cpm slow waves increased gradually over time to a value slightly lower than that in adults.[151] The rate of development was twice as fast in the first 2 months, and dominant peaks and an increase in power were not observed at birth in any of the infants but could be identified in 70% of the children at 6 months of age.[151] Patterson and colleagues studied 9 healthy neonates born at 34 weeks gestation and showed that their EGG differed from that of adults.[141] Tachygastria and bradygastria were seen more frequently, with fewer episodes of 3 cpm. There was an increase in 3 cpm episodes over time.[141]

Clinical Significance. Interest in EGG has been generated not only because it is a noninvasive technique but also because, in recent years, a correlation between disorders in gastric electrical rhythm and certain clinical syndromes characterized by alterations in gastrointestinal motility has been described.[138,140,146] Because normal motility of the stomach requires integrity of the enteric and extrinsic nerves and smooth muscle, any abnormality in them may result in dysfunction.[140] Therefore, there are some diseases in which EGG may be theoretically useful, and it is possible that it may be used as a noninvasive screening technique[140] or, most importantly, as a way to evaluate follow-up or the results of therapy, particularly when invasive techniques are the only other alternative. To date, however, no therapies have convincingly demonstrated in controlled studies that correcting abnormalities detected by EGG improves upper gastrointestinal symptoms.[138] Ideally, EGG could be used as a screening tool to detect those patients who may have underlying motility disorders. It may provide evidence that upper gastrointestinal symptoms are associated with gastric dysmotility. However, studies have shown that there are patients with gastric dysrhythmias who do not have abnormal motility or that not all patients with abnormal motility have dysrhythmias. In children, limited data have tried to validate the specificity and sensitivity of EGG to detect motility disorders in children. In a study in which simultaneous EGG was performed together with antroduodenal motility in 25 children, the authors found that EGG differentiated groups of children with normal manometry from others with neuropathic or myopathic change, but in some patients, there was an overlap of EGG results between children with normal and abnormal manometry.[55] The percentage of tachygastria time was higher in patients with mild ($44 \pm 16\%$) and severe neuropathy ($48 \pm 19\%$) compared with those with myopathy ($20 \pm 16\%$) or normal motility ($23 \pm 13\%$). There was considerable overlap in the percentage of tachygastria and total arrhythmia time among the different groups. Every child with a total arrhythmia time < 35% and a ratio of postprandial-to-preprandial power > 2.4 had normal motility.[55]

In children, EGG has also been used as a method to understand the physiopathology of upper gastrointestinal symptoms in patients with different medical problems, such as pseudo-obstruction,[152] GER after fundoplication,[153,154] with functional dyspepsia[139,140,145] or in children with systemic or generalized problems. Gastric dysrhythmias have been described in children with renal failure,[155] Noonan syndrome,[156] cyclic vomiting,[157] cystic fibrosis,[139] or neurologic handicaps.[154,158]

EGG has also been suggested as a noninvasive way in which to evaluate the effects of therapy for motor disorders. In a study to evaluate the effects of cisapride, Cucchiara and colleagues showed that after 8 weeks of therapy, the medication reversed the abnormal myoelectric activity in three children with nonulcer dyspepsia.[159]

Indications. Even though, at present, the use of EGG in children is still considered a research tool and future studies will be needed to continue to validate its usefulness, it is very likely that EGG will become a useful test in the evaluation and treatment of children with gastrointestinal motility disorders. The most likely indication will be in the evaluation of children with unexplained nausea, vomiting, and postprandial abdominal bloating or distention. It may also become a screening test to predict gastroparesis, to assess for gastric motor dysfunction in patients with other gastrointestinal symptoms (eg, constipation), to try to predict who will develop symptoms after fundoplication, or to follow the response to medications.[42,55,140,153,154,159] For now, however, the proposed clinical indications for the performance of the EGG in adult and pediatric patients with unexplained nausea, vomiting, and dyspeptic symptoms must be validated by prospective controlled investigations.[138]

OTHER FUTURE TECHNIQUES
Other gastrointestinal motility studies are currently being performed mostly in adult units or research laboratories that have the potential to become clinically useful in pediatrics. Therefore, a brief description follows, although, at present, there is very limited information in children, and these studies have no role in the routine treatment of children with motility problems.

Manometry of the SO. The evaluation of manometry of the SO has been used mainly to evaluate patients for SO dysfunction. The intraluminal pressure recording from the billiary tree requires intubation with the use of endoscopic retrograde cholangiopancreatography (ERCP), which makes the technique very invasive. Also, the effects of anesthesia or sedation on manometric results have not been well established. In addition to the technical difficulties involved, the performance of SO manometry increases the incidence of post-ERCP pancreatitis and may result in pancreatitis in up to 15 to 20% of patients.[160]

When SO manometry is performed, a perfused system is usually used. A catheter with three lumens of 0.5 mm internal diameter making up a catheter of 1.7 mm or a tapering catheter of 1.5 outer diameter is usually introduced using the biopsy channel of the duodenoscope through the papilla and into either the bile duct or the pancreatic duct. The catheter is then withdrawn until all three recording ports are situated in the SO. The SO is characterized by a basal pressure on which prominent pressure peaks representing phasic contractions are superimposed. Usually, the basal SO pressure ranges from 3 to 35, with a median of 15 mm Hg.[161,162]

Over the past decade, different abnormalities of the SO have been described,[160,161] and abnormal pressure is the parameter most often employed.[161] The clinical significance of SO manometric findings is still debated. Some authors recommend SO manometry for the evaluation of recurrent pancreatitis or unexplained biliary pain and for the selection of those patients who may benefit from endoscopic therapy (eg, sphincterotomy).[160,161] In children, there is very limited information,[162] and there are no normal controls or validation of its clinical utility. Because of those limitations and the high incidence of pancreatitis associated with its performance, SO manometry should still be considered only a research tool, although it is possible that, in the future, it may have a role in the evaluation and treatment of children with unexplained right upper quadrant pain or recurrent pancreatitis.[162]

Barostat. This technique allows the study of a component of motor activity that cannot be evaluated by conventional manometry or EMG. The barostat is mainly used to measure intraluminal volume or pressure relationships and helps to establish sensory thresholds.[163,164] The instrument requires a high-compliance balloon, and it measures tone by monitoring the volume of air required to maintain a constant preselected pressure level in a flaccid bag. The system uses an electronically regulated air injection/aspiration device. The volume of the bag increases or decreases depending on intraluminal pressure, which is determined by the motor activity of the organ being studied. When used in the stomach, it uses a balloon designed for the fundus/body, in which relaxations and contractions are relatively slow.

The barostat also allows the quantification of sensory thresholds triggered by intraluminal distention. In children, the use of the barostat has allowed some insight into the pathophysiology of irritable bowel syndrome and abdominal pain.[163,164] At this point, the barostat remains a research tool that is being used to understand the physiopathology of irritable bowel syndrome or other gastrointestinal disorders and to evaluate the effects of therapy, and it is difficult to predict what role it will play in the routine evaluation and treatment of patients with gastrointestinal motility disorders.

TRAINING IN GASTROINTESTINAL MANOMETRY

The North American Society for Pediatric Gastroenterology Hepatology and Nutrition (NASPGHAN) has approved and published guidelines for training in gastrointestinal motility.[165] The guidelines recommend two levels of training. Level 1, or basic training, is expected from all trainees and includes understanding the pathophysiology of motility disorders, treatment of an adequate number of patients with these problems, and understanding of the rationale, usefulness, and limitations of the common tests used in the evaluation of the patient. Level 2, or advanced training, is recommended for those who are planning to perform specialized motility studies or act as consultants to other gastroenterologists. Table 70-4 shows the number of procedures recommended to achieve proficiency in the performance of the common gastrointestinal manometry studies.[165]

SUMMARY

The study of gastrointestinal motility in children continues to evolve and has changed from being a research technique to becoming a useful diagnostic tool. There continues to be

TABLE 70-4   NUMBER OF PROCEDURES TO ACHIEVE COMPETENCE IN GASTROINTESTINAL MANOMETRY*

STUDY TYPE	THRESHOLD FOR COMPETENCE
Esophageal manometry	20
Anorectal manometry	20
Antroduodenal manometry	25
Colonic manometry	25
Electrogastrography	25

Adapted from Rudolph C et al.[165]
*NASPGHN guidelines.

a dichotomy between the use of manometry as an investigation technique or as a useful clinical test, and as new techniques are being developed and validated, the clinical indications are becoming better defined. The performance of gastrointestinal manometry in children is more challenging, and recent technical advances have allowed the study of younger and smaller babies, which has allowed the understanding of some developmental aspects.

The role of gastrointestinal manometry has been defined more clearly for anorectal and esophageal manometry, although small bowel motility is becoming clinically more accepted. Other studies are mainly performed in research laboratories and have still not been fully validated. Manometry is mainly useful for the diagnosis of primary motility disorders and can be useful in some cases in which the motility alterations are secondary to other illness. In general, the manometric evaluation may detect aberrations that may be clinically insignificant, so care needs to be exerted to avoid overinterpretation.

REFERENCES

1. DiLorenzo C, Hillemeier C, Hyman P, et al. Manometry studies in children: minimum standards for procedures. Neurogastroenterol Motil 2002;14:411–20.
2. Kaul A, Rudolph CD. Gastrointestinal manometry studies in children. J Clin Gastroenterol 1998;27:187–91.
3. Camilleri M. Study of human gastroduodenojejunal motility. Applied physiology in clinical practice. Dig Dis Sci 1993;38:785–94.
4. Kahrilas PJ, Clouse RE, Hogan WJ. American Gastroenterological Association technical review on the clinical use of esophageal manometry. Gastroenterology 1994;107:1865–84.
5. Baron HI, Beck DC, Vargas JH, Ament ME. Overinterpretation of gastroduodenal motility studies: two cases involving Munchausen syndrome by proxy. J Pediatr 1995;126:397–400.
6. Omari TI, Benninga MA, Barnett CP, et al. Characterization of esophageal body and lower esophageal motor function in the very premature neonate. J Pediatr 1999;135:517–21.
7. Hassan B, Butler R, Davidson G, et al. Patterns of antropyloric motility in fed healthy preterm infants. Arch Dis Child Fetal Neonatal Ed 2002;87:F95–9.
8. Omari T, Barnett C, Benninga M, et al. Mechanisms of gastroesophageal reflux in preterm and term infants with reflux disease. Gut 2002;51:475–9.
9. Vanderhoof JA, Rappaport PJ, Paxson CL. Manometric diagnosis of lower esophageal sphincter incompetence in infants: use of a small, single lumen perfused catheter. Pediatrics 1978;62:805–8.

10. Fung KP, Math MV, Ho CO, Yap KM. Midazolam as a sedative in esophageal manometry: a study of the effect on esophageal motility. J Pediatr Gastroenterol Nutr 1992;15:85–8.

11. Spechler SJ. AGA technical review on treatment of patients with dysphagia caused by benign disorders of the distal esophagus. Gastroenterology 1999;117:229–32.

12. American Gastroenterological Association medical position statement on treatment of patients with dysphagia caused by benign disorders of the distal esophagus. Gastroenterology 1999;117:229–32.

13. Gilger MA, Boyle JT, Sondheimer JM, Colletti RB. Indications for pediatric esophageal manometry. J Pediatr Gastroenterol Nutr 1997;24:616–8.

14. Sondeheimer JM. Upper esophageal sphincter and pharyngo-esophageal motor function in infants with and without gastroesophageal reflux. Gastroenterology 1983;85:301–5.

15. Kharilas PJ, Clouse RE, Hogan WJ. American Gastroenterological Association technical review on the clinical use of esophageal manometry. Gastroenterology 1994;107:1865–84.

16. Richter JE, Wu WC, et al. Esophageal manometry in 95 healthy adult volunteers. Dig Dis Sci 1987;32:583–92.

17. Tutuian R, Vela M, Balaji S, et al. Esophageal function testing with combined multichannel intraluminal impedance and manometry: multicenter study in healthy volunteers. Clin Gastroenterol Hepatol 2003;1:174–82.

18. Hillemeier C, Grill BB, McCallum R, Gryboski J. Esophageal and gastric motor abnormalities in gastroesophageal reflux during infancy. Gastroenterology 1983;84:741–6.

19. Cucchiara S, Staiano A, Di Lorenzo C, et al. Esophageal motor abnormalities in children with gastroesophageal relfux and peptic esophagitis. J Pediatr 1986;198:907–10.

20. Moroz S, Espinoza J, Cumming W, Diamant N. Lower esophageal sphincter function in children with and without gastroesophageal reflux. Gastroenterology 1976;71:236–41.

21. Orenstein SR, Gairrusso VS, Proujansky R, Kocoshis SA. The Santmeyer swallow: a new useful infant reflex. Lancet 1988;i:345–6.

22. Shanmuganthan G, Ritz M, Holloway R, et al. Evaluation of miniature manometric techniques for the measurement of esophageal body pressure waves. J Gastroenterol Hepatol 2000;15:1362–9.

23. Omari TI, Barnett C, Snel A, et al. Mechanisms of gastro-esophageal reflux in healthy premature infants. J Pediatr 1998;133:650–4.

24. Tovar JA, Prieto G, Molina M, Arana J. Esophageal function in achalasia: preoperative and postoperative manometric studies. J Pediatr Surg 1998;33:834–8.

25. Katz PO, Richter JE, Cowan R, Castell DO. Apparent complete lower esophageal sphincter relaxation in achalasia. Gastroenterology 1986;90:978–83.

26. Rosario JA, Medow MS, Halata MS, et al. Nonspecific esophageal motility disorders in children without gastroesophageal reflux. J Pediatr Gastroenterol Nutr 1999;28:480–5.

27. Katz PO, Dalton CB, Richter JE, et al. Esophageal testing of patients with noncardiac chest pain or dysphagia. Results of three years experience with 1161 patients. Ann Intern Med 1987;106:593–7.

28. Beckingham IJ, Cariem AK, Bornman PC, et al. Oesophageal dysmotility is not associated with poor outcome after laparoscopic Nissen fundoplication. Br J Surg 1998;85:1290–3.

29. Ceriati E, Guarino N, Zaccara A, et al. Gastroesophageal reflux in neurologically impaired children: partial or total fundoplication? Langenbecks Arch Surg 1998;383:317–9.

30. Snyder CL, Ramachandran V, Kennedy AP, et al. Efficacy of par-

31. Lock G, Pfeifer M, Straub RH, et al. Association of esophageal dysfunction and pulmonary function impairment in systemic sclerosis. Am J Gastroenterol 1998;93:341–5.

32. Flick JA, Boyle JT, Tuchman DN, et al. Esophageal motor abnormalities in children and adolescents with scleroderma and mixed connective tissue disease. Pediatrics 1988;82:107–11.

33. Lapadula G, Muolo P, Semeraro F, et al. Esophageal motility disorders in the rheumatic diseases: a review of 150 patients. Clin Exp Rheumatol 1994;12:515–21.

34. Netzer P, Gut A, Heer R, et al. Five-year audit of ambulatory 24-hour esophageal pH-manometry in clinical practice. Scand J Gastroenterol 1999;34:676–82.

35. Paterson WG, Beck IT, Wang H. Ambulatory esophageal manometry/pH-metry discriminates between patients with different esophageal symptoms. Dig Dis Sci 1996;41:357–64.

36. Guzman C, Nurko SS. Value of prolonged pH-motility in children with non-cardiac chest pain or dysphagia. Gastroenterology 1997;112:A878.

37. Tovar JA, Diez-Pardo JA, Murcia J, et al. Ambulatory 24-hour manometric and pH metric evidence of permanent impairment of clearance capacity in patients with esophageal atresia. J Pediatr Surg 1995;30:1224–31.

38. Tomamasa T, DiLorenzo C, Morikawa A, et al. Analysis of fasting antroduodenal manometry in children. Dig Dis Sci 1996;41:2195–203.

39. Boige N, Faure C, Cargill L, et al. Manometrical evaluation in visceral neuropathies in children. J Pediatr Gastroenterol Nutr 1994;19:71–7.

40. Uc A, Hoon A, Di Lorenzo C, Hyman PE. Antroduodenal manometry in children with no upper gastrointestinal symptoms. Scand J Gastroenterol 1997;32:681–5.

41. Quigley EM. Intestinal manometry—technical advances, clinical limitations. Dig Dis Sci 1992;37:10–3.

42. Camilleri M, Hasler WL, Parkman H, et al. Measurement of gastrointestinal motility in the GI laboratory. Gastroenterology 1998;115:747–62.

43. Berseth CL. Antral and duodenal motor responses to duodenal feeding in preterm and term infants. J Pediatr Gastronetrol Nutr 1992;14:182–6.

44. Berseth CL, Nordyke CR. Manometry can predict feeding readiness in preterm infants. Gastroenterology 1992;103:1523–8.

45. Soffer EE, Thongsawat S. Small bowel manometry: short or long recording sessions? Dig Dis Sci 1997;42:873–7.

46. Tomamasa T. Antroduodenal manometry. In: Hyman PE, editor. Pediatric gastrointestinal motility disorders. New York: Academy Professional Information Systems Inc; 1994. p. 195–214.

47. Soffer EE, Thongsawat S. The clinical value of duodeno-jejunal manometry; its usefulness in the diagnosis and management of patients with gastrointestinal symptoms. Dig Dis Sci 1996;41:859–63.

48. Tomamasa T, Itoh Z, Koizumi T, Kuroume T. Nonmigrating rhythmic activity in the stomach and duodenum of neonates. Biol Neonate 1985;48:1–9.

49. Di Lorenzo C, Hyman PE, Flores AF, et al. Antroduodenal manometry in children and adults with severe nonulcer dyspepsia. Scand J Gastroenterol 1994;29:766–806.

50. Camilleri M, Brown ML, Malagelada JR. Relationship between impaired gastric emptying and abnormal gastrointestinal motility. Gastroenterology 1986;91:94–9.

51. Soffer EE, Adrian TE. Effect of meal composition and sham

feeding on duodenojejunal motility in humans. Dig Dis Sci 1992;37:1009–14.

52. Di Lorenzo C, Flores A, Hymand PE. Intestinal motility in symptomatic children with fundoplication. J Pediatr Gastroenterol Nutr 1991;12:169–73.

53. Di Lorenzo C, Flores AF, Buie T, Hyman P. Intestinal motility and jejunal feeding in children with chronic intestinal pseudo-obstruction. Gastroenterology 1995;108:1379–85.

54. Tomamasa T, Hyman PE, Itoh K, et al. Gastroduodenal motility in neonates: response to human milk compared with milk formula. Pediatrics 1987;80:434–8.

55. Di Lorenzo C, Reddy SN, Flores AF, Hyman PE. Is electrogastrography a substitute for manometric studies in children with functional gastrointestinal disorders? Dig Dis Sci 1997;42:2310–6.

56. Baker JH, Berseth CL. Duodenal motor responses in preterm infants fed formula with varying concentrations and rates of infusion. Pediatr Res 1997;42:618–22.

57. Prather CM, Camilleri M, Thomforde GM, et al. Gastric axial forces in experimentally delayed and accelerated gastric emptying. Am J Physiol 1993;264:G928–34.

58. Greydanus MP, Camilleri M. Abnormal postcibal antral and small bowel motility due to neuropathy or myopathy in systemic sclerosis. Gastroenterology 1989;96:110–5.

59. Camilleri M, Carborne LD, Schuffler MD. Familial ebteric neuropathy with pseudo-obstruction. Dig Dis Sci 1991;36: 1168–71.

60. Frank JW, Sarr MG, Camilleri M. Use of gastroduodenal manometry to differentiate mechanical and functional intestinal obstruction. Am J Gastroenterol 1994;89:339–44.

61. Husebye E. The patterns of small bowel motility: physiology and implications in organic disease and functional disorders. Neurogastroenterol Motil 1999;11:141–61.

62. Kellow JE, Borody TJ, Phillips SF, et al. Human interdigestive motility: variations in patterns from esophagus to colon. Gastroenterology 1986;91:386–95.

63. Samsom M, Jebbink RJ, Akkermans LM, et al. Abnormalities of antroduodenal motility in type I diabetes. Diabetes Care 1996;19:21–7.

64. Quigley EM, Donovan JP, Lane MJ, Gallagher TF. Antroduodenal manometry. Usefulness and limitations as an outpatient study. Dig Dis Sci 1992;37:20–8.

65. Wilson P, Perdikis G, Hinder RA, et al. Prolonged ambulatory antroduodenal manometry in humans. Am J Gastroenterol 1994;89:1489–95.

66. DiLorenzo C, Flores A, Tomamasa T, Hyman PE. Effect of erythromycin on antroduodenal motility in children with chronic functional gastrointestinal symptoms. Dig Dis Sci 1994;39:1399–404.

67. Tomamasa T, Kuruome T, Arai H, et al. Erythromycin induces migrating motor complex in humans gastrointestinal tract. Dig Dis Sci 1986;31:157–61.

68. Cucchiara S, Minella R, Scoppa A, et al. Antroduodenal motor effects of intravenous erythromycin in children with abnormalities of gastrointestinal motility. J Pediatr Gastroenterol Nutr 1997;24:411–8.

69. Jadcherla SR, Berseth C, Klee G. Regulation of migrating motor complexes by motility and pancreatic polypeptide in human neonate. Pediatr Res 1997;42:365–9.

70. Jadcherla SR, Berseth C. Effect of erythromycin on gastroduodenal contractile activity in developing neonates. J Pediatr Gastroenterol Nutr 2002;34:16–22.

71. Hyman PE, Di Lorenzo C, McAdams L, et al. Predicting the clinical response to cisapride in children with chronic intestinal pseudo-obstruction. Am J Gastroenterol 1993;88:832–6.

72. Di Lorenzo C, Lucano C, Flores AF, et al. Effect of octreotide on gastrointestinal motility in children with functional gastrointestinal symptoms. J Pediatr Gastroenterol Nutr 1998;27: 508–12.

73. Perlemuter G, Cacoub P, Chaussade S, et al. Octreotide treatment of chronic intestinal pseudoobstruction secondary to connective tissue diseases. Arthritis Rheum 1999;42:1545–9.

74. Fell JM, Smith VV, Milla PJ. Infantile chronic idiopathic intestinal pseudo-obstruction: the role of small intestinal manometry as a diagnostic tool and prognostic indicator. Gut 1996;39:306–11.

75. Bassotti G, Iantorno G, Fiorella S, et al. Colonic motility in man: features in normal subjects and in patients with chronic idiopathic constipation. Am J Gastroenterol 1999;94:1760–70.

76. Di Lorenzo C. Colonic manometry. In: Hyman PE, editor. Pediatric gastrointestinal motility disorders. New York: Academy Professional Information Services, Inc; 1994. p. 215–30.

77. Di Lorenzo C, Flores AF, Hyman PE. Age-related changes in colon motility. J Pediatr 1995;127:593–6.

78. Hamid SA, Di Lorenzo C, Reddy SN, et al. Bisacodyl and high-amplitude-propagating colonic contractions in children. J Pediatr Gastroenterol Nutr 1998;27:398–402.

79. Di Lorenzo C, Flores AF, Reddy SN, Hyman PE. Use of colonic manometry to differentiate causes of intractable constipation in children. J Pediatr 1992;120:690–5.

80. Di Lorenzo C, Flores AF, Reddy SN, et al. Colonic manometry in children with chronic intestinal pseudo-obstruction. Gut 1993;34:803–7.

81. Di Lorenzo C, Solzi GF, Flores AF, et al. Colonic motility after surgery for Hirschsprung's disease. Am J Gastroenterol 2000;95:1759–64.

82. Heikenen JB, Werlin SL, Di Lorenzo C, et al. Colonic motility in children with repaired imperforate anus. Dig Dis Sci 1999; 44:1288–92.

83. Zaslavsky C, Loening-Baucke V. Anorectal manometric evaluation of children and adolescents postsurgery for Hirschsprung's disease. J Pediatr Surg 2003;38:191–5.

84. Frenckner B, Euler CV. Influence of pudendal block on the function of the anal sphincters. Gut 1975;16:482–9.

85. Diamant NE, Kamm MA, Wald A, Whitehead WE. AGA technical review on anorectal testing techniques. Gastroenterology 1999;116:735–60.

86. Loening-Baucke V, Pringle KC, Ekwo EE. Anorectal manometry for the exclusion of Hirschsprung's disease in neonates. J Pediatr Gastroenterol Nutr 1985;4:596–603.

87. Meunier PD. Anorectal manometry. A collective international experience. Gastroenterol Clin Biol 1991;15:697–702.

88. Nurko SS, Garcia-Aranda JA, Guerrero VY, Worona LB. Treatment of intractable constipation in children: experience with cisapride. J Pediatr Gastroenterol Nutr 1996;22:38–44.

89. Lopez-Alonso M, Ribas J, Hernandez A, et al. Efficiency of the anorectal manometry for the diagnosis of Hirschsprung's disease in the newborn period. Eur J Pediatr Surg 1995;5:160–3.

90. Benninga M, Omari T, Haslam R, et al. Characterization of anorectal pressure and the anorectal inhibitory reflex in healthy preterm and term infants. J Pediatr 2001;139:233–7.

91. Loening-Baucke VA. Modulation of abnormal defecation dynamics by biofeedback treatment in chronically constipated children with encopresis. J Pediatr 1990;116:214–22.

92. Baker S, Liptak G, Colletti R, et al. Constipation in infants and children: evaluation and treatment. A medical position statement of the North American Society for Pediatric Gastroenterology and Nutrition. J Pediatr Gastroenterol Nutr 1999;29:612–26.

93. Nolan T, Catto-Smith T, Coffey C, Wells J. Randomised controlled trial of biofeedback training in persistent encopresis with anismus. Arch Dis Child 1998;79:131–5.

94. Wald A, Cauana BJ, Freimanis MG, et al. Contributions of evacuation proctography and anorectal manometry to evaluation of adults with constipation and defecatory difficulty. Dig Dis Sci 1990;35:481–7.

95. Holschneider AM, Kellner E, Streibl P, et al. The development of anorectal continence and its significance in the diagnosis of Hirschsprung's disease. J Pediatr Surg 1976;11:151–6.

96. Ito Y, Donahue PK, Hendren WH. Maturation of the rectoanal response in premature and perinatal infants. J Pediatr Surg 1977;12:477–82.

97. Boston VE, Scott JES. Anorectal manometry as a diagnostic method in the neonatal period. J Pediatr Surg 1976;11:9–16.

98. Verder H, Krasilnikoff PA, Scheibel E. Anal tonometry in the neonatal period in mature and premature children. Acta Pediatr Scand 1974;64:592–6.

99. Rao SS, Hatfield R, Soffer E, et al. Manometric tests of anorectal function in healthy adults. Am J Gastroenterol 1999;94:773–83.

100. Loening-Baucke V. Anorectal manometry and biofeedback training. In: Hyman PE, editor. Pediatric gastrointestinal motility disorders. New York: Academy Professional Information Systems Inc; 1994. p. 231–52.

101. Meunier P, Marechal JM, Mollard P. Accuracy of the manometric diagnosis of Hirschsprung's disease. J Pediatr Surg 1978;13:411–5.

102. Ciamarra P, Nurko S, Barksdale E, et al. Successful use of botulinum toxin injection in anal sphincter achalasia. J Pediatr Gastroenterol Nutr 2000;31 Suppl 2:S131.

103. Emir H, Akman M, Sarimurat N, et al. Anorectal manometry during the neonatal period: its specificity in the diagnosis of Hirschsprung's disease. Eur J Pediatr Surg 1999;9:101–3.

104. Iwai N, Yanagihara J, Tokiwa K, et al. Reliability of anorectal manometry in the diagnosis of Hirschsprung's disease. Zschr Kinderchirurg 1988;43:405–7.

105. Lanfranchi GA, Bazzocchi G, Federici S, et al. Anorectal manometry in the diagnosis of Hirschsprung's disease—comparison with clinical and radiological criteria. Am J Gastroenterol 1984;79:270–5.

106. Low PS, Quak SH, Prabhakaran K, et al. Accuracy of anorectal manometry in the diagnosis of Hirschsprung's disease. J Pediatr Gastroenterol Nutr 1989;9:342–6.

107. Mahboubi S, Schnaufer L. The barium-enema examination and rectal manometry in Hirschsprung's disease. Radiology 1979;130:643–7.

108. Neilson IR, Yazbeck S. Ultrashort Hirschsprung's disease: myth or reality? J Pediatr Surg 1990;25:1135–8.

109. Puri P. Variant Hirshcsprung's disease. J Pediatr Surg 1997;32:149–57.

110. Oue T, Puri P. Altered intramuscular innervation and synapse formation in internal sphincter achalasia. Pediatr Surg Int 1999;15:192–4.

111. Benninga MA, Buller HA, Taminiau AJ. Biofeedback training in chronic constipation. Arch Dis Child 1993;68:126–9.

112. Loening-Baucke VA. Factors determining the outcome in children with chronic constipation and fecal soiling. Gut 1989;30:999–1006.

113. Loening-Baucke V. Biofeedback training in children with constipation: a critical review. Dig Dis Sci 1996;41:65–71.

114. Loening-Baucke V. Biofeedback therapy for chronic constipation and encopresis in childhood: long term outcome. Pediatrics 1995;96:105–10.

115. Van der Plas RN, Benninga MA, Buller HA, et al. Biofeedback training in treatment of childhood constipation: a randomized controlled study. Lancet 1996;348:776–80.

116. Borowitz SM, Sutphen J, Ling W, Cox DJ. Lack of correlation of anorectal manometry with symptoms of chronic childhood constipation and encopresis. Dis Colon Rectum 1996;39:400–5.

117. Loening-Baucke VA. Abnormal rectoanal function in children recovered from chronic constipation and encopresis. Gastroenterology 1984;87:1299–304.

118. Sutphen J, Borowitz S, Ling W, et al. Anorectal manometric examination in encopretic-constipated children. Dis Colon Rectum 1997;40:1051–5.

119. Mishalany HG, Wooley MM. Postoperative functional and manometric evaluation of patients with Hirschsprung's disease. J Pediatr Surg 1987;22:443–6.

120. Moore SW, Millar AJ, Cywes S. Long term clinical, manometric, and histologic evaluation of obstructive symptoms in the postoperative Hirschsprung's patient. J Pediatr Surg 1994;29:106–11.

121. Nagasaki A. Anorectal manometry after Ikeda Z-shaped anastomosis in Hirschsprung''s disease. Prog Pediatr Surg 1989;21:59–66.

122. Heikkinen M, Rintala R, Luukkonen P. Long-term anal sphincter performance after surgery for Hirschsprung's disease. J Pediatr Surg 1997;32:1443–6.

123. Abbas Banani S, Forootan H. Role of anorectal myectomy after failed endorectal pull-through in Hirschsprung's disease. J Pediatr Surg 1994;29:1307–9.

124. Langer JB, Birnbaum E. Preliminary experience with intrasphincteric botulinum toxin for persistent constipation after pull-through for Hirschsprung's disease. J Pediatr Surg 1997;32:1059–62.

125. Koletzko S, Ballauff A, Hadziselimovic F, Enck P. Is histological diagnosis of neuronal intestinal dysplasia related to clinical and manometric findings in constipated children? Results of a pilot study. J Pediatr Gastroenterol Nutr 1993;17:59–65.

126. Koletzko S, Jesch I, Faus-Kebler T, et al. Rectal biopsy for diagnosis of intestinal neuronal dysplasia in children: a prospective multicentre study on interobserver variation and clinical outcome. Gut 1999;44:853–61.

127. Krebs C, Silva C, Parra M. Anorectal electromanometry in the diagnosis of neuronal intestinal dysplasia in childhood. Eur J Pediatr Surg 1991;1:40–4.

128. Schmidt A. Electromanometrical investigations in patients with isolated neuronal intestinal dysplasia (NID). Eur J Pediatr Surg 1994;4:310–4.

129. Glia A, Gylin M, Akerlund JE, et al. Biofeedback training in patients with fecal incontinence. Dis Colon Rectum 1998;41:359–64.

130. Sun VM, Donnelly TC, Read NW. Utility of a combined test of anorectal manometry, electromyography and sensation in determining the mechanisms of "idiopathic" fecal incontinence. Gut 1992;33:807–13.

131. Nurko SS, Worona L. Anorectal function in children with imperforate anus. J Gastrointest Motil 1993;5:209.

132. Wald A, Tunuguntla AK. Anorectal sensorimotor dysfunction in fecal incontinence and diabetes mellitus. Modification with biofeedback. N Engl J Med 1984;310:1282–7.

133. Iwai N, Yanagihara J, Tokiwa K, et al. Voluntary anal continence after surgery for anorectal malformations. J Pediatr Surg 1988;23:393–7.

134. Hedlund H, Pena A, Rodriguez G, Maza J. Long-term anorectal function in imperforate anus treated by a posterior sagittal

anorectoplasty: manometric investigation. J Pediatr Surg 1992;27:906–9.

135. Lin CL, Chen CC. The rectoanal relaxation reflex and continence in repaired anorectal malformations with and without an internal sphincter-saving procedure. J Pediatr Surg 1996;31:630–3.

136. Menard C, Trudel C, Cloutier R. Anal reeducation for postoperative fecal incontinence in congenital diseases of the rectum and anus. J Pediatr Surg 1997;32:867–9.

137. Wu JS, Schoetz DJ Jr, Coller JA, Veidenheimer MC. Treatment of Hirschsprung's disease in the adult. Report of five cases. Dis Colon Rectum 1995;38:655–9.

138. Parkman H, Hasler W, Barnett L, Eaker E. Electrogastrography: a document prepared by the gastric section of the American Motility Society Clinical GI Motility Testing Task Force. Neurogastroenterol Motil 2003;15:89–102.

139. Aktay A, Splaingard M, Miller T, et al. Electrogastrography in children with cystic fibrosis. Dig Dis Sci 2002;47:699–703.

140. Levanon D, Chen JZ. Electrogastrography: its role in managing gastric disorders. J Pediatr Gastroenterol Nutr 1998;27:431–43.

141. Patterson M, Rintala R, Lloyd D. A longitudinal study of electrogastrography in normal neonates. J Pediatr Surg 2000;35:59–61.

142. Patterson M, Rintala R, Lloyd D, et al. Validation of electrode placement in neonatal electrogastrography. Dig Dis Sci 2001;46:2245–9.

143. Levy J, Harris J, Chen J, et al. Electrogastrographic norms in children: toward the development of standard methods, reproducible results, and reliable normative data. J Pediatr Gastroenterol Nutr 2001;33:455–61.

144. Chen J, McCallum RW. Clinical applications of electrogastrography. Am J Gastroenterol 1993;88:1324–36.

145. Cucchiara S, Riezzo G, Minella R, et al. Electrogastrography in non ulcer dyspepsia. Arch Dis Child 1992;67:613–7.

146. Riezzo G, Chiloiro M, Guerra V. Electrogastrography in healthy children: evaluation of normal values, influence of age, gender, and obesity. Dig Dis Sci 1998;43:1646–51.

147. Cheng W, Tam P. Gastric electrical activity normalises in the first decade of life. Eur J Pediatr Surg 2000;10:295–9.

148. Tomomasa T, Miyazaki M, Nako Y, Kuroume T. Electrogastrography in neonates. J Perinatol 1994;14:417–21.

149. Chen JD, Co E, Liang J, et al. Patterns of gastric myoelectrical activity in human subjects of different ages. Am J Physiol 1997;272(5 Pt 1):G1022–7.

150. Koch KL, Tran TN, Stern RM, et al. Gastric myoelectrical activity in premature and term infants. J Gastrointest Motil 1993;5:41–7.

151. Liang J, Co E, Zhang M, et al. Development of gastric slow waves in preterm infants measured by electrogastrography. Am J Physiol 1998;274(3 Pt 1):G503–8.

152. Devane SP, Ravelli AM, Bisset WM, et al. Gastric antral dysrhythmias in children with chronic idiopathic intestinal pseudoobstruction. Gut 1992;33:1477–81.

153. Richards CA, Andrews PL, Spitz L, Milla PJ. Nissen fundoplication may induce gastric myoelectrical disturbance in children. J Pediatr Surg 1998;33:1801–5.

154. Ravelli AM, Milla PJ. Vomiting and gastroesophageal motor activity in children with disorders of the central nervous system. J Pediatr Gastroenterol Nutr 1998;26:56–63.

155. Ravelli AM, Lederman SE, Bisset WM, et al. Foregut motor function in chronic renal failure. Arch Dis Child 1992;67:1343–7.

156. Shah N, Rodriguez M, Louis DS, et al. Feeding difficulties and foregut dysmotility in Noonan's syndrome. Arch Dis Child 1999;81:28–31.

157. Chong SK. Electrogastrography in cyclic vomiting syndrome. Dig Dis Sci 1999;44(8 Suppl):64S–73S.

158. Heikenen JB, Werlin SL, Brown CW. Electrogastrography in gastrostomy-tube-fed children. Dig Dis Sci 1999;44:1293–7.

159. Cucchiara S, Minella R, Riezzo G, et al. Reversal of gastric electrical dysrhythmias by cisapride in children with functional dyspepsia. Report of three cases. Dig Dis Sci 1992;37:1136–40.

160. Maldonado ME, Brady PG, Mamel JJ, Robinson B. Incidence of pancreatitis in patients undergoing sphincter of Oddi manometry (SOM). Am J Gastroenterol 1999;94:387–90.

161. Hogan WJ, Sherman S, Pasricha P, Carr-Locke D. Sphincter of Oddi manometry. Gastrointest Endosc 1997;45:342–8.

162. Guelrud M, Morera C, Rodriguez M, et al. Sphincter of Oddi dysfunction in children with recurrent pancreatitis and anomalous pancreaticobiliary union: an etiologic concept. Gastrointest Endosc 1999;50:194–9.

163. Di Lorenzo C, Youssef N, Sigurdsson L, et al. Visceral hyperalgesia in children with functional abdominal pain. J Pediatr 2001;139:838–43.

164. Van Ginkel R, Voskuijl WP, Benninga M, et al. Alterations in rectal sensitivity and motility in childhood irritable bowel syndrome. Gastroenterology 2001;120:31–8.

165. Rudolph C, Winter HS, NASPGN Executive Council, NASPGN Training and Education Committee, Contributing Authors. NASPGN guideliness for training in pediatric gastroenterology. J Pediatr Gastroenterol Nutr 1999;29 Suppl 1:S1–26.

166. Barham CP, Gotley DC, Fowler A, et al. Diffuse esophageal spasm: diagnosis by ambulatory 24 hour manometry. Gut 1997;41:151–5.

167. Richter JE. Diffuse esophageal spasm. In: Castell DO, Castell JA, editors. Esophageal motility testing. 2nd ed. Norwalk (CT): Appleton and Lange; 1994. p. 122–34.

168. Handa M, Mine K, Yamamoto H, et al. Antidepressant treatment of patients with diffuse esophageal spasm: a psychosomatic approach. J Clin Gastroenterol 1999;28:228–32.

CHAPTER 71

pH MEASUREMENT

Yvan Vandenplas, MD, PhD

WHY MONITOR THE PH IN THE ESOPHAGUS?

The idea that the measurement of the pH in the esophagus may be of great clinical importance started with the observation that acid perfusion–induced heartburn coincides with the fall of intraesophageal pH below 4.0.[1] Esophageal pH monitoring is often considered an investigation technique studying esophageal motility, which it obviously does not do because it does even not measure gastroesophageal reflux (GER). This being said, the major shortcoming of esophageal pH monitoring is obvious: the technique measures changes in esophageal pH, not GER. The first clinical tests were performed in the early 1960s by Miller.[2] Modern electronic technology has profoundly changed the practice of medicine, principally through its ability to monitor, record, and analyze large volumes of data. The introduction of computers has provided physicians with powerful tools to identify elusive and intermittent disorders, such as gastroesophageal reflux disease (GERD). Although a continuous investigation technique such as pH monitoring is extremely suitable for ambulatory outpatient application, many centers still hospitalize patients.

Major areas of indications for esophageal pH monitoring are (1) in clinical and laboratory research, (2) as a routine clinical procedure in the diagnosis of GERD, especially in children presenting with atypical GER manifestations (Table 71-1), and (3) in the evaluation of the efficacy of treatment of GERD on the frequency and duration of the presence of acid in the esophagus.[3,4]

HARDWARE AND SOFTWARE: PEDIATRIC NEEDS

DEVICE

Purchase costs, system abilities, costs in use, number of measurements, and durability of the material are factors to consider before purchasing equipment. Of importance for pediatric use are a time indication on the display (ie, the number of data recorded, the real time, the duration of the investigation) and the protection of the event marker(s) to avoid erroneous use by the child.[4] A system should refuse to work if it has not been calibrated properly

One of the advantages of pH monitoring is the possibility of realizing an ambulatory recording, even in young children. Therefore, the device should be small and light. Devices not larger than a credit card, although of course a little thicker, are commercially available.

ELECTRODE

pH sensors or "electrodes" exist in several forms, of which the two most popular are glass and antimony. Ion-sensitive field effect pH electrodes are modified field effect transistors. Glass electrodes are generally considered to be the most accurate.[5,6] Clinical studies require a pH sensor that is both economical and reliable. Glass electrodes with an internal reference are "the best" but are expensive and have a rather large diameter (3.0–4.5 mm). Although the passage of such an electrode through the nostrils of a young baby is, most of the time, technically possible, it does not mean that it is well

TABLE 71-1	SYMPTOMS OF GASTROESOPHAGEAL REFLUX DISEASE

ESOPHAGEAL MANIFESTATIONS
Specific symptoms
  Regurgitation
  Nausea
  Vomiting
Symptoms possibly related to reflux esophagitis
  Symptoms related to anemia (iron deficiency anemia)
  Hematemesis, melena
  Dysphagia (as a symptom of esophagitis and/or due to stricture formation)
  Weight loss and/or failure to thrive
  Epigastric or retrosternal pain
  "Noncardia angina-like" chest pain
  Pyrosis or heartburn, pharyngeal burning
  Belching, postprandial fullness
  Irritable esophagus
  General irritability in infants ("colic")

UNUSUAL PRESENTATIONS
GER related to chronic respiratory disease (eg, bronchitis, asthma, laryngitis, pharyngitis)
Cystic fibrosis
Sandifer Sutcliffe syndrome
Rumination
Apnea, apparent life-threatening event, sudden infant death syndrome

GER = gastroesophageal reflux

tolerated and that it is the best option. From recent experience with combined pressure-pH recordings, it became clear that the larger the diameter of the electrode(s), the more the patient had to swallow (personal data). Thus, the pharyngeal presence of an (large size) electrode has a decreasing effect on GER episodes because the more the patient has to swallow, the more primary peristalsis is induced, and the better esophageal clearance becomes.

Because of their smaller diameter, antimony (2.1 mm) (Synectics Medical, Queluz, Portugal) or glass microelectrodes (1.2 mm) are preferable in infants. Antimony electrodes also exist with a diameter of about 1.5 mm for use in premature babies; these electrodes are too flexible for older babies. Single esophageal pH monitoring cannot detect alkaline reflux.[7] Glass electrodes have only one pH sensor. Antimony electrodes with multiple pH sensors may help to detect alkaline reflux episodes. Antimony electrodes with two sensors can also be helpful to evaluate the therapeutic efficacy of acid-reducing medication: the esophageal sensor measures the incidence of acid GER, whereas a gastric sensor measures the efficacy of the medication. Antimony is only poorly resistant to gastric acid, but the fact that acid should be reduced or minimalized in these patients minimizes the impact of this shortcoming.

Most antimony and all glass microelectrodes need an external cutaneous reference electrode, which is a possible cause of erroneous measurement resulting from transmucosal potential differences. If the environmental temperature is high or the patient sweats a lot, the conductivity of the contact gel will change, resulting in a less accurate conduction of the electric potential. Antimony electrodes with a diameter of about 2.0 mm with an internal reference electrode have been developed, providing comparable results (personal data, 1997; Table 71-2). This electrode is accurate, thin, flexible, and easy to place in the esophagus, and there is no longer need for a cutaneous reference electrode. However, in clinical reality, the purchase cost of the electrode and income of the pH monitoring will substantially influence the type of electrode used. Whatever the type of electrode chosen, each center should preferentially use one type or a limited number of electrodes.

Prior to each study, an in vitro two-point calibration must be carried out. The electrode and reference are placed in two buffer solutions (usually pH 1.0 and 7.0) at either room or body temperature until stabilization is reached. This calibration should be repeated on return of the patient to rule out electrode failure and to check for slow pH drift. A drift of less than 0.5 pH over the 24-hour period is acceptable. Calibration needs to be corrected according to room and body temperature.

LOCATION OF THE ELECTRODE

There is abundant evidence in the literature that the esophageal location of the electrode is of critical importance regarding the number and duration of acid reflux episodes recorded. It seems logical that the closer the electrode is located to the lower esophageal sphincter (LES), the more acid reflux episodes will be detected.[8,9] In adults, the electrode is, by consensus, positioned 5 cm above the proximal border of the LES. Also in adults, determination of the position of the LES by means of a standard stationary esophageal manometry study is generally regarded as the optimum method for pH probe localization.[6] In children, several methods have been proposed to determine the location of the electrode: fluoroscopy, calculation of the esophageal length according to the Strobel formula (distance from the nose to the cardia = 5 + 0.252 [length in cm]), manometry, and endoscopy. Ideally, as in adults, the electrode should be sited in reference to the manometrically determined LES. However, this has several inconveniences: (1) manometry in infants and children is time consuming, rather invasive, or at least unpleasant, and (2) this method would have the inconvenience that the electrode is located at a fixed distance to the LES, whereas the length of the esophagus increases from less than 10 cm in a newborn to over 25 cm in an adult. Moreover, manometry cannot be performed in all centers. Therefore, the European Society for Paediatric Gastroenterology, Hepatology, and Nutrition Working Group on GER recommended the use of fluoroscopy to locate the electrode.[4] The radiation involved is minimal, and the method can be applied in each center. As the tip of the electrode moves with and during respiration, the tip should be positioned in such a way that it overlies the third vertebral body above the diaphragm throughout the respiration cycle (Figure 71-1). Dislocation by a curled electrode is also

TABLE 71-2   ADVANTAGES AND DISADVANTAGES OF PH MONITORING TO DIAGNOSE GASTROESOPHAGEAL REFLUX DISEASE

	ADVANTAGES	DISADVANTAGES
Technique	Physiologic conditions Normal ranges Good reproducibility Long duration (24 h)	Physiologic conditions Social discomfort (electrode)
Diagnosis	Quantification of number of pH changes Quantification of duration pH changes Time-relation symptom-pH change	pH change, not GER Alkaline GER (?) No neutral GER
Complications	Area under pH 4: related to esophagitis	No information tissue damage
Treatment	Contributes to choice of treatment Evaluation of treatment	No acid if H₂ blocker, PPI

GER = gastroesophageal reflux; PPI = proton pump inhibitor.

prevented with fluoroscopy. If the pH device is exposed to x-rays, the data and calibration may be erased.

PATIENT PREPARATION

No special patient preparation is required for pH monitoring, except for fasting. The patient should fast for at least 3 to 5 hours before the study, depending on the age, to avoid nausea and vomiting. If the child is able to communicate, it is important to reassure the child at the beginning of the study and explain what will happen. The child should understand that the passage of the catheter through the throat is uncomfortable, but after the first few swallows, it will feel better. To facilitate insertion, a silicone spray (eg, Silicone-spray, Alphamed, Brussels, Belgium) can be placed on the electrode (but not on the pH sensor!) and/or local anesthesia of the mucosa of the nostrils can be done. Sedation should not be used because the sedative may interfere with swallowing and influence pressures.

Histamine$_2$ (H$_2$) blockers or proton pump inhibitors should be stopped at least 3 or 7 days, respectively, before a diagnostic pH monitoring (on the condition that the investigation is not performed to evaluate the acid-buffering effect of the drug). Antacids are permitted up to 6 hours prior to the start of the recording. Prokinetics should be stopped at least 48 hours before the pH monitoring.[8] The continuation or discontinuation of drugs depends on the indication for the pH study: diagnosis of reflux or evaluation of efficacy of treatment.

It is best not to start a pH metry the same day an upper gastrointestinal tract endoscopy was performed because of the sedation, fasting, and inflated air. It is best to start pH metry at least 3 hours after a barium swallow or radionuclide gastric or esophageal studies.

PATIENT-RELATED INFLUENCING FACTORS: RECORDING CONDITIONS

Feeding, position, and physical activity are examples of patient-related factors influencing pH monitoring data. Patient-related factors that possibly influence the results of pH monitoring are a controversial topic.[4,8] The answer to the fundamental question if patient-related factors should be minimized and standardized is difficult and necessarily ambiguous. If the pH monitoring is performed as part of a diagnostic workup in a patient, it is interesting to study the patient during normal daily life, noting what is enhanced by unrestricted recording conditions. But if the pH monitoring is performed as part of a (clinical) research project, recording conditions should be standardized. Standardization of recording conditions inevitably causes a loss of patient-specific information.

DURATION OF THE RECORDING

The duration of the recording should be "as close as possible to 24 hours" and at least 18 hours, including a day and a night period.[4,10,11] If the pH monitoring is performed for diagnostic purpose, there is no indication for short-

duration pH tests (eg, Tuttle and Bernstein tests, 3-hour postprandial recording). The first reports on the clinical use of pH monitoring concerned esophageal tests of short duration. Tuttle and Grossman developed the "standard acid reflux test."[12] This test was modified by Skinner and Booth[13] and Kantrowitz and colleagues,[14] demonstrating that pH tests can contribute to define abnormal GER. The Tuttle test was reported to have a sensitivity of 70%.[15] After great initial enthusiasm for this test, criticism became more and more common. The test is unphysiologic in requiring intragastric instillation of acid and various artificial maneuvers to raise intragastric pressure. In the early 1980s, it was reported that the false-positive rate might be as high as 4 to 20% and the false-negative rate as high as 40%.[16–18] Bernstein and Baker demonstrated in 1958 that heartburn could be provoked by infusing diluted hydrochloric acid into the esophagus in susceptible individuals.[19] This test was shown to be 100% positive in reflux patients.[20] A modified Bernstein test was used to illustrate the relationship between GER and apnea and stridor and between nonspecific chest pain and GER.[21,22] Provocative testing can be used in particular conditions to demonstrate the relationship between GER and specific symptoms (bradycardia in relation to acid in the esophagus). However, provocative testing has always had the inconvenience that the investigation conditions are unphysiologic. The latter might explain some discrepancies in literature. Ramet and colleagues showed a prolongation of the R-R interval in infants during provocative testing with acid instillation in the esophagus,[23] whereas others could not reproduce these findings in 24-hour recordings in physiologic conditions.[24,25]

There is now substantial evidence that in controls and in the majority of infants and children with classic symp-

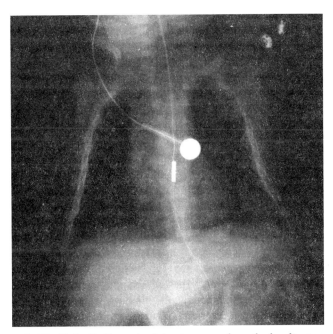

FIGURE 71-1 Radiograph of the thorax to show the localization of the pH electrode (third vertebra above the diaphragm). The radiograph shows a two-channel electrode with the distal electrode in the stomach and the proximal electrode at the third vertebra.

toms of GERD, esophageal acid exposure is highest during the day, probably because of provocation of GER by food ingestion and physical activity. Controls have more reflux upright than supine or more reflux awake than asleep.[26] The relationship between esophagitis and nocturnal reflux is far from clear.[27–29]

FEEDING

Feeding during pH monitoring has been and still is an area of controversy. On the one hand, it seems logical to forbid the intake of acidic foods and drinks. However, many popular foods and beverages have a pH of < 5.0 (eg, cola drinks, fruit juice, tea, soup), resulting in a quite restricted diet. A too restricted diet might alter the patient's normal daily habits in such a way that the investigation is no longer performed in physiologic conditions. Electrodes are temperature sensitive; therefore, very hot and ice cold beverages and food (eg, coffee, tea, ice cream) should be avoided.[4] Ask the older child not to chew gum or eat hard candy because these will increase saliva production and thus will induce swallowing and peristalsis and tend to normalize the test results. In older children, alcohol intake and smoking should be recorded on the diary.

In infants, it has been suggested to replace one or several feedings during pH monitoring with apple juice.[30] This would solve the problem of gastric anacidity after a milk feeding, but apple juice has a pH of about 4.0 and a very rapid gastric emptying and is not part of normal infant feeding. In our unit, feeding is free, but parents and children are asked not to exaggerate "acid" ingestion and to avoid very hot and cold food and beverages and chewing gum. Although the ingestion of acid such as a cola drink might simulate a reflux episode, the duration of ingestion is limited to a few minutes and most of the time is irrelevant to the total 24-hour data. To minimize this effect, it is possible to eliminate these false reflux episodes with the help of a diary.

All of the above is true for diagnostic investigations. However, in research, the opposite might be valid: all factors possibly influencing the pH data should be controlled and standardized as much as possible.

The influence of a particular food on the incidence of acid GER episodes detected by pH monitoring might be opposite to its influence on the incidence of reflux episodes: a fat meal is known to provoke GER because of its delayed gastric emptying. Because the duration of postprandial gastric anacidity after a fat meal is prolonged, a meal with a high fat content will result in delayed gastric emptying and thus less acid reflux episodes detected by pH monitoring.[31,32] Some drugs influencing gastric emptying (eg, prokinetic agents) have a comparable effect on pH monitoring data: prokinetic drugs enhance gastric emptying, shorten the period of postprandial gastric anacidity, and prolong the periods during which acid GER can be detected.

POSITION

Different patterns of GER (upright, supine, combined) have been reported in adults and older children.[33] Orenstein and colleagues. demonstrated that the prone sleeping position is the preferred position for infants as far as GER is concerned because crying time is decreased if compared with the supine position.[34–36] There is evidence that the prone anti-Trendelenburg 30° sleeping position reduces GER in normal subjects and patients, although the position is difficult to apply and maintain correctly (infants have to be tied up in their bed). Meanwhile, the literature on sudden infant death syndrome (SIDS) in infants shows that infant mortality decreases if infants are put to sleep in the supine position. Accordingly, the prone anti-Trendelenburg position is no longer recommended in infants at risk for SIDS.[37,38] Thus, the position of the infant should be recorded on the diary during pH monitoring.

DATA ANALYSIS

INTERPRETATION AND PARAMETERS

Interpretation starts with a visual appreciation of the pH tracing, what is subjective and difficult to standardize (Figure 71-2). Nevertheless, it is of the utmost importance "to have a look" at the tracing. The parameters that are classically analyzed are the total number of reflux episodes, the number of reflux episodes lasting more than 5 minutes, the duration of the longest reflux episode, and the reflux index that is the percentage of time of the entire duration of the investigation during which the pH is less than 4.0. From all "classic" parameters, the acid exposure time or reflux index is the most relevant. The correlation between all four parameters is good, and they are closely related to the reflux index.[39] Results should also be (automatically) calculated for periods of interest, such as sleep, wakefulness, feeding, postprandial fasting, and body position. A time relation between atypical manifestations (eg, cough, bradycardia, desaturation) and "changes" in pH (not necessarily a drop in pH below 4.0) should be searched for. The duration of reflux during sleep has been suggested to be a good selection criterion for reflux related to apnea in infancy (the "ZMD-score").[40] However, one should not forget that the response time of an electrode (the time needed to reach 95% of the exact pH) is at least about 5 seconds. The "area below pH 4.0" is a parameter considering the acidity of the reflux episodes,[41] which has been shown to correlate better with the presence of reflux esophagitis than with the reflux index.

Various complex reflux scoring systems (Johnson-Demeester Composite Score, Jolley, Branicki, Kaye, Boix-Ochoa scoring systems) have been developed. The majority of all of the parameters have been developed for assessing reflux esophagitis in adults. In marked contrast to these complex scoring systems is the simple recommendation by some investigators that the reflux index or total acid exposure time should be regarded as the most important, if not the only, variable in clinical practice.[39,41] Jolley and colleagues proposed a score for children.[42] Scores based on symptom indices are not applicable in infants and young children.

A major interfering factor in the interpretation of pH monitoring data is the "yes" or "no" interpretation of the data by computer software: a pH of 4.01 will be regarded as normal, whereas a pH of 3.99 will be considered as acid

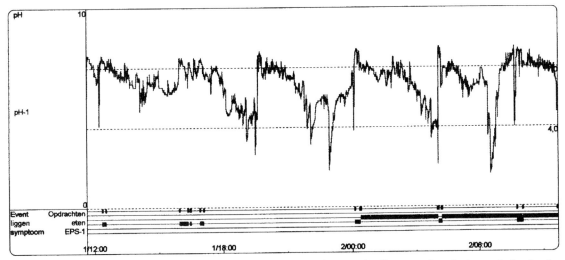

FIGURE 71-2   A 24-hour pH tracing, showing different acid and nonacid reflux episodes, during periods of wakefulness and sleep (*dark line*). Events (coughing) are either nonrelated or occur just after a reflux episode.

reflux. Minimal changes in esophageal pH around pH 4.0 can be at the origin of different software interpretations, although without difference in clinical meaning. The oscillatory index, a parameter measuring the time the pH oscillates around pH 4.0, was developed to evaluate this risk for erroneous computer interpretation.[43]

NORMAL RANGES

As for any measurement, normal ranges are mandatory. However, because there is a continuum between physiologic and pathologic GER, normal ranges should be regarded as a guideline for interpretation. Because GER is a naturally occurring phenomenon, there will inevitably be an overlap between "normal" and "abnormal" data. Excellent reproducibility has been shown for various parameters. Intrasubject reproducibility supports the diagnostic use of continuous pH monitoring. In general, it can be stated that a reflux index above 10% should be considered as abnormal, a reflux index below 5% as normal, and a reflux index between 5 and 10% as between normal and abnormal. However, normal ranges are developed to separate patients at risk for esophagitis from those not at risk, which is not the major indication of the procedure. Normal ranges proposed by one group can be used by another group only if the investigations are performed and interpreted in a comparable way. This means that materials and methodology should be identical (Tables 71-3 and 71-4). For some individuals and in some clinical situations, it may be more important to relate "events" (eg, coughing, wheezing, apnea) to pH changes rather than to know if the data are within the normal range. It should be borne in mind that normal ranges for a group are not always applicable to an individual.

pH MONITORING AND OTHER INVESTIGATIONS

Many different techniques to evaluate GER do exist, focusing on different aspects, such as postprandial reflux (scintiscan, barium swallow, ultrasonography), histologic abnormalities (endoscopy), continuous measurements that are pH dependent (pH monitoring) or not (impedance), and pathophysiology by measuring the relaxations of the LES (manometry). Because there is no one investigation for GER that is accepted to provide a clear-cut discrimination between normal and abnormal, there is no reason why pH monitoring should do so. Abnormal pH monitoring does not accurately predict the risk for esophagitis.[30,44] In a group of reflux patients with esophagitis, the sensitivity of pH metry is 88% and of scintigraphy is 36%.[45] In a group of patients with abnormal scintigraphy, the sensitivity of pH monitoring is 82%, of endoscopy is 64%, and of manometry of the LES is 33%.[46] Nonacid reflux my be inoffensive (postprandial) reflux at a neutral pH but may also contain bile, which is also toxic for the esophageal mucosa.[46] There is little experience with esophageal bile monitoring in children. The overall correlation between scintiscanning and pH monitoring is acceptable (r = .78).[47] However, during simultaneous pH recording and scintiscanning, only 6 of 123 reflux episodes were recorded simultaneously.[48] There is no correlation between the number of reflux episodes detected with scintigraphy and pH monitoring.[49] Barium studies seem to have a much lower sensitivity to pick up reflux episodes if pH monitor-

TABLE 71-3   COMPARISON BETWEEN DATA RECORDED WITH AN ANTIMONY ELECTRODE WITH INTERNAL REFERENCE ELECTRODE AND A GLASS MICROELECTRODE WITH EXTERNAL REFERENCE ELECTRODE IN 20 PATIENTS WITH TWO GASTROGRAPH MARK II* DEVICES

	ANTIMONY	GLASS
Reflux index	3.94 ± 3.68	3.61 ± 3.25
Number episodes	15.15 ± 11.09	17.45 ± 10.41
Mean pH/24 h	5.46 ± 0.39	5.33 ± 0.25

*Fresenius, Medical Intruments Corporation.
No significant difference between the different parameters studied.

TABLE 71-4   DEPENDABILITY OF ESOPHAGEAL PH MONITORING DATA ON THE
                SOFTWARE PROGRAM (37 RECORDINGS)

| | PROGRAM | | |
PARAMETER	1	2	3
Reflux index (% < 4.0)	4.85 ± 3.84	4.86 ± 3.90	5.02 ± 4.15
Number episodes/24 h	87.38 ± 149.14 (a)	16.05 ± 10.38 (b, c)	19.05 ± 9.85 (a, b, c)
N° Ep > 5 min/24 h	2.32 ± 2.42 (b)	2.27 ± 2.25 (c)	2.92 ± 2.78 (b, c)
Duration Lo Ep (min)	18.54 ± 18.07	17.45 ± 16.84	15.33 ± 11.17

Program 1: Medical Instruments Cooperation program for Gastrograph Mark II (Fresenius, Medical Instruments Corporation): four measurements per second; the program calculates 360 medians per 24 hours; program 2: MIC program for Gastrograph Mark II: four measurements per second; the program calculates 43,200 medians per 24 hours; program 3: program for Gastrograph Mark II, developed by another company.
(a) : $p < .001$; (b) and (c) : $p < .05$.

ing is regarded as the "gold standard."[48] According to many authors, there is a high incidence of false-positive and false-negative studies with barium studies that is related to the short investigation time on the one hand and the intensity of reflux-provoking maneuvers on the other hand. Fifteen-minute postprandial period color Doppler ultrasonography was compared with 24-hour pH monitoring, showing agreement in 81.5%.[50] However, if pH monitoring was considered the "gold standard," the specificity of the color Doppler ultrasonography was as low as 11%, and there was no correlation between the incidence of reflux episodes measured with both techniques.[50] A far higher number of reflux episodes is detected with impedance in comparison with pH monitoring because only 14.9% of all reflux episodes are acid.[52] But only 57% of acid reflux episodes are detected with impedance.[51]

CONCLUSION

Esophageal pH monitoring measures pH in the esophagus, not GER. The miniaturization of devices and electrodes has made pH monitoring a procedure that is easy to perform, even in the youngest children. Patient-related factors such as feeding and physical activity influence pH monitoring results. Hardware- and software-related factors, as well as patient-related factors and recording conditions, determine the results. In clinical practice, pH monitoring is of interest in those patients in whom GERD is suspected who present without clear regurgitation or emesis and to measure the efficacy of treatment.

REFERENCES

1. Tuttle SG, Grossman MI. Detection of gastroesophageal reflux by simultaneous measurements of intraluminal pressure and pH. Proc Soc Exp Biol 1958;98:224.
2. Miller FA. Utilization of inlying pH probe for evaluation of acid peptic diathesis. Arch Surg 1964;89:199–203.
3. Vandenplas Y, Ashkenazi A, Belli D, et al. A proposition for the diagnosis and treatment of gastro-oesophageal reflux disease in children: a report from a working group on gastro-oesophageal reflux disease. Eur J Pediatr 1993;152:704–11.
4. Vandenplas Y, Belli D, Boige N, et al. A standardized protocol for the methodology of esophageal pH monitoring and interpretation of the data for the diagnosis of gastro-esophageal reflux. J Pediatr Gastroenterol Nutr 1992;14:467–71.
5. Emde C. Basic principles of pH registration. Neth J Med 1989; 34:S3–9.
6. De Caestecker JS, Heading RC. Esophageal pH monitoring. Gastroenterol Clin North Am 1990;19:645.
7. Vandenplas Y, Loeb H. Alkaline gastroesophageal reflux in infants. J Pediatr Gastroenterol Nutr 1991;12:448–52.
8. Vandenplas Y, editor. Oesophageal pH monitoring for gastro-oesophageal reflux in infants and children. J. Wiley & Sons; 1992.
9. Cravens E, Lehman G, O'Connor K, et al. Placement of esophageal pH probes 5 cm above the lower esophageal sphincter: can we get closer? Gastroenterology 1987;92:1357–9.
10. Vandenplas Y, Casteels A, Naert M, et al. Abbreviated oesophageal pH monitoring in infants. Eur J Pediatr 1994;153:80–3.
11. Belli DC, Le Coultre D. Comparison in a same patient of short-, middle- and long-term pH metry recordings in the presence or absence of gastro-esophageal reflux. Pediatr Res 1989; 26:269.
12. Tuttle SG, Grossman MI. Detection of gastroesophageal reflux by simultaneous measurement of intraluminal pressure and pH. Proc Soc Exp Biol Med 1958;98:225–30.
13. Skinner DB, Booth DJ. Assessment of distal esophageal function in patients with hiatal hernia and or gastroesophageal refluc. Ann Surg 1970;172:627–36.
14. Kantrowitz PA, Corson JG, Fleischer DJ, Skinner DB. Measurement of gastroesophageal reflux. Gastroenterology 1969;56: 666–74.
15. Kaul B, Petersen H, Grette K, Myrvold HE. Scintigraphy, pH measurements, and radiography in the evaluation of gastro-esophageal reflux. Scand J Gastroenterol 1985;20:289–94.
16. Arasu TS. Gastroesophageal reflux in infants and children: comparative accuracy of diagnostic methods. J Pediatr 1979;94: 663–8.
17. Holloway RH, McCallum RW. New diagnostic techniques in esophageal disease. In: Cohen S, Soloway RD, editors. Diseases of the esophagus. New York: Churchill Livingstone; 1982. p. 75–95.
18. Richter JE, Castell DO. Gastroesophageal reflux disease: pathogenesis, diagnosis and therapy. Ann Intern Med 1982; 97:93–103.
19. Bernstein IM, Baker IA. A clinical test for esophagitis. Gastroenterology 1958;34:760–81.
20. Benz LJ. A comparison of clinical measurements of gastroesophageal reflux. Gastroenterology 1972;62:1–3.
21. Herbst JJ, Minton SD, Book LS. Gastroesophageal reflux causing respiratory distress and apnea in newborn infants. J Pediatr 1979;95:763–8.
22. Berezin S. Use of the intraesophageal acid perfusion test in pro-

voking non-specific chest pain in children. J Pediatr 1989; 115:709–12.

23. Ramet J, Egreteau L, Curzi-Dascalova L, et al. Cardia, respiratory and arousal responses to an esophageal acid infusion test in near-term infants during active sleep. J Pediatr Gastroenterol Nutr 1992;15:135–40.

24. Kahn A, Rebuffat E, Sottiaux M, et al. Lack of temporal relation between acid reflux in the proximal oesophagus and cardiorespiratory events in sleeping infants. Eur J Pediatr 1992; 151:208–12.

25. Suys B, DeWolf D, Hauser B, et al. Bradycardia and gastroesophageal reflux in term and preterm infants: is there any relation? J Pediatr Gastroenterol Nutr 1994;19;187–90.

26. Vandenplas Y, DeWolf D, Deneyer M, Sacré L. Incidence of gastro-esophageal reflux in sleep, awake, fasted and postcibal periods in asymptomatic and symptomatic infants. J Pediatr Gastroenterol Nutr 1988;7:177–81.

27. Schindlbeck NE, Heinrich C, König A, et al. Optimal thresholds, sensitivity, and specificity of long-term pH metry for the detection of gastroesophageal reflux disease. Gastroenterology 1985;93:85–90.

28. Armstrong D, Emde C, Bumm R, et al. Twenty-four hour pattern of esophageal motility in asymptomatic volunteers. Dig Dis Sci 1990;35:1190–7.

29. Avidan B, Sonnenberg A, Schnell TG, Sontag SJ. Acid reflux is a poor predictor for severity of erosive reflux esophagitis. Dig Dis Sci 2002;47:2565–73.

30. Vandenplas Y, Franckx-Goossens A, Pipeleers-Marichal M, et al. Area under pH 4: advantages of a new parameter in the interpretation of esophageal pH monitoring data in infants. J Pediatr Gastroenterol Nutr 1989;9:34–9.

31. Vandenplas Y, Sacré L, Loeb H. Effects of formula feeding on gastric acidity time and oesophageal pH monitoring data. Eur J Pediatr 1988;148:152–4.

32. Estevao-Costa J, Campos M, Dias JA, et al. Delayed gastric emptying and gastroesopheageal reflux: a pathophysiologic relationship. J Pediatr Gastroenterol Nutr 2001;32:471–4

33. DeMeester TR, Johnson LF, Joseph GJ, et al. Patterns of gastroesophageal reflux in health and disease. Ann Surg 1976; 184:459–66.

34. Orenstein SR, Whitington PF. Positioning for prevention of infant gastroesophageal reflux. Pediatrics 1982;69:768–72.

35. Orenstein SR, Whitington PF, Orenstein DM. The infant seat as treatment for gastroesophageal reflux. N Engl J Med 1983; 309:709–12.

36. Orenstein SR. Effects on behavior state of prone versus seated positioning for infants with gastroesophageal reflux. Pediatrics 1990;85:765–7.

37. Vandenplas Y, Belli D, Benhamou PH, et al. Current concepts and issues in the management of regurgitation of infants: a reappraisal. Acta Paediatr 1996;85:531–4

38. Vandenplas Y, Belli DC, Dupont C, et al. The relation between gastro-oesophageal reflux, sleeping position and sudden infant death syndrome and its impact on positional therapy. Eur J Pediatr 1997;156:104–6.

39. Vandenplas Y, Goyvaerts H, Helven R, Sacre L. Gastroesophageal reflux, as assessed by 24-hour pH monitoring, in 509 healthy infants screened for SIDS-risk. Pediatrics 1991; 88:834–40.

40. Jolley SG, Halpern LM, Tunell WP, et al. The risk of sudden infant death from gastroesophageal reflux. J Pediatr Surg 1991;26:691–6.

41. Johnson LF, DeMeester TR. Twenty-four hour pH monitoring of the distal esophagus: a quantitative measure of gastroesophageal reflux. Am J Gastroenterol 1974;62:325–32.

42. Jolley SG, Johnson DG, Herbst JJ, et al. An assessment of gastroesophageal reflux in children by extended pH monitoring of the distal esophagus. Surgery 1978;84:16–24.

43. Vandenplas Y, Lepoudre R, Helven R. Dependability of esophageal pH monitoring data in infants on cut-off limits: the oscillatory index. J Pediatr Gastroenterol Nutr 1990;11:304–9.

44. Heinre RG, Cameron DJ, Chow CW, et al. Esophagitis in distressed infants: poor diagnostic agreement between esophageal pH monitoring and histopathologic findings. J Pediatr 2002;140:3–4.

45. Shay SS, Abreu SH, Tsuchida A. Scintigraphy in gastroesophageal reflux disease: a comparison to endoscopy, LESP, and 24-h pH score, as well as to simultaneous pH monitoring. Am J Gastroenterol 1992;87:1094–101.

46. Marshall RE, Anggiansah A, Owen WJ. Bile in the oesophagus: clinical relevance and ambulatory detection. Br J Surg 1997; 84:21–8.

47. Ozcan Z, Ozcan C, Erinc R, et al. Scintigraphy in the detection of gastro-oesophageal reflux with caustic oesophageal burns: a comparative study with radiography and 24-h pH monitoring. Pediatr Radiol 2001;31:737–41.

48. Vandenplas Y, Derde MP, Piepsz A. Evaluation of reflux epsidoes during simultaneous esophageal pH monitoring and gastroesophageal reflux scintigraphy in children. J Pediatr Gastroenterol Nutr 1991;14:256–60.

49. Tolia V, Kuhns L, Kauffman RE. Comparison of simultaneous esophageal pH monitoring and scintigraphy in infants with gastroesophageal reflux. Am J Gastroenterol 1993;88: 661–4.

50. Jang HS, Lees JS, Lim GY, et al. Correlation of color Doppler sonographic findings with pH measurements in gastroesophageal reflux in children. J Clin Ultrasound 2001;29: 212–7.

51. Wenzl TG, Moroder C, Trachterna M, et al. Esophageal pH monitoring and impedance measurement: a comparison of two diagnostic tests for gastroesophageal reflux. J Pediatr Gastroenterol Nutr 2002;34:519–23.

CHAPTER 72

PANCREATIC FUNCTION TESTS

Richard T. Lee Couper, MD

Mark R. Oliver, MBBS, MD, FRACP

Exocrine pancreatic function is notoriously difficult to assess. In practical terms, the organ and its secretions are relatively inaccessible, and direct assessment requires duodenal intubation to collect pancreatic secretions. The other obstacle rendering assessment difficult is the enormous functional reserve capacity of the exocrine pancreas. Digestive enzymes are synthesized and secreted by the pancreatic acini in considerable excess. Marked reduction of exocrine pancreatic function must occur before nutrients are malassimilated and the functional loss becomes a homeostatic threat. In pediatric patients with cystic fibrosis and Shwachman-Diamond syndrome, Gaskin and colleagues found that lipase and colipase outputs had to be less than 2% and 1% of normal values, respectively, before steatorrhea was apparent.[1] The corollary is that between 98 and 99% of pancreatic reserve for lipase and colipase must be lost before fat maldigestion occurs.

Steatorrhea is a useful indicator of pancreatic function. Steatorrhea is defined as a fecal fat output in excess of 7% of ingested fat in patients over 6 months of age and in excess of 15% in patients under 6 months of age. Patients are pancreatic insufficient if steatorrhea is present. Patients are pancreatic sufficient if steatorrhea is absent and may have pancreatic function in excess of 2% of normal. Pancreatic-insufficient subjects can be detected reliably by a variety of tests. The challenge has been to develop a test that evaluates the range of function in pancreatic-sufficient subjects.

TESTS OF EXOCRINE PANCREATIC FUNCTION

TEST CATEGORIES

There are three categories of exocrine pancreatic function tests (Table 72-1). Direct tests assess the secretory capacity of the exocrine pancreas. Pancreatic secretions are collected via intubation of the small intestine, usually under stimulated conditions, and are analyzed for the output of water, ions, and enzymes. Stimulation of the pancreas allows the pancreatic functional reserve to be assessed. Collection of unstimulated secretions from a rested organ provides little information.

Indirect tests detect abnormalities secondary to loss of pancreatic function, such as the maldigestion and consequent malabsorption of fat and/or nitrogen. Alternatively, these tests depend on the ability of pancreatic enzymes to cleave specific synthetic substrates, generating absorbable, measurable end products that are detectable in breath, serum, or urine. Additionally, pancreatic enzymes such as chymotrypsin and elastase 1 are relatively biostable and can be detected in the stool.

Blood tests rely on the fact that small but significant amounts of the enzymes and enteroendocrine hormones synthesized by the pancreas are normally present in the systemic circulation. In certain circumstances, the serum concentration of specific pancreatic enzymes (such as immunoreactive trypsinogen) and specific hormones (such as pancreatic polypeptide) may reflect residual exocrine pancreatic function.

The criteria for an ideal pancreatic function test are listed in Table 72-2. All currently available tests have one drawback, and many have several. Direct tests provide the most sensitive and specific measurements of exocrine pancreatic function and are useful in the detection of mild to moderate dysfunction. However, these tests are invasive and expensive, and the results are poorly reproducible between laboratories owing to different study protocols. Indirect and blood tests, although cheaper and easier to administer, are less sensitive and specific and, as a whole, lack an ability to differentiate between mild and moderate exocrine dysfunction.

INDICATIONS FOR PANCREATIC FUNCTION TESTS

1. Differentiate pancreatogenous malabsorption from other causes of malabsorption.
2. Diagnose and study the natural history of disorders affecting exocrine pancreatic function.
3. Assess the efficacy of pancreatic enzyme replacement in children with malabsorption secondary to exocrine pancreatic dysfunction.

DIRECT TESTS

The exocrine pancreas secretes fluid and ions in response to endogenous secretin and enzymes in response to endogenous cholecystokinin (CCK). Endogenous secretin and CCK are released from small intestinal mucosa in response to nutrients and/or gastric acid. The pancreas is also stimulated by neural pathways. It is supplied by vagal efferents that act on muscarinic receptors. Intestinal nutrients provoke stimulation of enzyme secretion via this pathway as well as by CCK release. Stimulation of the exocrine

TABLE 72-1   TESTS OF EXOCRINE PANCREATIC
              FUNCTION

DIRECT TESTS
Exogenous hormonal stimulants
  Cholecystokinin*†
  Cerulein*
  Bombesin*
  Secretin†
Nutrient stimulants
  Lundh test meal
  Fatty acids
  Amino acids
Other
  Selenium 75 methionine incorporation and release
  Pure pancreatic juice

INDIRECT TESTS
Stool
  Microscopy—fat, meat fibers†
  Acid steatocrit†
  Fecal balance†
  Iodine 131 triolein excretion
  Dual-radiolabeled fat
  Trypsin,† chymotrypsin,† lipase, elastase†
Breath tests
  Carbon 14 lipids
  Carbon 13 lipids†
  Carbon 14 cholesterol octanoate
  Starch breath hydrogen
Urinary/plasma markers
  Bentiromide†
  Fluorescein dilaurate (pancreolauryl)†
  Oral tolerance (fat and vitamins)
  Dual-label Schilling
  Urinary lactulose

BLOOD TESTS
  Total amylase or lipase
  Isomylase
  Cationic/anionic trypsinogen†
  Pancreatic polypeptide
  Amino acids

*Used in various dose combinations with or without secretin.
†Test currently used in pediatric practice.

pancreas is undertaken by using one or both of these pathways by supplying either exogenous hormones or intestinal nutrients.

Successful quantitation of human pancreatic exocrine function is contingent on the following conditions:

1. The development of appropriate intravenously administered hormonal stimuli or appropriate nutrient delivery to the small intestine
2. The ability to quantitatively measure pancreatic secretions
3. The ability to exclude gastric acid and pepsin

EXOGENOUS HORMONAL STIMULATION

There is no standard method of hormonal stimulation. Consequently, techniques vary between centers, and each laboratory is required to establish its own range of normal values. The doses of hormones used, the mode of administration (intravenous bolus or intravenous infusion), the duration of infusion, and, in the case of a combined secretin CCK infusion, the sequence of administration may all differ. Little information exists regarding optimum doses in children, especially for synthetic secretin and CCK; in most cases, doses have been extrapolated from adult data on a weight per kilogram basis. Current sources of supply of pancreatic secretagogues are listed in Table 72-3. Synthetic preparations of secretin and CCK are preferable to animal extracts in that they are not contaminated with other gut-derived peptides and because they are less allergenic. Supply of agents approved for human use has been problematic in recent years. Combined stimulation is optimal because there is evidence that CCK or similar hormones act synergistically with secretin.[2] Other investigators have used cerulein (a decapeptide) or bombesin (a tetradecapeptide) alone or in combination with secretin because these peptides have effects on the exocrine pancreas similar to those of CCK. No published information exists regarding their use in children.

Quantification of secretions requires that precise volume data be obtained. Two approaches are used: distal occlusion of the duodenum by a balloon[3] or continuous perfusion of a nonabsorbable marker,[4] allowing correction for distal losses. Balloon occlusion techniques are less physiologic in that they may cause luminal distention and possible stimulation by this means. Similarly, gastric acid and pepsin can be excluded either by continuous nasogastric suction or by a pyloric balloon.

The technique used at The Hospital for Sick Children in Toronto and at Australian centers employs practical solutions to the above conditions and is readily adaptable. The test is a quantitative technique modified from Go and colleagues[5] and is represented diagrammatically in Figure 72-1. Subjects should be fasting, and in the case of patients on pancreatic enzyme supplements, these supplements should be discontinued at least 48 hours prior to the test to remove any suppression of the exocrine pancreas by negative-feedback inhibition. Under fluoroscopic control, a double-lumen tube is inserted into the duodenum. The tube is constructed so that one lumen opens proximally at the ampulla of Vater, and the other lumen, which has several distal ports, is positioned 5 to 12 cm distally at the ligament of Treitz. Through the proximal lumen, a nonabsorbable marker solution (gentamicin, 20 mg/mL in 5% mannitol) is infused into the duodenum at a constant rate. Pancreatic juice mixed with infused marker solution is aspirated distally by intermittent low-pressure suction and

TABLE 72-2   CRITERIA FOR THE IDEAL PANCREATIC
              FUNCTION TEST

Inexpensive and easily performed
Noninvasive
Specific for pancreatic disease and able to exclude patients with other digestive disorders owing to small bowel mucosal disease, inherited defects of fat transport, or cholestasis
Defines the exact level of pancreatic function in subjects with pancreatic sufficiency and in whom partial impairment of exocrine function is present but nutrient assimilation is unaffected
Repeatable, reproducible between laboratories and able to monitor exocrine function longitudinally
No interference from exogenous pancreatic supplements

TABLE 72-3   SOURCES OF PANCREATIC SECRETAGOGUES

SECRETAGOGUE	SUPPLIER
Secretin, natural porcine; Secretin, Secrepan	Eisai (Bungkyo-Ku, Tokyo, Japan)*; www.eisai.co.jp
Synthetic porcine secretion	ChiRhoClin (Silver Springs)*†; www.chirhoclin.com
	Goldham-Bioglan Pharma GMBH* (Zusmarshausen, Germany)
Synthetic human secretion	Bachem AG (Bubendorb, Switzerland)*; www.bachem.com
	Calbiochem (La Jolla, CA); www.calbiochem.com
	Repligen (Needham, MA)*; www.repligen.com
	Research Plus (Bayonne, NJ); www.researchplus.com
	Sigma Aldrich (St Louis, MO); www.sigma-aldrich.com
Cholecystokinin octapeptide	Anaspec (San Jose, CA); www.anaspec.com
	Sigma Aldrich (St Louis, MO); www.sigma-aldrich.com
	Research Plus; www.researchplus.com
	Calbiochem (La Jolla, CA); www.calbiochem.com
	Anaspec (San Jose, CA); www.anaspec.com
Cerulein	Sigma Aldrich; www.sigma-aldrich.com
	Anaspec (San Jose, CA); www.anaspec.com
	Research Plus (Bayonne, NJ); www.researchplus.com
Bombesin	Research Plus (Bayonne, NJ); www.researchplus.com
	Calbiochem (La Jolla, CA); www.calbiochem.com
	Anaspec (San Jose, CA); www.anaspec.com

*Sources approved for human use (not necessarily in United States).
†Licensed to Repligen.

is collected over four 20-minute collection periods into flasks on ice. The first period allows equilibration of marker solution with pancreatic juice and also allows residual luminal pancreatic enzymes to be washed out. During the subsequent three periods, duodenal juice mixed with marker is collected while continuously and simultaneously infusing intravenous secretin and CCK at doses known to achieve maximal pancreatic stimulation. A separate nasogastric tube facilitates aspiration of gastric juice and minimizes contamination of duodenal contents with acid and pepsin.

This technique allows both the collection and quantification of pancreatic secretions. Although the biliary tree and the duodenal mucosa contribute to fluid secretion, the vast bulk of the secretory response is generated by the action of secretin on pancreatic ductular epithelium and acini and by the effect of CCK on acini. This fact, coupled with the use of a nonabsorbable marker, allows correction for distal losses of fluid and enzyme by the assumption that once equilibration has been attained, the degree of distal loss of the marker is the same as the degree of enzyme and fluid loss.[6] A simple volume correction factor can be calculated as follows:

FIGURE 72-1 Scheme of the exogenous secretion/cholecystokinin pancreatic stimulation test with nonabsorbable marker perfusion. Gastric juice is removed via the nasogastric tube. Through the proximal lumen of the double-lumen intestinal tube, the nonabsorbable marker is perfused at a constant rate. Pancreatic secretions mix with the marker in the mixing segment, and the mixture is aspirated via the distal port. Pancreatic secretions are collected over a specific time period (60–80 minutes) while maximally stimulating pancreatic secretion with intravenous hormones (cholecystokinin and/or secretin). Adapted from Durie PR. Pancreatic function tests. Med Clin North Am 1988;20:3842–5.

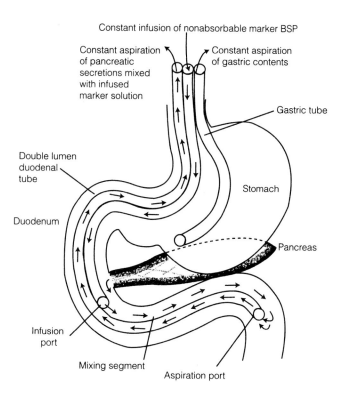

$$\frac{\text{gentamicin in μg per period infused}}{\text{gentamicin in μg per period recovered}}$$

The determination of fluid, electrolyte, and enzymatic output can be adjusted accordingly. Trypsin, colipase, and total lipase outputs are measured routinely by titrimetric techniques, and bicarbonate output is measured by a colorimetric technique. Sodium, potassium, and chloride outputs are also measured. Other investigators have measured total protein, amylase, chymotrypsin, carboxypeptidase, elastase, cholesterol esterase, and deoxyribonuclease.

The techniques employed for enzymatic determination, especially for amylase and lipase, may differ. The substrates used for the colorimetric determination of amylase activity vary; consequently, the units used to express activity differ. In the case of lipase, results vary depending on whether a short-chain triglyceride such as glycerol tributyrate or a long-chain triglyceride such as olive oil is used as the substrate.

The invasiveness of this test tends to discourage routine clinical use, particularly in pancreatic-sufficient patients, the group in which it is most helpful. It is worthwhile reiterating that this test has helped to delineate pancreatic function in both healthy and diseased individuals. For example, the fact that colipase is the rate-controlling factor for lipolysis became apparent with the analysis of stimulated secretions from both normal individuals and patients with steatorrhea.[7] Additionally, in patients with cystic fibrosis, deficits in electrolyte secretion, particularly chloride[8] and bicarbonate secretion,[9] have been identified, which, in turn, may lead to reduced fluid secretion.[10]

NUTRIENT STIMULATION

Nutrient stimulation of the exocrine pancreas can be undertaken by adapting the principles of the secretin-CCK stimulation test and substituting intraluminal nutrients for the intravenous secretagogues. This method is more physiologic in that the stimulus is provided both by the release of endogenous secretin and CCK directly into the splanchnic circulation and by a vagal mechanism that can be inhibited by atropine.

The most commonly used test meal has been that devised by Lundh for use in adult patients, consisting of milk powder, vegetable oil, and dextrose.[11] The total volume is 300 mL, with a final composition of 6% fat, 5% protein, and 15% carbohydrate. The Lundh meal is composed of intact nutrients. The presence of intact fat, protein, and carbohydrate renders the enzymatic determinations of lipase, protease, and amylase activity difficult. Lundh used a nonabsorbable marker to provide a reference for the absorption of nutrients, but the lack of continuous duodenal marker perfusion, coupled with the presence of salivary and gastric secretions, makes this test relatively qualitative. Although the test is more physiologic than exogenous hormonal stimulation, these practical difficulties have led other investigators to develop more quantitative methods of nutrient stimulation.

Alternative nutrients have been used. The most potent nutrient stimuli are essential amino acids, particularly phenylalanine, but methionine, valine, and tryptophan have also been shown to stimulate the pancreas.[12] Amino acids are usually given as duodenal infusions. Amino acids do not interfere with enzymatic or electrolyte determinations. For physiologic purposes, amino acid solutions should have a pH approximating that of the duodenal lumen because hydrogen ions neutralize bicarbonate, rendering assessment of secretin response difficult. A low-pH solution can also directly stimulate the pancreas through secretin release independent of the amino acid content. The volume of the infusions should be low because duodenogastric reflux of nutrients can stimulate the pancreas via gastrin release. The response of the pancreas to individual nutrients may depend in part on duodenal baroreceptors. Too low an infusion volume will result in a suboptimal stimulus.[13] With the exception of the Lundh meal, which is relatively unpalatable, nutrient stimulation has not been used clinically in children.

OTHER DIRECT TESTS

A variety of alternative approaches have been used in adult patients. These include the use of radioisotopes to assess uptake, incorporation, and release of amino acids; direct ductal sampling of secretions; and other methods employing microtechniques to assess protease activity. Pancreatic synthetic capacity is measured by the ability to incorporate selenium 75 (^{75}Se)-labeled methionine.[14] In response to a CCK stimulus, ^{75}Se-labeled methionine is released into pancreatic secretions as a constituent of enzymes and other proteins. Measurement of ^{75}Se activity serves as a guide to acinar function. ^{75}Se is a high-energy–emitting isotope, unsuitable for pediatric use. Endoscopic collections of pure pancreatic juice allow the assessment of uncontaminated samples.[15] Duodenal fluid collected at endoscopy and following intravenous infusion of secretin and CCK has been used to evaluate pancreatic function in children.[16] Unfortunately, a general anesthetic is required, and this may, in itself, suppress pancreatic function.

INDIRECT EXOCRINE PANCREATIC FUNCTION TESTS

The actions of individual pancreatic enzymes are assessed indirectly by quantifying the appearance of inappropriately increased amounts of specific nutrients in the feces (eg, fecal fat) or by measuring metabolic products in the blood, urine, or breath (eg, the bentiromide test and radiolabeled breath tests). Alternatively, the amount of enzymes such as chymotrypsin and elastase in the stool may reflect residual pancreatic function. Most of these tests cannot reliably assess the level of function in pancreatic-sufficient subjects or exclude biliary or intestinal causes of malabsorption. However, because they are relatively noninvasive and are indeed sometimes referred to as tubeless, some of the tests (such as that for fecal fat) can be used to evaluate the success of pancreatic enzyme supplementation in pancreatic-insufficient subjects.

FECAL TESTS

Microscopic Examination. Microscopic examination of the stools may reveal meat fibers, neutral fat droplets, or free fatty acid crystals, suggesting partial fat hydrolysis. Sudan III is the preferred stain for neutral fat, although the fat droplets can be seen quite easily without staining. Free fatty acid crystals are birefringent and are best visualized by a microscope with a polarizing filter. They can also be visualized by lowering the pH of the Sudan III stain.[17] If stool is obtained by rectal examination, lubricants containing oil or petroleum jelly should be avoided. Neutral fat droplets do not differentiate pancreatogenous steatorrhea from steatorrhea of intestinal or biliary origin.[18] Similarly, free fatty acid crystals do not rule out pancreatogenous malabsorption.

Attempts have been made to quantify the degree of steatorrhea by counting the number and determining the size of fat globules in a high-power field.[19] If, on cursory examination, steatorrhea is present, it is sensible to quantify fecal fat losses using balance studies. Microscopic examination of the stool should be mandatory in all cases of suspected malabsorption. However, it should not be regarded as more than a highly useful, albeit crude, screening test for malabsorption.

Steatocrit. The steatocrit, a measurement of fat malabsorption, works on the following principle: if homogenized feces are centrifuged, the lipid and liquid phases and stool residues separate, with the lipid phase on top of the liquid phase and the stool residue.[20] The lipid phase can be measured in a hematocrit tube if the tube is centrifuged at 15,000 rpm for 15 minutes. Reference values and ranges have recently been established for normal children.[21] The sensitivity of this test is markedly improved by the addition of perchloric acid to the fecal homogenate, and the acid steatocrit is determined.[22,23] This may prove to be a useful adjunct in laboratories with limited technical expertise, particularly in the third world, and may also provide a crude method for monitoring the response of patients receiving pancreatic enzyme supplements.

Pooled Stool Collections for Fat, Nitrogen, and Carbohydrate. Because of the functional reserve of the exocrine pancreas, these tests detect only pancreatic-insufficient subjects. All three nutrient classes—fat, protein, and carbohydrate—have been measured in stool to assess pancreatic function. Fecal fat analysis is the most widely used, the most informative, and the most homeostatically relevant of these tests. Pooled stool collections detect malabsorption but do not discriminate between patients with pancreatic and nonpancreatic malabsorption. Despite these limitations, fecal fat analysis is useful longitudinally, especially for assessing the efficacy of pancreatic enzyme supplements in patients with pancreatic insufficiency. Because of the odious nature of the test for both patients and laboratory technicians, it has fallen into disfavor in some circles. Alternative tests that rely on isotopic methods are more expensive, are almost as inconvenient, and still fail to differentiate the various causes of malassimilation.

The method most commonly used for the measurement of fecal fat is the titrimetric Van de Kamer method.[24] In adults, the test involves a diet containing 100 g of fat for 3 to 5 days.[25] Stools collected over 72 to 96 hours are pooled and refrigerated. The mechanics of collection can be improved by the use of a nonabsorbable marker at the start and the end of the diet. In children, the collection period is usually 3 days, although it is occasionally extended to 5 days. Because children find it difficult to adhere to a strictly regimented diet, meticulous weighing of food and careful dietary records are required to calculate the mean daily fat intake. Steatorrhea is present if more than 7% of ingested fat is excreted. Owing to the physiologic immaturity of the pancreatic and biliary secretions, infants under 6 months of age can excrete up to 15% of dietary fat.[26] The Van de Kamer method must be modified if the diet contains appreciable amounts of medium-chain triglycerides because these are not detected by the standard method. The potential for error is great because collections may be incomplete, fat intake may be inaccurately quantitated, and the occasional patient may have delayed intestinal transit. Other methods of estimating fat in feces, such as nuclear magnetic resonance spectrometry[27] and near-infrared reflectance spectroscopy,[28] may make laboratory analysis easier and less odious. The Van de Kamer method and these other methods potentially overestimate fecal fat excretion because they detect biliary lipids and complex lipids derived from intestinal cell turnover. Additionally, this test does not discriminate readily between mucosal, pancreatic, and other causes of fat absorption.

Fecal nitrogen has been used as an index of exocrine pancreatic function but does not provide further diagnostic information because it is unlikely that significant creatorrhea will occur if steatorrhea is absent. The same criticism can be made of fecal carbohydrate measurements. The most commonly used assessment of carbohydrate relies on the measurement of reducing sugars and does not assess total carbohydrate. The anthrone method, which assesses all hexose carbohydrates, has provided better quantitation of carbohydrate losses.[29] Carbohydrate measurements are likely to be elevated with small intestinal mucosal disease, and both nitrogen and carbohydrate are subject to variable colonic absorption and substrate use by fecal flora. For the above reasons, they are less accurate than neutral fat as a guide to pancreatic insufficiency.

Stool Isotopic Methods. Most of these methods are inappropriate for pediatric use because they use gamma ray–emitting isotopes. Single isotopes (iodine 131, iodine 125) bound to triglycerides are expensive, and the test necessitates a 3-day stool collection, but the need for strict dietary records is eliminated. Dual-isotope methods append markers to a nonabsorbable lipid such as glycerol triether and to a lipid subject to hydrolysis and absorption such as glycerol trioleate. This technique allows fat malabsorption to be estimated from single stool samples. Although some of the dual-labeling systems use β-emitting isotopes,[30] none of these methods has been adapted for pediatric use.

Fecal Trypsin, Chymotrypsin, Lipase, and Elastase 1. The capacity to measure both fecal trypsin and chymotrypsin has existed for 30 years. Fecal elastase 1 has been widely used only for the last decade. The initial tests measured enzymatic activity by means of a laborious titrimetric estimation using low-molecular-weight substrates. A number of problems existed with these tests. The enzymes are subject to proteolytic degradation by both pancreatic and bacterial proteases; thus, interpretation varies with intestinal transit. Chymotrypsin was preferentially measured instead of trypsin because it is more resistant to inactivation by colonic bacteria. However, a high proportion of chymotrypsin is strongly bound to insoluble stool residue,[31] and this thwarted attempts to develop accurate and more convenient photometric methods. The early tests have been superseded by a photometric method, the BMC test developed by Boehringer Mannheim Corporation (Mannheim, Germany), which employs a detergent to solubilize chymotrypsin in stool[32] and is convenient, reproducible, and sensitive. Patients receiving pancreatic enzyme supplements should discontinue them at least 5 days prior to measurement. Fecal chymotrypsin reliably differentiates between pancreatic-insufficient and pancreatic-sufficient patients. However, it does not reliably discriminate between pancreatic-sufficient patients and normal subjects. Patients with pancreatic insufficiency can be differentiated from those with intestinal or biliary disease. This method has been validated for pediatric use by showing a good correlation between the 72-hour fecal output of chymotrypsin and the CCK-secretin–stimulated duodenal output of chymotrypsin.[33] Other observers have shown a good correlation in children between duodenal chymotrypsin output following CCK stimulation and three random stool samples collected within 72 hours of pancreatic stimulation with CCK.[34] Fecal chymotrypsin is relatively stable at 18°C for up to 72 hours and can thus be sent from peripheral centers to a reference laboratory. If random stool samples are used and a low value is obtained, repeating the test will eliminate most false-negative results.

Fecal immunoreactive lipase can be measured by using an enzyme-linked immunosorbent assay (ELISA) technique.[35,36] The test has limitations similar to those of the fecal chymotrypsin test and is both sensitive (87%) and specific (97%) in pediatric patients with cystic fibrosis.[36]

The sensitivity is reduced comparably, presumably because of the inclusion of pancreatic-sufficient subjects. The technique is absolutely specific for human pancreatic lipase, and the results are not confounded by concomitant use of pancreatic enzyme supplements. It has also been found to be useful in the first 6 months of life, when lipase secretion is traditionally held to be low owing to ontogenic immaturity of the acini.

Elastase 1 is a member of the acidic elastase family. It is a sterol-binding protein as well as an endoprotease.[37] Elastase 1 is both a human- and pancreas-specific enzyme that is stable during abnormal intestinal transport.[38] Consequently, porcine pancreatic enzyme supplements do not alter the measurement of elastase 1. Age-related increase of elastase occurs only in the first 3 months of life, probably because the ontogenic development of elastase 1 is completed in early postnatal life.[39] An ELISA has been used to assess elastase 1 as an indirect measure of pancreatic function in both children and adults. This test is both more sensitive and specific than fecal chymotrypsin in detecting pancreatic insufficiency, but it will not delineate patients who are pancreatic sufficient.[40,41] However a decline in fecal elastase concentrations precedes fat malabsorption in patients with pancreatic-sufficient cystic fibrosis who become pancreatic insufficient.[42] False-positive results may occur as a result of villous damage secondary to several conditions, including celiac disease, cow's milk protein, enteropathy, and bacterial overgrowth.[43] It is possible that these patients may have a secondary pancreatic insufficiency owing to impairment of mucosal release of pancreatic secretagogues. Diarrheal disease and short-gut syndrome may result in false-negatives owing to a dilutional effect.[44,45] This problem can be overcome by lyophilization of stool samples, which removes stool water content as a confounding variable.[46] False-negatives are occasionally seen in pancreatic-sufficient patients with Shwachman-Diamond syndrome.[45] Despite these limitations, the stability of this enzyme allows storage at room temperature for at least a week, which facilitates mailing of fecal samples, and the absolute specificity of this test makes it one of the most attractive "tubeless" pancreatic function tests.[37,40] The use of this test is becoming more prevalent in pediatric practice.

BREATH TESTS

Radiolabeled and Stable Isotope Breath Tests. The technique and principles of breath testing are described in Chapter 73, "Breath Analysis." Ingested lipids are predominantly hydrolyzed by pancreatic lipases in the small intestine, absorbed as free fatty acids and monoglycerides, and transported to the liver, where oxidative metabolism liberates carbon dioxide (CO_2). The radiolabeled breath tests take advantage of this fact by substituting either carbon 14 (^{14}C) or 13 (^{13}C) for carbon 12 in a triglyceride molecule. The three triglycerides of different carbon chain lengths that have been commonly used are trioctanoin, tripalmitate, and triolein. All three substrates labeled with ^{14}C are sensitive in detecting fat malabsorption.[47] Triolein is more specific than either trioctanoin or tripalmitate for fat malabsorption; however, it does not differentiate between pancreatic and nonpancreatic causes of fat malabsorption. Normal release of CO_2 from triolein and tripalmitate requires adequate lipolysis, bile salt solubilization, and an adequate mucosal surface and transport capability. The release of CO_2 from trioctanoin is limited by lipolysis alone and can distinguish pancreatic insufficiency from bile salt deficiency and mucosal defects. Using these substrates in combination with one another (eg, testing with triolein and repeating the test with trioctanoin) improves specificity but not sensitivity. Other confounding variables are the action of lingual and gastric lipases on the substrate, varying individual lipid pool sizes, and the variable respiratory excretion of CO_2 in chronic respiratory disease. ^{14}C labeling mandates that these tests not be used in children.

The specificity of these tests may be improved by repeating them after administering pancreatic enzyme supplements. The same compounds have been labeled with ^{13}C, a stable isotope that is measurable by mass spectroscopy, and similar results have been obtained in children.[48] These tests have also recently been adapted to assess gastric emptying in children. Recently, ^{14}C cholesteryl octanoate, which is hydrolyzed by the pancreatic-specific cholesterol esterase, has been used as a substrate.[49] Studies suggest that hydrolysis by cholesterol esterase is the rate-limiting step.[50] The test is adaptable to ^{13}C labeling, allowing its use in children.[50] A synthetic mixed triglyceride (1,3-distearyl 2[^{13}C] octanolyl glycerol) has also been used as a substrate.[51] Excretion of ^{13}C-labeled CO_2 ([13]CO_2) is slower than that seen with cholesteryl octanoate. Stearyl hydrolysis by pancreatic lipase is the rate-limiting step.

Release of CO_2 from ^{13}C-labeled starch has been assessed in adults.[52] This test works on the principle that hydrolysis of starch by pancreatic isoamylase is the rate-limiting step in carbohydrate metabolism. Test specificity is improved by also measuring CO_2 release after ^{13}C-labeled glucose. The ratio of [13]CO_2 excretion after starch ingestion to [13]CO_2 excretion after glucose ingestion corrects for differences in oxidative metabolism. Even after correction, the test is relatively insensitive and will only detect pancreatic-insufficient subjects.

Release of CO^2 from ^{13}C-labeled egg white has been assessed in adults with pancreatic disease. This test is a crude test of proteolytic activity and could be adapted to pediatric subjects.[53]

Because stable isotopes and mass spectroscopy are expensive, these breath tests have not found a niche for routine pediatric use. However, benchtop devices for measuring ^{13}C have become more affordable, making these tests more accessible.

Hydrogen Breath Test. This test measures breath hydrogen excretion following starch ingestion. Starch is normally cleaved enzymatically into oligosaccharides by pancreatic isoamylase prior to further cleavage by brush border disaccharidases. When amylase secretion is impaired, undigested starch is digested by colonic bacteria, generating hydrogen, which is absorbed and excreted in the breath. A two-stage test with concomitant ingestion of oral pancreatic enzymes results in reduced breath hydrogen. This test is extremely nonspecific; false-positive results may occur in blind loop syndromes and also when small intestinal transit time is reduced. False-negative results may occur when the colon is colonized with non–hydrogen-producing bacteria and in subjects who have recently received antibiotics. Currently, there are no pediatric data.

URINARY/PLASMA MARKERS

Bentiromide Test. Bentiromide is a nonabsorbable synthetic peptide (N-benzoyl-L-tyrosyl-p-aminobenzoic acid) that is specifically cleaved by pancreatic chymotrypsin in the upper small intestine. This results in the release of p-aminobenzoic acid (PABA), which serves as a marker and which is rapidly absorbed, conjugated in the liver, and excreted in the urine. Colorimetric assay can measure PABA in both blood and urine, and the detection and quantification of PABA form the basis of the test. Falsely abnormal results have been demonstrated in subjects with bowel,

liver, or renal disease owing to defects in the absorption, conjugation, or excretion of PABA. Additionally, both intestinal bacteria and the intestinal brush border may demonstrate chymotrypsin-like activity, reducing specificity. Ingestion of a number of drugs such as sulfonamides, diuretics, acetaminophen, and chloramphenicol and foods such as prunes and cranberries may result in elevated aromatic amines that may interfere with laboratory determinations of PABA.[54] Recently, high-pressure liquid chromatography techniques have been developed to sensitively detect PABA and its metabolites, and these techniques may prove to be superior to colorimetric assay because they eliminate interference from drug and dietary amines.[55]

The bentiromide test was introduced in 1972, and initial reports relied on a one-stage test with a urinary collection.[56] The method involved collections over varying time periods and varying doses of substrate. Consequently, reports of test specificity and sensitivity varied widely. In North America, the recommended method for adults entails the patient receiving a 500 mg dose of bentiromide (170 mg of PABA), ingesting sufficient fluid to maintain an adequate diuresis, and collecting urine for a period of 6 hours.[57] The urinary recovery of PABA is expressed as a percentage of the orally ingested PABA. Less than 50% PABA excretion purportedly reflects pancreatic insufficiency. To correct for potential defects of absorption, hepatic conjugation, or excretion, a two-stage test has been suggested with an equivalent dose of free PABA administered subsequently and the urine collected for an identical time period.[58] This allows the urinary recovery of PABA after bentiromide to be corrected for the urinary recovery of equimolar free PABA. The results are expressed as a PABA excretion index (PEI):

$$PEI = \frac{\text{PABA recovered after bentiromide (\%)}}{\text{PABA recovered after free PABA (\%)}}$$

This maneuver improves sensitivity and specificity, but the test is cumbersome and time-consuming. Additionally, timed urine collections make the test awkward to perform in infants. In adults, this drawback has been circumvented by the simultaneous administration of ^{14}C-free PABA[59] or a free structural analog of PABA, p-aminosalicylic acid (PAS).[60] The ^{14}C-PABA method is impractical for pediatric use. A ^{13}C-PABA method that could be adapted for use in children has been described.[61] The PAS method has been used in the pediatric age group and has improved the sensitivity of the test.[62]

The initial pediatric experience with the bentiromide test concentrated on timed urine collections.[63] However, the specificity and sensitivity of the test have been improved with the development of methods to measure plasma PABA,[55] and the need for dual collections and urinary collections has been eliminated. The recommended pediatric dose of bentiromide (15 mg/kg) has been used in older children and is based on extrapolation from adult data. For the first 3 hours following ingestion of the dose, plasma PABA concentrations rise, and optimal discrimination between normal adolescent controls and patients with pancreatic insufficiency is obtained at the 90- and 120-minute points.[64] Reliable detection was not obtained in patients with cystic fibrosis and pancreatic sufficiency (between 5 and 10% of normal pancreatic chymotrypsin output as measured by the secretin-CCK test). In patients with Shwachman-Diamond syndrome, none of whom had malabsorption, the plasma test failed to detect pancreatic dysfunction in those patients with an enzyme output as low as 1% of normal. Bentiromide (15 mg/kg) is not useful for assessment in infants if clear fluids are given with the dose. Test sensitivity is improved by using a liquid meal and by increasing the dose to 30 mg/kg.[65] The bentiromide test may discriminate between pancreatic steatorrhea and steatorrhea from other causes and could potentially provide a method of monitoring the effect of pancreatic enzyme supplementation.

4-(N-Acetyl-L-tyrosyl) aminobenzoic acid has been used in adults and children[66,67] and has reportedly allowed better differentiation between controls and patients with chronic pancreatitis in comparison with the standard bentiromide test.[66] A modified Lundh meal was used in the pediatric study, and extremely good separation was obtained between normal controls and patients with cystic fibrosis.[67] However, no information exists on its usefulness in subjects who have pancreatic sufficiency but reduced functional reserve.

Fluorescein Dilaurate (Pancreolauryl) Test. This test is based on a principle similar to that of the bentiromide test. Orally administered fluorescein dilaurate is hydrolyzed by pancreatic cholesterol esterase, liberating lauric acid and free water-soluble fluorescein. Fluorescein is readily absorbed in the small intestine, partially conjugated in the liver, and excreted in the urine, predominantly as fluorescein diglucuronide. Fluorescein is nontoxic and can be easily measured in both serum and urine by spectrophotometric or fluorometric techniques.

The commercial version of this test in adult patients involves the ingestion of 0.5 mmol of fluorescein dilaurate with a standard meal. To enhance diuresis, 1 L of unsweetened tea is consumed between the third and fifth hour of the test. All urine is collected over a 10-hour period. To correct for individual differences in intestinal absorption, conjugation, and urinary excretion, the test is repeated using equimolar free fluorescein after an interval of at least 24 hours. The results are expressed as a ratio of the fluorescein detected on the test and the control days. A ratio of greater than 30% is considered normal, a ratio of between 20 and 30% is equivocal, and a ratio of less than 20% is abnormal.[54] Equivocal results should be repeated. The dose can be modified for pediatric purposes.[68] Caution should be used in interpreting this test in diabetic patients in whom glucose interferes owing to the formation of fluorescein glucuronide.[69]

The serum test is more convenient because it is less time-consuming and because the need for urine collection is eliminated. Peak serum levels occur at approximately 210 minutes after absorption, and the best cutoff point for discriminating between pancreatic exocrine-insufficient patients and controls appears to be between 240 and 300 minutes.[70] Concomitant administration of mannitol,

which is transported in a similar fashion to free fluorescein, permits completion of the test in 1 day. The results are expressed as a fluorescein-to-mannitol ratio and are equivalent to those of the more cumbersome 2-day test. This method has been used successfully in pediatric subjects.[71] This test has some advantages over the bentiromide test but is not capable of detecting subtle impairment of function in pancreatic-sufficient subjects. Analysis is easier, and there is less interference by exogenous compounds, although it is recommended that niacin and sulfasalazine be avoided prior to the test.[68] False-positive results can occur in patients with biliary tract and mucosal disorders. Cholesterol esterase is pancreatic specific, and the test is therefore not subject to the influence of brush border enzymes. However, bacterial overgrowth can influence the results because some bacteria (in particular, streptococci) are able to hydrolyze fluorescein dilaurate.[68]

ORAL TOLERANCE TESTS

Oral fat-loading tests may provide useful information in patients from whom a reliable stool sample cannot be obtained. Serum triglycerides and chylomicron levels are measured at 2, 3, and 5 hours following the ingestion of a meal consisting of 50 g of fat, containing equal amounts of butter and margarine, emulsified in 70 mL of water. Serum triglycerides usually peak at 3 hours after ingestion. An abnormal result consists of a serum triglyceride rise of less than 1.13 mmol/L, or less than 100% above the fasting level, and/or the appearance of less than 7% chylomicrons.[72] This test does not differentiate among patients with pancreatic disease, intestinal mucosal defects, and bile salt deficiency.

Attempts have been made to improve test specificity by using radiolabeled lipids. Initial tests in adults employed triolein labeled with iodine 131 (^{131}I). Subsequently, a dual-label lipid system was evaluated using a tritium (^{3}H)-labeled free fatty acid (oleic acid) and a ^{14}C-labeled triglyceride (triolein). The substrates are administered simultaneously, and the serum ^{3}H-to-^{14}C ratio is calculated.[72] Patients with pancreatic insufficiency have a higher ratio than normal patients or patients with mucosal disease. However, this test does not exclude patients with defects of bile salt delivery or synthesis. Labeling with radioisotopes precludes using this test in children.

DUAL-LABEL SCHILLING TEST

Patients with exocrine pancreatic insufficiency often have an abnormal Schilling test. Pancreatic enzymes are responsible for the cleavage of intrinsic factor from the R protein–intrinsic factor complex secreted by the gastric parietal cells. This step is required for intrinsic factor–cyanocobalamin binding to occur before ileal absorption. A dual-label Schilling test using this principle has been developed.[73] Cobalt 57 (^{57}Co) cobalamin–intrinsic factor complex is administered with cobalt 58 (^{58}Co) cobalamin–hog R protein complex. Free human intrinsic factor and a cobalamin analog are administered to prevent endogenous human R protein from stripping ^{57}Co cobalamin from intrinsic factor. The excretion of ^{58}Co and ^{57}Co is measured in the urine and expressed as a ratio. A low ratio is said to denote severe pancreatic insufficiency. Because transfer of cobalamin from R protein to intrinsic factor is pH dependent, this test is capable of detecting pancreatic-sufficient patients with impaired pancreatic bicarbonate secretion.[74] Unfortunately, this test is not suitable for pediatric use owing to the radiation dose.

Urinary Lactulose. Lactulose is a poorly absorbed and nonmetabolized disaccharide. Increased small intestinal permeability to lactulose, reflected by increased urinary lactulose excretion as measured by thin-layer chromatography, has been demonstrated in patients with pancreatic insufficiency owing to cystic fibrosis and Shwachman-Diamond syndrome.[75] Less pronounced increases in lactulose excretion were also seen in pancreatic-sufficient patients. The mechanisms responsible for this finding are unknown, but the test could prove to be a useful screening test for pancreatic exocrine insufficiency. Unfortunately, it does not exclude mucosal defects such as celiac disease. Lactulose excretion could also vary with intestinal transit; this could be a problem in cystic fibrosis, where increased intestinal transit time has been noted. Although intestinal transit should be factored into this test, altered intestinal transit has been shown to be a major contributor to increased urinary lactulose excretion.[76]

BLOOD TESTS

All pancreatic enzymes are detectable in small quantities (ng/mL) in the sera of normal individuals. Some enzymes, such as lipase and amylase, are released as active enzymes, whereas others, such as trypsin, are released as the zymogen or proenzyme trypsinogen. Excessive quantities of circulated pancreatic enzymes are seen in the following three circumstances:

1. *Acute pancreatitis.* Enzymes and proenzymes may be released directly into the circulation as a consequence of inflammation.
2. *Ductal obstruction.* Obstruction of pancreatic enzymatic outflow may result in elevated levels of pancreatic enzymes in sera in the absence of inflammation. The mechanism responsible is thought to be regurgitant release of enzymes from the acini or ducts.
3. *Impaired renal function.* Pancreatic enzymes are cleared from the circulation by the kidneys. Impaired renal function may result in significant elevations of pancreatic enzymes in the absence of pancreatic disease.

Theoretically, in the absence of inflammation, ductal obstruction, or impaired renal function, the serum level of a particular enzyme should reflect the amount of functioning acinar tissue, and this consideration forms the rationale for enzyme determination in sera. However, until recently, two considerations have prevented this goal from being attained. The first is a lack of test specificity. Biochemical determinations of enzymes in sera (total amylase, in particular) have been used for many years as a crude screening test for acute pancreatitis. The major limitation of enzymatic techniques has been the lack of substrate specificity.

For example, the traditional starch and iodine method does not distinguish between salivary and pancreatic isoamylases. Similarly, trypsin substrates are subject to degradation by other circulating serine proteases. Immunoassay techniques have been developed that sensitively detect and measure specific pancreatic enzymes and that should circumvent these problems. Because techniques vary, it is vital that each laboratory establish its own normative data.

The second constraint on serum enzyme determination is the variable maturation (ontogeny) of pancreatic enzymes. Concentration of serum enzymes varies with age, especially in early infancy. In most instances, serum enzyme levels increase with age and reflect the ongoing maturation of the exocrine pancreas and consequent pancreatic parenchymal enzyme levels. For example, at birth, the pancreas synthesizes and secretes very little amylase and continues to produce very little during the first year of life. In contrast, trypsin(ogen) production is relatively mature, and comparatively larger amounts of trypsin are secreted.[77] Serum trypsinogen levels change relatively little during childhood, whereas serum amylase levels increase markedly. The different rates of maturation of pancreatic enzymes lead to varying degrees of usefulness of serum enzyme determinations for diagnosing pancreatic disease or for determining function. An appreciation of the dynamics of enzyme maturation helps in the interpretation of serum enzyme data. These considerations are best addressed by detailed examination of the various tests.

SERUM AMYLASE

Total amylase measurements are extremely nonspecific because the enzymatic determination does not distinguish between salivary and pancreatic isoenzymes. Refinement of amylase measurement has concentrated on distinguishing between pancreatic and salivary isoamylase. Biochemical methods include column chromatography, electrophoresis, isoelectric focusing, salivary isoenzyme inhibitors derived from wheat, and differential thermolability. In addition, highly specific monoclonal antibodies to the pancreatic isoenzyme have been raised, permitting the development of immunoassay techniques. The pancreatic isoenzyme peak on isoelectric focusing or electrophoresis appears to correlate with the level of function in older patients with cystic fibrosis and Shwachman-Diamond syndrome.[78] However, in patients with slight or moderate reduction of function, values are within the normal range. This test is therefore of little use in pancreatic-sufficient individuals. In addition, levels of pancreatic isoenzyme are low in both normal neonates and neonates with cystic fibrosis, and the levels rise throughout childhood.[79] This finding limits the interpretability of the test in younger patients.

SERUM LIPASE

The enzymatic measurement of serum lipase relies on a titrimetric or turbidometric method in which lipase hydrolyzes a triglyceride substrate, producing free fatty acids and glycerol. These methods are not conducive to the assessment of large sample numbers. A sensitive ELISA is available commercially and allows rapid determination of lipase in sera from multiple patients. Cross-sectional evaluation of the usefulness of serum lipase as a measure of pancreatic exocrine function was undertaken in a population with cystic fibrosis and was compared with normal controls. The results were validated by fecal fat evaluation and/or a secretin-CCK stimulation test in younger patients (less than 5 years of age) and in older patients (greater than 5 years of age) with cystic fibrosis.[80,81] The patterns seen in each group are distinctive. In all cystic fibrosis patients, serum lipase is much higher than control values during the first year of life. In pancreatic-insufficient patients, the levels decline after the first year of life, gradually reaching a nadir of 25% of control values after 5 years of age. In pancreatic-sufficient subjects, levels also decline during early childhood, but after 5 years of age, they remain elevated approximately threefold above control levels. There is a wide scatter, however, and some pancreatic-sufficient patients have levels within the normal range. The elevated serum lipase in the first year of life has encouraged the adaptation of serum lipase as a screening test for cystic fibrosis. However, the test has not attained the same popularity as cationic trypsinogen. It is less sensitive, with a detection rate of 76% in the first year of life as opposed to a 90% detection rate with cationic trypsinogen. After 5 years of age, the test is reasonably sensitive and specific for the detection of pancreatic insufficiency (95% and 85%, respectively) but remains relatively imprecise for the detection of pancreatic-sufficient subjects. There is no information about the usefulness of serum lipase in delineating pancreatic insufficiency in other pancreatic diseases of childhood.

SERUM IMMUNOREACTIVE TRYPSIN(OGEN)

Two forms of trypsin(ogen) (cationic and anionic trypsinogen) exist and are detectable in sera. Specific radioimmunoassays, particularly for the cationic form, have permitted the population screening of pediatric groups at risk for pancreatic disease. An ELISA method using a monoclonal antibody specific for the zymogen (proenzyme) trypsinogen is quicker, easier to perform, and less labor intensive.[82] Neonatal screening for cystic fibrosis by measuring immunoreactive trypsinogen in dried blood spots is now routine in some parts of the world.[83,84]

Serum immunoreactive trypsinogen levels have been evaluated both cross-sectionally and longitudinally in pediatric patients with cystic fibrosis[85] and also in children with exocrine pancreatic functional impairment attributable to other causes.[86] The findings have been validated in comparison with those in normal controls. In cystic fibrosis, two patterns emerge. In all individuals with cystic fibrosis, the serum immunoreactive trypsinogen level is grossly elevated during the first year of life.[87] In pancreatic-insufficient patients, a rapid decline is noted during the second year of life, with levels becoming subnormal by 6 years of age.[87] In pancreatic-sufficient patients with cystic fibrosis, no consistent pattern of decline is seen; indeed, many older patients continue to have elevated serum levels.[80] However, there is a wide scatter, and the test is of little value for predicting the degree of functional impairment in this group. The control group provides a

reasonably narrow normal range, with individual values being unrelated to age. Serum immunoreactive trypsinogen measurement in cystic fibrosis is useful in two circumstances. In infants less than 1 year of age, the test is a sensitive diagnostic screening test; the detection rate is 90%. In patients over 7 years of age, depressed serum levels are highly predictive of pancreatic insufficiency. In 199 patients with cystic fibrosis over 7 years of age who had pancreatic insufficiency, only 9 had normal values and 3 had elevated values, resulting in a predictive rate of 94%.[85] Although this test does not distinguish pancreatic-sufficient subjects from normal individuals, it is a sensitive, relatively noninvasive method of screening for pancreatic insufficiency in older subjects. Below 7 years of age, a fecal fat determination is recommended.

In patients with other pancreatic diseases of childhood, this test has proved useful in distinguishing pancreatic steatorrhea from nonpancreatic steatorrhea. At The Hospital for Sick Children, this test provided absolute separation of 10 children with pancreatic steatorrhea from 22 children with other causes of steatorrhea (Figure 72-2).

The other causes of pancreatic steatorrhea included Shwachman-Diamond syndrome, insulin-dependent diabetes mellitus, idiopathic pancreatic insufficiency, and celiac disease with primary pancreatic insufficiency.

SERUM PANCREATIC POLYPEPTIDE

Pancreatic polypeptide, a 36–amino acid straight-chain peptide, is predominantly confined to the pancreatic islets of Langerhans and is also located between acinar cells. Pancreatic polypeptide is an inhibitor of pancreatic enzyme secretion and is released into the circulation in response to various stimuli, particularly protein meals and CCK.

A radioimmunoassay technique has been used to assess fasting pancreatic polypeptide levels or to assess serial responses of plasma pancreatic polypeptide evoked by CCK infusions or in response to various nutrients.[88,89] In adult patients with chronic pancreatitis, fasting plasma pancreatic polypeptide levels are low. Additionally, in response to CCK octapeptide, patients with chronic pancreatitis display either no rise in pancreatic polypeptide or a greatly limited rise compared with both normal controls and patients with other causes of steatorrhea. Thus, the test is capable of differentiating between patients with pancreatic steatorrhea and those with nonpancreatic steatorrhea. However, the test fails to discriminate between pancreatic-sufficient and pancreatic-insufficient subjects with chronic pancreatitis and, as such, gives no indication of actual pancreatic function.[89] This test has not been used in pediatric practice.

AMINO ACIDS

Plasma amino acid levels decrease if the exocrine pancreas is stimulated. The amino acids are incorporated into enzymatic protein within minutes of hormonal stimulation. Both CCK and cerulein stimulation coupled with secretin result in a decrease of plasma amino acid levels in humans.[90,91] The magnitude of this decrease at 45 minutes after stimulation appears to be directly related to pancreatic function and can differentiate patients who are pancreatic sufficient with decreased functional reserve as measured by stimulated chymotrypsin output.[91] Serine, valine, isoleucine, and histidine reduction may discriminate mild impairment of function better than total plasma amino acid reduction. More recently, others have not been able to replicate these results by using CCK alone.[92] This test is time-consuming and expensive and has not been used in pediatric practice.

FUTURE DIRECTIONS

Fecal elastase is the only new widely used pancreatic function test to be developed in the last 15 years. It is becoming increasingly unlikely that new stool urine and breath tests more specific and sensitive than current tests will be developed. Functional imaging techniques using new imaging technology have been developed and trialed in adult patients. These tests, which both image the pancreas and allow an estimate of function, may be adaptable in the future to pediatric patients.

The first of these tests to be reported uses magnetic resonance cholangiopancreatography after secretin stimulation.[93] This technique, which employs a negative bowel contrast agent, was evaluated in 34 adult patients who had undergone prior pancreatoduodenectomy. The caliber of the main pancreatic duct can be graded on a scale of 1 to 3, reflecting secretion. More recently, the technique has been further refined to calculate water secretion rates by correcting for signal intensity.[94] These gradings correlate well with clinical symptoms but do not correlate well with a urine bentiromide test. The poor correlation with the bentiromide test, the necessity for the patient to cooperate and stay still, and the expense of the technique suggest that it will not be adaptable for pediatric use.

More recently, biliary excretion has been assessed by secretin stimulation after injection of sodium bicarbonate ($NaH^{11}CO_3$) in adult patients.[95] This test, which is adaptable to pancreatic function, requires a cyclotron (to generate carbon 11) and a positron emission tomography scanner. Patients need to stay still for 10 minutes. Most pediatric units do not have access to this technology. Carbon 11 is radioactive but has a short half-life, which may allow the adaptation of this test to selected older pediatric patients.

SUMMARY, CONCLUSION, AND RECOMMENDATIONS

Clinical use of pancreatic function tests depends on three major variables: (1) the indications for pancreatic function testing, (2) how the test satisfies the criteria for ideal pancreatic function in the clinical circumstance in which it is being used, and (3) the age of the patient. If useful clinical information can be obtained that subverts the need for a pancreatic function test, this information should be obtained. For example, if a mucosal cause of malabsorption is suspected, it is sensible to perform an intestinal biopsy as the primary investigation. Similarly, if biliary disease is suspected, there are usually good clinical signs that

will point in this direction, and pancreatic function testing is usually inappropriate.

Invasive tests are now used much less frequently in pediatric practice. The major use of the direct pancreatic function tests in pediatric practice was to delineate pancreatic-insufficient from pancreatic-sufficient cystic fibrosis and also to establish a diagnosis of cystic fibrosis in those cystic fibrosis patients in whom sweat tests and clinical signs were equivocal. Genetic testing and, to a lesser extent, nasal potential difference have rendered this indication partially obsolete. If we know a patient's genotype, we can, with a degree of certainty, predict whether they have cystic fibrosis and whether they either have or will develop pancreatic sufficiency.[96] The genetic diagnosis of other disorders, coupled with an awareness of the clinic constellation, also means that direct pancreatic function testing is seldom required. Genetic diagnosis is possible for lipase,[97] colipase,[98] trypsinogen,[99] and enterokinase[100] deficiency; Pearson bone marrow pancreas syndrome[101]; some forms of pancreatic aplasia[102]; and Shwachman syndrome.[103] It should soon be possible for Johanson-Blizzard syndrome. In these circumstances, the diagnosis should be sought, and the presence of malabsorption should be sought either by microscopy for fecal fat or a 3-day fecal fat collection in an older child or by fecal elastase 1 determination in a younger child.

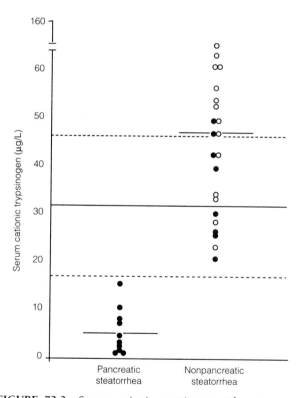

FIGURE 72-2   Serum cationic trypsinogen values in patients with pancreatic and nonpancreatic steatorrhea. The solid and interrupted horizontal lines indicate mean normal cationic trypsinogen of ±2 SD, respectively (31.4 ± 14.8 g/L). *Closed circles* = patients who underwent a pancreatic stimulation test. *Open circles* = patients with nonpancreatic steatorrhea who did not have a pancreatic stimulation test. Reproduced with permission from Moore DJ et al.[86]

TABLE 72-4 RECOMMENDED PANCREATIC FUNCTION TEST: CLINICAL INDICATIONS

Determination of pancreatogenous malabsorption
  Fecal elastase 1
  ^{13}C octanoin breath test
  ^{13}C cholesterol octanoate
  ^{13}C mixed synthetic triglyceride
  Serum fluorescein dilaurate/mannitol collection
  Serum bentiromide/PAS collection or ^{13}C label
  Direct pancreatic stimulation—CCK
  Direct pancreatic stimulation—CCK + secretion

Natural history of disease
  Fecal elastase
  Serum cationic trypsinogen
  Acid steatocrit
  Fecal fat 3 or 5 d (near-infrared reflectance spectroscopy or magnetic resonance spectrometry analysis)
  ^{13}C octanoin breath test
  ^{13}C cholesterol octanoate
  ^{13}C mixed synthetic triglyceride
  Serum fluorescein dilaurate/mannitol
  Serum bentiromide/PAS collection
  Direct pancreatic stimulation

Effectiveness of pancreatic enzyme supplements
  Acid steatocrit
  3- to 5-d fecal fat
  ^{13}C octanoin and other breath tests
  Serum fluorescein dilaurate/mannitol collection
  Serum bentiromide/PAS collection or ^{13}C PABA

CCK = cholecystokinin; PABA = *p*-aminobenzoic acid; PAS = *p*-aminosalicylic acid.

TABLE 72-5 RECOMMENDED PANCREATIC TESTS BY AGE GROUP

Age < 1 yr
  Fecal elastase
  Serum cationic trypsinogen
  ^{13}C-labeled breath tests

Age > 1 yr–toilet training
  Fecal elastase
  ^{13}C-labeled breath tests
  Acid steatocrit
  Direct pancreatic function tests

Toilet training to 7 yr of age
  Fecal elastase
  ^{13}C-labeled breath tests
  Acid steatocrit
  3- to 5-d fecal fat
  Fluorescein dilaurate test bentiromide + PAS or ^{13}C PABA modification
  Direct pancreatic function tests

Seven yr of age and older
  Fecal elastase
  ^{3}C-labeled breath tests
  Acid steatocrit
  3- to 5-d fecal fat
  Fluorescein dilaurate
  Serum bentiromide/PAS collection or ^{13}C PABA
  Direct pancreatic function test
  Lundh meal

Teenagers
  All the above tests and MRCP with secretin

MRCP = magnetic resonance cholangiopancreatography; PABA = *p*-aminobenzoic acid; PAS = *p*-aminosalicylic acid.

The other major consideration for pancreatic function testing is to assess the efficacy of enzyme supplements, and in these circumstances, the more dynamic tests that rely on proteolysis or lipolysis, such as the bentiromide tests, the pancreolauryl tests, and breath-stable isotope-labeled tests, are more appropriate.

The most appropriate tests for the clinical indications are listed in Table 72-4, and the most appropriate tests for the various pediatric age groups are listed in Table 72-5. The principle employed in listing these tests is the axiom *primum non nocere*. The tests are listed pragmatically, with the easiest and most applicable test listed first and the most difficult, invasive, and expensive test last.

REFERENCES

1. Gaskin KJ, et al. Colipase and lipase secretion in childhood-onset pancreatic insufficiency. Gastroenterology 1984;86:1–7.
2. Meyer JH, Spingola LJ, Grossman MI. Endogenous cholecystokinin potentiates exogenous secretin on pancreas of dog. Am J Physiol 1971;221:742–7.
3. Hadorn B, et al. Quantitative assessment of exocrine pancreatic function in infants and children. J Pediatr 1968;73:39–50.
4. Lagerlöf HO, Schütz HB, Holmer S. A secretin test with high doses of secretin and correction for incomplete recovery of duodenal juice. Gastroenterology 1967;52:67–82.
5. Go VLW, Hofmann AF, Summerskill WHJ. Simultaneous measurements of total pancreatic, biliary and gastric outputs in man using a perfusion technique. Gastroenterology 1970;50:321–0.
6. Soergel KH, Hogan WJ. On the suitability of poorly absorbed markers as dilution indicators in the gastrointestinal tract. Gastroenterology 1967;52:1056–7.
7. Borgstrom B, Hildebrand H. Lipase and colipase activities of human small intestinal contents after a liquid test meal. Scand J Gastroenterol 1975;10:585–91.
8. Kopelman H, et al. Impaired chloride secretion, as well as bicarbonate secretion, underlies the fluid secretory defect in the cystic fibrosis pancreas. Gastroenterology 1988;95:349–55.
9. Gaskin KJ, et al. Evidence for a primary defect of pancreatic HCO^{3-} secretion in cystic fibrosis. Pediatr Res 1982;16:554–7.
10. Kopelman H, et al. Pancreatic fluid secretion and protein hyperconcentration in cystic fibrosis. N Engl J Med 1985;313:329–34.
11. Lundh G. Pancreatic exocrine function in neoplastic and inflammatory disease: a simple and reliable new test. Gastroenterology 1962;42:275–80.
12. Go VLW, Hofmann AF, Summerskill WHJ. Pancreozymin bioassay in man based on pancreatic enzyme secretion: potency of specific amino acids and other digestive products. J Clin Invest 1970;49:1558–64.
13. Dooley CP, Valenzuela JE. Duodenal volume and osmoreceptors in the stimulation of human pancreatic secretion. Gastroenterology 1984;86:23–7.
14. Shichiri M, et al. Radioselenium pancreozyminecretin test for pancreatic exocrine function. Am J Dig Dis 1975;20:460–8.
15. Denyer ME, Cotton PB. Pure pancreatic juice studies in normal subjects and patients with chronic pancreatitis. Gut 1978;20:89–97.
16. Del Rosario MA, et al. Direct measurement of pancreatic

enzymes alter stimulation with secretin versus secretin plus cholecystokinin. J Pediatr Gastroenterol Nutr 2000;31:28–32.

17. Khouri MR, Huang G, Shiau YF. Sudan stain of fecal fat: new insight into an old test. Gastroenterology 1989;96:421–7.

18. Khouri MR, et al. Fecal triglyceride excretion is not excessive in pancreatic insufficiency. Gastroenterology 1989;96:848–52.

19. Drummey GD, Benson JA Jr, Jones CM. Microscopic examination of the stool for steatorrhea. N Engl J Med 1961;264:85–7.

20. Colombo C, et al. The steatocrit: a simple method for monitoring fat malabsorption in patients with cystic fibrosis. J Pediatr Gastroenterol Nutr 1987;6:926–30.

21. Guarino A, et al. Reference values of the steatocrit and its modifications in diarrheal disease. J Pediatr Gastroenterol Nutr 1992;14:268–74.

22. Van den Neucker AM, et al. Acid steatocrit: a reliable screening tool for steatorrhoea. Acta Paediatr 2001;90:873–5.

23. Wagner MH, et al. Comparison of steatocrit and fat absorption in persons with cystic fibrosis. J Pediatr Gastroenterol Nutr 2002;35:202–5.

24. Van de Kamer JK, ten Bokkel Huinink H, Weyers HA. Rapid method for the determination of fat in feces. J Biol Chem 1949;177:347–55.

25. Thompson JB, et al. Fecal triglycerides. II. Digestive vs absorptive steatorrhea. J Lab Clin Med 1969;73:521–30.

26. Fomon SJ, et al. Excretion of fat by normal full-term infants fed various milks and formulas. Am J Clin Nutr 1970;23:1299–313.

27. Schnieder MU, et al. NMR spectrometry: a new method for total stool fat quantification in chronic pancreatitis. Dig Dis Sci 1987;32:494–9.

28. Koumentakis G, Radcliff PJ. Estimating fat in feces by near infrared reflectance spectroscopy. Clin Chem 1987;33:502–6.

29. Green VZ, Powel GK. A simple spectrophotometric method for quantitative fecal carbohydrate measurement. Clin Chim Acta 1985;152:3–9.

30. Nelson LM, Mackenzie JF, Russell RI. Measurement of fat absorption using [^{3}H] glycerol triether and [^{14}C] glycerol trioleate in man. Clin Chim Acta 1980;103:325–34.

31. Goldberg DM, Campbell R, Roy AD. Fate of trypsin and chymotrypsin in the human small intestine. Gut 1969;10:477–83.

32. Kaspar P, Möller G, Wahlfield A. New photometric assay for chymotrypsin in stool. Clin Chem 1984;30:1753–7.

33. Bonin A, et al. Fecal chymotrypsin: a reliable index of exocrine pancreatic function in children. J Pediatr 1973;83:594–600.

34. Brown GA, et al. Fecal chymotrypsin: a reliable index of exocrine pancreatic function. Arch Dis Child 1988;63:785–9.

35. Münch R, Ammann R. Faecal immunoreactive lipase: a new tubeless pancreatic function test. Scand J Gastroenterol 1992;27:289–94.

36. Münch R, et al. Faecal immunoreactive lipase: a simple diagnostic test for cystic fibrosis. Eur J Pediatr 1998;157:282–6.

37. Sziegoleit A, Linder D. Studies on the sterol-binding capacity of human pancreatic elastase 1. Gastroenterology 1991;100:768–74.

38. Sziegoleit A, et al. Elastase 1 and chymotrypsin B in pancreatic juice and feces. Clin Biochem 1989;22:85–9.

39. Stein J, et al. Immunoreactive elastase 1: clinical evaluation of a new noninvasive test of pancreatic function. Clin Chem 1996;42:222–6.

40. Glasbrenner B, et al. Clinical evaluation of the fecal elastase test in the diagnosis and staging of chronic pancreatitis. Eur J Gastroenterol Hepatol 1996;8:1117–20.

41. Loser C, Mollgarrd A, Folsch UR. Faecal elastase 1: a novel, highly sensitive and specific tubeless pancreatic function test. Gut 1996;39:580–6.

42. Walkowiak J, et al. Longitudinal follow-up of exocrine pancre-

atic function in pancreatic sufficient cystic fibrosis patients using the fecal elastase-1 test. J Pediatr Gastroenterol Nutr 2003;36:474–8.

43. Nousia-Arvantakis S. Fecal elastase-1 concentration: an indirect test of exocrine pancreatic function and a marker of enteropathy regardless of cause. J Pediatr Gastroenterol Nutr 2003;36:314–5.

44. Salvatore S, et al. Low fecal elastase: potentially related to transient small bowel damage related to enteric petrogens. J Pediatr Gastroenterol Nutr 2003;36:392–6.

45. Beharry S, et al. How useful is fecal pancreatic elastase-1 as a marker of exocrine pancreatic disease? J Pediatr 2002;141:84–90.

46. Fischer B, et al. Faecal elastase lyophilization of stool samples prevents false low results in diarrhoea. Scand J Gastroenterol 2002;36:771–4.

47. Newcomer AD, et al. Triolein breath test: a sensitive and specific test for fat malabsorption. Gastroenterology 1979;76:6–13.

48. Watkins JB, et al. Diagnosis and differentiation of fat malabsorption in children using ^{13}C-labelled lipids: tricanoin, triolein and palmitic acid breath tests. Gastroenterology 1982;82:922–17.

49. Cole SG, et al. Cholesteryl octanoate breath test: preliminary studies on a new noninvasive test of human pancreatic exocrine function. Gastroenterology 1987;93:1372–80.

50. Ventrucci M, et al. ^{13}C labelled cholesteryl octanoate breath test for assessing pancreatic exocrine insufficiency. Gut 1998;42:81–7.

51. Vantrappen GR, et al. Mixed triglyceride breath test of pancreatic lipase activity in the duodenum. Gastroenterology 1989;96:1126–34.

52. Hiele M, et al. Starch digestion in normal subjects and patients with pancreatic disease using a $^{13}CO_2$ breath test. Gastroenterology 1989;96:503–9.

53. Evenepoel P, et al. ^{13}C egg white breath tests: a non-invasive test of pancreatic trypsin activity in the small intestine. Gut 2000;46:52–7.

54. Scharpé S, Iliano L. Two indirect tests of exocrine pancreatic function evaluated. Clin Chem 1987;33:5–12.

55. Durie PR, et al. Bentiromide test using liquid chromatographic measurement of p-aminobenzoic acid and its metabolites for diagnosing pancreatic insufficiency in childhood. J Pediatr 1992;121:413–6.

56. Imondi AR, Stradley RP, Wolgemuth R. Synthetic peptides in the diagnosis of exocrine pancreatic insufficiency in animals. Gut 1972;13:726–31.

57. Toskes PP. Bentiromide as a test of exocrine pancreatic function in adult patients with pancreatic exocrine insufficiency: determination of appropriate dose and urinary collection interval. Gastroenterology 1983;85:565–9.

58. Mitchell CJ, et al. Improved diagnostic accuracy of a modified oral pancreatic function test. Scand J Gastroenterol 1979;14:737–41.

59. Mitchell CJ, et al. Preliminary evaluation of a single day tubeless test of pancreatic function. BMJ 1981;282:1751–3.

60. Hoek FJ, et al. Improved specificity of the PABA test with p-aminosalicylic acid (PAS). Gut 1987;28:468–73.

61. Larsen B, Ekelund S, Jorgensen L, Bremmelgaard A. Determination of the exocrine pancreatic function with the NBT-PABA test using a novel dual isotope technique and gas chromatography—mass spectrometry. Scand J Clin Lab Invest 1997;57:159–66.

62. Puntis JWL, et al. Simplied oral pancreatic function test. Arch Dis Child 1988;63:780–4.

63. Sacher M, Kobsa A, Schmerling DH. PABA screening test for

exocrine pancreatic function in infants and children. Arch Dis Child 1979;53:639–41.

64. Weizman Z, et al. Bentiromide test for assessing pancreatic dysfunction using analysis of para-aminobenzoic acid in plasma and urine: studies in cystic fibrosis and Shwachman's syndrome. Gastroenterology 1985;89:596–604.

65. Laufer D, et al. The bentiromide test using plasma PABA for diagnosing pancreatic insufficiency in young children: the effect of different dose and a liquid meal. Gastroenterology 1991;101:207–13.

66. Malis F, et al. Comparative study of the estimation of exocrine pancreatic function using p-(N-acetyl-L-tyrosyl) and p-(N-benzoyl-L-tyrosyl) aminobenzoic acid. Hepatogastroenterology 1983;30:99–101.

67. Malis F, et al. A peroral test of pancreatic insufficiency with 4-(N-acetyl-L-tyrosyl) aminobenzoic acid in children with cystic fibrosis. J Pediatr 1979;94:942–4.

68. Lankisch PG, et al. Pancreolauryl and NBT-PABA tests: are serum tests a more practicable alternative to urine tests in the diagnosis of exocrine pancreatic insufficiency? Gastroenterology 1986;90:350–4.

69. Trewick AL. Glucose interference in the pancreolauryl test. Ann Clin Biochem 1998;35:274–8.

70. Cumming JGR, et al. Diagnosis of exocrine insufficiency in cystic fibrosis by use of fluorescein dilaurate test. Arch Dis Child 1986;61:573–5.

71. Green MR, Austin S, Weaver LT. Dual marker one day pancreolauryl test. Arch Dis Child 1993;68:649–52.

72. Goldstein R, et al. The fatty meal test: an alternative to stool fat analysis. Am J Clin Nutr 1983;38:763–8.

73. Brugge WR, et al. Development of a dual label Schilling test for pancreatic exocrine function based on the differential absorption of cobalamin bound to intrinsic factor and R protein. Gastroenterology 1980;78:937–49.

74. Chen W-L, et al. Clinical usefulness of dual-label Schilling test for pancreatic exocrine function. Gastroenterology 1989;96:1337–45.

75. Mack DR, et al. Correlation of intestinal lactulose permeability with exocrine pancreatic dysfunction. J Pediatr 1992;120:696–701.

76. Glick JA, et al. Effect of pancreatic function on intestinal transit and kinetics of hydrogen production. Gastroenterology 1990;98:A351.

77. Lebenthal E, Lee PC. Development of functional response in human exocrine pancreas. Pediatrics 1980;55:556–60.

78. Davidson GP, Koheil A, Forstner GG. Salivary amylase in cystic fibrosis: a marker of disordered autoimmune function. Pediatr Res 1978;12:967–70.

79. O'Donnell MD, Miller NJ. Plasma pancreatic and salivary type amylase and immunoreactive trypsin concentrations: variations with age and reference ranges for children. Clin Chim Acta 1980;104:265–73.

80. Cleghorn G, et al. Age-related alterations of immunoreactive pancreatic lipase and cationic trypsinogen in young children with cystic fibrosis. J Pediatr 1985;107:377–81.

81. Cleghorn G, et al. Serum immunoreactive pancreatic lipase and cationic trypsinogen for the assessment of exocrine pancreatic function in older patients with cystic fibrosis. Pediatrics 1986;77:301–6.

82. Bowling FG, et al. Monoclonal antibody-based enzyme immunoassay for trypsinogen in neonatal screening for cystic fibrosis. Lancet 1987;i:826–7.

83. Crossley JR, et al. Neonatal screening for cystic fibrosis using immunoreactive trypsin assay in dried blood spots. Clin Chim Acta 1981;113:111–21.

84. Wilcken B, et al. Cystic fibrosis screening by dried blood spot trypsin assay: results in 75,000 newborn infants. J Pediatr 1983;102:383–7.

85. Durie PR, et al. Age-related alterations of immunoreactive pancreatic cationic trypsinogen in sera from cystic fibrosis patients with and without pancreatic insufficiency. Pediatr Res 1986;20:209–13.

86. Moore DJ, et al. Serum immunoreactive cationic trypsinogen: a useful indicator of severe exocrine dysfunction in the pediatric patient without cystic fibrosis. Gut 1986;27:1362–8.

87. Couper RT, et al. Longitudinal evaluation of serum trypsinogen measurement in pancreatic insufficient and pancreatic sufficient patients with cystic fibrosis. J Pediatr 1995;127:408–13.

88. Owyang C, Scarpello JH, Vinik AI. Correlation between pancreatic enzyme secretion and plasma concentration of human pancreatic polypeptide in health and in chronic pancreatitis. Gastroenterology 1982;83:55–62.

89. Koch MB, Go VLW, Di Magno EP. Can plasma amino acid level after secretin and pancreatic polypeptide be used to detect diseases of the exocrine pancreas? Mayo Clin Proc 1985;60:259–65.

90. Domschke S, et al. Decrease in plasma amino acid level after secretin and pancreozymin as an indicator of exocrine pancreatic function. Gastroenterology 1986;90:1031–8.

91. Gullo L, et al. Caerulein induced plasma amino acid decrease: a simple, sensitive and specific test of pancreatic function. Gut 1990;31:926–9.

92. Maringhini A, Nelson DK, Jones JD, Di Magno EP. Is the plasma amino acid constipation test an accurate test of exocrine pancreatic insufficiency? Gastroenterology 1994;106:488–93.

93. Sho M, et al. A new evaluation of pancreatic function after pancreatoduodenectomy using secretin magnetic resonance cholangiopancreatography. Am J Surg 1998;176:279–82.

94. Punwani S, Gillam AR, Lees WR. Non-invasive quantification of pancreatic exocrine function using secretin-stimulated MRCP. Eur Radiol 2002;13:273–6.

95. Preto J, et al. Assessment of biliary bicarbonate secretion in humans by positron emission tomography. Gastroenterology 1999;117:167–72.

96. Wilschanski M, et al. Correction of sweat chloride concentration with classes of the cystic fibrosis transmembrane conductance regulator gene mutations. J Pediatr 1995;127:705–10.

97. Sims HF, Jennens ML, Lowe ME. The human pancreatic lipase-encoding gene: structure and conservation of an Alu sequence in the lipase gene family. Gene 1993;131:281–5.

98. Sims HF, Lowe ME. The human colipase gene: isolation, chromosomal location and tissue-specific expression. Biochemistry 1992;31:7120–5.

99. Whitcomb DC, et al. Hereditary pancreatitis is caused by a mutation in the cationic trypsinogen gene. Nat Genet 1996;14:141–5.

100. Holzinger A, et al. Mutations in the proenteropeptidase gene are the molecular cause of congenital enteropeptidase deficiency. Am J Hum Genet 2002;70:20–5.

101. Rotig A, et al. Site-specific deletions of the mitochondrial genome in the Pearson Marrow–pancreas syndrome. Genomics 1991;10:502–4.

102. Stoffers DA, et al. Pancreatic agenesis attributable to a single nucleotide deletion in the IPF1 gene coding sequence. Nat Genet 1997;15:106–10.

103. Popovic M, et al. Fine mapping of the locus for Shwachman-Diamond syndrome at 7qll, identification of shared disease haplotypes, and of TPST1 as a candidate gene. Eur J Hum Genet 2002;10:250–8.

CHAPTER 73

BREATH ANALYSIS

Geoffrey P. Davidson, MBBS, MD, FRACP
Ross N. Butler, PhD

The analysis of components of the breath to assess gastrointestinal function has undergone a resurgence in recent years. Dynamic function testing using expired breath to better understand both physiology and pathology depends on the measurement of freely diffusible gases that are either produced endogenously or in response to an orally administered substrate. In the former case, the gas is produced as either a bacterial metabolite or in response to cellular damage following oxidant stress or inflammation. The gas detected can then indicate the presence or absence of an infection or an inflammatory process and the intactness of digestive processes such as fat absorption or gut motility (Figure 73-1).

This chapter discusses the current status of breath testing, which is rapidly evolving; thus, many of the tests discussed are not yet in routine clinical practice.

HISTORY

The noninvasive nature of breath tests makes them particularly useful for application in pediatric settings; nonetheless, no clinical applications were to be realized for almost 40 years after alveolar carbon dioxide (CO_2) was first measured.[1] The two major gases in expired air for understanding and investigating gastrointestinal function are hydrogen (H_2) and CO_2. However, other gases, such as methane (CH_4), ethane, pentane, and mercaptans, are also likely to be important indicators of disease and gastrointestinal malfunction in the future. The principles of measuring labeled CO_2 using radioactive substrates tagged with carbon (^{14}C) were introduced in the 1960s.[2] In the early 1970s, use of nonradioactive breath tests, led by H_2 assessment,[3] ushered in a new era for diagnosis, particularly in childhood for the assessment of lactose and other carbohydrate intolerances. For breath tests using expired CO_2 as the end point, several technological advances and observations have redefined the potential scope of clinical use. The first was the observation that an individual at rest produces a roughly constant amount of CO_2 output per unit time.[4] This allowed interval breath sampling for estimating labeled CO_2 in expired breath as a paradigm for the determination of absorption and subsequent metabolism of a test substrate. The second was the availability of a wide variety of substrates labeled with the radioactive isotope of carbon, ^{14}C. The third more recent development has been the introduction of user-friendly mass spectrometers (isotope ratio mass spectrometry) for the detection of the stable isotope of carbon, ^{13}C, in expired air. For H_2 breath testing, the important demonstration of a direct relationship between expired H_2 and H_2 produced by the microflora in the large bowel formed the basis of this test for diagnosis of sugar intolerances.[5]

ANALYTIC TECHNIQUES

The variety of techniques for measurement of particular gases primarily rely on gas chromatography to separate the gases as a first step prior to detection by selected detectors (eg, thermal conductivity, mass spectrometry). This is not the case for detection of radioactively labeled ^{14}C, in which the CO_2 is trapped using an alkaline liquid scintillation fluid for adsorption of the CO_2 to a solid substrate, and the disintegrations per minute are subsequently assessed using a scintillation counter or similar device. The implications of using the radioactive ^{14}C versus the stable isotope (^{13}C) are discussed below. For mea-

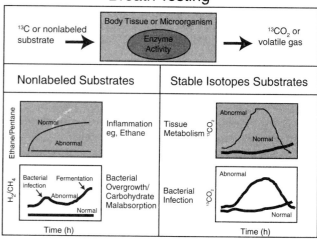

FIGURE 73-1 Principles of $^{13}CO_2$ breath tests, nonlabeled substrate breath tests, and volatile gas breath tests. Theoretic curves are presented for presence or absence of various gases where nonlabeled substrates or no substrates (eg, ethane) are used. Where ^{13}C substrates are used, the curves presented are $^{13}CO_2$ expiration. Ideal excretion curves are illustrated for tissue tests, inflammation, bacterial overgrowth, and fermentation.

surement of H_2, CH_4, and other hydrocarbons (eg, ethane and pentane), gas chromatography followed by flame ionization detection, thermal conductivity, or solid-state sensing devices is commonly used.

BREATH SAMPLING AND COLLECTION TECHNIQUES

Although interval sampling methods are less precise than closed continuous collection techniques, they are certainly adequate for patient management and clinical research. Most clinical applications only need the concentration of the specific gas at particular time points from which an estimate of output over time can be made (usually expressed as an area under the curve generated) and not the absolute quantity excreted. In pediatric populations, well-tolerated collection systems have been developed that can be used in infants and toddlers who cannot actively cooperate. The most successful method for this is the nasal prong, which is held at the nostril by the patient or collector.[6] As the patient expires, the collector aspirates 2 to 4 mL during the latter period of expiration until a sample sufficient for analysis has been obtained. Correction for contamination with ambient air using either O_2 or CO_2 is mandatory when collecting expired gases using this technique.[7,8] For older children and adults, samples can be collected by simply blowing through a straw into an evacuated glass tube or a suitable gas-tight bag (eg, Mylar, Teflon).

SAFETY ISSUES

Depending on the substrate, a wide variety of breath tests are unquestionably safe. For breath tests that do not involve the ingestion of an isotopically labeled substrate, the major probes used to date have been sugars, both natural and synthetic. Of the synthetic sugars, the disaccharide lactulose (constituent sugars galactose and fructose), generally derived from lactose, is the most studied carbohydrate probe. This sugar is a laxative and therefore requires some care in the dose used. This has been well characterized in more than 20 years of use as a diagnostic tool. Routinely, a dose of less than 10 g is administered to children.

For isotopic studies, the situation is different, particularly in women of childbearing age and children in whom the use of a radioactive substrate is contraindicated. This is both on environmental grounds and to protect the patient from unnecessary exposure to radiation no matter how

small the actual measured and the biologically active dose. Thus, ^{13}C substrates should be used for breath testing. The instruments required for measurement of $^{13}CO_2$ are now much more user-friendly and are becoming more widely available. Indeed, more stable isotopes are also now on the market, and the use of naturally enriched substrates is likely to open up many more possibilities for studies in nutrition[9] and in the clinical setting (lactose).[10]

SAMPLE STORAGE

In many cases, sample storage is not required; however, where collection is carried out remotely from the analytic unit, then evacuated glass tubes that have not been irradiated (because this releases gases into the evacuated glass tubes from the rubber seals) can be employed. Indeed, these collection tubes are used in most isotope ratio mass spectrometers and thus afford a standardized system for collection of H_2, CH_4, and ^{13}C-labeled CO_2. Other hydrocarbons may also be stored and collected in these containers provided that special attention is paid to the type of seal used (eg, silicon or silicon plus Teflon seals may be necessary for storing samples other than H_2 and CH_4).

H_2, CH_4, and $^{13}CO_2$ can be collected and stored at room temperature for at least 30 days[6] and, in our experience in the latter case, for 6 months or longer.

NONLABELED COMPONENTS OF BREATH

The clinical applications of nonlabeled components of breath H_2 testing are outlined in Table 73-1. This does not include tests such as breath CH_4, which is still being evaluated. The use of breath H_2 test for carbohydrate malabsorption was the first clinical application of breath testing and is still the only one used continually in clinical practice. Most of the information on the efficacy of breath H_2 testing relates to lactose malabsorption owing to its high prevalence in most parts of the world. Other components of the breath, such as methane, ethane, and pentane, have been studied but have not yet been validated for use in routine clinical practice.

HYDROGEN BREATH TEST

The criterion for H_2 breath test positivity is a sustained rise in H_2 of greater than 10 ppm above baseline, which is usually seen 60 to 120 minutes after sugar ingestion.[7,11] Others have suggested a rise of 20 ppm, but this may lead to decreased sensitivity.[3]

TABLE 73-1   CLINICAL APPLICATIONS OF NONLABELED COMPONENTS OF BREATH

CLINICAL QUESTION	SUBSTRATE	DOSE	INTERVAL/DURATION	REFERENCE
Lactose malabsorption	Lactose	2 g/kg; maximum 20 g in 20% solution	Every 30 min for 3 h	7, 11
Sucrose malabsorption	Sucrose	2 g/kg; maximum 20 g in 20% solution	Every 30 min for 3 h	6, 27–29
Glucose malabsorption	Glucose	1 g/kg; maximum 20 g in 20% solution	Every 30 min for 4 h	41
Fructose malabsorption	Fructose	0.3–0.5 g/kg; maximum 20 g in 20% solution	Every 30 min for 3 h	33
Bacterial overgrowth	Glucose	20 g	Every 20 min for first hour then every 30 min for 2 h	51, 46, 47
	Lactulose	6.68 g (10 mL Duphalac)		

In some cases, the baseline H_2 is high (> 10 ppm) but drops to lower levels within the first 30 minutes. In this situation, the 30-minute sample is considered as the baseline. A persistently elevated fasting H_2 may indicate either inadequate fasting or a high nonabsorbable carbohydrate diet in the previous 24 hours.[12] The possibility of gastrointestinal stasis and bacterial overgrowth also needs to be considered, as discussed below.[13]

A false-negative result may be obtained because of factors affecting H_2 production, which requires a colonic bacterial flora capable of fermenting carbohydrate. Failure to detect H_2 occurs in 2 to 40% of subjects.[3,7,14,15] The prevalence of true nonhydrogen detection in breath may, however, be quite low and dependent on the time of collection, as shown by Strocchi and colleagues, who collected for up to 8 hours.[12] Antibiotics may also suppress H_2 production, which may last for several months, although, again, this may be questioned.[12] In a recent study of patients with bacterial overgrowth, H_2 production was significantly decreased after 1 week of antibiotic therapy.[16] Rapid ventilation can also reduce H_2 in expired air,[17] whereas cigarette smoking can produce a falsely elevated H_2.[18] To avoid a false-negative result, any subject on recent antibiotic therapy and all negative results should have a lactulose breath test to confirm H_2 detection.

CARBOHYDRATE MALABSORPTION

LACTOSE

The principal clinical use of the breath H_2 test is for the diagnosis of lactose malabsorption, and it has been clearly shown to be the most accurate indirect test of lactase deficiency[19] and is used widely in pediatric practice.[20,21] Because it assesses the function of the small intestine as a whole, it is also more reliable than the rather invasive small intestinal biopsy,[22] which is probably required only to prove a congenital absence of lactase.

The importance of testing for carbohydrate malabsorption rather than relying on clinical symptoms (abdominal pain, distention, and diarrhea) is highlighted by studies showing that patients with these symptoms were unaware that they were due to lactose ingestion,[23] and, alternatively, those who believed themselves to be severely intolerant were shown to be breath test negative.[24] The use of clinical symptoms as the basis to invoke dietary change is thus unreliable and may contribute to unnecessary parental anxiety and the possibility of dietary insufficiency.[25,26] It is, therefore, best clinical practice to prove the diagnosis of lactase deficiency before embarking on dietary change.

SUCROSE

Both primary and secondary sucrase deficiency can be diagnosed using breath H_2 testing.[6,27-29] In primary sucrose malabsorption (congenital sucrase-isomaltase deficiency), the diagnosis can be suspected with clinical improvement following removal of sucrose from the diet but needs to be proven by showing sucrase deficiency in an intestinal mucosal biopsy sample. In a recent study of children with cystic fibrosis and abnormal bowel function, breath testing showed a high prevalence of secondary sucrose malabsorption.[29]

MONOSACCHARIDES

Fructose malabsorption has been demonstrated in children with diarrhea and abdominal pain using the breath H_2 test.[30,31] Both children and adults may physiologically malabsorb fructose owing to a limited absorptive capacity.[31-33] Fructose absorption can be facilitated by equimolar doses of glucose and especially L-alanine, although the mechanism remains unclear.[34] Without the underlying knowledge of the rate-limiting step in fructose absorption, it is difficult to apply a standardized breath H_2 test to investigate for possible fructose malabsorption.[33,35]

Sorbitol, which is present naturally in fruits and juices and is also used as a sweetener in low-joule products, has a similar structure to fructose and has also been shown to be malabsorbed in children.[36] Like fructose, sorbitol is commonly malabsorbed in healthy individuals; therefore, a breath H_2 test cannot be used to simply demonstrate abnormality.[37] Although the demonstration of fructose or sorbitol malabsorption, even in patients with abdominal symptoms, cannot of itself be considered pathologic,[38,39] there may be a subgroup of patients with functional bowel symptoms who can be identified and improved by a fructose-sorbitol–free diet.[40] Breath testing with fructose and sorbitol may help identify those patients.

Glucose malabsorption as an isolated event is extremely rare and probably occurs only in association with severe mucosal injury except in the case of congenital glucose-galactose malabsorption. Douwes and colleagues were able to use the breath H_2 test to confirm this diagnosis in a breastfed infant with severe diarrhea.[41]

BACTERIAL OVERGROWTH

Its noninvasive nature and lack of a radioactive label prompted the use of the H_2 breath test for diagnosis of bacterial overgrowth. Lactulose was used as the initial substrate because it is fermented rapidly, appearing in the breath within 8 minutes of bacterial contact. The first study in adults showed an early peak within 30 minutes of lactulose administration followed by a later peak when the rest of the lactulose bolus reached the colon.[42] Several subsequent studies in children confirmed the double peak as a diagnostic feature.[15,43] These children presented with symptoms of chronic diarrhea and abdominal pain, and bacterial overgrowth was unsuspected.[43] Lactulose was given in a dose of 6.68 g (10 mL) in 100 mL of water, and samples were collected every 20 minutes for the first 60 minutes and at 30-minute intervals for the next 2 hours. The finding in this study and others of an elevated fasting breath H_2 may be a useful indicator of small bowel bacterial overgrowth, but it is not specific, and the diagnosis needs to be confirmed with an oral glucose or lactulose challenge.[43-45] The combination of an elevated fasting breath H_2 concentration and increased breath H_2 excretion after a sugar load has been reported to have a 100% specificity for small bowel bacterial overgrowth.[44]

Most recently, Pimentel and colleagues have shown evidence of small bowel bacterial overgrowth in patients with irritable bowel syndrome using lactulose as the substrate.[45]

Glucose has also been shown to be an effective substrate for the diagnosis of bacterial overgrowth in both adults[46] and children.[47] In the latter study, glucose was given in a dose of 1 g/kg, and samples were collected at 20, 40, 60, and 90 minutes after ingestion. Recently, glucose has been used as the substrate to diagnose small bowel strictures and secondary bacterial overgrowth in Crohn disease.[48]

As with other breath H_2 tests, the major limitation is the possibility of non-H_2 detection, which is quite variable, occurring in 5 to 42% of patients.[7,14] The sensitivities of both lactulose (68%) and glucose (52%) breath H_2 tests to detect bacterial overgrowth have also been shown to be low when compared to jejunal culture in one study.[46] Despite these potential shortcomings, the noninvasive nature of the test, the ease of performance, the ability to repeat the test following therapy, and the lack of a suitable alternative make this approach worthwhile until more accurate tests become available.

METHANE

Methane is produced in the left colon by reduction of H_2 and CO_2. Thus, delivery of an increased carbohydrate load to the colon may provide extra substrate for H_2 and CO_2 production in intolerant individuals, thus increasing the substrate for methanogenic bacteria and hence an increase in breath CH_4. Some studies have suggested that low or absent H_2 production following lactulose ingestion is related to H_2 consumption by methanogenic bacteria.[49] At present, it is unclear whether CH_4 measurement can usefully contribute to routine studies of carbohydrate malabsorption, particularly lactose. It has been shown that the prevalence of CH_4 production in lactose absorbers and malabsorbers was identical, and the same proportion of subjects were lactose malabsorbers regardless of methane status.[50] It has also been reported that the percentage of children with lactose intolerance who produce CH_4 is similar to that of normal children.[51] Most recently, Myo-Khin and colleagues showed breath CH_4 to be ineffective as a test for lactose malabsorption.[52]

Although the role of CH_4 as a useful tool in assessing large bowel bacterial metabolism is unclear, an interesting recent report showed that CH_4 production during a lactulose breath test was positive in 100% of constipation-predominant irritable bowel syndrome patients compared with diarrheal conditions such as ulcerative colitis and Crohn disease.[53]

ETHANE/PENTANE

The alkanes ethane and pentane are the major volatile hydrocarbons resulting from in vivo peroxidation of unsaturated fatty acids, especially those in lipid bilayers of cell membranes, and can be measured in breath. Ethane may be the better marker of lipid peroxidation because it passes through the liver intact, whereas pentane undergoes extensive hepatic oxidation. Both of these gases have been used to study the conditions that could affect lipid peroxidation

in intact animals and humans. Vitamin E status in children has been studied noninvasively using both ethane[54] and pentane[55] as markers. More recently, an adult study has shown a reduction in oxidative stress in Crohn disease following vitamin E and C supplementation using ethane and pentane as breath markers.[56]

Excessive lipid peroxidation is probably an important pathogenic factor in inflammatory bowel disease that can now be assessed noninvasively by breath measurement.[57] Both breath ethane[58] and pentane[59] have also been shown to correlate with disease activity in ulcerative colitis.

STABLE ISOTOPE BREATH TESTS

The majority of stable isotope breath tests depend on the measurement of changes in labeled breath CO_2 concentration. CO_2 can be labeled radioactively with ^{14}C or ^{13}C, which is the nonradioactive stable isotope of carbon. The latter is the preferred isotope in children and women of childbearing age. ^{13}C is a naturally occurring isotope consisting of approximately 1.1% of total carbon. It is not radioactive and can be detected by a number of techniques (isotope ratio mass spectrometry, infrared spectroscopy, laser resonance spectroscopy), of which isotope ratio mass spectrometry is the traditional method used for breath tests because it has a high accuracy for a low level of enrichment (0.001–0.01 atom %). To enable suitable precision, stability, and comparable data, the ^{13}C abundance is always measured against a universal reference standard, which is carbon from Pee Dee Belemnite limestone.

The substrates most commonly used for CO_2 breath tests include carbohydrate, starch, fatty acids, bile acids, amino acids, and urea. The only test currently used widely in clinical practice is the ^{13}C urea breath test (UBT) for the diagnosis of *Helicobacter pylori* infection. Other potential clinical applications include evaluation of mucosal function, bacterial overgrowth, gastrointestinal motility, carbohydrate absorption, bile acid absorption, lipid absorption and pancreatic lipase activity, hepatic function, and protein absorption (Table 73-2). This review only discusses the ^{13}C breath tests because they are safe and suitable for use in children, unlike the radioactively labeled isotopes.

^{13}C UREA BREATH TEST

H. pylori is a gastric infection acquired in childhood that has been shown to be the major cause of gastritis in humans. The mode of acquisition and the evolution of the infection and disease associations must be studied in childhood and therefore require a safe, reliable, noninvasive diagnostic test. The ^{13}C UBT meets these requirements because it has been demonstrated to have a sensitivity of 100% and a specificity from 90 to 98%.[60]

The principle of the test relies on the presence of *H. pylori* infection in the gastric mucosa, a urease-producing organism that splits the orally administered ^{13}C-labeled urea into ammonia and labeled bicarbonate. The bicarbonate is absorbed, and labeled CO_2 is excreted in expired breath. Expired breath samples can be collected either using a nasal prong or by blowing through a straw into an evacuated glass tube. Analysis of the ^{13}C content of breath

TABLE 73-2   STABLE ISOTOPE BREATH TESTS IN CURRENT USE

FUNCTIONAL TEST	SUBSTRATE	REFERENCES
Motility		
Gastric emptying	^{13}C-octanoate	80–83
Orocecal transit	^{13}C–lactose ureide	86
Digestion and absorption		
Lipase	^{13}C–mixed triglyceride	69, 72, 76, 77
Amylase	^{13}C-starch	9, 74, 87, 88
Lactase	^{13}C-lactose	10, 78, 79
Sucrase	^{13}C-sucrose	No published information
Protein	^{13}C–L-leucine-enriched proteins	97–99
Carbohydrate	^{13}C-fructose, glucose, galactose	33, 35, 78
Lipid	^{13}C-triolein	66, 67
Malabsorption		
Protein	^{13}C-labeled protein (^{13}C-leucine)	97–99
Lipids	^{13}C–lipids	66, 67–73
Hepatic		
Liver glycogen storage	^{13}C-carbohydrate	95, 96
Hepatic cytochrome P-450	^{13}C-aminopyrine	95, 96
Hepatic cytochrome P-448	^{13}C-caffeine	95, 96
Infection		
Helicobacter pylori*	^{13}Urea	60–65
Small intestinal bacterial overgrowth	^{13}C-xylose	94

*Only test currently widely accepted in clinical practice.

can be carried out using isotope ratio mass spectrometry. Other techniques, such as laser or infrared spectroscopy, may prove to be cheaper but have the disadvantage of requiring larger breath samples.[61]

The test can be performed after a 2-hour fast, and no test meal is required.[61] The oral dose of urea varies between 50 and 100 mg ^{13}C urea and can be administered dissolved in 10 mL of glucose polymer solution or citric acid solution. Citric acid is preferred to orange juice because the latter reduces the diagnostic accuracy of the tests.[62] Citric acid may also reduce contamination of the test by oral flora. Samples are collected before and 30 minutes after ingestion of the substrate. The ratio of ^{13}C to ^{12}C in the two samples is measured, with a positive test being above a cut-off value of 3.5%.

One of the most important advantages of the ^{13}C UBT, apart from its safety, is that it samples the whole stomach and is thus not prone to sampling error, as are biopsy-based tests. More experience is now being acquired with the use of this test in younger children[63] and children in developing countries.[64] It is suitable for epidemiologic studies, in any clinical condition in which endoscopy is not required and for assessing the efficacy of eradication therapy. It is also possible that the level of ^{13}CO$_2$ in expired breath using the ^{13}C UBT may be a predictor of *H. pylori* bacterial load and the severity of gastritis.[65]

PANCREATIC FUNCTION AND FAT MALABSORPTION

^{13}C-labeled substrates offer a safe, noninvasive, attractive alternative to 3-day fecal fat collections because they provide a simple test that can be performed in a single day with minimal discomfort to the child.

The tests use lipids labeled with ^{13}C in the carboxyl moiety using either triolein,[66] hiolein,[67] or mixed triglyceride (MTG).[68–70] Recovery of labeled CO$_2$ in breath in amounts within a range established in healthy individuals is assumed to indicate normal fat digestion and absorption and, as such, an indirect measure of lipolysis within the small intestine.

A number of factors can theoretically affect the absorption or metabolism of labeled triglycerides and hence cause discordant or false results. These include gastric emptying, lung disorders reducing CO$_2$ excretion, disorders affecting fat metabolism, or oxidations such as obesity, hyperlipidemia, hepatic disease, thyroid disease, and small bowel transit time.

The MTG breath test molecule contains both long- and medium-chain fatty acids with stearic acid in the 1 and 3 position forming free fatty acids after lipase hydrolysis and ^{13}C octanoic acid at the 2 position forming the monoglyceride. MTG has advantages over other triglycerides such as trioctanoin and triolein because the rate-limiting step in its digestion is hydrolysis of the two stearyl groups by pancreatic lipase. Octanoic acid is rapidly absorbed and oxidized by the liver and in adults has been shown to correlate closely with pancreatic lipase activity. Normal values for this test have been obtained in children[69] and adults.[71] It may be used to compare the level of fat digestion of patients with pancreatic disease with healthy controls[71] and optimize the use of pancreatic enzyme replacement therapy in children with steatorrhea or poor growth.[72] The ^{13}C hiolein breath test, on the other hand, will assess pancreatic steatorrhea but does not reflect pancreatic function, and its primary clinical value would be in diagnosing pancreatic steatorrhea and monitoring efficacy of pancreatic enzyme replacement therapy.[68] This probably also applies to the ^{13}C triolein breath test. The ^{13}C cholesteryl-octanoate breath test has also been used to study pancreatic insufficiency, which, as in the MTG breath test, uses octanoic acid, in this case released by pancreatic cholesterol esterase activity.[73] Its specificity and sensitivity for pancreatic insufficiency are similar to those of other tubeless pancreatic function tests. Unlike the other breath tests, it can be shortened to 3 hours.

The ^{13}C starch breath test has also been used in children to assess starch digestion in cystic fibrosis.[74] Corn provides a naturally enriched ^{13}C labeled starch and is thus cheaply and readily available. The study showed evidence of impaired starch digestion[74] but is not a suitable test for pancreatic function in clinical practice because of limited specificity and sensitivity.[75]

The above breath tests, particularly the ^{13}C MTG, represent a simple, safe, noninvasive, and repeatable method to study fat digestion and monitor pancreatic enzyme replacement therapy in children.[68,69,72] There is a need for studies aimed at standardizing the test parameters, which include the dose of isotope, type of meal, collection periods, exercise, and the length of fasting required.[76] Another unresolved issue is the significant discrepancy between the dose of isotope given and the percentage recovered, which can be as high as 80%.[77]

CARBOHYDRATE ABSORPTION

Unlike the H_2 breath test, which measures carbohydrate malabsorption, ^{13}C-labeled carbohydrates can measure carbohydrate absorption, providing a noninvasive analysis of enzyme or transport activity. Naturally enriched ^{13}C lactose has been the most widely used, with studies in both adults and children.[10,78,79] The test has also been used in combination with the H_2 breath test and was found to be more sensitive than the H_2 breath test alone.[79]

Fructose absorption has also been studied using combined breath H_2 and breath $^{13}CO_2$ using ^{13}C-labeled fructose.[35] Unfortunately, $^{13}CO_2$ in breath reflects both the absorbed fructose fraction and also the fraction formed as a result of colonic fermentation of unabsorbed fructose, and because of the inability to separate these over time, the test is of limited value in studies of fructose absorption. Thus, the H_2 breath test, although it only reflects malabsorption, may provide a more reproducible method for studying intestinal fructose transport.[35] The ^{13}C breath tests to study carbohydrate absorption are simple to use in clinical practice but are only in their infancy at present. They do, however, have the potential to provide the information needed to allow breath tests to stand alone as routine diagnostic tools.[78]

MOTILITY

GASTRIC EMPTYING

The understanding of both normal and aberrant gastrointestinal motility has been hampered by the invasiveness and lack of portability of scintigraphic techniques. Impaired gastric emptying causes significant morbidity in the pediatric population, with different presentations in various age groups. For example, determining the optimum time to institute enteral feeding in premature infants and in children and adolescents dyspepsia may involve altered gastric emptying.[80] Methods to study gastric emptying used in adults are not readily applicable to pediatrics. The results of noninvasive techniques such as applied potential tomography and ultrasonography are difficult to quantify. Breath testing to probe gut motility using ^{13}C-labeled substrates is now being increasingly applied to infants and children to measure gastric emptying.

Ghoos and colleagues pioneered the use of ^{13}C octanoic acid in adults and children,[81] and this has now been used in neonates[80] and premature infants.[82] Gastric emptying of liquids initially received more attention largely because it is easier to assess than gastric emptying of solids.[83] However, studies on the development of reproducible techniques for estimating emptying of solids have now increased.[84] Specific aspects of the methodology, including the test meal and sampling techniques, require standardization for different age groups. Research on gastric emptying in cystic fibrosis and other diseases is progressing but is not yet completely standardized for routine clinical use outside specialist centers.[77]

SMALL INTESTINAL TRANSIT TIME

Although administration of lactulose and measurement of breath H_2 has been widely used to obtain an estimate of small intestinal transit time, because it is a laxative, at the doses administered, the probe accelerates transit time.[85] The stable isotope probe lactose ^{13}C ureide, at a dose lacking the osmotic properties of lactulose, is likely to be more applicable in the future in a clinical setting.[86]

The use of naturally enriched substrates is also likely to become important for nutritional studies in children in which the ability to follow the transit of functional foods such as labeled starch[87] and nonstarch polysaccharides[88] will enable us to understand both normal and pathologic dynamics of handling and assimilation of different components of a meal. Furthermore, the development of naturally derived substrates with sufficient enrichment for detection may also provide a more affordable array of useful substrates for a variety of different breath tests.[87]

BACTERIAL OVERGROWTH

The efficacy of breath tests to detect small intestinal bacterial overgrowth is, at present, controversial. The ^{14}C-labeled bile acid breath test was originally designed to demonstrate bacterial overgrowth in the jejunum and ileum but also measures ileal function[89]; its efficacy as a marker of small intestinal bacterial overgrowth has been questioned,[90] and it is largely not used. However, significant differences between young and old individuals with respect to bile acid metabolism have been shown using this test. Whether a ^{13}C-labeled bile acid breath test can also be used to assess either bacterial overgrowth or ileal dysfunction has also been questioned.[91] The most acceptable labeled breath test is the use of xylose.[92,93] This has also been performed with ^{13}C xylose, and results are promising, but more studies need to be done.[94]

Combination breath tests have been suggested where, for example, ^{13}C xylose is combined with lactulose and the measurement of $^{13}CO_2$ and products of bacterial fermentation is assessed simultaneously. This potentially enhances the precision and accuracy of a test for bacterial overgrowth. Application of stable isotope breath tests has been limited in pediatrics.[94]

LIVER FUNCTION

A number of different stable isotope probes of liver function have been assessed experimentally in children (and adults), but none has yet been adopted in routine clinical practice. These tests assess liver function by determining the integrity of different metabolic pathways.[95] However, before application to clinical practice, tests need to be validated for normality, specific liver function, and variability.[96] The challenge now is to identify substrates that can be used to measure liver function validly and to compare these in prospective studies with conventional liver function tests.

PROTEIN ABSORPTION

Labeled amino acids have been used for some time to study protein metabolism in vivo in animals and humans. These studies mainly involved the measurement of protein synthesis and breakdown. Only recently have stable isotope labeled proteins become available for the study of protein digestion and absorption following a meal. Milk[97] and egg proteins[98] have been labelled with L-(1-^{13}C) leucine. Simultaneous measurement of ^{13}C enrichment of breath and enrichment of plasma in L-(1-^{13}C) leucine after ingestion of a ^{13}C-labeled egg white protein meal in healthy volunteers and patients with pancreatic insufficiency has confirmed that assimilation kinetics are accurately reflected by the breath test.[99] Although this test can be considered as showing promise for the evaluation and follow-up of patients with pancreatic insufficiency and studies of protein absorption in other disease states, more work is required. This relates particularly to an appropriately labeled test meal and establishing the sensitivity and specificity of the test and the effects of other parameters, such as gastric emptying.

SUMMARY

Because of their simplicity in application, particularly in the pediatric age group, breath tests provide the ideal noninvasive investigative modality for gastrointestinal function in health and disease. It is apparent that they are significantly underused in routine practice despite the amount of information supporting their veracity. This has been recently highlighted in a review of all English language abstracts from 1966 to March 2001, suggesting that breath tests are valuable tools and are generally underused, particularly in the pediatric setting.[100]

REFERENCES

1. Dodds EC. Variations in alveolar carbon dioxide pressure in relation to meals. J Physiol 1920;54:342.
2. Schwabe AD, Cozzetto FJ, Bennett RL, Mellinkoff SM. Estimation of fat absorption by monitoring of expired radioactive carbon dioxide after feeding a radioactive fat. Gastroenterology 1962;42:285–91.
3. Bond JH, Levitt MD. Investigation of small bowel transit time in man utilising pulmonary (H$_2$) measurement. J Lab Invest 1975;85:546–55.
4. Abt AF, Von Schuching SL. Fat utilization test in disorders of fat metabolism. A new diagnostic method applied to patients suffering with malabsorption syndrome, chronic pancreatitis and arteriosclerotic cardiovascular disease. Bull Johns Hopkins Hosp 1966;119:316–30.
5. Perman JA, Modler S, Olson AC. Role of pH in production of hydrogen from carbohydrates by colonic bacterial flora. J Clin Invest 1981;67:643–50.
6. Perman JA, Barr RB, Watkins JB. Sucrose malabsorption in children: non-invasive diagnosis by interval breath hydrogen determination. J Pediatr 1978;93:17–22.
7. Robb TA, Davidson GP. Advances in breath hydrogen quantitation in paediatrics: sample collection and normalisation to constant oxygen and nitrogen levels. Clin Chim Acta 1981;111:281–3.
8. Niu H, Schoeller DA, Klein PD. Improved gas chromatographic quantitation of breath hydrogen by normalization to respiratory carbon dioxide. J Lab Clin Med 1979;94:755–63.
9. Koletzko B, Demmelmair H, Hartl M. The use of stable isotope techniques for nutritional and metabolic research in paediatrics. Early Hum Dev 1998;53 Suppl:577–97.
10. Hiele M, Ghoos Y, Rutgeerts P, et al. $^{13}CO_2$ breath test using naturally enriched ^{13}C-lactose for detection of lactase deficiency in patients with gastrointestinal symptoms. J Lab Clin Med 1988;112:193–200.
11. Barr RG, Watkins JB, Perman JA. Mucosal function and breath hydrogen excretion: comparative studies in the clinical evaluation of children with non-specific abdominal complaints. Pediatrics 1981;68:526–33.
12. Strocchi A, Corazza GR, Ellis CJ, et al. Detection of malabsorption of low doses of carbohydrate: accuracy of various breath H$_2$ criteria. Gastroenterology 1993;105:1404–10.
13. Perman JA, Modler S, Barr RG, Rosenthal P. Fasting breath hydrogen concentration: normal values and clinical applications. Gastroenterology 1984;97:1358–63.
14. Gilat T, Ben Hur H, Gelman-Malachi E, et al. Alterations of the colonic flora and their effect on the hydrogen breath test. Gut 1978;19:602–5.
15. Pereira SP. A pattern of breath hydrogen excretion suggesting small bowel bacterial overgrowth in Burmese village children. J Pediatr Gastroenterol Nutr 1991;13:32–8.
16. Attar A, Flourie B, Rambaud JC, et al. Antibiotic efficacy in small intestinal bacterial overgrowth-related chronic diarrhoea: a crossover randomised trial. Gastroenterology 1999;117:794–7.
17. Perman JA, Modler S, Engel RR, Heldt G. Effect of ventilation on breath hydrogen measurement. J Lab Clin Med 1985;105:436–9.
18. Bjortneklett A, Jensen E. Relationship between hydrogen and methane production in man. Scand J Gastroenterol 1982;17:985–92.
19. Newcomer AD, McGill DB, Thomas PJ, Hofman AF. Prospective comparison of indirect methods for detailing lactose deficiency. N Engl J Med 1975;293:1232–6.
20. Douwes AC, Fernandes J, Degenhart HJ. Improved accuracy of lactose tolerance test in children, using expired H$_2$ measurement. Arch Dis Child 1978;53:939–42.
21. Davidson GP. The breath hydrogen test—an evaluation. Aust Paediatr J 1988;24:1–2.
22. Davidson GP, Robb TA. Value of breath hydrogen analysis in management of diarrhoeal illness in childhood: comparison with duodenal biopsy. J Pediatr Gastroenterol Nutr 1985;4:381–7.
23. Di Palma JA, Narvaez RM. Prediction of lactose malabsorption in referral patients. Dig Dis Sci 1988;33:303–7.
24. Suarez FL, Savaiano DA, Levitt MD. A comparison of symptoms after the consumption of milk or lactose-hydrolysed milk by

people with self-reported severe lactose intolerance. N Engl J Med 1995;333:1–4.

25. Lloyd-Still JD. Chronic diarrhea of childhood and the misuse of elimination diets. J Pediatr 1979;95:10–3.

26. Ulrich CM, Georgiou CC, Snow-Harter CM, Gillis DE. Bone mineral density in mother-daughter pairs: relations to life-time exercise, life-time milk consumption and calcium supplements. Am J Clin Nutr 1996;63:72–9.

27. Douwes AC, Fernandez J, Jongbloed AA. Diagnostic value of sucrose tolerance test in children evaluated by breath hydrogen measurement. Acta Paediatr Scand 1980;69:79–82.

28. Davidson GP, Robb TA. Detection of primary and secondary sucrose malabsorption in children by means of the breath hydrogen technique. Med J Aust 1983;2:29–32.

29. Lewindon PJ, Robb TA, Moore DJ, et al. Bowel dysfunction in cystic fibrosis: importance of breath testing. J Paediatr Child Health 1998;34:79–82.

30. Barnes GL, McKellar W, Lawrence S. Detection of fructose malabsorption by breath hydrogen test in a child with diarrhea. J Pediatr 1983;103:575–7.

31. Kneepkens CMF, Jakobs C, Douwes AC. Apple juice, fructose and chronic non-specific diarrhoea. Eur J Paediatr 1989;148:51–73.

32. Hockstra JH, Van Kampen AAMW, Bijl SB, Kneepkens CMF. Fructose breath hydrogen tests. Arch Dis Child 1993;68:136–8.

33. Choi YK, Johlin FC, Summers RW, et al. Fructose intolerance: an underrecognized problem. Am J Gastroenterol 2003;98:1348–53.

34. Hoekstra JH, Van Kampen AAMW. Facilitating effect of amino acids on fructose and sorbitol absorption in children. J Pediatr Gastroenterol Nutr 1996;23:118–24.

35. Corpe CP, Burant CF, Hoekstra JH. Intestinal fructose absorption: clinical and molecular aspects. J Pediatr Gastroenterol Nutr 1999;28:364–74.

36. Hyams JS. Chronic abdominal pain caused by sorbitol malabsorption. J Pediatr 1982;100:772–3.

37. Hyams JS. Sorbitol intolerance: an unappreciated cause of functional gastrointestinal complaints. Gastroenterology 1983;84:30–3.

38. Rumessen JJ, Gudmand-Hoyer E. Functional bowel disease: the role of fructose and sorbitol. Gastroenterology 1991;101:1452–3.

39. Rumessen JJ. Functional bowel disease: the role of dietary carbohydrates. Eur J Gastroenterol Hepatol 1993;12:999–1008.

40. Mishkin D, Sablauskas L, Yalousky M, Mishin S. Fructose and sorbitol malabsorption in ambulatory patients with functional dyspepsia. Dig Dis Sci 1997;42:2591–8.

41. Douwes AC, van Caillie M, Fernandes J, et al. Interval breath hydrogen test in glucose-galactose malabsorption. Eur J Pediatr 1981;137:273–6.

42. Rhodes JM, Middleton P, Jewell DP. The lactulose hydrogen breath test as a diagnostic test for small-bowel bacterial overgrowth. Scand J Gastroenterol 1979;14:333–6.

43. Davidson GP, Robb TA, Kirubakaran CP. Bacterial contamination of the small intestine as an important cause of chronic diarrhoea and abdominal pain: diagnosis by breath hydrogen test. Pediatrics 1984;74:229–35.

44. Kerlin P, Wong L. Breath hydrogen testing in bacterial overgrowth. Gastroenterology 1988;95:982–8.

45. Pimentel M, Soffer EE, Chow ET, et al. Lower frequency MMC is found in IBS subjects with abnormal lactulose breath test, suggesting bacterial overgrowth. Dig Dis Sci 2002;21:27–42.

46. Corazza GR, Menozzi MG, Strocchi A, et al. The diagnosis of small bowel bacterial overgrowth. Reliability of jejunal cul-

47. De Boissieu D, Chaussain M, Badoual J, et al. Small bowel bacterial overgrowth in children with chronic diarrhea, abdominal pain or both. J Pediatr 1996;128:203–7.

48. Mishkin D, Boston FM, Blank D, et al. The glucose breath test: a diagnostic test for small bowel strictures in Crohn's disease. Dig Dis Sci 2002;47:489–94.

49. Cloarec D, Bornet F, Gouilloud S, et al. Breath hydrogen response to lactulose in healthy subjects: relationship to methane production status. Gut 1990;31:300–4.

50. Montes RG, Saavedra JM, Perman JA. Relationship between methane production and breath hydrogen excretion in lactose malabsorbing individuals. Dig Dis Sci 1993;38:445–8.

51. Medow MS, Glassman MS, Schwarz SM, Newman LJ. Respiratory methane excretion in children with lactose intolerance. Dig Dis Sci 1993;8:328–32.

52. Myo-Khin, Bolin TD, Khin-Mar-OO, et al. Ineffectiveness of breath methane excretion as a diagnostic test of lactose malabsorption. J Pediatr Gastroenterol Nutr 1999;28:474–9.

53. Pimentel M, Mayer AG, Park S, et al. Methane production during lactulose breath test is associated with gastrointestinal disease presentation. Dig Dis Sci 2003;48:86–92.

54. Refat M Moore TJ, Kazui M, et al. Utility of breath ethane as a non-invasive biomarker of vitamin E status in children. Pediatr Res 1991;30:396–403.

55. Lemoyne M, Van Gossum A, Kurian R, et al. Breath pentane analysis as an index of lipid peroxidation: a functional test of vitamin E status. Am J Clin Nutr 1987;41:267–72.

56. Aghdessi E, Wendland BE, Steinhart AH, et al. Antioxidant vitamin supplementation in Crohn's disease decreases oxidative stress, a randomized controlled trial. Am J Gastroenterol 2003;98:348–53.

57. Pelli MA, Trovarelli G, Capodicasa E, et al. Breath alkanes determination in ulcerative colitis and Crohn's disease. Dis Colon Rectum 1999;42:71–76.

58. Sedghi S, Keshavarzian A, Klamut M, et al. Elevated breath ethane levels in active ulcerative colitis: evidence of excessive lipid peroxidation. Am J Gastroenterol 1994;89:2217–21.

59. Kokaszka J, Nelson RL, Swedler WI, et al. Determination of inflammatory bowel disease activity by breath pentane analysis. Dis Colon Rectum 1993;36:597–601.

60. Savarino V, Vigneri S, Celle V. The ^{13}C urea breath test in the diagnosis of Helicobacter pylori infection. Gut 1999;45 Suppl 1:118–22.

61. Rowland M, Lambert I, Gormally S, et al. Carbon 13-labeled urea breath test for the diagnosis of Helicobacter pylori infection in children. J Pediatr 1997;131:815–20.

62. Dominguez-Munoz J, Leodolter A, Sauerbruch T, Malfertheiner P. A citric acid solution is an optimal test drink in the ^{13}C urea breath test for the diagnosis of Helicobacter pylori infection. Gut 1997;40:459–62.

63. Imrie C, Rowland M, Bourke B, Drumm B. Limitations to carbon 13-labelled urea breath testing for Helicobacter pylori in infants. J Pediatr 2001;139:734–7.

64. Thomas JE, Dale A, Harding M, et al. Interpreting the ^{13}C urea breath test among a large population of young children from a developing country. Pediatr Res 1999;46:147–51.

65. Perri F, Clemente R, Pastore M, et al. ^{13}C urea breath test as a predictor of intragastric bacterial load and severity of Helicobacter pylori gastritis. Scand J Clin Lab Invest 1998;58:19–28.

66. Watkins J, Klein PD, Schoellar DA, et al. Diagnosis and differentiation of fat malabsorption in children using ^{13}C-labelled

lipids: trioctanoin triolein and palmitic acid breath tests. Gastroenterology 1982;82:911–7.

67. Lembcke B, Braden B, Caspary WF. Exocrine pancreatic insufficiency: accuracy and clinical value of the uniformly labelled ^{13}C hiolein breath test. Gut 1996;39:668–74.

68. DeBoeck K, Delbeke I, Eggermont E, et al. Lipid digestion in cystic fibrosis: comparison of conventional and high lipase enzyme therapy using the mixed triglyceride breath test. J Pediatr Gastroenterol Nutr 1998;26:408–11.

69. van Dijk-van Aalst K, van Den Driessche M, van Der Schoor S, et al. ^{13}C mixed triglyceride breath test: a non-invasive method to assess lipase activity in children. J Pediatr Gastroenterol Nutr 2001;32:579–85.

70. Van Trappen GR, Rutgeerts PJ, Ghoos YF, Hiele MI. Mixed triglyceride breath test: a noninvasive test of pancreatic lipase activity in the duodenum. Gastroenterology 1989;96:1126–34.

71. Seal S, McClean P, Walters M, et al. Stable isotope studies of pancreatic enzyme release in vivo. Postgrad Med J 1996;72 Suppl 2:S37–8.

72. Amarri S, Harding M, Goward WA, et al. ^{13}C mixed triglyceride breath test and pancreatic enzyme supplementation in children with cystic fibrosis. Arch Dis Child 1997;6:349–51.

73. Ventrucci M, Cipolla A, Ubalducci GM, et al. ^{13}C-labelled cholesteryl octanoate breath test for assessing pancreatic exocrine insufficiency. Gut 1998;42:81–7.

74. Dewitt O, Prentice A, Coward A, Weaver LT. Starch digestion in young children with cystic fibrosis measured using a ^{13}C starch breath test. Pediatr Res 1992;32:45–9.

75. Loser C, Mollgaard A, Aygen S, et al. ^{13}C starch breath test—comparative clinical evaluation of an indirect pancreatic function test. Z Gastroenterol 1997;35:187–94.

76. Kalivianakis M, Verkade IIJ, Stellaard F, et al. The ^{13}C mixed triglyceride breath test in healthy adults: determinants of the CO_2 response. Eur J Clin Invest 1997;27:434–42.

77. Weaver LT, Amarri S, Swart GR. ^{13}C mixed triglyceride breath test. Gut 1998;43 Suppl 3:S13–9.

78. Vonk RJ, Stellaard F, Hoekstra JH, Koetse HA. ^{13}C carbohydrate breath tests. Gut 1998;43 Suppl 3:S20–2.

79. Vonk RJ, Stellaard F, Driebe MG, et al. The $^{13}C/H_2$ glucose test for determination of small intestinal lactase activity. Eur J Clin Invest 2001;31:226–33.

80. Van Den Driessche M, Peeters K, Marien P, et al. Gastric emptying in formula fed and breast fed infants measured with the ^{13}C–octanoic acid breath test. J Pediatr Gastroenterol Nutr 1999;29:46–51.

81. Ghoos Y, Mars BD, Geypens B, et al. Measurement of gastric emptying rate of solids by means of carbon labelled octanoic breath test. Gastroenterology 1993;104:1640–7.

82. Barnett C, Omari T, Davidson GP, et al. Effect of cisapride on gastric emptying in premature infants with feed intolerance. J Pediatr Child Health 2001;37:559–63.

83. Maes BD, Ghoos Y, Geypens B, et al. Combined carbon-13-glycine/carbon-14-octanoic acid breath test to monitor gastric emptying rates of liquids and solids. J Nucl Med 1994;35:824–31.

84. Choi MG, Camilleri M, Burton DD, et al. 13C octanoic acid

breath test for gastric emptying of solids: accuracy, reproducibility, and comparison with scintigraphy. Gastroenterology 1997;112:1155–62.

85. Miller MA, Parkman HP, Urbain JL, et al. Comparison of scintigraphy and lactulose breath hydrogen test for assessment of orocecal transit time: lactulose accelerates small bowel transit. Dig Dis Sci 1997;41:10–8.

86. Van Den Driessche M, Van Malderen N, Geypens B, et al. Lactose–[^{13}C] ureide breath test: a new noninvasive technique to determine orocecal transit time in children. J Pediatr Gastroenterol Nutr 2000;31:433–8.

87. Christian MJ, Amari S, Franchini F, et al. Modeling ^{13}C breath curves to determine site and extent of starch digestion and fermentation in infants. J Pediatr Gastroenterol Nutr 2002;34:158–64.

88. Achour L, Flourie B, Briet F, et al. Metabolic effects of digestible and partially indigestible cornstarch: a study in the absorptive and postabsorptive periods in healthy humans. Am J Clin Nutr 1997;66:1151–9.

89. Fromm HS, Hofmann AF. Breath test for altered bile acid metabolism. Lancet 1971;ii:621–5.

90. Lauterburg BH, Newcomer AD, Hofmann AF. Clinical value of the bile acid breath tests: evaluations of Mayo Clinic experience. Mayo Clin Proc 1978;53:227–33.

91. Hofmann AF. Breath tests as diagnostic tests in gastroenterology. In: Current topics in gastroenterology and hepatology. Stuttgart: Gray Thieme Verlog; 1990. p. 545–61.

92. Saltzman JR. Bacterial overgrowth without clinical malabsorption in elderly hypochlorhydric subjects. Gastroenterology 1994;106:615–23.

93. King CE, Toskes PP. Comparison of the 1-gram (^{14}C) xylose, 10-gram lactulose–H_2 and 80-gram glucose–H_2 breath tests in patients with small intestinal bacterial overgrowth. Gastroenterology 1986;91:1447–51.

94. Dellert SF, Nowicki MJ, Farrell MK, et al. The ^{13}C-xylose breath test for the diagnosis of small bowel bacterial overgrowth in children. J Pediatr Gastroenterol Nutr 1997;25:153–8.

95. Amuzzi A, Candelli MA, Zocco MA, et al. Review article: breath testing for human liver assessment. Aliment Pharmacol Ther 2002;16:1977–96.

96. Rating D, Langhans CD. Breath tests: concepts applications and limitations. Eur J Pediatr 1997;156 Suppl 1:S18–23.

97. Boirie Y, Gachon P, Corny S, et al. Acute postprandial changes in leucine metabolism as assessed with an intrinsically labelled milk protein. Am J Physiol 1996;271:E1083–91.

98. Evenepoel P, Geypens B, Luypaerts A, et al. Digestibility of cooked and raw egg protein in humans as assessed by stable isotope techniques. J Nutr 1998;128:1716–22.

99. Evenepoel P, Hiele M, Geypens B, et al. ^{13}C–egg white breath test: a non-invasive test of pancreatic trypsin activity in the small intestine. Gut 2000;46:52–7.

100. Rmagnuolo J, Schiller D, Bailey RJ. Using breath tests wisely in a gastroenterology practice: an evidence-based review of indications and pitfalls in interpretation. Am J Gastroenterol 2002;97:1113–26.

CHAPTER 74

IMAGING

1. *Plain Radiographs and Contrast Studies*

Ghislaine Sayer, MRCP, DMRD, FRCR
Helen Carty, FRCR, FRCPI, FRCP, FRCPCH, FFRRCSI(Hon)

Radiologic investigations are frequently required in the diagnosis of pediatric gastrointestinal disease. Close cooperation between clinicians and radiologists is essential in selecting and interpreting those tests, which will contribute meaningful information to the diagnostic process. To avoid unnecessary repeat examinations, all of the patient's previous imaging should be available for review. The motto should be do it once, properly. To comply with radiation exposure regulations, each medical exposure should be justified. The referring clinician is obliged to provide sufficient and accurate clinical information.[1]

All radiologic modalities (including plain films, fluoroscopy, ultrasonography, computed tomography [CT], magnetic resonance imaging [MRI], and radioisotope studies) have applications in pediatric gastroenterology. This chapter outlines the use of plain radiographs and contrast studies of the gastrointestinal tract.

Although not strictly a gastroenterologic investigation, a plain chest radiograph is an important part of the initial assessment of an ill child. It should be remembered that erect chest radiography is not possible in very young children; therefore, the absence of free subdiaphragmatic air on the chest film cannot always rule out a perforation.

Children with chest infections do not expectorate but swallow sputum, subsequently presenting with vomiting. Abdominal pain, mimicking appendicitis, may be the clinical presentation of basal lung consolidation (Figure 74.1-1).

ABDOMINAL RADIOGRAPH

INDICATIONS

An abdominal radiograph is a useful starting point in the investigation of acute abdominal pain,[2] although it may be unhelpful in up to half of such cases.[3] It is essential in suspected intestinal obstruction or perforation. Ingestion of foreign bodies does not necessitate an abdominal radiograph unless the object is sharp or potentially dangerous

(eg, batteries, which may leak),[4,5] although a chest film is important to exclude aspiration (Figure 74.1-2).

The plain film is particularly useful in neonates with obstruction, in whom the distribution of bowel gas is a

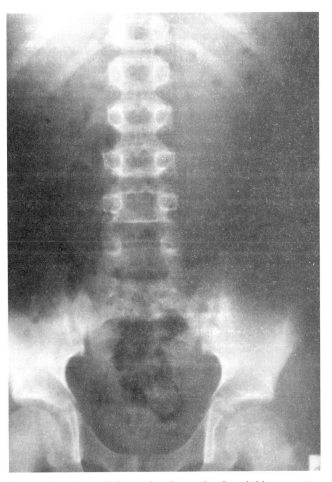

FIGURE 74.1-1 Abdominal radiograph of a child presenting with abdominal pain. There is right lower lobe consolidation

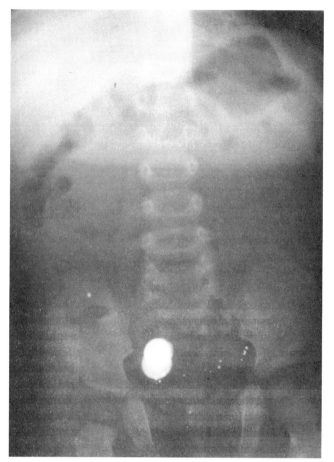

FIGURE 74.1-2 Foreign body ingestion: this patient had swallowed a battery.

clue to the level of obstruction, for example, differentiating esophageal from distal atresia. Associated findings such as the bubbly appearance of gas in meconium ileus, calcification following antenatal perforation, or gas in the bladder in a high anorectal malformation may give further clues as to the cause of the obstruction.[6] In modern practice, ultrasonography is often used in addition to the plain film and can be particularly useful in the diagnosis of intussusception, hypertrophic pyloric stenosis, and appendicitis.

The role of the plain film in chronic abdominal pain is less certain. Its main use here is to exclude pathology such as calcification in the renal tracts or biliary tree. It is diagnostically helpful when such calcification is found. Other features that may be suspected on the plain abdominal film are malrotation (easily missed on ultrasonography), impacted foreign bodies in a Meckel diverticulum, foreign bodies in the colon from compulsive pica, bezoars, and, rarely, duplication cysts seen as a mass or air-fluid levels in a focal area of ileal dysgenesis, which is sometimes called a giant Meckel diverticulum.[7]

Technique

A supine film is adequate in the majority of cases. The lung bases and hernial orifices must be included on the film.[2,3] The radiation dose can be reduced by the use of computed radiography,[8] the addition of extra filtration,[9] and not using antiscatter grids.[10] Specialized pediatric departments

consistently record lower doses than do general hospitals,[10] not least because of familiarity with the unique challenges involved in gaining the cooperation of children and their parents: getting it right the first time avoids repeat films and unnecessary additional radiation.

Gonad shielding should not be used in girls because it may obscure important signs within the pelvis.[2] Indeed, studies have shown that lead shields are seldom appropriately placed to protect the ovaries in any case.[11,12]

In adult practice, erect films of the abdomen are sometimes performed to identify free intraperitoneal air and to look for fluid levels in intestinal obstruction. The incidence of intestinal perforation after the neonatal period is extremely low in children. Free air in the neonate is usually of large volume and easy to see on a supine film. Intestinal obstruction, after the neonatal period, usually occurs only with intussusception, postoperative adhesive obstruction, inguinal hernias, and sepsis. In most instances, the diagnosis is clinically obvious—hence the relatively limited value of a routine additional erect or decubitus film. If the diagnosis of intestinal perforation is in doubt, a lateral decubitus film (or, in neonates, a horizontal beam "shoot-through" with the patient supine) should clearly delineate free intraperitoneal gas, which will "float" above dependent fluid levels in the peritoneal space.

Interpretation

All abdominal radiographs should be reviewed in a systematic fashion. The following approach will ensure that nothing is missed:

1. Check the name, date, and left and right markers.
2. Identify the liver and stomach bubble to exclude situs inversus.
3. Check bowel gas distribution: masses or fluid collections will displace the bowel from its normal position. Identify, if possible, the cecum in the right iliac fossa (Figure 74.1-3).
4. Look for any gas that does not lie within the stomach or bowel; triangles, arcs, or straight lines of gas usually denote a perforation. The falciform ligament may be seen near the midline, outlined, or either side with free gas (Figures 74.1-4 and 74.1-5). Mottled or patchy areas of gas may lie within an abscess. Retroperitoneal air is notoriously difficult to see on a plain film but may be seen outlining the kidneys (Figures 74.1-6 and 74.1-7).
5. If distended bowel loops are present, identify the level to which they extend and the presence of any distal gas. In general, the jejunum has a feathery pattern owing to the plenitude of mucosal folds, whereas the ileum is more featureless. Haustral folds are present in the colon. An important caveat in neonates is that the colon has poorly developed haustral folds and can be mistaken for small bowel.[13] Owing to the absence of a pelvic cavity in an infant, the sigmoid colon may lie on the right side of the abdomen or even abut the liver. Assess the thickness of the bowel wall and the separation of bowel loops.
6. Identify both renal outlines, the liver and the spleen. Are there any unexplained masses? Renal outlines are

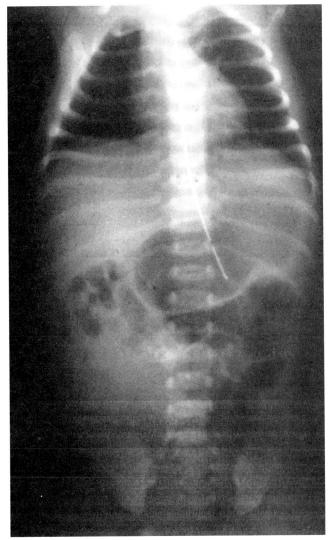

FIGURE 74.1-3 Malrotation: abnormal distribution of bowel gas with the small bowel lying to the right of the midline and the cecum clearly in the left iliac fossa.

poorly seen in children owing to the paucity of perirenal fat, but, as a rule of thumb, the kidneys should each measure about three and a half vertebral bodies in length. Liver size is poorly assessed on abdominal radiography. A Riedel lobe is a normal variant that may extend to the right iliac fossa. Spleen size may be reliably assessed; if the tip of the spleen is seen below the ribs, it is likely to be enlarged (Figure 74.1-8).

7. Look for any calcifications and decide on their location: renal tract, a mass lesion, lymph nodes?

8. Check the corners of the film (ie, lung bases and hernial orifices). Abdominal pain may be referred from above the diaphragm, and strangulated hernias are a common cause of bowel obstruction.

9. Examine the bones: vertebral anomalies are a clue to congenital anomalies such as tracheoesophageal fistulae and renal and anorectal malformations (Figure 74.1-9). Check sites of tubes and lines (see below).

10. Identify the properitoneal fat lines, which are normally convex medially beyond infant age. Distention of these, particularly if coupled with separation from bowel

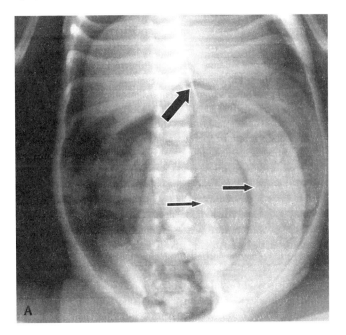

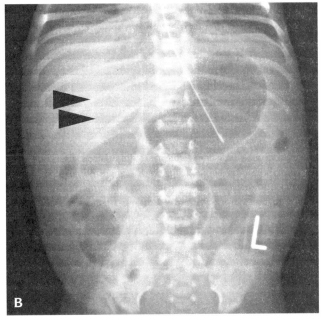

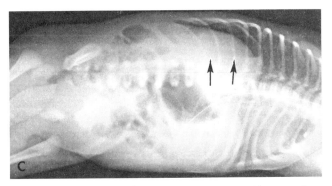

FIGURE 74.1-4 *A*, Perforation in a neonate with meconium ileus. Gas outlines the liver and the falciform ligament (*large arrow*) and distends the flanks (so-called "football sign"). Loops of bowel filled with granular-looking meconium are seen (*small arrows*). *B*, A more subtle example of perforation: an abnormal gas lucency lies centrally in the abdomen (*arrows*). Again, the falciform ligament is clearly seen. *C*, Decubitus film of the baby in *B*. A horizontal air-fluid level is now visible (*arrows*).

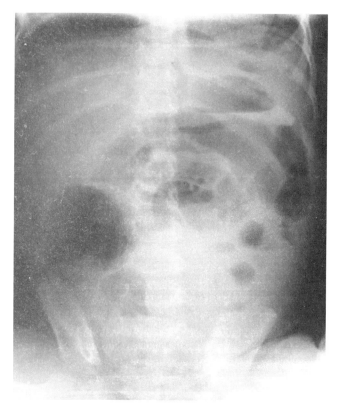

FIGURE 74.1-5   Perforation: crescents of air are seen beneath both hemidiaphragms.

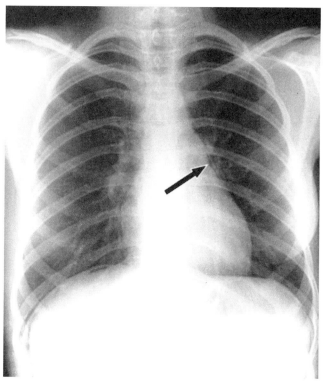

FIGURE 74.1-7   Chest radiograph of the patient in Figure 74.1-6. Air has tracked through the diaphragmatic hiatus into the mediastinum (*arrow*).

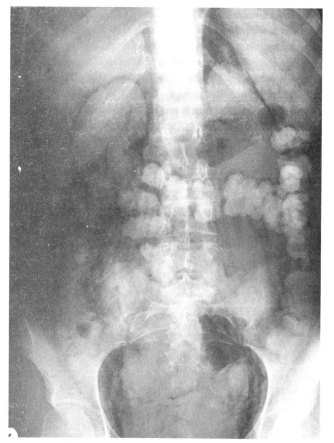

FIGURE 74.1-6   Retroperitoneal air following iatrogenic duodenal perforation. (Contrast in the colon is from a recent fluoroscopic examination.)

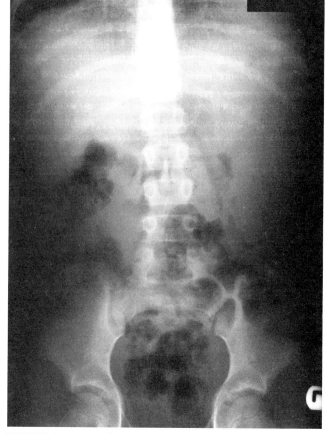

FIGURE 74.1-8   Splenomegaly in a patient with liver cirrhosis owing to cystic fibrosis.

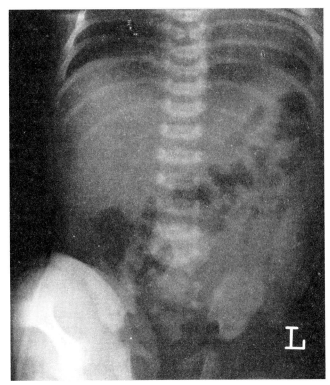

FIGURE 74.1-9 Vertebral anomalies in a patient with an anorectal malformation.

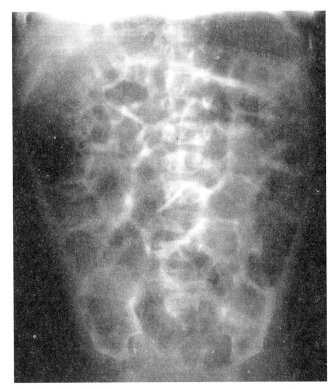

FIGURE 74.1-10 Gaseous distention in a patient with a tracheoesophageal fistula.

loops, may indicate ascites (although this is much more easily identified on ultrasonography). Look for the psoas outline, which is rendered visible by a fat plane. This may become obscured in intra-abdominal sepsis, which is classically described with perforated appendix. However, the psoas outline may be obscured in normal children owing to rotation of the film.

The following conditions have characteristic appearances and may be diagnosed on plain films:

Congenital Obstruction. The level of obstruction can usually be deduced from the plain film. Esophageal atresia could be expected to produce a gasless abdomen, but in practice, there is often a large amount of bowel gas present owing to a tracheoesophageal fistula distal to the esophageal atresia (Figure 74.1-10). Duodenal atresia produces the "double bubble" sign, with air in the distended stomach and proximal duodenum (Figure 74.1-11). Jejunal obstruction produces several dilated loops of small bowel in the left upper quadrant (Figure 74.1-12). The more distal the obstruction, the more loops of distended bowel are seen. Distal small bowel obstruction may be difficult to distinguish from large bowel obstruction.[14]

Anorectal Anomalies. The diagnosis of anorectal anomalies is clinical. However, a plain abdominal film is required to assess the sacrum for associated anomalies. A prone lateral "shoot-through" of the rectum will help to delineate the level of the anorectal atresia, but meticulous technique is essential. The baby should be laid prone with its bottom elevated for 30 minutes prior to the film being

taken to allow air to rise to the most distal portion of the rectum. A radiopaque marker should be placed on the skin at the anal dimple. Rarely, there is air in the bladder owing to a colovesical fistula.

Acquired Bowel Obstruction. The plain film in acquired obstruction typically shows dilated loops of

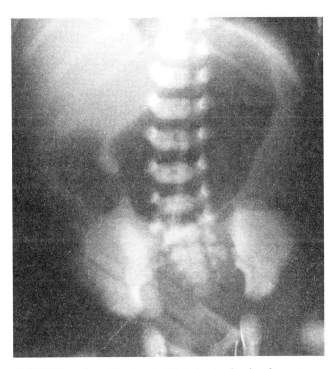

FIGURE 74.1-11 "Double bubble" sign in duodenal atresia.

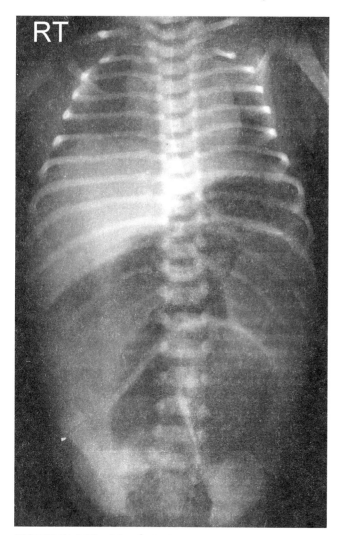

FIGURE 74.1-12   Jejunal atresia.

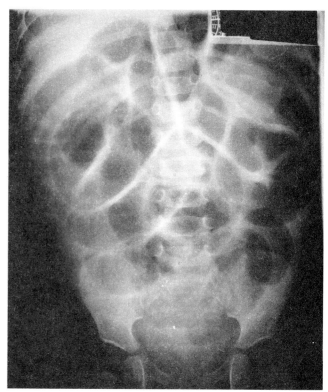

FIGURE 74.1-13   Small bowel obstruction. Note absence of gas in the rectum.

bowel proximal to the obstruction (Figure 74.1-13). If the obstruction is of recent onset, there may still be gas in the bowel distal to the obstruction. Multiple fluid levels within dilated loops form a "ladder" pattern.[2] In high-level obstruction, or when the bowel is very full of fluid, such as in closed-loop obstruction, air-fluid levels may not be present. Nasogastric suction may also alter the pattern of fluid levels.

Ileus.   In paralytic ileus, there is an absence of peristalsis rather than mechanical obstruction. Therefore, both small and large bowel are dilated (Figure 74.1-14). The individual loops tend to be less distended than in mechanical obstruction, and fluid levels are longer.[2] Gas is seen as far as the rectum. Confusion may arise, however, in cases of prolonged mechanical obstruction, when ileus may ensue. Since sepsis is a common cause of ileus in children, ultrasonography is supplementary to identify any intra-abdominal or pelvic collections.

Intra-abdominal Abscess.   Large abscesses will be visible on the plain radiograph as mass lesions with displacement of bowel loops. There is often gas within the abscess; depending on its location, this may be a subtle finding,

such as in a subphrenic collection, in which the gas overlies the dome of the liver, and may form a gas-fluid level. A localized ileus may cause a few loops of distended bowel adjacent to the abscess.

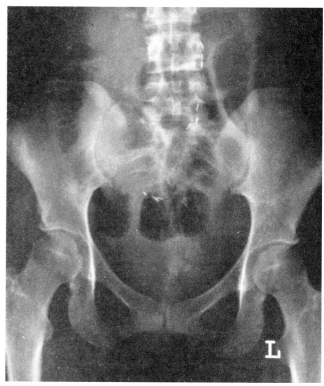

FIGURE 74.1-14   Postoperative ileus. Note the surgical clips and several loops of dilated small bowel.

Necrotizing Enterocolitis. The abdominal radiograph in the neonate with necrotizing enterocolitis will display nonspecific signs such as widespread dilatation of bowel loops and separation of loops. The radiologic hallmark, however, is intramural gas. This may be present at any level from the esophagus to the rectum and may be linear or bubbly in appearance (Figure 74.1-15). Portal venous gas may be present and is no longer regarded as an ominous prognostic sign.[13,15] It must be differentiated from air in the biliary tree, which tends to be more centrally located (around the porta hepatis) and displays a branching pattern. Portal venous gas occasionally may be introduced via an umbilical vein catheter.

Bowel Wall Thickening. Edematous, inflamed bowel wall appears thickened, and loops lie slightly separated from one another. "Thumbprinting" occurs with ischemia and may also be due to hemorrhage into the bowel wall, such as occurs in hemolytic uremic syndrome, Henoch-Schönlein purpura, or thrombocytopenia (Figure 74.1-16). Toxic megacolon, when the transverse colon is unduly dilated and inflamed, is rare in children.

Hernias. Gas within the scrotal sac in boys (or below the inguinal ligament in girls) indicates a hernia; however, in strangulated hernias, the gas may be absent, but there will be asymmetry of the scrotal shadow (Figure 74.1-17). Umbilical hernias may cause unusual gas shadows on plain films owing to air interposed between the hernial sac and the anterior abdominal wall (Figure 74.1-18).

Foreign Bodies. Incidental foreign bodies are frequently seen in children, particularly in the colon. Most will pass without incident. Swallowed dental amalgam

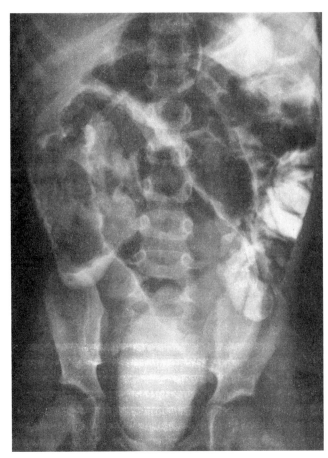

FIGURE 74.1-16 "Thumbprinting" of the colonic mucosa in a patient with Hirschsprung disease and necrotizing enterocolitis.

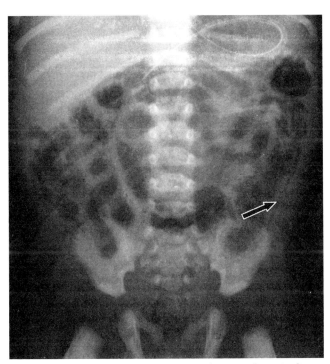

FIGURE 74.1-15 Necrotizing enterocolitis resulting in linear gas lucencies within the thickened bowel wall (*arrow*).

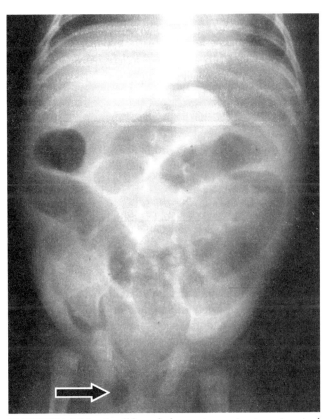

FIGURE 74.1-17 Small bowel obstruction owing to an inguinal hernia. There is gas in the scrotum (*arrow*).

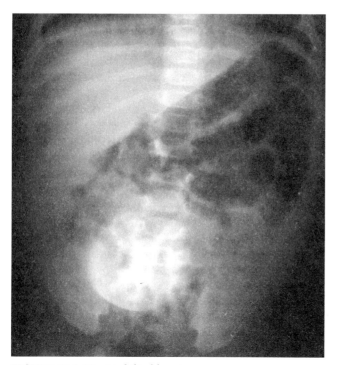

FIGURE 74.1-18   Umbilical hernia.

results in a characteristic pattern of small flakes distributed throughout the colon.

Tubes and Lines.   The tip of a nasogastric tube should lie in the body of the stomach.

An umbilical vein catheter should lie in the right atrium[16]; a lateral film may be required to confirm this because malposition in the left atrium is associated with an increased incidence of intracardiac thrombus formation.[17] An umbilical artery catheter should lie between T6 and T10 (or L3–L5 if the low position is used) (Figures 74.1-19 and 74.1-20).[16] The positions of lines will vary in neonates with congenital diaphragmatic hernias and may give clues as to the contents of the hernia.[18] Ventriculoperitoneal shunts should terminate within the peritoneal cavity but may migrate upward as the child grows. If there is doubt as to the position of the line tip, a lateral film may be useful. If the tip is projected below the costal margin on the frontal radiograph, a lateral radiograph may show it to be superficial to the liver, where it may pass in and out of the peritoneal cavity, creating a valve effect, resulting in intermittent hydrocephalus.

Calcification.   It is important to determine exactly where calcification on an abdominal radiograph is and to decide on its cause. Adrenal calcification commonly follows neonatal adrenal hemorrhage and is seen on either side of the vertebral column, at the top of the renal outlines. Antenatal intestinal perforation results in calcified meconium in the peritoneal cavity. Calcification within a mass lesion should always raise suspicion: neuroblastomas commonly calcify, and calcification is seen rarely in Wilms tumor, hepatoblastoma, and liver hemangioma (Figure 74.1-21).[19] In older children with cystic fibrosis, pancreatic calcification may be

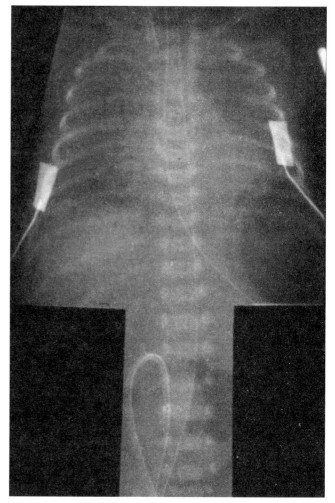

FIGURE 74.1-19   The umbilical vein catheter has been placed too high; its tip lies in a neck vein. Note endotracheal tube and nasogastric tube in a satisfactory position.

seen extending across the midline at the L1 level. Previous tuberculous infection may cause calcification in mesenteric lymph nodes, liver, and spleen; treatment of lymphoma with radiotherapy may also result in lymph node calcification. Fecoliths are common incidental findings, but their presence should be reported because elective appendectomy is indicated.[2] Renal calcification should be differentiated into parenchymal versus pelvic: medullary sponge kidney, renal papillary necrosis, and hyperparathyroidism are among the causes of the former, whereas calcification within the lumen of the renal pelvis, ureters, or bladder is likely to represent a true "stone." A transplant kidney may calcify owing to chronic rejection. In older children, phleboliths within the pelvic veins are easily mistaken for ureteric stones. In general, phleboliths are rounded with a slightly lucent center, whereas urinary tract calculi tend to be more angular in shape. An intravenous urogram, possibly including an oblique film of the bladder area, may be required to show whether a calcific focus lies along the path of the ureter.

Appendicitis.   A child with unequivocal clinical signs of appendicitis does not require imaging. However, in cases in which the diagnosis is in doubt, radiologic input may be

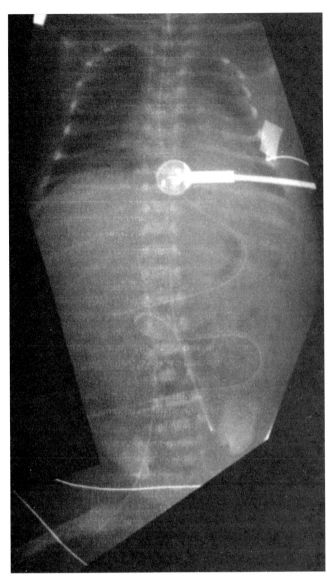

FIGURE 74.1-20 The umbilical artery catheter has been placed too low.

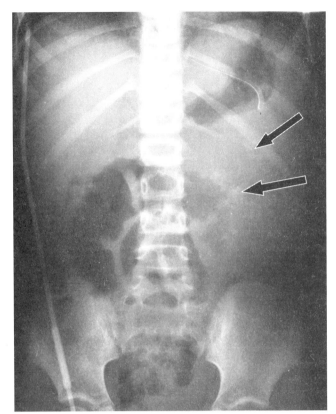

FIGURE 74.1-21 Left-sided abdominal mass containing calcification (*arrows*). This was a neuroblastoma.

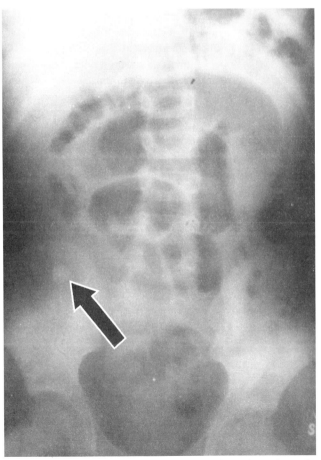

FIGURE 74.1-22 Appendicitis: there is a fecolith in the right iliac fossa (*arrow*).

valuable. The plain abdominal film is frequently normal in appendicitis. In about 10% of cases, a calcified fecolith in the right iliac fossa will confirm the diagnosis (Figure 74.1-22).[2] If the appendix is retrocecal, the fecolith may lie more superiorly and may even mimic a gallstone. Other plain film findings that have been described in appendicitis include a mass in the right iliac fossa with displacement of bowel loops and possibly containing gas (Figure 74.1-23), a localized ileus or even complete small bowel obstruction, and blurring of the peritoneal fat lines. In modern practice, ultrasonography is the first-line investigation in suspected appendicitis[20] and has the considerable advantage of not using ionizing radiation. There is also increasing evidence that CT in selected cases can significantly reduce the rate of negative appendectomies (Figure 74.1-24).[21,22]

Typhlitis. This severe form of colitis is seen in neutropenic and immunocompromised children. The name strictly refers to cecal inflammation, but the whole colon may be involved. Plain film signs include bowel wall edema

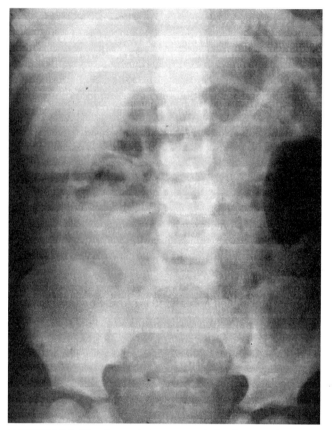

FIGURE 74.1-23 Appendicitis: a rounded soft tissue density in the right iliac fossa displaces bowel loops.

and "thumbprinting"; in severe cases, intramural gas may be present. Secondary dilatation of the small bowel may occur.[2] As with appendicitis, ultrasonography and CT are playing an increasingly important role in the diagnosis of typhlitis. It is particularly important to distinguish this condition from appendicitis because surgical intervention is not required in typhlitis unless complications (such as perforation) occur.[23,24]

Intussusception. The plain film may be entirely normal in cases of intussusception. The typical finding of a soft tissue mass indenting the colon (usually seen in the trans-

verse colon) is seen in only about 25% of patients (Figure 74.1-25).[2,25] Less specific findings include the absence of gas in the right upper quadrant (with failure to identify the cecum and the typical hepatic flexure gas pattern) and a vague right-sided mass. Varying degrees of small bowel obstruction may be present, depending on the time elapsed since the onset of symptoms. Ultrasonography is sensitive in the diagnosis of intussusception and should be performed before proceeding to a contrast study and attempts at reduction.[26]

Pitfalls for the Unwary. While assessing a pediatric abdominal radiograph, the clinician should be aware of several "oddities" that may masquerade as pathology. Films taken on the intensive care unit often include various tubes and equipment, which, in fact, lie outside the patient. The access hatch of an incubator may cause a mysterious circular lucency in the center of the film. Similarly, the umbilical cord, particularly if there is no clamp, may simulate a mass. The same effect can be produced by the penis seen end on. The tip of the normal coccyx may be misinterpreted as abnormal calcification within the pelvis. When assessing suspected intestinal obstruction, it is important to remember that air seen in the rectum may have been introduced by digital rectal examination and therefore cannot be relied on as a sign of patency of the distal bowel.

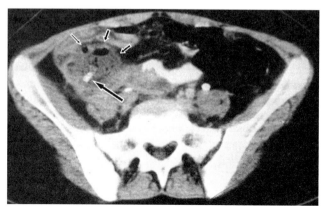

FIGURE 74.1-24 Computed tomographic scan of appendicitis: there is a fecolith (*large arrow*) and a rounded fluid collection (*small arrows*) containing flecks of gas.

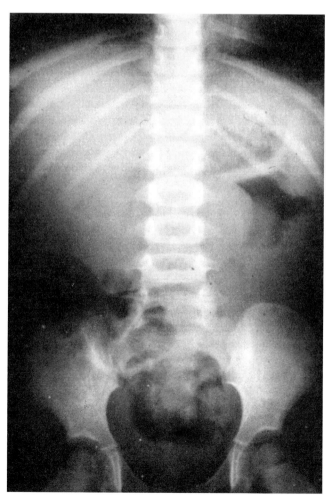

FIGURE 74.1-25 Intussusception.

CONTRAST STUDIES

INDICATIONS

Contrast studies of the gastrointestinal tract, when tailored specifically to the clinical indications, can provide the clinician with anatomic detail and functional information about motility and gastric emptying. The spectrum of disease in children differs from that in adults; ulcers and tumors are rare, and congenital anomalies, such as malrotation, are more frequent. Thus, the emphasis is on anatomy and function rather than mucosal detail, making a fluoroscopic contrast study a potentially more useful diagnostic tool than endoscopy in many cases. Contrast studies are well tolerated by the vast majority of children, whereas endoscopy requires sedation or a general anesthetic. However, contrast studies of the esophagus, stomach and duodenum, and colon have largely been replaced by endoscopy in specialist pediatric units. Contrast studies of the small bowel now make up a larger proportion of the work in a pediatric radiology department, although ultrasonography and CT are often complementary investigations in the diagnosis of small bowel lesions (Table 74.1-1 and Figure 74.1-26).

As well as the conventional techniques listed above, there is frequently the need for specific investigations in specific circumstances: "loopograms" or sinograms, which are intended to answer a particular clinical question, most often in surgical patients (Figure 74.1-27). It cannot be overemphasized that communication between the clinician and the radiologist is of the utmost importance to ensure that the appropriate test is performed. In some cases, CT may be used in conjunction with fluoroscopy, for example, giving more detail about the track of a sinus or fistula in three dimensions.

Contrast studies have been used in the past for the investigation of the gallbladder and biliary tract in children. Ultrasonography is extremely reliable in the diagnosis of biliary tract dilatation, choledochal cysts, and gallstones. More recently, MRI has advanced to the point where magnetic resonance cholangiopancreatography (MRCP) can provide high-resolution images of the biliary tree, gallbladder, and pancreatic duct, obviating the need for invasive procedures such as percutaneous transhepatic cholangiography or endoscopic retrograde cholangiopancreatography. MRCP has proved useful in the investigation of acute pancreatitis, primary sclerosing cholangitis, choledochal cyst, and congenital anomalies, such as pancreas divisum.[27–30] New techniques are continually being explored in this exciting field, and in the near future, virtual endoscopy of the pancreatic and biliary ducts using data from MRCP studies is likely to become routinely available.[31]

CHOICE OF CONTRAST

Barium sulfate is the traditional gastrointestinal contrast medium of choice. It is cheap and readily available, and its high density provides excellent contrast and definition. It is not absorbed by the gut and can, therefore, be used anywhere in the bowel. It remains the contrast medium of choice for small bowel studies and for double-contrast ene-

TABLE 74.1-1 GASTROINTESTINAL CONTRAST STUDIES PERFORMED IN CHILDREN AND SOME OF THEIR INDICATIONS

SPEECH STUDY/PHONETICS
Identification of palatal movement and choanal closure
Pre- and postsurgical repair of cleft palate
Speech problems with nasal escape
Nasal reflux of food

SWALLOWING STUDY
Oropharyngeal incoordination, mainly in children with neurologic impairment

CONTRAST SWALLOW
Vascular rings and other extrinsic masses affecting swallowing
Tracheoesophageal fistula (including follow-up postsurgical repair) (see Figure 74.1-26)
Gastroesophageal reflux
Foreign body ingestion
Strictures

UPPER GASTROINTESTINAL STUDY
Usually follows contrast swallow
Demonstrates anatomy (eg, duodenojejunal flexure) and motility
Pyloric stenosis (now largely replaced by ultrasonography)

GASTROSTOMY STUDY
Contrast instilled via gastrostomy tube
Assesses gastric emptying and reflux

SMALL BOWEL STUDIES
Assesses the bowel, which is not within reach of endoscopy
Performed as follow-through or enteroclysis (see below)
Crohn disease
Small bowel strictures (traumatic/postsurgical)
Dysmotility

BARIUM ENEMA
Now rarely performed
A limited study may be performed in severe constipation to exclude Hirschsprung disease

DEFECATING PROCTOGRAPHY
To assess pelvic floor dysfunction in obstructed defecation

FISTULOGRAPHY/SINOGRAPHY
Identification of tracks

WATER-SOLUBLE CONTRAST ENEMA
Performed in neonates
To identify cause of intestinal obstruction, eg, Hirschsprung disease, meconium ileus, meconium plug, intussusception

mas on the rare occasions that these are done. However, if any of the following contraindications exist, a water-soluble contrast medium (see below) should be used:

- Suspected perforation (barium excites an aggressive inflammatory response if allowed to escape into the mediastinum or peritoneum).
- Possibility of aspiration, for example, in neurologically impaired children (although aspirated barium is usually well tolerated, serious respiratory impairment can occur).
- Because barium is contraindicated, water-soluble media are now the contrast of choice for neonates.
- Barium may become inspissated in defunctioned bowel (eg, loopograms postsurgical resection), and there is a risk of impaction in Hirschsprung disease and cystic fibrosis.

Gastrografin should not be used in the upper gastrointestinal tract because it is very hyperosmolar and can precipitate pulmonary edema if aspirated. It is used for

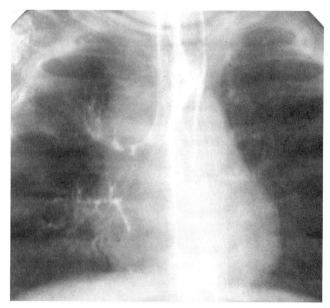

FIGURE 74.1-26   Contrast swallow in a patient with H-type tracheoesophageal fistula. Contrast is seen outlining the trachea and bronchial tree.

therapeutic enemas in meconium ileus, where it draws fluid into the bowel lumen to aid disimpaction of the sticky meconium. However, it may cause dehydration by drawing excessive amounts of water into the bowel,[6] particularly in a vulnerable neonate, and great care should be taken to ensure adequate fluid replacement. The radiologist must inform the clinician that Gastrografin has been used.

The iso-osmolar contrast agents are more expensive than Gastrografin but are safe if aspirated and have no effect on the peritoneum or mediastinum. Perhaps surprisingly, there is no evidence that iso-osmolar agents are any less effective in the treatment of meconium ileus than hyperosmolar media.[6]

Double-contrast studies of the gastrointestinal tract are performed in adult practice and provide excellent mucosal detail. The technique uses a thin coating of barium to define the mucosa, combined with distention of the viscus with air. With the advent of endoscopy, double-contrast studies are now rarely required in children.

Air is now the medium of choice for intussusception reduction.[32,33] It is introduced into the colon at pressures of up to 120 mm of mercury. Perforation is a rare complication, but if it occurs, a large pneumoperitoneum will result, with respiratory compromise. Accordingly, a large trochar should be available for immediate decompression of the peritoneum.[2]

TECHNIQUE

General Considerations.   A pediatric "barium" list presents a unique challenge. Flexibility and ingenuity are essential so that each study is specifically tailored to the patient and the clinical problem.

Steps should always be taken to minimize the radiation dose to children undergoing fluoroscopic examinations. Digital fluoroscopy delivers a lower dose than older cine-film systems, and the dose can be reduced further by using

pulsed screening.[34,35] A last-image-hold ("frame grab") facility allows images to be recorded without a static exposure being made. Grids should not be used routinely.

Video recordings should be made of all gastrointestinal contrast studies. This allows dynamic processes such as swallowing, gastroesophageal reflux, or gastric transit to be viewed in real time, or frame by frame. If an uncooperative child has allowed only an incomplete study to be performed, the video footage will often contain sufficient information even if no static images have been recorded, thus obviating the need for a repeat study.

Specific Techniques.   *Speech and Swallowing Studies.*
Speech and swallowing difficulties frequently coexist in neurologically impaired children. A multidisciplinary approach is essential in their management, and videofluoroscopy swallowing studies should be carried out with the speech therapist. Videofluoroscopy swallowing studies provide more detailed and objective evidence of swallowing dysfunction than traditional bedside evaluation.[36] The aim is to assess the phases of swallowing and to ensure that there is complete glottic closure without aspiration. Specific observable problems include poor tongue movements, delayed swallow reflex, reduced laryngeal elevation, and silent aspiration.[37] Aspiration is more likely to occur with thin fluids; therefore, swallowing of thicker consistencies should be assessed first, using, for example, bread or bis-

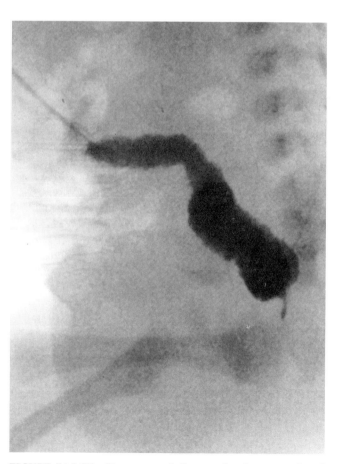

FIGURE 74.1-27   "Loopogram." Contrast has been introduced via the defunctioning stoma to demonstrate the level of the anorectal atresia.

cuits dipped in barium or yogurt mixed with barium for infants who cannot yet manage solids. Appropriate commercial thickening agents are available. The result of these studies can be of vital importance in the future management of the child, for example, determining the safest position for feeding, which will help prevent long-term aspiration and malnutrition.[38,39]

Upper Gastrointestinal Studies. Infants whose last feed has been withheld are usually quite willing to drink unflavored barium or (amazingly!) Omnipaque from a bottle. For older children, barium can be flavored to make a relatively pleasant milkshake-style drink; Omnipaque is effectively disguised in orange juice. To assess swallowing of solids, marshmallows can be soaked in barium.

Contrast swallows have historically been performed mainly for the detection of gastroesophageal reflux. However, the sensitivity of radiologic studies for reflux has been reported to be as low as 52%[40]; therefore, a negative study is of little diagnostic value. Barium swallows continue to be useful in the diagnosis of structural causes of dysphagia, such as vascular rings, strictures following caustic ingestion, longstanding reflux disease, or postsurgical repair of tracheoesophageal fistulae, as well as functional disorders such as achalasia and globus hystericus. Views should always be taken in the supine oblique position to fully distend the lower esophagus. A careful history is important: establish exactly what provokes the child's symptoms and try to reproduce these conditions as closely as possible during the study.

In children with feeding gastrostomies, the parent or caregiver should be asked to replicate the child's usual feeding process, using contrast mixed with food. Again, the conditions that produce symptoms should be reproduced; for example, if the patient habitually vomits after 200 mL of food have been given, a study using only a small volume of contrast will not be helpful.

The radiologist should take the opportunity during all upper gastrointestinal studies in children to observe the passage of contrast around the duodenal loop to the duodenojejunal flexure. An image of the correctly sited flexure (to the left of the spinal column, at the level of L1) will rule out 98% of cases of malrotation (Figure 74.1-28). In some centers, a contrast enema (rather than an upper gastrointestinal study) is the investigation of choice to rule out malrotation; however, in 16% of children with malrotation, the cecum is normally sited in the right iliac fossa. Furthermore, the cecum may be displaced from the right iliac fossa in 15% of normal children.[6] In cases of strong clinical suspicion of malrotation, where the duodenal position appears normal or equivocal, it is logical to proceed to an enema study to evaluate the cecal position.

All radiologic studies for malrotation are limited by the fact that only the bowel is imaged, not the mesenteric fixation, which is what actually determines the malrotation. It is also well recognized that the normal duodenum may be markedly mobile, especially in neonates, and this may lead to further confusion.[41]

Small Bowel Follow-through. Most would agree that the initial investigation of the small bowel should be by follow-through, with enteroclysis (see below) being

reserved for selected difficult cases in which a follow-through study has failed to make a diagnosis.[42] In the follow-through technique, the child drinks about 500 mL of dilute barium after a 6-hour fast. An immediate supine film is taken, followed by prone films (the prone position separates bowel loops) at intervals until the ileocecal junction has been visualized. The films should be carefully examined as they are done, and fluoroscopy should be performed to clarify any doubtful areas, for example, to confirm fixation or separation of bowel loops. The terminal ileum should always be screened to ensure that underfilling is not misinterpreted as a stricture. If the colon is loaded with feces, the passage of barium will be slowed; this may often be overcome by giving the child a meal once contrast has reached the ileum.

Enteroclysis. Enteroclysis (or small bowel enema) involves introduction of contrast directly into the proximal jejunum via a long, wide-bore oro- or nasojejunal tube. A bolus of dilute barium is used, followed by water or methylcellulose for a double-contrast effect, and is monitored with fluoroscopy throughout the small bowel. The technique is more sensitive than follow-through studies, particularly for the demonstration of polyps, but is often poorly tolerated by children. Intubation may be difficult, and if the tube is too proximal, barium will reflux into the stomach and result in vomiting.

Peroral Pneumocolon. This technique is supplementary to a small bowel follow-through study. Once barium has reached the terminal ileum, air is insufflated per rectum to distend the colon and terminal ileum. This gives good mucosal detail of the terminal ileum but is relatively more invasive.

Characteristic Appearances of Selected Conditions on Contrast Studies. The reader is referred to the individual chapters for a more complete discussion of these conditions.

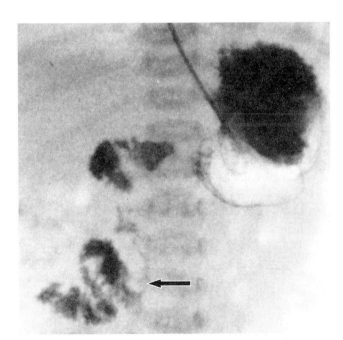

FIGURE 74.1-28 Malrotation: upper gastrointestinal contrast study showing abnormal position of the duodenojejunal flexure, which lies to the right of the midline (arrow).

Vascular Rings. The lateral view of the esophagus during a contrast swallow can predict the type of vascular anomaly in most cases. The plain chest radiograph will provide additional information about the aortic arch and tracheal position. In modern practice, the definitive diagnosis is usually made by MRI.

There are four patterns of esophageal and/or tracheal compression on the contrast swallow; these correspond to four major vascular anomalies. A double aortic arch causes posterior esophageal compression together with anterior tracheal compression. (A similar pattern occurs with a right-sided arch in combination with a left ductus arteriosus and aberrant left subclavian artery.) Compression of the trachea by a prominent innominate artery causes an anterior impression on the trachea but a normal esophagus. Aberrant right subclavian artery (the most common anomaly of the aortic arch) results in a posterior impression on the esophagus with a normal trachea. Finally, a posterior impression on the trachea, coupled with anterior compression of the esophagus, is caused by an aberrant left pulmonary artery, arising from the right pulmonary artery and passing between the trachea and esophagus.[14,43]

Achalasia. Videofluoroscopy in achalasia shows abnormal motility and failure of relaxation of the lower esophageal sphincter. The esophagus becomes dilated in long-standing cases and may be filled with food debris. The narrowed lower esophageal sphincter has a characteristic "rat-tail" appearance.[14]

Hiatal Hernia and Gastroesophageal Reflux. If the gastroesophageal junction lies above the diaphragm, a hiatal hernia is present. The significance of hiatal hernia in reflux disease has yet to be established.[44] A small amount of reflux is a normal finding in children. A clinical history of repeated vomiting, failure to thrive, and recurrent chest infections (owing to aspiration) are clues that significant reflux is present. If the gastroesophageal junction is widened and the esophagus appears "baggy," significant reflux is likely to be present. Any contrast refluxing above the gastroesophageal junction should be noted, as well as the level to which it ascends and the frequency of episodes during the study.[2] Failure to demonstrate reflux on videofluoroscopy does not exclude the diagnosis (see under "Technique" above). In chronic reflux disease, an esophageal stricture may develop, which is usually smooth and tapering in appearance.

Duodenal Obstruction. Complete duodenal atresia is usually diagnosed on the plain film, which typically shows the "double bubble" sign. Partial duodenal obstruction may be due to congenital webs, annular pancreas, Ladd bands, or a preduodenal portal vein. A web may appear as a linear filling defect within the duodenum, and the dilated, barium-filled distal duodenum with a convex end has been described as a "wind sock." Other causes of partial duodenal obstruction are difficult to distinguish from webs on barium studies (Figures 74.1-29 and 74.1-30). Cross-sectional imaging will be helpful in demonstrating

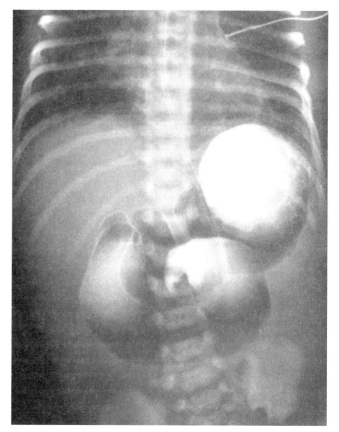

FIGURE 74.1-29   Contrast study demonstrating duodenal atresia.

pancreatic and portal vein anomalies.[14] However, pragmatically, this is not done in neonates because these children require surgery.

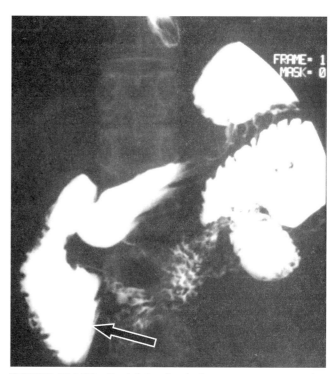

FIGURE 74.1-30   Partial duodenal obstruction, owing in this case to compression by the superior mesenteric artery. There is dilatation of the duodenum proximal to the obstruction (*arrow*).

Malrotation and Volvulus. As discussed under "Technique" above, contrast studies are not infallible in the diagnosis of malrotation. The major life-threatening complication of malrotation is volvulus of the small bowel around the superior mesenteric artery. If this is present, the contrast study may demonstrate a corkscrew or "twisted ribbon" appearance of the duodenum and jejunum, with thickened mucosal folds owing to edema of the bowel wall. Classically, the contrast terminates in a "bird's beak" at the point of obstruction; however, the obstruction may be rounded and appear to be similar to duodenal atresia.[14]

Malabsorption. Malabsorption attributable to any cause characteristically results in nonspecific changes in the small bowel contrast study: fragmentation of the barium column, flocculation of barium, and mild dilatation of the small bowel. Celiac disease is classically described as causing a featureless, smooth jejunum with an increase in mucosal folds in the ileum (so-called "jejunization" of the ileum) (Figure 74.1-31). Transient intussusceptions may be seen during the small bowel study.[2,45] There is an increased risk of small bowel lymphoma, so any mass should be treated with suspicion.

Crohn Disease. Crohn disease may affect any part of the gastrointestinal tract. In the small bowel, the terminal ileum is the most commonly affected region; however, up to 20% of children with small bowel Crohn disease will have a normal terminal ileum on imaging.[14,46] More typically, there is a segment of narrowed, rigid bowel with mucosal nodularity or "cobblestoning" and deep ulcers (Figure 74.1-32). If the stricture is tight, the proximal portion of bowel may be dilated. Several sections of bowel may be affected, with the intervening areas appearing normal ("skip lesions"). Fistulae may occur between adjacent loops of small bowel or between small bowel and colon or even stomach. In long-standing disease, eccentric scarring occurs, resulting in "pseudosacculations" on the antimesenteric border of the bowel. CT and ultrasonography have an important supplementary role in delineating thickened bowel loops and inflammatory masses.[47] In difficult cases, an isotope-labeled white cell scan may be required to identify an intra-abdominal site of inflammation.[2]

Crohn disease of the colon can be demonstrated on a double-contrast barium enema; however, these are rarely performed in modern pediatric practice because endoscopy is the mainstay of diagnosis for inflammatory diseases of the colon. The colon is usually asymmetrically involved (in contrast to ulcerative colitis), with predominantly the right colon being affected and less commonly the rectum.[14] In early Crohn colitis, there may be discrete aphthae (ulcers with a smooth raised edge); these later coalesce to form

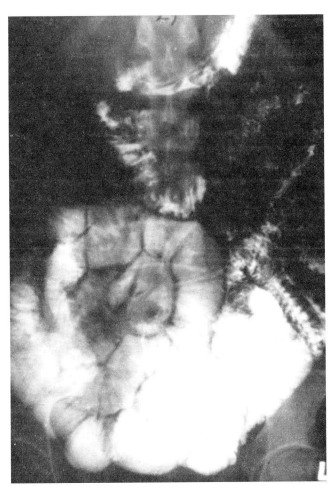

FIGURE 74.1-31 Small bowel meal in celiac disease. The jejunum is mildly dilated, smooth, and relatively featureless.

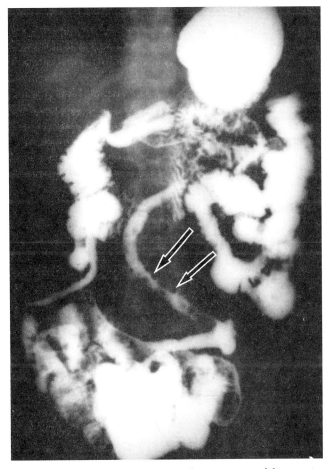

FIGURE 74.1-32 Crohn disease. There are several long strictures of the small bowel with "cobblestoning" and "rose-thorn" ulcers (arrows).

linear ulceration and may penetrate the bowel wall to form sinuses or fistulae. As in the small bowel, skip lesions are characteristic, and pseudosacculations may occur.

Intussusception. Intussusception may be ileoileal, ileo-colic, or ileoileocolic (in which an ileoileal intussusception then invaginates into the colon). In all of these cases, the intussusceptum will be seen as a filling defect indenting the column of contrast or air (Figure 74.1-33). Following successful reduction, a residual filling defect is often seen in the cecum: this is the edematous ileocecal valve.[2,14]

Meconium Ileus. A contrast enema in meconium ileus will show a microcolon, and contrast refluxing into the terminal ileum will outline inspissated meconium (Figure 74.1-34). The colon is also of very small caliber in distal ileal atresia but tends to be of near-normal caliber in proximal ileal or jejunal atresia owing to a larger quantity of small intestinal secretions reaching the colon in fetal life.[14,48] However, in practice, the colon is seldom examined radiologically.

Meconium Plug. In meconium plug syndrome, there is functional immaturity of the colon. A contrast enema will demonstrate the meconium in a normal-caliber colon. A caliber change at or proximal to the splenic flexure, with the descending colon being narrowed, is known as small left colon syndrome but is a variant of meconium plug syndrome. A therapeutic enema with water-soluble contrast medium will aid the passage of meconium.[14]

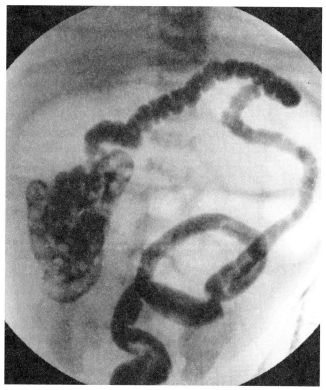

FIGURE 74.1-34 Contrast enema in meconium ileus. Note meconium within the terminal ileum.

Hirschsprung Disease. The characteristic indicator of Hirschsprung disease is a transitional zone between the proximal, dilated (normal) bowel and the distal, small-caliber aganglionic segment (Figure 74.1-35). Irregular

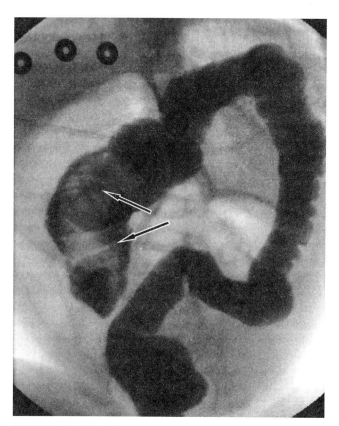

FIGURE 74.1-33 Contrast enema in intussusception. The intussusceptum shows as a filling defect (*arrows*).

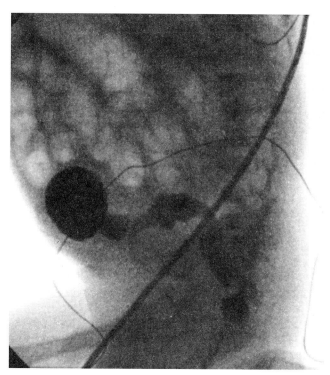

FIGURE 74.1-35 Contrast enema in Hirschsprung disease showing sharp caliber change at the transitional zone.

"sawtooth" contractions in the aganglionic segment may be seen.[14] A rectum that is narrower in caliber than the sigmoid colon is also highly suggestive of the diagnosis, although the value of this sign is debatable.[49] In rare cases of total colonic aganglionosis, there will be no transitional zone.

Ulcerative Colitis.   As with Crohn colitis, endoscopy has largely replaced double-contrast barium enema in the diagnosis of ulcerative colitis in children. Barium studies show diffusely granular mucosa in early colitis. Unlike Crohn disease, involvement of the colon is continuous, usually extending proximally from the rectum. As the disease progresses, there is haustral thickening owing to edema, and deepening ulcers result in islands of normal mucosa appearing as "pseudopolyps." In long-standing cases, the colon may appear shortened and tubular—the "lead pipe" colon. Reflux ileitis may result in a patulous terminal ileum.[50]

Polyps.   Polyps appear as sessile or pedunculated filling defects on barium studies. The appearances of the polyps in the various polyposis syndromes are nonspecific, but their distribution in the gastrointestinal tract, together with the associated clinical features, may suggest the diagnosis.[51] However, fiberoptic endoscopy is now the preferred diagnostic technique.

REFERENCES

1. Teunen D. The European Directive on health protection of individuals against the dangers of ionising radiation in relation to medical exposures. J Radiol Prot 1998;18:133–7.
2. Carty H. Non-neonatal gastrointestinal tract. In: Carty H, Brunelle F, Shaw D, Kendall B, editors. Imaging children. Edinburgh: Churchill Livingstone; 1994. p. 303–454.
3. Grier D. Radiology of paediatric gastrointestinal emergencies. In: Carty H, editor. Emergency pediatric radiology. Berlin: Springer; 1999. p. 118, 142.
4. RCR Working Party. Making the best use of a department of clinical radiololgy: guidelines for doctors. 5th ed. London: The Royal College of Radiologists; 2003.
5. Boothroyd AE, Carty HM, Robson WJ. "Hunt the thimble": a study of the radiology of ingested foreign bodies. Arch Emerg Med 1987;4:33–8.
6. Stringer DA, Babyn PS. Pediatric gastrointestinal imaging and intervention. Hamilton (ON): BC Decker; 2000.
7. Bell M, Ternberg J, Bowen R. Ileal dysgenesis in infants and children. J Pediatr Surg 1982;17:395–9.
8. Hufton AP, Doyle SM, Carty HM. Digital radiography in pediatrics: radiation dose considerations and magnitude of possible dose reduction. Br J Radiol 1998;71:186–99.
9. Mooney R, Thomas PS. Dose reduction in a pediatric x-ray department following optimisation of radiographic technique. Br J Radiol 1998;71:852–60.
10. Kyriou JC, Fitzgerald M, Pettett A, et al. A comparison of doses and techniques between specialist and non-specialist centres in the diagnostic x-ray imaging of children. Br J Radiol 1996;69:437–50.
11. Liakos P, Schoenecker PL, Lyons D, Gordon JE. Evaluation of the efficacy of pelvic shielding in preadolescent girls. J Pediatr Orthoped 2001;21:433–5.
12. Wainwright AM. Shielding reproductive organs of orthopaedic patients during pelvic radiography. Ann R Coll Surg Engl 2000;82:318–21.
13. Donoghue V. Neonatal gastrointestinal tract. In: Carty H, Brunelle F, Shaw D, Kendall B, editors. Imaging children. Edinburgh: Churchill Livingstone; 1994. p. 250–302.
14. Liu PCF, Stringer DA. Radiographic contrast studies. In: Walker WA, Durie PR, Hamilton JR, et al, editors. Pediatric gastrointestinal disease. 3rd ed. Hamilton (ON): BC Decker; 2000. p. 1555–90.
15. Donoghue V, Kelwan CG. Transient portal venous gas in necrotizing enterocolitis. Br J Radiol 1982;55:681–3.
16. Narla LD, Hom M, Lofland GK, Moskowitz WB. Evaluation of umbilical catheter and tube placement in premature infants. Radiographics 1991;11:849–63.
17. Raval NC, Gonzalez E, Bhat AM, et al. Umbilical venous catheters: evaluation of radiographs to determine position and associated complications of malpositioned umbilical venous catheters. Am J Perinatol 1995;12:201–4.
18. Sakurai M, Donnelly LF, Klosterman LA, Strife JL. Congenital diaphragmatic hernia in neonates: variations in umbilical catheter and enteric tube positions. Radiology 2000;216:112–6.
19. Chapman S, Nakielny R. Aids to radiological differential diagnosis. London: WB Saunders; 1995.
20. Jeffrey R, Laing F, Lewis F. Acute appendicitis: high resolution real time ultrasound findings. Radiology 1987;163:11–4.
21. Callahan MJ, Rodriguez DP, Taylor GA. CT of appendicitis in children. Radiology 2002;224:325–32.
22. Pena BM, Taylor GA, Fishman SJ, Mandi KD. Effect of imaging protocol on clinical outcomes among pediatric patients with appendicitis. Pediatrics 2002;110:1088–93.
23. Schlatter M, Snyder K, Freyer D. Successful nonoperative management of typhlitis in pediatric oncology patients. J Pediatr Surg 2002;37:1151–5.
24. McNamara MJ, Chalmers AG, Morgan M, Smith SE. Typhlitis in acute childhood leukaemia: radiological features. Clin Radiol 1986;37:83–6.
25. Bisset G, Kirby D. Intussusception in infants and children: diagnosis and therapy. Radiology 1988;168:141–5.
26. Swischuk L, Hayden C, Boulden T. Intussusception: indications for ultrasonography and explanation of the doughnut and pseudokidney signs. Pediatr Radiol 1985;15:388–91.
27. Ferrara C, Valeri G, Salvolini L, Giovagnoni A. Magnetic resonance cholangiopancreatography in primary sclerosing cholangitis in children. Pediatr Radiol 2002;32:413–7.
28. Shimizu T, Suzuki R, Yanashiro Y, et al. Magnetic resonance cholangiopancreatography in assessing the cause of acute pancreatitis in children. Pancreas 2001;22:196–9.
29. Arcement CM, Meza MP, Arumania S, Towbin RB. MRCP in the evaluation of pancreaticobiliary disease in children. Pediatr Radiol 2001;31:92–7.
30. van Heurn-Nijsten EW, Snoep G, Kootstra G, et al. Preoperative imaging of a choledochal cyst in children: non-breath-holding magnetic resonance cholangiopancreatography. Pediatr Surg 1999;15:546–8.
31. Neri E, Boraschi P, Braccini G, et al. MR virtual endoscopy of the pancreaticobiliary tract. Magn Reson Imaging 1999;17:59–67.
32. Paes R, Hyde I, Griffiths D. The management of intussusception. Br J Radiol 1988;61:187–9.
33. Stringer D, Ein S. Pneumatic reduction: advantages, risks and indications. Pediatr Radiol 1990;20:475–7.
34. Hernandez RJ, Goodsitt MM. Reduction of radiation dose in pediatric patients using pulsed fluoroscopy. AJR Am J Roentgenol 1996;167:1247–53.
35. Mooney RB, McKinstry J. Pediatric dose reduction with the introduction of digital fluorography. Radiat Protect Dosim 2001;94:117–20.

36. Zerilli KS, Stefans VA, DiPetro MA. Protocol for the use of video-fluoroscopy in pediatric swallowing dysfunction. Am J Occup Ther 1990;44:441–6.

37. Morgan A, Ward E, Murdoch B, Bilbie K. Acute characteristics of pediatric dysphagia subsequent to traumatic brain injury: videofluoroscopic assessment. J Head Trauma Rehabil 2002; 17:220–41.

38. Morton RE, Bonas R, Fourie B, Minford J. Videofluoroscopy in the assessment of feeding disorders of children with neurological problems. Dev Med Child Neurol 1993;35: 388–95.

39. Wright RE, Wright FR, Carson CA. Videofluoroscopic assessment in children with severe cerebral palsy presenting with dysphagia. Pediatr Radiol 1996;26:720–2.

40. Aksglaede K, Funch-Jensen P, Thommesen P. Radiological demonstration of gastroesophageal reflux. Diagnostic value of barium and bread studies compared with 24-hour pH monitoring. Acta Radiol 1999;40:652–5.

41. Katz ME, Siegel MJ, Shackelford GD, McAlister WH. The position and mobility of the duodenum in children. AJR Am J Roentgenol 1987;148:947–51.

42. Stringer DA, Clouter S, Daneman A, et al. The value of the small bowel enema in children. J Can Assoc Radiol 1986;37:13–6.

43. Klinkhamer AC. Esophagography in anomalies of the aortic arch system. Baltimore: Williams and Wilkins; 1969.

44. Steiner GM. Review article: gastro-oesophageal reflux, hiatus hernia and the radiologist, with special reference to children. Br J Radiol 1977;50:164–74.

45. Howarth E, Hodson C, Pringle E, Young W. The value of radiological investigations of the alimentary tract in children with the coeliac syndrome. Clin Radiol 1986;19:65–76.

46. Kirks D, Curranino G. Regional enteritis in children: small bowel disease with normal terminal ileum. Pediatr Radiol 1978;7:10–4.

47. Siegel M, Evans S, Balfe D. Small bowel disease in children: diagnosis with CT. Radiology 1988;169:127–30.

48. Berdon WE, Baker DH, Santulli TV, et al. Microcolon in newborn infants with intestinal obstruction: its correlation with the level and time of onset of obstruction. Radiology 1968; 90:878–85.

49. Siegel MJ, Shackelford GD, McAlister WH. The rectosigmoid index. Radiology 1981;139:497–9.

50. Stringer DA. Imaging inflammatory bowel disease in the pediatric patient. Radiol Clin North Am 1987;25:93–113.

51. Dodds WJ. Clinical and roentgen features of the intestinal polyposis syndromes. Gastrointest Radiol 1976;1:127–42.

2. Cross-Sectional Imaging: Ultrasonography, Computed Tomography, Magnetic Resonance Imaging

Karen Norton, MD

Keith J. Benkov, MD

The subspecialty of pediatric gastroenterology began almost 30 years ago, coinciding with revolutionary technological advances being made in the field of diagnostic imaging. Concurrent with the introduction of ultrasonography (US) in the early 1970s, gastrointestinal endoscopy was introduced. Rapidly following the introduction of US, computed tomography (CT) and then magnetic resonance imaging (MRI) were developed. These advances in imaging, which allow complex images to be stored, manipulated, and retrieved in microseconds, have now become routine radiology procedures rather than what might have been envisioned in science fiction stories 30 years ago. The detail of anatomic information gathered by these radiology examinations often approaches what is depicted at direct surgical exploration or pathology. Pediatric-sized endoscopes have made direct visualization and intervention possible even in very small children. It is now implausible to envision practicing the subspecialty of pediatric gastroenterology without these remarkable complementary technologies.

To successfully practice pediatric gastroenterology requires more than casual familiarity with cross-sectional imaging modalities. Although the clinical gastroenterologist is usually not required to perform or independently interpret these studies, an understanding of the indications, strengths, and limitations of particular investigative studies is extremely useful. In a rapidly evolving field, it is sometimes difficult to know the true benefit of a new technique until years later, when it has been fully applied and compared with other techniques. Especially important is to know when to use these often expensive technologies, which may involve exposure to ionizing radiation, the injection of potentially nephrotoxic contrast agents, and the risks of conscious sedation or general anesthesia. In this regard, there is no substitute for a good history and physical examination, and there is probably no more important a colleague than a trusted pediatric radiologist to help direct the imaging evaluation.

ULTRASONOGRAPHY

In children, US is often the initial choice of radiologic investigation because it does not require ionizing radiation, is not painful, requires little or no preparation, and is a relatively inexpensive examination. In children, especially younger infants, it is ideal because the general lack of internal body fat facilitates imaging. In certain settings, US is superior to other modalities, especially for delineation of cystic lesions. Generally, no sedation is needed, and even with young infants and children, little or no restraint is required.[1]

Technically, US uses sound above the audible range of frequencies of 20 kHz or 20,000 cycles per second. In practice, diagnostic US uses a much higher frequency, from 1 to 20 MHz (a million cycles per second). These sound waves are emitted from a transducer that contains crystals with piezoelectric properties. When the crystals are subjected to an electric current, they emit sound waves at a particular frequency depending on the size of the crystals and the current. Once the sound is emitted, it is directed through the body and is either reflected, refracted, scattered, or absorbed, depending on the properties of the tissues that are encountered, producing the equivalent of a reflected echo. This reflected echo, when returned to the transducer crystal, causes a vibration that generates an interpretable electric pulse. The returning sound beam will have a different speed and intensity from the original, which is referred to as attenuation, which depends on the properties of the encountered tissues.[2] "Real-time" images can be generated if rapid sound emissions are done at a rate of at least 15 image frames per second.[3]

US can also be used to determine blood flow moving through vessels and structures, based on the "Doppler shift principle." Sound reflecting off a moving target will change in frequency, proportional to the speed of the moving target. The returning echo can be detected as audible sound or as a traceable wave pattern depending on velocity. The use of color allows determination of direction of flow, conventionally with red indicating flow toward the transducer and blue indicating flow away from the transducer. Some investigators are using contrast agents such as stabilized intravascular microbubbles to accentuate detection of blood flow, but these techniques are not widely used in clinical practice.[4]

US has limitations that should be addressed and understood. US cannot penetrate air-containing structures well, as in bowel or lungs. Structures underlying bowel gas may be completely obscured. US has little ability to penetrate bone, other calcified structures, and metal, such as sutures or plates.[5] The images are obtained in small sectors or wedges of information, and depth of penetration is limited, especially in older and larger patients. The spatial relationships and resolution are not as great as in CT or MRI, which sometimes leads nonradiologists to not fully understand or trust and therefore not fully appreciate the anatomic information offered by US.[3]

COMPUTED TOMOGRAPHY

Similar to routine radiographic studies, CT uses electromagnetic radiation to obtain images. A well-collimated beam is passed through the subject and, depending on the characteristics of the tissues and spaces, the x-ray will be subject to differing attenuation, making it possible to reconstruct an image via complex computer programs to create a cross-sectional image. Sophisticated hardware and software advances have enabled finely detailed images to be displayed by a grayscale, with a spectrum from air, seen as black, to water, seen as gray, to bone, seen as white. With use of the newer spiral and helical technology, the image is generated quickly and accurately as the table moves while the scan is being done. Now with the advent of multislice CT, the images can be acquired so quickly that CT "fluoroscopy" to assist biopsies and catheter insertions are possible. Vascular studies can be obtained from a single rapid injection in a matter of seconds. Traditionally, CT images are obtained in the axial plane, but images can be reconstructed in any plane desired at modern workstations after processing.[6]

Before ordering a CT scan, the clinician should be aware of several issues related to the risks versus the benefits of the modality. CT does involve exposure to radiation, raising important safety concerns that should be carefully considered, especially in children. Recent evidence postulating an increased cancer risk in adulthood in children exposed to diagnostic CT[7] has led to a complete revamping of the CT protocols used in pediatric studies to minimize dosage while still delivering high-quality images. Newer multislice CT scanners are now capable of better imaging with less radiation exposure than older machines and are preferable. Motion degrades the images, usually making some form of sedation or even anesthesia necessary in younger children. Intravenous injection of iodinated contrast is useful in most body cases, requiring adequate venous access. Although relatively safe, these agents can be nephrotoxic, and occasional allergic and anaphylactoid reactions are reported. Adequate ingestion of oral contrast, which is difficult to obtain in children who require sedation, increases the accuracy of the study. Young children and sedated subjects cannot maintain rectal contrast. The lack of internal body fat in children often makes interpretation of CT of the abdomen and pelvis challenging. CT is a more expensive test than US. The greatest advantage of CT is the high-resolution images it produces, including the ability to evaluate air-containing structures such as bowel that are relatively deep to the surface and may not be readily palpable or accessible to US.[8]

MAGNETIC RESONANCE IMAGING

This technique is based on the interaction between atomic nuclei of various tissues and radio waves that are directed through the body in a strong magnetic field. How the mobile nuclei are modified is labeled magnetic relaxation times (T_1 and T_2), which can be measured as a change in the electromagnetic field. The hydrogen atom is used for imaging purposes because it is the most abundant nucleus with a strong magnetic signal. A superconductor-type magnet generates the electromagnetic field by use of large coils reduced to near absolute zero to offer no resistance. In the presence of the strong magnetic field, the randomly oriented protons are aligned in the longitudinal axis. When subjected to a radio frequency in a perpendicular transverse axis, the protons are disrupted in their alignment. Once the pulse is discontinued, they will precess until they resume their alignment in the magnetized field, which can be detected as a voltage.[9] The rate of return to the magnetized state is the T_1 relaxation time and the rate of decay of the transverse signal is the T_2 parameter.[10]

Variations can be added to the magnetic field or the radio waves to highlight various features of the scan. The detail afforded by MRI allows precise characterization in different planes. With the injection of materials with distinct spectroscopic qualities, detailed images can be obtained. The most commonly used agent, gadolinium chelate, is useful in evaluation of solid organs, and enhancement characteristics often aid in differential diagnosis. With rapid injection of gadolinium, blood flow through various vessels can be highlighted, producing an angiography-like study.[11]

No ionizing radiation is involved in MRI, and there are no known biologic side effects from this imaging modality, making it excellent for pediatric applications. Images are, however, very affected by movement, often requiring conscious sedation or anesthesia, and, at times, extended breath-holding is needed to optimize certain acquisitions, something many young children cannot do. Even peristalsis from bowel can produce artifacts. Recent advances have reduced the acquisition times for MRI substantially, making MRI a more practical modality in pediatric settings.[12] Finally, MRI examinations are relatively expensive and sometimes less readily available than CT.

NORMAL APPEARANCE AND ANATOMY AS SEEN WITH CROSS-SECTIONAL IMAGING

Some baseline findings need to be appreciated before looking for abnormalities on any of these imaging modalities. Each modality has some advantages when compared with the other modalities, and they are very often complementary.

LIVER

Normal hepatic parenchyma appears homogeneous on US, with relative increased echogenicity compared with the renal cortex and echogenicity similar to that of the spleen. The vessels of the liver are determined by their point of origin and course.[13] Color Doppler US easily separates vessels, which have slightly echogenic walls, from the biliary tree. On nonenhanced CT, normal liver parenchyma is slightly higher in attenuation than the spleen, with contrasting hypodense vessels. With contrast, the parenchyma enhances uniformly, with vessels that become hyperdense compared with the parenchyma. On MRI, the hepatic parenchyma varies with imaging sequences, with T_1-weighted images showing a higher signal intensity than the spleen and the reverse being true with T_2-weighted images.[14]

On previous classification schemata, the liver was broken down by anatomic lobar divisions; however, a more useful subdivision for the surgeon is based on the vessels that supply the various segments.[15] The right and left hepatic ducts are seen on all cross-sectional imaging studies, anterior to the portal vein bifurcation. The extrahepatic ducts should not measure more than 4 to 7 mm in diameter. In fact, the range within the pediatric population is substantially smaller, with normal ducts usually less than 4 mm.[16] The common bile duct is important to identify and can be seen at the level of the pancreas on MRI or CT. With US or magnetic resonance cholangiopancreatography (MRCP), the entire course of the common duct can be determined, although it is technically often difficult with US owing to overlying bowel gas. The gallbladder is generally pear shaped at the inferior border of the liver and in its normal state is thin walled and enhances after intravenous contrast on CT. On MRI, bile has the same signal as water but may have a higher intensity if it is concentrated in the gallbladder.[17] On heavily T_2-weighted images, the entire biliary tree can be imaged without the use of any contrast agents, producing MRCP of striking detail (Figure 74.2-1).

SPLEEN

The normal spleen on US shows a homogeneous echogenicity, similar to that of the liver, and lies adjacent to the left hemidiaphragm and stomach. The hilum is generally directed medially, and both the splenic vein and artery are easily seen on US. CT will also show homogeneous density with attenuation equal to or slightly lower than that of the liver. Rapid injection of contrast will show heteregeneous uptake initially as a manifestation of variable flow patterns.[18] On MRI, T_1-weighted images show signals of lower intensity than the liver, and T_2-weighted images will show brighter intensity. Intravenous gadolinium causes a similar enhancement pattern of the spleen, as seen on CT scan.

PANCREAS

In children, the entire pancreas is usually not well defined on US because it lies obliquely or transversely in the retroperitoneum and is often obscured in parts by gas in the bowel. The normal pancreas is of uniform, cross-hatched echo-texture and of an echogenicity similar to that of the liver, but it can also be normal and hyperechoic or hypoechoic, especially in children. The normal pancreatic duct, if visualized, is a 2 mm or less tubular structure that runs through the pancreatic body and tail. The common bile duct, as well as either one or two gastroduodenal arteries[19] within the head of the pancreas, can be seen. On

CT, the pancreas is better defined, with borders well highlighted when the adjacent bowel is opacified with oral contrast and blood vessels are highlighted by intravenous contrast, especially if there is retroperitoneal fat. The splenic vein and superior mesenteric vein can be seen posterior to the body. The lateral aspect of the head is nestled by the second and third portions of the duodenum, with the third and fourth portions of the duodenum extending inferior to the pancreas. The attenuation of the pancreas on CT is less than that of the liver.[20] On MRI, the pancreas can also be well displayed; however, thin-section CT is usually easier to obtain and requires shorter study times to produce high-resolution images.

GASTROINTESTINAL TRACT

The gastrointestinal tract is a hollow tube that is either fluid or air filled, and the gas pattern on plain film often dictates the imaging plan. On US, the mucosa of the bowel will appear as an echogenic interface with the echolucent muscularis. Bowel wall thickening can be appreciated, especially if the bowel is fluid filled. Although, more traditionally, the bowel is studied by upper gastrointestinal (UGI) and small bowel follow-through (SBFT) or by barium enema (BE), the bowel can be well studied by CT after the administration of oral and sometimes intravenous contrast. On CT, bowel wall thickening may be appreciated, and inflamed mucosa will enhance after the administration of intravenous contrast. The lumen can be delineated by oral contrast, but mucosal details are better

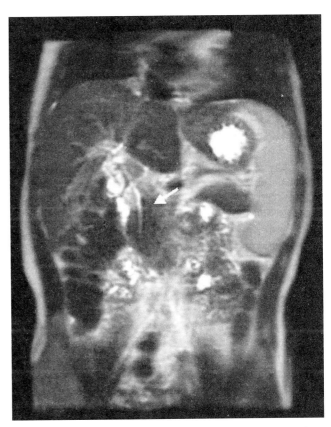

FIGURE 74.2-1 Normal coronal magnetic resonance cholangiopancreatogram reveals a normal extrahepatic bile duct (arrow).

defined by UGI, SBFT, or BE. Inflammatory changes in the mesentery and associated lymphadenopathy are well displayed. MRI is less useful at present for evaluating the bowel, but newer MRI techniques are being investigated to help better define the bowel.

CONGENITAL HEPATOBILIARY ANOMALIES

Anatomic anomalies of the hepatic lobar structure do exist but generally are not of great clinical significance and can be evaluated by CT, US, or MRI. Atresia of a specific lobe of the liver is usually associated with hypertrophy of the remaining lobes and can be an isolated finding or may be associated with other anomalies.[21] Venous anomalies most frequently involve variations in the branching of the portal vein, with the only real clinical significance reserved for the technical aspects that arise during liver transplant. Color Doppler US is probably the best modality for demonstrating most of these vascular variations.[22] Congenital absence of the portal vein, which can also be documented by color Doppler US, is rare and is associated with a multitude of clinical associations, including cardiac defects, extrahepatic biliary atresia, and polysplenia.[23]

Also included under congenital vascular anomalies are vascular malformations, which consist mostly of hemangiomas and, less frequently, arteriovenous malformations. Both can present with high-output heart failure in the newborn period. Infantile hemangiotheliomas and cavernous hemangiomas are both mesenchymal tumors that demonstrate a considerable amount of variability of endothelial proliferation—hence their potential for both growth and involution.[24] Hemangioendotheliomas are the more common vascular liver tumors in infants, almost always presenting before 6 months of age with hepatomegaly and sometimes heart failure, massive bleeding, and uncontrollable coagulopathy. Hemangioendotheliomas can occur as solitary lesions or as multiple hepatic lesions, and probably half are associated with cutaneous hemangiomas.[25–27] Hemangioendotheliomas (Figure 74.2-

2) on US are predominantly hypoechoic, whereas cavernous hemangiomas are hyperechoic, with a very high-velocity flow that can be demonstrated by color flow Doppler US.[28] On unenhanced CT scan, hemangioendotheliomas will show calcification in 40%. After the intravenous injection of contrast, both hemangioendotheliomas and hemangiomas classically show peripheral enhancement and delayed enhancement of the central areas (Figure 74.2-3).[29] Infarction can create considerable variations in enhancement patterns. Small lesions demonstrate homogeneous low signal intensity on T_1-weighted MRI, but larger lesions can be more heterogeneous (Figure 74.2-4). A T_2-weighted MRI will show high signal intensity of small lesions and more heterogeneity of large lesions (Figures 74.2-5 and 74.2-6).[30]

Anomalies of gallbladder position and number are more common than total agenesis, hypoplasia, duplication, and left-sided position. Although US is still the modality of choice to screen for biliary anomalies,[31] radionuclide scans and MRI can also be useful.

Choledochal cysts can be diagnosed at any age and are classified by location and shape. The most common are fusiform dilatation of the common duct (type I), but other variants, such as saccular diverticulum, choledochoceles that extend into the wall of the duodenum, and multiple cystic dilatations, as in Caroli disease (Figure 74.2-7), occur.[32] US is the study of choice for suspected cases (Figures 74.2-8 and 74.2-9), with MRCP used for confirmation and pre-preoperative definition, replacing percutaneous transhepatic cholangiography and endoscopic retrograde cholangiography (Figure 74.2-10).[33] The presentation of choledochal cysts during the neonatal period can be confused with biliary atresia, in which a cystic remnant of the atretic biliary system can remain. Choledochal cysts in later childhood can present with significant obstruction, and other causes of biliary dilatation, such as stone, stricture, or tumor, need to be excluded.[34]

US is often the preliminary study done when biliary

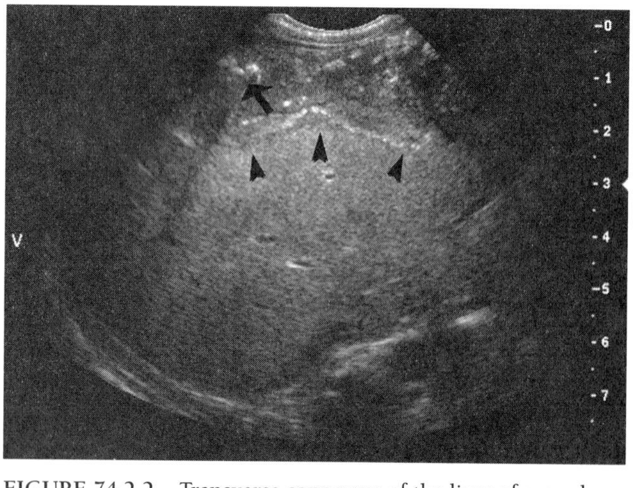

FIGURE 74.2-2   Transverse sonogram of the liver of a newborn infant with a hemangioendothelioma reveals a well-defined hypoechogenic mass with echogenic borders (*arrowheads*). Several echogenic foci with associated shadowing within the mass represent areas of calcification (*arrow*).

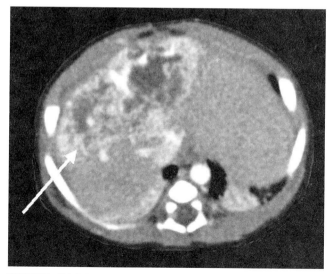

FIGURE 74.2-3   Contrast-enhanced axial computed tomographic scan of an infant with hemangioendothelioma reveals a large mass in the liver with peripheral enhancement (*arrow*).

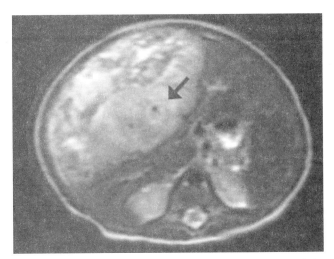

FIGURE 74.2-4 T$_2$-weighted magnetic resonance image of the infant in Figure 74.2-2 reveals the large, well-defined mass to have variable signal characteristics. Calcification appears as a signal void (*arrow*).

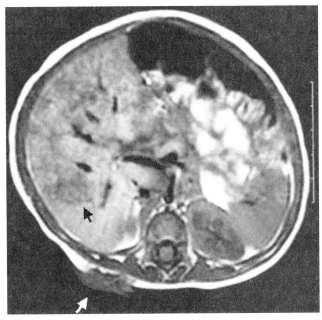

FIGURE 74.2-5 Axial T$_1$-weighted image of the liver of an infant with disseminated hemangiomas reveals multiple soft tissue masses in the liver (one indicated by a *black arrow*) and a soft tissue mass that arises from the posterior back (*white arrow*).

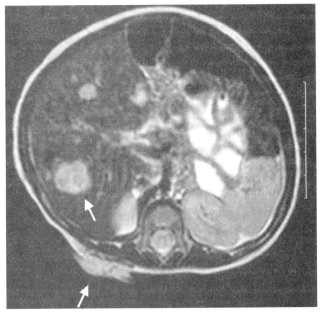

FIGURE 74.2-6 Axial T$_2$-weighted magnetic resonance image reveals that the lesions are of bright signal intensity (*arrows*).

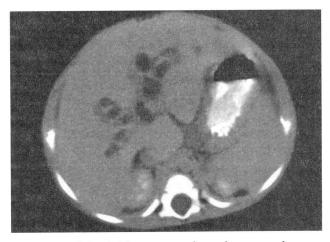

FIGURE 74.2-7 Axial contrast-enhanced computed tomographic scan of the abdomen shows multiple cystic branching structures within the liver in this patient with Caroli disease.

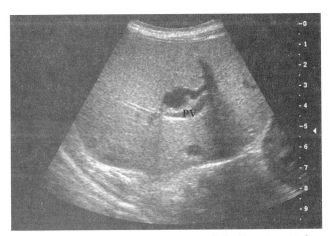

FIGURE 74.2-8 Transverse sonogram of the liver in an infant with a choledochal cyst reveals significant intrahepatic biliary dilatation, seen anterior to the portal vein (PV).

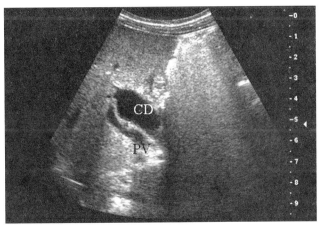

FIGURE 74.2-9 Sagittal sonogram of an infant with cholestasis reveals enlargement of the common duct (CD), consistent with a choledochal abnormality. PV = portal vein.

atresia is suspected; however, the absence of a normal-size gallbladder and failure to delineate the extrahepatic duct on US is suggestive but not conclusive. Documentation of the triangular cord, a periportal band of fibrotic tissue, both on US[35] and more recently on CT,[36] has been shown to correlate well with the documentation of biliary atresia at the time of surgical exploration. There was initial enthusiasm for MRCP for evaluating infants with cholestasis, but MRI is no more sensitive or specific than other modalities, including radionucleotide scanning, with a 75% positive predictive rate and roughly a 90% negative predictive rate[37] for biliary atresia. MRCP (Figure 74.2-11) does have the advantages of not requiring pretreatment and not using ionizing radiation,[38] and it has been shown to be extremely helpful in supporting the diagnosis of biliary atresia in late-presenters, in whom the morbidity and mortality of exploratory laparotomy are especially increased.[37]

Congenital Splenic Anomalies

The shape and position of the spleen can be quite variable and are not of clinical significance. Splenic clefts are common, as is persistent fetal lobulation, and both can occasionally be confused with lacerations.[39] US is generally adequate for most examinations, but CT will yield better images. The orientation of the hilum can be variable, and laxity of the ligamentous attachment can result in a mobile spleen. Occasionally, a "wandering spleen" can be confused for a neoplasm or can result in torsion.[40] Accessory spleens or splenules (Figure 74.2-12) occur in 10% or more of healthy individuals and are typically near the splenic hilum.[39] These are usually at least 2 cm in diameter to be visualized by radionucleotide scanning. Although not clinically significant,

accessory spleens can hypertrophy after splenectomy or in patients with splenomegaly (Figure 74.2-13). Primary asplenia is not common and with polysplenia falls into the category of situs anomalies or heterotaxy syndromes (Figure 74.2-14), half of which are associated with cardiac and renal malformations and many with immunodeficiency. Because of the complexity and variability of the heterotaxy syndromes, US, followed by MRI, CT, and sometimes red blood cell–tagged radionuclide scanning, is helpful for full delineation.[41] True congenital splenic cysts are extremely rare, and those less than 5 cm can be managed conservatively.[42]

Pancreas

Most congenital anomalies of the pancreas involve anatomic variations of the ductal system. Numerous series have reported the inadequacies of US and CT and the need for endoscopic retrograde cholangiopancreatography (ERCP) to delineate ductal anatomy. Most recently, MRCP has proved useful in defining pancreatic duct anatomy.[43] Pancreas divisum (Figure 74.2-15) is a common anomaly that arguably may predispose the patient to pancreatitis.[44] Hypoplasia and agenesis of the pancreas have been reported but are extremely rare. Isolated congenital cysts and cystic disease of the pancreas are associated with polycystic disease of the kidneys and liver,[45] as well as the rare case of von Hippel-Lindau disease (Figures 74.2-16 and 74.2-17). Annular pancreas, which typically presents in the newborn period with bilious vomiting, is generally not diagnosed by cross-sectional imaging but rather by UGI series. Variations of annular pancreas have been reported in adults and can be imaged by MRI.

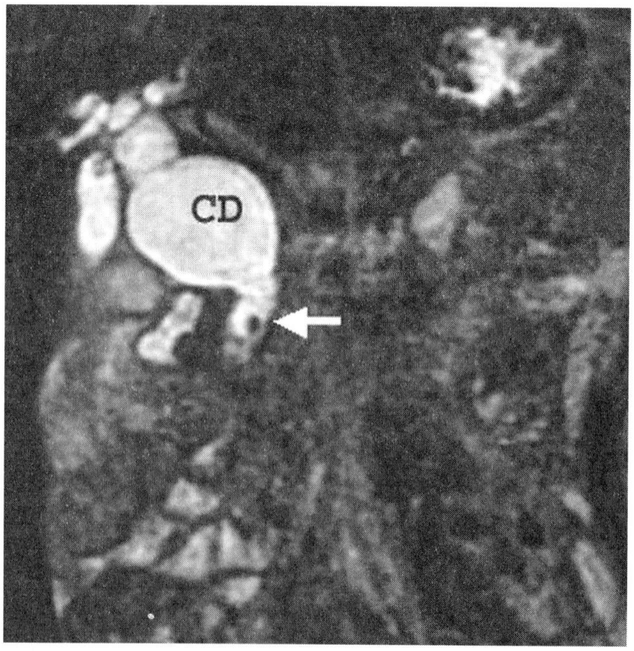

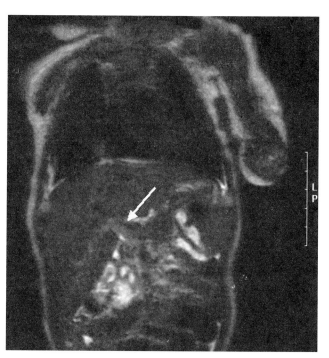

FIGURE 74.2-10 *Coronal magnetic resonance cholangiopancreatogram of an infant with jaundice reveals marked enlargement of the extrahepatic bile duct consistent with a type I choledochal cyst. A signal void in the distal end was caused by a stone* (arrow). *CD = common duct.*

FIGURE 74.2-11 *Coronal magnetic resonance cholangiopancreatography failed to reveal the extrahepatic biliary system in this infant evaluated for cholestasis. A chord of tissue was present in the anticipated location* (arrow). *Biliary atresia was confirmed at laparotomy.*

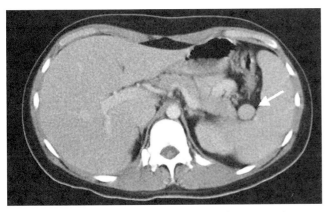

FIGURE 74.2-12 Axial contrast-enhanced computed tomographic scan of the abdomen reveals a small, well-defined mass (*arrow*) in the splenic hilum, of identical attenuation to normal spleen.

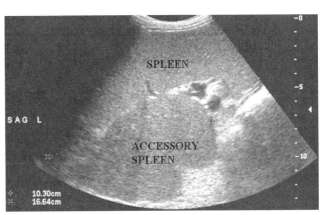

FIGURE 74.2-13 Sagittal sonogram of the left upper quadrant of a patient with Jeune syndrome, a rare cause of hepatic fibrosis, reveals an enlarged spleen. A large mass of identical echogenicity in the splenic hilum is consistent with an accessory spleen.

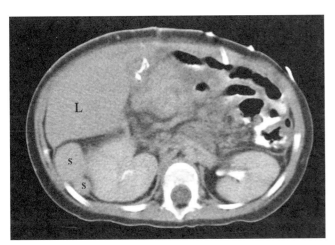

FIGURE 74.2-14 Axial contrast-enhanced computed tomographic scan of the abdomen reveals several small spleens (s) on the right, inferior to the liver (L) in this patient with heterotaxy syndrome.

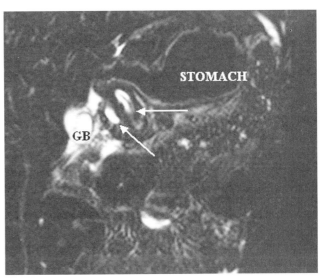

FIGURE 74.2-15 Coronal magnetic resonance cholangiopancreatography was performed in this 5-year-old female with recurrent pancreatitis. A dual drainage (*arrows*) system was seen in the head of the pancreas consistent with pancreas divisum. GB = gallbladder.

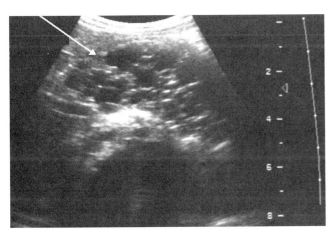

FIGURE 74.2-16 Transverse sonogram of a 7-month-old male with a palpable mass reveals that the pancreas is replaced by multiple cysts (*arrow*).

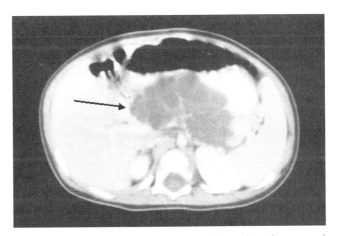

FIGURE 74.2-17 Follow-up contrast-enhanced axial computed tomographic scan of a 7-month-old boy confirms that the pancreas is replaced by multiple cysts (*arrow*) and no other cysts were present in other intra-abdominal organs. A diagnosis of von Hippel-Lindau disease was subsequently made.

GASTROINTESTINAL TRACT

Numerous congenital malformations of the esophagus and the remaining gastrointestinal tract exist, including esophageal duplication cysts, which may be detected on CT (Figure 74.2-18).[46] Vascular rings and impinging vessels, traditionally suggested by UGI series and confirmed by angiography, can now be well demonstrated by either CT or MRI (Figure 74.2-19).[47] Although antral webs and pyloric atresia can occasionally be seen on US as an intraluminal diaphragm of linear echo density within a fluid-filled cavity,[48] UGI or endoscopy remains the mainstay of diagnosis. High obstructions of the gastrointestinal tract, such as duodenal atresia, are readily suggested by a fluid-filled "double bubble" on prenatal US but are typically confirmed in the newborn period by UGI and not cross-sectional imaging. Low obstruction in the neonatal period may be caused by intrauterine perforation, resulting in meconium peritonitis, which calcifies and is evident on plain film. In this clinical situation, US is extremely useful in distinguishing active peritonitis and surgical emergency from a healed perforation by the detection of intra-abdominal fluid. Absence of fluid suggests recannalization and resolution in utero, allowing these infants to be fed and clinically monitored. Encysted collections of meconium will show a heterogeneous appearance on US.[49] Duplication and intestinal cysts, unless detected on prenatal US, generally present later in childhood. Duplication cysts most commonly occur in the distal ileum and esophagus, usually do not communicate with the intestinal lumen, and may or may not cause obstruction. US can be useful to define these fluid-filled lesions when intra-abdominal, and the presence of a double-walled sign helps distinguish gastrointestinal cysts from single-walled simple mesenteric cysts (Figure 74.2-20).[50] MRCP is helpful in distinguishing gastric duplication cysts from cysts of biliary origin (Figure 74.2-21).

Although hypertrophic pyloric stenosis does not usually present at birth but typically after the first month of

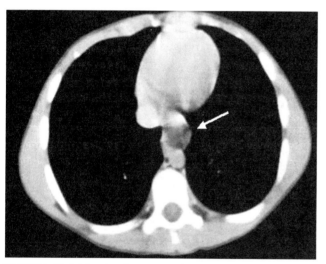

FIGURE 74.2-18   Axial computed tomographic scan of the lower chest of a 5-year-old boy with a history of dysphasia reveals a cystic mass adjacent to the esophagus (*arrow*), consistent with a duplication.

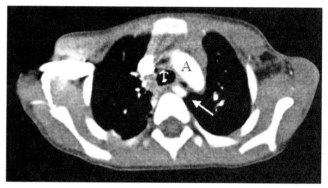

FIGURE 74.2-19   Contrast-enhanced multislice computed tomographic angiography demonstrating an aberrant subclavian artery.

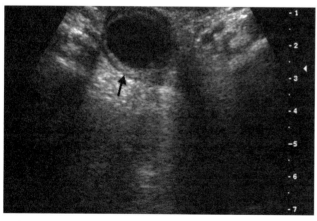

FIGURE 74.2-20   Sonogram of the right lower quadrant was performed on a newborn infant because of an abnormal prenatal sonogram. The presence of a cystic mass (*arrow*) was confirmed. The double wall suggests that it arises from the bowel as opposed to a simple cyst of another origin, such as the ovary or mesentery.

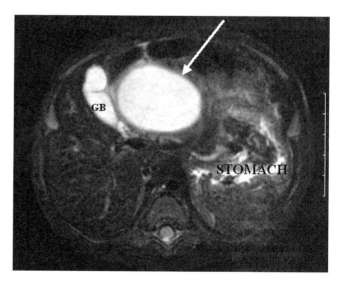

FIGURE 74.2-21   Axial magnetic resonance cholangiopancreatogram of a 4-month-old girl with a history of vomiting and cystic mass seen on ultrasonography demonstrates that the mass (*arrow*) arises in close proximity to the lesser curvature of the stomach and appeared separate from the gallbladder (GB), biliary system, and liver. A gastric duplication cyst was successfully resected.

life, it can be classified under congenital lesions of the stomach. The condition results from hypertrophy of the circular muscle of the pylorus, causing both thickening and elongating. The typical finding on physical examination is the palpated "olive" of hypertrophied muscle. When this cannot be felt, US is the study of choice to demonstrate the increased thickness and the increased length of the pyloric muscle (Figure 74.2-22).[51]

CROSS-SECTIONAL IMAGING IN ABDOMINAL TRAUMA

In pediatric settings, there is much less experience with penetrating injuries than with blunt trauma. With the increasing tendency toward conservative, nonoperative management of abdominal trauma, precise imaging of the abdomen is of the utmost importance. The liver is still the most frequently injured organ; however, in 20% of cases, multiple organs are involved. In general, contrast-enhanced CT is the recommended modality for diagnosing traumatic injury, with US reserved for serial follow-up examinations.[52] The use of imaging is both to detect specific injuries such as lacerations and subcapsular hematomas and to search for peritoneal fluid that might indicate impending clinical compromise.

Parenchymal disruption to the liver can vary from small lacerations to extensive fractures with significant extravasation of blood. Lacerations can be simple or complex and on CT (Figure 74.2-23) appear hypodense in either a linear, round, or stellate shape. Subscapular hematomas (Figure 74.2-24) vary in density according to the amount of blood loss and hematocrit, and tears in the capsule will allow blood to fill the peritoneal spaces. Traumatic injuries to the spleen (Figure 74.2-25) are very

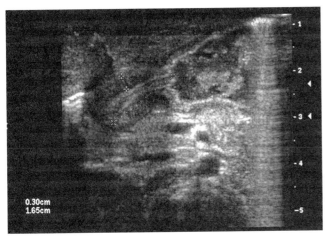

FIGURE 74.2-22 Hypertrophic pyloric stenosis. Transverse sonogram of the abdomen in an infant with nonbilious vomiting reveals both elongation of the pyloric channel (x) and thickening of the muscle (+), consistent with the diagnosis of hypertrophic pyloric stenosis.

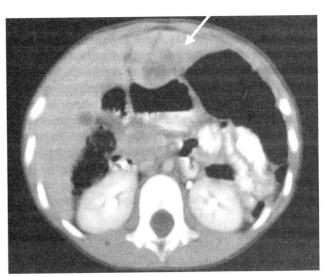

FIGURE 74.2-23 Axial contrast-enhanced computed tomographic scan of the abdomen was performed in this 11-year-old boy after a fall. Laceration of the left lobe of the liver is evident (arrow).

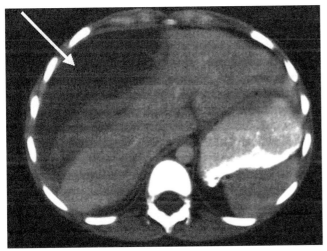

FIGURE 74.2-24 Contrast-enhanced computed tomographic scan of the liver of a 10 year old after a sledding accident reveals a large subcapsular hematoma peripheral to a lacerated liver (arrow).

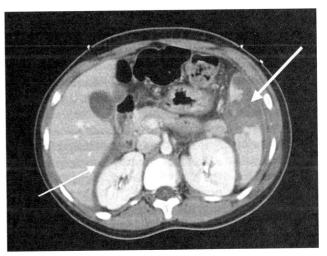

FIGURE 74.2-25 Contrast-enhanced axial computed tomographic scan performed after a motor vehicle accident on this 11-year-old boy reveals a fractured spleen (thick arrow) and free ascites, presumably blood, in Morrison pouch (thin arrow).

similar in CT appearance and are easily missed on initial US because acute injuries may appear isoechoic. US should be reserved for serial examinations of known injuries (Figure 74.2-26).

Much debate has surrounded the management of patients with blunt abdominal trauma. Most clinicians agree that in clinical settings in which surgical intervention is not necessary, there is little need for follow-up CT scans.[53] US is usually adequate for following the evolution from poorly defined and iso- or hyperechoic to less echoic and smaller because liquefaction and organization occur over time.[54] Complications, such as the formation of cysts, bile lakes, infarctions, and calcifications, can also be determined by US[55] but are best defined by CT with contrast.

Contrast-enhanced multidetector CT angiography[56] has largely replaced angiography in the screening for arterial vascular injury, and interventional angiography with embolization has reduced the need for surgery in a significant number of cases.[57] Contrast-enhanced multidetector CT can be very useful in determining active hemorrhage but is inadequate in diagnosing disruption of the bile ducts, whereas radionucleotide scanning is useful in diagnosing suspected bile leaks.[58]

CT is the modality of choice for detecting trauma to the pancreas, which can be manifested by enlargement, edema, or complete transection (Figure 74.2-27), as well as pseudocyst formation. US is useful to follow pseudocysts, but pancreatic duct injury is best seen on MRCP.[59]

Hollow viscus gastrointestinal tract, namely the stomach and small and large intestine, is also subject to blunt trauma. CT is able to detect bowel and mesenteric injuries in greater than 90% of cases but cannot necessarily differentiate the need for surgical intervention.[60] Free air from perforation is readily identified on CT. Bowel wall hematomas are sometimes more readily seen on UGI and SBFT, and water-soluble studies should be obtained if clinically suspect.[61] Focused abdominal US for trauma has been advocated, but the high false-negative rate supports the use of CT for all significant injuries.[62]

TUMORS

Approximately 5% of all intra-abdominal masses, benign and malignant, occur in the liver, and of all pediatric malignancies, almost 2% are primary hepatic.[15] US is the preferred initial examination for lesions that are either purely cystic or typical for benign hemangiomata, seen as small, well-defined, echogenic masses. Serial US is recommended to follow these benign findings. Contrast-enhanced CT and MRI both provide further definition of all other liver masses. CT-guided biopsies may be used for diagnosis.[62,63]

MALIGNANT HEPATIC TUMORS

Hepatoblastoma is the most common primary malignancy of the gastrointestinal tract in children and is the third most common abdominal malignancy after Wilms tumor and neuroblastoma.[15] Hepatoblastoma usually presents at a median of 1 year of age as a painless, solitary lesion, but it may be multifocal. Serum α-fetoprotein is elevated in 90% of patients, and metastasis occurs in up to 20%. Plain films will show calcifications in up to 55%. On US, there is usually a large, well-outlined, predominantly echogenic mass. CT will show any calcifications present in the mass well, and with intravenous contrast, there will be heterogeneous enhancement, usually related to hemorrhage and/or necrosis within the tumor. MRI also reveals a solid mass that typically enhances irregularly after the administration of gadolinium (Figures 74.2-28 and 74.2-29). Calcifications are not well seen on MRI but rather appear as signal voids.[64]

Hepatocellular carcinoma (HCC) (Figure 74.2-30) is more common in older children and is typically associated with some progressive, preexisting liver disease, such as chronic hepatitis, tyrosinemia, or glycogen storage disease. HCC is more often multifocal and infiltrative. In the setting of end-stage liver disease, it can be difficult to distinguish from diseased parenchyma on all imaging modalities. Small lesions are typically hyperechoic on US, whereas larger lesions are generally mixed. Color Doppler US is useful to demonstrate low-resistance tumor flow, as

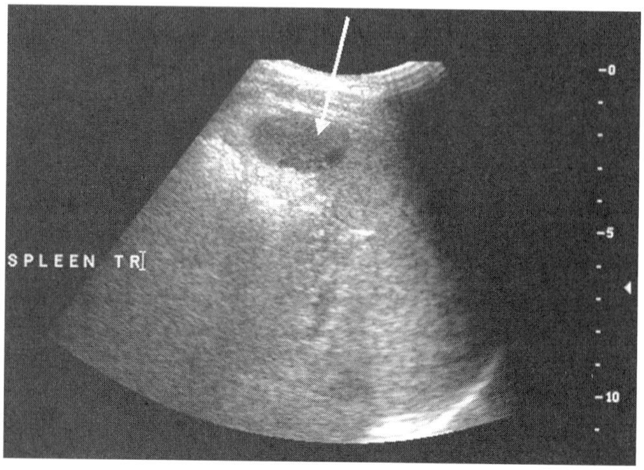

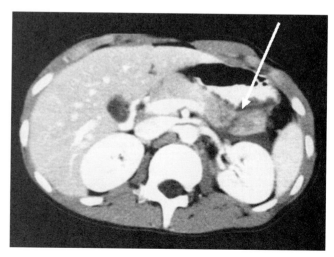

FIGURE 74.2-26   Transverse ultrasonography was used to follow the fractured spleen serially. Six months after the initial trauma, a hypoechoic area was still visualized (*arrow*) consistent with an organizing hematoma.

FIGURE 74.2-27   Contrast-enhanced axial computed tomographic scan of a 10-year-old boy who was struck by an automobile reveals a complete transection of the pancreas (*arrow*).

well as thrombosis of the adjacent veins by tumor extension if present.[65,66] Nonenhanced CT will show poorly defined masses, but after the intravenous administration of contrast, HCC usually demonstrates intense enhancement secondary to its hypervascular nature. Calcifications are unusual.[67] HCC is typically of low signal intensity on T_1-weighted MRI and hyperintense on T_2-weighted imaging. Gadolinium-enhanced imaging demonstrates a hypervascular tumor, similar to a contrast-enhanced CT scan.[68,69]

Fibrolamellar carcinoma is a very rare hepatic neoplasm but is often discussed in the differential diagnosis of HCC, despite very different features and presentation. In contrast to HCC, patients with fibrolamellar carcinoma are usually symptomatic, have normal serum α-fetoprotein, do not have predisposing liver disease, and carry a much poorer prognosis.[70] The tumors are usually solitary and lobulated, with a distinguishing central

fibrous scar that is typically hyperechoic on US and at times calcified. On nonenhanced CT, the lesion, and especially the central scar, is well demarcated and of low attenuation relative to the surrounding normal liver. With the administration of intravenous contrast, the entire tumor, but not the central scar, will enhance. On MRI, the lesion will appear of low signal intensity on T_1-weighted images and of high signal intensity on T_2-weighted images, with failure of the central scar to enhance after the injection of gadolinium (Figure 74.2-31).[71] The presence of a central scar, although help-

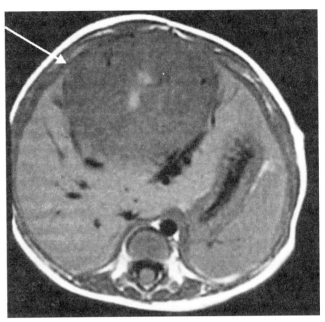

FIGURE 74.2-29 T_1-weighted axial magnetic resonance image of the abdomen of an infant reveals a large, well-defined mass (*arrow*) with a central area of high signal, which was proven to represent a hepatoblastoma with central hemorrhage.

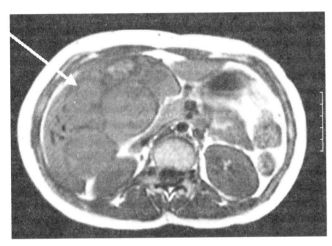

FIGURE 74.2-28 Axial T_1-weighted magnetic resonance image of an 11-year-old girl with a firm liver reveals a multilobulated solid mass within the liver (*arrow*), which was subsequently proven to be a hepatoblastoma.

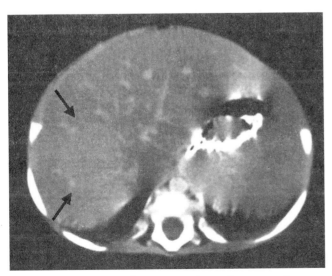

FIGURE 74.2-30 Axial contrast-enhanced computed tomographic scan of the abdomen of a 12-year-old girl who was hepatitis B positive reveals a well-defined mass in the posterior right lobe (*arrows*). Biopsy revealed hepatocellular carcinoma.

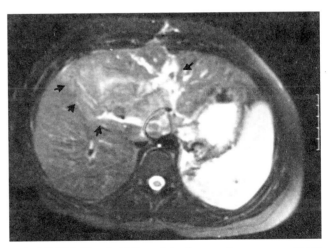

FIGURE 74.2-31 Axial T_2-weighted magnetic resonance image of a 16-year-old girl with a firm liver mass reveals a poorly defined mass (*arrows*) with a large central scar of increased signal after the administration of gadolinium. The patient underwent a computed tomography–guided biopsy that confirmed fibrolamellar carcinoma. Enhancement of the central scar is more typical for focal nodular hyperplasia.

ful, is not diagnostic because it can also be seen in focal nodular hyperplasia (FNH) and giant hemangiomas.

The fourth most common pediatric hepatic tumor is the undifferentiated embryonal sarcoma, which may be difficult to differentiate from a mesenchymal hamartoma. Unlike the latter, embryonal sarcoma often presents with symptoms of pain or mass. On US, it is usually solitary and echogenic, with small anechoic areas that probably represent cystic necrosis.[72] Nonenhanced CT shows a well-demarcated, low-attenuation mass. On contrast-enhanced CT, septations become evident. The lesion tends to be of low signal intensity on both T_1- and T_2-weighted MRIs, with enhancement of the tumor contrasting with low signal of the septa[73] after gadolinium administration.

As in adults, tumors of the biliary tree are much less common than hepatic tumors, and the prognosis is much worse. Embryonal rhabdomyosarcoma is probably the only one in this category that is seen at all in children, and it usually presents with jaundice. US will show biliary obstruction as well as an inhomogeneous echogenic mass, typically in the porta hepatis. CT shows a low-attenuation mass with some enhancement with contrast, and MRCP will show irregular, berry-like filling defects within the biliary system.[74]

Secondary malignant tumors of the liver occur, most commonly from neuroblastoma, Wilms tumor, lymphoma (Figure 74.2-32), and leukemia. All can be diffuse or focal. Immunosuppressed patients can develop post-transplant lymphoproliferative disease (PTLD) with various lesions that range from polyclonal B-cell hyperplasia to malignant lymphoma. Hepatic metastases from other tumors occur rather late in the disease process and carry a poor prognosis. The value of US in detecting lesions depends on the primary tumor and the pattern of metastasis, and even the presence of hepatomegaly is not useful.[75] CT with contrast can be more useful but may require dual-phase arterial and venous scanning for full evaluation. MRI with and without gadolinium is also sensitive for detection of focal liver lesions.

BENIGN HEPATIC TUMORS

FNH is an uncommon epithelial lesion in childhood, more often seen in middle-aged women. In children, it is usually an incidental finding, as a solitary lesion of less than 5 cm in size, without internal hemorrhage or necrosis. The distinguishing feature is a central fibrous scar, which is vascular and extends outward into fibrous septa. On US, FNH is a well-demarcated, either iso- or hyperechoic lesion, with a central scar demonstrated in 20% of cases. Associated calcifications are rare enough to suggest another pathology.[76] On nonenhanced CT, the lesion appears as a hypo- or isodense lesion that enhances after the administration of contrast but becomes isodense on delayed scans. The central scar in FNH will enhance in 70% of cases, helping to distinguish FNH from fibrolamellar carcinoma, in which the scar typically does not enhance. On T_1-weighted MRIs, FNH appears as a lesion of decreased or isointensity, and on T_2-weighted images, the signal intensity increases. After the administration of gadolinium, over 80% of cases will show enhancement of the central scar,[48] again distinguishing FNH from fibrolamellar carcinoma (Figures 74.2-33 and 74.2-34).

Hepatocellular adenoma is a rare epithelial tumor with an increasing incidence secondary to oral contraceptive and androgen use. Hepatocellular adenomas are also reported in association with glycogen storage disease type Ia and diabetes. In 80% of cases, hepatocellular adenoma is a solitary, well-circumscribed, and encapsulated mass. The US appearance can be variable, depending on the presence of lipid or internal hemorrhage.[77] On nonenhanced CT, the lesions are generally of decreased attenuation, with 50% containing calcifications (Figure 74.2-35). After the injection of intravenous contrast, feeding vessels may be identified.[78] The lesions have a variable appearance on MRI. Gadolinium is useful to identify feeding vessels.[79] Serial US

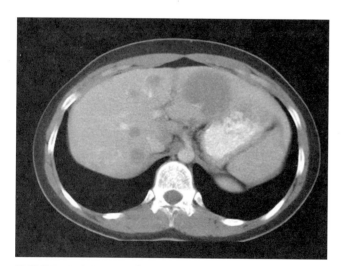

FIGURE 74.2-32 Axial contrast-enhanced computed tomographic scan of the abdomen of an 18-year-old female patient with night sweats reveals multiple low-attenuation masses within the liver. Bone marrow biopsy was consistent with B-cell lymphoma.

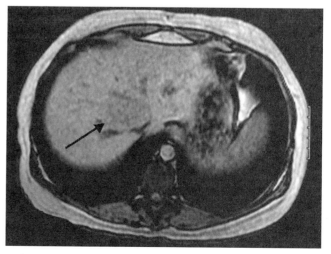

FIGURE 74.2-33 Axial magnetic resonance image of a 14-year-old asymptomatic girl followed for a liver mass discovered incidentally during renal ultrasonography shows a well-defined low signal lesion (*arrow*) with a central scar. Differential diagnosis was fibrolamellar carcinoma versus focal nodular hyperplasia.

examinations, in conjunction with monitoring the serum α-fetoprotein level, are recommended to screen for malignant degeneration, seen as sudden growth, necrosis, or a change to a heterogeneous appearance.[80]

Mesenchymal hamartomas, like most hamartomas, should probably be considered as developmental anomalies rather than true neoplasms. They contain gelatinous serous fluid in cystic spaces, intermixed with biliary ductal and connective tissue. On US, mesenchymal hamartomas are predominantly cystic, with multiple echogenic septa (Figure 74.2-36). Their appearance is similar on CT scan (Figure 74.2-37) and MRI (Figure 74.2-38).[81] Occasionally, mesenchymal hamartomas present as purely cystic lesions (Figure 74.2-39). Serial US examinations aid in distinguishing simple liver cysts (Figures 74.2-40 and 74.2-41) from cystic hamartoma; the latter tend to grow

and change in appearance, and may develop more solid components with time.[82]

Related and more common entities are mesenchymal tumors, which include hemangiomas, hemangioendotheliomas, and lipomas. The first two have been discussed in part above. Cavernous hemangiomas are more commonly seen in adults than in children. Lipomas, benign masses of mature adipose tissue, are rarely seen in children.

SPLENIC TUMORS

Splenic tumors are in general rare and can be divided between cystic lesions and solid neoplasia. Cysts are classified as true cysts, pseudocysts, and parasitic cysts. True cysts (Figures 74.2-42 and 74.2-43) have an epithelial lin-

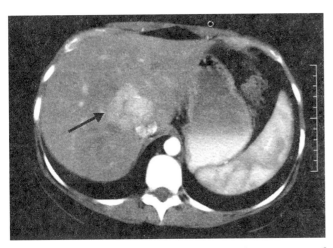

FIGURE 74.2-34   After the intravenous administration of gadolinium, there is intense enhancement of the mass (*arrow*) but not the central scar, a finding suggestive of fibrolamellar carcinoma rather than focal nodular hyperplasia. α-Fetoprotein remained normal, and the mass has remained stable in size for 5 years, findings more suggestive of focal nodular hyperplasia.

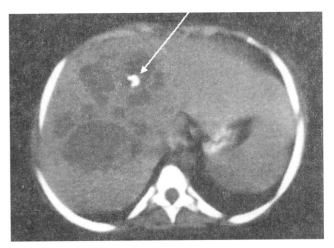

FIGURE 74.2-35   Non–contrast-enhanced computed tomographic scan of a 10-year-old girl with type IV glycogen storage disease reveals a large low-attenuation mass within the liver. A central calcification (*arrow*) was present. It was resected, and the diagnosis of giant adenoma was made.

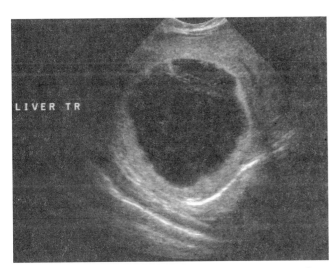

FIGURE 74.2-36   Sonogram of the liver of a newborn with an enlarged liver reveals a complex cyst within the liver, containing multiple septations. It was resected, and histopathology revealed a cystic hamartoma.

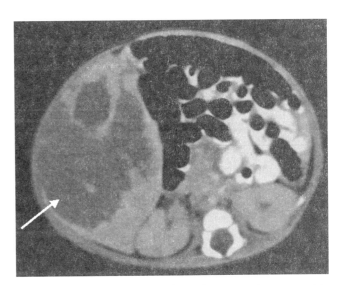

FIGURE 74.2-37   Contrast-enhanced computed tomographic scan of the liver demonstrates that a large portion of the liver has been replaced by cystic and solid tumor. Peripheral enhancement was seen. The patient underwent a three-quadrant resection for this hamartoma. The arrow demonstrates the cystic hamartoma within normal liver parenchyma.

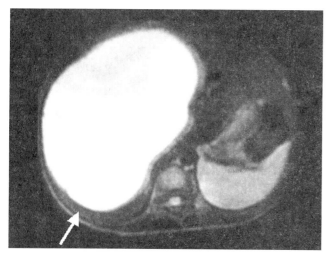

FIGURE 74.2-38 T₂-weighted axial magnetic resonance image of the abdomen of this infant with an enlarged liver reveals a large cystic mass (*arrow*). It was unroofed, but pathology was consistent with a cystic hamartoma rather than a simple liver cyst. It regrew with more solid components, and the patient underwent a successful wide resection of this tumor.

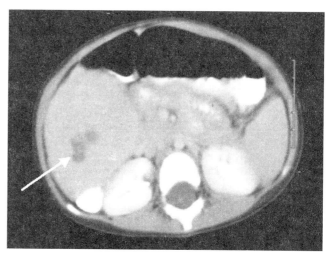

FIGURE 74.2-39 Axial contrast-enhanced computed tomographic scan of the abdomen of a 5 year old with right upper quadrant pain reveals a multilobulated cystic mass within the liver, which was subsequently proven to be a mesenchymal hamartoma.

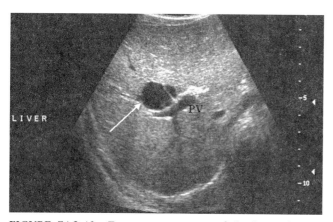

FIGURE 74.2-40 Transverse sonogram of the liver of an 8-month-old girl shows a multilobulated cyst within the liver above the portal vein (PV).

ing and are sometimes termed congenital epidermoids (Figure 74.2-44). They may contain brightly reflective echoes within them from floating crystals. Pseudocysts, which contain no epithelial lining, are believed to be secondary to infection, trauma, or infarction and cannot be distinguished from true cysts radiologically. Some neoplasms, such as lymphangioma, hemangioma, and hamartoma, may appear largely cystic on US. Septations and rim calcifications may be present.[83] Hemorrhage or protein content can increase the attenuation on CT. MRI will also demonstrate true solid lesions (Figure 74.2-45).

Splenic involvement by lymphoma and leukemia presents in several ways. On US, homogeneous enlargement with normal echogenicity, solitary or multifocal hypoechoic lesions, or diffuse infiltration with heterogeneous echogenicity can be seen. CT and MRI demonstrate similar findings, although MRI may be less useful because lymphomatous tissue can have signal intensity similar to that of normal splenic tissue.[55]

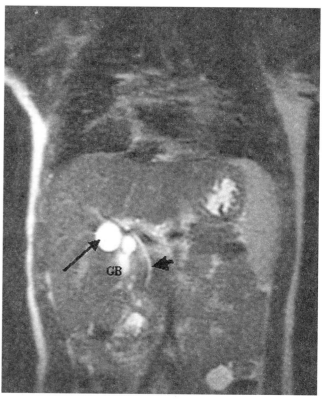

FIGURE 74.2-41 Follow-up coronal magnetic resonance cholangiopancreatogram confirms that the cysts (long *arrow*) are within the liver and separate from the biliary system. The normal extrahepatic duct is demarcated by the *short arrow*. A portion of the gallbladder (GB) is also seen.

PANCREATIC TUMORS

Pancreatic tumors are a very small percentage of pediatric intra-abdominal tumors and usually present with either a mass, abdominal distention, or a variety of endocrine abnormalities. Atypically, they present with the more usual adult presentation of bowel obstruction, weight loss, or jaundice.[84] These tumors can be classified into nonfunc-

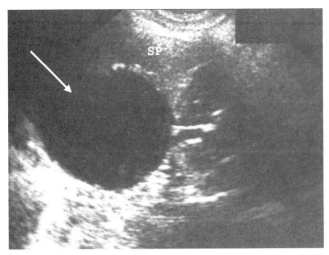

FIGURE 74.2-42 Sagittal sonogram of the left upper quadrant reveals a simple cyst (*arrow*) arising from the spleen (SP).

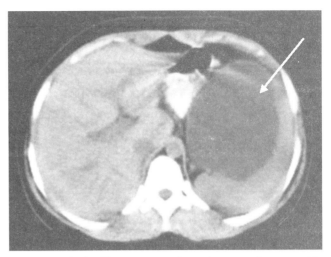

FIGURE 74.2-43 Non–contrast enhanced computed tomographic scan demonstrates a large cyst arising from the spleen (*arrow*).

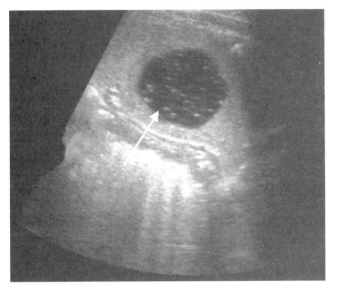

FIGURE 74.2-44 Sagittal sonogram of the spleen reveals a central cyst with particular echoes dispersed throughout. This is a typical appearance for an epidermoid cyst (*arrow*).

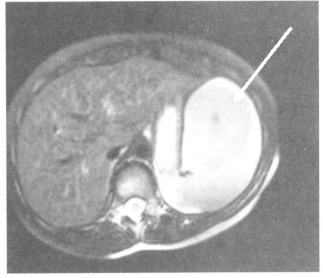

FIGURE 74.2-45 Axial T_2-weighted magnetic resonance image of the abdomen reveals a solid mass with a central scar arising from the spleen, which was subsequently proven to be a hamartoma (*arrow*).

tioning and functioning tumors, as well as malignant or benign tumors.[85] Pancreatoblastomas usually occur before 8 years of age as large, well-defined masses, with both cystic and solid components arising from the body or tail. Although pancreatoblastomas can be seen on US, CT is better at fully defining these tumors and demonstrating any associated calcifications.[86] Solid and papillary epithelial neoplasm is a rare, low-grade malignancy that typically occurs in young adult women, but a third of cases are described in adolescents. These tumors typically have cystic areas, as well as areas of hemorrhage and calcification, producing a very heterogeneous appearance on imaging studies (Figure 74.2-46).[87] Acute lymphocytic leukeumia is a rare cause of diffuse pancreatic infiltration and enlargement (Figure 74.2-47).[88] Thin-section contrast-enhanced CT is the best modality to image the pancreas because it is unaffected by overlying bowel gas, which can obscure the pancreas on US. Functioning pancreatic tumors, including

insulinoma, gastrinoma, and VIPoma, are notoriously difficult to image, especially because these lesions may be very small. Gadolinium-enhanced MRI, which can depict subtle changes in tissue planes, may be of benefit in the detection of small tumors.[89]

GASTROINTESTINAL TUMORS

Primary malignancies such as adenocarcinoma, lymphoma, and sarcoma are rarely reported in childhood. Cross-sectional imaging is most useful for staging to determine the extent of tumor and the presence of metastatic disease. In general, intra-abdominal lymph nodes in excess of 1 cm should raise suspicion.[90] Primary lymphoma is rare, occurring most commonly in the ileocecal region, followed by gastric origin.[91] Polyps can sometimes be detected on US as incidental findings. The use of compression US in unprepared patients can be useful. Juvenile polyps may appear almost cystic on US but vascular on color flow

Doppler US.[92] Desmoid tumors, encountered in association with familial polyposis, are not malignant but can be quite aggressive (Figure 74.2-48).[93] PTLD can present in the immunosuppressed patient as nonspecific hepatosplenomegaly or focal masses within the bowel wall, organs, or lymph nodes. US and CT combined will detect up to three-quarters of cases of PTLD (Figure 74.2-49).[94]

INFECTIOUS PROCESSES

The most common infectious processes that affect the liver are abscesses and hepatitis. Fungal, bacterial, or other infectious abscesses are more commonly seen in immunocompromised children, those with human immunodeficiency virus (HIV), chronic granulomatous disease, or leukemia or on immunosuppression therapy following organ transplant or for treatment of diseases

such as inflammatory bowel disease (IBD). US is an excellent initial study and a useful guide for diagnostic biopsy. Fungal abscesses are usually small and multiple and appear on US as "target" lesions, with a central echogenic focus surrounded by a hypochoic rim. On contrast-enhanced CT, the central area enhances within the low-attenuation lesions.[95] Bacterial abscesses tend to be singular, round, and located in the periphery. A hypoechoic halo may be seen on US.[96] Similarly on CT and MRI, pyogenic abscesses are well-defined, low-density lesions that demonstrate peripheral enhancement after contrast administration.[97] Staphylococcal abscesses can also present as target lesions. Amebic or hydatid abscesses can be difficult to diffentiate from pyogenic abscesses.[98] Echinococcosis is endemic in certain parts of the world, and two-thirds of cases will involve only the liver. US, CT, or MRI will show either single or a few very large cysts,

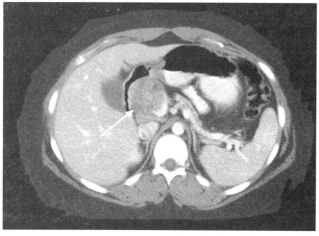

FIGURE 74.2-46   Contrast-enhanced axial computed tomographic scan of the abdomen of a 13-year-old girl with abdominal pain reveals a solid tumor in the head of the pancreas (*arrow*). The patient underwent a modified Whipple procedure for what proved to be a cystadenoma.

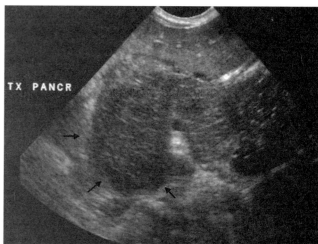

FIGURE 74.2-47   Transverse sonogram of a 3-week-old female infant showed marked enlargement of the pancreas. The echotexture appears decreased. The patient was diagnosed with acute lymphocytic leukemia. *Arrows* indicate the leukemic infiltration.

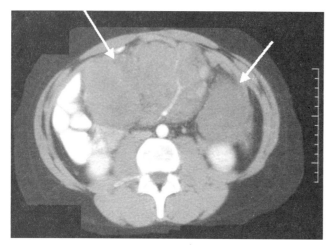

FIGURE 74.2-48   Axial contrast-enhanced computed tomographic scan of the lower abdomen of a 14-year-old boy who underwent a total colectomy for familial polyposis demonstrates bulky soft tissue masses (*arrows*). The patient was diagnosed with Gardner syndrome and desmoid tumors.

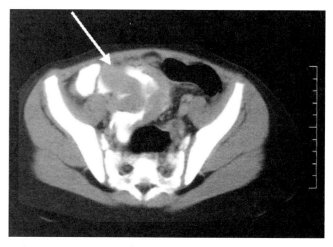

FIGURE 74.2-49   Axial contrast-enhanced computed tomographic scan of the pelvis of a 6-year-old female heart recipient on immunosuppression shows a large soft tissue mass encasing loops of bowel (*arrow*). Biopsy confirmed the diagnosis of monoclonal lymphoproliferative disease.

sometimes with calcifications (Figure 74.2-50). Perforation into the biliary tree has been reported.[99]

In general, most children with acute hepatitis have a normal US examination, although diffuse hepatomegaly may be present and echogenicity may be either increased or decreased.[31] Thickening of the gallbladder wall is sometimes seen in acute hepatitis as well as a contraction of the total volume of the gallbladder.[100] In certain settings, as with ingestion of a fatty meal, paradoxical dilatation of the gallbladder can also be seen on US.[101] CT and MRI will show similar nonspecific changes. Assorted neonatal infections, including cytomegalovirus, toxoplasmosis, and coxsackievirus, have been associated with parenchymal liver calcifications. Interestingly, infections in older children rarely result in calcifications.[102]

Splenic abscesses appear hypoechoic on US, with low attenuation on CT and with high fluid content on MRI. Peripheral enhancement after contrast administration is seen on CT and MRI. Fungal abscess may be very small, multiple, and occasionally calcified and is seen better on CT scan.[103,104] The spleen is subject to opportunistic infections, including *Pneumocystis* and *Mycobacterium*, especially in immunocompromised patients.[105]

Primary pancreatic abscesses do not occur, but there can be secondary infection of pseudocysts, usually occurring 4 to 6 weeks after acute pancreatitis and appearing as well-circumscribed complex cysts on imaging studies. This occurrence usually requires surgical débridement.[106]

Intra-abdominal abscesses occur with some frequency in children and are usually secondary to ruptured appendicitis. They can also be secondary to trauma and Crohn disease.[107] US has limited usefulness in searching for intra-abdominal abscess, and contrast-enhanced CT of the abdomen and pelvis with both oral and rectal contrast is the modality of choice.

Various bacterial enteritides, including *Campylobacter jejuni* and *Yersinia enterocolitica*, can also cause thickening and inflammation of the bowel wall, especially in the ileum, and may be associated with mesenteric adenitis, making them difficult to distinguish from Crohn disease.[108]

ACQUIRED CONDITIONS

LIVER

Parenchymal disease from various processes, including metabolic diseases, drug and environmental toxicities, and congenital hepatic fibrosis, does not offer specific imaging findings. Some of these processes cause fatty infiltration, fibrosis, and even cirrhosis, all of which have further imaging findings, albeit nonspecific. Fatty infiltration with enlargement of the organ is a common finding in early liver disease, seen on US as diffuse increased echogenicity (Figure 74.2-51). On CT, the liver with fatty infiltration has lower attenuation to the spleen rather than the normally expected similar or increased attenuation (Figure 74.2-52). As liver parenchyma is destroyed and the organ becomes fibrotic, there is a commensurate decrease in size and a heterogeneous increase in echogenicity on US.

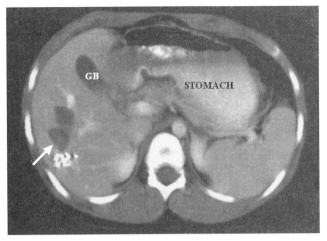

FIGURE 74.2-50 Contrast-enhanced computed tomographic scan of a 14-year-old boy reveals recurrent cystic masses (*arrow*) arising anterior to multiple clips, status postresection of ecchinococcal cysts.

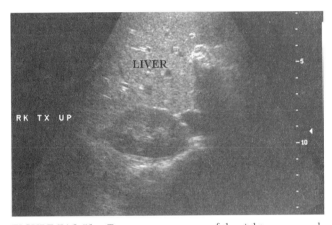

FIGURE 74.2-51 Transverse sonogram of the right upper quadrant shows the liver to be of increased echogenicity compared with the right kidney, suggesting fatty infiltration. Normally, the liver is of decreased attenuation compared with the kidney.

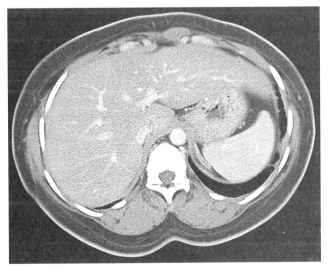

FIGURE 74.2-52 Axial contrast-enhanced computed tomographic scan of the abdomen of an 18 year old with cystic fibrosis reveals that the liver has lower attenuation to the spleen rather than the normally expected similar or increased attenuation, a finding suggestive of fatty infiltration. The spleen is mildly enlarged.

US, CT, or MRI can also demonstrate changes associated with chronic liver disease and cirrhosis. Such findings include macronodular contours, regenerating relative enlargement of the caudate and left lobes,[109] and sclerotic nodules (Figure 74.2-53), as well as the development of portal hypertension, with splenomegaly, varices (Figure 74.2-54), and ascites. Recannalization of the umbilical vein, hypertrophy of the hepatic artery signal, and biphasic and eventual reversal of flow in the portal vein are demonstrated by color Doppler US. Enlarged coronary veins and retroperitoneal varices can be seen with portal vein thrombosis and cavernous transformation. CT and MRI can show collaterals and clots extending into vessels.[110] Increased attenuation of parenchyma can be seen with iron deposition, with glycogen storage disease, and after the administration of cisplatinum for chemotherapy.[111] MRI may be more sensitive than CT for detecting early deposition. Because deposition can be preceded by the accumulation of fat, the liver may initially appear of decreased attenuation on CT.[112] Budd-Chiari syndrome is a relatively rare disorder caused by the acute or chronic obstruction of the hepatic veins, usually by membranous obstruction. It may also be caused by hypercoagulability associated with hematologic and systemic disease. The presentation of Budd-Chiari syndrome is similar to other liver diseases, with right upper quadrant pain, tender hepatomegaly, and possibly ascites. Astute clinical suspicion and proper imaging are essential for diagnosis. Angiography had been the principal diagnostic modality; however, noninvasive duplex Doppler US is now preferred to show the venous anomalies, with a sensitivity that approaches angiography.[113] Contrast-enhanced CT and MRI do not demonstrate venous obstruction as well but do detect the associated parenchymal disease, the relative preservation of the caudate lobe, and large regenerative nodules (Figures 74.2-55 and 74.2-56). [114]

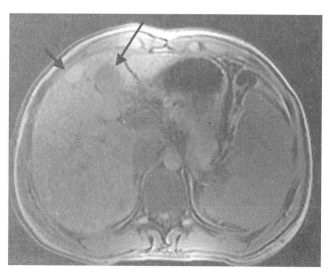

FIGURE 74.2-53 Spoiled gradient axial magnetic resonance image of the liver in an 18-year-old male patient with chronic active hepatitis B demonstrates multiple nodules within the liver. Most were of low signal characteristic and did not enhance after gadolinium, similar to the nodule demarcated by the *thin arrow*. These were presumed to represent siderotic type nodules. One lesion was of bright signal on multiple sequences but also did not enhance (*short arrow*) and was thought to represent a regenerating nodule. All nodules remained stable over a 3-year follow-up.

LIVER TRANSPLANT

The most significant and dramatic acquired condition of the liver is transplant. Accurate imaging is crucial for both pre- and post-transplant evaluations. Potential recipients are typically followed by serial US examinations to document progression of disease, the development of portal hypertension, and the patency of vessels essential for graft anastomosis. Congenital anomalies that might complicate the surgical procedure, such as a preduodenal portal vein, are documented. CT and MRI are reserved for

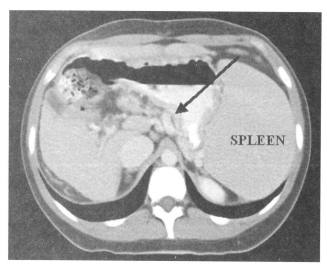

FIGURE 74.2-54 Axial contrast-enhanced computed tomographic scan of the abdomen of a 16-year-old female patient with autoimmune hepatitis reveals splenomegaly, varices (*arrow*), and the inferior portion of a small liver. Clinically, the patient had portal hypertension.

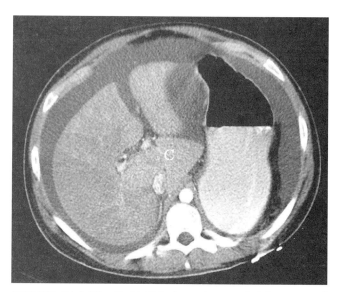

FIGURE 74.2-55 Budd-Chiari syndrome. Axial computed tomographic scan after the intravenous administration of contrast reveals heterogeneous enhancement of the liver, except for the caudate lobe (c), which appears preserved.

excluding the possibility of malignancy[115] and establishing accurate liver volume for surgical planning. MRCP, in conjunction with liver biopsy, is particularly important in excluding large duct primary sclerosing cholangitis as the cause of liver failure because this diagnosis requires that a Roux-en-Y portoenterostomy be performed rather than a duct-to-duct anastomosis.

Serial US examinations are crucial in the postoperative period to access for patency of the newly anastomosed vessels. Vascular complications of stenosis or occlusion, if diagnosed promptly and corrected in the immediate postoperative period, can significantly improve graft success and decrease the incidence of biliary compromise. Bile duct dilatation can be related to vascular compromise or anastomotic stricture. Dilatation or beading of the biliary system on a chronic basis may also be related to prolonged cold-ischemia at the time of transplant. Biliary dilatation will be seen on US or CT if moderate to severe[116] and on MRCP even if mild (Figure 74.2-57). Small focal areas of infarction are not uncommon in the immediate postoper-

ative period and can be detected on US as hypoechoic, peripheral, wedge-shaped areas of decreased perfusion but may be more evident on CT scan, where they appear to be of decreased attenuation.[117] US-guided biopsies and interventional percutaneous transhepatic drainage of bilomas or abscesses[118] play an important role in the postsurgical management. Contrast-enhanced CT of the abdomen and pelvis remains the mainstay of evaluating for posttransplant abscess, collections, and PTLD.

BILIARY DISEASE

The most common form of acquired biliary disease is cholelithiasis, and although the incidence is not as common as in adults, it does occur with some frequency in children, especially in the setting of sickle cell disease, hereditary spherocytosis, and related hematologic diseases (Figure 74.2-58). In children, both gallstones and sludge can be well seen on US (Figure 74.2-59), although the clinical significance of each is different. Sludge is more often associated with prior parenteral nutrition or antibi-

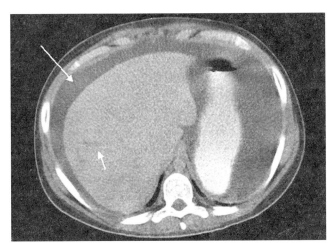

FIGURE 74.2-56   Delayed axial computed tomographic scan after the intravenous administration of contrast reveals filling defects in the liver corresponding to thrombosed hepatic veins (*short arrow*) in this 16-year-old patient with Budd-Chiari syndrome. The *long arrow* demonstrates ascitic fluid surrounding the liver.

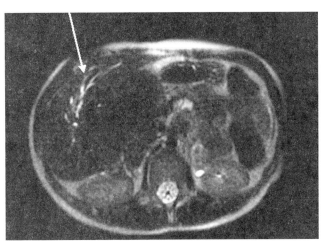

FIGURE 74.2-57   Axial magnetic resonance cholangiopancreatography performed on a 6-year-old girl with rising liver enzymes 5 years following a segmented liver transplant reveals mild intrahepatic biliary dilatation and beading (*arrow*).

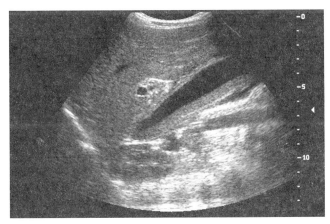

FIGURE 74.2-58   Acute cholecystitis. Sagittal sonogram of the gallbladder reveals a thick wall and a scant amount of percholecystic fluid (*arrow*).

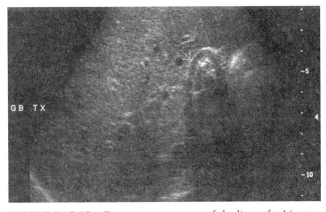

FIGURE 74.2-59   Transverse sonogram of the liver of a 16-year-old female patient with right upper quadrant pain reveals a thick-walled, contracted gallbladder (*arrow*) filled with shadowing stones. The patient was treated for acute cholecystitis.

otics and can appear and resolve in a matter of days. Most stones are related to hemolytic processes and, unlike in adults, do not necessarily require surgery.[119] Common duct stones are rare in children (Figure 74.2-60). Acalculous cholecystitis may show thickening of the gallbladder wall on US, although hypoalbuminemia and infections may cause similar findings.[32]

Primary sclerosing cholangitis, a chronic inflammatory process affecting the extrahepatic and/or medium to large bile ducts, is seen in children and has features suggesting an autoimmune pathogenesis. It is associated with IBD, histiocytosis, and, less commonly, lymphoma and infections related to immunodeficiencies.[120] MRCP is as sensi-

tive as ERCP in demonstrating large duct primary sclerosing cholangitis in children by demonstrating beading of the ducts (Figure 74.2-61).[121]

SPLEEN

The spleen is not usually the primary organ of disease processes, but it is frequently secondarily enlarged by neoplasia, infection, venous engorgement from portal hypertension, or infiltrative disease as in storage diseases. Gaucher disease is associated with some of the largest documented spleens (Figure 74.2-62). On all modalities, the parenchyma is usually uniform. Complicating splenomegaly, infarction appears as hypoperfused, wedge-shaped, round, or irregular areas on US and as low-attenuation areas on contrast-enhanced CT unless superimposed hemorrhage causes an increase in attenuation. When followed serially, infarcts tend to contract and progressively liquefy, and may calcify. In sickle cell disease, multiple, recurrent infarctions result in eventual destruction of the entire spleen.[122]

PANCREAS

Of the identifiable causes of pancreatitis, trauma is the most common in childhood, and abuse should always be excluded. Nontraumatic pancreatitis may be caused by viral infection, hypercholesterolemia, and obstruction. Obstruction as an etiology is much less common in children than in adults. It may appear as focal or diffuse enlargement, which is sometimes difficult to define because there is great variability in the size of the normal pancreas. US is an excellent modality for the initial study; however, owing to obscuring bowel gas, demonstration of the entire pancreas can present challenges. Associated findings of acute pancreatitis include ductal enlargement, either decreased or increased echogenicity of the entire gland, or heterogeneous echogenicity within the same gland. Peripancreatic fluid can be detected loculated

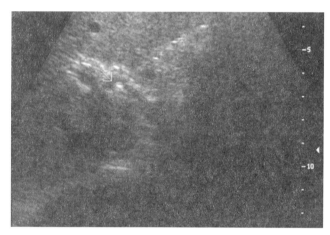

FIGURE 74.2-60   Sagittal sonogram of the porta hepatis reveals an echogenic focus within the common duct (*arrow*), consistent with a stone.

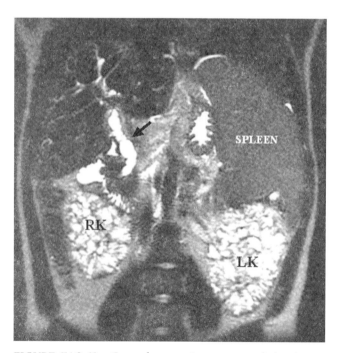

FIGURE 74.2-61   Coronal magnetic resonance cholangiopancreatogram of an 8-year-old boy with autosomal dominant polycystic kidney disease reveals dilatation and beading of the extrahepatic bile duct (*arrow*), as well as milder intrahepatic biliary beading, suggesting the appearance of primary sclerosing cholangitis. Note the multicystic enlarged kidneys and splenomegaly.

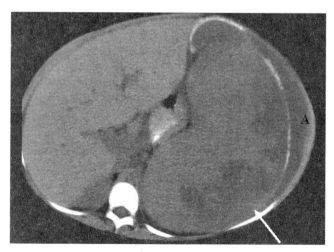

FIGURE 74.2-62   Axial non–contrast-enhanced computed tomographic scan of the abdomen of a 16-year-old female patient with Gaucher disease demonstrates marked splenomegaly with multiple peripheral low-attenuation areas consistent with infarcts (*arrow*). A thin calcified rim is present. Free ascites (A) is also present.

adjacent to the pancreas or free in the peritoneal space as ascites and pleural effusions (Figure 74.2-63). Phlegmons, fistulae, infarctions, and pseudocysts[123] can complicate pancreatitis. CT with contrast has been used to evaluate pancreatic morphology, detect pancreatic necrosis, and depict retroperitoneal complications, resulting in a CT staging severity index that has proven to be a reliable indicator of prognosis (Figure 74.2-64).[124] In children with recurrent episodes of idiopathic acute pancreatitis, MRCP allows visualization of the pancreatic duct anatomy, including side branches, ductal narrowing, endoluminal filling defects, irregular ductal contour, cavities, and pancreas divisum, thus increasing the ability to diagnose risk factors associated with chronic pancreatitis (Figure 74.2-65).[125]

Chronic pancreatitis, relatively rare in childhood, shows ductal dilatation, irregularity, calcification, pseudocyst formation, and, ultimately, a smaller gland. In cystic fibrosis, pancreatic atrophy and fatty infiltration may be dramatic (Figure 74.2-66).[126] Diffuse enlargement or focal alteration of the gland is seen in fibrosing pancreatitis and may result in biliary obstruction.[127]

GASTROINTESTINAL TRACT

Cross-sectional imaging of the gastrointestinal tract has dramatically altered the standard of care in gastrointestinal disorders over the past several decades. Various imaging studies are routinely ordered for diagnosing entities such as appendicitis, intussusception, IBD, and even bowel obstruction, although plain films and contrast studies, coupled with clinical judgment, still play a very large role in the diagnosis and management of these disorders.

Up to 20% of small bowel obstruction will not be evident on plain films,[128] but it is unclear whether these undetected cases can be managed conservatively or indeed need surgical management. Contrast studies are at times not useful owing to delayed transit time and dilution of contrast. US examination of small bowel obstruction will demonstrate either hyperactive or hypoactive, atonic and dilated, fluid-filled bowel, but the same findings can be seen in gastroenteritis.[129] US may suggest malrotation based on demonstrating the superior mesenteric vein to the left of the superior mesenteric artery.[130] CT can reveal

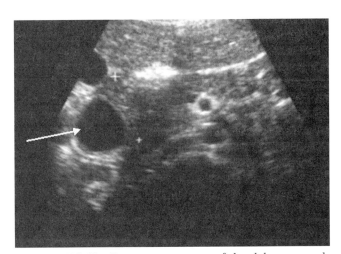

FIGURE 74.2-63   Transverse sonogram of the abdomen reveals an enlarged head of the pancreas with a central pseudocyst (*arrow*).

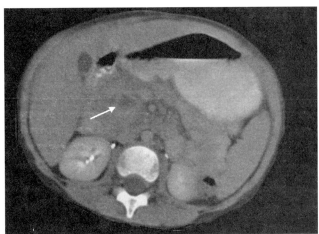

FIGURE 74.2-64   Axial contrast-enhanced computed tomographic scan of a 12-year-old boy with familial hypercholesterolemia and pancreatitis reveals an enlarged head of the pancreas and a central pseudocyst (*arrow*).

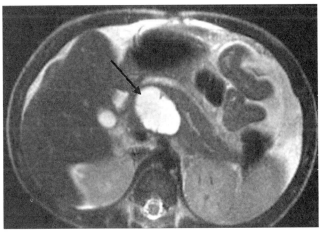

FIGURE 74.2-65   Axial magnetic resonance cholangiopancreatogram of a 5-year-old boy with a history of abuse demonstrates a large pseudocyst in the pancreas (*arrow*).

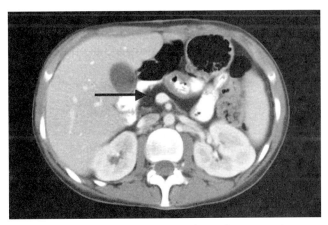

FIGURE 74.2-66   Axial contrast-enhanced computed tomographic scan of an 18-year-old female patient with cystic fibrosis reveals complete fatty replacement of the pancreas (*arrow*). The patient clinically had insulin dependent diabetes.

high-grade obstruction with dilated loops of bowel and closed-loop strangulating obstruction, and some authors advocate CT as the investigative modality of choice. Specific causes of small bowel obstruction can be seen on cross-sectional imaging studies, although traditional SBFT remains helpful.[128]

Causes of obstruction include congenital duplication and mesenteric cysts. If the cyst contains gastric mucosa, it can ulcerate, bleed, or even perforate.[129] Another cause of intestinal obstruction is Meckel diverticulum, which can contain gastric mucosa and therefore can be detected by radionucleotide scan. Occasionally, the diverticulum can be imaged by US or CT[131] as the lead point for an intussusception, with a blind-ended, thick-walled bowel segment projecting beyond the apex of the intussusceptum.[132]

APPENDICITIS

The diagnosis of appendicitis,[133] once a clinical one with a large margin of error, has been considerably changed by advances in cross-sectional imaging. The US finding of an appendix greater than 6 mm in diameter, with a blind-ending lumen that is noncompressible and hyperemic, became the hallmark of acute appendicitis, with up to a 90% sensitivity and 95% specificity.[134] The presence of a appendicolith and periappendiceal fluid supports the diagnosis,[135] although documentation of an appendicolith may be associated with normal appendices in up to 14% of surgically explored cases.[136] US is useful to exclude ovarian pathology in female patients and can demonstrate abscess formation suggesting perforation. Unfortunately, as in physical examination, US is limited by overlying bowel gas and the fact that many appendices are not in a typical location. The inability to demonstrate an inflamed appendix does not exclude acute appendicitis on US. Because the technique uses graded compression, US is uncomfortable and can be difficult to perform in uncooperative children. Furthermore, US of the appendix is highly operator dependent.

Because of these limitations, CT of the abdomen and pelvis has largely replaced US for the diagnosis of acute appendicitis. Various techniques are advocated, including contrast- and noncontrast-enhanced techniques. Some radiologists prefer oral, rectal, and intravenous contrast, whereas others perform the examination with only rectal contrast. Despite these differences in technique, the objective is to visualize the enlarged and inflamed appendix (Figure 74.2-67) and an appendicolith if present (Figure 74.2-68) and to identify any associated findings of pericecal fluid and inflammation. CT is also used extensively to document suspected complications such as abscess formation both pre- and postoperatively (Figure 74.2-69). With the widespread use of US and CT, the negative appendectomy rate has dropped from 15 to 4%, whereas the rate of perforation has decreased from 35 to 16% in one reporting institution.[137]

INTUSSUSCEPTION

The most common cause of intestinal obstruction from 6 months to 6 years of age is intussusception, which most commonly occurs before age 2 years, with a peak incidence between 3 and 9 months. Of the intussusceptions that

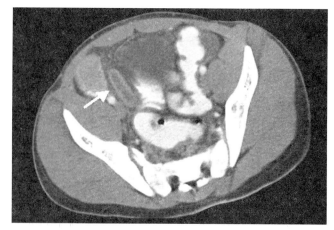

FIGURE 74.2-67 Axial contrast-enhanced computed tomographic scan with oral and rectal contrast reveals a fluid-filled, swollen appendix in the right lower quandrant (*arrow*). The inflammed appendix wall is enhancing.

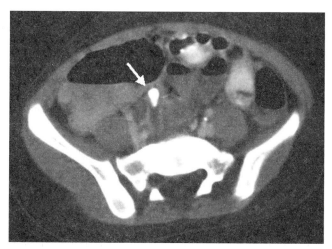

FIGURE 74.2-68 Axial computed tomographic scan of the pelvis reveals a thick tubular structure in the right lower quandrant consistent with a swollen appendix. A calcified appendicolith (*arrow*) is present.

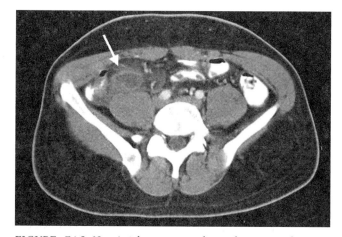

FIGURE 74.2-69 Axial contrast-enhanced computed tomographic scan of the pelvis reveals a fluid collection with a thin enhancing rim in the right lower quandrant (*arrow*) adjacent to thick-walled bowel. At surgery, a perforated appendix with a periappendiceal abscess was found.

occur in the typical age group, 90% are ileocolic and probably only 5% have a lead point, whereas the occurrence under the age of 6 months and over 3 years of age can be located in other segments of the bowel and may have a lead point.[138] Not all children will have the typical clinical presentation of episodic cramps, currant jelly stools, and abdominal pain, making it most important to maintain a high clinical suspicion and have sensitive imaging techniques to confirm. Findings of intussusception may be evident on plain film radiographs, but in 25% of cases, the bowel pattern is normal. Enema, using either barium or air, is the gold standard, both for diagnosis and treatment.

US is a reliable study for diagnosing intussusception, although it may not reach the high sensitivity and 100% negative predictive values that have been reported.[139] The characteristic finding is an intra-abdominal mass that demonstrates a hypoechoic ring of bowel wall mucosa surrounding an echogenic center of trapped mesenteric fat and vessels, the "doughnut sign" (Figure 74.2-70).[140] Multiple concentric circles may be seen when there are multiple layers of both intussusceptum and intussuscipiens. In the plane longitudinal to the mass, there are alternating hypoechogenic and echogenic layers, the "sandwich" or "pseudokidney" sign.[141] Thickening of the echolucent rim greater than 8 mm and fluid within the intussusceptum, especially if there is a dilated apex, have been suggested as indications of significant ischemia and irreducibility by enema reduction.[142] Free intraperitoneal fluid and bowel thickness did not alter outcome of reduction in another large series; however, the presence of small bowel obstruction on plain film reduced the success rate from 90 to 65%.[143]

Clinical peritonitis is a contraindication to hydrostatic or air reduction. An intussusception present for greater than 48 hours or one in an infant less than 6 months with bowel obstruction on plain films has a high likelihood of perforation.[144] Lead points have included most polyps, Meckel diverticulum, duplication cysts, and submucosal bleeds associated with Henoch-Schönlein purpura. Although the vast majority of intussusceptions are reduced under conventional fluoroscopic guidance, recent attempts at air reduction under US guidance have been met with some success.[145]

INFLAMMATORY CONDITIONS

Various inflammatory processes demonstrate bowel wall thickening on cross-sectional imaging. Although this is usually caused by an infectious process and is accompanied by mesenteric adenitis, IBD can cause similar findings. Using bowel wall thickness as a criterion for diagnosing IBD on US and comparing it with colonoscopic findings as the gold standard, US showed a sensitivity of 88% and a specificity of 93%.[146] In addition, CT can demonstrate transmesenteric disease associated with Crohn disease, such as creeping apposition of fat, mesenteric lymphadenopathy, and fistula formation helping to distinguish Crohn disease from ulcerative colitis (Figures 74.2-71 and 74.2-72). Intravenous contrast will enhance the margins of inflamed bowel wall or an inflammatory mass (Figure 74.2-73), whereas oral or rectal contrast will identify lumen. Another study, which looked at a combined group of IBD, infectious colitis, pseudomembranous colitis, Henoch-Schönlein purpura, and hemolytic syndrome, could not differentiate one condition from another.[147] Bowel thickening without transmesenteric disease is, however, more typical of colitis from causes other than Crohn disease (Figure 74.2-74).[148] Currently, MRI is less effective in demonstrating bowel pathology.[149]

In necrotizing enterocolitis, US has been demonstrated to be sensitive in detecting bowel wall thickening, pneumatosis intestinalis, portal venous gas, and perforation causing inflammatory mass[150]; however, serial plain films

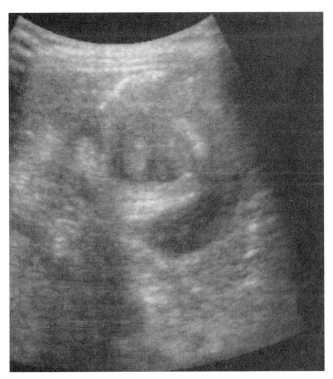

FIGURE 74.2-70 Sonogram of the abdomen in a 2 year old with crampy abdominal pain reveals a soft tissue mass in the right upper quadrant. The alternating echogenic and hypoechoic layers are typical for an intussusception.

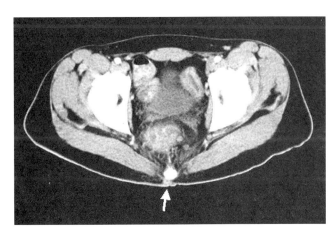

FIGURE 74.2-71 Contrast-enhanced computed tomographic scan of the pelvis in this 15-year-old male patient with Crohn colitis reveals contrast extending into a perirectal fistula (arrow).

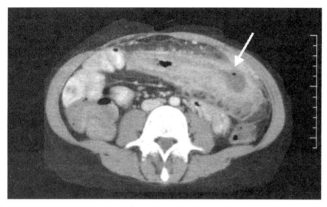

FIGURE 74.2-72 Axial contrast-enhanced computed tomographic scan of the abdomen in an adolescent female with Crohn disease reveals an abscess arising from the wall of the transverse colon (*arrow*).

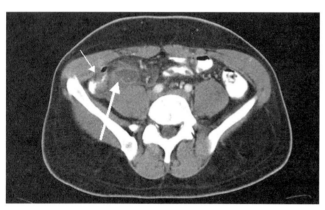

FIGURE 74.2-73 Axial contrast-enhanced computed tomographic scan of the pelvis reveals a collection with an enhancing rim abutting the psoas muscle (*long arrow*) in this adolescent male with Crohn disease and right lower quadrant pain. Note the thick-walled bowel adjacent to the abscess (*short arrow*).

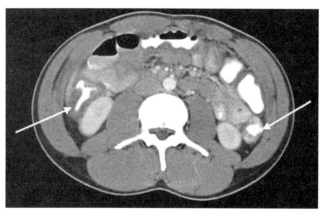

FIGURE 74.2-74 Contrast-enhanced computed tomographic scan of the lower abdomen reveals a thick-walled ascending colon (*up arrow*) and a descending colon (*down arrow*) in this teenager with known colitis.

remain the mainstay of diagnosis. In an investigative study, MRI showed good correlation with operative findings in a small group of premature infants determined to have necrotizing enterocolitis.[151] However, in view of the tech-

nical and practical considerations, cross-sectional imaging probably does not have a great deal to contribute to the care of these critically ill infants.

CONCLUSION

Imaging technology has markedly altered the traditional workup of gastrointestinal disorders. Ongoing advances in US, CT, and MRI have revolutionized the approach to many common diseases and greatly increased the accuracy of diagnosis. The risks of radiation exposure, contrast toxicity, and sedation should always be considerations, especially when a pediatric patient is concerned. As with any modality, an understanding of the risks, benefits, and limitations of a procedure is needed to effectively use these sophisticated technologies.

REFERENCES

1. Cremin BJ. Real time ultrasonic evaluation of the paediatric abdomen: technique and anatomical variations: a personal view. Br J Radiol 1985;58:859–68.
2. Merritt CRB. The physics of ultrasound. In: Rumack CM, Wilson SR, Charboneau JW, editors. Diagnostic ultrasound. St. Louis (MO): Mosby Year Book; 1998. p. 3–33.
3. Ralls PW, Jeffrey RB Jr, Kane RA, Robbin M. Ultrasonography. Gastroenterol Clin North Am 2002;3:801–25.
4. Scatamacchia SA, Raptopoulos V, Davidson RI. Saline microbubbles monitoring sonography-assisted abscess drainage. Invest Radiol 1987;22:868–70.
5. Brasch RC, Abols IB, Gooding CA, Filly RA. Abdominal disease in children: a comparison of computed tomography and ultrasound. AJR Am J Roentgenol 1980;134:153–8.
6. Danemen A. Pediatric body CT. 1st ed. London: Springer-Verlag; 1986.
7. Brenner D, Elliston C, Hall E, Berdon W. Estimated risks of radiation-induced fatal cancer from pediatric CT. AJR Am J Roentgenol 2001;176:289–96.
8. Kirks DR. Practical techniques for pediatric computed tomography. Pediatr Radiol 1983;13:148–55.
9. Leonard JC, Younkin DP, Chance B, et al. Nuclear magnetic resonance: an overview of its spectroscopic and imaging applications in pediatric patients. J Pediatr 1985;106:756–61.
10. Cohen MD. Magnetic resonance imaging techniques in children. In: Cohen MD, editor. Pediatric magnetic resonance imaging. 1st ed. Philadephia: WB Saunders; 1986. p. 8–17.
11. Cohen MD, et al. The visualization of major blood vessels by magnetic resonance imaging in children with malignant tumors. Radiographics 1985;5:441–5.
12. Siegel MJ. MR imaging of the pediatric abdomen. Magn Reson Imaging Clin N Am 1995;3:161–82.
13. Abbitt PL. Ultrasonography. Update on liver technique. Radiol Clin North Am 1998;36:299–307.
14. Laing AD, Gibson RN. MRI of the liver. J Magn Reson Imaging 1998;8:337–45.
15. Donnelly LF, Bisset GS. Pediatric hepatic imaging. Radiol Clin North Am 1998;36:413–27.
16. Hernanz-Schulman M, Ambrosino MM, Freeman PC, Quinn CB. Common bile duct in children: sonographic dimensions. Radiology 1995;195:193–5.
17. Schneck CD. Part II: the gallbladder and biliary tract. Embryology, histology, gross anatomy, and normal imaging anatomy of the gallbladder and biliary tract. In: Friedman AC,

Dachman AH, Farrell RJ, editors. Radiology of the liver, biliary tract, and pancreas. St. Louis (MO): Mosby Year Book; 1994. p. 355–407.

18. Kasales CJ, Patel S, Hopper KD, et al. Imaging variants of the liver, pancreas, and spleen. Crit Rev Diagn Imaging 1994;35:485–543.

19. Siegel MJ, Martin KW, Worthington JL. Normal and abnormal pancreas in children: US studies. Radiology 1987;165:15–8.

20. Vaughn DD, Jabra AA, Fishman EK. Pancreatic disease in children and young adults: evaluation with CT. Radiographics 1998;18:171–87.

21. Radin DR, Colletti PM, Ralls PW, et al. Agenesis of the right lobe of the liver. Radiology 1987;164:639–42.

22. Gallego C, Velasco M, Marcuello P, et al. Congenital and acquired anomalies of the portal venous system. Radiographics 2002;22:141–59.

23. Niwa T, Aida N, Tachibana K, et al. Congenital absence of the portal vein: clinical and radiologic findings. J Comput Assist Tomogr 2002;26:681–6.

24. Mulliken JB, Glowacki J. Hemangiomas and vascular malformations in infants and children: a classification based on endothelial characteristics. Plast Reconstr Surg 1982;69:412–20.

25. Dachman AH, Lichtenstein JE, Friedman AC, Hartman DS. Infantile hemangioendothelioma of the liver: a radiologic-pathologic-clinical correlation. AJR Am J Roentgenol 1983;140:1091–6.

26. Keslar PJ, Buck JL, Selby DM. From the archives of the AFIP. Infantile hemangioendothelioma of the liver revisited. Radiographics 1993;13:657–70.

27. Boon LM, Enjolras O, Mulliken JB. Hepatic vascular anomalies in infancy: a twenty-seven-year experience. J Pediatr 1996;129:346–54.

28. Taylor KJ, Ramos I, Morse SS, et al. Focal liver masses: differential diagnosis with pulsed Doppler US. Radiology 1987;164:643–7.

29. Lucaya J, Enriquez G, Amat L, Gonzalez-Rivero MA. Computed tomography of infantile hepatic hemangioendothelioma. AJR Am J Roentgenol 1985;144:821–6.

30. Chung T, Hoffer FA, Burrows PE, Paltiel HJ. MR imaging of hepatic hemangiomas of infancy and changes seen with interferon alpha-2a treatment. Pediatr Radiol 1996;26:341–8.

31. Ozgen A, Akata D, Arat A, et al. Gallbladder duplication: imaging findings and differential considerations. Abdom Imaging 1999;24:285–8.

32. Siegel MJ. Pediatric sonography. 2nd ed. New York: Raven Press; 1995. p. 171–236.

33. Lam WW, Lam TP, Saing H, et al. MR cholangiography and CT cholangiography of pediatric patients with choledochal cysts. AJR Am J Roentgenol 1999;173:401–5.

34. Torrisi JM, Haller JO, Velcek FT. Choledochal cyst and biliary atresia in the neonate: imaging findings in five cases. AJR Am J Roentgenol 1990;155:1273–6.

35. Park WH, Choi SO, Lee HJ. Technical innovation for noninvasive and early diagnosis of biliary atresia: the ultrasonographic "triangular cord" sign. J Hepatobiliary Pancreat Surg 2001;8:337–41.

36. Kotb MA, Kotb A, Sheba MF, et al. Evaluation of the triangular cord sign in the diagnosis of biliary atresia. Pediatrics 2001;108:416–20.

37. Norton KI, Glass RB, Kogan D, et al. MR cholangiography in the evaluation of neonatal cholestasis: initial results. Radiology 2002;222:687–91.

38. Jaw TS, Kuo YT, Liu GC, et al. MR cholangiography in the evaluation of neonatal cholestasis. Radiology 1999;212:249–56.

39. Gayer G, Zissin R, Apter S, et al. CT findings in congenital anomalies of the spleen. Br J Radiol 2001;74:767–72.

40. Danaci M, Belet U, Yalin T, et al. Power Doppler sonographic diagnosis of torsion in a wandering spleen. J Clin Ultrasound 2000;28:246–8.

41. Applegate KE, Goske MJ, Pierce G, Murphy D. Situs revisited: imaging of the heterotaxy syndrome. Radiographics 1999;19:837–52.

42. Morgenstern L. Nonparasitic splenic cysts: pathogenesis, classification, and treatment. J Am Coll Surg 2002;194:306–14.

43. Takehara Y. Can MRCP replace ERCP? J Magn Reson Imaging 1998;3:517–34.

44. Kim HJ, Kim MH, Lee SK, et al. Normal structure, variations, and anomalies of the pancreaticobiliary ducts of Koreans: a nationwide cooperative prospective study. Gastrointest Endosc 2002;55:889–96.

45. Benya EC. Pancreas and biliary system: imaging of developmental anomalies and diseases unique to children. Radiol Clin North Am 2002;40:1355–62.

46. Kitano Y, Iwanaka T, Tsuchida Y, Oka T. Esophageal duplication cyst associated with pulmonary cystic malformations. J Pediatr Surg 1995;30:1724–7.

47. Berdon WE. Rings, slings, and other things: vascular compression of the infant trachea updated from the midcentury to the millennium—the legacy of Robert E. Gross, MD, and Edward B. D. Neuhauser, MD. Radiology 2000;216:624–32.

48. Mathieu D, Rahmouni A, Anglade MC, et al. Focal nodular hyperplasia of the liver: assessment with contrast-enhanced turboFLASH MR imaging. Radiology 1991;180:25–30.

49. Berrocal T, Lamas M, Gutieerrez J, et al. Congenital anomalies of the small intestine, colon, and rectum. Radiographics 1999;19:1219–36.

50. Macpherson RI. Gastrointestinal tract duplications: clinical, pathologic, etiologic, and radiologic considerations. Radiographics 1993;13:1063–80.

51. Hulka F, Campbell TJ, Campbell JR, Harrison MW. Evolution in the recognition of infantile hypertrophic pyloric stenosis. Pediatrics 1997;100(2):E9.

52. Henderson SO, Sung J, Mandavia D. Serial abdominal ultrasound in the setting of trauma. J Emerg Med 2000;18:79–81.

53. Mizzi A, Shabani A, Watt A. The role of follow-up imaging in paediatric blunt abdominal trauma. Clin Radiol 2002;57:908–12.

54. Brick SH, Taylor GA, Potter BM, Eichelberger MR. Hepatic and splenic injury in children: role of CT in the decision for laparotomy. Radiology 1987;165:643–6.

55. Stringer DA. Pediatric gastrointestinal tract imaging. Philadelphia: BC Decker; 1989.

56. Willmann JK, Roos JE, Platz A, et al. Multidetector CT: detection of active hemorrhage in patients with blunt abdominal trauma. AJR Am J Roentgenol 2002;179:437–44.

57. Poletti PA, Mirvis SE, Shanmuganathan K, et al. CT criteria for management of blunt liver trauma: correlation with angiographic and surgical findings. Radiology 2000;216:418–27.

58. Sharif K, Pimpalwar AP, John P, et al. Benefits of early diagnosis and preemptive treatment of biliary tract complications after major blunt liver trauma in children. J Pediatr Surg 2002;37:1287–92.

59. Fulcher AS, Turner MA, Yelon JA, et al. Magnetic resonance cholangiopancreatography (MRCP) in the assessment of pancreatic duct trauma and its sequelae: preliminary findings. J Trauma 2000;48:1001–7.

60. Killeen KL, Shanmuganathan K, Poletti PA, et al. Helical computed tomography of bowel and mesenteric injuries. J Trauma 2001;51:26–36.

61. Ciftci AO, Tanyel FC, Salman AB, et al. Gastrointestinal tract perforation due to blunt abdominal trauma. Pediatr Surg Int 1998;13:259–64.

62. Stassen NA, Lukan JK, Carrillo EH, et al. Abdominal seat belt marks in the era of focused abdominal sonography for trauma. Arch Surg 2002;137:718–22; discussion 722–3.

63. Guo Z, Kurtycz DF, Salem R, et al. Radiologically guided percutaneous fine-needle aspiration biopsy of the liver: retrospective study of 119 cases evaluating diagnostic effectiveness and clinical complications. Diagn Cytopathol 2002;26:283–9.

64. Pobiel RS, Bisset BS III. Pictorial essay: imaging of liver tumors in the infant and child. Pediatr Radiol 1995;25:495–506.

65. Choi BI, Kim CW, Han MC, et al. Sonographic characteristics of small hepatocellular carcinoma. Gastrointest Radiol 1989; 14:255–61.

66. Furuse J, Matsutani S, Yoshikawa M, et al. Diagnosis of portal vein tumor thrombus by pulsed Doppler ultrasonography. J Clin Ultrasound 1992;20:439–46.

67. Fernandez MDP, Redvanly RD. Primary hepatic malignant neoplasms. Radiol Clin North Am 1998;36:333–48.

68. Itoh K, Nishimura K, Togashi K, et al. Hepatocellular carcinoma: MR imaging. Radiology 1987;164:21–5.

69. Yamashita Y, Mitsuzaki K, Yi T, et al. Small hepatocellular carcinoma in patients with chronic liver damage: prospective comparison of detection with dynamic MR imaging and helical CT of the whole liver. Radiology 1996;200:79–84.

70. Farhi DC, Shikes RH, Murari PJ, Silverberg SG. Hepatocellular carcinoma in young people. Cancer 1983;52:1516–25.

71. Corrigan K, Semelka RC. Dynamic contrast-enhanced MR imaging of fibrolamellar hepatocellular carcinoma. Abdom Imaging 1995;20:122–5.

72. Moon WK, Kim WS, Kim IO, et al. Undifferentiated embryonal sarcoma of the liver: US and CT findings. Pediatr Radiol 1994;24:500–3.

73. Marti-Bonmati L, Ferrer D, Menor F, Galant J. Hepatic mesenchymal sarcoma: MRI findings. Abdom Imaging 1993;18: 176–9.

74. Geoffray A, Couanet D, Montagne JP, et al. Ultrasonography and computed tomography for diagnosis and follow-up of biliary duct rhabdomyosarcomas in children. Pediatr Radiol 1987;17:127–31.

75. Soyer P, Van Beers B, Teillet-Thiebaud F, et al. Hodgkin's and non-Hodgkin's hepatic lymphoma: sonographic findings. Abdom Imaging 1993;18:339–43.

76. Shamsi K, De Schepper A, Degryse H, Deckers F. Focal nodular hyperplasia of the liver: radiologic findings. Abdom Imaging 1993;18:32–8.

77. Golli M, Van Nhieu JT, Mathieu D, et al. Hepatocellular adenoma. Colour Doppler US and pathologic correlations. Radiology 1994;190:741–4.

78. Welch TJ, Sheedy PF II, Johnson CM, et al. Focal nodular hyperplasia and hepatic adenoma: comparison of angiography, CT, ultrasound and scintigraphy. Radiology 1985;150:593–5.

79. Arrivé L, Flejou JF, Vilgrain V, et al. Hepatic adenoma: MR findings in 51 pathologically proved lesions. Radiology 1994;193:507–12.

80. Miller JH, Greenspan BS. Integrated imaging of hepatic tumors in childhood. Part I. Malignant lesions (primary and metastatic). Radiology 1985;154:91–100.

81. Ros PR, Goodman ZD, Ishak KG, et al. Mesenchymal hamartoma of the liver: radiologic-pathologic correlation. Radiology 1986;158:619–24.

82. Sato M, Ishida H, Konno K, et al. Liver tumors in children and young patients: sonographic and color Doppler findings. Abdom Imaging 2000;25:596–601.

83. Rabushka LS, Kawashima A, Fishman EK. Imaging of the spleen: CT with supplemental MR examination. Radiographics 1994;14:307–32.

84. Jaksic T, Yaman M, Thorner P, et al. A 20-year review of pediatric pancreatic tumors. J Pediatr Surg 1992;27:1315–7.

85. Kissane JM. Tumors of the exocrine pancreas in childhood. In: Humphrey GB, et al, editors. Pancreatic tumors in children. The Hague: Martinus Nijhoff; 1982. p. 99–129.

86. Cohen MD. Imaging of children with cancer. 1st ed. St. Louis (MO): Mosby Year Book; 1992.

87. Robey G, Daneman A, Martin DJ. Pancreatic carcinoma in a neonate. Pediatr Radiol 1983;13:284–7.

88. Rausch DR, Norton KI, Glass RB, Kogan D. Infantile leukemia presenting with cholestasis secondary to massive pancreatic infiltration. Pediatr Radiol 2002;32:360–1.

89. Semelka RC, Cumming MJ, Shoenut JP, et al. Islet cell tumors: comparison of dynamic contrast-enhanced CT and MR imaging with dynamic gadolinium enhancement and fat suppression. Radiology 1993;186:799–802.

90. Siegel M, Evan SJ, Balfe DM. Small bowel disease in children: diagnosis with CT. Radiology 1988;169:127–30.

91. Bethel CA, Bhattacharyya N, Hutchinson C, et al. Alimentary tract malignancies in children. J Pediatr Surg 1997;32:1004–9.

92. Baldisserotto M, Spolidoro JV, Bahu M. Graded compression sonography of the colon in the diagnosis of polyps in pediatric patients. AJR Am J Roentgenol 2002;179:201–5.

93. Soravia C, Berk T, McLeod RS, Cohen Z. Desmoid disease in patients with familial adenomatous polyposis. Dis Colon Rectum 2000;43:363–9.

94. Wu L, Rappaport DC, Hanbidge A, et al. Lymphoproliferative disorders after liver transplantation: imaging features. Abdom Imaging 2001;26:200–6.

95. Pastakia B, Shawker TH, Thaler M, O'Leary T, Pizzo PA. Hepatosplenic candidiasis: wheels within wheels. Radiology 1988;166:417–21.

96. Oleszczuk-Raszke K, Cremin BJ, Fisher RM, et al. Ultrasonic features of pyogenic and amebic hepatic abscesses. Pediatr Radiol 1988;19:230–3.

97. Francis IR, Glazer GM, Amendola MA, Trenkner SW. Hepatic abscesses in the immunocompromised patient: role of CT in detection, diagnosis, management and follow-up. Gastrointest Radiol 1986;257–62.

98. Merten DF, Kirks DR. Amebic liver abscess in children: the role of diagnostic imaging. AJR Am J Roentgenol 1984;143:1325–9.

99. Warmann S, Meier PN, Kardorff R, Fuchs J. Cystic echinococcosis with perforation into the biliary tract in an eight-year-old girl. Eur J Pediatr Surg 2002;12:134–7.

100. Maresca G, De Gaetano AM, Mirk P, et al. Sonographic patterns of the gallbladder in acute viral hepatitis. J Clin Ultrasound 1984;12:141–6.

101. David V, Laing FC. Paradoxical dilatation of the gallbladder after fat ingestion in patients with acute hepatitis. J Ultrasound Med 1996;15:179–82.

102. Konen O, Rathaus V, Bauer S, et al. Progressive liver calcifications in neonatal coxsackievirus infection. Pediatr Radiol 2000;30:343–5.

103. Laurin S, Kaude JV. Diagnosis of liver and spleen abscess in children with emphasis on ultrasound for the initial and follow-up examinations. Pediatr Radiol 1984;14:198–204.

104. Tikkakoski T, Siniluoto T, Paivansalo M, et al. Splenic abscess. Imaging and intervention. Acta Radiol 1992;33:561–5.

105. Rabushka LS, Kawashima A, Fishman EK. Imaging of the spleen: CT with supplemental MR examination. Radiographics 1994;14:307–32.

106. Tsiotos GG, Sarr MG. Management of fluid collections and necrosis in acute pancreatitis. Curr Gastroenterol Rep 1999;1:87–8.

107. Blachar A, Federle MP. Gastrointestinal complications of laparo-

scopic Roux-en-Y gastric bypass surgery in patients who are morbidly obese: findings on radiography and CT. AJR Am J Roentgenol 2002;179:1437–42.

108. Puylaert JB. Mesenteric adenitis and acute terminal ileitis: US evaluation using graded compression. Radiology 1986;161:691–5.

109. Torres WE, Whitmire LF, Gedgaudas-McClees K, Bernardino ME. Computed tomography of hepatic morphologic changes in cirrhosis of the liver. J Comput Assist Tomogr 1986;10:47–50.

110. Friedman AC, et al. Cirrhosis, other diffuse diseases, portal hypertension, and vascular diseases. In: Friedman AC, editor. Radiology of the liver, biliary tract, pancreas and spleen. Baltimore: Williams & Wilkins; 1987. p. 69–75.

111. Taylor KJW. Gastrointestinal Doppler ultrasound. In: Taylor KJW, Burns PN, Wells PNT, editors. Clinical applications of Doppler ultrasound. New York: Raven Press; 1986. p. 162–200.

112. Mergo PJ, Ros PR. Imaging of diffuse liver disease. Radiol Clin North Am 1998;36:365–75.

113. Chawla Y, Kumar S, Dhiman RK, et al. Duplex Doppler sonography in patients with Budd-Chiari syndrome. J Gastroenterol Hepatol 1999;14:904–7.

114. Brancatelli G, Federle MP, Grazioli L, et al. Large regenerative nodules in Budd-Chiari syndrome and other vascular disorders of the liver: CT and MR imaging findings with clinicopathologic correlation. AJR Am J Roentgenol 2002;178:877–83.

115. Letourneau JG, Maile CW, Sutherland DE, Feinberg SB. Ultrasound and computed tomography in the evaluation of pancreatic transplantation. Radiol Clin North Am 1987;25:345–55.

116. Marincek B, Barbier PA, Becker CD, et al. CT appearance of impaired lymphatic drainage in liver transplants. AJR Am J Roentgenol 1986;147:519–23.

117. Letourneau JG, Day DL, Maile CW, et al. Liver allograft transplantation: postoperative CT findings. AJR Am J Roentgenol 1987;148:1099–103.

118. Rose SC, Andre MP, Roberts AC, et al. Integral role of interventional radiology in the development of a pediatric liver transplantation program. Pediatr Transplant 2001;5:331–8.

119. Wesdorp I, Bosman D, de Graaff A, et al. Clinical presentations and predisposing factors of cholelithiasis and sludge in children. J Pediatr Gastroenterol Nutr 2000;31:411–7.

120. Roberts EA. Primary sclerosing cholangitis in children. J Gastroenterol Hepatol 1999;14:588–93.

121. Ferrara C, Valeri G, Salvolini L, Giovagnoni A. Magnetic resonance cholangiopancreatography in primary sclerosing cholangitis in children. Pediatr Radiol 2002;32:413–7.

122. Paterson A, Frush DP, Donnelly LF, et al. A pattern-oriented approach to splenic imaging in infants and children. Radiographics 1999;19:1465–85.

123. Fishman EK, Siegelman SS. Pancreatitis and its complications. In: Taveras JM, Ferrucci JT, editors. Radiology—diagnosis imaging—intervention. Vol. 4. Philadelphia: Lippincott; 1988.

124. Balthazar EJ. Staging of acute pancreatitis. Radiol Clin North Am 2002;40:1199–209.

125. Manfredi R, Lucidi V, Gui B, et al. Idiopathic chronic pancreatitis in children: MR cholangiopancreatography after secretin administration. Radiology 2002;224:675–82.

126. Liu P, Daneman A, Stringer DA, Durie PR. Pancreatic cysts and calcification in cystic fibrosis. Can Assoc Radiol J 1986;37:279–82.

127. Sylvester FA, Shuckett B, Cutz E, et al. Management of fibrosing pancreatitis in children presenting with obstructive jaundice. Gut 1998;43:715–20.

128. Megibow AJ. Bowel obstruction. Evaluation with CT. Radiol Clin North Am 1994;32:861–70.

129. McAlister WH. Gastrointestinal tract. In: Siegel MJ, editor. Pediatric sonography. 2nd ed. New York: Raven Press; 1995.

130. Dufour D, Delaet MH, Dassonville M, et al. Midgut malrotation, the reliability of sonographic diagnosis. Pediatr Radiol 1992;22:21–3.

131. Pantongrag-Brown L, Levine MS, Elsayed AM, et al. Inverted Meckel diverticulum: clinical, radiologic, and pathologic findings. Radiology 1996;199:693–6.

132. Daneman A, Myers M, Shuckett B, Alton DJ. Sonographic appearances of inverted Meckel diverticulum with intussusception. Pediatr Radiol 1997;27:295–8.

133. Puylaert JB. Acute appendicitis: US evaluation using graded compression. Radiology 1986;158:355–60.

134. Jeffrey RB Jr, Laing FC, Townsend RR. Acute appendicitis: sonographic criteria based on 250 cases. Radiology 1988;167:327–9.

135. Sivit CJ. Diagnosis of acute appendicitis in children: spectrum of sonographic findings. AJR Am J Roentgenol 1996;161:147–52.

136. Lowe LH, Penney MW, Scheker LE, et al. Appendicolith revealed on CT in children with suspected appendicitis: how specific is it in the diagnosis of appendicitis? AJR Am J Roentgenol 2000;175:981–4.

137. Pena BM, Taylor GA, Fishman SJ, Mandl KD. Effect of an imaging protocol on clinical outcomes among pediatric patients with appendicitis. Pediatrics 2002;110:1088–93.

138. Hutchinson IF, Olayiwola B, Young DG. Intussusception infancy and childhood. Br J Surg 1980;67:209–12.

139. Verschelden P, Filiatrault D, Garel L, et al. Intussusception in children: reliability of US in diagnosis—a prospective study. Radiology 1992;184:741–4.

140. del-Pozo G, Albillos JC, Tejedor D. Intussusception: US findings with pathologic correlation—the crescent-in-doughnut sign. Radiology 1996;199:688–92.

141. Swischuk LE, Hayden CK, Boulden T. Intussusception: indications for ultrasonography and an explanation of the doughnut and pseudokidney signs. Pediatr Radiol 1985;15:388–91.

142. del-Pozo G, Gonzalez-Spinola J, Gomez-Anson B, et al. Intussusception: trapped peritoneal fluid detected with US—relationship to reducibility and ischemia. Radiology 1996;201:379–83.

143. Britton I, Wilkinson AG. Ultrasound features of intussusception predicting outcome of air enema. Pediatr Radiol 1999;29:705–10.

144. Stein M, Alton DJ, Daneman A. Pneumatic reduction of intussusception: 5-year experience. Radiology 1992;183:681–4.

145. Gu L, Zhu H, Wang S, et al. Sonographic guidance of air enema for intussusception reduction in children. Pediatr Radiol 2000;30:339–42.

146. Faure C, Belarbi N, Mougenot JF, et al. Ultrasonographic assessment of inflammatory bowel disease in children: comparison with ileocolonoscopy. J Pediatr 1997;130:147–51.

147. Siegel MJ, Friedland JA, Hildebolt CF. Bowel wall thickening in children: differentiation with US. Radiology 1997;203:631–5.

148. Sarrazin J, Wilson SR. Manifestations of Crohn disease at US. Radiographics 1996;16:499–520.

149. Miao YM, Koh DM, Amin Z, et al. Ultrasound and magnetic resonance imaging assessment of active bowel segments in Crohn's disease. Clin Radiol 2002;57:913–8.

150. Bomelburg T, von Lengerke HJ. Sonographic findings in infants with suspected necrotizing enterocolitis. Eur J Radiol 1992;15:149–53.

151. Maalouf EF, Fagbemi A, Duggan PJ, et al. Magnetic resonance imaging of intestinal necrosis in preterm infants. Pediatrics 2000;105(3 Pt 1):510–4.

3. *Interventional Gastrointestinal Radiology*

Peter G. Chait, MBBCh(Rand)(D), SA, FRCPR(Eng)

Pediatric interventional radiology[1,2] has expanded in the last 5 to 10 years as a direct result of the improvement in cross-sectional imaging, including ultrasonography, computed tomography (CT), and magnetic resonance imaging (MRI), as well as rapid biotechnologic advancement in the development of catheter materials, balloons, wires, stents, filters, retrieval devices, and embolic and sclerosing agents.[3,4] The development of this subspecialty has been facilitated by the emergence of pediatric radiologists specifically trained in interventional procedures. To perform these procedures, a fully equipped, dedicated interventional facility must be established. This facility would include anesthetic equipment and monitoring for sedation, color Doppler ultrasonography with a variety of high-resolution interventional probes, a CT scanner, and, finally, a C-arm interventional fluoroscopic table with digital subtraction.

INTERVENTIONAL RADIOLOGY SERVICE

To provide a highly successful service that achieves excellence in patient care, a team approach is stressed.[3,5] Dedicated professionals should include a pediatric interventional radiologist; a fellow or resident in training; pediatric radiology nurses with training in patient assessment, sedation, and postsedation recovery; and technologists trained in angiography, interventional procedures, CT, and ultrasonography. It is important for the team members to liaise with referring physicians, other radiologists, the parent, and the patient to provide the best care possible.[5] The development of the interventional radiology service provides both inpatient and outpatient care and establishes interventional radiology as an important primary service.[4,6]

The following overview is based largely on the experience at The Hospital for Sick Children, Toronto, during the past 4 years. In this period, there has been significant growth and development of interventional procedures, with approximately 1,500 interventional procedures being performed per year. Gastrointestinal (GI) and biliary procedures represent almost half of these procedures. Gastrostomy tube (G tube) placement, follow-up studies, and G-tube changes represent the largest single technique performed at our hospital.

PREPROCEDURE PLANNING

Careful assessment of all patients prior to performing procedures is an essential prerequisite. This includes discussion with the referring physician with respect to the indications and specifics of the procedure required; assessment of the patient; and review of previous imaging studies and laboratory findings, including prothrombin time, partial thromboplastin time, platelets, and hemoglobin, the patient's medical history, drug allergies, and response to previous sedation. Where necessary, further imaging or laboratory studies are ordered and other services are consulted, particularly with regard to patient safety and the suitability of the procedure.[7,8] If sedation or anesthesia is required, intravenous access is placed prior to the procedure. According to the guidelines of the American Society of Pediatrics, presedation or anesthetic orders should include no solid food for 6 hours prior to the procedure, but clear fluids up to 2 hours are permissible.[9] We strictly enforce these guidelines and delay the procedure if necessary. At least 1 hour prior to the procedure, Emla cream (Astra, Mississauga, ON), a topical anesthetic, is applied to the area where percutaneous entry is to be performed. This significantly decreases the pain experienced when local anesthetic is administered.

SEDATION AND ANALGESIA

During the past year, 45% of procedures were performed with a local anesthetic alone, 50% with a local anesthetic plus sedation, and 5% with a general anesthetic. The need for a general anesthetic is determined by the status of the patient, the nature of the procedure, and, in some cases, the needs of the physician.

Patients are categorized according to the American Society of Anesthesiologists' classification[10]:

I. Normal healthy patient
II. Patient with mild systemic disease
III. Patient with severe systemic disease that limits activity but is not incapacitating
IV. Patient with incapacitating systemic disease that is a constant threat to life
V. Moribund patient not expected to survive 24 hours with or without intervention

Class I and II patients are candidates for conscious deep sedation. Patients in class III or IV require special considerations; they generally require general anesthesia but should be dealt with on an individual basis. Patients who have airway anomalies or who have experienced airway complications during past anesthesia or sedation should be thoroughly assessed prior to the administration of any sedative or anesthetic agent. In neonates with oropharyngeal or airway problems, the procedures may be performed with a local anesthetic alone. In older, cooperative children, a local anesthetic alone or combined with sedation may be all that is needed. General anesthetic is also indicated for (1) lengthy procedures, (2) complete patient cooperation, (3) an area of interest close to vital structures, and (4) procedures requiring a high degree of technical expertise and accuracy.

Numerous drugs are available for sedation and pain control.[11–19] Individuals ordering and administering the drugs and those monitoring the patient should be comfortable with the drugs in use; their effective use is best accomplished by using a carefully described protocol. We use a combination of drugs for sedation and pain control (Table 74.3-1).

We do not use intramuscular sedation. If sedation is required, intravenous access is essential, whereas the response to intramuscular injection is variable. The pain experienced during the introduction of 1% lidocaine into subcutaneous tissues is thought to be due to its low pH. Premixing the lidocaine with bicarbonate prior to injection increases the pH and appears to effectively reduce the pain.[20] It is also helpful to inject the lidocaine with a 27- or 30-gauge needle at a slow rate. Patients are monitored with pulse oximetry, blood pressure, and electrocardiography (ECG) throughout the procedure and following the procedure until they are fully responsive.[21] Postprocedure vital signs are recorded every 5 minutes until the patient awakes and then every 15 minutes. The patient is discharged from the radiology department when cardiovascular and airway stability is ensured and the patient is alert and can talk, sit unattended, and ambulate with assistance.

PATIENT PREPARATION

It is important to predetermine the best position for the patient undergoing the procedure, whether it be supine, oblique, decubitus, or prone. The position of the head of the patient, the ultrasound machine, the intravenous (IV) pole, the anesthetist (if present), and the radiologist should all be predetermined prior to placing the patient on the table. The position of the patient's arms, monitors, and ECG wires is optimized for the procedure and for patient comfort, which is always a high priority. For smaller patients, a restraining device (Figure 74.3-1) is useful to reduce the need for sedation and improve patient control. The body temperature of the neonate or small child is maintained by either increasing the room temperature, placing the child on heating blankets, covering the child with blankets or plastic wrap, using radiant heat from a baby warmer, or blowing hot air over the infant. Most gastrointestinal procedures accessed percutaneously require antibiotic coverage. For upper gastrointestinal procedures, a first-generation cephalosporin (cefazolin 20–30 mg/kg)

is used as a single dose prior to the procedure.[22] For small bowel and colorectal procedures, we use cefoxitin (25 mg/kg) and for biliary procedures cefazolin (20 mg/kg).

IMAGING GUIDING SYSTEMS

Interventional procedures may be performed under fluoroscopic, ultrasonographic, or CT guidance or a combination of these modalities. The relative merits of the various guidance systems are listed in Table 74.3-2. Pediatric patients are ideally suited to ultrasonography guidance because of the small size of the patient and the decreased subcutaneous and intraperitoneal fat.[23,24] Furthermore, ultrasonography uses no ionizing radiation, is portable, and provides a real-time image. It is not suitable for structures that are poorly visualized or obscured by overlying bone or air-filled structures. Therefore, structures that can be clearly visualized, such as abdominal solid organs and masses, are ideally suited for ultrasonography guidance. Fluoroscopy is generally used for guidance in areas in which there are differences in x-ray density, such as needle placement into a gas-filled stomach. When ultrasonography guidance is used to place a needle in the correct position, fluoroscopy is often used to allow further intervention, whether this is wire placement, stent deployment, or merely injection of contrast. CT is infrequently used in the pediatric setting. It is indicated primarily when lesions are small or not well visualized by ultrasonography or fluoroscopy.[25] The prime disadvantage of this modality is that it is not portable and fails to provide real-time images. Furthermore, it is time-consuming and therefore expensive and exposes the patient to significant radiation. It is, however, often used in the diagnostic evaluation to exclude other pathologies and to define anatomy and structural relationships, thereby allowing planning of a procedure. After prior imaging and laboratory studies have been adequately reviewed, the optimal guidance method is chosen to provide the safest, easiest, and least invasive approach. Intervening structures such as bowel loops, fluid-filled bladder, vessels, and other sterile spaces, particularly the pleura and the peritoneal cavity, are avoided to reduce complications.

CONTRAST MEDIA

Water-soluble contrast media are used for all interventional procedures performed under fluoroscopy or those requiring fluoroscopic guidance after ultrasonography or CT placement of a needle. High osmolar contrast media are hypertonic ionic triodinated fully substituted benzene derivatives with osmolalities of 1,200 to 2,000 mOsm/L (four to seven times the osmolality of blood). Low osmolar

TABLE 74.3-1   DRUGS AND DOSAGES FOR SEDATION AND PAIN CONTROL

0–5 KG	5–20 KG	> 20 KG
Chloral hydrate 50–80 mg/kg (oral) then meperidine (IV) 1 mg/kg or morphine (IV) 0.05 mg/kg	Pentobarbital 3 mg/kg (IV) then 5 min meperidine 1 mg/kg (IV) then repeat if necessary	Diazepam 0.1 mg/kg (IV) then meperidine 1 mg/kg (IV) then repeat if necessary

IV = intravenous.

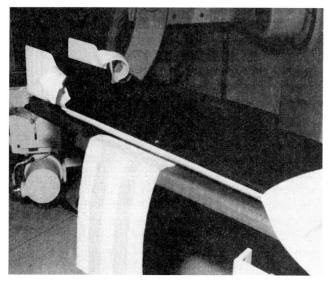

FIGURE 74.3-1   General Electric restraining device designed primarily for computed tomography.

contrast media (LOCM) are significantly more expensive, with significantly less osmolar composition,[7] with an osmolality of approximately 470 mOsm/L. Numerous studies have documented a reduction in overall adverse reactions with the use of LOCM in childhood.[8–12] LOCM also offer a reduction in side effects, especially nausea and vomiting. All water-soluble contrast media are absorbed from the GI tract and other tissues. The high osmolar agents cause significant pain if introduced into the subcutaneous tissue, may cause tissue necrosis,[26] and, obviously, produce an increased risk of pulmonary edema if aspirated. Because of these considerations, low-osmolar, nonionic contrast media are uniformly used for procedures in our institution. Barium sulfate and other varieties of barium suspensions are rarely used, and they are contraindicated if there is any risk of peritoneal spill,[27] extravasation into tissues, or aspiration.[28] Barium is used to do G- or gastroje-

junostomy (GJ) tube checks to confirm positions provided that there is no risk of intraperitoneal spillage.[29]

SPECIFIC PROCEDURES

PERCUTANEOUS GASTROSTOMY AND GASTROENTEROSTOMY

Percutaneous G tube and GJ tube are by far the most common procedures performed in our diagnostic imaging department. Before 1980, the only approach to G-tube placement was surgical.[30] In 1980, Gauderer and colleagues described G-tube placement by a percutaneous endoscopic gastrostomy (PEG) technique.[31] Most pediatric institutions now use this technique.[32–36] A radiologically guided retrograde technique was described a few years later,[37–44] followed by a radiologically guided antegrade technique similar to the PEG1 (Table 74.3-3[45–58]). More recently, laparoscopically performed gastrostomy has been described as a safe alternative to open surgical gastrostomy in patients who cannot undergo percutaneous gastrostomy.[59–64] All approaches to nonsurgical G-tube placement have proved to be cost-effective, with reduced morbidity and mortality.[32,65–67]

There has been a concomitant increase in the number and variety of replacement tubes (Figure 74.3-2) and types of enteral feeding formulas. This has allowed provision for nutrition support on an ambulatory basis using pump-regulated overnight enteral feeding. Currently, the Home Feeding Program at The Hospital for Sick Children, Toronto, monitors approximately 200 patients on overnight enteral feeds compared with only 8 to 10 patients on home total parenteral nutrition. Almost all G tubes are placed in diagnostic imaging; approximately 120 new G tubes are inserted annually. This large patient group requires specialized care, which is best approached by a medical team including interventional radiologists, nutritionists, gastroenterologists, dietitians, and trained enterostomy nursing staff.[68]

Informed consent is obtained either from the patient (if over 16 years and able to give consent) or from the parent or

TABLE 74.3-2   RELATIVE MERITS OF DIFFERENT IMAGING GUIDING SYSTEMS

ADVANTAGES		
FLUOROSCOPY	**ULTRASONOGRAPHY**	**COMPUTED TOMOGRAPHY**
Availability	Rapid localization	Small lesions shown
Rapid localization	Flexible imaging	Needle tip easily seen
Needle tip easy to identify	Flexible patient positioning	Precise anatomic relationship revealed
Diaphragm easily seen	No radiation	Precise target sampling
Modality of choice for further imaging and intervention after needle placement	Ideal for superficial structures or solid organs or masses	No interference because of overlying bowel or gas images, easy to comprehend in three dimensions
Real time	Portable	
	Real time	
DISADVANTAGES		
FLUOROSCOPY	**ULTRASONOGRAPHY**	**COMPUTED TOMOGRAPHY**
Poor target visibility	Needle difficult to see	Time-consuming
Radiation exposure	Limited anatomic information	Expensive
Not portable	Obscured by gas or bone	Radiation exposure
	More difficult technically with significant learning curve	Not portable
		Not real time

TABLE 74.3-3   RELATIVE MERITS OF ANTEGRADE AND RETROGRADE GASTROSTOMY TECHNIQUES

ADVANTAGES	
ANTEGRADE	RETROGRADE
Stable catheter	Seldom needs general anesthetic—can be performed on unstable patient with airway instability with local anesthetic alone[45]
	Catheters are smaller and less bulky
	Can be performed in patient with esophageal strictures or atresia
	No risk to upper airway or esophagus
	Change, removal, or manipulation of catheter is easily performed on an outpatient basis
	Versatile

DISADVANTAGES	
ANTEGRADE	RETROGRADE
May go through other loops of bowel (colon)[46]	Easier to dislodge
Potential esophageal damage[47]	Catheter smaller
Not possible if esophageal stricture or atresia	
Pulls down bacteria and infection from the mouth, pharynx, and esophagus[47,48]	
Difficult to remove (may need repeat gastroscopy)[47–51]	
Requires nasogastric and orogastric tubes for radiologic placement[49,52–54]	
If catheter is cut, it may cause obstruction[55,56]	
Catheters are bulky[57,58]	

guardian. The various risks of the procedure are explained, including gastric leak with associated cellulitis or peritonitis, which is the most significant complication. Other complications include the risk of hemorrhage and some discomfort and pain after the procedure.[69] Six hours before the procedure, a nasogastric tube is inserted and barium is administered so that the colon will be outlined. Prior to the procedure, antibiotics (cefazolin 30 mg/kg) and an analgesia (rectal acetaminophen 15 mg/kg) are administered and Emla cream is applied to the left upper quadrant to reduce the discomfort during introduction of a local anesthetic. The position of the lower edge of the liver and spleen is marked using ultrasonography (Figure 74.3-3). The patient is assessed to determine the need for sedation, a general anesthetic, or a local anesthetic alone. The choice of drugs and the doses used are outlined in the previous section on sedation.

PROCEDURE

The patient is placed on a C-arm fluoroscopic table (Figure 74.3-4).[44] Fluoroscopy is used to identify the contrast-filled colon (Figure 74.3-5). If this is not adequately filled with contrast, a dilute barium single-contrast enema is performed. The patient is given IV glucagon (0.2–0.5 mg). Stomach contents are aspirated via the nasogastric tube. Air is then injected into the stomach under direct vision, and the chosen site for placement of the G tube (lateral to the left rectus muscle and below the costal margin) is marked with a metallic object. Safe access at this site is ascertained prior to skin cleansing and introduction of a local anesthetic. The C-arm table is tilted as necessary to ensure a safe route into the stomach. The stomach is then deflated. Using standard sterile technique, with operating room gowns and gloves, the anterior abdominal wall is prepared and draped.

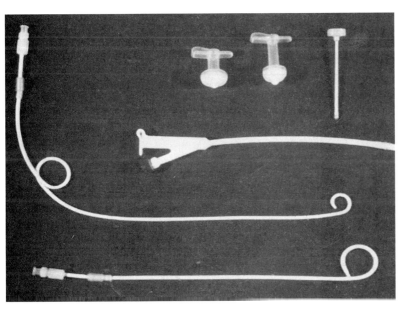

FIGURE 74.3-2 A variety of feeding tubes. *A*, Cope loop gastrostomy tube. *B*, Chait gastrojejunostomy tube. *C*, Balloon gastrostomy tube. *D*, Bard low-profile button gastrostomy tube.

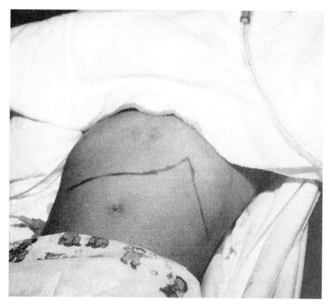

FIGURE 74.3-3 Ultrasonography is used to mark the lower limits of the liver and spleen on a patient prior to gastrostomy placement.

The chosen site for puncture is then infiltrated with 1% lidocaine (maximum dose of 0.5 cc/kg) using a 27-gauge needle. A spinal needle is used if the depth to the stomach is of significant distance. An incision is made with a number 11 scalpel blade to approximately equal the size of the catheter that is to be introduced. Usually, an 8.5 French catheter is used in the neonate; in infants and slightly older children, a 10 French catheter is used, whereas in children over 5 years of age, a 12 French catheter is introduced. The stomach is then reinflated with air, and the distended stomach is punctured percutaneously with a 19-gauge single-wall puncture needle (Cook, Bloomington, IN) using rapid entry. Contrast is then injected to confirm the position, and the retention suture, which is loaded within the access needle, is deposited in the stomach using an 0.25-inch guidewire (Figure 74.3-6).[70–72] The needle is then removed, and the reten-

tion suture is pulled up to maintain the stomach against the anterior abdominal wall. A second puncture is then performed with a 19-gauge Seldinger-type needle (Inrad, Kentwood, MI), through which a 0.35-inch straight guidewire (Cook; 70 cm) is introduced. A Coons dilator (Cook) is then used to dilate the tract (Figure 74.3-7).

Dilatation is assisted by using muco jelly on the tip of the dilator and by viewing the dilatation under fluoroscopy to reduce the risk of the retention suture breaking. The dilator is then removed, and the G tube (15 cm Dawson Mueller Mac-Loc, Cook) of chosen size is introduced. The locking loop is tied, and the loop is pulled up to the anterior abdominal wall. The position is checked with contrast to confirm placement and to check for leaks (Figure 74.3-8). If indicated, a GJ catheter can be placed as a primary procedure.[73] In this situation, once access has been obtained with the Seldinger needle, a 5 French dilator is then introduced, followed by a 5 French directional catheter (JB-1, Cook). A Benston wire (0.035 inch) is then introduced through the directional catheter, and the catheter and wire are manipulated into the pylorus and down the duodenum into the proximal jejunum. Once the wire is in position, the catheter is removed and the tract is dilated to the required size. An 8.5 or 10 French GJ catheter (Chait, GJ tube, Cook) (see Figure 74.3-7) is then introduced with a stiffener (Figure 74.3-9). The position of the GJ tube is confirmed prior to returning the patient to the ward.

POSTPROCEDURE ORDERS

Patients fast for 12 hours after the procedure. IV fluids are given to maintain hydration and to replace fluids lost via GI drainage. Nasogastric and G tubes are left to gravity drainage. Antibiotics are continued if there was any difficulty with the procedure or if there is an increased risk of infection. However, in 99% of cases, a single dose of antibiotics given at the time of the procedure is all that is needed. Analgesia in the form of morphine (0.05 mg/kg IV for the first 24 hours) and then acetaminophen (15 mg/kg) is given.

FIGURE 74.3-4 Patient is placed in the restraining device on the C-arm fluoroscopic table with a nasogastric tube, electrocardiograph, and pulse oximetry in position, as well as peripheral intravenous access in the left foot. The position of the liver has been outlined with ultrasonography and the site for gastrostomy placement outlined.

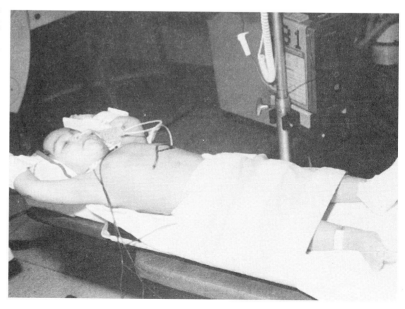

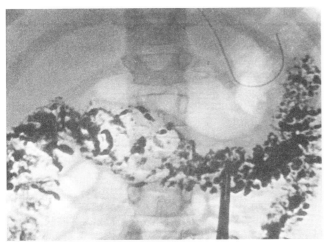

FIGURE 74.3-5 Contrast-filled transverse colon is seen in a patient with a nasogastric tube in position. The side position of a gastrostomy tube is marked with forceps, and the stomach is undistended.

At 12 hours, tube feeding is begun if the patient is clinically well and bowel sounds are present. Initially, clear fluids (Pedialyte) are given either intermittently or continuously, followed by half-strength feed and, finally, full-strength feed. Patients are usually kept in hospital for 72 hours and then discharged. Patients are assessed at 6 weeks, at which time long-term nutritional needs are assessed. At this stage, the Cope loop catheter is exchanged for a balloon type G catheter (see Figure 74.3-2) (MICC, Milpitas, CA). The balloon catheter permits the parent to replace it at home without the need to return to the hospital. Second, the size of the catheter can be increased over the ensuing 3 months to allow placement of a button G tube.

Some patients require gastric drainage and GJ feeding. This can be achieved by placing two catheters, one as a GJ tube and the other as a draining G tube. Alternatively, a balloon type G catheter containing a central jejunostomy feeding catheter can be placed, thereby allowing for feeding and gastric drainage through the same G tube site (MICC).

The indications for this procedure are to maintain the nutritional support of patients who are unable to maintain adequate nutrition by mouth or are unable to tolerate nasogastric tubes or for gastric decompression.[74–78] The vast majority of patients have neurologic deficits,[79] have swallowing disorders, or suffer from malignancies. We also use the G tube for gastric decompression in patients with small bowel obstruction or GI dysmotility.

RESULTS AND FOLLOW-UP STUDIES

Our interventional service has placed an average of 160 new G and 25 primary GJ tubes per year since 1995. There were no major complications of bowel perforation or catheter placement through another loop of bowel. In one patient, the catheter was malpositioned, and peritonitis developed, requiring laparotomy. Initially, a small number of patients developed local cellulitis, but routine use of antibiotics before the procedure has almost completely eliminated this complication.[55]

Two types of low-profile silicon button type G catheters are available. These are not placed before 3 months.[80,81] In most cases, the procedure is performed without difficulty by the enterostomy nurse in the outpatient clinic, but if there is any difficulty or if the patient requires sedation, it is performed in the radiology department. The indwelling G tube is removed, and a wire is left in position in the stomach. Lidocaine jelly is applied to the G tube site. Dilatation of the tract is performed if necessary. The more popular Bard button catheter (see Figure 74.3-2) is placed in boiling water, and then with the stiffener in place, the button is introduced into the stomach under fluoroscopic control using the wire in the tract as a guide. Dilatation of the tract may be needed because this is an 18 French catheter. The position is then confirmed radiologically. The other balloon low-profile catheter (MICC) is used usually in smaller children when dilatation is thought to be a problem. This catheter has the advantage of being small (14 French) and can be placed over a wire because it has a central opening. This catheter is best used as a replacement catheter rather than as a primary catheter because it is not

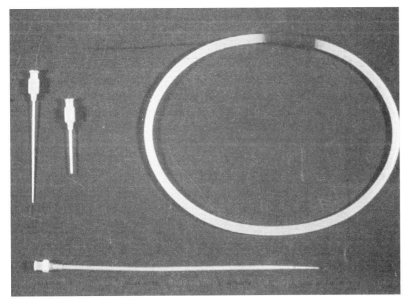

FIGURE 74.3-6 Retention suture is seen with the 19-gauge needle and wire introducer, as well as a Coons fascial dilator.

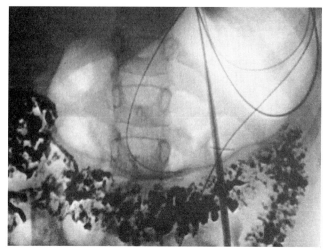

FIGURE 74.3-7   After a second puncture with a Seldinger needle, the tract was dilated with a Coons fascial dilator under fluoroscopic control.

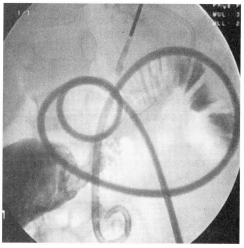

FIGURE 74.3-9   Example of the gastrojejunostomy catheter with the proximal loop in the stomach and the distal catheter in the proximal jejunum with a distal tight pigtail.

very well tapered. The MICC balloon catheter is not as durable as the Bard button catheter because it is more prone to rupture or leakage of the balloon. It is used in selected cases or because of parent preference.

In the small number of patients with proximal small bowel dysmotility, a gastrojejunal feeding tube and a gastric drainage tube are needed; in this situation, we favor the placement of two catheters at separate sites (Figure 74.3-10).

PERCUTANEOUS CECOSTOMY

Percutaneous cecostomy, commonly used in adults for decompression,[82–85] is less frequently performed in children. A surgically described technique of performing reversed appendicocecostomy for performing antegrade enemas has been described.[83] On occasion, a cecostomy is required in patients with severe intestinal pseudo-obstruction or in those with spina bifida and meningomyelocele who have severe constipation or fecal incontinence. The cecostomy permits introduction of a catheter to allow for direct ene-

mas to the large bowel or to allow decompression. The percutaneous procedures can be performed under sedation. Before the procedure, the patient is kept on oral fluids for 2 days. Then, prior to the procedure, a balanced electrolyte lavage solution is infused via a nasogastric tube at a rate of 25 mL/kg/h until rectal effluent is clear of solid fecal material. Antibiotics are given prior to the procedure. A large Foley catheter is introduced into the rectum, and air is introduced to fill the cecum. The technique is similar to that described for placement of a G tube using a transperitoneal or retroperitoneal approach (Figure 74.3-11).[83] There has been a single report of abdominal wall cellulitis secondary to percutaneous cecostomy.[86]

PLACEMENT OF NASODUODENAL TUBES

Catheters used primarily for duodenal manometry or pancreatic function tests are placed nasojejunally, but if a G tube is present, a gastrojejunal approach is feasible. The latter approach is less invasive and easier. Initially, a direc-

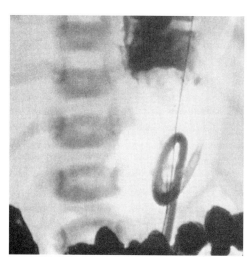

FIGURE 74.3-8   Cope loop gastrostomy tube is tightened and pulled up against the anterior abdominal wall and its position confirmed with contrast.

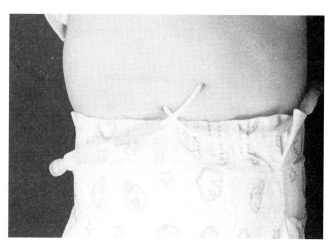

FIGURE 74.3-10   Gastrostomy and gastrojejunostomy tubes shown in a patient with separate entrance site, with the gastrostomy tube used for gastric aspiration and drainage and the gastrojejunostomy tube for feeding.

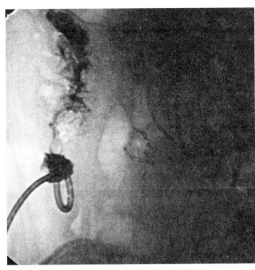

FIGURE 74.3-11 Cecostomy showing a catheter in the right iliac fossa with contrast filling the cecum.

tional catheter and wire are used to get into the proximal jejunum. The manometry catheter has multiple ports and a very small central lumen requiring an 0.018- or 0.025-inch wire over which the catheter is introduced.

DILATATION PROCEDURES

Esophageal Dilatation. Traditionally, esophageal strictures are dilated blindly following the introduction of bougie dilators through the mouth. However, the introduction of balloon catheters for angioplasty has resulted in the development of catheters for dilatation of esophageal strictures.[87] Larger balloons have also been developed for use in the GI tract. Balloon dilatation appears to carry a

reduced risk of complications in comparison with traditional bougie dilatation, particularly when used with fluoroscopic guidance. Over a 3-year period, we have done 70 esophageal dilatations in 30 patients carrying a variety of diagnoses, including achalasia,[88] strictures owing to caustic ingestion or radiation,[89] and gastroesophageal reflux. The choice of catheter size depends on the patient and the diameter of the esophagus above and below the stricture. In patients with achalasia, balloons of 25, 30, and 35 mm are routinely used, and a variety of balloon diameters from 4 mm up are used for other cases.

The procedure is performed under sedation or, if indicated, under general anesthetic. Local anesthetic is sprayed into the back of the throat. A nasogastric tube is placed to aspirate any residual gastric contents and to introduce contrast. A bite block is used to keep the teeth apart, and a directional catheter (JB-1) stabilized by a Benston 0.035-inch wire is directed down the esophagus. This procedure can be done through either the transoral or nasal approach. Occasionally, oblique or lateral fluoroscopy is required to direct the wire into the correct position. The length and diameter of the stricture and its relationship to the rest of the esophagus are assessed with contrast. The wire and catheter are placed through the stricture with little risk of damage or perforation. The correct-sized balloon catheter is introduced over the wire. Dilatations are performed by inflating the balloon for 30 seconds, and then, after deflation, the procedure is repeated three times at each level (Figure 74.3-12). Contrast is then injected to assess for any leaks, and the proximal esophagus is aspirated during withdrawal of the nasogastric tube. After the procedure, the patient is kept with nothing per mouth for 24 hours and is monitored for any complications. Occasionally, combined radiologic and endoscopic procedures are performed, and,

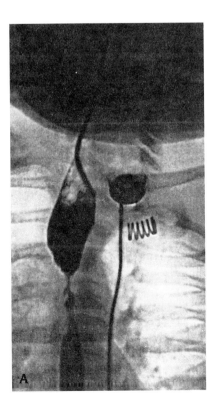
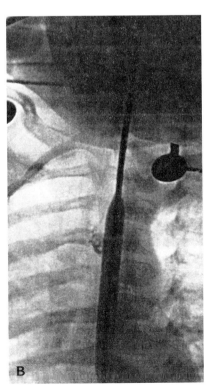

FIGURE 74.3-12 *A*, Esophageal stricture post tracheoesophageal fistula. *B*, Stricture dilatation using a balloon.

if indicated, a corticosteroid is injected directly into the wall of the esophagus to reduce the risk of scarring and inflammation. Repeat dilatation is performed as necessary. In patients with a G tube, esophageal strictures can be dilated via the G-tube site instead of the more traditional oral or nasal approach. Treatment of the underlying cause of the stricture must also be considered, which might include antireflux surgery for reflux esophagitis or chemotherapy or radiotherapy for malignant strictures. Recently, expandable metallic stents have been used for esophageal strictures, particularly in strictures caused by malignancies. We have not had any experience with this technique.

Using the aforementioned approach, no patients have developed mediastinitis or an esophageal leak.[90] However, we have treated several patients who experienced complications from bougie dilatation who required percutaneous drainage of abscesses and leaks.

Dilatation of Other Intestinal Strictures. Occasionally, prepyloric strictures develop following the ingestion of corrosive materials. These patients are usually treated with gastroenterostomy. However, in those patients deemed unsuitable for operative treatment, dilatation may be considered. This technique, which requires the use of a balloon catheter, is very similar to that used for esophageal dilatation. The correct size of the balloon may be difficult to determine because the pylorus is a dynamic channel. Similarly, the technique for the dilatation of the esophageal strictures may be applied to anastomotic strictures elsewhere in the intestinal tract provided that they are accessible.

Colonic strictures may be treated by balloon dilatation via the rectal approach or, if present, through a colostomy (Figure 74.3-13).[91,92] Owing to the higher risk of infection, antibiotic coverage is required. These procedures are not commonly performed in the pediatric setting.

PERCUTANEOUS BIOPSY OF ABDOMINAL MASSES

Percutaneous biopsy of abdominal masses is a commonly performed procedure using ultrasonography or CT guidance.[24,93–96] Increased availability and use of image-guided biopsy is a direct result of the development of various cross-sectional imaging modalities, including fluoroscopy, ultrasonography, CT, and MRI.[97,98] As well, thin-walled fine-gauge needles possessing a variety of tips have been developed, which allows for obtaining larger tissue specimens. At the same time, great advances in the histopathologic methods for identifying and grading tumor material determine the need for larger tissue specimens.[99–101] A high proportion of intra-abdominal tumors in the pediatric population are sarcomas, and aspiration biopsies or small-core biopsies fail to provide sufficient tissue for diagnosis. Furthermore, in patients with known primary malignancies, fine-needle biopsies are ideal for confirmation of malignancy, to document metastases, or to identify recurrent tumors.

Prior review of the patient's imaging studies is required, which, together with consultation with responsible physicians, surgeons, and pathologists, will predetermine the probable identity of the tumor, the amount of tissue required, and the potential risks and benefits of using a percutaneous approach. Patient preparation is similar to that with other interventional procedures, and choice of sedation versus a general anesthetic is made on an individual basis. The primary contraindications to percutaneous biopsy include a significant, uncorrectible coagulopathy and/or lack of a safe pathway for needle placement and guidance. The most accessible lesion is identified if they are multiple, and a skin entrance site is chosen. If it is a large lesion, the periphery of the lesion is biopsied preferentially to avoid the risk of biopsying a central necrotic area. Most intra-abdominal biopsies are performed under

FIGURE 74.3-13 *A,* Colonic strictures following necrotizing enterocolitis. *B,* Stricture dilated via the colostomy with a 10 mm balloon.

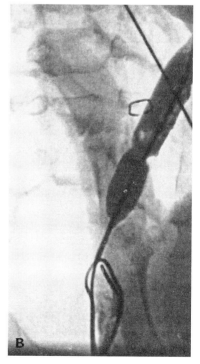

ultrasonography guidance (Figure 74.3-14). CT is seldom used because it is time-consuming and expensive and requires patient cooperation or a general anesthetic. Ultrasonography is ideal for biopsies of solid organs such as the liver, accessible solid lesions arising from the pancreas or spleen, or other intra-abdominal masses. The chosen puncture site is marked prior to the procedure using a permanent marker. The patient is positioned for the procedure to allow optimum access. The overlying skin is then prepared and draped using sterile technique. After lidocaine is introduced in the subcutaneous tissues, a small nick is made in the skin with a scalpel blade.

A variety of needles are available for percutaneous biopsies. They differ in gauge, length, and mechanism of obtaining tissue. They can be categorized into aspiration or cutting mechanisms and automated or manual devices.

The Chiba and Turner needles are both aspiration biopsy needles (20–23 gauge). The Chiba needle has a beveled edge of 25° and the Turner needle of 45°. Aspiration needles can be used for obtaining cytologic and bacteriologic material. Occasionally, histologic material may be obtained, especially with the Turner needle, owing to the acutely beveled edge.

Cutting needles, categorized as end-cutting and side-cutting types, are designed to increase the probability of obtaining histologic material. The end-cutting needles either have an end-cutting bevel or a serrated edge, which allows for optimal cutting and retention of core material. The side-cutting needles include the Truecut, the automated, reusable Biopty (Bard, Murray Hill, NJ) (Figure 74.3-15), and minopty guns (Meditech, Westwood, MA) (Figure 74.3-16). The Autovac needle (Angiomed, Karlsruhe, Germany), an end-cutting needle, is automated to allow a variety of depths of tissues to be biopsied, ranging from 1 to 4 cm (see Figure 74.3-16). This needle, which permits the operator to guide the needle with ultrasonography, is ideally suited for most abdominal core biopsies. In general, fine needles (20–23 gauge) should be used when

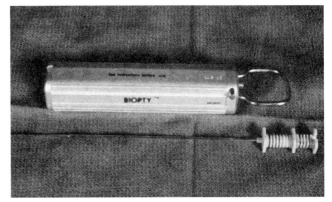

FIGURE 74.3-15   Bard resterilizable Biopty gun with disposable needles in (14, 16, and 18 gauge) and a 2.3 cm throw.

there is a risk of entering vital structures such as blood vessels or bowel loops.[102] Larger needles may be selected for percutaneous biopsy in certain situations in which there is no intervening vital structure, when a retroperitoneal or a posterior extraperitoneal approach is used, or when round cell tumors are suspected.

Percutaneous Liver Biopsy.   Blind percutaneous biopsy of the liver has been performed for a number of years, with a high success rate. However, biopsies of focal hepatic lesions are best performed with image guidance using either ultrasonography or CT. It is possible to biopsy a lesion as small as a few millimeters in size under ultrasonography control (Figure 74.3-17). We routinely use an 18-gauge Surecut (TSK Laboratory, Tochigi, Japan) needle for biopsy of diffuse parenchymal lesions and a Surecut, Autovac (Angiomed), or Biopty gun for the biopsy of focal lesions.[103–105]

In patients with coagulopathies, transcutaneous biopsy of liver lesions can be performed coaxially with removal of the biopsy needle and then introduction of Gelfoam or coils to reduce the risk of bleeding.[106–108]

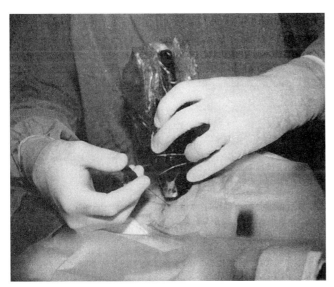

FIGURE 74.3-14   Ultrasonography guidance is shown using an ultrasound probe with a sterile cover and freehand guidance.

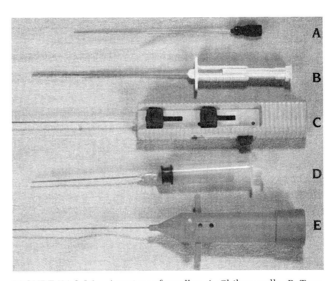

FIGURE 74.3-16   A variety of needles. *A,* Chiba needle. *B,* Truecut needle. *C,* Minopty gun (disposable). *D,* Surecut needle. *E,* Angiomed autovac needle.

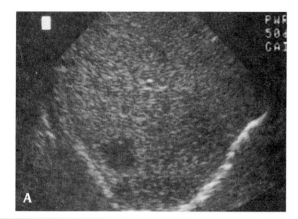

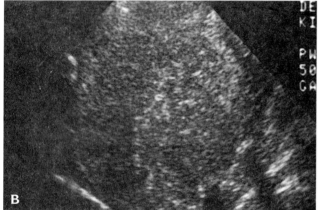

FIGURE 74.3-17   *A*, Deep 5 mm lesion is seen in the posterior aspect of the right lobe of the liver on ultrasonography. *B*, Biopsy under ultrasonography guidance is performed successfully with the needle seen traversing the lesion.

Transjugular Liver Biopsy. Transjugular biopsy is reserved for patients with severe coagulopathies that are uncorrectable.[109–111] This procedure is usually performed under a general anesthetic with the patient in the supine Trendelenberg position. The right internal jugular vein is accessed percutaneously, and a wire and sheath are introduced. Selective catheterization of the right hepatic vein is performed. Wedge pressures and free hepatic and inferior vena cava pressures are taken. A wedge of hepatic and free hepatic venogram is performed. The biopsy is performed with a Colapinto (Cook)-type biopsy needle with the tip of the needle directed posteriorly and a sheath placed within the right hepatic vein (Figure 74.3-18). The biopsy technique involves rapid puncture with aspiration. Saline is injected to release the core of liver tissues. Postprocedure venograms are performed to exclude perforation of the liver capsule (Figure 74.3-19). Transvenous biopsies can also be performed from a femoral approach using a claw-type biopsy forceps through a sheath and catheter.

Transcatheter biopsy of hepatic lesions is not commonly required in the pediatric setting because primary hilar lesions are rare. These are performed using a brush biopsy technique or by introducing a needle through the biliary drainage catheter, and biopsies are made at the site of the mass.[112] Fluoroscopy can also be used to guide a biopsy needle to a presumed tumor site shown with percutaneous transhepatic cholangiography (PTC) or as an area of stricture or mass.

Pancreatic Biopsy. Primary pancreatic tumors are relatively rare in pediatric patients. The principles for obtaining a biopsy are similar to those for other solid masses. The decision to perform a percutaneous biopsy depends on the extent of the primary lesion, the presence of secondary pathology, and the surgical alternatives. Direct visualization with ultrasonography or CT[111] is usually required to allow accurate placement of needles for small pancreatic lesions.[106,113,114]

Lymph Node Biopsy. Percutaneous biopsy of intra-abdominal lymph nodes can be accomplished with fluoroscopic guidance following opacification by lymphangiography. In the case of suspected lymphoma, percutaneous lymph node biopsy can be performed using ultrasonography or CT guidance. The results obtained from percutaneous lymph node biopsy are generally not as rewarding as those of biopsies of other organs.

Splenic Biopsy. Splenic aspiration and biopsy under ultrasonography or CT guidance are usually indicated for the histologic diagnosis of the etiology of diffuse splenomegaly[115] or focal masses. Fine-needle biopsy may be sufficient for the confirmation of known tumors or identifying an organism, but core biopsy with either 20- or 18-gauge needles provides a much better yield. In our experience in those patients with normal clotting, there is little risk of intraperitoneal hemorrhage, even with the larger needles.

PERCUTANEOUS ASPIRATION AND DRAINAGE

Percutaneous drainage of abdominal abscesses has proved to be one of the most successful and gratifying of all interventional procedures. In a relatively short time, it has achieved a remarkable degree of acceptance within the surgical community.[116] Intra-abdominal abscesses can now be

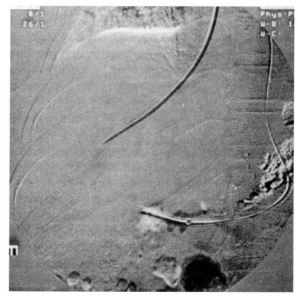

FIGURE 74.3-18   Subtracted image with a sheath seen in the right hepatic vein in the position ready for placement of the Colapinto biopsy needle.

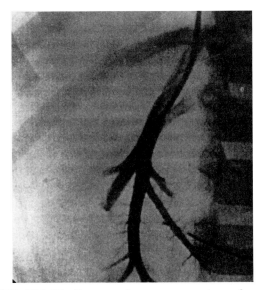

FIGURE 74.3-19 Postprocedure venogram is performed to exclude extravasation of contrast and perforation.

aspirated and drained percutaneously, with a "cure" rate approaching 85%.[117-121] A variety of other intra-abdominal fluid collections can be safely aspirated and drained percutaneously, including hematomas, seromas, lymphoceles, bilomas, pancreatic pseudocysts, and loculated ascites. In general, the technique is similar for all fluid collections. This involves guided introduction of a needle and aspiration of the material. If drainage is required, the needle is exchanged over a wire with a catheter. Contraindications to aspiration and drainage include the absence of a safe access route, which would include the transgression of major organs such as liver, spleen, or kidney; the presence of overlying blood vessels and nerves; or sterile spaces such as the peritoneum or pleura. The presence of coagulation abnormalities is a relative contraindication.

The procedure is performed under sterile conditions. The skin is prepared and draped, and 1% lidocaine is introduced. The technique usually involves placement of a 22-gauge Chiba needle into the collection under ultrasonography guidance. The collection is aspirated, and if drainage is required, a 0.018-inch wire is exchanged using a Neff introducer system (Cook) for a 0.035-inch wire. The tract is dilated, and a catheter is introduced. An 8.5 or 10 French all-purpose drainage catheter (Meditech) is usually sufficient for most fluid collections. A larger-caliber catheter such as a Sump drain or a Thalquick (Cook) abscess drainage catheter is used if necessary. The abscess or fluid collection is drained using a closed system drainage bag (Medics, Hilliard, OH) either by gravity drainage or suction using a Hemovac (Zimmer, Dover, OH). For large or superficial lesions, a trocar technique can be used with direct introduction of an all-purpose drain (Meditech), which is supplied with a sharp inner stylet.

Monitoring Drainage Procedures. Regular saline irrigation is used to help clear the cavity of pus or particulate debris. Antibiotics are continued postprocedure until the signs and symptoms of infection have resolved.

The volume of drainage is reviewed daily, and if there is a sudden drop in volume, a block in the catheter should be suspected. If the volume increases dramatically, this might represent development of a fistula or leak. A sinogram, using dilute water-soluble contrast medium, should be performed 1 to 2 days after the initial drainage. This will define the extent of the abscess and its communication with other structures. Ultrasonography or CT should be repeated 3 to 4 days after the procedure and again immediately before the catheter is removed. Percutaneous drainage may not be successful because of a persistent fistula, necrotic material within the collection, viscous pus, multiloculated (or multiple) abscesses, or a large abscess cavity. To improve the success of drainage and to minimize complications, bowel loops should be avoided and sterile spaces should not be contaminated. Catheter manipulation should be minimized to reduce the spread of infection. Tissue trauma should also be kept to a minimum to reduce complications, and a large catheter should be used if the collection is viscous or contains cellular debris.

Abscesses. Hepatic Abscess. Primary hepatic abscesses are relatively uncommon in pediatrics. Pyogenic abscesses are most commonly seen in children with chronic granulomatous disease or those immunocompromised owing to treatment.[122] They are also seen as a complication of appendicitis with portal vein thrombophlebitis.

Amebic liver abscesses are seen in Southeast Asia, Africa, and South America and are typically single and loculated in the posterosuperior or anteroinferior aspect of the right lobe of the liver. These can be complicated by rupture intra-abdominally or even into the pleural space. Depending on the size of the abscess, they can be treated either by antibiotics (metronidazole) or by percutaneous drainage (Figure 74.3-20).

In the immunocompromised patient, microabscesses of fungal origin are often present. These are usually too small to require drainage but may be aspirated to make the diagnosis.[123]

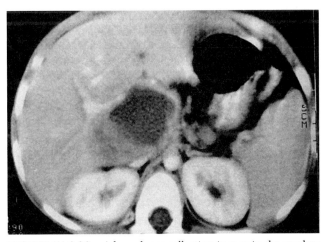

FIGURE 74.3-20 A hypodense collection is seen in the caudate lobe of the liver, which is well seen on computed tomography and is best drained under ultrasonography and fluoroscopic guidance.

Subphrenic Abscess. Subphrenic abscesses arise postoperatively or occur quite commonly in childhood following a ruptured appendix. Subphrenic abscesses are frequently difficult to access, and a transhepatic or intercostal route may be necessary (Figure 74.3-21). A combination of CT and ultrasonography guidance may be required.[124,125]

Splenic Abscesses. Splenic abscesses can be aspirated or drained successfully under ultrasonography control.[126] Most cases can be treated effectively with repeated aspiration or catheter drainage with a relatively low rate of complication (13%) (Figure 74.3-22).[127] Splenectomy should be performed only in splenic abscesses that are not accessible percutaneously and in those cases with percutaneous drainage failure.[127]

Pelvic Abscess. Pelvic abscesses are often deep and obscured by overlying bowel, vessels, urinary bladder, and bony pelvis (Figure 74.3-23). If they are superficial and easily visualized under ultrasonography or CT guidance, transabdominal access for drainage can be performed. If

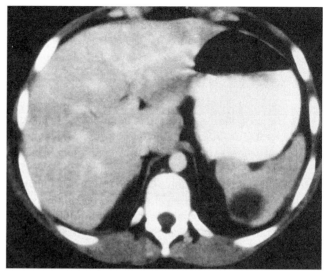

FIGURE 74.3-22   A posterior hypodense lesion seen in the spleen, which was aspirated successfully under ultrasonography guidance.

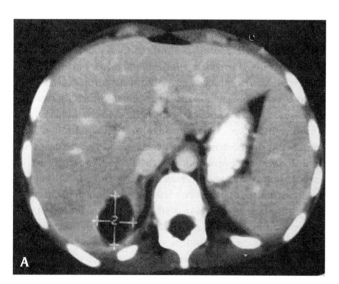
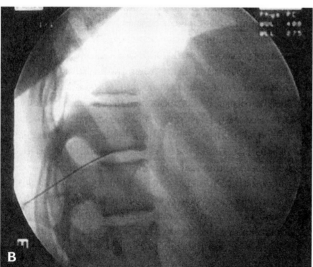

FIGURE 74.3-21   *A,* Subphrenic abscesses on computed tomography just below the right hemidiaphragm posterior to the liver. *B,* Lateral view of fluoroscopy seen with a needle entering the abscess. Guidance was performed under ultrasonography and further wire and catheter placement was performed under fluoroscopy.

the lesions are deep and anterior to the rectum, a transrectal approach can be used.[128] The patient is placed in the decubitus position. Ultrasonography is performed transabdominally to identify the abscess and to place the needle (Figure 74.3-24). Guidance can also be obtained with a transrectal ultrasound probe.[129–131] An enema tip catheter is introduced into the rectum, and a trocar needle is advanced to the tip of the catheter. Under ultrasonography control, the needle and stylet are advanced through the anterior rectum into the abscess. This is followed by placement of a wire, dilatation, and catheter placement. We have performed this procedure in 30 patients and have shown that we can achieve a significant reduction in the time of recovery when compared with the traditional transabdominal or surgical approach (Figure 74.3-25). These deep abscesses can also be drained under CT guidance via the paracoccygeal route.[132]

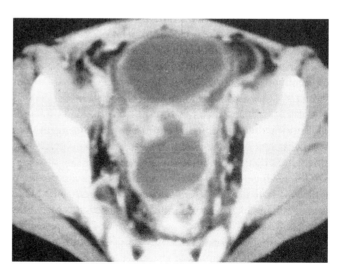

FIGURE 74.3-23   Deep pelvic abscess seen posterior to the bladder (*arrow*) with enhancing rim and the rectum seen posteriorly.

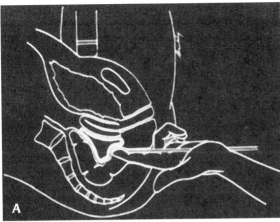

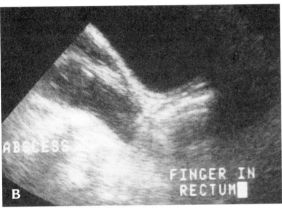

FIGURE 74.3-24 *A,* Diagram of transabdominal ultrasonography with rectal placement of the index finger with a trocar needle anterior to the index finger seen through the distended urinary bladder. *B,* Ultrasonographic view of the same patient with the finger seen in the rectum. The abscess posterior to the bladder is seen in the longitudinal section.

Interloop Abscess. Because of the position and the overlying bowel loops, these abscesses are difficult to access. It is best to assess interloop abscesses with CT to determine the precise location. Aspiration can be performed under CT or ultrasonography guidance, transgressing bowel with a 22-gauge Chiba needle.[133]

Pancreatic Pseudocyst. Pseudocysts develop following acute pancreatitis, which in the pediatric age group can be due to multiple etiologies.[134] They present as low-density collections on CT and hypoechoic masses on ultrasonography (Figure 74.3-26). Most pseudocysts resolve spontaneously over a period of weeks or months. If the patient is asymptomatic, a pseudocyst can be drained percutaneously or preferably transgastrically. Under ultrasonography guidance, the position of the pseudocyst is marked on the skin of the patient. The stomach is then inflated using a nasogastric tube, and a trocar needle (18 gauge) is introduced through the anterior and posterior stomach walls into the pseudocyst behind. After the pseudocyst has been drained, the needle is replaced with a wire, the tract is dilated, and a Cope loop catheter is introduced into the pseudocyst. The pseudocyst is left to drain for 4 to 6 weeks. A cystogram may be performed to assess communication with the pancreatic duct. Once the catheter is removed, residual

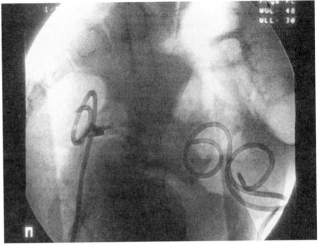

FIGURE 74.3-25 Lateral radiograph of a patient who has a transrectal drain in position and two transpercutaneous drains seen anteriorly for the treatment of a ruptured appendix.

drainage will continue through the fistulous tract into the stomach (Figure 74.3-27).

Pancreatic Abscesses. Abscesses related to pancreatitis can be treated percutaneously if a safe access route is available. Percutaneous aspiration of these lesions can also be performed for diagnostic purposes. Phlegmonous pancreatitis does not respond to simple drainage and is not suited to simple percutaneous drainage because of the nature of the tissues (Figure 74.3-28).

BILIARY INTERVENTION

PTC, percutaneous transhepatic transcholecystic cholangiography (PTTC), percutaneous biliary drainage, dilatation of biliary strictures, and stone removal are established interventional techniques in the diagnosis and management of biliary tract disease.[135–140] Owing to the advent of liver transplant, there has been an increase in the need for

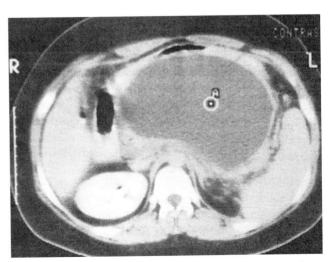

FIGURE 74.3-26 A computed tomographic scan of an abdomen showing a large, relatively hypodense collection in the midabdomen posterior to the stomach consistent with a large pseudocyst.

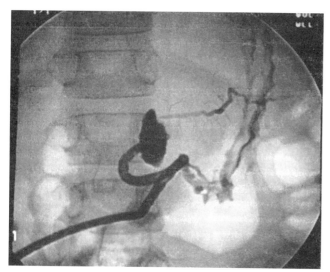

FIGURE 74.3-27 Transgastric drainage of a pseudocyst had been performed, with 6 weeks of drainage. A contrast study through the tube demonstrates filling of the small remaining cyst and the distal part of the pancreatic duct. Some contrast is draining into the stomach.

these procedures in the pediatric population.[141–143] Endoscopic retrograde cholangiographic procedures are indicated in those patients with intact common bile ducts and where access is possible.[144]

PERCUTANEOUS TRANSHEPATIC CHOLANGIOGRAPHY

The primary indications for PTC or PTTC include the differentiation of medically treatable from surgically treatable causes of cholestasis, demonstration of intrahepatic calculi, or extrahepatic choledocholithiasis. In addition, cholangiographic investigations are invaluable to diagnose a congenital abnormality such as biliary atresia or choledochal cyst and inflammatory conditions such as sclerosing or ascending cholangitis. They can also be used to evaluate surgical conditions such as biliary-enteric anastomoses and to assess if intrahepatic abscesses communicate with the bil-

iary radical. Contraindications include uncorrectable bleeding disorders or a previous life-threatening reaction to iodinated contrast material. Vascular hepatic tumors and vascular malformations, as well as ascites, are relative contraindications.

General anesthesia is used for most children because the procedure requires significant patient control, especially in those with small biliary radicals. If there is a strong suggestion of cholangitis, triple antibiotics (ampicillin, gentamicin, and metronidazole) are started 6 hours before the procedure. If there is no obvious cholangitis, a single IV dose of cefazolin (30 mg/kg) is given prior to the procedure.

Cholangiograms are performed with a 22-gauge Chiba needle with ultrasonography guidance.[145] We make use of a hiliter needle (Inrad), which is better seen on ultrasonography. All procedures are performed under ultrasonography guidance (Figure 74.3-29). After prior imaging investigation has been reviewed, a choice is made between a right hepatic, left hepatic, or transcholecystic approach. The right hepatic approach at the midaxillary line is most commonly used (Figure 74.3-30). Fluoroscopy of the upper abdomen is performed to identify the position of the chest cavity. The right-sided approach has the disadvantages of transgressing pleura, increased pain owing to the intercostal approach, and the possibility of intervening bowel. The left-sided approach is more vertical and may allow easier access to the common bile duct via the common hepatic duct. This is a safer approach because the pleura is not being transgressed.

Transcholecystic studies are performed in patients who do not have dilated bile ducts or if repeated attempts at transhepatic cholangiography have been unsuccessful. This procedure is also performed using a 22-gauge needle under ultrasonography guidance, with a transhepatic route (Figure 74.3-31). Once the gallbladder is penetrated, a specimen is obtained, and dilute contrast is injected. After completion of the procedure, it is important to drain the gallbladder completely to reduce the risk of bowel peritonitis. In my own experience, the success rate with trans-

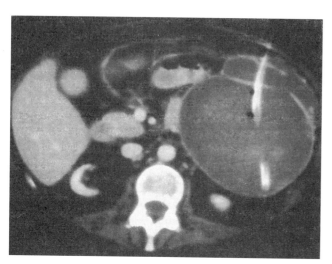

FIGURE 74.3-28 A complicated pancreatic pseudocyst with hemorrhage and infection. Percutaneous drainage was attempted but was unsuccessful owing to the thickness of the materials.

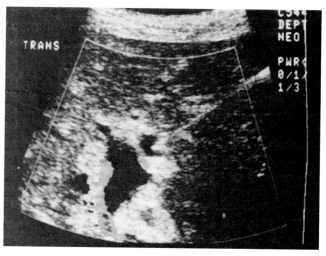

FIGURE 74.3-29 Ultrasonography guidance is used to place a 22-gauge Chiba needle into mildly dilated bile duct seen close to the portal vein and hepatic artery.

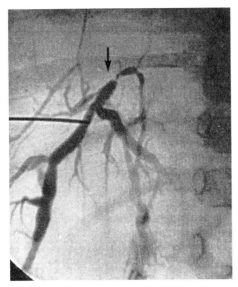

FIGURE 74.3-30 Right hepatic approach into transplanted reduced left hepatic lobe. A relatively normal-sized duct is seen with a focal biliary stricture just distal to the puncture site (*arrow*).

hepatic cholangiography in the patient with undilated intrahepatic ducts is approximately 70%, whereas the success rate of transcholecystic cholangiography approaches 100%. Our experience with 30 PTTCs has been very successful, with only one complication in our first patient, who developed a bile leak. In this case, the procedure was not performed under a general anesthetic.

BILIARY DRAINAGE

The decision to perform biliary drainage depends on the nature of the pathology. Indications include malignant obstruction with associated cholangitis, pruritus with liver dysfunction, biliary stricture owing to previous surgery, or sclerosing cholangitis. Drainage is also performed in patients with bile leaks, which is a relatively frequent postoperative complication following hepatic transplant.[146–148]

After cholangiography has been performed, it is important to carefully select the correct duct to drain. The duct should be entered peripherally, thus reducing the risk of damage to major vessels and increasing the purchase (ie, the length of catheter within the ductal system). The puncture site should be chosen so that there is a minimum of curvature, thus allowing for the forces during dilatation to be directed inferiorly. A 22-gauge Chiba needle is introduced into the selected duct, either under fluoroscopic guidance with a C-arm unit or with ultrasonography. Bile is aspirated, and a 0.018 Mandril (Cook) wire is introduced. The stricture is usually transgressed using selective wires and dilators. If there is evidence of cholangitis, manipulation should be kept to a minimum and drainage achieved as soon as possible. Further manipulation can occur once infection has resolved.

The ultimate goal of biliary drainage is to place a 10 French or larger catheter in position. We use a Cope loop catheter and hole punch to fashion the catheter according to the patient's size. After the stricture has been dilated or the obstruction has been transgressed, the tube should be allowed to drain externally until the bile is clear. Subsequent daily irrigations can be done with the catheter closed (Figure 74.3-32).

BILIARY DILATATION

Dilatation of a biliary stricture is usually performed with a balloon catheter (Figure 74.3-33).[149] The size of the dilatation should be gauged from the size of the normal duct proximal and distal to the obstruction. The dilatation is performed, and a catheter with multiple side holes is inserted. Occasionally, an internal stent may be used. The polyethylene type of internal stent should be considered only in patients with a short life expectancy or irreversible hepatic dysfunction.[150] We have made use of a wall-expandable stainless steel stent in a patient who developed an anastomotic stricture after hepatic transplant. The patient has remained symptom free, with no evidence of obstruction for a period of 18 months (Figure 74.3-34).[151]

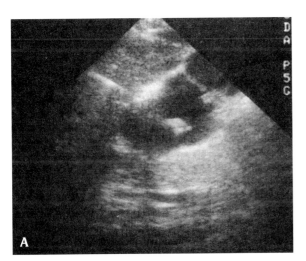
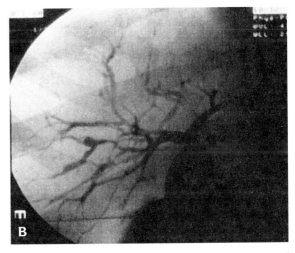

FIGURE 74.3-31 *A*, Sonogram of transhepatic placement of a Chiba needle into the gallbladder for the performance of a cholecystic cholangiogram. *B*, Contrast is injected through the catheter, and this demonstrates filling of the intrahepatic radicals, which demonstrate the features of sclerosing cholangitis with bleeding and irregularity of the bile ducts.

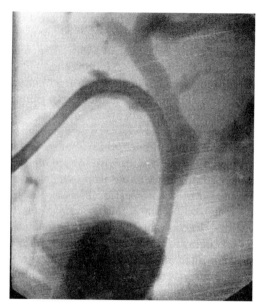

FIGURE 74.3-32 Internal and external biliary drainage has been performed in a patient with a focal stricture at the site of the choledochal jejunostomy anastomosis.

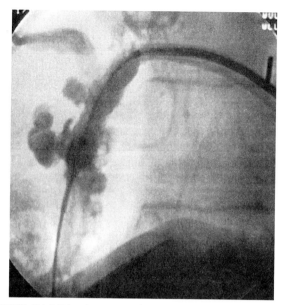

FIGURE 74.3-34 An internal metallic wall stent has been placed in a patient with a persistent choledochal jejunostomy stricture that was not responsive to repeated biliary dilatation.

T-TUBE CHOLANGIOGRAPHY
AND BILIARY INTERVENTION

T-tube cholangiography is performed in patients who have a T tube following surgical removal of the gallbladder or in patients who have had a total liver transplant with a bile duct anastomosis. Retained stones or debris can be removed via the tract. The tube is usually left in place for 6 weeks to form a fistulous tract. The T tube is then removed over a wire, a catheter is introduced, and the calculi or debris is removed with a basket. This is best performed using a steerable Burhenne (Cook)-type catheter.

Biliary debris or calculi can be removed percutaneously. After the correct duct has been accessed, a sheath is introduced followed by a basket, which is then used to grab or

crush the calculi prior to removal (Figure 74.3-35).[152] Debris can be removed in a similar manner.

TRANSHEPATIC PORTAL VENOUS INTERVENTION

The portal venous system can be accessed percutaneously quite easily using ultrasonography guidance. The technique is similar to that used for biliary cannulation using a 22-gauge Chiba needle followed by a 0.018 wire and then an exchange system. This allows for measurement of pressures, embolization of bleeding varices, and dilatation of portal venous anastomotic strictures. It can also be used to embolize portal venous to hepatic venous malformations. Dilatation of portal venous strictures after hepatic transplant can also be achieved (Figure 74.3-36).

TRANSJUGULAR INTRAHEPATIC
PORTOSYSTEMIC SHUNTS

Transjugular intrahepatic portosystemic shunting (TIPSS) is a recently developed procedure for the treatment of GI bleeding from varices owing to portal hypertension. It involves the creation of a parenchymal tract from the hepatic to portal vein, which is given support by the insertion of a metallic stent.[153–155]

TIPSS is described as a safe, effective, short-term procedure for the reduction of portal pressure. The short-term success rate is reported to be over 90%. The long-term outlook for the procedure will ultimately depend on the treatment and prevention of intimal hyperplasia within the shunt and draining veins.

The procedure is highly effective in lowering portal pressure and controlling acute variceal bleeding. However, its long-term effectiveness in preventing recurrent bleeding and as a treatment for ascites has not been clearly established when compared with conventional therapy. In addition, acute and chronic complications of the procedure are not insubstantial.

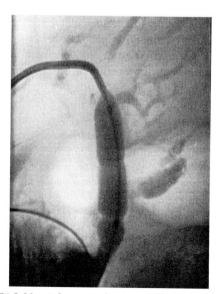

FIGURE 74.3-33 Dilatation of a choledochal jejunostomy stricture with a balloon dilator, with areas of narrowing seen in the balloon.

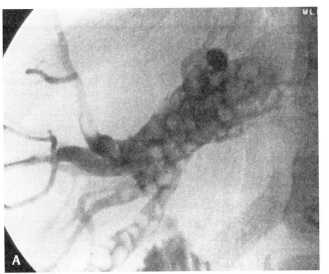
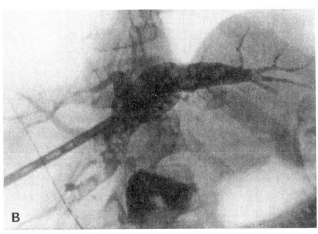

FIGURE 74.3-35 *A*, Cholangiogram demonstrating the biliary system of a patient with numerous calculi. *B*, Calculi were removed with the placement of a sheath and basket. This required repeated removal of calculi.

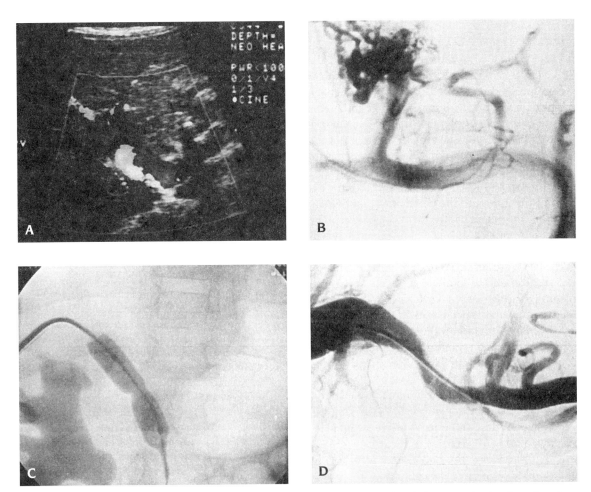

FIGURE 74.3-36 *A*, Ultrasonography of the portal venous system showed turbulence, and color Doppler ultrasonography showed changes consistent with a portal venous stricture. *B*, Transhepatic placement of a catheter in the portal venous system demonstrated gastric varices and prominence of the cardinal veins and esophageal varices. Portal hypertension was due to a portal venous anastomotic stricture. *C*, Balloon dilatation of the portal-venous stricture. *D*, Postdilatation venogram demonstrated resolution of the portal hypertension and pressure differential and antegrade flow into the liver.

The two main indications are (1) acute variceal bleeding uncontrolled by medical treatment, including sclerotherapy, and (2) recurrent variceal bleeding in patients who are refractory or intolerant to conventional management.[156] TIPSS is preferable to surgical shunting in Child's class C patients for both indications and in patients with refractory bleeding awaiting liver transplant.

Unproven indications are initial therapy of acute variceal hemorrhage, prophylactic therapy to prevent recurrent variceal hemorrhage, refractory ascites, and Budd-Chiari syndrome and to reduce intraoperative morbidity during liver transplant surgery. Contraindications include heart failure, polycystic liver disease, infection, severe hepatic encephalopathy, and fulminant liver failure.

Minor procedural complications occur in 10% of cases. Severe, life-threatening complications occur 1 to 2% of the time and include hemoperitoneum, hemobilia, acute hepatic ischemia, and pulmonary edema. Chronic complications include portal vein thrombosis, hemolysis, shunt stenosis, and hepatic encephalopathy. The latter may occur in 15 to 30% of cases and is associated with prior history of hepatic encephalopathy, severe liver disease, an older age group, large shunt diameters, and low final portosystemic gradient. Most respond to medical therapy, although the occasional shunt has to be occluded.[156]

The procedure is approached via puncture of the right internal jugular vein. A wire is then introduced, and the right hepatic vein is selectively catheterized. The catheter is wedged, and pressures are recorded. A wedged hepatic venogram may demonstrate the portal vein. The catheter is replaced by a sheath, and a Colapinto transjugular biopsy needle is introduced into the sheath and into the hepatic vein. The needle is directed anteromedially 2 to 3 cm into the parenchyma. Gentle aspiration is applied as the needle is slowly withdrawn, and when blood appears, contrast is injected to confirm entry into the portal vein or a branch. A wire is then introduced into the portal vein. The parenchymal tract is dilated with an 8 mm angioplasty balloon. The balloon is deflated, and the transjugular catheter and 9 French sheath are advanced into the portal vein. The transjugular catheter and balloon are removed, and a wall stent catheter, with a balloon attached, is introduced over the wire across from the hepatic vein to the portal vein. The balloon is inflated to distend the stent. Portal venous pressures are recorded, and venography is performed. This usually demonstrates the shunt and shows hepatopedal flow to the inferior vena cava with collapse of the varices. Rarely, the varices persist despite a well-functioning shunt, in which case, embolization is performed. If the shunt is felt to be open but the pressure remains above 12 mm Hg, the stent is dilated up to 10 mm.

Problems with accessing the portal vein do occur. In these circumstances, use of ultrasonography or the placement of a wire into the portal vein under ultrasonography control may help to direct the portal venous transjugular puncture. Some pain may be experienced during the procedure; for this reason, the procedure is best performed under a general anesthetic. If the stent is not long enough or does not cover the entire length of the parenchymal tract, an additional stent can be deployed to complete the shunt; parallel shunts may be used in patients with persistent portal hypertension. Doppler ultrasonography is used to monitor shunt patency approximately every 3 months, and venography is performed twice yearly. If shunt stenosis or occlusion is suspected, the patient is restudied. Stenosis is treated by angioplasty first and, in some cases, by additional stent placement. Thrombus within the shunt can be easily pushed into the portal vein using a soft occlusion balloon catheter. The clot presumably passes into the reopened varices and occludes them.[157–159]

REFERENCES

1. Towbin RB, Ball WS Jr. Pediatric interventional radiology. Radiol Clin North Am 1988;26:419–40.
2. Van Sonnenberg E, et al. Percutaneous diagnostic and therapeutic interventional radiologic procedures in children: experience in 100 patients. Radiology 1987;162:601–5.
3. White RI Jr, Rizer DM, Shuman KR, et al. Streamlining operation of an admitting service for interventional radiology. Radiology 1988;168:127–30.
4. Ring EJ, Kerlan RK Jr. Inpatient management: a new role for interventional radiologists. Radiology 1985;154:543.
5. Katzen BT, Kaplan JO, Dake MD. Developing an interventional radiology practice in a community hospital: the interventional radiologist as an equal partner in patient care. Radiology 1989;170:955–8.
6. Goldberg MA, Mueller PR, Saini S, et al. Importance of daily rounds by the radiologist after interventional procedures of the abdomen and chest. Radiology 1991;180:767–70.
7. Bisset GS, Ball WS Jr. Preparation, sedation, and monitoring of the pediatric patient in the magnetic resonance suite. Semin Ultrasound CT MR 1991;12:376–8.
8. Fisher DM. Sedation of pediatric patients: an anesthesiologist's perspective. Radiology 1990;175:745–52.
9. Piuitt AW. Committee on Drugs, Section on Anesthesiology. Guidelines for the elective use of conscious sedation, deep sedation, and general anesthesia in pediatric patients. Pediatrics 1985;76:317–21.
10. Dripps RD, Lamont A. ASA classification. JAMA 1961;178: 261–6.
11. Boyer RS. Sedation in pediatric neuroimaging: the science and the art. AJNR Am J Neuroradiol 1992;13:777–83.
12. Weiss S. Sedation of pediatric patients for nuclear medicine procedures. Semin Nucl Med 1993;23:190–8.
13. Lefever EB, Potter PS, Seeley NR. Propofol sedation for pediatric MRI. Anesth Analg 1993;76:919–20.
14. Cook BA, Bass JW, Nomizu S, et al. Sedation of children for technical procedures: current standard of practice. Clin Pediatr 1992;31:137–42.
15. Sievers TD, et al. Midazolam for conscious sedation during pediatric oncology procedures: safety and recovery parameters. Pediatrics 1992;88:1172–9.
16. Strain JD, et al. Intravenously administered pentobarbital sodium for sedation in pediatric CT. Radiology 1986;161: 105–8.
17. Ronchera CL, et al. Administration of oral chloral hydrate to paediatric patients undergoing magnetic resonance imaging. Pharm Weekbl [Sci] 1992;14:349–52.
18. American Academy of Pediatrics, Committee on Drugs and Committee on Environmental Health. Use of chloral hydrate for sedation in children. Pediatrics 1993;92:471–3.

19. Strain JD, et al. IV Nembutal: safe sedation for children undergoing CT. AJR Am J Roentgenol 1988;151:975–9.
20. Christoph RA, et al. Pain reduction in local anesthetic administration through pH buffering. Ann Emerg Med 1988;17:27–30.
21. American Academy of Pediatrics, Committee on Drugs. Guidelines for monitoring and management of pediatric patients during and after sedation for diagnostic and therapeutic procedures. Pediatrics 1992;89:1110–5.
22. Kowalczyk A, Smith J. The 1994 formulary. 13th ed. Toronto: The Hospital for Sick Children; 1994.
23. Sawhney S, Berry M, Bhargava S. Percutaneous real-time ultrasonic guided biopsy in the diagnosis of deep-seated, non-palpable intra-abdominal masses. Australas Radiol 1987;31:295–9.
24. Reading CC, et al. Sonographically guided percutaneous biopsy of small (3 cm or less) masses. AJR Am J Roentgenol 1988;1:189–92.
25. Reddy VB, et al. Computed tomography-guided fine needle aspiration biopsy of deep-seated lesions: a four-year experience. Acta Cytol 1991;35:753–6.
26. Elam E, et al. Cutaneous ulceration due to contrast extravasation: experimental assessment of injury and potential antidotes. Invest Radiol 1991;26:13–21.
27. Foley MJ, Chahremani GG, Rogers LF. Reappraisal of contrast media used to detect upper gastrointestinal perforations: comparison of ionic water-soluble media with barium sulfate. Radiology 1982;144:231–7.
28. Dodds WJ, Stewart ET, Vlyment WJ. Appropriate contrast media for evaluation of oesophageal disruption. Radiology 1982;144:439–41.
29. Cohen MD. Choosing contrast media for the evaluation of the gastrointestinal tract of neonates and infants. Radiology 1987;162:447–56.
30. Cunha F. Gastrostomy: its inception and evaluation. Am J Surg 1946;72:610–34.
31. Gauderer MWL, Ponsky JL, Izant RJ Jr. Gastrostomy without laparotomy: a percutaneous endoscopic technique. J Pediatr Surg 1980;15:872–5.
32. Marin OE, et al. Safety and efficacy of percutaneous endoscopic gastrostomy in children. Am J Gastroenterol 1994;89:357–61.
33. Di Abriola GF, et al. Nutritional stomas in children—experience with an antireflux percutaneous endoscopic gastrostomy: the right percutaneous endoscopic gastrostomy. Transplant Proc 1994;26:1468–9.
34. Gauderer MWL. Percutaneous endoscopic gastrostomy: a 10-year experience with 220 children. J Pediatr Surg 1991;26:288–94.
35. Caulfield M. Percutaneous endoscopic gastrostomy placement in children. Gastrointest Endosc Clin N Am 1994;4:179–93.
36. Mellinger JD, Ponsky JL. Percutaneous endoscopic gastrostomy. Endoscopy 1994;26:55–9.
37. Brown AS, Mueller PR, Ferruci JT Jr. Controlled percutaneous gastrostomy: nylon T-fasteners for fixation of the anterior gastric wall. Radiology 1986;158:543–5.
38. Van Sonneberg E, et al. Percutaneous gastrostomy and gastroenterostomy 2: clinical experience. AJR Am J Roentgenol 1986;146:581–6.
39. Varney RA, et al. Balloon techniques for percutaneous gastrostomy in a patient with partial gastrectomy. Radiology 1988;1:167–9.
40. Cory DA, Fitzgerald JF, Cohen MD. Percutaneous nonendo-
scopic gastrostomy in children. AJR Am J Roentgenol 1988;151:995–7.
41. Gray RR, St Louis EL, Grosman H. Percutaneous gastrostomy and gastrojejunostomy. Br J Radiol 1987;60:1067–70.
42. Malden ES, et al. Fluoroscopically guided percutaneous gastrostomy in children. J Vasc Intervent Radiol 1992;3:673–7.
43. Keller MS, Lai S, Wagner DK. Percutaneous gastrostomy in a child. Radiology 1986;160:261–2.
44. King SJ, et al. Retrograde percutaneous gastrostomy: a prospective study in 57 children. Pediatr Radiol 1993;23:23–5.
45. Halkier BK, Ho CS, Yee AC. Percutaneous feeding gastrostomy with the Seldinger technique: review of 252 patients. Radiology 1989;171:359–62.
46. Scapa E, et al. Colocutaneous fistula—a rare complication of percutaneous endoscopic gastrostomy. Surg Laparosc Endosc 1993;3:430–2.
47. Crombleholme TM, Jacir NN. Simplified "push" technique for percutaneous endoscopic gastrostomy in children. J Pediatr Surg 1993;28:1393–5.
48. Gottlieb K, et al. Oral *Candida* colonizes the stomach and gastrostomy feeding tubes. JPEN J Parenter Enteral Nutr 1994;18:264–7.
49. Bender JS, Levison MA. Complications after percutaneous endoscopic gastrostomy removal. Surg Laparosc Endosc 1991;1:101–3.
50. Laccourreye O, et al. Implantation metastasis following percutaneous endoscopic gastrostomy. J Laryngol Otol 1993;107:946–9.
51. Schiano TD, et al. Neoplastic seeding as a complication of percutaneous endoscopic gastrostomy. Am J Gastroenterol 1994;89:131–3.
52. Towbin RB, Ball WS Jr, Bissett GS. Percutaneous gastrostomy and percutaneous gastrojejunostomy in children: antegrade approach. Radiology 1988;168:473–6.
53. Cappell MS, Godil A. A multicenter case-controlled study of percutaneous endoscopic gastrostomy in HIV-seropositive patients. Am J Gastroenterol 1993;88:2059–66.
54. Goodman P, Levine MS, Parkman HP. Extrusion of PEG tube from the stomach with fistula formation: an unusual complication of percutaneous endoscopic gastrostomy. Gastrointest Radiol 1991;16:286–8.
55. Conventry BJ, et al. Intestinal passage of the PEG endpiece: is it safe? J Gastroenterol Hepatol 1994;9:311–3.
56. Duckworth PF Jr, et al. Percutaneous endoscopic gastrojejunostomy made easy: a new over-the-wire technique. Gastrointest Endosc 1994;40:350–3.
57. Riley DA, Strauss M. Airway and other complications of percutaneous endoscopic gastrostomy in head and neck cancer patients. Ann Otol Rhinol Laryngol 1992;101:310–3.
58. Gibson SE, Wenig BL, Watkins JL. Complications of percutaneous endoscopic gastrostomy in head and neck cancer patients. Ann Otol Rhinol Laryngol 1992;101:46–50.
59. Edelman DS, Unger SW, Russin DR. Laparoscopic gastrostomy. Surg Laparosc Endosc 1991;1:251–3.
60. Edelman DS, Arroyo PJ, Unger SW. Laparoscopic gastrostomy versus percutaneous endoscopic gastrostomy: a comparison. Surg Endosc 1994;8:47–9.
61. Lee WJ, et al. Laparoscopic-guided gastrostomy. J Formos Med Assoc 1993;92:911–3.
62. Raaf JH, et al. Laparoscopic placement of a percutaneous endoscopic gastrostomy (PEG) feeding tube. J Laparoendosc Surg 1993;3:411–44.

63. Bessell JR, Stanley B, Maddern GJ. The emerging role for laparoscopic gastrostomy. Aust N Z J Surg 1994;64:515–7.

64. Modesto VL, et al. Laparoscopic gastrostomy using four-point fixation. Am J Surg 1994;167:273–6.

65. Kaw M, Sekas G. Long-term follow-up of consequences of percutaneous endoscopic gastrostomy (PEG) tubes in nursing home patients. Dig Dis Sci 1994;39:738–43.

66. O'Keeffe F, et al. Percutaneous drainage and feeding gastrostomies in 100 patients. Radiology 1989;172:341–3.

67. Long B, Rafert J, Cory D. Percutaneous feeding tube method for use in children. Radiol Technol 1991;62:274–8.

68. D'Amelio LF, et al. Tracheostomy and percutaneous endoscopic gastrostomy in the management of the head-injured trauma patient. Am Surg 1994;60:180–5.

69. McLoughlin RF, Gibney RG. Fluoroscopically guided percutaneous gastrostomy: tube function and malfunction. Abdom Imaging 1994;19:195–200.

70. Saini S, et al. Percutaneous gastrostomy with gastropexy: experience in 125 patients. AJR Am J Roentgenol 1990;154:1003–6.

71. Moote DJ, Ho CS, Felice V. Fluoroscopically guided percutaneous gastrostomy: is gastric fixation necessary? Can Assoc Radiol J 1991;42:113–8.

72. Deutsch LS, et al. Simplified percutaneous gastrostomy. Radiology 1992;184:181–3.

73. Gray RR, St Louis EL, Grosman H. Percutaneous conversion of surgical gastrostomy to jejunostomy: indications and technique. Can Assoc Radiol J 1987;38:275–7.

74. Ghosh S, Eastwood MA, Palmer KR. Acute gastric dilatation—a delayed complication of percutaneous endoscopic gastrostomy. Gut 1993;34:859–60.

75. Ganga UR, Ryan JJ, Schafer LW. Indications, complications, and long-term results of percutaneous endoscopic gastrostomy: a retrospective study. S D J Med 1994;47:149–52.

76. Sant SM, et al. Percutaneous endoscopic gastrostomy—its application in patients with neurological disease. Ir J Med Sci 1993;162:449.

77. Boyd KJ, Beeken L. Tube feeding in palliative care: benefits and problems. Palliat Med 1994;8:156–8.

78. Steinkamp G, von der Hardt H. Improvement of nutritional status and lung function after long-term nocturnal gastrostomy feedings in cystic fibrosis. J Pediatr 1994;124:244–9.

79. Nutrition Committee, Canadian Paediatric Society. Undernutrition in children with a neurodevelopment disability. Can Med Assoc J 1994;151:753–9.

80. Faller N, Lawrence KG. Comparing low-profile gastrostomy tubes. Nursing 1993;23:46–8.

81. Haas-Beckert B, Heyman MB. Comparison of two skin-level gastrostomy feeding tubes for infants and children. Pediatr Nurs 1993;19:351–4.

82. Morrison MC, et al. Percutaneous cecostomy: controlled transperitoneal approach. Radiology 1990;176:574–6.

83. Squire R, et al. The clinical application of the Malone antegrade colonic enema. J Pediatr Surg 1993;28:1012–5.

84. Van Sonnenberg E, et al. Percutaneous cecostomy for Ogilvie syndrome: laboratory observations and clinical experience. Radiology 1990;175:679–82.

85. Casola G, et al. Percutaneous cecostomy for decompression of the massively distended cecum. Radiology 1986;158:793–4.

86. Maginot TJ, Cascade PN. Abdominal wall cellulitis and sepsis secondary to percutaneous cecostomy. Cardiovasc Intervent Radiol 1993;16:328–31.

87. Cox JG, et al. Balloon of bougie for dilatation of benign esophageal stricture? Dig Dis Sci 1994;39:776–81.

88. Ciarolla DA, Traube M. Achalasia: short-term clinical monitoring after pneumatic dilation. Dig Dis Sci 1993;38:1905–8.

89. Swaroop VS, et al. Dilation of esophageal strictures induced by radiation therapy for cancer of the esophagus. Gastrointest Endosc 1994;40:311–5.

90. Kim IO, et al. Perforation complicating balloon dilation of esophageal strictures in infants and children. Radiology 1993;189:741–4.

91. Johnson DL, Lang E. Technical aspects of nonoperative dilation of a complex colon anastomotic stricture. Dig Dis Sci 1993;38:1929–32.

92. Peer A, Lin B, Vinograd I. Balloon catheter dilatation of focal colonic strictures following necrotizing enterocolitis. Cardiovasc Intervent Radiol 1993;16:248–50.

93. Yeung EY. Percutaneous abdominal biopsy. Baillieres Clin Gastroenterol 1992;6:219–44.

94. Gazelle GS, Haaga JR. Guided percutaneous biopsy of intraabdominal lesions. AJR Am J Roentgenol 1989;153:929–35.

95. Jaeger HJ, et al. Diagnosis of abdominal masses with percutaneous biopsy guided by ultrasound. BMJ 1990;301:1188–91.

96. Bernardino ME. Percutaneous biopsy. AJR Am J Roentgenol 1984;142:41–5.

97. Silverman SG, et al. Needle-tip localization during CT-guided abdominal biopsy: comparison of conventional and spiral CT. AJR Am J Roentgenol 1992;159:1095–7.

98. Hammers LW, et al. Computed tomographic (CT) guided percutaneous fine-needle aspiration biopsy: the Yale experience. Yale J Biol Med 1986;59:425–34.

99. Bocking A. Cytological vs. histological evaluation of percutaneous biopsies. Cardiovasc Intervent Radiol 1991;14:5–12.

100. Somers JM, et al. Radiologically-guided cutting needle biopsy for suspected malignancy in childhood. Clin Radiol 1993;48:236–40.

101. Smith MB, et al. A rational approach to the use of fine-needle aspiration biopsy in the evaluation of primary and recurrent neoplasms in children. J Pediatr Surg 1993;28:1245–47.

102. Smith EH. Complications of percutaneous abdominal fine-needle biopsy. Radiology 1991;178:253–8.

103. Chezmar JL, et al. Liver transplant biopsies with a biopsy gun. Radiology 1991;179:447–8.

104. Sheets PW, et al. Safety and efficacy of a spring-propelled 18 gauge needle for US guided liver biopsy. J Vasc Intervent Radiol 1991;2:147–9.

105. Don S, et al. Ultrasound-guided pediatric liver transplant biopsy using a spring-propelled cutting needle (biopsy gun). Pediatr Radiol 1994;24:21–4.

106. Chuang VP, Alspaugh JP. Sheath needle for liver biopsy in high-risk patients. Radiology 1988;166:261–2.

107. Zins M, et al. US guided percutaneous liver biopsy with plugging of the needle track: a prospective study in 72 high risk patients. Radiology 1992;184:841–3.

108. Judmaier G, et al. A combined biopsy plugging device based on the Menghini or Trucut needle for percutaneous liver biopsy: clinical experience. Z Gastroenterol 1993;31:614–6.

109. Gamble P, et al. Transjugular liver biopsy: a review of 461 biopsies. Radiology 1985;157:589–93.

110. Corr P, Beningfield SJ, Davey N. Transjugular liver biopsy: a review of 200 biopsies. Clin Radiol 1992;45:238–9.

111. Furuya KN, et al. Transjugular liver biopsy in children. Hepatology 1992;15:1036–42.

112. Mewissen MW, et al. Liver biopsy through the femoral vein. Radiology 1988;169:842–3.

113. Sperti C, et al. Percutaneous CT-guided fine needle aspiration cytology in the differential diagnosis of pancreatic lesions. Ital J Gastroenterol 1994;26:126–31.

114. Graham RA, et al. Fine-needle aspiration biopsy of pancreatic ductal adenocarcinoma: loss of diagnostic accuracy with small tumors. J Surg Oncol 1994;55:92–4.

115. Zeppa P, Vetrani A, Luciano L. Fine needle aspiration biopsy of the spleen: a useful procedure in the diagnosis of splenomegaly. Acta Cytol 1994;38:299–309.

116. Hemming A, Davis NL, Robins RE. Surgical versus percutaneous drainage of intra-abdominal abscesses. Am J Surg 1991;161:593–5.

117. Van Sonnenberg E, Mueller PR, Ferrucci JT. Percutaneous drainage of 250 abdominal abscesses and fluid collections. 1. Results, failures and complications. Radiology 1984;151:337–41.

118. Mueller PR, Van Sonnenberg E, Ferrucci JT. Percutaneous drainage of 250 abdominal abscesses and fluid collections. Radiology 1984;147:57–63.

119. Gazelle GS, Mueller PR. Abdominal abscess: imaging and intervention. Radiol Clin North Am 1994;32:913–32.

120. Lambiase RE, et al. Percutaneous drainage of 335 consecutive abscesses: results of primary drainage with 1 year follow-up. Radiology 1992;184:167–79.

121. Brolin RE, et al. Limitations of percutaneous catheter drainage of abdominal abscesses. Surg Gynecol Obstet 1991;173:203–10.

122. Kong MS, Lin JN. Pyogenic liver abscess in children. J Formos Med Assoc 1994;93:45–50.

123. Moore SW, Millar AJ, Cywes S. Conservative initial treatment for liver abscesses in children. Br J Surg 1994;81:872–4.

124. Eisenberg PJ, et al. Percutaneous drainage of a subphrenic abscess with gastric fistula. AJR Am J Roentgenol 1994;162:1233–7.

125. Van Gansbeke D, et al. Percutaneous drainage of subphrenic abscesses. Br J Radiol 1989;62:127–33.

126. Schwerk WB, et al. Ultrasound guided percutaneous drainage of pyogenic splenic abscesses. J Clin Ultrasound 1994;22:161–6.

127. Tikkakoski T, et al. Splenic abscess: imaging and intervention. Acta Radiol 1992;33:561–5.

128. Yeung EY, Ho CS. Percutaneous radiologic drainage of pelvic abscesses. Ann Acad Med Singapore 1993;22:663–9.

129. Alexander AA, et al. Transrectal sonographically guided drainage of deep pelvic abscesses. AJR Am J Roentgenol 1994;162:1227–30.

130. Carmody E, et al. Transrectal drainage of deep pelvic collections under fluoroscopic guidance. Can Assoc Radiol J 1993;44:429–33.

131. Bennett JD, et al. Deep pelvic abscesses: transrectal drainage with radiologic guidance. Radiology 1992;185:825–8.

132. Longo JM, et al. CT guided paracoccygeal drainage of pelvic abscess. J Comput Assist Tomogr 1993;17:909–14.

133. Murphy FB, Bernardino ME. Interventional computed tomography. Curr Probl Diagn Radiol 1988;17:121–54.

134. Sunday ML, et al. Management of infected pancreatic fluid collections. Am Surg 1994;60:63–7.

135. Venbrux AC. Interventional radiology in the biliary tract. Curr Opin Radiol 1992;4:83–92.

136. Burke DR. Biliary and other gastrointestinal interventions. Curr Opin Radiol 1991;392:151–9.

137. Gordon RL, Ring EJ. Combined radiologic and retrograde endoscopic and biliary interventions. Radiol Clin North Am 1990;28:1289–95.

138. Coons H. Biliary intervention—technique and devices: a commentary. Cardiovasc Intervent Radiol 1990;13:211–6.

139. Burhenne HJ. The history of interventional radiology of the biliary tract. Radiol Clin North Am 1990;28:1139–44.

140. Ring EJ, Kerlan RK Jr. Interventional biliary radiology. AJR Am J Roentgenol 1984;142:31–4.

141. Letourneau JG, et al. Pictorial essay: imaging of and intervention for biliary complications after hepatic transplantation. AJR Am J Roentgenol 1990;154:729–33.

142. Letourneau JG, et al. Biliary complications after liver transplantation in children. Radiology 1989;170:1095–9.

143. Peclet MH, et al. The spectrum of bile duct complications in pediatric liver transplantation. J Pediatr Surg 1994;29:214–9.

144. Roy AF, et al. Bile duct injury during laparoscopic cholecystectomy. Can J Surg 1993;36:509–16.

145. Skukigara M, et al. Percutaneous transhepatic biliary drainage guided by color Doppler echography. Abdom Imaging 1994;19:147–9.

146. Kelin AS, et al. Reduction of morbidity and mortality from biliary complications after liver transplantation. Hepatology 1991;14:818–23.

147. Hoffer FA, et al. Infected bilomas and hepatic artery thrombosis in infant recipients of liver transplants: interventional radiology and medical therapy as an alternative to retransplantation. Radiology 1988;169:435–8.

148. Sheng R, et al. Bile leak after hepatic transplantation: cholangiographic features, prevalence, and clinical outcome. Radiology 1994;192:413–6.

149. Morrison MC, et al. Percutaneous balloon dilatation of benign biliary strictures. Radiol Clin North Am 1990;28:1191–1201.

150. Citron SJ, Martin LG. Benign biliary strictures: treatment with percutaneous cholangiography. Radiology 1991;178:339–41.

151. Maccioni F, et al. Metallic stents in benign biliary strictures: three-year follow-up. Cardiovasc Intervent Radiol 1992;15:360–6.

152. Pitt HA, et al. Intrahepatic stones: the transhepatic team approach. Ann Surg 1994;219:527–35.

153. LaBerge JM, et al. Creation of transjugular intrahepatic portosystemic shunts (TIPS) with the wallstent endoprosthesis: results in 100 patients. Radiology 1993;187:413–20.

154. Rossle M, et al. The transjugular intrahepatic portosystemic stent shunt procedure for variceal bleeding. N Engl J Med 1994;330:165–71.

155. Haskal ZJ, et al. Transjugular intrahepatic portosystemic shunt stenosis and revision: early and midterm results. AJR Am J Roentgenol 1994;163:439–44.

156. Boyer TD. Transjugular intrahepatic portosystemic shunt: current status. Gastroenterology 2003;124:1700–10.

157. Rosado B, Kamath PS. Transjugular intrahepatic portosystemic shunts: an update. Liver Transpl 2003;9:207–17.

158. Bilbao JI, Quiroga J, Herrero JI, Benito A. Transjugular intrahepatic portosystemic shunt (TIPS): current status and future possibilities. Cardiovasc Intervent Radiol 2002;25:251–69.

159. Ong JP, Sands M, Younossi ZM. Transjugular intrahepatic portosystemic shunts (TIPS): a decade later. J Clin Gastroenterol 2000;30:14–28.

ADDITIONAL READINGS

Angtuaco TL, Lal SK, Banaad-Omiotek GD, et al. Current liver biopsy practices for suspected parenchymal liver diseases in the United States: the evolving role of radiologists. Am J Gastroenterol 2002;97:1468–71.

Chait PG, Temple M, Connolly B, et al. Pediatric interventional venous access. Tech Vasc Interv Radiol 2002;5:95–102.

Civelli EM, Meroni R, Cozzi G, et al. The role of interventional radiology in biliary complications after orthotopic liver transplantation: a single-center experience. Eur Radiol 2003;21:63–7.

Dite P, Lata J, Novotny I. Intestinal obstruction and perforation—the role of the gastroenterologist. Dig Dis 2003;21:63–7.

Gulati MS, Batra Y, Paul SB, et al. Radiofrequency ablation: a new therapeutic modality for the management of hepatocellular cancer. Trop Gastroenterol 2002;23:183–5.

Heffron TG, Pillen T, Welch D, et al. Biliary complications after pediatric liver transplantation revisited. Transplant Proc 2003;35:1461–2.

John P. Thoracic interventional radiology in children. Paediatr Respir Rev 2001;2:131–44.

Juno RJ, Knott AW, Racadio J, Warner BW. Reoperative venous access. Semin Pediatr Surg 2003;12:132–9.

Lavine JE, Hart ME, Khanna A. Integral role of interventional radiology in the development of a pediatric liver transplantation program. Pediatr Transplant 2001;5:331–8.

Mason KP, Michna E, DiNardo JA, et al. Evolution of a protocol for ketamine-induced sedation as an alternative to general anesthesia for interventional radiologic procedures in pediatric patients. Radiology 2002;225:457–65.

Roberts TP, Hassenzahl WV, Hetts SW, Arenson RL. Remote control of catheter tip deflection: an opportunity for interventional MRI. Magn Reson Med 2002;48:1091–5.

Rose SC, Andre MP, Roberts AC, et al. Imaging and radiological interventional techniques for gastrointestinal bleeding in children. Semin Pediatr Surg 1999;8:181–92.

Sze DY, Esquivel CO. The role of interventional radiology in a pediatric liver transplant program. Pediatr Transplant. 2002;6:1–4.

4. Radionuclide Diagnosis

David Casson, BA, MBBS, MRCPI
Helen J. Williams, MB, ChB, MRCP, FRCR

GENERAL ASPECTS OF PEDIATRIC NUCLEAR MEDICINE

Nuclear medicine is the branch of medicine and imaging that uses radionuclides (radioisotopes) for diagnostic and therapeutic purposes. The radioisotope is bound to a compound to form a radiopharmaceutical that is often organ specific. Images are produced by mapping the distribution of radioactivity of the administered radiopharmaceutical in the body using radioactivity detectors. The most commonly used detector is the gamma camera. In most studies, planar images are produced, but by moving the gamma camera around the patient, a three-dimensional data set is obtained and can be reconstructed and viewed in different planes, a technique known as single photon emission computed tomography (SPECT). This technique is used routinely in certain areas of nuclear medicine (eg, cardiac and brain imaging). In gastrointestinal radionuclide imaging, SPECT may be used to detect small amounts of isotope uptake or excreted isotope not visible on planar scans, perhaps owing to overlying structures.

Nuclear medicine studies provide information about organ function, and although they give some anatomic information, this is often limited, as is their ability to differentiate between pathologies, which ultimately have the same effect on organ function. There are few situations in pediatric gastroenterology in which nuclear medicine should be used as a first-line investigation, but the role of nuclear medicine in gastrointestinal diagnosis is often to provide the answer to a specific question, and the results must be interpreted in the context of other investigations.

The underlying principles of nuclear medicine are parallel in both adult and pediatric practice. However, certain aspects of pediatric nuclear medicine are unique. Indications for some investigations in pediatrics are different because of the different spectrum of pathology in children compared with adults (Table 74.4-1), and there is frequently a requirement for modification of technique.

In all cases, obtaining a high-quality diagnostic nuclear medicine study is dependent on the cooperation of the child, parent, or other caregiver and staff in the nuclear medicine department. In nuclear medicine departments dealing primarily with adult patients, it is essential that staff carrying out procedures on children are familiar with handling and communicating with children and understand their special needs. A full explanation of the procedure to both the child and parent or carer is mandatory and will often allay any fears and misconceptions early. Many departments supply information leaflets with the appointment letter or on arrival in the department, which can answer a number of frequently asked questions. The patient and their parent should be aware of what the investigation entails, including the anticipated length of time that they will need to be in the hospital. This is often several hours for a nuclear medicine study, and advice should be given to bring toys or books to keep a young child amused. The unpleasant aspects of the study, such as the intravenous injection of isotope, should also be fully explained. This is usually acceptable to both child and parent when a local anesthetic cream is applied to the skin before the injection, rendering it a relatively painless procedure. When venipuncture is required, it must be done by trained staff, skilled in obtaining intravenous access in children to minimize discomfort and stress to the child.[1]

During the nuclear medicine study, parents should be allowed to remain with the child at all times. Immobiliza-

TABLE 74.4-1 CURRENT INDICATIONS FOR RADIONUCLIDE IMAGING IN PEDIATRIC GASTROENTEROLOGY

99mTc SULFUR COLLOID OR PHYTATE COLLOIDS
Assessment of esophageal dysmotility and gastric emptying
Evaluation of gastroesophageal reflux
Investigation of suspected pulmonary aspiration

99mTc IDA COMPOUNDS
Investigation of neonatal jaundice
Confirmation of biliary origin of choledochal cysts
Assessment of hepatobiliary function in acquired liver disease
Postoperative and post-trauma assessment of bile duct integrity
Heat-denatured red blood cells
Detection of functioning splenic tissue (heterotopic or ectopic)
Labeled white cell scans
Diagnosis of inflammatory bowel disease, detection of active disease

99mTc HUMAN SERUM ALBUMIN
Diagnosis of protein-losing enteropathy

99mTc-LABELED RED BLOOD CELLS AND 99mTc PERTECHNETATE
Investigation of gastrointestinal bleeding
Labeled somatostatin analogues
Detection of somatostatin receptor positive tumors
Labeled bile acid analogues
Diagnosis of bile acid malabsorption in cases of unexplained chronic diarrhea

IDA = iminodiacetic acid; 99mTc = technetium 99m.

tion is an essential requirement for obtaining high-quality images, and this can be a particular challenge, given the length of time taken to obtain views for some nuclear medicine studies. For neonates and children up to the age of 2 years, it is usually sufficient to hold the child in place or use sandbags and padding to aid immobilization. Sleep deprivation prior to the procedure and feeding the child while lying on the gamma camera table may also be useful. In many departments, music and television are used to help prevent the child from becoming bored and restless. Provided that the procedure is carried out in a calm environment and the child is accompanied and kept amused throughout, sedation is seldom required. During the scan, whenever possible, the gamma camera should be positioned underneath the child on the table because positioning the camera above children tends to frighten them. It is also customary to obtain the most important images first.[2,3]

Most pediatric nuclear medicine studies use the isotope technetium 99m (^{99m}Tc), which emits gamma rays and has a half-life of 6 hours. ^{99m}Tc can be bound to several substances, which are taken up by specific organs. The dose of the radiopharmaceutical should be scaled down according to the child's body surface area or weight (Table 74.4-2). Age is not used because of the wide variation in body surface area and weight, which would result in a variation in dose that may not necessarily be appropriate. There is also a minimum dose of radiopharmaceutical for each examination, below which the injected activity is too low to obtain adequate images no matter how small the child (Table 74.4-3). Absorbed radiation doses from gastrointestinal radionuclide examinations are usually lower than from radiographic procedures such as fluoroscopy or computed tomography (CT) of the abdomen. After the injection, where possible, patients should be encouraged to void frequently for those examinations in which the radiopharmaceutical is excreted by the kidneys so as to reduce the radiation burden to the pelvic organs.

TABLE 74.4-2   FRACTION OF ADULT ADMINISTERED ACTIVITY FOR CHILDREN BASED ON BODY WEIGHT*

KG	FRACTION OF ADULT-ADMINISTERED ACTIVITY	KG	FRACTION OF ADULT-ADMINISTERED ACTIVITY
3	0.1	30	0.62
4	0.14	32	0.65
6	0.19	34	0.68
8	0.23	36	0.71
10	0.27	38	0.73
12	0.32	40	0.76
14	0.36	42	0.78
16	0.40	44	0.80
18	0.44	46	0.82
20	0.46	48	0.85
22	0.50	50	0.88
24	0.53	52–54	0.90
26	0.56	56–58	0.95
28	0.58	60–62	1.00

*Recommended by the Pediatric Task Group of the European Association of Nuclear Medicine.[90]

TABLE 74.4-3   MINIMUM AMOUNTS OF ADMINISTERED ACTIVITIES FOR CHILDREN FOR GASTROINTESTINAL SCINTIGRAPHY*

RADIOPHARMACEUTICAL	MINIMUM ADMINISTERED ACTIVITY FOR CHILDREN (MBq)
^{99m}Tc colloid (liver and spleen)	15
^{99m}Tc colloid (gastric reflux)	10
^{99m}Tc spleen (denatured RBCs)	20
^{99m}Tc HIDA (biliary)	20
^{99m}Tc HMPAO (WBC)	40
^{99m}Tc pertechnetate (Meckel diverticulum)	20
^{99m}Tc RBCs (blood pool)	80

HIDA = hepatobiliary iminodiacetic acid; HMPAO = hexamethylpropyleneamine oxime; RBCs = red blood cells; ^{99m}Tc = technetium 99m.
*Recommended by the Pediatric Task Group of the European Association of Nuclear Medicine.[90]

SCINTIGRAPHIC ASSESSMENT OF GASTROESOPHAGEAL DYSFUNCTION AND REFLUX

Many techniques are used for the diagnosis of esophageal disorders, gastroesophageal reflux, and gastric emptying in children. These include pH studies, barium radiology, manometry, ultrasonography, impedance studies, endoscopy with biopsy, and scintigraphy. Each of these techniques has its own merits and limitations, and each may be informative about different aspects of esophagogastric physiology and pathophysiology. There is little recent published work comparing these methodologies and their relative contributions.

In this field, the main symptoms of relevance to pediatric practice are related to gastroesophageal reflux. Esophageal dysfunction and delay in gastric emptying are thought to contribute to reflux, as well as representing disease entities in their own right. The assessment of each is difficult for several reasons. There is no consensus as to what represents the reference or "gold standard." Additionally, the presence of gastroesophageal reflux in itself does not necessarily equate with a disease state. Thus, a distinction should be made between gastroesophageal reflux and gastroesophageal reflux disease. This is further complicated in pediatric practice by marked clinical and physiologic differences between age groups and between those children who seem to have reflux disease as an isolated problem and those in whom it is associated with another disorder, such as cerebral palsy or chronic lung disease. Because gastroesophageal reflux is mostly intermittent, methods of investigation must be longitudinal. Such limitations must be borne in mind when considering the role of scintigraphy.

Oral ^{99m}Tc sulfur colloid or phytate colloids are used in gastroesophageal scintigraphy because they are not absorbed from the gastrointestinal tract. Also, if aspirated, they remain localized, are readily detectable, and are eventually cleared without sequel.[4] The labeled colloid is mixed with the feed to be administered, residual activity is cleared from the mouth and esophagus with an unlabeled liquid or feed, and the patient is imaged for 1 hour. Ideally, milk should be used because this does not enhance gastric emptying. Dynamic images are taken at regular intervals (eg, every 10 seconds with the child lying comfortably on the scanning table). The stomach activity is masked by the use of lead shields to maximize esophageal visualization. Both images and time-activity curves are recorded. This enables the identification of the frequency of reflux episodes together with their proximal extent (Figure 74.4-1).

Using this method, the results obtained can be considered to represent only the postprandial situation. This

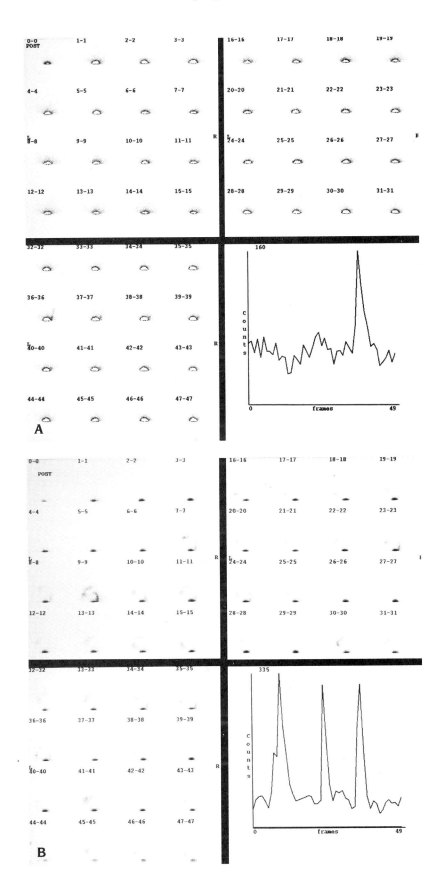

FIGURE 74.4-1   Gastroesophageal reflux studies using labeled sulfur colloid mixed with milk feed. Episodes of gastroesophageal reflux are indicated by the peaks on the activity curves. These represent individual reflux episodes, one in *A* and three in *B*. The proximal extent of the reflux is assessed from the accompanying images.

offers certain advantages over pH studies because gastric acidity may be neutralized by food, especially milk, in the immediate postprandial period, making pH studies unreliable.[5,6] Although scintigraphy is unable to delineate anatomic features, such as hiatus hernia, the radiation exposure is considerably less than that with barium studies. In addition, it has the advantage of allowing longer periods of observation to detect reflux. Piepsz and colleagues performed gastroesophageal scintigraphy in 35 children of varying ages who were felt clinically to have gastroesophageal reflux.[7] Compared with barium studies and findings on endoscopy with esophageal histology, gastroesophageal scintigraphy is more likely to detect reflux episodes than barium studies. However, there was no consistent correlation of scintigraphic results with findings at endoscopy. A second study compared several different methodologies in the diagnosis of 30 infants and children with symptoms of gastroesophageal reflux.[8] Gastroesophageal scintigraphy was positive in only 17 (56.6%) patients. The authors suggest that barium studies and scintigraphy are complementary evaluations and that a combination of the two increases sensitivity.

Images of the thorax taken 1 and 4 hours after the reflux study occasionally detect pulmonary aspiration, but this method of detecting aspiration is generally unreliable.[9] A salivagram has been developed in which a small amount of labeled colloid is placed on the tongue and is allowed to mix with saliva. Subsequent images of the tracheobronchial tree collected up to an hour afterward may indicate aspiration of saliva.[10] However, the accuracy of this method has not been assessed, and it is specific for aspiration of saliva as opposed to refluxate.

SCINTIGRAPHIC ASSESSMENT OF GASTRIC EMPTYING

The concept of abnormal gastric emptying as a disease entity and its possible relationship to gastroesophageal reflux disease has not been well validated. It has been suggested that delayed gastric emptying predisposes infants to reflux and to aspiration,[11] but this point was not confirmed in other studies.[12] Much of the uncertainty is due to the number of variables that can affect gastric emptying, such as age, feed type, and the lack of standardized normal values. Therefore, although scintigraphic assessment of gastric emptying in association with the assessment of reflux is feasible, its value must be considered questionable.

Gastric emptying studies may be useful in selected patients, for example, when considering gastrostomy placement or evaluation of patients with dumping syndrome. The patient's usual volume of milk or food is labeled with ^{99m}Tc sulfur colloid and is administered either orally or by nasogastric or gastric tube. Patients are imaged supine for 1 hour. If gastric emptying is roughly 50% at 1 hour, the study can be terminated. If there is delayed emptying at 1 hour, the patient is allowed to sit upright or walk around before delayed images are acquired at 90 minutes and 2 hours. If emptying is graphically displayed, then certain patterns may be recognized. These include plateau

phase seen in pylorospasm or antral web, increasing gastric counts owing to overlapping duodenum, and a rapid fall in activity seen in dumping syndrome.[13]

SCINTIGRAPHIC ASSESSMENT OF THE ESOPHAGUS

Scintigraphy can be used to assess esophageal motility and transit time. It is a dynamic method and so allows appropriate physiologic analysis. The technique can be performed only in cooperative children. A labeled colloid is used, as in the assessment of reflux, and is delivered as small oral boluses, which can be observed individually and summated to allow activity in any particular segment. Generalized dysmotility can be distinguished from focal areas of abnormality, such as a stricture.[14] As with many scintigraphic techniques, this approach has not been well validated compared with other methods, and its place in the routine investigation of children is not established. Esophageal scintigraphy may be considered in children with persistent symptoms of dysphagia in whom contrast studies are normal.

HEPATOBILIARY SCINTIGRAPHY

Hepatobiliary scintigraphy is used to assess hepatocyte function and the excretion of bile into the small intestine. There are many uses of hepatobiliary scintigraphy, but in pediatric practice, the most frequent one is to help determine the etiology of jaundice in the neonatal period.

The radiopharmaceuticals employed in hepatobiliary scintigraphy are those of the ^{99m}Tc-labeled iminodiacetic acid (IDA) group. The agent is given intravenously and is then transported to the liver bound to albumin, where it is taken up by the hepatocytes via an active process. Excretion into the bile ducts is by a combination of active and passive transport mechanisms. The kidneys excrete a proportion of the agent, but with increasing hepatocellular dysfunction, a higher percentage is renally excreted.[15] ^{99m}Tc diisopropryl-IDA (DISIDA) is the radiopharmaceutical most frequently used in hepatobiliary scintigraphy. In the normal patient, ^{99m}Tc DISIDA has a hepatic extraction of 88% and urinary excretion of 11%. ^{99m}Tc trimethylbromo-IDA (TBIDA; mebrofenin) has a hepatic extraction of 98% and urinary excretion of 1.5% and is currently the best agent for use in patients with high bilirubin levels because it has a higher resistance to displacement by bilirubin, which is also carried in the blood bound to albumin.[16] ^{99m}Tc TBIDA has a greater than 70% hepatic extraction with bilirubin levels over 20 mg/dL, whereas ^{99m}Tc DISIDA has a lower hepatic extraction at 36% with bilirubin levels of 10 mg/dL.[15]

INVESTIGATION OF NEONATAL JAUNDICE

Hyperbilirubinemia is common in the neonatal period and in the majority of cases is due to benign physiologic jaundice. Prolonged neonatal jaundice is defined as jaundice lasting more than 14 to 21 days. The immediate priority in prolonged neonatal jaundice is to differentiate between pathologic neonatal cholestasis (conjugated hyperbilirubinemia) and unconjugated hyperbilirubinemia, which is usually benign. More than 15% conjugated hyperbilirubinemia is considered to be significant rather than the absolute bilirubin level.[17] Cholestasis can be due to multiple intrahepatic causes such as infection, metabolic or genetic conditions, or extrahepatic abnormalities causing mechanical obstruction to bile flow. Early recognition of extrahepatic causes is vital because early surgical intervention in extrahepatic biliary atresia (EHBA) is associated with a better outcome.[18,19] In EHBA, all or part of the extrahepatic bile ducts are obliterated, leading to complete biliary obstruction. In approximately 5% of cases, the gallbladder or parts of the common bile duct are patent. Treatment is by the formation of a Kasai portoenterostomy in which the atretic extrahepatic biliary tissue is removed and a Roux-en-Y jejunal loop is anastomosed to the hepatic hilum to try to establish biliary drainage into the intestine. The likelihood of this surgery being successful is reduced after 60 days of age[20]; therefore, early diagnosis of EHBA is vital.

The complete workup of an infant with cholestasis will include laboratory tests of liver function, serologic tests for infection, metabolic screening tests, and imaging investigations, which are all correlated with clinical information. Ultrasonography is the primary imaging modality used to visualize the hepatobiliary anatomy and exclude congenital abnormalities of the liver and biliary system and other abdominal organs. Congenital bile duct dilatation, or choledochal cyst, is the disorder most commonly diagnosed by ultrasonography. Gallstones or sludge in the biliary system may be detected, sometimes in association with proximal biliary dilatation. Biliary dilatation is not a feature of EHBA. Ultrasonography is unable to diagnose EHBA, although many series report certain ultrasound findings that increase or decrease the likelihood of EHBA. These include the "triangular cord sign," which is a triangular- or tubular-shaped echogenic structure seen ultrasonographically in the vicinity of the portal vein at the porta hepatis and is said to represent the fibrous cone of atretic extrahepatic biliary tissue in patients with EHBA.[21] Although this is a helpful sign, it is not considered to be a reliable method of detecting or diagnosing EHBA.[22] A small or absent gallbladder in a fasting infant is suggestive of EHBA. Visualization of a normal-sized gallbladder makes the diagnosis of EHBA less likely, but appearances of the gallbladder at ultrasonography cannot be accurately relied on.[23]

The role of hepatobiliary scintigraphy in the investigation of neonatal cholestasis is primarily to exclude EHBA, but it cannot differentiate between other forms of cholestasis. Hepatobiliary scintigraphy demonstrates the ability of the hepatocytes to take up isotope, as a measure of hepatocyte function, and demonstrates patency of the biliary tree by the visualization of excretion of isotope into the gut. In neonates being investigated to differentiate between intrahepatic and extrahepatic causes of cholestasis, premedication with phenobarbital at a dose of 5 mg/kg/d orally is used for at least 3 days to induce hepatocyte microsomal enzymes, thereby increasing bilirubin conjugation and excretion. This approach increases the speci-

ficity of the test in distinguishing EHBA from other causes of neonatal cholestasis by ensuring the best possible excretion of hepatobiliary agents. If the test is performed urgently without premedication, it may have to be repeated following phenobarbital premedication if excretion of isotope into the bowel is not seen. Patients should be fasted for 3 to 4 hours prior to the study. Following injection of a radiopharmaceutical, dynamic imaging is performed for the first 5 minutes to visualize the distribution of tracer in the blood pool and to assess hepatic uptake. The gamma camera is placed anteriorly over the abdomen and positioned to include the heart, liver, and bowel. Thereafter, static images are acquired at intervals up to 1 hour after the injection. A suggested regimen is to obtain static images at 5, 10, 15, 30, and 45 minutes and 1 hour. If there is no excretion into the bowel at 1 hour, then further imaging is performed at later intervals, for example, at 3 to 4 hours until activity is seen in the bowel. If bowel activity remains undetectable, imaging at 24 hours is undertaken with anterior and lateral images to detect activity in the bowel or rectum. If the gallbladder has been visualized but fails to empty significantly during the first 60 minutes, an additional series of images should be taken following a normal feed to stimulate gallbladder contraction. Cholecystokinin can also be used to stimulate gallbladder emptying.[24]

Images can be interpreted to assess the following parameters: blood flow and extraction of isotope by the liver, time of excretion and visualization of the biliary tree, time of visualization of isotope in the duodenum, parenchymal clearance of isotope, gallbladder contractility, duodenogastric reflux, delayed images of bowel or rectal activity, and position of the small bowel. However, there are two main phases: hepatic extraction (uptake) and excretion of isotope into the bowel. In normal neonates, hepatic extraction of isotope is prompt, with a uniform distribution. Maximum hepatic accumulation is usually seen within 5 minutes. The gallbladder may be visualized as early as 10 minutes into the study but is not always seen. Bowel activity is usually observed by 30 to 40 minutes. The hepatic, cystic, and common bile ducts are not normally visualized in the neonatal period but become more obvious after 12 months of age. Over the age of 8 years and in adulthood, the left hepatic bile ducts become prominent on hepatobiliary scintigraphy (Figure 74.4-2).[25] The hepatic extraction function (HEF) is defined by the extraction of isotope by the liver and reflects hepatocyte function. It can be assessed visually and quantitatively by analysis of the initial hepatic uptake phase of the study. The normal pediatric HEF is over 92%.[26] Hepatic half clearance times ($t_{1/2}$) are defined as hepatic parenchymal clearance divided by excretion and can be quantitatively assessed. The hepatic $t_{1/2}$ is normally less than 37 minutes.[25] However, there is a large overlap in the neonatal period, and determination of the hepatic $t_{1/2}$ has not been found helpful in differentiating between EHBA and other forms of cholestasis.

Typically, patients with EHBA presenting in the first 2 months of life show prompt hepatic extraction with a normal HEF (over 92%), nonvisualization of the gallbladder, prolonged retention of isotope in the liver, and absent

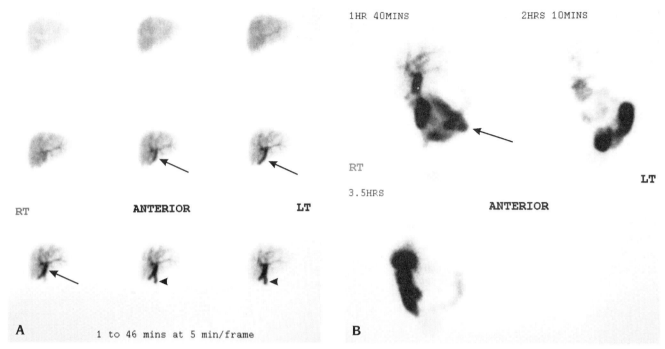

FIGURE 74.4-2 Normal hepatobiliary scintigraphy in a 9-year-old child. *A,* Initial images taken over the first hour of the study demonstrate normal uptake of isotope with good visualization of the intrahepatic bile ducts. The second and third rows of three images also demonstrate gallbladder filling (*arrows*) and the common bile duct (*arrowheads*). *B,* By 1 hour and 40 minutes, isotope has been excreted into the bowel (*arrow*). Subsequent images demonstrate gallbladder emptying and increased isotope excretion into the bowel.

excretion into the bowel even at 24 hours. Patients presenting after 3 months of age usually have compromised hepatocyte function and show reduced hepatic extraction, with reduced HEF and no biliary excretion. With this picture, differentiation from severe neonatal hepatitis or cholestasis may prove difficult. There are reports of patients with EHBA in whom excretion of isotope into the bowel was seen on scintigraphy in the early neonatal period, but repeat studies showed no excretion.[27] This may be due to progressive obliteration of the extrahepatic ducts continuing after birth. Therefore, it is appropriate to carefully monitor infants who show good extraction of isotope but only minimal excretion into the bowel.

Three patterns of hepatobiliary scintigraphic findings are described in neonatal hepatitis.[28] There may be normal hepatic extraction with visualization of isotope in the bowel, which excludes biliary atresia. Reduced hepatic extraction with absent excretion indicates severe parenchymal liver damage but would be inconsistent with EHBA in the first 3 months of life. Normal or near-normal hepatic uptake with no excretion is consistent with EHBA, but this pattern has been described in cases of severe neonatal hepatitis, cystic fibrosis (CF), α_1-antitrypsin deficiency, and syndromes with paucity of intrahepatic bile ducts.

In patients with neonatal hepatitis, the HEF is generally reduced, reflecting reduced hepatocyte function. There is persistent blood pool activity with delayed clearance because of reduced hepatocyte extraction. If there is severe hepatocyte dysfunction, there is reduced or absent excretion into the bowel and concurrent increased renal excretion of isotope (Figure 74.4-3). Any excretion of isotope into the bowel excludes EHBA.

The single most informative investigation in neonatal cholestasis is a liver biopsy. In experienced hands, liver biopsy has over 90% diagnostic accuracy, but it must be performed in a specialist pediatric center because it is not without risk, and the histopathology must be interpreted in the context of clinical information and other laboratory investigations.[29] The diagnosis of EHBA is ultimately confirmed at laparotomy and intraoperative cholangiography.

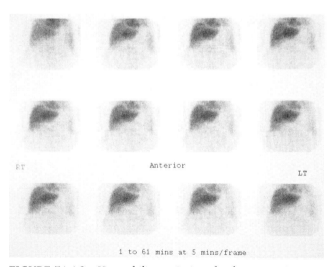

FIGURE 74.4-3 Hepatobiliary scintigraphy demonstrating generalized poor hepatic uptake of isotope, with persistent high background activity. The gallbladder is not visualized, and there is no excretion of isotope into the bowel. These findings reflect severe hepatocyte dysfunction in a patient with neonatal hepatitis, but extrahepatic biliary atresia cannot be excluded on the basis of this scan.

Spontaneous rupture of the common bile duct usually occurs in the first 1 to 2 weeks of life, and the cause is unknown. Infants present with jaundice and abdominal distention owing to ascites, which is bile stained on aspiration. Hepatobiliary ultrasonography may be normal in these children but often demonstrates a pseudocyst at the porta hepatis, usually without biliary dilatation. Occasionally, sludge or stones are seen in the common bile duct distal to the site of perforation, which is at the junction of the cystic duct and common bile duct. Hepatobiliary scintigraphy may show a photopenic area owing to the pseudocyst or extravasation of isotope into the peritoneal cavity. Intraoperative cholangiography confirms the diagnosis at the time of surgery.[25]

USE OF HEPATOBILIARY SCINTIGRAPHY BEYOND THE NEONATAL PERIOD

Patients with congenital bile duct dilatation (choledochal cyst) may present with cholestatic jaundice and acholic stools in the first few months of life. Most cases of choledochal cyst present under the age of 10 years, with 30% under 1 year of age. Presentation can even be delayed into adulthood, although this is uncommon. The diagnosis is usually made with ultrasonography at all ages. Following ultrasound examination, ^{99m}Tc IDA scintigraphy can be used to confirm the biliary origin of the cyst if thought clinically necessary. There is a known association of choledochal cysts with EHBA. Scintigraphy may help to determine the type of cystic dilatation and whether the cystic structure communicates with the biliary system. The scintigraphic appearance will depend partly on the degree of biliary obstruction caused by the cyst because extremely large cysts may obstruct biliary flow completely. There may be normal hepatic extraction and excretion of isotope, or, alternatively, isotope may accumulate in dilated ducts or cysts. A photopenic defect may be seen in the region of the porta hepatis depending on the size of the cyst. Complete obstruction with negligible biliary flow and nonfilling of the mass may occur. Rarely, activity is seen in the peritoneal cavity after cyst rupture. Like the gallbladder, choledochal cysts may contract after a fatty meal or cholecystokinin. Caroli disease (type 5 choledochal cyst) may present in infancy and shows an irregular pattern of cystic dilatation, with accumulation of isotope in the intrahepatic bile ducts on delayed images.[25] Although these findings are well described, with the advent of high-resolution ultrasonography and magnetic resonance cholangiography, radionuclides are currently seldom used in these clinical situations.

Patients with increased bile viscosity are at risk of developing bile plugs (inspissated bile syndrome), which can cause biliary obstruction. These include patients with CF, patients on total parenteral nutrition, and following extensive ileal resection. Appearances on ^{99m}Tc IDA scintigraphy are variable because there may be secondary liver damage, but there is typically good hepatic extraction of isotope and poor excretion into the gut. Occasionally, absent excretion is found in the neonatal period or in infancy, and the study is unable to exclude EHBA.[30] In Alagille syndrome, which

is characterized by a paucity of interlobular bile ducts in association with certain phenotypic features and congenital cardiac and vertebral abnormalities, patients develop cholestasis, and ^{99m}Tc IDA scintigraphy demonstrates good extraction of isotope by the liver with marked retention of isotope in the hepatic parenchyma and usually minimal excretion into the gut. Occasionally, absent excretion is shown, and EHBA cannot be excluded.

HEPATOBILIARY SCINTIGRAPHY IN CF

^{99m}Tc IDA scintigraphy may be incorporated in the assessment and follow-up of patients who develop CF-related liver disease and is complementary to ultrasonography. Deficiency of the CF transmembrane regulator in the bile duct epithelial cells of these patients causes increased viscosity of bile that becomes inspissated, leading to plugging of intrahepatic bile ducts. Impairment of both intra- and extrahepatic biliary drainage contributes to the development of liver disease in these patients, with the development of fatty liver, chronic cholestasis, and, eventually, cirrhosis. Peak onset is during adolescence. ^{99m}Tc IDA scintigraphy allows assessment of hepatic extraction, clearance of isotope from the hepatic parenchyma, and biliary drainage and may have a role in monitoring disease progression and the success of treatment.[31]

POSTOPERATIVE AND POST-TRAUMATIC HEPATOBILIARY SCINTIGRAPHY

Postoperative evaluation of biliary drainage using ^{99m}Tc IDA scintigraphy is useful in patients who have undergone portoenterostomy (Kasai procedure) and also following liver transplant. The main indications for performing scintigraphy are to assess hepatic perfusion, parenchymal function, detect bile leaks, and assess transit of radiopharmaceutical from the liver into the intestine.[32]

In cases of liver trauma, CT scanning is the best method of assessing liver injury acutely. ^{99m}Tc TBIDA scintigraphy is useful in the early detection of bile duct injuries and biliary leaks.[33] The technique demonstrates active leakage of isotope into the peritoneal cavity or focal abnormal areas of activity owing to bile collections (Figure 74.4-4).

RADIONUCLIDE IMAGING OF THE LIVER AND SPLEEN

Radionuclide imaging of the liver and spleen can be performed using ^{99m}Tc sulfur colloid by virtue of the reticuloendothelial activity of these organs. This technique was used to provide structural information and to evaluate focal or diffuse disorders affecting the liver or spleen, but it has now been superseded by ultrasonography, CT, and magnetic resonance imaging (MRI), which provide excellent anatomic information and better resolution. Injected ^{99m}Tc sulfur colloid particles are phagocytosed by the reticuloendothelial cells of the liver, spleen, and bone marrow. The bone marrow of normal patients is not visualized owing to greater concentration of reticuloendothelial activity in the

---

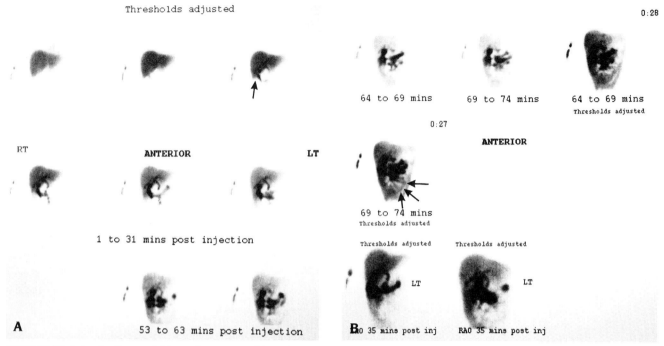

FIGURE 74.4-4 An 8-year-old boy who sustained liver lacerations in a road traffic accident. *A*, Hepatobiliary scintigraphy demonstrates normal hepatic uptake of isotope with visualization of main intrahepatic ducts. Focal collections of isotope around the porta hepatis on the far right image of the top row (*arrow*), and subsequent images are due to focal bile collections as a result of biliary leakage. There is excretion of isotope into the bowel but on images taken at 53 to 63 minutes (*bottom row*) and subsequently (*B*), peritoneal reflections are outlined by free isotope within the peritoneal cavity (*arrows*). This is better demonstrated following adjustment of the gamma camera parameters (threshold adjustment). Biliary leakage was confirmed at surgery.

liver and spleen. ^{99m}Tc sulfur colloid particles are cleared rapidly from the bloodstream following intravenous injection (typical $t_{1/2}$ of less than 3 minutes). Rapid sequence (dynamic) imaging is performed to show blood flow to the organs. There is earlier and more rapid uptake in the spleen and kidneys because the majority of the hepatic blood flow is via the portal vein. Static views are then obtained in multiple projections to visualize the organs and separate overlapping structures. SPECT images may improve resolution.

Imaging of primary and secondary hepatic tumors is now primarily with CT and MRI, and radionuclide imaging is not indicated. When performed, these studies show increased blood flow to the tumor on dynamic imaging, with photopenic defects on delayed static imaging using ^{99m}Tc sulfur colloid or ^{99m}Tc IDA compounds.[13] Vascular lesions, such as hepatic hemangiomas or hemangioendotheliomas, can be differentiated from hypervascular tumors because although both demonstrate increased perfusion during dynamic imaging using ^{99m}Tc sulfur colloid, there is prolonged retention of activity in the vascular spaces of hepatic vascular lesions (which does not occur in tumors). Both vascular lesions and tumors show photopenic defects on delayed static images owing to the absence of reticuloendothelial cells. The use of ^{99m}Tc-labeled red blood cells (RBCs) has been advocated in the case of suspected hepatic vascular lesions because of the overlap in scintigraphic findings with hypervascular tumors. However, three-phase CT and MRI have been shown to have greater sensitivity and accuracy and have therefore replaced scintigraphy in the evaluation of such lesions.

Hepatic infection, either diffuse hepatitis or focal infection with abscess formation, may show hepatomegaly with heterogeneous distribution of isotope. However, radionuclide imaging is not used routinely or as the primary method of imaging in these conditions. ^{99m}Tc sulfur colloid has been used as a screening or monitoring tool in patients with diffuse liver disease such as cirrhosis, α_1-antitrypsin deficiency, CF, storage diseases, or congenital hepatic fibrosis. In these disorders, the primary findings are diminished or heterogeneous uptake by the liver, with relatively increased uptake in the spleen and bone marrow in the setting of progressive disease. Hepatomegaly or reduction in liver size will depend on the stage of the disease.[32] In hepatic venous occlusion (Budd-Chiari syndrome), there is typically caudate lobe hypertrophy with increased uptake of ^{99m}Tc sulfur colloid and reduced uptake in the remainder of the liver, although other patterns are described.[34] Again, ultrasonography, CT, and MRI have replaced radionuclide imaging in screening for veno-occlusive disorders.

RADIONUCLIDE IMAGING OF THE SPLEEN

The spleen alone can be anatomically and physiologically imaged using ^{99m}Tc-labeled heat-denatured RBCs. The main indication for performing splenic scintigraphy is to identify functioning splenic tissue in patients with visceral heterotaxy syndromes and disorders that affect splenic function, such as sickle cell disease. Demonstration of splenic tissue on ultrasonography or cross-sectional imaging does not indicate splenic function, and this is particularly true for patients with visceral heterotaxy or abnormalities of isomerism associated with congenital cardiac disease. Functional asplenia may be suspected from the detection of Howell-Jolly bodies in the circulating blood. It is important to identify patients with asplenia or functional asplenia because they are susceptible to overwhelming bacterial sepsis and require vaccination and antibiotic prophylaxis. However, when functional asplenia is suspected, the necessary precautions against sepsis are usually instituted, without risk and without resorting to splenic scintigraphy for confirmation.

Splenic scintigraphy may be employed in the detection of abnormally sited splenic tissue, which can be implanted in the chest, abdomen, or pelvis following trauma to the native spleen (splenosis). The extrasplenic tissue accumulates ^{99m}Tc-labeled RBCs in the same manner as the spleen, and this finding is useful in identifying apparently abnormally sited masses, which are, in fact, implanted splenic tissue. A further related use of splenic scintigraphy is in the identification of accessory spleens or splenunculi. These are considered to be a normal variant, but their identification is important in patients undergoing splenectomy for hematologic reasons.

Heat-denatured RBCs are injected intravenously and are avidly sequestered by the normal spleen, thereby demonstrating splenic function in addition to showing the position and size of the organ. This is accompanied by only faint uptake in the liver. If no functioning splenic tissue is present, there will be hepatic uptake owing to its reticuloendothelial activity and some excretion of free pertechnetate by the kidneys.

Between 3 and 8 mL of blood are taken from the patient depending on chronologic age and body weight. Under sterile conditions, the cells are labeled with ^{99m}Tc pertechnetate and then heated in a water bath at 49.5°C for 12 to 15 minutes.[32] The ^{99m}Tc-labeled RBCs are then reinjected intravenously, and static scans are performed in a number of planes after at least 30 minutes. SPECT scanning can be performed to improve localization, particularly if only small volumes of splenic tissue are present.

LEUKOCYTE SCINTIGRAPHY IN INFLAMMATORY BOWEL DISEASE

Leukocyte scintigraphy is a well-established technique that has a role in the detection of inflammation and sepsis. Its initial use in the investigation of inflammatory bowel diseases (IBDs) was reported in 1981.[35,36] Since that time, the place of labeled white cell scans (WCSs) has not been well defined in existing guidelines for the investigation of IBD, and use seems to reflect preferences in personal practice.[37] The technique has been evaluated as part of the routine investigation of suspected IBD, as a method for assessing both disease location and disease activity, and as a tool for following disease progression.

White cell scanning offers several advantages over other techniques commonly used to investigate IBD. The technique is noninvasive, does not require any patient preparation, and is well tolerated. It also allows whole-bowel exam-

ination with low radiation exposure,[38] and patients prefer WCSs to barium follow-through studies or enteroclysis.[39] These features suggest that white cell scanning is a technique that could be applied more frequently than either barium imaging or endoscopy and, more specifically, that it might be a more appropriate technique for children.

As the migration of leukocytes into tissues is a direct manifestation of a pathophysiologic process, it has been suggested that WCSs represent a direct measure of disease activity. Assessment of mucosal inflammation is otherwise possible only for areas of bowel that can be directly visualized and biopsied.

Several different indices of scintigraphic activity have been published. Broadly, these encompass visual grading systems requiring comparison of bowel activity with that of bone marrow, liver, or spleen[40,41] and computer-based methods with or without background subtraction.[42] Visual assessment has been demonstrated to have a high degree of interobserver variability.[43] Currently, there is no apparent consensus between studies as to how various areas of the bowel should be divided for an assessment of disease activity. Commonly, segmental analysis is reported according to uptake in the small bowel; ileum; cecum; right, transverse, and left colon; sigmoid colon; and rectum. A lack of universally accepted measures likely contributes to the variability of reported results and the lack of a generally agreed on role for use of WCSs in the assessment of disease activity in IBD.

There are two main isotopes used in leukocyte imaging. White cells may be labeled with [111]indium (^{111}In) oxime or ^{99m}Tc hexamethylpropyleneamine oxime (^{99m}Tc HMPAO). [111]In is cyclotron produced, whereas ^{99m}Tc is generator produced and is therefore more readily available. [111]In also gives a relatively higher bone marrow dose to children compared with adults owing to the greater proportion of red marrow in children.[44] HMPAO has the advantage of having a longer shelf life of 5.5 months and is more specific for granulocytes in a mixed cell population. [99m]Tc HMPAO also generates a superior image quality. Therefore, this compound has become the most widely used radioisotope in current practice.[45,46] Using ^{111}In or ^{99m}Tc HMPAO, the labeling process is relatively simple, but the leukocytes must first be separated from whole blood using sedimentation, centrifugation, and washing. The leukocyte pellet is then resuspended in sterile saline. When using ^{99m}Tc HMPAO, the preparation is simply added to the leukocyte suspension and is gently mixed. Following a short period of incubation at room temperature, washing, and resuspension in a small quantity of plasma, the labeled leukocytes are ready for reinjection. The labeling yield is usually about 50%.[47]

After injection, the labeled granulocytes migrate into the inflamed area. Using ^{99m}Tc, the most reliable images are generated soon after injection of labeled cells, generally at 30 to 60 minutes, although delayed scans, at 2 to 4 hours, may also be helpful (Figure 74.4-5).[48] Careful interpretation of the images is important because activity occurring in the bowel on later images can represent normal "physiologic" bowel activity. The process underlying this is uncertain, although there is some suggestion that it may represent cells being shed into the bowel lumen.

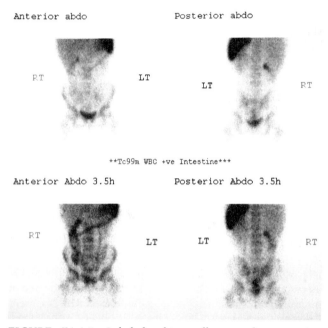

Anterior abdo   Posterior abdo

Tc99m WBC +ve Intestine

Anterior Abdo 3.5h   Posterior Abdo 3.5h

FIGURE 74.4-5 Labeled white cell scan demonstrating increased uptake in the cecum, ascending colon, and transverse colon in a 12-year-old boy with Crohn disease.

WCSs have obvious limitations. They cannot define anatomic features such as stricture, fistula, or prestenotic dilatation, although they may assist in distinguishing an inflammatory from a noninflammatory stricture. In interpretation of the images, potential causes of a false-positive WCS also must be considered. These include the presence of gastrointestinal bleeding, stoma sites, wounds, hematomas, deep vein thrombosis, and ischemic and infective bowel disease.[49] Other causes of bowel inflammation, such as infection or chronic granulomatous disease, may also generate positive studies.[50] Interpretation of anatomic distribution may be limited by bone, liver, spleen, and renal uptake, which can impair accurate assessment of small bowel involvement, and by urinary excretion because isotope within the bladder can affect assessment of uptake by rectal mucosa.

Several studies in children have compared the results of WCSs with histologic analysis of mucosal biopsies taken at colonoscopy. Such studies allow an assessment of the accuracy of the technique compared with the accepted diagnostic gold standard. A prospective investigation of 39 cases demonstrated that white cell scanning was able to diagnose IBD with a sensitivity of 90% and a specificity of 75% compared with colonic histology.[51] A similar prospective study compared scintigraphy in 137 children in whom colonoscopy and biopsy were also performed within 30 days and reported a sensitivity of 90%, a specificity of 97%, a positive predictive value of 97%, and a negative predictive value of 93% for WCSs.[39] However, endoscopic findings and histology remain the cornerstones for the diagnosis of pediatric IBD. It is not envisaged that these techniques would be replaced by scintigraphy.

Studies comparing WCSs and barium radiology demonstrate that scintigraphy has a higher accuracy for identifying

IBD.[51,52] This suggests that the role of barium studies needs re-evaluation, particularly in screening for IBD. However, studies report less enthusiastic results for the scintigraphic diagnosis of IBD.[53,54] Reported differences in reliability likely reflect several factors, including different patient populations and differences in the severity of disease activity.

Bowel scintigraphy examines the whole of the bowel during one procedure. However, disease location is not always accurate when assessed by WCSs. Charron and colleagues assessed the accuracy of scintigraphy compared with endoscopy and biopsy for identifying colonic or ileal disease and found that scintigraphic location of disease activity limited to the colon yielded sensitivity and a positive predictive value of 97% and 97%, respectively.[55] For locating disease activity to the ileum, scintigraphy was less sensitive and specific. Inflammation within the terminal ileum is frequently difficult to distinguish from lymphoid nodular hyperplasia seen in up to 24% of barium studies when investigating IBD.[56] Furthermore, direct endoscopic visualization of the terminal ileum is not always possible for technical reasons. Studies in patients being investigated for IBD or for nonspecific gastrointestinal symptoms and other unrelated medical reasons have not reported terminal ileal uptake in any children without a final diagnosis of IBD, even in the presence of lymphoid nodular hyperplasia.[54,55]

Very few studies comment on the ability of scintigraphy to distinguish Crohn disease from ulcerative colitis on the appearance of activity within the colon. With continuous colonic activity, a distinction between Crohn disease and ulcerative colitis is not possible. Demonstration of discontinuous activity does not indicate Crohn disease with absolute certainty because discontinuous uptake has also been found in patients with ulcerative colitis, perhaps related to the attenuation of already minimal disease activity.[53,57] In this respect, WCSs are not sufficiently accurate and cannot be considered an alternative to endoscopic evaluation.

The accuracy of scintigraphy in the evaluation of small bowel disease is uncertain. Activity in overlying liver, spleen, transverse colon, and skeletal structures makes WCSs less sensitive in detecting upper gastrointestinal disease, and localization of proximal small bowel disease is poor. Reduced sensitivity of WCSs may also be related to the absence of active disease, with only the sequel of previous inflammation evident on barium studies.[58] The timing of scans is also important to avoid errors of interpretation owing to the normal hepatobiliary excretion of ^{99m}Tc.[59] Scintigraphy cannot be as informative as barium radiology in the definition of anatomic detail such as stricture formation. However, WCSs may provide information, allowing a distinction to be made between an inflammatory and a fixed stricture.

Currently, the role of scintigraphy in the routine investigation and monitoring of IBD is not well established. However, an understanding of the principles underlying these investigations and knowledge of the advantages and disadvantages of the technique allow the practitioner to decide whether scintigraphy could contribute to the optimal management of individual patients. Demonstration of florid disease activity, for example, would reinforce a decision to use more aggressive medical and surgical treatment.[60]

WCSs might have a role in the detection of postoperative disease activity, thus avoiding invasive tests in such patients. However, there are only limited reports in the pediatric literature, many of which are anecdotal. In a study of adults, Biancone and colleagues reported using leukocyte scintigraphy for the early detection of postoperative recurrence in Crohn disease.[61] Anastomosis-related activity was controlled for by comparison with patients who had undergone ileocecal resection for cecal carcinoma, and the findings were compared with those noted at endoscopy. There was good correlation between the endoscopic and the 30-minute scintigraphy scores at both 6 and 12 months postoperatively, suggesting that white cell scanning may prove to be a sensitive technique for this purpose.

The relatively noninvasive nature of leukocyte scintigraphy recommends its use for the screening of IBD. As with other indications for these investigations, there is uncertainty about its exact role and the advantages it has over endoscopy, biopsy, and barium radiology. Several studies in adults have looked at the role of WCSs in the screening of patients with suspected irritable bowel syndrome. Some authors express concerns over the high rates of false-positive results.[62] Shah and colleagues evaluated the accuracy of WCSs in screening children with suspected IBD and found false-positive scans in patients with postenteritis syndrome, infectious colitis, and anorexia nervosa, but there were no false-negative WCSs.[49] In clinical practice, if the clinical suspicion of IBD is high, it is likely that even with a negative WCS, further investigation should be recommended. Concerns over the possible inadequacies of WCSs in identifying small bowel disease also mitigate against the use of WCSs as a screening tool.

Leukocyte scintigraphy has also been used for identifying bowel inflammation associated with other disease entities. Hoare and colleagues reported a positive scan in a child with colitis owing to chronic granulomatous disease.[50] WCSs have been used following bone marrow transplant and cord cell infusion as treatment for chronic granulomatous disease to assess whether there is recurrence of colonic inflammation, without recourse to more invasive diagnostic tests.

Overall, it appears that there is currently no generally accepted role for leukocyte scintigraphy in pediatric IBDs. Nevertheless, WCSs are of value in certain situations, and the clinician should be aware of their potential. Wider use may well lead to a better understanding of their place in the diagnostic armamentarium.

ROLE OF SCINTIGRAPHY IN PROTEIN-LOSING ENTEROPATHY

Protein-losing enteropathy (PLE) is defined as a condition in which excess protein loss into the gastrointestinal lumen is severe enough to produce hypoproteinemia. PLE can occur in conditions such as ulcerative colitis, Ménétrier disease, celiac disease, and intestinal lymphangiectasia.[63] Most proteins lost into the bowel undergo proteolysis and are thus unreliable as a generalized measurement of PLE. α_1-Antitrypsin is resistant to intestinal proteolysis and thus its fecal level is indicative of the degree of loss of serum protein into the gastrointestinal tract.[64] Although this test provides a quantitative measure of intestinal protein losses, it does not allow localization of the site where this loss is occurring. Studies with ^{99m}Tc-labeled human serum albumin suggest that it is stable in the gut and that it is impermeable to normal bowel, making it an appropriate nucleotide for scintigraphic detection of PLE.[65] After intravenous injection of freshly prepared ^{99m}Tc human serum albumin, serial images of the abdomen are obtained from 10 minutes up to 24 hours after injection. A ^{99m}Tc human serum albumin scan is considered positive for PLE if there is visible tracer exudation in the gut (Figure 74.4-6).

Lan and colleagues presented two cases of PLE in children in which the loss was localized to the stomach in one child with transient Ménétrier disease and the small bowel in another child with primary oxalosis.[66] The diagnosis was confirmed in both cases by elevated 72-hour fecal α_1-antitrypsin levels. Halaby and colleagues reported a retrospective review of ^{99m}Tc human serum albumin scans in 18 children.[67] Scans were positive in 12 children, of whom 10 had primary intestinal lymphangiectasia, 1 had active *Salmonella* enterocolitis, and 1 had giardiasis. Scans were normal in the remaining 6 children, of whom 5 were subsequently demonstrated to have a primary intestinal lymphangiectasia. The authors noted that serum indices of PLE were less decreased than in those with positive scans, suggesting that a lower rate of protein loss might explain the false-negative scans. Chiu and colleagues stressed the importance of obtaining images up to 24 hours following the administration of the labeled albumin.[63] In summary, labeled albumin scintigraphy may be a useful tool in establishing a PLE. However, owing to concerns about accuracy, it is most appropriately used in association with other investigations.

NUCLEAR MEDICINE IN THE INVESTIGATION OF GASTROINTESTINAL TRACT BLEEDING

The causes of gastrointestinal bleeding in children are numerous, and radiology has a role in detecting the origin of the blood loss, defining associated pathology, and, in certain cases, intervening to control hemorrhage. There are two main techniques in nuclear medicine used to localize the site of gastrointestinal bleeding. Administration of ^{99m}Tc sulfur colloid or radiolabeled RBCs during active bleeding can localize the source of hemorrhage. It is said that RBC scans have detection rates higher than angiography at lower rates of blood loss—even as little as 0.1 mL per minute.[68] RBC and sulfur colloid scans have the advantage of being less invasive than angiography. The second technique, the so-called Meckel scan, involves administration of radiolabeled pertechnetate, which localizes in gastric mucosa and can identify ectopic sites of gastric mucosa as the source of blood loss. This type of scan is more frequently used when bleeding is intermittent and more occult.

GASTROINTESTINAL BLEEDING SCANS

There is an important difference between the two agents used to perform gastrointestinal bleeding studies. ^{99m}Tc sulfur colloid is a non–blood pool agent, which is cleared rapidly from the blood following injection. ^{99m}Tc-labeled RBCs are a blood pool agent that circulate in the blood for hours. When ^{99m}Tc sulfur colloid is injected intravenously, the particles circulate through the mesenteric vascular supply before being cleared by the liver and reticuloendothelial system. Any site of bleeding, vascular leak, or tear will allow the ^{99m}Tc sulfur colloid particles to extravasate, and this is detected using the gamma camera as a site of focal

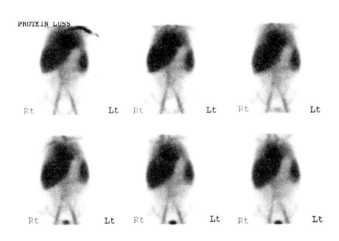

A

0-30 minutes post injection

6 frames 5 minutes each

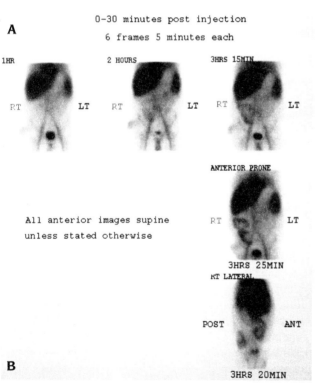

All anterior images supine
unless stated otherwise

B

FIGURE 74.4-6 Protein-losing enteropathy. *A* demonstrates normal isotope uptake in the liver and spleen, normal activity in the vascular system, and renal excretion of isotope with activity in the bladder. *B*, By 2 hours, activity is seen within the gut in the right side of the abdomen and becomes more prominent on later images. This is due to loss of labeled albumin into the gut lumen.

accumulation of isotope. Very small amounts of hemorrhage can be detected, but the patient must be actively bleeding between the time of injection and clearance of tracer, a window of approximately 15 to 20 minutes. For this reason, there is a high incidence of false-negative scans.[69] Bleeding near the liver or spleen may be obscured by activity in these organs, with a false-negative test result.

The use of ^{99m}Tc-labeled RBCs is the preferred method for investigating acute gastrointestinal bleeding in children using radioisotope. It is more suitable for patients who are bleeding slowly or intermittently. However, this method requires more preparation time for labeling the RBCs and careful handling of the patient's blood. The labeling process can occur in vivo or in vitro. With in vivo labeling, an initial intravenous injection of nonradioactive stannous (tin) ion is given, followed 10 to 20 minutes later by an injection of ^{99m}Tc pertechnetate. The RBCs react first with the stannous ion and then the pertechnetate. Pertechnetate is reduced by the intracellular stannous ion, forming a complex with intracellular hemoglobin. Images can be acquired for several hours after the injection. However, high background activity reduces the sensitivity of in vivo labeled RBCs. Therefore, an in vitro labeling method is more commonly employed with a sample of approximately 5 mL blood taken into a syringe containing acid citrate dextrose to which stannous chloride is added.[70] The blood is then re-injected, and the patient is imaged immediately to demonstrate initial blood flow, followed by imaging for up to 2 hours. A normal ^{99m}Tc RBC study (both in vivo or in vitro labeled RBCs) will demonstrate tracer within the blood pools of the aorta, inferior vena cava, iliac vessels, and portal, renal, and mesenteric vessels. Tracer activity also persists in the kidneys and penis. Free pertechnetate can be seen in the kidneys, ureters, and urinary bladder. These are normal scintigraphic features and, most importantly, do not change over time. Sites of active bleeding are seen as focal, increasing accumulation of tracer that does move over time owing to gut peristalsis. Peristaltic movement may lead to erroneous impression of the exact site of bleeding. Computerized acquisition with dynamic cinescintigraphic display of sequential images is reported to improve the localization of bleeding sites.[71]

MECKEL SCAN

A Meckel diverticulum is a remnant of the omphalomesenteric (vitelline) duct, which is normally obliterated between the fifth and ninth week of gestation. It is present in approximately 2% of the population on the antimesenteric border of the small intestine, approximately 2 feet proximal to the ileocecal valve. Approximately half of Meckel diverticula contain ectopic mucosa, 80% of which contain gastric mucosa and therefore may become symptomatic owing to mucosal ulceration and intestinal bleeding. Ectopic pancreatic mucosa is present in approximately 5%, and this can occur concomitantly with gastric mucosa.[72]

^{99m}Tc pertechnetate is used to evaluate patients with lower gastrointestinal bleeding and abdominal pain and in whom a Meckel diverticulum is suspected. ^{99m}Tc pertechnetate is taken up by the gastric mucin-producing cells and is then secreted into the gut lumen. Excretion of ^{99m}Tc pertechnetate is not dependent on the presence of parietal (acid producing) cells. It therefore detects the presence of gastric mucosa contained within a Meckel diverticulum rather than the diverticulum itself. In large case series, the test has a surgically proven sensitivity up to 85% and specificities as high as 95% for the detection of ectopic gastric mucosa.[73,74]

Ectopic gastric mucosa is visible as a focal area of isotope uptake simultaneous with uptake in eutopic gastric mucosa, usually within 10 minutes of injection of ^{99m}Tc pertechnetate (Figure 74.4-7). The intensity of the tracer accumulation may be less than that within the stomach, depending on the amount of mucosa present within the diverticulum and its secretory activity. Meckel diverticula are typically located in the right lower quadrant but may be found in different quadrants of the abdomen and can even move during the examination (Figure 74.4-8).[75] Normal excretion of ^{99m}Tc pertechnetate in the kidneys, ureters, and bladder should not be confused with pathology. Hydronephrosis, hydroureter, a pelvic kidney, and communicating urachal cysts can be mistaken for a Meckel diverticulum.[76] The bladder should be included on the abdominal images and postvoid images should be taken to ensure that a focal area of uptake is not obscured by activity within a full bladder.

Drugs that increase uptake or decrease the secretory activity of gastric mucosa can enhance the detection of a Meckel diverticulum. Pentagastrin given subcutaneously prior to the injection of ^{99m}Tc pertechnetate stimulates gastric mucosal uptake, whereas histamine$_2$-receptor antago-

nists inhibit the secretion of ^{99m}Tc pertechnetate from the mucin cells into the gut lumen. Glucagon acts to decrease gut peristalsis, thereby increasing retention of isotope within a diverticulum. In some institutions, pharmacologic enhancement is reserved for patients with a negative scan and a persisting high index of clinical suspicion.[13]

False-negative scans do occur and may be due to a number of factors, including suboptimal examination technique, impaired blood supply to the bowel, or insufficient mass of gastric tissue in the Meckel diverticulum to take up isotope. Continued bleeding or excessive secretions may cause washout of the isotope, leading to a false-negative test result. Repeat scanning, up to three times, is justified in patients with lower intestinal tract bleeding that is highly suspicious for originating from ectopic gastric mucosa and an initial negative ^{99m}Tc pertechnetate scan.[77] The use of SPECT has been advocated to increase the diagnostic accuracy of Meckel scans, particularly if the scan result is equivocal or if there is a strong clinical suspicion together with a negative Meckel scan.[78] Barium and contrast can interfere with visualization on scintigraphic examination. Therefore, Meckel scans or ^{99m}Tc RBC studies should be performed before barium studies or angiography. If both Meckel scan and ^{99m}Tc RBC imaging are to be performed, then Meckel scan should be performed first because stannous-containing agents affect the distribution of ^{99m}Tc pertechnetate within the body.[79]

False-positive scans may be seen with intestinal duplications that contain gastric mucosa. The presence of ectopic mucosa predisposes the patient to peptic ulceration, bleeding, and, occasionally, perforation as observed with Meckel diverticula. If a communication between the

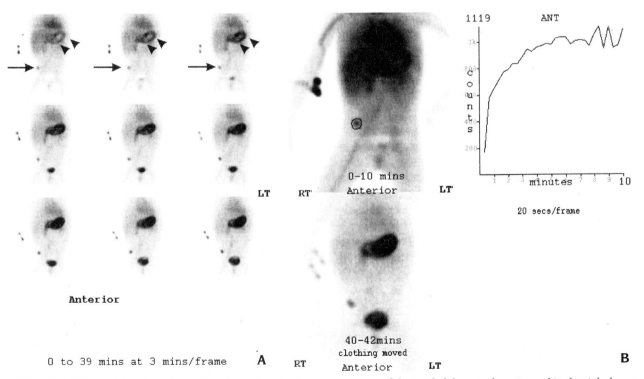

FIGURE 74.4-7   Positive Meckel scan. Uptake in the ectopic gastric mucosa of the Meckel diverticulum situated in the right lower quadrant (*arrow*) is simultaneous with uptake in gastric mucosa of the stomach (*arrowheads*). By drawing a region of interest around the ectopic gastric mucosa and plotting the count rate, maximum uptake is seen at approximately 5 minutes (*B*).

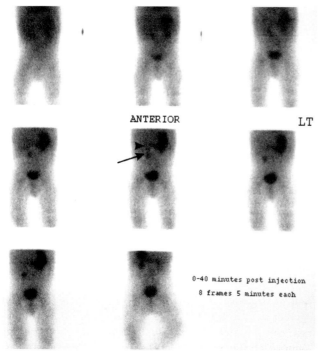

ANTERIOR   LT

0-40 minutes post injection
8 frames 5 minutes each

FIGURE 74.4-8   Positive Meckel scan. The Meckel diverticulum in this patient is located in the right upper quadrant (*arrow*), inferior to secreted activity in the first part of the duodenum (*arrowhead*).

cyst and the bowel exists, then bleeding will be intraluminal. If there is no communication, blood can accumulate within the cyst, and the patients present with a painful, rapidly enlarging abdominal mass.[72] Barrett esophagus, peptic ulcers, IBD, intussusception, vascular malformations, and neoplasms can also cause false-positive scans owing to the nonspecific accumulation of isotope.[13,72]

SOMATOSTATIN RECEPTOR SCINTIGRAPHY

Although neuroendocrine tumors affecting the gastrointestinal tract are uncommon in children, the gastrinoma (Zollinger-Ellison) syndrome and the VIPoma (Verner-Morrison) syndrome are well described (see Chapter 47, "Secretory Tumors Affecting the Gut"). These neuroendocrine tumors predominantly overexpress the somatostatin receptor SSTR2, which has a high affinity for synthetic analogues of somatostatin, such as octreotide.[80] This property has been exploited to allow accurate localization of the tumors. Radiolabeled peptides, such as ^{111}In pentreotide, bind to the SSTR expressed on the tumor, thereby allowing identification and localization.[81] Compared with other imaging techniques, including ultrasonography, CT, MRI, and angiography, somatostatin receptor scintigraphy is the most sensitive.[82,83] The ability of scintigraphy to image the whole body allows identification of both primary lesions and sites of metastatic spread. The technique has been further developed to allow tumor localization at surgery by use of a probe that detects preoperatively injected labeled octreotide.[84] Consideration has also been given to using receptor expression to target radiotherapy.

SCINTIGRAPHY IN BILE ACID MALABSORPTION

Bile acids are reabsorbed by an active transport mechanism in the terminal ileum as part of the enterohepatic circulation. Bile acid malabsorption is described as a rare cause of chronic diarrhea in infants owing to the effect of the bile acids on the colonic ability to reabsorb sodium.[85] Malabsorption of bile acids can also arise as a result of ileal resection (eg, in Crohn disease) and has been observed in association with cholecystectomy, chronic pancreatitis, celiac disease, and diabetes mellitus.[86] [75]Selenium (Se)-labeled homocholic acid conjugated with taurine ([75]SeHCAT) can be used to measure bile acid losses from the gut. Tauroselcholic acid does not occur naturally but is an analogue of the naturally occurring bile acid conjugate taurocholic acid. [75]SeHCAT is administered intravenously and, through hepatobiliary excretion, becomes mixed with the endogenous bile acid pool. Malabsorption is assessed either by regular fecal collections or by assessing the 7-day retention, which is measured as a whole-body gamma camera count. The effective dose for this study in adults is 0.3 mSv, but there are no equivalent pediatric data. For comparison, the effective dose of a posteroanterior chest radiograph is 0.02 mSv and for a CT scan of the abdomen, 10 mSv. The average effective dose from natural background radiation per year is 3 mSv.[87]

In adults, normal retention at 7 days is over 10%.[88] Unfortunately, no lower limit has been determined for use in pediatric practice. However, this has not prevented its use in the diagnosis of primary bile acid malabsorption as a cause of protracted diarrhea in infants.[89] In this report, two sisters with chronic diarrhea are described in whom the [75]SeHCAT retention over 7 days was less than 0.1%. Subsequent investigations confirmed the absence of the bile acid transporter in the apical membrane of ileal enterocytes. Thus, although experience is still quite limited in children, the use of [75]SeHCAT can be justified in the investigation of children with unexplained chronic diarrhea and impaired growth.

ACKNOWLEDGMENT

All figures, except Figure 74.4-1, are courtesy of Dr. Karl Johnson, Birmingham Children's Hospital, Birmingham, UK.

REFERENCES

1. Gordon I. Issues surrounding preparation, information and handling the child and parent in nuclear medicine. J Nucl Med 1998;39:490–4.
2. Piepsz A, Gordon I, Hahn K. Pediatric nuclear medicine. Eur J Nucl Med 1991;18:41–66.
3. Piepsz A. Recent advances in pediatric nuclear medicine. Semin Nucl Med 1995;2:165–82.
4. Stringer DA, Nadel H. Techniques for investigation of the pediatric gastrointestinal tract. In: Stringer DA, Babyn PS, editors. Pediatric gastrointestinal imaging and intervention. 2nd ed. Hamilton (ON): BC Decker Inc; 2000. p. 15–74.
5. Vandenplas Y, Derde MP, Piepsz A. Evaluation of reflux episodes during simultaneous esophageal pH monitoring and gastroesophageal reflux scintigraphy in children. J Pediatr Gastroenterol Nutr 1992;14:256–60.

6. Orenstein SR, Klein HA, Rosenthal MS. Scintigraphy versus pH probe for quantification of pediatric reflux: a study using concurrent multiplexed data and acid feedings. J Nucl Med 1993;34:1228–34.

7. Piepsz A, Georges B, Perlmutter N, et al. Gastro-esophageal scintiscanning in children. Pediatr Radiol 1981;11:71–4.

8. Arasu TS, Wyllie R, Fitzgerald JF, et al. Gastroesophageal reflux in infants and children—comparative accuracy of diagnostic methods. J Pediatr 1980;96:798–803.

9. Sambasiva R, Kottamasu MD, Stringer DA. Diaphragm and oesophagogastric junction. In: Stringer DA, Babyn PS, editors. Pediatric gastrointestinal imaging and intervention. 2nd ed. Hamilton (ON): BC Decker Inc; 2000. p. 237–68.

10. Heyman S, Respondek M. Detection of pulmonary aspiration in children by radionuclide "salivagram." J Nucl Med 1989;30:697–9.

11. Hillemeier AC, Lange R, McCallum R, et al. Delayed gastric emptying in infants with gastroesophageal reflux. J Pediatr 1981;98:190–3.

12. Billeaud C, Guillet J, Sandler B. Gastric emptying in infants with or without gastro-esophageal reflux according to the type of milk. Eur J Clin Nutr 1990;44:577–83.

13. O'Hara SM. Pediatric gastrointestinal nuclear imaging. Radiol Clin North Am 1996;4:845–62.

14. Heyman S. Gastric emptying in children. J Nucl Med 1998;39:865–9.

15. Krishnamurphy S, Krishnamurphy K. Quantitative assessment of hepatobiliary diseases with ^{99m}Tc-IDA scintigraphy. In: Freeman LM, Weissmann HS, editors. Nuclear medicine annual. New York: Raven Press; 1988. p. 309–13.

16. Krishnamurphy GT, Turner FE. Pharmacokinetics and clinical application of technetium 99m-labelled hepatobiliary agents. Semin Nucl Med 1990;20:130–49.

17. Kelly D, Green A. Investigation of pediatric liver disease. J Inherit Metab Dis 1991;14:531–7.

18. Mieli-Vergani G, Howard ER, Portman B, Mowat AP. Late referral for biliary atresia—missed opportunities for effective surgery. Lancet 1989;i:421–3.

19. Ohi R, Nio M, Chiba T. Long term follow up after surgery for patients with biliary atresia. J Pediatr Surg 1990;25:442–5.

20. Davenport M, Kerkar N, Mieli-Vergani G, et al. Biliary atresia: the King's College Hospital experience (1974-1995). J Pediatr Surg 1997;32:479–85.

21. Choi SO, Perk WH, Lee HJ. Ultrasonographic 'triangular cord': the most definitive finding for non-invasive diagnosis of extrahepatic biliary atresia. Eur J Pediatr Surg 1998;8:12–6.

22. Kotb MA, Kotb A, Sheba MF, et al. Evaluation of the triangular cord sign in the diagnosis of biliary atresia. Pediatrics 2001;108:416–20.

23. Farrant P, Meire HB, Mieli-Vergani G. Ultrasound features of the gallbladder in infants presenting with conjugated hyperbilirubinaemia. Br J Radiol 2000;73:1154–8.

24. Nadel H. Hepatobiliary scintigraphy in children. Semin Nucl Med 1996;26:25–42.

25. Howman-Giles R, Uren R, Bernard E, Dorney S. Hepatobiliary scintigraphy in infancy. J Nucl Med 1998;39:311–9.

26. Howman-Giles R, Moase A, Gaskin K, Uren R. Hepatobiliary scintigraphy in a pediatric population: determination of hepatic extraction by deconvolutional analysis. J Nucl Med 1993;34:214–21.

27. Williamson SL, Siebert JJ, Butler HL, Golladay ES. Apparent gut excretion of ^{99m}Tc-DISIDA in a case of extrahepatic biliary atresia. Pediatr Radiol 1986;16:245–7.

28. Majd M, Reba RC Altman RP. Effect of phenobarbitol on ^{99m}Tc-IDA scintigraphy in the evaluation of neonatal jaundice. Semin Nucl Med 1981;11:194 201.

29. McKiernan PJ. Neonatal cholestasis. Semin Neonatol 2002;7:153–65.

30. Sty JR, Wells RG, Schroeder BA. Comparative imaging. Bile-plug syndrome. Clin Nucl Med 1987;12:489–90.

31. Foster JA, Ramsden WH, Conway SP, et al. The role of IDA scintigraphy in the follow-up of liver disease in patients with cystic fibrosis. Nucl Med Commun 2002;23:673–81.

32. Treves ST, Jones AG, Markisz J. Liver and spleen. In: Treves ST, editor. Pediatric nuclear medicine. 2nd ed. New York: Springer-Verlag; 1994. p. 466–95.

33. Sharif K, Pimpalwar AP, John P, et al. Benefits of early diagnosis and pre-emptive treatment of biliary tract complications after major blunt liver trauma in children. J Pediatr Surg 2002;37:1287–92.

34. Picard M, Carrier L, Chartrand R, et al. Budd-Chiari syndrome: typical and atypical scintigraphic aspects. J Nucl Med 1987;28:803–9.

35. Segal AW, Ensell J, Munro JM, Sarner M. ^{111}Indium-tagged leukocytes in the diagnosis of inflammatory bowel disease. Lancet 1981;ii:230–2.

36. Saverymuttu SH, Peters AM, Lavander JP, et al. ^{111}In-labelled autologous leukocytes in inflammatory bowel disease. Gastroenterology 1981;80:1273.

37. British Society of Gastroenterology guideline: inflammatory bowel disease. London: The Society; 1996.

38. Sheilds RA, Lawson RS. Effective dose equivalent. Nucl Med Commun 1987;8:851–5.

39. Charron M, Del Rosario FJ, Kocoshis SA. Pediatric inflammatory bowel disease: assessment with scintigraphy with 99mTc white blood cells. Radiology 1999;212:507–13.

40. Park RHR, McKillop JH, Duncan A, et al. Can ^{111}indium autologous mixed leukocyte scanning accurately access disease extent and activity in Crohn's disease? Gut 1988;29:821–3.

41. Papos M, Nagy F, Lang J, Csernay L. Technetium-99m hexamethyl propylene amine oxime labeled leukocyte scintigraphy in ulcerative colitis and Crohn's disease. Eur J Nucl Med 1993;20:766–9.

42. Giaffer MH, Tindale WB, Senior S, et al. Quantification of disease activity in Crohn's disease by computer analysis of Tc-99m hexamethyl propylene amine oxime (HMPAO) labeled leukocyte images. Gut 1993;34:68–74.

43. Giaffer MH, Tindale WB, Holdswort CD. Background subtraction: a new approach to the assessment of disease activity in Crohn's disease using 99m-Tc-HMPAO labeled leucocytes. Scand J Gastroenterol 1994;29 Suppl 203:55–60.

44. Allan RA. Imaging in inflammatory bowel disease. Imaging 2001;13:272–84.

45. Mansfield JC, Giaffer MH, Tindale WB, et al. Quantitative assessment of overall inflammatory bowel disease activity using labeled leucocytes: a direct comparison between indium-111 and technetium-99m HMPAO methods. Gut 1995;37:679–83.

46. Arndt JW, Van der Sluys Veer A, Blok D, et al. Prospective comparative study of technetium-99m white blood cells and indium-111 granulocytes for the examination of patients with inflammatory bowel disease. J Nucl Med 1993;34:1052–7.

47. Buonomo C, Van den Abbeele AD. Infection and inflammation. In: Treves ST, editor. Pediatric nuclear medicine. 2nd ed. New York: Springer-Verlag; 1995. p. 546–55.

48. Giaffer MH. Labeled leukocyte scintigraphy in inflammatory bowel disease: clinical applications. Gut 1996;38:1–5.

49. Shah DB, Cosgrove M, Rees JIS, Jenkins HR. The technetium white cell scan as an initial imaging investigation for evaluating suspected childhood inflammatory bowel disease. J Pediatr Gastroenterol Nutr 1997;25:524–8.

50. Hoare S, Walch JE, Eactham E, et al. Abnormal technetium

labeled white cell scan in the colitis of chronic granulomatous disease. Arch Dis Child 1997;77:50–1.

51. Jobling JC, Lindley KJ, Yousef Y, et al. Investigating inflammatory bowel disease-white cell scanning, radiology and colonoscopy. Arch Dis Child 1996;74:22–6.

52. Charron M, Di Lorenzo C, Kocoshis S. Are 99mTc leukocyte scintigraphy and SBFT studies useful in children suspected of having inflammatory bowel disease? Am J Gastroenterol 2000;95:1208–12.

53. Alberini J, Badran A, Freneaux E, et al. Technetium-99m HMPAO-labeled leukocyte imaging compared with endoscopy, ultrasonography, and contrast radiology in children with inflammatory bowel disease. J Pediatr Gastroenterol Nutr 2001; 32:278–86.

54. Cucchiara S, Celentano L, de Magistris TM, et al. Colonoscopy and technietium-99m white cell scan in children with suspected inflammatory bowel disease. J Pediatr 1999;135:727–32.

55. Charron M, Del Rosario F, Kocoshis S. Assessment of terminal ileal and colonic inflammation in Crohn's disease with 99mTc-WBC. Acta Paediatr 1999;88:193–8.

56. Lipson A, Bartram CI, Williams CB, et al. Barium studies and ileoscopy compared in children with suspected Crohn's disease. Clin Radiol 1990;41:5–8.

57. Charron M, Del Rosario F, Kocoshis S. Use of technetium-tagged white blood cells in patients with Crohn's disease and ulcerative colitis: is differential diagnosis possible? Pediatr Radiol 1998;28:871–7.

58. Davison SM, Chapman S, Murphy MS. 99mTc-HMPAO leukocyte scintigraphy fails to detect Crohn's disease in the proximal gastrointestinal tract. Arch Dis Child 2001;85:43–6.

59. Kennan N, Hayward M. Tc HMPAO-labeled white cell scintigraphy in Crohn's disease of the small bowel. Clin Radiol 1992;45:331–4.

60. Del Rosario MA, Fitzgerald JF, Siddiqui AR, et al. Clinical applications of technetium Tc 99m hexamethyl propylene amine oxime leukocyte scan in children with inflammatory bowel disease. J Pediatr Gastroenterol Nutr 1999;28:63–70.

61. Biancone L, Scopinaro F, Ierardi M, et al. 99mTc-HMPAO granulocyte scintigraphy in the early detection of postoperative asymptomatic recurrence in Crohn's disease. Dig Dis Sci 1997;42:1549–56.

62. Gibson P, Lichtenstein M, Salehi N, et al. Value of positive technetium-99m leukocyte scans in predicting intestinal inflammation. Gut 1991;32:1502–7.

63. Chiu N, Lee B, Hwang S, et al. Protein-losing enteropathy: diagnosis with ^{99m}Tc-labelled human serum albumin scintigraphy. Radiology 2001;219:86–90.

64. Durie PR. Intestinal protein loss and faecal α_1-antitrypsin. J Pediatr Gastroenterol Nutr 1985;4:345–7.

65. Divgi CR, Lisann NM, Yeh SD, Benua RS. Technetium-99m albumin scintigraphy in the diagnosis of protein-losing enteropathy. J Nucl Med 1986;27:1710–2.

66. Lan JA, Chervu LR, Marans Z, Colloins JC. Protein-losing enteropathy detected by ^{99m}Tc-labelled human serum albumin abdominal scintigraphy. J Pediatr Gastroenterol Nutr 1988;7:872–6.

67. Halaby H, Bakheet S, Shabib S, et al. 99m-Tc-human labeled albumin scans in children with protein-losing enteropathy. J Nucl Med 2000;41:215–9.

68. Orella P, Vial I, Prieto C, et al. Tc-99m red blood cell scintigraphy for the assessment of active gastrointestinal bleeding. Rev Med Child 1998;126:413–8.

69. Racadio JM, Agha AKM, Johnson ND, Warner BW. Imaging and radiological interventional techniques for gastrointestinal bleeding in children. Semin Pediatr Surg 1999;8:181–92.

70. Landry A, Hartshorne MF, Bunker SR, et al. Optimal technetium 99m RBC labeling for gastrointestinal hemorrhage study. Clin Nucl Med 1985;10:491–3.

71. Maurer AH, Rodman MS, Vitti RA, et al. Gastrointestinal bleeding: improved localization with cine scintigraphy. Radiology 1992;185:187–92.

72. Brown R, Azizkhan RG. Gastrointestinal bleeding in infants and children: Meckel's diverticulum and intestinal duplication. Semin Pediatr Surg 1999;8:202–9.

73. Sfakianakis GN, Conway JJ. Detection of ectopic gastric mucosa in Meckel's diverticulum and other aberrations by scintigraphy: I. Pathophysiology and 10-year clinical experience. J Nucl Med 1981;22:647–54.

74. St-Vil D, Brandt ML, Panic S, et al. Meckel's diverticulum in children: a 20-year review. J Pediatr Surg 1991;26:1289–92.

75. Nadel HR. Where are we with nuclear medicine in pediatrics? Eur J Nucl Med 1995;22:1433–51.

76. Schussheim A, Moskowitz GW, Levy LM. Radionuclide diagnosis of bleeding Meckel's diverticulum in children. Am J Gastroenterol 1977;68:25–9.

77. Kong M-S, Huang S-C, Tzen K-Y, Lin J-N. Repeated technetium-99m pertechnetate scanning for children with obscure gastrointestinal bleeding. J Pediatr Gastroenterol Nutr 1994;18:284–7.

78. Connolly LP, Treves ST, Bozorgi F, O'Connor SC. Meckel's diverticulum: demonstration of heterotopic gastric mucosa with technetium-99m-pertechnetate SPECT. J Nucl Med 1998; 39:1458–60.

79. Yen C, Lanoie Y. Effect of stannous pyrophosphate red blood cell gastrointestinal bleeding studies on subsequent Meckel's scan. Clin Nucl Med 1992;17:454–6.

80. Krenning EP, Kwekkeboom DJ, Oei HY, et al. Somatostatin-receptor scintigraphy in gastroenteropancreatic tumors. An overview of European results. Ann N Y Acad Sci 1994;733: 416–24.

81. Seregni E, Chiti A, Bombardieri E. Radionuclide imaging of neuroendocrine tumors: biological basis and diagnostic results. Eur J Nucl Med 1998;25:639–58.

82. Jamar F, Fiasse R, Leners N, et al. Somatostatin receptor imaging with indium-111-pentreoctide in gastroenteropancreatic tumors: safety, efficacy, and impact on patient management. J Nucl Med 1995;36:542–9.

83. Termanini B, Gibril F, Reynolds JC, et al. Value of somatostatin receptor scintigraphy: a prospective study in gastrinoma of its effect on clinical management. Gastroenterology 1997; 112:335–47.

84. Kwekkeboom D, Krenning EP, de Long M. Peptide receptor imaging and therapy. J Nucl Med 2000;41:1704–13.

85. Oelkers P, Kirby LC, Heubi JE, et al Primary bile acid malabsorption caused by mutations in the ileal sodium-dependent bile acid transporter gene (SLC10A2). J Clin Invest 1997; 99:1880–7.

86. Bile acids, diarrhea and Se-HCAT. Lancet 1991;338:1563–4.

87. Hall EJ. Lessons we have learned from our children: cancer risks from diagnostic radiology. Pediatr Radiol 2002;32:700–6.

88. Smith MJ, Cherian P, Raju GS, et al. Bile acid malabsorption in persistent diarrhoea. J R Coll Physicians Lond 2000;34: 448–51.

89. Casson DH, Wood IS, Dawson PA, Shirazi-Beechy SP. Absence of the bile-acid transporter in the apical membrane of ileal enterocytes as a cause of intractable diarrhea of infancy. Presented at ESPGHAN 2002; 2002 June 5–8; Taormina, Italy.

90. Piepz A, Hahn K, Roca I, et al. A radiopharmaceutical schedule for imaging in paediatrics. Paediatric Task Group European Association of Nuclear Medicine. Eur J Nucl Med 1990;17: 127–9.

CHAPTER 75

1. Fluid and Dietary Therapy of Diarrhea

Dilip Mahalanabis, MBBS, FRCP

John D. Snyder, MD

Because diarrheal diseases have long been a major cause of morbidity and mortality,[1] the development of oral rehydration therapy (ORT) solutions has been hailed as one of the most important medical advances of the twentieth century.[2] This therapy is a rare but important example of the reverse transfer of technology from developing countries to developed countries. The initial trials of ORT were carried out primarily in less developed populations, where its effectiveness was established in children and adults with acute diarrhea from many etiologies.[3–6] The impact of ORT was established early in its development when it was used with dramatic effect during a cholera epidemic in West Bengal refugee camps in 1971.[7] ORT has been estimated to save about 1 million lives each year in the developing world.[8]

Although many of the basic science studies that provided the foundation of ORT were carried out in industrialized countries, these countries were slow to use ORT despite its successful use in the developing world.[9,10] The low rate of use of ORT occurred despite the endorsement of organizations including the American Academy of Pediatrics (AAP), the US Centers for Disease Control and Prevention (CDC), and the European Society for Pediatrics, Gastroenterology, Hepatology, and Nutrition.[11–13]

Optimal oral therapy has continued to evolve and now includes appropriate feeding during and after diarrhea in addition to the use of fluid and electrolyte solutions.[1,8] The emphasis on early feeding has helped to address the problem of malnutrition, which is often a major accompanying problem of diarrheal illness in developing countries.

This chapter discusses the continuing evolution of oral therapy, with special emphasis on dietary management of diarrhea. The principles of care established in developing countries now provide the basis for treatment in all parts of the world.

PHYSIOLOGIC BASIS OF ORAL THERAPY

To understand the concepts involved in effective oral therapy, it is helpful to review the physiology of intestinal fluid

movement. Each day, about 9 L of fluid are processed by the adult intestine.[8,10] These fluids dilute food and are essential to the digestive process.

Reabsorption of that large volume of fluid occurs through the villous cells of the small intestine and the epithelial cells of the colon. The main driving force for water absorption is the osmotic response to the absorption of electrolytes and solutes, especially sodium and glucose. The bulk of sodium and water absorption from the small intestine results from coupled transport, in which the absorption of sodium molecules is linked to glucose or other small organic molecules such as amino acids, short-chain polypeptides, bile acids, or water-soluble vitamins by a variety of sodium-solute cotransporters expressed in the enterocyte apical membrane.[8] Sodium uptake in the small intestine can also occur passively down a concentration gradient created by active pumping of the ion out of the enterocyte by several ion-coupled mechanisms, facilitated by sodium/potassium-exchanging adenosine triphosphatase.[14] In addition to coupled transport, sodium transport occurs by solvent drag through the paracellular pathway.[14,15]

Diarrhea results when these secretion or reabsorption mechanisms are disrupted, causing dehydration by depletion of intravascular fluid and electrolytes. Diarrhea-causing organisms can increase the chloride-secreting activity of the crypt cells (toxigenic), can disrupt the absorption of sodium by villous cells (invasion or adherence), or can affect both mechanisms (see Chapter 2, "Microbial Interactions with Gut Epithelium"). Coupled transport of sodium and glucose or other organic solutes is not affected in toxigenic diarrhea and is at least partially competent in other types of diarrhea, such as that caused by *Rotavirus*.[8] The key physiologic foundation for successful ORT is a functioning sodium-glucose transporter.[2]

In 1964, Phillips was the first to show that glucose-linked sodium absorption is retained during severe diarrhea owing to cholera.[3] The initial success of ORT for adult cholera patients was soon tested under controlled conditions in the treatment of children with cholera, *Rotavirus*, enterotoxigenic *Escherichia coli*, and other etiologic agents.[6,16–18] ORT emerged as a powerful therapeutic tool to correct dehydration resulting from acute diarrhea in all but the most severe cases and in all ages, irrespective of etiologic agents.[1,8] In severe cases, such as *Rotavirus* enteritis in infants, insufficient glucose-sodium absorptive capacity may be present to support ORT, perhaps because the infection involves all or most of the small intestine.

In addition to sodium and glucose, ORT also contains potassium, chloride, bicarbonate or citrate, and water (Table 75.1-1). Clinical balance studies have provided guidelines for the optimal concentration of the five components of ORT solutions and resulted in the formulation recommended by the World Health Organization/United Nations International Children's Emergency Fund (WHO/UNICEF) for over 30 years (see Table 75.1-1).[8] Maximal cotransport occurs when the molar ratio of glucose to sodium approaches 1.[8,10] Potassium is required because diarrheal dehydration can cause substantial loss of the ion, especially in infants and small children.[10] Chloride losses also occur during diarrhea, and the ion is required to balance the positive sodium and potassium ions. Varying degrees of base-deficit acidosis occur in diarrheal dehydration, and base replacement can speed the therapeutic response.[10] These other ions follow passively the coupled transport of sodium and glucose.

In North America, several commercial sugar-electrolyte solutions similar to the WHO/UNICEF formulation are widely available (see Table 75.1-1). They differ primarily in having slightly higher glucose and lower sodium concentrations than the WHO/UNICEF solution and are supplied in the more costly reconstituted form. In controlled trials in the United States, sugar-electrolyte solutions with sodium concentrations of 45 to 75 μmol/L have proven to be effective in the treatment of well-nourished children with mild to severe dehydration.[18–21] However, such solutions with sodium concentrations < 75 μmol/L are not suitable for use in adults and older children with cholera and similar secretory diarrheas.[10,11]

CONTINUING EVOLUTION OF ORAL THERAPY FOR DIARRHEA

Since 1971, WHO has recommended a single formulation of oral rehydration salts (ORS) to treat dehydration from diarrhea of any cause, including cholera, in all age groups.[1,8]

Although ORS has been immensely successful,[1,8] it has not been used as widely as anticipated, primarily because it has no effect on shortening the duration or volume of diarrhea[9]; in fact, stool volume may increase on ORS. To help address this important limitation, a variety of strategies have been tried to add antidiarrheal properties to oral therapy.

POLYMERS AND ADDED SOLUTES

Efforts to replace glucose with more effective cotransport molecules have included trials of amino acids, including glycine, glycyl-glycine, alanine, and glutamine.[22] These solutions have performed no better than ORS, especially in noncholera diarrhea, and have some important limitations, including the limited availability and high cost of amino acids and peptides, the development of metabolic abnormalities, and instability during storage.[22] The use of glucose polymers, including maltodextrins, permits the inclusion of additional cotransport molecules without incurring an osmotic penalty.[23] However, the reduced-osmolarity maltodextrin solutions resulted in no appreciable improvement over ORS.[22]

CEREAL-BASED ORAL THERAPY

A more effective approach to improving absorption of solutes and water proved to be the use of cereal-based solutions that use the complex carbohydrates and simple proteins of cereals as cotransport molecules.[23] Many of the studies of cereal-based therapy have used cooked rice and salts added in concentrations identical to the standard ORS.[24–26] Other cereals that have been used effectively include wheat, corn, sorghum, and millet.[26,27] A meta-analysis of randomized clinical trials of cereal-based ORT, especially rice-based ORT, has demonstrated that this form of ORT is superior to glucose ORT in adults and children with cholera and other high-purging diarrheas.[28] These solutions produced a mean reduction in stool output in the first 24 hours of therapy of ~ 30 to 40%. For children with acute noncholera diarrhea, the reduction in stool output was ~ 18%.[28] Despite these impressive results, cereal-based ORT has not been widely used, probably for a combination of reasons. One important constraint relates to the ease of preparation. Most studies of cereal-based ORT used cooked cereals, which require time and fuel to prepare, making these solutions less attractive than the easy-to-prepare packets of ORS. However, commercially prepackaged cereal-based ORT

TABLE 75.1-1   COMPOSITION OF GLUCOSE ELECTROLYTE SOLUTIONS

SOLUTION	CONCENTRATION (mmol/L)				
	CHO	NA	K	BASE	OSMOLALITY
KaoLectolyte (Pharmacia/Pfizer, New York, NY, USA)	112	48	28	20	240
Pediatric Electrolyte (PharmaScience, Montreal, QC, Canada)	140	45	20	30	250
Pedialyte (Ross, Columbus, OH, USA)	140	45	20	30	250
Infalyte (Mead Johnson Evansville, ID, USA)	70	50	25	30	200
Rehydralyte (Ross Columbus, OH, USA)	140	75	20	30	301
Cera-lyte (Cera Products, Jessup, MD, USA)	80	70	20	30	235
Reduced osmolar ORS (WHO/UNICEF)	75	75	20	30	245
Previously recommended WHO/UNICEF ORS	111	90	20	30	310

CHO = carbohydrate; ORS = oral rehydration solution.

solutions that dissolve easily in water are now available (see Table 75.1-1). Perhaps more importantly, the use of these solutions was affected by the nearly simultaneous introduction of early appropriate feeding along with ORS. The interest in feeding as an integral part of oral therapy arose from the same potential advantages of enhanced solute uptake from easily digested foods that stimulated the development of cereal-based ORT and is discussed below.

HYPO-OSMOLAR SOLUTIONS

The renewed interest in oral hypo-osmolar solutions for the treatment of diarrhea stems from perfusion studies that demonstrate a significant inverse correlation between ORT osmolality and water absorption in animals and humans.[29] Recent studies in children have demonstrated that hypo-osmolar ORT formulations can result in lower stool output (~ 20%), less vomiting (~ 30%), and less need for intravenous therapy for failures of ORT (~ 33%) compared with standard ORS.[30–34] A meta-analysis of 15 randomized controlled studies has helped to confirm the superiority of the reduced-osmolarity ORS over the standard WHO/UNICEF ORS.[35] However, concern exists for the development of hyponatremia when the reduced-osmolarity ORS is used in patients with high purging rates such as those caused by cholera because of the reduced sodium concentration. In the clinical trials, asymptomatic hyponatremia was reported in some patients, and WHO/UNICEF recommends that careful monitoring of electrolytes be done for patients with high purging rates who receive the new reduced-osmolarity solution.[36] Because of less need for intravenous therapy, decreased vomiting, and lower stool output, WHO/UNICEF now recommends the use of the reduced-osmolarity solution (see Table 75.1-1) as the single ORS for use in persons with diarrhea.[36]

EARLY APPROPRIATE FEEDING

Theoretical Considerations. The inclusion of early appropriate feeding along with ORT required the overturning of the common practice, used in many countries and cultures, of withholding feedings during diarrhea.[37] The rationale for withholding food during diarrhea was based primarily on the concern for malabsorption, which can occur because of an altered intestinal mucosa, decreased brush border enzymes, and a more rapid intestinal transit time.[38] The theoretical risk of increased macromolecular uptake across the damaged mucosa leading to intestinal allergy has been postulated but has never been shown to be of practical importance in diarrhea.[39] In contrast, the several important potential benefits of early feeding became a strong stimulus to study its safety and efficacy. These benefits include the chance to provide nutritional therapy to malnourished patients with diarrhea, especially in developing countries.[37,38] In addition, nutrient uptake plays an important role in intestinal repair.[40]

Nutrient Absorption during Diarrhea. Although some element of malabsorption is often associated with diarrhea, it is rarely complete, and substantial amounts of nutrients can be absorbed.[37,38,41,42] This is especially true for the digestion and absorption of complex carbohydrates in staple foods because the luminal concentrations of amylases and pancreatic enzymes appear to be largely unaffected during diarrhea.[37,38] Balance studies of nutrient absorption of staple foods have demonstrated that as much as 90% of complex carbohydrates, 70% of protein, and 60% of fat can be absorbed during acute diarrheal episodes.[41–43] Factors that influence the success of feeding include the age of the child, the etiology of the diarrhea, the severity of the stooling, and the composition of the diet.

Impact of Feeding on Diarrhea. Feeding is usually well tolerated in acute infectious diarrhea and can have a direct beneficial effect on diarrhea when combined with ORT.[38] Controlled clinical trials have shown that appropriate early feeding combined with ORT can reduce stool output[44–49] and the duration of diarrhea[46,48–53] compared with ORT or intravenous therapy alone.

Effective Feeding Regimens. Cereal-based staple-food diets have been among the most effective diets studied, but if cereals or legumes provide the sole source of protein, an amino acid profile deficient in essential amino acids is likely to result.[54] Also, a greater proportion of protein may be required in cereal- or legume-based diets because of their digestibility.[54] A solution to this problem is to include milk, a more complete protein source, along with cereals to improve the amino acid profile and digestibility. Ideally, milk can provide these essential amino acids, but because brush border lactase levels are often reduced during diarrhea, milk has often been avoided or diluted because of concerns about possible lactose intolerance.[37] The amount of lactose that can be tolerated by children with diarrhea is still a subject of controversy, but several principles have become clear.[54] Breastfed infants, who receive a higher concentration of lactose than children receiving cow's milk or cow's milk formula, can be fed safely through diarrhea.[37,38] Full-strength animal milk or animal milk formula is usually well tolerated by children who have mild, self-limited diarrhea, which is very common in the United States.[50] A meta-analysis on the use of lactose in children with acute diarrhea found that most children can safely tolerate full-strength animal milk, especially when combined with staple foods.[55] These mixed diets are better tolerated than milk alone[43] and are thought to be successful in part because of the smaller total lactose load and because solid foods help delay gastric emptying and thus slow transit time.[56]

Banana, Rice, Applesauce, and Toast Diet. This diet, commonly referred to as the BRAT diet, has long been used in North America to begin refeeding children who have had diarrhea. However, this diet is no longer recommended because it is low in energy density, protein, and fat and because the banana and applesauce may add an excessive load of sugars to the gut.[11] In addition, diets high in simple sugars (including sweet tea, juices, and soft drinks) (Table 75.1-2)[57] or fats should be avoided.[12] Optimal diets should provide a nutritionally acceptable balance of carbohydrate, protein, and fat.

TABLE 75.1-2   COMPOSITION OF REPRESENTATIVE CLEAR LIQUIDS NOT APPROPRIATE FOR ORAL REHYDRATION THERAPY*

LIQUID	CHO, mmol/L	Na, mmol/L	K, mol/L	BASE, mmol/L	OSMOLALITY, mmol/L
Cola	700 (F, G)	2	0	13	750
Apple juice	690 (F, G, S)	3	32	0	730
Chicken broth	0	250	8	0	500
Sports beverage	255 (S, G)	20	3	3	330

*Adapted from Snyder JD.[69]
CHO = carbohydrate; F = fructose; G = glucose; K = potassium; Na = sodium; S = sucrose.

Soy Formulas. Many practitioners in North America have switched their pediatric patients with diarrhea to soy formulas because of concerns for malabsorption of lactose in cow's milk and cow's milk formulas. However, data from controlled clinical trials demonstrate no benefit in soy formulas compared with cow's milk, especially when used with staple-food diets.[55] In addition, recent studies show that soy formulas were not as well tolerated in children with acute diarrhea as mixed staple-food diets[47] or soy formula with fiber.[58]

MANAGEMENT GUIDELINES

ORT can be administered to infants with a cup and spoon, a cup alone, or a feeding bottle. For weak small babies, a dropper or a syringe can be used to put small volumes of solution into the mouth. A nasogastric tube can be used to administer the ORT in babies or children who cannot drink because of fatigue or drowsiness but who are not in shock. In the vomiting child, small volumes, often 5 mL at a time, can be given frequently, as often as every few minutes (see below).

Early appropriate feeding, which has become an integral component of oral therapy, is the component that has the potential for the greatest impact on stool volume and duration.[11] Successful feeding trials have been carried out using breast milk, dilute or full-strength animal milk or animal milk formulas, dilute and full-strength lactose-free formulas, and mixed diets of staple foods with milk.[44–56] Recent studies indicate that diets of naturally occurring, culturally acceptable, inexpensive foods can be effective in diarrhea.[54] The implications of these findings are enormous from a health policy standpoint because they provide hope that the important ingredients of successful feeding therapy are already present, even in developing countries.

The specific recommendations for treatment depend on the severity of the diarrhea (Table 75.1-3).

NO DEHYDRATION
Intake of ORT is often low, in part because of the potentially salty taste of ORT.[9,11] Fortunately, if the stool output remains modest, ORT may not be required. If no dehydration develops, which is the case for the great majority of diarrhea patients in the United States, continued age-appropriate feeding is the only therapy required. Controlled clinical trials have demonstrated a number of foods that can be used safely and effectively in most children with diarrhea (Table 75.1-4). Unweaned infants should receive breast milk or continue to receive the regular formula. The formula does not require dilution if the diarrhea remains mild. If a diluted formula is used, the concentration should be increased rapidly if the diarrhea does not worsen. Weaned infants and children should have their regular nutritionally balanced diet continued, emphasizing complex carbohydrates (such as rice, wheat, and potatoes), meats (especially chicken), and the child's regular milk or formula. Diets high in simple sugars and fats should be avoided.[11,12]

MILD, MODERATE, OR SEVERE DEHYDRATION
After dehydration is corrected, appropriate feeding is begun, using the guidelines above (see Table 75.1-3). Children with severe dehydration, which is a shock or a shock-like condition,[11,12] should be treated as an emergency. A large-bore catheter should be used for the infusion of Ringer lactate, normal saline, or similar solution, and boluses of 20 to 40 mL/kg should be administered until signs of shock resolve. Fluid and electrolyte resuscitation may require more than one intravenous site, and alternate access sites (including venous cutdown, femoral vein, or interosseous locations) may be needed.[11,12] As the patient's level of consciousness improves, ORT can be instituted. The hydration status must be frequently reassessed to monitor the effectiveness of the therapy. When rehydration is complete, feeding is continued as directed above.

TABLE 75.1-3   EFFECTIVE FOODS FOR USE DURING DIARRHEA

FOOD	OUTCOME
Breast milk[44] + ORT	↓ Stool volume compared with ORT alone
Cow's milk + staples[43] + ORT	No difference compared with ORT alone
Rice-based diet[26,28,42] + ORT	↓ Stool volume and duration compared with ORT alone
Wheat-based diet[27] + ORT	↓ Stool volume and duration compared with ORT alone
Wheat-pea diet[45] + ORT	↓ Stool volume and duration compared with ORT alone
Potato diet[43] + ORT	↓ Stool volume and duration compared with ORT alone
Chicken[51] + ORT	↓ Stool volume and duration compared with ORT alone
Egg[53] + ORT	↓ Stool volume and duration compared with ORT alone

ORT = oral rehydration therapy.

TABLE 75.1-4   MANAGEMENT OF ACUTE DIARRHEA

TREATMENT	MILD DIARRHEA, NO DEHYDRATION	MILD DEHYDRATION (< 5%)	MODERATE DEHYDRATION (5–9%)	SEVERE DEHYDRATION (> 10%)
ORT	Rehydration: may not be required	Rehydration: 50 mL/kg over 4 h	Rehydration: 100 mL/kg over 4 h	Rehydration: IV therapy with solution like normal saline or Ringer lactate, 20–40 mL/kg/h until rehydrated; then may begin ORT
	Continuing losses: if required: 10 mL/kg/ each stool	Continuing losses: 10 mL/kg for each stool and estimated emesis volume	Continuing losses: same as for mild dehydration	
Early appropriate feeding	Continue age-appropriate diet (see Table 75.1-3)	Begin age-appropriate diet when dehydration corrected	Begin age-appropriate diet when dehydration corrected	Begin age-appropriate diet when dehydration corrected and patient stabilized

Adapted from American Academy of Pediatrics, Subcommittee on Acute Gastroenteritis.[11]
ORT = oral rehydration therapy.

SPECIAL CONSIDERATIONS

Vomiting. Vomiting, commonly associated with acute diarrhea, can make ORT more challenging, but almost all children with vomiting can be treated successfully with ORT.[11,12] When small volumes (eg, 5 mL) are given frequently (eg, every 1 to 2 minutes), an effective volume of ORT can be administered to a vomiting child.[11,12] Although this technique is labor intensive, as much as 150 to 300 mL/h of fluid can be administered.

Correction of fluid and electrolyte deficits by balanced-electrolyte ORT can help speed recovery from vomiting.[11,12] As vomiting decreases, ORT can be given in larger volumes, and when rehydration is complete, feeding can begin.

Nasogastric tubes can sometimes be of benefit in administering ORT to vomiting children. Continuous infusion of ORT can result in improved absorption of fluid and electrolytes and may permit more aggressive therapy in a child with poor intravenous access. Nasogastric infusion cannot be considered in children who are comatose or who have ileus or evidence of intestinal obstruction.

Zinc Supplementation. Several recent studies have identified zinc supplementation to have a significant impact on the duration and severity of acute and persistent diarrhea in children in nonindustrialized countries.[59–61] The mechanisms for this effect are not yet known but may include the effect of zinc on the absorption of water and electrolytes, improvement of intestinal function and enzyme activities, or enhanced immunocompetence.[62]

Hypernatremia. A long-standing concern, especially in developed countries, is the perceived risk of hypernatremia from ORT, especially with a relatively high sodium concentration in rehydration solutions.[8,10,11] However, a large body of data has clearly shown that oral rehydration solutions are an effective treatment for hypernatremia, given normal renal function.[63,64] These studies demonstrate that ORT can result in better outcomes than the best results reported with intravenous therapy.

Refusal to Take ORT. Refusal of pediatric patients to take ORT is a common complaint of practitioners in North America,[11] but children who are dehydrated rarely refuse ORT because they usually crave salt and water. The problem is usually found in children who have little or no dehydration. Most children do not require ORT if their diarrhea is mild, if they remain stable, and if they show no evidence of dehydration.[11]

Methods for increasing ORT intake include the use of flavored ORT, which does not alter the composition of fluid and electrolytes but which improves taste.[11] These flavored solutions are now the most popular forms of ORT sold in North America. Another effective way to increase intake is to freeze the ORT solution in an ice-pop form.

Management at Home. The principles for the effective household treatment of diarrhea, which have been developed primarily from extensive experience in developing countries, are the same for all settings.[9,11,12] As mentioned above, the most essential principles are the use of ORT to replace fluid and electrolyte losses and the continuation of appropriate feeding as soon as dehydration has been corrected. This is true both for developing and developed countries, but greater educational efforts are needed in all settings to help parents and caretakers provide effective therapy and to recognize the development of serious conditions.[65] The need for better education is underscored by the fact that approximately 10% of preventable infant deaths in the United States are caused by improper recognition and inappropriate treatment of acute diarrhea.[66]

Severe Malnutrition and ORT. Diarrhea is a serious and often fatal event in children with severe malnutrition. Although treatment and prevention of dehydration are essential, care must also focus on careful management of malnutrition and on treatment of other infections. Dehydration owing to acute diarrhea in children with severe protein-energy malnutrition (eg, marasmus, kwashiorkor) can be managed with ORT as described above.[1,12] In children with kwashiorkor, ORT must be closely supervised because of the increased risk of edema and congestive heart failure, especially with intravenous therapy.

Use of Antibiotics or Nonspecific Antidiarrheal Agents. The message that neither antibiotics nor nonspecific antidiarrheal agents are indicated for most diarrheal episodes also requires emphasis.[11,12,67] However, antibiotics are indicated for a few specific infections, including cholera *Shigella* with systemic spread, *Clostridium difficile*, *Salmonella* in children < 3 months old, *Giardia*, and *Entamoeba histolytica*.[68]

Drugs that alter intestinal motility, secretion, adsorption of fluid and toxins, or intestinal microflora have little or no data to support their use in children.[11,12,68] The AAP, CDC, and WHO all recommend that such drugs not be used to treat acute diarrhea.[11,12,68]

Low Use Rates for ORT. Low use rates continue to be an important problem in both the developing and the developed world. Despite its unquestioned success in saving lives, only about 40% of diarrheal episodes are treated with ORT in the developing world,[67] and the estimates for use in North America are far lower.[9,65,69] The efforts to improve the antidiarrheal properties of ORT may have an important impact on use. In the United States, the cost of ORT is often 20 to 50 times higher than the $0.10 to $0.15 per-packet cost for ORS in the developing world, limiting its use in the most disadvantaged portions of the population, who are at the greatest risk for morbidity and mortality from diarrhea.[66] In countries without state-sponsored health care, many third-party payers do not reimburse clinicians and hospitals for oral fluid therapy despite its proven ability to reduce unnecessary medical visits and hospitalization.[65]

Persistent Diarrhea. Persistent diarrhea, defined operationally as episodes that continue for 14 days or longer, is responsible for a large proportion of deaths in young children with diarrhea.[70–73] General treatment guidelines include the use of appropriate fluids to prevent or treat dehydration, a nutritionally effective diet that does not worsen the diarrhea, and supplementary vitamins, minerals, and antimicrobial agents to treat concurrent infections such as pneumonia, sepsis, and urinary tract infections.

A spectrum of illness exists for persistent diarrhea, but a common pattern is for affected children to pass several liquid stools in a day, without much dehydration. Growth failure and adverse nutritional consequences may result. In other cases, children may have severe and persistent watery diarrhea with dehydration. When more severe diarrhea is present, the principles of ORT are the same as for acute diarrhea except for the few children who will exhibit evidence of temporary glucose malabsorption. These children may require intravenous fluids until their glucose malabsorption resolves.

The feeding principles described earlier also apply to children with persistent diarrhea. A multicenter study that evaluated a diet algorithm for the treatment of persistent diarrhea in young children in developing countries provided several practical guidelines.[73] In this study, the initial diet used locally available staple foods (rice or corn), milk or yogurt (< 4 g lactose/150 kcal), vegetable oil, and sugar. The children who did not improve were given a lactose- and sucrose-free cereal-based diet. Most of the children had resolution of or improvement in their diarrhea while on these nutritional therapies even though this was a population of very compromised children, including many who had extraintestinal infections. Influenced by this study, the current guidelines on nutritional therapy for persistent diarrhea include (1) breastfeeding whenever possible, (2) animal milk (limited to 50 mL/kg/d) mixed with cereal for non-breastfed children, (3) a daily intake of at least 110 calories/kg, and (4) supplemental vitamins and minerals.[73]

REFERENCES

1. Cleason M, Merson MH. Global progress in the control of diarrheal diseases. Pediatr Infect Dis J 1990;9:345–55.
2. Oral glucose/electrolyte losses in cholera [editorial]. Lancet 1975;i:75.
3. Phillips RA. Water and electrolyte losses in cholera. Fed Proc 1964;23:705–12.
4. Hirschhorn NB, Kinzie JL, Sachar DB, et al. Decrease in net stool output in cholera during intestinal perfusion with glucose-containing solutions. N Engl J Med 1968;279:174–81.
5. Pierce NF, Sack RB, Mitra RC, et al. Replacement of water and electrolyte losses in cholera by an oral glucose-electrolyte solution. Ann Intern Med 1969;70:1173.
6. Hirschhorn NB, Cash RA, Woodward WE, et al. Oral fluid therapy of Apache children with infectious diarrhea. Lancet 1971;ii:15.
7. Mahalanalis D, Choudri AB, Bagchi NG, et al. Oral fluid therapy of cholera among Bangladesh refugees. Johns Hopkins Med J 1973;132:197–205.
8. Hirschhorn N, Greenough WB III. Progress in oral rehydration therapy. Sci Am 1991;264:50–6.
9. Avery ME, Snyder JD. Oral therapy for acute diarrhea: the underused simple solution. N Engl J Med 1990;323:891–4.
10. Hirschhorn N. The treatment of acute diarrhea in children: an historical and physiological perspective. Am J Clin Nutr 1980;33:637–63.
11. American Academy of Pediatrics, Subcommittee on Acute Gastroenteritis. Practice parameter: the management of acute gastroenteritis in young children. Pediatrics 1996;97:424–35.
12. Duggan C, Santosham M, Glass R. The management of acute diarrhea in children: oral rehydration, maintenance and nutritional therapy. MMWR Morb Mortal Wkly Rep 1992;41:1–20.
13. European Society of Pediatric Gastroenterology and Nutrition Working Group. Recommendations for composition of oral rehydration solutions for the children of Europe. J Pediatr Gastroenterol Nutr 1992;14:113.
14. Fordtran JS. Stimulation of active and passive sodium absorption by sugars in the human jejunum. J Clin Invest 1975;55:728–37.
15. Pappenheimer JR, Reiss KZ. Contribution of solvent drag through intercellular junctions to absorption of nutrients by the small intestine of the rat. J Membr Biol 1987;100:123–36.
16. Chatterjee A, Mahalanabis D, Jalan KN, et al. Evaluation of a sucrose/electrolyte solution for oral rehydration in acute infantile diarrhoea. Lancet 1979;i:133.

17. Pizarro D. Oral rehydration of neonates with dehydrating diarrheas. Lancet 1979;12:1209–10.

18. Santosham M, Daum RS, Dillman L, et al. Oral rehydration therapy of infantile diarrhea: a controlled study of well-nourished children hospitalized in the United States and Panama. N Engl J Med 1982;306:1070–6.

19. Tamer AM, Friedman LB, Maxwell SRW, et al. Oral rehydration of infants in a large urban U.S. medical center. J Pediatr 1986;107:14–9.

20. Santosham M, Burns B, Nadkarni V, et al. Oral rehydration therapy for acute diarrhea in ambulatory children in the United States: a double-blind comparison of four different solutions. Pediatrics 1985;76:159–66.

21. Listernick R, Zieseri E, Davis AT. Outpatient oral rehydration in the United States. Am J Dis Child 1986;140:211–5.

22. Bhan MK, Mahalanabis D, Fontaine O, Pierce NF. Clinical trials of improved oral rehydration salt formulations: a review. Bull World Health Organ 1994;72:945–55.

23. Carpenter CCJ, Greenough WB, Pierce NF. Oral rehydration therapy—the role of polymeric substrates. N Engl J Med 1988;319:1346–8.

24. Molla AM, Sarker SA, Hossain M, et al. Rice-powder electrolyte solution oral therapy in diarrhoea due to Vibrio cholerae and Escherichia coli. Lancet 1982;i:1317–9.

25. Patra FC, Mahalanabis D, Jalan KN, et al. Is oral rice electrolyte solution superior to glucose electrolyte solution in infantile diarrhoea? Arch Dis Child 1982;57:910–2.

26. Molla AM, Molla A, Nath SK, et al. Food-based oral rehydration salt solution for acute childhood diarrhea. Lancet 1989;ii:429–31.

27. Alam AN, Sarker SA, Molla AM, et al. Hydrolyzed wheat based oral rehydration solution for acute diarrhea. Arch Dis Child 1987;62:440–2.

28. Gore SM, Fontaine O, Pierce NF. Impact of rice based oral rehydration solution on stool output and duration of diarrhoea: meta-analysis of 13 clinical trials. BMJ 1992;304:287–91.

29. Thillainayagam AV, Hunt JB, Farthing MJG. Enhancing clinical efficacy of oral rehydration therapy: is low osmolality the key? Gastroenterology 1998;114:197–210.

30. Rautanen T, El-Radhi S, Vesikari T. Clinical experience with hypotonic oral rehydration solution in acute diarrhoea. Acta Paediatr 1993;82:52–4.

31. El-Mougi M, El Akkad N, Hendawi A, et al. Is a low-osmolarity ORS solution more efficacious than standard WHO ORS solution? J Paediatr Gastroentrol Nutr 1994;19:83–6

32. International Study Group on Reduced Osmolarity ORS Solution. Multicentre evaluation of reduced-osmolarity oral rehydration salts solution. Lancet 1995;345:282–5.

33. Mahalanabis D, Faruque ASG, Haque SS, Faruque SM. Hypotonic oral rehydration solution in acute diarrhoea: a controlled clinical trial. Acta Paediatr 1995;84:289–93.

34. Faruque ASG, Mahalanabis D. Reduced osmolarity oral rehydration salt in cholera. Scand J Infect Dis 1996;28:87–90.

35. Hahn S, Kim YJ, Garner P. Reduced osmolarity oral rehydration solution for treating dehydration due to diarrhoea in children: systematic review. BMJ 2002;323:81–5.

36. Reduced osmolarity oral rehydration salts (ORS) formulation. Report from a meeting of experts jointly organised by UNICEF and WHO. WHO/CAH/01.22 2002. Available at: http: // www.who.int/child-adolescenthealth/NewPublications/ChildHealth/Expert consulation.htm (accessed May 2002).

37. Brown KH, MacLean WL Jr. Nutritional management of acute diarrhea; an appraisal of the alternatives. Pediatrics 1984;73:119–28.

38. Duggan C, Nurko S. "Feeding the gut": the scientific basis for continued enteral nutriton during acute diarrhea. J Pediatr 1997;131:801–8.

39. Snyder JD. Dietary protein sensitivity: is it an important risk factor for persistent diarrhea? Acta Paediatr 1992;81 Suppl 381:78–81.

40. Vanderhoof JA. Short bowel syndrome. In: Lebenthal E, editor. Textbook of gastroenterology and nutrition in infancy. 2nd ed. New York: Raven Press; 1989. p. 794.

41. Chung AW. The effect of oral feeding at different levels on the absorption of foodstuffs in infantile diarrhea. J Pediatr 1948;33:14–22.

42. Molla A, Molla AM, Sarker S, et al. Absorption of nutrients during diarrhea due to V. cholerae, E. coli, Rotavirus and Shigella. In: Chen LC, Scrimshaw HA, editors. Diarrhea and malnutrition: interactions, mechanisms and interventions. New York: Plenum Publishing; 1981. p. 114–23.

43. Brown KH, Perez R, Gastanaduy AS. Clinical trial of modified whole milk, lactose-hydrolyzed whole milk, or cereal-milk mixtures for the dietary management of acute childhood diarrhea. J Pediatr Gastroenterol Nutr 1991;12:224–32.

44. Khin MU, Hyunt-Nyunt-Wai, Myo-Khin, et al. Effect of clinical outcome of breast feeding during acute diarrhoea. BMJ 1985;290:587–9.

45. Brown KH, Gastanaduay AS, Saaverdrea JM, et al. Effect of continued oral feeding on clinical and nutritional outcomes of acute diarrhea in children. J Pediatr 1988;112:191–200.

46. Hjelt K, Paerrgard A, Petersen W, et al. Rapid versus gradual refeeding in acute gastroenteritis in childhood: energy intake and weight gain. J Pediatr Gastroenterol Nutr 1989;8:75–80.

47. Alarcon P, Montoya R, Perez F, et al. Clinical trial of home available, mixed diets versus a lactose-free, soy-protein formula for the dietary management of acute childhood diarrhea. J Pediatr Gastroenterol Nutr 1991;12:224–32.

48. Santosham M, Fayad IM, Hashem M, et al. A comparison of rice-based oral rehydration solution and "early feeding" for the treatment of acute diarrhea in infants. J Pediatr 1990;116:868–75.

49. Fayad IM, Hashaem M, Duggan C, et al. Comparative efficacy of rice-based and glucose-based oral rehydration salts plus early reintroduction of food. Lancet 1993;342:772–5.

50. Margolis PA, Litteer T. Effects of unrestricted diet on mild infantile diarrhea. Am J Dis Child 1990;144:162–4.

51. Maulen-Radovan I, Brown KH, Acosta MA, Fernandez-Varela H. Comparison of a rice-based mixed diet versus a lactose-free, soy-protein isolate formula for young children with acute diarrhea. J Pediatr 1994;125:699–706.

52. Santosham M, Fister S, Reid R, et al. Role of soy-based, lactose-free formula during treatment of acute diarrhea. Pediatrics 1985;76:292–8.

53. Torun B, Chew F. Recent developments in the nutritional management of diarrhoea. Practical approaches towards dietary management of acute diarrhoea in developing communities. Trans R Soc Trop Med Hyg 1991;85:12–7.

54. Brown KH. Appropriate diets for the rehabilitation of malnourished children in the community setting. Acta Paediatr Scand 1991;374 Suppl:151–9.

55. Brown KH, Peerson JM, Fontaine O. Use of non-human milks in the dietary management of young children with acute diarrhea: a meta-analysis of clinical trials. Pediatrics 1994;93:17–27.

56. Martini MC, Savaiano DA. Reduced intolerance symptoms from lactose consumed during a meal. Am J Clin Nutr 1988;47:57–60.

57. Snyder J. The continuing evolution of oral therapy for diarrhea. Semin Pediatr Infect Dis 1994;5:231–5.

58. Brown KH, Perez F, Peerson J, et al. Effect of dietary fiber (soy polysaccharide) on the severity, duration, and nutritional outcome of acute, watery diarrhea in children. Pediatrics 1993;92:241–7.

59. Zinc Investigators' Collaborative Group. Therapeutic effects of oral zinc in acute and persistent diarrhoea in children in developing countries: pooled analysis of randomized controlled trials. Am J Clin Nutr 2000;72:1516–22.

60. Sazawal S, Black R, Bhan M, et al. Zinc supplementation in young children with acute diarrhea in India. N Engl J Med 1995;333:839–44.

61. Rahaman MM, Vermund SH, Wahed MA, et al. Simultaneous zinc and vitamin A supplementation in Bangladeshi children: randomized double blind controlled trial. BMJ 2001;323:314–8.

62. Hambidge MK. Zinc deficiency in young children. Am J Clin Nutr 1997;65:160–1.

63. Pizarro D, Posada G, Levine MM, et al. Hypernatremic diarrheal dehydration treated with "slow" (12 hour) oral rehydration therapy: a preliminary report. J Pediatr 1984;104:316–9.

64. Pizarro D, Posada G, Mata L, et al. Treatment of 242 neonates with dehydrating diarrhea with an oral glucose-electrolyte solution. J Pediatr 1983;102:153–6.

65. Santosham M, Keenan EM Tulloch J, et al. Oral rehydration therapy for diarrhea: an example of reverse transfer of technology. Pediatrics 1997;100:542–4.

66. Ho MS, Glass RI, Pinsky PF. Diarrheal deaths in American children: are they preventable? JAMA 1988;260:3281.

67. World Health Organization. The state of the world's children, 1988–1997. Geneva: WHO; 1997.

68. World Health Organization. The rational use of drugs in the management of acute diarrhoea in children. Geneva: World Health Organization; 1990.

69. Snyder JD. Use and misuse of oral therapy for diarrhea: comparison of U.S. practices with American Academy of Pediatrics recommendations. Pediatrics 1991;87:28–33.

70. Fauveau V, Henry FJ, Briend A, et al. Persistent diarrhoea as a cause of childhood mortality in rural Bangladesh. Acta Paediatr 1992;81 Suppl 381:12–4.

71. Victoria CG, Bhandari N, Sazawal S, et al. Deaths due to dysentery, acute and persistent diarrhoea among Brazilian infants. Acta Paediatr 1992;81 Suppl 381:7–11.

72. Bhan ML, Bhandari N, Sazawal S, et al. Descriptive epidemiology of persistent diarrhoea among young children in rural northern India. Bull World Health Organ 1989;67:281–8.

73. International Working Group on Persistent Diarrhoea. Evaluation of an algorithm for treatment of persistent diarrhoea: a multicentre study. Bull World Health Organization 1996;74:479–89.

2. Feeding Difficulties

Thomas M. Foy, MD

Danita I. Czyzewski, PhD

Although primary nutrient deficiencies are now rare in developed countries,[1] feeding difficulties are a continuing challenge for those who care for infants and children. It is estimated that up to 54% of infants and toddlers have problematic feeding behavior and that in 25% of children, feeding problems prompt parents to seek professional advice.[2,3] Feeding difficulties may persist and in 1 to 2% of infants will lead to retarded growth.[4–6] A survey of children with cerebral palsy found that in the first 12 months of life, 38% had problems with swallowing, 57% had problems with sucking, and more than 90% had significant oral-motor dysfunction.[7]

Disorders of the gastrointestinal tract will interfere with adequate intake of nutrients and may compromise the nutritional status of the infant at several levels. Poor intake owing to anorexia, fatigue, or dysphagia may add to the dilemma of increased losses from vomiting or malabsorption. The goals of nutritional therapy are to restore the patient to normal nutritional status, to enhance recovery from the underlying disease process, and, ultimately, to attain nutritionally adequate and developmentally appropriate feedings. This chapter examines the basis of feeding disorders in infants and children and current approaches to their evaluation and treatment.

NORMAL DEVELOPMENT AND MECHANICS

Feeding problems represent a deviation from normal feeding skill development and mechanics.[8–10] Maturation of deglutition, which begins in utero and is completed by 3 years of age, depends on integration of oral-motor, fine-motor, gross-motor, sensory, and behavioral skills. An outline of feeding development in normal infants is seen in Table 75.2-1. Whereas sucking movements can be seen at 15 to 18 weeks gestation, adequate coordination of suck, swallow, and breathing to permit significant nutrient intake is not present until 34 to 35 weeks gestation. Reflex behaviors present at term may disappear later in infancy (rooting, phasic bite) or may persist (gag, swallow).[11]

For the infant, successful feeding depends on coordination of suck, swallow, and breathing. Sucking itself has a developmental progression, with the earliest tongue movements described as "suckling" and characterized by an in-out horizonmental movement. "Sucking" appears later in infancy, indicates an up-down tongue movement with firm lip approximation, and is used in a general sense in this discussion. Swallowing, or deglutition, occurs in at least three phases, as shown in Figure 75.2-1.[11,12] The oral phase includes bolus formation of solid food or liquid by the

TABLE 75.2-1 NORMAL FEEDING DEVELOPMENT

AGE	REFLEXES	ORAL-MOTOR SKILLS	SELF-FEEDING
15–18 wk gestation		Sucking movement	
34–35 wk gestation		Adequate suck-swallow coordination	
Term	Rooting, gag, phasic bite	Jaw and tongue move up and down; air swallowing common	
3–4 mo	Phasic bite disappearing	Tongue protrudes in anticipation of feeding	Visual recognition of bottle/nipple
5–6 mo	Rooting diminishes	Munching begins, smacks lips together, strained foods begin	Puts hands on bottle, begins finger-feeding
7 mo	Mature gag		May insert spoon in mouth
9 mo		Lip closure, lateral tongue movement	
12 mo		Rotary chewing, controlled, sustained bite	Finger-feeds independently, brings spoon to mouth
18 mo		Swallows without food loss, tongue elevates intermittently or consistently	Cup drinking with two hands, spoon-feeds messily
24 months		Lips contain food/saliva within mouth, tongue transfers food one side to other side	Fills spoon with finger or spoon to mouth without inversion

Adapted from Glass RP and Wolf LS[8] and Cloud H.[9]

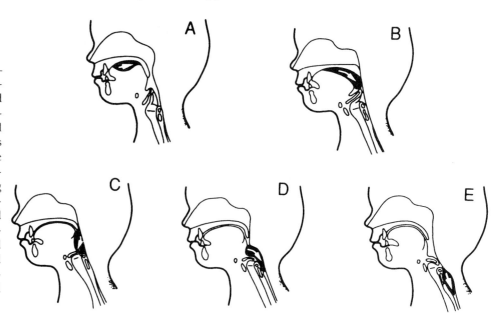

FIGURE 75.2-1 Schematic drawing to show oral, pharyngeal, and esophageal phases of normal swallow in a young child. *A*, Oral phase showing formed bolus moving posteriorly through the oral cavity. *B*, Beginning of pharyngeal phase. *C*, Bolus moving through the pharynx with adequate airway protection. *D*, End of pharyngeal phase as cricopharyngeus opens. *E*, Esophageal phase with bolus in the cervical esophagus. Reproduced with permission from Arvedson J and Brodsky L.[11]

tongue, with the soft palate lowering to prevent food from entering the pharynx and initiating a swallow. The pharyngeal phase is both voluntary and involuntary and begins as a swallow is initiated. As food enters the pharynx, the soft palate elevates to protect the nasopharynx and the larynx elevates and closes to protect the airway. The final or esophageal phase begins with relaxation of the upper esophageal sphincter (cricopharyngeus muscle) and carries the bolus to the stomach under involuntary control. The return of the upper esophageal sphincter to its tonically contracted state prevents laryngeal penetration or aspiration of esophageal contents or reflux of the bolus back into the pharynx.

ETIOLOGY

Infants with feeding problems are usually referred for evaluation when inadequate intake has led to growth faltering or eventually failure to thrive, or perhaps less frequently when a caregiver perceives significant difficulty in feeding the infant even if weight has not dropped off. The feeding problem may be the primary cause of poor growth, secondary to other disease processes, or both. Understanding which patients are at risk for feeding disorders will promote early intervention.[13]

Table 75.2-2 presents selected etiologies for feeding difficulties. Appetite will be altered if the timing or volume of feedings is inappropriate, an example being the "grazing" behavior of toddlers.[14] A common iatrogenic alteration of appetite occurs with the use of supplemental tube feedings. Although these may be necessary for adequate weight gain, they eventually interfere with normal hunger-satiety cycles. Anorexia is common in disorders of the urea cycle and organic acid metabolism, whereas a major cause of weight loss in Crohn disease is decreased intake owing to poor appetite.[15,16]

A child's diet can lead to feeding difficulties, and food allergy is one cause of vomiting or irritability associated with feeds.[17] Age-appropriate foods are essential to acquiring normal feeding behaviors.[18]

Dysphagia specifically refers to difficulty with swallowing and implies an organic basis.[19] Illingworth distinguished between anatomic, neuromuscular, and inflammatory factors for dysphagia.[20] Anatomic lesions range from the cleft lip and palate that present at birth to the more subtle anomalies such as submucous cleft palate or vascular ring. The neurologic immaturity of the premature infant results in predictable feeding concerns based on the gestational age and general medical conditions.[21] Other neuromuscular disorders may affect coordination of suck and swallow or esophageal peristalsis (pseudo-obstruction, repaired tracheoesophageal fistula).[22] Although not specifically related to difficulty in producing a swallow, as with neuromuscular and anatomic causes, the term dysphagia is also applied when the act of eating or swallowing produces pain or other discomfort. Acute inflammatory disorders are usually infectious, and chronic conditions are likely acid related (peptic esophagitis). A review of 600 infants with gastroesophageal reflux found that 4% had severe feeding resistance sufficient to warrant tube feedings, and this feeding resistance was often the initial or only symptom.[23] Dysphagia may be the first complaint in older children with gastroesophageal reflux disease (GERD).[24]

Systemic conditions, such as cardiovascular or pulmonary disease, may require extra work of breathing and stress the feeding infant. Such illnesses place greater caloric demand on the patient while also interfering with intake.[25–27]

Successful feeding results from appropriate infant responses to food and nurturing caregivers in a dynamic interaction. Not surprisingly, many infant feeding problems involve primarily nonorganic or behavioral factors.[13] These nonorganic feeding problems have been categorized or described by several authors. One categorization is tripartite: young infants (2–8 months) with an attachment disorder owing to poor parent–infant interaction, the older infant or toddler (6–36 months) with "infantile anorexia" and struggles around autonomy, and the less affected "picky eater" who is not yet malnourished.[28] Others describe early nonorganic failure to thrive as "failure to

TABLE 75.2-2   CAUSES OF FEEDING DIFFICULTIES

DECREASED APPETITE
Abnormal feeding patterns
Supplemental feedings
Metabolic disorders
Inflammatory bowel disease

DIET
Inappropriate foods
Food allergy

DYSPHAGIA
Anatomic
  Macroglossia
  Cleft lip and palate
  Submucous cleft palate
  Pierre Robin sequence
  Laryngeal cleft
  Tracheoesophageal fistula
  Vascular ring
  Foreign body
Neuromuscular
  Prematurity
  Cerebral palsy
  Bulbar palsy
  Infant botulism
  Muscular dystrophy
  Pseudo-obstruction
  Connective tissue disease
  Repaired tracheoesophageal fistula
Inflammatory
  Viral stomatitis
  Candida stomatitis, pharyngitis
  Peptic esophagitis
  Mucositis (graft-versus-host disease)
Systemic
  Cardiac disease
  Pulmonary disease

BEHAVIORAL
Attachment disorder
Infantile anorexia
Picky eater
Failure to imbibe
Delayed introduction of solids
Oral aversion
Conditioned dysphagia
Post-traumatic eating disorder
Vulnerable child
Parental responses

Adapted from Rudolph CD,[10] Kedesdy JH and Budd KS,[14] and Illingworth RS.[20]

imbibe" in young infants with poor intake and no apparent problems with mother–infant interactions.[29–31]

When the introduction of feedings is delayed beyond a sensitive or critical period, later acquisition of feeding skills may be difficult.[32] Medical or surgical disorders early in life may necessitate the use of nasogastric or gastrostomy feedings or parenteral nutrition to maintain adequate nutrition. If supplemental feeding is required on a short-term basis, growth is maintained, and generally the infant quickly resumes normal feeding behavior. However, if long-term tube feeding or intravenous alimentation is required, especially if the infant has had little previous positive experience with normal feeding, the child is at risk for the development of an aversion to oral feedings. Intrusive oral procedures such as nasogastric tube placement, endo-

tracheal intubation, and oropharyngeal suctioning have been associated with aversion to oral feedings.[33] The long-term pairing of eating and pain, as occurs in GERD, may establish a negative feeding experience and a "conditioned dysphagia."[23,34,35] Older children who experience an episode of choking have developed an acute food refusal, described as a post-traumatic eating disorder.[36]

Even in the case in which medical conditions impact nutrition, the parental reaction to feeding can play a pivotal role. Parents may be faced with innumerable negative feeding interactions because of the need to focus on the child's nutrient intake. These experiences can change feeding from a satisfying parent–child interaction to a grim, anxiety-producing chore. Further, infants with early medical problems may be perceived as "vulnerable" by their parents, who consequently may have difficulty setting age-appropriate limits, in this case around eating.[3,37] Therefore, even after an organic disorder is resolved, the feeding interaction remains stressed.

Multiple etiologies are often present in the child being evaluated for poor feeding. In 50 infants with feeding disorders, Budd and colleagues found that 64% had problems with both organic and nonorganic symptoms, contributing to their insufficient food intake.[38] Burklow and colleagues reviewed 103 children with complex feeding problems, identifying 80% with a significant behavioral component and 85% with multiple conditions leading to the feeding disorder.[39] Careful study of infants with a diagnosis of nonorganic failure to thrive has revealed that subtle oral-motor dysfunction may be responsible for inadequate feeding skills, contributing to their poor weight gain.[40,41] In children with multiple risk factors, these problems may coexist or evolve separately in time, with the nonorganic component remaining after the organic problem is resolved.

EVALUATION

The presence of feeding difficulties may be first noted by the infant's caregiver, primary care physician, early intervention specialist, or other health care personnel. The type and severity of the feeding problem will usually lead to the involvement of several allied professionals (Figure 75.2-2). Often an interdisciplinary team approach facilitates an efficient evaluation.[14,42]

The first step in evaluating feeding difficulties is a complete history and physical examination. The prenatal history, gestational age, birth weight, and neonatal course may suggest particular risk factors. The answers to questions regarding general psychomotor developmental progress will inform an understanding of feeding progress and why it might be delayed. The review of systems can identify those infants with chronic lung disease, cardiac malformations, or neurologic conditions that are likely to affect feeding (see Table 75.2-2). Symptoms of GERD should be sought because feeding resistance may be one of the early manifestations.[23] The nutritionist has a major role in obtaining the diet history, which will include the type, amount, and nutritional value of what is offered to the infant or child, as well as what is actually ingested. A 24-hour diet recall or a more formal 3-day diet record assists in calculating fluid, calorie,

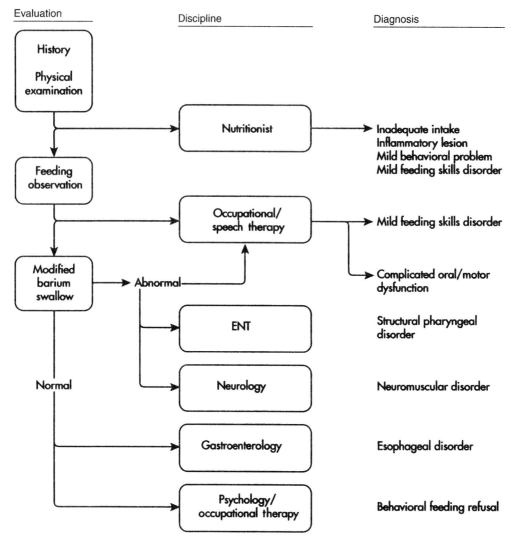

FIGURE 75.2-2   Steps in the evaluation of feeding difficulties. ENT = otorhinolaryngology.

mineral, and vitamin intake. This information, together with a review of feeding methods, will often suggest inadequate calorie intake or developmentally inappropriate food choices indicative of a feeding skill disorder.

Physical examination begins with careful anthropometric measurement, which can be plotted on the appropriate growth charts.[43] Progressive movement away from previous growth percentiles may indicate inadequate intake and the need for further investigation. Weight-for-length ratio is a sensitive measure of acute malnutrition.[44]

Oral examination should evaluate lip closure, tongue position and movement, and palatal movement. Nonnutritive sucking can be evaluated by allowing the infant to suck on the examiner's gloved finger. Infants with oral-motor problems may have poor coordination of suck, swallow, and breathing; poor mouth closure; decreased tongue movement; decreased jaw stability; or sustained or prolonged jaw closure. Oral hypersensitivity with increased gag reflex is common after mechanical ventilation or tube feeding.[45] Further neurologic examination may reveal cranial nerve deficits associated with dysphagia, as well as problems with posture, head and neck control, muscle tone, and persistence of primitive reflexes.[46]

The feeding observation is the central element of the clinical evaluation. The occupational therapist or speech-language pathologist can assist in assessing nutritive sucking and feeding by the primary caregiver, which may detect subtle disorders of feeding skills.[40,47] A prospective study of neonates found that those with disorganized or dysfunctional sucking patterns were more likely to have feeding problems at 6 and 12 months of age.[48] When observing parent–child interactions around feeding, the clinician should notice how the food is presented, which foods an infant prefers, and the parental responses to good and inappropriate feeding behaviors.

Several imaging methods are available to evaluate more complex oral-motor dysfunction. The primary technique is the modified barium swallow, also referred to as a videofluoroscopic swallow study.[49] It requires involvement of a feeding specialist (occupational therapist or speech-language pathologist) and radiologist. Unlike standard upper gastrointestinal barium contrast radiographs, in this study, the infant is placed in a standard feeding position and presented with a variety of textures (see Chapter 23, "Disorders of Deglutition"). This study is the best method of evaluating the pharyngeal phase of swallowing. Clinically inapparent difficulties with suck and swallow, nasopharyngeal reflux, ineffective pharyngeal closure, and aspiration can be seen and taped for later review. Aspiration is often subclinical. It is present in up to 40% of adults without previously identified aspiration undergoing modified barium swallow.[50] Knowledge of aspiration risk and the ability to handle food of different consistencies will assist in developing a safe feeding program.

Ultrasonography is ideal for evaluating the oral preparatory phase of swallow.[51,52] The infant and feeder can be studied in a more physiologic state, with repeated observations of swallow possible. No contrast material is needed, and there is no radiation exposure. Ultrasound study of the pharyngeal phase is difficult owing to air-filled spaces, and aspiration will not be detected.

Flexible endoscopic evaluation of swallowing is another technique that allows for evaluation of swallowing, particularly the pharyngeal phase.[53] After topical anesthesia of nasal tissues, a nasopharyngoscope is passed transnasally for observation of the anatomy and function of the palate, pharynx, and larynx. Next, swallowing function is evaluated with administration of food. The ability to handle liquids and risk of aspiration can be directly assessed. The study can be repeated as often as necessary because there is no preparation needed and no radiation exposure.[54]

Manometry is used to assess the esophageal phase of swallowing. It will detect abnormalities of upper esophageal sphincter relaxation or esophageal peristalsis but may be impractical during early infancy or childhood.

For the infant with behavioral refusal to feed, the presence of a psychologist on the treatment team can be crucial to understanding the development of the problem and the best way to approach the family. Behavioral assessment includes a thorough feeding history, including details of both the infant's feeding and the parental responses, intake history over several days to demonstrate the pattern of feedings, and feeding observation live or on videotape.[55]

TREATMENT

Treatment of feeding problems, which are often complex, should emanate from the interdisciplinary assessment.

Generally, not all aspects of the plan are begun simultaneously. Medical conditions causing pain or discomfort during eating should be resolved. Initial attention should be directed to providing sufficient intake for maintenance and catch-up growth. As nutritional status improves, the occupational therapist, speech therapist, and psychologist can help develop a program to establish normal feeding skills and parent–child interactions.

Whenever possible, oral feeding should be maintained even if alternative feeding is also used. This preserves the sensory function of taste and smell and the neuromotor skills of suck and swallow. Oral feeding promotes speech development and provides what should be a pleasurable social experience for the infant. Sucking appears to increase the concentration of lingual lipase, which, together with breast milk lipase, is important for digestion of lipid in the neonatal period.[56,57] Salivary amylase, along with small intestinal glucoamylase, is primarily responsible for starch digestion in early infancy because pancreatic amylase activity is low until 4 months of age.[58] Swallowing initiates primary peristalsis in the esophagus, enhancing esophageal acid clearance.

If nutritional support beyond oral supplementation is required, the route for provision of supplements can be chosen and therapy initiated (Figure 75.2-3). No advantage is achieved in delaying nutritional therapy in children with feeding problems because malnutrition is the primary cause of growth retardation and altered body composition in chronic illness.[59] Details of enteral and parenteral feeding are described in Chapter 75.4, "Nutrition Support."

Nutrient administration is based on patient needs and limitations. Nasogastric or orogastric tubes are easy to place, with feedings given on an intermittent (bolus) or continuous basis. Bolus feeds are more physiologic in preserving hunger-satiety cycles and allow greater mobility for the patient and family. Continuous feedings may be preferable when there is delayed gastric emptying or decreased gut absorptive capacity.[60,61]

Although gastric feeding is preferable, transpyloric tube placement is indicated when there is a high risk of aspiration.[62,63] The type of gastric tube used should be based on the length of time the tube is required. Polyvinylchloride tubes are relatively easy to pass but must be changed every 3 to 4 days. For many clinical situations, a flexible silicone

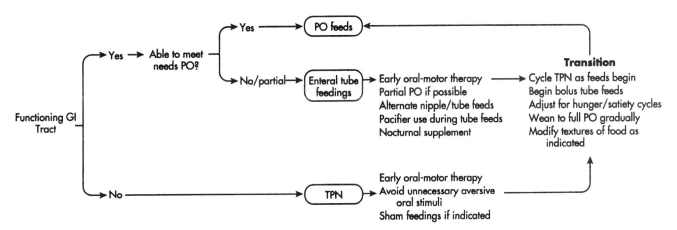

FIGURE 75.2-3 Treatment of feeding difficulties. GI = gastrointestinal; PO = per os; TPN = total parenteral nutrition.

elastic tube is more comfortable for the patient. These tubes produce less sensation when the child swallows, interfere less with feeding, and can remain in place for up to several weeks.[64] Fewer tube changes decrease noxious oral-facial stimuli for the child, which may help reduce the likelihood of future negative feeding behaviors.

Nocturnal feedings have been shown to provide excellent nutritional support while not interfering with daytime activities.[65–68] Percutaneous endoscopic gastrostomy and use of low-profile gastrostomy buttons facilitate the care of patients on long-term enteral support.[69] Families have often had significant distress regarding feedings by the time a gastrostomy is placed and need support and understanding when the decision is finally made.[70]

Various approaches to advancing feedings are available.[62,71] Tolerance can be assessed by gastric residuals and the absence of vomiting, diarrhea, or abdominal pain. Infants with chronic diarrhea and malnutrition can be successfully managed with enteral therapy, but the volume of the infusion should be increased gradually.[72] Attention to adequate water intake will prevent problems of dehydration owing to formulas with a high renal solute load.[73]

Gastrostomy tube feedings should not be considered an obstacle to overcoming feeding problems. A review of 100 infants fed by nasogastric tube indicated that earlier placement of a gastrostomy tube for the poor feeders was associated with improved success in transition to oral feeding.[74] In a study of 19 patients with severe feeding refusal, those gastrostomy-fed infants took slightly longer than the nasogastric tube–fed infants to achieve oral feeding, but use of gastrostomy feedings did not adversely affect eventual transition to oral feeds.[75]

Careful attention to appropriate techniques for the provision of proper diets can be of great benefit to children with major feeding difficulties. Two examples of such clinical problems are discussed below. Other dietary issues encountered in a range of gastrointestinal disorders are discussed in Chapter 75.5, "Special Dietary Therapy."

ORAL-FACIAL ANOMALIES

The newborn with cleft lip or palate has an immediate feeding problem. With a minor cleft lip or palate, the feeding problem is usually related to the inability to generate adequate negative pressure for suction. Apart from its nutritional advantages, breastfeeding may best facilitate intake because the soft tissue of the breast can help seal the cleft during feedings. When there is cleft lip and palate, the breastfed infant may be unable to generate sufficient negative pressure to hold the nipple and areola in place for compression, and the bottle-fed infant may not develop efficient suction on a nipple. Breastfeeding may be assisted with use of the Supplemental Nursing System (Medela, Inc., McHenry, IL); feeding devices for bottle-fed cleft lip and palate infants should deliver an adequate volume of milk into the mouth while allowing time for the infant to swallow (Table 75.2-3).[76,77]

Oral feeding of the infant with cleft lip or palate may be facilitated by upright positioning, small frequent feedings, careful burping, and applying pressure to the infant's cheek

and beneath the jaw to assist lip closure and sucking.[78] Nonoral feedings become necessary if significant risk of aspiration is present or if the infant fails to thrive because of either inadequate volume intake or prolonged feeding sessions. When micrognathia and glossoptosis occur with cleft palate (the Robin sequence), respiratory distress may preclude oral feeding. These infants have feeding difficulties caused by inadequate suction, swallowing difficulties, and compromised breathing owing to airway obstruction by the tongue.[79] Some infants will require surgical tongue-lip adhesion, use of a nasopharyngeal airway, or even tracheostomy.[80,81] These operative procedures are reserved for patients with the inability to maintain a stable airway using conversative measures. The incidence of failure to thrive was reduced when the families of infants with Robin sequence received assistance from a feeding-support nurse and supervised airway management.[82]

CEREBRAL PALSY

Cerebral palsy is a chronic, nonprogressive disorder of the nervous system, with an estimated incidence of 1 in 500 infants.[83] Cerebral palsy is a disorder of movement and posture, and most patients demonstrate spasticity of the extremities. Swallowing difficulties result from supranuclear bulbar palsies, and more severely affected children may have language and intellectual deficits and seizures. In a large survey of families with children with neurologic impairment, prolonged feeding times of 3 or more hours per day were common.[84] Early on, affected infants may have decreased sucking reflex and weak or uncoordinated sucking behavior; later, they can have tonic bite, tongue thrust or lip retraction, and lip pursing.[85,86]

Before oral feeds are begun, non-nutritive sucking can be encouraged at the breast (emptied by pumping) or with a pacifier. Non-nutritive sucking during gavage feeds has been shown to help the maturation of the sucking reflex in premature infants and may improve integration of oral and pharyngeal reflexes in the infant with an immature nervous system.[87]

Treatment techniques are available to enhance oral feeding at the breast and with bottle-feeding.[77,86,88] For the older

TABLE 75.2-3   SPECIAL NIPPLES
                 AND FEEDING DEVICES

NIPPLE/DEVICE	CHARACTERISTICS
Supplemental Nursing System	For breastfeeding infants; allows control of volume of milk from reservoir
Ross red premature nipple	Soft, durable
Mead-Johnson cleft palate feeder	Squeeze bottle helps with control of milk delivery; cross-cut nipple
Haberman feeder	Easy to use, with nipple the feeder can compress to help express milk
Any broad-based nipple	May conform to a cleft lip and help attain suction
Feeding obturator (prosthesis)	To stabilize wide cleft

Adapted from Case-Smith J and Humphry R.[86]

infant, the texture of foods can be adjusted, and with thicker liquids passing more slowly from mouth to throat, they often will be better tolerated. The use of a spoon requires that the infant open the mouth wide enough so that lateral tongue movements are adequate to remove the food and that jaw control is adequate. Spoons are designed with narrow, shallow bowls and are made of durable, plastic material; they may have specialized handles to help with the grasp. Cups are available with cut-out rims (to allow easier lifting), covers to decrease spillage, and wide bases to prevent tipping. The feeder can use techniques to provide external jaw and cheek support and to stabilize head position. Adaptive equipment is available to improve postural alignment during feedings. The feeder may hold an infant in the lap or use a foam-filled Tumble-Forms (Sammons Preston Rolyan, Bolingbrook, IL) seat. The older infant or toddler with fair sitting stability can use the Rifton chair (Rifton Equipment, Chester, NY) or other adaptive seating device for upright positioning with foot rests, arm supports, and pelvic strapping.[86] As noted above, some children with an inability to meet nutritional needs orally will require a feeding gastrostomy. The safety of oral feedings and risk of aspiration can be evaluated with videofluoroscopy of swallowing. Early attention to treatment of feeding disorders in these patients can result in significantly improved nutritional status.[89,90]

BEHAVIORAL APPROACHES TO FEEDING

Principles of learning are used to understand the development of feeding disorders and to design treatment programs for children with feeding problems when there is no apparent organic disease or when correction of an organic disorder or oral-motor deficit does not result in normal feeding.[14,91–99] Respondent learning or classic conditioning posits that the occurrence of some behaviors is increased or decreased based on their association with normal physiologic reactions, in this case hunger or pain. Specifically, eating may have been associated with pain in the development of the disorder. Further, in children with feeding disorders, the positive association between hunger, eating, and satiety is inconsistent. Often interventions for feeding disorders manipulate hunger to prompt eating behaviors. The rationale is that children are more likely to emit eating behaviors (show interest in food, accept food put into their mouth, put food into the mouth, swallow food) when they are hungry.

Hunger may be manipulated in several ways.[91] For the child fed by the mouth, the timing of meals should be regulated, and between-meal eating and drinking should be minimized or eliminated so that the child is hungry at mealtime. The length of meals is also regulated, so that meals last only 20 to 30 minutes, regardless of the amount of food ingested. After 20 to 30 minutes, it is assumed that rising blood sugar from the food that has been consumed leads to diminished sensation of hunger. From the respondent learning perspective, keeping meals short continues to reinforce the association of hunger-eating-satiety.

For children who are tube-fed, the timing and amount of the feeding should be regulated to maximize hunger. Bolus, rather than continuous, feeding and daytime, rather than nighttime, feeding will more closely mimic meals and thus move the child toward normal eating patterns. Tube feeding after, rather than before, an oral feeding session is generally recommended. Modestly decreasing the calories received by tube will, in many patients, increase appetite and better motivate the child to eat by mouth.

One caveat is necessary with respect to the manipulation of hunger. Although a modest amount of calorie restriction is typically helpful to encouraging eating behavior, severe calorie restriction is not. Many naive interveners, both lay and professional, have found that the statement "He'll eat when he gets hungry enough" is not true for those feeding disorders usually seen in a tertiary care center.

Operant learning principles posit that behaviors are increased or decreased based on the responses to the behaviors. Operant techniques are used to increase desired behaviors and decrease undesirable behaviors.[92] In the treatment of feeding problems, the most commonly used and effective operant treatment technique is differential attention.[93–98] During the meal, the child receives positive reinforcement or attention for specific behaviors related to feeding and no attention for inappropriate or off-task behaviors. Positive attention is often social interaction and praise from the caregiver, but depending on the child, it can be music or access to a preferred food. Inappropriate and off-task behaviors include tantrums, not approaching the food, and playing with the food. The target behaviors (behaviors to be increased) are changed as the treatment progresses. For example, the child may initially be reinforced for allowing food to be put in his mouth, then for swallowing the food, then for self-feeding, and, finally, for self-feeding a sufficient quantity in a specified time. Depending on the child's feeding problem, physical guidance of appropriate feeding behaviors may be used along with differential attention.[100–105] The physical guidance is decreased and then stopped as the child progresses through the program.

Extinction is the operant principle that suggests that a behavior will eventually cease if it is never reinforced. Extinction-based techniques have been used in the treatment of severe feeding refusal. Most typically, these are children who, for medical reasons and from a very early age, have not been fed by mouth and/or have experienced very aversive oral procedures, such as intubation. When faced with oral feeding these children produce strong rejecting behaviors such as screaming, spitting food, and physically resisting placement of food in the mouth. When the caregiver stops the feeding in response to these rejecting behaviors, the child's behaviors have been reinforced (by escaping the negative situation). Extinction techniques dictate that feeding should not stop in response to rejecting behaviors. Thus, spoonfuls of food (sometimes very little food) are put into the child's mouth repeatedly despite the child's protest. Eventually, when the child's protest behavior does not stop the feeding (ie, the protest behavior is not reinforced), the protest behavior stops. Although these extinction techniques have been successful in cases of severe feeding refusal,[75,105–109] they must be carefully planned and executed in an inpatient setting.

The role of parents in carrying out behavioral treatment programs for feeding must be fully appreciated and supported.[14] As discussed earlier in this chapter, parental anxiety about nutrition is an important factor in the development and maintenance of many feeding problems. For parents to decrease unhelpful behavior that is motivated by their own anxiety, their concerns and anxiety must by addressed specifically. The entire treatment team should know and agree on the treatment plan for the child's nutritional and behavioral feeding problem, and this consensus plan should be presented to the family. Most parents need help to understand that the multiple components of their child's feeding problem cannot all be addressed at once. They need to understand that the team has a plan to resolve all of the concerns in time and that the child's physical health will not be in danger during this process. Parental lack of understanding of this process can severely impede the progress of treatment. For example, parents will not follow guidelines to stop meals after 30 minutes and may give in to inappropriate feeding rituals if they fear that the child's nutritional status will be irretrievably harmed.

For the child with mild to moderate feeding problems, most parents can be taught behavioral treatment techniques. The behavioral feeding plan needs to be carried out consistently, that is, at every meal, to change the child's negative feeding behaviors. Thus, training the parent to carry out the treatment at each meal is far superior to an "expert feeder" who treats the child weekly or even several times per week. Parents will need to understand the behavioral principles and the importance of consistency in applying these techniques and that the target behaviors will more closely approximate normal eating as the child progresses. For children with very severe feeding refusal, especially if extinction procedures are used, inpatient treatment with alternative feeders may be most appropriate. In these cases, parents must initially understand and support the treatment and then must be taught to carry out the procedures themselves as feeding is transferred to the more normal parent–child interaction and home environment.

TRANSITION TO ORAL FEEDS

When medical or surgical disorders necessitate nonoral feedings or parenteral nutrition, planning for transition to oral feedings should begin early. Oral-motor skills should be assessed and swallowing ability documented. Oral feedings, even in small amounts, should continue, if at all possible, to maintain oral-motor skills. Total parenteral nutrition can be cycled while enteral feedings are advanced, even in the young infant.[110] Sham feedings for children with esophageal atresia and esophagostomies facilitate the return to normal feedings.[111] Other useful techniques include non-nutritive sucking during tube feeding of premature infants and giving nipple feeds during the daytime, with the balance of the feeding volume delivered by tube at night.[112] Attention to eating-related behaviors, the feeding environment, and hunger-satiety cycles will help normalize feedings.[113] Ongoing communication between the family and involved professionals will enhance the transition to normal eating behavior.

REFERENCES

1. Maclean W, Lucas A. Pediatric nutrition: a distinct subspecialty? In: Walker WA, Watkins JB, editors. Nutrition in pediatrics: basic science and clinical applications. 2nd ed. Hamilton (ON): BC Decker; 1997, p. 3–6.
2. Reau N, Senturia Y, Lebailly S, Christoffel K. Infant and toddler feeding patterns and problems: normative data and a new direction. J Dev Behav Pediatr 1996;17:149–53.
3. Singer L. When a child won't-or can't eat. Contemp Pediatr 1990;7:60–76.
4. Iwata BA, Riordan MM, Wohl MK, Finney JW. Pediatric feeding disorders: behavioral analysis and treatment. In: Accardo PJ, editor. Failure to thrive in infancy and early childhood. Baltimore: University Park Press; 1982. p. 297–329.
5. Dahl M, Sundelin C. Early feeding problems in an affluent society. I. Categories and clinical signs. Acta Paediatr Scand 1986;75:370–9.
6. Babbitt RL, Hoch T, Coe D, et al. Behavioral assessment and treatment of pediatric feeding disorders. J Dev Behav Pediatr 1994;15:278–291.
7. Reilly S, Skuse D, Poblete X. Prevalence of feeding problems and oral motor dysfunction in children with cerebral palsy: a community survey. J Pediatr 1996;129:877–82.
8. Glass RP, Wolf LS. Feeding and oral-motor skills. In: Case-Smith J, editor. Pediatric occupational therapy and early intervention. Boston: Andover Medical Publishers; 1993. p. 225.
9. Cloud H. Feeding problems of the child with special health care needs. In: Edvall SW, editor. Pediatric nutrition in chronic diseased and developmental disorders. New York: Oxford University Press; 1993. p. 203–18.
10. Rudolph CD. Feeding disorders in infants and children. J Pediatr 1994;125:S116–24.
11. Arvedson J, Brodsky L. Pediatric swallowing and feeding: assessment and management. 2nd ed. San Diego: Singular Publishing Group; 2002.
12. Logan WJ, Bosma JF. Oral and pharyngeal dysphagia in infancy. Pediatr Clin North Am 1967;14:47–61.
13. Blackman J. Children who refuse food. Contemp Pediatr 1998; 15:198–216.
14. Kedesdy JH, Budd KS. Childhood feeding disorders: biobehavioral assessment and intervention. Baltimore: Paul H. Brookes Publishing; 1998.
15. Hyman SL, Porter C, Page T, et al. Behavior management of feeding disturbances in urea cycle and organic acid disorders. J Pediatr 1987;111:558–62.
16. Seidman E. Nutritional treatment of growth failure and disease activity in children with inflammatory bowel disease. In: Suskind RM, Lewinter-Suskind L, editors. Textbook of pediatric nutrition. 2nd ed. New York: Raven Press; 1993. p. 341–52.
17. Iacono G, Carroccio A, Montalto G, et al. Gastroesophageal reflux and cow's milk allergy in infants: a prospective study. J Allergy Clin Immunol 1996;97:822–7.
18. American Academy of Pediatrics, Committee on Nutrition. Assessment of nutritional status. In: Kleinman R, editor. Pediatric nutrition handbook. 4th ed. Elk Grove Village (IL): American Academy of Pediatrics; 1998. p. 165–84.
19. Green M. Pediatric diagnosis: interpretation of symptoms and signs in infants, children, and adolescents. 5th ed. Philadelphia: WB Saunders; 1992.
20. Illingworth RS. Sucking and swallowing difficulties in infancy: diagnostic problem of dysphagia. Arch Dis Child 1969; 44:655–65.
21. Wolf LS, Glass RP. Feeding and swallowing disorders in infancy: assessment and management. Tucson (AZ): Therapy Skill Builders; 1992.

22. Tilton A, Miller M, Khoshoo V. Nutrition and swallowing in pediatric neuromuscular patients. Semin Pediatr Neurol 1998;5:106–15.

23. Dellert S, Hyams J, Treem W, Geertsma MA. Feeding resistance and gastroesophageal reflux in infancy. J Pediatr Gastroenterol Nutr 1993;17:66–71.

24. Catto-Smith AG, Machida H, Butzner J, et al. The role of gastroesophageal reflux in pediatric dysphagia. J Pediatr Gastroenterol Nutr 1991;12:159–65.

25. Hall K. Pediatric dysphagia: resource guide. San Diego: Singular Publishing Group; 2001.

26. Ford CF, Pietsch JB. Home enteral tube feeding in children after chemotherapy or bone marrow transplantation. Nutr Clin Pract 1999;14:19–22.

27. Morris B, Miller-Loncar C, Landry S, et al. Feeding, medical factors, and developmental outcome in premature infants. Clin Pediatr 1999;38:451–7.

28. Chatoor I, Ganiban J, Colin V, et al. Attachment and feeding problems: a reexamination of nonorganic failure to thrive and attachment insecurity. J Am Acad Child Adolesc Psychiatry 1998;37:1217–24.

29. Tolia V. Very early onset nonorganic failure to thrive in infants. J Pediatr Gastroenterol Nutr 1995;20:73–80.

30. Gremse D, Lytle JM, Sacks A, Balistreri W. Characterization of failure to imbibe in infants. Clin Pediatr 1998;37:305–10.

31. Lichtman S, Maynor A, Rhoads J. Failure to imbibe in otherwise normal infants. J Pediatr Gastroenterol Nutr 2000;30:467–71.

32. Illingworth RS, Lister J. The critical or sensitive period, with special reference to certain feeding problems in infants and children. J Pediatr 1964;65:839–48.

33. Geertsma MA, Hyams JS, Pelletier JM, Reiter S. Feeding resistance after parenteral hyperalimentation. Am J Dis Child 1985;139:255–6.

34. DiScipio WJ, Kaslon K, Ruben RJ. Traumatically acquired conditioned dysphagia in children. Ann Otol 1978;87:509–14.

35. Manikam R, Perman J. Pediatric feeding disorders. J Clin Gastroenterol 2000;30:34–46.

36. Chatoor I, Conley C, Dickson L. Food refusal after an incident of choking: a posttraumatic eating disorder. J Am Acad Child Adolesc Psychiatry 1988;27:1005–10.

37. Green M, Solnit A. Reactions to the threatened loss of a child: a vulnerable child syndrome. Pediatrics 1964;65:538–66.

38. Budd KS, McGraw T, Farbisz R, et al. Psychosocial concomitants of children's feeding disorders. J Pediatr Psychol 1992;17:81–94.

39. Burklow K, Phelps A, Schultz J, et al. Classifying pediatric feeding disorders. J Pediatr Gastroenterol Nutr 1998;27:143–7.

40. Ramsay M, Gisel E, Boutry M. Non-organic failure to thrive: growth failure secondary to feeding-skills disorder. Dev Med Child Neurol 1993;35:285–97.

41. Reilly S, Skuse D, Wolke D, Stevenson J. Oral-motor dysfunction in children who fail to thrive: organic or non-organic? Dev Med Child Neurol 1999;41:115–22.

42. Bithoney W, McJunkin J, Michalek J, et al. Prospective evaluation of weight gain in both nonorganic and organic failure-to-thrive children: an outpatient trial of a multidisciplinary team intervention strategy. J Dev Behav Pediatr 1989;10:27–31.

43. Centers for Disease Control and Prevention, National Center for Health Statistics. CDC growth charts. United States. Available at: http://www.cdc.gov/growthcharts/ (accessed May 30, 2000).

44. Hendricks K. Nutritional assessment. In: Hendricks K, Walker WA, editors. Manual of pediatric nutrition. 2nd ed. Toronto: BC Decker; 1990. p. 1–58.

45. Baker S, Boullard-Backunas K, Davis A. Common oral motor and gastrointestinal-nutritional problems in children

46. Hill A, Volpe J. Disorders of sucking and swallowing in the newborn infant: clinicopathological correlations. Prog Perinatal Neurol 1981;33:157–81.

47. Arvedson J, Brodsky L. Pediatric swallowing and feeding: assessment and management. 2nd ed. San Diego: Singular Publishing Group; 2002.

48. Hawdon J, Beauregard N, Slattery J, Kennedy G. Identification of neonates at risk of developing feeding problems in infancy. Dev Med Child Neurol 2000;42:235–9.

49. Benson J, Lefton-Greif M. Videofluoroscopy of swallowing in pediatric patients: a component of the total feeding evaluation. In: Tuchman D, Walter R, editors. Disorders of feeding and swallowing in infants and children. San Diego: Singular Publishing Group; 1994. p. 187–200.

50. Logeman J. Treatment for aspiration related to dysphagia: an overview. Dysphagia 1986;1:34–8.

51. Bu'Lock R, Woolridge M, Baum J. Development of coordination of sucking, swallowing and breathing: ultrasound study of term and preterm infants. Dev Med Child Neurol 1990;32:669–78.

52. Yang W, Loveday E, Metreweli C, Sullivan P. Ultrasound assessment of swallowing in malnourished disabled children. Br J Radiol 1997;992–4.

53. Willging J, Miller C, Hogan M, Rudolph C. Fiberoptic evaluation of swallowing in children: a preliminary report of 100 procedures. Dysphagia 1996;11:162.

54. Bastian R. The videoendoscopic swallowing study: an alternative and partner to the videofluoroscopic swallowing study. Dysphagia 1993;8:359–67.

55. Czyzewski D. Feeding and eating disorders in young children. In: Roberts M, Walker C, editors. Casebook of child and pediatric psychology. New York: Guilford Press; 1989. p. 255–80.

56. Smith L, Kaminsky S, D'Souza S. Neonatal fat digestion and lingual lipase. Acta Paediatr Scand 1986;75:913–8.

57. Hamosh M. Lipid metabolism in premature infants. Biol Neonate 1987;52:50–64.

58. Lebenthal E, Leung Y. The impact of development of the gut on infant nutrition. Pediatr Ann 1987;16:233–40.

59. Motil K. Aggressive nutritional therapy in growth retardation. Clin Nutr 1985;4:75–84.

60. Moore M, Greene H. Tube feeding of infants and children. Pediatr Clin North Am 1985;32:401–17.

61. Ghishan F. Nutritional management of pediatric gastrointestinal disorders. Pediatr Ann 1999;28:123–8.

62. Wilson S, Dietz W, Grand R. An algorithm for pediatric enteral alimentation. Pediatr Ann 1987;16:233–40.

63. Panadero E, Lopez-Herce J, Caro L, et al. Transpyloric enteral feeding in critically ill children. J Pediatr Gastroenterol Nutr 1998;26:43–8.

64. Fuchs G. Enteral support of the hospitalized child. In: Suskind R, Lewinter-Suskind L, editors. Textbook of pediatric nutrition. New York: Raven Press; 1993. p. 239–46.

65. Erdman S. Nutritional imperatives in cystic fibrosis therapy. Pediatr Ann 1999;28:129–36.

66. Motil K, Altchuler S, Grand R. Mineral balance during nutritional supplementation in adolescents with Crohn disease and growth failure. J Pediatr 1985;107:473–9.

67. Polk D, Hattner J, Kerner J. Improved growth and disease activity after intermittent administration of a defined formula diet in children with Crohn's disease. J Parenter Enteral Nutr 1992;16:499–504.

68. Claris-Appiani A, Ardissino G, Dacco V, et al. Catch-up growth in children with chronic renal failure treated with long-term enteral nutrition. J Parenter Enteral Nutr 1995;19:175–8.

69. Brant C, Stanich P, Ferrari A. Improvement of children's nutritional status after enteral feeding by PEG: an interim report. Gastrointest Endosc 1999;50:183–8.

70. Spalding K, McKeever P. Mothers' experiences caring for children with disabilities who require a gastrostomy tube. J Pediatr Nurs 1998;13:234–43.

71. Warman K. Enteral nutrition: support of the pediatric patient. In: Hendricks K, Walker WA, editors. Manual of pediatric nutrition. Philadelphia: BC Decker; 1990. p. 72–109.

72. Maclean W, Lopez de Romana G, Massa E, Graham G. Nutritional management of chronic diarrhea and malnutrition: primary reliance on oral feeding. J Pediatr 1980;97:316–23.

73. Pardoe E. Tube feeding syndrome revisited. Nutr Clin Pract 2001;16:144–6.

74. Bazyk S. Factors associated with the transition to oral feeding in infants fed by nasogastric tubes. Am J Occup Ther 1990; 44:1070–8.

75. Foy T, Czyzewski D, Phillips S, et al. Treatment of severe feeding refusal in infants and toddlers. Inf Young Child 1997;9:26–35.

76. Clarren SK, Anderson B, Wolf LS. Feeding infants with cleft lip, cleft palate, or cleft lip and palate. Cleft Palate J 1987;24:244–9.

77. Lawrence RA. Breastfeeding: a guide for the medical profession. 5th ed. St. Louis: Mosby;1999.

78. Balluf M. Nutritional needs of an infant or child with a cleft lip or palate. Ear Nose Throat J 1986;65:44–9.

79. Wolf L, Glass R. Feeding and swallowing disorders in infancy: assessment and management. Tucson (AZ): Therapy Skill Builders; 1992.

80. Heaf DP, Helms PJ, Dinwiddie R, Matthew DJ. Nasopharyngeal airways in Pierre Robin syndrome. J Pediatr 1982;100:698–703.

81. Lewis MB, Pashayan HM. Management of infants with Robin anomaly. Clin Pediatr 1980;19:519–28.

82. Pandya A, Boorman J. Failure to thrive in babies with cleft lip and palate. Br J Plast Surg 2001;54:471–5.

83. Haslam RH. Encephalopathies. In: Behrman RE, Kliegman RM, Arvin AM, editors. Nelson textbook of pediatrics. 15th ed. Philadelphia: WB Saunders; 1996. p. 1713–6.

84. Sullivan PB, Lambert B, Rose M, et al. Prevalence and severity of feeding and nutritional problems in children with neurological impairment: Oxford feeding study. Dev Med Child Neurol 2000;42:674–80.

85. McBride MC, Danner SC. Sucking disorders in neurologically impaired infants: assessment and facilitation of breastfeeding. Clin Perinatol 1987;14:109–30.

86. Case-Smith J, Humphry R. Feeding and oral motor skills. In: Case-Smith J, Allen AS, Pratt PN, editors. Occupational therapy for children. 3rd ed. St. Louis: Mosby; 1996. p. 430–60.

87. Bernbaum JC, Pereira GR, Watkins JB, Peckham GJ. Nonnutritive sucking during gavage feeding enhances growth and maturation in premature infants. Pediatrics 1983;71:41–5.

88. Camp KM, Kalscheur MC. Nutritional approach to diagnosis and management of pediatric feeding and swallowing disorders. In: Tuchman DN, Walter RS, editors. Disorders of feeding and swallowing in infants and children. San Diego: Singular Publishing; 1994. p. 153–86.

89. Sanders K, Cox K, Cannon R, et al. Growth response to enteral feeding by children with cerebral palsy. J Parenter Enteral Nutr 1990;14:23–6.

90. Schwarz S, Corredor J, Fisher-Medina J, et al. Diagnosis and treatment of feeding disorders in children with development disabilities. Pediatrics 2001;108:671–6.

91. Linscheid TR, Budd KS, Rasnake LK. Pediatric feeding disorders. In: Roberts MC, editor. Handbok of pediatric psychology. New York: Guilford Press; 1995. p. 501–15.

92. Kerwin MLE. Empirically supported treatments in pediatric psychology: severe feeding problems. J Pediatr Psychol 1999; 24:193–214.

93. Thompson RJ, Palmer S, Linscheid TR. Single subject design and interaction analysis in the behavioral treatment of a child with a feeding problem. Child Psychiatry Hum Dev 1977;8:43–53.

94. Linscheid TR, Tarnowski KJ, Rasnake LK, Brams JS. Behavioral treatment of food refusal in a child with short-gut syndrome. J Pediatr Psychol 1987;12:451–9.

95. Stark LJ, Bowen AM, Tyc VL, et al. A behavioral approach to increasing caloric consumption in children with cystic fibrosis. J Pediatr Psychol 1990;15:309–26.

96. Stark LJ, Powers SW, Jelalian E, et al. Modifying problematic mealtime interactions of children with cystic fibrosis and their parents via behavioral parent training. J Pediatr Psychol 1994;19:751–68.

97. Werle MA, Murphy TB, Budd KS. Treating chronic food refusal in young children: home-based parent training. J Appl Behav Anal 1993;26:421–33.

98. Turner KM, Sanders MR, Wall CR. Behavioral parent training versus dietary education in the treatment of children with persistent feeding difficulties. Behav Change 1994;11:242–58.

99. Lindscheid T, Murphy L. Feeding disorders in infancy and early childhood. In: Netherton D, Holmes D, Walker CE, editors. Child and adolescent psychological disorders: a comprehensive textbook. New York: Oxford; 1999. p. 139–55.

100. O'Brien F, Bugle C, Azrin NH. Training and maintaining a retarded child's proper eating. J Appl Behav Anal 1972;5:67–72.

101. Stimbert VE, Minor JW, McCoy JF. Intensive feeding training with retarded. Behav Modif 1977;1:517–30.

102. Reidy TJ. Training appropriate eating behavior in a pediatric rehabilitation setting: case study. Arch Phys Med Rehabil 1979;60:226–30.

103. Riordan MM, Iwata BA, Finney JW, et al. Behavioral assessment and treatment of chronic food refusal in handicapped children. J Appl Behav Anal 1984;17:327–41.

104. Sisson LA, Dixon MJ. Improving mealtime behaviors through token reinforcement. Behav Modif 1986;10:333–54.

105. Ahearn WH, Kerwin MLE, Eicher PS, et al. An alternating treatments comparison of two intensive interventions for food refusal. J Appl Behav Anal 1996;29:321–32.

106. Blackman JA, Nelson C. Rapid introduction of oral feedings to tube-fed patients. J Dev Behav Pediatr 1987;8:63–7.

107. Kerwin MLE, Ahearn WH, Eicher PS, Burd DM. The costs of eating: a behavioral economic analysis of food refusal. J Appl Behav Anal 1995;28:245–60.

108. Hoch TA, Babbitt RL, Coe DA, et al. Contingency contracting: combining positive reinforcement and escape extinction procedures to treat persistent food refusal. Behav Modif 1994;18:106–28.

109. Benoit D, Wang E, Zlotkin S. Discontinuation of enterostomy tube feeding by behavioral treatment in early childhood: a randomized controlled trial. J Pediatr 2000;137:498–503.

110. Collier S, Crough J, Hendricks K, Caballero B. Use of cyclic parenteral nutrition in infants less than 6 months of age. Nutr Clin Pract 1994;9:65–8.

111. Zisserman L. Feeding problems: weaning an infant from a transpyloric tube. Pediatr Nurs 1986;12:33–7.

112. Field T, Ignatoff E, Stringer S, et al. Nonnutritive sucking during tube feedings: effects on preterm neonates in an intensive care unit. Pediatrics 1982;70:381–4.

113. Schauster H, Dwyer J. Transition from tube feedings to feedings by mouth in children: preventing eating dysfunction. J Am Diet Assoc 1996;96:277–81.

3. Nutritional Assessment and Requirements

Christopher Duggan, MD, MPH

Children with gastrointestinal diseases are uniquely susceptible to many forms of malnutrition (Table 75.3-1), including acute and chronic protein-energy malnutrition,[1,2] micronutrient deficiencies,[3,4] and hypoalbuminemic malnutrition.[5] Patients who are force-fed (either enterally or parenterally) are even liable to overnutrition or obesity.[6] Although nutritional management of children with gastrointestinal disease is often considered a secondary therapeutic goal behind primary medical or surgical care, there is an increasing appreciation that nutritional therapy can and should be the prime focus. Gastrointestinal diseases for which nutritional management assumes primary importance include inflammatory bowel disease, cow's milk protein and other allergic enteropathies, celiac disease, short-bowel syndrome (and any condition in which parenteral nutrition is employed), and a wide variety of metabolic diseases of the liver. Further, many studies have shown that malnourished patients are more prone to both infectious and noninfectious complications of their disease or therapy[7] and require longer lengths of stay in hospital and more resources.[8,9] It is therefore essential that pediatric practitioners understand the principles of nutritional assessment, as well as the scientific basis of nutritional requirements, for effective medical and nutritional care of their patients.

TABLE 75.3-1   SUSCEPTIBILITY OF THE PEDIATRIC GASTROINTESTINAL PATIENT TO MALNUTRITION

DECREASED INTAKE/ANOREXIA
Primary anorexia nervosa
Secondary anorexia owing to chronic disease, inflammation, infection, micronutrient deficiencies, abdominal pain
Dysphagia

MALABSORPTION/MALDIGESTION
Mucosal, hepatobiliary, or pancreatic disease
Drug–nutrient interactions
Short-gut syndrome
Congenital transport defects

ALTERED NUTRIENT REQUIREMENTS
Fever, stress, malabsorption, recovery from malnutrition, prematurity
Immobility, decreased energy expenditure, hypothyroidism
Congenital metabolic defects or conditions requiring pharmacologic doses of some nutrients and/or dietary avoidance of others

DEPENDENCE ON CARETAKERS FOR NUTRIENT INTAKE
Parenteral/enteral nutrition is "force-feeding"
Neglect/maltreatment

NUTRITIONAL ASSESSMENT TECHNIQUES

The medical history, physical examination, and selective laboratory testing form the basis of nutritional assessment. Increasingly sophisticated biologic methodologies are also available for nutritional assessment,[10] especially in the area of body composition analysis. This chapter reviews those aspects of nutritional assessment that are most germane to the care of children with gastrointestinal diseases.

HISTORY

A detailed medical history is essential to the nutritional evaluation of a patient. In addition to recording the type and onset of gastrointestinal symptoms, the physician should document the following:

- Current symptoms and their effect on nutrient intake, absorption, and retention
- Past history, including neonatal history, duration of breastfeeding versus formula-feeding, past growth data, gastrointestinal surgery
- Chronic illnesses with known risk factors for malnutrition
- Developmental status, with special attention to milestones of swallowing function
- Known or perceived food allergies
- Medications, with special attention to those with known drug–nutrient interactions (eg, sulfasalazine and folate, corticosteroids and calcium)
- Family history, parental heights, and sibling growth patterns
- Social history, food preferences/beliefs, and food availability

A careful history, in conjunction with a physical examination, is an effective method to diagnose and evaluate patients with idiopathic growth failure,[11] but in patients with chronic gastrointestinal diseases, more detailed assessment techniques are often indicated.

DIETARY INTAKE METHODS

Techniques of dietary assessment range from the straightforward recall of recent intake to the detailed and methodical measuring and weighing of all intake during a 7- to 14-day period.[12] Semiquantitative food frequency questionnaires have been developed and validated in adults[13] and, more recently, in children.[14] From a population perspective, food disappearance and agricultural data may be used, but, of course, they offer no insight into individual nutrient intake. A comprehensive discussion of dietary assessment techniques is provided elsewhere.[15]

In the clinical setting, a 24-hour dietary recall, which is the most rapid dietary intake method, sheds light on family eating patterns and food availability; it can be easily incorporated into the general history and physical examination. Problems of recall bias and under- or overreporting of intake[16] limit the validity of this technique.

A prospective food diary, in which a patient measures and writes down all intake for 3 to 5 days, is probably the most reliable and valid clinical tool. Proper interpretation of these diet records requires consultation with a qualified dietitian. The nutritional composition of these foods is determined by using one of the common nutritional databases, often with the use of proprietary software.[17] An average daily intake of energy, macronutrients, and micronutrients can then be calculated and compared with published reference data. Prospective diet records should generally be performed while the patient is feeling well, free of the effects of acute illness, and should include at least one weekend day in school-age children.

PHYSICAL EXAMINATION AND ANTHROPOMETRIC DATA

The examination of all patients with growth failure should be thorough (Table 75.3-2). Careful inspection and palpation of tissues such as hair, skin, oral mucosa, and subcutaneous fat and muscle stores are particularly important in the physical examination. Formal measures of arm anthropometrics are possible, but encircling the patient's upper arm with the examiner's hand can provide informal assessment of arm muscle and fat stores.

Basic anthropometric data include body weight and height (or length in those children less than age 2 years). When compared with age- and sex-appropriate standards, these data can provide objective measures of nutritional status. The weight of infants should be recorded to the nearest gram with the child wearing no clothes or a diaper. In older children, shoes and heavy clothing should not be worn, and the scale should be accurate to the nearest 0.1 kg. Length should be measured on a length board with a tape measure attached and a moveable foot board. Children older than age 2 years should be measured with a stadiometer while standing erect. The average of three readings should be obtained for accurate height/length measurements and should be recorded to the nearest 0.1 cm.

TABLE 75.3-2   CLINICAL SIGNS ASSOCIATED WITH NUTRITIONAL DEFICIENCIES.

ORGAN	CLINICAL SIGN(S)	NUTRIENT DEFICIENCY
Hair	Thin, sparse, easily pluckable	Protein energy, zinc
Face	Diffuse pigmentation	Protein energy
	Moon face	Protein
	Nasolabial seborrhea	Riboflavin, niacin, or pyridoxine
Eyes	Pale conjunctivae	Iron, folate, or vitamin B_{12}
	Bitôt spots, conjunctival or corneal xerosis, or keratomalacia	Vitamin A
	Angular palpebritis	Riboflavin or niacin
Lips	Angular stomatitis or cheilosis	Riboflavin, niacin, iron, or pyridoxine
Mouth	Ageusia, dysgeusia	Zinc
Tongue	Magenta tongue	Riboflavin
	Atrophic filiform papillae	Folate, niacin, riboflavin, iron, or vitamin B_{12}
	Glossitis	Niacin, folate, riboflavin, iron, vitamin B_{12}, pyridoxine, tryptophan
Teeth	Caries	Fluoride
Gums	Swollen, bleeding	Vitamin C
Glands	Thyromegaly	Iodine
	Parotid enlargement	Protein energy
Skin	Xerosis, follicular keratosis	Vitamin A or essential fatty acids
	Perifolliculosis with blood or pigment	Vitamin C
	Petechiae, ecchymoses	Vitamin C or K
	Pellagrous dermatosis	Niacin, tryptophan
	Scrotal or vulval dermatosis	Riboflavin
Nails	Koilonychia	Iron
Subcutaneous tissues	Edema	Protein, thiamine
	Decreased subcutaneous fat	Protein energy
Musculoskeletal system	Muscle wasting	Protein energy
	Craniotabes, frontal bossing, rachitic rosary, epiphyseal enlargement	Vitamin D
	Epiphyseal enlargement, subperiosteal hemorrhage	Vitamin C
Hepatobiliary system	Hepatomegaly	Protein energy
Nervous system	Psychomotor changes, confusion, irritability	Protein
	Sensory loss, motor weakness, calf tenderness	Thiamine
	Loss of vibratory sense, decreased deep tendon reflexes	Vitamin B_{12} or E
Cardiovascular system	Cardiomegaly, tachycardia	Thiamine

Adapted from Suskind R and Varma R.[96]

Detailed methodologies are given elsewhere[18,19]; recent studies have confirmed that body length is often poorly measured in practice.[20]

Raw data are then plotted on reference curves for age and sex, and the corresponding percentile is determined. The 2000 release of updated growth curves was a welcome advance in the field of pediatric nutrition assessment. The previously used curves were criticized for the homogeneous genetic, geographic, and socioeconomic background of the participants less than age 2 years.[21] In addition, these infants were generally fed infant formulas, whereas breastfed infants show significantly different patterns of weight and length gain.[22,23]

The major differences between the 2000 US Centers for Disease Control and Prevention (CDC) growth charts and the 1977 National Center for Health Statistics (NCHS) charts were (1) inclusion of breastfed infants proportional to their distribution in the US population during the past 30 years; (2) wider representation of a cross-section of children living in the United States between 1971 and 1994 (versus primarily white, middle-class infants); (3) expansion to include up to 20 years of age; (4) body mass index (BMI) percentile curves for 2 to 20 years; and (5) using one data source to decrease the disjunction between recumbent length and stature when changing from the infant (0–36 months) to the older child growth chart.[24] The NCHS has prepared curves for the visual display of the data that are widely available in general pediatric texts, wards, and clinics.

Although deficits in weight for age were originally proposed as criteria for malnutrition by Gomez in the 1950s, the currently accepted standard for anthropometric screening is the criteria of Waterlow (Table 75.3-3).[25] These criteria recognize that children who are underweight may be either short and well proportioned (so-called "stunted") or truly underweight for their height (so-called "wasted"). Wasted children have an acute deficit of body mass that is more amenable to immediate nutritional therapy, whereas stunted children are more chronically undernourished. Acutely wasted patients suffer a variety of functional deficits (eg, decreased muscle strength, impaired immune function, and decreased organ mass, among others); the physiologic impairment of stunting is less obvious and is controversial.[26] Aggressive feeding in either case can actually lead to accumulation of excess body fat.

TABLE 75.3-3 WATERLOW CRITERIA FOR CATEGORIZING TYPE AND CHRONICITY OF MALNUTRITION

	ACUTE MALNUTRITION (WEIGHT FOR HEIGHT; % OF MEDIAN)	CHRONIC MALNUTRITION (HEIGHT FOR AGE) (% OF MEDIAN)
Normal	> 90	> 95
Mild	80–90	90–95
Moderate	70–80	85–90
Severe	< 70	< 85

Adapted from Waterlow J.[25]
Deficits of weight for height are termed "wasting" and those of height for age are called "stunting."

The statistical analysis of groups of patients, especially those whose anthropometric data place them at less than the 5th or greater than the 95th percentile, has been improved by the use of standard deviation scores (also termed z-scores).[27] By definition, a z-score of +2 represents a value 2 SD above the mean, +3 is 3 SD above the mean, etc. The calculation of a z-score is as follows:

$$z\text{-score} = \frac{(\text{actual value} - \text{median value for age and sex})}{\text{standard deviation of value for age and sex}}$$

Because the mean weight and standard deviation of boys aged 12 months are 10.1 kg and 1.0, respectively, a boy weighing 7 kg at this age has a z-score of $(7 - 10.1)/1.0 = -3.1$. His weight is therefore more than 3 SD below the mean. Z-scores can be calculated for patients with the use of software distributed free of charge by the CDC (<http://www.cdc.gov/epo/epi/epiinfo.htm>).

An increasingly used anthropometric index is the BMI.[28,29] The value, calculated by dividing weight in kilograms by height in meters squared, was shown by Quetelet in the nineteenth century to be a good measure of body mass but only minimally correlated with height, and therefore was a good candidate variable to measure body fatness. As the incidence of obesity has reached epidemic proportions in the United States and other industrialized countries,[30] assessment of BMI has been recommended as a valid and reliable screening tool for obesity. Children with BMIs greater than the 85th percentile for age and sex are termed overweight, and those with BMIs greater than the 95th percentile are obese. Reference values for BMIs are available, and the new growth curves include a visual display of BMI reference curves instead of weight-for-height curves of preadolescents. Because of the dramatic increase in obesity in childhood, the more recent survey data (Third National Health and Nutrition Examination Survey [NHANES III]) were not included in the weight-for-age and BMI-for-age curves for children age 6 years and older.

More sensitive than attained weight and height in diagnosing malnutrition are weight gain and growth velocity data. Serial growth data are very helpful in establishing a patient's previous growth pattern and interpreting its change with medical or nutritional interventions. For example, a substantial number of children with Crohn disease demonstrate a reduction in height velocity in the months preceding their diagnosis,[1] suggesting that malnutrition can be a presenting feature of this disease. Graphs are available for displaying height velocity data. Table 75.3-4 provides data on average rates of weight and height gain for a US sample of healthy children.[31] Determining an infant's or toddler's growth velocity between outpatient visits or in response to a nutritional intervention can help confirm or refute subjective clinical impressions of improved well-being.

BODY COMPOSITION METHODOLOGIES

Perhaps the most significant limitation of the anthropometric techniques summarized above is their inability to precisely measure body composition, namely the amount of body weight that is either fat mass or fat-free mass

TABLE 75.3-4　　MEAN INCREMENTS IN WEIGHT AND
　　　　　　　　　LENGTH FOR HEALTH US CHILDREN

AGE (MO)	WEIGHT (g/d)		LENGTH (mm/d)	
	BOYS	GIRLS	BOYS	GIRLS
Up to 3	31	26	1.07	0.99
1–4	27	24	1.00	0.95
2–5	21	20	0.84	0.80
3–6	18	17	0.69	0.67
4-7	16	15	0.62	0.60
5–8	14	14	0.56	0.56
6–9	13	13	0.52	0.52
7–10	12	12	0.48	0.48
8–11	11	11	0.45	0.46
9–12	11	11	0.43	0.44
10–13	10	10	0.41	0.42
11–14	10	9	0.39	0.40
12–15	9	9	0.37	0.38
13–16	9	9	0.36	0.37
14–17	8	8	0.35	0.36
15–18	8	8	0.33	0.34
16–19	8	8	0.32	0.33
17–20	8	8	0.31	0.32
18–21	7	8	0.30	0.32
19–21	7	7	0.30	0.31
20–23	7	7	0.29	0.30
21–24	7	7	0.28	0.29

Adapted from Guo SM et al.[31]

(FFM). The accepted standard test for body composition is hydrodensitometry (so-called underwater weighing). This technique relies on the principle that body composition can be known from measurements of body density, using assumptions about the average density of fat mass (0.9 g/cm^3) and FFM (1.1 g/cm^3). Weighing the subject in air and then while underwater allows calculations of body density. Obviously, this method is not feasible for infants and young children. Among the available clinical techniques for children are skinfold measurements, bioelectrical impedance analysis (BIA), and dual-energy x-ray absorptiometry (DXA).

Skinfold measurements, which offer the advantage of directly measuring body fat, have been widely used in clinical and epidemiologic studies. They are commonly obtained at four sites: the triceps, biceps, subscapular, and suprailiac. In addition to comparing individual skinfold measurements with published data for age and sex, some investigators have proposed the arithmetic sum of four skinfold measurements as a valid measure of body fatness.[32,33] Triceps skinfold measurement can be used in conjunction with mid–upper arm circumference measures to estimate measures of fat and lean body mass via nomograms[34] or equations:

$$MAMA = \frac{(MUAC - \pi {}^*TSF)^2}{4{}^*\pi}$$

where MAMA = midarm muscle area (cm^2), MUAC = mid–upper arm circumference (cm), TSF = triceps skinfold (cm), and π = 3.1416. This equation assumes that the midarm muscle is circular, that the triceps skinfold gives a good measure of the total rim of midarm fat, and that bone area is negligible. Because these are all questionable

assumptions, others have made modifications in the equation, using either computed tomography[35] or magnetic resonance imaging[36] as gold standards.

Skinfold measurements are prone to significant inter- and intraobserver variation. As a measure of total body fat, they do not measure intra-abdominal fat, and it is therefore not surprising to note the relatively low correlation between skinfold measures and total body fat. Skinfold thickness, as a measure of peripheral versus truncal obesity, may be helpful in the evaluation of some patients. The optimal use of skinfold measurements continues to be debated.[37]

BIA is a noninvasive, nonradioactive measure of body composition analysis. The technique relies on the principle that FFM, being composed of water and ions, conducts an electrical charge better than fat mass.[38] Lean body mass therefore has a lower resistance to current. Reactance, a measure of cell membrane capacitance, is also measured by BIA and, together with resistance, can be used to measure total body water, both intra- and extracellular. Using assumptions about the water content of FFM, FFM is calculated. In patients with human immunodeficiency virus (HIV) infection, BIA has been widely used as a measure of fat and FFM.[39,40] BIA has also been performed in children and compared with anthropometric measures of body fat,[41,42] as well as deuterium dilution[43] and underwater weighing.[44] Because the total body water content of infants and young children is not stable, there are inherent difficulties with using BIA in this age group. Nonetheless, this technique holds promise as a bedside measure of lean body mass. More recent validation of BIA has been performed using larger datasets and a multicomponent body composition model.[45]

The primary role of DXA scanning is to measure bone mineral content, bone mineral density, and total body bone mineral content. Some instruments also measure total body bone mineral content, nonbone lean tissue, and fat, thereby providing body composition information using a three-compartment model. A number of studies have compared measurements of fat mass with DXA versus results obtained from hydrodensitometry,[46] and the correlation between the methods has generally been high. Unlike hydrodensitometry, DXA also measures the composition of particular body parts, thereby allowing one to compare visceral and subcutaneous adiposity. Adults with inflammatory bowel disease have been reported to have lower fat mass and altered ratios of intracellular water to FFM than age-matched healthy controls.[47] DXA scanning has also been used to document the high prevalence of osteopenia in children with inflammatory bowel disease[48] and cerebral palsy.[49] The ultimate applicability of DXA scanning to human body composition is still evolving.[50,51]

LABORATORY ASSESSMENT OF NUTRITIONAL STATUS
Laboratory tests are useful in confirming the assessment made initially by history and physical examination, as well as in diagnosing subclinical nutritional deficiencies. As with any assessment technique, knowledge of the normal

range of parameters and confidence in the reliability and validity of the technique used are crucial.

GENERAL LABORATORY MEASURES
A complete blood count with differential is perhaps the most useful and least expensive laboratory measure of nutritional status. Lymphopenia is a well-known feature of protein-energy malnutrition owing to a reduction in circulating T lymphocytes. Total lymphocyte count (TLC) can be calculated as follows:

$$TLC \ (cells/mm^3) = \frac{white \ blood \ cell \ count \times}{percentage \ of \ lymphocytes}$$

With mild malnutrition, TLC is < 1,500/mm^3; with moderate malnutrition, TLC is 800 to 1,200/mm^3; and with severe malnutrition, TLC is < 800/mm^3. TLC is both a nonspecific and an insensitive measure of nutritional status, however.

Another common functional test of immunocompetence and, therefore, adequate nutritional status is delayed-type hypersensitivity testing. Cutaneous anergy, a delayed or absent response to intradermal injection of antigens, is a consistent finding in moderate to severe malnutrition and has been associated with an increased risk of complications of surgery. Anergy is also a nonspecific measure of nutritional status; other factors, such as the use of immunosuppressive agents, radiotherapy, and critical illness, may be associated with anergy as well.

Nitrogen (N) balance is one of the oldest and best-known methods of assessing nutritional status,[52] having been described as early as the 1830s. It has generally been used as a technique to measure the adequacy of dietary protein. Because negative N balance will ensue if an essential amino acid is ingested in inadequate amounts, the method has also been used to define requirements for specific amino acids and to define which amino acids are essential or nonessential.[53] The N balance technique has also been used to evaluate the response of amino acid supplements to the diet and to determine how exercise or other interventions impact on protein metabolism. Children and adults who are actively gaining lean body mass should be in positive N balance, whereas healthy adults may be said to be in nitrogen equilibrium if N loss is within 5% of N intake.

The concept of the N balance technique is straightforward: N intake is compared to N output to calculate net N balance. The difficulties of the test reside in the full and complete collection of all intake and output. These efforts require cooperative subjects and intensive monitoring. In addition, a stabilization phase of several days to weeks is needed to truly measure the effect of diet on N balance owing to the body's adaptation to the altered intake. Thus, a full N balance is best considered a research tool.

Clinical application of a N balance technique, measuring urine urea N only, has been proposed as an easy method to estimate protein nutriture and the adequacy of nutritional support in hospitalized patients.[54] Urea is the main excretory product of N metabolism, and approximately 85% of the body's N is lost in the urine, the major-

ity via urine urea N. Other sources of N loss include fecal losses, integumental losses (eg, desquamating skin, sweat, hair and nail growth), and miscellaneous losses (eg, saliva, vomitus, blood drawing and menstrual losses, etc). Some of these losses can be high in patients with wounds, burn injuries, or exudative gastrointestinal disease such as ulcerative colitis. Healthy adults excrete 7 to 10 g of urinary urea N per day. Because most proteins contain 16% N, dietary protein intake is customarily divided by a factor of 6.25 to estimate N intake. The equation for calculating N balance is therefore:

$$\begin{aligned} N \ balance &= N \ intake - N \ output \\ &= (24\text{-hour dietary protein intake in g}/ \ 6.25) \\ &\quad - 24\text{-hour UUN} - factor \end{aligned}$$

where UUN = urine urea nitrogen (in grams) and factor = allowance made for uncollected N loss in stool, skin, and miscellaneous sources. In adults, this factor is 2 to 4 g/d, and in children, an estimate of 10 mg/kg/d may be used.

Negative N balance can result from inadequate energy intake, inadequate protein intake, or catabolic stress and lean body mass breakdown. Positive N balance implies adequate energy and/or protein intake and, generally, an anabolic state. Nonetheless, the conceptual and methodologic problems in N balance studies should be recognized. The mere demonstration of positive N balance does not disclose information about N distribution throughout the body or about accumulation of lean body mass. Moreover, a positive N balance can occur despite the presence of other important nutrient deficiencies (eg, some micronutrients).

VISCERAL PROTEIN LEVELS
The blood concentrations of visceral proteins synthesized by the liver are often used to assess nutritional status because decreased levels presumably reflect a reduced supply of amino acid precursors and/or decreased hepatic (and other visceral) mass. The blood levels of these proteins, however, depend on their rates of synthesis, degradation, and escape from the circulatory system. Stable isotopes have been used to measure the rate of visceral protein synthesis, which is generally of greatest interest.[55,56]

Serum proteins are also affected by infectious or catabolic processes (Table 75.3-5). The concentrations of positive acute-phase proteins are increased in infectious or

TABLE 75.3-5   SERUM PROTEINS AND ACUTE ILLNESS

POSITIVE ACUTE-PHASE PROTEINS	NEGATIVE ACUTE-PHASE PROTEINS
C-reactive protein	Albumin
Fibrinogen	Prealbumin
Ferritin	Retinol binding protein
Ceruloplasmin	Transferrin
α_1-Antitrypsin	
α_1-Glycoprotein	

The blood concentrations of positive acute-phase proteins increase with fever, infection, or other catabolic stresses, whereas those of the negative acute-phase proteins generally decline.

other catabolic illnesses, whereas negative acute-phase proteins are decreased in these circumstances.

Albumin is the most abundant serum protein, making up nearly 5 of the 10 g/dL of total protein in the serum. It is the least expensive and easiest protein to measure and therefore is the most commonly used biochemical marker to assess protein status. Because more than half of body albumin is extravascular (primarily in skin and muscle), maintenance of normal serum levels can occur from mobilization of these stores despite prolonged energy or protein inadequacy. Combined with its long half-life of 20 days, these factors make serum albumin a relatively insensitive marker of nutritional status or a marker to follow nutritional interventions. Nonetheless, hypoalbuminemia is quite common among hospitalized pediatric patients[57] and is a surprisingly good predictor of mortality in hospitalized adults. Healthy adults with low normal concentrations of serum albumin have an increased risk of death than do those with higher levels,[58] although this may be a reflection of acute-phase protein shifts in visceral protein synthesis.[59]

Hypoalbuminemia is not necessarily diagnostic of malnutrition; it can occur in situations of decreased synthesis (eg, liver disease, age over 70 years, malignancy), increased losses (eg, nephrosis, protein-losing enteropathy, burn injuries), or redistribution between intra- and extravascular spaces (eg, acute catabolic stress with capillary leak syndrome). Fluid overload can also dilute albumin concentrations, and bed rest can decrease levels 0.5 g/dL.

Prealbumin is another visceral protein, named because of its proximity to albumin on an electrophoretic strip. It functions as a transport molecule for thyroxine—hence its alternative name, transthyretin. Prealbumin circulates in plasma in a 1:1 ratio with retinol binding protein (RBP). Its short half-life (2 days) and high ratio of essential to nonessential amino acids make it a good measure of visceral protein status, more sensitive than albumin as a measure of nutritional recovery. Studies have shown prealbumin to correlate well with N balance,[60,61] and it is likely the best available serum marker of nutritional status. Like albumin, concentrations fall with an acute-phase protein response or liver disease. Levels increase with renal failure.

Like prealbumin, RBP has a small body pool and a rapid response to protein-energy depletion and repletion. Its half-life is 12 hours. Because RBP is metabolized in the kidneys, levels will be artificially high in renal failure. RBP concentrations are lowered in vitamin A deficiency and, as with albumin and prealbumin, with infectious or other catabolic stresses.

Transferrin is another serum protein sometimes used to assess visceral protein status. It is synthesized primarily in the liver and has a half-life of 8 days. Transferrin concentrations are decreased in all situations that depress serum albumin (see above), as well as with steroid therapy, iron overload, and anemia of chronic disease. Increased concentrations are seen in pregnancy, oral contraceptive use, and iron deficiency anemia.

Other serum proteins of possible use in assessing nutritional status include insulin-like growth factor I (IGF-I),

which is the mediator for the anabolic effects of growth hormone. Although IGF-I levels vary with liver and kidney disease, the levels seem to correlate with N balance reasonably well. Fibronectin, a plasma protein with a half-life of 15 hours, has also been used as a marker for nutritional repletion in some studies.

INDIRECT CALORIMETRY AND ENERGY REQUIREMENTS

When considering energy requirements in the pediatric patient, it is helpful to review the components of total energy expenditure (TEE):

$$TEE = BMR + SDA + E_{activity} + E_{growth} + E_{losses}$$

where BMR = basal metabolic rate (the amount of energy required by the body at rest and while fasted), SDA = the specific dynamic action of food or thermic effect of food (the energy produced as heat during digestion and metabolism of food), $E_{activity}$ = energy required for physical activity, E_{growth} = energy needed for somatic growth, and E_{losses} = obligatory energy lost in urine and stool owing to inefficiencies of absorption and metabolism.

BMR is the largest component of TEE, and several equations have been published to calculate BMR from readily available anthropometric data, age and sex. The oldest and best known of these are the Harris Benedict equations for adults (Table 75.3-6). In children, it has been reported that the correlation between measured and predicted BMR is highest for the equations of Schofield (Table 75.3-7).[62,63]

The technique of indirect calorimetry to measure a patient's resting energy expenditure (REE) has recently shed much light on the subject of the energy requirements in health and disease. As the name implies (calor is the Latin word for heat), indirect calorimetry is the determination of heat production of a biochemical reaction by measuring uptake of oxygen and liberation of carbon dioxide. With direct calorimetry, the heat produced by the body at rest is measured. Oxygen consumption and carbon dioxide production measured by the calorimeter are entered into the Weir equation to calculate REE:

$$REE = (3.94 \times VO_2) + (1.06 \times VCO_2) - (2.17 \times UUN)$$

where UUN = urinary urea N excretion (g), used as a correction factor for protein oxidation, VO_2 = oxygen consumption (mL/min), and VCO_2 = carbon dioxide production (mL/min).

Note that although REE measurements are usually taken to approximate BMR, REE actually includes BMR, as well as nonshivering thermogenesis and stress hyper-

TABLE 75.3-6   HARRIS BENEDICT EQUATIONS FOR CALCULATING BMR IN ADULTS

Males:
  BMR = 66 + (13.7 × weight [kg]) + (5 × height [cm]) − (6.9 × age [yr])
Females:
  BMR = 665 + (9.6 × weight [kg]) + (1.8 × height [cm]) − (4.7 × age [yr])

Adapted from Harris JA and Benedict FG. A biometric study of basal metabolism. Washington (DC): Carnegie Institution of Washington; 1919. Publication No.: 279. BMR = basal metabolic rate.

TABLE 75.3-7   SCHOFIELD EQUATIONS FOR CALCULATING BASAL METABOLIC RATE IN CHILDREN

GROUP (AGE IN YR)	EQUATION
Males	
0–3	REE = 0.167W + 151.74H – 617.6
3–10	REE = 19.59W + 13.03H + 414.9
10–18	REE = 16.25W + 13.72H + 515.5
> 18	REE = 15.057W + 1.004H + 705.8
Females	
0–3	REE = 16.252W + 10.232H – 413.5
3–10	REE = 16.969W + 1.618H + 371.2
10–18	REE = 8.365W + 4.65H + 200
> 18	REE = 13.623W + 23.8H + 98.2

Adapted from Schofield W.[63]
REE = kcal/day, W = weight (kg), and H = height (cm).

metabolism. The difference between REE and BMR is estimated to be 10% or less.

The utility of indirect calorimetry in assessing energy needs has been evaluated by many investigators in adult[64] and pediatric patients[62,65]; these and other studies have generally confirmed that predictive equations have limited validity in hospitalized or sick patients. Among children with neurodevelopmental delay, studies of REE have shown that their basal energy needs are significantly lower than those predicted by a variety of methods.[6,66] These data have serious implications for a patient population often fed by gastrostomy tube and may explain their tendency to become overweight. A recent study of energy expenditure in children undergoing stem cell transplant has also suggested that these patients are not as hypermetabolic as previously thought.[67] Another study of patients with inflammatory bowel disease reported an increased REE in Crohn disease patients as opposed to healthy controls and those with ulcerative colitis.[68] More studies will be needed to determine whether patients with inflammatory bowel disease truly have an increased energy expenditure and, if so, whether this contributes to their undernutrition.

Indirect calorimetry can also help determine whether a patient is being overfed. The ratio of VCO_2 to VO_2 is termed the respiratory quotient (RQ), which is used to estimate substrate oxidation. For example, in the case of pure glucose oxidation, one mole of carbohydrate reacts with 6 moles of oxygen to create 6 moles each of water and carbon dioxide:

$$C_6H_{12}O_6 + 6\ O_2 \rightarrow 6\ CO_2 + 6\ H_2O$$

The RQ would then be 6/6 = 1.0. When long-chain fat such as palmitic acid is oxidized,

$$CH_3(CH_2CH_2)_7COOH + 23\ O_2 \rightarrow 16\ CO_2 + 16\ H_2O$$

The RQ = 16/23 = 0.695. Thus, the RQ in a fasted state is normally 0.70 to 1.00, and the RQ in this range usually represents a mixed substrate oxidation. The lower RQ noted for lipid oxidation has been used as a rationale for feeding patients with advanced lung disease a diet higher in fat than

in glucose to avoid an increased carbon dioxide load to excrete, although this strategy remains controversial.[69] When excess energy is provided and lipogenesis results,

$$9\ C_6H_{12}O_6 + 8\ O_2 \rightarrow 2\ CH_3(CH_2CH_2)_7COOH + 22\ CO_2 + 22\ H_2O$$

The resulting RQ = 22/8 = 2.75. Therefore, the finding of an RQ significantly greater than 1.0 is consistent with energy intake in excess of energy requirements. Other reasons would include hyperventilation (wherein CO_2 is excreted at high rates) or failure to achieve a steady state in gas measurement.

STABLE ISOTOPES AND ENERGY REQUIREMENTS

The advent in the 1950s of using doubly labeled water (two stable isotopes of water: ^2H_2O and $H_2^{18}O$) to measure TEE was a breakthrough in nutritional science. For the first time, TEE in free-living individuals could be validly and reliably measured, and the technique was applied widely in the 1980s and continues to be an important tool for determining energy requirements and validating epidemiologic questionnaires.[70] The method relies on the fact that ^2H_2O is excreted solely in body water, but $H_2^{18}O$ is excreted via water losses but also via the carbonic anhydrase system, so that measuring the differential decay rates of the two isotopes provides a measure of CO_2 production from which TEE can be calculated.

The advantages of this technique include the fact that it is noninvasive and safe, requires only serial urine collection, and provides data over a 7- to 14-day period. It has been widely used in pediatric studies.[71–73]

An alternative isotopic approach is the use of labeled bicarbonate (eg, $NaH^{13}CO_3$), which measures energy expenditure in an analogous fashion to doubly labeled water but over a shorter time frame. Studies in neonates and other pediatric subjects have confirmed the validity of this technique,[74] and it is generally less costly than doubly labeled water.

NUTRITIONAL REQUIREMENTS

DEFINITIONS OF ESSENTIAL AND NONESSENTIAL NUTRIENTS

Perhaps the most revolutionary concept in modern nutritional science has been the change in our appreciation of what makes a nutrient "essential."[75] As noted above, the classic experiments of Rose and colleagues defined an essential amino acid as one that is required in the diet of healthy human adults to maintain N equilibrium. Largely using this definition, the 20 amino acids were defined as either essential or nonessential. Indeed, the first half of the twentieth century was marked by a tremendous outpouring of scientific knowledge in the field of nutrition, with the essential nature of most vitamins (Table 75.3-8) and minerals (Table 75.3-9) being determined.

However, the practical and theoretical limitations of balance experiments, as well as their inapplicability to sick or pediatric patients, have been noted. A variety of techniques have therefore been applied to augment how nutrients have come to be defined as essential and what the precise

TABLE 75.3-8   VITAMINS: FUNCTION, DEFICIENCY STATES, AND LABORATORY ASSESSMENT TECHNIQUES

VITAMIN	FUNCTION	CLINICAL DEFICIENCY STATE	LABORATORY ASSESSMENT
Vitamin A (retinol [β-carotene is dietary precursor])	Retinal in rhodopsin and iodopsin Carbohydrate transfer to glycoprotein Maintains epithelial integrity Required for cell proliferation	Night blindness Xerophthalmia Bitot spots Keratomalacia	Plasma retinol (HPLC) Plasma retinol binding protein Relative dose response Dark adaptation test Liver biopsy concentration
Vitamin D (cholecalciferol D_3 [endogenous], ergocalciferol D_2 [synthetic])	Regulates calcium and phosphate Gut absorption, excretion by kidney, and bone resorption	Rickets/osteomalacia Dental caries Hypocalcemia/hypophosphatemia Increased alkaline phosphatase Phosphaturia, aminoaciduria	Plasma 25-hydroxyvitamin D (HPLC) Serum alkaline phosphatase, calcium, and phosphate Radiography Bone densitometry
Vitamin E (α-tocopherol)	Cell membrane antioxidant Inhibits polyunsaturated fatty acid oxidation	Anemia/hemolysis Neurologic deficit (ocular palsy, wide-based gait, decreased DTRs) Altered prostaglandin synthesis	Plasma tocopherol (HPLC) (corrected for total or LDL cholesterol) Hydrogen peroxide hemolysis
Vitamin K (phylloquinone, menadione [synthetic])	Carboxylation of clotting factors Affects bone formation	Coagulopathy/prolonged PT Abnormal bone matrix synthesis	PT (prolonged) Plasma phylloquinone Clotting factor levels Proteins induced by vitamin K absence or antagonists II
Vitamin B_1 (thiamine)	Oxidative phosphorylation Pentose phosphate shunt Aldehyde transferase Triosephosphate isomerase	Beriberi ("wet" or "dry") Cardiac failure/neuropathy Korsakoff syndrome Wernicke encephalopathy Lactic acidosis	Red cell transketolase activity Whole blood level (HPLC) Urine thiamine-to-creatinine ratio
Vitamin B_2 (riboflavin)	Oxidation/reduction reactions	Seborrheic dermatitis/cheilosis/glossitis Decreased fatty acid oxidation Altered vitamin B_6 activation to coenzyme Decreased tryptophan to niacin conversion	Red cell glutathione reductase activity Red cell flavine adenine dinucleotide Urine riboflavin-to-creatinine ratio
Vitamin B_6 (pyridoxine)	Aminotransferase reactions Irritability/convulsions Decreased tryptophan to niacin conversion	Dermatitis/cheilosis/glossitis Microcytic anemia/weight loss Decreased serum transaminases Peripheral neuritis/irritability/convulsions	Red cell aminotransferase activity Plasma pyridoxal phosphate (HPLC) Tryptophan loading test Urine 4-pyridoxic acid
Vitamin B_{12} (cyanocobalamin)	Methyl group donor Sulfur amino acid conversion Branched-chain amino acid catabolism	Megaloblastic anemia Hypersegmented neutrophils Demyelination/posterior spinal column changes Methylmalonicacidemia Hyperhomocysteinemia	Plasma level (RIA or microbiologic) Schilling test Plasma homocysteine Deoxyuridine suppression test
Vitamin C (ascorbate)	Reducing agent (regenerates vitamin E) Cofactor for hydroxylators Noradrenaline/carnitine synthesis? Cholesterol synthesis? Leukocyte function	Scurvy Perifollicular/petechial hemorrhages Hematologic abnormalities Poor wound healing Impaired collagen synthesis Psychological disturbances	Plasma level (enzyme assay/HPLC) Leukocyte concentration (longer term) Whole blood concentration Urine concentration
Folic acid	Methyl group donor DNA/RNA synthesis Amino acid metabolism	Megaloblastic anemia, neutropenia Altered amino acid metabolism Impaired growth Diarrhea	Plasma level (RIA/microbiologic) Red cell level
Biotin	Coenzyme for carboxylases, decarboxylases, and transcarboxylases	Multiple carboxylase deficiency Organic acidemia/acidosis Dermatitis/alopecia CNS: seizures/ataxia/depression	Plasma (microbiologic assay) Plasma lactate Urine organic acids Lymphocyte carboxylase

(continues)

TABLE 75.3-8   Continued

VITAMIN	FUNCTION	CLINICAL DEFICIENCY STATE	LABORATORY ASSESSMENT
Niacin	Dehydrogenase activity	Pellagra: diarrhea/dermatitis/ dementia Glossitis/stomatitis/vaginitis Impaired absorption of fat, carbohydrate, and vitamin B_{12} Achlorhydria	Urine ratio of metabolites (N-methylnicotinamide: 2-pyridone) Tryptophan load Red cell NAD or NAD:NADP ratio
Pantothenic acid	Pyruvate dehydrogenase cofactor Carrier of acyl groups Acetylation of alcohol/amines	Postural hypotension Anorexia and vomiting Reduced acetylation Neuromuscular defects/hyperreflexia	Urine excretion Whole blood level (RIA/microbiologic)

Adapted from Loughrey C and Duggan C.[97]

CNS = central nervous system; DNA = deoxyribonucleic acid; DTR = deep tendon reflex; HPLC = high-performance liquid chromatography; LDL = low-density lipoprotein; NAD = nicotinamide adenine dinucleotide; NADP = nicotinamide adenine dinucleotide phosphate; PT = prothrombin time; RIA = radioimmunoassay; RNA = ribonucleic acid.

requirements are in health and disease. In addition to balance studies, investigators have used the "factorial approach" to estimate requirements. This method, which was pioneered in estimating protein requirements in children,[76] is a theoretical approach that relies on the following factors: the body content of a nutrient needed for normal body growth; the amount lost in skin, urine, and other secretions; and the efficiency of gastrointestinal absorption.

Another approach to define optimal nutrient intakes, especially well suited for infants, has been the "analogy to breast milk" approach. This approach starts with the assumption that the types and amounts of nutrients commonly found in human breast milk are reasonable starting points in estimating human nutrient requirements. Although for many nutrients, and perhaps more significantly non-nutrients, this concept has considerable merit, the very low vitamin D content of human milk points out the limitations of this approach alone.[77]

Among the more recent and attractive options are studies in which the metabolic pathways of nutrients are measured using stable isotopes.[78] These experiments employ nonradioactive probes to quantify rates of nutrient synthesis, absorption, excretion, and flux into the bloodstream and have allowed better and more precise estimates of nutrient requirements. Important examples of this work include the use of $^2H_2^{18}O$ (so-called doubly labeled water) to measure TEE[79]; ^{13}C-leucine to measure oxidation rates of a large number of amino acids[80]; ^{67}Zn, ^{68}Zn, and ^{70}Zn for studies of zinc nutriture[81,82]; ^{44}Ca, ^{46}Ca, and other calcium isotopes for the assessment of calcium absorption[83]; and many others.

Well-conducted clinical trials of nutrient supplementation have also been used to more fully define nutrient requirements, especially in a variety of disease states. The finding of an improved clinical or metabolic outcome with supplementation of a nutrient normally considered nonessential has led to the introduction of the term "conditionally essential." Conditionally essential nutrients have been defined as those nutrients that normally are synthesized endogenously by the body but whose synthetic rates may be inadequate to meet needs in times of disease, stress, or developmental stages. Examples of nutrients thought to be conditionally essential include several amino acids (cysteine,[84] taurine, and glutamine[85]), inositol, nucleotides,[86] and others.[75] Other nutrients well known to be essential but increasingly appreciated in optimizing health include folate (which prevents neural tube defects[87] and lowers plasma homocysteine levels[88]), vitamin A (which reduces mortality rates in communities at risk of deficiency[89]), and zinc (which reduces rates of diarrheal diseases and respiratory infections[90,91]).

Finally, the use of nutrients and other biologic substances in high, perhaps pharmacologic, doses has spawned the terms "nutritional pharmacology" or "nutraceuticals" to describe their use.[92] Among nutrients used in this fashion are precursors of nutrients (eg, organic phosphates, dipeptides), probiotics (eg, lactobacilli), prebiotics (eg, fructose oligosaccharides), and various growth factors (eg, growth hormone, IGF, epidermal growth factor).

NEW DEFINITIONS

In concert with the increasing appreciation of essential and conditionally essential nutrients has been a change in how nutrient requirements are set. Previous levels of requirements had largely been derived from the observations of the metabolic derangements and/or clinical signs of deficiency states that would ensue when otherwise healthy subjects consumed a diet with inadequate amounts of the nutrient in question. Indeed, the genesis of the Food and Nutrition Board in the 1940s was in part due to the finding of a high frequency of malnutrition among draftees for the US armed forces,[93] and vitamin and mineral enrichment of wheat flour soon followed. With the growing realization of the importance of diet in influencing long-term health outcomes as well, published nutrient requirements have been rethought and redesigned. In the 1990s, nutrition scientists in the United States and Canada embarked on a thorough revision of the Recommended Dietary Allowances (RDAs; United States) and Recommended Nutrient Intakes (Canada) and published new definitions more suitable to optimizing health. These efforts were spearheaded by the Institute of Medicine of the National Academy of Science, a private, nongovernmental organization chartered by the US federal government to provide advice on scientific matters.

TABLE 75.3-9   MINERALS AND TRACE ELEMENTS: FUNCTION, DEFICIENCY STATES, AND LABORATORY
ASSESSMENT TECHNIQUES

MINERAL/ TRACE ELEMENT	FUNCTION	CLINICAL DEFICIENCY STATE	LABORATORY ASSESSMENT
Calcium	Bone structure Cell metabolic regulator Nerve excitation threshold	Bone demineralization Tetany/seizures Cardiac arrhythmias	Plasma total calcium Plasma free calcium in altered protein binding (eg, hypoalbuminemia, acidosis) Radiographs CT and photon densitometry
Chromium	Glucose tolerance factor Metabolism of nucleic acids ? Iodine/thyroid function	Glucose intolerance Neuropathy/encephalopathy Altered nitrogen metabolism Increased free fatty acids	Plasma chromium Glucose tolerance
Copper	Cofactor for several enzymes including superoxide dismutase, tyrosinase, ferrochelatase, cytochrome c oxidase	Hypochromic anemia, neutropenia Skin depigmentation Dyslipidemia CNS problems	Plasma copper Plasma ceruloplasmin (ferrochelatase) Liver biopsy concentration Superoxide dismutase activity
Iodide	Component of thyroid hormones	Goiter Cretinism	Thyroid hormones, TSH Urinary iodide-to-creatinine ratio
Iron	Heme synthesis Component of cytochromes	Hypochromic microcytic anemia Altered oxidative phosphorylation Diminished concentrative ability Decreased exercise tolerance	Plasma iron and ferritin Total iron-binding capacity Hemoglobin/hematocrit, red cell indices RBC zinc protoporphyrin-to-heme ratio Bone marrow aspirate stain
Magnesium	Cofactor for hexokinase and phosphokinase Alters ribosomal aggregation in protein synthesis Increases nerve excitation threshold	Cardiac dysrhythmias Neuromuscular excitability Decreased PTH level/activity Hypocalcemia/hypokalemia Convulsions	Plasma total or free magnesium Magnesium loading test
Manganese	Mucopolysaccharide synthesis Cholesterol synthesis Cartilage/bone formation Pyruvate carboxylase cofactor Superoxide dismutase cofactor	Dermatitis Decreased clotting factors Decreased nail/hair growth ?Hair color change	Plasma level Whole blood level Mitochondrial superoxide dismutase
Phosphorus	Bone structure Cell membrane structure Energy use Glycogen deposition Acid-base balance: buffering Oxygen release (2,3-DPG)	Tissue hypoxia Respiratory failure (ventilatory dependence) Hemolytic anemia Rickets CNS abnormalities	Serum/plasma levels Alkaline phosphatase activity Radiography Densitometry Renal tubular excretion threshold
Selenium	Glutathione peroxidase constituent Thyroid hormone metabolism	Myositis Cardiomyopathy Nail bed changes Macrocytic anemia?	Plasma concentration Glutathione peroxidase acitivity Nail/hair selenium
Zinc	Cofactor for > 70 enzymes Immune function Cell replication Vision	Skin lesions/poor wound healing Immune dysfunction (especially T cell) Anorexia/dysgeusia Growth failure/nitrogen wasting Hypogonadism/delayed puberty Diarrhea	Plasma concentration Alkaline phosphatase activity Urinary excretion Leukocyte concentration

Adapted from Loughrey C and Duggan C.[97]

CNS = central nervous system; CT = computed tomography; DPG = 2,3-diphosphoglycerate; PTH = parathyroid hormone; RBC = red blood cell; TSH = thyroid-stimulating hormone.

The mere prevention of a deficiency state is no longer the gold standard in setting nutrient requirement levels; instead, a broader concept of nutrition health has been taken. Nutritional requirements are those levels of intakes that are most consistent with optimal physiologic functioning and well-being at all life stages. Examples include using bone mineral accretion data in setting dietary calcium intake levels and dental caries protection data in setting reference intakes of fluoride.[94] Table 75.3-10 outlines the definitions now used to describe nutrient requirements since the publication of these new standards in 1994. Figure 75.3-1 shows the relationship between the three Dietary Reference Intakes (DRIs) and the risks of dietary inadequacy and adverse effects at various levels of dietary intake.

TABLE 75.3-10 DEFINITIONS OF NUTRITIONAL REQUIREMENTS TO SET STANDARDS OF INTAKE (FNB/IOM/NAS)

TERM	ABBREVIATION	YEAR INTRODUCED	DEFINITION/USE
Old			
Recommended Dietary Allowances	RDAs	1943	Average daily dietary intake value sufficient to meet the requirement of nearly all (97–98%) healthy individuals in a group; more recently, the term has been calculated as EAR plus 2 SD of the EAR (see below)
New			
Dietary Reference Intakes	DRIs	1994	Umbrella term including RDA, EAR, AI, and UL (see below)
Estimated Average Requirement	EAR	1994	Nutrient intake value that is estimated to meet the requirement of half the individuals in a group
Adequate Intake	AI	1994	Used when no EAR is available and therefore no RDA can be calculated; nutrient intake value based on observed or experimentally determined approximations of nutrient intakes by a group or groups of healthy people
Tolerable Upper Intake Level	UI	1994	Highest level of a daily nutrient intake that is likely to pose no risks of adverse health effects to almost all individuals in the general population

FNB/IOM/NAS = Food and Nutrition Board of the Institute of Medicine/National Academy of Sciences.

Of the new DRIs, RDAs are still the most appropriate measure to use when reviewing an individual's dietary intake (because, by definition, dietary intake at or above the RDA is likely to be adequate for healthy persons). Conversely, because an individual's specific requirement for each nutrient cannot be easily determined, the fact that his/her intake does not meet the RDA is not a sufficient cause to conclude that the diet is deficient. Dietary intake patterns in healthy individuals follow a distribution curve showing a range of intake levels associated with normal health. The risks of dietary inadequacy increase significantly as intake falls to less than 2 SD below the Estimated Average Requirement (EAR). In contrast to the RDAs, Adequate Intakes (AIs) and EARs are better suited to evaluating dietary patterns of groups of subjects rather than individuals alone.

Tables 75.3-11 through 75.3-14 present the most recently published data from the Food and Nutrition Board for a variety of micronutrients, protein, and energy. In cases for which no EAR has been set, the AI is used instead.

Concurrent with the new terminology proposed by the Food and Nutrition Board, new definitions from the US Food and Drug Administration (FDA) used for food labeling have been published (Table 75.3-15). The similarity between these sets of abbreviations may lead to some confusion, but their functions are distinct. The DRIs of the Food and Nutrition Board are published as proposed reference dietary intakes for healthy US and Canadian persons by a nongovernmental institute. In contrast, the Daily Reference Values (DRVs) and Reference Daily Intakes (RDIs) are published by the FDA and are designed to help consumers use food information to plan a healthy diet. Using an estimated energy intake of 2,000 or 2,500 calories per day, the DRVs express nutrient content as a proportion of generally recommended guidelines for a healthy diet (eg, less than 30% of calories as fat, less than 10% of calories as saturated fat, 11.5 g of fiber per 1,000 calories, etc). A second role of these new terms is to allow objective assessment and regulation of foods marketed as "low fat" or "high fiber." For example,

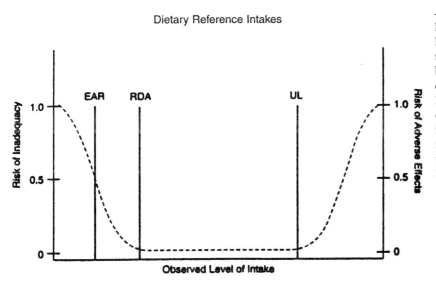

Dietary Reference Intakes

FIGURE 75.3-1 The relationship between Estimated Average Requirement (EAR), Recommended Dietary Allowance (RDA), and Tolerable Upper Intake Level (UL). The risk of inadequate intake is 50% at the EAR, 2 to 3% at the RDA, and close to 0% at the UL. Risks of adverse effects are close to 0% at the UL but increase with increasing intake. Reproduced with permission from Standing Committee on the Scientific Evaluation of Dietary Reference Intakes, Food and Nutrition Board, Institute of Medicine.[94]

TABLE 75.3-11   CRITERIA AND DIETARY REFERENCE INTAKE VALUES FOR PROTEIN BY LIFE STAGE GROUP

LIFE STAGE GROUP	CRITERION	AI OR RDA FOR REFERENCE INDIVIDUAL (g/d)		EAR (g/kg/d)		RDA (g/kg/d)		AI (g/kg/d)
		MALES	FEMALES	MALES	FEMALES	MALES	FEMALES	
0–6 mo	Average consumption of protein from human milk	9.1 (AI)	9.1 (AI)					1.52
7–12 mo	Nitrogen equilibrium + protein deposition	13.5	13.5	1.1	1.1	1.5	1.5	
1–3 yr	Nitrogen equilibrium + protein deposition	13	13	0.88	0.88	1.10	1.10	
4–8 yr	Nitrogen equilibrium + protein deposition	19	19	0.76	0.76	0.95	0.95	
9–13 yr	Nitrogen equilibrium + protein deposition	34	34	0.76	0.76	0.95	0.95	
14–18 yr	Nitrogen equilibrium + protein deposition	52	46	0.73	0.71	0.85	0.85	
>18 yr	Nitrogen equilibrium	56	46	0.66	0.66	0.80	0.80	

Adapted from Standing Committee on the Scientific Evaluation of Dietary Reference Intakes, Food and Nutrition Board, Institute of Medicine.[98]
EAR = Estimated Average Requirement: the intake that meets the estimated nutrient needs of half of the individuals in a group.
RDA = Recommended Dietary Allowance: the intake that meets the nutrient need of almost all (97–98%) of individuals in a group.
AI = Adequate Intake: the observed average or experimentally determined intake by a defined population or subgroup that appears to sustain a defined nutritional status, such as growth rate, normal circulating nutrient values, or other functional indicators of health. The AI is used if sufficient scientific evidence is not available to derive an EAR. For healthy infants receiving human milk, the AI is the mean intake. The AI is not equivalent to an RDA.

TABLE 75.3-12   CRITERIA AND DIETARY REFERENCE INTAKE VALUES FOR ENERGY BY ACTIVE INDIVIDUALS BY LIFE STAGE GROUP (FOR HEALTHY MODERATELY ACTIVE AMERICANS AND CANADIANS)

LIFE STAGE GROUP	CRITERION	ACTIVE PAL EER (kcal/d)	
		MALE	FEMALE
0–6 mo	Average consumption of protein from human milk	570	520 (3 mo)
7–12 mo	Nitrogen equilibrium + protein deposition	743	676 (9 mo)
1–2 yr	Nitrogen equilibrium + protein deposition	1,046	992 (24 mo)
3–8 yr	Nitrogen equilibrium + protein deposition	1,742	1,642 (6 yr)
9–13 yr	Nitrogen equilibrium + protein deposition	2,279	2,071 (11 yr)
14–18 yr	Nitrogen equilibrium + protein deposition	3,152	2,368 (16 yr)
> 18 yr	Nitrogen equilibrium	3,067*	2,403* (19 yr)
Pregnancy			
14–18 yr	Adolescent female EER plus change in TEE plus pregnancy energy deposition		
	1st trimester		2,368 (16 yr)
	2nd trimester		2,708 (16 yr)
	3rd trimester		2,820 (16 yr)
19–50 yr	Adult female EER plus change in TEE plus pregnancy energy deposition		
	1st trimester		2,403† (19 yr)
	2nd trimester		2,743† (19 yr)
	3rd trimester		2,855† (19 yr)
Lactation			
14–18 yr	Adolescent female EER plus milk energy output minus weight loss		
	1st 6 mo		2,698 (16 yr)
	2nd 6 mo		2,768 (16 yr)
19–50 yr	Adult female EER plus milk energy output minus weight loss		
	1st 6 mo		2,733‡ (19 yr)
	2nd 6 mo		2,803‡ (19 yr)

Adapted from Standing Committee on the Scientific Evaluation of Dietary Reference Intakes, Food and Nutrition Board, Institute of Medicine.[98]
EER = estimated energy requirement; PAL = physical activity level; TEE = total energy expenditure. The intake that meets the average energy expenditure of individuals at the reference height, weight, and age.
*Subtract 10 kcal/d for males and 7 kcal/d for females for each year of age above 19 years.
†The Estimated Average Requirement (EAR) and Recommended Dietary Allowance (RDA) for pregnancy are only for the second half of pregnancy. For the first half of pregnancy, the protein requirements are the same as those of the nonpregnant woman.
‡In addition to the EAR and RDA of the nonlactating adolescent or woman.

TABLE 75.3-13   DIETARY REFERENCE INTAKES FOR MINERALS

LIFE STAGE GROUP	CALCIUM (mg/d)	CHROMIUM (mg/d)	COPPER (mg/d)	FLUORIDE (mg/d)	IODINE (mg/d)	IRON (mg/d)	MAGNESIUM (mg/d)	MANGANESE (mg/d)	MOLYBDENUM (mg/d)	PHOSPHORUS (mg/d)	SELENIUM (mg/d)	ZINC (mg/d)
Infants												
0–6 mo	210*	0.2*	200*	0.01*	110*	0.27*	30*	0.003*	2*	100*	15*	2*
7–12 mo	270*	5.5*	220*	0.5*	130*	11*	75*	0.6*	3*	275*	20*	3
Children												
1–3 yr	500*	11*	340	0.7*	90	7	80	1.2*	17	460	20	3
4–8 y	800*	15*	440	1*	90	10	130	1.5*	22	500	30	5
Males												
9–13 yr	1,300*	25*	700	2*	120	8	240	1.9*	34	1,250	40	8
14–18 yr	1,300*	35*	890	3*	150	11	410	2.2*	43	1,250	55	11
19–30 yr	1,000*	35*	900	4*	150	8	400	2.3*	45	700	55	11
31–50 yr	1,000*	35*	900	4*	150	8	420	2.3*	45	700	55	11
51–70 yr	1,200*	30*	900	4*	150	8	420	2.3*	45	700	55	11
> 70 yr	1,200*	30*	900	4*	150	8	420	2.3*	45	700	55	11
Females												
9–13 yr	1,300*	21*	700	2*	120	8	240	1.6*	34	1,250	40	8
14–18 yr	1,300*	24*	890	3*	150	15	360	1.6*	43	1,250	55	9
19–30 yr	1,000*	25*	900	3*	150	18	310	1.8*	45	700	55	8
31–50 yr	1,000*	25*	900	3*	150	18	320	1.8*	45	700	5	8
51–70 yr	1,200*	20*	900	3*	150	8	320	1.8*	45	700	55	8
> 70 yr	1,200*	20*	900	3*	150	8	320	1.8*	45	700	55	8
Pregnancy												
≤ 18 yr	1,300*	29*	1,000	3*	220	27	400	2.0*	50	1,250	60	13
19–30 yr	1,000*	30*	1,000	3*	220	27	350	2.0*	50	700	60	11
31–50 yr	1,000*	30*	1,000	3*	220	27	360	2.0*	50	700	60	11
Lactation												
≤ 18 yr	1,300*	44*	1,300	3*	290	10	360	2.6*	50	1,250	70	14
19–30 yr	1,000*	45*	1,300	3*	290	9	310	2.6*	50	700	70	12
31–50 yr	1,000*	45*	1,300	3*	290	9	320	2.6*	50	700	70	12

Adapted from Standing Committee on the Scientific Evaluation of Dietary Reference Intakes, Food and Nutrition Board, Institute of Medicine.[94,99–101]

This table (taken from the Dietary Reference Intake reports (see <www.nap.edu>) presents Recommended Dietary Allowances (RDAs) in bold type and Adequate Intakes (AIs) in ordinary type followed by an asterisk. RDAs and AIs may both be used as goals for individual intake. RDAs are set to meet the needs of almost all (97–98%) individuals in a group. For healthy breastfed infants, the AI is the mean intake. The AI for other life stage and gender groups is believed to cover the needs of all individuals in the group, but lack of data or uncertainty in the data prevents specifying with confidence the percentage of individuals covered by this intake.

†As retinol activity equivalents (RAEs). 1 RAE = 1 mg retinol, 12 mg β-carotene, 24 mg α-carotene, or 24 mg β-cryptoxanthin. The RAE for dietary provitamin A carotenoids is twofold greater than retinol equivalent (RE), whereas the RAE for preformed vitamin A is the same as RE.

‡Cholecalciferol. 1 mg cholecalciferol = 40 IU vitamin D.

§In the absence of adequate exposure to sunlight.

‖As α-tocopherol. α-Tocopherol includes RRR-α-tocopherol, the only form of α-tocopherol that occurs naturally in foods, and the 2R-stereoisomeric forms of α-tocopherol (RRR-, RSR-, RRS-, and RRS-α-tocopherol) that occur in fortified foods and supplements. It does not include the 2S-stereoisomeric forms of α-tocopherol (SRR-, SSR, SRS-, and SSS-α-tocopherol), also found in fortified foods and supplements.

#As niacin equivalents (NE). 1 mg of niacin = 60 mg of tryptophan; 0–6 mo = preformed niacin (not NE).

**As dietary folate equivalents (DFE). 1 DFE = 1 mg food folate = 0.6 mg of folic acid from fortified food or as a supplement consumed with food = 0.5 mg of a supplement taken on an empty stomach.

††Although AIs have been set for choline, there are few data to assess whether a dietary supply of choline is needed at all stages of the life cycle, and it may be that the choline requirement can be met by endogenous synthesis at some of these stages.

‡‡Because 10 to 30% of older people may malabsorb food-bound vitamin B_{12}, it is advisable for those older than 50 years to meet their RDA mainly by consuming foods fortified with vitamin B_{12} or a supplement containing vitamin B_{12}.

§§In view of evidence linking folate intake with neural tube defects in the fetus, it is recommended that all women capable of becoming pregnant consume 400 mg from supplements or fortified foods in addition to intake of food folate from a varied diet.

TABLE 75.3-14 DIETARY REFERENCE INTAKES FOR VITAMINS

LIFE STAGE GROUP	VITAMIN A (mg/d)†	VITAMIN C (mg/d)	VITAMIN D (mg/d)†,§	VITAMIN E (mg/d)‖	VITAMIN K (mg/d)	THIAMINE (mg/d)	RIBOFLAVIN (mg/d)	NIACIN (mg/d)#	VITAMIN B₆ (mg/d)	FOLATE (mg/d)*,**	VITAMIN B₁₂ (mg/d)	PANTOTHENIC ACID (mg/d)	BIOTIN (mg/d)	CHOLINE†† (mg/d)
Infants														
0–6 mo	400*	40*	5*	4*	2.0*	0.2*	0.3*	2*	0.1*	65*	0.4*	1.7*	5*	125*
7–12 mo	500*	50*	5*	5*	2.5*	0.3*	0.4*	4*	0.3*	80*	0.5*	1.8*	6*	150*
Children														
1–3 yr	300	15	5*	6	30*	0.5	0.5	6	0.5	150	0.9	2*	8*	200*
4–8 yr	400	25	5*	7	55*	0.6	0.6	8	0.6	200	1.2	3*	12*	250*
Males														
9–13 yr	600	45	5*	11	60*	0.9	0.9	12	1.0	300	1.8	4*	20*	375*
14–18 yr	900	75	5*	15	75*	1.2	1.3	16	1.3	400	2.4	5*	25*	550*
19–30 yr	900	90	5*	15	120*	1.2	1.3	16	1.3	400	2.4	5*	30*	550*
31–50 yr	900	90	5*	15	120*	1.2	1.3	16	1.3	400	2.4	5*	30*	550*
51–70 yr	900	90	10*	15	120*	1.2	1.3	16	1.7	400	2.4‡‡	5*	30*	550*
> 70 yr	900	90	15*	15	120*	1.2	1.3	16	1.7	400	2.4‡‡	5*	30*	550*
Females														
9–13 yr	600	45	5*	11	60*	0.9	0.9	12	1.0	300	1.8	4*	20*	375*
14–18 yr	700	65	5*	15	75*	1.0	1.0	14	1.2	400	2.4	5*	25*	400*
19–30 yr	700	75	5*	15	90*	1.1	1.1	14	1.3	400	2.4	5*	30*	425*
31–50 yr	700	75	5*	15	90*	1.1	1.1	14	1.3	400	2.4	5*	30*	425*
51–70 yr	700	75	10*	15	90*	1.1	1.1	14	1.5	400§§	2.4	5*	30*	425*
> 70 yr	700	75	15*	15	90*	1.1	1.1	14	1.5	400§§	2.4	5*	30*	425*
Pregnancy														
≤ 18 yr	750	80	5*	15	75*	1.4	1.4	18	1.9	600***	2.6	6*	30*	450*
19–30 yr	770	85	5*	15	90*	1.4	1.4	18	1.9	600***	2.6	6*	30*	450*
31–50 yr	750	85	5*	15	90*	1.4	1.4	18	1.9	600***	2.6	6*	30*	450*
Lactation														
≤ 18 yr	1,200	115	5*	19	75*	1.4	1.6	17	2.0	500	2.8	7*	35*	550*
19–30 yr	1,300	120	5*	19	90*	1.4	1.6	17	2.0	500	2.8	7*	35*	550*
31–50 yr	1,300	120	5*	19	90*	1.4	1.6	17	2.0	500	2.8	7*	35*	550*

Adapted from Standing Committee on the Scientific Evaluation of Dietary Reference Intakes, Food and Nutrition Board, Institute of Medicine.[94,99–101]
This table presents Recommended Dietary Allowances (RDAs) in bold type and Adequate Intakes (AIs) in ordinary type followed by an asterisk. RDAs are set to meet the needs of almost all (97–98%) individuals in a group. For healthy breastfed infants, the AI is the mean intake. The AI for other life stage and gender groups is believed to cover the needs of all individuals in the group, but lack of data or uncertainty in the data prevents specifying with confidence the percentage of individuals covered by this intake.
Adapted from Dietary Reference Intakes for calcium, phosphorous, magnesium, vitamin D, and fluoride (1997); Dietary Reference Intakes for thiamine, riboflavin, niacin, vitamin B₆, folate, vitamin B₁₂, pantothenic acid, biotin, and choline (1998); Dietary Reference Intakes for vitamin C, vitamin E, selenium, and carotenoids (2000); and Dietary Reference Intakes for vitamin A, vitamin K, arsenic, boron, chromium, copper, iodine, iron, manganese, molybdenum, nickel, silicon, vanadium, and zinc (2001). These reports may be accessed at <www.nap.edu>.

TABLE 75.3-15   DEFINITIONS OF NUTRITIONAL REQUIREMENT USED FOR FOOD LABELING (FDA)

TERM	ABBREVIATION	YEAR INTRODUCED	DEFINITION/USE
Old			
US Recommended Daily Allowances	USRDAs	1973	Reference values for vitamins, minerals, and protein used in food labeling; based on RDAs (see Table 75.3-10)
New			
Reference Daily Intakes	RDIs	1994	Replaces the term "USRDAs"; values are generally comparable to them
Daily Reference Values	DRVs	1994	Dietary references applying to fat, saturated fat, cholesterol, carbohydrate, protein, fiber, sodium, and potassium; a 2,000- or 2,500-calorie reference diet is assumed

FDA = US Food and Drug Administration.

foods labeled as "high fiber" must contain at least 20% of the DRV for fiber per serving.

CONCLUSION

The precise nutrient needs of healthy persons is still a matter of intense scientific inquiry and debate, so it is not surprising that those of children with gastrointestinal disease are not well known. Despite the uncertainties of the field, clinicians must still use appropriate tools to accurately assess the dietary intake, anthropometric status, and biochemical profile of their patients. Significant malnutrition with functional and biochemical deficits can exist in patients with gastrointestinal disease even in the absence of overt symptoms or signs of active disease.[95] Advances in the technology of body composition analysis hold promise to further evaluate strategies to preserve and augment lean body mass. A heightened awareness of the susceptibility of the pediatric gastrointestinal patient to malnutrition and constant efforts to improve nutritional status are of paramount importance in patient care.

REFERENCES

1. Kanof M, Lake A, Bayless T. Decreased height velocity in children and adolescents before the diagnosis of Crohn's disease. Gastroenterology 1988;95:1523–7.
2. Motil KJ, Grand RJ, Davis-Kraft L, et al. Growth failure in children with inflammatory bowel disease: a prospective study. Gastroenterology 1993;105:681–91.
3. Jones M, Campbell KA, Duggan C, et al. Multiple micronutrient deficiencies in a child fed an elemental formula. J Pediatr Gastroenterol Nutr 2001;33:602–5.
4. Bousvaros A, Zurakowski D, Duggan C, et al. Vitamins A and E serum levels in children and young adults with inflammatory bowel disease: effect of disease activity. J Pediatr Gastroenterol Nutr 1998;26:129–35.
5. Baker SS, Davis AM. Hypocaloric oral therapy during an episode of diarrhea and vomiting can lead to severe malnutrition. J Pediatr Gastroenterol Nutr 1998;27:1–5.
6. Dickerson RN, Brown RO, Gervasio JG, et al. Measured energy expenditure of tube-fed patients with severe neurodevelopmental disabilities. J Am Coll Nutr 1999;18:61–8.
7. Naber TH, Schermer T, de Bree A, et al. Prevalence of malnutrition in nonsurgical hospitalized patients and its association with disease complications. Am J Clin Nutr 1997;66:1232–9.
0. Martyn CN, Winter PD, Coles SJ, Edington J. Effect of nutri-

tional status on use of health care resources by patients with chronic disease living in the community. Clin Nutr 1998; 17:119–23.
9. Chima CS, Barco K, Dewitt ML, et al. Relationship of nutritional status to length of stay, hospital costs, and discharge status of patients hospitalized in the medicine service. J Am Diet Assoc 1997;97:975–8.
10. Carlson-Newberry S, Costello R, editors. Emerging technologies for nutrition research: potential for assessing military performance capability. Washington (DC): National Academy Press; 1997.
11. Sills RH. Failure to thrive. The role of clinical and laboratory evaluation. Am J Dis Child 1978;132:967–9.
12. Beaton GH, Burema J, Ritenbaugh C. Errors in the interpretation of dietary assessments. Am J Clin Nutr 1997;65 Suppl 4: 1100S–7S.
13. Willett WC, Sampson L, Stampfer MJ, et al. Reproducibility and validity of a semiquantitative food frequency questionnaire. Am J Epidemiol 1985;122:51–65.
14. Rockett HR, Colditz GA. Assessing diets of children and adolescents. Am J Clin Nutr 1997;65 Suppl 4:1116S–22S.
15. Willett W. Nutritional epidemiology. 2nd ed. New York: Oxford University Press; 1998.
16. Briefel R, Sempos C, McDowell M, et al. Dietary methods research in the Third National Health and Nutrition Examination Survey: underreporting of energy intake. Am J Clin Nutr 1997;65 Suppl 4:1203S–9S.
17. Lee R, Nieman D, Rainwater M. Comparison of eight microcomputer dietary analysis programs with the USDA nutrient data base for standard reference. J Am Diet Assoc 1995;95: 858–67.
18. Guide to the growth assessment of infants in clinical studies. Columbus (OH): Ross Laboratories; 1992.
19. Rombeau J, Caldwell M, Forlaw L, et al. Atlas of nutritional support techniques. Boston: Little, Brown and Company; 1989.
20. Corkins MR, Lewis P, Cruse W, et al. Accuracy of infant admission lengths. Pediatrics 2002;109:1108–11.
21. de Onis M, Garza C, Habicht JP. Time for a new growth reference. Pediatrics 1997;100:E8.
22. Dewey K, Heinig M, Nommsen L, et al. Growth of breast-fed and formula-fed infants from 0 to 18 months: the DARLING study. Pediatrics 1992;89:1035–41.
23. Dewey K, Peerson J, Brown K, et al. Growth of breast-fed infants deviates from current reference data: a pooled analysis of US, Canadian, and European data sets. Pediatrics 1995;96: 495–503.
24. Ogden CL, Kuczmarski RJ, Flegal KM, et al. Centers for Disease Control and Prevention 2000 growth charts for the United

States: improvements to the 1977 National Center for Health Statistics version. Pediatrics 2002;109:45–60.

25. Waterlow J. Classification and definition of protein-calorie malnutrition. BMJ 1972;3:566–9.

26. Waterlow JC. Introduction. Causes and mechanisms of linear growth retardation (stunting). Eur J Clin Nutr 1994;48 Suppl 1:S1–4.

27. Dibley M, Staehling N, Nieburg P, Trowbridge F. Interpretation of Z-score anthropometric indicators derived from the international growth reference. Am J Clin Nutr 1987;46:749–62.

28. Dietz WH, Bellizzi MC. Introduction: the use of body mass index to assess obesity in children. Am J Clin Nutr 1999;70 Suppl 1:123S–5S.

29. Willett WC, Dietz WH, Colditz GA. Guidelines for healthy weight. N Engl J Med 1999;341:427–34.

30. Strauss RS, Pollack HA. Epidemic increase in childhood overweight, 1986-1998. JAMA 2001;286:2845–8.

31. Guo SM, Roche AF, Fomon SJ, et al. Reference data on gains in weight and length during the first two years of life. J Pediatr 1991;119:355–62.

32. Durnin J, Rahaman M. The assessment of the amount of fat in the human body from measurements of the skinfold thickness. Br J Nutr 1967;21:681–9.

33. Brook C. Determination of body composition of children from skinfold measurements. Arch Dis Child 1971;46:182–4.

34. Gurney JM, Jelliffe DB. Arm anthropometry in nutritional assessment: nomogram for rapid calculation of muscle circumference and cross-sectional muscle and fat areas. Am J Clin Nutr 1973;26:912–5.

35. Heymsfield S, McManus C, Smith J, et al. Anthropometric measurement of muscle mass: revised equations for calculating bone-free arm muscle area. Am J Clin Nutr 1982;36:680–90.

36. Rolland-Cachera MF, Brambilla P, Manzoni P, et al. Body composition assessed on the basis of arm circumference and triceps skinfold thickness: a new index validated in children by magnetic resonance imaging. Am J Clin Nutr 1997;65:1709–13.

37. Malina RM, Katzmarzyk PT. Validity of the body mass index as an indicator of the risk and presence of overweight in adolescents. Am J Clin Nutr 1999;70 Suppl 1:131S–6S.

38. Yanovski S, Hubbard V, Heymsfield S, Lukaski H. Bioelectrical impedance analysis in body composition measurement. Am J Clin Nutr 1994;64 Suppl 3:387S–532S.

39. Paton NI, Macallan DC, Jebb SA, et al. Longitudinal changes in body composition measured with a variety of methods in patients with AIDS. J Acquir Immune Defic Syndr Hum Retrovirol 1997;14:119–27.

40. Kotler DP, Fogleman L, Tierney AR. Comparison of total parenteral nutrition and an oral, semielemental diet on body composition, physical function, and nutrition-related costs in patients with malabsorption due to acquired immunodeficiency syndrome. JPEN J Parenter Enteral Nutr 1998;22:120–6.

41. Houtkooper LB, Lohman TG, Going SB, Hall MC. Validity of bioelectric impedance for body composition assessment in children. J Appl Physiol 1989;66:814–21.

42. Guo SM, Roche AF, Houtkooper L. Fat-free mass in children and young adults predicted from bioelectric impedance and anthropometric variables. Am J Clin Nutr 1989;50:435–43.

43. Davies PS, Preece MA, Hicks CJ, Halliday D. The prediction of total body water using bioelectrical impedance in children and adolescents. Ann Hum Biol 1988;15:237–40.

44. Houtkooper LB, Going SB, Lohman TG, et al. Bioelectrical impedance estimation of fat-free body mass in children and youth: a cross-validation study. J Appl Physiol 1992;72:366–73.

45. Sun SS, Chumlea WC, Heymsfield SB, et al. Development of bioelectrical impedance analysis prediction equations for body composition with the use of a multicomponent model for use in epidemiologic surveys. Am J Clin Nutr 2003;77:331–40.

46. Kohrt W. Dual-energy x-ray absorptiometry: research issues and equipment. In: Carlson-Newberry S, Costello R, editors. Emerging technologies for nutrition research. Washington (DC): National Academy Press; 1997. p. 151–67.

47. Geerling BJ, Lichtenbelt WD, Stockbrugger RW, Brummer RJ. Gender specific alterations of body composition in patients with inflammatory bowel disease compared with controls. Eur J Clin Nutr 1999;53:479–85.

48. Cowan FJ, Warner JT, Dunstan FD, et al. Inflammatory bowel disease and predisposition to osteopenia. Arch Dis Child 1997;76:325–9.

49. Henderson RC, Lark RK, Gurka MJ, et al. Bone density and metabolism in children and adolescents with moderate to severe cerebral palsy. Pediatrics 2002;110:e5.

50. Roubenoff R, Kehayias J, Dawson-Hughes B, Heymsfield S. Use of dual-energy x-ray absorptiometry in body-composition studies: not yet a "gold standard." Am J Clin Nutr 1993;58:589–91.

51. Leonard MB, Propert KJ, Zemel BS, et al. Discrepancies in pediatric bone mineral density reference data: potential for misdiagnosis of osteopenia. J Pediatr 1999;135:182–8.

52. Manatt M, Garcia P. Nitrogen balance: concepts and techniques. In: Nissen S, editor. Modern methods in protein nutrition and metabolism. New York: Academic Press; 1992. p. 9–66.

53. Rose W. The amino acid requirements of adult man. Nutr Abstr Rev 1957;27:631–47.

54. Blackburn G, Bistrian B, Maini B, et al. Nutritional and metabolic assessment of the hospitalized patient. JPEN J Parenter Enteral Nutr 1977;1:11–22.

55. Garlick P, McNurlan M, Essen P, Wernerman J. Measurement of tissue protein synthesis rates in vivo: a critical analysis of contrasting methods. Am J Physiol 1994;266:E287–97.

56. Rennie M, Smith K, Watt P. Measurement of human tissue protein synthesis: an optimal approach. Am J Physiol 1994;266:E298–307.

57. Hendricks KM, Duggan C, Gallagher L, et al. Malnutrition in hospitalized pediatric patients. Current prevalence. Arch Pediatr Adolesc Med 1995;149:1118–22.

58. Phillips A, Shaper AG, Whincup PH. Association between serum albumin and mortality from cardiovascular disease, cancer, and other causes. Lancet 1989;ii:1434–6.

59. Danesh J, Muir J, Wong YK, et al. Risk factors for coronary heart disease and acute-phase proteins. A population-based study. Eur Heart J 1999;20:954–9.

60. Fletcher J, Little J, Guest P. A comparison of serum transferrin and serum prealbumin as nutritional parameters. JPEN J Parenter Enteral Nutr 1987;11:144–7.

61. Hawker FH, Stewart PM, Baxter RC, et al. Relationship of somatomedin-C/insulin-like growth factor I levels to conventional nutritional indices in critically ill patients. Crit Care Med 1987;15:732–6.

62. Kaplan A, Zemel B, Neiswender K, Stallings V. Resting energy expenditure in clinical pediatrics: measured versus predicted equations. J Pediatr 1995;127:200–5.

63. Schofield W. Predicting basal metabolic rate, new standards and review of previous work. Hum Nutr Clin Nutr 1985;39C:5–41.

64. Flancbaum L, Choban PS, Sambucco S, et al. Comparison of indirect calorimetry, the Fick method, and prediction equations in estimating the energy requirements of critically ill patients. Am J Clin Nutr 1999;69:461–6.

65. Cross-Bu J, Jefferson L, Walding D, et al. Resting energy expenditure in children in a pediatric intensive acre unit: comparison of Harris-Benedict and Talbot predictions with indirect calorimetry values. Am J Clin Nutr 1998;67:74–80.

66. Bandini LG, Puelzl-Quinn H, Morelli JA, Fukagawa NK. Estimation of energy requirements in persons with severe central nervous system impairment. J Pediatr 1995;126:828–32.

67. Duggan C, Bechard L, Donovan K, et al. Resting energy expenditure changes among children undergoing allogeneic stem cell transplantation. Am J Clin Nutr 2003;78:104–9.

68. Capristo E, Mingrone G, Addolorato G, et al. Metabolic features of inflammatory bowel disease in a remission phase of the disease activity. J Int Med 1998;243:339–47.

69. Silberman H, Silberman A. Parenteral nutrition, biochemistry, and respiratory gas exchange. JPEN J Parenter Enteral Nutr 1986;10:151–4.

70. Schoeller DA. Recent advances from application of doubly labeled water to measurement of human energy expenditure. J Nutr 1999;129:1765–8.

71. Perks SM, Roemmich JN, Sandow-Pajewski M, et al. Alterations in growth and body composition during puberty. IV. Energy intake estimated by the Youth-Adolescent Food-Frequency Questionnaire: validation by the doubly labeled water method. Am J Clin Nutr 2000;72:1455–60.

72. Butte NF, Hopkinson JM, Wong WW, et al. Body composition during the first 2 years of life: an updated reference. Pediatr Res 2000;47:578–85.

73. Bodamer OA, Hoffmann GF, Visser GH, et al. Assessment of energy expenditure in metabolic disorders. Eur J Pediatr 1997;156 Suppl 1:S24–8.

74. Shew SB, Beckett PR, Keshen TH, et al. Validation of a [13C]bicarbonate tracer technique to measure neonatal energy expenditure. Pediatr Res 2000;47:787–91.

75. Furst P. Old and new substrates in clinical nutrition. J Nutr 1998;128:789–96.

76. Hegsted D. Theoretical estimates of the protein requirements of children. J Am Diet Assoc 1957;33:225–32.

77. Fomon S. Nutrition of normal infants. St. Louis: Mosby; 1993.

78. Bier D, Young VR. A kinetic approach to assessment of amino acid and protein replacement needs of individual sick patients. JPEN J Parenter Enteral Nutr 1987;11 Suppl 5:95S–7S.

79. Davies PS, Wells JC, Hinds A, et al. Total energy expenditure in 9 month and 12 month infants. Eur J Clin Nutr 1997;51:249–52.

80. Young VR. Human amino acid requirements: counterpoint to Millward and the importance of tentative revised estimates. J Nutr 1998;128:1570–3.

81. Krebs NF, Reidinger CJ, Miller LV, Borschel MW. Zinc homeostasis in healthy infants fed a casein hydrolysate formula. J Pediatr Gastroenterol Nutr 2000;30:29–33.

82. Hambidge KM, Krebs NF, Miller L. Evaluation of zinc metabolism with use of stable-isotope techniques: implications for the assessment of zinc status. Am J Clin Nutr 1998;68 Suppl 2:410S–3S.

83. Abrams SA, Griffin IJ, Davila PM. Calcium and zinc absorption from lactose-containing and lactose-free infant formulas. Am J Clin Nutr 2002;76:442–6.

84. Imura K, Okada A. Amino acid metabolism in pediatric patients. Nutrition 1998;14:143–8.

85. Lacey J, Wilmore D. Is glutamine a conditionally essential amino acid? Nutr Rev 1990;48:297–309.

86. Pickering LK, Granoff DM, Erickson JR, et al. Modulation of the immune system by human milk and infant formula containing nucleotides. Pediatrics 1998;101:242–9.

87. MRC Vitamin Study Research Group. Prevention of neural tube defects: results of the Medical Research Council Vitamin Study. Lancet 1991;338:131–7.

88. Brouwer IA, van Dusseldorp M, Thomas CM, et al. Low-dose folic acid supplementation decreases plasma homocysteine concentrations: a randomized trial. Am J Clin Nutr 1999;69:99–104.

89. Fawzi W, Chalmers T, Herrera M, Mosteller F. Vitamin A supplementation and child mortality: a meta-analysis. JAMA 1993;269:898–903.

90. Zinc Investigators Collaborative Group. Therapeutic effects of oral zinc in acute and persistent diarrhea in children in developing countries: pooled analysis of randomized controlled trials. Am J Clin Nutr 2000;72:1516–22.

91. Zinc Investigators' Collaborative Group, Bhutta ZA, Black RE, et al. Prevention of diarrhea and pneumonia by zinc supplementation in children in developing countries: pooled analysis of randomized controlled trials. J Pediatr 1999; 135:689–97.

92. Elia M. Changing concepts of nutrient requirements in disease: implications for artificial nutritional support. Lancet 1995; 345:1279–84.

93. Centers for Disease Control and Prevention. Lactic acidosis traced to thiamine deficiency related to nationwide shortage of multivitamins for total parenteral nutrition—United States, 1997. MMWR Morb Mortal Wkly Rep 1997;46:523–8.

94. Standing Committee on the Scientific Evaluation of Dietary Reference Intakes, Food and Nutrition Board, Institute of Medicine. Dietary Reference Intakes for calcium, phosphorus, magnesium, vitamin D, and fluoride. Washington (DC): National Academy Press; 1997.

95. Geerling BJ, Badart-Smook A, Stockbrugger RW, Brummer RJ. Comprehensive nutritional status in patients with long-standing Crohn disease currently in remission. Am J Clin Nutr 1998;67:919–26.

96. Suskind R, Varma R. Assessment of nutritional status of children. Pediatr Rev 1984;5:195–202.

97. Loughrey C, Duggan C. Assessment of nutritional status: the role of the laboratory. In: Soldin S, Rifai N, Hicks J, editors. Biochemical basis of pediatric disease. Washington (DC): AACC Press; 1998. p. 588–91.

98. Standing Committee on the Scientific Evaluation of Dietary Reference Intakes, Food and Nutrition Board, Institute of Medicine. Dietary Reference Intakes for energy, carbohydrate, fiber, fat, fatty acids, cholesterol, protein, and amino acids (macronutrients). Washington (DC): National Academy Press; 2002.

99. Standing Committee on the Scientific Evaluation of Dietary Reference Intakes, Food and Nutrition Board, Institute of Medicine. Dietary Reference Intakes for vitamin C, vitamin E, selenium, and carotenoids. Washington (DC): National Academy Press; 2000.

100. Standing Committee on the Scientific Evaluation of Dietary Reference Intakes, Food and Nutrition Board, Institute of Medicine. Dietary Reference Intakes for thiamin, riboflavin, niacin, vitamin B6, folate, vitamin B_{12}, pantothenic acid, biotin, and choline. Washington (DC): National Academy Press; 2000.

101. Standing Committee on the Scientific Evaluation of Dietary Reference Intakes, Food and Nutrition Board, Institute of Medicine. Dietary Reference Intakes for vitamin A, vitamin K, arsenic, boron, chromium, copper, iodine, iron, manganese, molybdenum, nickel, silicon, vanadium, and zinc. Washington (DC): National Academy Press; 2002.

4A. Parenteral Nutrition

Susan S. Baker, MD, PhD

Robert D. Baker, MD, PhD

In 1968, Dudrick and colleagues reported that exclusive intravenous feeding via a central vein could support the long-term survival and growth of puppies.[1] This breakthrough in technology was quickly applied to adult humans[2] and then children.[3] Subsequently, parenteral nutrition (PN) solutions have been widely used. However, knowledge to support this technology dates to the 1600s, when the circulation of blood was discovered and the first infusion of a liquid, wine, was accomplished.[4] Approximately 200 years later, the practice of starving ill patients began to change. In the twentieth century, safe infusates of fats, carbohydrates, and proteins were synthesized, production processes for the manufacture of components arose, and nutritional scientists began to develop an understanding of nutritional requirements. Knowledge of the requirements for micronutrients and metabolic changes associated with infection, injury, or surgery permitted the tailoring of infusions for specific situations. The identification of nutrients that may be essential under specific situations, the compatibility of PN solutions with medications, and the use of pharmacologic substances to promote growth and healing, scavenge oxidants, and prevent or ameliorate metabolic changes associated with inflammation have permitted the treatment of patients who cannot fully support their nutritional requirements through their gastrointestinal (GI) tract. The design of backpacks, subcutaneously accessible central lines, and cycled nutrient delivery permits patients, especially children, to receive nutrition support while they attend school and engage in other age-appropriate activities. For patients who are critically ill or are not candidates for a small bowel transplant, PN can be lifesaving. Still, the technique is not free of complications. It was initially assumed that these complications could be overcome with further fine-tuning. Subsequent experience has shown this to be only partially true. For instance, there have been vast improvements in line technology that resulted in a decrease in line-related complications.[5] Amino acid solutions have been improved, and special solutions for special conditions have been developed.[6,7] The problem of fat administration and essential fatty acid deficiency (EFAD) has been largely solved.[8] Some complications have proven difficult to resolve, bone disease and cholestasis being among these. Because of evidence for the benefits of enteral feeds[9,10] and the serious complications associated with PN,[11–14] parenterally administered nutrition should be reserved only for specific indications when enteral nutrition is not possible or adequate. Table 75.4A-1 lists situations in which the GI tract is nonfunctional or partially functional. Figure 75.4A-1 is an algorithm for initiation of pediatric PN. PN can be partial, used as an adjunct when enteral nutrition cannot meet all nutrient needs, or total, supplying all nutritional needs. Total PN must supply all of the nutrients needed by an individual in amounts necessary to replete malnourished states, prevent muscle breakdown during metabolic stress, and support normal growth and development over the long term.

INDICATIONS FOR PN IN THE PEDIATRIC PATIENT

There are few absolute indications for PN. In some circumstances, such as prematurely born infants, severe malnutrition that is refractory to enteral feedings, pseudo-obstruction, short small bowel, and children who undergo surgery of the GI tract and are not able to be fed, PN is beneficial. In the premature infant, especially the very low birth weight infant, the GI tract may not be capable of processing the amount of nutrients needed for the infant to survive and grow. Over the past three decades, the use of PN in the pediatric population has shifted. In a recent review of 30 years experience with PN in a single institution for pediatric patients, the number of parenterally fed patients did not change; however, the

TABLE 75.4A-1   GASTROINTESTINAL FUNCTION

PARTIALLY FUNCTIONAL OR INADEQUATE FUNCTION
Cannot meet nutrient requirements after maximizing enteral support
Burns
Multiorgan failure
Malabsorption
Short bowel, intractable diarrhea, villous atrophy, dysmotility syndromes
Risk of aspiration when small bowel feeds are not possible
Malnutrition with hypoproteinemia

NONFUNCTIONAL
Paralytic ileus
Intractable vomiting when small bowel feedings are not possible
Small bowel ischemia
Necrotizing enterocolitis
Severe acute pancreatitis
Gastrointestinal surgery
Gastroschisis, omphalocele, multiple intestinal atresias, etc. until enteral route is accessible
Severe inflammatory bowel disease with possible impending surgery

Adapted from Baker SS.[123]

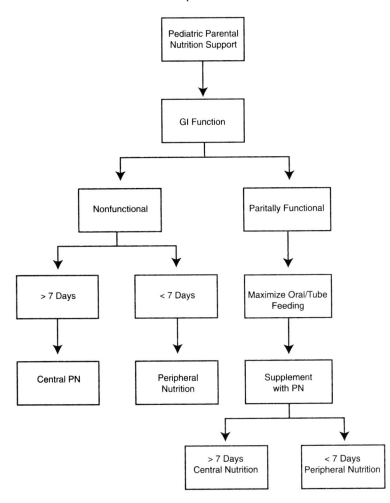

FIGURE 75.4A-1 Algorithm for initiating pediatric parenteral nutrition (PN) support. Adapted from Baker SS.[123] GI = gastrointestinal.

number of premature babies fed parenterally increased significantly, whereas the number of all other patients receiving PN decreased.[15] Severe malnutrition is associated with poor GI function, which is likely multifactorial in origin. Malnutrition causes atrophy of the GI tract in animals.[16] This phenomenon has not been demonstrated in humans, but "functional" atrophy is said to occur. Edema of the intestinal wall, radiographically visualized as separated loops of bowel, may impede nutrient absorption, as occurs in intestinal lymphangiectasia.[17] If of sufficient severity, pseudo-obstruction may require PN. However, intestinal pseudo-obstruction is a rare disease, and some cases of presumed pseudo-obstruction were shown to be Munchausen syndrome by proxy.[18] There is little evidence that nutrition support by itself is beneficial in pediatric oncologic disease. However, children in good nutritional status are better able to tolerate antitumor therapy. For a variety of reasons, children with cancer do not or cannot voluntarily consume adequate nutrition. Assisted enteral feeding in such cases should be considered before PN. PN, either pre- or post-surgery, has not been definitively demonstrated to be beneficial.[19] When surgery involves the GI tract and the child will not be able to be fed, PN is required.

SOLUTION COMPOSITION

The essential nutrients are water, protein, carbohydrate, fat, minerals, trace elements, and vitamins. In general, PN

should not be used to correct acute fluid or electrolyte abnormalities. Parenteral solutions are compounded once a day. Over- or underestimates of electrolyte requirements that result in the need to change solutions more frequently than once every 24 hours could result in the patient receiving no nutrition support during part of the day and waste of an expensive therapeutic agent. PN solutions can be used to replace nutritional deficits over the long term. For example, PN solutions can be used to replete muscle mass, providing the extra protein, minerals, electrolytes, and calories that this process requires in addition to the needs for normal growth.

Fluid requirements for infants and children are based on seminal studies performed by Darrow.[20] The objective of fluid therapy is to provide water to meet the requirements for physiologic processes, including insensible and urinary losses. These requirements are based on healthy infants and children and do not take into account the increased losses that may occur with diarrhea, vomiting, fistula, burns, and fever; decreased losses that might occur with the use of mist tents; or altered patient states, as occurs with heart failure or renal disease. Fluid requirements roughly parallel energy metabolism and do not parallel body mass.[21] Although there are several methods to estimate fluid requirements (Table 75.4A-2), the most commonly used is that of Holliday, volume/weight.[21]

During fetal life, there is a gradual decrease in total-body water and extracellular fluid.[22] In the first trimester,

TABLE 75.4A-2 FLUID REQUIREMENTS PER DAY IN PEDIATRIC PATIENTS AS DETERMINED BY VARIOUS METHODS

METHOD	BODY WEIGHT (KG)	AMOUNT/D
Volume/weight	0–10	100 mL/kg
	10–20	1,000 + 50 mL/kg over 10 kg
	> 20	1,500 + 20 mL/kg over 20 kg
Volume/surface area	1–70	1,500–1,700 mL/m²
Volume/kcal	0–70	100 mL/100 kcal metabolized

body water accounts for 95% of body weight. Body water decreases to 80% by 32 weeks and 78% at term. This shift is interrupted when an infant is born prematurely. Care must be taken to provide adequate water for the increased insensible skin losses yet permit the normal diuresis that occurs after birth. Too much water is associated with an increased incidence of patent ductus arteriosus, bronchopulmonary dysplasia, intraventricular hemorrhage, and necrotizing enterocolitis.[23] Anderson recommends 60 to 140 mL/kg/d for the first day of life, the higher amount for infants nursed under a radiant warmer or dry incubator and the lower amount for infants nursed in a humidified incubator or under a radiant warmer with a plastic blanket.[24] As the infant matures, the fluid requirement increases to 120 to 150 mL/kg/d to allow for increases in renal solute load, stool water output, and infant growth.[25]

Electrolytes are critically important in PN for the short term but also long term because normal muscle accretion cannot occur in the presence of insufficient electrolytes and minerals.[25] Essentially, all electrolyte loss occurs via the urine unless there is an ongoing source of additional losses such as diarrhea, fistula, or stoma. Table 75.4A-3 lists parenteral electrolyte requirements. When GI fluid losses occur, electrolytes and fluids must be replaced. Table 75.4A-4 lists the approximate electrolyte content of GI fluids.

PROTEIN

Proteins are essential for all metabolic functions in the body and serve as the main structural element of the body, as biochemical catalysts, and as regulators of gene expression. Proteins are complex, and their function is influenced by the availability of energy and nutrients such as minerals, vitamins, and trace elements. The average content of nitrogen in dietary protein is 16% by weight, and nitrogen metabolism is often considered synonymous with protein metabolism. Proteins consist of amino acids that have been categorized as essential, or indispensable, and nonessential, or dispensable. The nine essential amino acids—histidine, isoleucine, leucine, lysine, methionine, phenylalanine, threonine, tryptophan, and valine—are those that cannot be synthesized from precursors and hence must be provided. However, as more information on protein and intermediary metabolism becomes available, the definition of essential becomes blurred. Laidlaw and Kopple propose adding a third category of amino acid, conditionally indispensable.[26] Conditionally indispensable amino acids are those amino acids that are synthesized from other amino acids or their synthesis is limited under special physiologic conditions.[26–28] These amino acids can be especially important in the neonate, for whom it is likely that alanine, aspartate, glutamate, serine, and perhaps asparagine are conditionally indispensable.[29]

Unlike energy and other nutrients, the body has little in the way of protein that can be mobilized during times of insufficient intake. In a 70 kg adult, the "reservoir" of labile protein is estimated at about 1% of total-body protein. More than half of the body protein is present as skeletal muscle, skin, and blood. The liver and kidney are metabolically active tissues that contain about 10% of total-body protein. Brain, heart, lung, and bone account for about 15% of whole-body protein. The distribution of protein among these organs varies with age because the newborn has proportionately more brain and visceral tissue and less muscle. Thus, when exogenous protein is inadequate, functional body proteins are used. The body can adapt to a wide range of protein intakes; however, patho-

TABLE 75.4A-3 PARENTERAL ELECTROLYTE AND MINERAL REQUIREMENTS

NUTRIENT	PRETERM INFANTS*	TERM INFANT*	CHILDREN > 1 YR
Sodium (mEq/kg/d)	3	3	3
Potassium (mEq/kg/d)	2	2	2
Chloride (mEq/kg/d)	5	5	5
Calcium† (mg/kg/d)	80–100†	60–90	24–60
Phosphorus† (mg/kg/d)	43–62	48–68	18–45
Magnesium† (mg/kg/d)	3–6	6–10.5	2.4–6.0

*Preterm infants have the same requirements as term infants.[24,65] For preterm infants, electrolytes are generally not administered on the first day of life.
†Adapted from Greene HL et al.[65] American Society for Parenteral and Enteral Nutrition (ASPEN) based its recommendations[39] on the National Academy of Science Dietary Reference Intake.[178]—210 mg/d for infants 0 to 6 months, 270 mg/d for ages 6 months to 1 year, 500 mg/d for ages 1 to 3 years, 800 mg/d for ages 4 to 8 years, and 1,300 mg/d for ages 9 to 18 years—but notes that these levels may be difficult to achieve because administration is often limited by its solubility. ASPEN clinical guidelines make no recommendations for phosphorus or magnesium.
‡Adapted from American Academy of Pediatrics, Committee on Nutrition.[47]

TABLE 75.4A-4   ESTIMATES OF GASTROINTESTINAL FLUID AND ELECTROLYTES

FLUID	SODIUM (MEQ/L)	POTASSIUM (MEQ/L)	CHLORIDE (MEQ/L)
Gastric	20–80	5–20	100–150
Pancreatic	120–140	5–15	40–80
Small bowel	100–140	5–15	90–130
Bile	120–140	5–15	80–120
Ileostomy*	45–135	3–15	20–115
Secretory diarrhea	120	40	94
Osmotic diarrhea	54	33	94

Adapted from Institute of Medicine, Food and Nutrition Board,[178] and Johnson KB.[179]
*Decreases in volume occur with time after resection. Also dependent on length of small bowel removed.

logic conditions such as infection or trauma can cause substantial protein loss as the demand for either amino acids increases or as amino acid carbon skeletons are used to meet energy demands. If these extra needs are not met, a serious depletion of body protein mass occurs. Skeletal muscle is the largest single contributor to protein loss.

Protein requirements are based on the assumptions that adequate energy is provided so that the carbon skeletons of amino acids are not needed as an energy source and the protein quality is high. Table 75.4A-5 lists estimates of protein requirements by age. Protein quality is determined by digestibility (not a factor in PN) and the indispensable amino acid composition of the protein. If the content of a single indispensable amino acid is less than the requirement, that amino acid limits the use of other amino acids, preventing normal rates of protein synthesis even when the total nitrogen is adequate. Proposed amino acid requirements of the nine indispensable amino acids for infants (based on the amino acid composition of human milk), children, and adults have been reviewed.[30] Data exist, however, to suggest that histidine is conditionally essential for infants to 6 months of age[31] and cysteine is conditionally essential in low birth weight infants.[32] Table 75.4A-6 lists examples of the amino acid composition of some PN solutions.

The most reliable method to assess the adequacy of dietary protein is nitrogen balance, the difference between nitrogen intake and the amount excreted in urine, feces, skin, and sweat. This measurement is not practical clinically, especially for children. There is no reliable clinical measure of protein nutritional status. In infants and children, failure to gain weight or length can be used to assess the overall nutritional adequacy of a diet, and failure to gain length occurs with borderline inadequate protein intake.[33] Other anthropometrics are less sensitive. The most commonly used clinical tools to assess protein status are albumin and prealbumin.

Most individuals can tolerate a wide range of protein intakes. Foman reviewed adverse outcomes with increased protein intakes in healthy formula- and breastfed infants.[34] Diets high in protein were associated with an increase in renal solute load, a potential safety concern for water balance in the infant. Transient tyrosinemia as a consequence of delay in maturation of p-hydroxyphenylpyruvic acid oxidase can occur. The elevated levels can last as long as 6 weeks, raising a concern for long-term sequelae.

High-protein diets can alter the serum amino acid profile. The significance of this in infants and children who are already ill and may have an abnormal profile secondary to

TABLE 75.4A-5   ESTIMATES OF PROTEIN REQUIREMENTS BY AGE

AGE	IOM RECOMMENDATIONS (G/KG/D)*	RDA (G/KG/D)†	ESTIMATE FOR HEALTHY PATIENTS (G/KG/D)‡
Low birth weight	None	None	3–4
Full term to 6 mo	1.52 (AI)		2–3
7–12 mo	1.1 (EAR)	1.5	2–3
1–3 yr	0.88	1.1	1–1.2
4–8 yr	0.76	0.95	1–1.2
Adolescence			
Boys	0.76	0.76	0.9
Girls	0.76	0.76	0.8
Critically ill	None	None	1.5

AI = adequate intake, a recommended average daily nutrient intake level based on observed or experimentally determined approximations or estimates of nutrient intake by a group (or groups) of apparently healthy people who are assumed to be adequate; used when an RDA cannot be determined[181]; EAR = estimated average requirement, the average daily nutrient intake level estimated to meet the requirement of half the healthy individuals in a particular life stage and gender group[181]; IOM = Institute of Medicine; RDA = Recommended Dietary Allowance.
*Adapted from Standing Committee on the Scientific Evaluation of Dietary Reference Intakes, Food and Nutrition Board, Institute of Medicine.[30]
†Adapted from Subcommittee on the Tenth Edition of the RDAs, Food and Nutrition Board.[181]
‡Adapted from American Society for Parenteral and Enteral Nutrition Board of Directors and the Clinical Guidelines Task Force.[39]

TABLE 75.4A-6   AMINO ACID COMPOSITION OF COMMONLY AVAILABLE PARENTERAL SOLUTIONS

	PRODUCT (VENDOR)					
	FOR INFANTS LESS THAN 1 YR		FOR CHILDREN OLDER THAN 1 YR THROUGH ADULTHOOD			
	TROPHAMINE (B. BRAUN, MELSUNGEN, GERMANY)	AMINOSYN-PF (ABBOTT, CHICAGO, IL, USA)	AMINOSYN-HBC (ABBOTT)	AMINOSYN-II (ABBOTT)	TRAVASOL (BAXTER, DEERFIELD, IL, USA)	NOVAMINE (BAXTER)
Total nitrogen (g/L of a 10% solution)	15.5	15.2	16	15.3	16.5	23.9
Protein equivalent (approximate g/L of a 10% solution)	97	100	100	100	100	100
pH (range)	5.5 (5.0–6.0)	5.0 (5.0–6.5)	5.2 (4.5–6.0)	5.8 (5.0–6.5)	6.0 (5.0–7.0)	5.6 (5.2–6.0)
Essential amino acids, mg/100 mL of a 10% solution						
Isoleucine	820	760	1127	660	600	500
Leucine	1,400	1,200	2251	1,000	730	693
Lysine	820	677	378	1,050	580	787
Methionine	340	180	294	172	400	500
Phenylalanine	480	427	325	298	580	693
Threonine	420	512	388	400	420	500
Tryptophan	200	180	126	200	180	167
Valine	780	673	1,127	500	580	640
Nonessential amino acids, mg/100 mL of a 10% solution						
Alanine	540	698	943	993	2,070	1,447
Arginine	1,200	1,227	717	1,018	1,150	980
Aspartic acid	320	527	—	700	—	289
Glutamic acid	500	820	—	738	—	500
Glycine	360	385	943	500	1030	693
Histidine	480	312	220	300	560	596
Proline	680	812	640	722	680	596
Serine	380	495	316	530	500	667
Taurine	25	70	—	—	—	—
Tyrosine	240	44	47	270	40	26

Manufacturers' product information, February 2003.

the primary disease is not known. In an assessment of the tolerable upper limits in healthy populations for individual amino acids recently published by the National Academy of Sciences, no adverse effects were noted for branched-chain amino acids prescribed for PN.[30] The report cautions, however, that the studies may not have carefully monitored for adverse outcomes. Similarly, there are few, if any, reports of adverse effects of glutamine in the doses generally prescribed in PN solutions.

Specialized amino acid solutions have been proposed for a variety of clinical situations, including trauma, liver failure, metabolic stress, and to improve immune function. Branched chain–enriched preparations, glutamine-enhanced solutions, and a solution specially designed for infants are most commonly used.

The term "immunonutrition" refers to the use of specific nutrients, arginine, glutamine, nucleotides, and ω-3 fatty acids, alone or in combination to influence nutritional, immunologic, and inflammatory parameters in laboratory and clinical studies. The use of immunonutrition was systematically reviewed.[35] The primary outcomes of interest were mortality and the number of patients with new infectious complications. In the 22 articles that met the inclusion criteria, the reviewers found no consistently used standard definition of what constitutes immunonutriton. Pneumonia, intra-abdominal abscess, sepsis, line sepsis, wound infection, and urinary tract infections were identified as primary adverse outcomes. Secondary outcomes included length of hospital and intensive care unit stays and duration of mechanical ventilation. From this review, the authors concluded that immunonutrition may decrease infectious complication rates, but the treatment effect varies depending on the patient population, the intervention, and the quality of the study. In surgical patients, immunonutrition was associated with a reduction in infectious complication rates and shorter length of hospital stay without adverse effects on mortality. In critically ill patients, immunonutrition was not associated with any apparent clinical benefit and may be harmful in some subgroups of patients. Thus, immunonutrition is not recommended for all critically ill patients.

The use of glutamine was systematically reviewed.[36] Fourteen randomized trials compared the use of glutamine supplementation in surgical and critically ill patients. The review concluded that in surgical patients, glutamine supplementation (doses > 0.20 g/kg/d) may be associated with a reduction in infectious complication rates and shorter hospital stay. In critically ill patients, glutamine supplementation may be associated with a reduction in complication and mortality rates. The authors caution, however, that further separate studies of the surgical and critically ill groups need to be performed and powered large enough to detect clinically important differences using parenterally delivered glutamine. There was no evidence of harm with glutamine supplementation.

Protein-energy malnutrition is common in patients with liver disease. As the disease progresses and encephalopathy ensues, branched chain–enriched PN solutions may offer benefits.[37] However, rigorous clinical studies are not available to support the use of branched chain–enriched PN

solutions in all patients with liver disease.[38] Branched chain–enriched amino acid solutions can offer benefit for patients who have hepatic encephalopathy, and these solutions are recommended for such patients.[39–41]

Two amino acid solutions are specifically designed for infants less than 1 year of age. Use of these solutions results in plasma amino acid concentrations that approximate the profile seen in breastfed infants. The differences between these two solutions and others is that they contain taurine, glutamate, and aspartate; reduced amounts of methionine, glycine, and alanine; and increased arginine and leucine. Although there are differences between the two solutions, both have shown benefits in term and preterm infants.[42–44] There appears to be no difference in occurrence or magnitude of cholestasis between children who receive either of the two solutions.[45] Use of these solutions is recommended for infants less than 1 year of age. In addition to the differing amino acid compositions, these solutions are more acidic and permit the solubilization of a higher concentration of calcium and phosphorus than the amino acid mixtures prepared for adults.

CARBOHYDRATES

Glucose is the major energy source in PN because it is safe, economic, and readily available. Other sugars—fructose, sorbitol, glycerol, and xylitol—have been suggested as useful energy sources for specific conditions such as diabetes or post-trauma but are not readily available or used. Glucose in PN solutions is in the monohydrous form containing 3.4 kcal/g and is available commercially in concentrations of 2.5 to 70%. The glucose concentration of PN solutions that can be safely administered is limited by osmolality. Concentrations higher than about 12.5% sclerose peripheral veins, increasing the incidence of phlebitis and shortening the time that a vein could be used for infusion. Glucose solutions higher than 12.5% must be administered in a central vein. Glucose is calculated to provide 60 to 75% of nonprotein calories. Estimated energy requirements are provided in Table 75.4A-7.

Initiation of glucose infusion should occur in an incremental fashion to prevent hyperosmolarity and hyperinsulinemia (Table 75.4A-8). The glucose infusion rate (GIR) can be calculated using the following equation:

$$GIR = \frac{g/kg/d\ dextrose \times 1{,}000}{1{,}440\ min/d}$$

A GIR of 12 to 14 mg/kg/min is tolerated in a healthy child, and infants can be safely given a GIR of 8 to 12 mg/kg/min. In adult patients, there is no apparent correlation between glucose clearance and the rate of oxidation of glucose.[46] Increases in the rate of glucose infusion from 4 to 7 mg/kg/min are associated with an increase in the rate of glucose oxidation. At higher rates, fat is synthesized without a further increase in oxidation. High glucose loads (ie, those containing more than 25% glucose and delivered at > 26 mg/kg/min) may not be beneficial to infants and may contribute to hepatosteatosis.

TABLE 75.4A-7   ESTIMATES OF PARENTERAL ENERGY REQUIREMENTS

AGE (YR)	ENERGY (KCAL/KG/D)	CARBOHYDRATE (MG/KG/MIN)*
Premature infant	80–120	10–18
Term infant	90–120	11–18
1–3	75–90	9–14
4–6	65–75	8–11
7–10	55–75	7–11
11–18	40–55	7–8.5

Reproduced with permission from Lee PC and Werlin SL.[182]
*Estimate based on 60–75% of nonprotein calories as glucose.

The American Academy of Pediatrics recommends that insulin not be routinely added to PN solutions because responses to the addition of this hormone by infants are unpredictable.[47] For persistently hyperglycemic infants, insulin may improve tolerance to glucose.[48] However, a limited number of studies assess the clinical outcomes of infants treated with insulin.[49–51] Concerns about the use of insulin in the neonate include the possibility that suppression of muscle proteolysis may be undesirable, the composition of the resultant weight gain is not clearly understood, serum glucose is driven to tissues other than brain, and the possibility that glucose is converted to fat rather than being oxidized.[47]

Glucose intolerance can develop in critically ill patients, such as those who have experienced trauma, burns, sepsis, or cancer. For these patients, the GIR is limited to 5 to 7 mg/kg/min.[52] Infusion of excess glucose causes hyperglycemia, glucosuria, dehydration, and the conversion of glucose to fat. When hyperglycemia occurs, the GIR can be decreased or insulin can be added to the therapy. Exogenous insulin enhances the movement of substrate from the periphery to the liver and increases fat synthesis and storage. This can lead to hepatosteatosis; hence, insulin is not commonly used in critically ill patients outside the neonatal age group.

Complications associated with glucose infusion are listed in Table 75.4A-9.

INTRAVENOUS FAT ADMINISTRATION

Lipids are administered to virtually all patients who receive PN. Initially, intravenous fats were given to patients who had no oral intake to overcome EFAD; however, because intravenous lipids are the most calorically dense component of PN, intravenous fats are considered an important source of calories, especially for patients who are fluid restricted. Thus, intravenous lipids have at least two roles: avoiding or treating EFAD and as a source of energy.

There are a number of reasons to choose fat-predominant PN solutions over glucose-predominant ones. Glucose results in a higher specific dynamic action and thus higher resting energy expenditures and higher metabolic rates. Glucose-predominant PN can result in a respiratory quotient (RQ) of greater than 1.0, indicating the use of energy for lipogenesis. Finally, glucose metabolism results in an increased carbon dioxide elimination by the lungs when compared with fat metabolism. This fact can be of importance to mechanically ventilated patients and those with marginal lung function. In general, the ratio of calories derived from glucose to the calories derived from fats in the range of 3:1 or 2:1 minimizes carbon dioxide stress.[53,54]

Fats are bioactive precursors of prostaglandins, leukotrienes, and other mediators of inflammation and metabolism. They are also an essential part of neural tissue and cell membranes. These facts are especially important for the child who is growing, laying down tissue and gaining cells. Thus, intravenous lipids act as more than a source of calories, and in the future, intravenous fats will be used in a more specialized and directed way.[55,56]

Intravenous fats consist of three components: an aqueous phase, a lipid phase, and an emulsifier. The lipid phase supplies the majority of the calories and the essential fatty acids. Glycerin is present in the aqueous phrase

TABLE 75.4A-8   GLUCOSE CONCENTRATION IN PARENTERAL SOLUTIONS

	PREMATURE INFANT (< 1,000 G OR 28 WK GESTATION)	INFANT	CHILD (1–10 YR)	ADOLESCENT (11–18 YR)
Begin infusion	5–7.5% or glucose concentration in current IV solution	5–7.5% or glucose concentration in current IV solution	10% or percent higher than concentration in current IV solution	10% or percent higher than concentration in current IV solution
Advance	2.5% each day as tolerated	2.5% each day as tolerated	5% each day as tolerated	5% each day as tolerated
Usual GIR upper limit (mg/kg/min)	8–12	12–14	8–10	5–6
Peripheral maximum concentration (%)	12	12.5	12.5	12.5
Central glucose concentration (%)	20–25	25	25	25
Monitor at initiation and with every increase	Urine glucose	Urine glucose	Urine glucose	Urine glucose

Adapted from Lee PC and Werlin SL.[182]
GIR = glucose infusion rate; IV = intravenous.

TABLE 75.4A-9   COMMONLY REPORTED COMPLICATIONS OF GLUCOSE

COMPLICATION	USUAL CAUSE	PREVENTION OR TREATMENT
Phelibitis	High osmolarity	Limit glucose concentration to 12.5% for peripheral administration
Refeeding syndrome	Rapid refeeding of a malnourished patient	Refeed slowly; monitor serum phosphorus, potassium, calcium, and magnesium
Hepatosteatosis	All nonprotein calories provided as carbohydrate or excessive calories	Provide 30% of calories as lipid
Cholestasis	Infant fed exclusively by PN	Enteral feeding
Carbon dioxide retention	High GIR in a patient with respiratory failure	Decrease GIR
Hypoglycemia	Abrupt discontinuation of PN or decrease in GIR	Taper PN
Hyperglycemia	High GIR, stress, burns, sepsis, incorrect glucose concentration	Decrease GIR, add insulin

Adapted from Lee PC and Werlin SL.[182]
GIR = glucose infusion rate; PN = parenteral nutrition.

and raises the tonicity as well as incidentally supplying calories. The emulsifier is usually egg phospholipid. Soybean oil, safflower oil, and mixtures of the two have been used as sources of lipid. The caloric density of 10% lipid emulsions is 1.1 kcal/mL, 20% emulsion is 2.0 kcal/mL, and 30% emulsion is 3.0 kcal/mL (available for three-in-one solutions only).

Preventing EFAD is one of the two major reasons for administering intravenous fats. The essential fats for humans are linoleic ($C_{18:2\,\omega-6}$) and linolenic ($C_{18:3\,\omega-3}$). EFAD has been described in children and adults who have no exogenous source of fats for 3 weeks or more. In the preterm infant, EFAD is seen after only 1 week without essential fatty acids. Symptoms of EFAD include scaly skin rash, sparse hair, susceptibility to infection, failure to thrive, hypotonia, increased red cell fragility, and electroencephalographic and electrocardiographic changes. In EFAD, the ratio of trienoic to tetraenoic acids increases to greater than 0.2.[57] In older children and adults, EFAD can be prevented by supplying 0.5 to 1.0 g/kg/d as intravenous lipid, and for premature infants, 0.6 to 0.8 g/kg/d prevents EFAD.

For the most part, fats supplied intravenously as a lipid emulsion are handled in the circulation in much the same fashion as very-low-density lipoprotein (VLDL) particles. Lipoprotein lipase, present in the capillary endothelium, reduces the triglycerides at the core of the particle, whereas the polar lipids, at the surface of the VLDL, are removed to form nascent high-density lipoprotein (HDL). Lecithin-cholesterol acyltransferase (LCAT), released into the circulation from the liver, converts the nascent HDL into mature HDL.[58] These two enzymes, lipoprotein lipase at the endothelial surface and LCAT in circulation, seem to be key in clearing the infused lipid from the circulation.

Lipids can be cleared by other mechanisms, such as endothelial cell endocytosis via cell-surface heparin sulfate proteoglycans in a receptor-independent manner.[59]

The amount of lipid that can be given safely by the intravenous route is limited by the rate of clearance of lipids from circulation. Two to three grams/kg/d of lipid can be safely administered to premature infants, term babies, and older children. Serum triglycerides must be monitored to ensure that the clearing mechanism has not been overwhelmed. It has been suggested that heparin might enhance clearance. In a randomized trial of two heparin doses, the drug caused an increase in circulating free fatty acids, presumably because of release of the lipoprotein lipase into circulation. There was no increase in lipid use.[60] It was concluded that heparin was of no benefit for fat metabolism. Administering intravenous lipid over 20 hours while allowing 4 hours for lipid clearing has been proposed as another method of facilitating lipid clearing. Evidence does not support this practice.[61]

Lipid emulsions used for parenteral administration contain phytosterols. These are plant-derived isoflavones that possess estrogenic properties. Their importance, either beneficial or detrimental, as part of PN is not known. Phytoestrogens, present in soy-based formulas, have been suggested as a cause of decreased bone mineral content in premature infants. Whether these compounds figure in PN-associated bone disease is unknown. No consistent effect of soy feeding on menarche and telarche has been found.[62,63] The importance of phytosterols in infused lipid emulsions as feminizing compounds has not been studied. To date, there is no proof that phytosterols play a role in PN-associated cholestasis, although this relationship has been suggested.[64]

MINERALS AND TRACE ELEMENTS

In the context of pediatric PN solutions, calcium, phosphorus, and magnesium are usually termed "minerals." Trace elements are those minerals found in the body in small amounts and include iron, zinc, copper, selenium, chromium, manganese, molybdenum iodine, fluoride, strontium, lithium, nickel, boron, vanadium, and arsenic. The discussion of trace elements will include those present in PN trace element solutions (zinc, copper, manganese, and chromium), as well as iodine, selenium, and iron. Deficiency of iodine, selenium, and iron has been described in children receiving long-term PN. These minerals are not included in trace element solutions, but they are frequently added in the solutions of children receiving long-term PN. Table 75.4A-3 provides estimates of PN mineral requirements, and Table 75.4A-10 lists PN requirements for trace elements.

In 1988, the American Society for Clinical Nutrition (ASCN) published recommendations for parenteral trace elements for the pediatric age range.[65] These recommendations are based on calculations using the factorial method. As this committee recognized, trace element requirements of children receiving PN are inadequately studied. When the ASCN recommendations were critically assessed, some of the recommendations were found to be inaccurate. For instance, Mouser and colleagues found that children receiving the ASCN recommended amount of chromium had 10 times the serum concentration of children consuming a normal diet.[66]

CALCIUM, PHOSPHORUS, AND MAGNESIUM

The minerals calcium, phosphorus, and magnesium are vital to intermediary metabolism serving in energy transfer. Calcium and phosphorus also serve a structural function, and calcium is a regulator for a variety of intracellular processes. Calcium and phosphorus are presumed to be actively transported across the placenta against a concentration gradient.[67] Between the time a fetus weighs 1,000 g and 4,400 g at term, whole-body calcium content increases by 86%, phosphorus by 82%, and magnesium by 78%.[68] Many chronic diseases that require PN support are associated with calcium depletion. Approximately 99% of total-body calcium is found in bone, whereas 85% of phosphorus is in bone, and 50 to 60% of magnesium is in bone. Bone acts as a reservoir for calcium, phosphorus, and magnesium, so serum levels often do not reflect total-body content. This makes it difficult to identify deficiency states. Less than 1% of the total-body calcium, phosphorus, and magnesium is in the circulation. Because serum calcium is tightly controlled at the expense of bone, calcium deficiency is a chronic problem of bone loss. Calcium circulates in three forms: 45% is in the biologically active ionized form, 45% is bound to protein, mainly albumin, and 10% is complexed to phosphate, lactate, and citrate.[69] Measurement of ionized calcium, because it is the active form, better reflects calcium homeostasis than does measuring total serum calcium. Fifty percent of phosphorus exists in circulation as free ions, 10% is protein bound, and 40% is complexed to calcium, magnesium, and sodium as salts. Phosphorus deficiency can be a serious acute problem when malnourished patients are refed and sufficient phosphorus is not provided.[70] Magnesium is mainly an intracellular anion, so serum magnesium levels may not accurately reflect total-body magnesium status.

The parenteral requirements for calcium and phosphorus can be tremendous, especially in small prematurely born infants and in children with a chronic disease. Peak bone mass is attained in late adolescence and is determined by nutritional factors, genetics, mechanical factors, and the environment.[71] PN should supply adequate minerals to attain optimal peak bone mass. Metabolic bone disease is common in premature infants and in children receiving long-term PN.[72,73] The hypocalcemia associated with meta-

TABLE 75.4A-10   BASAL DAILY PARENTERAL REQUIREMENTS BY AGE AND DEVELOPMENTAL STAGE

TRACE ELEMENT	DOSE/D
VERY LOW BIRTH WEIGHT INFANTS	
Iron	100 µg/kg
Zinc	350 µg/kg
Copper	60 µg/kg
LOW BIRTH WEIGHT AND PRETERM NEONATES	
Iron	100 µg/kg
Zinc	400 µg/kg
Copper	20 µg/kg
Selenium	2 µg/kg
Chromium	0.2 µg/kg
Manganese	0.1 µg/kg
Molybdenum	0.25 µg/kg
NORMAL INFANTS	
Iron	100 µg/kg
Zinc	250 µg/kg* 400 µg/kg†
Copper	20 µg/kg
Selenium	2.0 µg/kg
Chromium	0.2 µg/kg
Manganese	1.0 µg/kg
Molybdenum	0.25 µg/kg
Iodine	1.0 µg/kg
CHILDREN	
Iron	1.0 mg
Zinc	5.0 mg
Copper	300 µg
Selenium	30 µg
Chromium	5.0 µg
Manganese	50 µg
Molybdenum	5.0 µg
Iodine	50 µg
ADOLESCENTS	
Iron	1–3 mg‡
Zinc	2.5–4.0 mg
Copper	0.5–1.5 mg
Selenium	30–60 µg
Chromium	10–14 µg
Manganese	150–800 µg
Molybdenum	20–120 µg
Iodine	150 µg
Zinc	350 µg/kg
Copper	60 µg/kg

Adapted from Schanler RJ et al[183] for very low birth weight infants, Zlotkin SH et al[184] for low birth weight infants, Greene HL et al[65] for term infants, with the amount for children being the maximal daily dose, and the American Medical Association (AMA)[185] for adolescents. The nutrients not addressed by the AMA panel consensus levels from diverse literature as discussed by Solomons N[186] have been listed.
The table is adapted from Solomons NW and Ruz M.[187]
*For full-term infants 0–3 months.
†For infants 3–12 months.
‡Depends on gender; extra is needed in females to compensate for menstrual losses.

bolic bone disease results from not supplying adequate calcium and from urinary calcium losses. Because at varying concentrations, calcium and phosphorus will complex with each other in PN solutions and form a precipitate, there are limitations to the amounts of calcium and phosphorus that can be supplied in PN solutions.[74] These limitations caused nutritionists to seek creative ways of providing the minerals, such as alternating intravenous solutions of high calcium concentration with those of high phosphorus content. These strategies have no proven benefit. Amino acid solutions designed for children under 1 year have added cysteine. Cysteine lowers the pH enough to permit the addition of calcium and phosphorus in amounts that may meet daily requirements.[75] In premature infants, it may not be possible to deliver these minerals in quantities that simulate intrauterine mineral accretion, but severe bone disease can be reduced. Because the amount of calcium that can be delivered is limited, maneuvers that decrease urinary calcium losses have been explored. Factors that promote hypercalciuria are increased calcium intake,[76] decreased phosphate intake,[76] increased amino acid infusion,[77] metabolic acidosis,[78] and cycling PN infusions.[79]

Children on long-term PN do not experience bone pain or fractures because the metabolic disease associated with PN is mostly subclinical.[80] Aluminum present as a contaminant in PN solutions and in additives can lead to decreased bone mineralization.[81] Parenteral amino acid solutions prepared from casein hydrolysates were contaminated with aluminum. Aluminum contamination is associated with osteopenia, growth arrest, fractures, and pain.[82–84] Since the discontinuation of these solutions, metabolic bone disease has become less of an issue. However, osteopenia remains a problem for children.[85,86] A study of children who had bowel resections of varying length, necessitating PN support for 1 to 67 months, showed appropriate bone mineralization for their weight and height after the PN solutions were discontinued.[87] The bone mineralization was less than that of children of the same age. Although this observation is encouraging, the findings must be viewed with caution because more than half of the children had relatively small amounts of bowel removed and required PN for less than 8 months.

Refeeding syndrome frequently accompanies the nutritional rehabilitation of malnourished individuals. The refeeding syndrome is a set of metabolic and functional complications that occurs as a result of intracellular shifts of elements. During rapid nutritional rehabilitation, profound hypophosphatemia, hypomagnesemia, and hypokalemia can precipitate acute respiratory and circulatory collapse. Neurologic manifestations of the refeeding syndrome include weakness, lethargy, paralysis, and confusion. Deaths have been documented.[88] Phosphorus, magnesium, and potassium must be carefully monitored in malnourished patients. Aggressive supplementation and correction of low values prevent the adverse outcomes of refeeding syndrome.

ZINC

Zinc is essential for growth. It is involved in chromosome replication and regulation of the translation of genetic information, provides structure for "zinc finger" proteins, stabilizes ribosomes and membranes, and is a component of a number of enzymes.[89] Zinc deficiency in humans impairs cell-mediated immunity.[90] Signs of zinc deficiency include dermatitis, alopecia, diarrhea, and immune deficiency. Severe PN-associated zinc deficiency mimics acrodermatitis enteropathica.[91] With zinc deficiency, relatively more fat

accrues than lean tissue.[92] Zinc status is difficult to monitor. Stress, infections, and trauma all alter circulating zinc levels. Merely administering PN diminishes plasma zinc by about 30%.[92] Despite these shortcomings, serum zinc is commonly used to monitor zinc nutriture. Zinc is lost from the body through urine, sweat, and stool. Zinc status should be assessed and corrected if necessary in the face of extra loss, as in the case of diarrhea or high ostomy output. The composition of the tissue acquired during nutritional rehabilitation may be affected by zinc status. Acute zinc toxicity has resulted in pancreatitis.[93] Chronic toxicity has not been described in pediatric patients receiving PN.

COPPER

Copper is important in many enzyme systems, especially those that involve oxygen, hydrogen peroxide, and superoxide. It is necessary for the formation of melanin, catecholamine synthesis, and crosslinking of elastin and collage.[94] Copper circulates bound to ceruloplasmin, which may have antioxidant properties of its own. Copper deficiency has been described in long-term PN patients frequently.[95,96] Premature infants are at special risk of becoming copper deficient because copper accumulates in the fetus during the third trimester. Signs of copper deficiency include hypochromic, microcystic anemia, depigmentation of skin and hair, hypothermia, and hypotonia.

MANGANESE

Manganese has two known functions: as cofactor for the enzyme pyruvate carboxylase and as part of the mitochondrial enzyme superoxide dismutase. Manganese deficiency in long-term PN has not been described; however, toxicity has been described. High levels of manganese have been implicated as a causative factor in the cholestatic effect of PN and also in basal ganglia damage resulting in Parkinson disease in adults on long-term PN.[97] Fell and colleagues have monitored basal ganglia damage associated with manganese accumulation in children on long-term PN using magnetic resonance imaging. This group also followed the cholestatic effects of manganese in children. This study supports a causative role for manganese in both of these complications of PN.[98]

CHROMIUM

The metabolic role of chromium is poorly understood. Proof that chromium plays a part in a "glucose tolerance factor," thought to activate insulin, is lacking. Two cases of chromium deficiency have been described in adults receiving PN. The symptoms of the described cases include glucose intolerance, hyperosmolarity, dehydration, and glucosuria. Symptoms responded poorly to insulin, but insulin responsiveness was restored with administration of chromium.[99] Chromium deficiency in children receiving PN has not been described; however, chromium excess has been reported.[100] Chromium toxicity results in skin irritation and carcinogenesis in animals.[101] The trivalent chromic ions present in PN solutions are not highly toxic, so excessive chromium from PN is not likely to be harmful.

IODINE

Iodine is essential, and its deficiency has been described in children.[102] However, iodine deficiency had not been described in children receiving PN until recently. Ibrahim and colleagues studied a group of extremely premature infants on PN who were in negative iodine balance.[103] Because the absorption of iodine is good, the parenteral dose should be similar to the enteral recommendation. One microgram/kg/d administered parenterally is recommended for the very low birth weight infant, whereas the enteral recommendation is 30 μg/kg/day.[104,105] Iodine is a minor contaminating component of many PN solutions and is present in antiseptics used to cleanse the skin at the catheter insertion site. PN patients receive measurable iodine from both of these sources.[106] No toxicity has been found in subjects receiving 20 times the Recommended Dietary Allowance for iodine. Any pediatric patient receiving long-term PN requires supplemental iodine.

SELENIUM

Selenium is bound at the catalytic site of glutathione peroxidase, an enzyme that catalyzes the reduction of H_2O_2 to H_2O. Selenium is also at the active site of type 1 and 3 iodothyronine deiodinase, which is important in the synthesis and degradation of triiodothyronine.[107] However, one study did not show a correlation between selenium supplementation and thyroid function in very low birth weight infants receiving long-term PN.[108] Selenium deficiency has been reported in children receiving PN.[109–111] The ASCN guidelines list the parenteral selenium requirements at 2.0 μg/kg/d for preterm and term infants as well as children.[65] Selenium toxicity is described.[112]

CHOLESTASIS

Because copper and manganese are excreted in the bile, patients with cholestasis who require PN are at risk of developing increased levels of manganese and copper. Therefore, the blood levels of these micronutrients should be carefully monitored and the content of manganese and copper in the PN solutions adjusted as indicated. Similarly, selenium, chromium, and molybdenum should be monitored and the PN content of these minerals adjusted as needed in children with renal disease.

IRON

Iron deficiency is the most common cause of anemia in children.[113] However, anemia is a manifestation of the severe end of the iron deficiency spectrum because iron is used for erythropoiesis at the expense of other tissues, including brain. Iron deficiency adversely affects behavior and neurodevelopment.[114] Iron deficiency is common among children receiving long-term PN. It occurs as a result of the underlying condition necessitating PN rather than as a result of the PN itself. Long-term PN without iron supplementation results in iron deficiency and iron deficiency anemia. Causes of anemia other than iron deficiency may be present and should be searched for before assuming that anemia is due to iron deficiency. These include the anemia of chronic disease, zinc deficiency, vitamin E deficiency, and hemolysis.

Chronic blood loss from stool, urine, or vomitus can lead to iron deficiency. These losses should be corrected when possible. A number of tests are useful in assessing iron nuriture: ferritin, free erythrocyte protoporphyrin, zinc protoporphyrin, transferrin saturation, transferrin receptors, and hemoglobin and hematocrit. Hemoglobin and hematocrit are readily accessible but represent severe, end-stage iron deficiency. Ferritin is an early marker of iron deficiency, reflecting liver stores of iron; however, ferritin is also an acute-phase reactant, making interpretation of this test problematic. Changes in protoporphyrin levels reflect early alteration of erythropoiesis. In the context of a child receiving PN, a combination of these tests is recommended.[115]

Prematurely born infants are at particular risk for deficiency because iron is transferred to the fetus via the placenta during the last trimester. Iron precipitates as iron phosphate from lipid emulsions and three-in-one solutions. Iron dextrans are compatible with PN solutions that do not contain lipid.[116]

See Table 75.4A-10 for recommended daily amounts of iron for parenteral administration. Iron can be given either intravenously or intramuscularly as iron dextran.[117] Inorganic salts of iron are used in PN solution in Europe.[118] Some report increased infection rates in children receiving iron supplementation.[119] Other reports have not found this association.[120] Iron homeostasis is regulated at the level of GI absorption. Parenterally administered iron bypasses this control mechanism, making iron overload possible. Iron administration should be reduced or eliminated if overload is present.[121]

VITAMINS

Vitamins are essential nutrients and must be provided by the PN solution, with the possible exception of vitamin D, to avoid deficiency. For the purposes of PN, both water-soluble and fat-soluble vitamins are available in a single solution. Several parenteral vitamin preparations are available for children and adults. Table 75.4A-11 lists some of the preparations, the US Food and Drug Administration (FDA) requirements for adult vitamin solutions (there is no FDA guideline for pediatric multivitamins), and the recommendations of the Committee on Clinical Practice Issues of the ASCN. These recommendations are based on the requirements for stable patients. Adjustments may need to be made for patients who have specific vitamin deficiencies or organ dysfunction, require ventilatory support, or are catabolic. Carnitine is likely a conditionally essential nutrient in the neonate and should be provided after deficiency has been confirmed.[39] To avoid potential toxicity, vitamin preparations designed for preterm infants should not be formulated with propylene glycol or polysorbate.[65]

CENTRAL VERSUS PERIPHERAL ADMINISTRATION OF PN

Central administration of PN solution is required in the infant and the premature infant to deliver meaningful nutrition support.[122] In the older child, peripheral administration can be maintained for a few days, but central

TABLE 75.4A-11 VITAMINS FOR PARENTERAL NUTRITION

	ML	A (IU)	D (IU)	E (IU)	K (MG)	B1 (MG)	B2 (MG)	B3 (MG)	B6 (MG)	B12 (µG)	FOLIC ACID (µG)	PANTOTHENIC ACID (MG)	BIOTIN (µG)	C (MG)	CARNITINE (MG/KG)
FDA*		4,000–5,000	400	12–15	2–4/wk	1–1.5	1.1–1.9	12–20	1.6–2.0	3	400	5.0–10	130–300	45	—
Infuvite Adult (Sabex 2002, Boucherville, QC, Canada)†‡	10	3,300	200	10	150	6	3.6	40	6	5	600	15	60	200	—
M.V.I. Adult 12 (aaiPharma, Wilmington, NC, USA)†	10	3,300	200	10	0	3	3.6	40	4	5	400	15	60	100	—
ASPEN§		2,300	400	7	200	1.2	1.4	17	1.0	1.0	140	5	20	80	2–10||
M.V.I. Pediatric (aaiPharma, Wilmington, NC, USA)†#	5	2,300	400	7	200	1.2	1.4	17	1.0	1.0	140	5	20	80	—
Infuvite Pediatric (Sabex 2002, Boucherville, QC, Canada)†‡	5	2,300	400	7	200	1.2	1.4	17	1.0	1.0	140	5	20	80	—

* US Food and Drug Administration (FDA) conditions for marketing an effective adult (ages 11 years and older) parenteral multivitamin.[189]
† Manufacturer's product information.
‡ Baxter.
§ As recommended by American Society for Parenteral and Enteral Nutrition.[39]
|| May be conditionally essential in neonates.[190] Confirm deficiency.
Leosan.

access is necessary for long-term (greater than 1 week) administration of PN. Because PN is not recommended for a duration less than a week,[123] peripheral PN should be thought of as a bridge until a central line can be placed. Although it is possible to provide peripheral PN over a long period of time in children and adolescents, it requires multiple intravenous site changes, risks local complications, and is inconvenient for both the patient and the caregivers. Therefore, central intravenous access for PN should be sought. The technique of peripherally accessed central catheterization (PICC line) for establishing central lines is relatively easily accomplished.[124]

INTRAVENOUS CATHETERS

There are three categories of PN central lines: (1) tunneled lines such as the Broviac or Hickman lines, (2) subcutaneous port lines such as the Medi-port or Hide-a-Port, and (3) PICC lines. No one type of catheter is clearly superior to the others in all situations.[125] PICC lines are easily placed and removed but are associated with the highest incidence of malposition, inadvertent removal, thrombophlebitis, and mechanical obstruction.[126,127] Subcutaneous ports are associated with the least number of infections[128,129] and have a smaller risk of intraluminal thrombosis when compared with the tunneled catheters.[130] Ports are the most difficult to place and require repeated percutaneous access.

In general, reducing the number of lumens reduces the risk.[131] Double-lumen PICC lines are often too large to be of use in young children. Subcutaneous reservoir devices are available with double lumens and divided ports but may be too large to be practical, especially in the small child. It is possible to place a second separate central line if additional access is required.

Catheters should be placed into the superior vena cava or right atrium. The superior vena cava can be reached via the internal jugular vein, the subclavian vein, and peripheral veins. Use of the femoral vein is discouraged. Femoral lines are associated with higher rates of venous thrombosis and catheter-related sepsis.[132] With subclavian access, there is a greater risk of pneumothorax when compared with internal jugular access.[133] Internal jugular insertion is associated with higher rates of hematoma formation, arterial injury, and catheter-related infections.[134] In a large series, radiologic insertion technique was superior to surgical insertion. The radiologic insertion led to fewer infections (1.9 vs 4.0 per 1,000 catheter days), fewer pneumothoraces, and fewer complications overall.[135] Maintaining central venous access long term can be challenging. When all conventional sites have been exhausted, thoracotomy with cannulation of the azygos vein or direct right atrial cannulation[136] has been used. More recently, use of a transhepatic approach for establishing central access for PN has been described.[137]

COMPLICATIONS

Complications associated with PN fall into three general categories: mechanical, metabolic, and infectious. Mechanical complications include misplaced lines and lines that move, fall out, are pulled out, break, kink, or become occluded. Table 75.4A-12 lists some examples of the specific injuries that can occur with mechanical misadventures. Some mechanical complications represent significant life-threatening events, and their occurrence is evident almost immediately or within a short period of time. Others, such as development of a thrombus, occur over a longer time and are heralded by the progressive difficulty in aspirating blood through the catheter. Children experience higher catheter occlusion rates than adults: 10% of children receiving home PN support,[87] 13 to 16% of oncology patients,[138,139] 31% of infants,[140] and 41% of patients with cystic fibrosis.[141] Catheters can be occluded by a thrombus, a kink in the line, too tight sutures, deposition of drugs, mineral precipitation, and lipid deposition within the lumen of the line or abutment of the catheter tip against the vessel wall. Mechanical maneuvers should be attempted as soon as a line is identified as occluded to restore the patency of the line. These maneuvers are not often successful and can be associated with dislodgment of a thrombus and pulmonary embolization, line rupture, or malposition of the catheter.

Thrombosis in central catheters is relatively common. Clot may form as a fibrin sheath at the catheter tip, or a thrombus may form on the outside wall of the catheter and/or on the wall of the vessel adjacent to the catheter. The fibrin sheath is a consistent finding on all indwelling catheters regardless of the type of material, but the amount of sheath varies with the thrombogenicity of catheter material.[142] Mural thrombi occur within 48 hours of catheter insertion. Many strategies have been attempted to prevent the development of catheter-related thrombosis, including the administration of salicylates, dextran, and heparin. Catheters have also been coated with salicylates, heparin, and antibiotics. Some advocate the routine addition of heparin to infused solutions (500–2000 U/L) because this may decrease thrombotic complications with long-term catheter use.[143] But saline flushes are equally efficacious in maintaining catheter patency.[144] Although heparin has been used for many years, some caution is necessary. Heparin can cause a transient fall in platelet count 1 to 3 days after initiation of treatment. In most patients, this is of no clinical significance; the platelet levels return to normal within a few days of the discontinuation of heparin. In some patients, heparin-induced thrombocytopenia, a life- and limb-threatening complication of heparin therapy, can occur. Heparin-induced thrombocytopenia is likely an immune-mediated syndrome that can be precipitated even by minute quantities of heparin given to flush catheters.[145,146] To restore line patency to a fibrin-occluded catheter, streptokinase, urokinase, and tissue plasminogen activator have been used successfully. Currently, recombinant tissue plasminogen activator is the agent of choice to restore patency of thrombin-occluded catheters.[147] Treatment of thrombotic occlusions with tissue plasminogen activator has resulted in removing the obstruction in over 90% of catheters treated[148] and has a low complication rate compared with treatment with either streptokinase or urokinase. Catheter occlusions by some drugs and minerals may be resolved with the instillation of 0.2 to 1.0 mL of 0.1N HCl for 30 minutes to 1 hour.[149–151] More than one instillation may be required. For other drugs, an alkaline solution may be necessary. In clinical situations that do not respond to usual treatment, the possibility of fragmentation or disconnection of part of the indwelling catheter with embolization should be considered.[152] Figure 75.4A-2 is an algorithm for the diagnosis and treatment of catheter occlusion in adult patients with short small bowel syndrome.

Infections related to the catheter can occur systemically or locally at the insertion site. A number of maneuvers have been demonstrated to reduce the risk of infection. These include (1) cleansing the skin prior to insertion with chlorhexidine,[153] (2) avoiding catheter insertion in a febrile child, (3) radiologic insertion by an expert team,[135] and (4) using full-barrier precautions during insertion.[154] Prophylactic antibiotics at the time of insertion do not decrease the risk of infection, and antibiotic ointment at the insertion site should be avoided because it results in the acquisition of resistant organisms and does not decrease the risk of infection.[155] Catheters impregnated with antimicrobial materials such as chlorhexidine, silver sulfadiazine, minocycline, and rifampin are associated with a lower incidence of line infection, but their higher cost may limit their use.[153,156] Certainly, these special catheters do not obviate the need to use all other techniques to reduce infections. Systemic infections occur in 10 to 60% of patients, often require removal of the catheter to clear,[138,157–159] and can be complicated by urinary tract infection, osteomyelitis, and abscess formation. Infections can be caused by bacteria such as those that occur on the skin, populate the GI tract, or have no identifiable source or fungi, the most common of which is Candida. The most important route of catheter-related contamination is thought to be migration of organisms from the skin along the subcutaneous tract into the vein. Another important source of infection is catheter hub contamination during tubing manipulations. One study noted that the infectious agent was often found on the skin of nurses who changed the PN fluid bag.[160] Some have hypothesized that a GI tract injured by inflammation, ischemia, surgical manipulation, or malnutrition may be more permeable to infectious organisms.[139,161] If a child with a central line develops a significant fever (38°C), whether or not there is another source of infection, central and peripheral cultures should be obtained, and the child should be treated with intravenous antibiotics covering both gram-positive cocci and gram-negative bacteria. If a source of fever other than the catheter is identified, such as an ear infection or a urinary tract infection, neither the catheter nor the other site can be assumed to be the source of the fever; therefore, antibiotic coverage should include coverage for organisms associated with catheter infections and possible non–catheter-related sources. Catheter-related infections can be eradicated with appropriate antibiotics; however, tunnel-related infections are more difficult to eliminate.[128,162] Catheter removal is usually curative if antibiotic coverage is extended 48 hours after the catheter is

TABLE 75.4A-12 COMPLICATIONS ASSOCIATED WITH PARENTERAL NUTRITION

COMPLICATION	CAUSE	INTERVENTION
Catheter related		
Cardiac arrhythmia	Catheter tip in heart	Remove catheter
Air embolus	Inadvertent injection of air; accidental uncoupling of infusion system	Place patient on left side and lower the head of the bed; this may keep air within apex of the right ventricle until it is absorbed
Thrombosis of central vein	Uncoupling of infusion system; catheter induced	Anticoagulation therapy; remove catheter if unsuccessful (see figure75.4-2)
Catheter occlusion	Hypotension; failure to maintain line patency; formation of fibrin sheath outside the catheter; lipid or mineral precipitates	Anticoagulation therapy (see Figure 75.4A-2)
Perforation and/or infusion leak	More common with polyvinyl polyethylene catheters	Check device connection sites; replace faulty devices, tubing, catheter
Infusion system obstruction	Catheter kinking, clot; bacterial filter airlock; clamping of line	Attempt mechanical manipulation
Phlebitis	Peripheral administration of hypertonic solution (osmolarity $\geq$ 900 mOsm/kg); line infiltration	Change peripheral line site
Infectious		
Sepsis	Improper aseptic technique; catheter insertion; catheter care; mixing of parenteral solutions	Blood cultures; antimicrobial medication (see Figure 75.4A-3)
Local infection	Improper aseptic technique	Local and/or systemic antimicrobial medications (see Figure 75.4A-3)
Metabolic		
Osmotic diuresis	Hyperglycemia; increased glucose in urine	Reduce infusion rate or decrease dextrose concentration; give insulin
Hyperammonemia	Hepatic dysfunction; excess free ammonia; insufficient arginine; excessive amino acid infusion	Reduce protein concentration; increase nonprotein calorie-to-nitrogen ratio
Azotemia or elevated blood urea nitrogen	Dehydration; calorie-nitrogen imbalance; renal dysfunction	Correct dehydration; increase nonprotein calorie-to-nitrogen ratio or reduce amino acid concentration; give insulin if hyperglycemia is present
Hyperglycemia	Excessive infusion rate or concentration of glucose; concurrent steroid therapy; possible sepsis; insulin insufficiency	Reduce rate or concentration of dextrose; rule out sepsis; give insulin
Hypoglycemia	Abrupt interruption of infusion of a high glucose concentration	Start dextrose infusion; monitor for seizures
Metabolic acidosis	Renal or gastrointestinal losses; infusion of hydrogen ion; inadequate amount of base-producing substance in solutions to neutralize acid products of amino acid degradation; excessive protein and/or calories; acute postinjury phase with increased metabolic rate	Increase acetate in solutions; decrease chloride in solutions with hypochloremic acidosis; provide maintenance calories and protein
Metabolic alkalosis	Base introduction or nasogastric drainage	Provide additional fluid and NaCl, KCl, or NH_4Cl
Fluid overload	Cardiac or renal insufficiency or excessive infusion rate	Decrease fluid; can increase the nutrient concentration of nutrient solutions
Respiratory acidosis	Increased calorie load with high fraction of calories as dextrose	Decrease total caloric intake; decrease fraction of calories from dextrose and increase fraction of calories from lipid
Cholestasis	Idiopathic; lack of enteral feeding	Provide some enteral nutrition, even if only 1–2 mL/h
Hypophosphatemia	Inadequate phosphate; refeeding syndrome; increased losses (diarrhea); high dextrose concentration infusion may increase phosphorus needs	Increase phosphate in solution; monitor solution for compatibility; monitor serum levels
Hyperphosphatemia	Renal insufficiency	Decrease phosphorus in nutrient solution but do not omit; check for other phosphorus source
Hypocalcemia	Refeeding syndrome; inadequate calcium in solution	Increase calcium in solution; monitor compatibility; monitor serum levels
Hypomagnesemia	Inadequate magnesium in solution; refeeding syndrome; gastrointestinal or renal losses	Increase magnesium in solution; monitor solution compatibility; monitor serum levels
Hypokalemia	Gastrointestinal or renal losses; refeeding syndrome; inadequate potassium in solution; high dextrose infusion; hypomagnesemia	Increase potassium in solution; may require 4 mEq K/kg/d; monitor serum levels
Hyponatremia	Gastrointestinal or renal losses; inadequate sodium in solution; excessive fluid intake	Increase sodium in solution; decrease fluid volume; check all sources of intake; monitor intake and output, serum sodium and urine-specific gravity
Essential fatty acid deficiency	Fat-free solutions	Provide at least 2–4% of calories as fat (0.5–1.0 g/kg/d)
Hypertriglyceridemia	Lipid infusion dose too high; acute inflammatory state	Increase duration of infusion; decrease total g/kg/d lipid infused
Rash	Possible allergy	Discontinue lipid administration or change lipid preparation
Trace element deficiency	Inadequate or incomplete trace element supplementation; gastrointestinal losses (zinc)	Routine trace element supplementation, monitor nutritional trace element status
Vitamin disorders	Inadequate intake; excess needs	Monitor serum levels; provide additional vitamins

Adapted from Davis AM.[191]

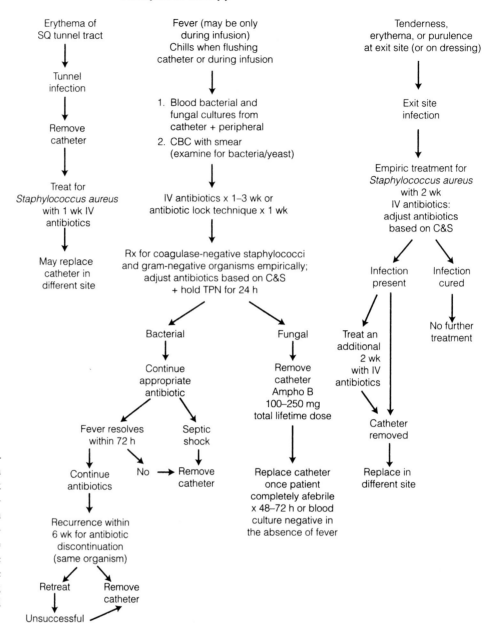

FIGURE 75.4A-2 Algorithm for the diagnosis and treatment of catheter occlusion. Reproduced with permission from the American Gastroenterological Association.[188] Ampho B = amphotericin B; C&S = culture and sensitivity; CBC = complete blood count; IV = intravenous; SQ = subcutaneous; TPN = total parenteral nutrition.

taken out. The catheter should be removed in the face of clinical deterioration, continued bacteremia, and suspected cardiac sepsis or after failing two courses of intravenous antibiotics. Figure 75.4A-3 is an algorithm for the diagnosis and treatment of catheter-related infection in adults with short small bowel syndrome.

The most common metabolic complications associated with PN are over- or underhydration. Too much fluid is sometimes administered when all fluid sources (other intravenous lines, enteral feedings, oral feedings, water flushes) are not considered. Underhydration can develop when inadequate fluids from all routes are provided, during extended periods of hyperglycemia, and when conditions arise that increase fluid requirements (ie, fever, increased renal solute load, ostomy losses, diarrhea). Other metabolic complications include hypoglycemia, electrolyte imbalances, inadequate growth, substrate intolerance, hypersensitivity reactions, and specific nutrient deficiencies. Hypoglycemia can occur if PN is abruptly stopped. Cholestasis associated with

PN support is a major problem. The etiology is unknown. Medications such as phenobarbital and ursodiol have been used with limited success. Factors associated with cholestasis include lack of enteral feeding; excessive carbohydrate, fat, and/or calories; inappropriate quality and quantity of amino acids; and deficient trace elements.[163] The only effective treatment is discontinuation of PN.

INITIATION

There is no standard pediatric patient. An individualized plan for initiation, advancement, and maintenance goals should be formulated before starting PN. The plan is based on estimates of requirements and should account for increased or decreased needs of each patient. Before starting PN, baseline laboratory values should be measured and electrolyte and mineral abnormalities corrected. The steps in devising a PN plan are as follows: (1) Determine fluid volume and rate. This determination is based on the fluid requirement and ability of

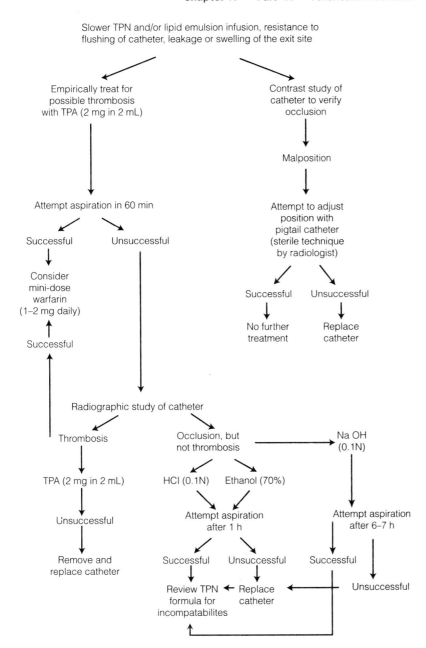

FIGURE 75.4A-3 Algorithm for the diagnosis and treatment of catheter-related infection. Reproduced with permission from the American Gastroenterological Association.[188] HCl = hydrochloric acid; Na OH = sodium hydroxide; TPA = tissue plasminogen activator; TPN = total parenteral nutrition.

the patient to tolerate a fluid load. (2) Calculate the amount of dextrose to be used initially, during advancement, and for maintenance. (3) Determine the amount of protein to be given at initiation, during advancement, and at maintenance. (4) Determine the dose of lipid, again taking into account the three phases, initiation, advancement, and maintenance. (5) Determine the amounts of micronutrients, electrolytes, minerals, trace elements, and vitamins. Vitamins and mineral and trace elements come as prepackaged units. Special consideration of acid-base balance is necessary. Increasing the amount of acetate while decreasing the chloride can shift the balance toward base.[164] Suggested ranges for macronutrient provision in pediatric PN solutions are given in Table 75.4A-13. The distribution of calories derived from macronutrients is quite flexible and depends on the clinical setting: from 7 to 20% of calories in the PN solution can be derived from protein, carbohydrate can account for 20 to 60% of calories, and lipid can range from 20 to 50%.

MONITORING

During initiation, while advancing, and at maintenance rates, patients need to be monitored for complications and to ensure that the goals of the PN are being achieved. A suggested list of laboratory determinations and a schedule for monitoring are provided in Table 75.4A-14. The PN plan as outlined in the previous section should be continually assessed and revised based on the results of monitoring and the changing clinical status of the patient.

DISCONTINUATION AND CYCLING

Sudden discontinuation of high glucose infusion has resulted in hypoglycemia, especially in children under 3 years of age.[165,166] Blood glucose levels should be monitored following cessation of high glucose infusions. PN should be tapered by decreasing to half the rate for 1 hour and to one fourth the

TABLE 75.4A-13 SUGGESTED PEDIATRIC PARENTERAL SUBSTRATE PROVISION

	NUTRIENT	AMOUNT
INITIATION	Carbohydrate	10% dextrose (6–8 mg/kg/min)
Amino acids	50–100% of goal	
Lipid		0.5–1.0 g/kg/d
ADVANCEMENT	Carbohydrate	5% dextrose per day (2–4 mg/kg/min)
Amino acid	100% of goal	
Lipid		0.5–1.0 g/kg/d
USUAL UPPER LIMIT	Carbohydrate	8–18 mg/kg/min
Peripheral	12.5% dextrose	
Central	25–35% dextrose	
Amino acid		3.0 g/kg/d

original rate for another hour before complete discontinuation. A similar strategy for tapering the PN and monitoring blood sugars should be followed when cycling PN.

There are physiologic and psychological advantages to cycling PN administration, that is, infusing the PN solution in less than 24 hours. For the older child, time without the infusion apparatus allows freedom for greater activity, more social interaction, and school attendance. Continuous PN infusion leads to continuously high serum insulin levels. This hyperinsulinemia causes hepatic lipid deposition and increased hepatic lipogenesis. EFAD may occur because insulin inhibits the release of free fatty acids from adipose tissue. These physiologic effects of continuous PN are reversed by cycling.[167] However, as discussed, cycling increases urinary calcium losses.

CRITICAL CARE

Changes in energy requirements in critically ill or injured children can be quite large, proportionately larger than the changes seen in adults. Especially during early childhood, the energy requirements for growth account for a significant proportion of total requirements. During growth, nutrients need to be supplied in amounts that accommodate tissue accretion, but during the catabolic response to illness or injury, somatic growth is not possible. At times when children are catabolic, overfeeding results from including a share for growth when calculating requirements. The dangers of overfeeding during critical illness are well recognized.[168] It remains a challenge to supply the correct nutrients for each phase of the acute response, allowing for changes in metabolic rate and for growth when it occurs while avoiding overfeeding.

The acute-phase response is proportional to the magnitude and duration of the injury. The response can be divided into three phases: the immediate response lasts minutes to hours and is characterized by autonomic stimulation, resulting in tachycardia, fever, and hypoglycemia. The second, or "ebb phase," is heralded by a sharp decrease in metabolic rate. Insulin levels and body temperature fall, whereas catecholamines, glucose, lactate, and free fatty acids increase. Cardiac output decreases. The second phase lasts from one to several days. The third phase is termed the "flow phase" and is characterized by hypermetabolism. The flow phase can be further subdivided into an early flow

phase characterized by hypermetabolism and a negative nitrogen balance. During the late flow phase, hypermetabolism persists, but anabolic repair of tissues and resumption of growth are signaled by a positive nitrogen balance.[169]

Nutritional assessment of a critically ill child includes measuring the constitutive protein pool, the acute-phase protein pool, nitrogen balance, and energy expenditure. All of these measurements can be easily accomplished in the pediatric intensive care unit setting. Prealbumin is a measure of the short-term status of constitutive proteins. C-reactive protein measures acute-phase reactants. These two tests, prealbumin and C-reactive protein, are inversely related and, when measured daily during an acute illness or injury, track the progression of the response. Levels of serum C-reactive protein less than 2 mg/dL are associated with a resumption of anabolic metabolism.[170] Prealbumin begins to rise once an anabolic state is achieved. There are a number of equations for calculating energy expenditure.[171] However, all of these equations are estimates and, especially in infants, can be inaccurate.[172] Indirect calorimetry, using a metabolic cart, measures oxygen consumption and carbon dioxide production. Resting energy expenditure (REE) can be calculated using the Weir equation:

Complete formula:
$$REE = [3.9(VO_2) + (VCO_2)]1.44 - 2.17(UN)$$

Abbreviated formula:
$$REE = [3.9(VO_2) + (VCO_2)]1.44$$

where REE is resting energy expenditure (kcal/d), VO_2 is oxygen consumption (mL/min), VCO_2 is carbon dioxide production (mL/min), and UN is urinary nitrogen (g/d). The RQ can be calculated from the measurements obtained by indirect calorimetry:

$$RQ = VCO_2/VO_2$$

The RQ is dependent on the substrate being used. Thus, when only fat is being oxidized, the RQ = 0.71. When only carbohydrates are oxidized, the RQ = 1.00. A mixed substrate yields an RQ of about 0.85. Some caution with regard to interpreting RQ; it does not reflect substrate oxidation during hyperventilation, metabolic alkalosis, or for about 6 to 8 hours after general anesthesia.[173]

A number of studies in adults suggest that in nutritional support of a critically ill patient, the enteral route is

TABLE 75.4A-14 SUGGESTED MONITORING PARAMETERS AND SCHEDULE DURING PARENTERAL NUTRITION IN PEDIATRICS

	SUGGESTED FREQUENCY	
PARAMETER	INITIAL/HOSPITALIZED	FOLLOW-UP/HOME
GROWTH		
Weight	Daily	Daily to monthly
Height/length	Weekly	Weekly to monthly
Head circumference	Weekly	Weekly to monthly
Body composition	Monthly	Monthly to annually
METABOLIC/SERUM*		
Electrolytes	Daily to weekly	Weekly to monthly
BUN/creatinine	Weekly	Monthly
Ca, PO₄, Mg	Twice weekly	Weekly to monthly
Acid-base status	Until stable	Weekly to monthly
Albumin/prealbumin	Weekly	Weekly to monthly
Glucose	Daily to weekly	Weekly to monthly
Triglycerides	Daily while increasing lipids	Weekly to monthly
Liver function tests	Weekly	Weekly to monthly
Complete blood count/differential	Weekly	Weekly to monthly
Platelets, PT/PTT	Weekly	As indicated
Iron indices	As indicated	Biannually to annually
Trace elements	Monthly	Biannually to annually
Fat-soluble vitamins	As indicated	Biannually to annually
Carnitine	As indicated	As indicated
Folate/vitamin B₁₂	As indicated	As indicated
Ammonia	As indicated	As indicated
Cultures	As indicated	As indicated
METABOLIC (URINE)		
Glucose	2 to 6 times/d	Daily to weekly
Ketones	2 to 6 times/d	Daily to weekly
Specific gravity	As indicated	As indicated
Urea nitrogen	As indicated	As indicated
CLINICAL OBSERVATION		
Vital signs†	Daily	Daily
Developmental milestones	As indicated	Annually
Intake and output	Daily	Daily to as indicated
Adminsitration system	6 to 12 times/d	6 to 12 times/d
Catheter site/dressing	6 to 12 times/d	6 to 12 times/d

Adapted from Davis AM.[191]
BUN = blood urea nitrogen; PT = prothrombin time; PTT = partial thromboplastin time.
Frequency depends on clinical conditions.
*For metabolically unstable patients, may need to check more frequently.
†Vital signs include respiratory rate, heart rate, temperature, and blood pressure.

preferred over PN.[174–176] In severe injury, enteral nutrition results in a greater and earlier visceral protein response.[177]

The aims of PN support in the critically ill child are to minimize the effects of catabolism and hypermetabolism that are part of the acute-phase response, to return the patient to positive nitrogen balance quickly, and, finally, to support growth when it resumes. In striving to achieve these aims, caution must be exercised to avoid both under- and overfeeding.

CONCLUSION

PN has saved lives and continues to do so. However, its use is fraught with complications: it is difficult to administer and requires knowledgeable personnel with technical expertise to design complete nutritional fluids, administer them, and monitor for complications. There are limited indications for PN. Its use has declined as medical personnel have become

more proficient in the use of enteral feedings, and evidence-based medicine that focuses on outcomes has shown that benefit is limited to defined groups of patients.

REFERENCES

1. Dudrick SJ, Wilmore DW, Vars HM, Rhoads JE. Long-term total PN with growth, development, and positive nitrogen balance. Surgery 1968;64:134–42.

2. Wilmore DW, Dudrick SJ. Safe long-term venous catheterization. Arch Surg 1968;98:256–8.

3. Wilmore DW, Dudrick SJ. Growth and development of an infant receiving all nutrients exclusively by vein. JAMA 1968; 203:860–4.

4. Wilmore DW. The history of PN. In: Baker RD, Baker SS, Davis AM, editors. Pediatric parenteral nutrition. New York: Chapman and Hall; 1997. p. 1–7.

5. Othersen HB, Hebra A, Chessman KH, Tagge GP. Central lines in parenteral nutrition. In: Baker RD, Baker SS, Davis AM,

editors. Pediatric parenteral nutrition. New York: Chapman and Hall; 1996. p. 259–72.

6. Mitton SG, Burston D, Brueton MJ, Kovar IZ. Plasma amino acid profiles in preterm infants receiving Vamin 9 glucose or Vamin infant. Early Hum Dev 1993;32:71–8.

7. Heyman MB. General and specialized parenteral amino acid formulations for nutrition support. J Am Diet Assoc 1990; 90:401–8, 411.

8. McClead RE Jr, Lentz ME, Coniglio JG, et al. The effect of three intravenous fat emulsions containing different concentrations of linoleic and alpha-linolenic acids on the plasma total fatty acid profile of neonates. J Pediatr Gastroenterol Nutr 1991;12:89–95.

9. de Lucas C, Moerna M, Lopez-Herce J, et al. Transpyloric enteral nutrition reduces the complication rate and cost in the critically ill child. J Pediatr Gastroenterol Nutr 2000;30:175–80.

10. Fish J, Sporay G, Beyer K, et al. A prospective randomized study of glutamine-enriched parenteral compared with enteral feeding in post operative patients. Am J Clin Nutr 1997;65:977–83.

11. Goplerud JM. Hyperalimentation associated hypertoxicity in the newborn. Am Clin Sci 1992;22:79–82.

12. Market AD, Lew DB, Schropp KP, Hak EB. Parenteral nutrition-associated anaphylaxis in a 4-year old child. J Pediatr Gastroenterol Nutr 1998;26:229–31.

13. Fell JME, Reynolds AP, Meadows N, et al. Manganese toxicity in children receiving long-term parenteral nutrition. Lancet 1996;347:1218–21.

14. Okada Y, Klein NJ, van Saene HKF, et al. Bactericidal activity against coagulase-negative staphylococci is impaired in infants receiving long-term parenteral nutrition. Ann Surg 2000;231:276–81.

15. Suita S, Yamanouchi T, Masumoto K, et al. Changing profile of parenteral nutrition in pediatric surgery: a 30-year experience at one institute. Surgery 2002;131(1 Pt 2):S275–82.

16. Feldman EJ, Dowling RH, McNaughton J, Peters TJ. Effects of oral versus intravenous nutrition on intestinal adaptation after small bowel resection in the dog. Gastroenterology 1976;70:712–9.

17. Stormon MO, Mitchell JD, Smoleniec JS, et al. Congenital intestinal lymphatic hypoplasia presenting as non-immune hydrops in utero, and subsequent neonatal protein-losing enteropathy. J Pediatr Gastroenterol Nutr 2002;35:691–4.

18. Hyman PE, Bursch B, Beck D, et al. Discriminating pediatric condition falsification from chronic intestinal pseudo-obstruction in toddlers. Child Maltreatment 2002;7:132–7.

19. Amii LA, Moss RL. Nutritional support of the pediatric surgical patient. Curr Opin Pediatr 1999;11:237–45.

20. Darrow DC. Physiologic basis for estimating requirements for parenteral fluids. Pediatr Clin North Am 1959;6:29–41.

21. Holliday MA, Segar WE. The maintenance need for water in parenteral fluid therapy. Pediatrics 1956;9:823.

22. Friis-Hansen B. Water distribution in the foetus and newborn infant. Acta Paediatr Scand 1983;305 Suppl:7–11.

23. El-Dahr SS, Chevalier RL. Special needs of the newborn infant in fluid therapy. Pediatr Clin North Am 1990;37:323–36.

24. Anderson DM. PN fluid and electrolytes In: Groh-Wargo S, Thompson M, Cox JH, Hartline JV, editors. Nutritional care for high-risk newborns, Chicago: Precept Press, Inc.; 2000. p. 109–18.

25. Rudman D, Millikan WJ, Richardson TJ, et al. Elemental balances during intravenous hyperalimentation of underweight adult subjects. J Clin Invest 1974;55:94–104.

26. Laidlaw SA, Kopple JD. Newer concepts of the indispensable amino acids. Am J Clin Nutr 1987;46:593–605.

27. Chipponi JX, Bleier JC, Santi MT, Rudman D. Deficiencies of essential and conditionally essential nutrients. Am J Clin Nutr 1982;35:1112–6.

28. Harper AE. Dispensable and indispensable amino acid relationships In: Blackburn GL, Grant JP, Young VR, editors. Amino acids. Metabolism and medical applications. Boston: John Wright-PSG; 1983. p. 105–21.

29. Pencharz BP, House JD, Wykes LJ, Ball RO. What are the essential amino acids for the preterm and term infant? In: Bindels JG, Goedhart A, Visser HKA, editors. Recent developments in infant nutrition. Nutricia symposia. Vol. 9. Dordrecht, the Netherlands: Kluwer Academic Publishers; 1996. p. 278–96.

30. Standing Committee on the Scientific Evaluation of Dietary Reference Intakes, Food and Nutrition Board, Institute of Medicine. Dietary reference intakes for energy, carbohydrate, fiber, fat, fatty acids, cholesterol, protein and amino acids (macronutrients). Washington (DC): National Academy Press; 2002.

31. Snyderman SE. The protein and amino acid requirements of the premature infant. In: Visser HKA, Toreistra JA, editors. Nutrica Symposium: Metabolic Processes in the Fetus and Newborn Infant. Leiden, the Netherlands: Stenfert Kroese; 1971. p. 128–43.

32. Sturman JA, Gaull GE, Raiha NCR. Absence of cystathionase in human fetal liver. Is cysteine essential? Science 1970;169:74–6.

33. Jelliffe DB. The assessment of the nutritional status of the community. WHO Monograph Series No. 53. Geneva: World Health Organization; 1966.

34. Fomon SJ. Nutrition of normal infants. St. Louis: Mosby-Year Book, Inc.; 1993.

35. Heyland, DK, Novak F, Drover JW, et al. Should immunonutrition become routine in critically ill patients? A systematic review of the evidence. JAMA 2001;286:944–53.

36. Frantisek N, Heyland D, Alison A, et al. Glutamine supplementation in serious illness: a systematic review of the evidence. Crit Care Med 2002;20:2022–9.

37. Naylor CD, O'Rourke K, Detsky A, Baker JP. PN with branched-chain amino acids in hepatic encephalopathy. Gastroenterology 1989;97:1033–42.

38. Nompleggi DJ, Bonkovsky HL. Nutritional supplementation in chronic liver disease: an analytical review. Hepatology 1994;19:518–33.

39. American Society for Parenteral and Enteral Nutrition Board of Directors and the Clinical Guidelines Task Force. Guidelines for the use of parenteral and enteral nutrition in adult and pediatric patients. JPEN J Parenter Enteral Nutr 2002;26 Suppl 1:1SA–138SA.

40. Korletz RL, Lipman TO, Klein S. AGA technical review on PN. Gastroenterology 2001;121:970–1001.

41. Klein S, Kinney J, Jeejeebhoy K, et al. Nutrition support in clinical practice: review of published data and recommendations for future research directions. JPEN J Parenter Enteral Nutr 1997;21:133–56.

42. Heird WC, Dell RB, Helms RA, et al. Amino acid mixture designed to maintain normal plasma amino acid patterns in infants and children requiring PN. Pediatrics 1987;80:401–8.

43. Heird WC, Hay W, Helms RA, et al. Pediatric parenteral amino acid mixture in low birth weight infants. Pediatrics 1988; 81:41–50.

44. Helms RA, Christensen ML, Mauer EC, Storm MC. Comparison of a pediatric versus standard amino acid formulation in preterm neonates requiring PN. J Pediatr 1987;110:466–70.

45. Forchielli ML, Gura KM, Sandler R, Lo C. Aminosyn PF or trophamine: which provides more protection from cholesta-

sis associated with total PN. J Pediatr Gastroenterol Nutr 1995;21:374–82.
46. Wolfe RR, Allsop JR, Burke JF. Glucose metabolism in man: responses to intravenous glucose infusion. Metabolism 1979;28:210–20.
47. American Academy of Pediatrics, Committee on Nutrition. Pediatric nutrition handbook. 4th ed. Elk Grove (IL): American Academy of Pediatrics; 1998.
48. Vaucher YE, Walson PD, Morrow G III. Continuous insulin infusion in hyperglycemic, very low birth weight infants. J Pediatr Gastroenterol Nutr 1982;1:211–5.
49. Binder ND, Raschko PK, Benda GI, et al. Insulin infusion with PN in extremely low birth weight infants with hyperglycemia. J Pediatr 1989;114:273.
50. Collins JW, Hoppe M, Brown K, et al. A controlled trial of insulin infusion with glucose intolerance. J Pediatr 1991;118:921.
51. Poindexter BB, Karn CA, Denne SC. Exogenous insulin reduces proteolysis and protein synthesis in extremely low birth weight infants. J Pediatr 1998;132:948.
52. Jeevanandam M, Mamias L, Schiller WR. Elevated urinary C-peptide excretion in multiple trauma patients. J Trauma 1991;31:334–8.
53. Nose O, Tipton JR, Ament ME. Administration of lipid improves nitrogen retention in children receiving isocaloric TPN. Pediatr Res 1985;19:228A.
54. Sauer P, Van Aerde J, Smith J, et al. Substrate utilization in newborn infants fed intravenously with or without a fat emulsion. Pediatr Res 1984;18:804A.
55. Donnell SC, Lloyd DA, Eaton S, Pierro A. The metabolic response to intravenous medium-chain triglycerides in infants after surgery. J Pediatr 2002;141:689–94.
56. Rubin M, Moser A, Vaserberg N, et al. Structured triacylglycerol emulsion, containing both medium- and long-chain fatty acids, in long-term home parenteral nutrition: a double-blind randomized cross-over study. Nutrition 2000;16:95–100.
57. Uauy R, Treen M, Hoffman D. Essential fatty acid metabolism and requirements during development. Semin Perinatol 1989;13:118.
58. Eisenberg S. Very low density lipoprotein metabolism. Prog Biochem Pharmacol 1979;15:139.
59. Olivecrona G, Olivecrona T. Clearance of artificial triacylglycerol particles. Curr Opin Clin Nutr Metab Care 1998;1:143–51.
60. Spear ML, Stahl GE, Hamossh M, et al. Effect of heparin dose and infusion rate on lipid clearance and bilirubin binding in premature infants receiving intravenous fat emulsions. J Pediatr 1988;112:94.
61. Kao LC, Cheng MH, Warburton D. Triglycerides, free fatty acids, free fatty acids/albumin molar ratio, and cholesterol levels in serum of neonates receiving long-term lipid infusions: controlled trial of continuous and intermittent regimens. J Pediatr 1984;104:429–35.
62. Freni-Titulaer LW, Cordero JF, Haddock L, et al. Premature telarche in Puerto Rico. A search for environmental factors. Am J Dis Child 1986;140:1263–77.
63. Strom BL, Schinnar R, Ziegler EE, et al. Exposure to soy-based formula in infancy and endocrinological and reproductive outcomes in young adulthood. JAMA 2001;286:807–14.
64. Clayton PT, Bowron A, Mills KA, et al. Phytosterolemia in children with parenteral nutrition-associated liver disease. Gastroenterology 1993;105:1808.
65. Greene HL, Hambidge KM, Schanler R, Tsang RC. Guidelines for the use of vitamins, trace elements, calcium, magnesium, and phosphorus in infants and children receiving total par-

enteral nutrition: report of the Subcommittee on Pediatric Parenteral Nutrient Requirements from the Committee on Clinical Practice Issues of the American Society for Clinical Nutrition [published erratum appears in Am J Clin Nutr 1989;49:1332]. Am J Clin Nutr 1988;48:1324–42.
66. Mouser JF, Hak EB, Helms RA, et al. Chromium and zinc concentrations in pediatric patients receiving long-term parenteral nutrition. Am J Health Syst Pharm 1999;56:1950–6.
67. Husain SM, Mughal MZ. Mineral transport across the placenta. Arch Dis Child 1992;67:874–78.
68. Widdowson EM, Spray CM. Chemical development in utero. Arch Dis Child 1951;26:205–14.
69. Koo W, Tsang RC. Calcium, magnesium and phosphorus. In: Tsang R, editor. Nutritional in infancy. Philadelphia: Henley and Belfus; 1988. p. 175–89.
70. Marinella MA. The refeeding syndrome. Nutr Rev 2003;61:320–3.
71. Matkovic V. Calcium intake and peak bone mass. N Engl J Med 1992;327:119–20.
72. Kien CL, Browning C, Jona J, Starshak RJ. Rickets in premature infants receiving parenteral nutrition: a case report and review of the literature. JPEN J Parenter Enteral Nutr 1982;6:152–6.
73. Shike M, Shils ME, Heller A, et al. Bone disease in prolonged parenteral nutrition: osteopenia without mineralization defect. Am J Clin Nutr 1986;44:89–98.
74. Dunham B, Marcuard S, Khazanie PG, et al. The solubility of calcium and phosphorus in neonatal total PN solutions. JPEN J Parenter Enteral Nutr 1991;15:608–11.
75. Heird WC, Hay W, Helms RA, et al. Pediatric parenteral amino acid mixture in low birth weight infants. Pediatrics 1988;81:41–50.
76. Larchet M, Garabedian M, Bourdeau A, et al. Calcium metabolism in children during long-term total parenteral nutrition: the influence of calcium, phosphorus, and vitamin D intakes. J Pediatr Gastroenterol Nutr 1991;13:367–75.
77. Lipkin EW, Ott SM, Chesnut CH III, Chait A. Mineral loss in the parenteral nutrition patient. Am J Clin Nutr 1988;47:515–23.
78. Karton MA, Rettmer R, Lipkin EW, et al. D-Lactate and metabolic bone disease in patients receiving long-term parenteral nutrition. JPEN J Parenter Enteral Nutr 1999;13:132–5.
79. Wood RJ, Bengoa JM, Sitrin MD, Rosenberg IH. Calciuretic effect of cyclic versus continuous total parenteral nutrition. Am J Clin Nutr 1985;41:614–9.
80. Ament ME. Bone mineral content in patients with short bowel syndrome: the impact of PN. J Pediatr 1998;132:386–8.
81. Klein GL. Metabolic bone disease of total parenteral nutrition. Nutrition 1998;14:149–52.
82. Ott SM, Maloney NA, Kleein GL, et al. Aluminum is associated with low bone formation in patients receiving chronic PN. Ann Intern Med 1983;98:910–4.
83. Klein GL, Ott SM, Alfrey AC, et al. Aluminum as a factor in the bone disease of long term PN. Trans Assoc Am Physicians 1982;15:155–64.
84. Klein GL, Alfrey AC, Miller NL, et al. Aluminum loading during total PN. Am J Clin Nutr 1982;35:1425–9.
85. Vargas JH, Klein GL, Ament ME, et al. Metabolic bone disease of total PN: course after changing from casein to amino acids in parenteral solutions with reduced aluminum content. Am J Clin Nutr 1988;48:1070–8.
86. Dellert SF, Farrelll MK, Specker BL, Heubi JE. Bone mineral content in children with short bowel syndrome after discontinuation of PN. J Pediatr 1998;132:516–9.
87. Schmidt-Sommerfeld E, Snyder G, Rotti TM, et al. Catheter-related complications in 35 children and adolescents with

gastrointestinal disease on home PN. JPEN J Parenter Enteral Nutr 1990;14:148–51.

88. Weinsier RL, Krumdieck CL. Death resulting from overzealous total parenteral nutrition: the refeeding syndrome revisited. Am J Clin Nutr 1981;34:393–9.

89. Prasad AS. Zinc: an overview. Nutrition 1995;11(1 Suppl):93–9.

90. Beck FW, Prasad AS, Kaplan J, et al. Changes in cytokine production and T cell subpopulations in experimentally induced zinc-deficient humans. Am J Physiol 1997;272(6 Pt 1):E1002–7.

91. Dibley MJ. Zinc. In: Bowman BA, Russell RM, editors. Present knowledge in nutrition. Washington: Ilsi Press; 2001. p. 329–43.

92. Golden BE, Golden MH. Plasma zinc, rate of weight gain, and the energy cost of tissue deposition in children recovering from severe malnutrition on a cow's milk or soya protein based diet. Am J Clin Nutr 1981;34:892–9.

93. Main AN, Hall MJ, Russell RI, et al. Clinical experience of zinc supplementation during intravenous nutrition in Crohn's disease: value of serum and urine zinc measurements. Gut 1982;23:984–91.

94. Solomon NW. Zinc and copper. In: Shils ME, Young VR, editors. Modern nutrition in health and disease. Philadelphia: Lea and Febiger; 1988. p. 238–42

95. Karpel JT, Peden VH. Copper deficiency in long-term parenteral nutrition. J Pediatr 1972;80:32–6.

96. Koo WW. Parenteral nutrition-related bone disease. JPEN J Parenter Enteral Nutr 1992;16:386–94.

97. Fitzgerald K, Mikalunas V, Rubin H, et al. Hypermanganesemia in patients receiving total parenteral nutrition. JPEN J Parenter Enteral Nutr 1999;23:333–6.

98. Fell JM, Reynolds AP, Meadows N, et al. Manganese toxicity in children receiving long-term parenteral nutrition. Lancet 1996;347:1218–21.

99. Freund H, Atamian S, Fischer JE. Chromium deficiency during total parenteral nutrition. JAMA. 1979;241:496–8.

100. Moukarzel AA, Song MK, Buchman AL, et al. Excessive chromium intake in children receiving total parenteral nutrition. Lancet 1992;339:385–8.

101. Katz SA, Salem H. The toxicology of chromium with respect to its chemical speciation: a review. J Appl Toxicol 1993;13:217–24.

102. Mirmiran P, Kimiagar M, Azizi F. Three-year survey of effects of iodized oil injection in schoolchildren with iodine deficiency disorders. Exp Clin Endocrinol Diabetes 2002;110:393–7.

103. Ibrahim M, de Escobar GM, Visser TJ, et al. Iodine deficiency associated with parenteral nutrition in extreme preterm infants. Arch Dis Child 2003;88(1):F56–7.

104. Ares S, Escobar-Morreale HF, Quero J, et al. Neonatal hypothyroxinemia: effects of iodine intake and premature birth. J Clin Endocrinol Metab 1997;82:1704–12.

105. Delange F. Iodine nutrition and neonatal hyperthyroidism. Rev Med Brux 1994;15:356–65.

106. Moukarzel AA, Buchman AL, Salas JS, et al. Iodine supplementation in children receiving long-term parenteral nutrition. J Pediatr 1992;121:252–4.

107. Larsen PR, Berry MJ. Nutritional and hormonal regulation of thyroid hormone deiodinases. Annu Rev Nutr 1995;15:323–52.

108. Klinger G, Shamir R, Singer P, et al. Parenteral selenium supplementation in extremely low birth weight infants: inadequate dosage but no correlation with hypothyroidism. J Perinatol 1999;19(8 Pt 1):568–72.

109. Kien CL, Ganther HE. Manifestations of chronic selenium deficiency in a child receiving total parenteral nutrition. Am J Clin Nutr 1983;37:319–28.

110. Van Caillie-Bertrand M, Degenhart HJ, Fernandes J. Selenium status of infants on nutritional support. Acta Paediatr Scand 1984;73:816–9.

111. Hatanaka N, Nakaden H, Yamamoto Y, et al. Selenium kinetics and changes in glutathione peroxidase activities in patients receiving long-term parenteral nutrition and effects of supplementation with selenite. Nutrition 2000;16:22–6.

112. Levander OA. A global view of human selenium nutrition. Annu Rev Nutr 1987;7:227–50.

113. Looker AC, Dallman PR, Carroll MD, et al. Prevalence of iron deficiency in the United States. JAMA 1997;277:973–6.

114. Nokes C, van den Bosch C, Bundy DAP. The effects of iron deficiency and anemia on mental and motor performance, educational achievement and behavior in children: a report of the International Nutrition Anemia Consultative Group. Washington (DC): International Nutrition Anemia Consultative Group; 1998.

115. Glader BE. Screening for anemia and erythrocyte disorders in children. Pediatrics 1986;78:368–9.

116. Mayhew SL, Quick MW. Compatibility of iron dextran with neonatal parenteral nutrient solutions. Am J Health Syst Pharm 1997;54:570–1.

117. Reed MD, Bertino JS Jr, Halpin TC Jr. Use of intravenous iron dextran injection in children receiving total parenteral nutrition. Am J Dis Child 1981;135:829–31.

118. Michaud L, Guimber D, Mention K, et al. Tolerance and efficacy of intravenous iron saccharate for iron deficiency anemia in children and adolescents receiving long-term parenteral nutrition. Clin Nutr 2002;21:403–7.

119. Murray MJ, Murray AB, Murray MB, Murray CJ. The adverse effect of iron repletion on the course of certain infections. BMJ 1978;2:1113–5.

120. Baltimore RS, Shedd DG, Pearson HA. Effect of iron saturation on the bacteriostasis of human serum: in vivo does not correlate with in vitro saturation. J Pediatr 1982;101:519–23.

121. Ben Hariz M, Goulet O, De Potter S, et al. Iron overload in children receiving prolonged parenteral nutrition. J Pediatr 1993;123:238–41.

122. Chowdary SK, Parashar K. Central venous access in neonates through the peripheral route. Curr Opin Clin Nutr Metab Care 2000;3:217–9.

123. Baker SS. Indications for parenteral nutrition. In: Baker RD, Baker SS, Davis AM, editors. Pediatric parenteral nutrition. New York: Chapman and Hall; 1996.

124. Alhimyary A, Fernandez C, Picard M, et al. Safety and efficacy of total parenteral nutrition delivered via a peripherially inserted central venous catheter. Nutr Clin Pract 1996;11:199.

125. Orr ME, Ryder MA. Vascular access devices: perspectives on designs, complications, and management. Nutr Clin Pract 1993;8:145–52.

126. Duerksen DR, Papineau N, Siemens J, Yaffe C. Peripherally inserted central catheters for parenteral nutrition: a comparison with centrally inserted catheters. JPEN J Parenter Enteral Nutr 1999;23:85–9.

127. Smith JR, Friedell ML, Cheatham ML, et al. Peripherally inserted central catheters revisited. Am J Surg 1998;176:208–11.

128. Severien C, Nelson JD. Frequency of infections associated with implanted systems vs cuffed, tunneled Silastic venous catheters in patients with acute leukemia. Am J Dis Child 1991;145:1433–8.

129. Ingram J, Weitzman S, Greenberg ML, et al. Complications of indwelling venous access lines in the pediatric hematology patient: a prospective comparison of external venous

catheters and subcutaneous ports. Am J Pediatr Hematol Oncol 1991;13:130–6.

130. Shulman RJ, Rahman S, Mahoney D, et al. A totally implanted venous access system used in pediatric patients with cancer. J Clin Oncol 1987;5:137–40.

131. Henriques HF III, Karmy-Jones R, Knoll SM, et al. Avoiding complications of long-term venous access. Am Surgeon 1993;59:555–8.

132. Trottier SJ, Veremakis C, O'Brien J, Auer AI. Femoral deep vein thrombosis associated with central venous catheterization: results from a prospective, randomized trial. Crit Care Med 1995;23:52–9.

133. Macdonald S, Gan J, McKay AJ, Edwards RD. Endovascular treatment of acute carotid blow-out syndrome. J Vasc Intervent Radiol 2000;11:1184–8.

134. Mermel L. Central venous catheter-related infections and their prevention: is there enough evidence to recommend tunneling for short-term use? Crit Care Med 1998;26:1315–6.

135. McBride KD, Fisher R, Warnock N, et al. A comparative analysis of radiological and surgical placement of central venous catheters. Cardiovasc Intervent Radiol 1997;20:17–22.

136. Oram-Smith JC, Mullen JL, Harken AH, Fitts WT Jr. Direct right atrial catheterization for total parenteral nutrition. Surgery 1978;83:274–6.

137. Sharif K, de Ville de Goyet J, Beath SV, et al. Transhepatic Hickman line placement: improving line stability by surgically assisted radiologic placement. J Pediatr Gastroenterol Nutr 2002;34:561–3.

138. Wiener ES, McGuire P, Stolar CJ, et al. The CCSG prospective study of venous access devices: an analysis of insertions and causes for removal. J Pediatr Surg 1992;27:155.

139. Hartman GE, Schochat SJ. Management of septic complications associated with Silastic R catheters in childhood malignancy. Pediatr Infect Dis J 1987;6:1042.

140. Bagnall HA, Comperts E, Atkinson JB. Continuous infusion of low-dose urokinase in the treatment of central venous catheter thrombosis in infants and children. Pediatrics 1989;83:1989.

141. Eppes SC, Troutman J, Gutman LT. Outcome of treatment of candidemia in children whose central catheters were removed or retained. Pediatr Infect Dis J 1989;8:99.

142. Borrow M, Crowley JG. Evaluation of central venous catheter thrombogenicity. Acta Anaesth Scand 1985;81:59.

143. Murphy LM, Lipman TO. Central venous catheter care in PN: a review. JPEN J Parenter Enteral Nutr 1987;11:190.

144. Smith S, Dawson S, Hennessey R, et al. Maintenance of the patency of indwelling central venous catheters: is heparin necessary? Am J Pediatr Hemat Oncol 1991;13:141.

145. Heeger PS, Backstrom JT. Heparin flushes and thrombocytopenia. Ann Intern Med 1986;105:143.

146. Ling E, Warkentin TE. Intraoperative heparin flushes and subsequent acute heparin-induced thrombocytopenia. Anesthesiology 1998;240:446–55.

147. Taketomo CK, Hodding JH, Kraus DM. Pediatric dosage handbook. 9th ed. Hudson (OH): Lexi-Comp, Inc; 2002–2003.

148. Jacobs BR, Haygood M, Hingl J. Recombinant tissue plasminogen activator in the treatment of central venous catheter occlusion in children. J Pediatr 2001;139:593–6.

149. Kupensky DT. Use of hydrochloric acid to restore patency in an occluded implantable port: a case report. J Intraven Nurs 1995;18:198.

150. Shulman RJ, Reed T, Pitre D, et al. Use of hydrochloric acid to clear obstructed central venous catheters. JPEN J Parenter Enteral Nutr 1988;12:509–10.

151. Duffy LF, Kerzner B, Gebus V, et al. Treatment of central venous catheter occlusions with hydrochloric acid. J Pediatr 1989;114:1002.

152. Monsuez JJ, Douard MC, Martin-Bouyer Y. Catheter fragments embolization. Angiology 1997;48:117–20.

153. Maki DG, Ringer M, Alvarado CJ. Prospective randomised trial of povidone-iodine, alcohol, and chlorhexidine for prevention of infection associated with central venous and arterial catheters. Lancet 1991;338:339–43.

154. Raad II, Hohn DC, Gilbreath BJ, et al. Prevention of central venous catheter-related infections by using maximal sterile barrier precautions during insertion. Infect Control Hosp Epidemiol 1994;15(4 Pt 1):231–8.

155. Soo RA, Gosbell IB, Gallo JH, et al. Hickman catheter complications in a haematology unit, 1996-98. Intern Med J 2002;32:100–3.

156. Jansen B, Ruiten D, Pulverer G. In-vitro activity of a catheter loaded with silver and teicoplanin to prevent bacterial and fungal colonization. J Hosp Infect 1995;31:238–41.

157. Johnson RR, Decker MD, Edwards KM, et al. Frequency of Broviac catheter infections in pediatric oncology patients. J Infect Dis 1986;154:670.

158. Keohane PP, Jones BJ, Attrill H, et al. Effect of catheter tunnelling and a nutrition nurse on catheter sepsis during parenteral nutrition. Lancet 1983;ii:1388–90.

159. Sitges-Serra A, Linaes J, Perez JL, et al. A randomized trial on the effect of tubing changes on hub contamination and catheter sepsis during PN. JPEN J Parenter Enteral Nutr 1985;9:322.

160. deCicco M, Chiaradia V, Veronisi A, et al. Source and route of microbial colonization of parenteral nutrition catheters. Lancet 1989;ii:1258–61.

161. Kurkchubasche AG, Smith SC, Rowe MI. Catheter sepsis in short-bowel syndrome. Arch Surg 1992;127:21.

162. Flynn PM, Shenep JL, Stokes DC, Barrett FF. In situ management of confirmed central venous catheter-related bacteremia. Pediatr Infect Dis J 1987;6:729–34.

163. Goplerud JM. Hyperalimentation associated hepatotoxicity in the newborn. Ann Clin Lab Sci 1992;22:79.

164. Peters O, Ryan S, Matthew L, et al. Randomised controlled trial of acetate in preterm neonates receiving parenteral nutrition. Arch Dis Child 1997;77:F12–5.

165. Werlin SL, Wyatt D, Camitta B. Effect of abrupt discontinuation of high glucose infusion rates during parenteral nutrition. J Pediatr 1994;124:441–4.

166. Bendorf K, Friesen CA, Roberts CC. Glucose response to discontinuation of parenteral nutrition in patients less than 3 years of age. JPEN J Parenter Enteral Nutr 1996;20:120–2.

167. Faubion WC, Baker WL, Iott BA, et al. Cyclic TPN for hospitalized pediatric patients. Nutr Suppl Serv 1981;1(4):24.

168. Chwals WJ, Lally KP, Woolley MM, Mahour GH. Measured energy expenditure in critically ill infants and young children. J Surg Res 1988;44:467–72.

169. Chwals WJ. Metabolism and nutritional frontiers in pediatric surgical patients. Surg Clin North Am 1992;72:1237–66.

170. Letton RW, Chwals WJ, Jamie A, Charles B. Early postoperative alterations in infant energy use increase the risk of overfeeding. J Pediatr Surg 1995;30:988–92; discussion 992–3.

171. White MS, Shepherd RW, McEniery JA. Energy expenditure in 100 ventilated, critically ill children: improving the accuracy of predictive equations. Crit Care Med 2000;28:2307–12.

172. Mayes T, Gottschlich MM, Khoury J, Warden GD. Evaluation of predicted and measured energy requirements in burned children. J Am Diet Assoc 1996;96:24–9.

173. Dietitians in Nutrition Support Newsletter 1990;12:15.

174. Moore FA, Feliciano DV, Andrassy RJ, et al. Early enteral feeding, compared with parenteral, reduces postoperative septic complications. The results of a meta-analysis. Ann Surg 1992;216:172–83.

175. Kudsk KA, Croce MA, Fabian TC, et al. Enteral versus parenteral feeding. Effects on septic morbidity after blunt and penetrating abdominal trauma. Ann Surg 1992;215:503–11; discussion 511–3.

176. Kudsk KA, Minard G, Croce MA, et al. A randomized trial of isonitrogenous enteral diets after severe trauma. An immune-enhancing diet reduces septic complications. Ann Surg 1996;224:531–40; discussion 540–3.

177. Kudsk KA, Minard G, Wojtysiak SL, et al. Visceral protein response to enteral versus parenteral nutrition and sepsis in patients with trauma. Surgery 1994;116:516–23.

178. Institute of Medicine, Food and Nutrition Board. Dietary reference intakes for calcium, phosphorus, magnesium, vitamin D, and fluoride. Washington (DC): National Academy Press; 1997.

179. Johnson KB. The Johns Hopkins Hospital Harriet Lane handbook. 13th ed. St. Louis: Mosby; 1993.

180. Roy CC, Silverman A, Alagille D. Pediatric clinical gastroenterology. 4th ed. St. Louis: Mosby; 1995.

181. Subcommittee on the Tenth Edition of the RDAs, Food and Nutrition Board. Recommended Dietary Allowances. Washington (DC): National Academy Press; 1989.

182. Lee PC, Werlin SL. Carbohydrates. In: Baker RD, Baker SS, Davis AM, editors. Pediatric parenteral nutrition. New York: Chapman and Hall; 1997. p. 99–107.

183. Schanler RJ, Shulman RJ, Prestridge LL. Parenteral nutrient needs of very low birth weight infants. J Pediatr 1994;125(6 Pt 1):961–8.

184. Zlotkin SH, Stallings VA, Pencharz PB. Total parenteral nutrition in children. Pediatr Clin North Am 1985;32:381–400.

185. American Medical Association. Guidelines for essential trace element preparation for parenteral use. JAMA 1979;241:2051.

186. Solomons N. Trace elements. In: Rombeau JL, Caldwell MD, editors. Parenteral nutrition. Philadelphia: WB Saunders; 1993. p. 150–83.

187. Solomons NW, Ruz M. Essential and beneficial trace elements in pediatric parenteral nutrition. In: Baker RD, Baker SS, Davis AM, editors. Pediatric parenteral nutrition. New York: Chapman and Hall; 1996. p. 175–96.

188. American Gastroenterological Association. American Gastroenterological Association medical position statement: short bowel syndrome and intestinal transplantation. Gastroenterology 2003;124:1105–10.

189. Department of Health and Human Services, Food and Drug Administration Parenteral multivitamin products; drugs for human use drug efficacy study implementations. Fed Reg 2000;65:21200–2. Docket No.: 79-013; DSE 2846.

190. Borum PR. Carnitine in neonatal nutrition. J Child Neurol 1995;10 Suppl 2:2S25–31.

191. Davis AM. Initiation, monitoring, and complications of pediatric parenteral nutrition. In: Baker RD, Baker SS, Davis AM, editors. Pediatric parenteral nutrition. New York: Chapman and Hall; 1996. p. 212–37.

4B. *Enteral Nutrition*

Ana Abad-Sinden, MS, RD, CNSD

James Sutphen, MD, PhD

Pediatric patients unable to tolerate adequate oral feedings may be nutritionally managed with enteral nutrition (EN). Commonly used EN routes include nasogastric (NG) tube, gastrostomy, nasojejunal (NJ) tube, and jejunostomy. The nutritional goal for pediatric patients with chronic illness should be the provision of nutrients appropriate to the patients' metabolic and physiologic limitations and capable of promoting continued growth and development. Although both enteral and parenteral nutrition can provide nutritional support to pediatric patients unable or unwilling to take in adequate oral feedings, EN support is generally considered the preferred modality for critically and chronically ill pediatric patients because they are more physiologic and economic and are easier and safer to administer than parenteral nutrition. Absence of a central venous catheter decreases infection and thrombotic complications. Delivery of nutrients to the intestine minimizes gut atrophy and decreases the risk for bacterial translocation. EN reduces the risk for infectious complications compared with parenteral nutrition.[1] Furthermore, EN allows for better physiologic control of electrolyte levels through endocrine modulation of intestinal absorption and serves as effective prophylaxis against stress-induced gastropathy and gastrointestinal (GI) hemorrhage. EN also offers more complete nutrient provision, including glutamine, nucleotides, trace elements, short-chain fatty acids, and fiber. EN avoids the hepatic complications associated with parenteral nutrition. In addition, EN provides trophic stimulation to the gut by promoting pancreatic and biliary secretions as well as endocrine, paracrine, and neural factors, which promote the physiologic and immunologic integrity of the GI tract.[2–4] Timely initiation of EN is also important, with the greatest metabolic benefits resulting from initiating early EN within less than 72 hours of injury or admission.[4]

Initial attempts at EN should be via the oral route. If the oral route is not emphasized during infancy, the suck reflex may be lost. Because it may take 8 to 9 months for the child to develop sufficiently for use of a cup, oral aversion and language delay may occur during this time interval. Some common indications for initiating EN include oral-motor or esophageal dysfunction owing to prematurity, morphologic abnormalities of the head or neck, or neurologic disease. Excessive respiratory demands from cardiorespiratory disease may compromise coordination of respiration and swallowing.[5] Although nasoenteric feedings are effective in the short-term support of these patients, long-term nutritional support often requires the placement of a feeding gastrostomy. This may be particularly important in the infant who develops oral aversion owing to the prolonged noxious stimulus of a NG tube and to minimize the risks associated with prolonged NG feedings, including sinusitis and otitis media.

This discussion reviews the pathophysiologic mechanisms and nutritional aspects of various pediatric disorders that have been successfully managed with EN. Formula selection and modification as well as enteral feeding techniques and equipment are presented. The administration and monitoring of pediatric EN techniques and the management of common complications are also discussed.

INDICATIONS FOR ENTERAL FEEDINGS: MANAGEMENT OF NUTRITION-RELATED DISORDERS

Table 75.4B-1 lists common conditions under which EN may be warranted in pediatric patients.

PRETERM INFANTS

Feeding methods for preterm infants should be individualized to gestational age, birth weight, and medical status.[6] Preterm infants present a unique nutritional challenge owing to their GI and immunologic immaturity; increased requirements for specific nutrients such as protein, fat, sodium, calcium, and phosphorus; limited renal function; and predisposition to specific metabolic and clinical com-

TABLE 75.4B-1 CONDITIONS UNDER WHICH ENTERAL NUTRITION MAY BE WARRANTED

PRETERM INFANTS
Cardiorespiratory disease
    Bronchopulmonary dysplasia
    Congenital heart disease
    Cystic fibrosis
Gastrointestinal disease and dysfunction
    Biliary atresia
    Inflammatory bowel disease
    Gastroesophageal reflux disease
    Pancreatitis
    Protacted diarrhea of infancy
    Short-gut syndrome
Critical illness and postoperative malnutrition
    Burn injury
    Cancer
    HIV/AIDS malnutrition
    Trauma/head injury
Renal disease
Neurologic disease and/or impairment

plications such as hypoglycemia, periodic dysmotility, and necrotizing enterocolitis.[6–8] As the coordination of sucking and swallowing appears at approximately 34 weeks gestation, intragastric or jejunal feedings are often used before this time, or beyond, in infants unable to tolerate adequate oral feedings. A number of studies in preterm infants suggest that minimal EN or trophic feedings, defined as the provision of low-volume feedings (10–24 cc/kg/d over 5–14 days) and administered within the first week of life, enhance intestinal adaptation to extrauterine conditions.[8–10] These feedings promote maturation of the mucosal lining, decrease cholestatic jaundice, aid maturation of intestinal motility, and allow earlier progression to full enteral feedings.[9–11] Intermittent bolus feedings may better promote gastrocolic reflexes, gallbladder emptying, and GI hormone release in preterm infants, thus promoting the trophic response,[12,13] and increase accommodation of the stomach to volume loads. Continuous feedings are reserved for neonates with short-gut syndrome, severe gastroesophageal reflux (GER) disease, or persistent feeding intolerance. Transpyloric feedings may promote less GER and overcome gastric dysmotility; however, they are technically more difficult and bypass the gastric phase of fat absorption promoted by lingual lipase and may therefore decrease total fat absorption.[6] This may be a particular concern when bile salt deficiency from prematurity or short-bowel syndrome exists. Early initiation of fat digestion in the stomach may partially offset the effect of bile salt deficiency by earlier formation of mixed micelles.

CARDIORESPIRATORY ILLNESS

Infants and children with cardiorespiratory disorders often require EN support during acute exacerbations of their primary disease, for nutritional rehabilitation of chronic secondary malnutrition, or for promotion of growth prior to surgical procedures. The etiology of growth failure and delayed neurointellectual development in patients with bronchopulmonary dysplasia (BPD) is related to the combined effects of prolonged hypoxia, elevated metabolic rates, inefficient suck and swallow mechanisms, poor appetite, prolonged periods of caloric and nutrient deficits, recurrent emesis, and GI dysmotility.[12–14] Potassium, sodium, and chloride supplementation of the formula is often required in conjunction with diuretic therapy. Increasing formula caloric and nutrient density through either formula concentration or the addition of carbohydrate and fat may be used to achieve caloric densities of 30 to 33 kcal per ounce (1.0 to 1.3 kcal per mL). Excess reliance on carbohydrate in infants who are fluid restricted, however, may result in CO_2 retention and suboptimal protein, vitamin, and mineral delivery if the base formula is excessively diluted.[15] Children with cystic fibrosis (CF) present additional challenges owing to maldigestion.[16] Although behavior modification techniques to improve intake and provision of appetizing high-calorie supplements should be instituted as routine components of medical nutrition therapy for children with CF, EN using semielemental or intact nutrient formulas supplemented with pancreatic enzymes is often necessary for

patients who have failed owing to noncompliance.[16,17] Pancreatic enzyme replacement is usually dosed based on lipase units per gram of long-chain triglycerides (mean of 1,800 lipase units). NG feedings have resulted in increased caloric intake and significant weight gain for patients with CF, but long-term effectiveness is hampered by noncompliance.[15] Nocturnal gastrostomy feedings provided over 8 to 10 hours for long-term management may be superior for selected patients.[16]

Infants with congenital heart disease are also at significant nutritional risk generally owing to inadequate calorie intake.[5] Growth failure results from poor nutritional intake, increased respiratory rates, and elevated energy expenditure. It may be exacerbated by tissue hypoxia, suboptimal nutrient absorption, delayed gastric emptying, or more generalized GI dysmotility.[18,19] Owing to their elevated nutritional needs and limited fluid tolerance, these infants often require high–caloric density formulas achieved through formula concentration to a maximum of 24 to 27 kcal per ounce, depending on GI tolerance. Concentration beyond 27 kcal per ounce may not allow enough free water for excretion of the renal osmotic load. Additional calories can be provided through the addition of carbohydrate or fat. Infants with congenital heart disease often benefit from the use of nocturnal continuous feeds while combined with oral intake ad libitum during the day. Alternatively, provision of oral feedings intermittently with NG supplementation of the remainder of the required intake volume may also facilitate provision of the nutritional goals.[5,20,21] Ultimately, effective EN can promote significant catch-up growth and facilitate surgical correction of cardiac defects.

GASTROINTESTINAL DISEASE

Pediatric patients with acute and chronic GI disease and dysfunction, such as inflammatory bowel disease, short-bowel syndrome, and pancreatitis, often benefit from EN regimens. The etiology of growth failure in children with Crohn disease is multifactorial but often related to inadequate nutrient intake. Semielemental and elemental diets administered orally and nasogastrically have been clinically demonstrated to induce remission in selected patients and produce a significant improvement in nutritional status.[22,23] Clinical remission is more likely in Crohn disease of the small bowel than of the colon.[23] Elemental, semielemental, and polymeric diets have been shown to produce similar clinical results.[24,25] Supplementation of an oral polymeric formula with transforming growth factor-β_2, a polypeptide normally found in human and cow's milk, resulted in clinical remission of 79% in 29 children with intestinal Crohn disease, as well as mucosal healing and a reduction in proinflammatory mediators.[26] For simple weight gain, however, emphasis on high-calorie appetizing food is the gold standard before implementation of less palatable enteral supplements.

The nutritional management of the infant or child with short-bowel syndrome involves the initial use of total parenteral nutrition with a gradually increasing amount of EN. The period of transition to complete EN may take weeks to years depending on the location and length of intestinal resection, associated dysmotility, presence of the ileocecal valve, and extent of colon preservation. Parenteral nutrition, however, must be continued until it is clinically evident that positive fluid and nutrient balance and weight gain can be maintained on EN alone.[27] Water and sodium may be considered the first limiting nutrients in short-bowel syndrome. Often stool sodium losses or negative water balance or both obscure weight gain. Important considerations for provision of adequate EN include the method of administration, volume, osmolality, and nutrient quality (polymeric versus elemental). Polymeric formulas with intact protein, long-chain fats, and complex carbohydrates may be less tolerated in the initial stages of the enteral feeding progression than glucose and glucose polymers, medium-chain triglycerides (MCTs), and hydrolyzed protein and dipeptides, which require less digestion, are less allergenic, and are more easily tolerated.[27,28] Long-term parenteral nutrition in these infants is associated with cholestatic liver disease, a significant cause of death in children with short-gut syndrome. To prevent liver disease, cyclic parenteral nutrition with provision of a 4- to 6-hour "window" in infants has been shown to reduce the incidence of cholestasis.[29] In older children and adolescents, provision of cyclic parenteral nutrition over 10 to 12 hours with continuous or intermittent enteral feedings, as tolerated, while promoting oral intake during the day can usually be managed in the home setting.[30] Furthermore, treatment of small bowel bacterial overgrowth, provision of supplemental ursodeoxycholic acid, and prevention of sepsis are also adjunctive therapies to decrease the risk of cholestatic liver disease. Prevention of oral aversion involves careful attention to persistent use of oral feedings and avoidance of noxious stimuli to the oral area. Proactive involvement of speech pathology experts during enteral feeding of infants is extremely helpful.

Several other GI diseases impacting nutritional intake and status can be successfully managed with EN. Infants with biliary atresia frequently experience reduced intake associated with liver disease and infection.[31] Following surgical procedures or liver transplant, nutritional support of these infants with continuous NG feedings using a semielemental formula rich in MCTs can promote energy and nitrogen balance.[31,32] Once the postoperative infant or child is clinically stable, transition to an intact nutrient formula or to an oral diet should be made.[33] Careful monitoring of fat-soluble vitamin levels and supplementation with water-soluble varieties using multiple doses during the day may help in the prevention of fat-soluble vitamin deficiency. Infants with GER disease who have failed conventional therapy with acid inhibition, thickened feeds, and upright positioning and have subsequently experienced growth failure have been shown to benefit from continuous NG feedings with improved intake, reduction or cessation of vomiting, and catch-up growth.[34] Children with acute and chronic pancreatitis may be nutritionally managed with NJ feedings of a standard pediatric or, if needed, semielemental formula administered beyond the ligament of Treitz. Clinical studies in adult patients with pancreati-

tis have demonstrated improved clinical outcomes with fewer infectious complications, decreased incidence of hyperglycemia, and decreased incidence of multiorgan failure and mortality in enterally fed patients compared with those on parenteral nutrition.[35,36]

CRITICAL ILLNESS AND POSTOPERATIVE MALNUTRITION

EN for the critically ill or postoperative pediatric patient has improved in recent years owing to improvements in EN products, equipment, and techniques.[3] Early EN within 48 hours of injury or surgery reduces sepsis and enhances GI immune function through maintenance of the gut mucosal barrier and enteric lymphoid tissue. Early postoperative EN helps prevent mucosal damage and bacterial translocation, results in decreased sepsis, and blunts the hypermetabolic response in some critically ill patients.[2,4] Clinical studies have demonstrated that GI function can be adequately maintained with improved nitrogen balance and nutritional status in the postsurgical trauma patient.[37,38]

Critically ill patients in hypermetabolic states, such as those with cancer or human immunodeficiency virus/acquired immune deficiency syndrome (HIV/AIDS), may also benefit from EN support. Cancer patients at high nutritional risk who have minimal GI symptoms and adequate platelet counts may be enterally fed via nocturnal or 24-hour feedings depending on the extent of oral intake.[39] Various studies have demonstrated the effectiveness and safety of gastrostomy tube feedings in malnourished children with cancer.[40,41] Pediatric HIV patients with protein-calorie malnutrition who are unable to meet their elevated energy requirements with oral intake alone may also benefit from enteral NG feedings with pediatric or other high–caloric density formulas. Nocturnal enteral feeding is the preferred method of EN in this patient population because it allows the child to eat during the day.[42] Gastrostomy tube feedings for the provision of supplemental nutrition have resulted in improvement in weight gain and reduced morbidity and mortality in pediatric HIV patients.[43]

RENAL DISEASE

Chronic renal failure in infants and children commonly results in growth failure and developmental delay, particularly in those patients with congenital renal disease early in life.[44] The etiology of growth failure in these children is thought to be related to protein-calorie deficiency, renal osteodystrophy, chronic metabolic acidosis, and endocrine dysfunction.[45] Despite aggressive medical management and use of specialized formulas of high caloric density, poor growth and development may persist. Early nutritional intervention and dialysis can result in improved growth and development.[44,45] Nocturnal NG feedings over a period of 8 to 12 hours in patients with renal insufficiency have resulted in catch-up growth.[45]

NEUROLOGIC DISEASE AND/OR IMPAIRMENT

The specific nutritional requirements and feeding approach for neurologically impaired children are highly variable and depend on the degree of impairment, oral-motor function, mobility, and muscular tone. Children with Down syndrome, Prader-Willi syndrome, or myelomeningocele have decreased energy needs, growth rates, and motor activity compared with healthy children.[46] Children with cerebral palsy, however, are generally underweight for height and may have increased energy needs, particularly if they are severely spastic or have choreoathetoid movements. Those patients who are severely affected often require high–caloric density enteral feedings and are often managed via continuous nocturnal gastrostomy feedings and intermittent bolus feedings during the day when oral intake is inadequate.[46] Important considerations for provision of EN to these patients include method of feeding, risk of aspiration, formula caloric density, osmolality and fiber content, fluid intake, and effect of enteral feeding therapy on current and future oral-motor function and intake.[47] Often daytime bolus feedings are preferred by caregivers because they are more easily given and avoid the risk of nighttime aspiration from continuous feedings. The goal of nutritional support for these children should not necessarily be persistent weight gain because increased weight may further compromise muscular ability and complicate the caregiver's ability to move the child. These children are also often at risk for constipation, which can compromise formula tolerance.

NUTRITIONAL NEEDS OF THE ENTERALLY FED CHILD

PRETERM INFANT

Caloric requirements to support a daily weight gain of 15 g/kg are estimated at 105 to 130 kcal/kg in the appropriate for gestational age preterm infant. Higher energy needs are required depending on the infant's thermal environment, cardiorespiratory status, presence of intrauterine growth retardation, and metabolic stress.[48,49] Infants who are small for gestational age or those with BPD may have caloric requirements of between 130 and 150 kcal/kg.[15] Intake of formulas with whey-to-casein ratios similar to those of breast milk results in metabolic indices and plasma amino acid profiles closer to those of breastfed infants.[50] Because of their GI immaturity, preterm infants demonstrate improved nutrient absorption when fed a mixture of MCT and long-chain unsaturated fatty acids and a mixture of lactose and glucose polymers as their fat and carbohydrate sources, respectively. Owing to the high accretion rates for calcium, phosphorus, and trace elements during the final trimester of gestation, preterm infants have elevated requirements for these nutrients.[8,49]

INFANTS AND CHILDREN

The nutritional requirements of infants and children are outlined elsewhere in the literarure.[48,49,51] It must be emphasized that these recommended allowances are intended for healthy active children and represent the average intake of nutrients that would maintain good health for an extended period.[51] As previously discussed, tube-fed children often have illnesses that result in malnutrition

and inactivity and thus require adjusted allowances for energy and other nutrients. The specialized nutritional requirements of nutrition-related illnesses have been reviewed extensively in the literature.[5,12–16,28,32,39,42,44,46,49]

EN support of critically ill pediatric patients requires careful attention to prevent overfeeding of calories with exacerbation of the underlying clinical status. Energy and protein requirements in the critically ill child are significantly different from those of healthy children. Although basal metabolic needs may be elevated owing to the stress response and its associated elevation of counterregulatory hormones and cytokines, inhibition of growth and reduced physical activity may result in an overall decrease in energy requirements.[52] Studies in critically ill pediatric patients have underscored the importance of not using the published Dietary Reference Intakes for estimating energy requirements but rather using the child's basic energy expenditure multiplied by a factor correlated to the underlying disease or injury process.[53] Overfeeding cannot reverse the catabolic process until the acute metabolic stress response resolves; furthermore, overfeeding of calories may result in iatrogenic hepatic and respiratory disease and decreased survival.[54]

In the child with failure to thrive, particular attention should be given to the estimation of the energy and protein for achievement of catch-up growth, which occurs when the cause of growth impairment is removed and requires the provision of calories and protein in excess of normal needs.[55] It is best to allow the child's appetite to be the determinant of intake whenever possible because overfeeding during the initial stages of rehabilitation may be associated with edema and refeeding syndrome in the severely malnourished child.[56] Estimated catch-up growth requirements can be calculated from the following equation[55]:

$$\frac{kcal}{kg} = \frac{RDA\ kcal/kg\ for\ weight\ age \times ideal\ body\ weight\ (kg)}{actual\ weight\ (kg)}$$

Weight age is the age at which the present weight is at the 50th percentile, ideal weight is at the 50th percentile for age or ideal weight for height, and RDA means Recommended Dietary Allowance.

Fluid requirements can be calculated by estimating normal water requirements adjusted for specific disease-related factors; special consideration must be given to monitoring the fluid balance of children receiving high-calorie, high-protein formulas; those who have short-bowel syndrome or severe neurologic impairment; or those with emesis, diarrhea, fever, or polyuria.[2,57] The provision of extra water to prevent slow dehydration or "tube feeding syndrome" is especially important for neurologically devastated or immature children who cannot communicate their thirst to the care provider.

INFANT AND PEDIATRIC FORMULA SELECTION FOR ENTERAL FEEDINGS

Selection of an optimal infant enteral formula depends on a number of factors, including diagnosis, associated nutritional problems and requirements, and GI function.

Important formula factors include osmolality, renal solute load, caloric density, viscosity, and composition. Figure 75.4B-1 presents an algorithm that identifies appropriate infant and pediatric formulas based on indication for use. Table 75.4B-2 lists and describes the nutrient sources of a variety of infant and pediatric formulas.

PRETERM INFANT FORMULAS

Specialized formulas have been developed that are uniquely suited to the physiologic needs of the preterm infant. Physiologic factors in the preterm infant that call for alterations in their nutritional management include limited oral-motor function, lactase deficiency, limited bile salt pool, decreased energy and nutrient stores, limited gastric volume, decreased intestinal motility, and limited renal function.[7,8]

There are several differences in nutrient content between preterm and term infant formulas. Preterm formulas provide a combination of both lactose and glucose polymers versus lactose alone in standard formulas, thus decreasing osmolality and improving digestibility and calcium absorption.[50,58] Preterm formulas use a fat blend containing both long-chain triglycerides, very-long-chain triglycerides such as docosahexaenoic acid (DHA) and arachidonic acid (ARA), and MCTs, which promote improved weight gain and fat, nitrogen, and calcium absorption.[59,60] Documented improvement in weight gain, linear growth, and central nervous system development in preterm infants fed DHA- and ARA-supplemented formula[61,62] has been observed and subsequently resulted in the addition of very-long-chain triglycerides to preterm and term infant formulas. An elevated protein content and 60:40 whey-to-casein formulation promote plasma amino acid profiles closer to those of the breastfed infant.[50,63] Increased amounts of sodium, calcium, and phosphorus compensate for the increased urinary sodium losses seen in the preterm infant and promote bone mineralization closer to intrauterine rates.[50] The concentration of various vitamins, including vitamin E, in preterm formula is greater than that found in term infant formula owing to preterm infants' limited stores and wide variability in absorption. Vitamin D content is also high for promotion of bone mineralization. Owing to the lower birth weight and initial hemoglobin concentration of preterm infants, iron has been added to preterm infant formulas to provide approximately 2 mg/kg of iron per day when fed at a level of 120 kcal/kg.[50]

Discharge preterm formulas for infants weighing less than 2,000 g provide additional calories and nutrients to promote optimal growth during the first year of life. Several studies have demonstrated benefits with their use, including improved weight gain and linear growth[64]; improved calorie, calcium, and phosphorus intakes[65]; and improved bone mineral content.[66] The use of discharge preterm formulas such as EnfaCare (Mead Johnson, Evansville, IN) and Similac NeoSure (Ross Products Division, Abbott Laboratories, Columbus, OH) has become standard practice in most neonatal intensive care units. These formulas are iron fortified and commercially available in the ready to feed 22 kcal/oz form for hospital use and in the powdered form for home use. Infants whose volume intakes continue to be limited owing to cardiorespiratory illness may be fed formulas concentrated to 24 to 30 kcal/oz using alternative mixing methods provided by the manufacturers. Both discharge preterm formulas contain a blend of lactose and glucose polymers and provide 20 to 25% of the fat as MCT oil. Vitamin and mineral levels are greater than those found in standard formulas. Preterm infants consuming a minimum of 165 cc/kg do not require additional multivitamin supplementation.[8]

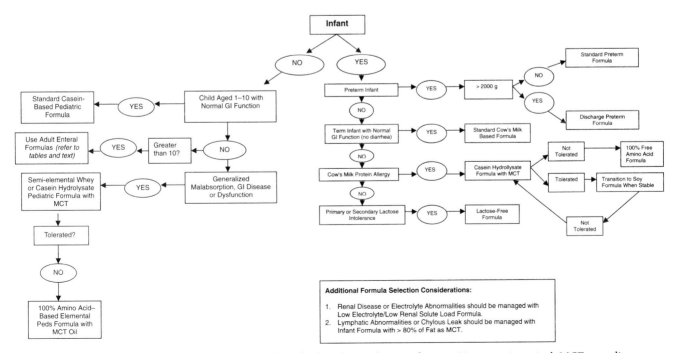

FIGURE 75.4B-1 Appropriate infant and pediatric formulas based on indication for use. GI = gastrointestinal; MCT = medium-chain triglycerides.

TABLE 75.4B-2   INFANT AND PEDIATRIC FORMULAS

PRODUCT NAME	KCAL/ OZ	CARBOHYDRATE (G/100 ML)	FAT (G/100 ML)	PROTEIN (G/100 ML)	MOSM/ KG	NUTRIENT SOURCES (CARBOHYDRATE; FAT; PROTEIN)
Preterm infant formulas						
Enfamil Premature Lipil	24	9.0	4.1	2.4	310	Corn syrup, lactose; MCT, soy, and sunflower oil; whey, casein
Similac Special Care 24	24	8.6	4.4	2.2	280	Corn syrup, lactose; MCT, soy and coconut oil; whey, casein
EnfaCare 22 Lipil	22	7.9	3.9	2.1	230	Maltodextrin, lactose; MCT, sunflower oil, soy, and coconut oil; whey, casein
Similac NeoSure 22	22	7.7	4.1	1.9	250	Maltodextrin, lactose; soy and coconut oil, MCT; whey, casein
Term infant formulas*						
Enfamil Lipil 20	20	7.3	3.5	1.4	300	Lactose; palm olein, soy, coconut, and sunflower oil; whey and casein
Similac Advance 20	20	7.2	3.6	1.4	300	Lactose; high-oleic safflower, coconut, and soy oil; whey, casein
Enfamil Lactofree	20	7.3	3.5	1.4	250	Corn syrup solids; palm olein, soy, coconut, and sunflower oil; whey and casein
Carnation Good Start	20	7.5	3.4	1.5	265	Lactose, maltodextrin; high-oleic safflower, palm olein, soy, and coconut oil; whey hydrolysates
Soy infant formulas†						
Prosobee 20	20	7.1	3.4	1.7	200	Corn syrup solids; palm olein, soy, coconut, and sunflower oils; soy protein + L-methionine
Isomil 20	20	6.9	3.4	1.6	200	Corn syrup, sucrose; high-oleic safflower, coconut, and soy oil; soy protein + L-methionine
Carnation Alsoy	20	7.4	3.3	1.9	200	Corn, maltodextrin, sucrose; palm olein, soy, coconut, and sunflower oil; soy protein + L-methionine
Specialized infant formulas†						
Nutramigen	20	7.4	3.4	1.9	320	Corn syrup, tapioca starch; palm olein, soy, coconut, and sunflower oil; casein hydrolysate
Pregestimil	20	6.9	3.8	1.9	320	Corn syrup, tapioca starch; MCT (55%), corn, soy, and sunflower oil; casein hydrolysates and amino acids
Alimentum	20	6.8	3.8	1.9	370	Tapioca starch, sucrose; MCT (50%), safflower and soy oil; casein hydrolysates and amino acids
Portagen	20	7.8	3.2	2.4	230	Corn syrup, lactose, sucrose; MCT (88%), corn oil (12%); sodium caseinate
Neocate	20	7.8	3.0	2.1	375	Corn syrup solids; safflower and soy oil, MCT (5%); free amino acids
Pediatric enteral formulas						
Kindercal with Fiber	31	13.5	4.4	3	325	Maltodextrin, sucrose; MCT, canola and high-oleic sunflower oil; calcium and potassium caseinates
PediaSure with Fiber	30	10.9	5.0	3	345	Corn syrup, sucrose, lactose; high oleic safflower and soy oil, MCT; sodium caseinate and whey
Peptamen Junior	30	13.7	3.9	3	260–360	Maltodextrin, corn starch; MCT, soy and canola, lecithin; hydrolyzed whey
Neocate Junior	30	10.4	5.0	3	607	Corn syrup solids; MCT, canola and safflower oil; free amino acids
EleCare	30	10.7	4.76	3	596	Corn syrup solids; high oleic safflower and soy oil, MCT; free amino acids

MCT = medium-chain triglyceride.

Enfamil products are Mead Johnson, Evansville, IN; Similac products are Ross Products Division, Abbott Laboratories, Columbus, OH; Carnation Infant Formula Products are Nestle Carnation, Wilkes Barre, PA.

*Term infant formulas are available in 24 kcal/oz ready to feed for hospital use.

†Can be prepared to 24 kcal/oz by adding less water to concentrate or powder base.

Breast milk continues to be the preferred EN source for preterm and sick neonates because it provides numerous nutritional, immunologic, and psychosocial advantages over formulas. Breast milk contains numerous trophic peptides, such as epidermal growth factor, which enhance GI growth and development.[67] Preterm breast milk is higher in protein, sodium, chloride, magnesium, and iron than mature human milk and is thus more suitable for the enteral feeding of the preterm infant.[50] Despite these advantages, preterm milk is still relatively deficient in calcium and phosphorus for the needs of the growing preterm infant.[8,50] Breast milk fortification is generally recommended for preterm infants (1) born at fewer than 34 weeks gestation, (2) born at less than 1,500 g, and (3) receiving parenteral nutrition for more than 2 weeks. Commercially available fortifiers include Enfamil Human Milk Fortifier (Mead Johnson), Similac Human Milk Fortifier (Ross Products Division, Abbott Laboratories), and Similac Natural Care (Ross Products Division, Abbott Laboratories), a liquid fortifier mixed 1:1 with pumped breast milk. The addition of one packet of Enfamil Human Milk Fortifier to 25 mL of human milk increases the caloric density by 4 kcal/oz and also increases the levels of protein, calcium, phosphorus, and other minerals. Most notably, the Enfamil fortifier contains added iron equal to that of iron-fortified term formulas and additional fat, 20% of which comes from MCTs. Beneficial outcomes in terms of infant growth, development, and nutritional status have resulted from fortification of breast milk.[68,69]

TERM INFANT FORMULAS: STANDARD, SOY, AND SPECIALIZED

Term infant formulas meet the nutritional requirements of term infants during the first year of life. The protein, carbohydrate, and lipid macronutrient sources vary depending on whether the formula is standard, soy based, or partially hydrolyzed. The protein source may be casein and whey, soy protein isolate, or hydrolysates of casein or whey.[70,71] Infant formulas contain a blend of vegetable oils as the fat source and either lactose, glucose polymers, sucrose, or a combination of these as the carbohydrate source.[72,73] Vitamins and minerals are added to all infant formulas in accordance with the recommendations set by the American Academy of Pediatrics (AAP) and the Infant Formula Act of 1980.[74,75] Specialized whey hydrolysate formulas have resulted in reduced incidence of intolerance in infants with a family history of allergy.[76–78] Follow-up formulas for infants 4 months or older follow the European Society of Pediatric Gastroenterology and Nutrition guidelines for follow-up formulas[79] and the US Food and Drug Administration (FDA) nutritional requirements guidelines. Specialized milk-based formulas such as lactose-free formulas and formulas with added rice starch such as Enfamil AR (Mead Johnson) have been introduced to manage GI intolerance and reflux. Infant formulas generally have a caloric density of 20 kcal/oz but can be concentrated to 24 kcal/oz or greater using both concentration and the addition of caloric additives to meet the needs of infants with cardiorespiratory illness or failure to thrive. The use of sterile liquid ready to feed or concentrate is recommended by the FDA for the preparation of infant formulas within the institutional setting.[80]

Specialized formulas such as soy formulas, partially hydrolyzed formulas, and elemental formulas are indicated for a variety of uses. Soy formulas are used in the management of primary and secondary lactase deficiency and galactosemia.[81–85] Specialized formulas such as Nutramigen (Mead Johnson), Pregestimil (Mead Johnson), and Alimentum (Ross Products Division, Abbot Laboratories) are indicated for infants with allergies to intact protein of cow's milk or soy and generalized malabsorption, respectively. Portagen (Mead Johnson), which contains 88% of the fat as MCT oil, is used in the management of severe steatorrhea or chylous leak.[82,86] Finally, elemental formulas such as Neocate (SHS North America, Gaithersburg, MD) are used in the management of infants with severe protein allergies who are intolerant of hydrolysate formulas.[87,88]

FORMULAS FOR CHILDREN 1 TO 10 YEARS OF AGE

Over the past 15 years, a number of pediatric enteral formulas, including polymeric, semielemental, and elemental formulas, have been developed for the support of children with a variety of disease states.[89] Figure 75.4B-1 presents an algorithm for selection of an appropriate pediatric formula based on GI function. Polymeric pediatric formulas meet the specialized needs of the 1- to 10-year-old child and are available in the tube feeding and flavored varieties and with or without fiber. The caloric and nutrient density and the osmolality and macronutrient sources can be found in Table 75.4B-2. Pediatric patients with GI disease or severe protein allergies may require EN support with a semielemental or an elemental formula. These formulas contain either peptides, free amino acids, or a combination of these, and part of the fat is provided as MCT. These formulas are also lactose and fructose free to optimize tolerance.

ADULT ENTERAL TUBE FEEDING FORMULAS

Children over the age of 10 years may be effectively managed with an adult enteral formula selected to meet the child's individual nutritional needs. Table 75.4B-3 lists the nutrient sources in a variety of selected adult formulas. These adult formulas are generally categorized into standard polymeric, semielemental, elemental, and specialized. Standard polymeric formulas contain mixtures of protein isolates, oligosaccharides, vegetable oil, MCTs, and added vitamins and minerals.[2,90,91] Soluble and insoluble fiber is added in a variety of forms. It serves as a fuel source for colonic mucosal cells and may also decrease the severity of diarrhea.[92] Older children and adolescents with markedly elevated calorie and protein requirements who require fluid restriction may be optimally managed with high-calorie, high-nitrogen formulations.[93] Semielemental and elemental formulas have been used effectively for the continuous enteral feeding support of patients with Crohn disease, CF, and short-gut syndrome[94–96] because nitrogen is more rapidly and effectively absorbed in the compromised bowel in the form of di- and tripeptides.[97,98]

TABLE 75.4B-3   SELECTED ADULT ENTERAL FORMULAS

PRODUCT NAME	KCAL/ CC	CARBOHYDRATE (G/1,000 ML)	FAT (G/1,000 ML)	PROTEIN (G/1,000 ML)	MOSM/ KG	NUTRIENT SOURCES (CARBOHYDRATE; FAT; PROTEIN)
Standard enteral formulas						
Isocal	1.06	135	44	34	270	Maltodextrin; soy, MCT; sodium and calcium caseinates and soy protein isolate
Osmolite	1.06	151	35	37	300	Maltodextrin; high-oleic safflower, canola, MCT; lecithin; sodium and calcium caseinates, soy protein
Nutren 1.5	1.5	169	68	60	510	Maltodextrin; MCT, canola, corn, soy lecithin; calcium and potassium caseinates
Nutren 2.0	2	196	106	80	745	Maltodextrin; MCT, canola, corn, soy lecithin; calcium and potassium caseinates
Osmolite HN	1.06	144	35	44	300	Maltodextrin; high-oleic safflower, canola, MCT; lecithin; sodium and calcium caseinates, soy protein
Osmolite HN Plus	1.2	139	35	49	360	Maltodextrin; high-oleic safflower, canola, MCT; lecithin; sodium and calcium caseinates, soy protein
Fiber-containing formulas						
Ultracal (cellulose and soy fiber)	1.06	142	39	44	360	Maltodextrin; canola, MCT, high-oleic sunflower, corn oil; milk protein concentrate and casein
Jevity (soy fiber)	1.06	155	35	44	300	Maltodextrin, corn syrup; high-oleic safflower, canola, MCT, lecithin; sodium and calcium caseinates
Nutren 1.0 with Fiber (soy polysaccharide)	1	127	38	40	320–380	Maltodextrin, corn syrup; canola, MCT, corn, soy, lecithin; calcium-potassium caseinates
Probalance (soy polysaccharide + gum arabic)	1.2	156	41	54	350–450	Maltodextrin, corn syrup solids; canola, MCT, corn, soy lecithin; calcium-potassium caseinates
IsoSource 1.5 (soy fiber + guar gum)	1.5	170	65	68	650	Hydrolyzed corn starch, sucrose; canola, MCT, soybean oil; sodium and calcium caseinates
Semielemental and elemental formulas						
Peptamen	1	127	39	40	270–380	Maltodextrin, corn starch; MCT, soybean, soy lecithin; enzymatically hydrolyzed whey
Peptamen 1.5	1.5	188	56	68	550	Maltodextrin, corn starch; MCT, soybean, soy lecithin; enzymatically hydrolyzed whey
Subdue	1	127	34	50	440–525	Maltodextrin, modified corn starch; MCT, canola, high-oleic sunflower, corn; hydrolyzed whey protein concentrate, casein hydrolysate
Vital HN	1	185	10.8	42	500	Maltodextrin, sucrose; safflower oil, MCT; partially hydrolyzed whey, meat, soy, free amino acids
Specialized adult enteral formulas						
Impact (immune enhancing)	1	130	28	56	375	Hydrolyzed corn starch; palm kernel, sunflower, menhaden oil; sodium and calcium caseinates, arginine
Crucial (immune enhancing)	1.5	135	68	94	490	Maltodextrin, corn starch; MCT, fish oil, soybean, soy lecithin; hydrolyzed casein, L-arginine
Nutri-Hep (hepatic)	1.5	290	21	40	690	Maltodextrin, modified corn starch; MCT, canola, soy lecithin, corn oil; amino acids, whey (50% branched-chain amino acids)
Suplena (renal—predialysis)	2	256	96	30	600	Maltodextrin, sucrose; high-oleic safflower, soy, lecithin; sodium and calcium caseinates
Nepro (renal—dialysis)	2	222	96	70	665	Corn syrup, sucrose, FOS; high-oleic safflower, canola, lecithin; calcium, magnesium and sodium caseinates
Respalor (pulmonary)	1.5	146	68	75	400	Corn syrup, sucrose; canola, MCT, high-oleic safflower, corn oil; calcium and sodium caseinates
Pulmocare (pulmonary)	1.5	106	93	63	475	Sucrose, maltodextrin; canola, MCT, corn, high-oleic safflower, lecithin (55% of kcal/fat); caseinates
Choice DM (glucose intolerance)	1.06	119	51	45	300	Maltodextrin; canola, high-oleic sunflower, corn oil; milk protein concentrate; fiber: soy fiber and cellulose
Glucerna (glucose intolerance)	1	96	54	42	355	Maltodextrin, fructose; high-oleic safflower, canola oil, lecithin; sodium and calcium caseinates

FOS = fructose oligosaccharide; MCT = medium-chain triglyceride.

Osmolite, Jevity, Vital HN, Glucerna, Pulmocare, Suplena, and Nepro products are Ross Products Division, Abbott Laboratories, Columbus, OH; Isocal, Ultracal, Subdue, Respalor, and Choice DM are Mead Johnson, Evansville, IN; the Nutren products, Probalance, Crucial, Nuri-Hep, and the Peptamen products are Nestle Clinical Nutrition, Deerfield, IL; Isosource products and Impact are Novartis Nutrition, Minneapolis, MN.

Specialized enteral formulas have been designed for the nutritional support of patients with a variety of specific diseases. Glutamine, arginine, ω-3 fatty acids, nucleotides, and other pharmacologic additives are provided in some formulas.[2] These formulas are expensive, and their clinical efficacy over standard polymeric formulas for the management of clinical conditions, including trauma, sepsis, diabetes, and renal failure, remains controversial.[99–108]

ORAL SUPPLEMENTS AND MODULAR COMPONENTS

Milk-based and polymeric formulas may be used as oral supplements and are usually of moderately high lactose and residue owing to their high lactose content. Oral supplements such as Carnation Instant Breakfast (Nestle Clinical Nutrition) mixed with milk are often better accepted by children than are the lactose-free commercial supplements. Flavored polymeric formulas such as Boost (Mead Johnson) and Ensure Plus (Ross Products Division, Abbott Laboratories) are well accepted and palatable. Table 75.4B-4 presents the nutrient content of a variety of oral supplements.

Owing to the unique and often elevated nutritional requirements of the enterally fed pediatric patient, modification of enteral formulas with modular components is often necessary.[109] In these clinical situations, standard and specialized infant and pediatric formulas may be supplemented with caloric modulars, including carbohydrate, fat, and protein modules. Table 75.4B-5 reviews the caloric density and nutrient composition of selected modular products.

GASTROSTOMY AND NG AND NJ FEEDINGS

When the requirement for EN support has been established, the optimal route of delivering nutrients must be determined. Many practitioners recommend the placement of NG or NJ tubes when the estimated course of therapy will not exceed 1 to 3 months. If the risk of aspiration is not significant, gastric feedings are preferable owing to the bactericidal effects of acid, the action of lingual lipase, ease of management, and ability to use bolus feedings. If GER is present, aspiration is a significant risk, and the duration of tube feeding may be relatively short. In this situation, NJ feeding is preferable to NG feeding. Tubes made of polyurethane and silicone rubber are soft and pliable and

may be left in place for indefinite periods of time. Polyvinyl chloride tubes become stiff and nonpliable when left in place for more than a few days; however, they are useful for intestinal decompression or short-term feeding. They should be changed every 2 to 3 days to avoid skin necrosis or intestinal perforation. Some feeding tubes made of polyurethane or silicone rubber have a weight at the tip that makes them useful for duodenal or jejunal feedings. Tube sizes of 5F to 8F are appropriate for most pediatric patients. The weight on tubes that are 7F or 8F may be too great for easy passage in a young infant.

Children who require long-term tube feeding are candidates for placement of a gastrostomy tube. GER, which may occur in neurologically disabled children or even in normal infants following gastrostomy tube placement, may necessitate an operative antireflux procedure (eg, Nissen fundoplication). Although the procedure is effective in reducing GER, postoperative complications can be troublesome. Intractable retching episodes, dumping syndrome, continued problems with swallowing, impaired esophageal emptying, slow feeding, and gas bloating have all been reported. Controversy currently exists over the necessity of an antireflux procedure in neurologically impaired children who require a feeding gastrostomy. Our current policy when there is a question of GER with continuous or bolus enteral feedings is to administer the feeding on a trial basis through a NG tube before a decision is made on the need for a Nissen fundoplication. We do not feel that preoperative endoscopy or pH probe studies allow one to predict who will have pulmonary complications with GER. Indeed, many times GER improves, especially with continuous feedings.

Percutaneous endoscopic gastrostomy (PEG) tubes can be placed without a laparotomy and, in some older adolescents, without general anesthesia. PEG tubes can also be placed fluoroscopically without endoscopy. The most frequent complication of percutaneous gastrostomies appears to be localized cellulitis. This may be controlled by careful attention to adjusting the tension on the external bolster, which will vary during the postoperative period depending on edema at the insertion sight. There is controversy as to whether preoperative antibiotics prevent postoperative

TABLE 75.4B-4   SELECTED ORAL SUPPLEMENTS

PRODUCT NAME	SERVING SIZE, ML (OZ)	KCAL PER SERVING	GRAMS PER SERVING		
			CARBOHYDRATE	FAT	PROTEIN
Boost Drink	237 (8)	240	40	4	10
Ensure	237 (8)	240	40	6	9
Resource Standard	237 (8)	240	40	6	9
Boost High Protein	237 (8)	240	33	6	15
Boost Plus	237 (8)	360	45	14	14
Ensure Plus	237 (8)	360	50	11.5	13
Carnation Instant Breakfast (mixed with low-fat milk)	270 (9)	250	39	5	12
Carnation Instant Breakfast (no sugar added)	270 (9)	190	24	5	12
Mighty Shake	120 (4)	200	32	5	6
Mighty Shake (sugar free)	120 (4)	200	18	10	8

Boost products are Mead Johnson, Evansville, IN; Ensure products are Ross Products Division, Abbott Laboratories, Columbus, OH; Carnation products are Nestle Clinical Nutrition, Deerfield, IL; Mighty Shakes are Hormel Healthlabs, Austin, MN.

TABLE 75.4B-5   SELECTED CALORIC AND NUTRIENT MODULAR PRODUCTS

PRODUCT NAME	CALORIC DENSITY	NUTRIENT COMPOSITION
Polycose Powder	8 kcal/tsp	Glucose polymers
Polycose Liquid	2 kcal/cc	Glucose polymers
Light Karo Syrup	4 kcal/cc	Corn syrup, sugar, vanilla
Microlipid	4.5 kcal/cc	Safflower oil emulsion
Vegetable oil	8.6 kcal/cc	Oleic, linoleic, linolenic acids
Resource BeneProtein	25 kcal/scoop	Whey protein isolate, 6 g/scoop
Duocal	14 kcal/tsp	Corn starch, vegetable oil, MCT

Polycose is Ross Products Division, Abbott Laboratories, Columbus, OH; Microlipid is Mead Johnson, Evansville, IN; Resource Beneprotein is Novartis Nutrition, Minneapolis, MN; Duocal is SHS NorthAmerica, Gaithersburg, MD.

local cellulites. PEGs are sometimes contraindicated after previous abdominal surgery, in the presence of an abdominal tumor or significant organomegaly, or when obesity complicates placement.

Another complication of PEG placement is inadvertent perforation of a loop of bowel, generally the transverse colon. The colon may be enlarged if there is preoperative constipation and also may enlarge owing to excessive gas production, generally from air swallowing. Occasionally, this occurs if a child cries and swallows air for an extended period just prior to the procedure. Skillful, rapid placement of intravenous lines for sedation and other placating tactics may minimize this. Careful observation of the gas pattern during transillumination of the stomach prior to tube placement can also hint at inadvertent colon enlargement.

The gastrostomy button is a feeding device that can be used to form an effective one-way valve at the gastrostomy site. These products fit flush with the skin and attach to commercial feeding tubes that lock onto the button in a variety of ways. The button is less prone to accidental removal. However, the valve system makes button devices difficult to use for decompression of the stomach unless a tube is inserted through the valve directly into the stomach. It is possible to modify the external PEG tube into a button using a commercial conversion kit. This temporary button may last up to a year after initial PEG placement. It must be removed endoscopically by pulling it out through the mouth. It can then be replaced with a standard button.

Two types of buttons are currently available on the market. One has an inner deformable bolster that must be stretched with a trocar and forcibly inserted into the gastrostomy orifice. There is a 2 to 5% risk of tearing or perforating the site during insertion. It has the advantage of being very durable and not prone to breakage. The other variety of button has an inflatable bolster that is easier to insert. After insertion, the balloon is inflated. The inner seal provided by the inflatable bolster products is somewhat adjustable by varying the amount of water used to inflate the bolster. A disadvantage is that the balloon or the button itself is more prone to breakage and generally must be changed every 3 months.

If short-term enteral support is necessary and GER, delayed gastric emptying, or chronic pancreatitis is present, transpyloric jejunal feedings are an alternative. Placement of transpyloric nasoduodenal or NJ tubes is more complicated than NG tube placement and requires confirmation of position by radiography or pH analysis of aspirates. Placement of transpyloric tubes can be facilitated by the use of fluoroscopy and intravenous metoclopramide. Special catheters that measure pH using an electrode system are also available to confirm placement. Transpyloric tubes can also be placed endoscopically through existing gastrostomies. Extreme care must be exercised to be certain that retching or emesis has not moved the tip of the tube into the esophagus. Retrograde continuous delivery of formula into the esophagus virtually ensures aspiration. When tubes are placed beyond the pylorus, gastric decompression may be required to prevent distention that could impair small bowel motility or lead to aspiration. Feeding jejunostomies generally do not tolerate large bolus feeding over short intervals without producing dumping syndrome.

Two different methods are employed for delivery of enteral feedings. Intermittent bolus feedings deliver the formula over a period of time similar to that for an oral feeding (ie, 10–20 minutes). This technique is simple, requires minimal supplies, and may facilitate the transition to home care. Intolerance of this method is indicated by gastric residuals, malabsorption, dumping syndrome, aspiration, or persistent regurgitation. Bolus feeding is not well tolerated when feedings are delivered distal to the pylorus. When there is intolerance of intermittent bolus feeding, continuous infusion using an infusion pump is an alternative. When compared with hourly bolus feeding in adult burn patients, continuous feeding resulted in fewer stools and reduced the time to reach nutritional goals. Continuous feeding appears to be particularly beneficial when used for patients with impaired absorption, such as chronic diarrhea or short-bowel syndrome.[110,111] For chronic diarrhea, the reason for success of continuous feeding may be related to decreased gastric distention, which, in turn, affects the gastrocolic reflex. In some patients, this lack of gastrocolic reflex may potentiate constipation, which is a frequent complication of enteral feedings. Also, lack of gastric distention may decrease the usual postcibal GER, which is directly correlated to increases in feeding volume.[112]

We have found that chronic constipation is often an occult complication of enteral feedings that is manifest by early satiety, distention, and poor gastric emptying or even emesis. Often it is unsuspected because overflow diarrhea is present. An abdominal radiograph and/or digital examination will often reveal large amounts of fecal material. Disimpaction with enemas and establishment of regular bowel movements using routine laxative administration is often extremely beneficial.

Similar symptoms of emesis and diarrhea during EN may also be observed with bacterial overgrowth. Bacterial overgrowth may occur as a result of altered anatomy, disorganized motility, and/or chronic acid inhibition. It may be diagnosed by enteral intubation and culture or inferred from high basal or early postcibal breath hydrogen analyses. However, neither of these measurements totally excludes bacterial overgrowth. Therefore, we prefer an empiric trial of treatment, generally with metronidazole for anaerobic bacteria or, less commonly, trimethoprim-sulfamethoxazole for gram-negative overgrowth. When the problem is recurrent, therapy with regular 3- or 4-day courses of treatment every 3 to 4 weeks allows for smoother progression of feedings. Alternatively, use of a probiotic such as *Lactobacillus* GG may be of benefit. We have also observed in two patients that use of a high-fat formula seemed to decrease the troublesome recurrent symptoms of bacterial overgrowth. This might be due to slower motility or less carbohydrate available as bacterial substrate.

WATER

It must be emphasized that the most important nutrient deficiency to be avoided is water deficiency (dehydration or tube feeding syndrome) Often this occurs insidiously over several days or even months. Those patients who are unable to voluntarily control their water intake, owing to limitations on absorption, developmental immaturity, or neuromuscular diseases, are at particular risk for the development of tube feeding syndrome. This deficiency will become particularly critical during times of increased water losses owing to fever, vomiting, or diarrhea. Even ambient weather conditions can contribute to deficiency. The patient discharged to a home without air-conditioning during the summer months may have an enormously increased requirement for water. If the patient wears diapers, it is useful to ask the caregiver how many urine voids there are during the day. If the diaper contents are always mixed urine and stool, it is important to ask how many "urine-only" diapers are changed during the day. During routine visits to the physician, urine-specific gravity, serum sodium, and blood urea to creatinine concentrations should be studied in a flowchart representation to help spot trends.

The practice of adding supplemental calories and electrolytes to feedings can exacerbate tube feeding syndrome water deficiency by producing increased GER[112] or diarrhea. Simplistically, clinicians often feed to the point of emesis or diarrhea in an attempt to maximize weight gain. This puts the patient at particular risk for tube feeding syndrome. The goal should be steady, modest weight gain with positive fluid balance.

Mechanical complications are also common with enteral feedings. The small-bore tubes can easily become clogged or kinked. Clogged feeding tubes can be a major problem, requiring repeated reinsertions. Newer enteral feeding tubes have wider openings to diminish clogging. Additional ports at the connection site allow for medication administration and flushing without interruption of the feeding

To prevent clogging, liquid medications should be used whenever available. If medication in tablet form is necessary, it should be crushed to a fine powder. Adequate suspension in solution can sometimes be achieved by allowing the tablet to dissolve in water rather than attempting to dissolve the crushed tablet. Medications that congeal, such as Metamucil or cholestyramine, easily clog small-bore tubes and should be avoided when possible. If they are necessary, these medications should be administered and cleared quickly. Cholestyramine products that have aspartame instead of sugar are often finer powders and less likely to clog the tube. Feeding tubes should be flushed with water before and after intermittent bolus feedings and periodically (every 4 to 6 hours) during continuous feeding. An investigation of nine nontoxic substances (including digestive enzymes, proteolytic enzymes, and cranberry juice) theoretically useful in clearing clogged feeding tubes demonstrated that successful declogging occurred with chymotrypsin, papain, and distilled water. Preventing feeding tubes from clogging is easier than attempting to clear them.[113] Other mechanical complications include irritation from transnasal tubes, which can produce sinusitis, otitis media, GER, and nasopharyngeal and gastric irritation.

SUMMARY AND CONCLUSIONS

We have discussed the indications for specialized enteral formulas and routes of administration. The enteral route is the preferred route of nutrient administration. Even in the face of relative compromise of the GI tract, specialized products and techniques promote positive nutrient balance. Partial use of the enteral route during parenteral nutrition prevents atrophy of the intestine and reduces the tendency toward the cholestasis associated with intravenous feeding. If possible, the oral route is preferable, and appetizing, nutritious foods should be emphasized. Enteral feeding is cheaper, simpler, more effective, and safer than parenteral feeding.

REFERENCES

1. Braunschweig CL, Levy P, Sheean PM, et al. Enteral compared with parenteral nutrition: a meta-analysis. Am J Clin Nutr 2001;74:534–42.
2. Charney P. Enteral nutrition: indications, options and formulations. In: Gottschlich MM, Fuhrman MP, Hammond KA, et al, editors. The science and practice of nutrition support. Dubuque (IA): Kendall/Hunt Publishing Company; 2002. p. 141–66.
3. Nevin-Folino N, Miller M. Enteral nutrition. In: Samour PQ, Helm KK, Lang CE, editors. Handbook of pediatric nutrition. Gaithersburg (MD): Aspen Publishers; 1999. p. 513–50.
4. McClave SA, Marsano LS, Lukan JK. Enteral access for nutritional support: rationale for utilzation. J Clin Gastroenterol 2002;35:209–13.
5. Abad-Sinden A, Sutphen JL. Growth and nutrition. In: Allen HD, Gutgesell HP, Clark EB, Driscoll DJ, editors. Moss and Adams' heart disease in infants, children, and adolescents. Philadelphia: Lippincott, Williams & Wilkins; 2001. p. 325–32.
6. Sapsford A. Human milk and enteral nutrition products. In:

Groh-Wargo S, Thompson M, Hovasi Cox J, editors. Nutritional care for high–risk newborns. Chicago: Precept Press; 2000. p. 265–302.

7. Anderson DA. Nutrition for premature infants. In: Samour PQ, Helm KK, Lang CE, editors. Handbook of pediatric nutrition. Gaithersburg (MD): Aspen Publishers; 1999. p. 43–64.

8. Abad-Sinden A, Bollinger R. Challenges and controversies in the nutrition support of the premature infant. Support Line 2002;24(2):5–16.

9. Schanler RJ, Shulman RJ, Lau C, et al. Feeding strategies for premature infants: randomized trial of gastrointestinal priming and tube-feeding method. Pediatrics 1999;103:434–9.

10. Tyson JE, Kennedy KA. Minimal enteral nutrition in parenterally fed neonates. Cochrane Database Syst Rev 1998;3:1–10.

11. Meetze W, Valentine C, McGuigan JE, et al. Gastrointestinal priming prior to full enteral nutrition in very low birth weight infants. J Pediatr Gastroenterol Nutr 1992;15:163–170.

12. Hovasi-Cox J. Bronchopulmonary dysplasia. In: Groh-Wargo S, Thompson M, Hovasi Cox J, editors. Nutritional care for high-risk newborns. Chicago: Precept Press; 2000. p. 369–91.

13. Johnson DB, Cheney C, Monsen ER. Nutrition and feeding in infants with bronchopulmonary dysplasia after initial hospital discharge: risk factors for growth failure. Am J Diet Assoc 1998;98:649–56.

14. Kurzner SI, Garg M, Bautista DB, et al. Growth failure in bronchopulmonary dysplasia; elevated metabolic rates and pulmonary mechanics. J Pediatr 1988;112:73–80.

15. Abad-Sinden A. Nutritional support and management in bronchopulmonary dysplasia. Building Block for Life 2002; 25(4):1–9.

16. Wooldridge NH. Pulmonary disease. In: Samour PQ, Helm KK, Lang CE, editors. Handbook of pediatric nutrition. Gaithersburg (MD): Aspen Publishers; 1999. p. 315–54.

17. Davis AM. Pediatrics. In: Matarese LE, Gottschlich MM, editors. Contemporary nutrition support practice—a clinical guide. Philadelphia: WB Saunders; 1998. p. 362–3.

18. Thomassen M, Heilberg A, Kase BF. Feeding problems in children with congenital heart disease: the impact on energy intake and growth outcome. Eur J Clin Nutr 1992;46:457–64.

19. Hansen SR, Dorup I. Energy and nutrient intakes in congenital heart disease. Acta Paediatr 1993;82:166–72.

20. Heymsfield SB, Casper K. Congestive heart failure: clinical management by use of continuous nasoenteric feeding. Am J Clin Nutr 1989;50:539–44.

21. Vanderhoof JA, Hofschire PJ, Baluff MA, et al. Continuous enteral feedings: an important adjunct to the management of complex congenital heart disease. Am J Dis Child 1982;136:825–7.

22. Morin CL, Roulet M, Weber A. Continuous elemental enteral alimentation in children with Crohn's disease and growth failure. Gastroenterology 1980;79:1205–10.

23. Morin CL, Roulet M, Roy CC, Lapointe N. Continuous elemental enteral alimentation in the treatment of children and adolescents with Crohn's disease. JPEN J Parenter Enteral Nutr 1982;6:194–9.

24. Ruemmele FM, Roy CC, Levy E, Seidman EG. Nutrition as primary therapy in pediatric Crohn's disease: fact or fantasy? Pediatrics 2000;136:285–91.

25. Cezard JP, Messing B. Enteral nutrition in inflammatory bowel disease: is there a special role for elemental diets? Clin Nutr 1993;12 Suppl 1:S75–81.

26. Fell JME, Paintin M, Arnaud-Battandier F, et al. Mucosal healing and a fall in mucosal pro-inflammatory cytokine mRNA induced by a specific oral polymeric diet in paediatric Crohn's disease. Aliment Pharmacol Ther 2000;14:281–89.

27. Vanderhoof JA, Langnas AN, Pinch LW, et al. Invited review: short bowel syndrome. J Pediatr Gastroenterol Nutr 1992; 14:359–70.

28. Jones-Wessel J. Short bowel syndrome. In: Groh-Wargo S, Thompson M, Hovasi Cox J, editors. Nutritional care for high-risk newborns. Chicago: Precept Press; 2000. p. 469–88.

29. Price P. Parenteral nutrition: administration and monitoring. In: Groh-Wargo S, Thompson M, Hovasi Cox J, editors. Nutritional care for high-risk newborns. Chicago: Precept Press; 2000. p. 91–108.

30. Mirtallo JM. Introduction to parenteral nutrition. In: Gottschlich MM, Fuhrman MP, Hammond KA, et al, editors. The science and practice of nutrition support. Dubuque (IA): Kendall/Hunt Publishing Company; 2002. p. 211–24.

31. Kaufman SS, Murray ND, Wood P, et al. Nutritional support for the infant with extrahepatic biliary atresia. J Pediatr 1987; 110:679–85.

32. Narkewicz MR. Biliary atresia: an update on our understanding of the disorder. Curr Opin Pediatr 2001;13:435–40.

33. Sutton M. Nutritional support in pediatric liver transplantation. Dietitians in Nutrition Support Newsletter 1989;11(1):1, 8–9.

34. Heubi JE, Heyman MB, Shulman RJ. The impact of liver disease on growth and nutrition. J Pediatr Gastroenterol Nutr 2002;35 Suppl 1:S55–9.

35. McClave S, Snider H, Owen N, et al. Clinical nutrition in pancreatitis. Dig Dis Sci 1997;42:2035–44.

36. Olah A, Pardavi G, Belagyi T, et al. Early nasojejunal feeding in acute pancreatitis is associated with a lower complication rate. Nutrition 2002;18:259–62.

37. Kudsk KA. Importance of enteral feeding in maintaining gut integrity. JPEN J Parenter Enteral Nutr 2001;25:S2–8.

38. Lewis SJ, Egger M, Sylvester PA, et al. Early enteral feeding versus "nil by mouth" after gastrointestinal surgery: systematic review and meta-analysis of controlled studies. BMJ 2001;323:1–5.

39. Barale KV, Charuhas PM. Oncology and marrow transplantation. In: Samour PQ, Helm KK, Lang CE, editors. Handbook of pediatric nutrition. Gaithersburg (MD): Aspen Publishers; 1999. p. 465–92.

40. Aquino VM, Smyrl CB, Hagg R, et al. Enteral nutritional support by gastrostomy tube in children with cancer. J Pediatr 1995;127:58–62.

41. Matthew P, Bowman L, Williams R, et al. Complications and effectiveness of gastrostomy feedings in pediatric cancer patients. J Pediatr Hematol Oncol 1996;18:81–5.

42. Gallagher Olsen L, Cutroni R, Furuta L. Pediatric acquired immunodeficiency syndrome. In: Samour PQ, Helm KK, Lang CE, editors. Handbook of pediatric nutrition. Gaithersburg (MD): Aspen Publishers; 1999. p. 453–64.

43. Miller TL, Awnetwant EL, Evans S, et al. Gastrostomy tube supplementation for HIV infected children. Pediatrics 1995;96: 696–702.

44. Spinozzi N. Chronic renal disease. In: Samour PQ, Helm KK, Lang CE, editors. Handbook of pediatric nutrition. Gaithersburg (MD): Aspen Publishers; 1999. p. 385–94.

45. Strife CF, Quinlan M, Mears K, et al. Improved growth of three uremic children by nocturnal nasogastric feedings. Am J Dis Child 1986;140:438–43.

46. Cloud HH. Developmental disabilities. In: Samour PQ, Helm KK, Lang CE, editors. Handbook of pediatric nutrition. Gaithersburg (MD): Aspen Publishers; 1999. p. 293–314.

47. Stevenson RD. Nutrition and feeding of children with developmental disabilities. Pediatr Ann 1995;24:255–60.

48. Tsang RC, Uauy R, Lucas A, Zlotkin S, editors. Nutritional needs of the preterm infant: scientific basis and practical guidelines. Baltimore: Williams and Wilkins; 1993. p. 288–95.

49. Groh-Wargo S. Recommended enteral nutrient intakes. In:

Groh-Wargo S, Thompson M, Hovasi Cox J, editors: Nutritional care for high-risk newborns. Chicago: Precept Press; 2000. p. 231–64.

50. Sapsford A. Human milk and enteral nutrition products. In: Groh-Wargo S, Thompson M, Hovasi Cox J, editors: Nutritional care for high-risk newborns. Chicago: Precept Press; 2000. p. 265–302.

51. Trumbo P, Yates AA, Schlicker S, Poos M. Dietary Reference Intakes: vitamin A, vitamin K, arsenic, boron, chromium, copper, iodine, iron, manganese, molybdenum, nickel, silicon, vanadium, and zinc. J Am Diet Assoc 2001;101:294–300.

52. Canete A, Duggan C. Nutritional support of the pediatric intensive care unit patient. Curr Opin Pediatr 1996;8:248–55.

53. Chwals WJ, Letton RW, Jamie A, Charles B. Stratification of injury severity using energy expenditure response in surgical infants. J Pediatr Surg 1995;30:1161–4.

54. Chwals WJ. Overfeeding the critically ill child: fact or fantasy? New Horizons 1994;2:147–55.

55. Peterson KE, Washington J, Rathbun JM. Team management of failure to thrive. J Am Diet Assoc 1984;84:810–5.

56. Salmon SM, Kirby DF. The refeeding syndrome: a review. JPEN J Parenter Enteral Nutr 1990;14:90–7.

57. Vanlandingham S, Simpson S, Daniel P, et al. Metabolic abnormalities in patients supported with enteral tube feeding. JPEN J Parenter Enteral Nutr 1981;5:322–4.

58. Strathos TJ, Shulman RJ, Schanler RJ, Abrams SA. Effect of carbohydrates on calcium absorption in premature infants. Pediatr Res 1996;39:666–79.

59. Tantibhedhyangkul P, Hashim SA. Medium chain triglyceride feeding in premature infants: effects on fat and nitrogen absorption. Pediatrics 1975;55:359–70.

60. Andrews BF, Lorch V. Improved fat and calcium absorption in LBW infants fed a medium chain triglyceride containing formula [abstract]. Pediatr Res 1974;8:104.

61. Clandinin M, VanAerde J, Antonson D, et al. Formulas with docosahexaenoic acid (DHA) and arachidonic acid (ARA) promote better growth and development scores in very low birth weight infants (VLBW). Pediatr Res 2002;51:187A–8A.

62. Innis SM, Adamkin DH, Hall RT, et al. Docosahexaenoic acid and arachidonic acid enhance growth with no adverse effects in preterm infants fed formula. J Pediatr 2002;140:547–54.

63. Kashyap S, Ikamoto E, Kanaya S, et al. Protein quality in feeding low birth weight infants: a comparison of whey predominant versus casein predominant formulas. Pediatrics 1987; 79:748–55.

64. Lucas A, Bishop NJ, King FJ, Cole TJ. Randomised trial of nutrition for preterm infants after discharge. Arch Dis Child 1992;67:324–7.

65. Friel JK, Andrews WL, Matthew JD, et al. Improved growth of very low birth weight infants. Nutr Res 1993;13:611–20.

66. Bishop NJ, King FJ, Lucas A. Increased bone mineral content of preterm infants fed a nutrient enriched formula after discharge from hospital. Arch Dis Child 1993;68:573–8.

67. Moran JR, Courtney ME, Orth DN, et al. Epidermal growth factor in human milk: daily production and diurnal variation during early lactation in mothers delivering at term and at premature gestation. J Pediatr 1983;103:402–5.

68. Lucas A, Fewtrell MS, Morley R, et al. Randomized outcome trial of human milk fortification and development outcome in preterm infants. Am J Clin Nutr 1996;64:142–51.

69. Reis BB, Hall RD, Schanler RJ, et al. Enhanced growth of preterm infants fed a new powdered human milk fortifier: a randomized controlled trial. Pediatrics 2000;106:581–8.

70. Akers SM, Groh-Wargo S. Normal nutrition from infancy. In:

Samour PQ, Helm KK, Lang CE, editors. Handbook of pediatric nutrition. Gaithersburg (MD): Aspen Publishers; 1999. p. 65–98.

71. Voltz VR, Book LS, Churella HR. Growth and plasma amino acid concentrations in term infants fed either whey predominant or human milk. J Pediatr 1983;102:27–33.

72. Benkov KJ, LeLeiko NS. A rational approach to infant formulas. Pediatr Ann 1987;16:225–30.

73. Clark KJ M, Makrides M, Neuman MA, Gibson PA. Determination of the optimal ratio of linoleic acid to alpha-linolenic acid in infant formulas. J Pediatr 1992;120:S129–38.

74. Committee on Nutrition, American Academy of Pediatrics. Kleiman RE, editor. Pediatric nutrition handbook. Elk Grove Village (IL): American Academy of Pediatrics; 1998.

75. US Congress. Infant Formulas Act of 1980, Pub. L. No. 96-359 (Sept. 26, 1980).

76. Chandra RK, Singh G, Shridhara B. Effects of feeding whey hydrolysate, soy and conventional cow milk formulas on incidence of atopic disease in high risk infants. Ann Allergy 1989;63:102–6.

77. Vandenplas Y, Malfroot A, Dab I. Short term prevention of cow's milk protein allergy in infants. Immunol Allergy Pract 1989;11:17–24.

78. Carnation Good Start Product [monograph]. Deerfield (IL): Nestle Clinical Nutrition; 2001.

79. Committee on Nutrition, European Society of Pediatric Gastroenterology and Nutrition. Guidelines on infant nutrition: recommendations for the composition of follow-own formula and beikost. Acta Paediatr Scand 1987;287:2–25.

80. American Academy of Pediatrics. Commentary: infant formula safety. Pediatrics 2002;110:833–5.

81. Commitee on Nutrition, American Academy of Pediatrics. Soy protein-based formulas: recommendations for use in infant feeding. Pediatrics 1998;101:148–53.

82. Brady MS, Rickard KA, Fitzgerald JF, Lemon JA. Specialized formulas and feedings for infants with malabsorption or formula intolerance. J Am Diet Assoc 1986;86:191–200.

83. Meeting the special feeding needs of infants with cow's milk and carbohydrate intolerance. Isomil product handbook. Columbus (OH): Ross Products Division, Abbott Laboratories; 1993.

84. Dietary management of diarrhea in infants and toddlers. Isomil DF product handbook. Columbus (OH): Ross Products Division, Abbott Laboratories; 1993.

85. Brown KH, Perez F, Peerson JM, et al. Effect of dietary fiber (soy polysaccharide) on the severity, duration, and nutritional outcome of acute, watery diarrhea in children. Pediatrics 1993;92:241–7.

86. Kaufman SS, Scrivner DJ, Murray ND, et al. Influence of Portagen and Pregestimil on essential fatty acid status in infantile liver disease. Pediatrics 1992;89:151–4.

87. Vanderhoof JA, Murray ND, Kaufman SS, et al. Intolerance to protein hydrolysate infant formulas: an underrecognized cause of gastrointestinal symptoms in infants. J Pediatr 1997;131:741–4.

88. Binder NB, Dupont C, Hadji C, et al. Prospective, controlled, multi-center study on the effect of an amino acid based formula in infants with cow's milk allergy/intolerance and atopic dermatitis. Pediatr Allergy Immunol 2001;12:78–82.

89. Enteral nutrition support of children. Pediasure and Pediasure With Fiber product handbook. Columbus (OH): Ross Products Division Abbott Laboratories; 1993.

90. Storm HM, Lin P. Forms of carbohydrate in enteral nutrition formulas. Support Line 1996;18(3):7–8.

91. Gottschlich MM, Shronts EP, Hutchins AM. Defined formula

diets. In: Rombeau JL, Rolandelli RH, editors. Enteral and tube feeding. Philadelphia: WB Saunders; 1997. p. 207–39.

92. Homann HH, Kemen M, Fuessenich C, et al. Reduction in diarrhea incidence by soluble fiber in patients receiving total or supplemental enteral nutrition. JPEN J Parenter Enteral Nutr 1994;18:486–90.

93. Taitz LS, Byers HB. Hich caloric osmolar feeding and hypertonic dehydration. Arch Dis Child 1972;47:257.

94. Park RHR, Galloway A, Danesh BSZ, et al. Double blinded controlled trial of elemental and polymeric diets as primary therapy in active Crohn's disease. Eur J Gastroenterol Hepatol 1991;3:483–90.

95. Raouf AH, Hildrey V, Daniel J, et al. Enteral feeding as sole treatment for Crohn's disease: controlled trial of whole protein vs. amino acid based feed and a case study of dietary challenge. Gut 1991;32:702–7.

96. Rigaud D, Cosnes J, LeQuintrec Y, et al. Controlled trial comparing two types of enteral nutrition in treatment of active Crohn's disease: elemental vs. polymeric diet. Gut 1991;32:1492–7.

97. Matthews DM, Adibi SA. Peptide absorption. Gastroenterology 1976;71:151–61.

98. Adibi SA, Fogel MR, Agrawal RM. Comparison of free amino acids and dipeptide absorption in the jejunum of sprue patients. Gastroenterology 1974;67:586–91.

99. Heys S, Walker L, Smith I, et al. Enteral nutritional supplementation with key nutrients in patients with critical illness and cander: a meta-analysis of randomized controlled clinical trials. Ann Surg 1999;229:467–77.

100. Moore FA, Moore EE, Kudsk KA, et al. Clinical benefits of an immune enhancing diet for early postinjury enteral feeding. J Trauma 1994;37:607–15.

101. Bower RH, Cerra FB, Bershadsky B, et al. Early enteral administration of a formula supplemented with arginine, nucleotides, and fish oil in intensive care unit patients: results of a multi-center, prospective, randomized clinical trial. Crit Care Med 1995;23:436–49.

102. Kudsk KA, Minard G, Croce MA, et al. A randomized trial of isonitrogenous enteral diets after severe trauma: an immune-enhancing diet reduces septic complications. Ann Surg 1996;224:531–40.

103. Fischer JE. Amino acids in hepatic coma. Dig Dis Sci 1982;27:97.

104. Kondrup J, Nielsen K, Hamberg O. Nutritional therapy in patients with liver cirrhosis. Eur J Clin Nutr 1992;46:239–46.

105. Otto C, Sonnichsen AC, Ritter MM, et al. Influence of fiber, xylitol, and fructose in enteral formulas on glucose and lipid metabolism in normal subjects. Clin Invest 1993;71:290–3.

106. Craig LD, Nicholson S, Silverstone FA, Kennedy RD. Use of a reduced carbohydrate, modified fat enteral formula for improving metabolic control and clinical outcomes in long-term care residents with type 2 diabetes: results of a pilot trial. Nutrition 1998;14:529–34.

107. Talpers SS, Romberger DJ, Bunce SB, Pingleton SK. Nutritionally associated increased carbon dioxide production: excess total calories vs. high proportion of carbohydrate calories. Chest 1992;102:551–5.

108. Ireton-Jones CS, Borman KR, Turner WW. Nutrition considerations in the management of ventilator-dependent patients. Nutr Clin Pract 1993;8:60–4.

109. Smith JL, Heymsfield SB. Enteral nutrition support: formula preparation from modular ingredients. JPEN J Parenter Enteral Nutr 1983;7:280–8.

110. Parker P, Stroop S, Greene H. A controlled comparison of continuous versus intermittent feeding in the treatment of infants with intestinal disease. J Pediatr 1981;99:360–4.

111. Orenstein SR. Enteral versus parenteral therapy for intractable diarrhea of infancy: a prospective, randomized trial. J Pediatr 1986;109:277–86.

112. Sutphen JL, Dillard VL. Effect of feeding volume on early post-cibal gastroesophageal reflux in infants. J Pediatr Gastroenterol Nutr 1988;7:185–8.

113. Nicholson LJ. Declogging small-bore feeding tubes. JPEN J Parenter Enteral Nutr 1987;11:594–7.

5. Special Dietary Therapy

Maria R. Mascarenhas, MBBS

Darla J. Bradshaw, BS, RD, CNSD

Virginia A. Stallings, MD

SPECIAL DIETARY NEEDS

Malnutrition in children with chronic gastrointestinal disorders includes underfeeding (protein-energy malnutrition [PEM]) and overfeeding (overweight or obesity). In childhood, malnutrition is characterized by growth failure (weight, height/length), behavioral and cognitive deficits, and increased susceptibility to infections secondary to immune system dysfunction. Repeated infections may further alter nutrient intake and requirements, making this a vicious cycle. PEM often occurs as a result of inadequate nutrient and energy supply or in response to an injury or illness with increased requirements in a marginally nourished child. Malnutrition is common in hospitalized pediatric patients, with an estimated prevalence of 25 to 60% in North America.[1,2] Therefore, it is essential to meet the special nutrition needs of children with significant medical conditions. An overview of the nutritional considerations for selected disease states is presented in Table 75.5-1.

In many disease states, PEM occurs as food intake fails to increase in response to the increased energy and nutritional demands of inflammation and/or malabsorption. Most illnesses exert some effect on nutrient status and requirements. In certain disorders, the ability of the body to use specific nutrients may be altered (eg, vitamin E deficiency seen in abetalipoproteinemia). Nutritional deficiencies can have long-lasting effects, especially in growing children. Therefore, it is important to thoroughly understand the pathophysiology of the patient's disorder and its impact on nutritional status as part of nutrition support planning. Because drug therapy is part of the management of many diseases, drug–nutrient interactions must be considered. Medication side effects, as well as therapeutic effects, may contribute to changes seen in nutritional status owing to anorexia, nausea, vomiting, diarrhea, malabsorption, and maldigestion.[3,4]

Previously, the 1989 Recommended Dietary Allowances (RDAs) guided macronutrient and micronutrient intake for healthy children and those with acute and chronic illness. The RDAs have been replaced by the new Dietary Reference Intakes (DRIs). The DRIs are evidence based and represent recommendations for healthy US and Canadian populations for nutrient intake for good health, as well as for the prevention of chronic disease.[5] Additional information on nutrient requirements of children is available in Chapter 75.3, "Nutritional Assessment and Requirements."

The role of nutrition in disease and disease prevention is recognized in the medical community. Studies have shown that poor nutritional status negatively affects health outcomes in chronic disorders of childhood such as pulmonary status in patients with cystic fibrosis[6] and survival rates following a liver transplant.[7] Additionally, foods such as those containing prebiotics and probiotics may be used to modulate disease activity and the immune system. Many children with chronic diseases require additional calories, as well as other specific dietary interventions, to achieve optimal growth and development. These therapeutic diets are modifications of a normal diet pattern and are intended to counteract specific nutrient inadequacies that are associated with the disease states. An example is the provision of a high-protein diet in patients with protein-losing enteropathy. Some disease states such as acute diarrhea require dietary modifications for a limited time. A lactose-free diet in patients with acute diarrhea may provide symptomatic relief. However, for the majority of children with chronic diseases, the dietary modifications will be long term and will require follow-up as well as ongoing age- and culturally appropriate education. Re-evaluation of the diet therapy and monitoring of nutrient and nutritional status are essential to ensure adherence and comprehension. The goal is optimization of micronutrient and macronutrient intake based on age, nutritional status, and medical condition. Nutritional assessment plays a key role in achieving this goal.

SPECIFIC ASPECTS OF NUTRITION ASSESSMENT

Detailed information on nutritional assessment in infants, children, and adolescents is available in Chapter 75.3. Nutrition assessment is a component of the medical physical examination for all children, especially for those with chronic disease. Monitoring nutrition status is critical to ensure that the patient's nutritional goals are met. A registered dietitian often contributes to this assessment, which includes nutrition-focused medical and nutrition history, including infant feeding history, typical current intake, food aversions, allergies or intolerances, recent weight loss or gain, chewing and swallowing difficulties, and dietary, vitamin, mineral, or herbal supplements. Physical examination and growth assessment include anthropometric measurements: weight, height or length, head circumference, body mass index (for children > 2 years), midarm muscle circumference, triceps skinfold thickness, an assessment of fat and muscle stores, and signs of

TABLE 75.5-1   SELECTED DISEASE CONDITIONS AND RELATED NUTRITIONAL CONSIDERATIONS

CYSTIC FIBROSIS High-calorie, high-fat diet Salt replacement, especially in hot weather Evaluation of essential fatty acids and bone health Fat-soluble vitamin supplementation Enzyme therapy for pancreatic insufficiency Oral supplements for calories	**LIVER DISEASE** Fluid restriction for end-stage disease Fat-soluble vitamin/multivitamin supplementation Fat malabsorption may occur with biliary atresia or Alagille syndrome Evaluation of essential fatty acid status Evaluation of bone health Protein restriction with encephalopathy Adequate calories and protein for growth
INFLAMMATORY BOWEL DISEASE High-calorie diet Lactose-free diet Vitamin B_{12} supplementation with ileal disease Vitamin D, calcium, iron, zinc, folic acid supplementation Multivitamin supplementation Elemental diet for inducing remission and providing caloric support Bone disease evaluation	**METABOLIC DISORDERS** Dietary restriction of the offending nutrients Adjusted intake of offending amino acids and fats to promote optimal growth and development Monitor compliance to diet Replacement of deficient coenzymes
CONGENITAL HEART DISEASE (in infants) High-calorie formula in infants Concentrated formulas Fortified breast milk in infants Tube feeds Sodium restriction Fluid restriction	**CEREBRAL PALSY** Supplemental tube feeds Fiber-containing formula Speech evaluation if chewing/swallowing difficulties May require modified diet (puree, thickened liquids, etc) Supplemental multivitamin and minerals Ketogenic diet (patients with intractable seizures) Bone disease evaluation
CANCER High-calorie diet Oral supplements Tube feeds Parenteral nutrition for extensive nausea and vomiting Appetite stimulants Small, frequent feedings	**DIABETES MELLITUS** Blood glucose control Dietary balance with regularly scheduled meals and snacks Meal planning, carbohydrate counting, insulin education when indicated Monitor cholesterol and triglycerides and recommend low-fat diet when indicated Adequate calories for proper growth and development
RENAL DISEASE Fluid restriction Fortified breast milk or concentrated formula Sodium restriction Provide RDA for protein Phosphorus restriction Phosphorus binder Supplement with vitamin D, calcium Bone disease evaluation	**CELIAC DISEASE** Gluten-free diet Lactose-free diet may be indicated until complete mucosal healing Possible infant sensitivity to cow's milk protein Vitamin and mineral therapy Adequate calories for catch-up growth Bone disease evaluation Monitor compliance to diet

RDA = Recommended Dietary Allowance.

micronutrient excesses and deficiencies. Alternative anthropometric measures for linear growth (lower leg length and upper arm length) should be performed on patients who are unable to stand. A midarm circumference may be a useful measure to follow in patients with significant dependent edema that results in an unreliable weight. This measurement can be done every 2 weeks in infants and every 4 weeks in children and adolescents as a gross estimate of growth and response to therapy. To ensure reliability and accuracy, an experienced clinician should obtain these measurements using quality calipers that have been maintained regularly. Signs of malnutrition may be identified with physical assessment of body fat and muscle stores, the oral cavity, skin, hair, and eyes.

Evaluating pubertal development is also an important part of nutritional assessment. For those patients at nutritional risk, resting energy expenditure measurements by indirect calorimetry are recommended to determine individual caloric needs. Obtaining a dual-energy x-ray absorptiometry (DXA) scan provides body composition information such as fat and muscle stores and bone health. Biochemical analysis, including prealbumin, albumin,

electrolytes, minerals (calcium, phosphorus, and magnesium), trace minerals, iron studies, and liver function tests, is important in selected clinical settings. Specific nutrient analysis will depend on the underlying disease state (eg, triene-to-tetraene ratio to evaluate for essential fatty acid deficiency in cystic fibrosis or serum alkaline phosphatase, parathormone, vitamin D [25-hydroxy and 1,25-dihydroxy], calcium, and phosphorus to evaluate for rickets).

SPECIFIC DIETARY THERAPY BY NUTRIENT GROUPS
Dietary therapy during chronic illness is directed at providing calories, macronutrients, and micronutrients to support normal growth and, in many cases, nutritional rehabilitation. In an effort to meet the increased nutritional needs associated with chronic illness, infants and children may require dietary modifications. Typically, infant formulas are calorically concentrated from the standard 20 calories per ounce to 27 calories per ounce by mixing with less water. When higher caloric content is required, additional macronutrients can be added, usually in the form of modular components. The addition of carbohydrate, protein, and fat modular components to increase the caloric density of a formula is a com-

mon practice in pediatric nutrition support and is indicated for patients who are unable to meet nutrient needs with standard amounts of formula. Attention must be paid to the renal solute load when concentrating formulas, especially for patients with renal dysfunction. Generally, caloric density should be advanced by 2 to 4 calories per ounce in a 24-hour period as tolerated. The selection of the modular component (carbohydrate, protein, or fat) is dependent on the clinical situation. See Table 75.5-2 for a list of some commonly used modular components and their indications.

CARBOHYDRATES

The DRIs state that 45 to 65% of total calories should come from carbohydrates (Tables 75.5-3 and 75.5-4).[5] No more than 25% of total calories is recommended as added sugars because more may result in reduced intakes of certain micronutrients.[5] A number of popular weight loss diets recommend very low intakes of carbohydrate. A growing body of scientific evidence has shown an increased risk for adverse health effects with chronic consumption of any diet that has a pattern of increased or decreased micronutrients. Therefore, low-carbohydrate weight loss diets are not recommended for growing children. An exception is the ketogenic diet, which provides the majority of calories from fat with minimal protein and carbohydrate and is used to treat children with intractable seizure disorders.

The DRIs recommend that children > 1 year consume at least 130 g of carbohydrates each day. Adequate intake of carbohydrate is specifically important for brain health and to spare metabolism of protein for energy.

Human milk and most infant formulas contain 40 to 50% carbohydrate, with lactose being the primary source. Lactose plays a key role in infant feeding because it maintains lactobacilli in the gut, thereby preventing the growth of less desirable bacteria. Lactose also lowers the pH of the intestinal contents, thereby providing the optimal calcium absorption environment. Lactose intolerance commonly occurs in older children and adolescents. In infancy, lactose intolerance is often secondary to damage to the intestinal epithelium following acute gastrointestinal infections and celiac disease. Symptoms include bloating, flatulence, and diarrhea with ingestion of lactose-containing foods. Treatment may include supplemental lactase enzymes, restrictions of dietary lactose (lactose-free formula, reduced-lactose diet), and provision of adequate calcium and vitamin D intake. These conditions are discussed in more detail elsewhere in this text. See Table 75.5-5 for a list of selected common infant and childhood formulas and indications for use.

A well-appreciated role of dietary carbohydrates is in blood glucose control in diabetes. Nutritional management for children with diabetes includes carbohydrate counting and distribution of carbohydrates evenly throughout each meal or snack of the day. The number of carbohydrate

TABLE 75.5-2   SELECTED THERAPEUTIC MODULAR DIET COMPONENTS

MODULAR COMPONENT	INDICATION	CARBOHYDRATE	PROTEIN	FAT	CALORIC DENSITY
Polycose liquid (glucose corn polymer)	Added to supplements and formulas or foods to increase calories	X			2 kcal/mL
Polycose powder (glucose corn polymer)	Added to supplements and formulas or foods to increase calories	X			23 kcal/tbsp
Duocal powder (SHS Ltd, Rockville, MD, USA) (corn syrup solids; vegetable, corn, coconut oil)	Added to supplements and formulas or foods to increase calories	X		X	42 kcal/tbsp
Promod powder (whey protein)	Added to oral supplements, enteral tube feedings, or food to increase protein		X		28 kcal/scoop; 5 g protein/scoop
Additions (must be mixed with hot food) (corn syrup solids, whey protein isolate, canola oil, soy lecithin)	Added to foods to increase calories and protein	X	X	X	43 kcal/tbsp; 2.5 g protein/tbsp
MCT oil (fractionated coconut oil)	Added to formulas or tube feedings to increase calories; often used for fat malabsorption disorders; does not contain essential fatty acids			X	7.7 kcal/mL
Microlipids (safflower oil)	Added to formulas or tube feedings to increase calories; also used in treatment or prevention of fatty acid deficiencies; contains essential fatty acids			X	4.5 kcal/mL
Vegetable oil (canola, corn, soybean, safflower, or sunflower)	Added to formulas and foods to increase calories			X	8.3 kcal/mL
Margarine, butter (long-chain triglycerides)	Added to foods to increase calories			X	102 kcal/tbsp

MCT = medium-chain triglyceride.

TABLE 75.5-3   DIETARY REFERENCE INTAKES:
                  RECOMMENDED INTAKES FOR
                  INDIVIDUALS FOR MACRONUTRIENTS

AGE GROUP	CARBOHYDRATE (g/d), AI OR RDA	FAT (g/d), AI	PROTEIN (g/d), AI OR RDA
Infants			
0–6 mo	60 (AI)	31	9.1 (AI)
7–12 mo	95 (AI)	30	13.5 (RDA)
Children			
1–3 yr	130 (RDA)	ND	13 (RDA)
4–8 yr	130 (RDA)	ND	19 (RDA)
Males			
9–13 yr	130 (RDA)	ND	34 (RDA)
14–18 yr	130 (RDA)	ND	52 (RDA)
19–30 yr	130 (RDA)	ND	56 (RDA)
Females			
9–13 yr	130 (RDA)	ND	34 (RDA)
14–18 yr	130 (RDA)	ND	46 (RDA)
19–30 yr	130 (RDA)	ND	46 (RDA)

Adapted from Institute of Medicine.[5]
AI = Adequate Intake; ND = not determinable; RDA = Recommended Dietary
Allowance.

servings is adjusted in relation to a child's growth and energy needs.

There are other clinical disorders in which digestion or absorption of carbohydrate is altered, resulting in carbohydrate intolerance. These can be seen in children with transient lactase deficiency owing to mucosal damage from an acute viral illness and newly diagnosed patients with celiac disease with villous atrophy and congenital/genetic disorders (eg, sucrase-isomaltase deficiency, alactasia, and glucose-galactose malabsorption). In addition, some metabolic disorders of carbohydrate metabolism such as aldolase-B deficiency, fructose 1-6-diphosphatase deficiency, and galactosemia require the elimination of certain carbohydrates. Table 75.5-5 lists selected enteral products that have been developed to accommodate these dietary restrictions.

Humans cannot digest and absorb many plant carbohydrates. The DRIs define fiber as the nondigestible carbohydrate and lignin components from the plant cell wall that are composed of soluble and insoluble fiber. This includes fiber contained in oat and wheat bran. Soluble fiber is fermented by colonic bacteria and converted into short-chain fatty acids that are subsequently absorbed by the colon. In this process, fructo-oligosaccharides (FOSs) are formed and promote the growth of probiotic bacteria. FOSs have been shown to be beneficial in inflammatory bowel disease (IBD). Functional fiber is the dietary fiber that has potential beneficial physiologic effects and includes FOS, pectins, and gums.[5]

The potential health benefits of certain dietary fibers include a role in the management of diabetes by delaying glucose uptake and reducing the insulin response. In addition, certain dietary and functional fibers may have a protective effect against coronary heart disease by decreasing serum cholesterol levels. Fiber also delays gastric emptying, which may play a key role in weight control by increasing satiety.[8–10] In children, the consumption of fiber is important to prevent constipation, which accounts for 25% of pediatric gastroenterology office visits.[11] The 2002

DRIs provide the first recommendation for dietary fiber intake and refer to total fiber (sum of dietary fiber and functional fiber) (Table 75.5-6). These recommendations were generated in response to evidence that shows an increased risk for heart disease when low-fiber diets are consumed.

PROTEIN

Protein intake should constitute 5 to 35% of total daily calories (see Tables 75.5-3 and 75.5-4). Protein requirements are altered in many pediatric illnesses. Inborn errors of amino acid metabolism require that certain dietary proteins be restricted to minimize exposure to indicated amino acids. Care must be taken in these conditions to ensure an adequate energy and total protein energy intake to support normal rates of growth. Examples include phenylketonuria, maple syrup urine disease, propionic acidemia, and methylmalonic acidemia. Table 75.5-5 lists selected enteral products that have been developed to accommodate these dietary restrictions.

In chronic renal failure not requiring dialysis, the DRI for protein should be provided to ensure adequate growth. No data exist to show that protein restriction below the DRI delays the progression of renal disease. Restricting dietary phosphorus also leads to protein restriction. For those children undergoing dialysis, it is important to supply adequate amounts of protein to compensate for protein lost in the dialysate.

Protein requirements are increased in the pediatric patient with burn injury owing to an accelerated breakdown of tissue and from protein losses from the wound before skin grafting. Failure to meet protein requirements can decrease wound healing and increase the risk for infection.

Selected amino acids may become conditionally essential during periods of rapid growth and serious illness (trauma, severe infection, and cancer). This occurs because synthetic rates do not adequately increase during periods of increased requirements. Arginine is a precursor of nitric oxide, and it modulates hepatic protein synthesis, mediates the vasodilatory effects of the endotoxins, and reduces tumor and bacterial growth.[12] Enteral arginine supplementation has been shown to be most beneficial in adult postoperative, critically ill, and trauma patients.

TABLE 75.5-4   DISTRIBUTION RANGES FOR
                  MACRONUTRIENT INTAKE

MACRONUTRIENT	RANGE (PERCENT ENERGY)	
	CHILDREN, AGE 1–3 YR	CHILDREN, AGE 4–18 YR
Fat	30–40	25–35
ω-6 Polyunsaturated fatty acids (linoleic acid)	5–10	5–10
ω-3 Polyunsaturated fatty acids (linolenic acid)	0.6–1.2	0.6–1.2
Carbohydrate	45–65	45–65
Protein	5–20	10–30

Adapted from Institute of Medicine.[5]

TABLE 75.5-5   SELECTED ENTERAL PRODUCTS AND COMMON INDICATIONS

FORMULA TYPE/INDICATION	PRODUCT	< 1 YR	AGE 1–10 YR	> 10 YR
HYPOALLERGENIC				
Cow's milk protein	Nutramigen* (Mead Johnson, Evansville, IN, USA)	X		
allergy, soy protein	Neocate (SHS Ltd, Rockville, MD, USA)	X		
allergy, impaired	Neocate One Plus		X	
GI function	Elecare (Ross, Columbus, OH, USA)		X	
	Pediatric E028*(SHS Ltd, Rockville, MD, USA)			X
SEMIELEMENTAL				
Malabsorption,	Nutramigen	X		
impaired GI function,	Pregestimil (Mead Johnson, Evansville, IN, USA)	X		
cow's milk protein	Alimentum (Ross, Columbus, OH, USA)	X		
allergy	Peptamen Jr. (Nestle, Deerfield, IL, USA)		X	
	Peptamen			X
	Peptamen 1.5			X
ELEMENTAL				
Pancreatitis	Vivonex T.E.N.(Novartis, Minneapolis, MN, USA)			X
(if enteral nutrition	Tolerex (Novartis, Minneapolis, MN, USA)			X
initiated)				
Malabsorption,				
impaired GI function,	Elecare		X	
protein allergy	Neocate	X		
	Neocate One Plus		X	
	Pediatric E028			X
	Pediatric Vivonex		X	
	Tolerex			X
	Vivonex T.E.N.			X
LOW LONG-CHAIN TRIGLYCERIDES				
Chylothorax	Portagen (Mead Johnson, Evansville, IN, USA)	X	X	
	Lipisorb (Mead Johnson, Evansville, IN, USA)			X
	Vivonex T.E.N.			X
	Tolerex			X
LIVER				
Biliary atresia, alagille	Alimentum	X		
syndrome, maldigestion,	Pregestimil	X		
malabsorption	Peptamen Jr.		X	
	Peptamen			X
	Peptamen 1.5			X
RENAL				
Alterations in electrolytes	Good Start Supreme (Nestle, Deerfield, IL, USA)	X		
and protein	Suplena (Ross, Columbus, OH, USA) (predialysis)			X
	Nepro (Ross, Columbus, OH, USA) (dialysis)			X
FIBER-CONTAINING FORMULAS				
To normalize bowel	Pediasure with Fiber (Ross, Columbus, OH, USA)		X	
function	Kindercal with Fiber (Mead Johnson, Evansville, IN, USA)		X	
	Nutren Junior with Fiber (Nestle, Deerfield, IL, USA)		X	
	Nutren 1.0 with Fiber			X
	Jevity 1 Cal (Ross, Columbus, OH, USA)			X
	Ensure with Fiber (Ross, Columbus, OH, USA)			X
STANDARD FORMULAS				
	Pediasure		X	
	Kindercal		X	
	Nutren Jr.		X	
	Nutren 1.0			X
	Ensure			X
	Isosource (Novartis, Minneapolis, MN, USA)			X
SPECIALTY FORMULAS				
Acute respiratory distress	Oxepa (Ross, Columbus, OH, USA)			X
syndrome				
Carbohydrate intolerance,	Mead Johnson 3232A (Mead Johnson, Evansville, IL, USA)	X	X	X
malabsorption fat/protein,				
Carbohydrate intolerance,	Ross Carbohydrate-Free (RCF) (Ross, Columbus, OH, USA)	X	X	X
ketogenic diet	Ketocal (SHS Ltd, Rockville, MD, USA)		X	X
Phenylketonuria	Phenex-1 (Ross, Columbus, OH, USA)	0–3 yr		
	Phenex 2		> 4 yr	

(continues)

TABLE 75.5-5　　Continued

FORMULA TYPE/INDICATION	PRODUCT	AGE		
		< 1 YR	1–10 YR	> 10 YR
Maple syrup urine disease	Ketonex-1 (Ross, Columbus, OH, USA)	0–3 yr		
	Ketonex-2		> 4 yr	
Propionic acidemia	Propimex-1 (Ross, Columbus, OH, USA)	0–3 yr		
	Propimex-2		> 4 yr	
Methylmalonic acidemia	Propimex-1	0–3 yr		
	Propimex-2		> 4 yr	
Tyrosinemia	Tyrex-1 (Ross, Columbus, OH, USA)	0–3 yr		
	Tyrex-2		> 4 yr	
Galactosemia	Isomil (Ross, Columbus, OH, USA)	X		
	Prosobee (Soy) (Mead Johnson, Evansville, IL, USA)	X		
	Fortified rice milk		X	
Glycogen storage disease	Prosobee	X		
Pyruvate dehydrogenase deficiency	Ross Carbohydrate-Free (RCF) + Microlipid (Mead Johnson, Evansville, IL, USA) + Polycose (Ross, Columbus, OH, USA) or Ketocal	X	X	X
VLCAD deficiency	Portagen (Mead Johnson, Evansville, IL, USA)	X	X	X
LCAD deficiency	Provimin (Ross, Columbus, OH, USA) + MCT oil + Polycose	X	X	X
CONCENTRATED FORMULAS				
Fluid restriction, increased energy needs or volume intolerant	Nutren 1.5			X
	Peptamen 1.5			X
	Crucial 1.5 (Nestle, Deerfield, IL, USA)			X
	Nutren 2.0			X
	Nu Basics 2.0 (Nestle, Deerfield, IL, USA)			X
	Deliver 2.0 (Mead Johnson, Evansville, IL, USA)			X
	Jevity 1.2 Cal (Ross, Columbus, OH, USA)			X
	Jevity 1.5 Cal			X
	Ensure Plus			X

GI = gastrointestinal; LCAD = long-chain hydroxyacyl CoA dehydrogenase deficiency; MCT = medium-chain triglyceride; VLCAD = very-long-chain acyl-CoA dehydrogenase deficiency.

*These products are not completely hypoallergenic.

This chart does not represent a comprehensive list of enteral products but rather a listing of commonly used enteral products. Note that in some special circumstances, an adult formula (used in children > 10 years old) may be used in children < 10 years old under the close supervision of a registered dietitian. Computerized diet analysis is required in these instances to determine nutrient imbalance.

Glutamine is the most abundant nonessential amino acid and is a precursor for glutathione, and it, too, may be conditionally essential during selected clinical conditions. It has a major role as an energy source for enterocytes, colonocytes, lymphocytes, and macrophages.[13,14] It may reduce bacterial translocation in the gut, thereby reducing the risk of bacteremia and consequent mortality in adult patients with cancer undergoing chemotherapy. Glutamine supplementation has been found to be safe in premature infants,[12,15,16] to be beneficial in patients with short-bowel syndrome, to improve nitrogen balance in critically ill and postsurgical patients,[17] to preserve gastrointestinal mucosal structure,[18] and to decrease sepsis and shorten the hospital stay in some adult bone marrow transplant patients.[19] Glutamine is currently added to some specialized enteral formulas and parenteral nutrition solutions for patients with short-bowel syndrome and those undergoing bone marrow transplants. It is unstable in solution, but newer formulations of glutamine dipeptides are stable, allowing its addition to enteral products.

Taurine is essential for the conjugation of bile acids early in infancy, especially in small premature infants. It is added to infant formulas at concentrations similar to those in breast milk and at higher levels in premature infant formulas. Carnitine is important for intracellular fatty acid oxidation and energy production. It is a nonessential amino acid but may become conditionally essential when requirements increase. Carnitine has been used in the treatment of various genetic defects in organic and fatty acid metabolism in pharmacologic doses. Nucleotides are important during periods of metabolic stress and rapid growth. Beneficial effects on the immune system have been observed,[20] and infant formulas are now supplemented with nucleotides at concentrations seen in human milk.

FAT

It is recommended that 20 to 40% of total daily calories come from dietary fat (see Tables 75.5-3 and 75.5-4). Certain inborn errors in fatty acid oxidation require restriction of dietary fats. Deficiency of the essential fatty acids linoleic and linolenic acids results when adequate long-chain fat is not provided in the diet. Table 75.5-5 lists selected enteral products that have been developed to accommodate these dietary restrictions. Recently, there has been an increased interest in two fatty acids that occur naturally in breast milk. Docosahexaenoic acid (fish and organ meat) and arachidonic acid (meat, eggs, and milk) are ω-3 and ω-6 polyunsaturated fatty acids that are important constituents of the brain and the

TABLE 75.5-6   DIETARY REFERENCE INTAKES:
RECOMMENDED INTAKES
FOR TOTAL FIBER

AGE GROUP	AVERAGE INTAKE (AI) TOTAL FIBER (g/d)
Children	
0–6 mo	ND
7–12 mo	ND
1–3 yr	19
4–8 yr	25
Males	
9–13 yr	31
14–18 yr	38
19–30 yr	38
Females	
9–13 yr	26
14–18 yr	26
19–30 yrs	25

Adapted from Institute of Medicine.[5]
AI = Adequate Intake; ND = not determinable. AI based on 14 g total fiber/1,000 kcal and average kcal intake for age range; decrease fiber goal if kcal intake is less than amount recommended for age.

retina. Arachidonic acid is essential for growth and functions as a precursor for eicosanoids. Several infant formulas are now supplemented with docosahexaenoic acid and arachidonic acid.

Essential fatty acid deficiency (EFAD) occurs in patients receiving long-term parenteral nutrition without adequate intravenous fat, with prolonged fasting, or with extended use of a formula predominantly containing medium-chain fats. In addition, EFAD may occur in patients who have fat malabsorption. Signs of EFAD include poor growth, thrombocytopenia, and rough, scaly skin. EFAD is commonly diagnosed by a serum triene-to-tetraene ratio of greater than 0.4. Fatty acids are precursors of prostaglandins and leukotrienes. The ω-3 fatty acids have been shown to affect the clinical course of patients with IBD, rheumatoid arthritis, cardiovascular disease, and respiratory distress syndrome.[21–24]

Medium-chain triglycerides (MCTs) are found in coconut oil and contain fatty acids with a chain length of 6 to 12 carbons. MCTs are absorbed directly into the portal system and do not require bile salts for absorption. Typical diets do not contain large amounts of MCTs; however, they are often used as an energy source and as a component of specialized diets for patients with fat malabsorption or pancreatic insufficiency.

MICRONUTRIENTS

Supplemental vitamin and mineral use is increasing,[25,26] and there is much interest in the role of the antioxidants (vitamins A, E, and C; selenium; and β-carotene) for disease prevention. Additionally, there is evidence to support increased use of specific vitamins and minerals in specific disease states. Examples include conditions in which deficiencies exist owing to malabsorption, as seen in patients with cystic fibrosis and cholestatic liver disease who need fat-soluble vitamin supplementation. Certain micronutrients are required as cofactors for enzyme reactions in a variety of metabolic disorders, such as the role of thiamine in Kearns-Sayre syndrome.[24] Supplemental micronutrients may also be required to counterbalance the depletion caused by medications, for example, folic acid and sulfasalazine in patients with IBD. Enhanced outcomes in certain disease states can also be related to supplemental micronutrients such as vitamin A supplementation of extremely low birth weight infants with bronchopulmonary dysplasia[27] and to treat ichthyosis and psoriasis.[28] The general public is using supplements in variable dose ranges without medical supervision, and the US Food and Drug Administration does not regulate these products. Serious adverse side effects have been reported with the use of these dietary supplements.[29]

Evidence is accumulating to support the use of specific micronutrients in the prevention and treatment of adult chronic disease. Many of these diseases, especially atherosclerotic cardiovascular disease and osteoporosis, begin in childhood. This leads to consideration of whether prevention measures should be initiated in children. The Dietary Guidelines for Americans recommend consuming a balanced diet and five servings of fruits and vegetables a day to provide sufficient levels of micronutrients.[30] Further research is required to evaluate whether dietary modifications in children may help prevent the development of adult chronic diseases.

The following examples help illustrate how certain micronutrients have been used to treat and prevent diseases. Vitamin E has been shown to decrease atherosclerotic heart disease[31] and lung cancer.[32] Riboflavin has been used to decrease migraine headaches.[33] Patients with infantile lactic acidosis, skeletal myopathy, and Leigh disease can improve following riboflavin administration.[34] Nicotinic acid is used to treat atherosclerotic heart disease.[35] The benefits of folic acid are seen not only in megaloblastic anemia but also in pregnancy, in which a decrease in spontaneous abortion is noted. Periconceptional folate decreases birth defects, especially neural tube defects. Public health policy worldwide recommends that women in the childbearing age group should be supplemented with folate.[36] Folate supplementation also reduces homocysteine levels, and trials are under way to see if this effect will reduce cardiovascular disease risk.[37] Folate has been shown to be effective in the prevention of certain types of cancer.[38] In the United States, grains intended for processed foods are fortified with folate.

Glucose tolerance has been shown to improve with the use of chromium. This effect is due to improved efficiency of insulin and improved blood lipid profiles. Adult subjects with some degree of impaired glucose tolerance were more responsive to the effects of chromium, and no effect was seen in those with normal glucose tolerance. Improved glucose control was also seen in patients with diabetes mellitus.[39] Zinc supplementation has been used in diarrhea and pneumonia prevention.[40] Beneficial effects of zinc supplementation are also seen in growth, neuropsychological performance, fetal growth, and birth outcomes.[13] The benefits of iron supplementation in infants and children with iron deficiency anemia are well known, with improvement in work capacity, behavior and cognitive function, body temperature regulation, immunity, and resistance to infections.[41] The use of calcium and vitamins in osteoporosis prevention is discussed later in the chapter.

Evidence suggests that antioxidant levels are decreased in chronic disease.[42,43] Oxidative stress that occurs in chronic inflammation leads to increased requirements of antioxidant vitamins and consequent depletion, resulting in a relative deficiency state. Vitamin A, β-carotene, and vitamin C are added to specialty formulas (for trauma, critical care, and IBD) to enhance healing and reduce inflammation.

Transforming growth factor-β_2 is a cytokine that is present in human milk and gut epithelial cells. It has anti-inflammatory effects, reduces epithelial permeability, and regulates cellular growth. It has been added to formulas used to treat children with IBD, with preliminary reports suggesting improved mucosal healing.[44–46]

COMPLEMENTARY AND ALTERNATIVE MEDICINE

Complementary and alternative medicine (CAM) covers a broad range of healing philosophies and therapies that are not commonly part of mainstream Western (conventional) medicine. This includes diet-based therapies that often employ herbal and botanical supplements. Concerns about the use of CAM in pediatric health care relate to the potential of CAM products to adversely influence growth and development. Limited efficacy and safety information is available. Dosing information for body size and herb–drug interaction is also unavailable.

CAM use in pediatric patients with IBD has been reviewed.[47] It was noted that 50% of patients used CAM therapies, which included nutritional supplements (43%), special diets (22%), alternative health systems (8%), and herb medicines (5%). No association was seen with a history of previous surgery and hospitalizations. Higher use was noted among patients receiving immunomodulatory therapy, suggesting that patients who are more ill may be more likely to seek adjunctive therapies. In an international CAM study, in patients with IBD, 41% used CAM (megavitamin therapy in 19%, dietary supplements in 17%, and herbal medicine in 14%). The reasons for CAM use included a history of previous side effects from conventional medications, hope for a cure, and prescribed medications not working as well as anticipated. Additionally, 59% of respondents not taking CAM were interested in learning about it, suggesting that patients with chronic illness are interested in CAM.[48]

The use of herbal compounds is increasing in pediatric and adolescent patients,[49] with limited scientific data to guide this use. Epogam (Scotia Pharmaceuticals Ltd, Auckland, Australia) evening primrose oil treatment was evaluated in pediatric patients with atopic dermatitis and asthma. Increased plasma essential fatty acid levels and significant improvement were seen with eczema symptoms in the subjects who received primrose oil, but no differences were seen between the control and treatment groups with reactive airways disease.[50] Certain oils (evening primrose,

borage, and black currant) have anti-inflammatory effects and have been used in rheumatoid arthritis. The active ingredient is γ-linolenic acid (18:3, ω-6), which is anti-inflammatory and immune regulating.[51,52] Trials of probiotics and fish oil in adult patients with IBD have suggested potential efficacy, but similar studies have yet to be done in children.

Probiotics are recognized as being beneficial in normal health (maintaining a healthy gastrointestinal ecosystem) and for immune modulation and disease prevention.[53,54] Probiotics help control gastrointestinal inflammation, normalize mucosal function, and down-regulate hypersensitivity reactions. They have been used for the treatment of infectious diarrhea, IBD, radiation-induced diarrhea, traveler's diarrhea, antibiotic-associated diarrhea, *Helicobacter pylori* infection, and food allergy, with varying success.[55,56] There are several proposed mechanisms of action. These include stimulation of the immune response to pathogens, competition for nutrients required for the growth of pathogens, synthesis of compounds that inhibit or destroy pathogens, competitive inhibition of bacterial adhesion, normalizing intestinal permeability, altering gut flora, decreasing intestinal inflammatory responses, and controlling the balance between pro- and anti-inflammatory cytokines. *Lactobacillus acidophilus*, *Lactobacillus* GG, *Lactobacillus planatarum* 299V, *Bifidobacterium bifidum*, *Bifidobacterium longum*, *Streptococcus thermophilus*, *Enterococcus faecium* SF68, and *Saccharomyces boulardii* are among the probiotics that have been studied.[13,57]

Prebiotic compounds (FOS) support the growth of probiotic organisms and are found in foods (eg, onions, artichokes, and bananas). They are not digested in the small bowel and pass into the colon, where they are metabolized into short-chain fatty acids, promote sodium and water absorption, and serve as an energy source for colonocytes. Their use has been studied in constipation, irritable bowel syndrome, and lipid metabolism and necrotizing enterocolitis.[58,59] They have a low cariogenic potential, improve lipid metabolism, protect against colorectal cancer and infectious colitis, increase the bioavailability of calcium and magnesium, and may enhance host defenses.[60–62] Fructans (inulin and oligofructose) and soybean oligosaccharides are among the prebiotics that have been added to foods.[63,64] In both human and animal studies, beneficial effects have also been seen in calcium, magnesium, zinc, and iron nutriture.[65,66]

BONE HEALTH

Bone tissue is continuously being laid down during infancy, childhood, and adolescence, so disease processes that affect the normal pattern of bone accretion will affect ultimate bone health. Peak bone mass (PBM) is the maximum amount of bone mineral that is achieved during the life cycle in all bones in the body. It determines bone health later on in life, and it has been noted that 90% of PBM is achieved by 18 years of age.[67,68] Childhood and adolescence are crucial periods for bone health, not only for healthy children but also for those with chronic disease. Factors adversely affecting bone development include poor weight and height gain, delayed puberty, immobilization, reduced weight-bearing activity, malnutrition, insufficient calcium intake, vitamin D deficiency, inflammatory conditions, high levels of circulating cytokines, and corticosteroid use.[69]

Bone disease is often suspected when a radiograph is obtained for an unrelated reason and is reported to be "osteopenic." Plain films should not be used to screen for bone disease because these radiographic changes represent a late effect. Indeed, bone disease should be suspected long before a radiograph shows "washed out" bones. In instances in which bone disease is suspected, a DXA assessment should be conducted. This is a safe test, with approximately only one-twentieth of the radiation of a chest radiograph and less radiation than a transcontinental airplane flight. The results are expressed in terms of bone mineral content in grams and bone mineral density (BMD) in g/cm^2. New technology allows for quick scanning of the patient. In children and adolescents, lumbar spine and whole-body scans are obtained. Sufficient normative data using the current technology do not exist for infants and children less than 4 years of age. Reference data are available for lumbar spine scans, and the results are expressed in terms of standard deviation or z-scores. Normative data do not exist for whole-body scans. DXA also evaluates body composition as fat and lean body mass. The use of DXA for body composition analysis has been validated, and DXA is an accepted modality to determine body composition.[70–73]

Although a valuable diagnostic tool, DXA does have some drawbacks. Interpretation of scans is sometimes difficult, especially if there is delayed growth and a significant difference between chronologic age and height age. This is especially true in the patient with delayed pubertal development. Additionally, the reference data for the lumbar spine scans are based on relatively small numbers of subjects. Studies are in progress to combine data sets, collect additional data, and thus improve the reference standards. DXA has clinical value in many disease states. There may be difficulty interpreting the DXA scan in the clinical setting of delayed puberty and growth. In these cases following BMD over time, taking into account that increases in BMD may just be due to maturation and growth and not necessarily due to therapy is important.

Therapy for bone disease is limited in pediatric patients. Important therapeutic options include (1) improving nutritional status and normalizing weight and height; (2) controlling the underlying chronic disease and decreasing inflammation and malabsorption; (3) ensuring adequate or therapeutic intake (diet and/or supplements) of calcium, vitamin D, magnesium, and vitamin K and monitoring levels as indicated; (4) monitoring pubertal status and optimizing pubertal development; and (5) increasing weight-bearing physical activity as appropriate. Those pediatric patients with significantly abnormal BMD and those with increased fracture risks should be prescribed noncontact, weight-bearing physical activity. There are limited data regarding intervention studies using the antiresorptive medications commonly used in adults, and routine use in pediatric patients is not advised at this time.

Osteopenia[74,75] and vertebral compression fractures[76] have been shown in children with IBD. Possible reasons for the osteopenia include malnutrition, poor dietary intake, malabsorption, inflammation, and elevated cytokine levels.[77] Medications can also affect BMD, for example, glucocorticoids and immunosuppressives, which are frequently used in children and adolescents with more severe forms of the disease.[74,75,78] Although lower BMD z-scores have been noted, once these results have been adjusted for bone age, the difference between control subjects and patients is less.[79] Similarly, bone disease has been noted in patients with chronic liver disease.[80] Possible factors include malnutrition, micronutrient deficiency, and malabsorption of vitamins D and K.[81,82] Despite normalizing vitamin D levels, some patients still persist in having bone disease.[83] Bone disease has also been noted in patients following liver transplant, but in children, improvement in BMD frequently occurs.[84–86] Bone disease is also seen in patients with celiac disease.[87] A gluten-free diet may result in some improvement in BMD.[88–90]

CONCLUSION

Nutritional therapy is important in the treatment and prevention of many disorders. This chapter has attempted to provide guidelines for nutritional therapy in selected pediatric disorders and to illustrate how the manipulation of macronutrients and micronutrients can be used in disease treatment and rehabilitation. There is an increase in the use of CAM in the United States, and many pediatric patients, including those with gastrointestinal diseases, are using CAM. Familiarity with these modalities and an open climate for discussion with patients are key to optimal patient care. The foundation for healthy bones is laid down in childhood and adolescence. Attention must be paid to the prevention and treatment of bone disease in those patients with chronic gastrointestinal disease.

REFERENCES

1. Hendricks KM, Duggan C, Gallagher L, et al. Malnutrition in hospitalized pediatric patients. Current prevalence. Arch Pediatr Adolesc Med 1995;149:1118–22.
2. Merritt RJ, Suskind RM. Nutritional survey of hospitalized pediatric patients. Am J Clin Nutr 1979;32:1320–5.
3. Roche AF, Mukherjee D, Guo S, Moore WM. Head circumference reference data: birth to 18 years. Pediatrics 1987;79:706–12.
4. Maka DA, Murphy LK. Drug-nutrient interactions: a review. AACN Clin Issues 2000;11:580–9.
5. Institute of Medicine. Dietary Reference Intakes for energy, carbohydrates, fiber, fat, fatty acids, cholesterol, protein and amino acids. Washington (DC): National Academies Press; 2002.
6. Zemel BS, Jawad AF, FitzSimmons S, Stallings VA. Longitudinal relationship among growth, nutritional status, and pulmonary function in children with cystic fibrosis: analysis of the Cystic Fibrosis Foundation National CF Patient Registry. J Pediatr 2000;137:374–80.
7. Moukarzel AA, Najm I, Vargas J, et al. Effect of nutritional status on outcome of orthotopic liver transplantation in pediatric patients. Transplant Proc 1990;22:1560–3.

8. Roberfroid M. Dietary fiber, inulin, and oligofructose: a review comparing their physiological effects. Crit Rev Food Sci Nutr 1993;33:103–48.

9. Low AG. Nutritional regulation of gastric secretion, digestion and emptying. Nutr Res Rev 1990;3:229–52.

10. Bergmann JF, Chassany O, Petit A, et al. Correlation between echographic gastric emptying and appetite: influence of psyllium. Gut 1992;33:1042–3.

11. Loening-Baucke V. Chronic constipation in children. Gastroenterology 1993;105:1557–64.

12. Barton RG. Immune-enhancing enteral formulas: are they beneficial in critically ill patients? Nutr Clin Pract 1997;12:51–62.

13. Duggan C, Gannon J, Walker WA. Protective nutrients and functional foods for the gastrointestinal tract. Am J Clin Nutr 2002;75:789–808.

14. Schloerb PR. Immune-enhancing diets: products, components and their rationales. JPEN J Parenter Enteral Nutr 2001;25 Suppl 2:S3–7.

15. Neu J, Roig JC, Meetze WH, et al. Enteral glutamine supplementation for very low birth weight infants decreases morbidity. J Pediatr 1997;131:691–9.

16. Lacey JM, Crouch JB, Benfell K, et al. The effects of glutamine-supplemented parenteral nutrition in premature infants. JPEN J Parenter Enteral Nutr 1996;20:74–80.

17. Vinnars E, Hammarqvist F, von der Decken A, Wernerman J. Role of glutamine and its analogs in posttraumatic muscle protein and amino acid metabolism. JPEN J Parenter Enteral Nutr 1990;14 Suppl 4:125S–29S.

18. van der Hulst RR, van Kreel KB, von Meyenfeldt MF, et al. Glutamine and the preservation of gut integrity. Lancet 1993;341:1363–5.

19. Ziegler TR, Young LS, Benfell K, et al. Clinical and metabolic efficacy of glutamine-supplemented parenteral nutrition after bone marrow transplantation. A randomized, double-blind, controlled study. Ann Intern Med 1992;116:821–8.

20. Pickering LK, Granoff DM, Erickson JR, et al. Modulation of the immune system by human milk and infant formula containing nucleotides. Pediatrics 1998;101:242–9.

21. Belluzzi A, Brignola C, Campieri M, et al. Effect of an enteric-coated fish-oil preparation on relapses in Crohn's disease. N Engl J Med 1996;334:1557–60.

22. Kremer JM, Bigauoette J, Michalek AV, et al. Effects of manipulation of dietary fatty acids on clinical manifestations of rheumatoid arthritis. Lancet 1985;i:184–7.

23. Gadek JE, DeMichele SJ, Karlstad MD, et al. Effect of enteral feeding with eicosapentaenoic acid, gamma-linolenic acid, and antioxidants in patients with acute respiratory distress syndrome. Enteral Nutrition in ARDS Study Group. Crit Care Med 1999;27:1409–20.

24. Lou HC. Correction of increased plasma pyruvate and plasma lactate levels using large doses of thiamine in patients with Kearns-Sayre syndrome. Arch Neurol 1981;38:469.

25. Eisenberg DM, Davis RB, Ettner SL, et al. Trends in alternative medicine use in the United States, 1990-1997: results of a follow-up national survey. JAMA 1998;280:1569–75.

26. Kessler RC, Davis RB, Foster DF, et al. Long-term trends in the use of complementary and alternative medical therapies in the United States. Ann Intern Med 2001;135:262–8.

27. Tyson JE, Wright LL, Oh W, et al. Vitamin A supplementation for extremely-low-birth-weight infants. National Institute of Child Health and Human Development Neonatal Research Network. N Engl J Med 1999;340:1962–8.

28. Solomons NW. Vitamin A and carotenoids. In: Bowman BA, Russell RM, editors. Present knowledge in nutrition. 8th ed. Washington (DC): ILSI Press; 2003. p. 127–45.

29. Palmer ME, Haller C, McKinney PE, et al. Adverse events associated with dietary supplements: an observational study. Lancet 2003;361:101–6.

30. Dietary Guidelines for Americans. Available at: http://www.nal.usda.gov/fnic/dga/index.html (accessed Oct 9, 2003).

31. Stephens NG, Parsons A, Schofield PM, et al. Randomised controlled trial of vitamin E in patients with coronary disease: Cambridge Heart Antioxidant Study (CHAOS). Lancet 1996;347:781–6.

32. Woodson K, Tangrea JA, Barrett MJ, et al. Serum alpha-tocopherol and subsequent risk of lung cancer among male smokers. J Natl Cancer Inst. 1999;91:1738–43.

33. Schoenen J, Jacquy J, Lenaerts M. Effectiveness of high-dose riboflavin in migraine prophylaxis. A randomized controlled trial. Neurology 1998;50:466–70.

34. Ogle RF, Christodoulou J, Fagan E, et al. Mitochondrial myopathy with tRNA(Leu(UUR)) mutation and complex I deficiency responsive to riboflavin. J Pediatr 1997;130:138–45.

35. Guyton JR. Effect of niacin on atherosclerotic cardiovascular disease. Am J Cardiol 1998;82:18U–23U.

36. Botto LD, Moore CA, Khoury MJ, Erickson JD. Neural-tube defects. N Engl J Med 1999;341:1509–19.

37. Selhub J. Homocysteine metabolism. Annu Rev Nutr 1999;19:217–46.

38. Kim YI. Folate and cancer prevention: a new medical application of folate beyond hyperhomocysteinemia and neural tube defects. Nutr Rev 1999;57:314–21.

39. Anderson RA, Cheng N, Bryden NA, et al. Elevated intakes of supplemental chromium improve glucose and insulin variables in individuals with type 2 diabetes. Diabetes 1997;46:1786–91.

40. Bhutta ZA, Black RE, Brown KH, et al. Prevention of diarrhea and pneumonia by zinc supplementation in children in developing countries: pooled analysis of randomized controlled trials. Zinc Investigators' Collaborative Group. J Pediatr 1999;135:689–97.

41. Yip R, Dallman PR. Iron. In: Bowman BA, Russell RM, editors. Present knowledge in nutrition. 8th ed. Washington (DC): ISLI Press; 2003. p. 311–28.

42. Floreani A, Baragiotta A, Martines D, et al. Plasma antioxidant levels in chronic cholestatic liver diseases. Aliment Pharmacol Ther 2000;14:353–8.

43. Wood LG, Fitzgerald DA, Gibson PG, et al. Oxidative stress in cystic fibrosis: dietary and metabolic factors. J Am Coll Nutr 2001;20(2 Suppl):157–65.

44. Cox DA, Burk RR. Isolation and characterisation of milk growth factor, a transforming-growth-factor-beta 2-related polypeptide, from bovine milk. Eur J Biochem 1991;197:353–8.

45. Donnet-Hughes A, Schiffrin EJ, Huggett AC. Expression of MHC antigens by intestinal epithelial cells. Effect of transforming growth factor-beta 2 (TGF-beta 2). Clin Exp Immunol 1995;99:240–4.

46. Fell JM, Paintin M, Arnaud-Battandier F, et al. Mucosal healing and a fall in mucosal pro-inflammatory cytokine mRNA induced by a specific oral polymeric diet in paediatric Crohn's disease. Aliment Pharmacol Ther 2000;14:281–9.

47. Markowitz JE, Culton K, Mamula P, et al. Complementary and alternative medicine use among pediatric patients with inflammatory bowel disease [abstract]. J Pediatr Gastroenterol Nutr 2002;35:409.

48. Heuschkel R, Afzal N, Wuerth A, et al. Complementary medicine use in children and young adults with inflammatory bowel disease. Am J Gastroenterol 2002;97:382–8.

49. Gardiner P, Wornham W. Recent review of complementary and alternative medicine used by adolescents. Curr Opin Pediatr 2000;12:298–302.

50. Hederos CA, Berg A. Epogam evening primrose oil treatment in atopic dermatitis and asthma. Arch Dis Child 1996;75:494–7.

51. Leventhal LJ, Boyce EG, Zurier RB. Treatment of rheumatoid arthritis with gammalinolenic acid. Ann Intern Med 1993; 119:867–73.

52. Brzeski M, Madhok R, Capell HA. Evening primrose oil in patients with rheumatoid arthritis and side-effects of non-steroidal anti-inflammatory drugs. Br J Rheumatol 1991;30:370–2.

53. Newburg DS. Oligosaccharides and glycoconjugates in human milk: their role in host defense. J Mammary Gland Biol Neoplasia 1996;1:271–83.

54. Roberfroid MB. Prebiotics: preferential substrates for specific germs? Am J Clin Nutr 2001;73(2 Suppl):406S–9S.

55. Marteau PR, de Vrese M, Cellier CJ, Schrezenmeir J. Protection from gastrointestinal diseases with the use of probiotics. Am J Clin Nutr 2001;73(2 Suppl):430S–6S.

56. Vanderhoof JA. Probiotics and intestinal inflammatory disorders in infants and children. J Pediatr Gastroenterol Nutr 2000;30 Suppl 2:S34–8.

57. Markowitz JE, Bengmark S. Probiotics in health and disease in the pediatric patient. Pediatr Clin North Am 2002;49:127–41.

58. Danan C, Huret Y, Tessedre AC, et al. Could oligosaccharide supplementation promote gut colonization with a beneficial flora in preterm infants? J Pediatr Gastroenterol Nutr 2000; 30:217–9.

59. Caplan MS, Jilling T. Neonatal necrotizing enterocolitis: possible role of probiotic supplementation. J Pediatr Gastroenterol Nutr 2000;30 Suppl 2:S18–22.

60. Grizard D, Barthomeuf C. Non-digestible oligosaccharides used as prebiotic agents: mode of production and beneficial effects on animal and human health. Reprod Nutr Dev 1999;39: 563–88.

61. Gibson GR, Beatty ER, Wang X, Cummings JH. Selective stimulation of bifidobacteria in the human colon by oligofructose and inulin. Gastroenterology 1995;108:975–82.

62. Dai D, Nanthkumar NN, Newburg DS, Walker WA. Role of oligosaccharides and glycoconjugates in intestinal host defense. J Pediatr Gastroenterol Nutr 2000;30 Suppl 2:S23–33.

63. Roberfroid MB. Concepts in functional foods: the case of inulin and oligofructose. J Nutr 1999;129:1398S–401S.

64. Gnoth MJ, Kunz C, Kinne-Saffran E, Rudloff S. Human milk oligosaccharides are minimally digested in vitro. J Nutr 2000;130:3014 –20.

65. Carabin IG, Flamm WG. Evaluation of safety of inulin and oligofructose as dietary fiber. Regul Toxicol Pharmacol 1999; 30:268–82.

66. Scholz-Ahrens KE, Schaafsma G, van den Heuvel EG, Schrezenmeir J. Effects of prebiotics on mineral metabolism. Am J Clin Nutr 2001;73(2 Suppl):459S–64S.

67. Bailey DA, McKay HA, Mirwald RL, et al. A six-year longitudinal study of the relationship of physical activity to bone mineral accrual in growing children: the University of Saskatchewan bone mineral accrual study. J Bone Miner Res 1999;14:1672–9.

68. Matkovic V, Heaney RP. Calcium balance during human growth: evidence for threshold behavior. Am J Clin Nutr 1992;55: 992–6.

69. Leonard MB, Zemel BS. Current concepts in pediatric bone disease. Pediatr Clin North Am 2002;49:143–73.

70. Fors H, Gelander L, Bjarnason R, et al. Body composition, as assessed by bioelectrical impedance spectroscopy and dual-energy x-ray absorptiometry, in a healthy paediatric population. Acta Paediatr 2002;91:755–60.

71. Fuller NJ, Wells JC, Elia M. Evaluation of a model for total body protein mass based on dual-energy x-ray absorptiometry: comparison with a reference four-component model. Br J Nutr 2001;86:45–52.

72. Treuth MS, Butte NF, Wong WW, Ellis KJ. Body composition in prepubertal girls: comparison of six methods. Int J Obes Relat Metab Disord 2001;25:1352–9.

73. Wong WW, Hergenroeder AC, Stuff JE, et al. Evaluating body fat in girls and female adolescents: advantages and disadvantages of dual-energy x-ray absorptiometry. Am J Clin Nutr 2002;76:384–9.

74. Gokhale R, Favus MJ, Karrison T, et al. Bone mineral density assessment in children with inflammatory bowel disease. Gastroenterology 1998;114:902–11.

75. Hyams JS, Wyzga N, Kreutzer DL, et al. Alterations in bone metabolism in children with inflammatory bowel disease: an in vitro study. J Pediatr Gastroenterol Nutr 1997;24:289–95.

76. Semeao EJ, Stallings VA, Peck SN, Piccoli DA. Vertebral compression fractures in pediatric patients with Crohn's disease. Gastroenterology 1997;112:1710–3.

77. Papadakis KA, Targan SR. Role of cytokines in the pathogenesis of inflammatory bowel disease. Annu Rev Med 2000;51: 289–98.

78. Semeao EJ, Jawad AF, Stouffer NO, et al. Risk factors for low bone mineral density in children and young adults with Crohn's disease. J Pediatr 1999;135:593–600.

79. Semeao EJ, Jawad AF, Zemel BS, et al. Bone mineral density in children and young adults with Crohn's disease. Inflamm Bowel Dis 1999;5:161–6.

80. Argao EA, Specker BL, Heubi JE. Bone mineral content in infants and children with chronic cholestatic liver disease. Pediatrics 1993;91:1151–4.

81. Heubi JE, Hollis BW, Specker B, Tsang RC. Bone disease in chronic childhood cholestasis. I. Vitamin D absorption and metabolism. Hepatology 1989;9:258–64.

82. Heubi JE, Hollis BW, Tsang RC. Bone disease in chronic childhood cholestasis. II. Better absorption of 25-OH vitamin D than vitamin D in extrahepatic biliary atresia. Pediatr Res 1990;27:26–31.

83. Argao EA, Heubi JE, Hollis BW, Tsang RC. d-Alpha-tocopheryl polyethylene glycol-1000 succinate enhances the absorption of vitamin D in chronic cholestatic liver disease of infancy and childhood. Pediatr Res 1992;31:146–50.

84. D'Antiga L, Moniz C, Buxton-Thomas M, et al. Bone mineral density and height gain in children with chronic cholestatic liver disease undergoing transplantation. Transplantation 2002;73:1788–93.

85. Argao EA, Balistreri WF, Hollis BW, et al. Effect of orthotopic liver transplantation on bone mineral content and serum vitamin D metabolites in infants and children with chronic cholestasis. Hepatology 1994;20:598–603.

86. Holt RI, Broide E, Buchanan CR, et al. Orthotopic liver transplantation reverses the adverse nutritional changes of end-stage liver disease in children. Am J Clin Nutr 1997;65:534–42.

87. Fickling WE, McFarlane XA, Bhalla AK, Robertson DA. The clinical impact of metabolic bone disease in coeliac disease. Postgrad Med J 2001;77:33–6.

88. Mora S, Weber G, Barera G, et al. Effect of gluten-free diet on bone mineral content in growing patients with celiac disease. Am J Clin Nutr 1993;57:224–8.

89. Kemppainen T, Kroger H, Janatuinen E, et al. Bone recovery after a gluten-free diet: a 5-year follow-up study. Bone 1999; 25:355–60.

90. Molteni N, Caraceni MP, Bardella MT, et al. Bone mineral density in adult celiac patients and the effect of gluten-free diet from childhood. Am J Gastroenterol 1990;85:51–3.

6. Protective Nutrients

Judith A. O'Connor, MD, MS

Elizabeth C. Utterson, MD

Nancy F. Krebs, MD, MS

The gastrointestinal (GI) tract is a major interface between the host and the environment. It has a dual function, acting as the portal of entry for nutrients used for cell growth and function while serving as a barrier for noxious agents. The epithelial cells and other cells of the GI mucosa rely on nutrients supplied from both the bloodstream and intestinal lumen. These nutrients serve to preserve the integrity and function of the GI mucosa. Protective nutrients or "functional foods" are terms used to describe nutrients or foods that have an effect on the physiologic function of the GI mucosa that is separate from their established nutritional functions.[1] The cells of the GI tract are capable of specific adaptive responses to ingested nutrients. Undernutrition, starvation, inflammation, and noxious agents impair intestinal adaptation and mucosal integrity. The physiologic function of the GI mucosa also varies with age, specifically the premature intestine, infantile intestine, and adult GI tract.[2] Thus, human adult clinical trials may not be relevant to infants or children. Animal studies have suggested that the presence of luminal nutrients is important to intestinal mucosal metabolism, regardless of overall nutritional status.[3,4] Human studies have often not been conclusive and suffer from uncontrolled variables. This chapter reviews the basic physiologic development of the gut and the purported effect of protective nutrients on cell function and immunity. Candidate protective nutrients reviewed include glutamine, arginine, polyunsaturated fatty acids (PUFAs), nucleotides, and zinc. The roles of prebiotics, non-nutritive ingredients in foods that foster growth of beneficial bacteria, and transforming growth factor-β (TGF-β) are briefly explored.

EFFECT OF NUTRITION OR INFLAMMATION ON GUT DEVELOPMENT AND FUNCTION

Because the GI tract undergoes postnatal maturation, the importance of protective nutrients on mucosal integrity may vary with postgestational age. The basic structure of the GI tract is the crypt-villus unit. Mucosal cells are formed at the base of the crypt and, once formed, migrate to the villus tip. During this migration, the cell functionally matures and develops a thick microvillus membrane with numerous glycoprotein enzymes.[2,5,6] These enzymes function in digestion, absorption, and antigen recognition. When the cell reaches the villus tip,

programmed cell death occurs, and the cell is extruded. Cell division requires 24 hours, whereas cell migration requires 3 to 6 days.[6] In states of malnutrition, inflammation, or toxins, there is an imbalance of cell renewal and cell death.

Malnutrition resulting from starvation results in a thinning of the mucosa and muscularis. There is a marked increase in the cell-cycle time, which decreases crypt cell proliferation or cell renewal, resulting in a shortening of both the villi and crypts.[7] As a consequence of reduced protein synthesis, there is a decrease in disaccharidase activity.[8] Additionally, decreased cellular immunity and secretory immunoglobulin A produce an environment conducive to bacterial overgrowth.[9] Bacterial overgrowth may produce mucosal injury and bile salt deconjugation, resulting in steatorrhea, diarrhea, and increased nutrient loss.[10] Many chronic disorders, such as Crohn disease, liver or renal disease, malignancy, cystic fibrosis, and celiac disease, are exacerbated by undernutrition and produce a lesion morphologically similar to marasmus.

Diseases that result in protein deficiency often cause a flat villus lesion. The mucosal thickness appears normal owing to marked elongation of the crypt.[11] This flattening results from alterations in protein metabolism, such as hypoalbuminemic protein-calorie malnutrition (kwashiorkor), or an inflammatory response to a specific protein, as in celiac disease, allergic enteropathy, or severe cow's milk or soy protein intolerance. Additionally, profound inflammation or infection may produce a similar lesion. Morphologically, there is an increase in the crypt-to-villus ratio. Physiologically, there is a reduction of the absorptive surface, resulting in a loss of disaccharidase activity and of mucosal integrity. Clinically, this is manifested as malabsorption of macro- and micronutrients.

The intestinal mucosa is highly dynamic in terms of cell renewal and response to nutrients, circulating or local hormones, and neurohumoral influences.[12] The presence of specific glycoprotein enzymes varies with gestational age, and gene expression can also be affected by diet. Expression of the disaccharidase sucrase-isomaltase is modulated by dietary source. Diets high in sucrose and fructose induce gene transcription, whereas diets low in these nutrients have a decreased enzymatic specific activity.[13] Mucosal development and integrity of the gut are dependent on numerous endogenous factors, such as thyroxine, cortisol, gastrin, enteroglucagon, pancreatic glucagon, growth hormone, and epidermal growth factor.[14] Neurohumoral influences include enteroglucagon, gastrointestinal inhibitory peptide, motilin, and neurotensin. These agents also influence gastric, pancreatic, and biliary secretion.

Human clinical trials cannot control for the various factors affecting gut development and integrity; therefore, the results of clinical studies are often difficult to interpret. Nutrients that may be advantageous in a preterm infant may have no observable advantage for children or adults. Nutrient supplements may be beneficial, harmful, or unhelpful depending on the underlying status of the GI mucosa and the specific disease. Intestinal mucosal requirements may be different in disorders resulting from intestinal inflammation or septic shock compared with requirements for recovery from massive surgical resection, ischemia, toxic injury, or physiologic stress from severe burns. Thus, published human studies evaluating protective nutrients and factors must be interpreted cautiously, and the results cannot be extrapolated to patients of different ages or disease states. Additionally, animal models used to study these factors may not be applicable for human requirements or disease states.

PROTECTIVE NUTRIENTS

Functional food ingredients and nutrients may influence intestinal growth, maturation, and adaptation. Essential nutrients are those that are required for physiologic function and cannot be endogenously synthesized. In states of immaturity or severe catabolism, intracellular stores of specific essential nutrients may become depleted and lead to deficiency, and/or existing biosynthetic pathways of normally nonessential nutrients cannot meet increased metabolic demands. These nonessential nutrients then may become "conditionally essential" and may be potentially useful ingredients in functional foods.

GLUTAMINE

Glutamine is the most abundant amino acid in the human body. It is defined as a nonessential amino acid because it can be synthesized by a wide variety of tissues rich in glutamine synthetase. Glutamine, a structural component of proteins, functions in nitrogen transfer between tissues, is a precursor in the synthesis of nucleotides, and serves as an important nutrient for renal excretion of ammonia.[15] Importantly, glutamine also serves as the substrate for production of glutathione, a crucial antioxidant found in high concentrations in the GI mucosa. Inhibition of its synthesis results in mucosa degeneration, diarrhea, and growth failure.[16,17] Animal studies suggest that GI epithelial cells are highly dependent on glutathione, and oral or intravenous administration of glutathione may be protective against toxicity associated with inflammatory disease, ischemia, oxidative damage, chemotherapy, and radiation.[18]

Glutamine is of interest as a protective nutrient because it is the major fuel source for rapidly dividing cells such as GI epithelial cells, lymphocytes, fibroblasts, and reticulocytes.[16] Although glutamine is an abundant nonessential amino acid, it has been proposed to become a conditionally essential amino acid in catabolic conditions. In severe catabolic stress, humans show an increased efflux of glutamine from skeletal muscle and hepatocytes.[18] Severely ill patients nutritionally dependent on total parenteral nutrition (TPN) are at risk for glutamine deficiency owing to the combination of increased turnover, reduced dietary intake, and absence of this amino acid in parenteral solutions. Glutamine is relatively unstable and is therefore not included in standard intravenous protein solutions.[19] Premature or very low birth weight infants are also at risk for nutritional insufficiency and catabolism. Sparse energy reserves are rapidly depleted, and enteral sufficiency is delayed owing to the immaturity of the GI tract. Additionally, full enteral feeding is often delayed owing to the risk of necrotizing enterocolitis (NEC).

Some adult human studies have shown that glutamine-supplemented TPN has significantly reduced hospital-acquired infection, decreased gut permeability to lactulose, and improved nitrogen balance and protein synthesis after bone marrow transplant.[20,21] Other studies have shown no advantage from enteral or parenteral glutamine supplementation on clinical infections after bone marrow transplant in adults[22] or children (Krebs N, et al, unpublished data, 2000). Enteral supplementation of very low birth weight infants resulted in improved tolerance to enteral feedings and a decrease in the incidence of hospital-acquired infection.[23]

Numerous animal and human studies support a benefit of supplemental glutamine on gut function, including reversal of gut atrophy associated with TPN, radio- or chemotherapy, improved immune function, and reduced episodes of bacterial translocation and sepsis.[16] Although several studies suggest that glutamine supplementation is advantageous, problems with sample size, randomization, and comparable control groups limit interpretation. For example, studies using glutamine-supplemented TPN have been designed to provide isonitrogenous amino acid solutions to patients, but different amino acid admixtures were also used to ensure adequate intake of essential amino acids without excessive nitrogen intake in the test groups. A recent review of clinical trials of glutamine supplementation highlights the challenges of conducting adequately controlled human studies.[24] Short-term studies using intravenous glutamine have generally reported no safety concerns. An exception may be with preexisting liver disease, in which case, further elevation of transaminases has been observed.[24,25] With the putative beneficial effects from controlled trials, glutamine-supplemented enteral formulas are now available (Table 75.6-1). Although glutamine supplementation in parenteral nutrition remains investigational, newer approaches using glutamine dipetides, which have better solubility and heat stability, are expected to enable the development of glutamine-enriched enteral formulas. Well-designed and -controlled trials will be necessary, however, to determine whether such formulations will benefit clinical outcomes.

TABLE 75.6-1   COMMERCIALLY AVAILABLE FORMULAS CONTAINING PROTECTIVE NUTRIENTS

FORMULA	MANUFACTURER	FORM	AMINO ACID SUPPLEMENT	OMEGA-3 PUFA
Vivonex–Pediatric Vivonex–Plus Vivonex–TEN	Novartis Nutrition	Powder	L-Glutamine + L-arginine	–
Impact–1.0/1.5 calories/cc Impact–Fiber Impact–glutamine	Novartis Nutrition	Liquid	L-Arginine	+
Impact–Recover	Novartis Nutrition	Powder	L-Glutamine + L-arginine	–
Immune-Aid	McGraw	Powder	L-Arginine + L-glutamine	–
Crucial	Nestle Nutrition	Liquid	L-Arginine	+
Internical	Mead Johnson	Liquid	L-Arginine	+
Optimental	Ross Laboratories	Liquid	L-Arginine	+
Periactive	Ross Laboratories	Liquid	L-Arginine	–
Resource–Arginade Extra	Novartis Nutrition	Liquid	L-Arginine	NA
Resource–Gluta Solve	Novartis Nutrition	Powder	L-Glutamine	NA
Ristope-X	Cambridge Neutraceuticals	Powder	L-Glutamine + L-arginine + N-acetylcysteine	NA

NA = not added; PUFA = polyunsaturated fatty acid.

ARGININE

Arginine is a nonessential amino acid important in the transport, storage, and excretion of nitrogen. Similar to glutamine, arginine has been postulated to be a conditionally essential amino acid under conditions of catabolic stress.[26] The importance of arginine as a protective nutrient is related to its role as a precursor of nitric oxide (NO). Arginine is converted to NO via a family of enzymes, the nitric oxide synthases (NOSs). There are two identified forms of NOS: the constitutive form (cNOS) and the inducible form (iNOS). Calcium and calmodulin activate cNOS, whereas iNOS is calcium independent. cNOS produces small amounts of NO, which acts as a biologic mediator previously referred to as endothelium-derived relaxing factor. NO derived from vascular endothelium plays an important role in maintaining baseline vasodilator tone. NO derived from cNOS is secreted from peripheral nonadrenergic-noncholinergic neurons mediating neurogenic vasodilatation and regulating various GI, respiratory, and genitourinary tract functions.[27] Compared with cNOS, iNOS is found in a wide variety of cells, including macrophages, neutrophils, mast cells, fibroblasts, hepatocytes, vascular endothelial cells, smooth muscle cells, and cardiac myocytes. Inflammatory cytokines and bacterial endotoxins induce iNOS, whereas glucocorticoids inhibit the induction of iNOS but have no effect on the activity of either the constitutive or the inducible enzyme.

The role of arginine and NO and its relation to immunity and inflammation have been studied in various animal models. Animals supplemented with arginine have higher thymic weight and thymic lymphocyte counts and improved wound healing.[28,29] Tumor-bearing rat models have decreased tumor protein synthesis with improved whole-body protein synthesis. Intestinal integrity was improved with arginine supplementation in rodents subjected to intestinal ischemia, radiation, resection, or transplant.[16] Additionally, bacterial translocation was decreased in rats recovering from radiation enteritis receiving supplemental arginine.[26]

Inflammatory bowel disease (IBD) and neonatal NEC are examples of two human disease states marked by inflammation and increased intestinal permeability. The role of iNOS in adult chronic IBD has been investigated using surgically resected intestine obtained from patients suffering from active ulcerative or Crohn colitis. When compared with intestine resected from adults for other reasons, there was a marked increase in iNOS expression in patients with colitis compared with control specimens.[30] Low levels of serum arginine[31] and glutamine have been demonstrated in premature infants prior to and during an episode of NEC. Using a hypoxia-reoxygenation–induced NEC model in young mice, supplemental arginine or carnitine greatly attenuated hypoxia-induced tissue damage.[32] In a recent prospective double-blind randomized placebo-controlled arginine supplementation trial, 152 premature infants were followed for 28 days. There was a significantly lower incidence of NEC in the arginine-supplemented group. Serum arginine levels decreased in all infants who developed NEC; however, they were significantly higher in the supplemented group than in the control group.[33] Although NEC resembles IBD microscopically, the histopathologic response may result from different mechanisms. Additionally, the apparent protective role of arginine in NEC may not be related to NO production but to other functions of arginine, such as the production of glutamine, nucleotides, and polyamines. Thus, the role of NO and its production from cNOS or iNOS is not completely defined because it appears that NO has both anti- and proinflammatory effects.

Human clinical trials have evaluated arginine supplementation in healthy adults and healthy adult surgical patients. Dietary supplementation in these patients increased lymphocytic immune response and increased exhaled NO.[34] Many clinical trials using arginine supplementation in adult patients at risk of intestinal stress because of trauma, cancer, or critical illnesses have been reported.[16] It is difficult to compare results owing to the variety of other nutrients supplied in these so-called "immune-enhancing" formulations. Two meta-analyses comparing commercially available formulas have been published. An analysis of 12 trials with a total of 1,557 patients[35] and 22 trials among 2,419 patients[36] showed a decrease in the length of hospitalization, duration of ventilator support, and lower overall infection rates in patients receiving an arginine-supplemented diet. The effect on mortality was not clear. In planned subgroup analysis, patients who were undergoing elective surgery benefited more than did critically ill patients. These studies suggest that the use of arginine-supplemented formulas may be beneficial for discreet patient conditions such as surgical or cancer patients. Further studies are needed to ensure that there is no detrimental effect from such formulas in septic patients or solid organ transplant recipients. Although several supplemented formulas designed to enhance immune function are commercially available (see Table 75.6-1), indiscriminate use of these formulas is not justified.

LONG-CHAIN PUFAS

Long-chain PUFAs are essential for membrane structure, fluidity, and function, specifically in neural and retinal tissues. PUFAs are precursors for the production of prostaglandins, prostacyclins, thromboxanes, and leukotrienes. PUFAs are divided into two broad classes: ω-3 and ω-6 fatty acids. Omega-3 fatty acids are represented by α-linolenic acid (ALA), whereas ω-6 fatty acids are represented by linoleic acid. This nomenclature refers to the location of the first double bond from the methyl terminus. Mammals are unable to insert double bonds into fatty acid molecules closer than the 9 position and thus are dependent on dietary consumption of these essential fatty acids (EFAs). Linoleic acid is found abundantly in the seeds of most plants and is especially high in corn, safflower, and soy oils but is present in only limited amounts in coconut, cocoa, and palm oils. ALA is found in soy and canola oils, as well as marine plants, algae, and phytoplankton. ALA is transformed in the marine food chain, and its derivatives are present in large quantities in some fish oils. Omega-6 fatty acids are the most abundant PUFAs in the Western diet. It is estimated that over the last 100 years, the ratio of consumption between ω-6 and ω-3 PUFAs has changed from 1 to 20:1. This change is associated with the increased use of vegetable oil and changes in agriculture practices. Domestic beef are fed grain rich in ω-6 fatty acids, and modern aquaculture produces fish that contain less ω-3 fatty acids than fish grown in the wild.[37]

Animal cells modify these EFAs into long-chain PUFAs by elongation, desaturation, and β-oxidation. Linoleic acid is modified to arachidonic acid (AA). ALA is modified to eicosapentaenoic acid (EPA) and docosahexaenoic acid (DHA). Premature infants may be limited in their ability to make EPA and DHA from ALA,[38] although quantitative data are very limited. Importantly, ω-6 long-chain PUFA derivatives induce a stronger inflammatory response than ω-3 fatty acid derivatives.

The nutritional importance of specific fatty acids was first reported in weanling rats fed a fat-free diet. These animals developed scaly skin, tail necrosis, impaired fertility and growth retardation, which was reversed or prevented with the addition of either linoleic acid or ALA to their diet.[39] EFAs were initially considered of marginal importance for humans. Infants fed either a fat-free milk–based formula or lipid-free parenteral nutrition developed growth failure and dry thickened skin, which was primarily associated with linoleic acid. ALA deficiency resulted in more subtle clinical symptoms affecting neurodevelopment, visual function, and a peripheral neuropathy.[40]

EFA concentrations in breast milk vary with diet. In breast milk from women in most Western countries, the ratio of AA to DHA is 2:1, whereas in women in Asian or fish-eating communities, the ratio is 1:1 or lower.[37] Determination of the optimal ratio of EFAs awaits further studies. Although the addition of PUFAs to commercially available formulas (Table 75.6-2) may better mimic human breast milk and increase measured fatty acids in plasma and erythrocyte membrane phospholipids, the long-term functional significance of these findings is presently unclear.

Laboratory studies on animal models and clinical trials in human adults suffering from IBD have investigated the immunomodulatory effects of ω-3 PUFAs. The conflicting results in reducing inflammation, prolonging remission, or decreasing steroid requirements are likely due to the multifactorial nature of the disease and the complexity of the immune system.[38] Clinical studies vary in the disease type (Crohn disease or ulcerative colitis), disease location and activity, and the composition and dose of fatty acids supplied. The role of ω-3 fatty acids for the treatment of IBD has yet to be defined.

The role of PUFAs as a protective nutrient in NEC has been investigated in a hypoxia-induced mouse model of NEC. Mice fed a diet deficient in ω-3 fatty acids developed more severe ischemia and had increased levels of platelet activating factor and leukotriene B_4 than did control animals.[41] In a human clinical trial, preterm infants were fed a diet supplemented with egg phospholipids, which contain increased levels of esterified choline, AA, and DHA. When compared with infants fed a nonsupplemented formula, there was significantly less stage II and III NEC.[42] The advantages of routine supplementation for gastrointestinal protection are not clearly defined for preterm and term infants. Special conditions such as NEC and IBD warrant further carefully designed studies.

TABLE 75.6-2   PEDIATRIC FORMULAS CONTAINING POLYUNSATURATED FATTY ACIDS VERSUS HUMAN MILK*

POLYUNSATURATED FATTY ACID	HUMAN MILK	ENFAMIL LIPIL	SIMILAC ADVANCE	PREMATURE ENFAMIL LIPIL
Docosahexaenoic acid	0.15–0.3	0.32	0.15	0.33
Arachidonic acid	0.5–0.6	0.64	0.40	0.67

*Numbers represent percentage of fatty acid content.

NUCLEOTIDES

Nucleotides are nonprotein nitrogen compounds composed of a nitrogenous base, a pentose sugar, and one or more phosphate groups. Nucleotides serve as nucleic acid precursors, physiologic mediators, components of coenzymes, and sources of cellular energy and participate in immunity. Nucleotides can be synthesized de novo, but the process is metabolically costly. An alternative mechanism is the salvage pathway, where preformed nitrogen bases or nucleosides are converted to nucleotides. Nucleotides have been postulated to be conditionally essential during severe malnutrition, rapid cellular growth, or severe disease states. Therefore, nucleotides may also be conditionally essential in conditions such as prematurity, small for gestational age infants, severe diarrhea, short-gut syndrome, NEC, intestinal transplant, or IBD.

Much of the interest in nucleotides arose from the observation that the nucleotide content of human breast milk is significantly higher than that of cow's milk protein formulas. The nonprotein nitrogen content of human milk is approximately 25 to 30% of the total nitrogen content. Nucleotides comprise 2 to 5% of the nonprotein nitrogen. In contrast, nonprotein nitrogen accounts for only 2% of the nitrogen content of cow's milk.[43] Additionally, the nucleotide profile differs in cow's milk compared with human milk, with a lower proportion of cytidine and adenosine derivatives in cow's milk.

Beneficial effects of dietary nucleotides have been demonstrated in several animal models. Dietary nucleotides have been associated with increased mucosal deoxyribonucleic acid (DNA), protein synthesis, villus height, enterocyte proliferation and maturation, and reduced bacterial translocation during recovery from malnutrition.[44–46] Dietary nucleotides promote healing of small bowel ulcers in experimental ulcerative ileitis, decrease the inflammatory response to ischemia and reperfusion, and improve morphologic development of small intestinal mucosa after transplant.[47–49]

The beneficial effects of supplemental dietary nucleotides in humans are less certain. Initial reports suggested that infants fed a nucleotide-supplemented formula (NSF) had an increase in stool bifidobacteria and enterobacteria that mimicked human milk–fed infant stool microflora.[50] In contrast, a more recent study reported that infants fed NSF had reduced amounts of bifidobacteria and enterococci and increased amounts of Bacteroides and Escherichia coli when compared with human milk–fed infants.[51] Increased postprandial mesenteric artery blood flow has been demonstrated in both term and preterm infants following NSF formula compared with either human milk–fed or nonsupplemented formula-fed infants.[52] Infants fed NSF had an increased antibody response to Haemophilus influenzae type b and diphtheria but not to tetanus or oral polio vaccine.[53]

NSF first became available in Japan in 1965 and in the United States in 1989.[53] Currently, most infant formulas contain supplemental nucleotides. To date, no deleterious effects have been reported. The European Commission's Scientific Committee for Food has provided several published guidelines for nucleotide supplementation suggesting that the total nucleotide concentration should be less than 1.2 mg/100 J, which is the same order of magnitude as the free nucleotides in human milk. The latest recommendations from the United States suggest a maximum of 5 mg/100 J for term infant formula and 7 mg/100 J for preterm infant formula.[54] Human milk is considered to be the gold standard for infant nutrition. Thus, the rationale for nucleotide supplementation of infant formula is to mimic the composition of human milk. Because the role of human milk nucleotides for breastfed infants is not known, the indications for nucleotide supplementation of infant formula and the optimal amounts remain somewhat controversial.[55]

ZINC

As an essential trace element, zinc is second only to iron in its abundance in the human body and has a very broad range of functions. For example, approximately 80% of total-body iron in the human is localized to the erythrocyte mass alone, whereas similar total amounts of zinc are spread among thousands of proteins.[56] Zinc functions as a cofactor to more than 100 metalloenzymes involved in DNA synthesis and repair, cellular integrity, bone and liver metabolism, and multiple dehydrogenase and carboxypeptidase reactions.[57] As a component of the zinc finger transcription factors, zinc is critical to both transcription and regulation of gene expression and to cell differentiation and proliferation in rapidly turning over tissues such as the bone marrow, thymus, and GI tract. Acrodermatitis enteropathica is a congenital defect of zinc absorption and transport and represents the prototype of severe zinc deficiency. Affected infants have a characteristic erythematous, vesiculobullous, pustular rash, which is most prominent around the orifices, along with mucous membrane damage, alopecia, nail loss, growth retardation, diarrhea, and recurrent infections. Acquired zinc deficiency is often of mild to moderate severity and typically results from inadequate intake of bioavailable zinc or from excessive losses. Mild zinc deficiency is associated with growth impairment, anorexia, and immune dysfunction, with impairment of both T- and B-cell function in animal models and pediatric populations. Zinc deficiency has been associated with a wide range of malabsorptive conditions, including protein-energy malnutrition, short-gut syndrome, celiac disease, cystic fibrosis, or IBD. Zinc deficiency is associated with decreased resistance to parasitic, fungal, and viral infections.[58] Complicating the assessment of zinc status in disease conditions are the lack of a sensitive biomarker of zinc status and the hypozincemia resulting from redistribution of circulating zinc in conjunction with the acute-phase response. These realities result in dependence on response to carefully controlled zinc supplementation trials to demonstrate preexisting zinc deficiency.[59]

Consideration of the role of zinc as a protective nutrient for the GI tract is particularly complex owing to the circular relationship between zinc deficiency, which causes diarrhea, and diarrhea, which may cause zinc deficiency. The critical role of the GI tract in normal zinc homeostasis is well established, both in terms of absorption of dietary zinc and modulation of secretion and reabsorption of endogenous intestinal zinc. Thus, pathologic conditions of the GI tract predictably perturb zinc homeostasis and predispose the individual to zinc deficiency, possibly by morphologic changes that alter transit, permeability, and/or absorptive surface, thereby interfering with absorption of exogenous zinc and reabsorption of endogenous zinc. On the other hand, zinc deficiency is associated with induction of proteins that may increase fluid and possibly endogenous zinc secretion into the GI tract. Candidate proteins that have been proposed include uroguanylin and iNOS, both of which reportedly have increased expression during zinc deficiency. The effects of zinc deficiency on the immune system or on the integrity of the mucosal surface may also have adverse effects on the GI tract and predispose the individual to diarrhea.[60]

Regardless of the questions remaining about mechanisms, there is now little doubt that zinc supplementation in vulnerable populations reduces the severity of diarrhea. In a pooled analysis of randomized blinded controlled zinc supplementation trials conducted in developing countries, infants and children who received zinc supplements had a significant reduction in the length of an episode of acute diarrhea, a decreased probability of developing chronic diarrhea, and a lower probability of associated morbidity compared with children who did not receive supplemental zinc.[61] Although the dietary intake and the nutritional status of the subjects in these studies were generally not characterized in detail, they were presumed to have a high prevalence of zinc deficiency, and the positive response was interpreted to be due to correction of the deficiency rather than a pharmacologic effect of the supplement. Since this pooled analysis, similar findings have been reported in other settings of poverty and high infectious burden.[62,63] Ongoing studies are also investigating the role of zinc-supplemented oral rehydration formulas for the treatment of acute diarrhea in developing countries.[16]

Among the most urgent remaining issues are identification of the populations at most risk for zinc deficiency and therefore to be targeted for interventions; the optimal doses, modes, and schedules of supplemental and therapeutic zinc; and, ultimately, identification of sustainable and culturally appropriate strategies to reduce the prevalence of zinc deficiency through changes in dietary practices. In addition to the exigency for eradication of zinc deficiency on a global basis, there is also substantial need for investigations to clarify the potential contribution of perturbations in zinc homeostasis to some of the clinical manifestations of other GI diseases, including especially those with chronic inflammatory components. Investigations to better characterize mechanisms of altered GI function in relation to zinc metabolism and homeostasis will be especially important to optimally define the role of zinc in therapy.

PREBIOTICS

Prebiotics are nondigestible food ingredients that promote the growth and/or activity of natural or supplemented beneficial bacteria residing in the colon, thus enhancing the health of the host (see Chapter 77.2, "The Pediatric Ostomy").[64] Criteria for a classification as a prebiotic are as follows: the substance should not be hydrolyzed or absorbed in the upper GI tract; it is selectively beneficial for growth of commensal bacteria in the colon; and it alters the flora to a healthy balance by inducing favorable luminal or systemic effects in the host.[65] Prebiotics have many of the same attributes of dietary fiber, with an added benefit for selective colonic bacteria, and include short-chain carbohydrates such as inulin and fructo-oligosaccharides (FOSs), soybean oligosaccharides, and galacto-oligosaccharides (GOSs).[65] The putative nutritional and physiologic effects of prebiotics include alteration of the composition of colonic flora, effects on bowel function, enhanced bioavailability of minerals (especially calcium), and possibly beneficial effects on lipid metabolism and on the risk of colon cancer.[66]

The fructans, which include inulin and FOS, have been extensively studied and are naturally present in more than 36,000 plant species as storage carbohydrates.[65] The most popular natural sources of these indigestible ingredients include wheat, onion, bananas, garlic, tomatoes, and chicory. In addition to their natural availability in foods, prebiotics have been used in food manufacturing for calorie reduction. Used as a replacement for fat and sugar in foods such as ice cream, dairy products, confections, and baked goods, they not only add fiber but also maintain a creamy, fat-like feel in the mouth of the consumer.[16]

GOSs are among numerous disaccharides primarily found in human milk,[67] and it seems likely that they survive digestion in the GI tract of the human infant.[68–70] Colonic bifidobacteria possess an enzyme that facilitates preferential use of the oligosaccharide and thereby allow a prebiotic effect of the GOSs. The GOSs thus comprise one of the components of breast milk that facilitates the preferential growth of *Bifidobacterium* and *Lactobacillus* in the colon[67] and may also provide anti-inflammatory effects in the intestine.[71] These protective colonic bacteria ferment the prebiotic substance to release lactic and acetic acid and thus create a desirable acidic environment. There is intense interest in the potential for addition of oligosaccharides to infant formula to provide some of the protective function of human milk. One randomized, double-blinded trial comparing an infant formula containing a mixture of GOSs and FOSs to a similar standard formula without these additives found a higher proportion of bifidobacteria in the infants' stools after 6 weeks of consuming the supplemented formula.[72]

There are few studies of prebiotic therapeutic efficacy in children. A double-blind, randomized, controlled study compared the use of oligofructose-supplemented formula and unsupplemented formula among 123 nonbreastfed infants. The supplemented formula group had a decrease in both the severity and duration of acute diarrhea episodes.[73] A large-scale community-based randomized controlled trial of oligofructose-supplemented infant cereal conducted in infants from a shantytown near Lima, Peru, was not associated with any benefit on the prevalence of diarrhea, use of health care resources, or response to immunization. The Peruvian infants were between 6 and 12 months of age and were receiving both human milk and complementary foods. The authors concluded that the effects of breastfeeding may mitigate the potential benefit of prebiotic supplementation.[74] Thus, despite the purported benefits of prebiotic consumption, large-scale clinical studies demonstrating the beneficial effects of prebiotics in children are currently lacking.[67] This is likely to remain an area of strong clinical interest, however, because of the potential positive effects on GI health and function.

TRANSFORMING GROWTH FACTOR-β

TGF-β has been shown to antagonize certain proinflammatory cytokines, including interferon-γ, tumor necrosis factor-α, and interleukin-2.[75] Many different authors have proposed that the intestinal mucosa is under a state of "controlled inflammation" owing to exposure to a large variety of antigens.[76] Interferon-γ is known to stimulate the expression of major histocompatibility (MHC) class II proteins on the surfaces of cells. This expression attracts inflammatory mediators to the location of the MHC class II proteins within the small intestine, resulting in inflammation. Enteral formulas that contain certain bioactive molecules may be therapeutic by stimulating the maturation and differentiation of cells and by modulating the immune and inflammatory responses.[75]

Enteral nutrition may pose fewer potential side effects than the current medication treatments used for IBD. Formulas that include bioactive molecules such as TGF-β have been developed for this purpose. In an uncontrolled study, 29 children with active Crohn disease received a TGF-β–supplemented formula. Clinical remission was achieved in 79% of children after 8 weeks of therapy. There was a reduction of interferon-γ and interleukin-8 messenger ribonucleic acid, suggesting an immunologic downregulation.[76] Randomized controlled clinical trials are needed to confirm these findings and to support the routine use of TGF-β–supplemented formulas as a primary treatment for IBD.

SUMMARY

This chapter summarized some of the published animal and human studies evaluating various protective nutrients and substances in relation to maintaining health and function in the GI tract. Some nutrients seem promising for specific disease states, whereas others appear safe but have minimal clinical impact. Despite great strides in medical molecular biology over the last decade, particularly in genomics and proteomics, the ability to detect clinically important changes in GI function remains limited. Clinical trials are often poorly designed and suffer from inadequate numbers and a lack of appropriate control population. Despite the relative lack of controlled studies and questionable clinical efficacy, commercial products containing "protective nutrients" are actively marketed. Indiscriminate use of these products is not warranted. Large carefully designed randomized multi-

center studies are needed to further investigate the health claims of these products and to better quantify their potential for primary or adjunctive clinical treatments.

REFERENCES

1. Koletzko B, Aggett PJ, Bindels JG, et al. Growth, development and differentiation: a functional food science approach. Br J Nutr 1998;80 Suppl 1:S5–45.
2. Montgomery RK, Grand RJ. Development of gastrointestinal tract structure and function. In: Chandra RK, editor. Food intolerance. New York: Elsevier North-Holland; 1984. p. 67–100.
3. Feldman EJ, Dowling RH, McNaughton J, Peters TJ. Effects of oral versus intravenous nutrition on intestinal adaptation after small bowel resection in the dog. Gastroenterology 1976;70(5 Pt1):712–9.
4. Johnson LR, Copeland EM, Dudrick SJ, et al. Structural and hormonal alterations in the gastrointestinal tract of parenterally fed rats. Gastroenterology 1975;68(5 Pt 1):1177–83.
5. Klein RM, McKenzie JC. The role of cell renewal in the ontogeny of the intestine. I. Cell proliferation patterns in adult, fetal, and neonatal intestine. J Pediatr Gastroenterol Nutr 1983;2:10–43.
6. Lipkin M. Proliferation and differentiation of normal and diseased gastrointestinal cells. In: Johnson LR, editor. Physiology of the gastrointestinal tract. 2nd ed. New York: Raven Press; 1987. p. 255–84.
7. Brown HO, Levine ML, Lipkin M. Inhibition of intestinal epithelial cell renewal and migration induced by starvation. Am J Physiol 1963;205:868–72.
8. McNeill LK, Hamilton JR. The effect of fasting on disaccharidase activity in the rat small intestine. Pediatrics 1971;47:65–72.
9. Reddy V, Raghuramulu N, Bhaskaram C. Secretory IgA in protein-calorie malnutrition. Arch Dis Child 1976;51:871–4.
10. Heyman M, Perman J. Nutrition in bacterial overgrowth syndromes of the gastrointestinal tract. In: Sutphen J, Diets W, editors. Pediatric nutrition. Stoneham (MA): Butterworth; 1987. p. 445–53.
11. Brunser O. Effects of malnutrition on intestinal structure and function in children. Clin Gastroenterol 1977;6:341–53.
12. Jackson WD, Grand RJ. The human intestinal response to enteral nutrients: a review. J Am Coll Nutr 1991;10:500–9.
13. Rosensweig NS, Herman RH. Control of jejunal sucrase and maltase activity by dietary sucrose or fructose in man. A model for the study of enzyme regulation in man. J Clin Invest 1968;47:2253–62.
14. Weisbrodt N. Neural and humoral regulation of enteral function. In: Sutphen J, Dietz W, editors. Pediatric nutrition. Stoneham (MA): Butterworth; 1987. p. 185–201.
15. Bulus N, Cersosimo E, Ghishan F, Abumrad NN. Physiologic importance of glutamine. Metabolism 1989;38(8 Suppl 1):1–5.
16. Duggan C, Gannon J, Walker WA. Protective nutrients and functional foods for the gastrointestinal tract. Am J Clin Nutr 2002;75:789–808.
17. Martensson J, Jain A, Meister A. Glutathione is required for intestinal function. Proc Natl Acad Sci U S A 1990;87:1715–9.
18. Stehle P, Zander J, Mertes N, et al. Effect of parenteral glutamine peptide supplements on muscle glutamine loss and nitrogen balance after major surgery. Lancet 1989;i:231–3.
19. Hardy G, Wiggins D, Aima P, et al. The effect of temperature on glutamine-containing TPN mixtures [abstract]. Clin Nutr 1992;11 Suppl:33.
20. Ziegler TR, Young LS, Benfell K, et al. Clinical and metabolic

efficacy of glutamine-supplemented parenteral nutrition after bone marrow transplantation. A randomized, double-blind, controlled study. Ann Intern Med 1992;116:821–8.

21. van der Hulst RR, van Kreel BK, von Meyenfeldt MF, et al. Glutamine and the preservation of gut integrity. Lancet 1993; 341:1363–5.

22. Schloerb PR, Skikne BS. Oral and parenteral glutamine in bone marrow transplantation: a randomized, double-blind study. JPEN J Parenter Enteral Nutr 1999;23:117–22.

23. Neu J, Roig JC, Meetze WH, et al. Enteral glutamine supplementation for very low birth weight infants decreases morbidity. J Pediatr 1997;131:691–9.

24. Buchman AL. Glutamine: commercially essential or conditionally essential? A critical appraisal of the human data. Am J Clin Nutr 2001;74:25–32.

25. Fidanza S, Smith S, Ybarra R, et al. Apparent glutamine toxicity in an infant with short bowel syndrome and liver disease. Nutr Clin Pract 1997;12:91–6.

26. Gurbuz AT, Kunzelman J, Ratzer EE. Supplemental dietary arginine accelerates intestinal mucosal regeneration and enhances bacterial clearance following radiation enteritis in rats. J Surg Res 1998;74:149–54.

27. Moncada S, Higgs A. The L-arginine-nitric oxide pathway. N Engl J Med 1993;329:2002–12.

28. Barbul A, Rettura G, Levenson SM, Seifter E. Arginine: a thymotropic and wound-healing promoting agent. Surg Forum 1977;28:101–3.

29. Seifter E, Rettura G, Barbul A, Levenson SM. Arginine: an essential amino acid for injured rats. Surgery 1978;84:224–30.

30. Boughton-Smith NK, Evans SM, Hawkey CJ, et al. Nitric oxide synthase activity in ulcerative colitis and Crohn's disease. Lancet 1993;342:338–40.

31. Zamora SA, Amin HJ, McMillan DD, et al. Plasma L-arginine concentrations in premature infants with necrotizing enterocolitis. J Pediatr 1997;131:226–32.

32. Akisu M, Ozmen D, Baka M, et al. Protective effect of dietary supplementation with L-arginine and L-carnitine on hypoxia/reoxygenation-induced necrotizing enterocolitis in young mice. Biol Neonate 2002;81:260–5.

33. Amin HJ, Zamora SA, McMillan DD, et al. Arginine supplementation prevents necrotizing enterocolitis in the premature infant. J Pediatr 2002;140:425–31.

34. Daly JM, Reynolds J, Thom A, et al. Immune and metabolic effects of arginine in the surgical patient. Ann Surg 1988;208:512–23.

35. Beale RJ, Bryg DJ, Bihari DJ. Immunonutrition in the critically ill: a systematic review of clinical outcome. Crit Care Med 1999;27:2799–805.

36. Heyland DK, Novak F, Drover JW, et al. Should immunonutrition become routine in critically ill patients? A systematic review of the evidence. JAMA 2001;286:944–53.

37. Gibson RA, Chen W, Makrides M. Randomized trials with polyunsaturated fatty acid interventions in preterm and term infants: functional and clinical outcomes. Lipids 2001;36:873–83.

38. Teitelbaum JE, Allan Walker W. Review: the role of omega 3 fatty acids in intestinal inflammation. J Nutr Biochem 2001; 12:21–32.

39. Uauy R, Hoffman DR. Essential fat requirements of preterm infants. Am J Clin Nutr 2000;71(1 Suppl):245S–50S.

40. Carlson SE, Rhodes PG, Ferguson MG. Docosahexaenoic acid status of preterm infants at birth and following feeding with human milk or formula. Am J Clin Nutr 1986;44:798–804.

41. Akisu M, Baka M, Coker I, et al. Effect of dietary n-3 fatty acids on hypoxia-induced necrotizing enterocolitis in young mice.

n-3 fatty acids alter platelet-activating factor and leukotriene B$_4$ production in the intestine. Biol Neonate 1998;74:31–8.

42. Carlson SE, Montalto MB, Ponder DL, et al. Lower incidence of necrotizing enterocolitis in infants fed a preterm formula with egg phospholipids. Pediatr Res 1998;44:491–8.

43. Donovan SM, Lonnerdal B. Non-protein nitrogen and true protein in infant formulas. Acta Paediatr Scand 1989;78:497–504.

44. Uauy R, Stringel G, Thomas R, Quan R. Effect of dietary nucleosides on growth and maturation of the developing gut in the rat. J Pediatr Gastroenterol Nutr 1990;10:497–503.

45. Sato N, Nakano T, Kawakami H, Idota T. In vitro and in vivo effects of exogenous nucleotides on the proliferation and maturation of intestinal epithelial cells. J Nutr Sci Vitaminol (Tokyo) 1999;45:107–18.

46. Adjei AA, Yamamoto S. A dietary nucleoside-nucleotide mixture inhibits endotoxin-induced bacterial translocation in mice fed protein-free diet. J Nutr 1995;125:42–8.

47. Lopez-Navarro AT, Ortega MA, Peragon J, et al. Deprivation of dietary nucleotides decreases protein synthesis in the liver and small intestine in rats. Gastroenterology 1996;110:1760–9.

48. Bustamante SA, Sanches N, Crosier J, et al. Dietary nucleotides: effects on the gastrointestinal system in swine. J Nutr 1994;124(1 Suppl):149S–56S.

49. Ogita K, Suita S, Taguchi T, et al. Benefit of nucleosides and nucleotide mixture in small bowel transplantation. Transplant Proc 2002;34:1027.

50. Gil A, Pita M, Martinez A, et al. Effect of dietary nucleotides on the plasma fatty acids in at-term neonates. Hum Nutr Clin Nutr 1986;40:185–95.

51. Balmer SE, Hanvey LS, Wharton BA. Diet and faecal flora in the newborn: nucleotides. Arch Dis Child 1994;70:F137–40.

52. Carver JD, Saste M, Sosa R, et al. The effects of dietary nucleotides on intestinal blood flow in preterm infants. Pediatr Res 2002;52:425–9.

53. Yu VY. Scientific rationale and benefits of nucleotide supplementation of infant formula. J Paediatr Child Health 2002; 38:543–9.

54. Klein C. Nutrient requirements for preterm infant formulas. FDA Contract No. 223-92-2185. Task order 11 and 13. Washington (DC): Department of Health and Human Services; 2001.

55. Rudloff S, Kunz C. Protein and nonprotein nitrogen components in human milk, bovine milk, and infant formula: quantitative and qualitative aspects in infant nutrition. J Pediatr Gastroenterol Nutr 1997;24:328–44.

56. Maret W. Editorial: zinc biochemistry, physiology, and homeostasis—recent insights and current trends. Biometals 2001;14:187–90.

57. Sandstead HH. Understanding zinc: recent observations and interpretations. J Lab Clin Med 1994;124:322–7.

58. Shankar AH, Prasad AS. Zinc and immune function: the biological basis of altered resistance to infection. Am J Clin Nutr 1998;68(2 Suppl):447S–63S.

59. Krebs N, Hambidge K. Trace elements in human nutrition. In: Walker W, Watkins J, editors. Nutrition in pediatrics, basic science and clinical applications. 3rd ed. Hamilton (ON): BC Decker, Inc.; 2003. p. 86–110.

60. Krebs NE, Hambidge KM. Zinc metabolism and homeostasis: the application of tracer techniques to human zinc physiology. Biometals 2001;14:397–412.

61. Bhutta ZA, Black RE, Brown KH, et al. Prevention of diarrhea and pneumonia by zinc supplementation in children in developing countries: pooled analysis of randomized controlled trials. Zinc Investigators' Collaborative Group. J Pediatr 1999;135:689–97.

62. Baqui AH, Black RE, El Arifeen S, et al. Effect of zinc supplementation started during diarrhoea on morbidity and mortality in Bangladeshi children: community randomised trial. BMJ 2002;325:1059.

63. Strand TA, Chandyo RK, Bahl R, et al. Effectiveness and efficacy of zinc for the treatment of acute diarrhea in young children. Pediatrics 2002;109:898–903.

64. Gibson GR, Roberfroid MB. Dietary modulation of the human colonic microbiota: introducing the concept of prebiotics. J Nutr 1995;125:1401–12.

65. Gibson GR, Fuller R. Aspects of in vitro and in vivo research approaches directed toward identifying probiotics and prebiotics for human use. J Nutr 2000;130(2S Suppl):391S–5S.

66. Roberfroid MB. Prebiotics: preferential substrates for specific germs? Am J Clin Nutr 2001;73(2 Suppl):406S–9S.

67. Sentongo T, Mascarenhas MR. Newer components of enteral formulas. Pediatr Clin North Am 2002;49:113–25.

68. Gnoth MJ, Kunz C, Kinne-Saffran E, Rudloff S. Human milk oligosaccharides are minimally digested in vitro. J Nutr 2000;130:3014–20.

69. Obermeier S, Rudloff S, Pohlentz G, et al. Secretion of 13C-labelled oligosaccharides into human milk and infant's urine after an oral [13C]galactose load. Isotopes Environ Health Stud 1999;35:119–25.

70. Sabharwal H, Nilsson B, Gronberg G, et al. Oligosaccharides from feces of preterm infants fed on breast milk. Arch Biochem Biophys 1988;265:390–406.

71. Kunz C, Rudloff S, Baier W, et al. Oligosaccharides in human milk: structural, functional, and metabolic aspects. Annu Rev Nutr 2000;20:699–722.

72. Schmelzle H, Wirth S, Skopnik H, et al. Randomized double-blind study of the nutritional efficacy and bifidogenicity of a new infant formula containing partially hydrolyzed protein, a high beta-palmitic acid level, and nondigestible oligosaccharides. J Pediatr Gastroenterol Nutr 2003;36:343–51.

73. Saavedra J, Tschernia A, Moore N, et al. Gastro-intestinal function in infants consuming a weaning food supplemented with oligofructose, a prebiotic. J Pediatr Gastroenterol Nutr 1999;29:513.

74. Duggan C, Penny ME, Hibberd P, et al. Oligofructose-supplemented infant cereal: 2 randomized, blinded, community-based trials in Peruvian infants. Am J Clin Nutr 2003;77:937–42.

75. Donnet-Hughes A, Duc N, Serrant P, et al. Bioactive molecules in milk and their role in health and disease: the role of transforming growth factor-beta. Immunol Cell Biol 2000;78:74–9.

76. Fell JM, Paintin M, Arnaud-Battandier F, et al. Mucosal healing and a fall in mucosal pro-inflammatory cytokine mRNA induced by a specific oral polymeric diet in paediatric Crohn's disease. Aliment Pharmacol Ther 2000;14:281–9.

CHAPTER 76

DRUG THERAPY

1. *Immunosuppressive Therapies*

Sue J. Rhee, MD

Athos Bousvaros, MD

Significant progress continues to occur in the medical treatment of autoimmune diseases and graft rejection. Drugs previously studied in clinical trials (eg, mycopheno-late, infliximab, sirolimus) have now received regulatory approval from the US Food and Drug Administration (FDA) and are being increasingly used in the treatment of a variety of autoimmune diseases and transplant rejection. Genotyping and blood level metabolite monitoring of 6-mercaptopurine (6-MP) and azathioprine now enable the clinician to improve efficacy and decrease the risk of side effects such as pancytopenia. In addition, basic scientists have continued to elucidate the cellular and molecular mechanisms of T-lymphocyte activation, graft rejection, and tolerance to foreign antigens.

There are three principal uses of immunosuppressive therapies in medicine: prevention of organ transplant rejection, treatment of diseases with a presumed autoimmune etiology, and treatment of graft-versus-host disease. In the case of organ rejection, the primary goal of immunosuppression is to abolish the normal host response against foreign tissues. In contrast, the treatment of autoimmune diseases involves the control of an aberrant immune response that has developed against the host's own tissues.

This chapter first reviews components of the immune response that are potential targets for immunosuppressive therapies. The second portion of the chapter reviews currently available and commonly used immunosuppressive agents. The emphasis is on the mechanisms of action and the pharmacology of these agents. Clinical uses in pediatric gastrointestinal disease are discussed in a limited manner. For further information regarding the therapy of specific diseases, the reader is referred to other chapters within this textbook. Lastly, novel immunotherapies not currently in widespread use are considered.

COMPONENTS OF THE IMMUNE RESPONSE

Immunosuppressive medications block both "classic" immune responses (ie, the response of the immune system

to a foreign pathogen or self-antigen) and "nonclassic" immune responses (ie, those seen in rejection, the response of the host's immune system to an allogeneic graft). Classic immune responses are characterized by major histocompatibility complex (MHC)-associated antigen presentation (Figure 76.1-1): CD4 T lymphocytes (which include most T helper [Th] cells) recognize peptides presented by antigen-presenting cells (APCs) expressing MHC class II molecules, whereas CD8 T lymphocytes (which include most suppressor and cytotoxic T cells) recognize antigenic peptides in association with MHC class I expressing cells.[1] In contrast, transplant rejection involves alternative immune responses, including the attack of graft tissue and endothelium by preformed immunoglobulin (Ig)G antibodies (hyperacute rejection), attack of donor tissues by CD4 and CD8 T cells (acute rejection), and the stimulation of fibrosis by leukocytes producing fibrogenic cytokines (chronic rejection). The modes of T-lymphocyte activation also vary in rejection and may include antigen presentation by APCs of the donor graft, and direct recognition by T lymphocytes of MHC molecules without antigen.[2] In general, the magnitude of the immunologic response observed in rejection (allogeneic response) is much greater than that seen in an immune response to microbial infections.

COMPONENTS OF THE CLASSIC IMMUNE RESPONSE

Antigen Uptake and Delivery. An immune response is a humoral and cellular response to either a self- or a foreign antigen, with most antigens being protein fragments (peptides), proteins, or polysaccharides. The classic immune response is summarized in Table 76.1-1 and described in the following subsections. Foreign antigens, including bacteria and viruses, inhaled antigens (pollen), or ingested antigens (foods or toxins), can be prevented from eliciting an immune response by the barrier function of mucosal epithelia. In the digestive tract, gastric acid and pancreatic enzymes degrade bacterial and food antigens,

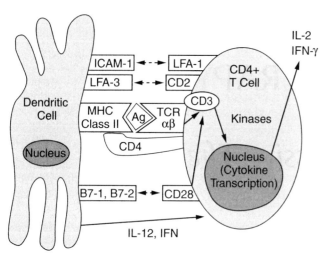

FIGURE 76.1-1 Molecular interactions involved acquired immunity: antigen presentation and helper (CD4) T-cell activation. An antigen-presenting cell (APC; eg, a dendritic cell) endocytoses a dietary or bacterial antigen, digests the protein via endosomes into smaller peptides, and binds the antigen (Ag) to major histocompatibility complex (MHC) class II molecules. The MHC-Ag complex travels to the surface of the APC. Here the MHC-Ag complex binds to the CD4 T cell via the T-cell receptor (TCR). The CD4 molecule strengthens the APC–T-cell interaction by binding to MHC class II. Additional binding occurs by the association of accessory molecules on the APC and T cell, respectively, including intercellular adhesion molecule 1 (ICAM-1)–lymphocyte function–associated antigen (LFA-1), LFA-3–CD2, and B7–CD28. Additional cytokines released by the dendritic cell may determine which cytokines the T cell produces (eg, secretion of interleukin [IL]-12 and interferon [IFN] may promote a T helper 1 cytokine [IL-2, IFN-γ] pattern). The MHC-TCR reaction is the first signal initiating T-cell activation, and B7-CD28 costimulation provides the second signal. If these two events occur, cell signaling via the T cell–CD3 complex and ζ chain occurs (see Figure 76.1-2), resulting in phosphorylation of kinases, cytokine gene transcription through nuclear factor κB, and cytokine synthesis and release.

and intestinal mucin and epithelial cells physically block the passage of antigen. In addition to a simple barrier function, intestinal epithelial cells digest pathogens via intracellular lysosomes and secrete chemokines such as interleukin (IL)-8, which, in turn, recruit polymorphonuclear leukocytes and other cells of the immune system.[3,4] The barrier function of human mucosal epithelia is augmented by secretory IgA, by the cytotoxic properties of intraepithelial lymphocytes, and by the secretion of antimicrobial cryptdins by Paneth cells.[5,6] Both transplanted organs and tissues attacked in autoimmune disease are already located within the host. Therefore, prevention of antigen passage across epithelia will not ameliorate the immune response seen in these disorders.

Antigen Processing and Presentation. The two principal classes of mature T lymphocytes are CD4 cells (which help recruit and activate calls that kill extracellular pathogens) and CD8 cells (which kill cells infected with intracellular pathogens). Helper T cells of the CD4 phenotype are essential in stimulating the inflammatory response to antigen, regulating antibody production, stimulating

cytotoxic (CD8) T-cell responses, and recruiting effector cells (such as cytotoxic T cells, neutrophils, and eosinophils). However, CD4 T lymphocytes do not directly bind or respond to antigen unless the antigen is bound to the surface of an APC. APCs are characterized by their ability to phagocytose proteins or peptides, degrade them intracellularly, complex these peptides with proteins of the MHC class II (human leukocyte antigen [HLA] molecules -DP, -DQ, and -DR), and transport these proteins in association with MHC class II molecules to the cell surface of the APC.

The "professional" APC of the body is the dendritic cell. Dendritic cells endocytose antigen and present to T cells via MHC class II molecules (adaptive immunity; see below) and also recognize bacterial constituents (eg, lipopolysaccharide) via either Toll-like receptors present on the plasma membrane or caspase-recruitment domain/nucleotide-binding oligomerization domain receptors in the cell cytoplasm (innate immunity).[7,8] In either case, a dendritic cell stimulated with antigen will express increased levels of costimulatory molecules on the cell surface and also produce cytokines that down-regulate or up-regulate inflammation. The dendritic cell is perceived as a gatekeeper cell, which determines whether an antigen generates an immune response or tolerance (ie, the absence of an immune response).[7] In addition to dendritic cells, other APCs include B lymphocytes, monocytes, and macrophages.[1]

Once ingested, antigen is degraded by proteases in intracellular vesicles termed endosomes. Simultaneously, class II molecules manufactured in the endoplasmic reticulum are transported into the endosomes in association with a transport protein called the invariant chain. Once inside the endosome, invariant chain is cleaved, the MHC class II molecule binds to the antigenic peptide, and the MHCII-peptide complex is transported to the surface of the dendritic or other APC.[9]

Once the antigen-MHC complex has been transported to the surface of the APC, the complex then interacts with the T-cell receptor (TCR) on the surface of the CD4 Th cell (see Figure 76.1-1). The principal component of the TCR is a heterodimeric complex consisting of two covalently linked chains (either the α/β chain or the γδ chain). The other components of the TCR complex are the CD3 molecule and the TCR ζ protein; these two proteins mediate intracellular signaling by activation of tyrosine kinases. Binding between the T cell and the APC is strengthened by accessory molecules on the surface of the T cell (eg, CD4, CD28, leukocyte

TABLE 76.1-1   COMPONENTS OF THE IMMUNE
                RESPONSE

Antigen uptake across mucosal surfaces
Antigen processing
Antigen presentation to T cells
T-lymphocyte activation
B-cell activation and immunoglobulin production
Leukocyte homing and adhesion to tissues
Effector cell recruitment
Cytokine and chemokine production
Release of inflammatory mediators
   (eg, prostaglandin, leukotriene, complement)

function-associated antigen [LFA]-1, and CD2), which bind to corresponding ligands on the surface of the APC (class II MHC, B7, intercellular adhesin molecule 1 [ICAM-1], and LFA-3, respectively; see Figure 76.1-1).[10,11]

To initiate intracellular events that result in CD4 T-lymphocyte activation, at least two binding events (signals) must occur between the molecules on the surface of the APC and the T cell. The first signal is initiated by binding between the peptide-MHC complex on the APC and the TCR-CD4-CD3 complex on the T cell (Figure 76.1-2). Antigen binding to the TCR initiates a cellular signal transmitted through the CD3 molecular complex to intracellular tyrosine kinases. However, stimulation of a T cell by this signal alone does not induce an immune response and may even result in anergy (ie, the absence of an immune response). The second signal in T-cell activation is a co-

stimulatory signal provided by other APC–T-cell membrane interactions. Although a number of costimulatory signals have been identified, the most important is the interaction between B7 (CD80 or CD86) on the APC with CD28 on the T cell. This interaction promotes T-cell differentiation and cytokine secretion. Additional events include the binding of CD40 on APCs with CD40 ligand on T cells, which may serve to increase the expression of B7 molecules on the APC surface. Cell-cell adhesion is strengthened by binding between ICAM-1 (CD54) on the APC with LFA-1 (CD11a/CD18) on the T cell.[12,13]

T-Lymphocyte Activation. If antigenic stimulation and costimulation occur, a signal is transduced through the CD3 complex, characterized by phosphorylation of tyrosine molecules in the CD3 and ζ chains (see Figure 76.1-2).[14] Subsequently, tyrosine kinases, including lymphocyte protein tyrosine kinase (Lck) and ζ-associated 70 (ZAP-70), are activated and induce phosphorylation of phospholipase Cγ1, which, in turn, converts inositol 4,5-biphosphate to inositol 1,4,5-triphosphate (IP$_3$).[13,15] IP$_3$ formation results in increased cytosolic free calcium from intracellular stores and activation of the molecule calcineurin.

A second intracellular signal transduction pathway initiated by phospholipase Cγ1 involves the molecules diacylglycerol and protein kinase C (see Figure 76.1-2).[16,17] These pathways are separate but synergistic, and inhibition of one or the other may abrogate T-cell activation. Calcineurin and protein kinase C enzymes, in turn, promote increased transcription of cytokine gene products mediated by nuclear binding factors, including nuclear factor of activated T cell (NFAT) and nuclear factor κB (NFκB). A third T-cell activation pathway triggered by antigen recognition involves a group of kinases termed mitogen-activated protein (MAP) kinases, which, in turn, activate the transcription factor activator protein 1(AP-1).[18]

Activation of T cells is characterized by increased T-cell deoxyribonucleic acid (DNA) synthesis and proliferation, increased protein synthesis, increased production of cytokines, and increased production of cytokine receptors. Cell membrane proteins (activation markers) present on the surface of activated T cells include the IL-2 receptor CD154 (ie, CD40 ligand, a molecule that promotes B-cell differentiation), CD45RO (a marker for memory T cells), trace amine receptor 1, and signalling lymphocyte activation molecule (a transmembrane receptor that, when activated, induces interferon [IFN]-γ production).[17,19] In addition, activated T cells express a ligand for the protein Fas. Binding of Fas to Fas ligand results in caspase activation and T-cell apoptosis, thereby helping to clear kill activated T cells that have been repeatedly stimulated by antigen.[20] Of importance in immunosuppression, the molecules cyclosporine and tacrolimus (FK506) both inhibit T-lymphocyte activation by decreasing the activity of calcineurin and intranuclear levels of NFAT (see Figure 76.1-2).[21]

Based on studies performed with murine T-lymphocyte clones, Th (CD4) lymphocytes have been categorized into two broad types. Th1 cells promote cellular immune responses and delayed-type hypersensitivity by secreting

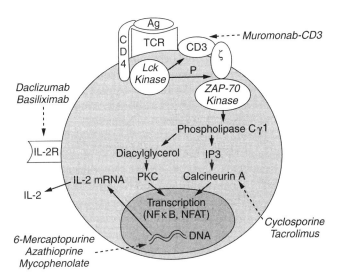

FIGURE 76.1-2 Signal transduction pathways involved in T-lymphocyte activation and sites of action of immunosuppressive therapies. Binding of antigen (Ag) (in association with major histocompatibility complex proteins) to the T-cell receptor (TCR)-CD4-CD3 complex activates intracellular tyrosine kinases. The CD4 molecule is closely associated with the lymphocyte-specific protein tyrosine kinase (Lck), which, in turn, phosphorylates intracellular portions of the CD3 molecule and the ζ chain. The ζ chain, in turn, activates the ZAP-70 kinase, which results in the activation of phospholipase Cγ1. The activated phospholipase converts inositol biphosphate into inositol 1,4,5-triphosphate (IP$_3$), which, in turn, activates calcineurin A in the cytosol. Calcineurin A is essential in dephosphorylating transcription factors such as nuclear factor κB (NFκB) and nuclear factor of activated T cell (NFAT), which allows the factors to travel to the nucleus. A second pathway activated by phospholipase C and important in promoting transcription involves diacylglycerol and protein kinase C (PKC). The end result is increased intranuclear transcription factor activity, deoxyribonucleic acid (DNA) synthesis, and cytokine (eg, interleukin [IL]-2) production. Cyclosporine and tacrolimus inactivate calcineurin A and inhibit cytokine transcription. Azathioprine, 6-mercaptopurine, and mycophenolate inhibit DNA synthesis. Muromonab-CD3 (OKT3) is a monoclonal antibody that binds to the CD3 molecule, resulting in removal of T lymphocytes from the circulation in vivo. In contrast, the antibodies daclizumab and basiliximab bind to IL-2 receptors (IL-2R) that are present only on activated T lymphocytes. mRNA = messenger ribonucleic acid.

IL-2, IFN-γ, and tumor necrosis factor (TNF)-β, whereas Th2 cells promote humoral responses by secreting IL-4, -5, -10, and -13.[22] IL-4, -5, and -13, in turn, promote B-lymphocyte differentiation into plasma cells and antibody synthesis. Both Th1 and Th2 T-cell subsets develop from naive CD4 cells, depending on the type of antigens processed by dendritic cells or macrophages. A Th1 cytokine response promotes macrophage activation with the aim of eliminating intracellular microbes, whereas a Th2 response results in mast cell activation, clearing of parasites, and allergic reactions.[23] Two other groups of regulatory T-cell subsets, Th3 and CD4+CD25+ cells, decrease inflammation and promote tolerance by secreting anti-inflammatory cytokines, such as transforming growth factor-β (TGF-β) and IL-10.[23] Th1 cells are implicated in the pathogenesis of Crohn disease, whereas Th2 cells have been implicated in the pathogenesis of ulcerative colitis and allergic disorders.

Development of Humoral Immunity. In contrast to T lymphocytes, which require processed antigen presented through peptide and MHC, B lymphocytes recognize protein antigen via Ig molecules directly on the cell surface (Figure 76.1-3). Mature B lymphocytes with surface Ig are present in the peripheral blood, spleen, lymph nodes, and lymphoid follicles. Surface Ig on the B-cell membrane binds antigen and provides an initial stimulus for B-cell lymphocyte activation. The antigen–surface Ig complex results in tyrosine phosphorylation, activation of downstream kinases and phospholipase C, and activation of transcription factors. If an activated B cell is to further differentiate into an Ig-producing plasma cell, it requires both physical contact with a T-cell membrane and stimulation by exogenous cytokines produced by T cells (see Figure 76.1-3). IL-2, -4, and -5 promote B-cell proliferation and differentiation, whereas IL-6 perpetuates proliferation of antibody-secreting B cells.[24]

All B cells are initially programmed to synthesize IgM. For a B cell to switch its class of antibody produced to IgG or IgA (isotype switching), several other molecular stimuli need to occur. The CD40 ligand (glycoprotein 39, CD154) is a molecule on the surface of the T cell that binds to CD40 on B cells. This interaction promotes B-cell activation and differentiation and isotype switching from IgM to IgG, IgA, or IgE (see Figure 76.1-3). Conversely, the CD40-CD154 interaction also promotes activation of CD4 T cells. Deficiency of this molecule results in an unusual form of immunodeficiency, termed the hyper-IgM syndrome.[25] Cytokines such as IL-4 are responsible in switching B cells from IgM to IgE production, and TGF-β has been shown to play a role in B-cell switching to IgA production.[26]

Homing and Adhesion. Immune cells that react to a tissue protein must leave the systemic circulation and bind to the tissue or region where they exert their effects. A large number of molecules mediate adhesion between the circulating lymphocytes and the vascular endothelium, extracellular matrix proteins, and tissues. These molecules have been divided into three superfamilies based on their protein structure: the integrin superfamily (including the molecules very late activation [VLA]-1 through VLA-6 and LFA-1), the Ig

superfamily (including the molecule ICAM-1), and the selectin superfamily (including the molecules L-selectin and E-selectin).[27,28] Among the more important interactions mediated by adhesion molecules, the β1 integrin VLA-4 binds the protein vascular cell adhesion molecule 1 (VCAM-1) on the surface of activated endothelial cells. This reaction is blocked by the monoclonal antibody natalizumab (see section entitled "Natalizumab [Antegren]"). The selectin family of molecules, including L-selectin and E-selectin, also promotes binding of lymphocytes to vascular endothelial cells.[27] Soluble cytokines and chemokines promote stronger cell adhesion by increasing the expression of integrins on the cell surface.[29]

Cytokine and Chemokine Production. Activated cells of the immune system, including macrophages, monocytes, and B and T lymphocytes, produce a large number of multifunctional cytokines and chemokines. These can be functionally categorized into Th1-type cytokines, which stimulate cell-mediated immunity and cytotoxicity, and Th2-type cytokines, which stimulate humoral immunity and allergic responses.[30,31] These molecules promote activation of cells of the immune system, recruitment of effector

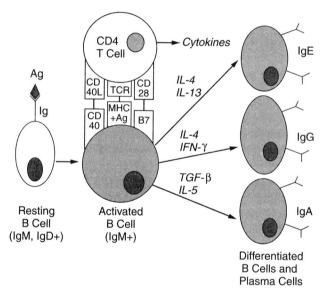

FIGURE 76.1-3 B-cell differentiation and the role of T helper cells. For a resting B cell to differentiate into an antibody-producing plasma cell, three steps are necessary. The first step involves binding of antigen (Ag) onto immunoglobulin (Ig) molecules on the surface of the B cell, which provides an initial signal for B-cell activation. The second step involves physical contact with a T helper lymphocyte, which further activates both the B and the T cell. The three major molecular interactions mediating the B- and T-cell contact involve the CD40-CD40 ligand, major histocompatibility complex (MHC) + antigen with the T-cell receptor (TCR), and B7-CD28. This physical contact promotes B-cell proliferation and differentiation. The third step in B-cell differentiation involves cytokine stimulation. The activated T cell may produce different cytokines, which promote Ig class switching (isotype switching). Differentiation into IgE-producing B cells and plasma cells are promoted by interleukin (IL)-4 and IL-13, IgG-producing B cells are promoted by IL-4 and interferon-γ (IFN-γ), and IgA-producing B cells are promoted by transforming growth factor-β (TGF-β) and IL-5.

cells such as neutrophils and eosinophils, and the production of acute-phase reactants by the liver. Many cytokines have both proinflammatory and anti-inflammatory effects. For example, IL-2 promotes differentiation of Th1 cells, which, in turn, mediate macrophage activation. However, IL-2 can also have anti-inflammatory effects, such as promoting lymphocyte apoptosis and increasing the population of CD4+CD25+ (suppressor type) T cells.[32] Cytokines such as IL-1 and TNF-α mediate the clinical effects (including fever, diarrhea, and hypotension) seen in rejection, shock, and sepsis.[33] IL-5 recruits eosinophils, whereas IFN-γ activates macrophages to phagocytose and kill microbes. Regulatory T lymphocytes release molecules that inhibit inflammation, including IL-10 and TGF-β.[34] Oral tolerance to an antigen develops when dendritic cells exposed to dietary antigens produce IL-10 and TGF-β.[35]

Other Inflammatory Events.   The recruitment of effector cells, including eosinophils and neutrophils, together with complement fixation by IgG, follows B- and T-lymphocyte activation. A group of soluble chemoattractant molecules termed chemokines (eg, eotaxin, IL-8) are released by dendritic cells and T cells to recruit eosinophils and neutrophils to the site of inflammation.[36,37] Chemokines also promote the growth of new blood vessels (angiogenesis) and secretion of matrix metalloproteinases.[38] Neutrophils, mast cells, and eosinophils are considered effector cells. Their products (including prostaglandins and leukotrienes by neutrophils, prostaglandins and histamine by mast cells, and eosinophilic chemotactic factor and major basic protein by eosinophils) cause many of the end-stage characteristics of inflammation, including fever, pain, swelling, erythema, cramping, and diarrhea.[39] However, because these events occur late in the inflammatory cascade, therapies targeted against these late manifestations of inflammation (eg, 5-aminosalicylate derivatives, sodium cromolyn, or lipoxygenase inhibitors) are generally less effective at controlling inflammation than immunosuppressive agents that work earlier in the proinflammatory cascade.

ALLOGENEIC IMMUNE RESPONSE

The allogeneic immune response to a foreign allograft is a far stronger immune reaction than the classic response to an antigen, involving up to 2% of the total T-lymphocyte population.[40] Multiple mechanisms occur by which a transplanted organ is rejected. First, CD8 cytotoxic lymphocytes from the recipient recognize MHC class I molecules on the surface of the donor tissue. These MHC class I (HLA-A, -B, and -C) molecules differentiate self from nonself, and, in the case of transplant rejection, the HLA molecules of the donor graft are inevitably different from those of the host. The cytotoxic CD8 lymphocytes then bind and destroy foreign cells through the release of cytotoxic molecules (including perforins and granzymes).

Whereas CD8 T cells mediate much of the tissue damage seen in rejection, CD4 T cells are probably even more important. In CD4 knockout mice, allografts are retained indefinitely.[41] In contrast, CD8 knockout mice can still reject allografts. This suggests that CD4 T cells mediate

allograft rejection via either stimulation of antibody production or the generation of other cytotoxic leukocytes. The rejection effects of CD4 T cells include enhancing antigen presentation by APCs and promoting the survival and proliferation of cytotoxic T cells and the secretion of proinflammatory cytokines. In addition, CD4 T cells induce dendritic cells to produce IL-12, which induces the proliferation of CD4 cells with a Th1 phenotype.[40,41]

In allograft rejection, CD4 Th cells produce lymphokines such as IL-2 and IFN-γ, which recruit and activate more cytotoxic T cells, thereby propagating both cellular and humoral immune responses. CD4 cells can be activated in one of two ways. The indirect pathway (classic antigen-presenting pathway) involves antigen presentation of foreign (donor) antigens by recipient APCs to recipient CD4 cells. In the indirect pathway, the donor antigens are bound to recipient MHC and are presented to recipient T cells in a way similar to that of a microbial peptide. The second (direct) pathway is unique to transplant recipients and involves recognition of the intact unprocessed MHC of donor APCs by recipient CD4 T cells. The direct T-cell recognition of allogeneic MHC molecules is evaluated by using a mixed lymphocyte reaction.[42]

Despite the complexities and differences between the classic immune response to tissues seen in autoimmune disease and the allogeneic immune response seen in rejection, the final common pathway of both responses involves mononuclear cell activation, generation of proinflammatory lymphokines, and generation and recruitment of cytotoxic effector cells (including macrophages, killer T cells, neutrophils, mast cells, and eosinophils). The most potent immunosuppressive agents currently in use (including cyclosporine, tacrolimus, and monoclonal anti-CD3) either remove host T-lymphocyte populations or inhibit T-lymphocyte activation.

Some individuals, however, develop the ability to tolerate a foreign graft with minimal or no immunosuppression, a condition termed chimerism or transplant tolerance. Tolerance is an ideal outcome because it allows retention of a graft without the long-term toxicity of immunosuppression. Potential mechanisms for inducing tolerance in the host include stimulation of the TCR without the delivery of a second costimulatory signal, infusion of immunosuppressive cytokines at the time of graft delivery, and the promotion of T-cell apoptosis via the Fas–Fas ligand interaction. Another approach to promoting graft tolerance involves the infusion of donor bone marrow cells at the time of solid organ transplant.[43,44] Although the exact mechanism of chimerism or tolerance is not known, it most likely involves the development of a population of CD4 T cells that down-regulate the immune response.[41] At this time, no reliable method exists to consistently promote tolerance in human liver and small bowel transplant recipients.

COMMONLY USED IMMUNOSUPPRESSIVE THERAPIES

CORTICOSTEROIDS

Corticosteroids are natural or pharmacologically modified molecules that are derivatives of cortisol, which is synthesized from its precursors cholesterol and pregnenolone in the adrenal cortex. Corticosteroids have 21-carbon atoms, with a 2-carbon chain attached at position C_{17} of the sterol molecule; they differ from androgenic steroids, which are 19-carbon steroids.[45] Corticosteroids have a wide variety of endocrinologic, anti-inflammatory, and immunosuppressive effects. Commonly used immunosuppressive corticosteroids, their half-lives, and relative potencies are shown in Table 76.1-2.

Mechanism of Action. Corticosteroids are transported through the circulation to tissues by steroid binding proteins. They then dissociate from the binding protein, cross the cell membrane, and bind to nuclear receptors. The steroid-receptor complex stimulates the production of the NFκB inhibitor IκB, which down-regulates NFκB (the transcription factor that is critical in promoting synthesis of cytokines; see Figure 76.1-3). The end result is decreased synthesis of a wide variety of proinflammatory cytokines, including IL-1, IL-2, TNF-α, and IFN-γ.[46]

Corticosteroids reduce the numbers of lymphocytes in the circulation. In addition, corticosteroids decrease prostaglandin and leukotriene production by blocking arachidonic acid synthesis through effects on the enzyme phospholipase A_2.[47] Corticosteroids do not inhibit phospholipase A_2 directly but rather potentiate the release of lipocortin, a powerful inhibitor of phospholipase A_2.[48] Corticosteroids also down-regulate leukocyte recruitment into inflamed areas by modulating chemokine production.[49] Therefore, corticosteroids have multiple immunosuppressive and anti-inflammatory effects and act on multiple levels of the proinflammatory cascade.

Pharmacology. Corticosteroids are well absorbed from the gastrointestinal tract, principally from the proximal jejunum[50]; up to 30% of corticosteroids are absorbed from retention enemas.[51] In the systemic circulation, 90% of cortisol is bound to serum albumin and corticosteroid binding globulin. Cortisol and other corticosteroids are metabolized by both reduction and glucuronidation in the liver. Inducers of hepatic conjugation, including phenobarbital and rifampin, increase hepatic metabolism and excretion of steroids.[45] Although the plasma half-life of cortisol and other steroids is less than 5 hours, the biologic half-life (as measured by adrenal suppression and tissue effects) is far longer (see Table 76.1-2).[45] The most prominent pharmacologic effect of corticosteroids, suppression of the hypothalamic-pituitary adrenal axis, can occur with as little as 5 days of high-dose (50 mg/d) oral prednisone and is almost universally seen with 14 days of therapy.[50,51]

Adrenal suppression with corticosteroid therapy is assessed by screening of morning cortisol levels or more formal assessment after adrenal stimulation with metyrapone or corticotropin.[52] The degree of adrenal suppression is a function of the dose of the steroid, the mode of delivery, the half-life of the steroid, and the frequency of the doses given. Therefore, twice-daily dosing of prednisone, even with a lower dose, increases the degree of adrenal suppression, and alternate-day prednisone therapy reduces the adrenal suppression. In contrast, alternate-day treatment with dexamethasone has significant side effects because of its longer half-life.[45,51] Inhaled corticosteroids, such as beclomethasone, which are given twice per day to asthmatics, can suppress pituitary function and inhibit linear growth.[52,53] As little as 3 mg/m² of prednisone given daily for any longer than 6 months may decrease growth.[54] In contrast, there is no evidence that low-dose alternate-day prednisone therapy results in suppression of growth velocity.

Adverse Events. The large number of side effects (Table 76.1-3) seen with chronic high-dose steroids limits both the dose and duration of therapy.[50] Some side effects (eg, hypertension, fluid retention, diabetes mellitus) may be seen within 2 weeks of the onset of treatment, but most side effects are seen with prolonged (> 1 month) treatment. Loss of trabecular bone and a decrease in bone density occurs in adults treated with more than 7.5 mg/d of prednisone, with the greatest degree of bone loss occurring during the first

TABLE 76.1-2   COMMONLY USED GLUCOCORTICOID PREPARATIONS

STEROID PREPARATIONS	EQUIVALENT DOSE (MG)	PLASMA HALF-LIFE (MIN)	TISSUE HALF-LIFE (H)
SHORT ACTING			
Cortisone*	25	30	8–12
Hydrocortisone*	20	90	8–12
INTERMEDIATE ACTING			
Prednisone	5	60	12–36
Prednisolone	5	200	12–36
Methylprednisolone	4	180	12–36
Budesonide†	1.25†	180	??
LONG ACTING			
Dexamethasone	0.5	100–300	36–54
Betamethasone	0.6		

Adapted from Yang Y and Lichtenstein G,[46] Truhan A and Ahmed A,[50] and Spencer C and McTavish D.[82]
*Strongest mineralocorticoid (sodium retaining) effects.
†Locally acting preparation, with high first-pass metabolism and 15% or less systemic absorption. In clinical trials, 9 mg of enteric-coated budesonide has been compared with 40 mg prednisone.

few weeks of therapy, when dosages are highest.[55,56] Aseptic necrosis of the hip is also reported to complicate long-term corticosteroid use, but this may be related, in fact, to the

TABLE 76.1-3   SIDE EFFECTS OF CORTICOSTEROID THERAPY

CARDIOVASCULAR
Hypertension
? Atherosclerosis

DERMATOLOGIC
Cushingoid appearance
Moon facies
Striae
Alopecia
Hirsutism
Acne
Thinning/friability of skin
Telangiectasia
Impaired wound healing

ENDOCRINOLOGIC
Adrenal suppression
Impaired stress response
Growth failure
Diabetes mellitus/glucose intolerance
Hyperlipidemia

GASTROINTESTINAL
Nausea/vomiting
Fatty liver
Gastritis
Peptic ulcer
Pneumatosis intestinalis
Pancreatitis

HEMATOLOGIC
Leukocytosis
Lymphocytopenia

INFECTIOUS
Viral: especially varicella, herpes zoster
Bacterial: staphylococcal/pseudomonal
Fungal: especially *Candida, Aspergillus*
Parasitic: *Pneumocystis*
Mycobacterial: reactivation of tuberculosis

NEUROLOGIC
Headache
Pseudotumor cerebri

MUSCULAR
Proximal myopathy

OPHTHALMOLOGIC
Posterior subcapsular cataracts
Increased intraocular pressure
Papilledema
Exophthalmos
Eyelid swelling

ORTHOPEDIC
Osteoporosis
Fractures
Aseptic necrosis
Spontaneous tendon rupture

PSYCHIATRIC
Depression
Mania

RENAL
Sodium retention
Nephrocalcinosis
Hypercalciuria

Adapted from Swartz S and Dluhy R,[57] Truhan A and Ahmed A,[70] and Flevy S.[77]

underlying disease process.[57] The child on chronic steroid therapy is at increased risk for opportunistic infection, such as disseminated varicella. Ideally, children should be immunized against varicella prior to the institution of corticosteroid therapy. An unexposed, unimmunized child should receive zoster Ig after exposure and acyclovir for active infection. Gastrointestinal side effects (peptic ulcers and pancreatitis) occur only rarely.[58]

Another adverse event of corticosteroid therapy is the development of corticosteroid dependence or corticosteroid resistance. In both autoimmune hepatitis (AIH) and inflammatory bowel disease, the proportion of patients relapsing after weaning or cessation of corticosteroids is greater than 70%.[59,60] In adults with asthma, corticosteroid resistance is associated with decreased levels of the glucocorticoid receptor and increased expression of the cytokine transcription factor AP-1 and other phosphorylated signaling proteins.[61,62] Thus, patients who are corticosteroid resistant may acquire a population of leukocytes resistant to the pharmacologic effects.[63]

Clinical Indications.   Corticosteroids are used to treat a wide variety of gastrointestinal diseases, including allergic and eosinophilic gastroenteritis, graft-versus-host disease, liver transplant rejection, inflammatory bowel disease, and AIH. Corticosteroids have no proven efficacy in the therapy of many gastrointestinal diseases, including Reye syndrome, fulminant liver failure, primary sclerosing cholangitis (PSC), Ménétrier disease, and Whipple disease.

Inflammatory Bowel Disease.   Corticosteroids are used as induction therapy in moderate to severe active ulcerative colitis. For patients with severe colitis, intravenous methylprednisolone twice daily in a total daily dose of 40 to 60 mg (or 1–2 mg/kg/d) is used, whereas for patients with moderate colitis, 1 mg/kg/d up to 40 mg/d of prednisone is used. Assuming that remission is achieved, one author recommends that the prednisone dosage be reduced by 5 to 10 mg/wk to 20 mg/d and then decreased by 2.5 to 5 mg each week until complete withdrawal of the prednisone.[55] Some clinicians prefer to taper to a dose of between 10 and 20 mg and then wean to an alternate-day regimen. For patients with ulcerative proctitis or left-sided colitis, the use of topical hydrocortisone enemas or foam preparations (Cortenema, Cortifoam) may induce and maintain remission with fewer systemic side effects.[64]

Two large studies in adults have demonstrated the superiority of corticosteroids over placebo in the treatment of active Crohn ileitis and ileocolitis.[65,66] In both the National Cooperative Crohn's Disease Study and the European Cooperative Crohn's Disease Study, 60 to 80% of patients treated with prednisone for approximately 4 months entered remission compared with 30 to 40% of patients given placebo. However, up to 30% of patients persist with active disease despite steroid treatment (ie, corticosteroid resistance), and another 30% of patients will relapse within 1 to 3 months of steroid discontinuation (corticosteroid dependence).[60,67] Risk factors for the development of corticosteroid dependence include smoking, young age, and colonic Crohn disease.[68]

Whether alternate-day steroid administration helps prevent the relapse of Crohn disease is controversial. Early studies suggested that alternate-day prednisone was useful in preventing relapse in Crohn disease or ulcerative colitis, but this approach has not been validated in a long-term prospective placebo-controlled trial.[69,70] Given the availability of other effective maintenance therapies, such as 6-MP, this strategy is unlikely to become the subject of a randomized controlled trial.

Autoimmune Hepatitis.

AIH is characterized by a mixed cellular inflammatory infiltrate of the hepatic portal areas and parenchyma and by the presence of hypergammaglobulinemia. Older children and teenagers often have anti–smooth muscle antibodies in the serum, whereas younger children frequently present with anti–liver-kidney microsomal antibodies.[71] Prednisone at a dose of 40 mg/d in adults or 1 mg/kg/d in children will improve both symptoms and biochemical parameters of AIH and prolong survival. The response rate to corticosteroid induction in AIH exceeds 80%.[72,73] As with inflammatory bowel disease, AIH has a high rate of relapse once steroids are either tapered or discontinued.[59,74] Therefore, steroids should be slowly tapered over a 2- to 3-month period to a low daily dose while monitoring liver biochemistries and serum Ig levels. To maintain remission once corticosteroid weaning is undertaken, physicians frequently add azathioprine (1.5–2 mg/kg/d) to the therapeutic regimen because azathioprine has been shown to be effective in preventing relapse.[75] Cyclosporine and tacrolimus have been used with success to treat corticosteroid-resistant cases of AIH.[76,77]

Eosinophilic Esophagitis.

This increasingly recognized condition presents in children with symptoms of solid food dysphagia, heartburn, and dyspeptic symptoms. Affected individuals frequently have an atopic history. Endoscopy demonstrates a thick, irregular esophageal wall, and biopsies demonstrate large numbers of eosinophils.[78] Both oral prednisone and swallowed fluticasone successfully treat this condition.[79] Teitelbaum and colleagues demonstrated that induction therapy with fluticasone results in improved symptoms and decreased numbers of antigen-presenting T cells.[80] Although fluticasone therapy relieves symptoms, it may be complicated by the development of Candida esophagitis. Moreover, relapse following the cessation of therapy is frequent.

BUDESONIDE (ENTOCORT)

Budesonide is a synthetic corticosteroid structurally related to 16α-hydroxyprednisolone. An enteric-coated form designed for controlled ileal release is available in the United States, whereas budesonide enemas also are available in Canada and many European countries. The mechanism of action is similar to other corticosteroids, but because of the rapid first-pass metabolism, budesonide may have fewer corticosteroid-associated side effects.

Pharmacology. Budesonide is available in two principal forms: an oral form (3 mg controlled ileal release capsule), which provides controlled release into the ileum and cecum, and an enema (2 mg/100 mL) designed for drug delivery into the left colon. In both children and adults, budesonide has a low systemic bioavailability (approximately 10 to 15% of the ingested dose). However, following ingestion of a single 9 mg dose of budesonide, plasma cortisol is decreased by approximately 50% in adults and 60% in children.[81] After enema infusion, maximum plasma concentrations of 3 nmol/L are achieved 90 minutes after rectal administration. In the body, budesonide is rapidly metabolized to 6β-hydroxybudesonide and 16α-hydroxyprednisolone, which have 1 to 10% the glucocorticoid activity of budesonide. The elimination half-life of budesonide is approximately 3 hours.[82]

Adverse Effects. Because of the low systemic bioavailability and rapid metabolism of budesonide, it has been proposed to have fewer side effects than conventional corticosteroids. Volovitz and colleagues found no growth suppression in 15 children with asthma who inhaled 100 μg of budesonide 4 times daily for 3 years or longer.[83] In contrast, two asthma studies documented decreased adrenal cortisol output following a 1.2 mg oral dose of budesonide.[84,85] A number of studies in adults with ulcerative colitis suggest that the enema form of budesonide does not decrease basal plasma cortisol levels but may decrease adrenal gland reserve, as measured by adrenocorticotropic hormone testing.[82]

A number of clinical trials in adults using oral budesonide as induction and maintenance therapy in Crohn disease suggest that steroid side effects (moon face, acne, hirsutism) are reduced, but not eliminated, in patients receiving budesonide.[86] In one multicenter study, 67% of patients receiving prednisone (40 mg/d) compared with 44% of patients receiving budesonide (9 mg/day) reported cushingoid side effects.[87] The long-term effects of budesonide on bone density are unclear. In one study, methylprednisolone was noted to impair osteoblast activity (as measured by serum osteocalcin), whereas budesonide did not.[88]

Clinical Use. The principal gastrointestinal indication for use of budesonide has been in the therapy of Crohn disease and ulcerative colitis. Budesonide enemas (2 mg/100 mL) are effective in treating distal ulcerative colitis.[89] For Crohn disease in adults limited to the ileocecal region, 9 mg of budesonide given orally has comparable efficacy to 40 mg/d of prednisone.[90] However, oral budesonide may be less effective than prednisone for disease involving the distal colon and rectum.[87] Lower-dose budesonide (either 3 mg or 6 mg/d) may have some efficacy in the maintenance of remission, but this is controversial. In three identically designed studies, patients were randomized to placebo, budesonide 3 mg/d, or budesonide 6 mg/d. Two studies noted that budesonide prolonged the time to relapse, with the 6 mg/d dose being more effective.[91,92] However, a third study showed no difference in the median time to relapse between groups.[86]

There are extensive data on inhaled budesonide in children with asthma but less information on children with inflammatory bowel disease. In an initial randomized comparison of budesonide and prednisone for the treatment of children with active Crohn disease, budesonide 9 mg/d and prednisone 40 mg/d had comparable response rates after 12 weeks of therapy.[93] However, a subsequent retrospective study by the same investigators suggested that prednisone was more effective induction therapy for active Crohn disease, with a response rate of 77% for prednisone versus 48% for budesonide. In addition, prednisone was effective as rescue therapy in 73% of children who did not achieve a remission with budesonide.[94]

Although budesonide may be less effective as an induction agent, it has the benefit of producing fewer cosmetic side effects, such as moon face, acne, and hirsutism.[93] Whether budesonide suppresses growth with long-term use remains unclear. A large cohort of asthma patients treated with inhaled budesonide and followed for a mean of 9 years demonstrated reduced growth velocity initially but achieved normal final adult height.[95] Kundhal and colleagues described a cohort of children with Crohn disease treated with budesonide who demonstrated a reduced height velocity (mean 2.3 cm/yr) while on therapy.[96] It is unclear from this study, however, whether the growth suppression was secondary to the drug itself or subclinical disease activity. There are limited data on bone turnover and osteoporosis in budesonide-treated children, but results from asthmatics suggest that budesonide likely causes less bone resorption than prednisone.[97]

CYCLOSPORINE (SANDIMMUNE, NEORAL)

Cyclosporine is a cyclic 11–amino acid peptide produced by the fungus *Tolypocladium inflatum Gams*. Its potent immunosuppressive properties revolutionized the field of transplant in the early 1980s and made it possible for solid organ transplant (including liver and small bowel transplant) to become a recognized mode of therapy for specific illnesses. Dosages, adverse effects, and pharmacokinetics of cyclosporine and other immunomodulatory agents are summarized in Table 76.1-4.

Mechanism of Action. Cyclosporine enters the cytosol of T cells and binds to the cytosolic protein cyclophilin A (Cyp-A). In the cytoplasm, the cyclosporin A–cyclophilia complex binds to the calcium-dependent phosphatase calcineurin (see Figure 76.1-2). The calcineurin molecule is essential in T-lymphocyte activation and in the transcription of cytokines by Th cells because it dephosphorylates the transcription factor NFAT, thereby facilitating migration of NFATs across the nuclear membrane, leading to decreased transcription and release of IL-2 and other proinflammatory cytokines.[21,98] Of note, only calcium-dependent pathways of T-lymphocyte activation are affected by cyclosporin A. Activation of T lymphocytes via the cell surface molecule CD28 (a calcium-independent process) is not inhibited by cyclosporin A.[99]

The most prominent immunologic effect of cyclosporine is the suppression of IL-2 release by Th cells,

resulting in marked inhibition of cell-mediated immunity. The synthesis and release of other cytokines, including IL-6 and -8, are also impaired.[98] Cyclosporin A exhibits a wide variety of other effects on nonhelper T cells (Table 76.1-5). Cyclosporin A impairs the cytotoxic action of CD8 (killer) T cells.[100] Paradoxically, in some animal models, cyclosporin A prevents the development of tolerance and can exacerbate autoimmune disease by blocking the suppressive effects of CD8 suppressor T cells.[101] Cyclosporine also modulates antibody production by B lymphocytes, as well as the release of proinflammatory and chemotactic cytokines by mast cells. Although the in vitro effects of cyclosporine are varied, the net effect of cyclosporine administration to humans is to suppress the cellular immune response without lowering antibody levels.[98,102]

Pharmacology. Cyclosporine is a highly lipophilic molecule. The initial formulation of cyclosporine (Sandimmune, Sandoz Pharmaceuticals Corporation, East Hanover, NJ) consisted of cyclosporine in an oil base. Thus, the oral absorption was dependent on intact fat absorption and bile flow, and the bioavailability of this formulation was quite low (approximately 20–30%). The bioavailability was further impaired in conditions that reduced fat absorption, such as cholestasis and enteropathies.[103] Coadministration of oral D-α-tocopheryl polyethylene glycol 1000 succinate (TPGS) (the water-soluble vitamin E derivative) increases the oral bioavailability of oil-based cyclosporine.[104]

In the late 1990s, an oral-microemulsion formulation of cyclosporine (Neoral, Sandoz Pharmaceuticals Corporation) was made available and is now almost exclusively used by liver and renal transplant centers.[105] The new formulation has improved bioavailability, thus necessitating a reduction in drug dosage of approximately 10 to 15% when patients are converted from the oil-based product.[98] In liver transplant recipients, the frequency of graft survival and patient survival is similar regardless of the formulation.[98] Adverse effects are also comparable in both Sandimmune- and Neoral-treated patients.[106]

Cyclosporine has a large volume of distribution (ranging from 3 to 5 L/kg in adults) and is 90% bound to plasma proteins and erythrocytes. Cyclosporine is hydroxylated and demethylated in the liver and excreted in the bile, with less than 10% of each dose excreted in the urine. Clearance of the drug is biphasic, with an initial elimination half-life ($t_{1/2\alpha}$) of 1.2 hours and a terminal elimination half-life ($t_{1/2\beta}$) of 8 to 27 hours. As a result of dependence on hepatic metabolism, cyclosporine can be used even in patients with renal failure. However, drugs that induce P-450 microsomal enzymes (including phenobarbital, phenytoin, and carbamazepine) decrease cyclosporin A concentrations, whereas compounds that inhibit P-450 enzymes (including ketoconazole, erythromycin, and grapefruit juice) increase cyclosporin A concentrations (Table 76.1-6).[98,103]

The exact protocol for monitoring of cyclosporine levels varies between transplant centers. Traditionally, trough values of cyclosporin A levels are obtained, with a target

TABLE 76.1-4   COMMONLY USED IMMUNOSUPPRESSIVES (PHARMACOLOGY)

DRUG	DOSAGES	HALF-LIFE	METABOLISM AND EXCRETION	ABSORPTION/ BIOAVAILABILITY	DRUG INTERACTIONS	COMMENTS
Cyclosporin A (CyA)	5–10 mg/kg/d orally twice a day (adjust by blood levels); intravenous dose approximately 30% of oral dose	10 h (range 4–48 h)	Hydroxylation and methylation; 95% biliary excretion < 5% urinary excretion	Poor (~ 30%); dependent on bile flow, intestinal absorption; microemulsion (Neoral) has improved absorption.	See Table 76.1-6; multiple medications will either increase or decrease half-life	Liver failure increases half-life
Tacrolimus (FK-506)	0.2–0.4 mg/kg/d orally twice a day (adjust by blood levels)	9 h (range 5–16 h)	Bound to erythrocytes; whole blood levels are 10 times serum levels; 99% hepatic metabolism (hydroxylation/ demethylation) absorption	Poor (~ 30%); less dependent on bile flow or mucosal integrity than CyA	See Table 76.1-6; multiple medications will either increase or decrease half-life	Intravenous form is more toxic than oral; useful in liver bowel transplant because of more reliable oral absorption
Methotrexate	15 mg/m²/wk intramuscular or subcutaneous	Biphasic: initial phase 1.5–3.5 h; final phase 8–15 h	Hepatic 7-hydroxylation; intracellular polyglutamate formation; 60–90% renal excretion; < 10% biliary excretion	Poor (30–50% absorbed by gut)	Sulfonamides, salicylates, tetracycline, phenytoin may displace methotrexate from plasma proteins	Bioavailability decreases with increasing oral dosage; may enter pleural or ascitic fluid
6-Mercaptopurine (6-MP)	1.5–2.0 mg/kg orally once a day	Triphasic 45 min, 2.5 h, and 10 h	Degradation by xanthine-oxidase S-methylation in liver; 40% renal excretion	Variable (10–50% absorbed)	Allopurinol, probenecid, increase level	Wide genetic variations in metabolism, determined by thiopurine methyltransferase activity
Azathioprine	2.–2.5 mg/kg/d orally once a day	5 h	Metabolized to 6-MP; 6-thioinosinic acid	Well absorbed from the gastrointestinal tract	See 6-MP	See 6-MP
Mycophenolate mofetil	20 mg/kg/d in 2 divided doses	18 h (adult)	Hepatic glucuronidation 90% renal excretion	99% bound to plasma albumin		Significant gastrointestinal side effects in 20–30% of patients
Sirolimus (rapamycin)	2–5 mg/d, adults 3 mg/m², children	60 h	Hepatic by CYP3A4; excretion by P-glycoprotein	15% oral bioavailability; food interferes with absorption	Multiple, including cyclosporine and other drugs metabolized by cytochrome 3A4	Hyperlipidemia and myelosuppression major side effects

CyA = cyclosporin A; 6-MP = 6-mercaptopurine.

TABLE 76.1-5   IMMUNOLOGIC EFFECTS OF CYCLOSPORIN A

CELL	EFFECTS
CD4 T cell	Decreases IL-2, IFN-γ release
	Decreases IL-2 receptor expression
Cytotoxic T cell	Decreases proliferation
	Decreases IL-2 responsiveness
	Possible decrease in cytotoxicity
B cells	Decreases activation gene expression
	Decreases anti-immunoglobulin responsiveness
Mast cells	Decreases TNF-α release

IFN = interferon; IL = interleukin; TNF = tumor necrosis factor.

therapeutic range of 150 to 400 µg/L. However, because the half-life is variable, trough values poorly predict the actual concentration of the drug over time (area under the curve [AUC]) and correlate less well than true AUC in predicting rejection or nephrotoxicity.[98] For this reason, many centers calculate AUC by performing a trough level and levels 2 hours and 4 hours after a dose.

Adverse Effects. Cyclosporine, even at therapeutic levels, has a wide variety of adverse effects and toxicities (Table 76.1-7). Nephrotoxicity, manifested by a decrease in creatinine clearance and a rise in serum creatinine, occurs in 25 to 75% of patients. Nephrotoxicity usually reverses on discontinuation of the drug or lowering of the dose. Other adverse effects include hypertension, neurotoxicity, insulin-dependent diabetes mellitus, elevated transaminases, hirsutism, and gingival hyperplasia.[102] In liver transplant recipients receiving cyclosporine, up to two-thirds of patients will have bacterial infection and up to 20% will have infections with opportunistic pathogens such as cytomegalovirus, Epstein-Barr virus, *Candida* species, and *Aspergillus*.[107] Lymphoproliferative disorders also occur in patients receiving cyclosporine, usually correlating with serologic or molecular evidence of Epstein-Barr virus infection.[108] Although lymphoproliferative disease can be reversible if immunosuppression is halted, in a minority of patients, the disease progresses to lymphoma.

Clinical Uses. Cyclosporine has been used primarily in the prevention of rejection in liver transplant recipients. More recently, it has been applied to autoimmune liver and bowel diseases, including AIH, ulcerative colitis, Crohn disease, and autoimmune enteropathy. In pediatric liver transplant recipients, cyclosporine is typically begun on the first postoperative day. Whereas the old preparation (Sandimmune) was given intravenously, the microemulsion preparation (Neoral) can be given orally or via nasogastric tube. In the early post-transplant period, clinicians adjust the cyclosporine dosage to maintain a trough level between 150 and 250 ng/mL, as determined by high-performance liquid chromatography. The oral maintenance dosage of cyclosporine is approximately 5 to 10 mg/kg/d in two divided doses, but higher doses may be necessary with the older preparation.[109] In one Canadian study, 32 children undergoing liver transplant were randomly assigned to receive either the lipid-soluble form or the microemulsion in the post-transplant period. Pharmacokinetic studies performed 3 weeks after transplant demonstrated that patients receiving the microemulsion had a mean 8-hour AUC of 950 µg/L/h compared with 300 µg/L/h with the standard formulation.[110] Thus, in children, the Neoral microemulsion gives higher levels of cyclosporine for a longer period of time. However, it remains unclear if this pharmacokinetic benefit translates into improved graft and patient survival.

Two studies emphasize the efficacy of cyclosporine in children with AIH. Debray and colleagues used cyclosporine (mean dose 4.7 mg/kg/d) alone as primary induction therapy in children with type 2 AIH and obtained remission in six children. In another portion of the same study, the authors successfully used cyclosporine (5.6 mg/kg/d) to induce remission in five patients with type 2 AIH resistant to steroids and azathioprine.[111] In another study, 30 patients with AIH were given cyclosporine as monotherapy for 6 months. Twenty-five of the 30 children had normal alanine transaminase (ALT) levels within 6 months.[112] Therefore, early use of cyclosporine can induce remission in AIH without the use of high-dose corticosteroids.

Dosages used in the therapy of Crohn disease and ulcerative colitis are lower. Brynskov and colleagues demonstrated that an oral dose of 5 to 7.5 mg/kg/d promotes remission of Crohn disease in 22 of 37 adults with steroid-refractory Crohn disease.[113] In contrast, a large multicenter placebo-controlled study using low-dose (2.5 mg/kg) cyclosporine as an adjunct to standard treatment for adults with Crohn disease did not demonstrate any benefit of low-dose cyclosporin A.[114]

For ulcerative colitis, Lichtiger and colleagues demonstrated that intravenous cyclosporin A was effec-

TABLE 76.1-6   IMPORTANT DRUG INTERACTIONS WITH CYCLOSPORINE OR TACROLIMUS

CLASS OF MEDICATION	RAISES CYCLOSPORINE AND TACROLIMUS LEVELS	LOWERS CYCLOSPORINE AND TACROLIMUS LEVELS
Antimicrobials	Erythromycin, clarithromycin, clotrimazole, ketoconazole, itraconazole, fluconazole, doxycycline	Isoniazid, nafcillin, rifampin
Antihypertensives	Diltiazem, verapamil, nicardipine	
Anticonvulsants		Phenobarbital, primidone, carbamazepine, phenytoin
Other	Amiodarone, methylprednisolone, danazol, grapefruit juice, sirolimus	Octreotide, St. John's wort

Adapted from Dunn C et al,[98] Kahan B,[102] Kosmach B et al,[109] and Peters D et al.[124]
Potential synergistic nephrotoxicity: acyclovir, aminoglycosides, nonsteroidal anti-inflammatory drugs, amphotericin, vancomycin, certain antineoplastic agents.

TABLE 76.1-7   SIDE EFFECTS OF CYCLOSPORIN A OR TACROLIMUS (FK506) THERAPY

ORGAN SYSTEM	ADVERSE EFFECT
Renal and electrolyte	Hypertension; nephrotoxicity: increased creatinine, oliguria, kidney failure; hypomagnesemia, hyper- and hypokalemia
Nervous system*	Tremor, headache, paresthesia, myalgias, muscle spasm
Gastrointestinal	Nausea, vomiting, diarrhea, anorexia, constipation
Endocrine and metabolic	Hyperglycemia and diabetes,* hypercholesterolemia[†]
Cardiovascular	Arrhythmia,[†] cardiomyopathy*
Infectious	Opportunistic infections: eg, herpes, CMV, EBV, parvovirus, *Pneumocystis*
Malignancy	EBV-associated lymphoproliferative disorder, lymphoma
Other	Gingivitis and gingival hyperplasia,[†] hirsutism,[†] anemia, pruritus

Adapted from Dunn C et al,[98] Kahan B,[102] Plosker G and Foster R,[123] Peters D et al,[124] and Atkison P et al.[131]
CMV = cytomegalovirus; EBV = Epstein-Barr virus.
*More common with tacrolimus.
[†]More common with cyclosporine therapy.

tive treatment in steroid-refractory fulminant colitis. In this trial, 9 of 11 adults treated with cyclosporin A responded within 7 days compared with 0 of 9 receiving placebo.[115] A subsequent study suggested that intravenous cyclosporine (4 mg/kg/d) is effective as monotherapy compared with corticosteroids in the treatment of ulcerative colitis, with a response rate of 60%.[116] In children, given either orally or intravenously at a dose of 4 mg/kg, cyclosporine will bring about remission of ulcerative colitis in up to 80% of children.[117] However, withdrawal of the medication both in children and in adults is associated with a high rate of relapse, even if azathioprine is added as maintenance therapy. Long-term remission rates (> 1 year) are less than 50%.[118] Because the remission induced by cyclosporine is short, it remains a matter of debate whether the benefits of short-term remission outweigh the complications of potent immunosuppressive therapy.

Cyclosporine also has been used to treat autoimmune enteropathy, an idiopathic intestinal inflammatory disease occurring in young children in association with antienterocyte antibodies and evidence of systemic autoimmunity (including renal disease, diabetes, and arthritis). Two groups have treated patients with autoimmune enteropathy with cyclosporin A and noted improved growth and increased nutrient absorption.[119]

Cyclosporine has been used in conjunction with corticosteroids for the treatment of graft-versus-host disease, although the benefit over corticosteroids alone is unclear.[120,121] However, in one study comparing tacrolimus with cyclosporine for prophylaxis of graft-versus-host disease, the incidence of graft-versus-host disease was 18% in the tacrolimus group compared with 48% in the cyclosporine group.[122]

TACROLIMUS (FK506, PROGRAF)

Tacrolimus is a macrolide lactone produced by the fungus *Streptomyces tsukubaensis*. The principal uses of tacrolimus include primary therapy in liver, bowel, and liver-bowel transplants; treatment of cyclosporine-refractory organ rejection; and treatment of graft-versus-host disease. Although the molecule is structurally different from cyclosporine, tacrolimus also works by inhibiting cytokine transcription via calcineurin (see Figure 76.1-3).

Mechanism of Action. Tacrolimus is a lipid-soluble molecule that is internalized into the intracellular compartment of the lymphocyte. Once in the cytosol, tacrolimus complexes with a group of proteins termed FK binding proteins (FKBP, especially FKBP-12). In a manner similar to that of cyclosporine, the tacrolimus-FKBP complex binds calcineurin to inhibit the calcium-dependent pathway of lymphocyte activation. Tacrolimus inhibition of calcineurin results in decreased levels of the NFAT and decreased transcription of T-cell activation genes.[123] Transcription of cytokines produced by activated T cells, such as IL-2, is also drastically decreased. Therefore, T-cell lymphocyte proliferation and cytokine production are blocked by tacrolimus.[124] As with cyclosporine, calcium-independent mechanisms of T-lymphocyte activation are not affected by tacrolimus. In addition to effects on T lymphocytes, tacrolimus inhibits B-cell proliferation and the production of IgM and IgG. At higher doses, tacrolimus also inhibits cytokine production by monocytes and prostaglandin production by mast cells.[125,126] Although tacrolimus and cyclosporine have similar immunologic effects, work in animal models and in humans suggests that tacrolimus also inhibits anti-inflammatory cytokines, such as IL-10, whereas cyclosporine has stronger effects on humoral immunity.[127,128]

Pharmacology. Tacrolimus is 10 to 100 times more potent than cyclosporine. The oral bioavailability of tacrolimus is similar to that of cyclosporine (approximately 30% absorption), but tacrolimus is less dependent on bile flow than cyclosporine for absorption. In fact, tacrolimus absorption is independent of the presence of bile acids, and absorption is less affected by enteropathies. However, coadministration with foods will decrease bioavailability. Once absorbed, tacrolimus is distributed in tissues and in erythrocytes, with a volume of distribution of approximately 1 L/kg.[123]

As with cyclosporine, metabolism of tacrolimus occurs almost exclusively in hepatocytes, with demethylation and hydroxylation occurring via the cytochrome P-450 system. The half-life of tacrolimus is variable, with a mean of 12 hours in both adult and pediatric transplant recipients. Although the half-life is unchanged in renal disease, even mild hepatic impairment will significantly prolong the half-life. Drugs that inhibit P-450 metabolism, such as ketoconazole and erythromycin (see Table 76.1-7), will raise tacrolimus levels, whereas drugs that accelerate P-450 metabolism decrease tacrolimus levels.[124] Children require higher mg/kg doses than adults because of more rapid drug clearance and higher volumes of distribution.[129] McDiarmid and colleagues compared the dose requirements and clearances of the pediatric and adult liver transplant patients. The overall mean pediatric oral dose for the first year was 0.46 mg/kg/d, a dose approximately three times the mean adult dose.[130]

Toxicities of tacrolimus are similar to those seen with cyclosporine (see Table 76.1-7). Side effects include nephrotoxicity, electrolyte abnormalities (hypokalemia, hypomagnesemia), diabetes mellitus, tremor, hypertension, diarrhea, post-transplant seizures, and lymphoproliferative disease. In addition, patients receiving tacrolimus are predisposed to opportunistic bacterial, viral, and fungal infections. Some side effects seen with cyclosporin A, including hirsutism, coarsening of facial features, and gingival hyperplasia, are not seen with tacrolimus.[124] Cardiomyopathy, a rare but serious complication of tacrolimus therapy, typically resolves after lowering the dose of tacrolimus or changing to cyclosporine.[131]

Clinical Uses. The principal indication for the use of tacrolimus is in the prevention of solid organ transplant rejection.[132] As primary therapy immediately after liver transplant in children, tacrolimus is usually given in a dose of 0.3 mg/kg/d, and the dosage is adjusted to give a whole blood level between 10 and 15 µg/L. Over the first few months after transplant, the drug dosage is weaned to achieve levels of 5 to 10 µg/L. Concomitant therapies include corticosteroids, azathioprine, or mycophenolate mofetil; corticosteroids are weaned over time. A European multicenter trial reported that patients treated with tacrolimus (vs cyclosporine) are more likely to wean off corticosteroids.[133] In one pediatric series, 233 children were given tacrolimus as primary therapy, and, when compared with historical controls treated with cyclosporine, the patient survival was 86% in the tacrolimus group versus 69% in the cyclosporine group. However, this difference may simply reflect improved care of liver transplant patients over time.[134] Histologic rejection rarely occurs in children receiving tacrolimus as primary therapy.[135] Tacrolimus has also been used as rescue therapy for children who have developed either chronic rejection despite cyclosporine therapy or adverse effects of cyclosporine.[136,137]

Tacrolimus has been the mainstay of antirejection therapy for patients having received bowel, combined liver and bowel transplants, or multivisceral transplants.[138] In these settings, tacrolimus is usually given with other concurrent immunosuppression, such as corticosteroids and monoclonal antibodies (eg, daclizumab). Initially, levels may need to be kept higher (eg, 15–25 µg/L) to prevent bowel rejection.[139] Both rejection and lymphoproliferative disease occur more commonly in this patient population.

Tacrolimus has also been employed in a wide variety of nontransplant conditions, including as an alternative to cyclosporine in both type 1 and type 2 AIH.[72,140] Children with autoimmune enteropathy that is resistant to cyclosporine can develop restoration of bowel function and histologic improvement after tacrolimus therapy.[141,142] Open-label studies suggest that tacrolimus is effective in treating severe mucosal and fistulizing Crohn disease, but the rate of adverse events is high.[143,144] In a multicenter open-label experience of tacrolimus in the treatment of severe ulcerative colitis and Crohn colitis in children, 70% of patients responded, but more than 50% underwent colectomy within a year.[145] In graft-versus-host disease, tacrolimus can stabilize or improve cases refractory to cyclosporine; however, in one open-label study of 39 patients, the long-term response was approximately 30%.[146]

AZATHIOPRINE (IMURAN) AND 6-MP (PURINETHOL)

Both azathioprine and 6-MP are purine derivatives that are incorporated into DNA and inhibit DNA synthesis. Azathioprine is metabolized in vivo to 6-MP, and its biologic effects are essentially identical to those of 6-MP; therefore, both the mechanisms of action and the toxicities of these drugs are identical. In contrast to 6-MP, azathioprine is metabolized more slowly and has a longer half-life. Therefore, azathioprine has been more widely used as an immunosuppressive agent in transplant recipients. Both drugs are useful in the treatment of liver transplant rejection, as well as in the therapy of inflammatory bowel disease and chronic active hepatitis.

Mechanism of Action. 6-MP is converted to 6-thioguanine (6-TG) ribonucleotides by the enzyme hypoxanthine-guanine phosphoribosyltransferase (HGPRT). The ribonucleotides produced by HGPRT are then incorporated into the DNA of rapidly dividing cells and are cytotoxic. In vitro, 6-MP can inhibit Th cell–dependent Ig production. In addition, 6-MP inhibits Ig production by IL-6–stimulated B-cell lines.[147,148]

Pharmacology. The absorption of 6-MP from the gastrointestinal tract is variable; as little as 10% or much as 50% may be absorbed. In contrast, azathioprine is well absorbed from the gastrointestinal tract. 6-MP is primarily metabolized in the liver, but up to 40% can be excreted in the urine.

There are three major pathways of 6-MP metabolism (Figure 76.1-4). The first route involves transformation by HGPRT and other enzymes into 6-TG nucleotides. Because inhibition of lymphocyte proliferation depends on 6-TG, concentrations of 6-TG in the body may predict the therapeutic efficacy of 6-TG. A second metabolic pathway involves breakdown of 6-MP via xanthine oxidase to 6-thiouric acid; because xanthine oxidase can be inhibited by allopurinol, this drug is relatively contraindicated by individuals taking 6-MP. The third pathway is the principal route of catabolism of 6-MP and involves S-methylation by the enzyme thiopurine methyltransferase (TPMT) to generate 6-methylmercaptopurine (6MMP).[147]

The half-life of 6-MP is triphasic, with the half-life of the final phase being 10 hours. Allopurinol increases levels of 6-MP by inhibiting xanthine oxidase metabolism. In

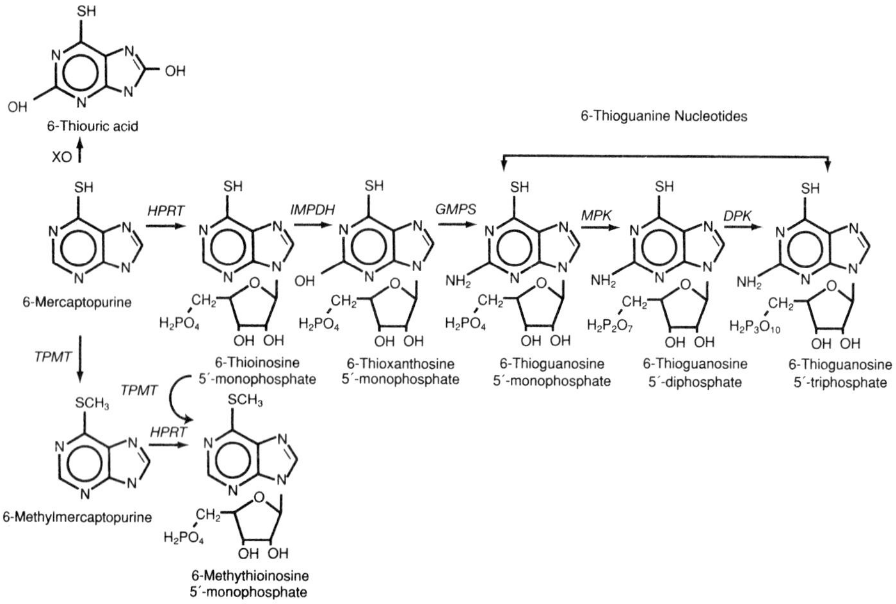

FIGURE 76.1-4 Metabolism of 6-mercaptopurine (6-MP). The initial metabolism of 6-MP may occur via one of three competing enzymatic pathways: thiopurine methyltransferase (TPMT), xanthine oxidase (XO), and hypoxanthine phosphoribosyltransferase (HPRT). Further metabolism of the thinucleotide is catalyzed by inosine monophosphate dehydrogenase (IMPDH) and guanosine monophosphate synthetase (GMPS) to produce 6-thioguanine nucleotides, which are principally responsible for the immunosuppressive effects of 6-MP. Reproduced from Cuffari C et al,[147] with permission of Dr. E. Seidman and BMJ Publishing Group.

addition, probenecid increases the level of 6-MP by inhibiting urinary excretion.[148] There is extensive variability in TPMT activity in human hepatocytes, presumably on the basis of genetic polymorphisms. Approximately 90% of individuals have normal or high TPMT activity and break down 6-MP at a normal rate. Those patients with high TPMT activity have lower concentrations of 6-TG. Lennard and colleagues reported that patients with higher TPMT activity have a higher relapse rate of acute lymphoblastic leukemia, suggesting that the more rapid metabolism of the drug leads to decreased efficacy.[149] Ten percent of individuals have low TPMT activity and have higher concentrations of 6-TG in their tissues and greater potency of the drug; however, this subset of patients may also be at increased risk of myelosuppression. Approximately 0.3% of individuals have negligible TPMT activity, this group is at the highest risk of developing myelosuppression associated with very high 6-TG levels.[147,150] Laboratory tests to determine TPMT genotype, blood TPMT activity, and 6-TG levels are now commercially available.

Adverse Effects and Toxicity. The principal toxic effects of 6-MP are myelosuppression, pancreatitis, elevated transaminases, increased risk of viral infection, and a theoretical increased risk of lymphoma. In one large series of inflammatory bowel disease patients taking 6-MP, 4% developed pancreatitis, up to 10% developed systemic infections, and 1 patient in 400 developed a cancer potentially attributable to the therapy.[151] Whether 6-MP increases the risk of lymphoma remains controversial. Connell and colleagues tracked 755 adults who received 2 mg/kg of azathioprine for up to 15 years (median 12.5 months) and found no increased risk of cancer.[152] However, an increased incidence of Epstein-Barr virus–associated lymphoma was reported in a cohort of 1,200 adults with inflammatory bowel disease treated with either 6-MP or azathioprine.[153] Kirschner described a case series of 95 children who received 6-MP or azathioprine for a mean of 2.2 years. Overall, 82% of children tolerated 6-MP, with the most

common complications being elevated aminotransferases (13% of patients), leukopenia (10%), infections (8%), nausea (5%), and pancreatitis (4%).[154]

Clinical Utility. *Inflammatory Bowel Disease.* 6-MP came into widespread use for the treatment of Crohn disease after 1980, when a randomized placebo-controlled trial demonstrated a 70% response rate in patients with steroid-refractory Crohn disease.[155] It is now recognized that 6-MP has multiple beneficial effects in the therapy of inflammatory bowel disease, including a decrease in disease activity, steroid-sparing effects, and the healing and closure of fistulae. In children and adolescents, treatment of Crohn disease with 6-MP (at a dose of 1.5 mg/kg/d) results in similar improvement and response rates.[156] However, there is a 3- to 4-month lag time between the initiation of 6-MP treatment and a clinical response. A 6-TG level of > 235 pmol/10^8 erythrocytes appears to correlate with an improved clinical response.[147,157,158] A subset of patients who may be resistant to treatment with 6-MP includes those with low levels of 6-TG nucleotides and a high ratio of 6MMP to 6-TG, suggesting rapid breakdown of 6-MP and a decrease in levels of active metabolites.[159] 6-TG has been associated with an increased risk of liver toxicity, so this drug cannot be recommended for use.[160]

Children with Crohn disease may benefit from the early use of 6-MP as a maintenance agent. In an important study by Markowitz and colleagues, 55 children with newly diagnosed Crohn disease were induced with prednisone and then randomized to either 6-MP or placebo as the steroid therapy was withdrawn. After 18 months, the relapse rate was 9% in the 6-MP group compared with 47% in the placebo group. In addition, the 6-MP–treated group received a lower cumulative dose of corticosteroids over the 18-month period.[161]

Another potential use of 6-MP in Crohn disease is the prevention of postoperative disease recurrence. One retrospective study in children suggested that early use of 6-MP decreases the recurrence risk in patients undergoing ileal or colonic resection.[162] Another study suggested that azathioprine heals recurrent ileitis developing in the neoterminal ileum.[163]

Azathioprine also has been widely used in the therapy of inflammatory bowel disease. The results suggest clinical efficacy comparable with that of 6-MP. In one study of the pharmacokinetics of azathioprine, oral azathioprine achieved 6-TG levels comparable to those of 6-MP, although name brand azathioprine (Imuran) gave higher 6-TG levels than the generic drug.[164] In adults with Crohn disease, high-dose intravenous azathioprine is reported to shorten the time to remission.[165] A case series reporting azathioprine use in children with steroid-refractory inflammatory bowel disease identified a response rate of 75%.[166]

Few controlled trials have been performed to evaluate the efficacy of 6-MP or azathioprine in ulcerative colitis. Roughly 60% of patients with ulcerative colitis refractory to steroid tapering demonstrate an apparent clinical response to 6-MP (as defined by both improvement in clinical symptoms and a decrease in steroid dosage).[167] Another study reported a comparable response rate to 6-MP in children with ulcerative colitis.[168] 6-MP and azathioprine maintenance therapy may be particularly useful following treatment of severe colitis with cyclosporine.[118] A small case series of three children suggested that intravenous azathioprine can be effective as primary therapy for fulminant colitis.[169] It is unclear whether therapy with immunosuppressive agents such as 6-MP and azathioprine increases the risk of colon cancer in children with ulcerative colitis. However, for some patients, such therapy is beneficial and can allow the children and the family to psychologically prepare themselves for colectomy.

Liver Disease. Azathioprine is used in liver transplant patients in conjunction with cyclosporine and prednisone (triple-drug immunosuppression); the usual dose used is 1 to 2 mg/kg/d. Azathioprine is not effective in treating acute rejection. The use of azathioprine and the duration of therapy varies with individual transplant centers; some centers discontinue use of the drug within a year of transplant.[170] A retrospective study by van Hoek and colleagues found that patients receiving azathioprine were less likely to develop ductopenic rejection and vanishing bile duct syndrome, 14 of 66 patients (21%) without azathioprine, compared with 1 of 98 patients (1%) receiving 2 mg/kg/d of azathioprine.[171]

Complicating the use of azathioprine in liver transplant recipients is the occasional development of azathioprine-induced hepatotoxicity, including cholestasis, peliosis hepatis, nodular regenerative hyperplasia, and veno-occlusive disease. Withdrawal of azathioprine in patients with azathioprine-associated induced hepatitis generally results in an improvement of liver enzyme tests within a week.[172]

Azathioprine also has been widely used in the treatment of steroid-refractory autoimmune chronic active hepatitis.[173] Traditionally, the therapy of this entity involved high-dose steroid therapy with a slow steroid taper. However,

many patients relapse once the steroid dose is tapered. Chronic active hepatitis can be kept in prolonged remission if patients continue to take azathioprine.[75] Thus, a commonly used alternative to prednisone as monotherapy for AIH involves the addition of 50 mg, or more, of azathioprine as a maintenance agent. In adults who relapse on low-dose azathioprine, the dose may be increased up to 150 mg/d.[72] Since up to 80 to 90% of children with autoimmune chronic active hepatitis relapse once corticosteroids are tapered, azathioprine is useful in the treatment of pediatric type I and type II AIH. The addition of azathioprine will also decrease the long-term toxicities and growth-impairing effects of chronic corticosteroid therapy in childhood.

METHOTREXATE

In 1948, methotrexate was used by Sidney Farber to treat pediatric leukemia. Since then, it has been discovered that lower doses of this drug could also be used to treat autoimmune diseases such as psoriasis, PSC, and primary biliary cirrhosis (PBC). In 1989, the first open trial using methotrexate in patients with refractory inflammatory bowel disease was conducted.

Mechanism of Action. Methotrexate is an inhibitor of the enzyme dihydrofolate reductase and decreases the synthesis of the reducing agent tetrahydrofolate. Tetrahydrofolate is essential in the synthesis of thymidylate, a pyrimidine nucleoside required for DNA synthesis. At high doses, methotrexate inhibits DNA synthesis and is cytotoxic to rapidly proliferating cells. At low dosages, however, methotrexate has no cytotoxic or antiproliferative effects. Instead, methotrexate polyglutamates increase intra- and extracellular levels of adenosine by indirectly inhibiting adenosine deaminase. In neutrophils, this effect leads to a diminished oxidative burst, decreased adhesion to endothelial cells, and decreased production of leukotriene B_4 and TNF-α. In monocytes and macrophages, adenosine inhibits expression of TNF-α, IL-6, and IL-8 and promotes transcription of the anti-inflammatory agents IL-10 and IL-1 receptor antagonist.[174,175]

Pharmacology. Methotrexate can be administered orally, subcutaneously, intramuscularly, or intravenously. The enteral bioavailability varies widely between 45 and 100%.[176] Although oral methotrexate generally has good bioavailability at doses < 15 mg, higher doses can result in poorer absorption. Therefore, high-dose methotrexate is traditionally administered parenterally. The steady-state volume of distribution is approximately 1 L/kg. Although methotrexate undergoes 7-hydroxylation in the liver, the bulk of its excretion (80–90%) occurs in the urine. Less than 10% of methotrexate is excreted into the bile, and there is essentially no extrahepatic circulation. Methotrexate has a biphasic half-life, with the initial phase being 1.5 to 3.5 hours and the terminal half-life 8 to 15 hours.[177] The half-life is increased in patients with renal failure. There is evidence that certain other chemotherapeutic agents, such as cytarabine, lower red blood cell methotrexate levels, but it is unclear whether lower blood levels decrease drug efficacy because methotrexate levels are not routinely monitored.[178]

Adverse Effects and Toxicity. The most common side effects of methotrexate include anorexia, nausea, stomatitis, diarrhea, hepatitis, renal toxicity, bone marrow suppression, opportunistic infections, and, possibly, neoplasm. Severe toxicity usually occurs when high-dose methotrexate is given to treat hematologic malignancies. If leucovorin rescue is not given to patients undergoing high-dose methotrexate therapy, the consequences can be fatal. For autoimmune diseases, however, far lower doses are used, and the primary toxicity of concern has been hepatic fibrosis.[179]

Several studies in patients with rheumatoid arthritis or psoriasis receiving low-dose methotrexate suggest that over a period of years, fatty change in the liver, hepatic lobular necrosis, fibrosis, and cirrhosis rarely occur. As the use of methotrexate has increased, it has become evident that clinically serious liver disease is far less common in patients with rheumatoid arthritis compared with those with psoriasis. Therefore, the recommendations for monitoring by the American College of Rheumatology differ from those of the American Association of Dermatology, with pretreatment liver biopsy recommended only if there is prior excessive alcohol consumption, chronic hepatitis B or C infection, or persistently abnormal baseline aspartate aminotransferase (AST). During therapy, serum AST, ALT, and albumin are monitored at 4- to 8-week intervals. Subsequent liver biopsy is recommended only if the AST is abnormal in 5 of 9 determinations within a 12-month period (6 of 12 determinations if tests are obtained monthly) or if the serum albumin is below normal.[180] Because there is a lack of correlation between liver function abnormalities and liver histology in patients with psoriasis, some physicians still suggest that a liver biopsy be performed after each cumulative dose of 1 to 1.5 g of methotrexate.[181] The effects of methotrexate on liver histology may be formally classified using published criteria.[181]

Until recently, few data regarding hepatotoxicity in patients receiving methotrexate for inflammatory bowel disease have been available.[182] In a study of 32 patients with inflammatory bowel disease receiving a cumulative methotrexate dose of $\geq$ 1,500 mg, liver chemistry tests were obtained before and during therapy. Twenty patients underwent liver biopsies and had little hepatoxicity despite cumulative doses up to 5.4 g. Although the majority of biopsied patients had mild to moderate steatosis or portal tract inflammation, only one had evidence of fibrosis.[183] In a recent review, it was recommended that liver function tests be checked every 3 months in patients with inflammatory bowel disease receiving methotrexate. If there is an elevation of transaminases, they should be checked monthly. If they are elevated on three consecutive tests or are > 120 IU/L on any one occasion, methotrexate should be stopped or a liver biopsy performed. Some still suggest that surveillance biopsies be considered after 1.5 g of methotrexate or 2 years after starting treatment, whichever is sooner.[184]

Guidelines for biopsy in children are not well established. In one study, 33 children with juvenile rheumatoid arthritis receiving methotrexate (duration of therapy 17–140 months) underwent liver biopsy; 18% had histologic changes, including hepatocellular inflammation or

mild fibrosis. In this study, elevated AST or ALT was the best predictor of histologic abnormalities.[185]

In addition to hepatotoxicity, hypersensitivity pneumonitis is a rare but potentially life-threatening event that occurs in < 1% of patients on methotrexate. The onset of fever, cough, shortness of breath, tachypnea, or hypoxia should prompt further evaluation with a chest radiograph and formal pulmonary function testing, and the methotrexate should be discontinued.[186] There have also been case reports of patients on low-dose methotrexate having an increased susceptibility to opportunistic infections, including herpes zoster and *Pneumocystis carinii*. Therefore, although methotrexate is considered to be a less potent immunosuppressive agent than cyclosporine or tacrolimus, the risk of opportunistic infection is still present.

Clinical Uses. In 1989, Kozarek and colleagues used parenteral methotrexate to treat 21 patients with steroid-refractory ulcerative colitis and Crohn disease. Sixteen of 21 subjects had clinical and endoscopic improvement with decreased diarrhea, lowering of the corticosteroid dose, and improvement in disease activity index parameters.[187] Subsequently, the same investigators demonstrated, in an open-label trial, that patients who failed 6-MP or azathioprine therapy could respond to parenteral methotrexate. Further follow-up studies suggest that Crohn disease patients can be maintained in remission with methotrexate, whereas ulcerative colitis patients tend to relapse and require colectomy.[187]

In 1995, Feagan and colleagues conducted a large multicenter trial of intramuscular methotrexate (25 mg weekly) for active Crohn disease. Methotrexate was more effective than placebo in achieving remission (39% vs 19%, respectively) and reducing requirements for prednisone.[188,189] A subsequent multicenter study was conducted to determine the use of methotrexate in the maintenance of remission in Crohn disease. Patients with chronically active Crohn disease who had entered remission after 16 to 24 weeks of treatment with 25 mg intramuscular methotrexate once weekly were included in this study. At week 40, 65% of the methotrexate-treated patients were in remission compared with 39% who received placebo (p = .01). Less than 50% of the patients in the methotrexate group had relapsed by the end of the 40 weeks. In addition, fewer patients in the methotrexate group required prednisone for relapse compared with the placebo group (28% vs 58%; p = .01). Although nausea and vomiting occurred more frequently among patients receiving methotrexate, none had a severe adverse event. Therefore, patients with Crohn disease can achieve remission with methotrexate therapy, and a low dose is effective in maintaining remission.[190]

In children, Mack and colleagues conducted an open-label trial of methotrexate (15 mg/m^2/wk subcutaneously) in 14 patients with inflammatory bowel disease who had failed 6-MP therapy. After 3 months of therapy, seven patients had inactive Pediatric Crohn's Disease Activity Index (P-CDAI) scores, six still had active P-CDAI scores, and one patient died (most likely unrelated to the methotrexate).[191]

Methotrexate also has been used to treat PBC and PSC. However, studies of methotrexate efficacy in the treatment of PBC have given conflicting results.[192–194]

In a randomized double-blind trial involving 24 patients with PSC, those on methotrexate had lowering of alkaline phosphatase levels but no improvement of liver histology. However, these patients had advanced liver disease, with 50% having cirrhosis at the start of therapy.[195] In another study of 19 patients with PSC, the use of methotrexate, in combination with ursodeoxycholic acid (UDCA), was associated with toxicity without further improvement in liver biochemistries compared with UDCA alone.[196] Therefore, there is little evidence that methotrexate is of benefit in the treatment of PBC or PSC.

MYCOPHENOLATE MOFETIL (CELLCEPT)

Mycophenolate mofetil (MMF) is an antiproliferative agent that inhibits lymphocyte DNA synthesis and that was given FDA approval in 1995 for the treatment of renal transplant rejection. The drug is now undergoing widespread use in renal, heart, and liver transplant recipients and has been preliminarily studied in inflammatory bowel disease.

Mechanism of Action. MMF is an ester prodrug of the immunosuppressant mycophenolic acid. MMF inhibits lymphocyte proliferation by blocking the de novo synthesis of guanosine nucleotides from inosine via reversible inhibition of the enzyme inosine monophosphate dehydrogenase (IMPDH). Mycophenolic acid is a more potent inhibitor of the type II isoform of IMPDH, which is found in activated lymphocytes, as opposed to the type I isoform, which is expressed in most cell types.[197] Unlike other cell types that can use a salvage pathway for synthesis of guanosine, B and T lymphocytes are dependent on the de novo pathway for generation of guanosine. The effects of this drug are wide ranging and include inhibition of cytotoxicity by T lymphocytes and the inhibition of antibody production by B cells. In vitro, MMF inhibits DNA synthesis and the proliferation of peripheral blood lymphocytes in response to both T- and B-cell mitogens. In addition, MMF alters cell adhesion and decreases the recruitment of inflammatory cells into target tissues by inhibiting glycosylation of adhesion molecules.[198]

Pharmacokinetics. Oral MMF is generally well absorbed, even though intake with food will decrease absorption. The volume of distribution is approximately 3.6 L/kg in healthy adults. In the body, MMF is rapidly converted to mycophenolic acid, the active metabolite. Enterohepatic cycling contributes about 40% to the AUC of mycophenolic acid.[199] Elimination of mycophenolic acid involves glucuronidation by the liver, with renal elimination of more than 90% of the glucuronidated compound and fecal excretion of the remainder. The half-life of the mycophenolic acid is approximately 18 hours in adults. Patients with renal failure ($Cr_{Cl} < 25$ mL/min) have an increased AUC and a prolonged half-life. In children, AUC increases with increasing age, suggesting that young children metabolize the drug more rapidly.[198,200] Most studies in adults agree that therapeutic drug monitoring can help to avoid adverse effects and optimize immunosuppression. There is increasing evidence that children may benefit from the same monitoring, particularly in the early postoperative period. A trough of 2 to 5 mg/L and an average AUC_{12} of 59 mg/L/h, corresponding to 50% inhibition of IMPDH, is proposed to be sufficient for immunosuppression.[199]

Adverse Effects. The principal side effects of MMF are gastrointestinal and hematologic. Gastrointestinal side effects, including diarrhea, constipation, nausea, dyspepsia, vomiting, esophagitis, and ulcers, occur in up to 30% of patients. Severe neutropenia may occur in up to 2% of patients receiving MMF. Anemia, thrombocytopenia, and leukopenia also occur in 10 to 25% of patients, a rate comparable to that seen with azathioprine.[198] Opportunistic infections (including cytomegalovirus, herpes zoster, and herpes simplex infections) and malignancies (including lymphoproliferative disease and lymphoma) also occur in transplant patients treated with MMF.

Clinical Use. MMF was first studied as a supplemental antirejection medication in renal transplant patients. In a multicenter trial, MMF at doses of 2 or 3 g/d combined with cyclosporine and steroids reduced the incidence of acute rejection to 31% compared with 47% in patients receiving azathioprine.[201] Multiple studies in liver transplant patients also suggest that MMF can provide effective rescue therapy in patients who develop chronic rejection.[202] In one study, 12 of 19 patients who had failed treatment with azathioprine, prednisone, and cyclosporine had complete histologic resolution of rejection when converted from azathioprine to MMF (from 0.25 to 2 g twice a day).[203]

In a study using MMF as part of induction therapy, 350 liver transplant patients were randomized to receive either double-drug therapy (tacrolimus and steroids) or triple-drug therapy (tacrolimus, steroids, and MMF 1 g twice a day). Patients in the double-drug arm who developed acute rejection received MMF as rescue therapy. The rate of rejection was significantly lower at 3 months in the group that received triple-drug therapy ($p < .03$). However, there was no difference in the overall rejection rate or graft survival at the end of follow-up (mean 33.8 ± 9.1 months). This study suggests that MMF does not need to be started immediately post-transplant but can be added to the drug regimen if rejection develops.[202,204] In a prospective study comparing the efficacy of MMF versus azathioprine in 63 liver transplant patients, who also received thymoglobulin and methylprednisolone, there was a trend toward a lower incidence of acute rejection in the MMF group ($p = .06$). There was, however, a decreased rate of thrombocytopenia in patients who received MMF compared with those who received azathioprine (19% vs 47%, respectively).[205] In a pediatric series of 26 patients, MMF (10–12.5 mg/kg/dose twice a day), the combination of microemulsion cyclosporine and prednisone, was found to be effective primary antirejection therapy, with only 20% of patients needing conversion to tacrolimus for persistent rejection.[206]

MMF also has been used as adjunctive therapy in adults with Crohn disease with variable success.[207,208] In one open-label trial involving six patients with refractory perianal or ileal Crohn disease unresponsive to azathio-prine, patients were given 1 g twice a day of MMF. All six patients improved, and four entered full remission.[207] A larger randomized trial involving 70 patients used MMF or azathioprine as a steroid-sparing agent. Response rates, tol-erability, and side effects were comparable in both arms of the trial.[208] In an open-label trial, 11 patients with Crohn disease and 13 with ulcerative colitis were treated with MMF 2 g/d and prednisone (starting dose of 60 mg/d fol-lowed by a taper of 5 mg/wk to reach a final dose of 5 mg/d). Four patients with Crohn disease and six with ulcerative colitis achieved remission at 3 months. How-ever, remission was maintained in only one Crohn disease patient at the end of the 6-month study.[209]

A pilot study comparing MMF versus azathioprine in 24 patients with active ulcerative colitis found that 42% (5 of 12) of patients who received MMF and prednisolone achieved remission in the first 4 weeks and remained in remission at 1 year. When compared with the azathioprine and prednisone group, however, the rates of remission were lower, the number of relapses higher, and the number of patients weaned off steroids lower. Current data suggest that in inflammatory bowel disease, MMF should only be used as a rescue therapy if more conventional immunomod-ulatory agents (eg, 6-MP, azathioprine, methotrexate, inflix-imab) are ineffective or not tolerated.[210]

Although the frequency of intestinal transplant is increas-ing, there still are limited data regarding the use of MMF in this setting. In one center's experience with 77 intestinal transplant patients, there did not appear to be improved graft survival with MMF compared with three other treatment arms. In addition, it was noted that patients who received MMF tended to have a higher incidence of graft-versus-host disease and post-transplant lymphoproliferative disease com-pared with the other treatment regimens.[211]

SIROLIMUS (RAPAMYCIN, RAPAMUNE)

Sirolimus is a hydrophobic macrocyclic lactone produced by *Streptomyces hygroscopicus*. Although structurally simi-lar to tacrolimus, the mechanism of action and adverse effect profiles of the two drugs are quite different. Sirolimus is a potent immunosuppressive drug that has been used in renal transplant and is being increasingly studied in liver transplant as well.

Mechanism of Action. Sirolimus, like tacrolimus, read-ily penetrates the plasma membrane and binds to FKBP12. Whereas tacrolimus blocks cytokine gene transcription by binding calcineurin, the sirolimus-FKBP12 complex binds to a specific cell-cycle regulatory protein, mammalian target of rapamycin (mTOR). This binding to mTOR then leads to suppression of cytokine-driven (IL-2, -4, -7, and -15) T-cell proliferation, interrupted progression from the G_1 to the S phase of the cell cycle, and inhibition of IL synthesis.[212]

Pharmacokinetics. Sirolimus is manufactured as an oral solution and as a tablet, which are bioequivalent in nature. The oral bioavailability is 14%, and there is rapid intestinal absorption. Intake with food and drugs such as cyclosporine, diltiazem, and ketoconazole will increase exposure to

sirolimus. There are interactions with drugs metabolized by cytochrome P-450 3A.[213] More than 90% of drug is excreted in feces, with urine representing only a minor route of elim-ination (2.2%). The mean half-life is 60 hours, but there is significant interpatient variation, particularly in patients with hepatic impairment and in children. For this reason, thera-peutic drug monitoring is recommended.[214]

Adverse Effects. The principal adverse effects associated with sirolimus include hyperlipidemia and bone marrow suppression. Sirolimus raises high-density lipoproteins in serum but also produces much greater elevations of low-density lipoproteins, cholesterol, and triglycerides.[215] Hyperlipidemia occurs in about 40% of renal transplant recipients receiving sirolimus.[214] Bone marrow suppression is reversible and concentration dependent and occurs in 61% of sirolimus-treated patients. Inhibition of critical cytokine signals that promote maturation and proliferation of bone marrow precursors are likely responsible for sirolimus-related myelosuppression. Patients with trough levels $\geq$ 15 ng/mL tend to have an increased risk for lipo-toxicity and myelotoxicity. Other less common adverse effects include diarrhea, epistaxis, noninfectious pneu-monitis, arthralgia, and potentiation of adverse reactions to cyclosporine, namely hypertension, acne, and hir-sutism.[214,215] The incidence of post-transplant lymphopro-liferative disorders in renal transplant patients receiving sirolimus was not significantly different compared with placebo (p = .162).[216]

Clinical Uses. Sirolimus has recently been studied in phase III trials in renal transplant and has been used in liver and small bowel transplant. In a multicenter, double-blind, placebo-controlled trial of 576 renal transplant patients, subjects treated with cyclosporine and corticosteroids were then randomly assigned to receive either placebo or sirolimus at either 2 mg/d or 5 mg/d. The primary compos-ite end point (ie, first occurrence for biopsy-confirmed acute rejection, graft loss, or death) at 6 months post-trans-plant was lower in the sirolimus-treated groups compared with the placebo group. Also, the incidence of biopsy-proven rejection at 12 months was lower in both of the sirolimus groups (2 mg/d and 5 mg/d) compared with the placebo group (24.7% and 19.2% vs 43.3%; $p \leq$ .002).[216]

Flechner and colleagues conducted a prospective ran-domized trial of sirolimus versus cyclosporine in 61 adult primary renal transplant patients treated with basiliximab and MMF.[217] There was no statistically significant difference in the 1-year patient survival, graft survival, and biopsy-confirmed acute rejection rates between the two study arms. At 6 and 12 months, the sirolimus-treated patients had significantly better serum creatinine levels and creati-nine clearances compared with cyclosporine-treated patients. This would suggest that calcineurin inhibitor drug avoidance with sirolimus provides comparable immuno-suppression while diminishing the nephrotoxic side effects.

A pilot study of 15 liver transplant patients suggested that sirolimus reduces the incidence of rejection when added to prednisone and cyclosporine.[217] In a retrospective review of 14 liver transplant patients with renal insufficiency or acute mental status impairment, immunosuppression with MMF, corticosteroids, and sirolimus (dose between 1 and 4 mg/d) was used. Six patients developed acute rejection; however, only one required antilymphocytic therapy. The findings suggest that sirolimus may be an alternative immunosuppressive agent when calcineurin inhibitors are undesirable or contraindicated.[218] In another study, 39 liver transplant patients were treated with either tacrolimus or cyclosporin A and sirolimus (dose 2 mg/d), with a 3-day tapered dose of steroids. Patient and graft survival rates were identical to those of historical controls. The incidence of rejection and muromonab-CD3 use was lower than that of historical controls. These findings suggest that liver transplant may be successfully performed with sirolimus and minimal corticosteroid use.[219]

Florman and colleagues have reported on intestinal transplant patients treated with tacrolimus-based immunosuppression and steroids. In addition, subjects received either sirolimus and basiliximab or daclizumab. There was a decreased incidence of rejection among the sirolimus-treated group both at 30 days ($p < .002$) and at 90 days ($p < .02$). There was no significant difference in actuarial 1-year patient survival or graft survival.[220]

INFLIXIMAB (ANTI-TNF, cA2, REMICADE)

Infliximab is a murine-human chimeric monoclonal antibody directed against TNF-α. Over the past decade, infliximab has been used extensively in the treatment of inflammatory conditions such as rheumatoid arthritis and Crohn disease.

Mechanism of Action. TNF-α is a potent proinflammatory cytokine whose effects are mediated by ligation to the receptors, tumor necrosis factor receptor (TNFR)-I and TNFR-II. In addition, both monocytes and lymphocytes express a membrane-bound form of TNF-α that is thought to activate other cells by direct cell-cell contact. When bound to soluble TNF-α, infliximab is able to neutralize its effects, preventing release of other cytokines, such as IL-6.[221] When bound to the membrane-bound form of TNF-α, infliximab is able to fix complement and mediate destruction of TNF-α–producing cells such as T lymphocytes and is thereby able to induce apoptosis of macrophages.[222,223]

Pharmacokinetics. Infliximab is administered as an intravenous infusion, usually given over 2 hours. Recommended adult dosing is as follows:

1. Fistulizing Crohn disease: 5 mg/kg given at weeks 0, 2, and 6

2. Moderate to severe Crohn disease, induction: 5 mg/kg given at weeks 0, 2, and 6

3. Moderate to severe Crohn disease, maintenance: 5 mg/kg every 8 weeks

Infliximab is distributed primarily within the vascular compartment. Serum concentrations of infliximab may be detected up to 8 to 12 weeks after infusion.[224]

Adverse Effects. Infusion reactions are a well-described complication of infliximab therapy, occurring in 4 to 13% of adult patients (Table 76.1-8). Reactions may be immediate or delayed and range in degree from a mild reaction to anaphylaxis. Typical immediate reactions include flushed sensation, shortness of breath, dizziness, hypotension, hives, nausea, vomiting, rash, and numbness. Delayed reactions include joint pain or swelling, rash, and fever. For immediate reactions, patients generally respond to a decreased rate of infusion. Occasionally, however, diphenhydramine or even epinephrine may be required.[225]

Other adverse effects include a risk for reactivation of tuberculosis (TB), development of autoantibodies, risk for infection, and risk of malignancy. Between 1998 and 2002, 101 cases of TB were reported in patients receiving infliximab.[226] Current recommendations include screening for TB prior to the initiation of infliximab therapy.

In the ACCENT I trial of 573 patients with Crohn disease receiving infliximab as a maintenance therapy, 32% had infections (most commonly, upper respiratory tract and urinary tract infections) requiring treatment. More serious infections occurred in 4% of patients.[227]

The development of antinuclear antibodies (ANAs) and rare cases of lupus-like syndrome have been reported. A recent report of 125 patients with Crohn disease receiving infliximab found that 56.8% of patients have developed a positive ANA (titer > 1:40) during treatment. To date, two patients developed symptoms, which resolved after the cessation of therapy.[228] The clinical implication of an elevated ANA in the absence of symptoms has yet to be determined. Eight cases of lymphoma, occurring a median of 6 weeks after initiation of the infliximab treatment, were reported to the FDA between May 1999 and December 2000. There are insufficient data to determine if infliximab directly contributed to the development of the malignancy.[229]

Clinical Use. Infliximab was first used for Crohn disease in 1993.[230] Since then, it has been employed in the treatment of adults with moderate to severe Crohn disease and/or fis-

TABLE 76.1-8	ADVERSE EFFECTS REPORTED IN INFLAMMATORY BOWEL DISEASE AND RHEUMATOID ARTHRITIS PATIENTS TREATED WITH INFLIXIMAB
Infusion reactions	Chest pain, dyspnea, vomiting, urticaria, anaphylaxis
Immune-mediated reactions	Aseptic meningitis
	Antinuclear antibodies and lupus-like syndrome
	Adult respiratory distress syndrome
Opportunistic infections	Tuberculosis, histoplasmosis, *Salmonella*, *Listeria*, *Cryptococcus*, cytomegalovirus, aspergillosis
Hematologic	Neutropenia, thrombocytopenia
Other	Headache, nausea, upper respiratory infection, pharyngitis, sinusitis

Adapted from Cunnane G et al,[275] Cheifetz A et al,[276] Lee JH et al,[277] and Lipsky PE et al.[278]

tulizing disease with inadequate response to more conventional therapies. In a retrospective review of 19 pediatric children with Crohn disease who received one to three infusions of infliximab at a dose of 5 mg/kg over a 12-week period, there was a reduction in the P-CDAI in all patients.[231] In a prospective open-label trial of a single 5 mg/kg infusion of infliximab in 15 children with medically refractory Crohn disease, 14 of 15 (94%) had a decrease of both P-CDAI and daily steroid use. Ten patients (67%) achieved complete remission by 10 weeks.[232] In a multicenter, open-label, dose-blinded trial, 21 pediatric patients received a single infusion of infliximab at a dose of 1, 5, or 10 mg/kg. Improvement in the P-CDAI was observed with all infliximab dosages (median improvement 50%). All achieved clinical response, and 10 of 21 (48%) achieved clinical remission. Adverse events included upper respiratory tract infection, pancreatitis, sinusitis, and appendicitis.[224]

Although infliximab has been effective in inducing clinical response and remission after a single infusion, the benefit of infliximab as maintenance therapy is not as well established. In a multicenter randomized controlled trial of 573 adults with active Crohn disease, subjects received an initial 5 mg/kg infusion and then were randomized to receive repeat infusions of placebo or 5 or 10 mg/kg of infliximab at 8-week intervals. Patients receiving infliximab as maintenance infusions were more likely to maintain remission and to discontinue steroids compared with those who received placebo. However, a cautionary note is highlighted by two patients who died from sepsis.[227]

Randomized trials have not yet established efficacy of infliximab in ulcerative colitis. Nonetheless, initial studies suggest that infliximab may be effective in the treatment of this disease. A double-blind placebo-controlled trial of infliximab conducted in 11 patients with severe, active, steroid-refractory ulcerative colitis was terminated early because of slow enrolment. Nevertheless, 4 of 8 patients who received infliximab were considered treatment successes compared with none of the 3 receiving placebo.[233] In another study, eight patients with refractory ulcerative colitis scheduled for surgical colectomy were treated with a single 5 mg/kg infusion of infliximab. All patients experienced marked improvement in clinical symptoms, colonoscopic findings, and histopathology.[234] Nine children with moderate to severe ulcerative colitis unresponsive to conventional therapies were treated with infliximab infusions. Seven (77%) patients had improvement in activity of their disease at a median follow-up of 20 weeks.[235]

The formation of antibodies to infliximab (ATI) is associated with an increased risk of infusion reactions and diminished efficacy of repeated infusions. The use of concurrent immunosuppressants and the administration of a second infusion of infliximab within 8 weeks of the first both reduce ATI formation.[236] In a cohort of 125 patients with Crohn disease treated with infliximab, ATI were detected in 61% of patients. The presence of antibody was associated with an increased risk of infusion reactions and a reduced duration of response to treatment.[237] Another study found that 19 of 53 patients (36%) developed ATI. Loss of initial response and incidence of infusion reactions were strongly related to ATI formation. Following this finding, 80 patients were randomized to receive intravenous hydrocortisone 200 mg or placebo prior to infusions of infliximab. At week 16, whereas ATI levels were lower among hydrocortisone-treated patients (1.6 vs 3.4 µg/mL, $p = .02$), there was no reduction in infusion reactions.

ANTILYMPHOCYTE ANTIBODY PREPARATION: MUROMONAB-CD3 (ORTHOCLONE, OKT3, MONOCLONAL ANTI-CD3)

Polyclonal antisera to human T cells (antilymphocyte globulins) were developed in the 1970s for the treatment of organ rejection and hematologic malignancies. However, such preparations were variable in their potency (because they were prepared by generating immune responses in vivo in animals) and contained extraneous antibodies. Muromonab-CD3 is a purified monoclonal IgG2a antibody obtained from murine ascites directed against the CD3 antigen on human T lymphocytes. Treatment with muromonab CD3 results in the short-term depletion of systemic T lymphocytes and a dramatic inhibition of lymphocyte cytotoxic reactions. This drug is now accepted therapy for the treatment of acute cellular graft rejection.

Mechanism of Action. Muromonab-CD3 binds to virtually all differentiated human T lymphocytes through the CD3 molecule. The CD3 complex is essential for signal transduction between the TCR and the intracellular kinases, resulting in T-lymphocyte activation. In vitro effects of anti-CD3 are complex; anti-CD3 can cause polyclonal T-lymphocyte activation, but only when a second signal (such as phorbol myristate acetate or a monocyte–T-cell interaction) is delivered in addition to the anti-CD3. In vivo, however, muromonab anti-CD3 opsonizes T cells; the coated T cells are subsequently removed by cells of the reticuloendothelial system or lysed by complement. Within 1 hour of muromonab-CD3 administration, CD3+ T lymphocytes are cleared from the systemic circulation.[238]

Pharmacologic Aspects. Muromonab-CD3 must be given intravenously to prevent degradation. Goldstein and colleagues demonstrated in adult renal transplant recipients treated for rejection that a once-daily dose of 5 mg maintains a steady-state level of 800 to 1,000 µg/L, a level adequate to block cytotoxic T-cell function and facilitate T-cell clearance.[239] Cessation of treatment results in a rapid return of peripheral blood CD3 T cells, which reach normal levels within a few days. Therefore, muromonab-CD3 must be administered for 10 to 14 days to have a sustained effect. Alloway and colleagues demonstrated that a lower dose of muromonab-CD3 (2 mg daily) as prophylactic therapy for rejection of renal allografts is as efficacious as the higher (5 mg) dose.[240] Dosage for smaller pediatric recipients is 2.5 mg/d (weight < 30 kg) and 5 mg/d for those with body weight > 30 kg.[241]

Adverse Effects. The adverse effects of muromonab-CD3 require that the first few doses be given in hospital and currently limit this therapy to transplant recipients

(Table 76.1-9). The administration of muromonab-CD3 is associated with a variety of adverse effects known as the cytokine release syndrome. This occurs as a result of the systemic release of cytokines (including TNF-α and IFN-γ) by activated or lysed T lymphocytes.[242] Symptoms generally include fever, chills, shortness of breath, nausea, vomiting, diarrhea, headaches, and myalgias. Less commonly, patients experience wheezing, thrombocytopenia, hypertension, and rash.[238] More serious, and rarer, complications of muromonab-CD3 include pulmonary edema (which generally develops in patients with fluid overload) and aseptic meningitis.[238]

Long-term side effects include overwhelming infection with conventional and opportunistic pathogens (particularly herpes simplex virus and cytomegalovirus).[243,244] In addition, treatment with anti-CD3 places transplant patients at increased risk for the development of lymphoproliferative disease or other hematologic malignancies.[245]

Clinical Use. Pediatric gastroenterologists use muromonab-CD3 almost exclusively in the treatment of liver transplant recipients. Currently, muromonab-CD3 is used to treat episodes of acute rejection usually after courses of high-dose steroid therapy have failed. The drug also is useful in patients who have renal dysfunction, which limits the use of cyclosporine.[243]

Treatment of acute rejection with muromonab-CD3 reverses rejection up to 70 to 80% of cases in adult series and improves allograft survival.[246] A randomized trial found muromonab-CD3 better than high-dose steroids (73% vs 23% response rate) in treating the first episode of rejection following liver transplant.[247] However, a large pediatric study using muromonab-CD3 to treat liver transplant rejection reported a success rate in treating rejection of only 59%. In addition, the majority of patients still had greater than 5% CD3+ cells in their peripheral blood during therapy. The investigators concluded that pediatric patients may be less responsive to muromonab-CD3 than are adults.[243]

Administration of a second course of muromonab-CD3 is less effective than the initial course of therapy owing to the development of anti-idiotype antibodies, which inactivate the molecule. Antibody production can be measured, however, and patients who develop only low-titer antibodies after the first course of muromonab-CD3 may be successfully treated with a second course.[238,248] Muromonab-CD3 also has been used as prophylaxis in the immediate postoperative period following liver transplant.

Although clearly effective in prevention of rejection, muronomab does not appear to offer any demonstrable benefit over conventional immunosuppression (calcineurin inhibitor, azathioprine, and prednisone). The cost and future risks of opportunistic infections and malignancy limit its use.[249]

IL-2 RECEPTOR ANTIBODIES

Another target for monoclonal antibodies is the IL-2 receptor (IL-2R). T cells involved in acute rejection are characterized by increased expression of activation markers such as IL-2R. The IL-2R is composed of three chains (a 55 kD

TABLE 76.1-9   ADVERSE EFFECTS OF MUROMONAB-CD3 (OKT3)

"First-dose syndrome": > 50% of patients
Fever
Chills
Tremor
Dyspnea
Wheezing
Nausea/vomiting
Diarrhea
Rash
Joint pain
Tachycardia, hypertension (rare)
Pulmonary edema (rare)
Aseptic meningitis
Interstitial nephritis
Infections (especially cytomegalovirus, adenovirus, herpes simplex)
Lymphoproliferative disease

Adapted from Todd P and Brogden R,[238] McDiarmid S et al,[243] and Fung J and Starzl T.[249]

α chain, a 75 kD β chain, and a 64 kD γ chain) and is present on activated T cells. Binding of IL-2 to IL-2R results in T-cell proliferation and clonal expansion of activated T lymphocytes. Anti–IL-2R antibodies (antibodies to the α chain of the IL-2R) are designed to provide greater selectivity against only those lymphocytes directly involved in the immune response because resting T lymphocytes express low levels of the IL-2R.

IL-2R antibodies were initially developed for use in induction protocols for renal transplant patients. There have been good results in this setting, with a decreased incidence of acute rejection and minimal side effects. More recently, use has been applied to the prophylaxis of acute rejection in liver transplant patients. Two antibodies are now commercially available, both of which contain the hypervariable regions of the murine anti–IL-2R antibody (anti-Tac) involved in binding the α subunit. The main differences between the two are the half-life, the proportion of murine to human sequences, and the affinity to its target.[250]

Daclizumab (Zenapax). In a study by Koch and colleagues, the pharmacokinetics and pharmacodynamics of daclizumab in liver transplant patients were investigated. Patients were given daclizumab at a dose of 1 mg/kg within 6 hours of graft reperfusion on day 0 and then a dose of 0.5 mg/kg on day 4 following transplant. This dosing regimen provided effective blockade of the IL-2Rα for at least 14 days after transplant. CD25+ cells are decreased for 28 days following administration of daclizumab. Whereas the half-life of daclizumab in renal transplant patients is 273 hours, in liver transplant patients, it is significantly shorter (99 hours). Drug clearance through drained ascites, postoperative blood loss, or loss of antibody into intercellular and extravascular spaces may account for this difference. To date, no human antibody responses against daclizumab have been reported.[250]

An initial study by Hirose and colleagues investigated the use of daclizumab (1 mg/kg on day 0 then at 2-week intervals for a total of five doses) as part of an induction therapy with mycophenolate and corticosteroids but without calcineurin inhibitors. Treatment with daclizumab in the absence of calcineurin inhibitors was ineffective, with a 100% acute rejection rate. One possible explanation was inadequate dosing of daclizumab.[251] In a subsequent study of 39 adult liver transplant patients, daclizumab was used as adjunctive therapy to an induction regimen of corticosteroids and cyclosporine or tacrolimus. The daclizumab group experienced less acute rejection (18% vs 40%; $p = .02$) in the first 6 months compared with the control group.[252] Heffron and colleagues conducted an open-label prospective study of daclizumab in pediatric liver transplant recipients. Twenty patients received a single dose of daclizumab (1 mg/kg) within 24 hours after liver transplant, and tacrolimus was withheld for 7 days following surgery. A historical control group of patients who received tacrolimus immediately following tranplant was used for comparison. Both groups of children also received mycophenolate and corticosteroids. There were fewer episodes of acute rejection in the daclizumab-treated group compared with historical controls ($p = .002$).[253]

Basiliximab (Simulect). In comparison with daclizumab, basiliximab has a shorter half-life (approximately 6.5 days in renal transplant patients) and is less humanized but has a higher affinity for IL-2Rα. The role of basiliximab in liver transplant is still being developed. In a multicenter randomized controlled trial, 381 adult liver transplant patients received basiliximab 20 mg on days 0 and 4 in addition to cyclosporine and corticosteroids. There was a decreased acute rejection rate in patients receiving basiliximab (33.1% vs 47.6%; $p = .034$).[254] In a smaller study, seven pediatric liver transplant recipients with steroid-resistant rejection received one or two doses of basiliximab (10 mg for patients < 30 kg, 20 mg for patients > 30 kg; doses were given 3 to 7 days apart). Primary antirejection therapy consisted of cyclosporine, azathioprine, and prednisolone in four patients and tacrolimus and prednisolone in three others. All had received high-dose steroids for acute rejection and were converted to tacrolimus, followed by the addition of mycophenolate. Five of the patients had improvement, as measured by biochemical responses and by liver biopsy. There were no immediate side effects associated with basiliximab. However, two children went on to develop chronic rejection and subsequently died.[255]

OTHER AGENTS

LEFLUNOMIDE (ARAVA)

Leflunomide is a relatively new immunosuppressive agent that inhibits dihydroorotate dehydrogenase.[256] It is an isoxazole derivative that is converted by first-pass metabolism in the liver and gut to an active metabolite, A77 1726, which inhibits de novo synthesis of pyrimidines.[257] In addition, leflunomide also inhibits lymphocyte activation by blocking intracellular tyrosine kinases.[258] In rat xenograft models, leflunomide is effective antirejection therapy.[259] More recently, the active metabolite of leflunomide was shown to halt the replication of herpes viruses, particularly cytomegalovirus and herpes simplex virus.[260]

In 1998, leflunomide was approved in the United States for the treatment of rheumatoid arthritis. A 2-year double-blind randomized controlled trial compared the efficacy of leflunomide versus methotrexate in 235 patients with rheumatoid arthritis. The results demonstrated that leflunomide is safe and equally effective treatment for active rheumatoid arthritis compared with methotrexate. Adverse effects reported include upper respiratory tract infections, diarrhea, nausea and vomiting, rash, reversible alopecia, and transient elevations in liver enzymes.[261]

Efficacy trials have not yet been reported in human transplant recipients. One study by Williams and colleagues, however, reports experience with leflunomide in both renal and liver transplant patients with regard to pharmacologic properties. There was marked interpatient variability (> 300%) in the dose required to reach a targeted serum level. The terminal half-life also varied between 5.2 and 15.1 days. In renal transplant patients, the principal side effect observed was anemia, and in those with liver transplants, there were elevations of serum transaminases.[262]

THALIDOMIDE (THALOMID)

Thalidomide (α-N-phthalimidoglutarimide) is a glutamic acid derivative with multiple biologic properties. It is a sedative, a teratogen, an inhibitor of angiogenesis, and an inhibitor of TNF-α production.[263] A number of open-label trials purport that thalidomide is efficacious in a variety of autoimmune and intestinal conditions, including erythema nodosum, aphthous stomatitis, Behçet syndrome, human immunodeficiency virus (HIV)-associated mucosal ulceration, and graft-versus-host disease.[263] Open-label trials also suggest that up to 50% of patients with Crohn disease refractory to other therapies will respond to thalidomide. The drug is typically started at a dose of 50 mg in adults and advanced as high as 200 mg, with clinical improvement usually occurring about 4 to 6 weeks after instituting therapy.[263,264] The primary side effect of thalidomide is neurotoxicity. In addition, the drug is contraindicated in women of childbearing age because of severe limb deformities (phocomelia) in the fetus. Because of the toxicities, this agent should be used with caution in patients with intestinal inflammation.[265,266]

ETANERCEPT (ENBREL)

Etanercept is a genetically engineered fusion protein composed of two identical chains of the recombinant human TNFR p75 monomer that is fused to the Fc domain of human IgG1. This protein binds to and inactivates TNF and lymphotoxin, a cytokine that activates lymphocytes. One of the potential benefits of etanercept is that it does not contain nonhuman material, thereby rendering it less immunogenic. There is extensive clinical experience in the treatment of rheumatoid arthritis with etanercept. More recently, its use in the treatment of refractory Crohn disease also has been studied. In an open-label trial, 10 patients with active Crohn disease were treated with subcutaneous etanercept (25 mg) twice weekly for 12 weeks. Although there was an improvement in CDAI in 6 of 10 patients ($p < .03$), there was no improvement in follow-up terminal ileal or colonic biopsies. In addition, all patients who initially responded to therapy reported relapse of symptoms within 4 weeks after discontinuation.[267] In a randomized, double-blinded, placebo-controlled trial of 43 patients with moderate to severe Crohn disease, subcutaneous etanercept (25 mg) was administered twice weekly. There was no difference in clinical response at week 4 in patients treated with etanercept compared with placebo (39% vs 45%; $p = .763$). In addition, there was no clear benefit for fistulizing Crohn disease. Common adverse events include injection-site reactions, headache, asthenia, abdominal pain, and skin rash.[268] A report of two patients with Crohn spondyloarthropathy found that although these patients experienced complete resolution of spinal pathology with etanercept, the activity of the Crohn disease did not improve. These findings indicate that binding of TNF alone is not sufficient to ameliorate the inflammatory response in the intestinal mucosa.[269]

NATALIZUMAB (ANTEGREN)

Natalizumab is humanized monoclonal antibody targeted against α_4 integrin. The integrins are a group of heterodimeric proteins composed of noncovalently bound α and β chains that promote cell-cell or cell-matrix adhesion. The α_4 integrins heterodimerize with either α_1 or α_7 subunits. Integrins containing the β_1 subunit are also known as the VLA antigens and are the predominant integrin found on the surface of T lymphocytes. $\alpha_4\beta_1$ (VLA-4) is expressed only on leukocytes and mediates their attachment to endothelial cells via binding to VCAM-1. VCAM-1 is expressed on cytokine-activated endothelial cells and is one of the principal surface proteins that regulates trafficking of lymphocytes to the endothelium. In the gut, the $\alpha_4\beta_7$ integrin binds to mucosal addressin cell adhesion molecule (MAdCAM-1), which mediates homing of T cells to sites of inflammation in the intestinal tract.[270] MadCAM-1 expression is enhanced in inflammatory bowel diseases.[271]

Natalizumab is effective in controlling the exacerbations of inflammatory bowel disease. In a double-blind placebo-controlled dose-ranging multicenter trial of natalizumab of 248 adults with active Crohn disease, clinical responses were higher in all three natalizumab groups at weeks 4, 6, and 8 than in the placebo group. The highest rate of remission (71%) occurred at 6 weeks in the group of patients given two infusions of 3 mg/kg. Drug-associated adverse events were mild; two patients had infusion reactions during the second infusion, and one of these patients developed antinatalizumab antibodies.[272] In a pilot study, 10 patients with ulcerative colitis had improved clinical scores 2 and 4 weeks after a single (3 mg/kg) infusion of natalizumab.[273]

RITUXIMAB (RITUXAN, MONOCLONAL ANTI-CD20)

Rituximab is a chimeric (mouse-human) monoclonal antibody that binds to the CD20 antigen on the surface of B lymphocytes. Binding results in antibody-dependent and complement-dependent cytotoxicity. Initially, rituximab was used to treat low-grade B-cell lymphomas but more recently has been used in the treatment of post-transplant lymphoproliferative disease. In one case series reporting six pediatric liver transplant recipients with Epstein Barr

virus–associated post-transplant lymphoproliferative disease, rituximab was given intravenously (375 mg/m² once a week for a total of 4 weeks in four patients and a total of 3 weeks in the other three). Infusion with rituximab was associated with complete remission in five patients. Disappearance of tumor masses occurred within 1 to 2.5 months after initiating treatment. Adverse effects included headaches, hypogammaglobulinemia, transient neutropenia, and one case of anaphylactic reaction.[274]

CONCLUSIONS

The optimal treatment of organ rejection and autoimmune diseases continues to evolve dramatically. Newer immunosuppressive agents are effective and potent and seem to have fewer adverse effects, at least in the short term. Instead of agents with broad physiologic and immunologic effects (eg, corticosteroids, azathioprine, calcineurin inhibitors, cyclosporine), the clinician can now use monoclonal antibodies that target one point in the T-cell activation pathway (eg, sirolimus), one cytokine (eg, infliximab, anti-TNFα), or one cell type (eg, rituximab, anti-CD20 B cells). The principal drawback of these new agents is that patients receiving the recombinant proteins develop antibodies, which puts them at risk for infusion reactions, decreased antibody efficacy, and, possibly, other autoimmune disorders. It remains to be seen whether the favorable safety profile of these new biologics will persist with long-term follow-up. Currently, however, these new medications have dramatically improved the quality of life for children and adolescents following organ transplant and those with refractory inflammatory bowel disease.

REFERENCES

1. Grey H, Sette A, Buus S. How T cells see antigen. Sci Am 1989; 261:56–64.
2. Gould D, Auchincloss H. Direct and indirect recognition: the role of MHC antigens in graft rejection. Immunol Today 1999;20:77–82.
3. Schreiber R, Walker W. The gastrointestinal barrier: antigen uptake and perinatal immunity. Ann Allergy 1988;61:3–12.
4. Walker W. Development of the intestinal mucosal barrier. J Pediatr Gastroenterol Nutr 2002;34 Suppl 1:S33–9.
5. Fellermann K, Stange E. Defensins—innate immunity at the epithelial frontier. Eur J Gastroenterol Hepatol 2001;13:771–6.
6. Yoshikai Y. The interaction of intestinal epithelial cells and intraepithelial lymphocytes in host defense. Immunol Res 1999;20:219–35.
7. Stagg AJ, Hart AL, Knight SC, Kamm MA. The dendritic cell: its role in intestinal inflammation and relationship with gut bacteria. Gut 2003;52:1522–9.
8. Medzhitov R. Toll-like receptors and innate immunity. Nat Rev Immunol 2001;1:135–45.
9. Abbas A, Lichtman A. Antigen processing and presentation to T lymphocytes, in cellular and molecular immunology. 5th ed. Philadelphia: Elsevier Science; 2003. p. 81–104.
10. Hennecke J, Wiley D. T cell receptor-MHC interactions up close. Cell 2001;104:1–4.
11. van der Merwe P, Davis S. Molecular interactions mediating T cell antigen recognition. Annu Rev Immunol 2003;21:659–84.

12. McAdam A, Schweitzer A, Sharpe A. The role of B7 co-stimulation in activation and differentiation of CD4+ and CD8+ T cells. Immunol Rev 1998;165:231–47.

13. Abbas A, Lichtman A, editors. Activation of T lymphocytes. In: Cellular and molecular immunology. Philadelphia: WB Saunders; 2003. p. 163–88.

14. Wecker H, Auchincloss H. Cellular mechanisms of rejection. Curr Opin Immunol 1992;4:561–6.

15. Ward S. The complexities of CD28 and CTLA-4 signalling: PI3K and beyond. Arch Immunol Ther Exp 1999;47:69–95.

16. Dumont F. The immunosuppressants, cyclosporin A and FK-506, and their mechanisms of action. In: Arias I, et al, editors. The liver: biology and pathobiology. Vol. I. New York: Raven Press; 1994. p. 1563–77.

17. Suthanthiran M, Morris R, Strom T. Immunosuppressants: cellular and molecular mechanisms of action. Am J Kidney Dis 1996;28:159–72.

18. Dong C, Davis R, Flavell R. MAP kinases in the immune response. Annu Rev Immunol 2002;20:55–72.

19. Aversa G, et al. SLAM and its role in T cell activation and Th cell responses. Immunol Cell Biol 1997;75:202–5.

20. Seigel R, Chan FM, Lenardo M. The multifaceted role of Fas signaling in immune cell homeostasis and autoimmunity. Nat Immunol 2000;1:469–74.

21. Jorgensen K, Koefoed-Nielsen P, Karamperis N. Calcineurin phosphatase activity and immunosuppression. A review on the role of calcineurin phosphatase activity and the immunosuppressive effect of cyclosporin A and tacrolimus. Scand J Immunol 2003;57:93–8.

22. Mosmann T, Coffman R. TH1 and TH2 cells: different patterns of lymphokine secretion lead to different functional properties. Annu Rev Immunol 1989;7:145–73.

23. Neurath M, Finotto S, Glimcher L. The role of Th1/Th2 polarization in mucosal immunity. Nat Med 2002;8:567–73.

24. Rudin C, Thompson C. B-cell development and maturation. Semin Oncol 1998;25:435–46.

25. Allen R, Armitaje R, Conley M, et al. CD40 ligand gene defects responsible for X-linked hyper-IgM syndrome. Science 1993;259:990–3.

26. Abbas A, Lichtman A, editors. B cell activation and antibody production. In: Cellular and molecular immunology. Philadelphia: WB Saunders; 2003. p. 189–215.

27. Patel K, Cuvelier S, Wiehler S. Selectins: critical mediators of leukocyte recruitment. Semin Immunol 2002;14:73–81.

28. Springer T. Adhesion receptors of the immune system. Nature 1990;346:425–34.

29. Laudanna C, Kim JY, Constantin G, et al. Rapid leukocyte integrin activation by chemokines. Immunol Rev 2002;186:37–46.

30. Yoshie O, Imai T, Nomiyama H. Chemokines in immunity. Adv Immunol 2001;78:57–110.

31. Hill N, Sarvetnick N. Cytokines: promoters and dampeners of autoimmunity. Curr Opin Immunol 2002;14:791–7.

32. O'Shea J, Ma A, Lipsky P. Cytokines and autoimmunity. Nat Immunol 2002;2:37–45.

33. Platanias L, Vogelzang N. Interleukin-1: biology, pathophysiology and clinical prospects. Am J Med 1990;89:621–9.

34. Miller A, Lider O, Roberts A, et al. Suppressor T cells generated by oral tolerization to myelin basic protein release TGF-β. Proc Natl Acad Sci U S A 1992;89:421–5.

35. Mowat A, Anatomical basis of tolerance and immunity to intestinal antigens. Nat Immunol 2003;3:331–41.

36. Baggiolini M, Dewald B, Moser B. Human chemokines: an update. Annu Rev Immunol 1997;15:675–705.

37. Zlotnik A, Morales J, Hedrick JA. Recent advances in chemokines and chemokine receptors. Crit Rev Immunol 1999;19:1–47.

38. Homey B, Muller A, Zotnik A. Chemokines: agents for the immunotherapy of cancer? Nat Immunol 2003;2:179–94.

39. Rocca B, FitzGerald G. Cyclooxygenases and prostaglandins: shaping up the immune response. Int Immunopharmacol 2002;2:603–30.

40. Auchincloss H, Sachs D. Transplantation and graft rejection. In: Paul W, editor. Fundamental immunology. New York: Raven Press; 1993. p. 1099–141.

41. Frasca L, Piazza C, Piccolella E. CD4+ T cells orchestrate both amplification and deletion of CD8+ T cells. Crit Rev Immunol 1998;18:569–94.

42. Buckley R. Transplantation immunology: organ and bone marrow. J Allergy Clin Immunol 2003;111(2 Suppl):S733–44.

43. Adler S, Turka L. Immunotherapy as a means to induce transplantation tolerance. Curr Opin Immunol 2002;14:660–5.

44. Goddard S, Adams D. New approaches to immunosuppression in liver transplantaion. J Gastroenterol Hepatol 2002;17:116–26.

45. Swartz S, Dluhy R. Corticosteroids: clinical pharmacology and therapeutic use. Drugs 1978;16:238–55.

46. Yang Y, Lichtenstein G. Corticosteroids in Crohn's disease. Am J Gastroenterol 2002;97:804–23.

47. Vane J, Botting R. Inflammation and the mechanism of action of anti-inflammatory drugs. FASEB J 1987;1:89–96.

48. Wallner B, Mattaliano R, Hession C, et al. Cloning and expression of human lipocortin, a phospholipase A_2 inhibitor with potent anti-inflammatory activity. Nature 1986;320:77–81.

49. Frieri M. Corticosteroid effects on cytokines and chemokines. Allergy Asthma Proc 1999;20:147–59.

50. Truhan A, Ahmed A. Corticosteroids: a review with emphasis on complications of prolonged systemic therapy. Ann Allergy 1989;5:375–90.

51. Helfer E, Rose L. Corticosteroids and adrenal suppression. Drugs 1989;38:838–45.

52. Levine L. Effect of inhaled corticosteroids on the hypothalamic-pituitary-adrenal axis and growth in children. J Pediatr 2000;137:450–4.

53. Simons F. A comparison of beclomethasone, salmetrol, and placebo in children with asthma. N Engl J Med 1997;337:1659–65.

54. Rimsza M. Complications of corticosteroid therapy. Am J Dis Child 1978;132:806–10.

55. Plevy S. Corticosteroid-sparing treatments in patients with Crohn's disease. Am J Gastroenterol 2002;97:1607–17.

56. Adachi J, Rostom A. Metabolic bone disease in adults with inflammatory bowel disease. Inflamm Bowel Dis 1999;5:200–11.

57. Vakil N, Sparberg M. Steroid related osteonecrosis in inflammatory bowel disease. Gastroenterology 1989;96:62–7.

58. Bialas M, Routledge P. Adverse effects of corticosteroids. Adverse Drug React Toxicol Rev 1998;17:227–35.

59. Czaja A, Menon K, Carpenter H. Sustained remission after corticosteroid therapy for type 1 autoimune hepatitis: a retrospective analysis. Hepatology 2002;35:890–7.

60. Faubion WJ, Loftus EJ, Harmsen W, et al. The natural history of corticosteroid therapy for inflammatory bowel disease: a population-based study. Gastroenterology 2001;121:255–60.

61. Lane S, Adcock I, Richards D, et al. Corticosteroid-resistant bronchial asthma is associated with increased c-fos expression in monocytes and T lymphocytes. J Clin Invest 1998;102:2156–64.

62. Sousa A, Lane S, Soh C, et al. In vivo resistance to corticosteroids in bronchial asthma is associated with enhanced

phosphorylation of JUN-N terminal kinase and failure of prednisolone to inhibit JUN N-terminal kinase phosphorylation. J Allergy Clin Immunol 1999;104:565–74.

63. Sousa A, Lano S, Cidloniski J, et al. Glucocorticoid resistance in asthma is associated with elevated in vivo expression of the glucocorticoid receptor beta-isoform. J Allergy Clin Immunol 2000;105:943–50.

64. Ruddell W, Dickinson R, Dixon M, Axon A. Treatment of distal ulcerative colitis in relapse: comparison of hydrocortisone enemas and rectal hydrocortisone foam. Gut 1980;21:885–9.

65. Malchow H, Ewe K, Brandes J, et al. European Cooperative Crohn's disease study: results of treatment. Gastroenterology 1984;86:249–66.

66. Summers R, Switz D, Sessions J, et al. National Cooperative Crohn's Disease Study: results of drug treatment. Gastroenterology 1979;77:847–69.

67. Munkholm P, Langholz V, Davidsen M, Binder V. Frequency of glucocorticoid resistance and dependency in Crohn's disease. Gut 1994;35:360–2.

68. Franchimont D, Louis E, Croes F, Belaiche J. Clinical pattern of corticosteroid dependent Crohn's disease. Eur J Gastroenterol Hepatol 1998;10:821–5.

69. Cocco A, Mendeloff A. Evaluation of intermittent corticosteroid therapy in management of ulcerative colitis. Johns Hopkins Med J 1967;120:162–9.

70. Bello C, Goldstein F, Thornton J. Alternate day prednisone treatment and treatment maintenance in Crohn's disease. Am J Gastroenterol 1991;86:460–6.

71. Mieli-Vergani G, Vergani D. Autoimmune hepatitis in children. Clin Liver Dis 2002;6:335–46.

72. Czaja A. Treatment of autoimmune hepatitis. Semin Liver Dis 2002;22:365–77.

73. Wright E, Seeff L, Berk P, et al. Treatment of chronic active hepatitis: an analysis of three controlled trials. Gastroenterology 1977;73:1422–30.

74. Maggiore G, Bernard O, Hadchouel M, et al. Treatment of autoimmune chronic active hepatitis in childhood. J Pediatr 1984;104: 839–44.

75. Stellon A, Keating J, Johnson P, et al. Maintenance of remission in autoimmune chronic active hepatitis with azathioprine after corticosteroid withdrawal. Hepatology 1988;8:781–4.

76. Medina J, Garcia-Buey L, Moreno-Otero R. Immunopathogenetic and therapeutic aspects of autoimmune hepatitis. Aliment Pharmacol Ther 2003;17:1–16.

77. Malekzadeh R, Nasseri-Moghaddam S, Kaviani M, et al. Cyclosporin A is a promising alternative to corticosteroids in autoimmune hepatitis. Dig Dis Sci 2001;46:1321–7.

78. Orenstein S, Shalaby T, Di Lorenzo C, et al. The spectrum of pediatric eosinophilic esophagitis beyond infancy: a clinical series of 30 children. Am J Gastroenterol 2000;95:1422–30.

79. Liacouras C, Wenner W, Brown K, et al. Primary eosinophilic esophagitis in children: successful treatment with oral corticosteroids. J Pediatr Gastroenterol Nutr 1998;26:380–5.

80. Teitelbaum J, Fox V, Twarog F, et al. Eosinophilic esophagitis in children: immunopathological analysis and response to fluticasone propionate. Gastroenterology 2002;122:1216–25.

81. Lundin P, Edsbacker S. Bergstrand M, et al. Pharmacokinetics of budesonide controlled ileal release capsules in children and adults with active Crohn's disease. Aliment Pharmacol Ther 2003;17:85–92.

82. Spencer C, McTavish D. Budesonide: a review of its pharmacological properties and therapeutic efficacy in inflammatory bowel disease. Drugs 1995;50:854–72.

83. Volovitz D, Amir J, Malik H, et al. Growth and pituitary-adrenal

function in children with severe asthma treated with inhaled budesonide. N Engl J Med 1993;329:1703–8.

84. Toogood J, Jennings B, Hodsman A, et al. Effects of dose and dosing schedule of inhaled budesonide on bone turnover. J Allergy Clin Immunol 1991;88:572–80.

85. Bisgaard H, Damjaer-Nielsen M, Andersen B, et al. Adrenal function in children with bronchial asthma treated with beclomethasone dipropionate or budesonide. J Allergy Clin Immunol 1988;81:1088–95.

86. Ferguson A, Campieri M, Doe W, et al. Oral budesonide as maintenance therapy in Crohn's disease—results of a 12-month study. Global Budesonide Study Group. Aliment Pharmacol Ther 1998;12:175–83.

87. Bar-Meir S, Chowers Y, Lavy A, et al. Budesonide versus prednisone in the treatment of active Crohn's disease. The Israeli Budesonide Study Group. Gastroenterology 1998;115: 835–40.

88. D'Haens G, et al. Bone turnover during short-term therapy with methylprednisolone or budesonide in Crohn's disease. Aliment Pharmacol Ther 1998;12:419–24.

89. Hanauer S, Robinson M, Pruitt R, et al. Budesonide enema for the treatment of active, distal ulcerative colitis and proctitis: a dose-ranging study. U.S. Budesonide Enema Study Group. Gastroenterology 1998;115:525–32.

90. Greenberg G, Feagan B, Martin F. Oral budesonide for active Crohn's disease. N Engl J Med 1994;331:842–5.

91. Greenberg GR, Feagan BG, Martin F, et al. Oral budesonide as maintenance treatment for Crohn's disease: a placebo-controlled, dose-ranging study. Canadian Inflammatory Bowel Disease Study Group. Gastroenterology 1996;110:45–51.

92. Lofberg R, Rutgeerts P, Malchow H, et al. Budesonide prolongs time to relapse in ileal and ileocacel Crohn's disease. Gut 1996;39:82–6.

93. Levine A, Broide E, Stein M, et al. Evaluation of oral budesonide for treatment of mild and moderate exacerbations of Crohn's disease in children. J Pediatr 2002;140:75–80.

94. Levine A, Weizman Z, Broide E, et al. A comparison of budesonide and prednisone for the treatment of active pediatric Crohn disease. J Pediatr Gastroenterol Nutr 2003;36:248–52.

95. Agertoft L, Pedersen S. Effect of long-term treatment with inhaled budesonide on adult height in children with asthma. N Engl J Med 2000;343:1064–9.

96. Kundhal P, Zachos M, Holmes JL, et al. Controlled ileal release budesonide in pediatric Crohn disease: efficacy and effect on growth. J Pediatr Gastroenterol Nutr 2001;33:75–80.

97. Agertoft L, Pedersen S. Bone mineral density in children with asthma receiving long-term treatment with inhaled budesonide. Am J Respir Crit Care Med 1998;157:178–83.

98. Dunn C, Wagstaff A, Perry C, et al. Cyclosporin. An updated review of the pharmacokinetic properties, clinical efficacy and tolerability of a microemulsion based formulation (Neoral) in organ transplantation. Drugs 2001;61:1957–2016.

99. June C, Ledbetter J, Gillespie M, et al. T cell proliferation involving the CD28 pathway is associated with cyclosporine resistant interleukin-2 gene expression. Mol Cell Biol 1987; 7:4472–81.

100. Hess A. Mechanisms of action of cyclosporine: considerations for the treatment of autoimmune diseases. Clin Immunol Immunopathol 1993;68:220–8.

101. Prud'Homme G, Vanier L. Cyclosporine, tolerance and autoimmunity. Clin Immunol Immunopathol 1993;66:185–92.

102. Kahan B. Cyclosporine. N Engl J Med 1989;321:1725–38.

103. Freeman D. Pharmacology and pharmacokinetics of cyclosporine. Clin Biochem 1991;24:9–14.

104. Sokol R, Johnson K, Karrer F, et al. Improvement of cyclosporin absorption in children after liver transplantation by means of water-soluble vitamin E. Lancet 1991;338:212–4.

105. Arumugam R, Soriano HE, Scheimann AO, et al. Immunosuppressive therapy with microemulsion cyclosporine A shortens the hospitalization of pediatric liver transplant recipients. Clin Transplant 1998;12:588–92.

106. Shah MB, Martin JE, Schroeder TJ, First MR. The evaluation of the safety and tolerability of two formulations of cyclosporine: Neoral and Sandimmune. A meta-analysis. Transplantation 1999;67:1411–7.

107. Gilbert J, Vacanti J. Infection and immunosuppression in children with cancer or organ transplants. In: Fonkalsrud E, editor. Infection in pediatric surgery and immunologic disorders. Orlando (FL): WB Saunders; 1992. p. 219–38.

108. Malatack J, Gartner J, Urbach A, et al. Orthotopic liver transplantation, Epstein-Barr virus cyclosporine and lymphoproliferative disease: a growing concern. J Pediatr 1991;118:667–5.

109. Kosmach B, Webber S, Reyes J. Care of the pediatric solid organ transplant recipient. Pediatr Clin North Am 1998;45:1395–418.

110. Alvarez F, Atkinson P, Grant D, et al. A one year pediatric randomized double-blind comparison of Neoral vs. Sandimmune in orthotopic liver transplantation. Transplantation 2000;69:87–92.

111. Debray D, Maggiore D, Girardet JP, et al. Efficacy of cyclosporin A in children with type 2 autoimmune hepatitis. J Pediatr 1999;135:111–4.

112. Alvarez F, Ciocca M, Canero-Velasco C, et al. Short-term cyclosporine induces a remission of autoimmune hepatitis in children. J Hepatol 1999;30:222–7.

113. Brynskov J, Freund L, Rasmussen S, et al. A placebo-controlled, double-blind, randomized trial of cyclosporine therapy in active chronic Crohn's disease. N Engl J Med 1989;321:845–50.

114. Feagan B, McDonald J, Rochon J, et al. Low-dose cyclosporine for the treatment of Crohn's disease. N Engl J Med 1994;330:1846–51.

115. Lichtiger S, Present D, Kornbluth A, et al. Cyclosporine in severe ulcerative colitis refractory to steroid therapy. N Engl J Med 1994;330:1841–5.

116. D'Haens G, Lemmens L, Geboes K, et al. Intravenous cyclosporine versus intravenous corticosteroids as single therapy for severe attacks of ulcerative colitis. Gastroenterology 2001;120:1323–9.

117. Treem W, Davis P, Hyams J. Cyclosporine treatment of severe ulcerative colitis in children. J Pediatr 1991;119:994–7.

118. Ramakrishna J, Langhans N, Calenda K, et al. Combined use of cyclosporine and azathioprine or 6-mercaptopurine in pediatric inflammatory bowel disease. J Pediatr Gastroenterol Nutr 1996;22:296–302.

119. Seidman E, Lacaille F, Russo P, et al. Successful treatment of autoimmune enteropathy with cyclosporine. J Pediatr 1990;117:929–32.

120. Mengarelli A, Iori P, Romano A, et al. One-year cyclosporine prophylaxis reduces the risk of developing extensive chronic graft-versus-host disease after allogeneic peripheral blood stem cell transplantation. Haematologica 2003;88:315–23.

121. Koc S, Leisenring W, Flowers ME, et al. Therapy for chronic graft-versus-host disease: a randomized trial comparing cyclosporine plus prednisone versus prednisone alone. Blood 2002;100:48–51.

122. Hiraoka A, Ohashi Y, Okamoto S, et al. Phase III study comparing tacrolimus (FK506) with cyclosporine for graft-versus-host disease prophylaxis after allogeneic bone marrow transplantation. Bone Marrow Transplant 2001;28:181–5.

123. Plosker G, Foster R. Tacrolimus: a further update of its pharmacology and therapeutic use in the management of organ transplantation. Drugs 2000;59:323–89.

124. Peters D, Fitton A, Plosker G, et al. Tacrolimus: a review of its pharmacology and therapeutic potential in hepatic and renal transplantation. Drugs 1993;46:746–94.

125. Keicho N, Sawada S, Kitamura K, et al. Effects of an immunosuppressant, FK506 on interleukin-1 production by human macrophages and a macrophage like cell line, U937. Cell Immunol 1991;132:285–94.

126. DePaulis A, Stellato C, Cirillo R, et al. Anti-inflammatory effect of FK-506 on human skin mast cells. J Invest Dermatol 1992;99:723–8.

127. Jiang H, Kobayashi M. Differences between cyclosporine A and tacrolimus in organ transplanatation. Transplant Proc 1999;31:1978–80.

128. Rayes M, Bechstein W, Volk H, et al. Distribution of lymphocyte subtypes in liver transplant recipients treated with tacrolimus. Transplant Proc 1997;29:501–2.

129. Wallemacq P, Furian V, Moller A, et al. Pharmacokinetics of tacrolimus in pediatric liver transplant recipients. Eur J Drug Metab Pharmacokinet 1998;23:367–70.

130. McDiarmid S, Colonna J, Shaked A, et al. Differences in oral FK-506 dose requirements between adult and pediatric liver transplant recipients. Transplantation 1993;55:1328–32.

131. Atkison P, Joubert G, Barron A, et al. Hypertrophic cardiomyopathy associated with tacrolimus in paediatric transplant patients. Lancet 1995;345:894–6.

132. McDiarmid SV. The use of tacrolimus in pediatric liver transplantation. J Pediatr Gastroenterol Nutr 1998;26:90–102.

133. Pichlmayr R, Winkler M, Neuhaus P, et al. Three year followup of the European Multicenter Tacrolimus (FK506) Liver Study. Transplant Proc 1997;29:2499–502.

134. Jain A, Mazariegos G, Kaskyap R, et al. Comparative long-term evaluation of tacrolimus and cyclosporine in pediatric liver transplantation. Transplantation 2000;70:617–25.

135. Jain A, Mazariegos G, Pokharna R, et al. The absence of chronic rejection in pediatric primary liver transplant patients who are maintained on tacrolimus-based immunosuppression: a long-term analysis. Transplantation 2003;75:1020–5.

136. Mazariegos G, Salzedas A, Jain A, et al. Conversion from cyclosporin to tacrolimus in paediatric liver transplant recipients. Paediatr Drugs 2001;3:661–72.

137. Reyes J, Jain A, Mazariegos G, et al. Long-term results after conversion from cyclosporine to tacrolimus in pediatric liver transplantation for acute and chronic rejection. Transplantation 2000;69:2573–80.

138. Tzakis A, Kato T, Nishida S, et al. Alemtuzumab (Campath-1H) combined with tacrolimus in intestinal and multivisceral transplantation. Transplantation 2003;75:1512–7.

139. Abu-Elmagd K, Reyes J, Bond G, et al. Clinical intestinal transplantation: a decade of experience at a single center. Ann Surg 2001;234:404–16; discussion 416–7.

140. vanThiel D, Wright H, Carroll P, et al. Tacrolimus: a potential new treatment for autoimmune chronic active hepatitis: results of an open-label preliminary trial. Am J Gastroenterol 1995;90:771–6.

141. Bousvaros A, Leichter A, Book L, et al. Treatment of pediatric autoimmune enteropathy with tacrolimus (FK506). Gastroenterology 1996;111:237–43.

142. Steffen R, Wyllie R, Kay M, et al. Autoimmune enteropathy in a pediatric patient: partial response to tacrolimus therapy. Clin Pediatr 1997;36:295–9.

143. Bousvaros A, Wang A, Leichtner AM. Tacrolimus (FK-506) treatment of fulminant colitis in a child. J Pediatr Gastroenterol Nutr 1996;23:329–33.

144. Sandborn WJ. Preliminary report on the use of oral tacrolimus (FK506) in the treatment of complicated proximal small bowel and fistulizing Crohn's disease. Am J Gastroenterol 1997;92:876–9.

145. Bousvaros A, Kirschner B, Day A, et al. Oral tacrolimus treatment of severe colitis in children. J Pediatr 2000;137:794–9.

146. Carnevale-Schianca F, Martin P, Sullivan K, et al. Changing from cyclosporine to tacrolimus as salvage therapy for chronic graft-versus-host disease. Biol Blood Marrow Transplant 2000;6:613–20.

147. Cuffari C, Theoret Y, Latour S, et al. 6-Mercaptopurine metabolism in Crohn's disease: correlation with efficacy and toxicity. Gut 1996;39:401–6.

148. Calabresi P, Chabner B. 6-Mercaptopurine. In: Gilman A, et al, editors. The pharmacological basis of therapeutics. New York: Pergamon Press; 1990. p. 1232–6.

149. Lennard L, Lilleyman J, Loon JV, et al. Genetic variation in response to 6-mercaptopurine for childhood acute lymphoblastic leukemia. Lancet 1993;336:225–9.

150. Rosen R, Integlia M, Bousvaros A. Severe pancytopenia from thiopurine methyltransferase deficiency: a preventable complication of 6-mercaptopurine therapy in children with Crohn's disease. J Pediatr Gastroenterol Nutr 2002;35:695–9.

151. Present D, Meltzer S, Krumholz M, et al. 6-Mercaptopurine in the management of inflammatory bowel disease: short- and long-term toxicity. Ann Intern Med 1989;111:641–9.

152. Connell W, Kamm M, Dickson M, et al. Long-term neoplasia risk after azathioprine treatment in Crohn's disease. Lancet 1994;343:1249–52.

153. Dayharsh GA, Loftus EV Jr, Sandborn WJ, et al. Epstein-Barr virus-positive lymphoma in patients with inflammatory bowel disease treated with azathioprine or 6-mercaptopurine. Gastroenterology 2002;122:72–7.

154. Kirschner BS. Safety of azathioprine and 6-mercaptopurine in pediatric patients with inflammatory bowel disease. Gastroenterology 1998;115:813–21.

155. Present D, et al. Treatment of Crohn's disease with 6-mercaptopurine. N Engl J Med 1980;302:981–7.

156. Markowitz J, Rosa J, Grancher K, et al. Long-term 6-mercaptopurine treatment in adolescents with Crohn's disease. Gastroenterology 1990;99:1347–51.

157. Dubinsky MC, Lamothe S, Yang HY, et al. Pharmacogenomics and metabolite measurement for 6-mercaptopurine therapy in inflammatory bowel disease. Gastroenterology 2000;118:05–13.

158. Cuffari C, Hunt S, Bayless T. Utilisation of erythrocyte 6-thioguanine metabolite levels to optimise azathioprine therapy in patients with inflammatory bowel disease. Gut 2001;48:642–6.

159. Dubinsky MC, Yang H, Hassard PV, et al. 6-MP metabolite profiles provide a biochemical explanation for 6-MP resistance in patients with inflammatory bowel disease. Gastroenterology 2002;122:904–15.

160. Dubinsky MC, Hassard PV, Seidman EG, et al. An open-label pilot study using thioguanine as a therapeutic alternative in Crohn's disease patients resistant to 6-mercaptopurine therapy. Inflamm Bowel Dis 2001;7:181–9.

161. Markowitz J, Grancher K, Kohn N, et al. A multicenter controlled trial of 6-mercaptopurine and prednisone in children with newly diagnosed Crohn's disease. Gastroenterology 2000;119:895–902.

162. Kader HA, Raynor SC, Young R, et al. Introduction of 6-mercaptopurine in Crohn's disease patients during the perioperative period: a preliminary evaluation of recurrence of disease. J Pediatr Gastroenterol Nutr 1997;25:93–7.

163. D'Haens G, Geboes K, Ponette E, et al. Healing of severe recurrent ileitis with azathioprine therapy in patients with Crohn's disease. Gastroenterology 1997;112:1475–81.

164. Cuffari C, Hunt S, Bayless TM. Enhanced bioavailability of azathioprine compared to 6-mercaptopurine therapy in inflammatory bowel disease: correlation with treatment efficacy. Aliment Pharmacol Ther 2000;14:1009–14.

165. Sandborn W, VanOs E, Zins B, et al. An intravenous loading dose of azathioprine decreases the time to response in patients with Crohn's disease. Gastroenterology 1995;109:1808–17.

166. Verhave M, Winter H, Grand R. Azathioprine in the treatment of children with inflammatory bowel disease. J Pediatr 1990;117:809–14.

167. Adler D, Korelitz B. The therapeutic efficacy of 6-mercaptopurine in refractory ulcerative colitis. Am J Gastroenterol 1990;85:717–22.

168. Kader HA, Mascarenhas MR, Piccoli DA, et al. Experiences with 6-mercaptopurine and azathioprine therapy in pediatric patients with severe ulcerative colitis. J Pediatr Gastroenterol Nutr1999;28:54–8.

169. Casson D, Davies S, Thompson M, et al. Low dose intravenous azathioprine may be effective in the management of acute fulminant colitis complicating inflammatory bowel disease. Aliment Pharmacol Ther 1999;13:891–5.

170. Dunn S, Falkenstein K, Lawrence J, et al. Monotherapy with cyclosporine for chronic immunosuppression in pediatric liver transplant recipients. Transplantation 1994;57:544–7.

171. vanHoek B, Weisner R, Ludwig J, et al. Combination immunosuppression with azathioprine reduces the incidence of ductopenic rejection and vanishing bile duct syndrome after liver transplantation. Transplant Proc 1991;23:1403–5.

172. Sterneck M, Wiesner R, Ascher N, et al. Azathioprine hepatotoxicity after liver transplantation. Hepatology 1991;14:806–10.

173. Czaja AJ. Drug therapy in the management of type 1 autoimmune hepatitis. Drugs 1999;57:49–68.

174. Rampton D. Methotrexate in Crohn's disease. Gut 2001;48:790–1.

175. Schroder O, Stein J. Low dose methotrexate in inflammatory bowel disease: current status and future directions. Am J Gastroenterol 2003;98:530–7.

176. Schnabel A, Gross W. Low dose methotrexate in rheumatic diseases—efficacy, side effects, and risk factors for side effects. Semin Arthritis Rheum 1994;23:310–27.

177. Schnabel A. Mechanisms of action, pharmacology and toxicology. In: Fellerman K, Jewell D, Sandborn W, editors. Immunosuppression in inflammatory bowel diseases. Standards, new developments, future trends. Dordrecht: Kluwer Academic Publishers; 2001. p. 113–8.

178. Balis FM, Holcenberg JS, Poplack DG, et al. Pharmacokinetics and pharmacodynamics of oral methotrexate and mercaptopurine in children with lower risk acute lymphoblastic leukemia: a joint Children's Cancer Group and Pediatric Oncology Branch study. Blood 1998;92:3569–77.

179. Evans W, Crom W, Yalowich J. Methotrexate. In: Evans W, Schentag, J, Jusko J, editors. Applied pharmacokinetics: principles of therapeutic drug monitoring. Spokane (WA): Applied Therapeutics; 1986. p. 1009–56.

180. Kremer J, Alarcon G, Lightfoot RW Jr, et al. Methotrexate for rheumatoid arthritis: suggested guidelines for monitoring liver toxicity. Arthritis Rheum 1994;32:316–28.

181. Roenigk H. Methotrexate in psoriasis: revised guidelines. J Am Acad Dermatol 1988;19:145–56.

182. Whiting-O'Keefe QE, Fye KH, Sack KD. Methotrexate and histologic hepatic abnormalities: a meta-analysis. Am J Med 1991;90:711–6.

183. Te HS, Schiano TD, Kuan SF, et al. Hepatic effects of long-term methotrexate use in the treatment of inflammatory bowel disease. Am J Gastroenterol 2000;95:3150–6.

184. Cunliffe RN, Scott BB. Review article: monitoring for drug side-effects in inflammatory bowel disease. Aliment Pharmacol Ther 2002;16:647–62.

185. Hashkes PJ, Balistreri WF, Bove KE, et al. The relationship of hepatotoxic risk factors and liver histology in methotrexate therapy for juvenile rheumatoid arthritis. J Pediatr 1999;134:47–52.

186. Imokawa S, Colby TV, Leslie KO, Helmers RA. Methotrexate pneumonitis: review of the literature and histopathological findings in nine patients. Eur Respir J 2000;15:373–81.

187. Kozarek R, Patterson D, Gelfand M, et al. Methotrexate induces clinical and histologic remission in patients with refractory inflammatory bowel disease. Ann Intern Med 1989;110:353–6.

188. Feagan B, Rochon J, Fedorak R, et al. Methotrexate for the treatment of Crohn's disease. N Engl J Med 1995;332:292–7.

189. Feagan BG. Methotrexate treatment for Crohn's disease. Inflamm Bowel Dis 1998;4:120–1.

190. Feagan BG, Fedorak RN, Irvine EJ, et al. A comparison of methotrexate with placebo for the maintenance of remission in Crohn's disease. North American Crohn's Study Group Investigators. N Engl J Med 2000;342:1627–32.

191. Mack DR, Young R, Kaufman SS, et al. Methotrexate in patients with Crohn's disease after 6-mercaptopurine. J Pediatr 1998;132:830–5.

192. Hendrickse M, Rigney E, Giaffer M, et al. Low dose methotrexate is ineffective in primary biliary cirrhosis: long-term results of a placebo-controlled trial. Gastroenterology 1999;117:400–7.

193. Bach N, Bodian C, Bodenheimer H, et al. Methotrexate therapy for primary biliary cirrhosis. Am J Gastroenterol 2003;98:187–93.

194. Bonis PA, Kaplan M. Methotrexate improves biochemical tests in patients with primary biliary cirrhosis who respond incompletely to ursodiol. Gastroenterology 1999;117:395–9.

195. Knox T, Kaplan M. A double-blind controlled trial of oral pulse methotrexate therapy in the treatment of primary sclerosing cholangitis. Gastroenterology 1994;106:494–9.

196. Lindor KD, Jorgensen RA, Anderson ML, et al. Ursodeoxycholic acid and methotrexate for primary sclerosing cholangitis: a pilot study. Am J Gastroenterol 1996;91:511–5.

197. Allison AC, Eugui EM. Mycophenolate mofetil and its mechanisms of action. Immunopharmacology 2000;47:85–118.

198. Fulton B, Markham A. Mycophenolate mofetil. Drugs 1996;51:278–98.

199. del Mar Fernandez De Gatta M, Santos-Buelga D, Dominguez-Gil A, Garcia MJ. Immunosuppressive therapy for paediatric transplant patients: pharmacokinetic considerations. Clin Pharmacokinet 2002;41:115–35.

200. Bullingham R, Nichols A, Hale M. Pharmacokinetics of mycophenolate mofetil: a short review. Transplant Proc 1996;28:925–9.

201. Sollinger H. Mycophenolate mofetil for prevention of acute rejection in primary renal allograft recipients. Transplantation 1995;60:225–32.

202. Jain AB, Hamad I, Rakela J, et al. A prospective randomized trial of tacrolimus and prednisone versus tacrolimus, prednisone, and mycophenolate mofetil in primary adult liver transplant recipients: an interim report. Transplantation 1998;66:1395–8.

203. Hebert MF, Asher NL, Lake JR, et al. Four-year follow-up of mycophenolate mofetil for graft rescue in liver allograft recipients. Transplantation 1999;67:707–12.

204. Jain A, Kashyap R, Dodson F, et al. A prospective randomized trial of tacrolimus and prednisone versus tacrolimus, prednisone and mycophenolate mofetil in primary adult liver transplantation: a single center report. Transplantation 2001;72:1091–7.

205. Fischer L, Sterneck M, Gahlemann CG, et al. A prospective study comparing safety and efficacy of mycophenolate mofetil versus azathioprine in primary liver transplant recipients. Transplant Proc 2000;32:2125–7.

206. Renz J, Lightdale J, Mudge C, et al. Mycophenolate mofetil, microemulsion cyclosporine and prednisone as primary immunosuppression for pediatric liver transplant recipients. Liver Transplant Surg 1999;5:136–43.

207. Fickert P, Hinterleitner TA, Wenzl HH, et al. Mycophenolate mofetil in patients with Crohn's disease. Am J Gastroenterol 1998;93:2529–32.

208. Neurath MF, Wanitschke R, Peters M, et al. Randomised trial of mycophenolate mofetil versus azathioprine for treatment of chronic active Crohn's disease. Gut 1999;44:625–8.

209. Fellermann K, Steffen M, Stein J, et al. Mycophenolate mofetil: lack of efficacy in chronic active inflammatory bowel disease. Aliment Pharmacol Ther 2000;14:171–6.

210. Orth T, Peters M, Schlaak JF, et al. Mycophenolate mofetil versus azathioprine in patients with chronic active ulcerative colitis: a 12-month pilot study. Am J Gastroenterol 2000;95:1201–7.

211. Pinna AD, Weppler D, Nery JR, et al. Induction therapy for clinical intestinal transplantation: comparison of four different regimens. Transplant Proc 2000;32:1193–4.

212. Sehgal SN. Rapamune (RAPA, rapamycin, sirolimus): mechanism of action immunosuppressive effect results from blockade of signal transduction and inhibition of cell cycle progression. Clin Biochem 1998;31:335–40.

213. Sattler M, Guengerich FP, Yun CH, et al. Cytochrome P-450 3A enzymes are responsible for biotransformation of FK506 and rapamycin in man and rat. Drug Metab Dispos 1992;20:753–61.

214. Kahan BD. Sirolimus: a comprehensive review. Exp Opin Pharmacother 2001;2:1903–17.

215. Kahan BD, Camardo JS. Rapamycin: clinical results and future opportunities. Transplantation 2001;72:1181–93.

216. MacDonald AS, RGS Group. A worldwide, phase III, randomized, controlled, safety and efficacy study of a sirolimus/cyclosporine regimen for prevention of acute rejection in recipients of primary mismatched renal allografts. Transplantation 2001;71:271–80.

217. Flechner SM, Goldfarb D, Modlin C, et al. Kidney transplantation without calcineurin inhibitor drugs: a prospective, randomized trial of sirolimus versus cyclosporine. Transplantation 2002;74:1070–6.

218. Chang GJ, Mahanty HD, Quan D, et al. Experience with the use of sirolimus in liver transplantation—use in patients for whom calcineurin inhibitors are contraindicated. Liver Transplant 2000;6:734–40.

219. Trotter JF, Wachs M, Bak T, et al. Liver transplantation using sirolimus and minimal corticosteroids (3-day taper). Liver Transplant 2001;7:343–51.

220. Florman S, Gondolesi G, Schiano T, et al. Improved results in small bowel transplantation using sirolimus. Transplant Proc 2002;34:936.

221. Knight D, Trinh H, Le J, et al. Construction and initial characteization of a mouse-human anti-TNF antibody. Mol Immunol 1993;30:1443–53.

222. van Deventer SJ. Transmembrane TNF-alpha, induction of apoptosis, and the efficacy of TNF-targeting therapies in Crohn's disease. Gastroenterology 2001;121:1242–6.

223. Sandborn WJ, Hanauer SB. Antitumor necrosis factor therapy for inflammatory bowel disease: a review of agents, pharmacology, clinical results, and safety. Inflamm Bowel Dis 1999; 5:119–33.

224. Baldassano R, Braegger CP, Escher JC, et al. Infliximab (Remicade) therapy in the treatment of pediatric Crohn's disease. Am J Gastroenterol 2003;98:833–8.

225. Crandall WV, Mackner LM. Infusion reactions to infliximab in children and adolescents: frequency, outcome and a predictive model. Aliment Pharmacol Ther 2003;17:75–84.

226. Baker D, Clark J, Keenan G, Jones S. Tuberculosis occurring in patients receiving the anti-TNF agent infliximab. Arthritis Rheum 2001;44 Suppl:S105.

227. Hanauer SB, Feagan BG, Lichtenstein GR, et al. Maintenance infliximab for Crohn's disease: the ACCENT I randomised trial. Lancet 2002;359:1541–9.

228. Vermeire S, Noman M, Van Assche G, et al. Autoimmunity associated with anti-tumor necrosis factor alpha treatment in Crohn's disease: a prospective cohort study. Gastroenterology 2003;125:32–9.

229. Brown SL, Greene MH, Gershon SK, et al. Tumor necrosis factor antagonist therapy and lymphoma development: twenty-six cases reported to the Food and Drug Administration. Arthritis Rheum 2002;46:3151–8.

230. Derkx B, Taminiau J, Radema S, et al. Tumour-necrosis-factor antibody treatment in Crohn's disease. Lancet 1993;342:173–4.

231. Hyams JS, Markowitz J, Wyllie R. Use of infliximab in the treatment of Crohn's disease in children and adolescents. J Pediatr 2000;137:192–6.

232. Kugathasan S, Werlin SL, Martinez A, et al. Prolonged duration of response to infliximab in early but not late pediatric Crohn's disease. Am J Gastroenterol 2000;95:3189–94.

233. Sands BE, Tremaine WJ, Sandborn WJ, et al. Infliximab in the treatment of severe, steroid-refractory ulcerative colitis: a pilot study. Inflamm Bowel Dis 2001;7:83–8.

234. Chey WY, Hussain A, Ryan C, et al. Infliximab for refractory ulcerative colitis. Am J Gastroenterol 2001;96:2373–81.

235. Mamula P, Markowitz JE, Brown KA, et al. Infliximab as a novel therapy for pediatric ulcerative colitis. J Pediatr Gastroenterol Nutr 2002;34:307–11.

236. Farrell RJ, Alsahli M, Jeen YT, et al. Intravenous hydrocortisone premedication reduces antibodies to infliximab in Crohn's disease: a randomized controlled trial. Gastroenterology 2003;124:917–24.

237. Baert F, Noman M, Vermeire S, et al. Influence of immunogenicity on the long-term efficacy of infliximab in Crohn's disease. N Engl J Med 2003;348:601–8.

238. Todd P, Brogden R. Muromonab CD3: a review of its pharmacology and therapeutic potential. Drugs 1989;37:871–99.

239. Goldstein G, Fuccello A, Norman D, et al. OKT3 monoclonal antibody plasma levels during therapy and the subsequent development of host antibodies to OKT3. Transplantation 1986;42:507–10.

240. Alloway R, Hathaway D, Gaber L, et al. Results of a prospective, randomized double-blind study comparing standard vs. low dose OKT3 induction therapy. Transplant Proc 1993;25:550–2.

241. Debray D, Furlan V, Baudouin V, et al. Therapy for acute rejection in pediatric organ transplant recipients. Paediatr Drugs 2003;5:81–93.

242. Chatenoud L, Feean C, Legendre L, et al. In vivo cell activation following OKT3 administration—systemic cytokine release and modulation by corticosteroids. Transplantation 1990;49 :697–702.

243. McDiarmid S, Busuttil R, Terasaki P, et al. OKT3 treatment of steroid-resistant rejection in pediatric liver transplant recipients. J Pediatr Gastroenterol Nutr 1992;14:86–91.

244. Stratta R, Shaefer M, Markin R, et al. Clinical patterns of cytomegalovirus disease after liver transplantation. Arch Surg 1989;124:1442–50.

245. Melosky B, Karim M, Chui A, et al. Lymphoproliferative disorders after renal transplantation in patients receiving triple or quadruple immunosuppression. J Am Soc Nephrol 1992;2 (12 Suppl):S290–4.

246. Kremer A, Barnes L, Hirsch R, Goldstein G. Orthoclone OKT3 monoclonal antibody reversal of hepatic and cardiac allograft rejection unresponsive to conventional immunosuppressive treatments. Transplant Proc1987;19 Suppl 1:54–7.

247. Cosimi A, Cho S, Delmonico F, et al. A randomized clinical trial comparing OKT3 and steroids for treatment of hepatic allograft rejection. Transplantation 1987;43:91–5.

248. First M, Schroeder T, Hurtubuise P, et al. Successful retreatment of allograft rejection with OKT3. Transplantation 1989;47:88–91.

249. Fung J, Starzl T. Prophylactic use of OKT3 in liver transplantation: a review. Dig Dis Sci 1991;36:1427–30.

250. Koch M, Niemeyer G, Patel I, et al. Pharmacokinetics, pharmacodynamics, and immunodynamics of daclizumab in a two-dose regimen in liver transplantation. Transplantation 2002;73:1640–6.

251. Hirose R, Roberts JP, Quan D, et al. Experience with daclizumab in liver transplantation: renal transplant dosing without calcineurin inhibitors is insufficient to prevent acute rejection in liver transplantation. Transplantation 2000;69:307–11.

252. Eckhoff DE, McGuire B, Sellers M, et al. The safety and efficacy of a two-dose daclizumab (Zenapax) induction therapy in liver transplant recipients. Transplantation 2000;69:1867–72.

253. Heffron TG, Smallwood GA, Pillen T, et al. Liver transplant induction trial of daclizumab to spare calcineurin inhibition. Transplant Proc 2002;34:1514–5.

254. Neuhaus P, Clavien PA, Kittur D, et al. Improved treatment response with basiliximab immunoprophylaxis after liver transplantation: results from a double-blind randomized placebo-controlled trial. Liver Transplant 2002;8:132–42.

255. Aw MM, Taylor RM, Verma A, et al. Basiliximab (Simulect) for the treatment of steroid-resistant rejection in pediatric liver transpland recipients: a preliminary experience. Transplantation 2003;75:796–9.

256. Gummert JF, Ikonen T, Morris RE. Newer immunosuppressive drugs: a review. J Am Soc Nephrol 1999;10:1366–80.

257. Davis JP, Cain GA, Pitts WJ, et al. The immunosuppressive metabolite of leflunomide is a potent inhibitor of human dihydroorotate dehydrogenase. Biochemistry 1996;35:1270–3.

258. Silva H, Morrris R. Leflunomide and malonitriloamides. Exp Opin Invest Drugs 1997;6:51.

259. Chong AS, Huang W, Liu W, et al. In vivo activity of leflunomide: pharmacokinetic analyses and mechanism of immunosuppression. Transplantation 1999;68:100–9.

260. Waldman WJ, Knight DA, Lurain NS, et al. Novel mechanism of inhibition of cytomegalovirus by the experimental immunosuppressive agent leflunomide. Transplantation 1999;68: 814–25.

261. Cohen S, Cannon GW, Schiff M, et al. Two-year, blinded, randomized, controlled trial of treatment of active rheumatoid arthritis with leflunomide compared with methotrexate. Utilization of Leflunomide in the Treatment of Rheumatoid Arthritis Trial Investigator Group. Arthritis Rheum 2001;44:1984–92.

262. Williams JW, Mital D, Chong A, et al. Experiences with leflunomide in solid organ transplantation. Transplantation 2002;73:358–66.

263. Sampaio E, Sarno E, Galilly R, et al. Thalidomide selectively inhibits tumor necrosis factor alpha production by stimulated human monocytes. J Exp Med 1991;173:699–703.

264. Bousvaros A, Mueller B. Thalidomide in gastrointestinal disorders. Drugs 2001;61:777–87.

265. Ehrenpreis ED, Kane SV, Cohen LB, et al. Thalidomide therapy for patients with refractory Crohn's disease: an open-label trial. Gastroenterology 1999;117:1271–7.

266. Vasiliauskas EA, Kam LY, Abreu-Martin MT, et al. An open-label pilot study of low-dose thalidomide in chronically active, steroid-dependent Crohn's disease. Gastroenterology 1999;117:1278–87.

267. D'Haens G, Swijsen C, Noman M, et al. Etanercept in the treatment of active refractory Crohn's disease: a single-center pilot trial. Am J Gastroenterol 2001;96:2564–8.

268. Sandborn WJ, Hanauer SB, Katz S, et al. Etanercept for active Crohn's disease: a randomized, double-blind, placebo-controlled trial. Gastroenterology 2001;121:1088–94.

269. Marzo-Ortega H, McGonagle D, O'Connor P, Emery P. Efficacy of etanercept for treatment of Crohn's related spondyloarthritis but not colitis. Ann Rheum Dis 2003;62:74–6.

270. von Andrian UH, Engelhardt B. Alpha4 integrins as therapeutic targets in autoimmune disease. N Engl J Med 2003;348:68–72.

271. Butcher EC, Picker LJ. Lymphocyte homing and homeostasis. Science 1996;272:60–6.

272. Ghosh S, Goldin E, Gordon FH, et al. Natalizumab for active Crohn's disease. N Engl J Med 2003;348:24–32.

273. Gordon FH, Hamilton MI, Donoghue S, et al. A pilot study of treatment of active ulcerative colitis with natalizumab, a humanized monoclonal antibody to alpha-4 integrin. Aliment Pharmacol Ther 2002;16:699–705.

274. Serinet MO, Jacquemin E, Habes D, et al. Anti-CD20 monoclonal antibody (rituximab) treatment for Epstein-Barr virus-associated, B-cell lymphoproliferative disease in pediatric liver transplant recipients. J Pediatr Gastroenterol Nutr 2002;34:389–93.

275. Cunnane G, Doran M, Bresnihan B. Infections and biological therapy in rheumatoid arthritis. Best Pract Res Clin Rheumatol 2003;17:345–63.

276. Cheifetz A, Smedley M, Martin S, et al. The incidence and management of infusion reactions to infliximab: a large center experience. Am J Gastroenterol 2003;98:1315–24.

277. Lee JH, Slifman NR, Gershon SK, et al. Life-threatening histoplasmosis complicating immunotherapy with tumor necrosis factor alpha antagonists infliximab and etanercept. Arthritis Rheum 2002;46:2565–70.

278. Lipsky PE, van der Heijde DM, St Clair EW, et al. Infliximab and methotrexate in the treatment of rheumatoid arthritis. Anti-Tumor Necrosis Factor Trial in Rheumatoid Arthritis with Concomitant Therapy Study Group. N Engl J Med 2000;343:1594–602.

2A. Antimicrobials

Michael R. Millar, MB, ChB, PhD, FRCPath

Mark Wilks, BSc, Dip Bacteriol, PhD

This section deals with antibiotic modulation of the pattern of colonization at a site or sites within the gastrointestinal tract. Eradication of single pathogens such as *Helicobacter pylori*, *Giardia lamblia*, and parasitic worms from the gastrointestinal tract by antimicrobials is covered in other sections.

The gastrointestinal tract provides the major reservoir of colonizing microorganisms. Determinants of bowel colonization are poorly understood but include mode of delivery (vaginal/cesarean), diet, health status, age, travel, and gastrointestinal physiology and pathology. The impact of the bowel flora on the human host is complex, with a wide range of metabolic, nutritional, and immunologic effects.[1] In health, the bowel flora provides many benefits for the host, including competitive exclusion of pathogens, the recovery of usable energy sources from cellulose, and provision of butyrate to the colonic mucosa. The gastrointestinal microflora and interactions with the mucosa are reviewed in Chapter 2, "Intestinal Flora and Microbial Epithelial Interactions."

Determinants of the resistance of the microflora to perturbation are poorly understood. There is broad agreement that increasing diversity of an ecosystem promotes stability and increases the resistance to perturbation,[2] yet administration of most antimicrobials, by a systemic route to most individuals, will lead to modulation of the bowel flora. Microbial colonization of the gut with commensal flora benefits the host by preventing colonization or overgrowth with pathogens,[3] so it follows that use of antimicrobials for the prevention or treatment of disease can lead to a detrimental change in colonization.[4] The concept of colonization resistance is often taken to imply that the intestinal flora, once established, is relatively static. However, molecular analysis of the bifidobacterial and lactobacillus composition of the microflora in humans suggests that this may not be so and that the pattern of bacterial flora is dynamic in healthy people, regardless of selection pressure caused by the use of antimicrobials.[5] Gastrointestinal side effects are a common consequence of use of antimicrobials. The most frequent side effects are changes in bowel habit and overgrowth with fungi, and a large proportion of these disturbances probably result from alterations of the bowel flora.

The clinical consequences of use of antimicrobials reflect not only modulation of the distribution of microorganisms in the gastrointestinal tract but also changes in microbial physiology and the production of microbial virulence determinants, such as lipopolysaccharide, toxins, and colonization factors.[6–10] Antimicrobials, by modifying microbial metabolic activities, can induce changes in intraluminal conditions, for example, pH, which may also have profound effects on microbial growth and physiology and modify the interaction with the host.[11] Acquisition of antibiotic resistance may be associated with changes in the production of microbial virulence or colonization factors.[12] Even a subinhibitory concentration of antibiotics can have major effects on the transcription of bacterial genes.[13]

There is increasing evidence that the early pattern of colonization is an important determinant of development of the intestine.[14,15] Gram-positive bacteria, such as *Lactobacillus* spp and *Bifidobacterium* spp, may have a role in the prevention of the development of atopy.[16] Neonatal antibiotic treatment of mice leads to a long-term T helper 2 skewed immunologic response, which can be prevented by the introduction of intestinal bacteria.[17]

The effect of administration of antimicrobials in the peripartum period on the early pattern of colonization in the newborn has not been extensively studied, but there is some support for the idea that use of antibiotics in the peripartum period alters the pattern of subsequent microbial colonization and the risk of systemic infection of the newborn.[18] The effects of antibiotic treatment may be more marked in infants than in adults. In a recent study of the fecal flora of 1- to 3-month-old infants, bifidobacteria and lactobacilli were suppressed to undetectable levels in most infants during treatment with amoxicillin, pivampicillin, cefaclor, cefadroxil, erythromycin, or cotrimoxazole.[19]

Antimicrobials may facilitate the acquisition of novel colonizers, a strategy that can be used to facilitate bowel colonization by probiotic strains, but can also reduce the infective inoculum of microbial pathogens.[20] Antimicrobials also provide a selection pressure for colonization or overgrowth of the gut with antimicrobial-resistant microorganisms. The density and diversity of the microflora facilitate the spread of transmissible genetic elements,[21] so the gastrointestinal tract can become a major reservoir for antimicrobial-resistant bacteria and resistance genes, with important consequences for both the colonized individual and others. This is particularly important in hospital environments, such as intensive care units. In preterm infants cared for in a neonatal intensive care unit, use of antibiotics for suspected or proven episodes of infection encourages colonization with a limited range of antibiotic-resistant bacteria, while at the same time the opportunities are reduced for acquisition of bacteria that normally colonize healthy infants. The intestine, as a major reservoir for antibiotic-resistant bacteria, can predispose the individual infant to systemic infection but also puts at risk other infants in the hospital setting.[22,23] The abnormal pattern of colonization also has been implicated in the pathogenesis of neonatal necrotizing enterocolitis (NEC).[24]

Older infants and children nursed in intensive care units generally arrive in the unit with a complex gastrointestinal microflora but while in hospital acquire novel colonizers, which are frequently antibiotic resistant. Changes in gastrointestinal motility, use of drugs that reduce gastric acid production, and use of biomedical devices such as nasogastric tubes also contribute to modification of the gut flora in children nursed in intensive care units.

CLASSES OF ANTIBIOTIC

A wide range of antimicrobials are available, including β-lactams (cephalosporins and penicillins), related compounds such as carbapenems and monobactams, and macrolides, quinolones, aminoglycosides, tetracyclines, and peptides. Few novel classes of antimicrobial agent have been marketed over the last 10 years, and most that are currently marketed are representative of classes of antimicrobial agents that have been available for over 20 years.

PENETRATION OF THE GASTROINTESTINAL TRACT BY ANTIMICROBIAL AGENTS

The main routes by which antimicrobial agents reach the lumen of the gastrointestinal tract are by oral ingestion, in bile, by transudation across the gut wall, and by rectal administration. Erythromycin, ampicillin-related drugs (including ureidopenicillins), and rifamycins are excreted in high concentrations in bile. In contrast, sulfonamides, chloramphenicol, and aminoglycosides are relatively poorly excreted in bile.

DETERMINANTS OF ANTIMICROBIAL ACTIVITY

Antimicrobial agents differ in the extent to which they impact on the gastrointestinal flora. Activity is dependent on a wide range of factors, including drug characteristics such as spectrum of activity, modes of administration, and routes of excretion (bile, urine) and the extent to which there is an enterobiliary circulation. Important factors specific to individuals include diet, transit time, intraluminal conditions (eg, pH, redox potential, ionic conditions, nonspecific binding to macromolecules such as proteins and mucins, presence of inhibitors, degrading enzymes, growth substrate availability, and bacterial growth phase), and bowel flora components and complexity. For example, the concentration of divalent cations, such as calcium, is an important determinant of the activity of gentamicin, iron may interfere with the activity of tetracyclines, and sulfonamides are inhibited

by para-aminobenzoic acid. Some antimicrobials, such as colistin, are rapidly inactivated.[25]

EFFECTS OF ANTIMICROBIAL AGENTS ON THE MICROBIAL FLORA OF THE GASTROINTESTINAL TRACT

The impact of antimicrobials on the culturable components of the oral and fecal flora has been extensively studied,[26–28] frequently in healthy adult volunteers. On the other hand, relatively little is known about the impact of antimicrobial agents in patients with specific disease states or at less accessible sites, such as the small intestine and proximal colon. Attempts to describe the impact of antimicrobials on the flora at inaccessible sites using both in vitro continuous culture and animal models demonstrate that the fecal flora does not accurately represent changes in other parts of the gastrointestinal tract.[29]

Recent molecular studies from subjects undergoing colonoscopy confirm that whereas the fecal flora is different from that of the colon, mucosa-associated bacteria are relatively uniformly distributed along the colon.[30] There is some evidence that host-related factors are important in determining the intestinal microflora, and, as a result, attempts to modulate the gut flora in different individuals may give quite variable results.[30]

In vitro models are an attractive approach for studies of bowel flora modulation by antimicrobials but also may not accurately describe changes in vivo. For example, studies of microbial responses in models of the gastrointestinal flora in vitro have historically used planktonic (ie, free floating) populations of bacteria.[31,32] In contrast, in vivo bacteria usually grow in surface-associated communities referred to as biofilms.[33] Biofilm growth may prove an important element in the pathogenesis of intestinal infections.[34] Bacteria growing in biofilms show important differences from planktonic cells in metabolic activity, gene transfer, and susceptibility to both antimicrobial agents and host defense factors.[35,36]

Another area of uncertainty is the impact of antimicrobials on the unculturable components of the gastrointestinal flora. Recent molecular studies suggest that 50 to 90% of the human fecal flora is unculturable using conventional techniques.[37,38] Current technology precludes studies of the unculturable components of the bowel flora of more than a few individuals. Accordingly, there is little information on the impact of antimicrobials on the uncultured components of the bowel flora. It may be that the use of nucleotide sequence arrays will facilitate further research in this area.

Most studies have concentrated on the impact of antimicrobials on facultative gram-positive cocci (such as staphylococci, enterococci, and streptococci), Enterobacteriaceae, anaerobic species (such as clostridia) and yeasts, and the emergence of antimicrobial resistance. In general, bacteria that are susceptible to the antimicrobial agent administered tend to decrease in numbers, and those that are resistant increase in numbers. For example, administration of penicillin reduces the numbers of streptococci in the mouth, whereas the numbers of Enterobacteriaceae increase. There is considerable interindividual variation in the effect of antimicrobial exposure on the microflora. In addition, antimicrobials within the same class may vary in their impact on the bowel flora.[39] The results of individual studies also will vary depending on the population studied and on the constituents of the microflora, such as the proportion of resistant components. Some of the effects of antimicrobial administration cannot be explained by antimicrobial susceptibility. For example, oral vancomycin reduces the numbers of *Bacteroides* spp despite poor antimicrobial activity in vitro.[40] Some antibiotics, such as macrolides, have effects on gastrointestinal motility through binding and activation of the motilin receptor,[41] and these changes can modify the bowel flora indirectly.

It is still widely assumed that there is a direct and exclusive relationship between the use of a particular antimicrobial agent and the development of resistance. This assumption underlies antibiotic use policies of clinics and hospitals and even national policies. However, it has been known for more than two decades that, at least in the case of Enterobacteriaceae, development of multidrug-resistant strains is generally not the result of accumulation of single point mutations. Instead, there is simultaneous acquisition of genetically linked resistance genes carried on transmissible genetic elements such as transposons, integrons, and plasmids.[42,43] Extensive horizontal gene transfer allows passage of resistance in the intestine between both closely related and distantly related bacteria.[21] Earlier assumptions that bacteria pay a fitness penalty in maintaining antimicrobial resistance in the absence of any selective pressure have proven to be incorrect.[42,44]

USE OF ANTIBIOTICS FOR PREVENTION OR TREATMENT OF DISEASE

Antimicrobials may be used to eradicate a specific pathogen from the gastrointestinal tract (see specific sections) or to modulate the pattern of colonization at a site or sites in the gastrointestinal tract. Antimicrobials may be

prescribed for the prevention or treatment of disease and may be used as a sole treatment strategy but are also commonly used in combination with other strategies. Some classes of antimicrobial have highly selective activities, so, for example, aztreonam is active only against gram-negative bacteria, and there are a number of agents with specific activity against gram-positive bacteria. These agents may have a particular role in elucidating the contribution of specific elements of the bowel flora to the pathogenesis of disease.

Table 76.2A-1 summarizes the bowel flora activities of selective antimicrobials and potential indications for their use in the prevention or treatment of disease. Some recently introduced antimicrobials have not been evaluated for bowel flora modulation, and some classes of agent have bowel flora activity only when administered orally or rectally, such as glycopeptides. Carbapenems do not reach high intraluminal concentrations so may have less impact on the bowel flora than antimicrobials such as cephalosporins, which have a similar spectrum of activity.

TREATMENT OF CONDITIONS ASSOCIATED WITH ABNORMAL DISTRIBUTION OF BACTERIA IN THE GASTROINTESTINAL TRACT

There is evidence that some groups of patients with small bowel bacterial overgrowth may benefit from use of antimicrobials over weeks or months.[45-48] However, there are few long-term follow-up studies of patients treated for small bowel stasis. Relapse of symptoms is common unless underlying defects can be corrected. Recent studies do not support the use of small bowel decontamination following liver transplant.[49,50]

Antimicrobials chosen for control of small bowel bacterial overgrowth include tetracyclines, quinolones such as ciprofloxacin, and metronidazole. Each of these classes of agent has a different spectrum of activity and produces a different range of effects on the fecal flora of healthy volunteers. There are no randomized trial data available regarding the comparative efficacy of agents used to treat and control small bowel bacterial overgrowth.

TABLE 76.2A-1 BOWEL FLORA ACTIVITIES OF SELECTIVE ANTIMICROBIALS AND POTENTIAL INDICATIONS FOR THEIR USE IN THE PREVENTION OR TREATMENT OF DISEASE

ANTIMICROBIAL AGENT	BOWEL FLORA ACTIVITY	POTENTIAL INDICATIONS
Cephalosporin	Broad (depends on cephalosporin); generally includes gram-negative bacilli; staphylococci	Prophylaxis of infection—surgery, intensive care (selective decontamination)
Monobactam (aztreonam)	Gram-negative bacilli	? Prophylaxis of necrotizing enterocolitis
Aminoglycosides	Oral administration—gram-negative bacilli; staphylococci	Prophylaxis of infection— surgery, ? neonatal necrotizing enterocolitis, intensive care (selective decontamination)
Penicillins	Broad (depends on penicillin); penicillinase inhibitors further broaden spectrum (tazobactam, clavulanate)	Same as for cephalosporins
Quinolones	Gram-positive bacilli; staphylococci	Small bowel overgrowth; prophylaxis of infection—surgery, immunocompromised
Tetracyclines	Broad	Small bowel overgrowth
Metronidazole	Anaerobes	Small bowel overgrowth
Azole antifungals		Prevention of fungal infection

PROPHYLAXIS OF INFECTION IN THE IMMUNOCOMPROMISED HOST

Antifungal agents have been used to prevent fungal overgrowth of the gastrointestinal tract and thereby reduce the risk of both local and systemic fungal infections in a wide variety of groups of immunocompromised patients, such as in patients being treated for malignancies and those with human immunodeficiency virus (HIV) infection. A recent systematic review concluded that systemic antifungal prophylaxis reduces the severity of oral mucositis and the frequency of oral candidiasis in patients treated with chemotherapy for cancer.[51] Systemic antifungal prophylaxis probably also prevents invasive fungal infection in patients with neutropenia.[52] Antimicrobials also have been used to prevent gram-negative sepsis in patients undergoing treatment for cancer, particularly hematologic malignancies.[53] However, there are concerns that this approach increases the likelihood of serious infection involving antimicrobial-resistant strains and modification in the pattern of infecting agents causing disease, with marginal benefit for patient outcomes.[54,55]

PROPHYLAXIS OF INFECTION IN THE INTENSIVE CARE UNIT

Selective decontamination of the digestive tract has been advocated as a strategy to reduce the risk of ventilator-associated pneumonia in patients undergoing intensive care. The aim of selective decontamination of the digestive tract is to reduce colonization of the upper gastrointestinal tract with aerobic gram-negative rods and Candida species. Selective decontamination of the digestive tract involves the administration of a topical antimicrobial preparation to the oropharynx, usually combined with a systemic antimicrobial agent. The use of selective decontamination of the digestive tract has been subject to a number of meta-analyses.[56] The implementation of a selective decontamination of the digestive tract strategy carries considerable costs. Between 13 and 39 patients would require selective decontamination of the digestive tract to prevent one death from ventilator-associated pneumonia.[57] The methodologic quality of these studies also has been criticized.[58] Moreover, there are concerns about the long-term consequences of selective decontamination of the digestive tract on levels of antimicrobial resistance.[59,60] Given that critically ill patients are so heterogeneous and that the antibiotic treatments may be quite different (in duration, type of antibiotic, and route of administration), it is hardly surprising that no overall consensus has emerged. In the largest single trial of selective decontamination of the digestive tract (546 predominantly surgical adult patients), mortality was reduced significantly (number needed to treat = 12). In this study, there was no observed increase in colonization by resistant gram-negative organisms, but there was increased colonization of all patients by ciprofloxacin-resistant coagulase-negative staphylococci and enterococci.[61] Concerns about antibiotic resistance could be reduced if oropharyngeal decontamination alone were enough to improve survival. In a recent study of oropharyngeal decontamination, the incidence of ventilator-associated pneumonia was reduced, but overall patient survival was not improved.[62]

PROPHYLAXIS AND/OR TREATMENT OF INFLAMMATORY BOWEL DISEASE

In animal models of inflammatory bowel disease, the colonizing microflora has an important etiologic role.[63,64] However, evidence supporting the role of antimicrobial agents in the treatment or prevention of inflammatory bowel diseases in humans is limited.[65–68] Metronidazole, in high doses, has been shown to modify the course of Crohn disease in some patients, such as those with perianal fistulae.[69] There is little evidence of a role for antimicrobial agents in the control or treatment of ulcerative colitis.[70] The use of live microbial feed supplements (probiotics) has been shown in one randomized controlled trial to benefit patients with pouchitis.[71] Antimicrobial agents also can be used to facilitate probiotic colonization, and it may be that in the future, attempts to modify the luminal flora to benefit patients with inflammatory bowel disease will use an approach in which antimicrobial agents are first used to facilitate subsequent colonization with probiotics.

PROPHYLAXIS OF INFECTION ASSOCIATED WITH ABDOMINAL SURGERY

There is an extensive literature and broad agreement on the benefit of antimicrobial agents for the prophylaxis of infection associated with gastrointestinal tract surgery.[72–74] Current recommendations are that there should be a suprainhibitory concentration of appropriate antimicrobial agents present at the site of operation and at the time of bacterial contamination of the operative site. There is little evidence that extending prophylaxis beyond the period of operation is of any benefit, and it may be of harm.[75] Antimicrobial agents chosen for prophylaxis should be active against both facultative bacteria and strict anaerobes. Metronidazole alone is less effective than when it is combined with an agent active against facultative bacteria, such as a cephalosporin. However, the optimum regimen for prophylaxis in the perioperative setting has not been defined.

NEONATAL NECROTIZING ENTEROCOLITIS

Attempts to reduce the incidence of NEC by the oral administration of antibiotics have not provided conclusive results. This subject has been systematically reviewed,[76] with the conclusion that the incidence of NEC may be reduced by the oral administration of antibiotics, but also concluding that there are concerns about the selection of antibiotic-resistant bacteria and identifying a need for further studies of sufficient size and duration to allow the risks and benefits to be assessed. The antibiotics used to treat infants for episodes of suspected sepsis may also modify the bowel flora and influence the incidence of NEC.[77] There are no randomized comparative studies of antimicrobial efficacy in the treatment of neonatal NEC.

SHIFTING THE FLORA TO A MORE HEALTHY COMPOSITION

Recent research suggests that the pattern of bowel colonization, particularly in early life, may have an important influence on subsequent health and disease, such as on the risk of development of atopy.[78] The use of antibiotics to modulate the bowel flora of healthy individuals with a view to long-term health benefits, however, has not been systematically investigated.

It is now well established that there are major differences between the intestinal flora of formula-fed and breast milk–fed infants. These differences are particularly marked in very low birth weight infants.[79] The mode of delivery also is important, and babies born by cesarean section have a different flora, which persists at least until 6 months after birth, presumably owing to the use of prophylactic antibiotics (a single dose of ampicillin) and reduced exposure to the mother's bacterial flora at the time of delivery.[80]

There is no agreement regarding the age at which the intestinal microflora becomes comparable to that of an adult. In a recent study using viable bacterial counts, 16S ribosomal ribonucleic acid, and generic probes, it was found that there were higher numbers of bifidobacteria and clostridial species in the pediatric population compared with healthy adults. Most strikingly, the carriage of Enterobacteriacae was 100-fold higher in children (16 months to 7 years) than in healthy adults (21–34 years).[81]

PROMOTING COLONIZATION OF PROBIOTICS

Antimicrobial agents may have a role in changing patterns of colonization to a more healthy composition and perhaps facilitate colonization of the intestinal tract by probiotic bacteria. There is a need for further research in this area.

CONCLUSIONS

Antimicrobial agents can be used to modify the gastrointestinal flora in ways that may benefit the host, such as for prophylaxis of infection associated with gastrointestinal tract surgery. Antibiotics may also have other indirect effects on the flora that are not readily apparent. Current strategies emphasize the eradication of pathogens or suppression of flora rather than modulation to a more healthy composition. Future strategies may well see the use of antimicrobial agents to facilitate colonization of the bowel with microbes that contribute to the maintenance of health (ie, probiotics) rather than simply for the eradication or suppression of those microbes that cause disease.

REFERENCES

1. Hooper LV, Gordon JI. Commensal host-bacterial relationships in the gut. Science 2001;292:1115–8.
2. Conway PL. Microbial ecology of the human large intestine. In: Gibson GR, Macfarlane GT, editors. Human colonic bacteria. Role in nutrition, physiology, and pathology. London: CRC Press; 1995. p. 1–24.
3. Ward PB, Young GP. Dynamics of Clostridium difficile infection. Control using diet. Adv Exp Med Biol 1997;412:63–75.
4. Trenschel R, Peceny R, Runde V, et al. Fungal colonization and invasive fungal infections following allogeneic BMT using metronidazole, ciprofloxacin and fluconazole or ciprofloxacin and fluconazole as intestinal decontamination. Bone Marrow Transplant 2000;26:993–7.
5. McCartney AL, Wenzhi W, Tannock GW. Molecular analysis of the composition of the bifidobacterial and lactobacillus microflora of humans. Appl Environ Microbiol 1996;62:4608–13.
6. Ginsburg I. Role of lipoteichoic acid in infection and inflammation. Lancet Infect Dis 2002;2:171–9.
7. Worlitzsch D, Kaygin H, Steinhuber A, et al. Effects of amoxicillin, gentamicin, and moxifloxacin on the hemolytic activity of Staphylococcus aureus in vitro and in vivo. Antimicrob Agents Chemother 2001;45:196–202.
8. Holzheimer RG, Hirte T, Reith B, et al. Different endotoxin release and IL-6 plasma levels after antibiotic administration in surgical intensive care patients. J Endotoxin Res 1996;3:261–267
9. Kobayashi T, Tateda K, Matsumoto T, et al. Initial macrolide-treated Pseudomonas aeruginosa induces paradoxical host responses in the lungs of mice and a high mortality rate. J Antimicrob Chemother 2002;50:59–66.
10. Tsuzuki T, Ina K, Ohta M. Clarithromycin increases the release of heat shock protein B from Helicobacter pylori. Aliment Pharmacol Ther 2002;16 Suppl 2:217–28.
11. Qa'Dan M, Spyres LM, Ballard JD. pH-enhanced cytopathic effects of Clostridium sordellii lethal toxin. Infect Immun 2001;69:5487–93.
12. Hirakata Y, Srikumar R, Poole K, et al. Multidrug efflux systems play an important role in the invasiveness of Pseudomonas aeruginosa. J Exp Med 2002;196:109–18.
13. Goh EB, Yim G, Tsui W, et al. Transcriptional modulation of bacterial gene expression by subinhibitory concentrations of antibiotics. Proc Natl Acad Sci U S A 2002;99:17025–30.
14. Bry L, Falk PG, Midtvedt T, Gordon JI. A model of host-microbial interactions in an open mammalian ecosystem. Science 1996;273:1380–3.
15. Stappenbeck TS, Hooper LV, Gordon JI. Developmental regulation of intestinal angiogenesis by indigenous microbes via Paneth cells. Proc Natl Acad Sci U S A 2002;99:15451–5.
16. Kirjavainen PV, Apostolou E, Arvola T, et al. Characterizing the composition of intestinal microflora as a prospective treatment target in infant allergic disease. FEMS Immunol Med Microbiol 2001;32(1):1–7.
17. Sudo N, Yu XN, Aiba Y, et al. An oral introduction of intestinal bacteria prevents the development of a long-term Th2-skewed immunological memory induced by neonatal antibiotic treatment in mice. Clin Exp Allergy 2002;32:1112–6.
18. Stoll BJ, Hansen N, Fanaroff AA, et al. Changes in pathogens causing early-onset sepsis in very-low-birth-weight infants. N Engl J Med 2002;347:240–7.
19. Bennet R, Eriksson M, Nord CE. The fecal microflora of 1-3-month-old infants during treatment with eight oral antibiotics. Infection 2002;30:158–60.
20. Lipson A. Infecting dose of Salmonella. Lancet 1976;i:969.
21. Shoemaker NB, Vlamakis H, Hayes K, Salyers AA. Evidence for extensive resistance gene transfer among Bacteroides spp. and among Bacteroides and other genera in the human colon. Appl Environ Microbiol 2001;67:561–8.
22. Gupta A. Hospital-acquired infections in the neonatal intensive care unit—Klebsiella pneumoniae. Semin Perinatol 2002;26:340–5.

23. Singh N, Patel KM, Leger MM, et al. Risk of resistant infections with Enterobacteriaceae in hospitalized neonates. Pediatr Infect Dis J 2002;21:1029–33.

24. Hoy CM. The role of infection in necrotising enterocolitis. Rev Med Microbiol 2001;12:121–9.

25. Veringa EM, van der Waaij D. Biological inactivation by faeces of antimicrobial drugs applicable in selective decontamination of the digestive tract. J Antimicrob Chemother 1984;14:605–12.

26. Nord CE, Heimdahl A, Kager L. Antimicrobial induced alterations of the human oropharyngeal and intestinal microflora. Scand J Infect Dis Suppl 1986;49:64–72.

27. Nord CE, Heimdahl A. Impact of orally-administered antimicrobial agents on human oropharyngeal and colonic microflora. J Antimicrob Chemother 1986;19 Suppl C:159–64.

28. Sullivan A, Edlund C, Nord CE. Effect of antimicrobial agents on the ecological balance of human microflora. Lancet Infect Dis 2001;1:101–14.

29. Itoh K, Freter R. Control of *Escherichia coli* populations by a combination of indigenous clostridia and lactobacilli in gnotobiotic mice and continuous-flow cultures. Infect Immun 1989;57:559–65.

30. Zoetendal EG, von Wright A, Vilpponen-Salmela T, et al. Mucosa-associated bacteria in the human gastrointestinal tract are uniformly distributed along the colon and differ from the community recovered from feces. Appl Environ Microbiol 2002;68:3401–7.

31. Freter R, Brickner H, Botney M, et al. Mechanisms that control bacterial populations in continuous-flow culture models of mouse large intestinal flora. Infect Immun 1983;39:676–85.

32. Freter R, Brickner H, Fekete J, et al. Survival and implantation of *Escherichia coli* in the intestinal tract. Infect Immunol 1983;39:686–703.

33. Costerton JW, Rozee KR, Cheng KJ. Colonization of particulates, mucous, and intestinal tissue. Prog Food Nutr Sci 1983;7:91–105.

34. Donnenberg MS, Whittam TS. Pathogenesis and evolution of virulence in enteropathogenic and enterohemorrhagic *Escherichia coli*. J Clin Invest 2001;107:539–48.

35. Stewart PS, Casterton JW. Antibiotic resistance of bacteria in biofilms. Lancet 2001;358:135–8.

36. Nichols WW. Susceptibility of biofilms to toxic compounds. In: Characklis WG, Wilderer PA, editors. Structure and function of biofilms. New York: John Wiley & Sons; 1989. p. 321–33.

37. Langendijk PS, Schut F, Jansen GJ, et al. Quantitative fluorescent in situ hybridization of *Bifidobacterium* spp. with genus-specific 16S rRNA-targeted probes and its application in fecal samples. Appl Environ Microbiol 1995;61:3069–75.

38. Suau A, Bonnet R, Sutren M, et al. Direct analysis of genes encoding 16S rDNA from complex communities reveals many novel molecular species within the human gut. Appl Environ Microbiol 1999;65:4799–807.

39. Nord CE. Studies on the ecological impact of antibiotics. Eur J Clin Microbiol Infect Dis 1990;9:517–8.

40. Lund B, Edlund C, Barkholt L, et al. Impact on human intestinal microflora of an *Enterococcus faecium* probiotic and vancomycin. Scand J Infect Dis 2000;32:627–32.

41. Feighner SD, Tan CP, McKee KK, et al. Receptor for motilin identified in the human gastrointestinal system. Science 1999;284:2184–8.

42. Summers AO. Generally overlooked fundamentals of bacterial genetics and ecology. Clin Infect Dis 2002;34 Suppl 3:S85–92.

43. O'Brien TF. Emergence, spread, and environmental effect of antimicrobial resistance: how use of an antimicrobial anywhere can increase resistance to any antimicrobial anywhere else. Clin Infect Dis 2002;34 Suppl 3:S78–84.

44. Millar MR, Walsh TR, Linton CJ, et al. Carriage of antibiotic-resistant bacteria by healthy children. J Antimicrob Chemother 2001;47:605–10.

45. Pimentel M, Chow EJ, Lin HC. Eradication of small intestinal bacterial overgrowth reduces symptoms of irritable bowel syndrome. Am J Gastroenterol 2000;95:3503–6.

46. Attar A, Flourie B, Rambaud JC, et al. Antibiotic efficacy in small intestinal bacterial overgrowth-related chronic diarrhea: a crossover, randomized trial. Gastroenterology 1999;117:794–7.

47. Di Stefano M, Malservisi S, Veneto G, et al. Rifaximin versus chlortetracycline in the short-term treatment of small intestinal bacterial overgrowth. Aliment Pharmacol Ther 2000;14:551–6.

48. De Boissieu D, Chaussain M, Badoual J, et al. Small-bowel bacteria overgrowth in children with chronic diarrhea, abdominal pain, or both. J Pediatr 1996;128:203–7.

49. Hellinger WC, Yao JD, Alvarez S, et al. A randomized, prospective, double-blinded evaluation of selective bowel decontamination in liver transplantation. Transplantation 2002;73:1904–9.

50. Zwaveling JH, Maring JK, Klompmaker IJ, et al. Selective decontamination of the digestive tract to prevent postoperative infection: a randomized placebo-controlled trial in liver transplant patients. Crit Care Med 2002;30:1204–9.

51. Worthington HV, Clarkson JE. Prevention of oral mucositis and oral candidiasis for patients with cancer treated with chemotherapy: Cochrane Systematic Review. J Dent Educ 2002;66:903–11.

52. Bow EJ, Laverdiere M, Lussier N, et al. Antifungal prophylaxis for severely neutropenic chemotherapy recipients: a meta analysis of randomized-controlled clinical trials. Cancer 2002;94:3230–46.

53. Baum HV, Franz U, Geiss HK. Prevalence of ciprofloxacin-resistant *Escherichia coli* in hematological-oncologic patients. Infection 2000;28:259–60.

54. Van Belkum A, Goessens W, van der Schee C. Rapid emergence of ciprofloxacin-resistant Enterobacteriaceae containing multiple gentamicin resistance-associated integrons in a Dutch hospital. Emerg Infect Dis 2001;7:862–71.

55. Jansen J, Cromer M, Akard L, et al. Infection prevention in severely myelosuppressed patients: a comparison between ciprofloxacin and a regimen of selective antibiotic modulation of the intestinal flora. Am J Med 1994;96:335–41.

56. D'Amico R, Pifferi S, Leonetti C, et al. Effectiveness of antibiotic prophylaxis in critically ill patients: systematic review of randomised controlled trials. BMJ 1998;316:1275–85.

57. Selective Decontamination of the Digestive Tract Triallists' Collaborative Group. Meta-analysis of randomised controlled trials of selective decontamination of the digestive tract. BMJ 1993;307:525–32.

58. van Nieuwenhoven CA, Buskens E, van Tiel FH, Bonten MJ. Relationship between methodological trial quality and the effects of selective digestive decontamination on pneumonia and mortality in critically ill patients. JAMA 2001;286:335–40.

59. Rocha LA, Martin MJ, Pita S, et al. Prevention of nosocomial infection in critically ill patients by selective decontamination of the digestive tract. Intensive Care Med 1992;18:398–404.

60. Bonten MJ, Kullberg BJ, van Dalen R, et al. Selective digestive decontamination in patients in intensive care. The Dutch Working Group on Antibiotic Policy. J Antimicrob Chemother 2000;46:351–62.

61. Krueger WA, Lenhart FP, Neeser G, et al. Influence of combined intravenous and topical antibiotic prophylaxis on the incidence of infections, organ dysfunctions, and mortality in critically ill surgical patients: a prospective, stratified, ran-

domized, double-blind, placebo-controlled clinical trial. Am J Respir Crit Care Med 2002;166:1029–37.

62. Bergmans DC, Bonten MJ, Gaillard CA, et al. Prevention of ventilator-associated pneumonia by oral decontamination: a prospective, randomized, double-blind, placebo-controlled study. Am J Respir Crit Care Med 2001;164:382–8.

63. Rath HC, Schultz M, Freitag R, et al. Different subsets of enteric bacteria induce and perpetuate experimental colitis in rats and mice. Infect Immun 2001;69:2277–85.

64. Swidsinski A, Ladhoff A, Pernthaler A. Mucosal flora in inflammatory bowel disease. Gastroenterology 2002;122:44–54.

65. Podolsky DK. Inflammatory bowel disease. N Engl J Med 2002;347:417–29.

66. Farrell RJ, LaMont JT. Microbial factors in inflammatory bowel disease. Gastroenterol Clin North Am 2002;31:41–62.

67. Shanahan F. Crohn's disease. Lancet 2002;359:62–9.

68. Linskens RK, Huijsdens XW, Savelkoul PH, et al. The bacterial flora in inflammatory bowel disease: current insights in pathogenesis and the influence of antibiotics and probiotics. Scand J Gastroenterol 2001;36 Suppl 234:29–40.

69. Sutherland L, Singleton J, Sessions J, et al. Double blind, placebo controlled trial of metronidazole in Crohn's disease. Gut 1991;32:1071–5.

70. Jani N, Regueiro MD. Medical therapy for ulcerative colitis. Gastrenterol Clin North Am 2002;31:147–66.

71. Gionchetti P, Rizzello F, Venturi A, et al. Oral bacteriotherapy as maintenance treatment in patients with chronic pouchitis: a double-blind, placebo-controlled trial. Gastroenterology 2002;119:305–9.

72. Song F, Glenny A. Antimicrobial prophylaxis in colorectal surgery: a systematic review of randomised controlled trials. Br J Surg 1998;85:1232–41.

73. Swedish-Norwegian Consensus Group. Antibiotic prophylaxis in surgery: summary of a Swedish-Norwegian consensus conference. Scand J Infect Dis 1998;30:547–57.

74. Antimicrobial prophylaxis in colorectal surgery. Effective Health Care Bulletins 1998;4(5):1–8.

75. Norrby S. Cost effective prophylaxis of surgical infections. Pharmacoeconomics 1996;10:129–39.

76. Bury RG, Tudehope D. Enteral antibiotics for preventing necrotizing enterocolitis in low birthweight or preterm infants. Cochrane Database Syst Rev 2001;(1):CD000405.

77. Millar R, MacKay P, Levene M, et al. Enterobacteriaceae and neonatal necrotising enterocolitis. Arch Dis Child 1992;67:53–6.

78. Hopkin JM. The rise of atopy and links to infection. Allergy 2002;57 Suppl 72:5–9.

79. Gewolb IH, Schwalbe RS, Taciak VL, et al. Stool microflora in extremely low birthweight infants. Arch Dis Child 1999;80:F167–73.

80. Gronlund MM, Lehtonen OP, Eerola E, Kero P. Fecal microflora in healthy infants born by different methods of delivery: permanent changes in intestinal flora after cesarean delivery. J Pediatr Gastroenterol Nutr 1999;28:19–25.

81. Hopkins MJ, Sharp R, Macfarlane GT. Age and disease related changes in intestinal bacterial populations assessed by cell culture, 16S rRNA abundance, and community cellular fatty acid profiles. Gut 2001;48:198–205.

2B. Probiotics

Erika Isolauri, MD, PhD

Seppo Salminen, PhD

Probiotics are live microbial food supplements or components of bacteria that have been demonstrated to have beneficial effects on human health. Oral introduction of probiotics reinforces various lines of gut defense, including immune exclusion, immune elimination, and immune regulation. Probiotics also stimulate nonspecific host resistance to microbial pathogens and thereby aid in their eradication. Correction of the properties of unbalanced indigenous microbiota forms the rationale of probiotic therapy. The application of probiotics currently lies in reducing the risk of diseases associated with gut barrier dysfunction; the most fully documented probiotic intervention is the treatment and prevention of acute infectious diarrhea. Recent clinical and nutritional studies and characterization of the immunomodulatory potential of specific strains of the gut microbiota, beyond the effect on the composition of the microbiota, may lead to future applications not only for different infectious diarrheas but also for allergic and inflammatory diseases.

The probiotic potential of strains differs; different bacterial species, and even strains of the same species, are each unique and have defined adherence sites, specific immunologic effects, and varied effects in the healthy versus the inflamed mucosal milieu. Current probiotic research aims at characterization of the healthy individual gut microbiota and understanding the microbe-microbe and host-microbe interactions. The goal is to use the defined microbiota both as a tool for nutritional management of specific gut-related diseases and as a source of novel microbes for future probiotic bacteriotherapy applications.

HEALTHY GUT MICROBIOTA

The human gastrointestinal tract harbors a complex collection of microorganisms, which form a typical individual microbiota for each person.[1] This specific microbiota is dependent on genetic factors and the environment. The total number of microbes in the intestinal tract is estimated to reach 10^{12} bacteria per gram of intestinal contents. Several hundred bacterial species can be identified using traditional culture methods.[1] The development of novel means of characterizing gut microbiota, in particular molecular methods, has uncovered new microbial species in intestinal mucosa and contents.[1,2]

The microbiota is metabolically active, and its composition is related to multiple disease states within the intestine and also beyond the gastrointestinal tract. Components of the human intestinal microbiota or organisms entering the intestine may, however, have both harmful or beneficial effects on human health.

The basis of healthy gut microbiota lies in early infancy and the initial process of intestinal colonization. The generation of immunophysiologic regulation in the gut depends on the establishment of indigenous microbiota.[3–5] The microbiota of a newborn develops rapidly after birth and is initially strongly dependent on the mother's microbiota, mode of delivery, and birth environment.[6] Subsequently, feeding practices and the home environment of the child influence the composition. Major changes in the composition occur during breastfeeding, weaning, and introduction of solid foods.[6,7]

The establishment of the gut microbiota has traditionally been considered a stepwise process with facultative anaerobics such as the enterobacteria, coliforms, and lactobacilli first colonizing the intestine with rapid succession by bifidobacteria and lactic acid bacteria.[7–9] New molecular methods indicate, however, that lactic acid–producing bacteria account for less than 1% of the total microbiota in infants, whereas bifidobacteria can range from 60 to 90% of the total fecal microbiota in breastfed infants.[2,10] Moreover, the new techniques indicate that the greatest difference in the microbiota of breastfed and formula-fed infants lies in the bifidobacterial composition of intestinal microbiota, whereas the lactic acid bacteria composition appears to be rather similar. *Bifidobacterium breve*, *Bifidobacterium infantis*, and *Bifidobacterium longum* are frequently found in fecal samples of breastfed infants, whereas the most common lactobacilli in breastfed and formula-fed infant feces constitute *Lactobacillus acidophilus* group microorganisms such as *L. acidophilus*, *L. gasseri*, and *L. johnsonii*.[10,11]

Healthy microbiota is defined as the normal microbiota of an individual that both preserves and promotes well-being and absence of disease, especially in the gastrointestinal tract.[12] The collective composition of the colonizing strains in infancy also provides the basis for healthy gut microbiota later in life. In addition, the development of the disease-free state of the gut lies in the host-microbe interaction in infancy.[13,14]

DEFINITIONS OF PROBIOTICS

The history of probiotics dates back to ancient times, but the scientific work on health benefits was initiated by Metchnikoff early last century.[15] Health-promoting fermented foods are used for the treatment and prevention of infant diarrhea in countries around the world without knowledge of the specific microbial composition of such products.[16] Beneficial bacteria in fermented foods that promote health have only more recently been called probiotics. These have been variously defined, according to their initial application, in animal feeds. For the purpose of human nutrition, a probiotic is currently defined as a live microbial food ingredient beneficial to health.[12] However, inactivated probiotic bacteria also may have beneficial health effects. The history of the definition and the current status are presented in Table 76.2B-1.[15,17–22]

Probiotics were initially selected to provide strains with good food-processing conditions, but, more recently, the physiologic properties of probiotics in the human gastrointestinal tract have formed the basis for selection. These criteria have been redefined to include the healthy human intestinal or mucosal microbiota as the main source of new strains. At present, emphasis is placed on survival in the gut, acid and bile stability, temporary colonization of the mucosal surfaces in the intestinal tract, and fecal recovery of the administered probiotic to define the dosage needed for individual target uses.[23] The most frequently used genera fulfilling these criteria are lactobacilli and bifidobacteria. Currently, most probiotics have been selected from members of normal healthy adult microbiota.

RATIONALE FOR PROBIOTIC INTERVENTION IN PEDIATRIC PRACTICE

The therapeutic and prophylactic interventions by probiotics derive from the concept of a well-functioning gut barrier and a normal balanced microbiota. In addition to its principal physiologic function, digestion and absorption of nutrients, the intestinal mucosa provides a protective interface between the internal environment and the constant challenge from antigens of the external environment, also carrying defense mechanisms against infectious and inflammatory diseases.

Gut microbiota as a component of intestinal barrier has been considered as a physiologic blockade to foreign substances such as antigens. One current view focuses on communication between the host and the resident commensal microbes.[22] This interaction manifests best during early infancy, when the colonization process governs the development of intestinal integrity and host immune defense mechanisms.[3–5] Conversely, the genetic background of the host and development of the immune system influence the collective composition of the intestinal microbiota.

In several gut-related inflammatory conditions, the healthy host-microbe interaction is disturbed, and inflammation is accompanied by an imbalance in the intestinal microbiota in such a way that an immune response may be generated against resident bacteria. For example, an altered gut microbiota is reported in patients with rotavirus diarrhea, inflammatory bowel diseases, rheumatoid arthritis, and allergic diseases,[23] implying that the normal gut microbiota constitutes an ecosystem responding to inflammation both in the gut and elsewhere in the human body. Normalization of the properties of an unbalanced indigenous microbiota by specific strains of the healthy gut microbiota constitutes the rationale for probiotic therapy. Such an approach with oral introduction of specific probiotics may halt the vicious circle in inflammation.

The probiotic effects in conditions involving impaired mucosal barrier function, particularly infectious and inflammatory diseases, lie in normalization of increased intestinal permeability and altered gut microecology, improvement of immunologic barrier functions of the intestine, and alleviation of intestinal inflammatory responses.[22,23]

Although it is well documented that balanced normal microbiota may become aberrant and immunogenic secondary to gut-related disease, it is not known whether changes in the composition of the microbiota can be a primary cause of disease. Such associations recently have been suggested in allergic disease[22] and autism.[24] Differences in the neonatal gut microbiota, in particular the bal-

TABLE 76.2B-1   CURRENT UNDERSTANDING AND HISTORY OF PROBIOTIC DEFINITIONS

DEFINITION	SOURCE
Specific bacteria in yoghurt fermentation balance intestinal microbiota	Metchnikoff (1907)[15]
Substances excreted by one protozoan to stimulate the growth of another	Lilly and Stillwell (1965)[17]
Substances that have a beneficial effect on animals by contributing to the balance of the intestinal biota	Parker (1974)[18]
Live microbial feed supplements that beneficially affect the host animal by improving the intestinal microbial balance	Fuller (1989)[19]
Mono- or mixed cultures of live microorganisms that, when applied to humans, affect beneficially the host by improving the properties of the indigenous microbiota	Huis in't Veld and Havenaar (1991)[20]
Live microbial food ingredients that are beneficial to health (efficacy and safety scientifically documented)	Salminen et al (1998)[12]
Live microbial cell preparations or components of cells that have a beneficial effect on human health	Salminen et al (1999)[21]
Specific live or inactivated microbial cultures that have documented targets in reducing the risk of human disease or in their adjunct treatment	Isolauri et al (2002)[22]

ance between *Bifidobacterium* and *Clostridium* microbiota, may precede the manifestation of the atopic responder type with heightened production of antigen-specific immunoglobulin E antibodies, suggesting a crucial role of the balance of the indigenous intestinal bacteria for the maturation of human immunity to a nonatopic mode.[25] These observations underline the importance of the need for precise characterization of healthy versus aberrant microbiota development and composition. This requires thorough investigation of the infant microbiota by up-to-date techniques; in particular those based on molecular techniques including ribosomal ribonucleic acid sequencing. Indirect methods, such as fecal microbial enzyme activities,[26] may also reflect differences in microbiota development.

CLINICAL EVIDENCE OF PROBIOTIC EFFECTS IN CHILDREN

The potential health effects of normal gut microbiota must be demonstrated by well-controlled clinical and nutritional studies in human subjects.[27] So far, several clinical studies have investigated the use of probiotics, principally lactobacilli and bifidobacteria, as dietary supplements for the prevention and treatment of various gastrointestinal infectious and inflammatory conditions (Table 76.2B-2).

ACUTE ENTERITIS

The currently accepted guidelines for treatment of acute diarrhea are based on correcting the dehydration by oral rehydration solutions. In addition, immediately after the completion of oral rehydration, full feedings of a previously tolerated diet can be reintroduced. Well-controlled clinical studies have shown that probiotics such as *Lactobacillus rhamnosus* GG, *Lactobacillus reuteri*, *Lactobacillus casei* Shirota, and *Bifidobacterium lactis* Bb12 can shorten the duration of acute rotavirus diarrhea,[23] above the beneficial effect of rapid refeeding, and thus constitute safe adjunct nutritional management of the condition.

In patients hospitalized for acute rotavirus diarrhea, *L. rhamnosus* strain GG (ATCC 53103) as a fermented milk or as a freeze-dried powder reduced the duration of diarrhea compared with the placebo group given a fermented and then pasteurized milk product.[28] This result has been confirmed in subsequent studies.[29,30] Moreover, probiotics reduce the duration of rotavirus excretion in stools.[31] A multicenter study by the European Society for Pediatric Gastroenterology, Hepatology, and Nutrition working group tested the clinical efficacy and safety of a probiotic administered in an oral rehydration solution.[32] In rotavirus diarrhea, but not in nonspecific or bacterial diarrhea, a decrease in the number of diarrhea episodes was observed. The study also confirmed the safety of administration of a probiotic in an oral rehydration solution and prevention of the evolution of rotavirus-induced diarrhea toward a protracted course. These studies have invariably evaluated patients with mild or moderate dehydration. A recent randomized placebo-controlled study in severely dehydrated male children under 2 years of age showed no clinical benefit of supplementing oral rehydration with *Lactobacillus* GG.[33]

Probiotics, specifically *Bifidobacterium bifidum* (later renamed *B. lactis*) and *Streptococcus thermophilus*, are also effective in the prevention of acute infantile diarrhea.[31] *Lactobacillus* GG supplementation resulted in a decrease in the incidence of diarrhea in undernourished, nonbreastfed Peruvian children followed for 15 months.[34] *Lactobacillus* GG also reduces the incidence of nosocomial diarrhea but has no effect on the prevalence of rotavirus infection.[35] Recently, Mastretta and colleagues confirmed the result when assessing the effects of *Lactobacillus* GG and breastfeeding on nosocomial rotavirus infections in 220 hospitalized infants during one rotavirus epidemic season.[36] The frequency of nosocomial rotavirus infection was 28%. This probiotic preparation was ineffective, whereas breastfeeding was effective in reducing the risk of rotavirus infection.

The effect of probiotic therapy (see Table 76.2B-2) in diarrhea has been explained by a reduction in the duration of rotavirus shedding, normalization of gut permeability

TABLE 76.2B-2   TARGETS OF PROBIOTIC THERAPY

EFFECT	METHOD OF ASSESSMENT	OUTCOME
Nutritional management of disease Diarrhea Allergic/inflammatory diseases	Randomized double-blind clinical studies	Reduction in the duration of symptoms Eradication of the infectious agent Symptom score
Control of disease activity/reactions/ relapses/inflammation	Clinical follow-up studies Crossover challenge studies (double blind, placebo controlled)	Reduction of disease activity indices specific for the condition Reduction of proinflammatory cytokines specific for the condition and site
Enhanced host defense	Intestinal permeability Immunomodulation in vitro/in vivo Gut microbiota aberrancy	Promotion of immunologic and nonimmunologic barrier function Generation of anti-inflammatory cytokines
Reduction in risk of disease Diarrhea Allergic disease	Randomized double-blind, placebo-controlled study	Reduction in the frequency of the condition after appropriate follow-up
Gut microbiota stabilization Regulation of bowel movement Comparative exclusion	Modern techniques of evaluation of the gut microecology	Balanced microbiota appropriate for age

Adapted from Isolauri E et al.[22,23]

caused by rotavirus infection, and an increase in immunoglobulin (Ig)A-secreting cells against rotavirus.[14,23] Moreover, the ability of specific probiotics to increase the expression of mucins may contribute to the barrier effect but also to inhibition of rotavirus replication.[37]

Antimicrobial treatment disturbs colonization resistance of the gut microbiota,[1] which may induce clinical symptoms, most frequently diarrhea. The incidence of diarrhea after single antimicrobial treatment and the effect of probiotics was evaluated in children with no history of antimicrobial use during the previous 3 months.[38] The frequency of diarrhea was 5% in the group given *Lactobacillus* GG and 16% in the placebo group ($p = .05$), supporting the efficacy of probiotics. *Lactobacillus* GG, compared with placebo, reduces stool frequency and increases stool consistency during antibiotic therapy in children aged 6 months to 10 years given oral antibiotics in an outpatient setting.[39] In addition, there are preliminary reports on resolution of *Clostridium difficile* diarrhea and colitis in adults.[40]

The value of probiotic preparations for the prophylaxis of traveler's diarrhea has been studied using *Lactobacillus acidophilus*, *B. bifidum*, *Lactobacillus bulgaricus*, and *S. thermophilus*, but the results have been conflicting, likely owing to differences in probiotic species and vehicles used, in dosage schedules, as well as varying travel destinations with different causes of diarrhea.[12]

INFLAMMATORY BOWEL DISEASES

An increasing number of clinical and experimental studies demonstrate the importance of constituents within the intestinal lumen, in particular the resident microbiota, in driving the inflammatory responses in these diseases. Intestinal microbiota appears to be responsible for deep colonic lesions and severe inflammatory response.[41] Probiotic bacteria may counteract the inflammatory process by stabilizing the gut microbial environment and the intestine's permeability barrier and by enhancing the degradation of enteral antigens and altering their immunogenicity. Another explanation for the gut-stabilizing effect could be improvement of the intestine's immunologic barrier, particularly intestinal IgA responses. Probiotic effects may also be mediated via control of the balance between pro- and anti-inflammatory cytokines.[14,23]

Preliminary reports indicate benefit in reversing some of the immunologic disturbances characteristic of Crohn disease.[23] In addition, reductions in disease activity and increased intestinal permeability have been achieved in pediatric patients with Crohn disease by probiotic intervention.[42] In adults operated on for the condition, however, *Lactobacillus* GG failed to prevent endoscopic recurrence during 1 year of follow-up.[43] A recent study provides evidence for treatment with a nonpathogenic *Escherichia coli* in maintaining remission in ulcerative colitis.[44] In a clinical trial in adults, a preparation containing four strains of lactobacilli (*L. casei*, *L. plantarum*, *L. acidophilus,* and *L. delbrückii* subsp. *bulgaricus*) and three bifidobacteria strains (*B. longum*, *B. breve*, and *B. infantis*), together with *Streptococcus salivarius* subsp. *thermophilus*, is encouraging for prevention of relapses of chronic pouchitis.[45]

Additional, controlled prospective data in human inflammatory bowel diseases are required to define the effects of specific probiotic strains on distinct forms of inflammatory bowel disease and attendant complications.

ALLERGIC DISEASES

The prevalence of atopic diseases, atopic eczema, allergic rhinoconjunctivitis, and asthma appears to have increased over this century throughout the industrialized world.[46] These conditions are associated with the generation of T helper (Th) cell 2–type cytokines, including interleukin (IL)-4, IL-5, and IL-13, which promote IgE production and eosinophilia.[46] Initial signals to counter IL-4, and thereby IgE and atopy, and IL-5–generated eosinophilic inflammation may stem from components of the innate immune system, which generates the necessary initial steps for the targeted and specific function of the adaptive immune system.[22,46]

Two structural components of bacteria, the lipopolysaccharide portion of gram-negative bacteria (endotoxin) and a specified CpG motif in bacterial deoxyribonucleic acid (DNA),[47,48] activate immunomodulatory genes via Toll-like receptors (TLR4 and TLR9, respectively) present on macrophages and dendritic and intestinal epithelial cells[49,50] and elicit an immunosuppressive effect on intestinal epithelial cells by inhibition of the transcription factor nuclear factor-κB signaling pathway.[51] Specific strains of the gut microbiota contribute to a T regulatory cell population amenable to oral tolerance induction[13] and counter allergy by the generation of IL-10 and transforming growth factor-β.[52,53] These activities are associated with suppression of proliferation of Th cells and reduced secretion of proinflammatory cytokines,[53–57] with control of IgE responses[58] and reduced allergic inflammation in the gut.[59] However, different *Lactobacillus* and *Bifidobacterium* strains appear to induce distinct and even opposing responses.[60,61] Thus, specific strains of the gut micobiota and probiotics may play a crucial role in determining the Th1/Th2-driving capacity of intestinal dendritic cells. In parallel, recent observations indicate that the cytokine production patterns induced by intestinal bifidobacteria are strain specific.[22] The results of clinical studies evaluating the effects of probiotics in allergic disease appear to substantiate this suggestion.

In one prospective study, the intestinal microbiota from 76 infants at high risk of atopic diseases was analyzed at 3 weeks of age by conventional bacterial cultivation and two culture-independent methods.[25] A positive skinprick reaction at 12 months was observed in 29% of the subjects. At 3 weeks of age, the bacterial cellular fatty acid profile in fecal samples differed between those infants later developing atopic sensitization and those not developing atopy. Fluorescence in situ hydridization was used to show that atopic subjects have more *Clostridium* species and fewer *Bifidobacterium* species in stools compared with nonatopic subjects.[25] Differences in the neonatal gut microbiota thus appear to precede the manifestations of atopy, suggesting a crucial role of the balance of indigenous intestinal bacteria for the maturation of human immunity to a nonatopic mode.

Improvement in the clinical course of atopic eczema and cow's milk allergy is observed in infants when given probiotic-supplemented extensively hydrolyzed formula compared with placebo-supplemented formula.[59,62] In parallel, markers of systemic[62] and intestinal[59] allergic inflammation were reduced (see Table 76.2B-2). Similar results have been obtained in milk-hypersensitive adults.[63] In these subjects, a milk challenge in conjunction with a probiotic strain prevented the immunoinflammatory response characteristic of the response without probiotics.

The preventive potential of probiotics in atopic diseases has been demonstrated in a double-blind, placebo-controlled study.[64] Probiotics administered pre- and postnatally for 6 months to children at high risk of atopic diseases reduced the prevalence of atopic eczema to half compared with infants receiving placebo.[64] Moreover, the effect extends beyond infancy.[65]

WHAT IS REQUIRED FOR FUTURE PROBIOTICS?

Research interest in the science of nutrition is currently directed toward improvement of defined physiologic functions beyond the nutritional impact of food, including the potential to reduce the risk of diseases. This is also the focus for probiotic research. Future probiotics must have more thoroughly defined mechanisms either to control specific physiologic processes in the evolution of disease for at-risk populations or in the dietary management of specific diseases (Figure 76.2B-1).

Prerequisites for probiotic action include survival in and adhesion to specific areas of the gastrointestinal tract and competitive exclusion of pathogens or harmful antigens.[66] These processes may depend first on specific strain characteristics and second on the age and the immunologic state of the host (Table 76.2B-3). Some probiotic strains adhere better to the small intestine, whereas others bind specifically to different parts of the large intestine.[67] It is likely that strains also adhere differently to healthy versus damaged mucosa.[68] It has also recently been demonstrated that strains with lower total in vitro binding capacity may still effect high competitive exclusion of pathogens or harmful bacteria,[66] indicating a need for further characterization of in vivo adhesion properties to develop preclinical selection methodologies for candidate probiotic strains.

Genetically modified bacteria evincing improved or added functional properties may also achieve probiotic effects. These include probiotics encoding mammalian genes to produce and secrete functional anti-inflammatory cytokines, such as *L. lactis* engineered to produce IL-10 locally.[69] Other methods of probiotic modification are exposure of the microorganism to sublethal stress such as acidic conditions or heat to improve survival in the gastrointestinal tract and tolerance to stress and thereby to furnish the organism with improved competitiveness against pathogens in the intestinal milieu.[70–72] Inactivation may also have potential in the modification of probiotics. The use of inactivated instead of viable microorganisms would have merit in terms of safety, longer shelf-life, and less interaction with other components in food products.

Owing to limited availability of controlled data in humans, more research is required on the effects of specific probiotic strains, in particular when there are modifications of components of these bacteria. Probiotic effects appear to be strain specific.[60,61] Indeed, the effects of even closely related strains can be counteractive. No single probiotic strain alone can influence all of the multifactorial processes controlling the intestinal milieu. Therefore, targets of probiotic intervention should be clearly identified and effective strains and specific strain combinations must be developed with desired properties for both nutritional management and the control of human diseases (see Figure 76.2B-1).

SAFETY ASPECTS OF PROBIOTIC THERAPY

Probiotic therapy forms a relatively new treatment modality for gastrointestinal disorders. The ingestion of large numbers of viable bacteria requires strict assurance of both acute and long-term safety. Probiotics currently used have been assessed as safe for use in fermented foods, but, generally, the safety assessment of microbial food supplements is not well developed.[73] The ability of probiotic strains to survive in gastric conditions and to strongly adhere to the intestinal epithelium may entail a risk of bacterial translocation,[74] bacteremia,[75] and sepsis.[76]

Reports from countries with high probiotic consumption suggest that current preparations are safe for their intended uses.[75,76] However, patients with severe underly-

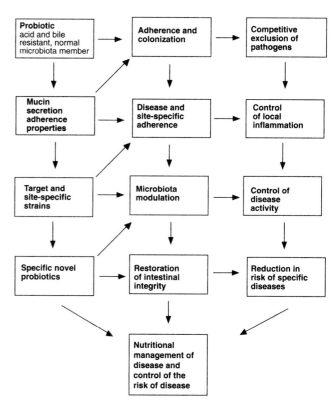

FIGURE 76.2B-1   The selection and use of specific probiotic strains and some targets in disease risk reduction symptom management.

TABLE 76.2B-3   PROPERTIES OF PROBIOTICS TO BE ASSESSED DURING THE DEVELOPMENT OF NEW STRAINS AND NEW APPLICATIONS

PROPERTY	TARGET AND METHOD
Species specificity	Source or origin; healthy human gut microbiota as the source
Resistance to pH	Model systems for gastric and bile effects
Adhesion to intestinal mucosa	Several model systems to be used (eg, cell cultures, mucus, intestinal segments)
	Fecal recovery in human subjects
Competitive exclusion	In vitro and in vivo model systems for pathogen adherence exclusion
Immune regulation	In vitro and human studies
Generation and balance of cytokines	Cytokine profile
	Contact with immune cells
	Adhesion related to immune effects
	Improvement of gut barrier and permeability disorders
Safety	Exclusion of antibiotic resistance and virulence factors and postmarket surveillance
Technological properties	Stability and activity throughout the processes
Efficacy assessment	Human clinical intervention studies with final product formulations; at least two independent studies to prove efficacy in target populations and safety in all consumer groups

Adapted from Salminen S et al[12] and Isolauri E et al.[22]

ing diseases, particularly immunocompromised subjects, appear to carry an increased risk of bacteremia associated with the use of some current probiotics.[75,76] Translocation of intraluminal bacteria may be one risk factor, but recent data also suggest that some probiotic strains directly interfere with host innate immune functions.[77]

Genetically modified microorganisms could be developed for use in foods. Developments in this area also may provide medical applications. However, a safety concern is the potential for the transfer of antibiotic resistance from modified organisms to gut pathogens.[78] Selection procedures have been developed to monitor the absence of antibiotic resistance, thus far specifically for Lactococcus.[79] The use of inactivated bacteria as probiotics has been advocated because their consumption may be safer than the use of viable bacteria.[23] However, information on the effects of inactivation methods on cell wall structure and composition is scarce. Such concerns are not limited to heat treatment; detrimental effects also may be expected in response to lyophilization and irradiation.[80]

To conclude, specific probiotics offer a tool for modification of the gut barrier and microbiota. The microbes used must be obtained from acceptable sources with scientifically proven safety and efficacy to guarantee their application in infectious, allergic, and inflammatory diseases.

REFERENCES

1. Guarner F, Malagelada JR. Gut flora in health and disease. Lancet 2003;361:512–9.
2. Favier C, Vaughan E, de Vos W, Akkermans A. Molecular monitoring of succession of bacterial communities in human neonates. Appl Environ Microbiol 2002;68:219–26.
3. Grönlund MM, Arvilommi H, Kero P, et al. Importance of intestinal colonisation in the maturation of humoral immunity in early infancy: a prospective follow up study of healthy infants aged 0-6 months. Arch Dis Child 2000;83:F186–92.
4. Cebra JJ. Influences of microbiota on intestinal immune system development. Am J Clin Nutr 1999;69 Suppl:1046–51.
5. Gaskins HR. Immunological aspects of host/microbiota interactions at the intestinal epithelium. In: Mackie RI, White DA, Isaacson RE, editors. Gastrointestinal microbiology. New York: International Thomson Publishing; 1997. p. 537–87.
6. Grönlund MM, Lehtonen OP, Eerola E, et al. Fecal microflora in healthy infants born by different methods of delivery: permanent changes in intestinal flora after cesarean delivery. J Pediatr Gastroenterol Nutr 1999;28:19–25.
7. Benno Y, Mitsuoka T. Development of intestinal microflora in humans and animals. Bifidobacteria Microfi 1986;5:13–25.
8. Berg RD. The indigenous gastrointestinal microflora. Trends Microbiol 1996;4:430–5.
9. Harmsen HJ, Wildeboer-Veloo AC, Raangs GC, et al. Analysis of intestinal flora development in breast-fed and formula-fed infants by using molecular identification and detection methods. J Pediatr Gastroenterol Nutr 2000;30:61–7.
10. Vaughan E, de Vries M, Zoetendal E, et al. The intestinal LABs. Anth Leeuwenh 2002;82:341–52.
11. Satokari RM, Vaughan EE, Akkermans AD, et al. Bifidobacterial diversity in human feces detected by genus-specific PCR and denaturing gradient gel electrophoresis. Appl Environ Microbiol 2001;67:504–13.
12. Salminen S, Bouley C, Boutron-Ruault MC, et al. Gastrointestinal physiology and function—targets for functional food development. Br J Nutr 1998;80 Suppl:147–71.
13. Sudo N, Sawamura S, Tanaka K, et al. The requirement of intestinal bacterial flora for the development of an IgE production system fully susceptible to oral tolerance induction. J Immunol 1997;159:1739–45.
14. Isolauri E, Sütas Y, Kankaanpää P, et al. Probiotics: effects on immunity. Am J Clin Nutr 2001;73 Suppl 2:S444–50.
15. Metchnikoff E. Prolongation of life. London: William Heinemann; 1907.
16. Jelliffe EF, Jelliffe DB, Feldon K, Ngokwey N. Traditional practices concerning feeding during and after diarrhoea (with special reference to acute dehydrating diarrhoea in young children). World Rev Nutr Diet 1987;53:218–95.
17. Lilly D, Stillwell E. Probiotics: growth promoting factors produced by microorganisms. Science 1965;147:747–8.
18. Parker RB. Probiotics: the other half of the antibiotics story. Anim Nutr Health 1974;29:4–8.
19. Fuller R. Probiotic in man and animals. Appl Bacteriol 1989;66:365–78.
20. Huis in't Veld J, Havenaar R. Probiotics and health in man and animal. J Chem Technol Biotechnol 1991;51:562–7.

21. Salminen S, Ouwehand A, Benno Y, Lee YK. Probiotics: how should they be defined? Trends Food Sci Technol 1999; 10:107–10.

22. Isolauri E, Rautava S, Kalliomäki M, et al. Role of probiotics in food hypersensitivity. Curr Opin Immunol Clin Allergy 2002;2:263–71.

23. Isolauri E, Kirjavainen PV, Salminen S. Probiotics: a role in the treatment of intestinal infection and inflammation? Gut 2002;50 Suppl III:iii54–9.

24. Finegold SM, Molitoris D, Song Y, et al. Gastrointestinal microflora studies in late-onset autism. Clin Infect Dis 2002;35 Suppl 1:S6–16.

25. Kalliomäki M, Kirjavainen P, Eerola E, et al. Distinct patterns of neonatal gut microflora in infants in whom atopy was and was not developing. J Allergy Clin Immunol 2001;107:129–34.

26. Isolauri E, Kaila M, Mykkänen H, et al. Oral bacteriotherapy for viral gastroenteritis. Dig Dis Sci 1994;39:2595–600.

27. Vanderhoof JA, Young RJ. Use of probiotics in childhood gastrointestinal disorders. J Pediatr Gastroenterol Nutr 1998;27:323–32.

28. Isolauri E, Juntunen M, Rautanen T, et al. A human Lactobacillus strain (Lactobacillus GG) promotes recovery from acute diarrhea in children. Pediatrics 1991;88:90–7.

29. Kaila M, Isolauri E, Soppi E, et al. Enhancement of the circulating antibody secreting cell response in human diarrhea by a human lactobacillus strain. Pediatr Res 1992;32:141–4.

30. Pant AR, Graham SM, Allen SJ, et al. Lactobacillus GG and acute diarrhoea in young children in the tropics. J Trop Pediatr 1996;42:162–5.

31. Saavedra JM, Bauman NA, Oung I, et al. Feeding of Bifidobacterium bifidum and Streptococcus thermophilus to infants in hospital for prevention of diarrhoea and shedding of rotavirus. Lancet 1994;344:1046–9.

32. Guandalini S, Pensabene L, Zikri MA, et al. Lactobacillus GG administered in oral rehydration solution to children with acute diarrhoea: a multicenter European trial. J Pediatr Gastroenterol Nutr 2000;30:54–60.

33. Costa-Ribeiro H, Ribeiro TC, Mattos AP, et al. Limitations of probiotic therapy in acute, severe dehydrating diarrhea. J Pediatr Gastroenterol Nutr 2003;36:112–5.

34. Oberhelman RA, Gilman RH, Sheen P, et al. A placebo-controlled trial of Lactobacillus GG to prevent diarrhea in undernourished Peruvian children. J Pediatr 1999;134:15–20.

35. Szajewska H, Kotowska M, Mrukowicz JZ, et al. Efficacy of Lactobacillus GG in prevention of nosocomial diarrhea in infants. J Pediatr 2001;138:361–5.

36. Mastretta E, Longo P, Laccisaglia A, et al. Effect of Lactobacillus GG and breast-feeding in the prevention of rotavirus nosocomial infection. J Pediatr Gastroenterol Nutr 2002;35:527–31.

37. Mack DR, Michail S, Wei S, et al. Probiotics inhibit enteropathogenic E. coli adherence in vitro by inducing intestinal mucin gene expression. Am J Physiol 1999;39:G941–50.

38. Arvola T, Laiho K, Torkkeli S, et al. Prophylactic Lactobacillus GG reduces antibiotic-associated diarrhea in children with respiratory infections: a randomized study. Pediatrics 1999; 104:e64.

39. Vanderhoof JA, Whitney DB, Antonson DL, et al. Lactobacillus GG in the prevention of antibiotic-associated diarrhea in children. J Pediatr 1999;135:564–8.

40. Elmer GW, Surawicz CM, McFarland LV. Biotherapeutic agents. A neglected modality for the treatment and prevention of selected intestinal and vaginal infections. JAMA 1996; 276:29–30.

41. Guarner F, Casellas F, Borruel N, et al. Role of microecology in chronic inflammatory bowel diseases. Eur J Clin Nutr 2002; 56 Suppl 4:S34–8.

42. Gupta P, Andrew H, Kirschner BS, Guandalini S. Is Lactobacillus GG helpful in children with Crohn's disease? Results of a preliminary, open-label study. J Pediatr Gastroenterol Nutr 2000;31:453–7.

43. Prantera C, Scribano ML, Falasco G, et al. Ineffectiveness of probiotics in preventing recurrence after curative resection for Crohn's disease: a randomised controlled trial with Lactobacillus GG. Gut 2002;51:405–9.

44. Rembacken BJ, Snelling AM, Hawkey PM, et al. Non-pathogenic Escherichia coli versus mesalazine for the treatment of ulcerative colitis: a randomised trial. Lancet 1999;354:635–9.

45. Gionchetti P, Rizzello F, Venturi A, et al. Oral bacteriotherapy as maintenance treatment in patients with chronic pouchitis: a double-blind, placebo-controlled trial. Gastroenterology 2000;119:305–9.

46. Yazdanbakhsh M, Kremsner PG, van Ree R. Allergy, parasites, and the hygiene hypothesis. Science 2002;296:490–4.

47. Hartmann G, Weiner GJ, Krieg AM. CpG DNA: a potent signal for growth, activation, and maturation of human dendritic cells. Proc Natl Acad Sci U S A 1999;96:9305–19.

48. Kranzer K, Bauer M, Lipford GB, et al. CpG-oligodeoxynucleotides enhance T-cell receptor-triggered interferon-gamma production and up-regulation of CD69 via induction of antigen-presenting cell-derived interferon type I and interleukin-12. Immunology 2000;99:170–8.

49. Cario E, Rosenberg IM, Brandwein SL, et al. Lipopolysaccharide activates distinct signaling pathways in intestinal epithelial cell lines expressing Toll-like receptors. J Immunol 2000; 164:966–72.

50. Hemmi H, Takeuchi O, Kawai T, et al. A Toll-like receptor recognizes bacterial DNA. Nature 2000;408:740–5.

51. Neish AS, Gewirtz AT, Zeng H, et al. Prokaryotic regulation of epithelial responses by inhibition of IkappaB-alpha ubiquitination. Science 2000;289:1560–3.

52. Pessi T, Sütas Y, Hurme M, et al. Interleukin-10 generation in atopic children following oral Lactobacillus rhamnosus GG. Clin Exp Allergy 2000;30:1804–8.

53. Rautava S, Kalliomaki M, Isolauri E. Probiotics during pregnancy and breast-feeding might confer immunomodulatory protection against atopic disease in the infant. J Allergy Clin Immunol 2002;109:119–21.

54. Sütas Y, Soppi E, Korhonen H, et al. Suppression of lymphocyte proliferation in vitro by bovine caseins hydrolysed with Lactobacillus GG-derived enzymes. J Allergy Clin Immunol 1996;98:216–24.

55. Sütas Y, Hurme M, Isolauri E. Downregulation of antiCD3 antibody-induced IL-4 production by bovine caseins hydrolysed with Lactobacillus GG-derived enzymes. Scand J Immunol 1996;43:687–9.

56. Pessi T, Sütas Y, Saxelin M, et al. Antiproliferative effects of homogenates derived from five strains of candidate probiotic bacteria. Appl Environ Microb 1999;65:4725–8.

57. von der Weid T, Bulliard C, Schiffrin EJ. Induction by a lactic acid bacterium of a population of CD4+ T cells with low proliferative capacity that produce transforming growth factor beta and interleukin-10. Clin Diagn Lab Immunol 2001; 8:695–701.

58. Shida K, Takahashi R, Iwadate E, et al. Lactobacillus casei strain Shirota suppresses serum immunoglobulin E and immunoglobulin G1 responses and systemic anaphylaxis in a food allergy model. Clin Exp Allergy 2002;32:563–70.

59. Majamaa H, Isolauri E. Probiotics: a novel approach in the man-

agement of food allergy. J Allergy Clin Immunol 1997;99: 179–86.

60. He F, Morita H, Hashimoto H, et al. Intestinal *Bifidobacterium* species induce varying cytokine production. J Allergy Clin Immunol 2002;109:1035–6.

61. Ibnou-Zekri N, Blum S, Schffrin EJ, von der Weid T. Divergent patterns of colonization and immune response elicited from two intestinal *Lactobacillus* strains that display similar properties in vitro. Infect Immun 2003;71:428–36.

62. Isolauri E, Arvola T, Sütas Y, et al. Probiotics in the management of atopic eczema. Clin Exp Allergy 2000;30:1605–10.

63. Pelto L, Isolauri E, Lilius EM, et al. Probiotic bacteria downregulate the milk-induced inflammatory response in milk-hypersensitive subjects but have an immunostimulatory effect in healthy subjects. Clin Exp Allergy 1998;28:1474–9.

64. Kalliomäki M, Salminen S, Kero P, et al. Probiotics in primary prevention of atopic disease: a randomised placebo-controlled trial. Lancet 2001;357:1076–9.

65. Kalliomäki M, Salminen S, Poussa T, et al. Probiotics and prevention of atopic disease—a 4-year follow-up of a randomised placebo-controlled trial. Lancet 2003;361;1869–71.

66. Lee YK, Lim CY, Teng WL, et al. Qualitative approach in the study of adhesion of lactic acid bacteria on intestinal cells and their competition with enterobacteria. Appl Environ Microbiol 2000;66:3692–7.

67. Ouwehand A, Salminen S, Tölkkö S, et al. Resected human colonic tissue: a new model for characterising adhesion of lactic acid bacteria. Clin Diagn Labor Immunol 2002;10:184–6.

68. Mao Y, Nobaek S, Kasravi B, et al. Effects of *Lactobacillus* strains and oat bran on methotrexate-induced enterocolitis in rats. Gastroenterology 1996;111:334–44.

69. Steidler L, Hans W, Schotte L, et al. Treatment of murine colitis by *Lactococcus lactis* secreting interleukin-10. Science 2000; 289:1352–5.

70. Hartke A, Bouché S, Giard JC, et al. The lactic acid stress response to *Lactococcus lactis* subsp. lactis. Curr Microbiol 1996;33:194–9.

71. Hartke A, Bouché S, Gansel X, et al. Starvation-induced stress resistance in *Lactococcus lactis* subsp. lactis IL1403. Appl Environ Microbiol 1994;60:3474–8.

72. Kets EPW, Teunissen PJM, de Bont JAM. Effect of compatible solutes on survival of lactic acid bacteria subjected to drying. Appl Environ Microbiol 1996;62:259–61.

73. Salminen S, von Wright A, Morelli L, et al. Demonstration of safety of probiotics—a review. Int J Food Microbiol 1998; 44:93–106.

74. Apostolou E, Kirjavainen, Saxelin M, et al. Good adhesion properties of probiotics: a potential risk for bacteremia? FEMS Immunol Med Microbiol 2001;67:2430–5.

75. Saxelin M, Chuang NH, Chassy B, et al. Lactobacilli and bacteremia in Southern Finland. 1989–1992. Clin Infect Dis 1996;22:564–6.

76. Salminen MK, Tynkkynen S, Rautelin H, et al. *Lactobacillus* bacteremia during a rapid increase in probiotic use of *Lactobacillus rhamnosus* GG in Finland. Clin Infect Dis 2002;35: 1155–60.

77. Asahara T, Takahashi M, Nomoto K, et al. Assessment of safety of lactobacillus strains based on resistance to host innate defense mechanisms. Clin Diagn Lab Immunol 2003;10: 169–73.

78. Salminen S, Isolauri E, von Wright A. Safety of probiotic bacteria. Rev Food Nutr Tox 2003;1:279–84.

79. de Vos W. Safe and sustainable systems for food grade fermentations by genetically modified lactic acid bacteria. Int Dairy J 1999;9:3–10.

80. Kulmala J, Salminen S, Salminen E. Adhesion of inactivated probiotic strains to intestinal mucus. Lett Appl Microbiol 2000;31:82–6.

3. Motility

Frances Laura Connor, MBBS, FRACP

Carlo Di Lorenzo, MD

As discussed in Chapter 4, "Motility," the mixing and propulsive actions of the gut are the result of coordinated activity in the enteric nervous system (ENS), modulated by hormones and central nervous system (CNS) input. The ENS contains complex motility "programs" for activities such as the interdigestive migrating motor complex (MMC) and the gastrointestinal components of emesis. Over 30 definite and putative neurotransmitters have been identified in the gut (see Table 4-2, Chapter 4). In many cases, a single neurotransmitter may stimulate several different receptors on different target tissues (nerves, smooth muscle) to produce different effects. As the rapidly advancing discipline of neurogastroenterology expands our understanding of motility and signaling within the gut, many new targets are being identified for specific therapeutic intervention.

This chapter provides an overview of the many drugs currently available and in development for modulating gastrointestinal motility. For each agent, the mechanism of action is briefly discussed, followed by a review of the currently available clinical experience. Wherever possible, data from pediatric trials are reported. However, in many cases, especially with newer medications, in which only scanty or no data exist for pediatric patients, data from trials in adults are discussed. The identification of effective pharmacologic therapies for pediatric gastrointestinal motility disorders using prospective randomized controlled trials has been identified as a research priority in the recently released research agenda of the North American Society of Pediatric Gastroenterology, Hepatology and Nutrition (NASPGHAN).[1]

Disorders of motility result in abnormalities of contraction amplitude, frequency, or coordination. Although many older motility drugs had nonspecific effects, affecting only contraction amplitude and/or frequency, newer agents also enhance the coordination of gastrointestinal contractions, greatly enhancing their therapeutic utility. The development of drugs targeting specific receptor subtypes in the ENS and enteric smooth muscle has reduced the incidence of systemic side effects that limited the use of previous agents. Drugs that alter motility fall into two broad categories: prokinetics and antimotility agents or antispasmodics. Also, it is increasingly apparent that many patients with motility disturbances also suffer from visceral hypersensitivity. Several of the newer motility drugs have additional antinociceptive qualities. The major drugs in each category are listed in Tables 76.3-1 (prokinetics) and 76.3-2 (antispasmodic and antimotility agents).

PROKINETICS

Prokinetic drugs may stimulate motility by direct actions on enteric smooth muscle or by interacting with the neurons of the ENS. Drugs currently in use include dopamine D_2 receptor antagonists, motilin agonists, 5-hydroxytryptamine subtype 4 (5-HT$_4$) agonists, and anticholinesterases. The final common pathway of all of these drugs is the M_3 muscarinic acetylcholine receptor on enteric smooth muscle cells.[2]

DOPAMINE ANTAGONISTS

Under normal physiologic conditions, dopamine inhibits the release of acetylcholine in the myenteric plexus by acting at presynaptic D_2 dopaminergic receptors. D_2 receptor antagonists such as metoclopramide and domperidone have prokinetic effects, enhancing the release of acetylcholine.[3] Domperidone is a specific D_2 antagonist, whereas metoclopramide also stimulates 5-HT$_4$ receptors and is an antagonist at 5-HT$_3$ receptors.[3]

Metoclopramide. The prokinetic effects of metoclopramide are primarily in the upper gut.[4] In addition to its peripheral effects, metoclopramide crosses the blood-brain barrier and exerts central antiemetic effects. This CNS activity may lead to side effects such as sedation, restlessness, and insomnia. Most concerning are dystonic reactions, such as oculogyric crisis and opisthotonos, which occur more frequently in children than in adults.[5] Tardive dyskinesia has been reported and may be permanent.[6] Rare side effects include neuroleptic malignant syndrome and methemoglobinemia. Despite its drawbacks, metoclopramide is one of the few prokinetic agents available at present. Although metoclopramide is widely used for its antiemetic action, the following focuses on its use as a prokinetic agent.

Randomized controlled trials of high-dose (1 mg/kg) intravenous metoclopramide have shown efficacy in improving delayed gastric emptying in children.[7] Recent experience in adult patients suggests that subcutaneous injection of metoclopramide may be effective in treating gastroparesis[8] and nausea.[9,10] Subcutaneous administration circumvents the problems of unpredictable oral drug bioavailability encountered in patients with severe motility disorders. Although this route of administration is less attractive in pediatric patients, it may well be acceptable to diabetic patients with symptomatic gastroparesis. However, further data from randomized double-blind placebo-controlled trials are required.

TABLE 76.3-1   PROKINETIC DRUGS

DRUG	RECEPTOR	EFFECT ON MOTILITY	REDUCES VISCERAL HYPERSENSITIVITY	POTENTIAL INDICATIONS
Metoclopramide	D₂ receptor antagonist, 5-HT₄ agonist, 5-HT₃ antagonist	↑Motility: proximal > distal[4]	Possible[178-180]	Foregut dysmotility syndromes: GERD, gastroparesis, nausea
Domperidone	D₂ receptor antagonist	↑Motility: proximal > distal gut[4]	Possible[181]	Foregut dysmotility syndromes: GERD, gastroparesis, nausea
Erythromycin	Motilin receptor agonist	↑Motility: proximal > distal[182]	No; possible worsening[183]	Foregut dysmotility syndromes: gastroparesis, postprandial hypomotility
Octreotide	Somatostatin receptor agonist	Stimulates phase III of MMC, beginning in duodenum[50]; antimotility effects (see Table 76.3-2)	Yes[55]	Small intestinal hypomotility, prevention of bacterial overgrowth, pseudo-obstruction, dumping syndrome, visceral hypersensitivity
Cisapride	5-HT₄ receptor agonist, 5-HT₃ receptor antagonist	↑Motility: proximal > distal gut[4]	No[184]	Foregut dysmotility syndromes: gastroparesis, postprandial hypomotility, pseudo-obstruction, possible role in constipation
Tegaserod	5-HT₄ receptor, potent partial agonist	↑Enhances gastric motility, stimulates peristaltic reflex and intestinal secretion, shortens colonic transit time[91,92]	Yes[92]	Constipation-predominant IBS in adult women
Bethanechol	Muscarinic receptor agonist	↑Contraction amplitude but not transit[97-99,185]	No; increased sensitivity[185]	GERD
Neostigmine	Anticholinesterase	↑Motility and transit: colonic > proximal[185-187]	No; increased sensitivity[185]	Acute colonic pseudo-obstruction, episodic pseudo-obstruction
Baclofen	GABA_B receptor agonist	↓Transient lower esophageal sphincter relaxations[107,108]	Possible (effective in neuropathic pain)[188,189]	GERD
Phenylephrine (topical)	α₁-Adrenergic agonist	↑Internal anal sphincter pressure[119,120]	No data	Fecal incontinence

GABA = γ-aminobutyric acid; GERD = gastroesophageal reflux disease; 5-HT = 5-hydroxytryptamine; MMC = migrating motor complex.

TABLE 76.3-2   ANTIMOTILITY AND ANTISPASMODIC DRUGS

DRUG	MECHANISM OF ACTION	EFFECT ON MOTILITY	REDUCES VISCERAL HYPERSENSITIVIY	POTENTIAL INDICATIONS
Loperamide	Mu opioid agonist	↓ Bowel motility and ↑ anal sphincter tone[4]	Yes[190]	Diarrhea, including IBS-D Hirschsprung disease post–pull-through surgery
Dicylomine, hyoscyamine	Nonspecific muscarinic antagonists	↓ Motility[4]	No data	Decreasing amplitude of painful/noxious visceral contractions, eg, visceral hypersensitivity, IBS, neuropathic pseudo-obstruction
Mebeverine	Complex actions at multiple receptors	Small intestine: mixed effects,[191] ↓ colonic motility[192]	No data	Decreasing amplitude of painful/noxious visceral contractions, eg, IBS
Nifedipine, verapamil, diltiazem	L-type calcium channel antagonists	↓ Amplitude contractions[149,150]	No data	Decreasing amplitude of painful/noxious visceral contractions, eg, nutcracker esophagus, diffuse esophageal spasm, esophageal achalasia
Pinaverium	Selective gastrointestinal calcium channel antagonist	↓ Colonic motility[193–195]	No data	Decreasing amplitude of painful/noxious visceral contractions
Peppermint oil	Calcium channel antagonist[157,196]	↓ Motility: upper and lower GIT Esophagus: ↓ simultaneous contractions, ↑ peristaltic contractions	Possible (anesthetic actions)[197]	Decreasing amplitude of painful/noxious visceral contractions, eg IBS, spastic esophageal disorders
Nitrates	Nitric oxide donors	Smooth muscle relaxation	No[198]	Decreasing amplitude of painful/noxious visceral contractions, eg, nutcracker esophagus, diffuse esophageal spasm, anal fissures
Ondansetron	5-HT₃ antagonist	↓ Motility[4,62]	Yes[4,62]	Decreasing visceral hypersensitivity and nausea
Granisetron	5-HT₃ antagonist	↓ Motility[4,62]	Yes[4,62]	Decreasing visceral hypersensitivity and nausea
Alosetron	5-HT₃ antagonist	↓ Motility and tone: slows colonic transit, ↑ fluid absorption[4,92]	Yes[4,92]	Intractable IBS-D in adult women, unresponsive to standard medical therapies
Sumatriptan	5-HT(1BD) receptor agonist	↑ Relaxation gastric fundus, colon ↓ gastric emptying[4,62]	No direct effect[199,200]	Increasing gastric receptive accommodation
Octreotide	Somatostatin receptor agonist	↓ Gastric emptying ↓ diarrhea, ↓ intestinal transit, ↓ secretions[54,201]	Yes[55]	Retarding gastric emptying, eg, in dumping syndrome; also reduces visceral hypersensitivity
Glucagon	Glucagon receptor agonist	↓ Motility smooth muscle relaxation	No data	Inhibiting gastrointestinal contractions, eg, during endoscopic procedures
Botulinum toxin	Prevents acetylcholine release from motoneurons	Denervation paralysis smooth muscle	No data	Reducing sphincter tone, eg, esophageal achalasia, anal achalasia, gastroparesis
Clonidine	α₂-Adrenergic agonist	↓ Motility and tone[198,202]	Yes[55,189,198,202]	Inhibiting noxious/painful gastrointestinal contractions and visceral hyperalgesia, eg, IBS-D
Salbutamol	β-Adrenergic agonist	Smooth muscle relaxation	No data	Inhibiting noxious/painful gastrointestinal contractions, eg, proctalgia fugax

GIT = gastrointestinal tract; 5-HT= 5-hydroxytryptamine; IBS = irritable bowel syndrome; IBS-D = diarrhea-predominant irritable bowel syndrome.

Metoclopramide has proven useful in accelerating the passage of small bowel biopsy capsules in children.[11] Similarly, metoclopramide has been used to assist the placement of transpyloric feeding tubes, although the results of clinical trials are contradictory.[12] Low-dose erythromycin (see below) is more effective for this indication.[12,13]

Although metoclopramide increases lower esophageal sphincter tone in children,[14] the majority of studies have shown little or no effect on gastroesophageal reflux disease (GERD) as measured by prolonged pH monitoring.[14–18] Also, metoclopramide was less well tolerated than placebo, with side effects including irritability and dystonic reactions.[14,15] The current position paper of the NASPGHAN states that although cisapride appears to be a marginally effective prokinetic agent for the treatment of GERD, the effectiveness in children of other prokinetic agents, including metoclopramide, is unproven.[19]

Domperidone. Another dopamine antagonist, domperidone, is available in most countries outside the United States. Unlike metoclopramide, domperidone does not pass the blood-brain barrier, and CNS side effects are rare.[20] Despite this, domperidone does have antiemetic effects, owing to the fact that the chemoreceptor trigger zone is outside the blood-brain barrier, and domperidone exerts its CNS effects here.[20] Domperidone raises lower esophageal sphincter pressure, increases the amplitude of gastric and duodenal contractions, and accelerates small intestinal transit.[21,22]

Domperidone seems effective in gastroparesis. A recent randomized controlled trial demonstrated that domperidone was more effective than cisapride in improving symptoms, diabetic control, gastric emptying, and electrogastrography variables in diabetic children with gastroparesis.[23] As with metoclopramide, there is minimal evidence that domperidone therapy is beneficial in GERD.[19]

MOTILIN AGONISTS

The peptide hormone motilin is released by enteroendocrine cells in the small intestine during fasting and has a role in initiating the interdigestive MMC. Motilin excites presynaptic neurons in the ENS to stimulate postsynaptic cholinergic motoneurons and induce phasic contractions in smooth muscle.[24] Motilin also has direct excitatory effects at motilin receptors on gastrointestinal smooth muscle cells, inducing an increase in intracellular calcium.[25] Motilin agonists (motilides) are a promising class of prokinetics that is currently the subject of intensive research.

Erythromycin. Erythromycin is a motilin receptor agonist that in low doses (1–3 mg/kg) stimulates phasic contractions in the stomach identical to spontaneous phase III of the MMC.[26] These activity fronts originate in the antrum and propagate into the small intestine and are inducible in adults and children over 32 weeks gestational age.[27] In premature babies less than 32 weeks gestational age, erythromycin increases antral motility but does not induce MMCs.[28] At higher doses, erythromycin produces uncoordinated high-amplitude antral contractions without propagation in healthy individuals.[29]

Low-dose erythromycin is an effective gastric prokinetic and is useful in the treatment of gastroparesis, as well as for placement of transpyloric feeding tubes[13,30] and for elimination of blood from the upper gastrointestinal tract prior to endoscopy for gastrointestinal hemorrhage.[31,32] In a recent systematic review of trials in adult patients, erythromycin was superior to cisapride, metoclopramide, and domperidone for treatment of gastroparesis.[33] In children, oral erythromycin 1 mg/kg is at least as effective as oral metoclopramide 0.15 mg/kg for emptying the stomach prior to emergency surgery.[34] At a higher dose, erythromycin was associated with increased postoperative vomiting,[35] although higher doses may be necessary in treatment of individuals with severely delayed gastric emptying.

Erythromycin has been extensively studied as treatment for feeding intolerance in patients in intensive care and in premature infants.[36–43] Despite the documented lack of effect on MMCs below 32 weeks, studies on premature babies under this gestation age indicate that low-dose erythromycin is effective in reducing the number of days until full enteral feeding is established.[39–41] The authors commented that this may result in a substantial saving on hyperalimentation.[39] Importantly, there were no significant adverse effects. In particular, no increase in necrotizing enterocolitis was seen. Trials of erythromycin in antimicrobial doses have yielded conflicting results but, in general, have also led to improved feed tolerance.[36,37,39,42]

Other Motilides. Current research aims to develop motilin agonists devoid of antibiotic activity. Clinical trials of ABT-229, an erythromycin derivative, demonstrated enhanced gastric emptying in healthy volunteers.[44] However, there was no symptomatic improvement in randomized double-blind placebo-controlled trials in adults with functional dyspepsia [45] or diabetes,[46] and research on ABT-229 as a gastrokinetic agent has been discontinued.[3] Other nonantibiotic erythromycin derivatives under investigation for their prokinetic effects include EM523,[47] EM574,[48] and GM-611.[49]

OCTREOTIDE

Somatostatin is a naturally occurring gastrointestinal peptide hormone that has complex actions in the gastrointestinal tract. It can augment or counteract a wide variety of other peptides and can have both prokinetic and antimotility effects. Octreotide is a long-acting synthetic analog of somatostatin that may be administered by intravenous, subcutaneous, or intramuscular injection.

In children with chronic gastrointestinal disorders, octreotide stimulates phase III of the MMC, beginning in the small intestine, and inhibits gastric contractions.[50] The inhibition of antral activity is reversed by feeding[50] or by pretreatment with erythromycin.[51] Octreotide may be of benefit in chronic intestinal pseudo-obstruction, although clinical trials have been limited to adults with connective tissue diseases.

Because octreotide retards gastric emptying, therapy should ideally be given to patients who are receiving post-gastric feeds, such as transpyloric or jejunostomy feeding.

Alternatively, combination therapy with erythromycin may be of benefit because the suppressant effect of octreotide on gastric motility is counteracted by erythromycin.[52] Conversely, octreotide enhances the prokinetic effects of erythromycin in patients with intestinal pseudo-obstruction[52] and on gastric emptying in normal subjects.[53]

Despite stimulating phase III of the MMC, octreotide also has antidiarrheal effects. It inhibits small bowel transit[54] and intestinal and pancreatic secretions. In the colon, octreotide inhibits the postprandial tonic response, whereas phasic pressure activity is increased. Octreotide also has antinociceptive effects that may increase its therapeutic utility in diseases with a component of visceral hyperalgesia.[55]

Because of its inhibitory effects on gastric emptying, octreotide is beneficial in dumping syndrome,[56] reducing the duration of the fed pattern and hastening the return of the MMC after a meal.[57] However, data in children are lacking.

The predominant adverse effects of octreotide include pain at injection sites and gastrointestinal disturbance. Occasionally, hyper- or hypoglycemia, hypertension, headache, dizziness, fatigue, hepatic dysfunction, and cholelithiasis may occur. Theoretically, long-term use of octreotide could inhibit growth by suppressing growth hormone secretion, although this has not occurred in several children treated with octreotide for gastrointestinal diseases.[58–61]

5-HT₄ AGONISTS

Serotonin (5-HT) is ubiquitous throughout the gastrointestinal tract and is important in modulating motility through its actions at several different receptors (Figure 76.3-1). There is currently intense research interest in developing drugs that manipulate motility by stimulating or antagonizing gastrointestinal serotonin receptors. Several classes of serotonergic agonists and antagonists are discussed in this chapter, including 5-HT₄ agonists and antagonists of 5-HT₃ and 5-HT₁B/D receptors. Stimulation of 5-HT₄ receptors initiates peristaltic contraction. These receptors are located on neurons in the myenteric plexus and on smooth muscle cells (see Figure 76.3-1).[62] Stimulation of cholinergic neurons at 5-HT₄ receptors results in acetylcholine release and enhanced contraction.[62]

Cisapride. Cisapride is a partial 5-HT₄ receptor agonist and a 5-HT3 antagonist with some affinity for dopamine D_2, 5-HT₂ receptors, and α-adrenoceptors.[63] Cisapride enhances gastric emptying in normals and in patients with gastroparesis. It increases lower esophageal sphincter tone and improves esophageal acid clearance, reducing esophageal acid exposure. Despite these effects, its clinical utility in unselected children with GERD is not supported by a recent systematic review.[64] This may be because cisapride has no effect on transient lower esophageal sphincter relaxations (TLESRs), the predominant mechanism of gastroesophageal

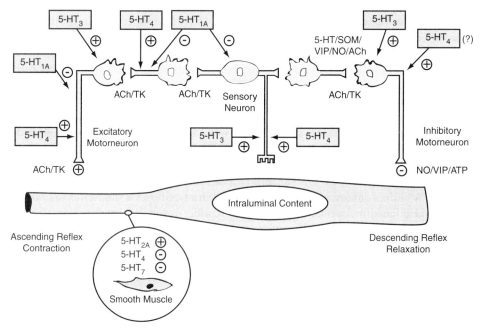

FIGURE 76.3-1 Modulation of intestinal motility by serotonergic receptors. Distention by intraluminal contents stimulates sensory neurons (intrinsic primary afferent neurons), which trigger an ascending excitatory reflex (leading to contraction) and a descending inhibitory reflex (leading to relaxation). Transmitters released by interneurons in the ascending reflex include acetylcholine (ACh) and substance P, whereas descending interneurons belonging to different subpopulations may use serotonin (5-hydroxytryptamine [5-HT]), somatostatin (SOM), vasoactive intestinal polypeptide (VIP), nitric oxide (NO), ACh, and other mediators as transmitters. Excitatory motoneurons release ACh and tachykinins (TK) at the neuromuscular junction, whereas inhibitory motoneurons may release NO, VIP, or adenosine triphosphate (ATP), depending on the gastrointestinal tract level and on the animal species. 5-HT₃ and 5-HT₄ receptors have an excitatory effect on enteric neurones, whereas 5-HT₁A receptors inhibit transmitter release. Serotonergic receptors may also directly contract or relax smooth muscle cells via 5-HT₂A, 5-HT₄, and 5-HT₇ receptors. + indicates stimulation; – indicates inhibition; (?) indicates limited data. Reproduced with permission from De Ponti F and Tonini M.[62]

reflux (GER).[65,66] Evidence for a beneficial effect of cisapride on reflux and feed intolerance in neonates is similarly contradictory.[67–71] In contrast, cisapride has proven effective in randomized trials in selected subsets of patients with reflux disease. In particular, cisapride improves symptoms, intraesophageal pH indices, and requirements for bronchodilator and steroid medication in patients with chronic respiratory symptoms and GER.[72–74]

Despite its documented efficacy in the treatment of gastroparesis,[33] a recent randomized trial demonstrated that domperidone is more effective for this indication in children.[23] Cisapride stimulates small intestinal motility and has been used in children with chronic intestinal pseudo-obstruction.[75–78] Response to therapy, as measured by the ability to tolerate enteral feeding, was predicted by the presence of phase III of the MMC in antroduodenal motility studies.[78] Cisapride is superior to placebo in the management of constipation.[79] However, owing to the risks of cardiac toxicity, use for this indication should be discouraged.

Cisapride Cardiotoxicity. Cisapride prolongs the Q–T interval in a dose-dependent manner, resulting in potentially fatal arrhythmias, including ventricular tachycardia, ventricular fibrillation, and torsades de pointes. From July 1993 to December 1999, 341 such cases were reported, including 80 deaths. In approximately 85% of these cases, the events occurred when cisapride was used in patients with known risk factors.[80] Patients most at risk include those who are receiving high doses or who have congenital or acquired long Q–T syndrome. Drugs that interfere with the metabolism of cisapride by the cytochrome P-450 (CYP)3A4 system potentiate cisapride cardiotoxicity and are contraindicated in patients on the medication. These include macrolide antibiotics, azole antifungals, and nonsedating antihistamines. Grapefruit juice also increases cisapride bioavailability by inhibiting CYP3A4.[81]

Until recently, it was unclear whether cisapride cardiotoxicity was a result of 5-HT$_4$ receptor stimulation or the molecular characteristics of cisapride and other members of the benzamide class. Clinical and experimental evidence now supports the latter theory. Clinical trials of tegaserod, a selective 5-HT$_4$ receptor agonist, showed no alteration of Q–T interval versus placebo in over 2,500 subjects.[82] In contrast, cisapride possesses class III antiarrhythmic properties and prolongs the action potential duration through blockade of distinct voltage-dependent K$^+$ channels, thus delaying cardiac repolarization and prolonging the Q–T interval.[83] Concurrent use of cisapride is therefore contraindicated in children receiving class III antiarrhythmic agents. To put the potential for cisapride cardiac toxicity in perspective, a critical analysis of safety data by Vandenplas showed that there were two instances of serious ventricular arrhythmia, Q–T prolongation, or sudden death reported for every million patients treated for a month, of which more than 85% could be related to known risk factors.[84]

Importantly, intravenous erythromycin at antimicrobial doses[85,86] and domperidone[87,88] have both been associated with prolongation of Q–Tc and cardiac arrhythmia.

Safety concerns about cisapride cardiotoxicity resulted in its withdrawal from sale in North America, most European countries, and Australasia. In some countries, including the United States, patient access to the drug is now restricted to investigational limited access programs. Patients must meet strict eligibility criteria, have failed other treatment options, and be stringently monitored. In pediatrics, cisapride is available under such programs for refractory GERD, pseudo-obstruction, and neonatal feeding intolerance, although specific details vary between countries.

Other side effects of cisapride include transient diarrhea; flatulence; borborygmi or abdominal cramps; CNS disturbances such as seizures, behavior disturbance, and extrapyramidal effects; and a dose-related increase in urinary frequency. Because of the importance of the liver and kidneys in its metabolism and excretion, the dosage should be reduced in patients with hepatic or renal insufficiency.

Other Benzamide Derivatives. Newer members of the benzamide class, all unavailable in the United States at present, include mosapride, renzapride, levosulpiride, and KDR-5169.[89] KDR-5169 is a 5-HT$_4$ agonist with dopamine D$_2$ receptor antagonist properties. In a recent animal study, it was extremely effective in treating gastroparesis, accelerating gastric emptying to supranormal levels.[89] The authors speculated that the increased efficacy of KDR-5169 over cisapride may have been due to more potent antagonism of D$_2$ receptors because combination therapy with cisapride and domperidone (a D$_2$ antagonist) has previously been shown to improve gastric emptying versus cisapride alone.[90]

Tegaserod. Tegaserod (HTF 919) is a specific 5-HT$_4$ antagonist recently licensed for the treatment of constipation-predominant irritable bowel syndrome (IBS-C) in adult women. Like cisapride, it accelerates gastric emptying and promotes gastrointestinal transit.[91,92] Unlike cisapride, tegaserod has no cardiotoxicity,[82] requires only twice-daily dosing, and does not cross the blood-brain barrier to cause CNS side effects. Clinical trials in adults with IBS-C indicate that tegaserod improves constipation, bloating, and overall symptom scores.[4,92] Diarrhea, abdominal cramping, headache, flatulence, and fatigue are the major associated adverse effects, resulting in discontinuation of the medication in 10 to 15% of patients.[93,94] The potential clinical use of tegaserod for GER was studied in adults with mild to moderate GERD. Tegaserod reduced esophageal acid exposure by 50%,[95] possibly by reducing the incidence of postprandial transient lower esophageal relaxations and/or by accelerating gastric emptying.

Prucalopride. Prucalopride (R0-93877) is another 5-HT$_4$ partial agonist that also accelerates gastrointestinal transit and has proven useful in treatment of constipation in adults. However, further clinical development of this compound has been suspended pending the results of toxicity studies owing to concerns about carcinogenesis in animals and possible cardiac effects.[96]

BETHANECOL

Bethanecol is a choline ester that stimulates muscarinic cholinergic receptors. It increases the amplitude of contractions throughout the gastrointestinal tract and raises lower esophageal sphincter tone.[97–99] Contrary to previous reports, it does not accelerate gastric emptying or gastrointestinal transit in adults or children.[7,99,100] Two trials evaluated its utility in pediatric GERD and demonstrated modest benefits, no greater than that achieved with antacids.[101,102] Its usefulness is also limited by side effects, including abdominal cramps, watery diarrhea, bradycardia, hypotension, urination, sweating, and bronchoconstriction.

NEOSTIGMINE

Neostigmine is a peripheral anticholinesterase. By inhibiting degradation of acetylcholine, it enhances cholinergic activity at nicotinic receptors in the myenteric plexus and muscarinic receptors on gastrointestinal smooth muscle. Neostigmine accelerates gastrointestinal transit, especially in the colon. It has proven efficacy in reversal of acute colonic pseudo-obstruction (Ogilvie syndrome), with colonic decompression occurring within minutes of drug administration in prospective randomized double-blind placebo-controlled studies.[103,104] Side effects were limited to mild abdominal cramping and bradycardia, which were responsive to atropine. This simple, effective therapy may now become the standard of care for acute colonic pseudo-obstruction in adults[105]; however, further data on pediatric patients are required. It has been suggested that the longer-acting anticholinesterase pyridostigmine may be beneficial for the outpatient management of gastrointestinal motility disturbances.[106]

BACLOFEN

Although not strictly a prokinetic, baclofen increases lower esophageal sphincter pressure and inhibits TLESRs by simulating the actions of the inhibitory neurotransmitter γ-aminobutyric acid in the brainstem.[107,108] This agent is being explored for its role in reducing gastroesophageal reflux. In the meantime, this mechanism is of potential benefit to neurologically handicapped children receiving baclofen for spasticity, possibly counteracting their known tendency to pathologic GER. Trials of baclofen in pediatric GERD are ongoing.

Other drugs have been shown to inhibit TLESRs and GER, including cholecystokinin A antagonists,[109] atropine,[110] morphine,[111] and nitric oxide synthase inhibitors.[112] The search for specific agents for pharmacologic suppression of TLESRs is currently the subject of intense research activity.

OPIOID AGONISTS

The Mu-opioid agonist fedotozine has both antinociceptive and promotility effects. Although the antinociceptive properties are mediated by stimulation of Mu-opioid receptors, it is likely that the prokinetic effects of fedotozine are due to a different mechanism, direct smooth muscle excitation.[113] In clinical trials of adults with IBS, fedotozine was superior to placebo in reducing abdominal pain and bloating.[114]

CHOLECYSTOKININ ANTAGONISTS

Although not currently available outside therapeutic trials, this class of agents is expected to reach the public some time in 2004.[4] Cholecystokinin (CCK) is released from the gut in response to fat and protein in food. CCK_A receptors on visceral afferents in the gut mediate sensations of satiety and gastric receptive relaxation via a vagal reflex. Stimulation of CCK_A receptors in the gallbladder and pancreas causes release of digestive juices. Whereas CCK_A receptors mediate stimulation of duodenal activity, CCK_A stimulation relaxes the lower esophageal sphincter, stomach, and colon via a nitric oxide–dependent mechanism.[115–117] CCK_A antagonists such as loxiglumide and dexloxiglumide reduce TLESR, promote gastric emptying, shorten colonic transit time, and increase the number of bowel movements.[4,109,118]

α-ADRENERGIC AGONIST: PHENYLEPHRINE

Topical phenylephrine increases anal sphincter tone in normals[119] and in patients with incontinence owing to low resting sphincter pressure.[120] In an initial trial, low concentration (10%) phenylephrine was ineffective in patients with incontinence owing to low resting anal sphincter pressure.[121] However, this concentration was effective in treating fecal incontinence after ileoanal anastomosis.[122] Research on the use of topical phenylephrine for fecal incontinence owing to internal anal sphincter incompetence is ongoing.

ANTISPASMODICS AND ANTIMOTILITY DRUGS

OPIOID AGONIST: LOPERAMIDE

Loperamide is a specific agonist at peripheral Mu-opioid receptors that has both antinociceptive and antimotility actions. Because it does not pass through the blood-brain barrier, CNS effects, including the potential for addiction, do not occur. The overall effect of loperamide is to delay gastrointestinal transit. Although loperamide stimulates gastrointestinal contractions, there is a disruption in the normal propulsive patterns of motility, leading to increased transit time.[3] The safety and efficacy of loperamide in treatment of diarrhea are well established, with the caveat that no hypomotility agent is recommended in the context of acute infective diarrhea in children or dysentery at any age.

ANTICHOLINERGICS

Anticholinergic medications have traditionally been used as antispasmodics. Blocking the action of acetylcholine at smooth muscle reduces the amplitude of gastrointestinal contractions, and this has been particularly useful in dysmotility syndromes characterized by excessive contractile activity. Older anticholinergic medications include scopolamine, dicyclomine, and hyoscyamine. Their therapeutic utility was limited by their nonspecific actions and unwanted side effects caused by antagonism of muscarinic receptors outside the gastrointestinal tract. These include dry mouth, tachycardia, blurred vision, and urinary difficulties. Toxicity has been a particular problem in children, with reports of serious side effects and anticholinergic poisoning.[123-127] Despite their widespread use, there are very few randomized controlled trials of anticholinergic drugs for gastrointestinal motility disorders in children.[128] A recent systematic review of 18 randomized controlled trials of antispasmodic and anticholinergic drugs in IBS concluded that, overall, the trials were of suboptimal methodologic quality. Evidence of effectiveness for these agents in IBS was inconsistent, and adverse effects limited their use.[92]

M3 MUSCARINIC ANTAGONISTS

Recently, more specific anticholinergic drugs have been developed that target the M3 muscarinic receptor responsible for gastrointestinal contraction.[129] M3 receptors are also found in the bladder (and these drugs have been employed in enuresis and urinary incontinence); however, they are not present in the heart, and cardiovascular side effects do not occur.[130] Examples are zamifenacin and darifenacin, which both inhibit contractile activity throughout the small and large bowel.[4] In a multicenter double-blind parallel-group placebo-controlled study of adult patients with IBS, zamifenacin profoundly inhibited colonic motor activity without significant extraintestinal side effects.[130]

MEBEVERINE

Although mebeverine has some antimuscarinic activity, it is far less potent than atropine. The spasmolytic action of mebeverine is the result of at least three additional mechanisms. Mebeverine has a direct musculotropic action involving calcium ion exchange and stabilization of excitable membranes, a local anesthetic action, and also potentiates sympathetic inhibition of gastrointestinal contraction owing to blockade of noradrenaline uptake into sympathetic nerve endings.[131-133] Mebeverine seems effective in reducing diarrhea and global symptom scores in adults with IBS; however, data from children are scant.[128]

5-HT3 ANTAGONISTS

Alosetron is a 5-HT3 antagonist that inhibits colonic transit and reduces colorectal hypersensitivity, probably by inhibiting 5-HT3 receptors on vagal afferents and in the CNS.[4] In the colon, it delays transit and decreases wall tension and sensitivity to distention.[4,92,134] It is effective in female adults with diarrhea-predominant IBS (IBS-D), improving stool consistency and frequency and reducing pain and urgency.[4,92] The most commonly reported side effect was constipation. Owing to reports of rare severe side effects, including ischemic colitis and severe constipation, alosetron was temporarily withdrawn from sale in 2000. In 2002, it was reintroduced for use in women with severe IBS-D who have failed to respond to conventional IBS therapy. The recommended adult dosage is 1 mg twice daily, and the agent should be avoided in patients with constipation.

5-HT1 ANTAGONIST

Originally developed to treat migraine headaches, the 5-HT1B/D antagonist sumatriptan also has effects on gastrointestinal motility. This agent enhances postprandial gastric fundic relaxation and reduces symptoms of early satiety in patients with functional dyspepsia.[135] Although sumatriptan inhibits gastric motility, it stimulates small intestinal contractions, causing premature phase III of the MMC after subcutaneous injection in fasting individuals.[136] Despite increasing lower esophageal sphincter tone, sumatriptan increases postprandial reflux episodes via an increased incidence of TLESRs and delayed gastric emptying.[137]

BOTULINUM TOXIN

Botulinum toxin (BT) type A is widely used for reduction of muscle spasticity in children with cerebral palsy or strabismus. The toxin binds irreversibly to presynaptic cholinergic nerve terminals, where it prevents the release of acetylcholine, causing paralysis by functional denervation. These effects persist for several months, with reversal dependent on sprouting of new terminal axons.

Gastrointestinal uses of BT revolve around the injection of sphincters[138] and include cricopharyngeal dysphagia,[139] achalasia of the esophagus,[140] spastic esophageal disorders,[141] gastroparesis (pyloric injection),[142] anal achalasia,[143] and fissure in ano.[144] In children with persistent obstructive symptoms after anal pull-through procedures for Hirschsprung disease, BT injection of the internal anal sphincter has been advocated as an effective and atraumatic alternative to myectomy.[145,146] Current pediatric data on the use of BT for gastrointestinal disorders are limited to individual case reports and small series. Larger randomized placebo-controlled trials are needed to fully define efficacy, dosage interval, side-effect profile, and cost effectiveness.

Clinical use of BT in thousands of patients for musculoskeletal disorders and cosmetic applications suggests that BT is extremely well tolerated. Repeated use has been associated with the development of antibodies to BT and reduction of the magnitude and duration of clinical effects. The possibility of distal or systemic paralysis is extremely unlikely given that the estimated lethal dose is 40 U/kg (intramuscularly or intravenously),[147] and doses of 100 U (one vial) or less are sufficient for gastrointestinal interventions. Even if inadvertently injected into the bloodstream, this dose is unlikely to have significant effects.[138] Adverse reactions related to the physiologic effect of BT include occurrence of GER symptoms after lower esophageal sphincter injection. Transient incontinence of flatus and stool has been reported after anal sphincter injection in children with anal hypertonia after surgery for Hirschsprung disease[146] and in adults treated for anal fissure.[148] Adjacent regions may be affected, for example, with the development of dysphagia after head and neck injections for cervical dystonia.

CALCIUM CHANNEL BLOCKERS

Nonselective: Nifedipine, Verapamil, and Diltiazem.

Calcium channel antagonists reduce the amplitude of gastrointestinal contractions.[149,150] There are anecdotal reports of their successful use in children with esophageal motility disorders, such as diffuse esophageal spasm and nutcracker esophagus, and with severe antral spasms.[151-153]

Selective: Pinaverium Bromide. This agent inhibits gastrointestinal contractions by preventing influx of calcium into myocytes. Most of the orally administered dose remains in the gut, resulting in antispasmodic effects at doses that do not cause cardiovascular disturbance.[154] Pinaverium reduces postprandial colonic activity in patients with IBS[155] and has been successful in reducing pain in trials of adult patients with IBS.[156]

PEPPERMINT OIL

In vitro, peppermint oil inhibits smooth muscle contraction in a manner similar to that of the dihydropyridine calcium antagonists by reducing calcium influx.[157] This results in reduced contraction amplitudes at the lower esophageal sphincter,[158] stomach,[159] and small intestine[159] and prevents colonic spasm.[160,161] However, other therapeutic effects are likely. In a study of adults with diffuse esophageal spasm, peppermint oil converted simultaneous to peristaltic contractions and alleviated chest pain, without any reduction of peristaltic amplitude.[162] In a manometric study of peppermint oil and caraway oil, the duration of phase III of the MMC was shortened, in addition to reductions in contraction amplitude and frequency. A nonenteric coated preparation had more rapid effects and more marked suppression of gastric contractions than an enteric coated preparation.[159] In recent systematic reviews, peppermint oil was found to be efficacious in the treatment of IBS in children and adults.[163,164]

NITRATES

Nitric oxide donors such as glyceryl trinitrate and isosorbide dinitrate have been used to reduce the intensity of gastrointestinal contractions in the treatment of fissure in ano, anal achalasia, and spastic disorders of the esophagus.[144,165,166] Side effects such as hypotension and headache are frequently reported and require careful dosage titration.[151] As a result, these agents are probably best used on a short-term or "as required" basis.

GLUCAGON

Glucagon relaxes smooth muscle throughout the gastrointestinal tract. Pharmacologic uses of glucagon as an antispasmodic include inhibition of small intestinal contractions during endoscopic retrograde cholangiopancreatography and relaxation of the esophagus in cases of impacted foreign bodies. Interestingly, recent prospective randomized double-blind placebo-controlled trials in children and adults failed to show any benefit of glucagon over placebo for this indication.[167,168]

ADRENERGIC AGONISTS AND ANTAGONISTS

α_2-Adrenoceptors mediate sympathetic nervous system inhibition of motility in vivo.[169] α_2-Adrenergic agonists such as clonidine are being investigated for their antidiarrheal and antinociceptive actions.[55] However, the use of clonidine in gastrointestinal motility disturbance has been limited by marked intraindividual variation in response[170] and the potential for systemic hypotension.

The β_2-receptor agonist salbutamol, when administered by an inhaler, is effective in reducing the duration of severe pain in proctalgia fugax.[171–173] However, this agent does not affect resting anal pressure between attacks,[171] and the mechanism of action of salbutamol in this condition is unknown. Because attacks of proctalgia fugax are associated with increased anal tone,[174] salbutamol probably acts to reduce abnormal excessive contractions during attacks.

OTHER ANTISPASMODIC DRUGS ON THE HORIZON

Other antispasmodic, motility-inhibiting drugs currently being developed include neurokinin$_2$ antagonists (such as MEN-10627 and MEN-11420) and β_3-adrenoreceptor agonists (eg, SR-58611A). Both groups are able to decrease painful contractile activity in the gut without significantly affecting other bodily functions.[175]

CONCLUSION

Owing to the recent explosion in knowledge about the ENS and gastrointestinal motility, therapeutic options for patients with motility disturbance are rapidly expanding. New agents are being tested, and many older drugs, previously used for diseases as diverse as asthma, depression, and arterial hypertension, are being assessed for their utility in the gastrointestinal system. Because symptoms of most gastrointestinal motility disorders fluctuate over time and there may be a significant placebo effect on both symptoms and motility indices,[176] any new therapies require thorough evaluation in appropriately sized randomized placebo-controlled trials. As with any chronic disease, the importance of an effective physician-patient relationship in caring for patients with motility disturbance cannot be overstated. Pharmacologic therapy for functional bowel disorders is best administered as part of a biopsychosocial approach.[177]

REFERENCES

1. Li BU, Altschuler SM, Berseth CL, et al. Research agenda for pediatric gastroenterology, hepatology and nutrition: motility disorders and functional gastrointestinal disorders: report of the North American Society for Pediatric Gastroenterology, Hepatology and Nutrition for the Children's Digestive Health and Nutrition Foundation. J Pediatr Gastroenterol Nutr 2002;35 Suppl:S263–7.
2. Goyal R. Muscarinic receptor subtypes. N Engl J Med 1989; 312:1022–29.
3. Galligan JJ. Motility and pharmacologic therapies. In: Schuster MM, Crowell MD, Koch KL, editors. Schuster atlas of gastrointestinal motility in health and disease. 2nd ed. Hamilton (ON): BC Decker Inc; 2002. p. 399–410.
4. Callahan MJ. Irritable bowel syndrome neuropharmacology. A review of approved and investigational compounds. J Clin Gastroenterol 2002;35 Suppl 1:S58–67.
5. Bateman D, Rawlins M, Simpson J. Extrapyramidal reactions with metoclopramide. BMJ Clin Res Ed 1985;291:930–2.
6. Putnam PE, Orenstein SR, Wessel HB, Stowe RM. Tardive dyskinesia associated with use of metoclopramide in a child. J Pediatr 1992;121:983–5.
7. Hyman PE, Abrams C, Dubois A. Effect of metoclopramide and bethanechol on gastric emptying in infants. Pediatr Res 1985;19:1029–32.
8. McCallum RW, Valenzuela G, Polepalle S, Spyker D. Subcuta-

neous metoclopramide in the treatment of symptomatic gastroparesis: clinical efficacy and pharmacokinetics. J Pharmacol Exp Ther 1991;258:136–42.

9. Drummond SH, Peterson GM, Galloway JG, Keefe PA. National survey of drug use in palliative care. Palliat Med 1996; 10:119–24.

10. Buttino L Jr, Coleman SK, Bergauer NK, et al. Home subcutaneous metoclopramide therapy for hyperemesis gravidarum. J Perinatol 2000;20:359–62.

11. Grunow JE, Howard S. A randomized study of oral metoclopramide in small bowel biopsy of infants and children. J Pediatr Gastroenterol Nutr 1988;7:64–7.

12. Booth CM, Heyland DK, Paterson WG. Gastrointestinal promotility drugs in the critical care setting: a systematic review of the evidence. Crit Care Med 2002;30:1429–35.

13. Di Lorenzo C, Lachman R, Hyman PE. Intravenous erythromycin for postpyloric intubation. J Pediatr Gastroenterol Nutr 1990;11:45–7.

14. Machida HM, Forbes DA, Gall DG, Scott RB. Metoclopramide in gastroesophageal reflux of infancy. J Pediatr 1988;112:483–7.

15. Hyams JS, Leichtner AM, Zamett LO, Walters JK. Effect of metoclopramide on prolonged intraesophageal pH testing in infants with gastroesophageal reflux. J Pediatr Gastroenterol Nutr 1986;5:716–20.

16. Tolia V, Calhoun J, Kuhns L, Kauffman RE. Randomized, prospective double-blind trial of metoclopramide and placebo for gastroesophageal reflux in infants. J Pediatr 1989;115:141–5.

17. Pons G, Duhamel JF, Guillot M, et al. Dose-response study of metoclopramide in gastroesophageal reflux in infancy. Fundam Clin Pharmacol 1993;7:161–6.

18. Bellissant E, Duhamel JF, Guillot M, et al. The triangular test to assess the efficacy of metoclopramide in gastroesophageal reflux. Clin Pharmacol Ther 1997;61:377–84.

19. Rudolph C, Mazur L, Liptak G, et al. Guidelines for evaluation and treatment of gastroesophageal reflux in infants and children: recommendations of the North American Society for Pediatric Gastroenterology and Nutrition. J Pediatr Gastroenterol Nutr 2001;32 Suppl 2:S1–31.

20. Barone JA. Domperidone: a peripherally acting dopamine₂-receptor antagonist. Ann Pharmacother 1999;33:429–40.

21. Weihrauch TR, Forster CF, Krieglstein J. Evaluation of the effect of domperidone on human oesophageal and gastroduodenal motility by intraluminal manometry. Postgrad Med J 1979; 55:7–10.

22. Baeyens R, van de Velde E, De Schepper A, et al. Effects of intravenous and oral domperidone on the motor function of the stomach and small intestine. Postgrad Med J 1979;55:19–23.

23. Franzese A, Borrelli O, Corrado G, et al. Domperidone is more effective than cisapride in children with diabetic gastroparesis. Aliment Pharmacol Ther 2002;16:951–7.

24. Sarna SK, Gonzalez A, Ryan RP. Enteric locus of action of prokinetics: ABT-229, motilin, and erythromycin. Am J Physiol Gastrointest Liver Physiol 2000;278:G744–52.

25. Van Assche G, Depoortere I, Thijs T, et al. Contractile effects and intracellular Ca2⁺ signalling induced by motilin and erythromycin in the circular smooth muscle of human colon. Neurogastroenterol Motil 2001;13:27–35.

26. Tomomasa T, Kuroume T, Arai H, et al. Erythromycin induces migrating motor complex in human gastrointestinal tract. Dig Dis Sci 1986;31:157–61.

27. Jadcherla SR, Berseth CL. Effect of erythromycin on gastroduodenal contractile activity in developing neonates. J Pediatr Gastroenterol Nutr 2002;34:16–22.

28. Tomomasa T, Miyazaki M, Koizumi T, Kuroume T. Erythromycin increases gastric antral motility in human premature infants. Biol Neonate 1993;63:349–52.

29. Tack J, Janssens J, Vantrappen G, et al. Effect of erythromycin on gastric motility in controls and in diabetic gastroparesis. Gastroenterology 1992;103:72–9.

30. Stern MA, Wolf DC. Erythromycin as a prokinetic agent: a prospective, randomized, controlled study of efficacy in nasoenteric tube placement. Am J Gastroenterol 1994;89:2011–3.

31. Coffin B, Pocard M, Panis Y, et al. Erythromycin improves the quality of EGD in patients with acute upper GI bleeding: a randomized controlled study. Gastrointest Endosc 2002;56:174–9.

32. Frossard JL, Spahr L, Queneau PE, et al. Erythromycin intravenous bolus infusion in acute upper gastrointestinal bleeding: a randomized, controlled, double-blind trial. Gastroenterology 2002;123:17–23.

33. Sturm A, Holtmann G, Goebell H, Gerken G. Prokinetics in patients with gastroparesis: a systematic analysis. Digestion 1999;60:422–7.

34. Zatman TF, Hall JE, Harmer M. Gastric residual volume in children: a study comparing efficiency of erythromycin and metoclopramide as prokinetic agents. Br J Anaesth 2001;86:869–71.

35. Hall JE, Harmer M. Erythromycin as a prokinetic agent in children. Anaesthesia 1996;51:503–4.

36. Ng PC, Fok TF, Lee CH, et al. Erythromycin treatment for gastrointestinal dysmotility in preterm infants. J Paediatr Child Health 1997;33:148–50.

37. Stenson BJ, Middlemist L, Lyon AJ. Influence of erythromycin on establishment of feeding in preterm infants: observations from a randomised controlled trial. Arch Dis Child Fetal Neonatal Ed 1998;79:F212–4.

38. Patole SK, Kadalraja R, Tuladhar R, et al. Benefits of a standardised feeding regimen during a clinical trial in preterm neonates. Int J Clin Pract 2000;54:429–31.

39. Ng PC, So KW, Fung KS, et al. Randomised controlled study of oral erythromycin for treatment of gastrointestinal dysmotility in preterm infants. Arch Dis Child Fetal Neonatal Ed 2001;84:F177–82.

40. Nogami K, Nishikubo T, Minowa H, et al. Intravenous low-dose erythromycin administration for infants with feeding intolerance. Pediatr Int 2001;43:605–10.

41. Oei J, Lui K. A placebo-controlled trial of low-dose erythromycin to promote feed tolerance in preterm infants. Acta Paediatr 2001;90:904–8.

42. Costalos C, Gounaris A, Varhalama E, et al. Erythromycin as a prokinetic agent in preterm infants. J Pediatr Gastroenterol Nutr 2002;34:23–5.

43. Dellagrammaticas HD, Iacovidou N, Megaloyanni E, et al. Effect of low-dose oral erythromycin on gastric aspirates in ventilated neonates less than 32 weeks of gestation. Preliminary results. Biol Neonate 2002;81:213–6.

44. Verhagen MA, Samsom M, Maes B, et al. Effects of a new motilide, ABT-229, on gastric emptying and postprandial antroduodenal motility in healthy volunteers. Aliment Pharmacol Ther 1997;11:1077–86.

45. Talley NJ, Verlinden M, Snape W, et al. Failure of a motilin receptor agonist (ABT-229) to relieve the symptoms of functional dyspepsia in patients with and without delayed gastric emptying: a randomized double-blind placebo-controlled trial. Aliment Pharmacol Ther 2000;14:1653–61.

46. Talley NJ, Verlinden M, Geenen DJ, et al. Effects of a motilin receptor agonist (ABT-229) on upper gastrointestinal symptoms in type 1 diabetes mellitus: a randomised, double blind, placebo controlled trial. Gut 2001;49:395–401.

47. Kawamura O, Sekiguchi T, Itoh Z, Omura S. Effect of erythromycin derivative EM523L on human interdigestive gastrointestinal tract. Dig Dis Sci 1993;38:1026–31.

48. Sato F, Marui S, Inatomi N, et al. EM574, an erythromycin derivative, improves delayed gastric emptying of semi-solid meals in conscious dogs. Eur J Pharmacol 2000;395:165–72.

49. Peeters TL. GM-611 (Chugai Pharmaceutical). Curr Opin Investig Drugs 2001;2:555–7.

50. Di Lorenzo C, Lucanto C, Flores AF, et al. Effect of octreotide on gastrointestinal motility in children with functional gastrointestinal symptoms. J Pediatr Gastroenterol Nutr 1998;27:508–12.

51. Di Lorenzo C, Lucanto C, Flores AF, et al. Effect of sequential erythromycin and octreotide on antroduodenal manometry. J Pediatr Gastroenterol Nutr 1999;29:293–6.

52. Verne GN, Eaker EY, Hardy E, Sninsky CA. Effect of octreotide and erythromycin on idiopathic and scleroderma-associated intestinal pseudoobstruction. Dig Dis Sci 1995;40:1892–901.

53. Athanasakis E, Chrysos E, Zoras OJ, et al. Octreotide enhances the accelerating effect of erythromycin on gastric emptying in healthy subjects. Aliment Pharmacol Ther 2002;16:1563–70.

54. von der Ohe MR, Camilleri M, Thomforde GM, Klee GG. Differential regional effects of octreotide on human gastrointestinal motor function. Gut 1995;36:743–8.

55. Spiller R. Pharmacotherapy: non-serotonergic mechanisms. Gut 2002;51:i87–90.

56. Li-Ling J, Irving M. Therapeutic value of octreotide for patients with severe dumping syndrome—a review of randomised controlled trials. Postgrad Med J 2001;77:441–2.

57. Richards WO, Geer R, O'Dorisio TM, et al. Octreotide acetate induces fasting small bowel motility in patients with dumping syndrome. J Surg Res 1990;49:483–7.

58. Couper RT, Berzen A, Berall G, Sherman PM. Clinical response to the long acting somatostatin analogue SMS 201-995 in a child with congenital microvillus atrophy. Gut 1989;30:1020–4.

59. Jaros W, Biller J, Greer S, et al. Successful treatment of idiopathic secretory diarrhea of infancy with the somatostatin analogue SMS 201-995. Gastroenterology 1988;94:189–93.

60. Rodriguez A, del Pozo E, Rodriguez-Arnao MD, Gomez-Pan A. Growth progression and 24-hour hormone profile in an infant treated chronically with a long-acting somatostatin derivative. Horm Res 1991;35:217–21.

61. Gonzalez D, Elizondo BJ, Haslag S, et al. Chronic subcutaneous octreotide decreases gastrointestinal blood loss in blue rubber-bleb nevus syndrome. J Pediatr Gastroenterol Nutr 2001;33:183–8.

62. De Ponti F, Tonini M. Irritable bowel syndrome: new agents targeting serotonin receptor subtypes. Drugs 2001;61:317–32.

63. Briejer MR, Akkermans LM, Schuurkes JA. Gastrointestinal prokinetic benzamides: the pharmacology underlying stimulation of motility. Pharmacol Rev 1995;47:631–51.

64. Augood C, Gilbert R, Logan S, MacLennan S. Cisapride treatment for gastrooesophageal reflux in children. Cochrane Database Syst Rev 2002;3.

65. Van Herwaarden MA, Samsom M, Van Nispen CH, et al. The effect of motilin agonist ABT-229 on gastro-oesophageal reflux, oesophageal motility and lower oesophageal sphincter characteristics in GERD patients. Aliment Pharmacol Ther 2000;14:453–62.

66. Finizia C, Lundell L, Cange L, Ruth M. The effect of cisapride on oesophageal motility and lower sphincter function in patients with gastro-oesophageal reflux disease. Eur J Gastroenterol Hepatol 2002;14:9–14.

67. Van Eygen M, Van Ravensteyn H. Effect of cisapride on excessive regurgitation in infants. Clin Ther 1989;11:669–77.

68. Enriquez A, Bolisetty S, Patole S, et al. Randomised controlled trial of cisapride in feed intolerance in preterm infants. Arch Dis Child Fetal Neonatal Ed 1998;79:F110–3.

69. McClure RJ, Kristensen JH, Grauaug A. Randomised controlled trial of cisapride in preterm infants. Arch Dis Child Fetal Neonatal Ed 1999;80:F174–7.

70. Reddy PS, Deorari AK, Bal CS, et al. A double-blind placebo-controlled study on prophylactic use of cisapride on feed intolerance and gastric emptying in preterm neonates. Indian Pediatr 2000;37:837–44.

71. Ariagno RL, Kikkert MA, Mirmiran M, et al. Cisapride decreases gastroesophageal reflux in preterm infants. Pediatrics 2001;107:E58.

72. Saye Z, Forget P, Geubelle F. Effect of cisapride on gastrooesophageal reflux in children with bronchopulmonary disease: a double-blind cross-over pH monitoring study. Pediatr Pulmonol 1987;3:8–12.

73. Tucci F, Resti M, Fontana R, et al. Gastroesophageal reflux and bronchial asthma: prevalence and effect of cisapride therapy. J Pediatr Gastroenterol Nutr 1993;17:265–70.

74. Ibero M, Ridao M, Artigas R, et al. Cisapride treatment changes the evolution of infant asthma with gastroesophageal reflux. J Investig Allergol Clin Immunol 1998;8:176–9.

75. Cohen NP, Booth IW, Parashar K, Corkery JJ. Successful management of idiopathic intestinal pseudo-obstruction with cisapride. J Pediatr Surg 1988;23:229–30.

76. Hyman PE, McDiarmid SV, Napolitano J, et al. Antroduodenal motility in children with chronic intestinal pseudo-obstruction. J Pediatr 1988;112:899–905.

77. Di Lorenzo C, Reddy SN, Villanueva-Meyer J, et al. Cisapride in children with chronic intestinal pseudoobstruction. An acute, double-blind, crossover, placebo-controlled trial. Gastroenterology 1991;101:1564–70.

78. Hyman PE, Di Lorenzo C, McAdams L, et al. Predicting the clinical response to cisapride in children with chronic intestinal pseudo-obstruction. Am J Gastroenterol 1993;88:832–6.

79. Nurko S, Garcia-Aranda JA, Worona LB, Zlochisty O. Cisapride for the treatment of constipation in children: a double-blind study. J Pediatr 2000;136:35–40.

80. Letter-Propulsid. Important Drug Warning. Available at: http://www.fda.gov/medwatch/safety/2000/propul.htm (accessed Oct 22, 2003).

81. Gross A, Goh Y, Addison R, Shenfield G. Influence of grapefruit juice on cisapride pharmacokinetics. Clin Pharmacol Ther 1999;65:395–401.

82. Morganroth J, Ruegg PC, Dunger-Baldauf C, et al. Tegaserod, a 5-hydroxytryptamine type 4 receptor partial agonist, is devoid of electrocardiographic effects. Am J Gastroenterol 2002;97:2321–7.

83. Tonini M, De Ponti F, Di Nucci A, Crema F. Review article: cardiac adverse effects of gastrointestinal prokinetics. Aliment Pharmacol Ther 1999;13:1585–91.

84. Vandenplas Y. Current pediatric indications for cisapride. ESPGHAN Cisapride Panel. European Society for Pediatric Gastroenterology, Hepatology and Nutrition. J Pediatr Gastroenterol Nutr 2000;31:480–9.

85. Oberg KC, Bauman JL. QT interval prolongation and torsades de pointes due to erythromycin lactobionate. Pharmacotherapy 1995;15:687–92.

86. Drici MD, Ebert SN, Wang WX, et al. Comparison of tegaserod (HTF 919) and its main human metabolite with cisapride and erythromycin on cardiac repolarization in the isolated rabbit heart. J Cardiovasc Pharmacol 1999;34:82–8.

87. Bruera E, Villamayor R, Roca E, et al. QT interval and ventricu-

lar fibrillation with i.v. domperidone. Cancer Treat Rep 1986;70:545–6.

88. Drolet B, Rousseau G, Daleau P, et al. Domperidone should not be considered a no-risk alternative to cisapride in the treatment of gastrointestinal motility disorders. Circulation 2000; 102:1883–5.

89. Tazawa S, Masuda N, Koizumi T, et al. KDR-5169: a new gastrointestinal prokinetic agent, enhances gastric contractile and emptying activities in dogs and rats. Eur J Pharmacol 2002;434:169–76.

90. Tatsuta M, Iishi H, Nakaizumi A, Okuda S. Effect of treatment with cisapride alone or in combination with domperidone on gastric emptying and gastrointestinal symptoms in dyspeptic patients. Aliment Pharmacol Ther 1992;6:221–8.

91. Degen L, Matzinger D, Merz M, et al. Tegaserod, a 5-HT₄ receptor partial agonist, accelerates gastric emptying and gastrointestinal transit in healthy male subjects. Aliment Pharmacol Ther 2001;15:1745–51.

92. Brandt LJ, Bjorkman D, Fennerty MB, et al. Systematic review on the management of irritable bowel syndrome in North America. Am J Gastroenterol 2002;97 Suppl 1:S7–26.

93. Fidelholtz J, Smith W, Rawls J, et al. Safety and tolerability of tegaserod in patients with irritable bowel syndrome and diarrhea symptoms. Am J Gastroenterol 2002;97:1176–81.

94. Jones BW, Moore DJ, Robinson SM, Song F. A systematic review of tegaserod for the treatment of irritable bowel syndrome. J Clin Pharm Ther 2002;27:343–52.

95. Kahrilas PJ, Quigley EM, Castell DO, Spechler SJ. The effects of tegaserod (HTF 919) on oesophageal acid exposure in gastro-oesophageal reflux disease. Aliment Pharmacol Ther 2000; 14:1503–9.

96. Kamm MA. Review article: the complexity of drug development for irritable bowel syndrome. Aliment Pharmacol Ther 2002; 16:343–51.

97. Phaosawasdi K, Malmud LS, Tolin RD, et al. Cholinergic effects on esophageal transit and clearance. Gastroenterology 1981; 81:915–20.

98. Sondheimer JM, Arnold GL. Early effects of bethanechol on the esophageal motor function of infants with gastroesophageal reflux. J Pediatr Gastroenterol Nutr 1986;5:47–51.

99. Parkman HP, Trate DM, Knight LC, et al. Cholinergic effects on human gastric motility. Gut 1999;45:346–54.

100. Kirby MG, Dukes GE, Heizer WD, et al. Effect of metoclopramide, bethanechol, and loperamide on gastric residence time, gastric emptying, and mouth-to-cecum transit time. Pharmacotherapy 1989;9:226–31.

101. Euler AR. Use of bethanechol for the treatment of gastro-esophageal reflux. J Pediatr 1980;96:321–4.

102. Levi P, Marmo F, Saluzzo C, et al. Bethanechol versus antacids in the treatment of gastroesophageal reflux. Helv Paediatr Acta 1985;40:349–59.

103. Amaro R, Rogers AI. Neostigmine infusion: new standard of care for acute colonic pseudo-obstruction? Am J Gastroenterol 2000;95:304–5.

104. van der Spoel JI, Oudemans-van Straaten HM, Stoutenbeek CP, et al. Neostigmine resolves critical illness-related colonic ileus in intensive care patients with multiple organ failure—a prospective, double-blind, placebo-controlled trial. Intensive Care Med 2001;27:822–7.

105. Eaker EY. Update on acute colonic pseudo-obstruction. Curr Gastroenterol Rep 2001;3:433–6.

106. Sadjadpour K. Chronic intestinal pseudo-obstruction. Mayo Clin Proc 1989;64:728.

107. Lidums I, Lehmann A, Checklin H, et al. Control of transient lower esophageal sphincter relaxations and reflux by the GABA(B) agonist baclofen in normal subjects. Gastroenterology 2000;118:7–13.

108. Zhang Q, Lehmann A, Rigda R, et al. Control of transient lower oesophageal sphincter relaxations and reflux by the GABA(B) agonist baclofen in patients with gastro-oesophageal reflux disease. Gut 2002;50:19–24.

109. Zerbib F, Bruley Des Varannes S, Scarpignato C, et al. Endogenous cholecystokinin in postprandial lower esophageal sphincter function and fundic tone in humans. Am J Physiol 1998;275:G1266–73.

110. Lidums I, Checklin H, Mittal RK, Holloway RH. Effect of atropine on gastro-oesophageal reflux and transient lower oesophageal sphincter relaxations in patients with gastro-oesophageal reflux disease. Gut 1998;43:12–6.

111. Dowlatshahi K, Evander A, Walther B, Skinner DB. Influence of morphine on the distal oesophagus and the lower oesophageal sphincter—a manometric study. Gut 1985;26:802–6.

112. Oliveira RB, Matsuda NM, Antoniolli AR, Ballejo G. Evidence for the involvement of nitric oxide in the electrically induced relaxations of human lower esophageal sphincter and distal pylorus. Braz J Med Biol Res 1992;25:853–5.

113. Coruzzi G, Morini G, Coppelli G, Bertaccini G. The contractile effect of fedotozine on guinea pig isolated intestinal cells is not mediated by kappa opioid receptors. Pharmacology 1998;56:281–4.

114. Dapoigny M, Abitbol JL, Fraitag B. Efficacy of peripheral kappa agonist fedotozine versus placebo in treatment of irritable bowel syndrome. A multicenter dose-response study. Dig Dis Sci 1995;40:2244–9.

115. Martinez V, Jimenez M, Gonalons E, Vergara P. Mechanism of action of CCK in avian gastroduodenal motility: evidence for nitric oxide involvement. Am J Physiol 1993;265:G842–50.

116. Machino H, Kobayashi H, Hayashi K, et al. Nitric oxide is involved in the inhibitory action of cholecystokinin octapeptide (CCK-OP) on proximal colonic motility. Regul Pept 1997;69:47–52.

117. Takahashi T, Owyang C. Mechanism of cholecystokinin-induced relaxation of the rat stomach. J Auton Nerv Syst 1999;75:123–30.

118. Chovet M. Gastrointestinal functional bowel disorders: new therapies. Curr Opin Chem Biol 2000;4:428–32.

119. Carapeti EA, Kamm MA, Evans BK, Phillips RK. Topical phenylephrine increases anal sphincter resting pressure. Br J Surg 1999;86:267–70.

120. Cheetham MJ, Kamm MA, Phillips RK. Topical phenylephrine increases anal canal resting pressure in patients with faecal incontinence. Gut 2001;48:356–9.

121. Carapeti EA, Kamm MA, Phillips RK. Randomized controlled trial of topical phenylephrine in the treatment of faecal incontinence. Br J Surg 2000;87:38–42.

122. Carapeti EA, Kamm MA, Nicholls RJ, Phillips RK. Randomized, controlled trial of topical phenylephrine for fecal incontinence in patients after ileoanal pouch construction. Dis Colon Rectum 2000;43:1059–63.

123. Williams J, Watkin-Jones R. Dicyclomine: worrying symptoms associated with its use in some small babies. BMJ 1984; 288:901.

124. Garriott JC, Rodriquez R, Norton LE. Two cases of death involving dicyclomine in infants. Measurement of therapeutic and toxic concentrations in blood. J Toxicol Clin Toxicol 1984; 22:455–62.

125. Altman PM. Merbentyl syrup caution. Med J Aust 1985;142: 579–80.

126. Hardoin RA, Henslee JA, Christenson CP, et al. Colic medica-

tion and apparent life-threatening events. Clin Pediatr 1991;30:281–5.

127. Myers JH, Moro-Sutherland D, Shook JE. Anticholinergic poisoning in colicky infants treated with hyoscyamine sulfate. Am J Emerg Med 1997;15:532–5.

128. Grillage MG, Nankani JN, Atkinson SN, Prescott P. A randomised, double-blind study of mebeverine versus dicyclomine in the treatment of functional abdominal pain in young adults. Br J Clin Pract 1990;44:176–9.

129. Alabaster VA. Discovery and development of selective M_3 antagonists for clinical use. Life Sci 1997;60:1053–60.

130. Houghton LA, Rogers J, Whorwell PJ, et al. Zamifenacin (UK-76, 654) a potent gut M_3 selective muscarinic antagonist, reduces colonic motor activity in patients with irritable bowel syndrome. Aliment Pharmacol Ther 1997;11:561–8.

131. Den Hertog A, Van den Akker J. Modification of alpha 1-receptor-operated channels by mebeverine in smooth muscle cells of guinea-pig taenia caeci. Eur J Pharmacol 1987;138:367–74.

132. Subissi A, Brunori P, Bachi M. Effects of spasmolytics on K^+-induced contraction of rat intestine in vivo. Eur J Pharmacol 1983;96:295–301.

133. Colofac, product information. In: Caswell A, editor. MIMS annual 2002. Sydney: MediMedia Australia; 2002. p. 1–26.

134. Delvaux M, Louvel D, Mamet JP, et al. Effect of alosetron on responses to colonic distension in patients with irritable bowel syndrome. Aliment Pharmacol Ther 1998;12:849–55.

135. Tack J, Piessevaux H, Coulie B, et al. Role of impaired gastric accommodation to a meal in functional dyspepsia. Gastroenterology 1998;115:1346–52.

136. Tack J, Coulie B, Wilmer A, et al. Actions of the 5-hydroxy-tryptamine 1 receptor agonist sumatriptan on interdigestive gastrointestinal motility in man. Gut 1998;42:36–41.

137. Sifrim D, Holloway RH, Tack J, et al. Effect of sumatriptan, a $5HT_1$ agonist, on the frequency of transient lower esophageal sphincter relaxations and gastroesophageal reflux in healthy subjects. Am J Gastroenterol 1999;94:3158–64.

138. Mandal A, Robinson RJ. Indications and efficacy of botulinum toxin in disorders of the gastrointestinal tract. Eur J Gastroenterol Hepatol 2001;13:603–9.

139. Schneider I, Thumfart WF, Pototschnig C, Eckel HE. Treatment of dysfunction of the cricopharyngeal muscle with botulinum A toxin: introduction of a new, noninvasive method. Ann Otol Rhinol Laryngol 1994;103:31–5.

140. Hurwitz M, Bahar RJ, Ament ME, et al. Evaluation of the use of botulinum toxin in children with achalasia. J Pediatr Gastroenterol Nutr 2000;30:509–14.

141. Miller LS, Pullela SV, Parkman HP, et al. Treatment of chest pain in patients with noncardiac, nonreflux, nonachalasia spastic esophageal motor disorders using botulinum toxin injection into the gastroesophageal. Am J Gastroenterol 2002;97:1640–6.

142. Miller LS, Szych GA, Kantor SB, et al. Treatment of idiopathic gastroparesis with injection of botulinum toxin into the pyloric sphincter muscle. Am J Gastroenterol 2002;97:1653–60.

143. Messineo A, Codrich D, Monai M, et al. The treatment of internal anal sphincter achalasia with botulinum toxin. Pediatr Surg Int 2001;17:521–3.

144. American Gastroenterology Association Clinical Practice Committee. American Gastroenterology Association technical review on the diagnosis and care of patients with anal fissure. Gastroenterology 2003;124:235–45.

145. Langer J, Birnbaum E. Preliminary experience with intrasphincteric botulinum toxin for persistent constipation after pull-through for Hirschsprung's disease. J Pediatr Surg 1997; 32:1059–61; discussion 1061–2.

146. Minkes RK, Langer JC. A prospective study of botulinum toxin for internal anal sphincter hypertonicity in children with Hirschsprung's disease. J Pediatr Surg 2000;35:1733–6.

147. Scott A, Suzuki D. Systemic toxicity of botulinum toxin by intramuscular injection in the monkey. Mov Disord 1988; 3:333–5.

148. Madalinski M, Slawek J, Duzynski W, et al. Side effects of botulinum toxin injection for benign anal disorders. Eur J Gastroenterol Hepatol 2002;14:853–6.

149. Short TP, Thomas E. An overview of the role of calcium antagonists in the treatment of achalasia and diffuse oesophageal spasm. Drugs 1992;43:177–84.

150. Chrysos E, Xynos E, Tzovaras G, et al. Effect of nifedipine on rectoanal motility. Dis Colon Rectum 1996;39:212–6.

151. Milov DE, Cynamon HA, Andres JM. Chest pain and dysphagia in adolescents caused by diffuse esophageal spasm. J Pediatr Gastroenterol Nutr 1989;9:450–3.

152. Glassman MS, Medow MS, Berezin S, Newman LJ. Spectrum of esophageal disorders in children with chest pain. Dig Dis Sci 1992;37:663–6.

153. Freeman L, Mazur LJ. Verapamil therapy for persistent antral spasms in a child. South Med J 1996;89:529–30.

154. Christen MO. Action of pinaverium bromide, a calcium-antagonist, on gastrointestinal motility disorders. Gen Pharmacol 1990;21:821–5.

155. Bouchoucha M, Faye A, Devroede G, Arsac M. Effects of oral pinaverium bromide on colonic response to food in irritable bowel syndrome patients. Biomed Pharmacother 2000;54: 381–7.

156. Poynard T, Regimbeau C, Benhamou Y. Meta-analysis of smooth muscle relaxants in the treatment of irritable bowel syndrome. Aliment Pharmacol Ther 2001;15:355–61.

157. Hills JM, Aaronson PI. The mechanism of action of peppermint oil on gastrointestinal smooth muscle. An analysis using patch clamp electrophysiology and isolated tissue pharmacology in rabbit and guinea pig. Gastroenterology 1991;101:55–65.

158. Dalvi SS, Nadkarni PM, Pardesi R, Gupta KC. Effect of peppermint oil on gastric emptying in man: a preliminary study using a radiolabelled solid test meal. Indian J Physiol Pharmacol 1991;35:212–4.

159. Micklefield GH, Greving I, May B. Effects of peppermint oil and caraway oil on gastroduodenal motility. Phytother Res 2000;14:20–3.

160. Sparks MJ, O'Sullivan P, Herrington AA, Morcos SK. Does peppermint oil relieve spasm during barium enema? Br J Radiol 1995;68:841–3.

161. Asao T, Mochiki E, Suzuki H, et al. An easy method for the intraluminal administration of peppermint oil before colonoscopy and its effectiveness in reducing colonic spasm. Gastrointest Endosc 2001;53:172–7.

162. Pimentel M, Bonorris GG, Chow EJ, Lin HC. Peppermint oil improves the manometric findings in diffuse esophageal spasm. J Clin Gastroenterol 2001;33:27–31.

163. Weydert JA, Ball TM, Davis MF. Systematic review of treatments for recurrent abdominal pain. Pediatrics 2003;111:e1–11.

164. Pittler MH, Ernst E. Peppermint oil for irritable bowel syndrome: a critical review and metaanalysis. Am J Gastroenterol 1998;93:1131–5.

165. Millar AJ, Steinberg RM, Raad J, Rode H. Anal achalasia after pull-through operations for Hirschsprung's disease—preliminary experience with topical nitric oxide. Eur J Pediatr Surg 2002;12:207–11.

166. Storr M, Allescher HD. Esophageal pharmacology and treatment of primary motility disorders. Dis Esophagus 1999;12:241–57.

167. Tibbling L, Bjorkhoel A, Jansson E, Stenkvist M. Effect of spasmolytic drugs on esophageal foreign bodies. Dysphagia 1995;10:126–7.

168. Mehta D, Attia M, Quintana E, Cronan K. Glucagon use for esophageal coin dislodgment in children: a prospective, double-blind, placebo-controlled trial. Acad Emerg Med 2001;8:200–3.

169. Scheibner J, Trendelenburg AU, Hein L, et al. Alpha 2-adrenoceptors in the enteric nervous system: a study in alpha 2A-adrenoceptor-deficient mice. Br J Pharmacol 2002; 135:697–704.

170. Viramontes BE, Malcolm A, Camilleri M, et al. Effects of an alpha(2)-adrenergic agonist on gastrointestinal transit, colonic motility, and sensation in humans. Am J Physiol Gastrointest Liver Physiol 2001;281:G1468–76.

171. Eckardt VF, Dodt O, Kanzler G, Bernhard G. Treatment of proctalgia fugax with salbutamol inhalation. Am J Gastroenterol 1996;91:686–9.

172. Wright JE. Inhaled salbutamol for proctalgia fugax. Lancet 1985;ii:659–60.

173. Wright JE. Trial of inhaled salbutamol for proctalgia fugax. Lancet 1991;337:359.

174. Eckardt VF, Dodt O, Kanzler G, Bernhard G. Anorectal function and morphology in patients with sporadic proctalgia fugax. Dis Colon Rectum 1996;39:755–62.

175. Scarpignato C, Pelosini I. Management of irritable bowel syndrome: novel approaches to the pharmacology of gut motility. Can J Gastroenterol 1999;13 Suppl A:50A–65A.

176. Mearin F, Balboa A, Zarate N, et al. Placebo in functional dyspepsia: symptomatic, gastrointestinal motor, and gastric sensorial responses. Am J Gastroenterol 1999;94:116–25.

177. Hyman PE. Functional gastrointestinal disorders and the biopsychosocial model of practice. J Pediatr Gastroenterol Nutr 2001;32 Suppl 1:S5–7.

178. Banner SE, Sanger GJ. Differences between 5-HT$_3$ receptor antagonists in modulation of visceral hypersensitivity. Br J Pharmacol 1995;114:558–62.

179. Cai B, Huang X, Wang G, Mo W. Potentiation of electroacupuncture analgesia on visceral pain by metoclopramide and its mechanism. Chen Tzu Yen Chiu Acupuncture Res 1994;19:66–70, 74.

180. Gibbs RD, Movinsky BA, Pellegrini J, Vacchiano CA. The morphine-sparing effect of metoclopramide on postoperative laparoscopic tubal ligation patients. AANA J 2002;70:27–32.

181. Bradette M, Pare P, Douville P, Morin A. Visceral perception in health and functional dyspepsia. Crossover study of gastric distension with placebo and domperidone. Dig Dis Sci 1991;36:52–8.

182. Curry JI, Lander TD, Stringer MD. Review article: erythromycin as a prokinetic agent in infants and children. Aliment Pharmacol Ther 2001;15:595–603.

183. Kamerling IM, van Haarst AD, Burggraaf J, et al. Exogenous motilin affects postprandial proximal gastric motor function and visceral sensation. Dig Dis Sci 2002;47:1732–6.

184. Manes G, Dominguez-Munoz JE, Leodolter A, Malfertheiner P. Effect of cisapride on gastric sensitivity to distension, gastric compliance and duodeno-gastric reflexes in healthy humans. Dig Liver Dis 2001;33:407–13.

185. Law NM, Bharucha AE, Undale AS, Zinsmeister AR. Cholinergic stimulation enhances colonic motor activity, transit, and sensation in humans. Am J Physiol Gastrointest Liver Physiol 2001;281:G1228–37.

186. Foschi D, Callioni F, Castoldi L, et al. Effects of intranasal neostigmine on oesophageal motility in man. Pharmacol Res 1992;25:311–6.

187. Bortolotti M, Cucchiara S, Sarti P, et al. Comparison between the effects of neostigmine and ranitidine on interdigestive gastroduodenal motility of patients with gastroparesis. Digestion 1995;56:96–9.

188. McQuay HJ. Pharmacological treatment of neuralgic and neuropathic pain. Cancer Surv 1988;7:141–59.

189. Holzer P. Gastrointestinal afferents as targets of novel drugs for the treatment of functional bowel disorders and visceral pain. Eur J Pharmacol 2001;429:177–93.

190. Reichert JA, Daughters RS, Rivard R, Simone DA. Peripheral and preemptive opioid antinociception in a mouse visceral pain model. Pain 2001;89:221–7.

191. Evans PR, Bak YT, Kellow JE. Mebeverine alters small bowel motility in irritable bowel syndrome. Aliment Pharmacol Ther 1996;10:787–93.

192. Washington N, Ridley P, Thomas C, et al. Mebeverine decreases mass movements and stool frequency in lactulose-induced diarrhoea. Aliment Pharmacol Ther 1998;12:583–8.

193. Passaretti S, Sorghi M, Colombo E, et al. Motor effects of locally administered pinaverium bromide in the sigmoid tract of patients with irritable bowel syndrome. Int J Clin Pharmacol Ther Toxicol 1989;27:47–50.

194. Bouchoucha M, Salles JP, Fallet M, et al. Effect of pinaverium bromide on jejunal motility and colonic transit time in healthy humans. Biomed Pharmacother 1992;46:161–5.

195. Lu CL, Chen CY, Chang FY, et al. Effect of a calcium channel blocker and antispasmodic in diarrhoea-predominant irritable bowel syndrome. J Gastroenterol Hepatol 2000;15:925–30.

196. Hawthorn M, Ferrante J, Luchowski E, et al. The actions of peppermint oil and menthol on calcium channel dependent processes in intestinal, neuronal and cardiac preparations. Aliment Pharmacol Ther 1988;2:101–18.

197. Kline RM, Kline JJ, Di Palma J, Barbero GJ. Enteric-coated, pH-dependent peppermint oil capsules for the treatment of irritable bowel syndrome in children. J Pediatr 2001;138:125–8.

198. Thumshirn M, Camilleri M, Choi MG, Zinsmeister AR. Modulation of gastric sensory and motor functions by nitrergic and alpha$_2$-adrenergic agents in humans. Gastroenterology 1999;116:573–85.

199. Tack J, Coulie B, Wilmer A, et al. Influence of sumatriptan on gastric fundus tone and on the perception of gastric distension in man. Gut 2000;46:468–73.

200. Sarnelli G, Janssens J, Tack J. Effect of intranasal sumatriptan on gastric tone and sensitivity to distension. Dig Dis Sci 2001;46:1591–5.

201. O'Donnell LJ, Watson AJ, Cameron D, Farthing MJ. Effect of octreotide on mouth-to-caecum transit time in healthy subjects and in the irritable bowel syndrome. Aliment Pharmacol Ther 1990;4:177–81.

202. Malcolm A, Camilleri M, Kost L, et al. Towards identifying optimal doses for alpha-2 adrenergic modulation of colonic and rectal motor and sensory function. Aliment Pharmacol Ther 2000;14:783–93.

4. Pharmacologic Therapy of Exocrine Pancreatic Insufficiency

Geoffrey Cleghorn, MBBS, FRACP, FACG

The exocrine pancreas is involved in both the digestion and absorption of orally ingested nutrients. Normally, the fluid and exocrine secretions from the pancreas are secreted in great excess following a meal, and, in fact, before clinical manifestations of exocrine pancreatic insufficiency become manifest, over 98% of the gland's function needs to be lost.

Pancreatic fluid has two major components: a fluid consisting primarily of a solution of sodium bicarbonate and an enzyme component consisting of about 20 digestive enzymes and cofactors. The alkaline fluid serves to neutralize gastric acid entering the duodenum and helps to provide an adequate intraluminal pH for the optimal function of the pancreatic digestive enzymes. These enzymes provide the major route for intraluminal digestion of dietary proteins, triglycerides, and carbohydrates and are also involved in the cleavage of certain vitamins, such as A and B_{12}. Therefore, failure of the exocrine pancreas to secrete adequately its enzyme- and electrolyte-rich fluid can lead to major nutritional disturbances that manifest clinically as steatorrhea and azotorrhea, with resultant growth failure.[1] In addition to the obvious lack of intraluminal digestive activity as a result of the enzyme deficiencies, the failure of bicarbonate secretion also has major effects on both intraluminal pH and enzyme activity. An abnormally low pH can be seen in the late postprandial period, which reduces lipid digestion by inactivating pancreatic lipase and also by precipitating bile salts.

Not all diseases involving the exocrine pancrease have equal effects on both the enzyme component and the electrolyte component of the gland's secretion. In general, patients with cystic fibrosis (CF) have major deficits in both enzyme and electrolyte secretion, although there is a wide range of abnormalities; however, patients with Shwachman-Diamond syndrome have intact fluid and electrolyte secretion with marked disturbances in enzyme output.

CF is the most common cause of exocrine pancreatic insufficiency in childhood. Therefore, it is patients with CF who most commonly require oral pancreatic replacement therapy with pancreatic enzymes. Irrespective of the etiology of pancreatic failure, current replacement therapy with oral pancreatic enzymes, although far from ideal in many patients, remains the most important method of correcting the nutritional effects of maldigestion. Despite considerable improvements in the efficacy of pancreatic replacement therapy, it remains difficult to correct malabsorption

completely in all patients owing to the many factors adversely affecting the function of exogenously administered enzymes.

Because the major clinical manifestation of pancreatic failure is steatorrhea with large, bulky, malodorous stools, early management protocols of patients with pancreatic insufficiency relied heavily on severe restriction of dietary fat. A low-fat diet did indeed produce socially more acceptable stools, but it also severely restricted calories and essential fatty acids, which contributed significantly to clinical malnutrition and disease morbidity. Use of a low-fat diet in the management of pancreatic failure is no longer considered acceptable; in fact, some centers advocate the use of a high-fat diet, in conjunction with optimal pancreatic enzyme replacement therapy, to maximize total energy absorption.

PANCREATIC ENZYME REPLACEMENT

Extracts of pancreatic enzymes from animal sources have been available for almost a century and have been used clinically for a variety of conditions. However, in spite of their recognized importance, the use of pancreatic enzymes is still not without its difficulties (Table 76.4-1). Commercial enzyme supplements do not have an indefinite shelf life, and, for this reason, patients should be warned not to stockpile large quantities of enzymes. In fact, many commercially available supplements are initially packed with much

TABLE 76.4–1   FACTORS ADVERSELY AFFECTING THE EFFICIENCY OF PANCREATIC ENZYME REPLACEMENT THERAPY

PHARMACOLOGIC PHASE
    Enzyme source (porcine, bovine, fungal)
    Enzyme stability
    Particle size of microspheres
    Inadequate enzyme concentration
    Inappropriate oral administration
    Poor compliance

GASTROINTESTINAL PHASE
    Inactivation by gastric acid
    Insufficient mixing with chyme
    Delay in gastric emptying
    Prolonged acidic intraluminal pH
    Bile acid precipitation
    Abnormal intestinal motility
    Proteolytic destruction of lipase

higher protease and lipase values than their listed potencies to allow for this decline. Thomson and colleagues showed a decline of up to 20% in enzyme activity over an 8-month period in several different enzyme preparations, even though all were within the expiration date quoted by the manufacturers.[2] The earliest pancreatic extracts contained low concentrations of active enzymes. Furthermore, only minimal amounts of these were available for intestinal digestion because of gastric inactivation with acid and pepsin, with degradation of lipase and trypsin occurring below pH 4.5 and 3.5, respectively. Even the more active preparations in current use are rapidly degraded in the stomach when unprotected; up to 90% of ingested lipase and 80% of ingested trypsin have been found to be degraded prior to entering the ligament of Treitz.[3]

Broadly speaking, research has focused on three avenues of approach in improving nutrient absorption in patients with pancreatic insufficiency. First, because the older enzyme preparations were highly variable in enzyme content, the more modern approach has been to provide increased concentration of enzyme (up to 20,000 lipase units) in a single capsule or tablet.[4] Second, methods of protecting enzymes from gastric inactivation have been refined. Intensive research has also been aimed at manipulating the acid-alkaline imbalance in both the gastric and intestinal phases of enzyme activity. Third, attempts have been made at improving bile salt function.

Protective barriers were first used to make the enzyme preparations more resistant to acid inactivation. Initially, this was attempted by coating enzyme tablets with an acid-resistant material, but it was soon discovered that these preparations were no better than conventional preparations, and, in some cases, the steatorrhea was worse. This was thought to be due to both inefficient mixing of the tablet with the ingested chyme in the stomach and failure of liberation of the active enzyme in the duodenum secondary to slow release of the active ingredients. In fact, these tablets were not infrequently seen intact in the stools of patients taking them.[5]

To improve delivery of enzymes to the small intestine, a number of commercial pharmaceutical companies developed techniques capable of coating small "microspheres" with an acid-resistant coating.[6–12] The microspheres, in turn, were packaged in a gelatin capsule. The rationale behind this preparation is that the acid-resistant layer around the small spheres prevents acid-peptic degradation within the stomach, but their small size permits passage with chyme into the duodenum. When exposed to duodenal contents with a pH in excess of 5.5, the acid-resistant coating breaks down, releasing active pancreatic enzymes. This exposure may not occur in the proximal duodenum, however, because in CF, the postprandial intraluminal duodenum pH can frequently be below 5.0 for long periods of time. Thus, continued enzyme protection from the highly acidic milieu in the duodenum by the acid-resistant coating may allow for more distal bioavailability. The size of the microspheres also appears to be very important for adequate function. Several groups have shown that digestion in pancreatic insufficiency is more effective with microspheres of less than 1.4 mm com

pared with larger preparations, supporting the belief that microspheres of this size or smaller will optimally mix with the meal and empty the stomach together with the chyme, improving their digestive efficacy.[4]

Despite these advances in the use of microspheres, there is still some doubt over the reliability of gastric emptying. A study of 12 CF patients has shown considerable variation in gastric emptying and intestinal transit for food and pancreatic microspheres, with enzyme pellets generally emptying from the stomach more rapidly than the food.[13] This mismatch of emptying can be as high as 60 minutes in some patients, which will have obvious ramifications on the amount and timing of the enzyme replacement therapy.

Use of these enteric-coated microspheres has resulted in considerable improvement in fat absorption over that with conventional enzyme therapy.[7] A study has shown that CF patients with refractory malabsorption on conventional enzyme therapy derive significant benefit, with decreased steatorrhea and creatorrhea, using fewer capsules.[7] Other studies have found better compliance and improved absorption with these preparations, except in a minority of patients who appear to have acidic small intestinal contents, thereby preventing dissolution of the acid-resistant coating. Thus, there are few current uses for noncoated enzyme replacement therapy, although even with these modern preparations, some patients still have significant malabsorption.

In addition to acid-peptic denaturation and particle size, rapid proteolytic degradation of lipase, particularly by chymotrypsin, in the proximal small intestine is another important factor that limits the efficacy of pancreatic enzyme replacement therapy. Attempts at protecting lipase from this degradation using protease inhibitors have shown enhancement of lipolysis throughout the entire length of the small intestine.

The number of capsules required depends on the amount of active enzymes in the particular commercial preparation and also on the type and quantity of the meal to be consumed. To abolish malabsorption, the amount and concentration of enzyme present in the duodenum must be 5 to 10% (40–60 IU/mL intraluminal lipase concentration) of the quantities of endogenously secreted enzymes usually present in normal individuals after postprandial stimulation of the pancreas.[3] In an adult, assuming no inactivation of enzymes in the stomach and duodenum, approximately 25,000 to 40,000 U of lipase must be taken with an average meal.[14] In reality, the quantity of enzymes required becomes much higher (perhaps up to 10-fold) if one considers the degree of gastric inactivation and the consumption of a high-energy diet. There is, however, enormous patient to patient variability, and each patient and meal must be considered individually. In general, however, in light of findings regarding fibrosing colonopathy,[15] the daily dose of pancreatic enzymes for most patients should remain below 10,000 U of lipase/kg (Table 76.4–2).

Enzymes derived from porcine sources are the current standard treatment of exocrine insufficiency. Supplementation with enzymes from different species has also been suggested as a method of achieving improved digestion

TABLE 77.4–2   SUGGESTED DAILY REQUIREMENTS OF PANCREATIC ENZYME REPLACEMENT THERAPY

AGE (YR)	APPROXIMATE DAILY FAT INTAKE (G)*†	DAILY LIPASE UNITS (000S)† (MAXIMUM DAILY DOSE 10,000 U LIPASE/KG/D)
0.0–0.5	25	12.5–25
0.5–1.0	30	15–30
1–3	35	17.5–140
4–6	50	25–200
7–10	60	30–240
11–14	90	45–360
15–18	110	55–440

*Assume 40% of total energy needs.
†In cystic fibrosis, multiply by a factor of 1.5.

Enzymes from bovine sources have been considered but discarded owing to their inferior lipase content and hence increased tablet requirement.[16] Acid-resistant lingual lipase has been proposed as an enzyme worthy of further consideration and investigation. In a preliminary study in animals, lingual lipase was found to be stable in the stomach under both fasting and fed conditions but to be less stable in the duodenum; however, to date no worthwhile clinical trials have been undertaken or reported.[17,18] Lipases derived from fungi have also been examined for their acid-resistant properties, with these experimental studies possibly becoming forerunners of in vivo human work examining pancreatic enzyme supplementation containing "foreign" enzymes. Fungi, such as *Rhizopus arrhizus*, *Candida cylinderaza*, and *Aspergillus niger*, are potential sources of lipase, which differs from lipases of animal origin in that fungi provide greater amounts of acid-stable lipase activity in the stomach; however, they appear to be highly sensitive to denaturation by even low concentrations of bile acids. Despite early promise in vitro, early in vivo studies have failed to extend their clinical usefulness.[19–21]

Lipases derived from bacteria are, however, more promising in their efficacy. Unlike fungal lipases, lipase of bacterial origin appears to be resistant to both acid and alkaline inactivation as well as being stable in the presence of both proteolytic enzymes and bile salts.[22–24] These recent studies have suggested that lipase derived from *Burkholderia plantarii* has far greater lipolytic activity than conventional porcine products, holding out the potential for a dramatic reduction in the quantity of individual tablets required for equivalent lipase activity, but, to date, no human trials have been reported.[23,24]

It is also now possible using recombinant deoxyribonucleic acid (DNA) techniques to produce human acid-stable lipases because the gene for human gastric lipase has now been transfected and expressed using recombinant adenovirus in a variety of animal models.[25,26] Similarly, application of bioengineered, acid-resistant human gastric lipase is also being actively explored in in vitro studies, but, to date, human trials are still pending in these areas.[27,28]

Irrespective of the enzyme preparation used and the amount given, it is imperative that the enzymes be delivered in sufficient amounts to the small intestine to facilitate digestion. It is insufficient simply to take a handful of enzymes at the beginning or end of a meal and hope that this will result in optimal pancreatic replacement. For optimal efficacy, it has been suggested that enzymes be distributed throughout the meal and taken in several small aliquots. This, in theory, allows for adequate dispersal within the stomach throughout the meal and therefore allows for maximum exposure of that particular meal to the ingested enzymes. However, as mentioned above, there is still no certainty that the enzymes will both mix completely with the food and also empty from the stomach uniformly.

MONITORING ENZYME EFFICACY

The simplest method of monitoring the effectiveness of the enzyme replacement therapy is to regularly monitor the patient's growth (in particular weight) and also the nature and consistency of the stools. In general, it is not very difficult to ascertain by history alone if a patient's enzyme dosage is insufficient on the basis of a stool history, but the associated history of abdominal pain is far less helpful. However, it is much more difficult to gauge on the basis of history alone whether a dosage is, in fact, excessive. More precise, yet still very qualitative, to perform is a quantitative assessment of fat absorption pre- and postenzymes with a fecal fat analysis. Each individual requires an objective, quantitative assessment of fecal fat losses as a percentage of fat intake at baseline and after any major adjustments in enzyme replacement therapy. Quantitative fecal fat estimation is the one reliable method, but there are practical limitations. Breath tests for the detection of pancreatic insufficiency have also been developed.[29,30] Cholesteryl octanoate breath testing using a carbon 14 or carbon 13 label has been shown to monitor intraluminal enzymatic activity in both controls and patients with pancreatic insufficiency after treatment with different forms of enzyme replacement. Fecal chymotrypsin and elastase 1 measurements have also been suggested but are still only in research use. Others have suggested that the pancreatic Schilling test is also a means of assessing replacement therapy.[31] This is based on the relationship between the pancreatic output of trypsin and the urinary excretion of cobalamin.

SIDE EFFECTS

Enzyme therapy is not without potential problems in that, being concentrated proteolytic packages, enzymes have the potential for causing quite marked oral excoriation if chewed or held within the mouth too long. This is a particular problem in small infants, in whom gum or mouth injury frequently occurs; with rapid transit through the intestinal tract, anal excoriation has also been observed.

Hyperuricemia and uricosuria are believed to result from the high purine content of the conventional enzyme preparation. Obviously, the greater the dose, the higher the incidence of these biochemical abnormalities. Allergic responses such as bronchospasm, nasal irritation, and repeated coughing may develop, not only in the patients receiving the enzymes but also in any susceptible caregiver coming into repeated close contact with the enzyme preparations. These allergic reactions were much more prevalent with the nonencapsulated forms of the enzyme preparations.

The antigenicity of the pancreatic extracts should not be underestimated. Anaphylaxis has been observed in patients and caregivers exposed to the enzymes, particularly in a powdered form. Each capsule is a potent source of foreign protein, and small but significant amounts are absorbed into the body. Couper and Quirk and their colleagues studied two groups of CF patients using an enzyme-linked immunosorbent assay[32,33] specifically to detect immunoglobulin G (IgG) antibody directed against porcine trypsin. No antibodies were detected in patients prior to commencement of enzyme replacement, but 96% had developed porcine trypsin-binding IgG within a few years. This antibody production may possibly accentuate immune complex disease progression, which is well known in CF.

After its initial description and significant concerns, fibrosing colonopathy continues to generate debate as to its true place in the cystic fibrosis arena. First reported in 1994, fibrosing colonopathy is characterized by marked submucosal fibrosis with thickening of the muscularis propria and chronic inflammation chiefly affecting the cecum and ascending colon.[34] Typically, fibrosing colonopathy occurs in younger children, although it has been described arising de novo in a young adult patient with CF. Symptoms suggestive of colonic obstruction (abdominal pain and vomiting) occur within a few months after starting high-dose pancreatic enzyme replacement therapy. A systematic review of 114 accredited CF care centers in the United States revealed 31 proven cases of fibrosing colonopathy, with a strong relationship found between the occurrence of the fibrosing colonopathy and the total daily dose of the enzyme replacement.[34] This study showed that for patients taking more than 50,000 U of lipase/kg/d, the incidence of fibrosing colonopathy requiring surgery was about 3.8 per 1,000 patients per year of use, suggesting that most patients should remain below 10,000 U of lipase/kg/d.

The exact etiology of fibrosing colonopathy remains obscure. The appearance of this condition in cystic fibrosis patients initially appeared to coincide with the introduction of the "high-dose" enzyme preparations, with some patients consuming in excess of 20,000 IU lipase/kg/d. Interestingly, since the more conservative use of pancreatic enzymes, in particular, the high-dose preparations, there has been a reduction in the reported frequency of the problem.

Initially, it was suggested that the acid-resistant coating of the microspheres and tablets containing a methacrylic acid copolymer coating, Eudragit L (Röhm GmbH & Co., Darmstadt, Germany), was implicated.[35] Eudragit L has been shown to be toxic to rat intestine, causing mucosal ulceration and submucosal edema and fibrosis identical to the lesions seen in patients described in the literature. More recently, however, fibrosing colonopathy has been reported in patients not using this coating[34] and, in fact, not using pancreatic enzymes at all,[36,37] which highlights the continuing uncertainty of its etiology.

ADJUNCTIVE THERAPY TO ACID-BASE EQUILIBRIUM

The alternative method of improving the efficiency of the ingested pancreatic enzymes has been to modify the acid-base balance within the gastrointestinal tract. The H_2 receptor antagonists, such as cimetidine or ranitidine, have been used to diminish the secretion of gastric acid, thereby successfully decreasing the gastric inactivation of the ingested enzymes with resultant improvement in nutrient absorption.[7,14,38–42] Because enteric-coated microspheres are pH dependent and rely on a luminal pH of greater than 5.5 for dissolution of the acid-resistant coating, it is possible that jejunal hyperacidity may further hinder their activity. It has been shown that postprandial jejunal "hyperacidity" does occur in patients with CF, with 40% of a test meal entering the jejunum at a pH below 5.[38] At this pH, bile acids precipitate out of the aqueous solution, leading to a reduction in the aqueous phase bile acid concentration. In addition, lipase activity, which is extremely pH sensitive, is considerably reduced.

Cimetidine has been shown to increase jejunal pH, thus increasing aqueous phase bile acid concentration.[40] In a study of adult CF patients receiving noncoated enzymes, 60% of the test meal entered the jejunum at a pH less than 5, compared with only 17% in healthy subjects. There was a significant decrease in lipase activity and a decrease in aqueous phase lipid concentration, but the decrease in bile acid precipitation did not reach statistical significance. With the introduction of cimetidine, however, there was significantly less bile acid precipitation, and this resulted in improved lipid solubilization, suggesting that the efficacy of pancreatic enzyme therapy is limited both by exogenous enzyme inactivation in the stomach and by the pH-dependent environment within the proximal small intestine and that these effects were both improved by the addition of cimetidine. Data suggest that patients who had significant steatorrhea while taking enteric-coated microspheres also had improved nutrient absorption with the addition of cimetidine.[41] This improvement could result from both the prevention of gastric inactivitation and the reduction in small bowel hyperacidity levels, thus affecting the solubilization of bile salts.

Because the major effect of the addition of cimetidine appears to be improvement of the small intestinal alkalinity, it is not unreasonable to presume that the addition of antacids of bicarbonate therapy may have some merit. Graham found that the concurrent administration of enzymes with either sodium bicarbonate or aluminium hydroxide yields a greater reduction in steatorrhea than do enzymes alone.[38] Durie and others reported 21 patients with CF in whom sodium bicarbonate (15 g/m²/24 h) was an effective adjunct to enzyme therapy. These workers found that sodium bicarbonate or cimetidine (20 mg/kg/d) had equivalent beneficial effects as adjuvant therapy, but when both drugs were given simultaneously, there was no further improvement in nutrient absorption.[41] The choice of antacid does appear to be critical.[38]

The proton pump inhibitors, with more potency and duration of action compared to H_2 receptor antagonists, have also been used as an adjunctive therapy.[43] They have been shown to increase the efficacy of enteric-coated enzyme capsules dramatically and achieve near-normalization of fat absorption.[44,45] In addition to their effect on gastric acid secretion, they also have a profound effect on gastric volume, which may help to prevent dilution of the enzymes. The marked reduction in gastric pH may also see an increased postprandial duodenal pH, assisting in the effectiveness of the enzyme therapy. Further studies have shown that adjuvant therapy with the protein pump inhibitor lansoprazole in young CF patients with persistent fat malabsorption decreased fat losses and improved total body fat. In addition, lung hyperinflation was also decreased in the study patients, which may partly explain the improvement in inspiratory muscle performance.[46]

Yet another approach to adjuvant therapy is with the use of prostaglandin agents.[47] Prostaglandins of the E and I series inhibit basal and stimulate gastric acid secretion both in vivo and in vitro. In the dog, either prostaglandin E_2 or PGI_2 inhibits gastric acid secretion stimulated by food, histamine, pentagastrin, or reserpine. The mechanism by which natural prostaglandins and their analogs inhibit gastric acid secretion is still unknown, but one possibility is that there is direct inhibition of parietal cells by prostaglandins acting from the gastric lumen.[48]

Another mechanism through which prostaglandins might affect gastric secretion is suppression of gastrin release. It has been shown that methylated prostaglandin E analogs given orally in dogs and humans cause a marked suppression of gastrin response to a meal.[49] An important addition to the effect of gastric acid secretion is the effect of prostaglandins, particularly the methylated analogs, in stimulating mucus and bicarbonate secretion. This may account for the reduction in luminal acidity observed with the administration of these prostaglandins.

Prostaglandin therapy may have some inherent advantages over certain H_2 receptor antagonists as adjuvant therapy in CF patients. Cimetidine may interfere with the metabolism of certain drugs by inhibiting cytochrome P-450 oxygenase in the liver.[38] In CF patients, these potential drug interactions may assume some clinical importance by inhibiting metabolism of certain bronchodilators, notably theophylline. Because it has no human interactions with cytochrome P-450, misoprostol may be superior as long-term adjuvant therapy in CF.

BILE ACID DYSFUNCTION

In addition to manipulating the acid-alkaline balance in the upper small intestine, other researchers have explored the possibility of improving nutrient absorption with the addition of exogenous taurine.[50–53] As a result of large fecal losses of bile acids, patients with CF develop an increased ratio of glycine to taurine in conjugated bile acids. It has been proposed that correction of this elevated ratio by oral taurine supplements may improve absorption and, ultimately, nutrition by potentiating bile salt micelle formation. Taurine, which is more soluble in an acidic environment,

has been administered to patients with CF in doses of 30 mg/kg/d, and there has been significant improvement in fat absorption in patients on enzyme supplementation.[51] Supplementation with taurine significantly reduced the glycine-to-taurine ratio and bile acid losses in the stools.[51] A further disadvantage of preponderant glycine bile salts conjugates is that they are partly and passively absorbed in the proximal portion of the small intestine. Because taurine conjugates are predominantly absorbed in the ileum and are more resistant to bacterial degradation, they are more available to form mixed micelles with fat that may have escaped intestinal absorption more proximally.

REFERENCES

1. DiMagno EP, Go VLW, Summerskill WHJ. Relations between pancreatic enzyme outputs and malabsorption in severe pancreatic insufficiency. N Engl J Med 1973;288:813–5.
2. Thomson M, Clague A, Cleghorn GJ, Shepherd RW. Comparative in vitro and in vivo studies of enteric-coated pancrelipase preparations for pancreatic insufficiency. J Pediatr Gastroenterol Nutr 1993;17:407–13.
3. Di Magno EP, Malagelada JR, Go VL, Moertel CG. Fate of orally ingested enzymes in pancreatic insufficiency: comparison of two dosage schedules. N Engl J Med 1977;1318–22.
4. Layer P, Groger G. Enzyme pellet size and luminal nutrient digestion in pancreatic insufficiency. Digestion 1992;52:100.
5. Graham DY. Enzyme replacement therapy of exocrine pancreatic insufficiency in man: relation between in vitro enzyme activities and in vivo potency in commercial pancreatic extracts. N Engl J Med 1977;296:1314–8.
6. Salen G, Prakash A. Evaluation of enteric coated micro-spheres for enzyme replacement therapy in adults with pancreatic insufficiency. Curr Ther Res 1979;25:650–6.
7. Gow R, Bradbear R, Francis P, Shepherd R, et al. Comparative study of varying regimens to improve steatorrhoea and creatorrhoea in cystic fibrosis: effectiveness of an enteric coated preparation with and without antacids and cimetidine. Lancet 1981;ii:1071–4.
8. Mischler EH, Parrell S, Farrell PM, Odell GB, et al. Comparison of effectiveness of pancreatic enzyme preparations in cystic fibrosis. Am J Dis Child 1982;136:1060–3.
9. Sinaasapel M, Bouquet J, Nijens HJ. Problems in the treatment of malabsorption in CF. Acta Paediatr Scand Suppl 1985;317:22–7.
10. Petersen W, Heilmann C, Garne S. Pancreatic enzyme supplementation as acid resistant microspheres versus enteric coated granules in cystic fibrosis. Acta Paediatr Scand Suppl 1987;76:66–9.
11. Beverley DW, Kelleher J, MacDonald A, et al. Comparison of four pancreatic extracts in cystic fibrosis. Arch Dis Child 1987;62:564–8.
12. Stead RJ, Skypala I, Hodson ME, Batten JC. Enteric coated microspheres with pancreatin in the treatment of cystic fibrosis: comparison with a standard enteric coated preparation. Thorax 1987;42:533–7.
13. Taylor CJ, Hillel PG, Ghosal S, et al. Gastric emptying and intestinal transit of pancreatic enzyme supplements in cystic fibrosis. Arch Dis Child 1999;80:149–152.
14. DiMagno EP. Controversies in the treatment of exocrine pancreatic insufficiency. Dig Dis Sci 1982;27:481–4
15. FitzSimmons SC, Burkhart GA, Borowitz D, et al. High dose pancreatic enzyme supplements and fibrosing colonopathy

in children with cystic fibrosis. N Eng J Med 1997;336: 1283–9.

16. Layer P, Keller J. Lipase supplementation therapy: standards, alternatives, and perspectives. Pancreas 2003;26:1–7.

17. Roberts IM, Hanel SI. Stability of lingual lipase in vivo: studies of the iodinated enzyme in the rat stomach and duodenum. Biochim Biophys Acta 1988;960:107–10.

18. Assoufi BA . Efficacy of acid resistant fungal lipase in the treatment of adult cystic fibrosis. Pediatr Pulmonol Suppl 1988;2:134.

19. Schneider MU, Knoll-Ruzicka ML, Domschke S, et al. Pancreatic enzyme replacement therapy: comparative effects of conventional and enteric-coated microspheric pancreatin and acid-stable fungal enzyme preparations on steatorrhea in chronic pancreatitis. Hepatogastroenterology 1985;32:97–102.

20. Moreau J, Bouisson M, Saint MGM, et al. Comparison of fungal lipase and pancreatic lipase in exocrine pancreatic insufficiency in man: study of their in vitro properties and intraduodenal bioavailability. Gastroenterol Clin Biol 1988;12:787–92.

21. Zentler-Munro PL, Assoufi BA, Balasubramanian K, et al. Therapeutic potential and clinical efficacy of acid-resistant fungal lipase in the treatment of pancreatic steatorrhoea due to cystic fibrosis. Pancreas 1992;7:311–9.

22. Raimondo M, DiMagno EP. Lipolytic activity of bacterial lipase survives better than that of porcine lipase in human gastric and duodenal content. Gastroenterology 1994;107:231–5.

23. Suzuki A, Mizumoto A, Sarr MG, et al. Bacterial lipase and high-fat diets in canine exocrine pancreatic insufficiency: a new therapy of steatorrhea? Gastroenterology 1997;112:2048–55.

24. Suzuki A, Mizumoto A, Rerknimitr R, et al. Effect of bacterial or porcine lipase with low- or high-fat diets on nutrient absorption in pancreatic-insufficient dogs. Gastroenterology 1999;116:431–7.

25. Kuhel DG, Zheng S, Tso P, et al. Adenovirus-mediated human pancreatic lipase gene transfer to rat bile: gene therapy of fat malabsorption. Am J Physiol Gastrointest Liver Physiol 2000;79:G1031–6.

26. Maeda H, Danel C, Crystal RG. Adenovirus-mediated transfer of human lipase complementary DNA to the gallbladder. Gastroenterology 1994;106:1638–44.

27. Layer P, Keller J. Pancreatic enzymes: secretion and luminal nutrient digestion in health and disease. J Clin Gastroenterol 1999;28:3–10.

28. Lankisch PG. Appropriate pancreatic function tests and indications for pancreatic enzyme therapy following surgical procedures on the pancreas. Pancreatology 2001;1:14–26.

29. Adler G, Mundlos S, Kuhnelt P, Dreyer E. New methods for assessment of enzyme activity: do they help to optimize enzyme treatment. Digestion 1993;54 Suppl 2:3–9.

30. Bang Jorgensen B, Thorsgaard Pedersen N, Worning H. Monitoring the effect of substitution therapy in patients with exocrine pancreatic insufficiency. Scand J Gastroenterol 1991;26:321–6.

31. Brugge WR, Goldberg HJ, Burke CA, Depping BJ. Use of pancreatic Schilling test to determine efficiency of pancreatic enzyme delivery in pancreatic insufficiency. Dig Dis Sci 1988;33:1266–32.

32. Couper R, Lichtman S, Cleghorn G. Serum immunoglobulin G directed against porcine trypsin in pancreatic insufficiency cystic fibrosis patients receiving pancreatic enzyme supplements. Pancreas 1991;6:558–63.

33. Quirk P, Greer R, Shepherd R, Cleghorn G. Serum immunoglobulin G directed against porcine trypsin in the serum of cystic fibrosis children receiving porcine pancreatic enzyme

supplements. J Paediatr Child Health 1993;79: 196–200.

34. Smyth RL, van Velzen D, Smyth AR, et al. Strictures of ascending colon in cystic fibrosis and high strength pancreatic enzymes. Lancet 1994;343:85–6.

35. van Velzen D, Ball LM, Dezfulian AR, et al. Comparative and experimental pathology of fibrosing colonopathy. Postgrad Med J 1996;72 Suppl 2:S39–48; discussion S49–51.

36. Waters BL. Cystic fibrosis with fibrosing colonopathy in the absence of pancreatic enzymes. Paediatr Dev Pathol 1998; 1:74–8.

37. Serban DE, Florescu P, Miu N. Fibrosing colonopathy revealing cystic fibrosis in a neonate before and pancreatic enzyme supplementation. J Pediatr Gastroenterol Nutr 2002;35:356–9.

38. Graham DY. Pancreatic enzyme replacement: the effects of antacids or cimetidine. Dig Dis Sci 1982;27:485–90.

39. Zentler-Munro PL, Fine DR, Batten JC, Northfield TC. Effect of cimetidine on enzyme inactivation, bile acid precipitation, and lipid solubilization in pancreatic steatorrhoea due to cystic fibrosis. Gut 1985;26:892–901.

40. Shepherd RW, McGuffie C, Bradbear R. Cimetidine kinetics in CF. Aust Paediatr J 1981;17:234.

41. Durie PR, Bell L, Linton W, et al. Effect of cimetidine and sodium bicarbonate on pancreatic replacement therapy in cystic fibrosis. Gut 1980;21:778–86.

42. Lamers CBHLW, Jansen JBMJ. Omeprazole as an adjunct to enzyme replacement treatment in severe pancreatic insufficiency. BMJ 1987;293:994.

43. Tran TM, Van den Neucker A, Hendriks JJ, et al. Effects of a proton-pump inhibitor in cystic fibrosis. Acta Paediatr 1998;87:553–8.

44. Heijerman HGM. New modalities in the treatment of exocrine pancreatic insufficiency in cystic fibrosis. Neth J Med 1992;41:105–9.

45. Cleghorn GJ, Shepherd RW, Holt TL. The use of synthetic prostaglandin E$_1$ analogue (misoprostol) as an adjunct to pancreatic enzyme replacement in cystic fibrosis. Scand J Gastroenterol 1988;23 Suppl 143:142–7.

46. Hendriks JJ, Kester AD, Donckerwolcke R, et al. Changes in pulmonary hyperinflation and bronchial hyperresponsiveness following treatment with lansoprazole in children with cystic fibrosis. Pediatr Pulmonol 2001;31:59–66.

47. Robert A. Prostaglandins in a gastrointestinal tract. In: Johnson LR, editor. Physiology of the gastrointestinal tract. New York: Raven Press; 1981. p. 1407.

48. Konturek SJ, Pawlik W, Walus KM, et al. Mechanisms of the inhibitory action of prostaglandins on meal induced gastric secretions. Digestion 1978;17:281–90.

49. Robb TAS, Davidson GP, Kirubakaran C. Conjugated bile acids in serum and secretions in response to cholecystokinin/secretin stimulation in children with cystic fibrosis. Gut 1985;26:1246–56.

50. Darling PB, Lepage G, Leroy C, et al. Effect of taurine supplements on fat absorption in cystic fibrosis. Pediatr Res 1985;19:578–82.

51. Harries JT, Muller DP, McCollum JP, et al. Intestinal bile salts in cystic fibrosis. Arch Dis Child 1979;54:19–24.

52. Roy CC, Weber AM, Morin CL, et al. Abnormal biliary lipid composition in cystic fibrosis: effect of pancreatic enzymes. N Engl J Med 1977;297:1301–5.

53. Thompson GN. Excessive fecal taurine loss predisposes to taurine deficiency in cystic fibrosis. J Pediatr Gastroenterol Nutr 1988;7:214–9.

5. Acid-Peptic Disease

Frédéric Gottrand, MD, PhD

Christophe Faure, MD

The clinical spectrum of acid-peptic disease in children includes reflux esophagitis,[1] gastric and duodenal peptic ulcer disease,[2] gastritis and gastropathy,[3] duodenitis, and rare entities such as Zollinger-Ellison syndrome. Several chapters of this book specifically address the pathogenesis, diagnosis, and treatment of some of these diseases (see Chapter 29.1, Helicobacter pylori and Peptic Ulcer Disease," and Chapter 29.2, "Other Causes"). The purpose of this chapter is to focus on the pharmacologic aspects of the principal drugs used for acid-peptic diseases, including the mechanism of action, pharmacokinetic and pharmacodynamic data, efficacy, and side effects based mainly on information available in studies on children.

Two major developments have been observed in the management of acid-related disorders during the last 15 years represented by proton pump inhibitors (PPIs) and Helicobacter pylori. PPIs irreversibly bind to the H^+-K^+ adenosine triphosphatase (ATPase) enzyme complex and extensively inhibit acid production, revolutionizing the management of hyperacidity diseases. H. pylori has been shown to be the leading cause of primary peptic ulcer and chronic-active (type B) antral gastritis.[4] The eradication of this organism dramatically reduces the recurrence of gastric and duodenal ulcers both in adults and in children. These two factors have profoundly changed the natural history and epidemiology of acid-peptic disease in adults, mainly gastroesophageal reflux and peptic ulcer diseases, as well as diagnostic tests and therapeutic strategies, demonstrated by the dramatic decrease of surgical indications in this group of diseases. However, several childhood peculiarities and as yet still unresolved questions limit extensive use of antisecretory drugs in children. Peptic ulcer disease is rare in children, and the role of H. pylori in nonulcer dyspepsia in this age group remains a matter of debate. Therefore, recommendations for treatment remain limited to a selected number of patients, and use of PPIs for long-term management of gastroesophageal reflux disease (GERD) is still not recommended in children.

PROTON PUMP INHIBITORS

PPIs (omeprazole, lansoprazole, pantoprazole, rabeprazole, and esomeprazole) inhibit gastric acid secretion by selectively acting on gastric parietal cell H^+-K^+ ATPase, which is the enzyme involved in the last step of acid secretion by parietal cells (Figure 76.5-1).[5]

In contrast to histamine2 (H_2) receptor antagonists, inhibition of gastric acid secretion by PPIs is independent of the pathway of stimulation. PPIs are highly selective and effective in their action and have a few short- and long-term adverse effects. These pharmacologic features have made the development of PPIs the most significant advancement in the management of acid-peptic–related disorders in the last two decades. Although numerous adult studies have been published, there are still few large studies with significant patients enrolled and no randomized controlled comparative studies in childhood.[6] It should be emphasized that almost no clinical or pharmacologic data are available in infants under 1 year of age. Although several different PPIs are available on the market (Table 76.5-1), only two of them, namely omeprazole and lansoprazole, have been studied in childhood. The following section focuses mainly on those drugs that are the only two approved for use in children (with restriction on age, indication, or type of administration according to different countries).

MODE OF ACTION

PPIs form a group of compounds called substituted benzimidazoles, which concentrate within the intracellular canaliculi of parietal cells, irreversibly bind to the H^+-K^+ ATPase enzyme complex, and extensively inhibit acid production. PPIs differ from each other by the molecular structures bound to the pyridine and benzimidazole components of the molecule (Figure 76.5-2).[7] This explains differences in pharmacologic properties, but all of the PPIs

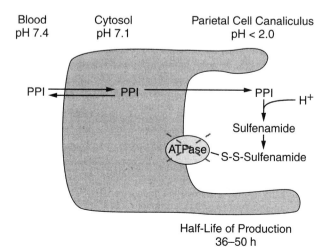

FIGURE 76.5-1 Mechanism of action of antisecretory drugs. ATPase = adenosine triphosphatase; PPI = proton pump inhibitor.

TABLE 76.5-1   DIFFERENT ANTISECRETORY DRUGS
                AVAILABLE

PROTON PUMP INHIBITORS
Omeprazole
Lansoprazole
Pantoprazole
Rabeprazole
Esomeprazole

H₂ BLOCKERS
Cimetidine
Ranitidine
Famotidine
Nizatidine

have the same mechanism of action. Because they are weakly basic compounds (the pKa value of the pyridine nitrogen being close to 4.0), they are maximally protonated in environments of high acidity (which is exclusively found in the intracellular canaliculi of actively secreting parietal cells and within the stomach cavity). PPIs can be considered prodrugs because in highly acidic environments, protonation of the molecule results in a series of reactions that ultimately produces the active form of the PPI (see Figure 76.5-2).[7] The active cyclic sulfenamide then binds permanently to exposed cysteine thiol groups on the luminal surface of the H^+-K^+ ATPase enzyme. Once covalently bound, the H^+-K^+ ATPase enzyme becomes nonfunctional, and activity returns only by parietal cell synthesis of new H^+-K^+ ATPase enzyme systems. The turnover of the H^+-K^+ ATPase is constant, with a half-life of about 48 hours in adults. The maturation of turnover is unknown in infants and children. The best access of the drug to the H^+-K^+ ATPase situated on the luminal side of the secretory membrane of the gastric parietal cells is provided by a meal, which is the strongest physiologic event inducing the exteriorization of the H^+-K^+ ATPase.[8]

Given orally, PPIs can be prematurely converted to the active form in the acidic environment of the stomach. They are prepared as capsules containing protective enteric-coated granules or as enteric-coated tablets. In these forms, absorption begins only in the higher pH environment of the duodenum. They are almost completely absorbed in the small intestine.[7]

PHARMACOKINETIC PROPERTIES
Most of the data on the pharmacokinetics of PPIs have been obtained in adult volunteers and adult patients with peptic ulcer disease. However, recent studies have provided extensive observations on the pharmacokinetics for omeprazole and lansoprazole in children.[9-16] Data are lacking on rabeprazole and esomeprazole in children; some data have recently been published on pantoprazole.[17]

PPIs are metabolized by the hepatocyte cytochrome P-450 isoforms CYP2C19 and CYP3A4 to inactive metabolites (sulfide, sulfone, and hydroxymetabolites) excreted in urine. A comprehensive comparative review on the pharmacokinetics of omeprazole, lansoprazole, pantoprazole, and rabeprazole has been published on adults.[7] Schematically, the drugs are quickly absorbed (T_{max} = 1–3 hours), with bioavailability varying between them (omeprazole 35–65%, lansoprazole 80–91%, and pantoprazole 57–100%). They are rapidly metabolized (half-time [$T_{\frac{1}{2}}$] = 0.6–2 hours). The antisecretory effect of PPIs is independent from plasma concentration but is correlated with the area under the plasma concentration time curve (AUC).[8] This has also been shown in children.[9]

In addition, in children and adolescents, the pharmacokinetic parameters have been reported in the same range as those in adults for omeprazole[10,11] and lansoprazole,[9,12–14] with variations according to age for omeprazole. Andersson and colleagues have reported a significant difference in $T_{\frac{1}{2}}$ between children aged 1 to 6 years and chil-

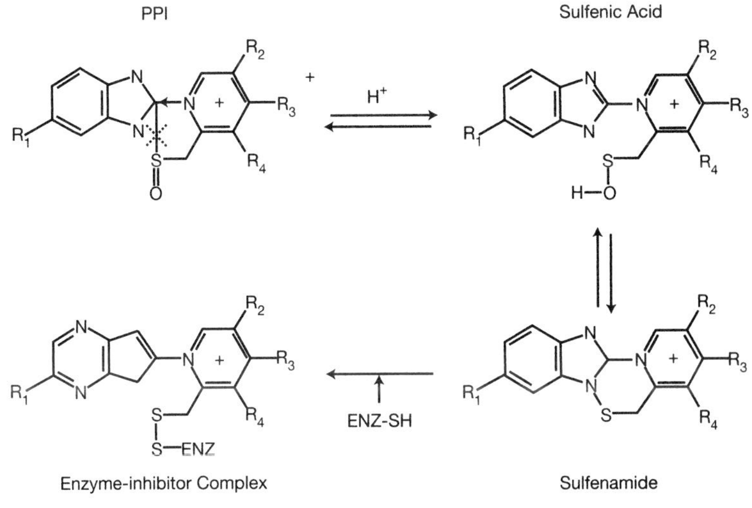

FIGURE 76.5-2 Chemical formula of proton pump inhibitors (PPIs) and the mechanisms of action of enzyme (H^+-K^+ adenosine triphosphatase [ATPase])-inhibitor complex formation. Reproduced with permission from Gibbons TE and Gold BD.[6]

	R_1	R_2	R_3	R_4
Omeprazole/Esomeprazole	CH₃O	CH₃	CH₃O	CH₃
Lansoprazole	H	H	CH₃F₂O	CH₃
Pantoprazole	CF₂HO	H	CH₃O	CH₃O
Rabeprazole	H	H	CH₃O(CH₂)₃O	CH₃

dren aged 7 to 12 years, with an increasing metabolism of omeprazole in the younger age group.[10] In neonates less than 10 days old, Anderson and colleagues reported a trend toward a prolonged $T_{\frac{1}{2}}$ for intravenous omeprazole.[15] This variability of metabolism related to age has not been reported with lansoprazole, for which data are available in children between the ages of 1 and 17 years.[9,12–14] All of these studies show a pharmacokinetic profile for lansoprazole similar to that of adults. Interindividual variability of pharmacokinetic parameters is wide in adults, as in children, and may explain to some extent the variations observed in the dosage requirement of the PPIs.

For both omeprazole and lansoprazole, there are almost no pharmacokinetic data available for neonates and infants under 1 year of age.

In addition to these maturation differences, pharmacokinetic parameters in children may be affected, as in adults, by genetic variability of the enzyme systems. Indeed, CYP2C19 displays a known genetic polymorphism,[18] and differences in pantoprazole, omeprazole, and lansoprazole disposition have been demonstrated with the AUC that are fivefold higher in poor metabolizers than in extensive metabolizers.[19] Clinically, poor metabolizers (a poor metabolizer phenotype occurs in 1% of blacks, 2–6% of whites, 15% of Chinese, and 23% of Japanese) have been shown to experience superior acid suppression (with omeprazole and lansoprazole) compared with extensive metabolizers, without an increase in the incidence of adverse effects.[7] Thus far, there is no toxicity issue that warrants dosage adjustment of pantoprazole in poor metabolizers.[20]

Other maturation factors may also affect the metabolism of PPIs, such as the rate of renewal of the proton pumps in the parietal cell. In patients with hepatic impairment, the AUC values increased to the same extent as observed in poor metabolizers, with no need to adjust the dosage, although caution should be exercised when giving PPIs to patients with severe hepatic insufficiency. No dosage adjustment of PPIs is required in patients with renal insufficiency[21] or on hemodialysis.[22]

PHARMACODYNAMIC PROPERTIES

Pharmacodynamic Efficacy of Omeprazole.
Omeprazole is available for oral and intravenous administration. In children, most data were obtained after oral administration, and a mean daily dose of 1 mg/kg body weight was required to obtain a sustained efficacy over 24 hours.[16,23–26] However, in a multicenter study of children aged 1 to 16 years using esophageal pH monitoring below a pH of < 4 for less than 6% of a 24-hour period, the healing dosage varied from 0.7 to 3.5 mg/kg/d. Overall, in this study, more than 75% of the patients required 1.4 mg/kg as the healing dosage.[10]

When the oral route cannot be used, it is necessary to inhibit acid secretion via intravenous administration of omeprazole, which is not approved for use in the United States and Canada. In children, the dose of 40 mg/1.73 m^2 (1.17 mg/kg) was required to achieve a gastric pH over 4 during more than 90% of a 24-hour period following omeprazole intravenous administration.[11]

Pharmacodynamic Efficacy of Lansoprazole.
In adults, a daily dosage of 30 mg of lansoprazole, that is, about 17 mg/m^2, has been found to be effective and safe in inhibiting gastric acid secretion and healing acid-related lesions. This dosage was effective in numerous randomized double-blind trials and has been recommended for the treatment of duodenal ulcer and reflux esophagitis in adults.[27] In children, as for omeprazole, the efficacy of lansoprazole on gastric acid secretion studied by gastric pH monitoring has been shown to vary widely among the patients studied: about 40% of children responded to the dose of 0.73 mg/kg (equivalent to the adult dose, ie, 17 mg/m^2), 26% responded to 1.44 mg/kg, and 35% failed to respond to this doubled dose.[9] This variability can be ascribed in part to differences in pharmacokinetics: the AUC of lansoprazole showed a significant positive correlation with gastric acid inhibition, and the AUC was significantly greater and the oral clearance was not significantly lower in the patients who did than in those who did not respond to the lower dose (0.73 mg/kg, ie, 17 mg/m^2). Thus, failure to respond to the lower dose may be ascribed to reduced bioavailability and/or to faster metabolism of the drug. Patients with these characteristics may require a higher dose to achieve the desired antisecretory effect.[9]

Pharmacodynamic Efficacy of Pantoprazole.
In a recent study, oral pantoprazole (20 mg daily) provided gastric acid control in 15 pediatric patients with reflux esophagitis.[17]

CLINICAL EFFICACY

The major use of PPIs in pediatrics has been the management of peptic esophagitis and peptic ulcer disease and for eradication of *H. pylori* infection. No controlled or open studies of the use of PPIs in the management of extraesophageal manifestations of gastroesophageal reflux such as otorhinolarygologic or respiratory symptoms have been performed.

PEPTIC ESOPHAGITIS

Most of the studies performed in children with gastroesophageal reflux assessed healing of esophagitis to define the efficacy of omeprazole[23–26,28–31] and lansoprazole.[9,13,32,33] In a review of omeprazole use in the treatment of acid-related disorders in children for the period 1986 to 2000, marketed and extemporaneous formulations of omeprazole were used at dosages of 5 to 80 mg/d (0.2–3.5 mg/kg/d) for periods ranging from 14 days to 36 months. The initial dose most consistently reported to heal esophagitis and provide relief of symptoms of gastroesophageal reflux appears to be 1 mg/kg/d.[34] A similar response was observed with omeprazole[26] among the responders to lansoprazole; 80% of children had healing of their esophagitis after 4 weeks of treatment.[9] Overall, for both omeprazole and lansoprazole, studies performed in children showed that in patients with adequate acid suppression (ie, receiving an appropriate dosage), the healing rate of peptic esophagitis is more than 75% after 4 to 8 weeks of treatment; the clinical symptoms improve in the same time period.[16,17,23–26,28,29,31,32] However, it should be emphasized that if one considers the initial dose (ie, 0.7–1 mg/kg) in these pediatric studies, the response rate is, as expected, lower (around 50%). In a recent small study, oral pantoprazole (20 mg daily) given to 15 pediatric patients with reflux esophagitis provided healing of the esophagitis in 52% of patients.[17]

Gastric and Duodenal Ulcers. Although rare in pediatrics, PPIs have been used in the treatment of gastric and duodenal peptic ulcers. Low doses (0.3–0.7 mg/kg) were required to achieve healing.[16,25]

H. *pylori* Eradication. Although there are still no clear recommendations on the treatment of *H. pylori* in childhood,[4,35–37] triple therapy using a PPI and two antibacterial agents is considered the treatment of choice.[35,38] However, several nonrandomized studies have also shown a high eradication rate with two antibiotics combining metronidazole or tinidazole and amoxicillin for 2 to 4 weeks.[39] As in adults, treatment failures are mainly explained by poor compliance and resistance of *H. pylori* to antibiotics. The only double-blind trial published in children showed an eradication rate of 74.2% with 1 week of triple therapy including omeprazole, clarithromycin, and amoxicillin compared with an eradication rate of 9.4% in children receiving placebo, clarithromycin, and amoxicillin.[40] This study demonstrated the low eradication rate with two antibiotics used for 1 week, including clarithromycin, and confirmed the efficacy of PPIs associated with antibiotics in *H. pylori* infection in children.

SAFETY

Short-Term Safety. PPIs are well tolerated by most patients. The principal side effects are mild to moderate headaches, abdominal pain, vomiting, and diarrhea (Table 76.5-2).[9] In the double-blind study previously mentioned comparing omeprazole, clarithromycin, and amoxicillin with placebo, clarithromycin, and amoxicillin in *H. pylori*–infected children, adverse events were reported in 24% of patients in both groups but remained mild.[40] No adverse effect was reported even in children who received a high dose of intravenous omeprazole.[11] A small reversible elevation of transaminases has been reported.

Prolonged periods of hypochlorhydria may lead to gastric bacterial overgrowth, as was noted in adults[41] and

neonates.[42] Although the clinical effect of this overgrowth remains unclear, this suggests that in critically ill patients and neonates, if required, the intravenous administration of PPIs should be as short as possible because of the prolonged inhibition of the gastric acid secretion.

Long-Term Safety. Although PPIs have been available for more than 15 years and are widely used in adults, with an excellent long-term safety profile, few data are available on infants and children regarding long-term use (eg, more than 6 months) of these potent acid-suppressing agents. Because of experimental data provided in newborn rats, there are concerns regarding the consequences and effects on the gastric mucosa of the increased gastrin levels (two- to fivefold rise in half of the treated patients). The trophic effects of gastrin lead to stimulation of the enterochromaffin-like cell population and hyperplastic changes in parietal cell mass. Carcinoid tumors have been observed in animals treated lifelong with high-dose omeprazole or an H_2 receptor antagonist. Although enterochromaffin-like hyperplasia has been observed in adults, carcinoid tumors have been reported only once in adults.[43] The trophic action of gastrin on digestive epithelium has not been implicated in the development of gastric or colonic adenocarcinoma in animal and adult safety studies.[44,45] However, fundic polyps and nodules have been reported in children who received omeprazole for more than 6 months.[46] The effect of long-term omeprazole therapy (4–7 years) on the ratio of G (gastrin secretion) to D cells (somatostatin secretion) was studied in 6 children.[47] The mean G-cell number and the ratio of G to D cells showed a significant increase for omeprazole compared with baseline levels. In adults, studies have shown an increased incidence of gastric atrophy associated with long-term use of PPIs, especially in the presence of *H. pylori* infection.[44] However, similar studies are still lacking in children.

Long-term acid suppression may promote the production of N-nitrosamine compounds in the stomach secondary to bacterial overgrowth. These compounds are considered carcinogenic.

Suppression of acid secretion may theoretically lead to malabsorption of vitamin B_{12} and maldigestion of proteins. Except for patients with Zollinger-Ellison syndrome, long-term treatment with PPIs is not considered a causal factor of vitamin B_{12} deficiency.[48] Moreover, Evenepoel and colleagues have shown the influence of PPIs on protein digestion.[49] Clinical consequences in children are currently unknown.[50]

In vitro data have shown that osteoclast activity may be inhibited by omeprazole without an influence on bone turnover in children during short-term treatment.[51]

Overall, one should consider that long-term use of PPIs in children is safe but requires careful long-term follow-up.[45]

Drug Interactions. Although most PPIs interact with the cytochrome P-450 system, no clinically important interactions have been observed between PPIs and other drugs.[8,52–55] However, omeprazole may increase the plasma concentration of diazepam, phenytoin, carbamazepine, and warfarin.[7]

TABLE 76.5-2   FREQUENCY OF SIDE EFFECTS ASSOCIATED WITH OMEPRAZOLE AND LANSOPRAZOLE IN CHILDREN

EVENT	OMEPRAZOLE (%)	LANSOPRAZOLE (%)
Headache	0–2	0–3
Constipation	0	0–5
Diarrhea	0–1	0–9
Vomiting	0–0.3	0–4
Dizziness	0	0–2
Insomnia	0	0–2
Total	0–2	0–15

Adapted from Faure C et al,[9] Hassall E et al,[26] Franco MT et al,[32] Tolia V,[33] and Hendriks HJ et al.[171]

DOSAGE AND ADMINISTRATION

PPIs are available per os in capsules containing protective enteric-coated granules or as an enteric-coated tablet. An intravenous formulation is available for omeprazole and pantoprazole. The granules and tablets should not be crushed, chewed, or dissolved because gastric acid secretion may alter the drug's action.

The capsules can be opened, and for children who are unable to swallow capsules or tablets, the microgranules may be administered per os or via a feeding tube, in suspension in an acidic medium such as fruit juice, yogurt, or applesauce. A "homemade" liquid formulation, produced by dissolving the drug in 8.4% bicarbonate solution, has been used in some reports.[56] However, a recent study performed in adults has shown that the pharmacokinetic parameters (absorption) of these simplified suspensions were altered when compared with the regular administration of a capsule. This was particularly true with the simplified omeprazole.[57] Pediatric pharmacokinetic, pharmacodynamic, and efficacy studies with these alternative oral preparations are lacking, preventing them from being recommended. Owing to the activation of the proton pumps in the pre- and postprandial periods, PPIs should be administered just before or during meals.

The intravenous formulation should not be administered per os because gastric acid secretion alters the drug.

Omeprazole. The usual recommended starting dosage of omeprazole is 1 mg/kg once daily (eg, 10 mg for children 10 to 20 kg and 20 mg for children weighing more than 20 kg).

Although not registered in all countries, intravenous omeprazole should be given once daily 40 mg/1.73 m^2 (eg, 1 mg/kg).[11] Because the benefit of a loading dose of intravenous omeprazole was demonstrated in adults,[58] it has been suggested to use a loading dose of 40 mg/0.73 m^2 repeated after 12 hours to achieve a rapid antisecretory effect in similar critical situations in pediatric patients.[11]

Lansoprazole. The usual recommended starting dosage is 1 mg/kg once daily (eg, 15 mg for children ≤ 30 kg in weight and 30 mg for those weighing > 30 kg[59]). This drug is not yet labeled in all countries for use in children.

For both omeprazole and lansoprazole, it should be emphasized that the optimal dose may vary among patients and that, in case of a lack of efficacy, one must be aware that almost 25% of patients may require a double dosage. In the absence of a clinical response to the starting recommended dose, it is suggested to check very carefully with caregivers regarding the mode of administration of the PPIs. If this is correct, doubling the dosage should be suggested.

Pantoprazole. Data are currently lacking on recommended dosages for intravenous pantoprazole in children.

H$_2$ RECEPTOR ANTAGONISTS

The first H$_2$ blocker licensed was cimetidine, in 1976, followed by ranitidine and later famotidine and nizatidine (see Table 76.5-1). Experience with other H$_2$ receptor antagonists, such as roxatidine and ebrotidine, is very limited or nonexistent in children. Although PPIs have now supplanted these drugs for the treatment of acid-peptic disease because of their higher efficacy and excellent tolerance, the large experience of more than 20 years of use of H$_2$ receptor antagonists on millions of patients has provided considerable insight into the efficacy, pharmacology, and long-term tolerance in adults and children.[60–67] A large number of studies in adults have established that PPIs are more effective in decreasing acid secretion and have better clinical efficacy than H$_2$ receptor antagonists; however, there are no published articles on children that specifically address this question. Ranitidine, famotidine, and nizatidine are preferred over cimetidine because cimetidine interferes with the cytochrome P-450 enzyme and demonstrates more central nervous system, gastrointestinal, and endocrine side effects than the other H$_2$ blockers. In parallel with the increase of self-medication of ranitidine in adults, there is also a movement toward the treatment of symptoms in children regardless of the presence or absence of esophagitis. However, the pharmacokinetic and pharmacodynamic effects of over-the-counter H$_2$ receptor antagonists in the pediatric population remain largely unknown.[63]

PHARMACODYNAMIC PROPERTIES

The H$_2$ receptor antagonists are competitive inhibitors of histamine-stimulated acid secretion; however, they have limited effects on acid secretion that is induced by meals or other stimuli. In most of the pediatric studies, a good correlation has been demonstrated between the median plasma ranitidine concentration and the pharmacodynamic parameter elevation of intragastric pH. The gastric pH typically rose above 4 when the plasma ranitidine concentration approached 100 ng/mL.[60,63,64] Pediatric subjects with suspected abnormal acid reflux aged 4 to 11 years received a single dose of 75 mg of ranitidine. The intragastric pH began to rise approximately 30 minutes after dosing with ranitidine to a peak of pH 4. Ranitidine, 75 mg, significantly increased the intragastric pH throughout the 6-hour evaluation period.[63] The return toward baseline after 5 hours suggests the potential utility of dosing more frequently than every 12 hours. In contrast to PPIs, tolerance and rebound effects may occur with the use of H$_2$ receptor antagonists. Tolerance to the antisecretory effects of H$_2$ receptor antagonists has been demonstrated in adults and appears to develop quickly in 3 days. The mechanisms are not fully understood but may be related to the upregulation of enterochromaffin-like cell activity.[68] However, no data are available in pediatrics. The occurrence of a rebound hypersecretion effect should be taken into account when discontinuing the drugs, which therefore should be progressively withdrawn.[69,70]

PHARMACOKINETIC PROPERTIES

Studies of pharmacokinetics of H$_2$ receptor antagonists have been conducted in infants and children.[60,64,65,67] Overall, the parameters are similar to those of adults, with a reasonable absorption after oral dosing. Absorption is not affected by food. Peak blood levels are achieved within 1 to 3 hours after an oral dose. These drugs are well distributed throughout the body and cross the blood-brain barrier. After oral administration, cimetidine, ranitidine, and famotidine undergo "first-pass" hepatic metabolic alteration that reduces their bioavailability by 50%. Protein binding is low (15%). H_2 receptor antagonists are eliminated by a combination of renal excretion and hepatic metabolic degradation. Sixty to 80% of orally administered cimetidine and ranitidine is cleared by the liver. In contrast, after intravenous administration, they are eliminated principally through renal excretion. Dose reductions are thus recommended for patients with renal insufficiency.

After a single dose of 75 mg of ranitidine in children aged 4 to 11 years, the median C_{max} value of 477 ng/mL occurred 2.5 hours after dosing, and the median half-life was 2.0 hours.[63] In infants, the half-life is higher (3.5 hours).

CLINICAL EFFICACY

Although no controlled trials are available in children, oral ranitidine therapy has been useful in pediatric practice for the treatment of GERD and peptic ulcer diseases.[60–62] Cucchiara and colleagues showed that high-dose (20 mg/kg/d) ranitidine was as effective as omeprazole in peptic esophagitis.[61]

TOLERABILITY

The side effects of H_2 receptor antagonist are reported in Table 76.5-3. The majority of pediatric clinical trials with ranitidine have reported few side effects or abnormal laboratory values. As for PPIs, raising the gastric pH may result in the overgrowth of pathogenic bacteria in the digestive tract.[41,42] It has been shown in neonates that the length of hospital stay, increased gastric pH, period of antibiotic therapy, and ranitidine use were independently associated with an increased colonization rate.[42]

Interactions between H_2 antagonists and other drugs have been extensively reviewed.[71] It is widely held that cimetidine is a more important antagonist of other drugs than the other H_2 antagonists (Table 76.5-4); however, the clinical relevance of many of the interactions with cimetidine is marginal. In neonates, cimetidine should be used cautiously in patients concurrently receiving theophylline, phenytoin, or caffeine because it may prolong the half-life of those drugs.[72]

DOSAGE AND ADMINISTRATION

The recommended oral dosage of H_2 blockers is summarized in Table 76.5-5. Ranitidine (5–10 mg/kg), given orally daily, divided into two or three doses, produces a symptomatic and endoscopic improvement in erosive esophagitis in children.[73] Pharmacodynamic data on ranitidine suggest that a dosing period of 6 to 9 hours may provide a more effective control of intragastric acidity.[63,73] In patients with renal impairment, the dosage should be adjusted: if the creatinine clearance is 10 to 50 mL/min, the dosage should be decreased to 75% of normal dosage; if the creatinine clearance is < 10 mL/min, the dosage should be decreased to 50% of normal dosage.

The recommended dosages of intravenous cimetidine are 5 to 10 mg/kg/d every 8 to 12 hours in neonates and 10 to 20 mg/kg/d every 6 to 12 hours in infants.[72] Intravenous cimetidine may be infused preferably over 15 to 30 minutes because rapid injection has been associated with cardiac arrhythmias and hypotension. It also may be given by continuous infusion. In premature infants and neonates, ranitidine is usually given intravenously or, rarely, intramuscularly at a dosage of 1 to 2 mg/kg/d divided every 6 hours. The maximal intravenous dosage is 6 mg/kg/d divided every 6 hours. Intravenous continuous infusion is

TABLE 76.5-3   SIDE EFFECTS OF H_2 RECEPTOR ANTAGONIST

SIDE EFFECT	CIMETIDINE	RANITIDINE	FAMOTIDINE	NIZATIDINE
HEMATOLOGY				
Thrombocytopenia	+		+	
Neutropenia	+	+		
Agranulocytosis	+	+		
CARDIAC				
Bradycardia	+	+		
Hypotension	+			
NEUROLOGIC				
Dizziness	+	+	+	+
Headache	+	+	+	+
Confusion	+	+	±	
Sleep disturbance	+			+
GYNECOMASTIA	+			
DIGESTIVE				
Vomiting	+	+	+	+
Diarrhea	+	+	+	+
Constipation		+	+	
Pancreatitis	+	+		
Hepatitis	+	+	+	+
CUTANEOUS				
Rash	+	+	+	+
RENAL				
Interstitial nephritis	+			

TABLE 76.5-4   CLINICALLY SIGNIFICANT DRUG INTERACTIONS WITH ACID-SUPPRESSING AGENTS

DRUGS INTERACTING	CIMETIDINE	OMEPRAZOLE	LANSOPRAZOLE
Cyclosporine	+		
Midazolam	+		
Phenytoin	+	+	+
Theophylline	+		
Warfarin	+	+	

Adapted from Flockhart DA et al[71] and Gold BD and Freston JW.[122]

preferred over intermittent dosing at a dosage of 1.44 to 4 mg/kg/d (maximum 6 mg/kg/d).[72] It can be administered in a parenteral nutrition solution. Famotidine can be given intravenously either at a dosage of 0.3 mg/kg every 8 hours (maximum 2.4 mg/kg/d) or by continuous infusion of 1 to 2 mg/kg/d over 24 hours. It can be administered in a parenteral nutrition solution.[72]

ANTACIDS

Antacids include carbonate and bicarbonate salts (eg, $NaHCO_3$ and Ca^- or $MgCO_3$), alkali complexes of aluminum and/or magnesium (eg, aluminum and magnesium hydroxides), aluminum and magnesium phosphates, magnesium trisilicate, and alginate-based raft-forming formulations. They are used for the symptomatic treatment of heartburn and esophagitis. Experience with antacids is limited in infants. Their efficacy in buffering the gastric acidity is strongly influenced by the time of administration and requires multiple administrations. Dimethicone is used in some regions for regurgitation, although there are no reliable studies demonstrating its efficacy in the treatment of gastroesophageal reflux in infants. Although often classified as an antacid, it acts more as a feed thickener because it contains more than 50% of bean gum and has hardly any acid-neutralizing properties.

PHARMACODYNAMIC PROPERTIES
All antacids have a nonsystemic mechanism of action. They chemically neutralize gastric acid. The key therapeutic advantage of antacids is their rapid onset of action. Antacids act within minutes to an elevated intragastric pH above 3.5 and provide symptomatic relief. Hence, their action is limited by the capacity to maintain an elevated pH in the presence of continued physiologic acid secretion and by normal gastric emptying. Alginate-based raft-forming preparations have a quite different mode of action. In the presence of gastric acid, alginates precipitate, forming a

gel. Alginate-based raft-forming formulations usually contain sodium or potassium bicarbonate; in the presence of gastric acid, the bicarbonate is converted to carbon dioxide, which becomes entrapped within the gel precipitate, converting it into a foam that floats on the surface of the gastric surface, providing a relative pH-neutral barrier.[74]

CLINICAL EFFICACY
Double-blind studies in adults have shown that alginate-based raft-forming preparations are superior to placebo in relieving the symptoms of heartburn.[74] However, studies in infants and children remain limited (six studies including a total of 303 patients, only one being double blind) and had various study designs (open-label prospective study, comparison of two different dosages of alginate, comparison of placebo, famotidine, or cisapride).[75–80] Their efficacy as monotherapy or in combination with prokinetics for gastroesophageal reflux is not convincing.[81,82]

TOLERABILITY
Because absorption from aluminum-containing antacids may cause serum aluminum concentrations to approach levels reported to cause osteopenia and neurotoxicity, chronic antacid therapy is not recommended.[83] Gaviscon contains a considerable amount of sodium carbonate, so its administration may increase the sodium content of the feeds to an undesirable level, especially in preterm infants (1 g of Gaviscon contains 46 mg of sodium, and the suspension contains twice this amount). Algicon, which has a better taste than Gaviscon, has a lower sodium load but a higher aluminum content. Occasional formation of large bezoar-like masses of agglutinated intragastric material has been reported in association with Gaviscon use.[81,82] Side effects include diarrhea with magnesium-rich preparations and excessive absorption of aluminum in infants.[81,82] The presence of aluminum and magnesium in the majority of antacids means that such products have the potential to chelate drugs in the upper gastrointestinal tract.[71] The

TABLE 76.5-5   RECOMMENDED ORAL DOSAGE OF H_2 RECEPTOR ANTAGONISTS

H^2 RECEPTOR ANTAGONIST	RECOMMENDED DOSAGE IN NEONATES	RECOMMENDED DOSAGE IN CHILDREN	RECOMMENDED DOSAGE IN ADULTS
Cimetidine	5–10 mg/kg/d bid or tid; 10–20 mg/kg/d bid or tid in infants	20–40 mg/kg/d bid or tid	600–1,600 mg/d once or bid or tid
Ranitidine	2–4 mg/kg/d divided every 6 h	5–10 mg/kg/d tid	150–600 mg/d once or bid
Nizatidine	—	10 mg/kg/d bid	150–300 mg/d once or bid
Famotidine	1 to 2 mg/kg/d tid	1 mg/kg/d bid	20–80 mg/d once or bid

Adapted from Bell SG[72] and Rudolph CD et al.[73]

drugs most frequently affected in this way include the quinolone antibacterial agents, didanosine, azithromycin, tetracycline, and the H_2 antagonists.[71] The effects of antacids on the pharmacokinetics of other drugs vary widely according to the type of antacid and time dosage of the administration of the other drug, ranging from no effect to an 85% decrease in bioavailability.[71] For example, a single dose of an aluminum-magnesium antacid was reported to reduce the area under the serum concentration time curve of cimetidine (23%), ranitidine (26%), famotidine (19%), and nizatidine (12%).[84] Separating the administration of antacid from that of another drug by 2 hours usually eliminated any interaction.

DOSAGE AND ADMINISTRATION

Because alginate-based raft-forming preparations need to float on the gastric contents for effectiveness, the time at which this medication is taken is of great importance. Optimal benefit is achieved when alginate-based raft-forming preparations are taken following a meal. Under fasting conditions or when taken just prior to or with a meal, alginate-based raft-forming preparations were reported to empty from the stomach with a $T_{\frac{1}{2}}$ of 20 to 30 minutes.[74] When dosed 30 minutes following a meal, alginate-based formulations empty from the stomach with a $T_{\frac{1}{2}}$ of 180 minutes.

PROSTAGLANDIN ANALOGUES

Misoprostol is a prostaglandin E_1 (PGE_1) analogue that is primarily used to prevent nonsteroidal anti-inflammatory drug (NSAID)-induced gastropathy in patients at high risk. Although initial animal studies showed considerable promise in the treatment of acid-peptic disease, studies in human have not confirmed any clear advantage of the PGE_1 analogues over the H_2 blockers, and their clinical efficacy is now attributed primarily to their antisecretory activity. Since the recent advent of cyclooxygenase 2–selective inhibitors, such drugs are now used less frequently in adults.

PHARMACODYNAMIC PROPERTIES

PGE_1 analogues bind to E-type receptors on basolateral parietal cell membranes, distinct from those at which the anti–H_2 receptor antagonists act, thereby inhibiting cyclic adenosine monophosphate–mediated acid production. In addition to blocking acid secretion and gastrin production, these agents may directly enhance mucosal protection through various mechanisms (increase of gastric mucus secretion, bicarbonate secretion, mucosal blood flow, and epithelial regeneration).

PHARMACOKINETIC PROPERTIES

At present, pharmacokinetic data for misoprostol derive from studies in animals and healthy adult volunteers only.[85] Following oral administration, it is rapidly absorbed and de-esterified to its acid form, with peak concentration being reached in 30 to 60 minutes. This free acid metabolite remains as potent as the parent drug in inhibiting acid secretion. It is 85% protein bound. Binding is not affected by age or other drugs. Further metabolism probably takes place in the liver and the kidneys. Biphasic elimination

occurs, with a terminal half-life of about 1.5 hours. By 8 hours, 90% of a single oral dose is excreted, mostly in the urine. No parent drug is recovered.[86]

CLINICAL EFFICACY

In adults, studies comparing omeprazole with misoprostol or ranitidine for NSAID ulcer prevention in true NSAID ulcers have shown that omeprazole is equal to full-dose misoprostol for ulcer healing and to the lowest useful dose of misoprostol for ulcer prevention.[87] Misoprostol (at dosages ranging from 400 to 800 µg/d in adults) is an effective form of therapy for preventing NSAID-induced gastroduodenal lesions. However, high-dose misoprostol seems adequate only for the prevention of ulcer complications, mainly in high-risk NSAID users.[88] An analysis of pooled data from comparative studies on omeprazole versus ranitidine, misoprostol, and sucralfate shows a therapeutic advantage in favor of the PPI, ranging from 10 to 40%.[88] In long-term prevention studies, omeprazole (20 mg/d) and pantoprazole (40 mg/d) have also been shown to reduce the risk of gastric and duodenal ulcers and NSAID-related dyspepsia. Current data from recent comparative studies of omeprazole (20 mg/d) versus ranitidine (150 mg/d) and misoprostol (200 µg/d) showed that after 6 months of follow-up, the PPI was significantly superior to control drugs in reducing the risk of both gastric and duodenal ulcers. Thus, available data are undoubtedly in favor of the PPIs as well-tolerated and effective drugs in the prophylaxis and treatment of NSAID-related mucosal lesions in the gastrointestinal tract.[88] Experience in children is much more limited and was mainly focused on children with rheumatologic disease.[89-91] Misoprostol appears to be effective in the treatment of gastrointestinal symptoms in children receiving NSAIDs and to result in a significant increase in the hemoglobin concentration.[90,91] Misoprostol was also shown to improve fat absorption in cystic fibrosis patients with pancreatic insufficiency with residual malabsorption on standard enzyme therapy.[92]

TOLERABILITY

In children, as in adults, misoprostol is usually well tolerated. The side effects are limited and mild. The most frequent adverse event is self-limited diarrhea,[89] and a significant elevation in the eosinophil count has been occasionally reported.[92] Prenatal exposure to misoprostol has been associated with Möbius disease and limb defects. Vascular disruption has been proposed as the mechanism for these teratogenic effects.[93] Apart from a possible interaction with propanolol, no major drug interactions have been reported.[94]

DOSAGE AND ADMINISTRATION

The recommended dosage in adults is 100 µg four times a day for prevention and 200 µg orally four times a day for treatment of NSAID digestive lesions. In children, a mean dosage of 300 µg/m²/d has been proposed.[89]

COATING AGENT

The coating agent sucralfate is a basic aluminum salt of sucrose octasulfate. At an acid pH, it polymerizes to form a white paste-like substance that adheres selectively to ulcer or erosions via an electrostatic attraction between the negatively charged sucralfate polyanions and the positively charged protein moieties exposed by the inflamed mucosa. At these specific sites, sucralfate acts as a protective barrier by slowing back-diffusion of acid, pepsin, and bile salts. It also directly inhibits the binding of pepsin to ulcer protein and, like cholestyramine, adsorbs free bile salts. Gastric pH does not appear to affect sucralfate binding to the ulcer bed. Other important effects of sucralfate include increased bicarbonate and mucus production, enhanced epithelial cell renewal, and restoration of a normal transmucosal potential difference. Sucralfate also protects the gastric mucosa against damage induced by ethanol, bile acids, and NSAIDs and prevents stress ulceration in critically ill patients. Despite its aluminum hydroxide components, sucralfate does not increase gastric pH or act as an antacid at the usual therapeutic doses. The drug has no apparent effects on gastric acid secretion, gastrin release, or upper gastrointestinal motility. Thus, hypochlorhydria and concomitant bacterial overgrowth do not occur.

PHARMACODYNAMIC PROPERTIES

Little, if any, sucralfate is absorbed after oral administration owing to its high polarity and poor solubility. It is absorbed as an aluminum base and sucrose octasulfate, with the latter excreted unchanged in urine because it cannot be metabolized.

PHARMACOKINETIC PROPERTIES

A study of the interaction of gastrointestinal agents in the presence of sucralfate has shown the adsorption of musculotropic and cholinolytic spasmolytic drugs on sucralfate.[95] Similarly, the absorption of certain drugs, such as warfarin, digoxin, and phenytoin, may be decreased when sucralfate is given concurrently. Although aluminum absorption is not significantly increased in patients with normal renal function, it has been shown that the use of sucralfate for stress ulcer prophylaxis in patients requiring hemofiltration results in toxic elevations in plasma aluminum levels.[96] Alternative agents should be considered for prophylaxis in these patients.

CLINICAL EFFICACY

Several studies in adults have shown that sucralfate (1 g orally before meals and at bedtime) is significantly better than placebo and equivalent to cimetidine and ranitidine in the healing of duodenal and gastric ulcers. Maintenance therapy with sucralfate decreases the recurrence rate of both gastric and duodenal ulcers. Sucralfate may also protect the patient from NSAID-induced gastroduodenal lesions. An analysis of pooled data from comparative studies on omeprazole versus ranitidine, misoprostol, and sucralfate shows a therapeutic advantage in favor of the PPI, ranging from 10 to 40% for preventing NSAID-induced gastroduodenal lesions.[88] Sucralfate is also superior to placebo and is as effective as cimetidine in the treatment of reflux esophagitis.[97] Sucralfate can prevent stress ulceration in critically ill patients. Recent data have also shown clinical efficacy of sucralfate topically to treat or prevent mucosal lesions from various origins (ie, stomatitis, mucositis, or pouchitis).[98,99]

TOLERABILITY

Sucralfate is relatively free of side effects, the only major one being constipation, which occurs in about 2 to 3% of patients. Nausea and headaches occur much less frequently. Sucralfate causes bezoars, especially when given to patients in intensive care units (especially in premature and neonates),[100] and diarrhea.[101] Patients with renal failure treated with sucralfate are exposed to aluminum toxicity.[102] Aluminum accumulation has been observed in critically ill children with acute renal failure.[103]

The presence of aluminum and magnesium in sucralfate means that this drug has the potential to chelate drugs in the upper gastrointestinal tract, as for other antacids (see above).[71] Hypophosphatemia may also result from sucralfate's action as a phosphate binder.

The influence of sucralfate on the incidence of ventilator-associated pneumonia and the incidence of upper airway colonization in critically ill children remains poorly studied in childhood.[104]

DOSAGE AND ADMINISTRATION

Sucralfate is available as tablets or suspension, both of which have better acceptance and compliance in children. To minimize the risk of decreased absorption of other drugs given concurrently, it is recommended to take sucralfate at least 2 hours apart from the other drugs.

BISMUTH

Bismuth compounds have been used for centuries to treat various diseases, from digestive diseases (gastric and duodenal ulcer, dyspepsia, infectious diarrhea) to infectious (scabies, malaria, syphilis), skin (eczema, pemphigus), and general disorders (lupus erythematosus, hypertension, edema).[105] Use of bismuth progressively declined in the last 30 to 40 years because its mode of action remained unknown and therapeutic benefits were unproved. Moreover, reports of encephalopathy associated with ingestion of various bismuth salts in large quantities over long periods in France and Australia in the early 1970s contributed to the dramatic reduction of its use and led to the interdiction of use both in adults and children in several countries by the appropriate national drug authorities. In the last decade, a renaissance of the use of some bismuth compounds has taken place. Bismuth subsalicylate and colloidal bismuth subcitrate have been demonstrated to effectively treat traveler's diarrhea[106–108] and *H. pylori* infection in association with antibiotics and/or antisecretory drugs.[39,109,110]

PHARMACODYNAMIC PROPERTIES

Bismuth acts to coat areas of mucosal ulceration and inflammation, thereby preventing further epithelial injury by luminal acid and pepsin. Bismuth preparations have also demonstrated inhibitory effects on the growth of *H. pylori* in vitro and in vivo.[105]

PHARMACOKINETIC PROPERTIES

Taken orally, bismuth salts are essentially insoluble in water. Bismuth salts are nearly completely hydrolyzed by gastric hydrochloric acid to form precipitate, namely Bi_2O_3 (oxide), $Bi(OH_3)$ (hydroxide), and $BiOCl$ (hydroxychloride). Small quantities of the ingested bismuth compounds remain nondissociated and enter the small intestine, where reactions with other anions take place to form bismuth subcarbonate and bismuth phosphate salts, which, like their parent compounds, are highly insoluble.[105] Delivered to the colon, the still nondissociated part of the ingested bismuth salts and the generated bismuth compounds react with hydrogen sulfide, which is also insoluble in water. Its black color is responsible for the darkening of the stool that occurs during bismuth salt medication. Because the ingested bismuth salts and the bismuth compounds formed in the gastrointestinal tract are highly insoluble in water, less than 1% of the bismuth is absorbed by the small intestine. The exact site and mechanisms by which bismuth is absorbed by the small intestinal mucosa are not known.[111] Some substances, such as the sulfhydryl group–containing compounds sorbitol and lactic acid, are able to enhance bismuth absorption. Ranitidine may enhance bismuth absorption from colloidal bismuth subcitrate by reducing gastric acidity, maintaining colloidal bismuth subcitrate as a soluble colloid.[112] Enhanced bismuth absorption has been reported in patients with colitis or other mucosal abnormalities.[113] Once absorbed, bismuth is distributed to different organs (kidney, lung, spleen, liver, brain, and muscle). Bismuth is eliminated from the body by two routes: two-thirds in the urine and one-third in the feces.

CLINICAL EFFICACY

Several studies have recently highlighted the therapeutic effects of bismuth salts on infectious diarrhea,[106–108,114] microscopic colitis, and pouchitis. Both bismuth subsalicylate and colloidal bismuth subcitrate have been shown to heal duodenal and gastric ulcers, but the relapse rate when these therapeutic agents are used alone is unacceptably high. In association with antibiotics, bismuth salts have been shown to eradicate *H. pylori* infection, and the relapse rate of primary ulcer is reduced when *H. pylori* is eradicated.[39,109,110] However, no controlled studies in children comparing bismuth association with other therapeutic regimens in *H. pylori* infection or peptic ulcer disease are yet available. Ranitidine bismuth citrate contains 128 mg of bismuth, 110 mg of citrate, and 162 mg of ranitidine in each tablet. The recommended dosage in adults is two tablets per day, in association with two antibiotics (amoxicillin and tinidazole or metronidazole). Experience in children remains very limited.[109]

TOLERABILITY

Bismuth encephalopathy has been reported in adults receiving large quantities of bismuth (most of the time as automedication) for months, even years, mainly with bismuth subgallate. All of these patients had high bismuth concentration in serum, but no relationship could be demonstrated between elevated blood concentrations and the severity of encephalopathy.[115] Individual susceptibility factors have been suggested, a hypothesis being that bacterial overgrowth proved or suspected in most of the cases reported could lead to conversion of bismuth salts to neurotoxic substances in the colon.[105] Observing that neurologic and psychiatric symptoms were described only in patients taking more than 1.5 g of bismuth metal per day, Lechat and Kisch arbitrarily stated that a dose less than 1.5 g of bismuth metal is safe in adults.[116] In the same way, comparing the bismuth blood concentration of asymptomatic adult patients on bismuth therapy with that of patients with bismuth encephalopathy, Hillemand and colleagues concluded that a bismuth blood concentration below 50 µg/L should be regarded as a safe level.[117] Such studies are completely lacking in childhood. Frequent side effects are dark stools, blackening of the tongue, and diarrhea.[109]

In children, rare cases of acute renal failure after overdose have been reported.[118,119]

DOSAGE AND ADMINISTRATION

Most of the national drug agencies in Europe and other developed countries prohibit the use of bismuth salts in children. Colloidal bismuth subcitrate and bismuth subsalicylate are, however, the most popular forms of bismuth used in children. A liquid 1.75% preparation of bismuth subsalicylate is usually prescribed at a dosage of 30 mL taken orally four times daily for a period of 6 weeks.[120] Colloidal bismuth subcitrate tablets are given at a dosage of 480 mg of $Bi_2O_3/1.73$ m^2 of body surface three to four times daily for 4 to 6 weeks.[110]

REFERENCES

1. Vandenplas Y. Reflux esophagitis in infants and children: a report from the Working Group on Gastro-Oesophageal Reflux Disease of the European Society of Paediatric Gastroenterology and Nutrition. J Pediatr Gastroenterol Nutr 1994;18:413–22.
2. Chelimsky G, Czinn S. Peptic ulcer disease in children. Pediatr Rev 2001;22:349–55.
3. Dohil R, Hassall E, Jevon G, Dimmick J. Gastritis and gastropathy of childhood. J Pediatr Gastroenterol Nutr 1999;29:378–94.
4. Sherman P, Czinn S, Drumm B, et al. *Helicobacter pylori* infection in children and adolescents: working group report of the First World Congress of Pediatric Gastroenterology, Hepatology, and Nutrition. J Pediatr Gastroenterol Nutr 2002;35 Suppl 2:S128–33.
5. Sachs G, Shin JM, Briving C, et al. The pharmacology of the gastric acid pump: the H$^+$,K$^+$ ATPase. Annu Rev Pharmacol Toxicol 1995;35:277–305.
6. Gibbons TE, Gold BD. The use of proton pump inhibitors in children: a comprehensive review. Paediatr Drugs 2003;5(1):25–40.
7. Stedman CA, Barclay ML. Review article: comparison of the pharmacokinetics, acid suppression and efficacy of proton pump inhibitors. Aliment Pharmacol Ther 2000;14:963–78.
8. Maton PN. Omeprazole. N Engl J Med 1991;324:965–75.
9. Faure C, Michaud L, Shaghaghi EK, et al. Lansoprazole in children: pharmacokinetics and efficacy in reflux oesophagitis. Aliment Pharmacol Ther 2001;15:1397–402.
10. Andersson T, Hassall E, Lundborg P, et al. Pharmacokinetics of

orally administered omeprazole in children. International Pediatric Omeprazole Pharmacokinetic Group. Am J Gastroenterol 2000;95:3101–6.

11. Faure C, Michaud L, Shaghaghi EK, et al. Intravenous omeprazole in children: pharmacokinetics and effect on 24-hour intragastric pH. J Pediatr Gastroenterol Nutr 2001;33:144–8.

12. Gremse D, Winter H, Tolia V, et al. Pharmacokinetics and pharmacodynamics of lansoprazole in children with gastroesophageal reflux disease. J Pediatr Gastroenterol Nutr 2002; 35 Suppl 4:S319–26.

13. Gunasekaran T, Gupta S, Gremse D, et al. Lansoprazole in adolescents with gastroesophageal reflux disease: pharmacokinetics, pharmacodynamics, symptom relief efficacy, and tolerability. J Pediatr Gastroenterol Nutr 2002;35 Suppl 4: S327–35.

14. Tran A, Rey E, Pons G, et al. Pharmacokinetic-pharmacodynamic study of oral lansoprazole in children. Clin Pharmacol Ther 2002;71:359–67.

15. Andersson T, Anderson G, Dasen S, et al. Pharmacokinetics and pharmacodynamics of oral omeprazole in infants [abstract]. J Pediatr Gastroenterol Nutr 2001;33:416.

16. Kato S, Shibuya H, Hayashi Y, et al. Effectiveness and pharmacokinetics of omeprazole in children with refractory duodenal ulcer. J Pediatr Gastroenterol Nutr 1992;15:184–8.

17. Madrazo-de la Garza A, Dibildox M, Vargas A, et al. Efficacy and safety of oral pantoprazole 20 mg given once daily for reflux esophagitis in children. J Pediatr Gastroenterol Nutr 2003; 36:261–5.

18. Furuta T, Ohashi K, Kosuge K, et al. CYP2C19 genotype status and effect of omeprazole on intragastric pH in humans. Clin Pharmacol Ther 1999;65:552–61.

19. Chang M, Tybring G, Dahl ML, et al. Interphenotype differences in disposition and effect on gastrin levels of omeprazole—suitability of omeprazole as a probe for CYP2C19. Br J Clin Pharmacol 1995;39:511–8.

20. Ferron GM, Preston RA, Noveck RJ, et al. Pharmacokinetics of pantoprazole in patients with moderate and severe hepatic dysfunction. Clin Ther 2001;23:1180–92.

21. Delhotal-Landes B, Flouvat B, Duchier J, et al. Pharmacokinetics of lansoprazole in patients with renal or liver disease of varying severity. Eur J Clin Pharmacol 1993;45:367–71.

22. Karol MD, Eason C. The pharmacokinetics of lansoprazole following administration of single daily doses to dialysis dependent subjects [abstract]. Pharm Res 1993;10(10 Suppl):S106.

23. Gunasekaran TS, Hassall EG. Efficacy and safety of omeprazole for severe gastroesophageal reflux in children. J Pediatr 1993;123:148–54.

24. Karjoo M, Kane R. Omeprazole treatment of children with peptic esophagitis refractory to ranitidine therapy. Arch Pediatr Adolesc Med 1995;149:267–71.

25. Kato S, Ebina K, Fujii K, et al. Effect of omeprazole in the treatment of refractory acid-related diseases in childhood: endoscopic healing and twenty-four-hour intragastric acidity. J Pediatr 1996;128:415–21.

26. Hassall E, Israel D, Shepherd R, et al. Omeprazole for treatment of chronic erosive esophagitis in children: a multicenter study of efficacy, safety, tolerability and dose requirements. International Pediatric Omeprazole Study Group. J Pediatr 2000;137:800–7.

27. Langtry HD, Wilde MI. Lansoprazole. An update of its pharmacological properties and clinical efficacy in the management of acid-related disorders. Drugs 1997;54:473–500.

28. Cucchiara S, Minella R, Iervolino C, et al. Omeprazole and high dose ranitidine in the treatment of refractory reflux oesophagitis. Arch Dis Child 1993;69:655–9.

29. Alliet P, Raes M, Bruneel E, Gillis P. Omeprazole in infants with cimetidine-resistant peptic esophagitis. J Pediatr 1998;132: 352–4.

30. Bohmer CJ, Niezen-de Boer RC, Klinkenberg-Knol EC, Meuwissen SG. Omeprazole: therapy of choice in intellectually disabled children. Arch Pediatr Adolesc Med 1998;152:1113–8.

31. Strauss RS, Calenda KA, Dayal Y, Mobassaleh M. Histological esophagitis: clinical and histological response to omeprazole in children. Dig Dis Sci 1999;44:134–9.

32. Franco MT, Salvia G, Terrin G, et al. Lansoprazole in the treatment of gastro-oesophageal reflux disease in childhood. Dig Liver Dis 2000;32:660–6.

33. Tolia V, Fitzgerald J, Hassall E, et al. Safety of lansoprazole in the treatment of gastroesophageal reflux disease in children. J Pediatr Gastroenterol Nutr 2002;35 Suppl 4:S300–7.

34. Zimmermann AE, Walters JK, Katona BG, et al. A review of omeprazole use in the treatment of acid-related disorders in children. Clin Ther 2001;23:660–79; discussion 645.

35. Gold BD, Colletti RB, Abbott M, et al. Helicobacter pylori infection in children: recommendations for diagnosis and treatment. J Pediatr Gastroenterol Nutr 2000;31:490–7.

36. Sherman P, Hassall E, Hunt RH, et al. Canadian Helicobacter Study Group Consensus Conference on the Approach to Helicobacter pylori Infection in Children and Adolescents. Can J Gastroenterol 1999;13:553–9.

37. Drumm B, Koletzko S, Oderda G. Helicobacter pylori infection in children: a consensus statement. European Paediatric Task Force on Helicobacter pylori. J Pediatr Gastroenterol Nutr 2000;30:207–13.

38. Gold BD. Current therapy for Helicobacter pylori infection in children and adolescents. Can J Gastroenterol 1999;13:571–9.

39. Oderda G, Rapa A, Bona G. A systematic review of Helicobacter pylori eradication treatment schedules in children. Aliment Pharmacol Ther 2000;14 Suppl 3:59–66.

40. Gottrand F, Kalach N, Spyckerelle C, et al. Omeprazole combined with amoxicillin and clarithromycin in the eradication of Helicobacter pylori in children with gastritis: a prospective randomized double-blind trial. J Pediatr 2001;139:664–8.

41. Osteyee JL, Banner W Jr. Effects of two dosing regimens of intravenous ranitidine on gastric pH in critically ill children. Am J Crit Care 1994;3:267–72.

42. Cothran DS, Borowitz SM, Sutphen JL, et al. Alteration of normal gastric flora in neonates receiving ranitidine. J Perinatol 1997;17:383–8.

43. Haga Y, Nakatsura T, Shibata Y, et al. Human gastric carcinoid detected during long-term antiulcer therapy of H$_2$ receptor antagonist and proton pump inhibitor. Dig Dis Sci 1998; 43:253–7.

44. Klinkenberg-Knol EC, Nelis F, Dent J, et al. Long-term omeprazole treatment in resistant gastroesophageal reflux disease: efficacy, safety, and influence on gastric mucosa. Gastroenterology 2000;118:661–9.

45. Youssef AF, Turck P, Fort FL. Safety and pharmacokinetics of oral lansoprazole in preadolescent rats exposed from weaning through sexual maturity. Reprod Toxicol 2003;17:109–16.

46. Pashankar DS, Israel DM. Gastric polyps and nodules in children receiving long-term omeprazole therapy. J Pediatr Gastroenterol Nutr 2002;35:658–62.

47. Pashankar DS, Israel DM, Jevon GP, Buchan AM. Effect of long-term omeprazole treatment on antral G and D cells in children. J Pediatr Gastroenterol Nutr 2001;33:537–42.

48. ter Heide H, Hendriks HJ, Heijmans H, et al. Are children with cystic fibrosis who are treated with a proton-pump inhibitor at risk for vitamin B$_{(12)}$ deficiency? J Pediatr Gastroenterol Nutr 2001;33:342–5.

49. Evenepoel P, Claus D, Geypens B, et al. Evidence for impaired assimilation and increased colonic fermentation of protein, related to gastric acid suppression therapy. Aliment Pharmacol Ther 1998;12:1011–9.

50. Cui GL, Syversen U, Zhao CM, et al. Long-term omeprazole treatment suppresses body weight gain and bone mineralization in young male rats. Scand J Gastroenterol 2001;36:1011–5.

51. Kocsis I, Arato A, Bodanszky H, et al. Short-term omeprazole treatment does not influence biochemical parameters of bone turnover in children. Calcif Tissue Int 2002;71:129–32.

52. Israel DM, Hassall E. Omerprazole and other proton pump inhibitors: pharmacology, efficacy, and safety, with special reference to use in children. J Pediatr Gastroenterol Nutr 1998;27:568–79.

53. Meyer UA. Metabolic interactions of the proton-pump inhibitors lansoprazole, omeprazole and pantoprazole with other drugs. Eur J Gastroenterol Hepatol 1996;8 Suppl 1:S21–5.

54. Andersson T, Rohss K, Bredberg E, Hassan-Alin M. Pharmacokinetics and pharmacodynamics of esomeprazole, the S-isomer of omeprazole. Aliment Pharmacol Ther 2001;15:1563–9.

55. Sachs G, Humphries TJ. Rabeprazole: pharmacology, pharmacokinetics, and potential for drug interactions. Introduction. Aliment Pharmacol Ther 1999;13 Suppl 3:1–2.

56. Phillips JO, Metzler MH, Palmieri MT, et al. A prospective study of simplified omeprazole suspension for the prophylaxis of stress-related mucosal damage. Crit Care Med 1996;24:1793–800.

57. Sharma VK, Peyton B, Spears T, et al. Oral pharmacokinetics of omeprazole and lansoprazole after single and repeated doses as intact capsules or as suspensions in sodium bicarbonate. Aliment Pharmacol Ther 2000;14:887–92.

58. Andersen J, Strom M, Naesdal J, et al. Intravenous omeprazole: effect of a loading dose on 24-h intragastric pH. Aliment Pharmacol Ther 1990;4:65–72.

59. Scott LJ. Lansoprazole: in the management of gastroesophageal reflux disease in children. Paediatr Drugs 2003;5:57–61; discussion 62.

60. Mallet E, Mouterde O, Dubois F, et al. Use of ranitidine in young infants with gastro-oesophageal reflux. Eur J Clin Pharmacol 1989;36:641–2.

61. Cucchiara S, Campanozzi A, Greco L, et al. Predictive value of esophageal manometry and gastroesophageal pH monitoring for responsiveness of reflux disease to medical therapy in children. Am J Gastroenterol 1996;91:680–5.

62. Kaufman SS, Loseke CA, Young RJ, Perry DA. Ranitidine therapy for esophagitis in children with developmental disabilities. Clin Pediatr (Phila) 1996;35:451–6.

63. Orenstein SR, Blumer JL, Faessel HM, et al. Ranitidine, 75 mg, over-the-counter dose: pharmacokinetic and pharmacodynamic effects in children with symptoms of gastro-oesophageal reflux. Aliment Pharmacol Ther 2002;16:899–907.

64. Blumer JL, Rothstein FC, Kaplan BS, et al. Pharmacokinetic determination of ranitidine pharmacodynamics in pediatric ulcer disease. J Pediatr 1985;107:301–6.

65. James LP, Stowe CD, Farrar HC, et al. The pharmacokinetics of oral ranitidine in children and adolescents with cystic fibrosis. J Clin Pharmacol 1999;39:1242–7.

66. Sutphen JL, Dillard VL. Effect of ranitidine on twenty-four-hour gastric acidity in infants. J Pediatr 1989;114:472–4.

67. Lugo RA, Harrison AM, Cash J, et al. Pharmacokinetics and pharmacodynamics of ranitidine in critically ill children. Crit Care Med 2001;29:759–64.

68. Lachman L, Howden CW. Twenty-four-hour intragastric pH: tolerance within 5 days of continuous ranitidine administration. Am J Gastroenterol 2000;95:57–61.

69. el-Omar E, Banerjee S, Wirz A, Penman I, et al. Marked rebound acid hypersecretion after treatment with ranitidine. Am J Gastroenterol 1996;91:355–9.

70. Smith AD, Gillen D, Cochran KM, et al. Dyspepsia on withdrawal of ranitidine in previously asymptomatic volunteers. Am J Gastroenterol 1999;94:1209–13.

71. Flockhart DA, Desta Z, Mahal SK. Selection of drugs to treat gastro-oesophageal reflux disease: the role of drug interactions. Clin Pharmacokinet 2000;39:295–309.

72. Bell SG. Gastroesophageal reflux and histamine2 antagonists. Neonatal Netw 2003;22:53–7.

73. Rudolph CD, Mazur LJ, Liptak GS, et al. Guidelines for evaluation and treatment of gastroesophageal reflux in infants and children: recommendations of the North American Society for Pediatric Gastroenterology and Nutrition. J Pediatr Gastroenterol Nutr 2001;32 Suppl 2:S1–31.

74. Mandel KG, Daggy BP, Brodie DA, Jacoby HI. Review article: alginate-raft formulations in the treatment of heartburn and acid reflux. Aliment Pharmacol Ther 2000;14:669–90.

75. Weldon AP, Robinson MJ. Trial of Gaviscon in the treatment of gastro-oesophageal reflux of infancy. Aust Paediatr J 1972;8:279–81.

76. Buts JP, Barudi C, Otte JB. Double-blind controlled study on the efficacy of sodium alginate (Gaviscon) in reducing gastro-esophageal reflux assessed by 24 h continuous pH monitoring in infants and children. Eur J Pediatr 1987;146:156–8.

77. LeLuyer P, Mougenot JF, Mashako L. Multicenter study of sodium alginate in the treatment of regurgitation in infants. Ann Pediatr (Paris) 1992;39:635–40.

78. Oderda G, Dell'Olio D, Forni M, et al. Treatment of childhood peptic oesophagitis with famotidine or alginate-antacid. Ital J Gastroenterol 1990;22:346–9.

79. Miller S. Comparison of the efficacy and safety of a new aluminium-free paediatric alginate preparation and placebo in infants with recurrent gastro-oesophageal reflux. Curr Med Res Opin 1999;15:160–8.

80. Greally P, Hampton FJ, MacFadyen UM, Simpson H. Gaviscon and Carobel compared with cisapride in gastro-oesophageal reflux. Arch Dis Child 1992;67:618–21.

81. Khoshoo V, Ross G, Brown S, Edell D. Smaller volume, thickened formulas in the management of gastroesophageal reflux in thriving infants. J Pediatr Gastroenterol Nutr 2000;31:554–6.

82. Vandenplas Y, Belli DC, Benatar A, et al. The role of cisapride in the treatment of pediatric gastroesophageal reflux. The European Society of Paediatric Gastroenterology, Hepatology and Nutrition. J Pediatr Gastroenterol Nutr 1999;28:518–28.

83. Tsou VM, Young RM, Hart MH, Vanderhoof JA. Elevated plasma aluminum levels in normal infants receiving antacids containing aluminum. Pediatrics 1991;87:148–51.

84. Sullivan TJ, Reese JH, Jauregui L, et al. Short report: a comparative study of the interaction between antacid and H2-receptor antagonists. Aliment Pharmacol Ther 1994;8:123–6.

85. Monk JP, Clissold SP. Misoprostol. A preliminary review of its pharmacodynamic and pharmacokinetic properties, and therapeutic efficacy in the treatment of peptic ulcer disease. Drugs 1987;33:1–30.

86. Schoenhard G, Oppermann J, Kohn FE. Metabolism and pharmacokinetic studies of misoprostol. Dig Dis Sci 1985;30 (11 Suppl):126S–8S.

87. Anand BS, Graham DY. Ulcer and gastritis. Endoscopy 1999;31:215–25.

88. Lazzaroni M, Bianchi Porro G. Prophylaxis and treatment of non-steroidal anti-inflammatory drug-induced upper gastrointestinal side-effects. Dig Liver Dis 2001;33 Suppl 2:S44–58.

89. Gazarian M, Berkovitch M, Koren G, et al. Experience with

misoprostol therapy for NSAID gastropathy in children. Ann Rheum Dis 1995;54:277–80.

90. Mulberg AE, Linz C, Bern E, et al. Identification of nonsteroidal antiinflammatory drug-induced gastroduodenal injury in children with juvenile rheumatoid arthritis. J Pediatr 1993;122:647–9.

91. Hermaszewski R, Hayllar J, Woo P. Gastro-duodenal damage due to non-steroidal anti-inflammatory drugs in children. Br J Rheumatol 1993;32:69–72.

92. Robinson P, Sly PD. Placebo-controlled trial of misoprostol in cystic fibrosis. J Pediatr Gastroenterol Nutr 1990;11:37–40.

93. Vargas FR, Schuler-Faccini L, Brunoni D, et al. Prenatal exposure to misoprostol and vascular disruption defects: a case-control study. Am J Med Genet 2000;95:302–6.

94. Herting RL, Clay GA. Overview of clinical safety with misoprostol. Dig Dis Sci 1985;30(11 Suppl):185S–93S.

95. Pluta J, Grimling B. Study of interaction of gastrointestinal agents in the presence of cytoprotective drugs. Part II. In vitro study on the adsorption of selected spasmolytic drugs on sucralfate. Acta Pol Pharm 2001;58:473–9.

96. Mulla H, Peek G, Upton D, et al. Plasma aluminum levels during sucralfate prophylaxis for stress ulceration in critically ill patients on continuous venovenous hemofiltration: a randomized, controlled trial. Crit Care Med 2001;29:267–71.

97. Arguelles-Martin F, Gonzalez-Fernandez F, Gentles MG. Sucralfate versus cimetidine in the treatment of reflux esophagitis in children. Am J Med 1989;86(6A):73–6.

98. Chiara S, Nobile MT, Vincenti M, et al. Sucralfate in the treatment of chemotherapy-induced stomatitis: a double-blind, placebo-controlled pilot study. Anticancer Res 2001;21:3707–10.

99. Marini I, Vecchiet F. Sucralfate: a help during oral management in patients with epidermolysis bullosa. J Periodontol 2001;72:691–5.

100. Guy C, Ollagnier M. [Sucralfate and bezoars: data from the system of pharmacologic vigilance and review of the literature]. Therapie 1999;54:55–8.

101. Amaro R, Montelongo PC, Barkin JS. Sucralfate-induced diarrhea in an enterally fed patient. Am J Gastroenterol 1999;94:2328–9.

102. Hemstreet BA. Use of sucralfate in renal failure. Ann Pharmacother 2001;35:360–4.

103. Thorburn K, Samuel M, Smith EA, Baines P. Aluminum accumulation in critically ill children on sucralfate therapy. Pediatr Crit Care Med 2001;2:247–9.

104. Lopriore E, Markhorst DG, Gemke RJ. Ventilator-associated pneumonia and upper airway colonisation with gram negative bacilli: the role of stress ulcer prophylaxis in children. Intensive Care Med 2002;28:763–7.

105. Menge H, Gregor M, Brosius B, Hopert R, Lang A. Pharmacology of bismuth. Eur J Gastroenterol Hepatol 1992;4 Suppl 2:S41–7.

106. Figueroa-Quintanilla D, Salazar-Lindo E, Sack RB, et al. A con-trolled trial of bismuth subsalicylate in infants with acute watery diarrheal disease. N Engl J Med 1993;328:1653–8.

107. Ericsson CD. Travellers' diarrhoea. Int J Antimicrob Agents 2003;21:116–24.

108. Cheng AC, Thielman NM. Update on traveler's diarrhea. Curr Infect Dis Rep 2002;4:70–7.

109. Nijevitch AA, Farztdinov KM, Sataev VU, et al. *Helicobacter pylori* infection in childhood: results of management with ranitidine bismuth citrate plus amoxicillin and tinidazole. J Gastroenterol Hepatol 2000;15:1243–50.

110. De Giacomo C, Fiocca R, Villani L, et al. *Helicobacter pylori* infection and chronic gastritis: clinical, serological, and histologic correlations in children treated with amoxicillin and colloidal bismuth subcitrate. J Pediatr Gastroenterol Nutr 1990;11:310–6.

111. Suarez FL, Furne J, Stiehm J, et al. Site of bismuth absorption from bismuth subsalicylate: implications for treatment of colonic conditions. Dig Dis Sci 2000;45:1444–6.

112. Nwokolo CU, Prewett EJ, Sawyerr AM, et al. The effect of histamine H_2-receptor blockade on bismuth absorption from three ulcer-healing compounds. Gastroenterology 1991;101:889–94.

113. Mendelowitz PC, Hoffman RS, Weber S. Bismuth absorption and myoclonic encephalopathy during bismuth subsalicylate therapy. Ann Intern Med 1990;112:140–1.

114. Chowdhury HR, Yunus M, Zaman K, et al. The efficacy of bismuth subsalicylate in the treatment of acute diarrhoea and the prevention of persistent diarrhoea. Acta Paediatr 2001; 90:605–10.

115. Teepker M, Hamer HM, Knake S, et al. Myoclonic encephalopathy caused by chronic bismuth abuse. Epileptic Disord 2002; 4:229–33.

116. Lechat P, Kisch R. [Bismuth encephalopathy: a reappraisal of risk factors]. Gastroenterol Clin Biol 1986;10:562–9.

117. Hillemand P, Palliere M, Laquais B, Bouvet P. Bismuth treatment and blood bismuth levels [in French]. Sem Hop Paris 1986; 53:1663–9.

118. Islek I, Uysal S, Gok F, et al. Reversible nephrotoxicity after overdose of colloidal bismuth subcitrate. Pediatr Nephrol 2001;16:510–4.

119. Sarikaya M, Sevinc A, Ulu R, et al. Bismuth subcitrate nephrotoxicity. A reversible cause of acute oliguric renal failure. Nephron 2002;90:501–2.

120. Drumm B, Sherman P, Chiasson D, et al. Treatment of *Campylobacter pylori*-associated antral gastritis in children with bismuth subsalicylate and ampicillin. J Pediatr 1988;113:908–12.

121. Hendriks HJ, van Kreel B, Forget PP. Effects of therapy with lansoprazole on intestinal permeability and inflammation in young cystic fibrosis patients. J Pediatr Gastroenterol Nutr 2001;33:260–5.

122. Gold BD, Freston JW. Gastroesophageal reflux in children: pathogenesis, prevalence, diagnosis, and role of proton pump inhibitors in treatment. Paediatr Drugs 2002;4:673–85.

6. Alternative Medical Treatment

Nadeem Ahmad Afzal, MBBS, MRCPCH, MRCP(UK)
Robert B. Heuschkel, MB, BS DRCOG, MRCPCH

The term complementary and alternative medicine (CAM) is commonly used to encompass approaches to health care not included in our understanding of "conventional" medicine. There is no sharp demarcation between the two, but perhaps it is easier to define CAM if we define what falls within the domain of conventional medicine. "Western," "mainstream," "orthodox," and "allopathic" medicine are all terms synonymous with conventional medicine. Interestingly, the boundaries of conventional medicine may vary greatly between countries, cultures, classes, and individuals. These boundaries also change with time because many alternative therapies are gradually adopted by conventional practitioners. Probably the best example of such change is the use of probiotics. These have become much more common in conventional medicine and are now considered much less of an "alternative" therapy. This ever-changing interface makes it all the more important for practitioners of conventional medicine to be alert to practices that may, in time, start appearing among their own therapies. Needless to say, there is an almost insatiable demand for therapies that lie just outside the domain of conventional medicine. Patients may place enormous, and frequently inappropriate, faith in these alternative therapies, which, by their very nature, may inspire hope beyond the rational expectations one might have of any conventional therapy.

Perhaps the most comprehensive definition of CAM was first coined by O'Connor, and it has since been adopted both by the National Centre for Complementary and Alternative Medicine (NCCAM) in the United States and the Cochrane database in the United Kingdom[1]:

> Complementary and Alternative Medicine (CAM) is a broad domain of healing resources that encompasses all health systems, modalities, and practices and their accompanying theories and beliefs, other than those intrinsic to the politically dominant health system of a particular society or culture in a given historical period. CAM includes all such practices and ideas self defined by their users as preventing or treating illness or promoting health and well-being. Boundaries within CAM and between the CAM domain and that of the dominant system are not always sharp or fixed.[1]

More recently, the term "integrative" medicine has been used. This style of practice combines the use of mainstream medical therapies with those CAM therapies for which there is high-quality scientific evidence on safety and efficacy. The focus is therefore more on the quality of available evidence for a particular therapy rather than on the type of therapy or the practitioner prescribing it.

Over the last decade, use of CAMs has increased worldwide. In 1990, the US population was making more visits to practitioners of alternative medicine than to their primary care physicians. By 1997, out of pocket expenditure for alternative medicines in the United States had increased by over 45% to about 27 billion dollars, similar to out of pocket expenditure for all US physician services.[2]

Whereas several studies have now addressed the use of CAM in adult patients, few have done so in children. Spigelblatt and colleagues showed that 11% of over 1,000 Canadian children attending routine outpatient clinics were using CAM, with chiropractic, homeopathy, naturopathy, and acupuncture accounting for more than 80% of use.[3] In this study, children who used CAM were older than nonusers, had better educated mothers, and tended to have parents who also used CAM. Almost 90% of parents opted to use conventional medicines first, suggesting that CAM be used in conjunction with it. In a review of Australian children with asthma aged 1 to 16 years, 55% used an additional alternative therapy, whereas 46% of those with childhood-onset malignancies used at least one form of CAM.[4,5]

For the purposes of this chapter, we are not including pre- and probiotic use in our definition of CAM. Both entities have, over the last few years, moved squarely into conventional gastroenterologic practice. However, in some fields, such as constipation, they are still felt to be complementary therapies, and, as such, we briefly discuss them. The maintenance of a normal healthy gut flora has become central to the management of many gastrointestinal pathologies, and the manipulation of gut flora with pre- and probiotics is dealt with elsewhere in the text in much greater detail.

USE OF CAM IN GASTROINTESTINAL DISORDERS

In this chapter, we focus on the currently available evidence for CAM use in the areas of inflammatory bowel disease (IBD), constipation, acute gastroenteritis, and liver disease.

SEARCH STRATEGY

We conducted a thorough search of the literature using the following on-line databases: MEDLINE, PsycINFO, Allied and Complementary Medicine, Psychological Abstracts, CINAHL, and the Cochrane Database of Systematic Reviews. The MeSH terms "homeopathy," "naturopathy," "comple mentary therapies," "alternative therapies," "acupuncture," "acupuncture therapy," "spiritual therapies," "music therapy," "laughter therapy," "aromatherapy," "medicine, herbal," "medicine, chinese traditional," "drugs, chinese herbal," "medicine, ayurvedic," "massage," and "phytotherapy" were used in a *MEDLINE* search, in conjunction with the term "gastrointestinal diseases." Almost 2,500 references were found, with 203 being clinical trials published in English with an available abstract. All of the latter were reviewed to select 58 articles that were felt to be relevant to this publication. These references were then reviewed in full where possible. Additional references were identified by manual searching of bibliographies from recent review articles, and further citations were received from experts in the field.

INFLAMMATORY BOWEL DISEASE

There is considerable evidence of CAM use in patients with IBD. However, there are very few studies documenting the efficacy in different disease types. There are no studies of efficacy in children with IBD, yet there is some preliminary information on the prevalence of its use in this population.

Heuschkel and colleagues carried out a survey of CAM use in children and young adults with IBD in three centers of pediatric gastroenterology (Boston, Detroit, and London, UK)[6]; 208 questionnaires were completed, and the frequency of CAM use in this population was 41%. The most common therapies were megavitamin therapy (19%), dietary supplements (17%), and herbal medicines (14%). Parental CAM use and the number of adverse effects from conventional medicines were predictors of CAM use (odds ratio [OR] = 1.9, 95% confidence interval [CI] = 1.2–3.1, $p = .02$; OR = 1.3, 95% CI = 1.2–1.5, $p < .001$, respectively). The most important reasons respondents gave for using CAM were side effects from prescribed medicines, prescribed medicines not working as well as they had hoped, and hoping for a cure. Almost 60% of respondents not taking CAM were interested in learning more about it. These results are broadly similar to those found in adults with IBD, in which 51% of patients reported some CAM use in the previous 2 years.[7]

Verhoef and colleagues recently explored how often CAM providers see patients with IBD and how ready they were to recommend therapies.[8] The group interviewed 66 chiropractors, 19 pharmacists, 16 herbalists, and 15 health food store employees in Calgary, Alberta. Most respondents had seen patients with IBD, and over 80% of each group, except pharmacists (only 10%), would treat these patients or recommend a therapy. Almost all chiropractors used spinal manipulation, whereas other practitioners recommended a wide variety of interventions. Most of the respondents viewed their own recommendations as moderate to very effective. It is clear from these types of data that a significant amount of information is being given to adults (and probably children) with IBD outside the physician-patient consultation.[9] Much of this information is also not discussed with the practitioners prescribing conventional therapies, potentially leading to significant drug interactions and to issues around long-term compliance with orthodox therapies.

Very few rigorous human intervention studies have been carried out with CAM, and almost all of these have been done with adult patients. There is also some limited laboratory and animal evidence accumulating, providing initial insights into the possible mechanisms underlying specific therapies.

Recently, Langmead and colleagues reviewed the in vitro antioxidant effects of six herbal remedies used by patients with IBD; these included slippery elm (derived from the bark of the slippery elm tree), fenugreek (an ayurvedic therapy), Mexican yam (a tropical staple), devil's claw (the root of an African flower), tormentil (a European flower), and Wei Tong Ning (a traditional Chinese herbal therapy).[10] All of these herbs are likely to contain numerous antioxidant compounds. Orange juice was used as a phytic control and 5-acetylsalicylic acid (5-ASA) as a positive control. Like 5-ASA, slippery elm, devil's claw, tormentil, and Wei Tong Ning all had dose-dependent antioxidant properties, whereas all of the herbs and 5-ASA also had dose-dependent peroxyl-radical scavenging effects. Detection of reactive oxygen metabolites was significantly reduced if inflamed mucosal biopsies were incubated with 1 in 100 dilutions of all herbs except Mexican yam and orange juice. This in vitro evidence provides intriguing evidence that substances present in certain diets or used as alternative therapies may have direct anti-inflammatory effects on an inflamed mucosa.

There is some work in animals focusing on individual herbs and plant compounds, assessing their efficacy in different mouse models of colitis. Among others, *Cordia myxa* fruit, polygalae root, and tryptanthrin all appear to have anti-inflammatory effects, with down-regulation of interferon-γ occurring in several disease models.[11–13]

There is further evidence from animal work that polyphenols in green tea, already thought to have some preventive role in carcinogenesis, may regulate tumor necrosis factor-α (TNF-α) production by their effect on the core molecule nuclear factor-κB.[14,15] A dose of 0.5 g/kg body weight of green tea polyphenols reduced the serum TNF-α concentrations by 80% and prevented induced lethality in mice. A further study has extended these findings, showing that the spontaneous colitis of interleukin-2 knockout mice is ameliorated by regular supplementation with green tea polyphenols over a 6-week period.[16]

Two studies report the efficacy of the Chinese herbal remedies Kui Jie Qing (KJQ) and Yukui Tang in the treatment of active ulcerative colitis (UC).[17] The authors used KJQ enemas for 20 days in 95 patients with UC, comparing the response with that of 11 controls. They showed 95% "effectiveness" compared with 53% using sulfasalazine, prednisolone tablets, and KJQ enemas. In a second study, 118 patients with UC received KJQ orally with herbal decoction enemas and 15 mg oral prednisolone, neomycin sulfate, and sulfasalazine. This group was compared with 86 patients receiving a similar treatment but without KJQ. Again, an "efficacy" rate of 84% was reported in the treated group compared with 60% in controls.

A randomized, double-blind study treated 153 patients with active UC in three different groups. Group 1 received

Jian Pi Ling and a retention enema of *Radix sophorae flavescentis* and Flos Sophora (RSF-FS) per night. Group 2 received sulfasalazine plus a retention enema of dexamethasone, whereas group 3 was randomized to placebo plus the same retention enema (RSF-FS) given to group 1.[18] The remission rates of groups 1 and 3 were 53.1% and 19.0%, respectively, with only 27.7% responding to treatment with conventional medications. The outcome measures in both of these studies were not clearly stated and were all recorded in an unblinded fashion, hence casting some doubt on the dramatic results.

An oral formulation of the Indian gum resin *Boswellia serrata* (900 mg/d) was compared with oral sulfasalazine (3 g/d) in the treatment of moderately active UC. Both treatments were effective in this study, with 14 of 20 of those receiving *B. serrata* achieving a clinical remission at 6 weeks compared with 4 of 10 given sulfasalazine.[19] Boswellic acids are thought to inhibit leukotriene synthesis by noncompetitive inhibition of 5-lipoxygenase, thereby leading to their anti-inflammatory effects on chronic inflammation in UC.[20]

Wheat grass juice has been reported as effective compared with placebo in a small but carefully conducted study on 24 adults with left-sided UC.[21] Patients treated with 100 mL of wheat grass juice for 1 month had significant improvements in rectal bleeding, abdominal pain, and disease activity scores. In addition, there was a trend toward sigmoidoscopic improvement at follow-up. Again, it is the antioxidant and anti-inflammatory properties of components such as the flavonoids, which are known to be active in the arachidonic acid pathway, that are felt to be responsible for the therapeutic effects.

There may be further mechanisms at play in some food derivatives. A pilot study, still awaiting placebo-controlled confirmation, has shown germinated barley foodstuff to be effective in achieving both clinical and endoscopic improvement in adults with treatment-resistant active UC. Much, if not all, of the effect of this treatment may be due to the inherent prebiotic properties, which increase colonic short-chain fatty acid concentrations significantly.[22]

There is an almost complete absence of well-controlled trials assessing the impact of neuromodulation on patients with IBD. Patients and their physicians have long been aware of the association between emotion, stress, and disease activity in IBD. An early randomized controlled trial on the impact of stress management in 80 patients with IBD did suggest a significant reduction in disease-specific activity. There was also a reduction in stress indices in adults who received six classes on stress management.[23]

There are only anecdotal reports of either mind-body influences or stress contributing to the degree of mucosal inflammation in IBD. Whorwell and colleagues did study the effect of three hypnotically induced emotions (excitement, anger, and happiness) on distal colonic motility in 18 adults with irritable bowel syndrome.[24] Anger and excitement increased the colonic motility index, pulse, and respiratory rate, providing some hard, albeit limited, data on this association. Further studies are required to identify suitable patients and provide more convincing evidence on the efficacy of these therapies.

CONSTIPATION

There is already a complete dearth of good-quality data on the conventional therapies used in the management of constipation in children, so it will come as no surprise that there are no controlled prospective trials on any complementary therapies and that all available evidence is anecdotal.

Anthraquinones are known to be the active components in senna and aloe (sap of aloe leaves) and have stimulant laxative properties. Their abuse, however, has been associated with an increased risk of colorectal cancer (OR = 3.4).[25] Ispaghula husk and the plant polysaccharide psyllium can be used as effective bulking agents. Odes and Madar compared capsules containing celandine, aloe vera, and psyllium with placebo in a randomized controlled trial of 35 adults over 28 days. The treated group had an increase in bowel movements, softer stools, and less laxative dependence than the placebo group, yet abdominal pain remained unchanged in both groups.[26]

A Thai plant containing anthraquinone, *Cassia alata*, was tested against *Mist. alba* and placebo in a blinded controlled multicenter trial. Eighty adults with a 72-hour history of constipation were randomized into three groups, and each received a single dose of treatment. Over 80% of adults in the *Cassia alata* and *Mist. alba* groups had passed stool within 24 hours compared with 18% in the placebo group.[27]

The centuries-old liquid ayurvedic medicine *Misrakasneham* (containing a mixture of herbs, castor oil, and ghee) was compared with a conventional senna-based laxative in a controlled trial for treatment of opioid-induced constipation in adults with advanced cancer.[28] Fifty patients were randomly allocated to the treatment group, receiving the treatment in incremental doses if necessary over 14 days. After the study period, 69% and 85% of the senna and the ayurvedic therapy groups, respectively, reported satisfactory bowel movements, a difference that was not statistically significant. However, the *Misrakasneham* was well tolerated, quicker acting, and cheaper than the senna.

Brazelli and Griffiths, in a Cochrane review, looked at the effects of behavioral and/or cognitive interventions for the management of defecation disorders in children.[29] Sixteen randomized trials with a total of 843 children met the inclusion criteria. Sample sizes were generally small. Interventions varied among trials, and few outcomes were shared by trials addressing the same comparisons. The synthesis of data from eight trials showed higher rather than lower rates of persisting problems up to 12 months when biofeedback was added to conventional treatment (OR = 1.34, 95% CI = 0.92–1.94). In two trials, significantly more encopretic children receiving behavioral intervention plus laxative therapy improved at both the 6-month (OR = 0.51, 95% CI = 0.29–0.89) and the 12-month follow-up (OR = 0.52, 95% CI = 0.30–0.93) compared with those receiving behavioral intervention alone. Similarly, in another trial, the addition of behavior modifications to laxative therapy was associated with a marked reduction in children's soiling episodes (OR = 0.14, 95% CI = 0.04–0.51). The reviewers concluded that there is no evidence that biofeedback training adds any benefit to conventional treatment in the management of encopre sis and constipation in children. However, there is some evidence that behavioral intervention plus laxative therapy, rather than behavioral intervention or laxative therapy alone, improves continence in children with primary and secondary encopresis.

Probiotics have been used for treatment of constipation, but there are no reports in the literature of their use in children. There is one randomized controlled trial reporting their use in the elderly. Ouwehand and colleagues enrolled 28 elderly subjects in an open-label parallel study.[30] In addition to a placebo group, two groups received different strains of probiotic over a 4-week period. The subjects receiving the *Lactobacillus rhamnosus/Propionibacterium freudenreichii*–supplemented juice exhibited a 24% increase in defecation frequency, although there was no overall reduction in laxative use. Trials are now in progress assessing the impact of nonabsorbable prebiotic sugars such as inulin and fructo-oligosaccharides on children with idiopathic constipation.

Abdominal massage has been used for centuries in the treatment of constipation. It has recently regained popularity, and Ernst completed a systematic review of controlled clinical trials of this therapy.[31] He was able to select only four studies from the available literature, yet even these were heterogeneous in trial design, patient sample, and type of massage used. He concluded that massage therapy may be a promising treatment for chronic constipation, yet, inevitably, more rigorous trials should evaluate its true value.

Dolk and colleagues assessed the effect of yoga on the puborectalis muscle in nine patients with severe defecation difficulties secondary to puborectalis dysfunction (puborectalis paradox).[32] Having had electromyography (EMG) of the striated anal sphincter muscles, patients were offered training in yogic techniques of relaxation and muscle control to change the activity of the pelvic floor muscles during attempted defecation. Five patients completed the training program of 20 2-hour sessions and were re-examined clinically and with EMG. One patient regained a normal EMG pattern, but none of the patients improved clinically.

Kesselring and colleagues reported on the role of foot reflexology (FR) on well-being, voiding, bowel movements, pain, and/or sleep in women who underwent an abdominal operation.[33] One hundred and thirty subjects were randomized into three groups. For 5 days, they were exposed to 15 minutes of FR, foot/leg massages (FMs), or interview alone, respectively. The results showed that women in the FR group were more able to void without problems after the indwelling catheter had been removed than were women in the comparison groups. There was also a tendency in the FR group for the indwelling catheter to be removed earlier than in the other groups. In comparison, the FR subjects slept worse than the others. FM showed significant results in subjective measurements of well-being, pain, and sleep.

LIVER DISEASE

Medicinal properties of the milk thistle plant (*Silybum marianum*) have been extensively researched. The active ingredient is silymarin, a mixture of at least four closely related flavonolignans, which appears to be antihepatotoxic owing to the antioxidant- and membrane-stabilizing properties of its components.[34]

The most dramatic reports of its use are in patients poisoned with the deathcap mushroom *Amanita phalloides*. In animal studies, dogs were given lethal doses of *A. phalloides*, 85 mg/kg, and were then randomized to receive either silymarin or placebo 5 to 24 hours after ingestion. None died in the treated group compared with 4 of 12 in the untreated group. This was supported in the treated group by improvement in hepatic enzymes and less necrosis on liver biopsy.[35] There are no randomized trials in humans, but there are various case series and retrospective studies supporting the usefulness of milk thistle in treatment of amanita poisoning.[36]

Liu and colleagues reported the efficacy and safety of Chinese herbal remedies in the treatment of asymptomatic carriers of hepatitis B.[37] Despite some methodologic problems, the "Jianpi Wenshen recipe" appeared to be significantly better than interferon for clearance of serum hepatitis B surface antigen (HBsAg) (relative risk [RR] = 2.40, 95% CI = 1.01–5.72) and hepatitis B e antigen (HBeAg) (RR = 2.03, 95% CI = 0.98–4.20), as well as in the seroconversion of HBeAg to anti-HB$_e$ (RR = 2.54, 95% CI = 1.13–5.70).

In a further Cochrane review of Chinese medicinal herbs in the treatment of chronic hepatitis B infection, of nine randomized trials included in the review, only one was considered to have adequate methodologic quality.[38] Ten different medicinal herbs were tested in these nine trials. Fuzheng Jiedu Tang was significantly better in clearing serum HBsAg, HBeAg, and hepatitis B virus deoxyribonucleic acid (DNA) compared with placebo. In a further randomized trial of 94 patients, kurorinone was found to be as effective as interferon-α in clearing HBeAg and hepatitis B virus DNA over a 12-month follow-up period.[39]

In the treatment of hepatitis C, 4 of 10 trials were considered to be of adequate quality for assessment.[40] When Bing Gan Tang was used in conjunction with interferon-α, it cleared serum hepatitis C virus ribonucleic acid (RNA) (RR = 2.54, 95% CI = 1.43–4.49) with normalization of serum alanine aminotransferase (ALT) (RR = 2.54, 95% CI = 1.43–4.49) better than interferon-α alone. The herbal mixture "Yi Zhu decoction," when compared with glycyrrhizin plus ribavirin, was significantly better at clearing serum hepatitis C virus RNA and normalizing ALT levels. In addition, Yi Er Gan Tang had a significant advantage over silymarin plus glucurolactone in normalizing serum ALT.

Although many of these data are intriguing, the lack of prospective randomized studies seriously limits any widespread clinical application. Caution is also indicated in view of the completely unknown adverse-effect profile of these medications.

Ayurvedic medications have also been used in the treatment of hepatitis. Despite initial hopes that the herb *Phyllanthus amarus* might reduce the carriage of surface antigen in carriers of hepatitis B, other studies have failed to show a similar improvement.[41,42] One study has shown *Phyllanthus urinaria* to be more effective than *P. amarus*.[43]

ACUTE GASTROENTERITIS

There is now extensive evidence in the literature about the use of probiotics in the treatment of acute gastroenteritis, especially in children. This is covered in greater detail elsewhere in the text.

Homeopathy is widely used in the treatment of gastroenteritis in children, and Jacobs and colleagues reported two double-blind placebo-controlled randomized trials to assess its efficacy in the treatment of childhood diarrhea.[44] Eighty-one children from Leon, Nicaragua, age 6 months to 5 years of age, received individualized homeopathic medicine daily over a period of 5 days. Standard treatment with oral rehydration treatment was also given. There was a statistically significant decrease in both the duration of diarrhea (less than three unformed stools daily for 2 consecutive days) and in the number of stools per day between the two groups after 72 hours of treatment. The same study was then repeated in 126 children from Kathmandu, Nepal.[45] This study revealed similar results, and a Kaplan-Meier survival analysis of the duration of diarrhea showed an 18.4% greater probability that a child would be free of diarrhea by day 5 with homeopathic treatment ($p = .036$).

Izadnia and colleagues reported the effective use of brewer's yeast for treatment of *Clostridium difficile* gastroenteritis in rats, with both brewer's yeast and *Saccharomyces boulardii* attenuating *C. difficile*–induced colonic secretion in the rat.[46] Hyperimmune cow's colostrum has also been used with some success in randomized trials of *Rotavirus* diarrhea in children.[47] However, bovine immunoglobulins are more easily digested by human trypsin and chymotrypsin and should thus have little or no effect on small intestinal function.[48]

Loeb and colleagues have shown, again in a randomized trial, that a tannin-rich carob pod, together with oral rehydration solution, led to a significantly quicker resolution of viral or bacterial diarrhea compared with oral rehydration solution alone.[49]

A combination of berberine and tetracycline was shown to significantly decrease the volume and frequency of diarrheal stools, the duration of diarrhea, and the requirement for intravenous and oral rehydration fluid in adults with cholera. However, neither berberine nor tetracycline was found to be better than placebo in treating noncholera diarrhea.[50]

Although not strictly used in acute infective gastroenteritis, psyllium was successful in reducing symptoms in 20 of 23 children with chronic nonspecific diarrhea.[51] Wenzl and colleagues showed that stool looseness is determined by the ratio of water to insoluble solids in the stools; therefore, diarrhea can also be the result of low output of insoluble solids, and psyllium may act by increasing these insoluble solids.[52]

ADVERSE EFFECTS

It is a popular belief that CAM therapies are natural products and therefore safe. Although this may apply to many CAM therapies, the recent explosion in CAM use has been paralleled by an increasing number of serious adverse events reported in the world literature. In the absence of any large prospective studies that systematically collect and report safety data, the vast majority of adverse events are reported as case reports, therefore clearly providing a gross underestimate of the actual incidence of adverse events related to CAM use.

Bensoussan and colleagues conducted a survey of reported adverse events in the use of traditional Chinese medicine in Australia.[53] Practitioners did report some adverse events with use of acupuncture (fainting, nausea and vomiting, and increased pain) and consumption of Chinese herbal medicines. However, these side effects were very uncommon when compared with those of practices in conventional medicine. An average of one adverse event was reported for 8 to 9 months of full-time practice (ie, 1 adverse event in 633 consultations). This type of study is clearly flawed in many ways, with significant bias again likely to significantly underestimate the incidence of adverse events. There is thus little reassurance both for practitioners of conventional medicine and for the consumers of CAM therapies that these therapies are as free from hazard as they are often purported to be.

Although most herbal remedies used in children at home appear to be safe, allergic reactions and cases of anaphylaxis have been reported.[54] The most frequently reported adverse effects include diarrhea, nausea, and vomiting, and although many herbs preferentially affect the digestive tract, most of their adverse effects are self-limiting.[55]

Adverse effects on liver function may be more serious, with hepatotoxicity secondary to ingestion of Chinese herbs being well described (Table 76.6-1). In Africa and Central America, toxicity can be endemic in areas where particular plants are consumed on a daily basis. Liver transplant has been necessary in cases of fulminant hepatic failure secondary to herbal remedies.[56]

The potential toxicity of pyrrolizidine alkaloids in herbal teas was recognized over 40 years ago. These can result in centrilobular necrosis, portal hypertension, veno-occlusive disease, and an increased risk of hepatocellular carcinoma.[57] In cases of suspected poisoning, it is important that some of the ingested product is retrieved and analyzed. It may be useful to save blood and urine for later analysis. Once the offending agent is identified and further intake is prevented, treatment of these cases is mostly supportive. Suspected poisoning should always be considered in patients presenting with unexplained hepatitis, although the offending constituent is identified in a minority of cases only.

In view of the widespread and self-directed use of herbal preparations, consumers and clinicians alike need to be increasingly aware of these potentially hepatotoxic products.

McGuire and colleagues reported a case of fatal hypermagnesemia secondary to the cardiac complications of high doses of magnesium oxide.[58] This had been given to a child with mental retardation, spastic quadriplegia, and seizures as part of a regimen of megavitamin and megamineral therapy and without the knowledge of the patient's physician.

Homeopathic medicines are generally considered to be nontoxic owing to the degree of dilution these medicines

TABLE 76.6-1   LIST OF HERBAL TREATMENTS WITH ADVERSE EFFECTS ON THE LIVER

BOTANICAL NAME	COMMON NAME	USE	SIDE EFFECTS	REFERENCE
Teucrium chamaedrys	Germander	Antipyretic, obesity	Hepatitis	69
Lycopodium serratum	Jin Bu Huan	Analgesic	Hepatitis	70
Cassia augustifolia	Senna	Laxative	Hepatitis	71
Atractylis gummifera	White chameleon	Antipyretic purgative	Hepatitis	72
Larrea trientata	Chapparal	Anti-inflammatory	Cholestatic hepatitis	73
Senecio crotolaria	Herbal tea	Tonic	Veno-occlusive disease	74

undergo. Massage therapies are also generally considered to be safe, although a hepatic hematoma has been reported after deep abdominal massage.[59]

In 1986, Stryker and colleagues reported six cases of acute hepatitis B after receiving acupuncture treatment in a chiropractic clinic over a period of 6 months.[60] In these cases, acupuncture needles were reused after overnight sterilization using 1:750 solution of benzalkonium chloride. Practitioners now use disposable needles to eliminate this risk.

Dunbabin and colleagues reported a case of lead poisoning in a 37-year-old man after the intake of some Indian ayurvedic medications. The tablets contained a very high concentration of lead, and the patient required chelation therapy.[61]

The majority of complementary therapies are taken as adjuncts to conventional therapies. As a result of this, and the fact that very few patients inform their physicians of concomitant use, there is now an increasing list of known interactions between certain remedies and commonly prescribed medications in pediatric gastroenterology (Table 76.6-2).

Plants undergo several processes before manufacturing of the final product. During this period, they are at risk of adulteration, deterioration, and contamination. Adulteration is more likely to occur with certain herbs, which are expensive and in short supply. Many countries of origin do not have a well-enforced code of good manufacturing practice, and remedies may be adulterated, with steroid and nonsteroidal anti-inflammatory drugs being the most commonly detected.

Plants may be misidentified at the time of picking, their true names misspelled or even mistranscribed during export. Proper identification of herbs is, of course, particularly important, particularly for the accurate reporting of adverse effects.[62]

The final concentration and quality of the active ingredient are determined by many different factors, not least of which are the local environmental conditions (availability of water, sunshine, and rainfall in some areas). Stringent collection and packaging measures with batch to batch analysis of the active ingredient in the final product are important.

Ginenoside is the biologically active glycosylated steroid in ginseng, which is commonly used and prescribed. It was examined in 50 commercial brands sold in 11 countries. In 44 of these products, the concentration of ginenoside ranged from 1.9 to 9% w/w; six products contained no ginenoside, with one of these six containing large amounts of ephedrine.[63] A series of five adults developed heavy metal poisoning in the United Kingdom from Indian ethnic remedies; the products used had lead concentrations varying from 6 to 60% w/w.[64]

In addition to the contamination of products, ingredients may be substituted without adequate research into their safety or efficacy. *Stephania tetrandra* was an active ingredient in a Belgian slimming treatment. This was, however, replaced by *Aristolochia fangchi* without a change in the brand name, and its use resulted in nine cases of rapidly progressive interstitial nephritis in young

TABLE 76.6-2   INTERACTIONS BETWEEN CONVENTIONAL DRUGS USED IN PEDIATRIC GASTROENTEROLOGY
AND HERBAL REMEDIES

HERB	CONVENTIONAL DRUG	CONSEQUENCE/EFFECT ON CONVENTIONAL THERAPY
Licorice	Spironolactone, prednisolone	Antagonistic effect; hypokalemia; increased salt and water retention
Echinacea	Anabolic steroids, methotrexate, immunosuppressants	Hepatotoxicity; theoretically may interfere because echinacea is an immune stimulant
St. John's wort	Cyclosporine	Reduced blood levels
Feverfew, garlic, ginkgo, ginger, and ginseng	Warfarin	Increased effect
St. John's wort, saw palmetto (containing tannic acid)	Iron	Inhibits absorption
Ephedra	Corticosteroids	Increased excretion
Xaio chai hu tang (sho-saiko-to)	Corticosteroids	Reduced blood levels

Adapted from Zou L et al,[75] Miller,[76] and Fugh-Berman A.[77]
Known herbal treatments that are cytochrome P-450 inhibitors: (1) ginkgo biloba (ginkgolic acids I and II); (2) kava (desmethoxyyangonin, dihydromethysticin, and methysticin); (3) garlic (allicin); (4) evening primrose oil (*cis*-linoleic acid); (5) St. John's wort (hyperforin and quercetin).

women. Laboratory analysis revealed it to contain a nephrotoxic component, aristolochic acid. To date, 80 cases have been identified. More than half of these patients have developed renal failure.[65]

Although the production of many CAM therapies is now more closely scrutinized, their final distribution can lead to further misinformation and subsequent confusion for the consumer. With the explosion of information sources on the Internet, it has become impossible to control or regulate many of the claims being made about remedies that are now sourced from around the world. Ernst and Schmidt investigated Internet advice offered by "medical herbalists" to a pregnant woman for the herbal treatment of morning sickness.[66] Search engines were used to find relevant Web sites, and all potential electronic mail addresses were contacted. Herbalists gave a wide range of differing advice, with less than one in three cautioning potential consumers about adverse effects.

Many complementary therapies, particularly those involving the administration of products encompassed by the term "dietary supplement," can continue to avoid the costly validation and safety studies that are required of conventional pharmaceutical products by relying on legislation passed in the United States in 1994 (Dietary Supplement Health and Education Act, 1994). Although this loophole exists, it is unlikely that manufacturers of dietary supplements will embrace the high cost of the formal drug trials and the research and development that are required of their colleagues in the pharmaceutical industry.

THE FUTURE OF CAM

LEGISLATION

United States.   CAM use has been increasing rapidly in the United States. The majority of expenditure for these therapies is made by individual third-party payers. This fact and the lack of evidence-based practice prompted Congress to create the NCCAM at the National Institutes of Health. NCCAM's mission is "to explore complementary and alternative healing practices in the context of rigorous science; to educate and train CAM researchers and to disseminate authoritative information to the public and professionals."[67] Although the budget for NCCAM has increased to 70 million dollars in the year 2000, it is still insufficient for exhaustive studies in all complementary therapies. Currently, scientific research is broadly aimed at publicly relevant therapies. These include, among others, characterizing the active components of cranberry that may help prevent urinary tract infections, finding out more about meditation through the use of functional magnetic resonance imaging, investigating the biologic and chemical activity of red clover for use in women's cardiovascular health, and studying the effects of ginseng in an animal model of diabetes.

United Kingdom.   In contrast to the United States and most European countries, there are almost no regulations governing the work of CAM practitioners in the United Kingdom. In 1997 and 2000, the Centre for Complementary Health Studies (UK) surveyed over 50,000 practitioners from 140 professional health bodies. There was a great variation in practicing standards. Homeopathic, osteopathic, and chiropractic practice have their own self-regulated professional bodies, and there has now been a move in the House of Lords that training courses for different CAM practitioners should become standardized and implemented by their respective professional bodies. There has also been a move to establish a body similar to the NCCAM to sponsor well-funded good-quality research into complementary therapies.

RESEARCH INTO CAM

Research in CAM generally suffers from different difficulties than does research into conventional medicines. Whereas in conventional medicine, direct comparison of the efficacy of two drugs is frequently possible, this is often not feasible with CAM therapies. Therapies in CAM may be based on whole systems; for example, ayurvedic medical therapy may include a combination of oral medicines, massage, and yoga exercises. This makes comparative studies very difficult because only certain aspects of a therapeutic approach are generally tested at any one time against a certain conventional medicine. Randomization leads to the paradox that much of CAM therapy relies on patient choice and individually tailored treatment programs, thereby making larger randomized studies extremely difficult to complete. Furthermore, diagnoses in CAM frequently rely on reported symptoms rather than on the pathogenesis of an underlying disease. Thus, two patients with the same disease process but differing symptoms might receive entirely different complementary therapies. Nonetheless, studies must continue to be carefully designed and carried out to overcome the above problems, thus ensuring that the best possible evidence informs our clinical decisions.

CONCLUSIONS

A Cochrane analysis of the literature for articles published on CAM from 1966 through 1996 shows that the total number of articles listed in *MEDLINE* rose to a peak of 400,000 additions by 1996, with only 1,500 per annum being indexed under alternative medicine.[68] Before 1986, only 2% of the latter were clinical trials in alternative medicine, with an increase to 10% by 1996. With the worldwide growth in interest, it is imperative that research on complementary medicines should be conducted using stringent criteria, as used in research on conventional therapies. Only in this way will it be possible to fully exploit the wealth of products and therapies at our disposal. The trend toward a more evidence-based approach in this discipline is vital if the move toward a more integrated type of health care provision is to occur.

It is now clear that clinicians can no longer ignore the potential benefits and occasional risks of CAM, making it necessary for us to familiarize ourselves with all of the therapies that our patients may be taking.

REFERENCES

1. Defining and describing complementary and alternative medicine. Panel on Definition and Description, CAM Research Methodology Conference, April 1995. Altern Ther Health Med 1997;3:49–57.

2. Neal R. Report by David M. Eisenberg, M.D., on complementary and alternative medicine in the United States: overview and patterns of use. J Altern Complement Med 2001;7 Suppl 1: S19–21.

3. Spigelblatt L, Laine-Ammara G, Pless IB, et al. The use of alternative medicine by children. Pediatrics 1994;94(6 Pt 1):811–4.

4. Andrews L, Lokuge S, Sawyer M, et al. The use of alternative therapies by children with asthma: a brief report. J Paediatr Child Health 1998;34:131–4.

5. Sawyer MG, Gannoni AF, Toogood IR, et al. The use of alternative therapies by children with cancer. Med J Aust 1994; 160:320–2.

6. Heuschkel R, Afzal N, Wuerth A, et al. Complementary medicine use in children and young adults with inflammatory bowel disease. Am J Gastroenterol 2002;97:382–8.

7. Hilsden RJ, Meddings JB, Verhoef MJ. Complementary and alternative medicine use by patients with inflammatory bowel disease: an Internet survey. Can J Gastroenterol 1999;13:327–32.

8. Verhoef MJ, Rapchuk I, Liew T, et al. Complementary practitioners' views of treatment for inflammatory bowel disease. Can J Gastroenterol 2002;16:95–100.

9. Calder J, Issenman R, Cawdron R. Health information provided by retail health food outlets. Can J Gastroenterol 2000;14:767–71.

10. Langmead L, Dawson C, Hawkins C, et al. Antioxidant effects of herbal therapies used by patients with inflammatory bowel disease: an in vitro study. Aliment Pharmacol Ther 2002;16:197–205.

11. Hong T, Jin GB, Yoshino G, et al. Protective effects of Polygalae root in experimental TNBS-induced colitis in mice. J Ethnopharmacol 2002;79:341–6.

12. Al Awadi FM, Srikumar TS, Anim JT, et al. Antiinflammatory effects of Cordia myxa fruit on experimentally induced colitis in rats. Nutrition 2001;17:391–6.

13. Micallef MJ, Iwaki K, Ishihara T, et al. The natural plant product tryptanthrin ameliorates dextran sodium sulfate-induced colitis in mice. Int Immunopharmacol 2002;2:565–78.

14. Gao YT, McLaughlin JK, Blot WJ, et al. Reduced risk of esophageal cancer associated with green tea consumption. J Natl Cancer Inst 1994;86:855–8.

15. Yang F, de Villiers WJ, McClain CJ, et al. Green tea polyphenols block endotoxin-induced tumor necrosis factor-production and lethality in a murine model. J Nutr 1998;128:2334–40.

16. Varilek GW, Yang F, Lee EY, et al. Green tea polyphenol extract attenuates inflammation in interleukin-2-deficient mice, a model of autoimmunity. J Nutr 2001;131:2034–9.

17. Wang B, Ren S, Feng W, et al. Kui jie qing in the treatment of chronic non-specific ulcerative colitis. J Tradit Chin Med 1997;17(1):10–3.

18. Chen ZS, Nie ZW, Sun QL. Clinical study in treating intractable ulcerative colitis with traditional Chinese medicine. Zhongguo Zhong Xi Yi Jie He Za Zhi 1994;14:400–2.

19. Gupta I, Parihar A, Malhotra P, et al. Effects of gum resin of Boswellia serrata in patients with chronic colitis. Planta Med 2001;67:391–5.

20. Ammon HP. Boswellic acids (components of frankincense) as the active principle in treatment of chronic inflammatory diseases. Wien Med Wochenschr 2002;152:373–8.

21. Ben Arye E, Goldin E, Wengrower D, et al. Wheat grass juice in the treatment of active distal ulcerative colitis: a randomized double-blind placebo-controlled trial. Scand J Gastroenterol 2002;37:444–9.

22. Mitsuyama K, Saiki T, Kanauchi O, et al. Treatment of ulcerative colitis with germinated barley foodstuff feeding: a pilot study. Aliment Pharmacol Ther 1998;12:1225–30.

23. Milne B, Joachim G, Niedhardt J. A stress management programme for inflammatory bowel disease patients. J Adv Nurs 1986;11:561–7.

24. Whorwell PJ, Houghton LA, Taylor EE, et al. Physiological effects of emotion: assessment via hypnosis. Lancet 1992;340:69–72.

25. Siegers CP, Hertzberg-Lottin E, Otte M, et al. Anthranoid laxative abuse—a risk for colorectal cancer? Gut 1993;34:1099–101.

26. Odes HS, Madar Z. A double-blind trial of a celandin, aloevera and psyllium laxative preparation in adult patients with constipation. Digestion 1991;49:65–71.

27. Thamlikitkul V, Bunyapraphatsara N, Dechatiwongse T, et al. Randomized controlled trial of Cassia alata Linn. for constipation. J Med Assoc Thai 1990;73:217–22.

28. Ramesh PR, Kumar KS, Rajagopal MR, et al. Managing morphine-induced constipation: a controlled comparison of an Ayurvedic formulation and senna. J Pain Symptom Manage 1998;16:240–4.

29. Brazelli M, Griffiths P. Behavioural and cognitive interventions with or without other treatments for defaecation disorders in children. Cochrane Database Syst Rev 2001;(4):CD002240.

30. Ouwehand AC, Lagstrom H, Suomalainen T, et al. Effect of probiotics on constipation, fecal azoreductase activity and fecal mucin content in the elderly. Ann Nutr Metab 2002;46:159–62.

31. Ernst E. Abdominal massage therapy for chronic constipation: a systematic review of controlled clinical trials. Forsch Komplementarmed 1999;6(3):149-51.

32. Dolk A, Holmstrom B, Johansson C, et al. The effect of yoga on puborectalis paradox. Int J Colorectal Dis 1991;6:139–42.

33. Kesselring A, Spichiger E, Muller M. Foot reflexology: an intervention study. Pflege 1998;11:213–8.

34. Saller R, Meier R, Brignoli R. The use of silymarin in the treatment of liver diseases. Drugs 2001;61:2035–63.

35. Vogel G, Tuchweber B, Trost W, et al. Protection by silibinin against Amanita phalloides intoxication in beagles. Toxicol Appl Pharmacol 1984;73:355–62.

36. Carducci R, Armellino MF, Volpe C, et al. Silibinin and acute poisoning with Amanita phalloides. Minerva Anestesiol 1996; 62:187–93.

37. Liu JP, McIntosh H, Lin H. Chinese medicinal herbs for asymptomatic carriers of hepatitis B virus infection. Cochrane Database Syst Rev 2001;(2):CD002231.

38. Liu JP, McIntosh H, Lin H. Chinese medicinal herbs for chronic hepatitis B. Cochrane Database Syst Rev 2001;(1):CD001940.

39. Chen C, Guo SM, Liu B. A randomized controlled trial of kurorinone versus interferon-alpha2a treatment in patients with chronic hepatitis B. J Viral Hepat 2000;7:225–9.

40. Liu JP, Manheimer E, Tsutani K, et al. Medicinal herbs for hepatitis C virus infection. Cochrane Database Syst Rev 2001;(4):CD003183.

41. Thyagarajan SP, Subramanian S, Thirunalasundari T, et al. Effect of Phyllanthus amarus on chronic carriers of hepatitis B virus. Lancet 1988;ii:764–6.

42. Doshi JC, Vaidya AB, Antarkar DS, et al. A two-stage clinical trial of Phyllanthus amarus in hepatitis B carriers: failure to eradicate the surface antigen. Indian J Gastroenterol 1994;13:7–8.

43. Wang M, Cheng H, Li Y, et al. Herbs of the genus Phyllanthus in the treatment of chronic hepatitis B: observations with three preparations from different geographic sites. J Lab Clin Med 1995;126:350–2.

44. Jacobs J, Jimenez LM, Gloyd SS, et al. Treatment of acute childhood diarrhea with homeopathic medicine: a randomized clinical trial in Nicaragua. Pediatrics 1994;93:719–25.

45. Jacobs J, Jimenez LM, Malthouse S, et al. Homeopathic treatment of acute childhood diarrhea: results from a clinical trial in Nepal. J Altern Complement Med 2000;6:131–9.

46. Izadnia F, Wong CT, Kocoshis SA. Brewer's yeast and *Saccharomyces boulardii* both attenuate *Clostridium difficile*-induced colonic secretion in the rat. Dig Dis Sci 1998;43:2055–60.

47. Sarker SA, Casswall TH, Mahalanabis D, et al. Successful treatment of *Rotavirus* diarrhea in children with immunoglobulin from immunized bovine colostrum. Pediatr Infect Dis J 1998;17:1149–54.

48. Petschow BW, Talbott RD. Reduction in virus-neutralizing activity of a bovine colostrum immunoglobulin concentrate by gastric acid and digestive enzymes. J Pediatr Gastroenterol Nutr 1994;19:228–35.

49. Loeb H, Vandenplas Y, Wursch P, et al. Tannin-rich carob pod for the treatment of acute-onset diarrhea. J Pediatr Gastroenterol Nutr 1989;8:480–5.

50. Khin MU, Myo K, Nyunt NW, et al. Clinical trial of berberine in acute watery diarrhoea. BMJ 1985;291:1601–5.

51. Smalley JR, Klish WJ, Campbell MA, et al. Use of psyllium in the management of chronic nonspecific diarrhea of childhood. J Pediatr Gastroenterol Nutr 1982;1:361–3.

52. Wenzl HH, Fine KD, Schiller LR, et al. Determinants of decreased fecal consistency in patients with diarrhea. Gastroenterology 1995;108:1729–38.

53. Bensoussan A, Myers SP, Carlton AL. Risks associated with the practice of traditional Chinese medicine: an Australian study. Arch Fam Med 2000;9:1071–8.

54. Fugh-Berman A. Herbal supplements: indications, clinical concerns, and safety. Nutr Today 2002;37:122–4.

55. Langmead L, Rampton DS. Review article: herbal treatment in gastrointestinal and liver disease—benefits and dangers. Aliment Pharmacol Ther 2001;15:1239–52.

56. Mattei A, Rucay P, Samuel D, et al. Liver transplantation for severe acute liver failure after herbal medicine (*Teucrium polium*) administration. J Hepatol 1995;22:597.

57. Haller CA, Dyer JE, Ko R, et al. Making a diagnosis of herbal-related toxic hepatitis. West J Med 2002;176:39–44.

58. McGuire JK, Kulkarni MS, Baden HP. Fatal hypermagnesemia in a child treated with megavitamin/megamineral therapy. Pediatrics 2000;105:E18.

59. Trotter JF. Hepatic hematoma after deep tissue massage. N Engl J Med 1999;341:2019–20.

60. Stryker WS, Gunn RA, Francis DP. Outbreak of hepatitis B associated with acupuncture. J Fam Pract 1986;22:155–8.

61. Dunbabin DW, Tallis GA, Popplewell PY, et al. Lead poisoning from Indian herbal medicine (Ayurveda). Med J Aust 1992; 157:835–6.

62. But PP. Need for correct identification of herbs in herbal poisoning. Lancet 1993;341:637.

63. Cui J, Garle M, Eneroth P, et al. What do commercial ginseng preparations contain? Lancet 1994;344:134.

64. Kew J, Morris C, Aihie A, et al. Arsenic and mercury intoxication due to Indian ethnic remedies. BMJ 1993;306:506–7.

65. Vanhaelen M, Vanhaelen-Fastre R, But P, et al. Identification of aristolochic acid in Chinese herbs. Lancet 1994;343:174.

66. Ernst E, Schmidt K. Health risks over the Internet: advice offered by "medical herbalists" to a pregnant woman. Wien Med Wochenschr 2002;152:190–2.

67. About the National Center for Complimentary and Alternative Medicine. Available at: http://nccam.nih.gov/about/aboutnccam/index.htm (accessed Nov 17, 2003).

68. Barnes J, Abbot NC, Harkness EF, et al. Articles on complementary medicine in the mainstream medical literature: an investigation of MEDLINE, 1966 through 1996. Arch Intern Med 1999;159:1721–5.

69. Larrey D, Vial T, Pauwels A, et al. Hepatitis after germander (*Teucrium chamaedrys*) administration: another instance of herbal medicine hepatotoxicity. Ann Intern Med 1992;117: 129–32.

70. Graham-Brown R. Toxicity of Chinese herbal remedies. Lancet 1992;340:673–4.

71. Beuers U, Spengler U, Pape GR. Hepatitis after chronic abuse of senna. Lancet 1991;337:372–3.

72. Georgiou M, Sianidou L, Hatzis T, et al. Hepatotoxicity due to *Atractylis gummifera*-L. J Toxicol Clin Toxicol 1988;26: 487–93.

73. Sheikh NM, Philen RM, Love LA. Chaparral-associated hepatotoxicity. Arch Intern Med 1997;157:913–9.

74. McDermott WV, Ridker PM. The Budd-Chiari syndrome and hepatic veno-occlusive disease. Recognition and treatment. Arch Surg 1990;125:525–7.

75. Zou L, Harkey MR, Henderson GL. Effects of herbal components on cDNA-expressed cytochrome P450 enzyme catalytic activity. Life Sci 2002;71:1579–89.

76. Miller LG. Herbal medicinals: selected clinical considerations focusing on known or potential drug-herb interactions. Arch Intern Med 1998;158:2200–11.

77. Fugh-Berman A. Herb-drug interactions. Lancet 2000;355:134–8.

7. Adherence to Medical Regimens

Eyal Shemesh, MD

Nonadherence to (noncompliance with) medical recommendations is a leading cause of morbidity and mortality in a wide array of disease processes and in all age groups.[1–8] These diseases include disorders of the gastrointestinal tract.[9–13] Nonadherence is specifically thought to be prevalent during the adolescent years.[1,10,11,14] Hence, it is frequently encountered by pediatricians. Adherence is especially important in patients who have a chronic medical illness, who need to adhere to medications and dietary regimens over a long period of time, and whose health outcome is closely related to following the recommendations.

Extant data strongly suggest that nonadherence is a significant cause of morbidity and mortality in several patient groups, such as post-transplant patients.[2,3,15–18] Yet the assessment and treatment of nonadherence are rarely approached in a systematic way in clinical practice.

This chapter reviews the definition and characteristics of nonadherence, its prevalence, ways to assess it, developmental considerations in adherence behavior, risk factors that predispose a patient to become nonadherent, and methods that are thought to improve adherence. Most of the discussion is not disease specific. However, specific examples, or a concise summary of issues that are unique to children who suffer from specific illnesses of the gastrointestinal tract, are included when relevant.

Nonadherence is a leading reason for poor outcome in a variety of disease processes. It can be improved in many cases. It is important to study it and to incorporate adherence assessments and interventions into routine practice. Very little has been done to date to address this important phenomenon in a concerted fashion. This chapter is intended to increase awareness of nonadherence as a mediator of outcome and to provide a framework for a rational approach to its assessment and treatment.

DEFINITION

Nonadherence to medical recommendations happens when a patient does not follow the recommendations that are given by physicians, nurses, or other medical professionals. Nonadherence could be related to a wide array of recommendations. These could be, for example, dietary recommendations, scheduling recommendations (clinic visits, imaging tests), and recommendations to take medications. Adherence to one type of recommendation (ie, coming to clinical visits as scheduled) does not necessarily imply adherence to another type of recommendation (ie, taking the medications as prescribed[19]). The treatment of gastrointestinal illnesses, such as celiac disease, frequently includes a dietary modification, which is a lifestyle change. Adherence to such lifestyle changes may be quite different from adherence to medications, which does not require a major change in lifestyle and habits. Even within one general type of recommendation, adherence may vary (ie, a patient may adhere to an immunosuppressant regimen but not to a prescribed vitamin pill, even though both are prescribed by the same clinician). Hence, adherence should be defined narrowly, in relation to a specific recommendation. I decided to focus the discussion in this chapter primarily on nonadherence to medications. This is done for clarity and also because more data are available on this particular type of adherence.

A strict definition of nonadherence is of very limited use in clinical practice. This is because it is quite likely that every once in a while, a patient who suffers from a chronic medical condition will not take the medications exactly as prescribed, and most clinicians will not call this behavior "nonadherence." The following example illustrates this principle: a patient who had a liver transplant has been prescribed tacrolimus every 12 hours. This patient occasionally (ie, every weekend) takes the medications on a slightly different schedule (ie, 8 am and 10 pm instead of 7 am and 7 pm). Most clinicians will not consider this slight variation to be nonadherence, and most would probably not think that this patient should be treated for it. Yet, by a strict definition, during the weekend this patient is nonadherent to the recommendation that the medication should be taken every 12 hours.

Hence, there should be a defined threshold beneath which a nonadherent behavior is acceptable. This threshold has not been prospectively determined in any gastrointestinal disease process. It is possible that certain illnesses require different levels of adherence. For example, a patient who is suffering from autoimmune hepatitis and has been transplanted will be expected to adhere to an immunosuppressant regimen more closely than a patient who had extrahepatic biliary atresia and was transplanted as well. This is because the disease process could recur in autoimmune hepatitis but not in extrahepatic biliary atresia, and strict adherence is mandatory to avert that possibility in the first, but not the second, patient.[18]

One way in which an adherence threshold level can be determined (ie, "it is okay for this patient to forget to take the medication once a week but not twice a week") is by determining at what point medical adverse events are likely. The danger of waiting for the actual occurrence of the adverse event to make this determination is obvious. Rather than waiting until some medical emergency has happened owing to nonadherence (ie, a flare of Crohn disease), a better method would be to predetermine a level of acceptable adherence for each patient or group of patients, assess it frequently, and try to act *before* the medical event has happened.

The way in which nonadherence is defined could have far-reaching consequences. For example, studies done by pharmaceutical companies sometimes set a threshold of 70% adherence for inclusion in a study that examines the effects of a certain medication against a placebo. Although it is indeed imperative to include only patients who actually take the medications in such studies, this approach is not supported by specific evidence as far as gastrointestinal illnesses in children are concerned. There are no data that demonstrate that 70%, or any particular percentage, should be the adherence threshold in any of these illnesses. Furthermore, this arbitrary cutoff point skews the study population by excluding nonadherent patients from the final analysis. Hence, if a medication seems less potent or not potent when used in standard practice rather than in the context of a research protocol, nonadherence could be a contributing factor.

To summarize, nonadherence should be defined in relation to a specific recommendation. It should include a threshold (ie, What degree of nonadherence is permissible?). In determining the threshold, the clinician should take the illness involved into account. Because no empiric data are available regarding the desirable threshold, clinicians must use their judgment and experience to decide what level of adherence is acceptable for each patient.

EXTENT OF THE PROBLEM

Nonadherence to medical recommendations has been reported to be a leading cause of morbidity and mortality in several chronic disease processes, such as ulcerative colitis,[12,13] celiac disease,[9–11] and survivors of liver transplant.[16] Nonadherence may be associated with grave consequences, and it may be quite frequent in children and adolescents (see below). A recent study reported 34 episodes of nonadherence among 28 pediatric liver transplant recipients, leading to acute cellular rejection and recurrent hepatitis in 16 patients, death in 2 patients, and loss of 5 transplants.[16] Our retrospective study of adolescent liver transplant recipients showed that a protracted course of nonadherence led to retransplant and death in several patients.[18] Interestingly, in that study, the rate of documented nonadherence exceeded 50% of the sampled adolescents. Among ulcerative colitis patients, nonadherence to medications was associated with a fivefold increase in the risk of recurrent disease by the end of 12 months of follow-up.[13] These and other data strongly suggest that nonadherence is a common and dangerous phenomenon in patients who are suffering from chronic illnesses of the gastrointestinal tract.

Yet nonadherence is rarely systematically addressed in clinical practice. The following sections review some of the difficulties that are encountered on the way to a rational approach to the detection and treatment of nonadherence.

DEVELOPMENTAL CONSIDERATIONS

A child's cognitive, emotional, and social development may alter adherence behavior. It is quite possible that the same child will be nonadherent at one point and adherent at another, in tandem with specific maturational and developmental stages. The following are a few specific examples of how different developmental stages[1,14] can affect nonadherence, its assessment, and its treatment.

One point is the shift of control, or responsibility, from parent to child. At a certain age or developmental stage, the child becomes responsible for taking his/her medications. Before that stage, it is the responsibility of the parent to administer them. It is obvious that in the treatment of an 8-month-old infant, the parents are the focus of assessment and treatment if nonadherence becomes a problem. In such a case, it is the parent's adherence to administering the medications that should be addressed. On the other hand, a parent may have very little input in affecting the adherence of an 18-year-old adolescent who is in college and is not living with the parent. Hence, somewhere between infancy and young adulthood, the main burden of adherence shifts from parent to child. Assessment and treatment of nonadherence should also shift their focus at that stage. Yet there are virtually no published empiric data about the average age at which this shift occurs. In a survey of 81 patients and their caretakers that was done at the Mount Sinai Medical Center's liver post-transplant clinic, the median age at which parents and children reported that the responsibility for taking the medications is in "transition" was 12 years old, but there was significant variability (range of reported age of transition = 9 to 16 years old). In this cohort, therefore, early adolescence is the time at which the shift in responsibility occurs. Therefore, it may be useful to review the medication regimen in detail with the child and family as the child approaches this age, perhaps even in the context of a dedicated "transitional" visit.

Another important aspect is the development of a child's body image as an essential part of emerging self-esteem during adolescence. Physically disabled children, who may suffer, for example, from disfiguring postoperative scars, reduced weight, or delayed hormonal maturation (as in cases of malnutrition or gut absorptive defects), may not be able to form a positive body image of themselves.[20–22] These patients may become nonadherent to recommendations that are perceived as disfiguring, such as prescriptions of steroid medications and surgery.[22]

Lastly, because of the significant psychosocial changes that children go through on the way to becoming young adults, nonadherence in a child should be viewed as a potentially transient problem. It depends on the child's particular circumstances, cognitive abilities, and emotional status at each point in time. Hence, the labeling of a patient, rather than the patient's behavior, as "nonadherent" is rarely justified. Therefore, clinicians should be encouraged to keep trying to improve adherence by offering counseling, advice, or sometimes specific psychiatric help. At some point, a child may become receptive to a treatment modality that has not been successful before because of different circumstances or cognitive abilities. The following case report illustrates this general principle:

Principles of Therapy

M is a 21-year-old patient who had her first liver transplant when she was 15 years old owing to fulminant hepatic failure caused by a psychoactive medication used to treat attention-deficit/hyperactivity disorder. Following the transplant, she was recovering well until about 1-year posttransplant, when a rejection episode was diagnosed by biopsy, following an elevation in hepatic enzymes. The patient's blood level of tacrolimus at admission was zero, and M disclosed that she was not taking her medication as prescribed. A psychiatric consultation was obtained, and a depressive disorder was diagnosed. The adoptive parents, at the time, were overwhelmed and stated that they could not be responsible for monitoring the child's adherence. Family sessions were conducted, an antidepressant was prescribed, and the patient was discharged. Following discharge, adherence was monitored closely by direct questioning at each clinic visit and medication blood levels. A psychosocial intervention included family sessions and educational efforts aimed at the parents and the child. For 2 years, the medical course was unremarkable. The psychiatric symptoms improved, and adherence was restored. However, when M approached 18 years of age, she moved out of her parents' home to live with her boyfriend. She started to miss clinic visits and seemed more depressed, and her medication blood levels became erratic. She was eventually admitted again for a second rejection episode related to nonadherence. Two more episodes followed in the span of less than a year. An antidepressant was prescribed but not taken. Because of progressive liver damage, retransplant became the only way to keep this patient alive. An extensive psychosocial evaluation was conducted again, and the patient was diagnosed with a depressive disorder (adjustment disorder with depressed mood). The boyfriend's parents, who were supportive but not well informed about the patient's condition, were engaged in sessions and encouraged to take an active supportive role. They ensured adherence to medications, including adherence to the antidepressant. The patient became adherent again for several months prior to a retransplant. One year following the second transplant, the patient was taking her medications and was doing well both medically and psychologically. A reevaluation found that her mood disorder was in remission.

ASSESSMENT

There is no gold standard for the measurement of adherence, and each proposed method has its shortcomings. Table 76.7-1 summarizes frequently used methods, their strengths, and their weaknesses. Below are specific comments about several methods that are in use.

SELF-REPORT

When compared with objective measures of adherence, data suggest that self-reports are not a sensitive and reliable way in which to assess adherence.[23–26] Self-reports that are obtained in the context of an interview may be an exception.[27,28] Self-reports may still have a place in assessment because a patient's report that he/she does not take the med-

ications is generally considered reliable.[26] The part that is not thought to be reliable is the patient's report that he/she is taking the medication. Hence, self-report measures may be considered a relatively easy screening method that will identify some but not all cases of nonadherence.

PILL COUNTS

Pill counts, obtained through a manual count at every clinic visit, are an objective method. A patient may engage in a variety of behaviors that would invalidate this method as a measure of adherence. For example, a patient may remove pills but not take them or take the correct number of pills at an incorrect time.[19] This method will therefore identify patients who are nonadherent, provided that they are not actively concealing it. Routine use of this method is time-consuming. It has not been empirically validated in children who suffer from gastrointestinal illnesses.

ELECTRONIC EVENT MONITORING DEVICES

Electronic event monitoring devices (eg, MEMS Caps, a product of AARDEX/APREX, Switzerland) are pill boxes with electronic caps that register each opening of the device (for dispensation of a pill). A dedicated software translates the pill box readings into an output chart that gives information about the number and timing of openings. Figure 76.7-1 represents the MEMS readings that were obtained for the patient who was described above shortly before retransplant. It is easy to note that adherence was restored in that patient in December 2001 following the intervention.

Although this method has been described as the state-of-the-art adherence monitoring method, it is not free of bias. Patients may open the pill box but not remove a pill, or they may discard the pill after removing it. Electronic monitoring provides a way to ascertain precisely when a bottle was opened. However, data are lacking about the importance of this precise information. It is possible that taking an immunosuppressant 10 hours as opposed to 12 hours apart does not really constitute a significant adherence problem. The precise threshold at which timing becomes important is not well defined. Finally, although electronic monitoring carries the promise of an objective method that is much harder to "fool" than pill counts, its use was not validated against other acceptable methods of adherence monitoring or clinical outcome in children who suffer from gastrointestinal illnesses.

PRESCRIPTION REFILL RATES

Prescription refill data have been used for the detection of nonadherence[29] and, in some instances, have been reported to be more reliable than patients' self-reports.[30] To use this method, the clinician needs to be able to communicate with the pharmacy, or pharmacies, that the patient is using. Patients are likely to request a refill a few days before they run out of their medications, so the refill rate is only a crude estimate of the time the patient ran out of his/her supply. Further, refilling a prescription is not synonymous with having taken the previously prescribed dose. Hence, prescription refill rates are an objective but crude, and sometimes inaccurate, method of detection.

TABLE 76.7-1　METHODS THAT ARE FREQUENTLY USED TO ASSESS ADHERENCE

ADHERENCE ASSESSMENT METHOD	STRENGTHS	WEAKNESSES	COMMENT
Subjective methods	Easy to obtain	Less reliable than objective methods	
Patient/parent self-report	(1) Easy to obtain; (2) specific (if the patient reports not taking the medication, this report is usually reliable)	Not sensitive (a report that the patient is taking the medication may not be reliable)	Interview results are probably more reliable than questionnaire results
Clinician report	Easy to obtain	(1) Not reliable in predicting nonadherence as judged by objective measures; (2) clinicians' disagreement is a problem (different adherence ratings by different clinicians)	Correlates with health outcome measures (clinicians are more likely to detect nonadherence after an adverse health event has happened as a result of the nonadherence)
Objective methods	More reliable than most subjective methods	Require time and resources	
Medication levels (in blood, urine, or saliva)	Indicates actual intake	(1) Costly; (2) some medications do not have a readily available assay; (3) requires obtaining a biologic specimen; (4) level may at times be affected by metabolic processes, not just by intake	Measurement of the degree of fluctuation between individual levels may be a more accurate representation of adherence over time
Measurement of metabolites of a medication	Reflects intake during a relatively long period of time (not just a single dose)	(1) Costly; (2) assay may not be available; (3) metabolism may be affected by factors other than intake	For example, azathioprine metabolites
Pill counts	Easy to perform and the least expensive method	Patients may discard pills without taking them	
Electronic monitoring devices	Provide specific data about the time in which a medication was taken	Patients may discard pills without taking them (but it is harder to "fool" the electronic device than it is to "fool" a pill counter)	May be too sensitive in some instances (ie, it does not really matter, sometimes, when exactly a patient has taken the medication)
Assessment of the biologic effect of the medication	Addresses the desired outcome of a medication and hence also assesses the effectiveness of the regimen	(1) A lack of biologic effect could be due to other factors (such as a biologic resistance to the medications); (2) assays may not be available	An example: an assessment of thromboxane production values in patients who are prescribed aspirin
Prescription refills	Inexpensive	May not reflect actual intake	

MEDICATION BLOOD LEVELS

Medication blood levels may be used for determination of nonadherence. The use of a blood level drawn only once may be misleading. This is because some fluctuation is permissible. An incidence of forgetting to take the medication once may be erroneously counted as nonadherence when using this method. My colleagues and I therefore previously argued that an evaluation of the fluctuation of medication blood levels over time is a better predictor of nonadherence, except in the rare case of a patient who is never taking the medication (this patient will have a consistent level of zero without any fluctuation).[31] We compared standard deviations of consecutive blood levels in pediatric liver transplant recipients.[31] A higher standard deviation and, therefore, more fluctuation between individual measures was deemed to be indicative of nonadherence and was shown to be consistent with a panel assessment of adherence in the same subjects. It is important to note that this method assumes that medication blood levels are closely related to intake. This was shown to be the case for tacrolimus but is not true for cyclosporine.[31] Hence, fluctuations in cyclosporine blood levels cannot be used as a reliable adherence detection method. This method will not identify

patients who take their medication only prior to clinic visits ("white coat adherence"[32]).

METABOLITES

Metabolites are levels of a medication degradation or metabolic products. Metabolite levels of azathioprine have been used to assess the degree of adherence to this medication.[33] The benefit of using this method is that metabolites accumulate over time, and hence their level reflects the level of medication intake over a period of time, not just recent intake (as is the case with medication blood levels). This method may be less sensitive than others in that only a significant deviation from the prescribed regimen will be detected. It is also usually quite expensive. Further, drug metabolism may be affected by factors other than intake (eg, level of activity of an enzyme that is responsible for the metabolite that is being measured) and may therefore differ between patients.

CLINICIANS' ASSESSMENT OF ADHERENCE

Clinicians' assessment of adherence, although used in a few adherence studies, was, in fact, not shown to be a particularly reliable method for the detection of nonadherence.[19,34] It may be more reliable in the most severe cases, and it does take into account the health status of these patients. My colleagues and I previously reported a perfect agreement in a post hoc blind assessment of the most severe cases of nonadherence in pediatric liver transplant patients among a clinician panel composed of two hepatologists and a nurse.[31] Agreement was reached only for the most severe cases, however. The use of clinicians' assessments of adherence has not been validated in children who suffer from gastrointestinal illness. Taken together, extant data suggest that clinicians' assessments are not a particularly reliable method of detection of nonadherence, with the possible exception of the detection of the most severe cases.

Finally, nonadherence has been described as dynamic in nature.[19] A patient may present as nonadherent at one point in time and adherent at another. Therefore, clinicians' assessments, or indeed any method used to measure adherence, must be examined repeatedly over time rather than at only one time point.

RISK FACTORS

Many risk factors have been reported to be associated with nonadherence to medications.[1,2,14,18] Only some of these are reviewed below. The factors are grouped into those that are associated with the illness, the treatment, the patient, the social milieu, and the clinic/clinician. These groups overlap, and factors may belong to more than one group.

FACTORS RELATED TO THE ILLNESS

Specific medical illnesses may predispose a patient to become nonadherent by virtue of their course or associated features. For example, some medical illnesses are associated with cognitive decline (eg, subacute hepatic encephalopathy as a complication of chronic liver disease). Nonadherence to medications was found to be increased in instances in which the cognitive abilities of a patient are diminished.[35–37] Therefore, diseases that are associated with cognitive decline may be associated with nonadherence owing to this decline. Another example relates to the course of the illness. The management of adherence in patients who suffer from a chronic (as opposed to acute) medical condition is thought to be different in focus and duration.[38] Thus, the characteristics of the illness process, such as chronicity, may influence the risk of nonadherence.

FACTORS RELATED TO THE TREATMENT

The characteristics of the treatment regimen may determine the likelihood that a patient will adhere to it. Treatments that are time-consuming, require a high level of organization (ie, multidrug regimens), and require a high level of motivation all carry an increased risk of nonadherence.[37,39,40] Treatments that have a severe spectrum of side effects were sometimes,[41–43] but not always,[18,44,45] reported to carry a higher risk of nonadherence; for specific regimens or illnesses, side effects may not independently constitute a significant risk factor for nonadherence. The nature of the recommendation is also important; lifestyle changes (ie, dietary) are thought to be hard to achieve, perhaps because lifestyle changes require a more complex behavior.[46]

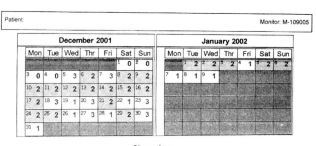

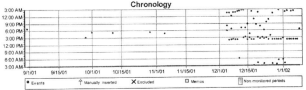

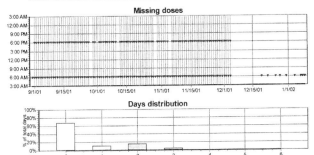

FIGURE 76.7-1 Output data from an electronic monitoring device (MEMS-IV, child resistant, a product of AARDEX/AAPREX). The device was used to monitor adherence to tacrolimus in the patient whose history is presented in the chapter. *A* includes basic patient information (deleted in this case), information about the medication that was used, basic statistics about the number and timing of doses, and data for September through November 2001. Each square represents the number of times the medication bottle was opened on a given day (should be twice a day for this regimen). *B* includes the calendar reports for December and January, the time-scatter (chronology) of the doses that were taken, and a representation of the missing doses. This patient was nonadherent until the beginning of December 2001, at which point she started taking the medications. An intensive psychosocial intervention occurred during the last week of November.

FACTORS RELATED TO THE PATIENT

Psychopathology, for example, the occurrence of depressive disorders[47–49] and post-traumatic stress disorder,[31,50] was consistently found to be related to nonadherence. A history of child abuse,[18] drug use,[18] reported feeling of "lack of control,"[51–53] and the use of avoidant coping[30,53] have all been implicated in nonadherence.

SOCIAL FACTORS

In young children, it is plausible that any of the above factors that apply to a child's parent will constitute a risk factor for the child's nonadherence (ie, parental psychopathology, depression, etc). A lower socioeconomic status is sometimes implicated as a risk factor.[54–57] A lack of social support (ie, only one parent lives at home or no caretaker lives at home) is also a predictor of nonadherence.[18,50,58]

FACTORS RELATED TO THE CLINIC OR THE CLINICIAN

A lack of empathy on the part of the clinician and a lack of trust between the patient and the clinician have been implicated in patient's nonadherence.[59–60] Lack of appropriate information about a medication is also a plausible reason for nonadherence, but lack of information alone may not be a sufficient cause for nonadherence in many cases.[61] Finally, the characteristics of the clinic itself (ie, time spent with patients, kind of illness that is addressed, awareness of adherence as a therapeutic goal, convenience of clinic hours, gender of clinicians) can be important to the development of adherence behavior in patients.[62]

TREATMENT

Treatment of nonadherence is best conceptualized as a stratified effort. It should begin with preventive efforts that are aimed at every patient and are expected to improve adherence in the clinic or practice as a whole. The preventive effort should also create a mechanism for early identification of nonadherence that needs to be further addressed. Specialized treatment strategies for identified or suspected cases that have not improved by using the general preventive model should then be offered.

PREVENTIVE MEASURES

The hallmarks of this part of an effort to improve adherence are (1) creation of a systematic method to assess patient's adherence as part of the general clinical care (ie, routinely asking about it, routine medication blood level determinations); (2) provision of general and specific education about medication-taking that is repeated frequently and targeted to the developmental stage of the child at the time the education is given; and (3) prospective assessment of risk factors that are known or suspected to be related to nonadherence and addressing these risk factors as they become known and before nonadherence develops.

SPECIALIZED TREATMENTS

Nonadherence can be managed in several ways once diagnosed or even when suspected but not confirmed. Available treatment strategies have been grouped below to

treatments that focus on patient education and awareness, treatments that focus on the adherence behavior itself, and treatments that seek to improve risk factors that are considered to be the main reason for nonadherence in a particular patient. These specialized treatment strategies are time-consuming and sometimes require a highly skilled individual to deliver it. However, the provision of such care may have a profound impact on adherence and outcome in selected patients.

PATIENT AND PARENT EDUCATION

It is hoped that education about the illness is provided to all patients, adherent or not, during the routine medical management of their illness. This section addresses a more intensive educational approach intended for confirmed or suspected nonadherent patients. The components of this approach are the assessment of the patient's (and parent's) actual understanding of the prescribed regimen, its administration, and the reasons for it; the correction of any misinformed notions that are discovered; and an open discussion about the ways in which the medication is being taken, how it can be better integrated into a patients' lifestyle, and what concessions or resources are needed to make medication-taking possible. Thus, education in this model is an interactive process in which the clinician tries to identify the cognitive and procedural needs of the patient and address them. Such an approach may also increase the patient's confidence in the clinician and enhance the collaboration between the two. Educational approaches have been shown to have limited but significant effects on adherence.[63,64] Because they are relatively straightforward and not labor intensive, they should be attempted in most cases as a first line of treatment. However, it should be emphasized that education alone is not sufficient in many instances.[61]

BEHAVIORAL MODIFICATION STRATEGIES

In this model, the adherence behavior itself is addressed. Behavior modification strategies can be used to implement a reward system for adherence (ie, a patient who is suffering from Crohn disease is rewarded with a sticker every day in which he is able to take his medications without being reminded, by an extra hour of play before bedtime on the weekend if all of the week's stickers have been collected). Parents are sometimes reluctant to implement behavioral techniques because they think that the child is suffering so much already and do not want to start being cruel or engage in strict disciplinary action against him/her. A medically ill child, however, frequently must follow very strict nutritional, medication-taking, and scheduling routines, for which a high level of discipline is required. The point to emphasize is that reinforcements are the best way to achieve a behavioral goal. Negative reinforcements or "strict discipline" is not always necessary.

Behavioral methods could also include a change in the frequency in which the patient is seen in the clinic to improve the physician's control on adherence (ie, more frequent assessments of medication metabolites and liver enzyme profiles in a pediatric hepatology clinic). Behavioral methods may sometimes necessitate the involvement of another caretaker or a therapist if the primary caretaker is unable to implement these methods consistently. For example, a school nurse may be enlisted to monitor and implement adherence to medications that are taken during school hours. Behavior modification strategies have been shown to dramatically improve an array of behaviors and have been reported as helpful in improving adherence.[65,66] However, these methods have not been rigorously evaluated in the improvement of adherence in children who are suffering from diseases of the gastrointestinal tract.

Although behavioral methods may well be successful in improving adherence, they require a specifically trained individual who is typically required to serve as a "coach" to patients and parents. This individual may not be readily available in many clinics. Also, the implementation of a successful behavioral plan may be harder to achieve in a context in which a child is chronically ill and a parent is reluctant to be "cruel," as mentioned above. Finally, because strict adherence to the behavioral intervention is required for success, it may at times be hard to implement these methods in patients who are nonadherent to recommendations to begin with.

STRATEGIES AIMED AT THE IMPROVEMENT OR ELIMINATION OF RISK FACTORS

There are many known or suspected risk factors for non-adherence, as mentioned above. A thorough discussion of methods that may be used to address each of these risks is well beyond the scope of the present review. The main point is that significant risk factors do exist and that these may be highly modifiable.

For example, the treatment of a specific psychiatric disorder such as a major depressive disorder or post-traumatic stress disorder[31,67] may improve adherence. Improvement of social stressors and provision of safety, such as the treatment of ongoing child abuse,[18] may be reasonably expected to improve adherence as well. The identification and management of risk factors related to the child and his/her environment should therefore be attempted. In a child, the assessment of risk should extend at least to the primary caretakers as well.

CONCLUSIONS

Nonadherence to medical recommendations is a significant, and mostly modifiable, risk factor for increased morbidity and poor outcome in many patient groups. The assessment of nonadherence and its management in children are complicated and not well standardized. The child's developmental stage affects adherence behavior, and the target for intervention frequently includes not only the child but also the caretakers. There are no "gold standard" methods for assessment of nonadherence. Yet several objective and subjective methods do exist. The management of nonadherence includes preventive, non-specific efforts that start with proper patient education and rapid identification of suspected cases and specialized treatment strategies that focus on education, behav-

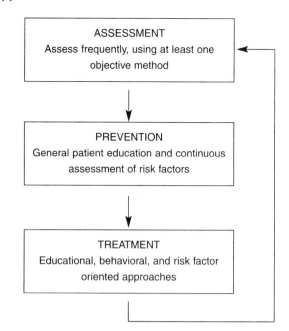

FIGURE 76.7-2 Suggested clinical approach to the management of nonadherence.

ior management, and addressing specific risk factors. Knowledge of the methods that are described in this review is expected to give practitioners the initial tools and confidence to deal with nonadherence as an important aspect of patient care.

The present textbook includes, in most chapters, a discussion of effective and sometimes innovative treatment strategies for children who suffer from gastrointestinal illnesses. These treatments include medications, dietary restrictions, surgical procedures, and other modalities. Although areas of medicine have advanced tremendously in the development of such strategies, these treatments will remain effective in practice only if they are adhered to. Extant data establish that complete adherence is, in fact, very hard to attain in clinical settings. Therefore, adherence should not be assumed. Rather, the attainment of adherence to recommendations must be included as a treatment goal. Figure 76.7-2 summarizes in a concise algorithm the clinical approach that was described in this chapter. Implementation of this approach would ensure a clinical focus on adherence. It could also facilitate research efforts that will provide crucial information about the validity and applicability of assessment and treatment methods that were discussed in this chapter.

REFERENCES

1. Cromer BA, Tarnowski KJ. Noncompliance in adolescents: a review. J Dev Behav Pediatr 1989;10:207–15.
2. De Geest S, Moons P, Dobbels F, et al. Profiles of patients who experienced a late acute rejection due to nonadherence with immunosuppressive therapy. J Cardiovasc Nurs 2001;16:1–14.
3. Dew MA, Kormos RL, Roth LH, et al. Early post-transplant medical compliance and mental health predict physical morbidity and mortality one to three years after heart transplantation. J Heart Lung Transplant 1999;18:549–62.

4. Didlake RH, Dreyfus K, Kerman RH, et al. Patient noncompliance: a major cause of late graft failure in cyclosporine-treated renal transplants. Transplant Proc 1988;20:63–9.

5. McDermott MM, Schmitt B, Wallner E. Impact of medication nonadherence on coronary heart disease outcomes. A critical review. Arch Intern Med 1997;157:1921–9.

6. Milgrom H, Bender B. Nonadherence to asthma treatment and failure of therapy. Curr Opin Pediatr 1997;9:590–5.

7. Murri R, Ammassari A, De Luca A, et al. Self-reported nonadherence with antiretroviral drugs predicts persistent condition. HIV Clin Trials 2001;2:323–9.

8. Rodgers PT, Ruffin DM. Medication nonadherence—part I: the health and humanistic consequences. Manag Care Interface 1998;11:58–60.

9. Colaco J, Egan-Mitchell B, Stevens FM, et al. Compliance with gluten free diet in coeliac disease. Arch Dis Child 1987;62: 706–8.

10. Fabiani E, Taccari LM, Ratsch IM, et al. Compliance with gluten-free diet in adolescents with screening-detected celiac disease: a 5-year follow-up study. J Pediatr 2000;136:841–3.

11. Greco L, Mayer M, Ciccarelli G, et al. Compliance to a gluten-free diet in adolescents, or "what do 300 coeliac adolescents eat every day?" Ital J Gastroenterol Hepatol 1997;29:305–10.

12. Kane SV, Cohen RD, Aikens JE, Hanauer SB. Prevalence of nonadherence with maintenance mesalamine in quiescent ulcerative colitis. Am J Gastroenterol 2001;96:2929–33.

13. Kane S, Huo D, Aikens J, Hanauer S. Medication nonadherence and the outcomes of patients with quiescent ulcerative colitis. Am J Med 2003;114:39–43.

14. Fotheringham MJ, Sawyer MG. Adherence to recommended medical regimens in childhood and adolescence. J Pediatr Child Health 1995;31:72–8.

15. Ringewald JM, Gidding SS, Crawford SE, et al. Nonadherence is associated with late rejection in pediatric heart transplant recipients. J Pediatr 2001;139:75–8.

16. Molmenti E, Mazariegos G, Bueno J, et al. Noncompliance after pediatric liver transplantation. Transplant Proc 1999;31:408.

17. Garcia V, Bittar A, Keitel E, et al. Patient noncompliance as a major cause of kidney graft failure. Transplant Proc 1997;29:252–4.

18. Lurie S, Shemesh E, Sheiner PA, et al. Non-adherence in pediatric liver transplant recipients—an assessment of risk factors and natural history. Pediatr Transplant 2000;4:200–6.

19. Johnson SB. Measuring adherence. Diabetes Care 1992;15: 1658–67.

20. Price B. The asthma experience: altered body image and noncompliance. J Clin Nurs 1994;3:139–45.

21. Bille DA. The role of body image in patient compliance and education. Heart Lung 1977;6:143–8.

22. Rayhorn N. Treatment of inflammatory bowel disease in the adolescent. J Infus Nurs 2001;24:255–62.

23. Burney KD, Krishnan K, Ruffin MT, et al. Adherence to single daily dose of aspirin in a chemoprevention trial. An evaluation of self-report and microelectronic monitoring. Arch Fam Med 1996;5:297–300.

24. Waterhouse DM, Calzone KA, Mele C, Brenner DE. Adherence to oral tamoxifen: a comparison of patient self-report, pill counts, and microelectronic monitoring. J Clin Oncol 1993; 11:1189–97.

25. Bender B, Wamboldt FS, O'Connor SL, et al. Measurement of children's asthma medication adherence by self report, mother report, canister weight, and Doser CT. Ann Allergy Asthma Immunol 2000;85:416–21.

26. Inui TS, Carter WB, Pecoraro RE. Screening for noncompliance

27. Dew MA, Roth LH, Thompson ME, et al. Medical compliance and its predictors in the first year after heart transplantation. J Heart Lung Transplant 1996;15:631–45.

28. Freund A, Johnson SB, Silverstein J, Thomas T. Assessing daily management of childhood diabetes using 24-hr recall interviews: reliability and stability. Health Psychol 1991;10: 200–8.

29. Galt KA, Backes J, Sondag LD. Identifying noncompliance by combining refill audits with telephone follow-up. Am J Health Syst Pharm 2000;57:219–20.

30. Choo PW, Rand CS, Inui TS, et al. Validation of patient reports, automated pharmacy records, and pill counts with electronic monitoring of adherence to antihypertensive therapy. Med Care 1999;37:846–57.

31. Shemesh E, Lurie S, Stuber ML, et al. A pilot study of posttraumatic stress and nonadherence in pediatric liver transplant recipients. Pediatrics 2000;105:E29.

32. De Geest S, Abraham I, Dunbar-Jacob J. Measuring transplant patients' compliance with immunosupressive therapy. West J Nurs Res 1996;18:595–605.

33. Rumbo C, Emerick KM, Emre S, Shneider BL. Azathioprine metabolite measurements in the treatment of autoimmune hepatitis in pediatric patients: a preliminary report. J Pediatr Gastroenterol Nutr 2002;35:391–8.

34. Matsui DR. Drug compliance in pediatrics—clinical and research issues. Pediatr Clin North Am 1997;44:1–14.

35. Ley P. Doctor-patient communication: some quantitative estimates of the role of cognitive factors in non-compliance. J Hypertens Suppl 1985;3(1):S51–5.

36. Salas M, In't Veld BA, van der Linden PD, et al. Impaired cognitive function and compliance with antihypertensive drugs in elderly: the Rotterdam Study. Clin Pharmacol Ther 2001;70: 561–6.

37. Hinkin CH, Castellon SA, Durvasula RS, et al. Medication adherence among HIV+ adults: effects of cognitive dysfunction and regimen complexity. Neurology 2002;59:1944–50.

38. Kieckhefer GM, Trahms CM. Supporting development of children with chronic conditions: from compliance toward shared management. Pediatr Nurs 2000;26:354–63.

39. Stone VE, Hogan JW, Schuman P, et al. Antiretroviral regimen complexity, self-reported adherence, and HIV patients' understanding of their regimens: survey of women in the her study. J Acquir Immune Defic Syndr 2001;28:124–31.

40. Schmier JK, Leidy NK. The complexity of treatment adherence in adults with asthma: challenges and opportunities. J Asthma 1998;35:455–72.

41. Ammassari A, Murri R, Pezzotti P, et al. Self-reported symptoms and medication side effects influence adherence to highly active antiretroviral therapy in persons with HIV infection. J Acquir Immune Defic Syndr 2001;28:445–9.

42. Hamano K, Ohta A, Masamura K, et al. Relationship between the experience of steroids side effects and noncompliance with oral steroids treatment in collagen disease patients. Kango Kenkyu 1997;30:47–54.

43. Bjorn I, Backsrom T. Drug related negative side-effects is a common reason for poor compliance in hormone replacement therapy. Maturitas 1999;32:77–86.

44. Richardson JL, Marks G, Levine A. The influence of symptoms of disease and side effects of treatment on compliance with cancer therapy. J Clin Oncol 1988;6:1746–52.

45. Hyder SM, Persson LA, Chowdhury AM, Ekstrom EC. Do side-effects reduce compliance to iron supplementation? A study

among patients with hypertension: is self-report the best available measure? Med Care 1981;19:1061–4.

of daily- and weekly-dose regimens in pregnancy. J Health Popul Nutr 2002;20:175–9.

46. Hsia J, Rodabough R, Rosal MC, et al. Compliance with National Cholesterol Education Program dietary and lifestyle guidelines among older women with self-reported hypercholesterolemia. The Women's Health Initiative. Am J Med 2002;113:384–92.

47. DiMatteo MR, Lepper HS, Croghan TW. Depression is a risk factor for noncompliance with medical treatment: meta-analysis of the effects of anxiety and depression on patient adherence. Arch Intern Med 2000;160:2101–7.

48. Lernmark B, Persson B, Fisher L, Rydelius PA. Symptoms of depression are important to psychological adaptation and metabolic control in children with diabetes mellitus. Diabet Med 1999;16:14–22.

49. DeGroot M, Jacobson AM, Samson JA, Welch G. Glycemic control and major depression in patients with type I and type II diabetes mellitus. J Psychosom Res 1999;46:425–35.

50. Shemesh E, Rudnick A, Kaluski E, et al. A prospective study of posttraumatic stress symptoms and nonadherence in survivors of a myocardial infarction. Gen Hosp Psychiatry 2001;23:215–222.

51. Raiz LR, Kilty KM, Henry ML, Ferguson RM. Medication compliance following renal transplantation. Transplantation 1999;68:51–5.

52. Wilson BM. Promoting compliance: the patient-provider partnership. Adv Ren Replace Ther 1995;2:199–206.

53. Reynaert C, Janne P, Donckier J, et al. Locus of control and metabolic control. Diabete Metab 1995;21:180–7.

54. Gacs G, Hosszu E. The effect of socio-economic conditions on the time of diagnosis and compliance during treatment in growth hormone deficiency. Acta Paediatr Hung 1991;31:215–21.

55. Reid V, Graham I, Hickey N, Mulcahy R. Factors affecting dietary compliance in coronary patients included in a secondary prevention programme. Hum Nutr Appl Nutr 1984;38:279–87.

56. Shobhana R, Begum R, Snehalatha C, et al. Patients' adherence to diabetes treatment. J Assoc Physicians India 1999;47:1173–5.

57. Swanson MA, Palmeri D, Vossler ED, et al. Noncompliance in organ transplant recipients. Pharmacotherapy 1991;11:173S–4S.

58. Morse EV, Simon PM, Coburn M, et al. Determinants of subject compliance within an experimental anti-HIV drug protocol. Soc Sci Med 1991;32:1161–7.

59. Rorer B, Tucker CM, Blake H. Long-term nurse-patient interactions: factors in patient compliance or noncompliance to the dietary regimen. Health Psychol 1988;7:35–46.

60. Wilson BM. Promoting compliance: the patient-provider partnership. Adv Ren Replace Ther 1995;2:199–206.

61. Katz RC, Ashmore J, Barboa E, et al. Knowledge of disease and dietary compliance in patients with end-stage renal disease. Psychol Rep 1998;82:331–6.

62. Abercrombie PD. Improving adherence to abnormal Pap smear follow-up. J Obstet Gynecol Neonatal Nurs 2001;30:80–8.

63. Bender BG. Overcoming barriers to nonadherence in asthma treatment. J Allergy Clin Immunol 2002;109(6 Suppl):S554–9.

64. Becker DM, Allen JK. Improving compliance in your dyslipidemic patient: an evidence-based approach. J Am Acad Nurs Pract 2001;13:200–7.

65. Lemanek KL, Kamps J, Chung NB. Empirically supported treatments in pediatric psychology: regimen adherence. J Pediatr Psychol 2001;26:253–75.

66. Dunbar-Jacob J, Erlen JA, Schlenk EA, et al. Adherence in chronic disease. Annu Rev Nurs Res 2000;18:48–90.

67. Nigro G, Angelini G, Grosso SB, et al. Psychiatric predictors of noncompliance in inflammatory bowel disease: psychiatry and compliance. J Clin Gastroenterol 2001;32:66–8.

CHAPTER 77

MANAGEMENT OF SURGICAL PATIENTS

1. *Complications after Gastrointestinal Surgery: A Medical Perspective*

Samuel Nurko, MD, MPH

Advances in pediatric surgery and in postoperative care have allowed the survival of children who were born with complex congenital anomalies. As more children survive and grow older, new long-term medical problems are arising, and new therapies are often needed. The pediatric gastroenterologist has to deal with some of these specific problems, particularly as they relate to the surgical correction of esophageal, hepatobilliary, intestinal, or anorectal malformations.

The purpose of this chapter is to describe some of the long-term medical complications seen in children after surgery in the alimentary tract. The following discussion deals specifically with representative problems after surgical therapy for gastroesophageal reflux (GER), imperforate anus, and Hirschsprung disease. The long-term problems after the correction of other surgical conditions such as tracheo-esophageal fistulae and hepatobiliary malformations, as well as the treatment of short gut, are dealt with in other chapters.

SURGERY FOR GER

Antireflux surgery is a successful way to treat intractable GER. Fundoplication is the third most commonly performed general surgical procedure in some institutions,[1,2] and the Nissen operation is the most common type performed (Figure 77.1-1).[3,4] In both children and adults, postoperative results after a Nissen operation are satisfactory in 74 to 94% of patients.[1–3,5–7] Operative mortality is low, usually less than 1%.[2] A substantial late death rate (16–24%) has been reported in some series, but this is usually secondary to the underlying diseases.[1–3,6,7]

Even though many centers report excellent results, it is known that antireflux surgery can have a significant amount of side effects, varying from minor to severe (Tables 77.1-1 and 77.1-2).[2,4,8–10] A recent multicenter retrospective review of 7,467 patients (56% neurologically

normal and 44% neurologically abnormal) operated on over 20 years reported that in the neurologically normal children, there was a good to excellent result in 95%, with major complications in 4.2%. These compared with a

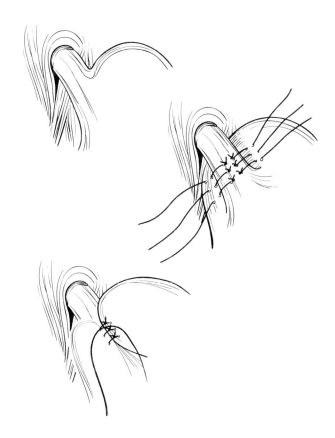

FIGURE 77.1-1 Nissen fundoplication. The fundus of the stomach is seen to be wrapped like a collar around the area of the lower esophageal sphincter. Adapted from Smout AJ, Akkermans LM. Normal and disturbed motility of the gastrointestinal tract. Petersfield, Hampshire (UK): Biomedical Publishing; 1992.

TABLE 77.1-1   LONG-TERM COMPLICATIONS AFTER
                FUNDOPLICATION

Small intestinal obstruction
Recurrence of symptoms and reappearance of gastroesophageal reflux
Dysphagia
Gas bloat syndrome
Herniation of the wrap
Fistula formation
Dumping syndrome

reported 84.6% good result in those with neurologic problems and a complication rate of 12.8%. The most common complications reported were recurrent reflux from wrap disruption in 7.1%, respiratory symptoms in 4.4%, gas bloat in 3.6%, and intestinal obstruction in 2.6%. Postoperative deaths occurred in 0.07% of normal versus 0.8% of neurologically abnormal children, whereas the incidence of reoperation was 3.6% in normal and 11.8% in neurologically abnormal patients.[2]

Children with underlying neurologic abnormalities have a higher incidence of complications.[1,2,4,8,11–14] Some authors have suggested that they have more than twice the complication rate, three times the morbidity, and four times the reoperation rate.[4,14] Some authors have attempted to do a direct comparison of the outcome between children with and without neurologic problems. Dedinsky and colleagues reported a large series of 429 fundoplications, of which 297 were done in children who were neurologically impaired.[15] This last group accounted for all 4 postoperative deaths, 24 of 28 wrap herniations, and most of the reoperations. Similar findings were reported by Pearl and colleagues when they compared the outcome in 81 normal children with the outcome in 153 patients who were neurologically impaired.[14] They showed that there was a morbidity of 12% versus 24%, a rate of reoperation for a failed fundoplication in 5% versus 19%, and an aspiration-induced mortality of 1% versus 9%. Because of all of the above findings, it has even been suggested that neurologic status is the major predictive factor of failure of antireflux surgery in children.[14]

Another high-risk population in which the outcome after fundoplication is not as good as that in neurologically normal children is those patients with esophageal atresia repair.[16] It has been reported that only 40% have excellent results and that many require reoperation.[3,4,17,18] The use of partial wraps has therefore been advocated in these patients.[17]

The surgical approach to children who require fundoplication has been changing in recent years with the advent of minimally invasive surgery.[19] The experience with laparoscopic procedures in children has been accumulating in recent years, and the results are similar to those found in adults.[19–26] Laparoscopic surgery has been successful even in small babies (3 kg), children less than 1 year,[24] children with neurologic problems,[22] and children with respiratory disease.[27] There are no prospective studies in children that have compared the open with the laparoscopic technique. There are limited studies in which the laparoscopic technique has been compared with retrospective "open" procedures.[20] Collins and colleagues, in a cohort of 120 children, compared the operative time, complication rate, and hospital stay between children who had a laparoscopic procedure and a retrospective control group who had undergone an open operation.[20] They found a slightly lower complication rate and a significant decrease in hospitalization after laparoscopy. In a large series of 220 patients aged 5 days to 18 years, an intraoperative complication rate of 2.6% and a postoperative complication rate of 7.3%, which included 7 patients with a breakdown of the fundoplication, 5 patients with gagging and retching, 2 patients with gastroparesis, and 4 patients with severe dysphagia, were reported.[19] It is becoming apparent that laparoscopic fundoplication is the procedure of choice in many centers and is slowly becoming the norm.

The most common problems after fundoplication are shown in Table 77.1-1 and are similar independently if the operation is open or performed laparoscopically.[20,21,28] The physiopathology of these symptoms may be multifactorial, and Table 77.1-2 suggests the different mechanisms by which some of the most common symptoms may be produced.

SMALL BOWEL OBSTRUCTION

This is one of the potentially serious complications after fundoplication.[2,3,15,29–31] Ashcraft reported in a recompilation of series with Nissen fundoplication that from a total of 1,319 patients, 43 had small bowel obstruction (3.2%),[29] and of 7,467 patients, Fonkalsrud and colleagues described it in 2.6%.[2] It has been suggested that the incidence of this complication is higher if other procedures are performed at the same time as the fundoplication. In these instances, the incidence has been reported to be as high as 10% compared with an incidence of 1.8% when only a fundoplication is performed.[29,32] This complication needs to be recognized promptly because it can be associated with significant morbidity and mortality. It has been reported that from one-third to one-fifth of patients who develop intestinal

TABLE 77.1-2   COMMON CLINICAL SYMPTOMS AFTER FUNDOPLICATION AND THE POSSIBILITIES THAT NEED TO BE
                CONSIDERED

VOMITING	DYSPHAGIA	GAS BLOAT	IRRITABILITY
Gastroesophageal reflux	Tight fundoplication	Tight fundoplication	Gastroesophageal reflux
Tight fundoplication	Peptic stricture	Delayed gastric emptying	Wrap herniation
Wrap herniation	Primary motility problem	Impaired gastric accommodation	Dumping syndrome
Small bowel obstruction		Visceral hyperalgesia	Small bowel obstruction
		Small bowel obstruction	Visceral hyperalgesia

obstruction may die if it is not promptly recognized. It can occur in the immediate postoperative period or many years thereafter. This complication has to be suspected when there is abdominal distention and pain, persistent vomiting (if the fundoplication is loose enough), and evidence of obstruction. Sometimes it is difficult to diagnose, particularly in severely impaired patients or when the patient cannot vomit, so there has to be a high index of suspicion. A delay in diagnosis and treatment will inevitably lead to bowel necrosis and death, and the treatment is surgical.

REAPPEARANCE OF GER

The return of symptoms compatible with GER usually indicates that the operation has failed. The incidence of GER can occur in the immediate postoperative period (surgical failure) or much later. The information about surgical failure is limited. In one series of 385 children evaluated by pH probe within 12 weeks postoperatively, GER was documented in 2.9%.[33] Most late cases in which symptoms recur happen in the first 1 to 2 years after the operation,[2,6,31] and it has been reported that in up to one-third of patients, the symptoms of GER become apparent after an episode of forceful emesis.[31] The incidence varies among series. It was described in 7.1% of 7,467 patients[2] and in 29 (12%) of 242 patients.[13]

Caniano and colleagues were able to identify the cause for the appearance of recurrent GER in 86% of children in their series: "slipped" fundoplication in 15, no fundoplication visualized in 2, and paraesophageal hernia in 1.[31] It is not known why wrap disruption occurs, but mental retardation, pulmonary dysfunction, and the presence of a seizure disorder are all risk factors.[13] It is also possible that the surgical technique may also have an influence, with the possibility that an inadequate mobilization of the gastroesophageal junction, fundus, and cardia has occurred, particularly in children with increased intra-abdominal pressure owing to movement disorders, aerophagia, or constipation.[13]

If the patient returns with symptoms that are compatible with reflux, an upper gastrointestinal (UGI) series needs to be obtained (Figure 77.1-2). The presence or absence of the wrap should be determined, and the functional integrity can be grossly examined. If there is evidence of wrap disruption (see Figure 77.1-2B) and of free-flowing reflux, it can be assumed that the fundoplication is not working, and antireflux therapy should be initiated. If it is necessary to judge the state of the esophageal mucosa, an endoscopy can then be performed. If, on the other hand, the UGI seems to show an intact wrap (see Figure 77.1-2A) and no evidence of GER, a pH probe study or an esophageal impedance will actually show the amount of reflux the patient is experiencing and give an assessment of acid clearance. An endoscopic procedure will then show if there has been esophageal damage. There is no need to perform esophageal manometry in these patients. Manometric studies should be performed, however, if a new surgical procedure is being contemplated or if there is the possibility that the patient has a primary esophageal motility disorder.

Once the diagnosis of recurrent GER is made, aggressive medical therapy needs to be instituted,[4,10] and a trial of gastrojejunal feeds may be necessary in those patients at risk of pulmonary complications, particularly in children with severe neurologic problems (see Figure 77.1-2).

If the reflux proves to be refractory, the patient seems to be aspirating, or new complications arise (eg, Barrett esophagus), a reoperation should be considered. In cases in which the main indication of a failed fundoplication and the need for reoperation is the presence of respiratory problems, a full assessment of oral motor function needs to be done because some of the symptoms may be due to inability to handle oral secretions, particularly in neurologically impaired children. The use of jejunal feedings can be used as a therapeutic trial before a reoperation is performed. Also, in those high-risk patients with recurrent GER and aspiration secondary to poor oral-motor function, the long-term use of jejunal feedings may be the best option because the performance of a fundoplication may alter esophageal clearance of saliva and exacerbate the problem. This is particularly important in patients with documented esophageal dysmotility.

Wheatley and colleagues described their experience in the treatment of 29 patients with recurrent GER after fundoplication.[13] They found that medical management was successful in controlling the symptoms in 11 of 29 (38%) patients. In another study, Caniano and colleagues reported that 21 of 364 (6%) patients who had a fundoplication required a reoperation because of GER recurrence.[31]

DYSPHAGIA

Dysphagia has been the most common problem after the Nissen operation and the symptom most commonly associated with long-term unsatisfactory results.[5,6,34] Some authors have suggested that more than 50% of patients have some degree of solid food dysphagia even after a follow-up of 20 years, but most report an incidence that varies from 0 to 40%.[6,35] The exact incidence of postoperative dysphagia is difficult to establish, but it has been suggested that its prevalence is higher in those children who have undergone a Nissen fundoplication when compared with those who have undergone fundoplications that are considered "more floppy," such as Thal, Toupet, or Rosetti.[36] In the largest pediatric series of 7,467 patients, dysphagia attributed to esophageal obstruction was reported in 2.4%.[2]

The dysphagia may be related to either a wrap that is too tight around an esophagus with good peristaltic function or secondary to a functional obstruction created by the inability of a damaged esophagus to produce enough force to propel the food into the stomach (see Table 77.1-2 and Figure 77.1-2A).

The role that preoperative esophageal peristalsis plays in the development of dysphagia has been controversial.[34,37] It has been suggested that even though there are no prospective data, care should be exercised when a fundoplication is performed in patients with abnormal esophageal peristalsis.[34,37] Low and colleagues reported in a series of patients who underwent secondary operations

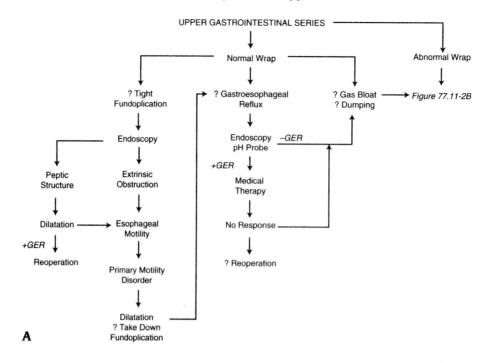

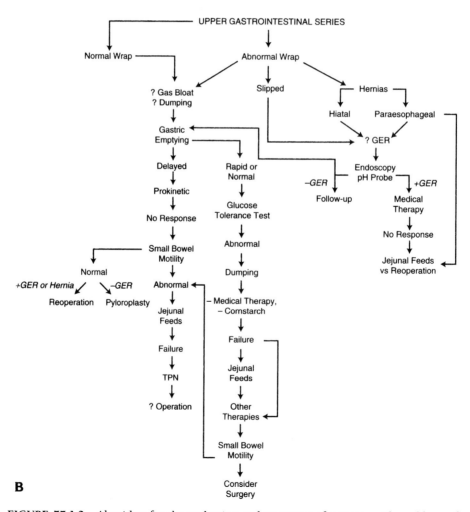

FIGURE 77.1-2   Algorithm for the evaluation and treatment of patients with problems after fundoplication. *A*, An approach in which the upper gastrointestinal series (UGI) has shown the presence of a normal wrap. *B*, This figure focuses on patients in whom the UGI has shown an abnormal wrap. GER = gastroesophageal reflux; TPN = total parenteral nutrition.

for failed Nissen procedures that six patients presenting with severe postoperative dysphagia had evidence of primary esophageal motility disorders (four with collagen vascular diseases and two with achalasia) that were not diagnosed before surgery,[38] indicating the importance of assessing esophageal motility before the operation.[37] In children, this problem is commonly found after patients with scleroderma or tracheoesophageal fistulae have undergone fundoplications.[17] Also, because of the possibility of creating a functional obstruction in a dysmotil esophagus, an esophageal motility test should be performed before the operation in those children in whom esophageal dysfunction is suspected.[37]

The relationship between preoperative esophageal motor abnormalities and postoperative dysphagia has been questioned.[34,39,40] A study after a laparoscopic Nissen operation in 81 adults who had baseline esophageal motility showed no difference in the prevalence of dysphagia up to a year after the operation (12.5% vs 15%) when comparing the 48 patients with normal motility with the 33 patients with abnormal esophageal function.[34] The authors suggested that there was poor correlation between the preoperative manometry and outcome and that abnormal esophageal peristalsis is not a contraindication to performing the operation.[34] Another recent prospective randomized clinical trial of 200 patients randomized either to Nissen (360°) or Toupet fundoplication (270°) studied esophageal motility before and after the surgery. They found that preoperative esophageal dismotility reflected more severe disease but did not affect postoperative clinical outcome. In 85%, the motility remained unchanged because it was not corrected by the fundoplication (independent of the surgical procedure performed). In 20 patients, the motility improved, whereas in 9 patients, it worsened. The authors concluded that preoperative esophageal dysmotility requires no tailoring of the surgical management.[39]

The dysphagia in many cases is transitory[5] but at times can be very severe, leading to significant dietary restrictions. The presence of dysphagia in the immediate postoperative period may be secondary to edema or transient esophageal hypoperistalsis (particularly if the operation is performed through the thoracic approach).[3] The management has to be conservative, allowing time for the edema to subside. However, if the dysphagia persists or is severe, it may be necessary to consider that the operation is too tight, and further evaluation will be necessary.

The best way to investigate patients with dysphagia is to perform a barium study to fully assess the anatomy (see Figure 77.1-2A). This study will help delineate the wrap and assess if there is obstruction. It can also detect the presence of peptic strictures. A better functional assessment of emptying can be performed with esophageal scintigraphy and can be a useful way to follow patients if dilatations are performed. An esophageal motility should be performed in cases with severe symptoms. This allows the definition of lower esophageal pressure and identifies the presence or lack of peristalsis. Endoscopy may be useful to assess if there is fibrosis or other complications from GER (eg, peptic stricture, esophagitis, Barrett adenocarcinoma). If there

is evidence of poor emptying and primary motility disorders, attempts to lower the functional obstruction should be undertaken. If the motility is normal, dilatation should be attempted, and if dilatation is necessary soon after the operation, great caution needs to be exerted because it has been shown that if done forcefully, it can lead to disruption of the repair.[35] The results after endoscopic dilatation in adults have been satisfactory.[35] In a series of 35 patients, dysphagia resolved in 52%, and there were no disruptions of the fundoplictions or GER. The results varied according to the radiologic appearance of the fundoplication. In those patients with a slipped operation, endoscopy relieved the dysphagia in only 27%, as opposed to 67% of those with intact fundoplication.[35] If symptoms persist after dilatation or the patient has other symptoms associated with a tight wrap (such as gas bloat), a revision of the surgery may be necessary. In general, this is not very common. Spitz and colleagues reported that only 1.2% of patients required a reoperation because of dysphagia.[12]

GAS BLOAT SYNDROME

Gas bloat syndrome is characterized by distention, inability to vomit, abdominal pain, and, in children, severe retching, gagging, and irritability.[11] Its duration is variable, but it can last for many hours and be severe enough for patients to seek medical attention. Many long-term studies of patients who have undergone Nissen fundoplication have reported that gas bloat syndrome can occur from 2.8%[3] to 50%[6] of cases. The exact incidence of this problem is difficult to assess, particularly because some surgeons routinely add a decompression gastrostomy at the time of the operation.[29] In one study of 106 patients, 2 required the placement of a late gastrostomy because of this problem,[41] and Fonkalsrud and colleagues reported that even though they routinely use a gastrostomy in children less than 3 years, gas bloat still developed in 12 patients following removal of the tube.[42] The problem with gastric distention cannot be minimized because it has been reported that death can occur secondary to gastric necrosis.[43] In their report of 7,467 patients, Fonkalsrud and colleagues reported gas bloat syndrome in 3.6% (2–10%) and suggested that the incidence was higher in those centers in which the gastric emptying procedure was rarely used.[2]

The physiopathology is not well characterized.[6] Patients who develop the syndrome tend to have GER associated with activation of the emetic reflex (pallor, sweating, retching, and forceful vomiting).[11] Most likely it is related to the presence of an increased amount of gastric air,[44] compounded by an inability to vomit or belch, impaired gastric accommodation,[5,45] gastric hypersensitivity,[5] and slow gastric emptying.[3,5,6]

It has been shown that many children with gas bloat syndrome have delayed gastric emptying (see Figure 77.1-2B).[3] In a retrospective review of fundoplications performed in 92 patients with delayed gastric emptying, the authors compared the outcome between those who also had a gastric emptying procedure and those who did not. They showed a higher incidence of recurrent reflux in those without a gastric emptying procedure (35 vs 18%).[46] Because of the possibility of this association, the performance of a pyloroplasty in conjunction with a fundoplication has been suggested when delayed gastric emptying is found preoperatively.[3,13,47]

It has also been shown that fundoplication may induce gastric myoelectrical disturbances that may correlate with the development of retching.[48] In one study, the authors showed that children who retch preoperatively were three times more likely to retch after the operation and that 25% of neurologically impaired children may start to retch after the operation. Sixty percent of neurologically impaired children had gastric dysrhythmias before the operation compared with 20% of neurologically normal children. These findings suggest a loss of central inhibitory mechanisms that may result in the inappropriate activation of the emetic reflex, which may be heightened by antireflux surgery.[48]

The role that small bowel motility plays in the development of this symptom is also not clear. In one study, 25 of 28 symptomatic children after fundoplication had abnormalities in antroduodenal motility. The most common abnormality found was an absence of the migrating motor complex in 12 children, whereas 6 children had postprandial hypomotility; other nonspecific abnormalities included clustered, retrograde, and tonic contractions.[49] It is unclear if the abnormalities were present before the operation or are a result of it, although the authors suggested that because the abnormalities found were similar to those seen in chronic intestinal pseudo-obstruction, it is likely that they predated the operation, suggesting that those children had a more generalized gastrointestinal dysfunction and not only GER. In that case, the performance of a fundoplication, with the elimination of the ability to vomit, could be expected to worsen symptoms such as retching and abdominal distention. This observation needs to be taken into account when the performance of a fundoplication is being considered in children with generalized symptoms of gastrointestinal dysfunction, and an antroduodenal motility may be a useful test to perform in those cases before the operation to exclude the possibility of pseudo-obstruction.

Recently, it has been suggested that gastric hypersensitivy may also play a role. Studies using the Barostat technique have documented that adult patients after fundoplication may have a lower threshold for postprandial discomfort and abnormal gastric postprandial relaxation.[5,50] This represents an emerging field of study, and treatments to decrease the hyperalgesia may be needed.

The medical therapy for gas bloat syndrome has included the use of motility and simethicone-containing agents. Cisapride has been used with success, particularly in children with delayed gastric emptying. Attempts to decrease air swallowing should be undertaken, and the status of vagal function can be determined by using sham feeding or Congo red testing. The tests have been found to be useful in adults, but no information is available in children.[6]

The inability to vomit and belch is rarely incapacitating enough to require another operation. At times, it may be necessary to perform a temporary gastrostomy.[3] It has been

reported that the symptoms disappear if the fundoplication is undone, although if the patient has underlying dysmotility or there was vagal nerve damage, they may persist after reoperation.[29] If there is evidence of delayed gastric emptying, it is possible to consider the performance of a pyloroplasty[3,42] without taking down the fundoplication (see Figure 77.1-2B).

Treatments to decrease the gastric hyperalgesia and improve gastric accommodation may be beneficial.[5] Because 5-hydroxytryptamine (HT)$_1$ receptors may be involved in gastric accommodation,[51] the use of 5-HT$_1$ agonists may be attempted. Cyproheptadine may be tried. In adults, 5-HT$_{1D}$ agonists such as sumatriptan or 5-HT$_{1DA}$ agonists such as buspirone have been attempted with some success in patients with dyspepsia as a way to increase postprandial fundic relaxation.[5,51,52] The visceral hyperalgesia may also be treated with medications such as anticholinergic agents.[5] Because tricyclic antidepressants such as amitriptyline have been shown to be useful in the treatment of the visceral hyperalgesia that can be seen in functional bowel disorders in adults,[5,53] they may be useful in children with severe hyperalgesia postfundoplication.[5] Future studies with new medications that change the threshold of sensation, such as 5-HT$_3$ antagonists or 5-HT$_4$ agonists, will be conducted in the coming years and will determine if these medications will be useful in the treatment of these children.[5]

HERNIAS AND OTHER PROBLEMS WITH THE FUNDOPLICATION

Herniation of the fundoplication is another common complication, and it represents the most common indication for late reoperation. Spitz and colleagues described their findings during reoperation of those patients in whom the initial operation failed and found that the most frequent finding in 25 patients (14%) was a prolapse of the wrap into the posterior mediastinum through an enlarged hiatus with or without a paraesophageal hernia.[12] In only two patients, the wrap was too tight, and in only two patients, the wrap was partially disrupted, leading to recurrent reflux. There are two principal types of herniation distinguished by the localization of the gastroesophageal junction.[54] In the first type, there is herniation of the entire wrap and gastroesophageal junction into the chest,[54] usually presenting as recurrent GER, and in the second or paraesophageal type, there is a posterolateral herniation of a portion of the wrap, with the gastroesophageal junction remaining within the abdomen (see Figure 77.1-2B). This latter type seems not to be associated with reflux but has the risk of incarceration/strangulation or bleeding.[30]

It can be argued that the herniation of the entire wrap usually indicates a failure of the surgery. Some studies, however, have shown that not all patients with this problem have recurrent symptoms of reflux.[6] If this type of hernia is found, the patient needs to be worked up for GER, and the presence of other symptoms should be ascertained (see Figure 77.1-2B). In the absence of any significant symptoms or of pathologic reflux, its presence is probably not important, but if significant problems are associated with its presence, a new operation may be necessary.

The significance of a paraesophageal hernia is more important. It is more common,[14] it is the primary reason for reoperation in some series,[3,14,30] and its appearance seems to be related to a failure to perform an adequate crural repair.[13,30,54] Pearl and colleagues reported after doing a recompilation of 2,142 cases postfundoplication that a wrap herniation occurred in 117 cases (18.3%) and accounted for 63% of reoperations.[14] Fonskalrud and colleagues reported that 11 (2.6%) of their patients developed this complication and that all required surgical correction.[42] It has also been reported that in neurologically impaired children, herniation occurred in 38%[14] and that the incidence of wrap breakdown/paraesophageal hernia and small bowel obstruction after Nissen fundoplication in this group of children is disturbingly high.[1,14]

The paraesophageal hernias usually increase over time and can produce symptoms, which may include GER, dysphagia, chest pain, bleeding from the hernia sac, or even ischemia of the gastric segment involving the hernia.[1,14] In smaller children or children with severe neurologic impairment, the only manifestation may be severe irritability. The demonstration of these hernias is done with the performance of a UGI (see Figure 77.1-2B). This test allows the visualization of any obstruction to esophageal emptying and will help delineate gastric anatomy; the presence, status, and location of the fundoplication; and any other gastric problem. Endoscopy may help evaluate the state of the herniated gastric mucosa and if there is ischemic damage.

The treatment of paraesophageal hernias has to be tailored to the individual patient (see Figure 77.1-2B). If there is evidence of recurrence of GER, aggressive medical therapy needs to be started, but if the associated symptoms are severe or there is evidence of inflammation or bleeding in the herniated segment, a reoperation needs to be performed. If the hernia is small and the patient is asymptomatic, conservative management with close follow-up should be undertaken.

FISTULA FORMATION

The performance of a Nissen fundoplication has been associated with the occurrence of fistula formation. The fistulae usually occur between the fundic wrap and other abdominal and mediastinal structures. Gastrodiaphragmatic, gastroaortic, gastrobronchial, gastrocardiac, and gastrocutaneous fistulae have been described.[14,55] The clinical presentation varies depending on the localization of the fistula, but it may be life-threatening when it involves the great vessels. When these are diagnosed, they need to be surgically treated.

DUMPING SYNDROME

Dumping syndrome refers to the symptom complex that results from the rapid transit of food into the small bowel[56–60] and is one of the most common causes of morbidity after gastric surgery.[61] It has been estimated that between 25 and 50% of all patients who have undergone some type of gastric surgery have some symptoms of dumping, although only 1 to 5% have serious disabling symptoms.[58,61] In children, dumping has been described almost exclusively as a postoperative complication of Nissen fundoplication, but the exact incidence is not known.[2,56,57,59–66] In the article by Fonskalrud and colleagues, they described a postoperative transient dumping syndrome in 0.9% of 7,467 fundoplications (0–5%).[2] In a study of 50 patients, Samuk and colleagues reported dumping in 30% (15 patients).[59]

The syndrome is characterized by both gastrointestinal and vasomotor complaints (see Table 77.1-2). Gastrointestinal symptoms include postprandial fullness, crampy abdominal pain, nausea, vomiting, and explosive diarrhea. In younger children, aversion to food, failure to thrive, and retching may be part of the clinical picture.[56,57,60,62] Vasomotor symptoms include diaphoresis, weakness, dizziness, flushing, palpitation, and a desire to lie down. In infants and children, the typical symptoms appear during or after feeding and include irritability, pallor, perspiration, tachycardia, lethargy, diarrhea, and vomiting.

Dumping has been classified into early and late forms based on the timing of onset of symptoms after a meal.[56,57,61] The early symptoms occur soon after eating (10–30 minutes) and can be a mixture of both gastrointestinal and vasomotor complaints. These include abdominal distention and discomfort, nausea, borborygmus, tachycardia, pallor, diaphoresis, somnolence, and, occasionally, syncope.[56–58] The late symptoms, in contrast, are mainly vasomotor and occur from 2 to 3 hours after eating. These include diaphoresis, weakness, dizziness, flushing, palpitations, and, usually, hypoglycemia.[56–58,60,61]

The pathophysiology of dumping syndrome is multifactorial. It seems to be related to alterations in gastric emptying, and its incidence and severity appear to be proportional to the rate of emptying.[56–58,60,61] The symptoms of early dumping are usually produced by the rapid emptying of hyperosmolar chyme into the small bowel. The osmotic effects of these foodstuffs drag large quantities of fluid from the intravascular space into the bowel, resulting in rapid small bowel distention and an increase in both the amplitude and the frequency of bowel contractions.[56,57,60,61] This bowel distention may be responsible for the gastrointestinal symptoms, such as diarrhea, bloating, and crampy abdominal pain. This sequestration of fluid into the bowel depletes circulating blood volume[60,61] and may be responsible for the vasomotor symptoms. The postprandial release of gut hormones is also enhanced,[56–58,60] and the release of enteroglucagon, glucose-dependent insulinotropic peptide, pancreatide polypeptide, vasoactive intestinal polypeptide, gastrin-releasing peptide, serotonin, bradykinin, motilin, and neurotensin is higher in patients with dumping syndrome than in asymptomatic patients after gastric surgery.[61]

Late dumping symptoms seem to be related to the development of hypoglycemia.[56–58,60,62] It has been suggested that the rapid gastric emptying results in the delivery of unusually high concentrations of carbohydrates to the small bowel, leading to hyperglycemia and to an exuberant postprandial insulin release.[58,60] This insulin release results in late hypoglycemia, which leads to vasomotor symptoms.[58,61] The hypoglycemia may persist after the disappearance of the circulating insulin, suggesting that the counterregulatory response to low blood sugar may also be inadequate.[56–58,60]

The reactive hypoglycemia that is observed is probably related to a continuing cellular glucose uptake after insulin has been cleared from the circulation.[58,60] Once the hypoglycemia has developed, spontaneous corrections do not generally occur, particularly in children.[58] Rivkees and Crawford showed that the glucagon levels did not increase in response to hypoglycemia during challenge tests, and their data suggest that the counterregulation was disturbed primarily because of the blunted response of glucagon.[58] This lack of glucagon response may be related to the release of other incretin hormones, such as glucagon-like peptide, which has been shown to be elevated in patients with dumping syndrome. The reactive hypoglycemia may also be related to the ingestion of other dietary components, such as protein.[60]

As can be appreciated, the symptoms of dumping syndrome are nonspecific. The diagnosis has to be suspected in patients who have had a Nissen fundoplication and present with any of the gastrointestinal or vasomotor complaints mentioned above (see Table 77.1-2). The possibility of late hypoglycemia has to be considered, and direct questions about the presence of diaphoresis, irritability, or lethargy need to be asked. In those patients who have a G tube, its position needs to be determined because if the tube has migrated into the duodenum, the patient may present with a dumping-like picture that is related to the administration of the feeds directly into the duodenum.[60] Because of the nonspecific nature of the symptoms, and particularly because dumping can present like other complications mentioned in this chapter, the workup has to include a UGI to evaluate the anatomy and the status of the fundoplication, as well as to establish if a pyloroplasty was performed (see Figure 77.1-2B). The measurement of gastric emptying is very useful.[56] A gastric emptying scan will show a rapid gastric emptying time, although it is worth mentioning that it may be normal if the test meal is of insufficient volume to reproduce the patient's symptoms.[56,59,67]

The measurement of serum glucose in the first hour after meals will usually reveal the presence of hyperglycemia and serves as a good screening measurement. The presence of late hypoglycemia is also an indicator that the patient may be suffering from "late dumping." The diagnosis can be made accurately by using a glucose tolerance test (see Figure 77.1-2B).[56–60,62] Ideally, it can be combined with simultaneous measurements of insulin, so the presence of the hypoglycemia can then be correlated to the insulin levels.

Once the diagnosis has been made, treatment needs to be instituted. Dietary manipulation is the mainstay of therapy and the most effective way to control the symptoms and avoid the late hypoglycemia.[56] When the symptoms are not very severe, it is recommended that the patients eat small frequent "dry" meals and avoid simple sugars. It has also been suggested to add fiber and to increase complex carbo-

hydrates (such as raw vegetables), dietary proteins (such as fish and chicken), and fat (to gain more calories and to decrease gastric emptying).[56,57,59–62] In children, particularly those with neurologic problems and an inability to eat complex meals and those who are fed mainly liquid diets through a gastrostomy tube, the dietary therapy is much more complicated.[60,62] Attempts to reduce the volume of the feeding, either by continuous infusion or by more frequent feedings, should be done first and can be successful in some patients.[58,60] At times, it is necessary to change the feeding regimen and give the infusions over 24 hours because the dumping may reappear if the feeding volume is increased to give only nightly feedings. Taking into account the proposed physiopathology for the occurrence of the delayed hypoglycemia, attempts to reduce the hyperinsulinism have been undertaken.[60] This has been successfully done with the use of formulas with added uncooked cornstarch, which permits the delivery of small amounts of glucose at a steady rate over a long period of time.[60,62,65] Gitzelmann and Hirsig compared the effects of the administration of a formula with cooked or uncooked starch in two infants with dumping and showed that only the uncooked starch controlled the late hypoglycemia and dumping syndrome.[65] Usually, the formula used has to contain the lowest amount of refined carbohydrate, and the uncooked corn starch is added to provide the equivalent to hepatic glucose production,[68] the same way it is added in patients with glycogen storage disease. The use of uncooked cornstarch usually allows the patient to be bolus fed, avoiding the initial hyperglycemia and the delayed hypoglycemia.[60,62,65,69] Other dietary additives, such as pectin, guar gum, and glucomannan, have also been tried.[60,61]

In an effort to reduce late hypoglycemia, acarbose, an α-glucosidase inhibitor, has been used.[57,70] Acarbose delays the conversion of oligosaccharides to monosaccharides and attenuates postprandial increases in blood glucose.[57,70] Ng and colleagues reported on the successful use of acarbose for the treatment of hypoglycemia.[57] They reported six children in whom acarbose was started at 12.5 mg and increased upward until hypoglycemia was controlled. The final dose ranged from 12.5 to 50 mg per feeding. The only side effect was flatulence, but other side effects can include diarrhea and abdominal distention.[57] It is recommended that if acarbose will be used, liver function tests need to be monitored because there have been reports of elevated enzymes during its administration.[57]

Because the physiopathology of dumping is multifactorial, it would be simplistic to think that if one deals only with the glucose homeostasis problems, most of the symptoms, particularly of early dumping, will be controlled. These are probably more related to the duodenal distention and to the gut hormone production mentioned above. Recently, octreotide acetate (Sandoz, East Hanover, NJ), a long-acting somatostatin analogue, has been used with some success in adults with severe dumping syndrome.[61,71] It probably acts by slowing gastric emptying, inhibiting insulin release, and decreasing enteric peptide secretion.[61,71] Several anecdotal reports and four controlled randomized trials have documented the short-term efficacy of octreotide treatment in patients with severe dumping syndrome.[61,71] In general, octreotide improves the symptoms in more than 90% of patients with severe symptoms. In all studies, the acute administration significantly reduced the symptoms and the scores, but it is unclear if the chronic administration will prove to be as beneficial as the acute therapy. No pediatric experience is available in dumping syndrome, but octreotide has been safely used for the treatment of other pediatric conditions, particularly gastrointestinal bleeding.[72]

If the symptoms are severe and intractable, a surgical option may be considered. Many different options have been designed, including procedures to decrease gastric emptying, such as a reconstruction of the pyloroplasty, or if the patient has had a gastroenteroanastomosis, a reduction of the size of the stoma.

REOPERATION FOR FAILED PRIMARY ANTIREFLUX REPAIRS

The selection of patients who need further surgical therapy remains a challenging problem.[2,6,46] Reoperative antireflux surgery is complicated and difficult and should be preceded by a complete investigation to ensure that symptom interpretation is correct and that no other coexistent abnormality in gastric emptying or antroduodenal or esophageal motility exists (see Figure 77.1-2). Preoperative investigation should include UGI, endoscopy, gastric emptying analysis, 24-hour pH probe, and esophageal motility. If a more diffuse motility problem is suspected, an antroduodenal motility test should also be performed, and a glucose tolerance test should be undertaken if dumping is a possibility. An assessment of oral pharyngeal coordination and the ability to swallow needs to be done, and a trial of jejunal feeds should be initiated when it is not clear if the symptoms are related only to GER or also to an inability to handle oral secretions. Frequently, it is beneficial to use jejunal feedings while the patient is being evaluated, and in some children, the use of gastrojejunal tubes may be a good long-term option.[46] Different authors have reported that a second operation is required from 1.6 to 12% in children without other underlying problems,[13,31,46,73] although in neurologically impaired children, the incidence of reoperation has been as high as 16%.[31,73] In a series of 7,467 children, Fonkalsrud and colleagues reported a reoperation rate in 3.6% (2–10%) of neurologically normal children and 11.8% (6–24%) in those with neurologic impairment.[2]

The results of a second operation will also vary depending on the underlying problem. Studies have shown that the increase in preoperative complications, including complete vagotomy, is significantly increased during the second procedure.[38] In children, the incidence of postoperative complications after reoperation also seems to be higher. Caniano and colleagues reported that a second operation was associated with a 14% incidence of intraoperative complications and a 43% incidence of postoperative morbidity.[31] The main complications were prolonged ileus, pneumonia, small bowel obstruction

(19%), wound infection, and pneumothorax, and intraoperative blood loss was substantially higher. Most authors report that for children who have undergone a second operation, the results have also been satisfactory from 70 to 80%.[2,13]

EVALUATION OF PATIENTS WITH PROBLEMS AFTER A FUNDOPLICATION

Table 77.1-2 presents the different possibilities that the clinician needs to entertain when confronted with a patient who has problems after fundoplication. Figure 77.1-2 shows an algorithm for the evaluation and treatment of children who present with complications after fundoplication.

Briefly, after a careful analysis of the symptoms, the workup can start with the performance of a UGI. As shown in Figure 77.1-2A, if there is evidence that the wrap is too tight and that there may be a functional obstruction to esophageal emptying, an endoscopy should be performed to see if there is a peptic stricture or an extrinsic compression. If there is no evidence of stricture, an esophageal motility should be performed to assess the possibility of a primary motility disorder. If after the UGI the wrap is intact and there does not seem to be a functional obstruction, the workup needs to proceed, depending on the main symptoms. If the symptoms are mainly those compatible with recurrence of GER, an endoscopy and pH probe or esophageal impedance should be performed (see Figure 77.1-2A). If, on the other hand, the main symptoms are related to gas bloat or possible dumping, gastric emptying should be performed first (see Figure 77.1-2B).

As shown in the algorithm, if there is evidence of GER, medical therapy should be undertaken, and if there is no response, a new operation should be considered. On the other hand, when evaluating for gas bloat (see Figure 77.1-2B), if the gastric emptying is delayed, a prokinetic agent should be tried. If there is no response, a pyloroplasty can be considered, but a small bowel motility study should be performed first to exclude the presence of pseudo-obstruction. If there is evidence of rapid emptying, the most likely diagnosis is dumping syndrome, and a glucose tolerance test should be done (see Figure 77.1-2B).

As can be appreciated in Figure 77.1-2B, if after the UGI there is evidence that the wrap has either slipped or there is evidence of a hernia, further evaluation for GER or the presence of complications should be undertaken, and if there is evidence of recurrence, bleeding, or mucosal compromise, a reoperation should be performed. In all cases, the administration of jejunal feedings needs to be carefully considered as an alternative to a reoperation, particularly in those children with severe esophageal dysmotility, high surgical risk, or chronic aspiration of their own oral secretions.

HIRSCHSPRUNG DISEASE

Hirschsprung disease is a congenital illness in which varying degrees of aganglionosis occur in distal segments of the intestinal tract.[74] Because these abnormal segments are unable to relax during peristalsis, they are spastic and produce mechanical obstruction.[75–77] The treatment of Hirschsprung disease is surgical.[78–81] The basic principle for definitive surgical therapy is resection of the aganglionic segment followed by a pull-through of ganglionic bowel down to the anus.[75,82] Surgery for Hirschsprung disease generally results in a satisfactory outcome,[79,82,83] and it has been suggested that the outcome after each commonly performed procedure is comparable.[79,82,83] There are, however, some patients who continue to have long-term difficulties (Table 77.1-3). Some studies have suggested that the prevalence of problems is much higher than previously anticipated.[84–87] The most common symptoms are diarrhea, constipation, and, sometimes, intermittent colitis (see Table 77.1-3).[84,87–89]

The most commonly used operations include the Swenson (rectosigmoidectomy), Duhamel (retrorectal transanal pull-through), and Soave (endorectal pull-through) (Figure 77.1-3). In the Swenson pull-through (rectosigmoidectomy), the rectum is removed and the normal ganglionic bowel is anastomosed to a 1 to 2 cm rectal cuff.[76,90,91] It requires a combined abdominoperineal approach, is probably the most difficult, and requires extensive pelvic dissection, so injury to the sacral innervation of the bladder and ejaculatory mechanisms is possible (see Figure 77.1-3). In the Duhamel (retrorectal transanal pull-through) procedure, the aganglionic rectum is left in place, and normal ganglionic bowel is pulled down behind the rectum and through an incision in the posterior rectal wall at the level of the internal sphincter.[92–94] The original Duhamel procedure was an anastomosis of the ganglionated proximal bowel to the closed native rectum at the anal verge. Dilatation of the defunctioned rectum by fecal retention in the blind loop led to the Martin modification, which added a proximal suture anastomosis of anterior native rectum to the pulled-through colon, following which the septum was crushed by a spur clamp.[82] A rectum of expanded size with an anterior aganglionic wall and a posterior ganglionic wall is therefore created.[82] This operation eliminates the need for much of the pelvic dissection needed in the Swenson procedure (see Figure 77.1-3).[94] The endorectal pull-through, as originally described by Soave and modified by

Bole, is the third alternative.[82] In the modified Soave procedure, there is no need to do any pelvic dissection. In this procedure, the mucosal lining of the rectum is removed, the ganglionic colon is pulled through the rectal muscular tube, and a primary anastomosis is done within 1 cm of the anal verge (see Figure 77.1-3).[82,95,96] The modified Soave procedure is easy to perform, and with it there is no need to do any pelvic dissection.

The outcome after these procedures is similar. It is difficult to compare the results obtained with the different operations because they have usually been done by different surgeons, in different institutions, and at different times, and it is possible that the incidence of complications after the different procedures is closely related to the skill of the individual surgeon.[89] There are some reports in which the experience with individual operations performed by the same surgeon have been reported, and these are useful to obtain an idea of the type of long-term complications that

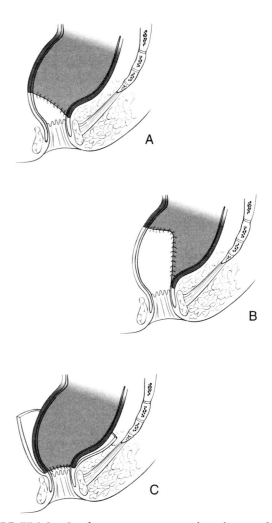

FIGURE 77.1-3 Graphic representation in lateral view of the three major operative procedures for Hirschsprung disease. *A*, Swenson; *B*, Duhamel/Martin; *C*, Soave/Boley. The unshaded native rectum is aganglionic, and the shaded pulled-through bowel contains ganglion cell. Adapted from Philippart AI.[82]

TABLE 77.1-3   COMMON SYMPTOMS AFTER REPAIR OF HIRSCHSPRUNG DISEASE

OBSTRUCTION
Anatomic
Anal stenosis
Functional
    Residual aganglionosis
    New aganglionosis
    Neuronal intestinal dysplasia
    Dysmotility

FECAL INCONTINENCE
Overflow incontinence from constipation
Abnormal sphincteric function after surgery
Diarrhea

ENTEROCOLITIS
Bacterial
Clostridium difficile
Other

can be seen with them. In a large multicenter report of 880 Swenson procedures that spanned four decades, it was reported that there was a 1% mortality, with a 6% incidence of an anastomotic leak and a late incidence of strictures of 8%.[97] Soiling was significant in 13%, and in 39%, enterocolitis was observed, leading to a 7% incidence of secondary sphincterotomies. They reported that 20 years after the operation, 90% had satisfactory bowel function.

There are several studies that describe the long-term results after Duhamel.[98–99] Ehrenpreis and colleagues reported their long-term experience after the Duhamel procedure.[98,99] The overall mortality rate in 352 operations was 2.8%, of which the late mortality was 1.1%. The most common postoperative complication was fecaloma formation, particularly in the early periods after the operation. In their first follow-up report, they found a fecaloma in 9 of 30 patients and fecal incontinence in 12 of 30 patients.[98] On long-term follow-up, however, 15 years later, fecaloma formation was not a significant problem (1/10), and fecal incontinence had decreased to 2 of 30 patients.[74] These findings suggest that over time, patients who undergo the Duhamel procedure tend to improve. In a recent long-term study, 91 children post–Duhamel procedure were compared with 22 healthy children. Outcome scores were significantly worse in the Hirschsprung disease group, and only 42% of patients overall and 79% of those above 14 years had a satisfactory outcome.[100] Some have suggested that the Duhamel procedure is associated with less risk of overall complications but may have a greater risk for postoperative enterocolitis.[92]

Tariq and colleagues described their long-term experience after the Soave procedure.[96] They described the follow-up of 53 survivors, and 18% had diarrhea with intermittent incontinence and 9.4% required a second pull-through, in this case a Duhamel procedure. Other series have described that up to 22% of the patients suffered from constipation at 3 years, with 18% with diarrhea and incontinence, although 82% had a satisfactory result.[101] After endorectal pull-through, it has also been reported that anastomotic stenosis occurs with an incidence that varies from 9 to 24%[96,101,102] and that even after dilatation, a mild residual stricture persists in 3%.[101]

As can be appreciated, it is difficult to directly compare the results of various operations. There are few truly comparative studies. Probably the largest compilation of patients, 1,196 children, and comparison between treatments were reported by Kleinhaus and colleagues.[89] They obtained information in an extensive survey of the members of the surgical section of the American Academy of Pediatrics. They reported results in 390 patients after the Swenson procedure, 339 patients after the Duhamel procedure, and 187 patients after the modified Soave procedure. Complications after the procedures included a disrupted anastomosis in 11.2% after the Swenson, 2.4% after the Duhamel, and 5.8% after the Soave procedure. This carried a mortality of 11% after the Swenson procedure, and 27% of patients with disrupted anastomosis after the Swenson procedure required a major surgical procedure. Anal stenosis was mild (requiring only dilatation) in 5.2% after the

Swenson, 2.9% after the Duhamel, and 5.2% after the Soave procedure and severe (requiring reoperation) in 4.3%, 2.6%, and 4.2%, respectively. After the Swenson procedure, there was a 15.6% incidence of postoperative enterocolitis and 3.2% of incontinence compared with 5.9% and 1.1% after the Duhamel procedure and 2.1% and 1.1% after the Soave procedure.

Most studies report short-term follow-up, and there are few long-term studies. Long-term survival is excellent, although sudden death from enterocolitis may occur years after successful surgical reconstruction.[103,104] Most series describe an overall good outcome in more than 90% of the patients, but many recent studies have shown a higher than anticipated incidence of problems, particularly persistent obstruction, fecal incontinence, or enterocolitis (see Table 77.1-3),[75,79,84,105] and they seem to indicate that any operation is associated with long-term morbidity.[100,106,107] In a series that followed patients from 1 to 30 years, Mishalany and Wooley reported the follow-up of 62 patients, of whom 14 had a Duhamel, 15 a Swenson, and 33 a Soave pull-through.[88] Approximately 23 to 50% felt that they had normal bowel movements, and the rest had various degrees of problems in defecation. Subjectively, half of the patients in the Duhamel and Soave groups and one-third in the Swenson group considered their stooling pattern normal. Of the whole group, 18 had one bowel movement per day, 15 had one every other or more days, and 29 had an increased frequency ranging from 2 to 7 per day. In 20 patients, there was evidence of postoperative enterocolitis, regardless of the type of operation (3 after the Duhamel, 7 after the Swenson, and 11 after the Soave procedure). Another study of the long-term quality of life in 178 patients showed that 76% had between one and five stools a day and 58% had normal stool consistency.[79] Full fecal continence was present in 75%, whereas 19% had minor degrees of leakage, and the rest had severe problems. The degree of stool control improved with age. Whereas 52% were fully continent below 4 years of age, 87.5% between age 9 and 12 years had full control. Neurologic impairment and length of the aganglitic segment beyond the rectosigmoid appeared to influence functional outcome. Enterocolitis was present in 16% at presentation and in 6% postoperatively. The long-term functional results were comparable for the Soave and Duhamel procedures, but children after the Swenson procedure had less favorable results. Growth was similar to the normal population, although younger patients had a tendency to be smaller. Delayed developmental milestones were present in 8%. Satisfactory school performance was achieved in 74%. Ninety-four percent of the patients appeared to be well adjusted, and five patients had severe behavioral problems. After the Soave procedure, there was a lower incidence of constipation, sexual dysfunction, and micturition problems. Duhamel patients tended to have more constipation, whereas the Swenson procedure was associated with more abdominal distention, micturition problems, and cuff strictures.

In another long-term study of 19 adolescents, it was found that 32% had significant impairment of continence but no more psychopathology or psychosocial dysfunction when compared with healthy controls. Fecal incontinence was associated with poorer psychosocial functioning and parental criticism, and psychosocial functioning was significantly correlated with the degree of fecal incontinence.[106] Another long-term follow-up of 45 patients after the Swenson procedure showed that 51.1% had bowel dysfunction, with 37.8% suffering from fecal soiling. Because of poor fecal continence, 55.7% had to restrict their foods, 13.3% had school absence, and 15.6% had problems with peer relationships.[84]

COMMON PROBLEMS FOUND AFTER SURGICAL TREATMENT FOR HIRSCHSPRUNG DISEASE

OBSTRUCTIVE SYMPTOMS

From the postoperative symptoms that can be found in children who have undergone surgical treatment for Hirschsprung disease, the presence of recurrent obstruction is one of the most common and difficult to manage (see Table 77.1-3).[75] Obstructive symptoms may be related either to an anatomic problem that is producing an obstruction[108] or to functional alterations (Figure 77.1-4).[79,109]

The most common anatomic problem that can be encountered is the presence of anal stenosis.[79,89] This complication seems to be more common after Soave pull-through and can usually be managed only with a dilatation program, although a secondary surgical procedure may be necessary.[89] Kleinhaus and colleagues reported that anal stenosis occurred in 5.2% after the Swenson procedure, 2.9% after the Duhamel procedure, and 19% after the Soave procedure.[89] The incidence of reoperation because of

the presence of stenosis also varied between techniques, being 4.3%, 2.6%, and 5.2% after the Swenson, Duhamel, and Soave procedures, respectively. Postoperative strictures can also occur at other sites, particularly in the segment that has been pulled through. These are most likely related to ischemic events; they respond rarely to dilatation and usually require surgical correction.

Most patients with obstructive symptoms do not have stenosis. A variety of functional problems that can be found are related to the residual abnormal function of the intestine after surgical correction (see Figure 77.1-4).[79,106] Moore and colleagues found that of 107 patients followed for at least 4 years, 14.9% had recurrent episodes of gaseous distention and symptoms suggestive of persisting obstruction in the absence of an anatomically defined problem.[83]

The first consideration must be that the patient continues to have the presence of residual aganglionosis because of an inadequate initial repair. The exact incidence of this complication is difficult to establish because it depends on the surgeon and the surgical technique. Soave found that in 5 of 271 patients, the aganglionic segment was not completely removed proximally at the time of the initial operation.[102] This possibility needs to be excluded early in the evaluation of these children, and a barium enema will show if there is evidence of a transition zone. Often it is necessary to perform rectal biopsies to establish the presence of ganglion cells. It is important to remember that in some corrective surgeries, such as the Duhamel, a piece of aganglionic segment is always left as part of the surgical technique, so I recommend obtaining biopsies in all four quadrants. It can therefore be appreciated that the decision about what to do if there are no ganglion cells in the biopsies depends on the type of initial operation that the patient

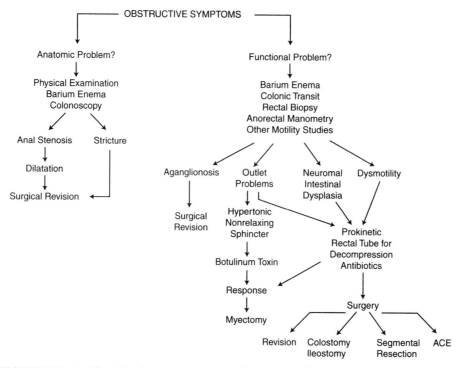

FIGURE 77.1-4   Algorithm for the evaluation and treatment of patients with obstructive symptoms after surgical repair for Hirschsprung disease. ACE = antegrade colonic enemas.

underwent. If there is evidence that a full aganglionic segment was left behind, the treatment needs to be surgical.

The finding of acquired or secondary aganglionosis following pull-through procedures is a rare occurrence, but it has been well described.[83,110] The patients described have developed obstructive symptoms that on evaluation were found to have aganglionosis in a pulled-through bowel that had previously been found to have ganglion cells. This complication has been reported following any of the different corrective procedures,[110] and it should be considered in any patient operated on for Hirschsprung disease in whom recurrent or obstructive symptoms persist. Multiple theories have been proposed for this development, but most authors believe that it is secondary to an increased susceptibility of neural tissues (including the plexuses of ganglion cells) to a hypoxic insult.[83,110] An alternative explanation is that there is postoperative cell death caused by the pull-through of abnormally innervated bowel (eg, the transitional zone or neuronal intestinal dysplasia [NID]).[109] If aganglionosis is suspected, a barium enema may show a transition zone, and rectal suction biopsies at different levels will be necessary to confirm it.

Some reports have suggested that NID type B may be present in more than 20% of cases with Hirschsprung disease.[83,109,111–114] Anorectal manometry is not useful in the diagnosis of NID,[115,116] so a full-thickness rectal biopsy is necessary.[111] The value of a suction rectal biopsy for the diagnosis of NID is controversial, and recent studies have shown that they may not be useful in its recognition.[111,117] Furthermore, there is still controversy regarding the significance of NID or if it truly represents a distinct clinicopathologic entity.[111,114,117] Of 47 cases of Hirschsprung disease, Hanimann and colleagues reported that 11 patients (23%) had associated NID and that after a mean follow-up of 5 years, there were no differences in the symptoms when comparing patients with NID with those without it.[112] Recent studies have reported that histologic criteria were not helpful in predicting clinical outcome and suggested that the finding of NID should not influence clinical management.[111,117]

Independent of the controversy, it is clear that some children may have abnormalities in the histologic examination of the residual colon and that these histologic abnormalities may be associated with symptoms.[113,117,118] Therefore, in children with obstructive symptoms after operation, it is advisable to perform a full-thickness rectal biopsy and to stain it with acetylcholinesterase or other special stainings. In these children, conservative management is indicated.[111,115,116] However, if symptoms are severe and dysmotility is clearly associated with the abnormal segment, surgical resection may be necessary.[118,119]

Persistent internal anal sphincter (IAS) dysfunction is another reason for the obstructive symptoms. This dysfunction is sometimes referred to as "internal sphincter achalasia"[120] and is related to specific abnormalities in IAS innervation. Some studies suggest that there is an intrinsic problem in the IAS in which there is an inability to respond to nitric oxide.[77] The above finding, namely that nitric oxide fails to relax the IAS of patients with Hirschsprung disease,

suggests that a primary defect within or around the myocytes of the sphincter and a separate abnormality of the IAS is compatible with some of the long-term obstructive symptoms that are frequently seen.[77,79,86,120,121] It is possible that the IAS pressure produces a functional outflow obstruction that, with time, leads to colonic dilatation and a less efficient peristalsis to expel stool.[83,120,122] The persistent chronic obstruction from the IAS may also lead to recurrent enterocolitis or bacterial overgrowth with stasis.[83,120,122] It is sometimes difficult to establish who are the patients in whom the symptoms are related to IAS problems. In one study in which children with obstructive symptoms were compared with those without symptoms, IAS pressure and other manometric findings were the same.[83] In some patients with obstructive symptoms, however, the high-pressure zone was longer, the sphincter pressure was higher, and there was evidence of prolonged transit times.[83] Because of these sphincteric abnormalities, some authors have suggested that an internal sphincter myotomy or myectomy needs to be performed in those patients with postoperative obstructive symptoms that have not responded to medical management.[100,22,123] Myectomy has been shown to significantly decrease IAS pressure.[123] Even though the initial experience reported a poor response after myectomy,[96] recent reports have shown it to be useful in the treatment of these children.[122,123] Sphincter-dividing procedures are not always effective; they affect the sphincter permanently and can rarely be associated with fecal incontinence. There is now growing experience that the injection of intrasphincteric botulinum toxin (Botox) can be used to temporarily decrease the pressure of the sphincter.[86,120] The mechanism of action of *Clostridium botulinum* toxin has been studied extensively.[86] Botulinum toxin has been used extensively in children with skeletal muscle problems and recently in the treatment of achalasia[124] and patients with chronic anal fissures.[125] Because it weakens the muscle in a transient fashion, it could be used to produce a "medical" myectomy, therefore allowing the evaluation of sphincter pressure reduction without permanent sphincter destruction.[86,120] In a prospective study of 18 children who were injected with botulinum toxin, the authors reported that 4 had no improvement in bowel function, 2 had improvement for less than 1 month, 7 had improvement for 1 to 6 months, and 5 had improvement more than 6 months. Nine of those with symptomatic improvement longer than 1 month had sphincter pressures measured, with a documented decrease in eight. Five with no significant clinical improvement had pressure measurements, with a decrease in three. There were no adverse effects associated with botulinum toxin injection. Four children had new encopresis postinjection, which was mild and resolved in each case. Repeated injections were often necessary.[86,120] The botulinum toxin injection seems to be safe, and no major side effects have been reported when it is used in skeletal muscle or the lower esophageal sphincter. Therefore, it is possible that botulinum toxin is useful as a way of predicting which children may benefit from myectomy or as a therapeutic modality in selected patients, in particular those with recurrent enterocolitis or intractable obstructive symptoms.

The obstructive symptoms may also be related to abnormal upper gastrointestinal motility.[87,126,127] It has been shown that years after the surgical resection, children with Hirschsprung disease can have evidence of esophageal, gastric, or small bowel dysfunction, suggesting that children with Hirschsprung disease may have underlying motility disorders in segments not involved by aganglionosis.[87,126–128]

The establishment of the cause of obstruction can usually be accomplished with the use of simple tests (see Figure 77.1-4). As can be appreciated, the treatment will depend on the etiology (see Figure 77.1-4). In general, and while the workup is in progress, close attention to rectal decompression and treatment of symptoms suggestive of enterocolitis are necessary. A barium enema will help define the anatomy and the appearance of the pull-through and determine if there is a stricture, a new transition zone, or a megacolon. Radiopaque transit studies will detect delays. A rectal biopsy with acetylcholinesterase staining will allow the detection of residual or new aganglionosis or neuronal dysplasia, and anorectal and colonic manometry will allow further assessment of motor function.[128,129]

Using the techniques mentioned above to evaluate patients with obstructive symptoms, Moore and colleagues found that of 107 patients followed at least 4 years, 14.9% had recurrent episodes of gaseous distention and symptoms suggestive of persisting obstruction, in the absence of an anatomically defined problem, and they all had evidence of radiologic megacolon and delayed colonic transit.[83] The reason for this delay was related not only to findings in anorectal function but also probably to abnormal or residual disease in the intestinal wall. Anorectal manometry detected four patients in whom the high-pressure zone was too long, and they all responded to myectomy. They performed histologic evaluation of rectal biopsies and found that in 56% of the patients with obstructive symptoms, there were changes compatible with NID,[109,118] and in another 25% of patients, they detected postoperative aganglionosis. The authors concluded that an aggressive and systematic approach for the evaluation of patients with obstructive symptoms allows the determination of the etiology in most patients and therefore guides their treatment. Recently, in an effort to define the physiology underlying the persistent symptoms in children with Hirschsprung disease, Di Lorenzo and colleagues suggested that colonic motility helps explain the pathophysiology and direct the treatment.[128] They studied 46 symptomatic patients and identified 4 motility patterns: (1) high-amplitude propagated contractions (HAPCs) migrating through the neorectum to the anal sphincter, associated with fecal soiling in 18 patients; (2) normal colonic motility associated with retentive posturing in 9 patients; (3) absence of HAPCs or persistent simultaneous contractions over two or more recording sites in 15 patients; and (4) normal colonic motility and a hypertensive anal sphincter (80 mm Hg) in 4 patients. As can be appreciated, the treatment of obstructive symptoms depends on the etiology (see Figure 77.1-4). If there is an anatomic problem (eg, a stricture), it needs to be corrected. If there is no evidence of anatomic problems and

the colonic transit study and anorectal manometry indicate that the obstruction is distal, aganglionosis needs to be considered.[83,102] Biopsies of the distal anastomotic site need to be performed. If aganglionosis is present, the aganglionic segment needs to be removed, or if it is short, a myectomy may be considered.[83] If the patient has neuronal dysplasia, I recommend the use of a prokinetic agent, and I and others have had good results with cisapride.[83] If the anorectal manometry indicates a nonrelaxing sphincter, suggesting that the obstruction is at the level of the IAS, steps to decrease sphincter pressure need to be undertaken.[83] A trial of botulinum toxin injection should be undertaken.[86,120] Repeated injections may be necessary. If the injection of botulinum toxin fails, a myectomy needs to be considered.[130] If there is evidence of aganglionosis, the segment needs to be resected.[130,131] At times, it may be necessary to perform a new pull-through procedure, particularly if there is residual aganglionosis, stricture, or a fistula or if the pull-through anastomosis is too high.[130] In one series, 23 of 68 patients after a Soave procedure and 15 of 39 after a Duhamel procedure required a reoperation. For unclear reasons in this series, the incidence of reoperation is very high, but, overall, 90% were cured after the reoperation.[130] In another report of 22 reoperations followed for a mean 6.5 years, 75% showed good results.[132]

Finally, it may also be necessary to resect dysfunctional bowel.[128] It has been postulated that colonic motility allows the detection of the abnormal segments guiding the surgical intervention.[128] In their series, 15 patients with abnormal colonic motility underwent colonic resection of the abnormal segment with good results. Long-term follow-up and larger studies are needed before the exact role that colonic resections will play in the management of these patients is defined. Finally, for patients with severe problems, it may be necessary at times to create a colostomy or ileostomy.

In recent years, antegrade colonic enemas (ACEs) have been developed as an effective way of treating constipation and fecal incontinence in different conditions, including Hirschsprung disease.[133–135] The ACE procedure produces a continent conduit from the skin to the cecum that can be catheterized for self-administration of enemas.[135–139] In short-term studies, the ACE has been shown to be very effective in children with Hirschsprung disease in whom a permanent colostomy was being considered for the treatment of refractory constipation or incontinence.[135,136] Data for long-term follow-up are not yet available, and close follow-up is needed because in some patients, the enemas may not give the desired results because they are working against a hypertonic, nonrelaxing sphincter.

FECAL INCONTINENCE

Another common problem that may be encountered is fecal incontinence in the absence of fecal impaction (see Table 77.1-3).[84,105,140] Even though long-term studies usually report fecal incontinence in 2.5 to 13% of patients,[75,104,140] a study designed specifically to establish the extent of incontinence found it in 80% of patients.[105] In 53%, it was significant, and in 27%, it was less severe. Contrary to other reports, the incontinence did not diminish with increasing age.[89] The mean age of the patients was 10.1 ± 3.6 years, and there were no differences in the age at the definitive surgery, sex, extent of aganglionosis, type of surgery, or early or late postoperative complications when comparing those with or without incontinence. The survey of the surgical section of the American Academy of Pediatrics reported that fecal incontinence occurred in 3.2% of patients after the Swenson procedure compared with 1.1% after Duhamel and 2.1% after Soave.[89] One long-term study has indicated that of 282 patients after the Swenson procedure, 90% had normal bowel habits, 3.2% had permanent soiling, and 2 patients had a permanent colostomy because of the incontinence,[90] whereas another study has found that in 185 cases after the Duhamel procedure, 8% had severe incontinence and 27% had used enemas in the past.[141] It has been reported that after the Soave procedure, 18% had diarrhea and incontinence, although 82% had a satisfactory result.[101] Mishalany and Wooley reported the follow-up of 62 patients after different procedures (14 Duhamel, 15 Swenson, and 33 Soave).[88] Approximately 23 to 50% felt that they had normal bowel movements, and the rest had various degrees of problems in defecation. Subjectively, half of the patients in the Duhamel and Soave groups and one-third in the Swenson group considered their stooling pattern normal. Approximately 50% were not totally continent. Half of the Duhamel, one-third of the Swenson, and slightly more than half of the Soave group considered themselves completely continent, and the incontinence ranged from moderate soiling several times a day in 28 patients to total incontinence in 3 patients.

The physiopathology of the incontinence not associated with constipation is not well understood. By doing anorectal manometry, Mishalany and Wooley found that 10% of patients were not able to increase external sphincter contraction and that 50% after the Duhamel or the Swenson procedure and 30% after the Soave procedure experienced an inability to have rectal sensation.[88] Both of those abnormalities have been shown in other populations to be associated with fecal incontinence.[142,143] In a study of 54 adult patients (mean age 29 years), there was a positive correlation between functional outcome and anal resting pressure. The low resting pressure reflects IAS dysfunction, which may be caused by operative trauma.[140] Other abnormalities that have been associated with incontinence in Hirschsprung disease patients are related to the ability of the IAS to relax after balloon distention. The presence of the rectoanal inhibitory reflex has been variable; it is usually absent and in most studies does not seem to be correlated with outcome.[83,88] Recently, Di Lorenzo and colleagues suggested that fecal incontinence can result from the presence of HAPCs that migrate all the way through the neorectum to the anal sphincter.[128] In normal patients, the HAPCs stop in the sigmoid, never reaching the rectum. In their series, 18 children had fecal soiling that occurred when an HAPC was present and migrated all the way down through the neorectum.

Independent of the physiopathology, the treatment of the fecal incontinence is complex. The main objective is to produce social continence. Biofeedback has been used successfully in these children and has focused on trying to improve sensation abnormalities and increase muscle strength. Other treatments that have been used have included the use of enemas, the bowel management tube,[144] or, recently, ACEs.[145]

When evaluating patients with fecal incontinence, the first thing that needs to be established is if this is related to overflow incontinence and encopresis or abnormalities in anorectal or colonic function. The use of physical examination, colonic transit studies, abdominal radiography, and particularly manometry will allow this differentiation. If constipation seems to be the cause, laxatives need to be initiated. On the other hand, if there is fecal incontinence not related to constipation, enemas to maintain the rectosigmoid empty, together with diet manipulation, and biofeedback therapy need to be instituted. In those patients in whom the HAPCs migrate all the way down through the neorectum, an anticholinergic agent or loperamide may be useful.[128] Particularly in patients with total colonic aganglionosis, the use of loperamide may be needed[146] at the same time as the use of rectal tubes allows complete evacuation.

ENTEROCOLITIS

Enterocolitis continues to be the major cause of both morbidity and mortality in Hirschsprung disease.[103,104,147–149] It has been shown that this can occur before or after surgical treatment[103,104,148,149] in 2 to 33% of patients, with a mortality that ranges from 0 to 30%.[75,147–150] In a retrospective review of 105 cases, enterocolitis occurred in 32%.[148,149] It has been suggested that postoperative development of this complication is the most reliable indicator of the successful relief of the low intestinal obstruction present in this patients.[89,148,149,151] In the survey of the surgical section of the American Academy of Pediatrics, it was reported to be present in 15% after Swenson repair, in 5.9% after Duhamel repair, and in 1 to 2% after a modified Soave procedure.[89] Klein and Phillipart reported that enterocolitis occurred a mean of 0.51 episodes per patient after the Swenson procedure, 1 episode per patient after the Duhamel procedure, and 0.21 episodes after the Soave procedure.[94] Enterocolitis tended to be more frequent in premature infants and patients with long-segment Hirschsprung disease. The usual clinical presentation consisted of fever, abdominal pain, and diarrhea. In a recent study of 168 patients with Hirschsprung disease, enterocolitis presented with abdominal distention in 83%, explosive diarrhea in 69%, vomiting in 51%, fever in 34%, lethargy in 27%, rectal bleeding in 5%, and colonic perforation in 2.5%.[150] Chronic diarrhea was present in 54% and delayed growth in 44%. The occurrence of explosive diarrhea in any patient with Hirschsprung disease should suggest the diagnosis, even in the absence of systemic symptoms.[103,104,147,149,150] The presence of postoperative enterocolitis needs to be recognized promptly because the child can present initially with mild symptoms that are followed by a rapid fulminating course that may lead to death.[103,104,147,149,150] The pathogenesis is not fully understood.[149,152] In a retrospective review of cases with postoper ative enterocolitis, the risk was significantly increased by mechanical factors related to anastomotic complications and intestinal obstruction.[148] In general, it appears that fecal stasis facilitates bacterial overgrowth and subsequent mucosal invasion. There may be an association between enterocolitis and the presence of *Clostridium difficile*,[149,151] although recent reports indicate that in up to two-thirds of patients, stool cultures are negative.[150] The enterocolitis secondary to *C. difficile* may be more fulminant,[103] with rapid progression, shock and prostration, and, eventually, death.[103,149,151] Other organisms that have been associated with enterocolitis include rotavirus, retrovirus, *Pseudomonas*, or *Escherichia coli*.

The diagnosis of enterocolitis needs to be suspected early. Appropriate stool tests for identification of *C. difficile* and stool cultures for other pathogens need to be obtained. The diagnosis may be helped by using abdominal radiographs, in which the presence of an intestinal cutoff sign and at least two air-fluid levels strongly suggests the diagnosis.[147,150] The barium enema usually shows colonic dilatation and modularity and speculation of the rectal mucosa, with significant narrowing.[147,150] Endoscopic examination will show colitis and will detect the presence of pseudomembranes. Conservative management in the hospital is usually necessary. The treatment of choice includes fluid and electrolyte support, antibiotics, and the use of transrectal decompression either by tube or by sphincter dilatation.[75,147,149,150,153] Antibiotics against *C. difficile* and bowel flora should be empirically started as soon as the appropriate cultures are obtained.[147,153] The rectal decompression may need to be accompanied with the use of saline irrigation to evacuate the retained stool and gas.[75,103,149,150,153] It has also been described that some patients have frequent relapses, and this is usually related to chronic obstruction from a nonrelaxing sphincter.[120,149] It has been suggested that in them, the chronic or intermittent use of metronidazole may be beneficial,[149] and the administration of botulinum toxin has been successful in the prevention of the recurrent episodes. Some authors have advocated the use of a myectomy.[149] If the problem persists, it may be necessary to consider a surgical approach, which may include a diverting ostomy.

TOTAL COLONIC HIRSCHSPRUNG DISEASE

Patients with transition zones in the small bowel account for 5 to 10% in most large series.[154,155] The complications found in patients with total colonic Hirschsprung disease are more severe when compared with those with shorter segments.[154,155] Preoperative complications continue to plague these patients,[154,155] and their mortality continues to be high.[89,154,155] In the survey of the American Academy of Pediatrics, there was a mortality of 47% (42 of 90).[89] Improvements in parenteral and enteral nutrition, as well as in surgical techniques, have recently decreased it.[154,155]

The surgical therapy initially includes and ileostomy. Later an endorectal pull-through, along with total colectomy, and the long side-to-side anastomosis with aganglionic bowel are the most commonly used procedures.[154,155] In a recent review of the treatment of 48 patients, 6% had died early, and 85% underwent a pull-

through (38 with the Duhamel procedure, with 13 having the Martin modification and 3 a Soave procedure).[155] Long-term follow-up was available in 27 patients, of whom 19 (70%) required additional surgical procedures. In six patients, a permanent stoma was necessary. Two patients who underwent the Martin modification required resection of the side-to-side anastomosis because of intractable diarrhea, and the authors concluded that there was no advantage to its performance. At 5-year follow-up, 82% had fecal incontinence, but by 10 and 15 years, the incontinence had decreased to 57% and 33%, respectively. At 15 years, over half of the patients were below the 2nd percentile for weight and one-quarter were below the second percentile for height.[155] Fecal incontinence is common, and failure to thrive and malnutrition have been described, as well as disturbances in electrolyte balance, lipid metabolism, and vitamin B_{12} absorption.[154] One of the main problems in these children is residual obstruction that leads to intestinal dilatation, diarrhea, and postoperative enterocolitis. In these patients, intermittent antibiotics and a rectal tube with irrigation need to be used chronically for decompression. If it is clear that the patient has a functional obstruction at the level of the sphincter, a procedure to relieve the obstruction may be indicated. Until recently, a myectomy was the procedure of choice, but the use of botulinum toxin is an alternative that will provide only a temporal effect.[120] These interventions need to be performed in patients who have been fully evaluated because fecal incontinence may result after the procedure. With aggressive follow-up and nutritional support, as well as treatment of obstructive episodes, most patients who survive will eventually attain normal growth and the ability to feed enterally.

IMPERFORATE ANUS

The treatment of children born with anorectal malformations continues to be a challenging problem.[156–158] The term "anorectal malformation" encompasses multiple congenital defects with varying degrees of involvement, and many authors have stressed the complexity of the anatomic, physiologic, psychological, and social aspects that come into play in the management of these children.[158–161] The main objective of treatment is to achieve fecal continence.[157] Proposed treatments for these malformations have included simple perineal operations for benign defects ("low"), abdominal pull-through for more complicated defects ("high"), the sacral approach devised to preserve the puborectalis muscle (Figure 77.1-5), and combined approaches such as the abdominoperineal, sacroabdominoperineal, or sacroperineal approaches.[161,162] Even though today's surgical management permits the survival of virtually all patients,[158,161] it has been reported that only 25 to 75% of the operated patients have an acceptable stool continence following surgery,[156,161,163] particularly those patients with the high-type anomalies.[157] The highest incidence of incontinence seems to occur in male patients who have a rectobladder-neck fistula.[156,158,164] These patients usually have very poor muscle structures, a flat (round) bottom, and a narrow pelvis, with little space for satisfactory levator reconstruction behind the rectum.[156–158] Recent developments in the surgical technique, particularly the development of the posterior sagittal anorectoplasty,[156,157,161,165–167] have improved some of the results, but fecal incontinence and stricture formation continue to be a problem after the newer operations.[156,158,168]

After long-term follow-up, postoperative results in children with imperforate anus vary according to the type of the original malformation and probably according to the age of the patient. It has usually been mentioned that fecal continence and bowel control improve with time and usually reach their maximum around puberty.[157–159] It has been the usual experience that patients with a good anatomy and adequate treatment become continent much earlier,[157,159] whereas those with the worst results usually do not improve spontaneously. In general, even after the new operations, it has been suggested that 25% of children will suffer from fecal incontinence, and 25 to 30% will have other forms of defecation disorders, such as constipation, soiling, and incontinence associated with episodes of diarrhea.[156,157] In the longest series, Pena and Hong described their experience with 1,192 children whose imperforate anus was repaired using the posterior sagittal approach.[158] They found that 75% had voluntary control of the bowel movements, with half of that group still soiling their underwear occasionally. Therefore, only 37.5% of all cases were considered totally continent.[158] Constipation was the most common sequela, and urinary incontinence was common after the repair of cloacas. Twenty-five percent suffered from fecal incontinence but improved once they were subjected to an aggressive bowel program, including an appendicostomy.[158] Molander and Frenckner described the long-term follow-up (18–35 years) of 29 patients operated on for high imperforate anus.[166] They found that 9 had a permanent colostomy as a consequence of severe fecal incontinence, 6 were the only totally continent patients, 6 had occasional accidents that made them wear sanitary napkins, 2 had constant incontinence, and 4 had a moderate degree of incontinence. In another report with an 8- to 20-year follow-up of 104 children with imperforate anus, Holschneider found that only 6 of 69 patients with a high anomaly had a normal or near-normal continence and that 20 of 104 children had uncorrectable urinary incontinence, suggesting also that a high percentage of these patients continues to have severe problems after long-term follow-up and does not improve spontaneously.[167]

Most information comes from those children with high malformations, and it has been suggested that those with low malformations have a better prognosis. Recent studies, however, suggest that they continue to have long-term problems, particularly constipation.[158,169–171] Ludman and Spitz reported that 28% had compromised continence, with up to 25% continuing to experience difficulty with constipation and 7% requiring enemas on a regular basis.[170] A recent long-term report of 44 girls with low malformations reported that 89% were successfully toilet trained but that 47% experience at least occasional soiling or episodes of fecal incontinence.[171] In a study that compared bowel function in 40 patients with low malforma-

tions with that of healthy controls, Rintala and colleagues found that 52% had a normal function indistinguishable from the controls.[169] Constipation requiring dietary or medical treatment was present in 42% compared with 7% of the controls, whereas soiling was present in 10%.

Long-term problems with fecal incontinence can have major effects on the development of the children.[107,161,163,172] In a recent long-term survey, Glinn-Pease and colleagues reported that almost half (47%) of parents report problems with bowel function (constipation, diarrhea, or soiling).[161] Most children had a normal growth and were of average intelligence, and scores for math and reading, as well as of adaptive behavior, were age appropriate. They found that 18% had learning disabilities and 18% had some degree of social maladjustment. Of interest is the fact that children with fecal incontinence represented 60% of the patients with behavior problems, suggesting that the frequent association of fecal incontinence with behavioral dysfunction may indicate that these children may benefit from psychological testing. In an interesting study in which 61 patients were observed for 2.5 to 24 years, Ditesehim and Templeton showed that in chil-

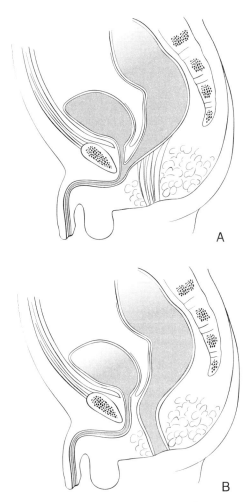

FIGURE 77.1-5 Schematic representation of a rectourethral fistula preoperatively and postoperatively. A, Rectourethral bulbar fistula. B, Repaired defect. Adapted from Pena A. Atlas: surgical management of anorectal malformations. Heidelberg (Germany): Springler Verlag; 1990.

dren older than 10 years, the quality of life was directly related to their fecal continence, whereas in younger children, their quality of life was better than their continence, indicating that in the younger children, the families tend to be more patient and use special stratagems to minimize incontinence problems: liners in the underpants, enemas, meticulous perineal hygiene, and avoidance of certain foods.[159] It seemed that after age 10, children with incontinence could not be shielded by parents and were not well tolerated by teachers and peers. In fact, in this older group, only 5 of 30 children had greater social adaptability scores than fecal continence scores, and children with a poor fecal continence score faced such severe social problems that they often requested aggressive medical or surgical interventions, including the performance of a colostomy. This study emphasizes the importance of continuing follow-up of these children and for aggressive evaluation of children with fecal incontinence. It is then clear that fecal incontinence is a socially disabling problem in children and remains a challenging problem.[107,156,157,159,163] A recent report of 33 adolescents status post repair of imperforate anus, with a median age of 15 years, found that 73% had flatus incontinence, whereas 70% had persistent dysfunction with staining. Fifty-eight percent met the criteria for a psychiatric diagnosis, and impairment of psychosocial function was found in 73%. The degree of psychosocial impairment correlated significantly with fecal incontinence and flatus incontinence.[163] The authors pointed out that in addition to soiling, staining and fear of flatus are associated with psychiatric and psychosocial dysfunction.[163]

The genesis of these problems is not clear.[107] In a study that compared outcome between children with Hirschsprung disease and children with low anorectal malformations, it was found that even though the degree of fecal dysfunction was similar in both groups, there were differences when comparing both groups. The duration of anal-invasive treatment procedures, particularly anal dilatation, was the most significant negative predictor of the adolescent's mental health, whereas chronic family difficulties and parental warmth, together with the current bowel function variables, best explained the variance in psychosocial outcome.[107] The authors concluded that anal dilatation and continence dysfunction have a negative impact on mental health and psychosocial functioning.[107] They suggest that the use of anal dilatations needs to be re-evaluated, particularly in older children.

A recent study of 160 children 6 to 18 years with fecal incontinence after surgery found that the way in which children dealt with the problem could be grouped into three phases.[172] In phase 1, around 6 to 7 years of age, boys were largely unaware of the unsociable nature of their condition, whereas girls were sensitive and withdrawn. In phase 2, between 8 and 11 years of age, boys used overt denial, whereas girls used secretiveness. In phase 3, from 12 years to adolescence, both sexes were marked by continued covert denial and eventual acceptance of their disability.[172] The authors pointed out that the coping mechanisms reflected a complex interrelationship between the charac-

teristics of the child, the family, the social environment, and the unsociable and embarrassing nature of fecal incontinence. Parents' perceptions of how others would react to a child with incontinence influence the children's coping behaviors. Frequently, the emphasis on the need to be secretive (to avoid ridicule) exacerbated the child's awareness of having a shameful disability.[172] Coping with children with fecal incontinence also poses a number of problems to teachers and schools. These children generally look healthy and do not have a visible handicap, and the condition is usually considered taboo. Despite efforts by all concerned, keeping the child's condition secret is difficult, and for a number of children, the problems at school become so acute that some children are removed from it.[172]

MANAGEMENT OF COMMON PROBLEMS

FECAL INCONTINENCE

The management of fecal incontinence is difficult.[135,156,157,160,161,173] Multiple attempts to control it have been done, starting with medical manipulations,[156,157,161] followed by surgical options such as colostomy, grafts, or reoperations.[156,157,164,174]

The physiopathology of fecal incontinence is multifactorial and is not well understood. It has been suggested that good bowel control is the result of the integrity of anatomic structures and the physiologic mechanisms involving three main factors: sensation, bowel motility, and voluntary muscles.[156,157] The presence of fecal incontinence could be related, on the one hand, to abnormalities in the muscle or its innervation[157,168,175] or intrarectal sensation but on the other hand to overflow incontinence from constipation and a lack of bowel motility.[156,176] Pena and colleagues suggested that patients with incontinence can be classified into the following groups: (1) those with a poor surgical repair who may require a reoperation, (2) those with poor functional prognosis who mostly have a tendency either to diarrhea or to constipation, and (3) those with overflow secondary to a dilated sigmoid colon. This distinction is important because the approach and treatment of the patient vary according to the nature of the problem (Figure 77.1-6).[157]

One of the main problems in the evaluation of fecal soiling is that even though there are many tests that try to obtain an objective assessment of anorectal function (eg, defecography, barium enema, manometry, anal endosonography, electromyography [EMG], nuclear medicine, computed tomography [CT], and magnetic resonance imaging [MRI]), each one studies only a specific aspect of a very complex function.[157,177] To evaluate the state of pelvic and anal muscles, as well as the position of the rectum after the operation, imaging techniques such as CT scan[168] and MRI have been used.[177,178] It has been suggested when comparing both techniques that MRI may be superior in the delineation of the pelvic muscles, and another advantage may be that it allows the detection of other unsuspected malformations, particularly tethered cord, or urinary tract problems and also because it does not involve ionizing radiation.[156,178] In general, it has been suggested that the main advantage of the imaging techniques rests in their ability to help evaluate patients who have been previously operated on and are having fecal incontinence because it allows the differentiation between poorly developed muscles and improper placement of the neorectum.[159,178]

Anal endosonography has also been shown to be useful in these patients.[177,179] In a study comparing anal endosonography with EMG and anorectal manometry in 15 patients, endosonography detected the external anal sphincter in all patients. The distribution image was inadequate in high anomalies. For the external anal sphincter, the endosonographic findings corresponded well to the EMG. The IAS was identified in five patients with high anomalies and in one patient with intermediate anomalies, although only one of the six patients had relaxation by manometry. The authors suggested that the IAS findings did not correspond to the manometry.[177]

However, even though these techniques are very useful in delineating the anatomy, there does not seem to be a good correlation between the anatomic findings and the degree of fecal continence.[158,180] Anorectal manometry is a useful technique to evaluate the state of intrarectal pressure and sensation, as well as of the voluntary muscles.[143,181–185] I and others have found that patients with repaired imperforate anus have significant abnormalities in anorectal function.[143,182–185] The threshold of sensation and the maximum tolerable pressure in the high type are sig-

nificantly higher than those in the low type were, and the rectal compliance in the high type is significantly lower than that in the low type. It has been found that patients with imperforate anus had a shorter and weaker intra-anal pressure and that patients with high anomalies had abnormalities in voluntary control and sensation.[183,186] Iwai showed an increase in the EMG activity of the external sphincter after voluntary contraction in the patients with imperforate anus, independent of the type of the malformation.[182] Molander and Frenckner suggested that in normal children, fecal continence correlated with the presence of the inflation reflex,[187] and they found that those postoperative patients in whom the inflation reflex was demonstrated had good Kelly scores, independent of the type of anorectal malformation. They also found that in contrast to normal subjects, the electrical activity of the external anal sphincter in children with high anomalies remained stationary in spite of further rectal filling. More sophisticated EMG studies showed that the number of spike bursts in the high and intermediate anomalies was significantly higher than those in the low type. A recent study of 45 patients measured pudendal nerve motor latency, spinoanal responses, and evoked potentials of the cauda equina.[85] The authors showed that patients with imperforate anus had latencies that were significantly prolonged when compared with controls.[85] Compared with normal values, the spinal central conduction time in patients was increased by 278%,

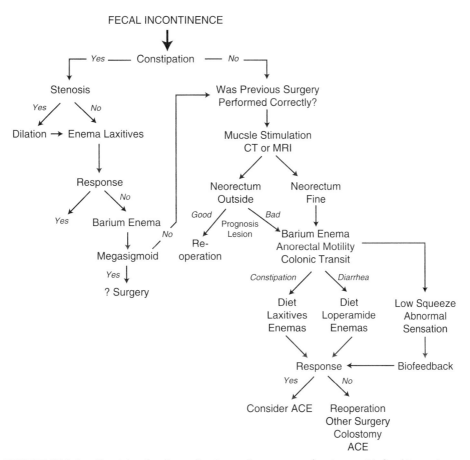

FIGURE 77.1-6   Algorithm for the evaluation and treatment of patients with fecal incontinence after surgery to correct imperforate anus. ACE = antegrade colonic enemas; CT = computed tomography; MRI = magnetic resonance imaging.

the latency of pudendoanal reflex by 232%, the latency of spinoanal response by 180%, and the latency of cauda equina evoked potential by 146%. There was also a negative correlation between the latencies and the clinical scores. The authors concluded that these patients have widespread and serious lumbar and sacral nerve lesions that probably have an impact on fecal continence.[85]

There are few long-term functional studies. Iwai and colleagues studied 27 patients and compared manometric results after surgery with those obtained 3 years later.[188] Manometrically, they found that 7 of 11 patients with a high anomaly had a high-pressure zone in the anal canal and only 1 of 11 patients had an anorectal reflex on the first examination and 3 on the second examination. All patients with intermediate and low anomalies had an anorectal reflex present. Overall, the authors concluded that incontinent patients had a lower anorectal pressure than controls or continent patients. Hedlund and colleagues described the long-term manometric investigation in 30 patients 5 to 10 years after posterior sagittal anorectoplasty.[184] They found that the sensation was within the normal range and that 9 of 30 patients had a rectoanal inhibitory reflex. They also found that soiling was common in patients with low anal resting tone and low squeeze pressures.

It can therefore be concluded from all of the above studies that fecal incontinence is usually related to low voluntary and intra-anal pressure and to abnormal sensation.[166] The role that colonic motility plays in these patients is also becoming increasingly more clear. It has been suggested that abnormal colonic transit is present in patients with either high or low anomalies.[189] The authors found that after using the saturation technique, patients had a significantly longer transit time compared with controls.[189] There was no difference when comparing total transit between those with low or high anomalies, but patients with low malformations have delays in the rectosigmoid segments, whereas those with high anomalies have a more generalized delay.[189] The authors found that the functional outcome was strongly related to the degree of these motility disturbances. Recently, by using colonic motility, it has been suggested that another mechanism that exacerbates incontinence is the presence of HAPCs that migrate in 80% of the subjects to the neorectum.[175] This suggests that it is possible that fecal soiling occurs when the HAPCs propel stool to a low-pressure anus that is unable to accommodate to maintain continence.[175]

Most of the above discussion has been related to the fact that the fecal incontinence of these children is usually the result of abnormalities in anorectal function. There are cases, however, in which there is fecal soiling as a result of overflow incontinence from constipation.

CONSTIPATION

Constipation can be a significant functional long-term problem after the posterior sagittal approach or in any operation in which the rectum has been preserved.[156–58,169,174,176,190] In a series of 1,192 patients, Pena and Hong found a 48% incidence of constipation.[158] This varied according to the type of malformation: vestibular fistula, 61%; bulbar urethral fis-

tula, 59%; rectal atresia/stenosis, 57%; imperforate anus without fistula, 55%; perineal fistula, 50%; long cloaca, 48%; prostatic fistula, 45%; short cloaca, 39%; and bladder-neck fistula, 15%.[158]

The physiopathology of the constipation is probably multifactorial.[157] Abnormal myenteric plexus innervation and smooth muscle have been described in rectal dissections.[190] There are cases in which the distal rectosigmoid may become atonic and baggy.[156,157,169,174,190,191] The degrees of rectal dilatation and dysfunction vary, and it has been shown by Rintala and colleagues that the grade of rectal dilatation prior to closure of the colostomy had a positive correlation with the severity of the constipation and that the occurrence of constipation was clearly related to the presence of a functioning IAS.[176] The main problem with the atonic rectum is that it is nonfunctional and has no peristaltic activity,[157,191] so in those patients with atonic rectum in which there is IAS activity, there may be a functional obstruction to rectal emptying causing significant constipation.

The presence of Hirschsprung disease needs to be excluded because aganglionosis has been observed in some patients with imperforate anus.[192]

Treatment of the Fecal Incontinence. The treatment of fecal incontinence has to be tailored to the specific problem presented by the patient. When examining a patient, one has to make the distinction between the different groups (see Figure 77.1-6). This distinction can usually be made on clinical grounds and using simple tests. If the subject has good bowel control potential, good sphincters, a good sacrum, and a malpositioned rectum, a reoperation needs to be considered. One must suspect that overflow incontinence from constipation is present when the child presents with a history of malformation with a "good" prognosis. A colonic transit study may be performed and a barium enema obtained to detect the presence of a megarectum and megasigmoids. On the other hand, if the impression is that the patient is suffering from fecal incontinence not related to constipation, it may be necessary to perform MRI or CT to further delineate the anatomy, to confirm that the neorectum is well placed, and to exclude a tethered cord.[193] If the previous operation is satisfactory, an anorectal manometry will then be necessary to delineate the degree of anorectal abnormalities and the possibility of performing biofeedback therapy.

If one suspects that the fecal soiling is secondary to overflow incontinence from constipation, then medical treatment with diet and bulk laxatives, followed by stimulant laxatives and enemas, needs to be instituted.[157,175] A multidisciplinary approach that also includes behavioral interventions has also been shown to be effective.[173] In those patients with megasigmoid and intractable symptoms even after aggressive medical therapy, resection of the baggy atonic rectosigmoid or sigmoid may be the only effective treatment.[156,157,174,191] Rintala and colleagues reported that 13 of 26 patients responded favorably to dietary manipulations and the use of bulk laxatives, and the researchers were later able to wean all medications.[176] In 11 patients, these measures failed, so enemas and stimulant laxatives were necessary; of those patients, 6 could not wean the medication without experiencing a relapse. Finally, two patients did not respond to medical therapy and underwent surgical resection, which relieved the constipation, although they continued to have inadequate fecal continence and to use enemas to stay clean. On the other hand, Cheu and Grosfeld reported three children with intractable constipation in whom the resection of the baggy rectum resulted in disappearance of the constipation and therefore in a normal fecal continence.[191] Pena and colleagues have questioned the wisdom of dissecting both the sigmoid and the rectum, and they reported the successful treatment of three patients in whom they only resected the sigmoid, preserving the rectum.[157,174] These authors suggested that all patients with fecal incontinence should have a barium enema, particularly those born with malformations and with the potential for good continence, and that if a megasigmoid is found and medical therapy fails, a sigmoid resection with rectal preservation should be performed without subjecting the patient to another pull-through.

On the other hand, if the soiling is the result of a lack of good muscles, an abnormal sacrum, a defect with poor prognosis, or an abnormal sensation, an aggressive bowel program needs to be instituted.[157,175] An attempt to make the stools more solid should be undertaken because liquid stools usually leak out without the patient's perception. The problem tends to be worse in those patients who were subjected to an operation in which the rectosigmoid was resected, such as after abdominoperineal procedures and endorectal dissections. These patients usually suffer from "diarrhea" and increased colonic motility and pass stool constantly. One approach to these patients involves the use of antimotility agents such as loperamide,[157,194,195] which decreases colonic transit and changes anorectal function, together with the use of bulking agents in the diet. In a study in which loperamide was administered to eight patients with fecal incontinence after rectoplasty for high imperforate anus, four had a significant decrease in the amount of soiling.[195]

Also, besides decreasing stool output, an attempt to keep the distal part of the colon empty needs to be undertaken, and the use of enemas and suppositories is useful.[157,158] At times, it is necessary to use large enemas or colonic irrigation.[157,158] Pena and colleagues have developed a program in which the parents are taught to clean the colon every day with the use of an enema or some form of colonic irrigation.[157,158] The problem is usually much more difficult to control in those children with absent sacrum and worse neurogenic abnormalities because they are unable to hold the enemas or the suppositories. For these patients, the use of a continence enema has proven very beneficial.[144] The success of the retrograde application of enemas or suppositories to achieve continence has changed the quality of life of these patients. However, the problem with this approach lies in the fact that a helper is needed, so independence is not achieved.

Pena and colleagues found that of 172 patients with fecal incontinence who were not candidates for a reoperation or a sigmoid resection, 44 had predominantly constipation and incontinence, whereas 128 had a tendency to diarrhea.[157] The first group was treated with enemas, with a 93% success rate, whereas those in the second group were treated with constipated diets and drugs to slow down the motility. The authors reported a success rate of 88%.

Another option for the treatment of fecal incontinence is biofeedback therapy.[196] Even though the mechanisms of fecal continence are still not well defined, studies in patients with fecal incontinence owing to a variety of different etiologies have suggested that it tends to occur in patients in whom the maximum squeeze pressure is low or in whom the sensation threshold is high. Attempts to correct both abnormalities have usually led to an improvement in the fecal incontinence.[142,156,181,197] Biofeedback for fecal incontinence has been successfully used in the treatment of patients with peripheral nerve impairment, such as diabetes mellitus and multiple sclerosis, myelomeningocele,[142] or after anorectal surgery.[181] In children, it has been successfully used for the treatment of myelomeningocele,[142] in patients with ileoanal anastomosis,[197] and, recently, in children with imperforate anus.[181,196] Most studies suggest that approximately 50 to 90% of patients with incontinence respond to biofeedback,[198,199] and in a review of all published studies in which biofeedback was performed in adults to treat fecal incontinence, the technique was successful in 79.8% (in 257/322 patients).[198]

The information on the use of biofeedback for the treatment of imperforate anus is limited. Arnbjornsson and colleagues performed biofeedback training in patients with incontinence.[165] They found a correlation between clinical improvement and EMG increase after voluntary contraction and EMG tonic activity, with 7 of 11 patients showing a decrease in fecal incontinence, 1 worsening, and 4 no change. No correlation was made with pressure changes. Worona and colleagues have also studied the effect of a biofeedback program on the manometric and clinical outcome of 54 patients with imperforate anus and fecal incontinence.[181] After multimodal treatment, including biofeedback, there was a significant improvement in 82% of the patients, and 34.5% became completely continent. There was a significant decrease in the number of accidents/day, laxatives/week used, number of enemas/week, and sensation threshold and a significant increase in squeeze pressure, total duration of squeeze, and duration of maximum squeeze. Ninety-two percent of the patients maintained their improvement for more than 6 months. Newer biofeedback techniques have used portable EMG machines with similar results.[196,200]

When all attempts to improve the fecal incontinence have failed, the option of a repeat surgical procedure needs to be considered.[201] This is particularly important in those children who were operated on years ago, for whom the performance of a posterior sagittal anorectoplasty may be beneficial, or in those in whom the initial repair might have been technically inadequate.[157] Candidates for a reoperation are those with good sphincters, a good sacrum, a good prognosis–type defect, and a mislocated rectum.[157] Brain and Kiely recently described 12 patients who underwent the procedure because of severe fecal incontinence after the original anal reconstruction.[202] They found that only two patients achieved good results, two others improved, and the rest remained incontinent. On the other hand, Pena and colleagues found that patients with a normal sacrum and fecal incontinence operated on elsewhere who underwent a posterior sagittal anorectoplasty achieved marked improvement in 45%, some improvement in 37%, and no improvement in 18%.[157,203] In contrast, a marked improvement in only 20%, some improvement in 30%, and no improvement in 50% were achieved in patients with an abnormal sacrum.[157] A report of 20 patients who were reoperated on showed that of 16 incontinent patients, 12 achieved continence and 4 some improvement; of those with fecal impaction, 2 achieved daily bowel movements, and 2 remain with mild constipation.[201] Resection of a dilated sigmoid (megasigmoid) has been suggested for those patients in whom there is overflow incontinence, good sphincters, a good sacrum, a good prognosis defect, and a preserved rectum.[157]

Knowing the success that the application of retrograde methods has on producing evacuation and continence, the idea of performing procedures that will allow the anterograde delivery of the enemas was brought forward, and the ACE procedure was proposed. As mentioned above, the ACE procedure has been developed to produce a continent conduit from the skin to the cecum that can be catheterized for self-administration of enemas.[131,139,145,157,204,205] The procedure can be performed with open surgery,[145,157] laparoscopically,[206] or percutaneously either by radiologic methods[131,135,136] or endoscopy.[137] The main disadvantage of the surgical approach is that it requires a laparoscopy or laparotomy, which, in many of the children who require this procedure, involves major surgery because they have usually had other surgical procedures. The advantage is that it can be done at the same time as the creation of a urinary conduit and that there is no indwelling device. The percutaneous approach can be done either radiologically[136] or endoscopically,[137] and its advantage is that it does not involve surgery, so the recovery time is very fast. The main disadvantage is that a device is left in place, which is not always acceptable to the patients.

Independently of the technique used, the patient is then able to administer an enema in an antegrade fashion. This allows the patient to be predictable and independent. The ACE procedure has been used in children with fecal incontinence secondary to different etiologies[135,136] but most commonly with spina bifida,[139,205,207] other neurogenic problems,[135] and also imperforate anus.[136,145,156–158,204,207] Even though some have suggested that the procedure should be performed only in those patients in whom the fecal incontinence and constipation have been controlled with bowel management,[156–158] recent experience has shown that it is also successful in those who do not respond to enema therapy[136] or even in those children with a poor prognosis.[204]

Overall success rates have been described as ranging from 60 to 90%. In a review of the literature, of 149 reported patients, 88% were completely continent and 12% were partially continent.[135] The most common solutions used are polyethylene glycol, tap water, saline, and phosphate enemas.[135,139,157,158,204] The use of tap water has been associated with hyponatremia,[133] so it is preferable to administer saline. The type, volume, and frequency must be individualized for each patient,[135] although they usually vary from 400 to 2,500 mL.[133,135] The patient sits on the toilet, administers the irrigation, and usually has complete evacuation in 30 to 60 minutes.[135] The most common complications have been stomal stenosis,[134] leakage at the surgical site,[145] or difficulty with catheterization.[208]

Recently, it has been suggested that the placement of an irrigation button in the sigmoid may be as effective as the ACE performed in the cecum.[138,209] The experience is very limited. The main theoretic disadvantage of pursuing that approach is that, most likely, laxatives will still be needed to allow the stool to move from the cecum to the sigmoid colon. More information is needed before this procedure can be recommended.

Several other surgical procedures have been recommended for patients with postoperative incontinence. Some are designed to increase the anorectal angle or reinforce the existing musculature.[210] Some authors have advocated the use of gracilis muscle transposition for the treatment of children with intractable fecal incontinence and evidence of a lack of muscle function.[210] The results have been mixed. In one series, however, Sonnino and colleagues reported their long-term experience in seven patients with gracilis transposition in whom there was severe fecal incontinence, a lack of adequate sphincteric function, and a properly positioned neorectum before the new procedure.[210] They all became continent after the procedure with a mean follow-up of 0.5 to 12.5 years. It is important to note, however, that this type of operation should not be performed if one determines that the neorectum is malpositioned, in which case, a posterior sagittal approach as a redo operation is still recommended.

For those patients who have failed all therapies and continue to have severe fecal incontinence, a permanent colostomy may be necessary.[157,158] Even though the performance of a colostomy may represent a chronic disability and loss of hope of a perfect cure; it may reduce the practical and emotional strain of soiling and invasive treatment procedures, both for the patients and the parents.[107] In fact, Lask and colleagues reported in a controlled study of psychosocial adjustment to stoma surgery for childhood inflammatory bowel disease that there was no evidence that the surgery was psychologically harmful to psychosocial adjustment, self-esteem, or quality of life.[211] They concluded that as long as children are well prepared and followed up carefully and sensitively, stoma surgery should not be deferred for fear of adverse psychological consequences.

It is difficult to estimate the exact incidence of children who have required colostomy. In a long-term follow-up reported by Molander and Frenckner, 9 of 29 patients had a permanent colostomy; the patients in this study, however, were operated on before the new techniques for the treatment of these children were available.[166] In a series of 348 patients, Pena and colleagues reported that they had to perform this procedure in 7 children.[157] Of those, 6 had diarrhea and incontinence as the main symptoms.

Summary on the Approach to the Patient with Fecal Incontinence. Figure 77.1-6 presents an algorithm for the treatment and evaluation of children with postoperative problems. When a patient is referred for the evaluation of fecal incontinence, the following questions need to be addressed:

1. Is the patient having overflow incontinence from constipation? If so, is there a massive dilatation of the rectosigmoid?
2. What is the status of the sacrum? Does the patient have more than two or three missing vertebrae?
3. What is the state of anorectal functioning? Is there a tethered spinal cord?
4. Was the original repair done properly? Is there evidence of stenosis or malposition of the neorectum?

In general, this information can be obtained from the history and physical examination and with the performance of some basic tests. The physical examination should provide information about the state of the anoplasty (particularly as it relates to stenosis), the presence of the midline groove and the anal dimple, and the status of the perineal musculature. A thorough neurologic examination will provide information about deficits in the sacral innervation. The abdominal examination will show the amount of fecal material that is present and should detect the presence of big stool masses.

A plain abdominal radiograph will provide information related to the amount of fecal material present. An anorectal manometry will be useful to evaluate intrarectal sensation, as well as the functioning of the IAS and the strength of the squeeze pressure.

If the patient has severe incontinence that is resistant to medical therapy and surgical options are being considered, the performance of a barium enema may be useful. This test will detect the presence of rectosigmoid dilatation in those patients with severe overflow incontinence from a nonfunctioning segment. In those patients in whom the sigmoid was resected in the initial pull-through, the barium enema will usually show a nondistended colon with normal haustration down to the perineum.

If it is necessary to establish the position of the neorectum in relation to the pelvic musculature, an MRI will be useful. An MRI will also show the presence of spinal cord tethering. At times, it may be necessary to perform electrical stimulation of the perineal region to try to identify where the muscle contractions are occurring in relation to the pull-through.

All of the information obtained after evaluation will allow a better understanding of the physiopathology of the fecal incontinence of the patient. If there is overflow incontinence, attempts to increase stool evacuation need to be undertaken. This may involve dilatation of the anus (if it is stenotic), the use of laxatives and particularly enemas, or sigmoid resection if the constipation is intractable and there is massive dilatation by barium enema. On the other hand, if the patient has fecal incontinence without constipation and a properly performed operation, a biofeedback and behavioral program should be undertaken. This should be accompanied by the use of bulking agents, colonic irrigations, and, usually, loperamide. If one is successful in maintaining a clean rectosigmoid, the incontinence will usually be controlled, independently of the muscle abnormalities. The performance of an ACE procedure needs to be considered, both in those who have achieved continence with enemas and in those in whom the bowel program has not been successful. In those patients with lesions that have been associated with a good prognosis, if the fecal incontinence persists or if there is evidence that the neorectum may not be positioned properly, a redo operation should be considered.[157] Finally, if the neorectum is in a good position but the patient has sacral abnormalities, poor muscles, and a flat perineum and continues to have incontinence independently of the therapy, the possibility of a different type of surgical procedure or the creation of a permanent colostomy will need to be considered.

SUMMARY AND CONCLUSIONS

As more children with complex congenital anomalies survive, new and long-term medical problems are arising. An attempt has been made in this chapter to analyze the long-term complications after surgery for some common and representative pediatric surgical procedures that are directly related to the gastrointestinal tract. The main focus has been to describe usual postoperative problems after surgery for gastroesophageal reflux, Hirschsprung disease, and imperforate anus. Practical aspects regarding their clinical presentation have been reviewed, and suggestions for the evaluation and therapy of these children have been proposed (see Figures 77.1-2, 77.1-4, and 77.1-6). Some general principles can be mentioned. Throughout the years, it has been learned that even though the surgical procedures are usually necessary, there has to be a balance between an attempt to follow physiologic principles and avoiding the creation of more problems. This may not always be possible, particularly when the patient's deficits are extensive, as in cases of fundoplication in children with severe neurologic impairment and esophageal dysmotility, patients with high imperforate anus without sacrum, or patients with total colonic aganglionosis. In most cases, however, recent advances have allowed for a better postoperative outcome, particularly in the area of anorectal malformations.

The pediatric gastroenterologist therefore needs to be familiar with the type of surgical procedures that can be performed, their indications, and their most common postoperative problems. An attempt should be made to participate with our surgical colleagues in deciding the best approach to therapy, particularly after the initial surgical procedures have failed.

REFERENCES

1. Smith CD, Othersen B, Gogan NJ, Walker JD. Nissen fundoplication in children with profound neutologic disability. Ann Surg 1992;215:654–9.

2. Fonkalsrud EW, Ashcraft KW, Coran AG, et al. Surgical treatment of gastroesophageal reflux in children: a combined hospital study of 7467 patients. Pediatrics 1998;101(3 Pt 1):419–22.

3. Fonkalsrud EW. Nissen fundoplication for gastroesophageal reflux disease in infants and children. Semin Pediatr Surg 1998;7:110–4.

4. Hassall E. Antireflux surgery in children: time for a harder look. Pediatrics 1998;101(3 Pt 1):467–8.

5. Di Lorenzo C, Orenstein S. Fundoplication: friend or foe? J Pediatr Gastroenterol Nutr 2002;34:117–24.

6. Low DE. Management of the problem patient after antireflux surgery. Gastroenterol Clin North Am 1994;23:371–89.

7. Hanimann B, Sacher P, Stauffer UG. Complications and long term results of the Nissen fundoplication. Eur J Pediatr Surg 1993;3:12–4.

8. Martinez DA, Ginn-Pease ME, Caniano DA. Sequelae of antireflux surgery in profoundly disabled children. J Pediatr Surg 1992;27:267–73.

9. Vane DW, Harmel RP, King DR, et al. The effectiveness of Nissen fundoplication in neurologically impaired children with gastroesophageal reflux. Surgery 1985;98:662–6.

10. Hassall E. Wrap session: is the Nissen slipping? Can medical treatment replace surgery for severe gastroesophageal reflux diseae in children? Am J Gastroenterol 1995;90:1212–20.

11. Richards CA, Milla P, Andrews PL, Spitz L. Retching and vomiting in neurologically impaired children after fundoplication: predictive preoperative factors. J Pediatr Surg 2001;36:1401–4.

12. Spitz L, Roth K, Kiely EM, et al. Operation for gastroesophageal reflux associated with severe mental retardation. Arch Dis Child 1993;68:347–51.

13. Wheatley MJ, Coran AG, Wesley JR, et al. Redo fundoplication in infants and childen with recurrent gastroesophageal reflux. J Pediatr Surg 1991;26:758–61.

14. Pearl RH, Robie DK, Ein SH, et al. Complications of gastroesophageal antireflux surgery in neurologically impaired versus neurologically normal children. J Pediatr Surg 1990;25:1169–73.

15. Dedinsky GK, Vane DW, Black T, et al. Complications and reoperation after Nissen fundoplication in childhood. Am J Surg 1987;153:177–83.

16. Bergmeijer JH, Tibboel FW, Hazerbroek J. Nissen fundoplication in the management of gastroesophageal reflux occurring after repair of esophageal atresia. J Pediatr Surg 2000;35:573–6.

17. Snyder CL, Ramachandran V, Kennedy AP, et al. Efficacy of partial wrap fundoplication for gastroesophageal reflux after repair of esophageal atresia. J Pediatr Surg 1997;32:1089–91; discussion 92.

18. Wheatley MJ, Coran AG, Wesley JR. Efficacy of the Nissen fundoplication in the management of gastroesophageal reflux following esophageal atresia repair. J Pediatr Surg 1993;28:53–5.

19. Rothenberg SS. Experience with 220 consecutive laparoscopic Nissen fundoplications in infants and children. J Pediatr Surg 1998;33:274–8.

20. Collins JB, Georgerson KE, Vicente Y, et al. Comparison of open and laparoscopic gastrostomy and fundoplication in 120 patients. Pediatr Surg 1995;30:1065–71.

21. Esposito C, Garipoli V, De Pasquale M, et al. Laparoscopic versus traditional fundoplication in the treatment of children with refractory gastro-oesophageal reflux. Ital J Gastroenterol Hepatol 1997;29:399–402.

22. Humphrey GM, Najmaldin AS. Laparoscopic Nissen fundoplication in disabled infants and children. J Pediatr Surg 1996;31:5969.

23. Rothenberg SS, Bratton D, Larsen G, et al. Laparoscopic fundoplication to enhance pulmonary function in children with severe reactive airway disease and gastroesophageal reflux disease. Surg Endosc 1997;11:1088–90.

24. Thompson WR, Hicks BA, Guzzetta PC Jr. Laparoscopic Nissen fundoplication in the infant. J Laparoendosc Surg 1996;6 Suppl 1:S5–7.

25. Tovar JA, Olivares P, Diaz M, et al. Functional results of laparoscopic fundoplication in children. J Pediatr Gastroenterol Nutr 1998;26:429–31.

26. van der Zee DC, Bax NM. Laparoscopic Thal fundoplication in mentally retarded children. Surg Endosc 1996;10:659–61.

27. Tashjan DB, Tirabassi MV, Moriarty KP, Salva PS. Laparoscopic Nissen fundoplication for reactive airway disease. J Pediatr Surg 2002;37:1021–3.

28. Heikkinen TJ, Haukipuro K, Koivukangas P, et al. Comparison of costs between laparoscopic and open Nissen fundoplication: a prospective randomized study with a 3-month followup. J Am Coll Surgeons 1999;188:368–76.

29. Ashcraft KM. Gastroesophageal reflux. In: Ashcraft KW, Holder TM, editors. Pediatric surgery. 2nd ed. Philadelphia: WB Saunders; 1993. p. 270–86.

30. Alrabeeah A, Giacomantonio M, Gillis D.. Paraesophageal hernia after Nissen fundoplication. A real complication in pediatric patients. J Pediatr Surg 1988;23:766–8.

31. Caniano DA, Ginn-Pease ME, King DR. The failed antireflux procedure. Analysis of risk factors and morbidity. J Pediatr Surg 1990;25:1022–6.

32. Wilkins BM, Spitz L. Adhesion obstruction following Nissen fundoplication in children. Br J Surg 1987;74:777–9.

33. Strecker-McGraw MK, Lorenz ML, Hendrickson M, et al. Persistent gastroesophageal reflux disease after antireflux surgery in children: I. Immediate postoperative evaluation using extended esophageal pH monitoring. J Pediatr Surg 1998;33:1623–7.

34. Beckingham IJ, Cariem AK, Bornman PC, et al. Oesophageal dysmotility is not associated with poor outcome after laparoscopic Nissen fundoplication. Br J Surg 1998;85:1290–3.

35. Wo JM, Trus TL, Richardson WS, et al. Evaluation and management of postfundoplication dysphagia. Am J Gastroenterol 1996;91:2318–22.

36. Weber TR. Toupet fundoplication for pediatric gastroesophageal reflux disease. Semin Pediatr Surg 1998;7:121–4.

37. Waring JP, Hunter JG, Oddsdittir M, et al. The preoperative evaluation of patients considered for laparoscopic antireflux surgery. Am J Gastroenterol 1995;90:35–8.

38. Low DE, Mercer CD, James EC, et al. Post Nissen syndrome. Surg Gynecol Obstet 1988;167:1–5.

39. Fibbe C, Layer P, Keller J, et al. Esophageal motility in reflux disease before and after fundoplication: a prospective, randomized, clinical and manometric study. Gastroenterology 2001;121:5–14.

40. Baigrie RJ, Watson DI, Myers JC, Jamieson GG. Outcome of laparoscopic Nissen fundoplication in patients with disordered preoperative peristalsis. Gut 1997;40:381–5.

41. Nyhus LM. Surgical treatment of gastroesophageal reflux in children. Surg Annu 1989;21:96–118.

42. Fonskalrud EW, Foglia RP, Ament M, et al. Operative treatment for the gastroesophageal reflux syndrome in children. J Pediatr Surg 1989;24:525–9.

43. Glick PL, Harrison MR. Gastric infarction secondary to small bowel obstruction: a preventable complication after Nissen fundoplication. J Pediatr Surg 1987;22:941–3.

44. DeMeester TR, Stein HJ. Minimizing the side effects of antireflux surgery. World J Surg 1992;16:335–6.

45. Vu MK, Straathof JW, v d Schaar PJ, et al. Motor and sensory function of the proximal stomach in reflux disease and after laparoscopic Nissen fundoplication. Am J Gastroenterol 1999;94:1481–9.

46. Dalla Vecchia LK, Grosfeld JL, West KW, et al. Reoperation after Nissen fundoplication in children with gastroesophageal reflux: experience with 130 patients. Ann Surg 1997;226: 315–21; discussion 21–3.

47. Bustorff-Silva J, Fonkalsrud EW, Perez CA, et al. Gastric emptying procedures decrease the risk of postoperative recurrent reflux in children with delayed gastric emptying. J Pediatr Surg 1999;34:79–82.

48. Richards CA, Andrews PL, Spitz L, Milla PJ. Nissen fundoplication may induce gastric myoelectrical disturbance in children. J Pediatr Surg 1998;33:1801–5.

49. DiLorenzo C, Flores A, Hyman PE. Intestinal motility in symptomatic children with fundoplication. J Pediatr Gastoenterol Nutr 1991;12:169–73.

50. Vu MK, Ringers J, Arndt JW, et al. Prospective study of the effect of laparoscopic hemifundoplication on motor and sensory function of the proximal stomach. Br J Surg 2000;87:338–43.

51. Tack J. Receptors of the enteric nervous system: potential targets for drug therapy. Gut 2000;47 Suppl 4:20–2.

52. Tack J. Functional dyspepsia. Curr Treat Options Gastroenterol 2000;3:287–94.

53. Jackson JL, O' Malley PG, Tomkins G, et al. Treatment of functional bowel disorders with antidepressant medications: a meta-analysis. Ann Intern Med 2000;108:65–72.

54. Festen C. Paraesophageal hernia: a major complication of Nissen's fundoplication. J Pediatr Surg 1981;16:496–9.

55. Wasvary H, Wease G, Bierema T, Glover J. Gastro-aortic fistula: an uncommon complication of Nissen fundoplication. Am Surgeon 1997;63:455–8.

56. Bufler P, Ehringhaus C, Koletzko S. Dumping syndrome: a common problem following Nissen fundoplication in young children. Pediatr Surg Int 2001;17:351–5.

57. Ng DD, Ferry RJ, Kelly A, et al. Acarbose treatment of postprandial hypoglycemia in children after Nissen fundoplication. J Pediatr 2001;139:877–9.

58. Rivkees SA, Crawford JD. Hypoglycemia pathogenesis in children with dumping syndrome. Pediatrics 1987;80:937–42.

59. Samuk I, Afriat R, Horne T, et al. Dumping syndrome following Nissen fundoplication, diagnosis, and treatment. J Pediatr Gastroenterol Nutr 1996;23:235–40.

60. Borovoy J, Furuta L, Nurko S. Benefit of uncooked corn starch in the management of children with dumping syndrome fed exclusively by gastrostomy. Am J Gastroenterol 1998;93:814–8.

61. Carvajal SH, Mulvihill SJ. Postgastrectomy syndromes: dumping and diarrhea. Gastroenterol Clin North Am 1994;23:261–79.

62. Khoshoo V, Roberts PL, Loe WA. Nutritional management of dumping syndrome associated with antireflux surgery. J Pediatr Surg 1994;29:1452–4.

63. Meyer S, Deckelbaum RJ, Lax E, Schiller M. Infant dumping syndrome after gastroesophageal reflux surgery. J Pediatr 1981;99:235–7.

64. Caulfield ME, Wylie R, Firor HV, Michener W. Dumping syndrome in children. J Pediatr 1987;110:212–5.

65. Gitzelmann R, Hirsig J. Infant dumping syndrome: reversal of symptoms by feeding uncooked corn starch. Eur J Pediatr 1986;145:504–6.

66. Kneepkens CM, Fernandes J, Vonk RJ. Dumping syndrome in children. Acta Paediatr Scand 1988;77:279–86.

67. Lavine JE, Hattner RS, Heyman M. Dumping in infancy diagnosed by radionuclide gastric emptying technique. J Pediatr Gastroenterol Nutr 1988;7:614–8.

68. Bier DM, Leake RD, Haymmond MW, et al. Measurement of "true" glucose production rates in infancy and childhood with 6,6-dideutero-glucose. Diabetes 1977;26:1016–23.

69. Khoshoo V, Reifen RR, Gold BD, et al. Nutritonal manipulation in the management of dumping syndrome. Arch Dis Child 1991;66:1447–8.

70. Hassegawa T, Yoneda M, Nakamura K, et al. Long term effect of alpha glucosidase inhibitor on late dumping syndrome. J Gastroenterol Hepatol 1998;13:1201–6.

71. Geer RJ, Richards WO, O'Diorisio TM, et al. Efficacy of octreotide acetate in the treatment of severe post gastrectomy dumping syndrome. Ann Surg 1990;212:678–81.

72. Siafakas C, Fox V, Nurko SS. Use of octreotide in severe gastrointestinal bleeding in children. J Pediatr Gastroenterol Nutr 1998;26:356–9.

73. Spitz L, Kirtane J. Results and complications of surgery for gastroesophageal reflux. Arch Dis Child 1985;60:743–7.

74. Puri P. Hirschsprung's disease: clinical and experimental observations. World J Surg 1993;17:374–84.

75. Reding R, Goyet JV, Gosseye S, et al. Hirschsprung's disease: a 20 year experience. J Pediatr Surg 1997;32:1221–5.

76. Swenson O. Early history of the therapy of Hirschsprung's disease: facts and personal observations over 50 years. J Pediatr Surg 1996;31:1003–8.

77. Bealer JF, Natuzzi ES, Flake AW, et al. Effect of nitric oxide on the colonic smooth muscle of patients with Hirschsprung's disease. J Pediatr Surg 1994;29:1025–9.

78. Barness PR, Lennard-Jones JE, Hawley PR, Todd IP. Hirschsprung's disease and idiopathic megacolon in adults and adolescents. Gut 1986;27:534–41.

79. Moore SW, Albertyn R, Cywes S. Clinical outcome and long term quality of life after surgical correction of Hirschsprung's disease. J Pediatr Surg 1996;31:1496–502.

80. Rudolph C, Benaroch L. Hirschsprung disease. Pediatr Rev 1995;16:5–11.

81. Teitelbaum MD. Hirschsprung's disease in children. Curr Opin Pediatr 1995;7:316–22.

82. Philippart AI. Hirschsprung's disease. In: Ashcraft KW, Holder TM, editors. Pediatric surgery. 2nd ed. Philadelphia: WB Saunders; 1993. p. 358–71.

83. Moore SW, Millar AJ, Cywes S. Long term clinical, manometric, and histologic evaluation of obstructive symptoms in the postoperative Hirschsprung's patient. J Pediatr Surg 1994;29: 106–11.

84. Bai Y, Chen H, Hao J, et al. Long term outcome and quality of life after Swenson procedure for Hirschsprung's disease. J Pediatr Surg 2002;37:639–42.

85. Yuan Z, Zhang Z, Zheng SJ, Wang W. Neural electrophysiological studies on the external anal sphincter in children with anorectal malformations. J Pediatr Surg 2000;35:1052–7.

86. Minkes RK, Langer JC. A prospective study of botulinum toxin for internal anal sphincter hypertonicity in children with Hirschsprung's disease. J Pediatr Surg 2000;35:1733–6.

87. Miele E, Tozzi A, Staiano A, et al. Persistence of abnormal gastrointestinal motility after operation for Hirschsprung's disease. Am J Gastroenterol 2002;95:1226–30.

88. Mishalany HG, Wooley MM. Postoperative functional and manometric evaluation of patients with Hirschsprung's disease. J Pediatr Surg 1987;22:443–6.

89. Kleinhaus S, Boley SJ, Sherman M, Sieber WK. Hirschsprung's disease: a survey of the surgical section of the American Academy of Pediatrics. J Pediatr Surg 1979;16:588–97.

90. Madonna MB, Luck SR, Reynolds M, et al. Swenson procedure for the treatment of Hirschsprung's disease. Semin Pediatr Surg 1998;7:85–8.

91. Swenson O, Sherman JO, Fisher JH. The treatment and postoperative complications of congenital megacolon: a 25 year follow up. Ann Surg 1975;182:266–72.

92. Stockmann PT, Philippart AI. The Duhamel procedure for Hirschsprung's disease. Semin Pediatr Surg 1998;7:89–95.

93. Duhamel B. Retrorectal and transanal pullthrough procedure for the treatment of Hirschsprung's disease. Dis Colon Rectum 1964;7:455–60.

94. Klein MD, Phillipart AI. Hirschsprung's disease: three decades' experience at a single institution. J Pediatr Surg 1993;10:1291–4.

95. Weinberg G, Boley SJ. Endorectal pull-through with primary anastomosis for Hirschsprung's disease. Semin Pediatr Surg 1998;7:96–102.

96. Tariq GM, Breteton RJ, Wright VM. Complications of endorectal pull-through for Hirschsprung's disease. J Pediatr Surg 1991;26:1202–8.

97. Sherman JO, Snyder ME, Witzman JJ, et al. A 40 year multinational retrospective study of 880 Swenson procedures. J Pediatr Surg 1989;24:833–8.

98. Ehrenpreis T, Livaditis A, Okmian L. Results of Duhamel's operation for Hirschsprung's disease. J Pediatr Surg 1966;1:40–6.

99. Livaditis A. Hirschsprung's disease: long term results of the original Duhamel operation. J Pediatr Surg 1981;16:484–6.

100. Baillie CT, Kenny SE, Rintala RJ, et al. Long-term outcome and colonic motility after the Duhamel procedure for Hirschsprung's disease. J Pediatr Surg 1999;34:325–9.

101. Ikeda K, Goto S. Diagnosis and treatment of Hirschsprung's disease in Japan. An analysis of 1628 patients. Ann Surg 1984;199:404–5.

102. Soave F. Endo-rectal pull-through: 20 years experience: address of the guest speaker, APSA. J Pediatr Surg 1985;20:568–79.

103. Marty TL, Matlak ME, Hendrickson M, et al. Unexpected death from enterocolitis after surgery for Hirschsprung's disease. Pediatrics 1995;96:118–21.

104. Marty TL, Seo T, Matalak ME, et al. Gastrointestinal function after surgical correction of Hirschsprung's disease: long term follow up in 135 patients. J Pediatr Surg 1995;30:655–8.

105. Catto-Smith AG, Coffey CM, Nolan T, Hutson JM. Fecal incontinence after the surgical treatment of Hirschsprung's disease. J Pediatr 1995;127:954–7.

106. Diseth T, Bjornland K, Novik T, Emblem R. Bowel function, mental health, and psychosocial function in adolescents with Hirschsprung's disease. Arch Dis Child 1997;76:100–6.

107. Diseth TH, Egeland T, Emblem R. Effects of anal invasive treatment and incontinence on mental health and psychosocial functioning of adolescents with Hirschsprung's disease and low anorectal anomalies. J Pediatr Surg 1998;33:468–75.

108. Holschneider AM. Treatment and functional results of anorectal continence in children with imperforate anus. Acta Chir Bel 1983;83:191–204.

109. Fadda B, Pistor G, Meier-Ruge W. Symptoms, diagnosis and therapy of neuronal intestinal dysplasia masked by Hirschsprung's disease. Pediatr Surg Int 1986;27:76–80.

110. Cohen MC, Moore SW, Neveling U, Kaschula RO. Acquired aganglionosis following surgery for Hirschsprung's disease: a report of five cases during a 33 year experience with pull-through procedures. Histopathology 1993;22:163–8.

111. Cord-Udy CL, Smith VV, Ahmed S, et al. An evaluation of the role of suction rectal biopsy in the diagnosis of intestinal neuronal dysplasia. J Pediatr Gastroenterol Nutr 1997;24:1–6.

112. Hanimann B, Inderbitzin D, Briner J, Sacher P. Clinical relevance of Hirschsprung-associated neuronal intestinal dysplasia. Eur J Pediatr Surg 1992;2:147–9.

113. Ure BM, Holschneider AM, Schulten D, Meier-Ruge W. Intestinal transit time in children with intestinal neuronal malformations mimicking Hirschsprung's disease. Eur J Pediatr Surg 1999;9:91–5.

114. Puri P. Variant Hirschsprung's disease. J Pediatr Surg 1997;32:149–57.

115. Koletzko S, Ballauff A, Hadziselimovic F, Enck P. Is histological diagnosis of neuronal intestinal dysplasia related to clinical and manometric findings in constipated children? Results of a pilot study. J Pediatr Gastroenterol Nutr 1993;17:59–65.

116. Holschneider AM, Meier-Ruge W, Ure BM. Hirschsprung's disease and allied disorders—a review. Eur J Pediatr Surg 1994;4:260–6.

117. Koletzko S, Jesch I, Faus-Kebler T, et al. Rectal biopsy for diagnosis of intestinal neuronal dysplasia in children: a prospective multicentre study on interobserver variation and clinical outcome. Gut 1999;44:853–61.

118. Scharli AF, Sossai R. Hypoganglionosis. Semin Pediatr Surg 1998;7:187–91.

119. Ryan DP. Neuronal intestinal dysplasia. Semin Pediatr Surg 1995;4:22–5.

120. Langer JB, Birnbaum E. Preliminary experience with intrasphincteric botulinum toxin for persistent constipation after pull-through for Hirschsprung's disease. J Pediatr Surg 1997;32:1059–62.

121. Bealer JF, Natuzzi ES, Buscher C, et al. Nitric oxide synthase is deficient in the aganglionic colon of patients with Hirschsprung's disease. Pediatrics 1994;93:647–51.

122. Blair GK, Murphy JJ, Fraser GC. Internal sphincterotomy in post-pull-through Hirschsprung's disease. J Pediatr Surg 1996;31:843–5.

123. Bannani SA, Forootan H. Role of anorectal myectomy after failed endorectal pull-through in Hirschsprung's disease. J Pediatr Surg 1994;29:1307–9.

124. Nurko S. Botulinum toxin for achalasia: are we witnessing the birth of a new era? J Pediatr Gastroenterol Nutr 1997;24:447–9.

125. Maria G, Cassetta E, Gui D, et al. A comparison of botulinum toxin and saline for the treatment of chronic anal fissure. N Engl J Med 1998;338:217–20.

126. Staiano A, Corazziari E, Andreotti M, et al. Esophageal motility in children with Hirschsprung's disease. Am J Dis Child 1991;145:310–3.

127. Faure C, Ategbo S, Ferreira GC, et al. Duodenal and esophageal manometry in total colonic aganglionosis. J Pediatr Gastroenterol Nutr 1994;18:193–9.

128. Di Lorenzo C, Solzi GF, Flores AF, et al. Colonic motility after surgery for Hirschsprung's disease. Am J Gastroenterol 2000;95:1759–64.

129. Zaslavsky C, Loening-Baucke V. Anorectal manometric evaluation of children and adolescents postsurgery for Hirschsprung's disease. J Pediatr Surg 2003;38:191–5.

130. Weber TR, Fortuna RS, Silen ML, Dillon PA. Reoperation for Hirschsprung's disease. J Pediatr Surg 1999;34:153–6; discussion 6–7.

131. Shandling B, Chait PG, Richards HF. Percutaneous cecostomy: a new technique in the management of fecal incontinence. J Pediatr Surg 1996;31:534–7.

132. Wilcox DT, Kiely EM. Repeat pull-through for Hirschsprung's disease. J Pediatr Surg 1998;33:1507–9.

133. Meier DE, Foster ME, Guzzetta PC, Coln D. Antegrade conti-

nent enema management of chronic fecal incontinence in children. J Pediatr Surg 1998;33:1149–51; discussion 51–2.

134. Wilcox DT, Kiely EM. The Malone (antegrade colonic enema) procedure: early experience. J Pediatr Surg 1998;33:204–6.

135. Graf JL, Strear C, Bratton B, et al. The antegrade continence enema procedure: a review of the literature. J Pediatr Surg 1998;33:1294–6.

136. Chait PG, Shandling B, Richards HM, Connolly BL. Fecal incontinence in children: treatment with percutaneous cecostomy tube placement—a prospective study. Radiology 1997;203:621–4.

137. Rivera M, Kugathasan S, Berger W, Werlin SL. Percutaneous colonoscopic cecostomy for management of chronic constipation in children. Gastrointest Endosc 2001;53:225–8.

138. Gauderer MW, Decou JM, Boyle JT. Sigmoid irrigation tube for the management of chronic evacuation disorders. J Pediatr Surg 2002;37:348–51.

139. Aksnes G, Diseth TH, Helseth A, et al. Appendicostomy for antegrade enema: effects on somatic and psychosocial functioning in children with myelomeningocele. Pediatrics 2002;109:484–9.

140. Heikkinen M, Rintala R, Luukkonen P. Long-term anal sphincter performance after surgery for Hirschsprung's disease. J Pediatr Surg 1997;32:1443–6.

141. Rescorla FJ, Morrison AM, Engles D, et al. Hirschsprung's disease. Evaluation of mortality and long-term function in 260 cases. Arch Surg 1992;127:934–41.

142. Loening-Baucke V, Desch L, Wolraich M. Biofeedback training for patients with myelomeningocele and fecal incontinence. Dev Med Child Neurol 1988;30:781–90.

143. Nurko SS, Worona L. Anorectal function in children with imperforate anus. J Gastrointest Motil 1993;5:209.

144. Blair GK, Djonlic K, Fraser GC, et al. The bowel management tube: an effective means for controlling fecal incontinence. J Pediatr Surg 1992;27:1269–72.

145. Levitt MA, Soffer SZ, Pena A. Continent appendicostomy in the bowel management of fecally incontinent children. J Pediatr Surg 1997;32:1630–3.

146. Bergmeijer JH, Tibboel D, Molenaar JC. Total colectomy and ileorectal anastomosis in the treatment of total colonic aganglionosis: a long term follow up study of six patients. J Pediatr Surg 1989;24:282–5.

147. Blane CE, Elhalaby E, Coran AG. Enterocolitis following endorectal pull-through procedure in children with Hirschsprung's disease. Pediatr Radiol 1994;24:164–6.

148. Hackam DJ, Filler RM, Pearl RH. Enterocolitis after the surgical treatment of Hirschsprung's disease: risk factors and financial impact. J Pediatr Surg 1998;33:830–3.

149. Teitelbaum DH, Coran AG. Enterocolitis. Semin Pediatr Surg 1998;7:162–9.

150. Elhalaby EA, Coran AG, Blane CE, et al. Enterocolitis associated with Hirschsprung's disease: a clinical-radiological characterization based on 168 patients. J Pediatr Surg 1995;30:76–83.

151. Bagwell CE, Langham MR, Mahaffey SM, et al. Pseudomembranous colitis following resection for Hirschsprung's disease. J Pediatr Surg 1992;27:1261–4.

152. Aslam A, Spicer RD, Corfield AP. Children with Hirschsprung's disease have an abnormal colonic mucus defensive barrier independent of the bowel innervation status. J Pediatr Surg 1997;32:1206–10.

153. Marty TL, Seo T, Sullivan JJ, et al. Rectal irrigations for the prevention of postoperative enterocolitis in Hirschsprung's disease. J Pediatr Surg 1995;30:652–4.

154. Hengster P, Pernthaler H, Gassner I, Menardi G. Twenty-three years of follow up in patients with total colonic aganglionosis. Klin Pediatr 1996;208:3–7.

155. Tsuji H, Spitz L, Kiely EM, et al. Management and long-term follow-up of infants with total colonic aganglionosis. J Pediatr Surg 1999;34:158–61; discussion 62.

156. Paidas CN. Fecal incontinence in children with anorectal malformations. Semin Pediatr Surg 1997;6:228–34.

157. Pena A, Guardino K, Tovilla JM, et al. Bowel management for fecal incontinence in patients with anorectal malformations. J Pediatr Surg 1998;33:133–7.

158. Pena A, Hong A. Advances in the management of anorectal malformations. Am J Surg 2000;180:370–6.

159. Ditesehim JA, Templeton JM. Short term vs long-term quality of life in children following repair of high imperforate anus. J Pediatr Surg 1987;22:581–7.

160. Templeton JM, Ditesheim JA. High imperforate anus: quantitative results of long term fecal continence. J Pediatr Surg 1985;20:645–52.

161. Glinn-Pease M, King DR, Tarnowski KJ, et al. Psychosocial adjustment and physical growth in children with imperforate anus or abdominal wall defects. J Pediatr Surg 1991;26:1129–35.

162. Pena A. Surgical management of anoectal malformations: a unified concept. Pediatr Surg Int 1988;3:82–93.

163. Diseth TH, Emblem R. Somatic function, mental health, and psychosocial adjustment of adolescents with anorectal anomalies. J Pediatr Surg 1996;31:638–43.

164. Pena A. Anorectal malformations. Semin Pediatr Surg 1995; 4:35–47.

165. Arnbjornsson E, Kullendorff CM, Okmian L, Rosen I. The value of physiotherapy for faecal continence after correction of high anal atresia. A clinical and electromyographic study. Acta Chir Scand 1988;154:467–70.

166. Molander ML, Frenckner B. Anal sphincter function after surgery for high imperforate anus. A long term follow up investigation. Z Kinderchirurg 1985;40:91–6.

167. Holschneider AM. Function of the sphincters in anorectal malformations and postoperative evaluation. In: Stephens D, Smith DE, editors. In: Anorectal malformations in children. Update 1988: March of Dimes Birth Defects Foundation. Birth defects: Original article series. New York: The Foundation; 1988. p. 425–45.

168. Doolin EJ, Black T, Donaldson JS, et al. Rectal manometry, computed tomography, and functional results of anal atresia surgery. J Pediatr Surg 1993;28:195–8.

169. Rintala RJ, Lindahl HG, Rasanen M. Do children with repaired low anorectal malformations have normal bowel function? J Pediatr Surg 1997;32:823–6.

170. Ludman L, Spitz L. Psychological adjustment of children treated for anorectal anomalies. J Pediatr Surg 1995;30:495–9.

171. Javid PJ, Barnhart DC, Hirschl RB, et al. Immediate and long-term results of surgical management of low imperforate anus in girls. J Pediatr Surg 1998;33:198–203.

172. Ludman L, Spitz L. Coping strategies of children with fecal incontinence. J Pediatr Surg 1996;31:563–7.

173. van Kuyk EM, Brugman-Boezeman AT, Wissink-Essink M, et al. Biopsychosocial treatment of defecation problems in children with anal atresia: a retrospective study. Pediatr Surg Int 2000;16:317–21.

174. Pena A, El Behery M. Megasigmoid: a source of pseudoincontinence in children with repaired anorectal malformations. J Pediatr Surg 1993;28:199–203.

175. Heikenen JB, Werlin SL, Di Lorenzo C, et al. Colonic motility in children with repaired imperforate anus. Dig Dis Sci 1999; 44:1288–92.

176. Rintala R, Lindhal H, Martinen E, Sariola H. Constipation is a major functional complication after internal sphincter-saving posterior sagittal anorectoplasty for high and intermediate anorectal malformations. J Pediatr Surg 1993;28:1054–8.

177. Fukata R, Iwai N, Yanagihara J, et al. A comparison of anal endosonography with electromyography and manometry in high and intermediate anorectal anomalies. J Pediatr Surg 1997;32:839–42.

178. Sachs TM, Applebaum H, Touran T, et al. Use of MRI in evaluation of anorectal anomalies. J Pediatr Surg 1990;28:817–21.

179. Emblem R, Diseth T, Morkird L, et al. Anal endosonography and physiology in adolescents with corrected low anorectal anomalies. J Pediatr Surg 1994;29:447–51.

180. Arnbjornsson E, Malmgren N, Mikaelsson C, et al. Computed tomography and magnetic resonance tomography findings in children operated for anal atresia. Z Kinderchirurg 1990; 45:178–81.

181. Worona L, Hernandez M, Consuelo A, et al. Successful use of biofeedback for the treatment of fecal incontinence in children with imperforate anus. J Pediatr Gastroenterol Nutr 2000;31:S243.

182. Iwai N, Yanagihara J, Tokiwa K, et al. Voluntary anal continence after surgery for anorectal malformations. J Pediatr Surg 1988;23:393–7.

183. Nagashima M, Iwai N, Yanagihara J, Shimotake T. Motility and sensation of the rectosigmoid and the rectum in patients with anorectal malformations. J Pediatr Surg 1992;27:1273–7.

184. Hedlund H, Pena A, Rodriguez G, Maza J. Long-term anorectal function in imperforate anus treated by a posterior sagittal anorectoplasty: manometric investigation. J Pediatr Surg 1992;27:906–9.

185. Lin CL, Chen CC. The rectoanal relaxation reflex and continence in repaired anorectal malformations with and without an internal sphincter-saving procedure. J Pediatr Surg 1996;31:630–3.

186. Rintala R. Postoperative internal sphincter function in anorectal malformations—a manometric study. Pediatr Surg Int 1990;5:127–30.

187. Molander ML, Frenckner B. Electrical activty of the external anal sphincter at different ages in childhood. Gut 1983;24:218–21.

188. Iwai N, Yanagihara J, Tsuto T, et al. Comparison of results of anorectal manometry performed after surgery for anorectal malformations and repeated three years later. Z Kinderchirurg 1986;41:97–100.

189. Rintala RJ, Marttinen E, Virkola K, et al. Segmental colonic motility in patients with anorectal malformations. J Pediatr Surg 1997;32:453–6.

190. Holschneider AM, Koebke J, Meier-Ruge W, et al. Pathophysiology of chronic constipation in anorectal malformations. Long-term results and preliminary anatomical investigations. Eur J Pediatr Surg 2001;11:305–10.

191. Cheu HW, Grosfeld JL. The atonic baggy rectum: a cause of intractable obstipation after imperforate anus repair. J Pediatr Surg 1992;27:1071–4.

192. Clarke SA, van der Avoirt A. Imperforate anus, Hirschsprung's disease, and trisomy 21: a rare combination. J Pediatr Surg 1999;34:1874.

193. Long FR, Hunter JV, Mahboubi S, et al. Tethered cord and associated vertebral anomalies in children and infants with imperforate anus: evaluation with MR imaging and plain radiography. Radiology 1996;200:377–82.

194. Arnbjornsson E, Breland U, Kullendorff CM, Okmian L. Effect of loperamide on fecal control after rectoplasty for high imperforate anus. Acta Chir Scand 1986;152:215–6.

195. Kekomaki M, Vikki P, Gordin A, Salo H. Loperamide as a symptomatic treatment in pediatric surgery: a double blind croosover study. Z Kinderchirurg 1981;32:237–43.

196. Menard C, Trudel C, Cloutier R. Anal reeducation for postoperative fecal incontinence in congenital diseases of the rectum and anus. J Pediatr Surg 1997;32:867–9.

197. Shamberger R, Lillhei C, Nurko SS, Winter H. Ano-rectal function in children following ileo-anal pull-through. J Pediatr Surg 1994;29:329–33.

198. Enck P. Biofeedback training in disordered defecation. A critical review. Dig Dis Sci 1993;38:1953–60.

199. Miner PB, Donnelly TC, Read NW. Investigation of mode of action of biofeedback in treatment of fecal incontinence. Dig Dis Sci 1990;35:1291–8.

200. Kirsch SE, Shandling B, Watson SL, et al. Continence following electrical stimulation and EMG biofeedback in a teenager with imperforate anus. J Pediatr Surg 1993;28:1408–10.

201. Tsugawa C, Hisano K, Nishijima E, et al. Posterior sagittal anorectoplasty for failed imperforate anus surgery: lessons learned from secondary repairs. J Pediatr Surg 2000;35: 1626–9.

202. Brain AJ, Kiely EM. Posterior sagittal anorectoplasty for reoperation in children with anorectal malformations. Br J Surg 1989;76:57–9.

203. Pena A. Current management of anorectal anomalies. Surg Clin North Am 1992;72:1393–416.

204. Lee SL, Rowell S, Greenholz SK. Therapeutic cecostomy tubes in infants with imperforate anus and caudal agenesis. J Pediatr Surg 2002;37:345–7.

205. Webb HW, Barraza MA, Stevens PS, et al. Bowel dysfunction in spina bifida—an American experience with the ACE procedure. Eur J Pediatr Surg 1998;8 Suppl 1:37–8.

206. Webb HW, Barraza MA, Crump JM. Laparoscopic appendicostomy for management of fecal incontinence. J Pediatr Surg 1997;32:457–8.

207. Malone PS, Curry JI, Osborne A. The antegrade continence enema procedure why, when and how? World J Urol 1998;16:274–8.

208. Marshall J, Anticich N, Stanton MP. Antegrade continence enemas in the treatment of slow transit constipation. J Pediatr Surg 2001;36:1227–30.

209. Whineray Kelly E, Bowkett B. Tube sigmoidostomy: a modification of the antegrade colonic evacuation. Aust N Z J Surg 2002;72:397–9.

210. Sonnino RE, Reinberg O, Bensoussan AL, et al. Gracilis muscle transposition for anal incontinence in children: long term follow up. J Pediatr Surg 1991;26:1219–23.

211. Lask B, Jenkins J, Nabarro L, et al. Psychosocial sequelae of stoma surgery for inflammatory bowel disease in childhood. Gut 1987;28:1257–60.

2. The Pediatric Ostomy

Catherine Cord-Udy, MBBS, FRACS(Paed Surg)
Erica Thomas, RGN, RSCN, DPNS, BSc(Hons)
Sarah Hotchkin, RN

A stoma can be a beneficial and life-changing surgical intervention for many chronic and acute gastrointestinal disease processes. It is a safe and effective way of diverting the fecal stream and allowing the bowel to heal while continuing enteral feeding. Indications vary depending on the age of the child, but a poorly created, poorly sited stoma can be a nightmare for both children and their family.

The first recorded formation of a colostomy on an infant was by the French surgeon Duret, in 1798,[1] when he successfully carried out the procedure on a 3-day-old infant with an imperforate anus. Although the basic principles and surgical technique have changed little over time, probably the single most significant development in pediatric stoma care has been the shift in emphasis from the earliest attempts of surgical intervention to cure or control the disease to the acknowledgment of the importance of the patient's quality of life after surgery. The identified need for education and support of the child and family before and after surgery has led to the creation of multidisciplinary teams of pediatric surgeons, pediatric stoma care nurses, dietitians, and gastroenterologists, all of whom play an important part in the rehabilitation of the child and family back into the community.

The aim of this chapter is to give an overview of the indications for stoma formation, describe the common types of stomas, and provide surgical tips for creating a good stoma. Practical advice will be included on coping with stomal complications and an understanding of the effect that a stoma has on both the child and the family, in particular the adolescent, who faces disturbance of body image and difficulty with emerging sexuality.

NUMBER OF PATIENTS

It is estimated that as many as 80,000 people in the United Kingdom have a stoma,[2] with only a small percentage of these being pediatric patients. Anecdotal evidence suggests that each regional center within the United Kingdom will see 40 to 100 new cases each year across the pediatric age range. The majority of stomas (76%) are formed in the first 6 weeks of life, 5% from 3 months to 1 year of age, 8% from 2 to 7 years of age, and the remaining 11% from the age of 8 to 16 years.[3]

TYPES OF STOMAS

The term *stoma* derives from the Greek meaning "mouth" or "opening" and is described as "an artificial opening established surgically between an organ and the exterior."[4]

JEJUNOSTOMY
The highest-output stoma is a jejunostomy, in which the stoma is sited in the jejunum. It is usually problematic owing to high fluid and electrolyte loss; therefore, enteral feeding cannot be established.

ILEOSTOMY
An ileostomy is a stoma formed in the ileum and can be either divided (ie, two ends spatially separated) or formed as a loop. It is our view that the bowel is not completely defunctioned by a loop because spillover of feces can occur, but it does give a blowhole effect.

COLOSTOMY
A colostomy is the formation of a stoma into the colon, and it is commonly sited in either the transverse or sigmoid colon and again can either be divided or formed as a loop. The lower down the bowel the stoma is placed, the less difficulty is faced with sodium and fluid imbalance because of the retained length of functioning bowel.

ANTEGRADE COLONIC ENEMA
The antegrade colonic enema was first developed by Malone in which one end of the appendix is reimplanted in a nonrefluxing manner into the cecum and the other end is brought out onto the abdominal wall as a continence stoma.[5] Surgical variations have been developed on this technique, but the basic function is to form an access port into the cecum. An alternative is the cecostomy button.[6] The procedure may be considered in children with anorectal anomalies, Hirschsprung disease, or spina bifida or in those children with chronic idiopathic constipation as an alternative to a permanent stoma or rectal washouts.

INDICATIONS FOR STOMA FORMATION

THE NEONATE
An acute stoma may be necessary in the following neonatal conditions: necrotizing enterocolitis, anorectal anom-

alies, Hirschsprung disease, complicated meconium ileus or failure to decompress the bowel after administration of Gastrografin, some intestinal atresias, and milk curd obstruction. Acute, short-term stomas may be situated within the wound to avoid a further site and therefore additional abdominal scars. Often the size of the abdomen in preterm babies makes siting near the umbilicus unavoidable, although still workable, and therefore avoids a second wound. Whatever the type of stoma, there needs to be an appreciation of the fragility of the blood supply to the mesentery of the neonatal bowel, with meticulous dissection and as limited as possible devascularization of the ends of the bowel. Historically this was why loop stomas were preferred.[7]

A neonate with gut dysmotility associated with, for example, gastroschisis or malrotation may need an end ileostomy to allow enteral nutrition to be established while the small bowel recovers function, without having to work against an ileocecal valve and unused colon. This may be required for several years and therefore should be properly sited by the stoma care nurse if possible.

THE OLDER CHILD

An acute stoma in the older child may be necessary in the following conditions: trauma sustained either rectally or abdominally; some intra-abdominal catastrophes such as intussusception or volvulus associated with malrotation, in which viability of the bowel is doubtful; ulcerative colitis with toxic megacolon or intractable bleeding; perianal sepsis in the immunocompromised oncology child or those with severe neutropenic enterocolitis associated with therapy; acute abdominal abscess; or perforation in Crohn disease.

A semiurgent stoma may be considered in the following conditions: chronic constipation, pseudo-obstruction, children with Hirschsprung disease in whom the bowel has not decompressed, and children born with anorectal anomalies who continue to have problems with constant soiling. Severe refractory ulcerative colitis will require a subtotal colectomy and formation of an end ileostomy, as will familial adenomatous polyposis[8] because of the risk of malignancy.

PREOPERATIVE CARE

STOMA SITING

It is important that, whenever practicable, patients have access to a stoma care nurse specialist for information, advice, and siting preoperatively. This is not always achievable because many stomas in children are formed as an emergency; therefore, there is little time for discussion and siting in relation to the position of the stoma, but the following principles of stoma siting should be adhered to whenever possible (Table 77.2-1).

Careful siting should involve the cooperation and consent of the patient (depending on the child's age). It is important to remember that the shape of the abdomen alters when the patient is lying, sitting, or standing and in thin or obese children. Each stoma site therefore needs to be tailored to the individual's needs, and, when possible,

patients should be given the chance to familiarize themselves with the stoma bag by applying it to the site, so as to predict any potential problems with positioning. As Black noted, "There is nothing that can compensate for a badly sited stoma, achieving the correct site will have an enormous influence on the individual's post-operative rehabilitation, ability to manage his/her own care and ultimately their quality of life."[9]

BOWEL PREPARATION

For the emergency stoma, there is no time to adequately prepare the bowel. For those children undergoing elective surgery, 24 to 48 hours of clear fluids and oral laxatives are often adequate; however, rectal washouts may be required to empty the bowel, but these should not be attempted on those at risk of perforation (eg, the immunocompromised child or the child with diffuse inflammatory bowel disease).

PSYCHOLOGICAL PREPARATION

The majority of congenital abnormalities requiring stoma formation are not apparent until after birth, therefore allowing parents no time to prepare for the consequences of giving birth to a baby with a disability.[10] It is often difficult for parents to understand the medical terminology being presented to them. Every family will have its own means of understanding the information provided, and, wherever possible, time should be allowed for questioning, preparation, and acceptance of the need for surgery. Sometimes this is realistically impossible when faced with a sick neonate or an adolescent trauma victim.

Even in these emergency situations, parents are entitled to feel that they have adequate information about the procedure to make an informed choice about their child's care. Parenthood can be traumatic and stressful at the best of times, and the support received from staff in the initial stages can make all the difference[11] as to their acceptance of the stoma after surgery.

When stoma surgery is planned, the method of preparation used should be related to the time frame available and the age of the child. A number of books and dolls are available through various organizations (see contact addresses) that can allow even a young child to come to some level of understanding of what is about to happen. Experienced play therapists and pediatric nurses can use play acting and painting to help the child become involved in the decision-making process.[12]

TABLE 77.2-1   AREAS TO AVOID IN STOMA SITING

Waistline
Hip bones
Previous scars
Groin area
Fat folds and bulges
Umbilicus
Under pendulous breasts
Areas of skin irritation (psoriasis, eczema, skin allergies)
Positioning of artificial limbs
Areas in which there would be difficulties if weight gain or loss occurred

---

Postoperatively, the older child who has suffered the consequences of inflammatory bowel disease, with pain, repeated hospitalization, polypharmacy, and exclusion from their peers, may see surgery as a relief and an opportunity to start living again. The desire for a cure often clouds many teenagers' judgment as to their true feelings about their altered body image, which tends to emerge months after surgery, when the true picture of their new life becomes apparent.

Access to the Internet can provide teenagers with information that they may feel too embarrassed to ask for (Table 77.2-2), and many self-help organizations have sites for the young adult ostomist. Approximately 20% of patients with a stoma experience clinically significant psychological symptoms postoperatively; commonly, these are anxiety and adjustment disorders.[13]

CULTURAL ISSUES

When caring for the child and family, it is important to take into account their religious, cultural, and individual needs. There may be a number of questions, such as "Is there any animal content in the makeup of the appliance being used?" According to Muslim culture, the left hand is used for cleansing and the right hand is used for meeting and greeting. This therefore requires special allowance when teaching stoma care if the left hand is the nondominant hand. The prolonged fasting during Ramadan can result in increased levels of dehydration and constipation. Children with a stoma can often be exempt from their religious duties at this time or at least be allowed some flexibility. Discussion with their religious leader can help in assistance and guidance.

COMPLICATIONS OF STOMA SURGERY: PRACTICAL ADVICE

Many of the complications listed below can be avoided by careful consideration of the site of the stoma and care being taken by the surgeon when surgically creating the stoma spout itself and its positioning in relation to the abdominal wound. Different complications can be seen at different time scales following surgery.

AVASCULAR NECROSIS
Stomas initially are often dusky and bruised in appearance, but many recover without any problems. Technical attention must be paid to preserving a good blood supply to the active stoma by not strangulating it either with a misplaced

suture, closing the abdomen too tightly, or by placing the mesentery under tension. The mucus fistula can be placed in slightly less healthy bowel, understanding that it may fibrose down, but it will preserve bowel length that would otherwise have been sacrificed in closure.

Stomas in neonates are usually covered only with a small piece of Jelonet (Smith and Nephew Healthcare Ltd, Hull, UK) and gauze to allow clear observation until the stoma becomes active. The first appliance in all age groups should always be clear-fronted and drainable with no flatus filter; this allows clear visual access and the ability to record the volume of stool passed and monitor any wind produced.

Care should be taken to protect the stoma in neonates when undergoing phototherapy because "sunburn" of the mucosa (black appearance) can result, and incubators can often dry out the stoma. Covering the stoma with Jelonet and gauze can prevent this.

DEHISCENCE
Complete dehiscence is when the stoma wound breaks open and a further portion of the bowel can extrude from the wound. This is unusual and requires surgical revision, and it is more likely to occur if the two stoma ends are crowded into too small a wound so that skin bridges between them fail to heal. Wound dehiscence is more likely if there is heavy soiling with fecal matter and a malnourished child or premature baby. A superficial dehiscence is more common and usually responds to topical packing, without revision being required.

BLEEDING
Bleeding can be peristomal, from erosions or ulcers (usually secondary to bag placement and local trauma). Parents should be warned to expect some bleeding when the stoma is wiped clean because of surface trauma or if the infant is crying when the appliance is being changed because tension on the sutures occurs owing to the increase in intra-abdominal pressure.

Bleeding may be a symptom of the intrinsic pathology of the sick child, but it is important to beware of parastomal varices that can accompany total parenteral nutrition–induced liver failure and portal hypertension. These can bleed exsanguinating amounts of blood rapidly. Local pressure and resuscitation with comprehensive blood products can be lifesaving.

STENOSIS
Ischemia to the bowel end is one of the most common causes of stenosis. Closing the abdominal wall too tightly

TABLE 77.2-2   WEB ORGANIZATIONS

ORGANIZATION	WEB SITE
United Ostomy Association	www.uoa.org
International Ostomy Association	www.ostomyinternational.org
Wound, Ostomy and Continence Nurses Association	www.wocn.org
The Mark Allen Group Organisation (specialist stoma care nursing)	www.internurse.com/stomacare.cfm
Living with a colostomy	www.ostomy.fsnet.co.uk
The Continence Foundation	www.continence-foundation.org.uk
The Simon Foundation for Continence	www.simonfoundation.org-html

around the stoma can cause an ischemic effect and can also tighten the abdominal exit site, causing stenosis.

A narrowing of the outlet of the stoma through the abdominal wall can cause an obstruction, often with output fluctuating from little to excessive. Translocation of bacteria can occur at the site, and the patient can become toxic and unwell, often with subsequent line sepsis. If this is suspected, the stoma should be digitally probed to check its patency and may require dilation (not in the neonate), although surgical revision is usually required.

A loopogram radiologic study can show dilatation, but it is a good precaution to cover the procedure with intravenous antibiotics to avoid translocation of bacteria and septicemia.

Necrosis following an infection around the stoma can result in narrowing at the entrance, causing acute abdominal pain and no activity or difficulty in passing stool. Colostomy patients should be advised to keep the stool soft by consuming additional fluids (especially in warm weather) and avoid a high-fiber or bulky diet.

PROLAPSE

Prolapse of the bowel can be quite dramatic (Figure 77.2-1). This is more common with loop enterostomies, especially in the distal limb, but can occur with end stomas, especially those in a very dilated bowel as it returns to normal size. Fixing the bowel to the muscle fascia in four quadrants goes some way to preventing prolapse.

Small prolapses can be ignored if easily reduced, but an irreducible stoma needs attention to avoid bowel compromise: application of fine sugar granules followed by manual reduction or warm saline gauze and slow pressure usually achieves a result. The sugar causes a fluid shift across the bowel wall via an osmotic gradient, causing the stoma to shrink.[14]

Failure to reduce the stoma requires urgent surgical intervention and, occasionally, revision. A chronic prolapse can be encircled with a nonabsorbable suture, as in a Thiersch suture for rectal prolapse. Refashioning of the stoma is sometimes the only option, and, if required, a new site is preferable. Adolescents who have difficulty with accepting their body image because of the prolapsed stoma may request revision.

When the stoma has prolapsed, it may be difficult to apply the original size appliance; therefore, increasing the size of the aperture can sometimes prevent the stoma from suffering trauma to its edges.

RETRACTION

Retraction of the stoma can be due to inadequate length of bowel pulled under tension, subsequent adhesions, or the disease process recurring, such as Crohn strictures. The stoma can become indrawn and flush with the skin, causing excoriation and problems with leakage. Although retraction can sometimes resolve spontaneously, revision may be required to make management of the stoma easier, and adequate spouting initially can make this less of a problem, even for colostomies.

Another cause can be from the child gaining a lot of weight after surgery, causing the stoma to become level with the abdominal wall; therefore, the feces has difficulty draining away from the appliance, causing pooling of stool (pancaking) under the appliance. In older children, a convex appliance can assist in pushing the stoma out and thus creating a moat effect to promote better drainage (pastes may help make the appliance stickier).

INCISIONAL OR PARASTOMAL HERNIA

This is not a big problem in young people because of the natural strength of the abdominal wall, but it may become a problem in those who have undergone repeated abdominal surgery or in those who are overweight.

The weakness in the closure of the abdominal wall adjacent to the stoma can result in an incisional hernia. This is more common in a very dilated bowel that returns to size, but it is also more frequently seen in children with Down syndrome who have required stoma formation owing to poor collagen and therefore poor healing. If troublesome, revision may be required; otherwise, it can be ignored, although bag application can be difficult.

INTESTINAL FISTULA

A leak of intestinal contents from a fistula adjacent to the stoma can result from an anchoring suture placed too deeply or from the disease process recurring in Crohn disease. Intra-abdominal fistulae need to be revised urgently, but a small external fistula can be of little consequence.

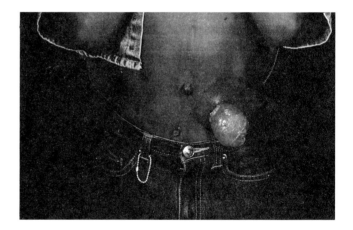

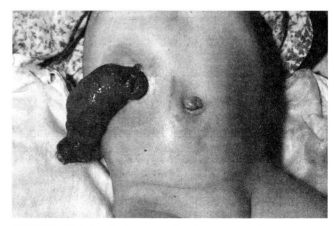

FIGURE 77.2-1   End sigmoid colostomy prolapse in two children.

MUCOCUTANEOUS SEPARATION

This results when the stoma edge comes away from the surrounding skin, leaving a shallow cavity around the stoma. It is a particular problem in neonates owing to insufficient bowel mobilization at the time of surgery, causing undue tension on the stoma sutures, which anchor it to the skin. Sore skin around the stoma can result from leakage of stool under the flange; the developing trough can be filled with hydrocolloid gel or paste to promote granulation tissue, and the appliance aperture can be cut to incorporate this.

DEHYDRATION AND ELECTROLYTE IMBALANCE

Every effort should be made to site the stoma as far as practicable down the bowel, and in the immediate postoperative period, close attention to fluid balance must be maintained to avoid electrolyte imbalance. Once on a full enteral diet, the urine should be monitored to ensure that adequate sodium levels are maintained. Supportive parenteral nutrition or fluids may be required for some time in children with acute high intestinal stomas. Enteral nutrition in children with jejunostomies should be given as a low continuous volume to keep the enterohepatic circulation going and decrease cholestasis; it also maintains nutrition to the enterocytes but avoids excessive fluid problems by limiting the input.

Oral sodium supplements are needed almost always in children with ileostomies and even with some colostomies. The infant's or child's growth can be severely impaired by low total-body sodium.

DIVERSIONAL COLITIS

This can occur in the defunctioning bowel owing to stagnation of the contents and a lack of topical nutrition to the enterocytes, with the child experiencing painful discharge and bleeding. Short-chain fatty acids can be instilled into the defunctioning limb with a good result; this is usually given daily for 1 week, with the amount dependent on the length of bowel involved, and then repeated as necessary until under control.[15]

The passage of mucus from the rectum is not uncommon, with older children reporting the urge to defecate. For the occasional rectal discharge, a plain saline washout through the defunctioning stoma or rectum may alleviate the problem, although too frequent washouts can have the undesirable effect of increasing mucus production. Bleeding from the rectum may be an indication of recurrence or continuation of active inflammatory bowel disease.

SKIN PROBLEMS

An entire atlas has been developed about abdominal stomas and their skin disorders.[16] Soreness can result from an allergic reaction or sensitivity to the adhesive part of the appliance (contact dermatitis), with the outline of the appliance clearly visible following removal. Changing the appliance used can usually resolve the problem; otherwise, barrier films or hydrocolloid dressing used under the appliance can reduce contact and therefore the likelihood of a reaction. Topical steroids should be used with extreme caution because they can result in the peristomal skin becoming very fragile.

Fungal infections often respond to topical nystatin or cotrimoxazole, or a single dose of fluconazole may be required orally if severe.

Effluent dermatitis, inflammation, or excoriation caused by leakage of stool directly onto the peristomal skin is more common in ileostomy patients owing to the liquid consistency damaging the skin on contact. Gut enzymes, particularly protease and amylase found in ileostomy output, can cause fecal irritation by damaging the horny layer of the skin.[17] The cause can be simply that the shape of the stoma has changed, thus allowing fecal fluid to leak under the flange. If this occurs, barrier films can be used to protect the skin.

Poor technique in the fitting of the appliance or the changing shape of the abdomen as children grow may result in the development of troughs and ridges, which prevent the appliance from lying flat against the skin. Pastes or seals can be used to fill uneven areas, allowing the appliance a flat, even surface to which to adhere.

Wet skin under an appliance can be dried using calamine lotion, also giving a soothing effect when the area is itchy. Preexisting skin conditions such as eczema can cause reactions and itchiness from some appliances, and often trial and error is the only way to achieve a solution.

The adhesive quality of the appliance can be increased by warming the appliance either in clasped hands, leaving it on a radiator for a short period of time, or by the use of a hairdryer before sticking it to the skin.

Overfull bags can increase the likelihood of leakage because the weight of the stool pulls the flange away from the skin. Patient education should include the importance of emptying the skin before it becomes no more than two-thirds full.

Granulation tissue may be "normal" and can be controlled with topical oxytetracycline and hydrocortisone (Terra-Cortril), silver nitrate application (with caution), or the regular use of dexamethasone, famycetin, and gramicidin (Sofradex) ointment.

CHOOSING THE RIGHT STOMA APPLIANCE

In the past decade, the choice of stoma appliances for the infant or child has increased dramatically. The following issues should be considered when offering advice to the new ostomist (Table 77.2-3):

- Stoma appliances are made either as a one-piece system; incorporating both the flange and bag (either drainable or closed), or a two-piece system with a separate flange and bag that connect together.

TABLE 77.2-3 FACTORS INFLUENCING CHOICE OF STOMA APPLIANCE

Age and size of the infant/child
Type of stoma: colostomy/ileostomy
Site/position of stoma
Physical/social activities
Dexterity of the child

- One-piece drainable appliances are particularly suitable for infants and younger children who do not have a high level of output. As children grow and their diet becomes more varied, the volume of effluent increases, and with increasing levels of activity, the support and flexibility of a two-piece system may be more suitable, allowing the bag to be changed without the need of the flange to be removed.
- Bags can be drainable for high-output stomas, or if the child has difficulty in emptying the bag, a nondrainable system may be more appropriate. The size or capacity of bags can be varied depending on the activities undertaken (a larger bag may be useful overnight to decrease the need for emptying).
- To combat the effects of flatulence, "flatus filters" are available in many drainable and nondrainable appliances. These do become ineffective when wet; therefore, the outlet should be covered when bathing or swimming.
- Convexity appliances have integral convexity and help create a seal for use with retracted stomas. This system is not recommended in young children because of the risk of pressure ulcer formation, and if used long term in young children, there is also some concern about interruption of muscle growth.
- A wide range of appliances and accessories is available that will cover the individual requirements of most patients. Before finalizing any appliance orders, the opportunity to try different products should be offered because the consumer should have ultimate choice on the system used.

DISCHARGE PLANNING

As the child recovers from surgery, plans should be made for the child to return home. Teaching should involve basic stoma care, knowledge of the practical skills required to change an appliance, possible complications, and whom to reach for advice (Table 77.2-4).

Regular contact should be maintained until the family has the necessary confidence to be totally independent at home. It should be clear to the family how and where additional supplies can be obtained from community services.

Ideally, home visits after discharge offer the family an opportunity to discuss issues that they may have felt unable to question while in the hospital environment. It also provides an opportunity to review bathroom facilities,

TABLE 77.2-4   DISCHARGE PLANNING

Discharge teaching should involve
  Normal stoma function
  Preparation, application, and removal of appliance
  Skin care
  Where to obtain supplies
  Disposal of used appliances
  Exemption from prescription charges
  Recognizing complications and whom to contact for advice
  Dealing with potential problems, eg, leakage, sore skin, odor, and flatus

which may need simple adaptation, and general storage advice for the new equipment.

EDUCATIONAL SUPPORT

Under the guidelines of The United Kingdom Education Act (1981), all children are entitled to an education, and it is the duty of their local educational authority to facilitate the necessary support. The reality is that parents are often "on call" to troubleshoot any problems that occur while the child is at school. The pediatric stoma nurse can offer the child and teachers support in terms of reintegration into the school environment and can educate teaching assistants and carers.

Most head teachers are only too willing to provide access to private toilets away from the main children's facilities, allowing the child to empty or change the appliance in private. The adolescent may have serious problems returning to school with a stoma, and avoidance behavior is common. Postoperative psychological support is often necessary to overcome this awkward period.

NUTRITIONAL CONSIDERATIONS

Concerns about eating and the associated reaction of the stoma are common among new ostomists. Initially, they are constantly aware when the stoma acts and, as a result, are cautious about eating certain foods. Flatus is produced more readily when eating pulses, baked beans, fizzy drinks, and, in some, chocolate. Eating slowly and chewing food well can reduce the amount of air swallowed.

Effluent will contain more fluid when eating spicy foods, fruit, and green vegetables. Eggs, boiled rice, sweetcorn, bananas, and mushrooms will thicken the stool and, in some children, lead to constipation. Foods that are known to cause problems should not be avoided, but by emptying the appliance more frequently or wearing an appliance to accommodate increased output, mealtimes should be more relaxed. It takes about 16 to 22 hours from food being swallowed to it being seen in a colostomy bag—less time with an ileostomy.

Children should be encouraged to experiment to see how their stoma reacts to different food items so that they can remain in control. A healthful balanced diet should always be encouraged. Useful tips in having a stoma can be gleaned from other patients and their families (Table 77.2-5).

TRANSITION OF CARE

The preparation to move from pediatric care to adult-based services can cause great anxiety to many families. For many parents, the security blanket of a pediatric service has enabled them to manage their children's chronic health needs and feel comfortable when attending clinic appointments. The handover of care should be planned and coordinated if possible in a combined adolescent clinic, giving the family the opportunity to meet the new team while maintaining links with the old.

TABLE 77.2-5   HELPFUL HINTS FROM OUR PATIENTS

When gaining confidence in fitting a new bag use a mirror so that you can see what you are doing.

Clean the stoma with gauze swabs because cotton wool balls can leave strands, preventing the bag from sticking.

Storage of appliances should be in a cool, dry area (steamy bathrooms affect the adhesive).

Always have some bags ready cut for those emergency changes; they will always happen.

It is up to you who you tell about your stoma!

To improve the stickiness of the appliance, warm it in clasped hands before applying.

To enable you to see what you are doing, use a clothes-peg to hold clothing out of the way.

If the smell is too offensive, use scented candles in the bathroom when changing the bag.

After the recovery phase of surgery, your stoma's activity will become more predictable. Often it is most active after breakfast.

Beer can give you wind!

REFERENCES

1. Duret C. Observations et reflexions sur une imperforation de l'anus. Recueil periodique de la Societe de Medecine de Paris; 3, 46. Reprinted in Amussat 1839. p. 88.

2. Coloplast. An introduction to stoma care: a guide for healthcare professionals. Peterborough (UK): Coloplast; 1999.

3. Fitzpatrick G. Stoma care in the community: a clinical resource for practitioners. Nurs Times 1999;33–56.

4. Barrett J, et al. Blackwell's dictionary of nursing. New York: Springer; 1994. Stoma.

5. Malone PS, Ransley PG, Kiely EM. Preliminary report: the antegrade continence enema. Lancet 1990;17:1217–8.

6. Fukunaga K, Kimura K, Lawrence JP, et al. Button device for antegrade enema in the treatment of incontinence and constipation. J Pediatr Surg 1996;31:1038–9.

7. Bishop HC. Ileostomy and colostomy. Paediatric surgery. 4th ed.

8. Arvanitis ML, Jagelmann DG, Fazio VW, et al. Mortality in patients with familial adenomatous polyposis. Dis Colon Rectum 1990;33:639–42.

9. Black P. An introduction to stoma care. Folkestone (UK): Clinical Pharmacology Research Institute; 1988.

10. Webster P. Special babies: community outlook. Nurs Times 1985;81:19–22.

11. Stewart AJ. Mums and dads need care too: supporting parents of babies in neonatal units. Prof Nurs 1990;5:660–5.

12. Ziegler DB, Prior MM. Preparation for surgery and adjustment to hospitalisation. Pediatr Surg Nurs 1994;29:655–69.

13. White C. Living with a stoma: a practical guide to coping with colostomy, ileostomy and urostomy. London: Sheldon Press; 1997.

14. Black P. Holistic stoma care. London: Bailliere Tindall; 2000.

15. Vernia P, et al. Butyrate enema therapy stimulates mucosal repair in experimental colitis in the rat. Bethesda (MD): National Library of Medicine; 1995.

16. Lyon CC, Smith JA. Abdominal stomas and their skin disorders: an atlas of diagnosis and management. Fredensborg: Dansac; 2001.

17. Collett K. Practical aspects of stoma management. Nurs Standard 2002;17:45–52.

ADDITIONAL READING

Andersen PH, Bucher AP, Saeed I, et al. Faecal enzymes: in vivo human skin irritation. Contact Dermatitis 1994;30:152–8.

Black PK. Colostomy. Prof Nurs 1998;13:851–7.

Bingham S, et al. Diet and health of people with an ileostomy: 1. Dietary assessment. Br J Nutr 1982;47:399–406.

Elcoat C. Stoma care nursing. London: Bailiere Tindall Myers; 1996.

Fitzpatrick TB, Eisen AZ, Wolff K, et al. Dermatology in general medicine. 4th ed. New York: McGraw-Hill; 1993.

Fligelsone L, Wanendeya N, Palmer BV. Osmotic therapy for acute irreducible stoma prolapse. Br J Surg 1997;84:390.

Kelly L. Patients becoming people. Journal of community: a clinical resource for practitioners. London: Nursing Times Books; 1995.

Porrett T, Daniel N. Essential coloproctology for nurses. London: Convatec; 1999.

Salter M. Altered body image: the nurse's role. London: Scutari Press; 1988.

Squire R, Kiely EM, Carr B, et al. Clinical application of the Malone antegrade colonic enema. J Pediatr Surg 1993;28:1012–5.

Stoma care nursing: a patient centred approach. London: Arnold.

Taylor P. Stoma care in the community. London: Nursing Times Books; 1999.

Wade B. A stoma is for life. Harrow (UK): Scutari Press; 1989.

White C, Hunt JC. Psychological factors in postoperative adjustment to stoma surgery. Ann R Coll Surg Engl 1997;79:3–7.

3. Psychological Aspects

Steven Schlozman, MD

Suzanne Bender, MD

The psychological effects on pediatric patients who are preparing for or have experienced gastrointestinal (GI) surgery are rich in scope and poor in documentation.[1] Although virtually all clinicians agree that GI surgery poses potentially significant psychological and emotional risks for children and adolescents, the medical and psychological literature addressing these issues continually emphasizes the need for more rigorous studies to ascertain which interventions are most useful for this patient population. Although pre- and postoperative preparations most often include a developmentally driven attempt to demystify the hospital and the operation itself, the existing studies lack methodologic consistency and concrete guidelines.[1,2] Indeed, consulting the existing literature alone leaves one uncertain of how best to help children and adolescents through the ordeals of major and minor GI surgeries.

However, the lack of methodologic consistency contrasts sharply with the wealth of clinical experience that many mental health clinicians have accrued in working with medically ill young people. With regard to GI surgery, a coherent picture of the psychic effects of surgical intervention on younger patients is complicated by the premorbid psychiatric and psychological state, which is itself often a function of the underlying chronic GI illness. Patients with inflammatory bowel disease (IBD), for example, will potentially suffer different psychological effects than patients who are awaiting liver transplant or who suffer from GI tumors. The variety of children in general and the breadth of medical illness in particular make generalizations about this patient population especially challenging.

Nevertheless, clinical experience and a growing appreciation for a biopsychosocial approach *do* yield important guidelines for the care of these young patients. With these concerns in mind, this chapter addresses both general developmentally based observations regarding pediatric patients undergoing GI surgery and specific psychological aspects of common surgical issues seen in patients with IBD and those who receive corticosteroid therapies.

DEVELOPMENTAL APPROACH

The most efficient and accurate approach to medically ill children and adolescents involves careful attention to developmental principles.[3] The effects of major surgical intervention will be different for toddlers than for teenagers, and clinicians must take these differences into account when assessing children in these settings. Although an exhaustive review of child and adolescent development is beyond the scope of this chapter, a brief summary of important differences among children of different ages is important.

Infants and toddlers lack the cognitive skills to understand the gravity of their condition. They rely on their parents and caregivers to relieve immediate suffering and discomfort, and they experience much of the surgical world in terms of the discomfort engendered and the limitations imposed.

Perhaps most importantly, the youngest patients rely on their parents and primary caregivers to keep them safe and to soothe them when they are troubled. Infant–parent attachment can be particularly compromised by severe medical illness, and the hospital staff should work to foster a milieu that allows for as much contact as possible between infant and parent. Parents should remain as close as possible and should interact as much as possible. In this light, fundamental issues such as parent–child physical contact, feeding, and, if possible, breastfeeding should be preserved as much as possible. However, potential exceptions include using parents to restrain older and struggling infants and toddlers during painful procedures. This practice is potentially extremely traumatic for the child and the parent and may prolong and make more dangerous the procedure in question.

As toddlers age, they develop the egocentrism that often defines younger children. They view all events as relating directly to themselves and interpret both bad and good experiences as a function of their own actions. Thus, the toddler often associates unrelated incidents as being causally related, a cognitive style that developmentalists refer to as associative thinking. In the setting of illness severe enough to warrant surgical intervention, toddlers (as well as older patients in more subtle ways) are particularly vulnerable to concluding that their own transgressions have led to their medical predicament. To protect against the damage that these conceptualizations can create, it is often helpful to clarify as much as possible the etiology of a given medical condition and to uncover and correct misconceptions about the cause of illness.

Separation from caregivers and anxieties around bedtime are some of the more common psychological stressors affecting toddlers as they prepare for or recover from surgical procedures. In addition, because they have only recently come to understand that they have control over their body, toddlers often experience insults such as blood draws and even physical examinations as assaults on their entire physical being. To the extent that they can be gently and consistently prepared before procedures and examinations, they will be protected from a state of constant hyperarousal as they prepare to defend themselves from the onslaught of physicians and technicians.

As children age, their cognitive capacities rapidly develop. They enjoy a growing sense of mastery in understanding the world around them, categorizing and labeling many of the central features of their lives. They will collect baseball cards, know their telephone number, and memorize the names of countless dinosaurs. Medically ill children will often take great pride and comfort in knowing the names of their diseases, of their medications, and of complicated surgical procedures. If a child in this setting expresses interest in what is happening medically, it is developmentally useful to answer as concretely as possible. Simple cause and effect are hallmarks of preadolescent cognitive development, and children in this age group understand, for example, that germs cause disease and that taking out something bad (like a splinter, in more benign settings) can lead to feeling better. However, this cognitive style can lead to psychological distress when there is no clear cause for a given illness. Always tuned into media and popular culture, children may wonder, for example, how they developed cancer without smoking or why they need to go back to the operating room if they diligently followed their postoperative instructions. Parents and clinicians must balance a child's desire to understand the world with helping the child to endure the ambiguities that we all find difficult to tolerate with regard to medical illness.

As children enter adolescence, they develop an increasing capacity to think abstractly and form multiple points of view. An appreciation for rules that more or less dominates preadolescent children develops into a tendency to question rules and restrictions. In this setting, adolescents begin to form a coherent sense of who they are and what matters to them. Although this sense of self seems constantly in flux to many adults, the intense exploration of different values and ideals is a normal adolescent obsession and should not necessarily be taken as a sign of serious difficulty. In addition, adolescents begin to separate themselves from their families of origin. For example, when they are in need, adolescents may increasingly turn to friends or mentors instead of parents. All of these forces can ultimately manifest themselves as apparent rebellion and "acting out" from the rules and values of their own families.

For medically ill children, it is vital that these normal adolescent tendencies not be expressed in terms of worsening medical compliance, both in and out of the hospital. The teenager with a new liver, for example, *must* take her medicines and must *never* experiment with alcohol. Helping adolescent patients to accept their limitations, to understand the necessities of their medical regimen, and to find alternative methods of expressing their individuality is absolutely essential to the successful management of the medically ill teenager.

Having stressed the discrete stages of normal development, it is paramount that one remember that developmental approaches are not static and often overlap. It is not unusual for teenagers to feel that their past transgressions

have caused their newly diagnosed malignancy. Indeed, it is their realization that such thoughts are juvenile and immature that compounds their shame as they try to make sense of their predicament. In a similar light, GI concerns such as bowel mastery and control of one's flatulence are mastered early in normal child development. To the extent that GI surgery can compromise bowel control, children and adolescents may find themselves with soiled pants and regressed anxieties. In this sense, earlier developmental concerns are revisited on the recovering patient.

Finally, children often compartmentalize their concerns. There is nothing that is necessarily worrisome about the youngster who worries more about a soccer game than his/her upcoming surgery. Only in rare and specific circumstances is it helpful to force a young patient who appears unbothered to discuss his/her medical condition.

SPECIFIC TREATMENT ISSUES

Given the number and variety of pediatric GI procedures, it is somewhat difficult to generalize with regard to the psychological effects of invasive GI surgery. However, a number of considerations specific to certain GI illnesses have a direct and discernable effect on the psychological well-being of pediatric patients.

For example, children who undergo surgery in the setting of IBD often take varying doses of steroids and immunosuppressing agents. Similar medication regimens exist for children who undergo liver transplant and a scattering of other autoimmune diseases that affect the GI system. Although these medications are extremely important to the medical well-being of the patient, they also carry the potential for substantial psychological risk. Furthermore, virtually every serious GI condition has, in and of itself, potential psychiatric sequelae. As IBD constitutes perhaps the most common indication for pediatric GI surgery, it is helpful for clinicians working with this population to familiarize themselves with both the psychological risks of this condition as they pertain to surgery and the risks associated with medication regimens.

UNIQUE EMOTIONAL STRESSORS IN PEDIATRIC IBD

Children and families coping with IBD face unique emotional stressors and social challenges. When a child with recurrent debilitating colitis has an increase in symptoms, including refractory diarrhea and possibly stooling accidents, it may be intermittently necessary for parents to help with their child's basic toileting hygiene for the first time since toilet-training. As parents feel increasingly helpless as the disease progresses, there is a risk that they may become overcontrolling and overinvolved in an attempt to manage the unmanageable. The pediatric patient with colitis also faces some unusual psychological challenges. For a child who is appropriately increasing her sense of independence as she gets older, a family focus on bowel habits and bowel control may feel overwhelming and humiliating. The familial stance that is most psychologically supportive balances the child's emotional needs, autonomy, and privacy. Often psychological support provided by a social worker, psychologist, or child psychiatrist can help the family refine an approach that best supports the patient's personal growth.

The social ramifications of colitis are unique. Compared with asthma, which is a common childhood disease that is well known and does not involve any specific toileting needs, colitis is not a disease familiar to most children. It is not an easy disease to explain to one's friends.

When the disease is active, the child's activities may be greatly curtailed owing to abdominal pain or frequent stooling. Embarrassed by their disorder, children may go to great lengths to hide their symptoms from their peers. Children with varied stages of disease, pre- and postoperatively, often worry about soiling their underwear if they do not make it to the bathroom on time. If bathroom access at school is limited, the child may start refusing to go to school to avoid the impending stooling disaster. Importantly, these symptoms can potentially worsen as a function of anxiety regarding an upcoming surgery or as a result of the surgery itself. It is extremely important, therefore, that clinicians be aware of these issues and facilitate the child's development in the context of his/her medical condition.

SCHOOL AND CAMP INTERVENTIONS THAT FACILITATE EMOTIONAL GROWTH AND MINIMIZE ANXIETY

A physician caring for a child with colitis can provide some sound advice about the basic social interventions that can increase a child's confidence at school. Children with IBD should be allowed open access to school bathrooms. They should also be allowed to use the bathroom in the nurse's office if necessary. (Whereas other bathrooms at school may have frequent toilet paper shortages, this one tends to be well equipped.) These children should not be required to ask the teacher or to obtain the one bathroom pass allotted for the classroom to leave the room; they may need every moment available to make it to the bathroom without soiling. Some schools provide a special hall/bathroom pass for these children that they can carry with them at all times.

In some cases, increased academic support may also be indicated. For children unable to carry heavy books back and forth from home to school, two sets of books should be provided. If the diarrhea or abdominal pain increases around a project due date, teachers should be flexible and provide due date extensions as needed. In addition, if a child needs to rush to a bathroom during a testing situation, he should not be penalized and should be allowed extra time to finish the examination.

Whatever unique setup is organized, the planning should be done privately with the children's teacher. If these safeguards are not in place, these children may worry about their bowel habits during the school day rather than focus on school activities. Knowing that they have open access to available restrooms and that the school will be appropriately flexible if their symptoms affect their academic availability can be a great relief that supports normal cognitive and social development.

For camping or portable toilet situations, children with IBD should be armed with flushable wipes and sterile gel hand cleanser to use as needed. For outside activities that may have limited toilet availability, such as rope courses in summer camps, children with IBD should be first in line to complete the activity so that they can make it to the bathroom after the event if necessary. For rowing or other boating events without available bathrooms, the counselor in charge needs to be informed of the patient's medical limitations before the activity rather than during the event because of an acute toilet need. In general, attention should be paid to anticipating and then preventing problems rather than ignoring the possible hazardous situations that may crop up.

POTENTIAL PSYCHIATRIC AND COGNITIVE EFFECTS OF CORTICOSTEROIDS

Many of the GI conditions that lead to surgical interventions are treated with corticosteroids. These medications often carry with them profound psychological impact secondary to side effects such as changes in facial characteristics and weight. Furthermore, these worries can be easily compounded if the child also suffers from psychiatric symptoms caused by the steroids themselves. Finally, patients can exhibit severe psychiatric symptoms as a result of steroid treatment without having a past history of psychiatric vulnerability or psychiatric family history.

Corticosteroids can cause a wide range of psychiatric symptoms that may occur at any stage of treatment, including treatment withdrawal.[4,5] Usually, the worst symptoms are dose related and notable within a few weeks of therapy. During steroid withdrawal, depression and fatigue have also been documented and are not always coincident with evidence of hypothalamic pituitary axis suppression.

Mood lability, irritability, depression, anxiety, and mania have been documented in children and adults during steroid treatment, even at modest doses. Depressed children may become more withdrawn and irritable and have trouble sleeping, eating, concentrating, and feeling motivated. Manic children may develop sleep difficulties and experience increased activity and impulsivity and worsening distractibility. Their mood can be euphoric or extremely irritable.

Patients with a history of post-traumatic stress disorder may have increased depressive symptoms or intrusive trauma memories during steroid treatment. Further, adolescent patients with a previously undisclosed trauma have been noted to become symptomatic during steroid therapy.

Finally, some children may experience cognitive difficulties as a result of steroid treatment. Difficulties with short-term memory and concentration have been reported in the absence of mood symptoms, and often these effects dissipate when the steroid dose is decreased.[4]

NUTRITIONAL SUPPORT

Patients who require GI surgical intervention will sometimes require some form of nutritional support for prolonged periods. Although one can imagine the potential psychological effects of these nutritional interventions, again, there is relatively little literature exploring these issues.

As noted above, children with illnesses such as severe IBD already run significant psychological risk. The developmental and emotional toll of these conditions is derived from a combination of the disease symptoms themselves, underlying psychiatric predispositions, and side effects to potentially psychotropic agents such as corticosteroids. Although it is clear that nutritional support can also affect emotional well-being, the etiology of psychic distress as a result of total parenteral nutrition or tube feedings is more subtle and poorly studied. Existing literature suggests relatively good emotional adjustment, although these studies are hampered by the lack of an adequate comparison group and by unclear measurements of psychological effects.[6]

Adequate exploration of these issues is also hampered by the lack of a clear etiologic connection between nutritional support and emotional well-being. Although corticosteroids, for example, directly affect mood and anxiety, evidence for a specific psychotropic effect related to successful nutritional support is somewhat lacking. However, for children who develop vitamin and mineral deficiencies during parenteral or enteral support, there is the possibility that psychological effects will develop as a direct consequence of these nutritional shortcomings.[7,8] In addition, for children already uncomfortable with the developmental and psychological burden of their GI illness, the motivation, patience, and perseverance necessary for successful total parenteral nutrition or enteral support can be particularly challenging.

PSYCHOLOGICAL EFFECTS OF OSTOMIES

Children whose medical conditions necessitate ostomy placement also may suffer emotionally and developmentally as a result of this intervention. Again, a developmental approach is necessary when understanding the potential psychological implications. For younger children, the growing sense of autonomy and pride with regard to appreciation of and control over one's own body is potentially compromised by the placement of ostomy itself. For older children, the growing emphasis on peer conformity and appearance is further threatened by this intervention. As with much of the psychiatric literature concerning severe GI illness, there is a relative shortage of systematic investigations into the effects of ostomy placement in pediatric populations. Nevertheless, much of the literature does support significant need for emotional support and psychoeducation to ensure favorable outcomes.[9–11]

MISCELLANEOUS TREATMENT ISSUES

Other important issues relevant to this patient population include the drug–drug interactions in children who are taking multiple medications. Although an exhaustive list of these interactions is beyond the scope of this discussion, some specific treatment issues deserve mentioning.

First, given the spread of alternative therapies, especially with regard to psychiatric symptoms, it is always important to ask parents and patients whether they take any agents that are categorized as herbal or homeopathic. Although both parents and patients alike may view these agents as benign, many of these therapies have the potential to complicate treatment. For example, St. John's wort, an extremely popular herbal medication purchased at health food stores and taken for depression, also interferes with cyclosporine metabolism.[12] Clinicians have worried about graft rejection in patients who began St. John's wort and subsequently increased the metabolism of their prescribed immunosuppressing agents.

In general, taking a careful psychosocial and medical history helps to make patients and their families more comfortable discussing psychological issues and allows the clinician to screen for psychological distress. Having said this, it is extremely important that seemingly psychological symptoms be examined from multiple perspectives. For example, the youngster who seems lethargic, even in the setting of active depression, should also be examined for a worsening medical condition. All of the antidepressants and psychotherapy in the world will not fully motivate an anemic or otherwise medically compromised child. To this end, a team approach is absolutely essential for the overall health of these young patients.

PRE- AND POSTOPERATIVE MANAGEMENT

As noted above, there is limited methodologic consistency with regard to how best to prepare children and adolescents for GI surgery. Investigations have focused on measurements of pre- and postoperative psychological distress, postoperative pain, overall psychological adjustment, and the extent to which parents effectively cope.[1,2,13]

Studies suggest that 40 to 60% of children experience significant psychological and behavioral distress prior to surgery.[1] However, many studies do not describe in detail the scope or characteristics of these behavioral difficulties. Nevertheless, although these percentages refer to the almost 3 million children per year who undergo any type of surgery, it is reasonable to conclude that all surgeries, including GI procedures, are potentially extremely distressing to children and adolescents.[1]

In spite of these findings, there is little consistency among the approaches used to help quell these concerns. Some institutions use preoperative anxiolytic pharmacologic management, whereas others pursue a psychoeducational approach, preparing youngsters as best as possible for what they can expect both pre- and post-operatively. Many institutions use some combination of behavioral and pharmacologic management, and regimens are often a function of individual preferences among clinicians and, hopefully, a careful assessment of the needs of patients and their families. One large meta-analysis notes that some institutions have favored an overall decrease in preoperative psychological management.[1] These hospitals and clinicians acknowledge that although some form of preoperative management is potentially very helpful, the lack of consistent data supporting any one method of intervention makes much of these endeavors somewhat suspect.[1]

Other investigations have centered on postsurgery analgesic requirements and use, as well as the relative characteristics of parents as they cope with their child's illness and procedures. For example, some small studies note that variables affecting pain medication requirements include the relative invasiveness of surgery, the preoperative psychological state of the patient, and the extent to which parents felt anxious or concerned about the upcoming procedure.[13]

As noted above, the heterogeneity of procedures that can be characterized as GI surgery makes generalizations difficult, and many smaller investigations suggest findings that one can cautiously extrapolate from the specific conditions that they discuss to the more general concerns of the surgical pediatric patient. For instance, a study examining 101 pediatric liver transplant patients found that earlier transplants correlated with increased aggressive behavior and sexual dysfunction.[14] Furthermore, this study found that the surgery itself continued to be an important psychological part of the child's sense of self many years after the procedure. A similar study examined results from psychological projective testing in post–liver transplant children, noting increased negative self-focus and depressive episodes in this patient population.[15] One study has found that children were relatively well psychologically and developmentally when the treating team used a multidisciplinary approach.[16] Although many of these findings seem specific to the extraordinary circumstances surrounding any transplant, it is reasonable to expect earlier major procedures in some instances to interrupt development sufficiently to confer significant and lasting psychological effects. More studies are badly needed to confirm these hypotheses.

Similarly, it is also possible to extrapolate information from other severe illnesses in children to the overall understanding of how pediatric patients might respond to GI surgery. An important finding over the last few years has been a growing recognition that pediatric patients who undergo invasive and side effect–laden treatments such as chemotherapy and massive surgeries are at risk for the development of post-traumatic syndromes, cognitive decline, and depression. In addition, because underlying psychiatric predispositions often express themselves in the setting of external stressors, it is likely that many children will experience their first presentation of major psychiatric conditions such as mood and anxiety disorders in the setting of the stress of a surgical procedure.[17,18] Indeed, one study examining risk factors for the development of post-traumatic stress disorder in children with cancer noted that the most robust predictor was the extent to which the parents felt traumatized. Thus, it behooves any treatment team to soothe the fears and anxieties of parents as well as patients.[19,20]

At this point, it should be noted that there are many relevant studies listed in psychological databases such as *PsychINFO* and relatively few studies in more medically oriented sites such as *MEDLINE* and *Index Medicus*. Indeed, many of the most intriguing investigations are listed as doctoral dissertations, unpublished in other formats as of yet. Clearly, the case can be made that the medical establishment has neglected a more systematic interest in the psychological effects of GI surgery on children.

CONCLUSION

Why the dearth of knowledge? Some clinicians suggest that recent improvements in the overall treatment of drastically ill children have spawned a new interest in understanding the psychosocial effects of severe medical illness in pediatric populations. There may have been a tendency in the past to simply ignore or pay little heed to psychological distress, given other, more pressing medical concerns.[21] After any medical condition serious enough to warrant surgery, many parents and clinicians are, understandably, delighted that the child is simply alive and functioning. This can lead to a relative lack of emphasis on psychological well-being, and many consultation-liaison psychiatrists, psychologists, and pediatricians are only now systematically examining the effects of major medical interventions, such as GI surgeries, on the psychological state of their younger patients. Future studies will undoubtedly yield more specific and important findings, filling an important gap in the understanding of a child's experience in the surgical setting.

REFERENCES

1. Kain ZN, Caldwell-Andrews A, Wang SM. Psychological preparation of the parent and pediatric surgical patient. Anesthesiol Clin North Am 2002;20:29–44

2. Palermo TM, Drotar D, Tripi PA. Current status of psychosocial intervention research for pediatric outpatient surgery. J Clin Psychol Med Sett 1999;6:405–26.

3. Rauch PK, Jellinek MS. Paediatric consultation. In: Rutter M, editor. Child and adolescent psychiatry. 4th ed. Malden (MA): Blackwell; 2002. p. 1051–66.

4. Brown ES, Khan DA, Nejtek VA. The psychiatric side effects of corticosteroids. Ann Allergy Asthma Immunol 1999;83: 495–503.

5. Patten SB, Neutel CI. Corticosteroid-induced adverse psychiatric effects: incidence, diagnosis and management. Drug Saf 2000;22:111–22.

6. Navarro J, Vargas J, Cezard JP, et al. Prolonged constant rate elemental enteral nutrition in Crohn's disease. J Pediatr Gastroenterol Nutr 1982;1:541–6.

7. Matarese LE. Enteral feeding solutions. Gastrointest Endosc Clin North Am 1998;8:593–609.

8. Benton D, Donohoe RT. The effects of nutrients on mood. Public Health Nutr 1999;2:403–9.

9. Bates-Jensen B. Psychological response to illness: exploring two reactions to ostomy surgery. Ostomy Wound Management 1989;23:24–30.

10. Borkowski S. Pediatric stomas, tubes, and appliances. Pediatr Clin North Am 1998;45:1419–35.

11. Garvin G. Caring for children with ostomies. Nurs Clin North Am 1994;2:645–54.

12. Henderson L, Yue QY, Bergquist C, et al. St John's wort (*Hypericum perforatum*): drug interactions and clinical outcomes. Br J Clin Pharmacol 2002;54:349–56.

13. Lilley CM. Psychological predictors of children's pain and parents' medication practices following pediatric day surgery. In: Dissertation Abstracts International: section B: the sciences & engineering. Vol. 62. US: Univ Microfilms International; 2001. p. 554.

14. Schwering KL, Febo-Mandl F, Finkenauer C, et al. Psychologi-

cal and social adjustment after pediatric liver transplantation as a function of age at surgery and of time elapsed since transplantation. Pediatr Transplant 1997;1:138–45.

15. Windsorova D, Stewart SM, Lovitt R, et al. Emotional adaptation in children after liver transplantation. J Pediatr 1991;119:880–7.

16. Stone RD, Beasley PJ, Treacy SJ, et al. Children and families can achieve normal psychological adjustment and a good quality of life following pediatric liver transplantation: a long-term study. Transplant Proc 1997;29:1571–2.

17. Walker AM, Harris G, Baker A, et al. Post-traumatic stress responses following liver transplantation in older children. J Child Psychol Psychiatry Allied Disciplines 1999;40:363–74.

18. Tarbell SE, Kosmach B. Parental psychosocial outcomes in pediatric liver and/or intestinal transplantation: pretransplantation and the early postoperative period. Liver Transplant Surg 1998;4:378–87.

19. Stuber ML, Christakis DA, Houskamp B, Kazak AE. Posttrauma symptoms in childhood leukemia survivors and their parents. Psychosomatics 1996;37:254–61.

20. Stuber ML, Kazak AE, Meeske K, et al. Predictors of posttraumatic stress symptoms in childhood cancer survivors. Pediatrics 1997;100:958–64.

21. Horner T, Liberthson R, Jellinek MS. Psychosocial profile of adults with complex congenital heart disease. Mayo Clin Proc 2000;75:31–6.

INDEX

In this index, page numbers in *italic* designate figures; page numbers followed by the letter "t" designate tables. *See also* cross-referenences indentify related topics or more detailed topic breakdowns.